D0866170

Ashcraft's
PEDIATRIC SURGERY

5th edition

Ashcraft's PEDIATRIC SURGERY

George Whitfield Holcomb III, MD, MBA
The Katharine B. Richardson Professor of Pediatric Surgery
University of Missouri–Kansas City
Surgeon-in-Chief
Director, Center for Minimally Invasive Surgery
Children's Mercy Hospital
Kansas City, Missouri

J. Patrick Murphy, MD
Professor of Surgery
University of Missouri–Kansas City
Section Chief, Urologic Surgery
Children's Mercy Hospital
Kansas City, Missouri

Associate Editor
Daniel J. Ostlie, MD
Associate Professor of Surgery
University of Missouri–Kansas City
Director, Surgical Critical Care
Children's Mercy Hospital
Kansas City, Missouri

SAUNDERS

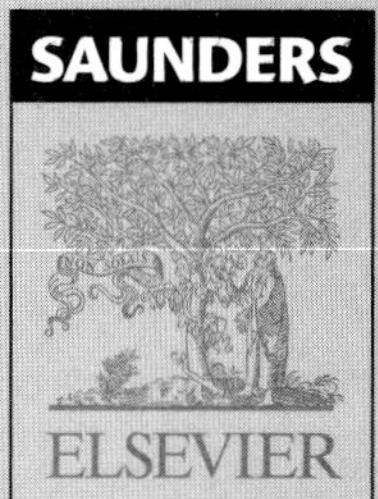

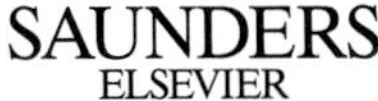

1600 John F. Kennedy Blvd.
Ste 1800
Philadelphia, PA 19103-2899

Ashcraft's Pediatric Surgery ISBN:978-1-4160-6127-4

Notice

Knowledge and best practice in this field are constantly changing. As new research and experience broaden our knowledge, changes in practice, treatment, and drug therapy may become necessary or appropriate. Readers are advised to check the most current information provided (i) on procedures featured or (ii) by the manufacturer of each product to be administered, to verify the recommended dose or formula, the method and duration of administration, and contraindications. It is the responsibility of practitioners, relying on their own experience and knowledge of the patient, to make diagnoses, to determine dosages and the best treatment for each individual patient, and to take all appropriate safety precautions. To the fullest extent of the law, neither the Publisher nor the Editors assume any liability for any injury and/or damage to persons or property arising out of or related to any use of the material contained in this book.

The Publisher

Library of Congress Cataloging-in-Publication Data

Ashcraft's pediatric surgery / [edited by] George Whitfield Holcomb III, J. Patrick Murphy ; associate editor, Daniel J. Ostlie. — 5th ed.
p. ; cm.
Rev. ed. of: Pediatric surgery / [edited by] Keith W. Ashcraft, George Whitfield Holcomb III, J. Patrick Murphy. 4th ed. c2005.
Includes bibliographical references and index.
ISBN 978-1-4160-6127-4
1. Children—Surgery. I. Ashcraft, Keith W. II. Holcomb, George W. III. Murphy, J. Patrick. IV. Ostlie, Daniel J. V. Pediatric surgery. VI. Title: Pediatric surgery.
[DNLM: 1. Surgical Procedures, Operative. 2. Child. 3. Infant. WO 925 A823 2009]
RD137.P43 2009
617.9'8—dc22 2009032713

Acquisitions Editor: Judith Fletcher
Developmental Editor: Arlene Chappelle
Publishing Services Manager: Tina Rebane
Project Manager: Norm Stellander
Design Direction: Lou Forgione

Printed in the United States of America

Last digit is the print number: 9 8 7 6 5 4 3 2 1

Dedication

Dr. Tom Holder
Dr. Keith Ashcraft
Master surgeons, teachers, mentors, and friends

CONTRIBUTORS

Stephanie P. Acierno, MD, MPH
Senior Pediatric Surgical Fellow
Seattle Children's Hospital
University of Washington School of Medicine
Seattle, Washington
75: Head and Neck Sinuses and Masses

Pablo Aguayo, MD
Instructor
Senior Resident
Department of Surgery
Kansas University Medical Center
Kansas City, Kansas
31: Duodenal and Intestinal Atresia and Stenosis

Craig T. Albanese, MD, MBA
Professor of Surgery and Pediatrics
Chief, Division of Pediatric Surgery
Stanford University School of Medicine
John A. and Cynthia Fry Gunn Director of Surgical Services
Lucile Packard Children's Hospital
Stanford, California
22: Congenital Bronchopulmonary Malformations

D. Adam Algren, MD
Assistant Professor
Departments of Emergency Medicine and Pediatrics
University of Missouri–Kansas City School of Medicine
Emergency Medicine Physician and Medical Toxicologist
Children's Mercy Hospital
Kansas City, Missouri
12: Bites

Uri S. Alon, MD
Professor of Pediatrics
University of Missouri–Kansas City School of Medicine
Pediatric Nephrologist
Children's Mercy Hospital
Kansas City, Missouri
4: Renal Impairment

Maria H. Alonso, MD
Assistant Professor of Surgery and Pediatrics
University of Cincinnati College of Medicine
Surgical Assistant Director, Liver Transplantation
Cincinnati Children's Hospital Medical Center
Cincinnati, Ohio
45: Solid Organ and Intestinal Transplantation

Richard J. Andrassy, MD
Professor and Chairman
Department of Surgery
University of Texas Medical School at Houston
Chief, Section of Pediatric Surgery
University of Texas M.D. Anderson Cancer Center
Surgeon-in-Chief
Memorial Hermann Hospital
Houston, Texas
72: Rhabdomyosarcoma

Walter S. Andrews, MD
Professor of Surgery
University of Missouri–Kansas City School of Medicine
Chief, Transplant Surgery
Children's Mercy Hospital
Kansas City, Missouri
69: Lesions of the Liver

Mara B. Antonoff, MD
Senior Resident
Department of Surgery
University of Minnesota Medical School
Minneapolis, Minnesota
1: Physiology of the Newborn

Jae-O Bae, MD
Pediatric Surgery Fellow
University of Texas Southwestern Medical Center
Dallas, Texas
78: Endocrine Disorders and Tumors

Klaas M. A. Bax, MD, PhD, FRCS(Ed)
Professor of Pediatric Surgery
Erasmus Medical School
University of Rotterdam
Head, Department of Pediatric Surgery
Sophia Children's Hospital
Rotterdam, The Netherlands
27: Esophageal Atresia and Tracheoesophageal Malformations

Robert E. Binda, Jr., MD
Associate Professor of Pediatric Anesthesiology
University of Missouri–Kansas City School of Medicine
Director, Pain Management
Children's Mercy Hospital
Kansas City, Missouri
3: Anesthetic Considerations

Casey M. Calkins, MD
Assistant Professor of Surgery
Medical College of Wisconsin
Pediatric General and Thoracic Surgery
Children's Hospital of Wisconsin
Milwaukee, Wisconsin
38: Acquired Anorectal Disorders

Patrick C. Cartwright, MD
Professor of Surgery
University of Utah School of Medicine
Chief, Division of Urology
Primary Children's Medical Center
Salt Lake City, Utah
57: Bladder and Urethra

Michael G. Caty, MD
Professor of Surgery and Pediatrics
Chief, Division of Pediatric Surgery
State University of New York at Buffalo
Surgeon-in-Chief
Department of Pediatric Surgical Services
Women and Children's Hospital of Buffalo
Buffalo, New York
33: Meconium Disease

Nicole M. Chandler, MD
Staff Surgeon
Pediatric General and Thoracic Surgery
All Children's Specialty Physicians
St. Petersburg, Florida
26: The Esophagus

Tyler L. Christensen, MD
Chief Resident in Urology
Department of Surgery
Washington University School of Medicine
Barnes Jewish Hospital
St. Louis Children's Hospital
St. Louis, Missouri
55: Ureteral Obstruction and Malformations

Dai H. Chung, MD
Professor and Vice-Chair
Department of Pediatric Surgery
Vanderbilt University School of Medicine
Nashville, Tennessee
13: Burns

Paul M. Colombani, MD, MBA
Professor of Surgery
Johns Hopkins University
Chief, Division of Pediatric Surgery
Johns Hopkins Hospital
Baltimore, Maryland
26: The Esophagus

Arthur Cooper, MD, MS
Professor of Surgery
Columbia University College of Physicians and Surgeons
Director of Trauma and Pediatric Surgical Services
Harlem Hospital Center
New York, New York
14: Early Assessment and Management of Trauma

Douglas E. Coplen, MD
Associate Professor of Surgery
Washington University School of Medicine
Director of Pediatric Urology
St. Louis Children's Hospital
St. Louis, Missouri
55: Ureteral Obstruction and Malformations

Hillary L. Copp, MD
Assistant Professor
Department of Urology
University of California, San Francisco
San Francisco, California
52: Undescended Testes and Testicular Tumors

Andrew M. Davidoff, MD
Associate Professor
Department of Surgery and Pediatrics
University of Tennessee School of Medicine
Chairman, Department of Surgery
St. Jude Children's Research Hospital
Memphis, Tennessee
68: Neuroblastoma

Romano T. DeMarco, MD
Associate Professor of Urology
University of Missouri–Kansas City School of Medicine
Director, Urology Research
Department of Surgery
Children's Mercy Hospital
Kansas City, Missouri
62: Prune-Belly Syndrome

Jack S. Elder, MD
Clinical Professor of Urology
Case Western Reserve University School of Medicine
Cleveland, Ohio
Chief, Department of Urology
Henry Ford Health System
Associate Director
Vattikuti Urology Institute
Department of Urology
Children's Hospital of Michigan
Detroit, Michigan
58: Posterior Urethral Valves

Mauricio A. Escobar, Jr., MD
Attending Surgeon
Mary Bridge Children's Hospital and Health Center
Tacoma, Washington
33: Meconium Disease

Mary E. Fallat, MD
Professor of Surgery
Director, Division of Pediatric Surgery
University of Louisville
Chief of Surgery
Kosair Children's Hospital
Louisville, Kentucky
39: Intussusception

Steven J. Fishman, MD
Associate Professor of Surgery
Harvard Medical School
Senior Associate in Surgery
Co-Director, Vascular Anomalies Center
Children's Hospital Boston
Boston, Massachusetts
74: Vascular Anomalies

Jason S. Frischer, MD
Assistant Professor
Department of Surgery
University of Cincinnati School of Medicine
Divison of Pediatric General and Thoracic Surgery
Cincinnati Children's Hospital Medical Center
Cincinnati, Ohio
6: Extracorporeal Membrane Oxygenation

Samir Gadepalli, MD
Clinical Lecturer
Department of Pediatric Surgery
University of Michigan
C.S. Mott Children's Hospital
Ann Arbor, Michigan
7: Mechanical Ventilation in Pediatric Surgical Disease

Alan S. Gamis, MD
Professor of Pediatrics
University of Missouri–Kansas City School of Medicine
Section Chief, Oncology
Children's Mercy Hospital
Kansas City, Missouri
71: Lymphomas

Victor F. Garcia, MD
Professor of Surgery
University of Cincinnati College of Medicine
Director, Trauma Services
Associate Surgical Director
Comprehensive Weight Management Center
Cincinnati Children's Hospital Medical Center
Cincinnati, Ohio
79: Bariatric Surgical Procedures in Adolescence

Carissa L. Garey, MD
Surgical Scholars Resident
Department of Surgery
Children's Mercy Hospital
Kansas City, Missouri
41: Meckel's Diverticulum

John M. Gatti, MD
Associate Professor of Surgery and Urology
University of Missouri–Kansas City School of Medicine
Director of Minimally Invasive Urology
Children's Mercy Hospital
Kansas City, Missouri
53: The Acute Scrotum
63: Disorders of Sexual Differentiation

Keith E. Georgeson, MD
Joseph M. Farley Professor of Surgery and Vice Chairman
Department of Surgery, Division of Pediatrics
Program Director, Pediatric Surgery Fellowship
University of Alabama School of Medicine at Birmingham
Director, Pediatric Surgical Sciences and Division of Pediatric Surgery
Children's Hospital of Alabama
Birmingham, Alabama
35: Hirschprung's Disease

Saif A. Ghole, MD
Department of Surgery
Stanford University School of Medicine
Stanford University Hospital and Clinics
Stanford, California
22: Congenital Bronchopulmonary Malformations

George K. Gittes, MD
Professor of Surgery
Chief, Division of Pediatric Surgery
University of Pittsburgh School of Medicine
Benjamin R. Fisher Chair of Pediatric Surgery and Surgeon-in-Chief
Children's Hospital of Pittsburgh
Pittsburgh, Pennsylvania
46: Lesions of the Pancreas

Richard W. Grady, MD
Associate Professor of Urology
University of Washington School of Medicine
Attending and Fellowship Program Director
Seattle Children's Hospital
Seattle, Washington
59: Bladder and Cloacal Exstrophy

Neil E. Green, MD
Professor of Orthopaedic Surgery
Vanderbilt School of Medicine
Department of Orthopaedics and Rehabilitation
Monroe Carell Jr. Children's Hospital at Vanderbilt
Nashville, Tennessee
18: Pediatric Orthopedic Trauma

Clarence S. Greene, Jr., MD
Associate Professor of Neurosurgery
University of Missouri–Kansas City School of Medicine
Attending Neurosurgeon
Children's Mercy Hospital
Kansas City, Missouri
19: Neurosurgical Conditions

Michael R. Harrison, MD
Director, Fetal Treatment Center
University of California, San Francisco Children's Hospital
San Francisco, California
10: Fetal Therapy

André Hebra, MD
Professor of Surgery and Pediatrics
Chief, Division of Pediatric Surgery
Medical University of South Carolina
Surgeon-in-Chief
The Children's Hospital
Charleston, South Carolina
21: Tracheal Obstruction and Repair

Marion C. W. Henry, MD, MPH
Attending Pediatric Surgeon
Section of Pediatric Surgery
Yale University School of Medicine
New Haven, Connecticut
34: Necrotizing Enterocolitis

David N. Herndon, MD
Professor and Jesse H. Jones Distinguished Chair in Surgery
Departments of Surgery and Pediatrics
University of Texas Medical Branch
Chief of Staff, Department of Surgery
Shriners Hospital for Children at Galveston
Galveston, Texas
13: Burns

Barry A. Hicks, MD
Professor of Surgery and Pediatrics
Division of Pediatric Surgery
University of Texas Southwestern Medical Center at Dallas
Children's Medical Center–Dallas
Dallas, Texas
16: Abdominal and Renal Trauma

Shinjiro Hirose, MD
Pediatric Surgeon
Fetal Treatment Center
University of California, San Francisco Children's Hospital
San Francisco, California
10: Fetal Therapy

Ronald B. Hirschl, MD
Arnold G. Coran Professor
Department of Pediatric Surgery
University of Michigan Health System
Section Head and Surgeon-in-Chief
C.S. Mott Children's Hospital
Ann Arbor, Michigan
7: Mechanical Ventilation in Pediatric Surgical Disease

George W. Holcomb III, MD, MBA
The Katharine B. Richardson Endowed Professor of Pediatric Surgery
University of Missouri–Kansas City School of Medicine
Surgeon-in-Chief
Director, Center for Minimally Invasive Surgery
Children's Mercy Hospital
Kansas City, Missouri
29: Gastroesophageal Reflux
40: Alimentary Tract Duplications
50: Laparoscopy

Gregory W. Hornig, MD
Clinical Assistant Professor of Neurosurgery
University of Missouri–Kansas City School of Medicine
Chief, Section of Neurosurgery
Children's Mercy Hospital
Kansas City, Missouri
19: Neurosurgical Conditions

Romeo C. Ignacio, Jr., MD
Pediatric Surgery Fellow
Division of Pediatric Surgery
University of Louisville
Kosair Children's Hospital
Louisville, Kentucky
39: Intussusception

Thomas H. Inge, MD, PhD
Associate Professor
Department of Pediatrics and Surgery
University of Cincinnati College of Medicine
Director, Surgical Weight Loss Program for Teens
Cincinnati Children's Hospital Medical Center
Cincinnati, Ohio
79: Bariatric Surgical Procedures in Adolescence

Tom Jaksic, MD, PhD
W. Hardy Hendren Professor of Surgery
Harvard Medical School
Vice Chairman of Pediatric Surgery
Children's Hospital Boston
Boston, Massachusetts
2: Nutritional Support of the Pediatric Patient

Yoshifumi Kato, MD, PhD
Associate Professor
Pediatric General and Urogenital Surgery
Juntendo University School of Medicine
Tokyo, Japan
44: Biliary Tract Disorders and Portal Hypertension

Scott J. Keckler, MD
Surgical Scholars Resident
Department of Surgery
Children's Mercy Hospital
Kansas City, Missouri
40: Alimentary Tract Duplications

Cassandra Kelleher, MD
Pediatric Surgery Fellow
Hospital for Sick Children
Toronto, Ontario, Canada
48: Congenital Abdominal Wall Defects

Robert E. Kelly, Jr., MD
Professor of Clinical Surgery and Pediatrics
Eastern Virginia Medical School
Chief, Department of Surgery
Children's Hospital of The King's Daughters
Norfolk, Virginia
20: Congenital Chest Wall Deformities

Curtis S. Koontz, MD
Assistant Professor of Surgery
University of Tennessee–Chattanooga
Chattanooga, Tennessee
30: Lesions of the Stomach

Thomas M. Krummel, MD
Emile Holman Professor and Chair
Department of Surgery
Stanford University School of Medicine
Susan B. Ford Surgeon-in-Chief
Lucile Packard Children's Hospital
Stanford, California
9: Surgical Infectious Disease

Arlet G. Kurkchubasche, MD
Associate Professor of Surgery and Pediatrics
Brown University Medical School
Hasbro Children's Hospital
Providence, Rhode Island
73: Nevus and Melanoma

Jean-Martin Laberge, MD, FRCSC, FACS
Professor of Surgery
McGill University
Senior Pediatric Surgeon
Montreal Children's Hospital
Montreal, Quebec, Canada
70: Teratomas, Dermoids, and Other Soft Tissue Tumors

Kevin P. Lally, MD, MS
A. G. McNeese Chair and Professor
Department of Pediatric Surgery
University of Texas Medical School at Houston
Surgeon-in-Chief
Children's Memorial Hermann Hospital
Houston, Texas
24: Congenital Diaphragmatic Hernia and Eventration

Jacob C. Langer, MD
Professor of Surgery
University of Toronto
Chief, Pediatric General and Thoracic Surgery
Hospital for Sick Children
Toronto, Ontario, Canada
48: Congenital Abdominal Wall Defects

Joseph L. Lelli, Jr., MD, MBA
Assistant Professor
Wayne State Medical School
Chief of Pediatric General and Thoracic Surgery
Children's Hospital of Michigan
Detroit, Michigan
11: Foreign Bodies

Marc A. Levitt, MD
Associate Professor
Department of Surgery
University of Cincinnati
Associate Director, Colorectal Center
Cincinnati Children's Hospital Medical Center
Cincinnati, Ohio
36: Imperforate Anus and Cloacal Malformations
37: Fecal Incontinence and Constipation

Karen B. Lewing, MD
Assistant Professor of Pediatrics
University of Missouri–Kansas City School of Medicine
Fellowship Program Director
Division of Hematology/Oncology
Children's Mercy Hospital
Kansas City, Missouri
71: Lymphomas

Charles M. Leys, MD
Assistant Professor of Surgery
Indiana University School of Medicine
Staff Surgeon
Riley Hospital for Children
Indianapolis, Indiana
53: The Acute Scrotum

Danny C. Little, MD
Assistant Professor of Surgery
Texas A&M University Health Center–College of Medicine
Chief of Pediatric Surgery
Children's Hospital at Scott & White
Temple, Texas
32: Malrotation

Jennifer A. Lowry, MD
Assistant Professor, Department of Pediatrics
University of Missouri–Kansas City School of Medicine
Medical Toxicologist and Clinical Pharmacologist
Children's Mercy Hospital
Kansas City, Missouri
12: Bites

Marcus M. Malek, MD
Surgical Research Fellow
Children's Hospital of Pittsburgh
Pittsburgh, Pennsylvania
46: Lesions of the Pancreas

Thao T. Marquez, MD
Senior Resident
Department of Surgery
University of Minnesota Medical School
Minneapolis, Minnesota
1: Physiology of the Newborn

Nilesh M. Mehta, MD, DCH
Instructor in Anesthesia
Harvard Medical School
Division of Critical Care Medicine
Children's Hospital Boston
Boston, Massachusetts
2: Nutritional Support of the Pediatric Patient

Gregory A. Mencio, MD
Professor and Chief
Pediatric Orthopaedics
Vanderbilt University School of Medicine
Monroe Carell Jr. Children's Hospital at Vanderbilt
Nashville, Tennessee
18: Pediatric Orthopedic Trauma

Marc P. Michalsky, MD
Assistant Professor of Clinical Surgery
Ohio University College of Medicine
Principal Investigator
Center for Clinical and Translational Research
Nationwide Children's Hospital
Columbus, Ohio
23: Acquired Lesions of the Lung and Pleura

Eugene A. Minevich, MD
Associate Professor of Surgery
University of Cincinnati College of Medicine
Cincinnati Children's Hospital Medical Center
Cincinnati, Ohio
56: Urinary Tract Infection and Vesicoureteral Reflux

Michael E. Mitchell, MD
Professor of Urology
Medical College of Wisconsin
Chief of Pediatric Urology
Children's Hospital of Wisconsin
Milwaukee, Wisconsin
59: Bladder and Cloacal Exstrophy

Go Miyano, MD
Department of Pediatric General and Urogenital Surgery
Juntendo University Hospital
Tokyo, Japan
79: Bariatric Surgical Procedures in Adolescence

Takeshi Miyano, MD, PhD
Emeritus Professor
Pediatric General and Urogenital Surgery
Juntendo University School of Medicine
Tokyo, Japan
44: Biliary Tract Disorders and Portal Hypertension

Christopher R. Moir, MD
Professor of Surgery
Mayo Clinic
Rochester, Minnesota
42: Inflammatory Bowel Disease and Intestinal Cancer

R. Lawrence Moss, MD, FACS
Robert Pritzker Professor and Chief
Pediatric Surgery
Yale University School of Medicine
Surgeon-in-Chief
Yale New Haven Children's Hospital
New Haven, Connecticut
34: Necrotizing Enterocolitis

J. Patrick Murphy, MD
Professor of Surgery and Urology
University of Missouri–Kansas City School of Medicine
Section Chief, Urologic Surgery
Children's Mercy Hospital
Kansas City, Missouri
60: Hypospadias

Don K. Nakayama, MD, MBA
Milford B. Hatcher Professor and Chair
Department of Surgery
Mercer University School of Medicine
Program Director, Residency in Surgery
Medical Center of Central Georgia
Macon, Georgia
77: Breast Diseases

Jaimie D. Nathan, MD, MS
Assistant Professor of Surgery and Pediatrics
University of Cincinnati College of Medicine
Cincinnati Children's Hospital Medical Center
Cincinnati, Ohio
45: Solid Organ and Intestinal Transplantation

Kathleen A. Neville, MD, MS
Assistant Professor of Pediatrics
Divisions of Pediatric Hematology/Oncology and Pediatric Pharmacology and Medical Toxicology
Children's Mercy Hospital
Kansas City, Missouri
5: Coagulopathies and Sickle Cell Disease

Donald Nuss, MB, ChB, FRCS(C), FACS
Professor of Surgery and Pediatrics
Eastern Virginia Medical School
Pediatric Surgeon
Children's Hospital of The King's Daughters
Norfolk, Virginia
20: Congenital Chest Wall Deformities

Keith T. Oldham, MD
Professor and Chief
Division of Pediatric Surgery
Medical College of Wisconsin
Marie Z. Uihlein Chair and Surgeon-in-Chief
Children's Hospital of Wisconsin
Milwaukee, Wisconsin
38: Acquired Anorectal Disorders

James A. O'Neill, Jr., MD
J. C. Foshee Distinguished Professor
Chairman Emeritus, Section of Surgical Sciences
Department of Pediatric Surgery
Vanderbilt University School of Medicine
Monroe Carell Jr. Children's Hospital at Vanderbilt
Nashville, Tennessee
65: Renovascular Hypertension

Daniel J. Ostlie, MD
Associate Professor of Surgery
University of Missouri–Kansas City School of Medicine
Director, Surgical Critical Care
Children's Mercy Hospital
Kansas City, Missouri
29: Gastroesophageal Reflux
31: Duodenal and Intestinal Atresia and Stenosis

H. Biemann Othersen, Jr., MD, BSM
Professor of Surgery and Pediatrics
Emeritus Head, Division of Pediatric Surgery
Medical University of South Carolina
Charleston, South Carolina
21: Tracheal Obstruction and Repair

Alberto Peña, MD
Professor, Department of Surgery
University of Cincinnati
Director, Colorectal Center
Cincinnati Children's Hospital Medical Center
Cincinnati, Ohio
36: Imperforate Anus and Cloacal Malformations
37: Fecal Incontinence and Constipation

Kathy M. Perryman, MD, FAAP
Associate Professor of Pediatric Anesthesiology
University of Missouri–Kansas City School of Medicine
Children's Mercy Hospital
Kansas City, Missouri
3: Anesthetic Considerations

Craig A. Peters, MD
John E. Cole Professor of Urology
University of Virginia School of Medicine
Chief, Division of Pediatric Urology
University of Virginia Children's Hospital
Charlottesville, Virginia
64: Urologic Laparoscopy

Devin P. Puapong, MD
Chief Resident in Pediatric Surgery
University of Oklahoma Health Sciences Center
Children's Hospital
Oklahoma City, Oklahoma
15: Thoracic Trauma

Pramod S. Puligandla, MD, FRCSC, FACS
Associate Professor of Surgery and Pediatrics
McGill University
Pediatric Surgery Training Program Director
Montreal Children's Hospital
Montreal, Quebec, Canada
70: Teratomas, Dermoids, and Other Soft Tissue Tumors

Stephen C. Raynor, MD
Chief of Pediatric Surgery
Children's Hospital & Medical Center
Omaha, Nebraska
61: Circumcision

Frederick J. Rescorla, MD
Lafayette L. Page Professor and Director
Section of Pediatric Surgery
Indiana University School of Medicine
Surgeon-in-Chief
Riley Hospital for Children
Indianapolis, Indiana
47: Splenic Conditions

Bradley M. Rodgers, MD
Professor of Surgery and Pediatrics
University of Virginia Health Sciences Center
Chief of Pediatric Surgery
University of Virginia Children's Hospital
Charlottesville, Virginia
23: Acquired Lesions of the Lung and Pleura

Michael T. Rohmiller, MD
Orthopedic Spine Surgeon
Cincinnati Spine Institute
Cincinnati, Ohio
18: Pediatric Orthopedic Trauma

Steven S. Rothenberg, MD
Clinical Professor of Surgery
Columbia University College of Physicians and Surgeons
New York, New York
Chief of Pediatric Surgery
The Rocky Mountain Hospital for Children
Denver, Colorado
28: Thoracoscopy in Infants and Children

Frederick C. Ryckman, MD
Professor of Surgery and Pediatrics
University of Cincinnati College of Medicine
Vice-President, System Capacity and Perioperative Operations
Cincinnati Children's Hospital Medical Center
Cincinnati, Ohio
45: Solid Organ and Intestinal Transplantation

Shawn D. St. Peter, MD
Assistant Professor of Surgery
University of Missouri–Kansas City School of Medicine
Director, Center for Prospective Clinical Trials
Children's Mercy Hospital
Kansas City, Missouri
43: Appendicitis
80: Evidence-Based Medicine

Daniel A. Saltzman, MD, PhD
Associate Professor of Surgery and Pediatrics
Dr. A.S. Leonard Endowed Chair in Pediatric Surgery
Chief, Division of Pediatric Surgery
University of Minnesota Medical School
Surgeon-in-Chief
University of Minnesota Amplatz Children's Hospital
Minneapolis, Minnesota
1: Physiology of the Newborn

Adam J. Schow, MD
Assistant Professor of Pediatric Anesthesiology
University of Missouri–Kansas City School of Medicine
Medical Director
Same Day Surgery and Post Anesthesia Care Unit
Children's Mercy Hospital
Kansas City, Missouri
3: Anesthetic Considerations

Kurt P. Schropp, MD
Associate Professor of Surgery
Program Director, General Surgery Residency
Kansas University School of Medicine
Kansas City, Kansas
41: Meckel's Diverticulum

Shinil K. Shah, DO
Senior Resident
Department of Surgery
University of Texas Medical School at Houston
Houston, Texas
72: Rhabdomyosarcoma

Robert C. Shamberger, MD
Robert E. Gross Professor of Surgery
Harvard Medical School
Chief of Surgery
Children's Hospital Boston
Boston, Massachusetts
67: Renal Tumors

Ellen Shapiro, MD
Professor of Urology
New York University School of Medicine
Director of Pediatric Urology
NYU Langone Medical Center
New York, New York
58: Posterior Urethral Valves

Kenneth Shaw, MD, FRCSE
Assistant Professor of Surgery
McGill University
Staff Pediatric Surgeon
Montreal Children's Hospital
Montreal, Quebec, Canada
70: Teratomas, Dermoids, and Other Soft Tissue Tumors

Curtis A. Sheldon, MD
Assistant Professor of Surgery
University of Cincinnati College of Medicine
Director, Pediatric Urology
Cincinnati Children's Hospital Medical Center
Cincinnati, Ohio
56: Urinary Tract Infection and Vesicoureteral Reflux

Stephen J. Shochat, MD
Department of Surgery
St. Jude Children's Research Hospital
Memphis, Tennessee
66: Principles of Adjuvant Therapy in Childhood Cancer

Linda D. Shortliffe, MD
Professor and Department Chair
Department of Urology
Stanford University School of Medicine
Pediatric Urology Service Chief
Department of Urology
Stanford University Medical Center
Stanford, California
52: Undescended Testes and Testicular Tumors

Michael A. Skinner, MD
Edwin Ide Smith, M.D. Professor of Pediatric Surgery
University of Texas-Southwestern Medical Center
Children's Medical Center–Dallas
Dallas, Texas
78: Endocrine Disorders and Tumors

Bethany J. Slater, MD
Senior Resident
Department of Surgery
Stanford University Medical Center
Stanford, California
9: Surgical Infectious Disease

Samuel D. Smith, MD
Professor of Surgery
University of Arkansas for Medical Sciences College of Medicine
Chief of Pediatric Surgery
Arkansas Children's Hospital
Little Rock, Arkansas
32: Malrotation

C. Jason Smithers, MD
Instructor in Surgery
Harvard Medical School
Assistant in Surgery
Children's Hospital Boston
Boston, Massachusetts
74: Vascular Anomalies

Brent W. Snow, MD, FACS, FAAP
Professor of Surgery
University of Utah School of Medicine
Chief, Division of Pediatric Urology
Primary Children's Medical Center
Salt Lake City, Utah
57: Bladder and Urethra

Charles L. Snyder, MD
Professor of Surgery
University of Missouri–Kansas City School of Medicine
Director of Clinical Research
Children's Mercy Hospital
Kansas City, Missouri
51: Inguinal Hernias and Hydroceles

Howard M. Snyder III, MD
Professor of Urology
Department of Surgery
University of Pennsylvania School of Medicine
Director of Surgical Teaching, Division of Pediatric Urology
Children's Hospital of Philadelphia
Philadelphia, Pennsylvania
54: Developmental and Positional Anomalies of the Kidneys

Charles J. H. Stolar, MD
Professor of Surgery and Pediatrics
Columbia University College of Physicians and Surgeons
Surgeon-in-Chief
Department of Pediatric Surgery
Morgan Stanley Children's Hospital of New York–Presbyterian
Columbia University Medical Center
New York, New York
6: Extracorporeal Membrane Oxygenation

Julie L. Strickland, MD, MPH
Associate Professor
Department of Obstetrics and Gynecology
University of Missouri–Kansas City School of Medicine
Section Chief, Gynecological Surgery
Children's Mercy Hospital
Kansas City, Missouri
76: Pediatric and Adolescent Gynecology

Steven Stylianos, MD
Clinical Professor of Surgery and Pediatrics
Florida International University College of Medicine
Voluntary Associate Professor of Surgery
University of Miami Miller School of Medicine
Chief, Department of Pediatric Surgery
Medical Director, Pediatric Training Program
Miami Children's Hospital
Miami, Florida
16: Abdominal and Renal Trauma

Karl G. Sylvester, MD
Associate Professor of Surgery and Pediatrics
Stanford University School of Medicine
Attending Surgeon
Lucile Packard Children's Hospital
Stanford, California
22: Congenital Bronchopulmonary Malformations

Greg M. Tiao, MD
Associate Professor of Surgery and Pediatrics
University of Cincinnati College of Medicine
Director, Liver/Intestine Transplant Program
Cincinnati Children's Hospital Medical Center
Cincinnati, Ohio
45: Solid Organ and Intestinal Transplantation

Kelly S. Tieves, DO, MS
Assistant Professor
Department of Pediatrics
University of Missouri–Kansas City School of Medicine
Pediatric Intensivist, Anesthesiology
Children's Mercy Hospital
Kansas City, Missouri
17: Pediatric Head Trauma

Juan A. Tovar, MD, PhD
Professor of Pediatric Surgery
Autonomous University of Madrid
Chief, Department of Pediatric Surgery
University Hospital of La Paz
Madrid, Spain
25: Mediastinal Tumors

Thomas F. Tracy, Jr., MD, MS
Professor of Surgery and Pediatrics
Vice Chairman, Department of Surgery
Brown University Medical School
Pediatric Surgeon-in-Chief
Hasbro Children's Hospital
Providence, Rhode Island
73: Nevus and Melanoma

KuoJen Tsao, MD
Assistant Professor of Surgery
Department of Pediatric Surgery
University of Texas Medical School at Houston
Children's Memorial Hermann Hospital
Houston, Texas
24: Congenital Diaphragmatic Hernia and Eventration

David W. Tuggle, MD
Professor and Vice-Chairman, Department of Surgery
Chief, Section of Pediatric Surgery
Paula Milburn Miller/Children's Medical Research Chair in Pediatric Surgery
University of Oklahoma Health Sciences Center
Children's Hospital
Oklahoma City, Oklahoma
15: Thoracic Trauma

Ravindra K. Vegunta, MD, MBBS
Associate Professor of Surgery and Pediatrics
University of Illinois College of Medicine at Peoria
Director, Pediatric Minimally Invasive Surgery
Children's Hospital of Illinois Pediatric Surgical Center
Peoria, Illinois
8: Vascular Access

Daniel von Allmen, MD
Professor of Surgery
University of Cincinnati College of Medicine
Director, Division of General and Thoracic Surgery
Cincinnati Children's Hospital Medical Center
Cincinnati, Ohio
66: Principles of Adjuvant Therapy in Childhood Cancer

John H. T. Waldhausen, MD
Professor of Surgery
University of Washington School of Medicine
Division Chief, Pediatric General and Thoracic Surgery
Seattle Children's Hospital
Seattle, Washington
75: Head and Neck Sinuses and Masses

Peter A. Walker, MD
Senior Resident
Department of Surgery
University of Texas Medical School at Houston
Houston, Texas
72: Rhabdomyosarcoma

M. Chad Wallis, MD
Clinical Assistant Professor
Department of Surgery
University of Utah School of Medicine
Primary Children's Medical Center
Salt Lake City, Utah
57: Bladder and Urethra

Bradley A. Warady, MD
Professor and Associate Chairman
Department of Pediatrics
University of Missouri–Kansas City School of Medicine
Section Chief, Nephrology
Director of Dialysis and Transplantation
Children's Mercy Hospital
Kansas City, Missouri
4: Renal Impairment

Gary S. Wasserman, DO
Professor
Department of Pediatrics
University of Missouri–Kansas City School of Medicine
Chief, Section of Medical Toxicology
Children's Mercy Hospital
Kansas City, Missouri
12: Bites

Thomas R. Weber, MD
Professor of Surgery and Pediatrics
University of Illinois College of Medicine
Director, Pediatric Surgery
Advocate Hope Children's Hospital
Chicago, Illinois
49: Umbilical and Other Abdominal Wall Hernias

Brian M. Wicklund, MD, CM, MPH
Associate Professor of Pediatrics
University of Missouri–Kansas City School of Medicine
Director, Hemophilia Treatment Center
Children's Mercy Hospital
Kansas City, Missouri
5: Coagulopathies and Sickle Cell Disease

Gerald M. Woods, MD
Professor of Pediatrics
University of Missouri–Kansas City School of Medicine
Chief, Division of Hematology/Oncology
Children's Mercy Hospital
Kansas City, Missouri
5: Coagulopathies and Sickle Cell Disease

Hsi-Yang Wu, MD
Associate Professor
Department of Urology
Stanford University School of Medicine
Pediatric Urologist
Lucile Packard Children's Hospital
Stanford, California
54: Developmental and Positional Anomalies of the Kidneys

Mark L. Wulkan, MD
Assistant Professor of Surgery and Pediatrics
Emory University School of Medicine
Director, Minimally Invasive Surgery
Children's Healthcare of Atlanta at Egleston
Atlanta, Georgia
30: Lesions of the Stomach

Atsuyuki Yamataka, MD, PhD
Professor and Head
Pediatric General and Urogenital Surgery
Juntendo University School of Medicine
Tokyo, Japan
44: Biliary Tract Disorders and Portal Hypertension

PREFACE

This is the fifth edition of *Pediatric Surgery*, but the first edition without the insights and efforts of either Dr. Tom Holder or Dr. Keith Ashcraft. In 1980, these two master surgeons had the foresight to develop a reference text focusing on infants and children with surgical conditions. The current editors would like to dedicate this fifth edition to our founding editors, Drs. Tom Holder and Keith Ashcraft.

Drs. Holder and Aschraft wanted to create a single-volume pediatric surgical work that was broad in scope and had some detail about each condition; however, they did not intend for this work to be encyclopedic. As they stated in their first Preface, "An effort has been made to provide sufficient information concerning physiology, embryology, and anatomy so that the reader may gain a thorough understanding of the patient, the disease process, its symptoms, diagnosis, and treatment. Authors were selected because they are acknowledged authorities in the area of their contribution."

This concept of a single-volume text has persisted over the subsequent editions. The current editors have tried to maintain this book in the style originally conceived by Drs. Holder and Ashcraft. Although most of the chapters in this edition have the same title as those in the first edition, the information and knowledge in the field of pediatric surgery have dramatically evolved. More than half the illustrations in this fifth edition are new. Management of urologic conditions remains an important part of this book because many pediatric surgeons around the world also perform urologic operations in children. An effort has been made to use experts from all over the world to write the chapters, as this book is read worldwide by surgeons, pediatricians, residents, and medical students.

Many, if not most, operations are now performed using a minimally invasive approach. Thus, operative technique is emphasized more in this edition than in previous ones. Prenatal diagnosis is an entity now commonly encountered by pediatric surgeons. In addition, so much more about genetic predisposition to certain conditions and cancers is known now versus 30 years ago. Finally, in this fifth edition, a chapter on "Evidence Based Medicine" has made its way into a pediatric surgical textbook for the first time. As previously emphasized, a concerted effort has been made to keep this book to a single volume. However, as there is so much more information that is important and known about pediatric surgical conditions than was available in 1980, we also need to allow for that growth. In an effort to limit the book to a single volume, references have been placed online on the associated *Expert Consult* website (www.expertconsult.com), rather than at the end of each chapter in the book itself. While some readers do not look at the references, those who do will find that they are easily accessible and linked to PubMed for easy access to abstracts and full text. By saving nearly 200 pages of text, we have helped to maintain the cost of the book. Also, the amount of paper needed was significantly reduced. In addition, the full text and color figures are also available on *Expert Consult*. Purchasers receive a PIN code and password with each copy of the book, making this edition the first pediatric surgery text that is available online. We hope our readers enjoy and appreciate this feature as we believe that a definite advantage of this book will be its portability. Whether in the office, the operating room, at home, or out of town, *Pediatric Surgery*, fifth edition, will be available online through a personal password.

In the fourth edition, videos were available on a DVD that accompanied the book. Since a companion book (*Atlas of Laparoscopy and Thoracoscopy*, Holcomb GW III, Georgeson KE, Rothenberg SS, editors) was recently published by Elsevier, access to videos from this atlas will also be available on *Expert Consult* to purchasers of this fifth edition.

The editors would like to thank all of the authors for their extraordinary efforts and time spent in writing their chapters. In addition, three of our colleagues (Kathy Smith, Linda Jankowski, and Barbara Juarez) have provided extraordinary technical support for this book. This book would not have been possible without their help. In addition, we would also like to thank the administration and leadership at The Children's Mercy Hospital for their continued full support for this book for the past 30 years. Finally, the editors would also like to thank our colleagues at Elsevier for their timeless attention to detail and support throughout the process of editing and publishing this textbook. This book was truly a team effort by a great many people. We hope you will enjoy this fifth edition and find it helpful in treating your patients.

GEORGE W. HOLCOMB III, MD, MBA

J. PATRICK MURPHY, MD

TABLE OF CONTENTS

SECTION 1 ■ GENERAL

SECTION 2 ■ TRAUMA

SECTION 3 ■ THORACIC

SECTION 4 ■ ABDOMEN

SECTION 5 ■ INGUINAL REGION AND SCROTUM

SECTION 6 ■ UROLOGY

section 1

GENERAL

chapter 1

PHYSIOLOGY OF THE NEWBORN

Mara Antonoff, MD • Thao Marquez, MD • Daniel Saltzman, MD, PhD

Newborns may be classified based on gestational age and weight. Preterm infants are those born before 37 weeks of gestation. Term infants are those born between 37 and 42 weeks of gestation, whereas post-term infants have a gestation that exceeds 42 weeks. Newborns whose weight is below the 10th percentile for age are considered small for gestational age (SGA), whereas those whose weight is at or above the 98th percentile are large for gestational age (LGA). The newborns whose weight falls between these extremes are appropriate for gestational age (AGA).

SGA newborns are thought to suffer intrauterine growth retardation as a result of placental, maternal, or fetal abnormalities. Conditions associated with deviation in intrauterine growth are shown in Figure 1-1. SGA infants have a body weight below what is appropriate for their age, yet their body length and head circumference are age appropriate. To classify an infant as SGA, the gestational age must be confirmed by the physical findings summarized in Table 1-1.

Although SGA infants may weigh the same as premature infants, they have different physiologic characteristics. Owing to intrauterine malnutrition, body fat levels are frequently below 1% of the total body weight. This lack of body fat increases the risk of cold stress with SGA infants. Hypoglycemia develops earlier in SGA infants owing to higher metabolic activity and reduced glycogen stores. The red blood cell (RBC) volume and the total blood volume are much higher in the SGA infant compared with the preterm average for gestational age or the non-SGA full-term infant. This rise in RBC volume frequently leads to polycythemia, with an associated rise in blood viscosity. Owing to the adequate length of gestation, the SGA infant has pulmonary function approaching that of a full-term infant or one who is average for gestational age.

Infants born before 37 weeks of gestation, regardless of birth weight, are considered premature. The physical examination of the premature infant reveals that the skin is thin and transparent with an absence of plantar creases. Fingers are soft and malleable, and ears have poorly developed cartilage. In females, the labia minora appear enlarged, but the labia majora are small. In males, the testes are usually undescended and the scrotum is undeveloped. Special problems with the preterm infant include the following:

- Weak suck reflex
- Inadequate gastrointestinal absorption
- Hyaline membrane disease
- Intraventricular hemorrhage
- Hypothermia
- Patent ductus arteriosus
- Apnea
- Hyperbilirubinemia

SPECIFIC PHYSIOLOGIC PROBLEMS OF THE NEWBORN

Fetal levels of glucose, calcium, and magnesium are carefully maintained by maternal regulation. The transition to extrauterine life can have profound effects on the physiologic well-being of the newborn.

Glucose Metabolism

The fetus maintains a blood glucose value 70% to 80% of the maternal value by facilitated diffusion across the placenta. There is a buildup of glycogen stores in the liver, skeleton, and cardiac muscles during the later stages of fetal development but little gluconeogenesis. The newborn must depend on glycolysis until exogenous glucose is supplied. After delivery, the newborn depletes his or her hepatic glycogen stores within 2 to 3 hours. Glycogen stores are more rapidly reduced in premature and SGA newborns. The newborn is severely limited in his or her ability to use fat and protein as substrates to synthesize glucose.

Hypoglycemia

Clinical signs of hypoglycemia are nonspecific and may include a weak or high-pitched cry, cyanosis, apnea, jitteriness, apathy, seizures, abnormal eye movements, temperature instability, hypotonia, and weak suck. Some infants, however, exhibit no signs, despite extremely low blood glucose levels.

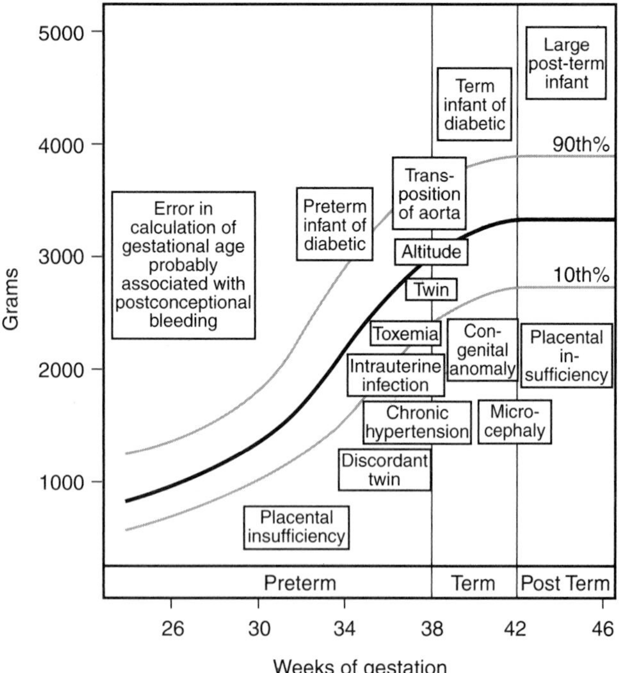

Figure 1-1. Graph of conditions associated with deviations in intrauterine growth. The boxes indicate the approximate birth weight and gestational age at which the condition is likely to occur. (Adapted from Avery ME, Villee D, Baker S, et al: Neonatology. In Avery ME, First LR [eds]: Pediatric Medicine. Baltimore, Williams & Wilkins, 1989, p 148.)

Neonatal hypoglycemia is generally defined as a glucose level lower than 40 mg/dL. After 72 hours of age, plasma glucose levels should be greater than or equal to 40 mg/dL.[1] Although there is not one specific threshold at which all infants will develop neurologic sequelae, features associated with adverse outcomes include blood glucose concentrations that are extremely low (<20 mg/dL) and/or persistently low (>1-2 hours).[2] Infants who are at high risk for developing hypoglycemia require frequent glucose monitoring. Because most newborns who require surgical procedures are at risk to develop hypoglycemia, a 10% glucose infusion is usually started on admission to the hospital and blood glucose levels are measured at the bedside and confirmed by periodic laboratory determinations. If the blood glucose level falls below 40 mg/dL or if any signs of hypoglycemia are present, an hourly bolus infusion of 1 to 2 mL/kg (4 to 8 mg/kg/min) of 10% glucose is given intravenously. If central venous access is present, concentrations of up to 50% glucose may be used. During the first 36 to 48 hours after a major surgical procedure, it is not uncommon to see wide variations in serum glucose levels. Therefore, frequent blood and urine glucose determinations should be performed. Rarely, hydrocortisone, glucagon, or somatostatin is needed to treat persistent hypoglycemia.

Hyperglycemia

Hyperglycemia is a common problem with the use of total parenteral nutrition (TPN) in very immature infants who are less than 30 weeks' gestation and weigh less than 1.1 kg at birth. These infants are usually younger than 3 days of age and are frequently septic.[3] This hyperglycemia appears to be associated with both insulin resistance and relative insulin deficiency, reflecting the prolonged catabolism seen in very low birth weight infants.[4] Hyperglycemia may cause intraventricular hemorrhage and water and electrolyte losses from glucosuria. The glucose concentration and infusion rate of the TPN must be adjusted based on serum glucose levels. Full parenteral caloric support is achieved with incremental increases in glucose, usually over several days. Occasionally, insulin, 0.001 to 0.01 U/kg/min, is given intravenously to maintain normoglycemia and may be helpful in achieving anabolism in infants of very low birth weight.[4]

Calcium

Calcium is continuously delivered to the fetus by active transport across the placenta. Of the total amount of calcium transferred, 75% occurs after 28 weeks' gestation.[5] This observation partially accounts for the high incidence of hypocalcemia in extremely preterm infants. Any neonate has a tendency for hypocalcemia due to limited calcium stores, renal immaturity, and relative hypoparathyroidism secondary to suppression by high fetal calcium levels. Some infants are at further risk for neonatal calcium disturbances due to

Table 1-1 Clinical Criteria for Classification of Low-Birth-Weight Infants

Criteria	36 Wk (Premature)	37-38 Wk (Borderline Premature)	39 Wk (Term)
Plantar creases	Rare, shallow	Heel remains smooth	Creases throughout sole
Size of breast nodule	Not palpable to < 3 mm	4 mm	Visible (7 mm)
Head hair	Cotton wool quality		Silky; each strand can be distinguished
Earlobe	Shapeless, pliable with little cartilage		Rigid with cartilage
Testicular descent and scrotal changes	Small scrotum with rugal patch; testes not completely descended	Gradual descent	Enlarged scrotum creased with rugae; fully descended testes

Adapted from Avery ME, Villee D, Baker S, et al: Neonatology. In Avery ME, First LR (eds): Pediatric Medicine. Baltimore, William & Wilkins, 1989, p148.

the presence of genetic defects, pathologic intrauterine conditions, or birth trauma.[6] Newborn calcium levels usually reach their nadir 24 to 48 hours after delivery, when parathyroid hormone responses become effective. Hypocalcemia is defined as an ionized calcium level of less than 1 mg/dL. At greatest risk for hypocalcemia are preterm infants, newborns requiring surgery, and infants of complicated pregnancies, such as those of diabetic mothers or those receiving bicarbonate infusions. Calcitonin, which inhibits calcium mobilization from the bone, is increased in premature and asphyxiated infants.

Exchange transfusions or massive transfusions of citrated blood can result in the formation of calcium citrate complexes, reducing the ionized serum calcium levels to dangerous or even fatal levels. Late-onset (>48 hours of age) hypocalcemia is less frequent now that most formulas are low in phosphate.

Signs of hypocalcemia may include jitteriness, seizures, cyanosis, vomiting, and myocardial depression, some of which are similar to the signs of hypoglycemia. Hypocalcemic infants have increased muscle tone, which helps differentiate infants with hypocalcemia from those with hypoglycemia. Ionized calcium levels are easily determined in most intensive care settings. Symptomatic hypocalcemia is treated with 10% calcium gluconate administered intravenously at a dosage of 1 to 2 mL/kg over 10 minutes while monitoring the electrocardiogram. Asymptomatic hypocalcemia is best treated with calcium gluconate in a dose of 50 mg of elemental calcium per kilogram per day added to the maintenance fluid; 1 mL of 10% calcium gluconate contains 9 mg of elemental calcium. Calcium mixed with sodium bicarbonate forms an insoluble precipitate. If possible, parenteral calcium should be given through a central venous line.

Magnesium

Magnesium is actively transported across the placenta. Half of the total-body magnesium is in the plasma and soft tissues. Hypomagnesemia is observed with growth retardation, maternal diabetes, after exchange transfusions, and with hypoparathyroidism. Magnesium and calcium metabolism are interrelated. The same infants at risk for hypocalcemia are also at risk for hypomagnesemia. Whenever an infant who has seizures that are believed to be associated with hypocalcemia does not respond to calcium therapy, magnesium deficiency should be suspected and confirmed by obtaining a serum magnesium level. Emergent treatment consists of magnesium sulfate solution, 25 to 50 mg/kg IV every 6 hours, until normal levels are obtained.

Blood Volume

Total RBC volume is at its highest point at delivery. Estimation of blood volume for premature infants, term neonates, and infants is summarized in Table 1-2. By about 3 months of age, total blood volume per kilogram is nearly equal to adult levels. The newborn blood volume is affected by shifts of blood between the placenta and the newborn before clamping the cord. Newborns with delayed cord clamping have higher hemoglobin levels.[7] A hematocrit greater than 50% suggests placental transfusion has occurred.

Table 1-2 Estimation of Blood Volume

Group	Blood Volume (mL/kg)
Premature infants	85-100
Term newborns	85
>1 mo	75
3 mo-adult	70

Adapted from Rowe PC (ed): The Harriet Lane Handbook, 11th eds. Chicago, Year Book Medical, 1987, p 25.

Polycythemia

A central venous hemoglobin level greater than 22 g/dL or a hematocrit value greater than 65% during the 1st week of life is defined as polycythemia. After the central venous hematocrit value reaches 65%, further increases result in rapid exponential increases in blood viscosity. Neonatal polycythemia occurs in infants of diabetic mothers, infants of mothers with toxemia of pregnancy, or SGA infants. Polycythemia is treated using a partial exchange of the infant's blood with fresh whole blood or 5% albumin. This is frequently done when the hematocrit is greater than 65%. Capillary hematocrits are poor predictors of viscosity. Therefore, decisions to perform exchange transfusions should be based on central hematocrits only.

Anemia

Anemia present at birth is due to hemolysis, blood loss, or decreased erythrocyte production.

HEMOLYTIC ANEMIA

Hemolytic anemia is most often a result of placental transfer of maternal antibodies that are destroying the infant's erythrocytes. This can be determined by the direct Coombs test. The most common severe anemia is Rh incompatibility. Hemolytic disease in the newborn produces jaundice, pallor, and hepatosplenomegaly. The most severely affected infants manifest hydrops. This massive edema is not strictly related to the hemoglobin level of these infants. ABO incompatibility frequently results in hyperbilirubinemia but rarely causes anemia.

Congenital infections, hemoglobinopathies (sickle cell disease), and thalassemias produce hemolytic anemia. In a severely affected infant with a positive-reacting direct Coombs test result, a cord hemoglobin level of less than 10.5 g/dL, or a cord bilirubin level of greater than 4.5 mg/dL, immediate exchange transfusion is indicated. For less severely affected infants, exchange transfusion is indicated when the total indirect bilirubin level is greater than 20 mg/dL.

HEMORRHAGIC ANEMIA

Significant anemia can develop from hemorrhage that occurs during placental abruption. Internal bleeding (intraventricular, subgaleal, mediastinal, intra-abdominal) in infants can also often lead to severe anemia. Usually, hemorrhage occurs acutely during delivery, and the newborn occasionally requires transfusion. Twin-twin transfusion reactions can produce polycythemia in one newborn and profound anemia in the other. Severe cases can lead to death in the donor and hydrops in the recipient.

ANEMIA OF PREMATURITY

Decreased RBC production frequently contributes to anemia of prematurity. Erythropoietin is not released until a gestational age of 30 to 34 weeks has been reached. These infants, however, have large numbers of erythropoietin-sensitive RBC progenitors. Research has focused on the role of recombinant erythropoietin in treating anemia in preterm infants.[8-10] Successful increases in hematocrit levels using recombinant erythropoietin may obviate the need for blood transfusions and reduce the risk of bloodborne infections and reactions. Studies suggest that routine use of erythropoietin is probably helpful for the very low birth weight infant (<750 g), but its regular use for other preterm infants does not likely significantly reduce the transfusion rate.

Hemoglobin

At birth, nearly 80% of circulating hemoglobin is fetal. When infant erythropoiesis resumes at about 2 to 3 months of age, most new hemoglobin is adult. When the oxygen level is 27 mm Hg, 50% of the bound oxygen is released from adult hemoglobin (P50). Therefore, the P50 of adult hemoglobin is 27 mm Hg. Reduction of hemoglobin's affinity for oxygen allows more oxygen to be released into the tissues at a given oxygen level.

Fetal hemoglobin has a P50 value 6 to 8 mm Hg higher than that of adult hemoglobin. This higher P50 value allows more efficient oxygen delivery from the placenta to the fetal tissues. In this situation, the hemoglobin equilibrium curve is considered to be shifted to the left of normal. This increase in P50 is believed to be due to the failure of fetal hemoglobin to bind 2,3-diphosphoglycerate to the same degree as does adult hemoglobin.[11] This is somewhat of a disadvantage to the newborn because lower peripheral oxygen levels are needed before oxygen is released from fetal hemoglobin. By 4 to 6 months of age in a term infant, the hemoglobin equilibrium curve gradually shifts to the right and the P50 value approximates that of a normal adult.

Jaundice

In the hepatocyte, bilirubin created by hemolysis is conjugated to glucuronic acid and rendered water soluble. Conjugated (also known as direct) bilirubin is excreted in bile. Unconjugated bilirubin interferes with cellular respiration and is toxic to neural cells. Subsequent neural damage is termed *kernicterus* and produces athetoid cerebral palsy, seizures, sensorineural hearing loss, and, rarely, death.

The newborn's liver has a metabolic excretory capacity for bilirubin that is not equal to its task. Even healthy full-term infants usually have an elevated unconjugated bilirubin level. This peaks about the third day of life at 6.5 to 7.0 mg/dL and does not return to normal until the 10th day of life. A total bilirubin level greater than 7 mg/dL in the first 24 hours or greater than 13 mg/dL at any time in full-term newborns often prompts an investigation for the cause. Breast-fed infants usually have serum bilirubin levels 1 to 2 mg/dL greater than formula-fed infants. The common causes of prolonged indirect hyperbilirubinemia are listed in Table 1-3.

Table 1-3 Causes of Prolonged Indirect Hyperbilirubinemia	
Breast milk jaundice	Pyloric stenosis
Hemolytic disease	Crigler-Najjar syndrome
Hypothyroidism	Extravascular blood

Data from Maisels MJ: Neonatal jaundice. In Avery GB (ed): Neonatology. Pathophysiology and Management of the Newborn. Philadelphia, JB Lippincott, 1987, p 566.

Pathologic jaundice within the first 36 hours of life is usually due to excessive production of bilirubin. Hyperbilirubinemia is managed based on the infant's weight. Although specific cutoffs defining the need for therapy have not been universally accepted, the following recommendations are consistent with most practice patterns.[12] Phototherapy is initiated for newborns (1) less than 1500 g, when the serum bilirubin level reaches 5 mg/dL; (2) 1500 to 2000 g, when the serum bilirubin level reaches 8 mg/dL; or (3) 2000 to 2500 g, when the serum bilirubin level reaches 10 mg/dL. Formula-fed term infants without hemolytic disease are treated by phototherapy when levels reach 13 mg/dL. For hemolytic-related hyperbilirubinemia, phototherapy is recommended when the serum bilirubin level exceeds 10 mg/dL by 12 hours of life, 12 mg/dL by 18 hours, 14 mg/dL by 24 hours, or 15 mg/dL by 36 hours.[13] An absolute bilirubin level that triggers exchange transfusion is still not established, but most exchange transfusion decisions are based on the serum bilirubin level and its rate of rise.

The use of transcutaneous devices for measurement of plasma bilirubin levels has become increasingly common. However, these devices have limited reliability and accuracy in determination of bilirubin levels for those infants who are less than 28 weeks of gestational age or weigh less than 1000 g.[14,15] In these patients, the total serum bilirubin measurement should still be utilized.

Retinopathy of Prematurity

Retinopathy of prematurity (ROP) develops during the active phases of retinal vascular development in the first 3 or 4 months of life. The exact causes are unknown, but oxygen exposure (>93%-95%)[16] and extreme prematurity are the only risk factors that have been repeatedly and convincingly demonstrated. The risk of ROP is probably related to the degree of immaturity, length of exposure, and oxygen concentration. ROP is found in 1.9% of premature infants in large neonatal units.[17] Retrolental fibroplasia is the pathologic change observed in the retina and overlying vitreous after the acute phases of ROP subsides. A study conducted by the National Institutes of Health found that cryotherapy was effective in preventing retinal detachment, macular fold, and retrolental fibroplasia.[18] Treatment of ROP more recently with laser photocoagulation has been shown to have the added benefit of superior visual acuity and less myopia when compared with cryotherapy in long-term follow-up studies.[19-21] Both treatments reduce the incidence of blindness by approximately 25% but do not increase the chance of good visual acuity (<20/40).

The American Academy of Pediatrics guidelines recommend that all infants who received oxygen therapy who weigh less than 1500 g and are fewer than 32 weeks' gestation, and selected infants with a birth weight between 1500 and 2000 g or gestational age of more than 32 weeks with an unstable clinical course, including those requiring cardiorespiratory support and who are believed by their attending pediatrician or neonatologist to be at high risk, should undergo a screening examination for ROP.[22] A re-examination schedule determined by the examining ophthalmologist, based on visual examination findings,[23] should be closely followed.[22]

Thermoregulation

A homeotherm is a mammal that can maintain a constant deep body temperature. Although humans are homeothermic, newborns have difficulty maintaining constant deep body temperature owing to their relatively large surface area, poor thermal regulation, and small mass to act as a heat sink. Heat loss may occur from (1) evaporation (a wet newborn or a newborn in contact with a wet surface), (2) conduction (direct skin contact with a cool surface), (3) convection (air currents blowing over the newborn), and (4) radiation (the newborn radiates heat to a cooler surface without contact with this surface).

Of these, radiation is the most difficult to control. Infants produce heat by increasing metabolic activity either by shivering like an adult or by nonshivering thermogenesis, using brown fat. Brown-fat thermogenesis may be involved in thermoregulatory feeding and sleep cycles in the infant, with an increase in body temperature signaling an increase in metabolic demand.[24] Brown-fat thermogenesis may be rendered inactive by vasopressors, by anesthetic agents, and through nutritional depletion.[25-28] Thermoneutrality (the optimal thermal environment for the newborn) is the range of ambient temperatures in which the newborn with a normal body temperature and a minimal metabolic rate can maintain a constant body temperature by vasomotor control. The *critical temperature* is the temperature below which a metabolic response to cold is necessary to replace lost heat. The appropriate incubator temperature is determined by the patient's weight and postnatal age (Figs. 1-2 and 1-3). For low birth weight infants, thermoneutrality is 34° to 35°C up to 6 weeks of age and 31° to 32°C until 12 weeks of age. Infants who weigh 2 to 3 kg have a thermoneutrality zone of 31° to 34°C on the first day of life and 29° to 31°C until 12 days. Double-walled incubators

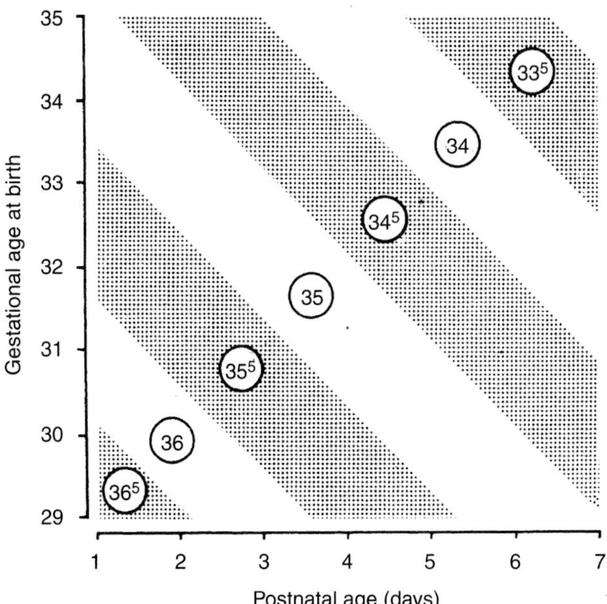

Figure 1-2. Neutral thermal environment (°C) during the first week of life calculated from these measurements: Dew point of the air, 18°C; flow, 10 L/min. (From Sauer PJJ, Dane HJ, Visser HKA: New standards for neutral thermal environment of healthy very low birthweight infants in week one of life. Arch Dis Child 59:18-22, 1984.)

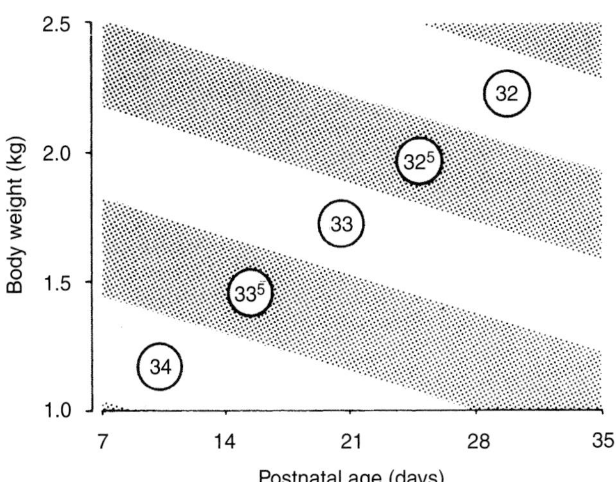

Figure 1-3. Neutral thermal environment (°C) from day 7 to 35. Dew point of air, 18°C; flow, 10 L/min. Body weight is current weight. Values for body weight greater than 2.0 kg are calculated by extrapolation. (From Sauer PJJ, Dane HJ, Visser HKA: New standards for neutral thermal environment of healthy very low birthweight infants in week one of life. Arch Dis Child 59:18-22, 1984.)

offer the best thermoneutral environment. Radiant warmers cannot prevent convection heat loss and lead to higher insensible water loss.

Failure to maintain thermoneutrality leads to serious metabolic and physiologic consequences. Special care must be exercised to maintain the body temperature within normal limits in the operating room.

Fluids and Electrolytes

At 12 weeks of gestation, the fetus has a total body water content that is 94% of body weight. This amount decreases to 80% by 32 weeks' gestation and 78% by term (Fig. 1-4). A further 3% to 5% reduction in total body water content occurs in the first 3 to 5 days of life. Body water continues to decline and reaches adult levels (approximately 60% of body weight) by 1½ years of age. Extracellular water also declines by 1 to 3 years of age. These water composition changes progress in an orderly fashion in utero. Premature delivery requires the newborn to complete both fetal and term water unloading tasks. Surprisingly, the premature infant can complete fetal water unloading by 1 week after birth. Postnatal reduction in extracellular fluid volume has such a high physiologic priority that it occurs even in the presence of relatively large variations of fluid intake.[29]

Glomerular Filtration Rate

The glomerular filtration rate (GFR) of newborns is slower than that of adults.[30] From 21 mL/min/1.73 m^2 at birth in the term infant, GFR quickly increases to 60 mL/min/1.73 m^2 by 2 weeks of age. GFR reaches adult levels by 1½ to 2 years of age. A preterm infant has a GFR that is only slightly slower than that of a full-term infant. In addition to this difference in GFR, the concentrating capacity of the preterm and the full-term infant is well below that of the adult. An infant responding to water deprivation increases urine osmolarity to a maximum of only 600 mOsm/kg. This is in contrast to the adult, whose urine concentration can reach 1200 mOsm/kg. It appears that the difference in concentrating capacity is due to the insensitivity of the collecting tubules of the newborn to antidiuretic hormone. Although the newborn cannot concentrate urine as efficiently as the adult, the newborn can excrete very dilute urine at 30 to 50 mOsm/kg. Newborns are unable to excrete excess sodium, an inability thought to be due to a tubular defect. Term infants are able to conserve sodium, but premature infants are considered "salt wasters" because they have an inappropriate urinary sodium excretion, even with restricted sodium intake.

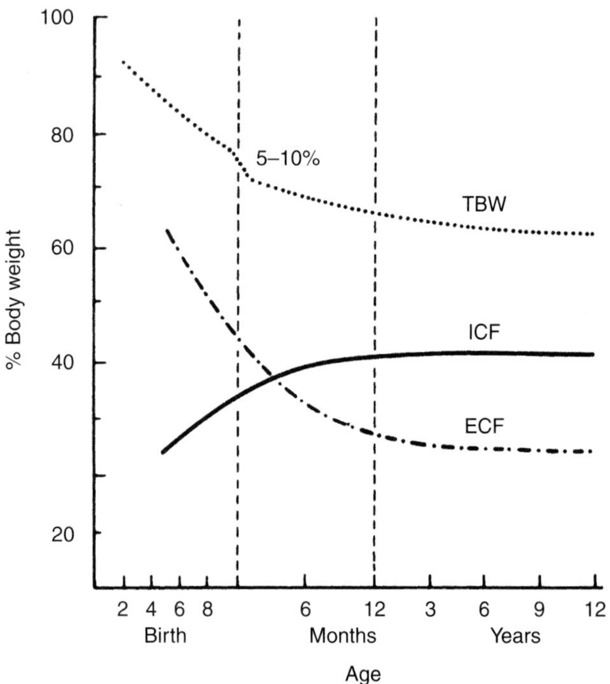

Figure 1-4. Friss-Hansen's classic chart relating total body weight (TBW) and extracellular (ECF) and intracellular fluid (ICF) to percentage of body weight, from early gestation to adolescence. (Adapted from Welch KJ, Randolph JG, Ravitch MM, et al [eds]: Pediatric Surgery, 4th ed. Chicago, Year Book Medical, 1986, p 24.)

Insensible Water Loss

Insensible water loss from the lungs can be essentially eliminated by humidification of inspired air. Transepithelial water loss occurs by the diffusion of water molecules through the stratum corneum of the skin. Owing to the immature skin, preterm infants of 25 to 27 weeks' gestation can lose more than 120 mL/kg/day of water by this mechanism. Transepithelial water loss decreases as age increases.

Neonatal Fluid Requirements

To estimate fluid requirements in the newborn requires an understanding of (1) preexisting fluid deficit or excess, (2) metabolic demands, and (3) losses.

Because these factors change quickly in the critically ill newborn, frequent adjustments in fluid management are necessary. Hourly monitoring of intake and output allows early recognition of fluid balance that will affect treatment decisions. This dynamic approach requires two components: an initial hourly fluid intake that is safe and a monitoring system to detect the patient's response to the treatment program selected. A table of initial volumes expressed in rates of milliliters per kilogram per 24 hours for various surgical conditions has been developed as a result of a study of a large group of infants followed during their first 3 postoperative days (Table 1-4). The patients were divided into three groups by condition: (1) moderate surgical conditions, such as colostomies, laparotomies, and intestinal atresia; (2) severe surgical conditions, such as midgut volvulus or gastroschisis; and (3) necrotizing enterocolitis with perforation of the bowel or bowel necrosis requiring exploration.

No "normal" urine output exists for a given neonate. Ideal urine output can be estimated by measuring the osmolar load presented to the kidney for excretion and calculating the amount of urine necessary to clear this load, if the urine is maintained at an isotonic level of 280 mOsm/dL (Table 1-5).

Table 1-4 Newborn Fluid Volume Requirements (mL/kg/24 hr) for Various Surgical Conditions

Group	Day 1	Day 2	Day 3
Moderate surgical conditions (e.g., colostomies, laparotomies for intestinal atresia, Hirschsprung's disease)	80 ± 25	80 ± 30	80 ± 30
Severe surgical conditions (e.g., gastroschisis, midgut volvulus, meconium peritonitis)	140 ± 45	90 ± 20	80 ± 15
Necrotizing enterocolitis with perforation	145 ± 70	135 ± 50	130 ± 40

Table 1-5 Minimum Newborn Ideal Urine Output (mL/kg/hr) for Various Surgical Conditions

Group	Day 1	Day 2	Day 3
Moderate surgical conditions (e.g., colostomies, laparotomies for intestinal atresia, Hirschsprung's disease)	2 ± 0.96	2.63 ± 1.71	2.38 ± 0.92
Severe surgical conditions (e.g., gastroschisis, midgut volvulus, meconium peritonitis)	2.67 ± 0.92	2.96 ± 0.54	2.96 ± 1.0
Necrotizing enterocolitis with perforation	2.58 ± 1.04	3.17 ± 1.67	3.46 ± 1.46

After administering the initial hourly volume for 4 to 8 hours, depending on the newborn's condition, he or she is reassessed by observing urine output and concentration. With these two factors, it is possible to determine the state of hydration of most newborns and their responses to the initial volume. In more difficult cases, changes in serial serum sodium (Na), blood urea nitrogen (BUN), creatinine, and osmolarity along with urine Na, creatinine, and osmolarity make it possible to assess the infant's response to the initial volume and to use fluid status to guide the next 4 to 8 hours' fluid intake.

Illustrative Examples

INSUFFICIENT FLUID

A 1-kg premature infant, during the first 8 hours postoperatively, has 0.3 mL/kg/hr of urine output. Specific gravity is 1.025. Previous initial volume was 5 mL/kg/hr. Serum BUN has increased from 4 mg/dL to 8 mg/dL; hematocrit value has increased from 35% to 37%, without transfusion. This child is dry. The treatment is to increase the hourly volume to 7 mL/kg/hr for the next 4 hours and to monitor the subsequent urine output and concentration to reassess fluid status.

INAPPROPRIATE ANTIDIURETIC HORMONE RESPONSE

A 3-kg newborn with congenital diaphragmatic hernia during the first 8 hours postoperatively has a urine output of 0.2 mL/kg/hr, with a urine osmolarity of 360 mOsm/L. The previous initial volume was 120 mL/kg/day (15 mL/hr). The serum osmolarity value has decreased from 300 mOsm preoperatively to 278 mOsm/L; and BUN has decreased from 12 to 8 mg/dL. The inappropriate antidiuretic hormone response requires reduction in fluid volume from 120 to 90 mL/kg/day for the next 4 to 8 hours. Repeat urine and serum measurements will guide the further adjustment of fluid administration.

OVERHYDRATION

A 3-kg newborn, 24 hours after operative closure of gastroschisis, had an average urine output of 3 mL/kg/hr over the previous 4 hours. During that time period, the infant received fluids at a rate of 180 mL/kg/day. The specific gravity of the urine has decreased to 1.006; serum BUN is 4 mg/dL; hematocrit value is 30%, down from 35% preoperatively. The total serum protein concentration is 4.0 mg/dL, down from 4.5 mg/dL. This child is being overhydrated. The treatment is to decrease the fluids to 3 mL/kg/hr for the next 4 hours and then to reassess urine output and concentration.

RENAL FAILURE

A 5-kg infant with severe sepsis secondary to Hirschsprung's enterocolitis has had a urine output of 0.1 mL/kg/hr for the past 8 hours. The specific gravity is 1.012; serum sodium, 150 mg/dL; BUN, 25 mg/dL; creatinine, 1.5 mg/dL; urine sodium, 130 mEq; and urine creatinine, 20 mg/dL.

Fractional Na excretion (FE Na) is shown by the following equation:

$$FE\,Na = \frac{(U\,Na \times P\,Cr)}{(P\,Na) \times (U\,Cr)} = \frac{130 \times 1.5}{150 \quad 20}$$
$$= 195/3000 \times 100$$
$$= 6.5\% (\text{normal} = 2\% \text{ to } 3\%)$$

FE Na less than 2% usually indicates a prerenal cause of oliguria, whereas greater than 3% usually implies a renal cause (e.g., acute tubular necrosis). This patient is in acute renal failure. The plan is to restrict fluids to insensible losses plus measured losses for the next 4 hours and to then reassess the plan using both urine and serum studies.

PULMONARY SYSTEM OF THE NEWBORN

The dichotomous branching of the bronchial tree is usually completed by 16 weeks' gestation. No actual alveoli are seen until 24 to 26 weeks' gestation. Therefore, should the fetus be delivered at this age, the air-blood surface area for gas diffusion is limited.

Between 24 and 28 weeks, the cuboidal and columnar cells become flatter and start differentiating into type I (lining cells) and/or type II (granular) pneumocytes. Between 26 and 32 weeks of gestation, terminal air sacs begin to give way to air spaces. From 32 to 36 weeks, further budding of these air spaces occurs and alveoli become numerous. At the same time, the phospholipids that constitute pulmonary surfactant begin to line the terminal lung air spaces. Surfactant is produced by type II pneumocytes and is extremely important in maintaining alveolar stability.

The change in the ratio of the amniotic phospholipids, lecithin and sphingomyelin, is used to assess fetal lung maturity. A ratio greater than 2 is considered compatible with mature lung function. Absence of adequate surfactant leads to hyaline membrane disease or respiratory distress syndrome. Hyaline membrane disease is present in nearly 10% of all premature infants and is the leading cause of morbidity and mortality (30%) among premature infants in the United States. Other conditions associated with pulmonary distress in the newborn include delayed fetal lung absorption (wet lung syndrome), intrauterine aspiration pneumonia (meconium aspiration), and intrapartum pneumonia. In all of these conditions, endotracheal intubation and mechanical ventilation may be required for hypoxia, CO_2 retention, or apnea. Ventilator options and management are discussed in Chapter 7.

Surfactant

Surfactant deficiency is believed to be the major cause of hyaline membrane disease. Surfactant replacement therapy improves effective oxygenation. Three surfactant preparations have been under investigation: (1) surfactant derived from bovine or porcine lung, (2) human surfactant extracted from amniotic fluid, and (3) artificial surfactant. Multicenter-based, randomized trials for modified bovine surfactant (Survanta)[31] and artificial surfactant (Exosurf Neonatal)[32] have been published.

In one study, Survanta was given as a single dose via an endotracheal tube an average of 12 minutes after birth. The patients who received Survanta demonstrated less severe radiographic changes at 24 hours of age compared with infants who received placebo. However, there was no clinical difference at 7 and 28 days after treatment compared with placebo.

In the Exosurf Neonatal study, the premature infants were randomized to receive one dose of the artificial surfactant or air placebo. In this study a significant reduction was noted in the surfactant-treated infants compared with the control group in all of the following: number of deaths attributed to hyaline membrane disease, incidence of pulmonary air leaks, oxygen requirements, and mean airway pressure.

An uncontrolled case series, in which surfactant was given to full-term newborns with pneumonia and meconium aspiration, showed a significant improvement in oxygenation after treatment.[33] Although these and other reports are promising, further studies are needed to determine the most effective dose, the number of doses, and the optimal timing for surfactant treatment. Regardless, surfactant therapy is an important addition to the pulmonary care of the preterm newborn.

One multicenter study reported that surfactant therapy early in the course of full-term newborn respiratory failure resulted in a significantly lower requirement for extracorporeal membrane oxygenation and produced no additional morbidity. Prophylactic treatment as well as rescue treatment with surfactant has proved to reduce the incidence and severity of respiratory distress syndrome, air leaks, and mortality in preterm infants (<30 weeks' gestational age).[34] Additionally, infants suspected of respiratory distress syndrome have been shown to have improved outcomes with early (<2 hour) administration of surfactant when compared with delayed treatment (2-6 hours).[35] This strategy has been shown to be particularly beneficial in those infants with a low rate of exposure to antenatal steroids.[36,37] Several recent multicenter studies compared the efficacy and complication rates of synthetic versus calf-lung cannula surfactant therapies for neonatal respiratory failure.[38-41]

Both natural and synthetic surfactant have been shown to be effective in the treatment and prevention of respiratory distress syndrome. In comparative trials with synthetic surfactant, natural surfactant has demonstrated earlier improvement in ventilator requirements, fewer pneumothoraces, a marginal decrease in bronchopulmonary dysplasia, and decreased mortality.[42] Natural surfactant has been noted to have a marginal increase in intraventricular hemorrhage, but without a difference in more serious (grade 3 to 4) intraventricular hemorrhage. However, support exists for the synthetic surfactant preparations. This support is based on the theoretical advantage of a possibly reduced risk of intraventricular hemorrhage, less exposure to animal antigen with subsequent reactions, and lower overall cost. Newer-generation synthetic surfactant preparations containing peptides that mimic the action of human surfactant protein-B (SP-B) are currently being investigated. In recent randomized, multi-center trials, Lucinactant (Discovery Laboratories, Warrington, PA), an SP-B protein–containing synthetic surfactant, was similar in efficacy and safety in the prevention and treatment of respiratory distress syndrome when compared with porcine-derived (poractant alpha) surfactant, was more effective than nonprotein synthetic preparations, and resulted in decreased respiratory distress syndrome–related mortality rates versus the bovine-derived Survanta.[43,44] It is hoped that future studies will provide additional insight into the appropriate applications of the available agents.

Monitoring

Continuous monitoring of physiologic indices provides data that assist in assessing response to therapy and trends that may be used to predict catastrophe. Many episodes of "sudden deterioration" in critically ill patients are viewed, in retrospect, as changes in the clinical condition that had been occurring for some time.

Arterial Blood Gases and Derived Indices

Arterial oxygen tension ($Pa{O_2}$) is most commonly measured by obtaining an arterial blood sample and by measuring the partial pressure of oxygen with a polarographic electrode. Defining normal parameters for $Pa{O_2}$ depends on the maturation and age of the patient. In the term newborn, the general definition for hypoxia is a $Pa{O_2}$ less than 55 mm Hg, whereas that for hyperoxia is a $Pa{O_2}$ greater than 80 mm Hg.

Capillary blood samples are "arterialized" by topical vasodilators or heat to increase blood flow to a peripheral site. Blood must be freely flowing and collected quickly to prevent exposure to the atmosphere. Blood flowing sluggishly and exposed to atmospheric oxygen falsely raises the $Pa{O_2}$ from a capillary sample, especially in the range of 40 to 60 mm Hg.[45] Capillary blood pH and carbon dioxide tension ($P{CO_2}$) correlate well with arterial samples, except when perfusion is poor. $Pa{O_2}$ is the least reliable of all capillary blood gas determinations. In patients receiving oxygen therapy in whom $Pa{O_2}$ exceeds 60 mm Hg, the capillary $Pa{O_2}$ correlates poorly with the arterial measurement.[46,47]

In newborns, umbilical artery catheterization can provide arterial access. The catheter tip should rest at the level of the diaphragm or below L3. The second most frequently used arterial site is the radial artery. Complications of arterial blood sampling include repeated blood loss and anemia. Changes in oxygenation are such that intermittent blood gas sampling may miss critical episodes of hypoxia or hyperoxia. Because of the drawbacks of ex-vivo monitoring, several in-vivo monitoring systems have been used.

Pulse Oximetry

The noninvasive determination of oxygen saturation ($Sa{O_2}$) gives moment-to-moment information regarding the availability of oxygen to the tissues. If the $Pa{O_2}$ is plotted against the oxygen saturation of hemoglobin, the S-shaped hemoglobin dissociation curve is obtained (Fig. 1-5). Referring to this curve, hemoglobin is 50% saturated at 25 mm Hg $Pa{O_2}$ and 90% saturated at 50 mm Hg. Pulse oximetry has a rapid (5 to 7 seconds) response time, requires no calibration, and may be left in place continuously.

Pulse oximetry is not possible if the patient is in shock, has peripheral vasospasm, or has vascular constriction due to hypothermia. Inaccurate readings may occur in the presence of jaundice, direct high-intensity light, dark skin pigmentation, and greater than 80% fetal hemoglobin. Oximetry is not a sensitive guide to gas exchange in patients with high $Pa{O_2}$ due to the shape of the oxygen dissociation curve. As an example, on the upper horizontal portion of the curve, large changes in $Pa{O_2}$ may occur with little change in $Sa{O_2}$. An oximeter reading of 95% could represent a $Pa{O_2}$ between 60 and 160 mm Hg.

A study to compare $Sa{O_2}$ from pulse oximetry with $Pa{O_2}$ determined from indwelling arterial catheters has shown that $Sa{O_2}$ greater than or equal to 85% corresponds to a $Pa{O_2}$ greater than 55 mm Hg and that $Sa{O_2}$ less than or equal to 90% corresponds to a $Pa{O_2}$ less than 80 mm Hg.[48] Guidelines for monitoring infants using pulse oximetry have been suggested for the following three conditions:

1. In the infant with acute respiratory distress without direct arterial access, saturation limits of 85% (lower) and 92% (upper) should be set.
2. In the older infant with chronic respiratory distress who is at low risk for retinopathy of prematurity, the upper saturation limit may be set at 95%; the lower limit should be set at 87% to avoid pulmonary vasoconstriction and pulmonary hypertension.
3. Because the concentration of fetal hemoglobin in newborns affects the accuracy of pulse oximetry, infants with arterial access should have both $Pa{O_2}$ and $Sa{O_2}$ monitored closely. A graph should be kept at the bedside documenting the $Sa{O_2}$ each time the $Pa{O_2}$ is measured. Limits for the $Sa{O_2}$ alarm can be changed because the characteristics of this relationship change.

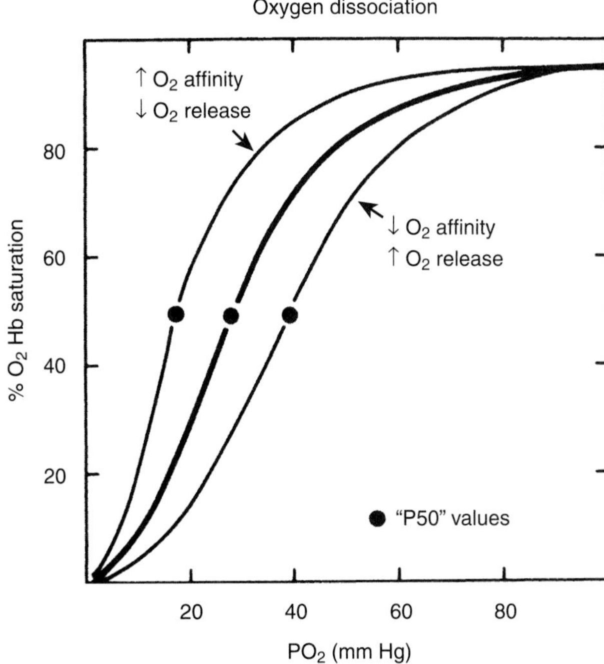

Figure 1-5. The oxygen dissociation curve of normal adult blood. The P50, the oxygen tension at 50% oxygen saturation, is approximately 27 mm Hg. As the curve shifts to the right, the oxygen affinity of hemoglobin decreases and more oxygen is released at a given oxygen tension. With a shift to the left, the opposite effects are observed. A decrease in pH or an increase in temperature reduces the affinity of hemoglobin for oxygen. (Modified from Glancette V, Zipursky A: Neonatal hematology. In Avery GB [ed]: Neonatology. Philadelphia, JB Lippincott, 1986, p 663.)

Carbon Dioxide Tension

Arterial carbon dioxide tension ($Pa{CO_2}$) is a direct reflection of gas exchange in the lungs and of the metabolic rate. In most clinical situations, changes in $Pa{CO_2}$ are due to changes in ventilation. For this reason, serial measurement of $Pa{CO_2}$ is a practical method to assess the adequacy of ventilation. The discrepancy among venous, capillary, and arterial carbon dioxide tensions is not great under most conditions, although one study noted a significant increase in $Paco_2$ in venous samples compared with simultaneous arterial samples.[49]

Because it is possible to monitor $Paco_2$ and pH satisfactorily with venous or capillary blood samples and because pulse oximetry is now commonly used to assess oxygenation, many infants with respiratory insufficiency no longer require arterial catheters for monitoring.

End-tidal Carbon Dioxide

Measuring expired CO_2 by capnography provides a noninvasive means of continuously monitoring alveolar Pco_2. Capnometry measures CO_2 by an infrared sensor either placed in line between the ventilator circuit and the endotracheal tube or off to the side of the air flow, both of which are applicable only to the intubated patient. A comparative study of end-tidal CO_2 in critically ill neonates demonstrated that both sidestream and mainstream end-tidal CO_2 measurements approximated $Paco_2$.[50] When the mainstream sensor was inserted into the breathing circuit, the $Paco_2$ increased an average of 2 mm Hg. Although this is not likely to significantly affect infants who are ventilated, it might create fatigue in weaning infants from mechanical ventilation. The accuracy of the end-tidal CO_2 is diminished with small endotracheal tubes.

Central Venous Catheter

Indications for central venous catheter placement include (1) hemodynamic monitoring, (2) inability to establish other venous access, (3) TPN, and (4) infusion of inotropic drugs or other medications that cannot be given peripherally. Measurement of central venous pressure to monitor volume status is frequently used in the resuscitation of a critically ill patient. A catheter placed in the superior vena cava or right atrium measures the filling pressure of the right side of the heart, which usually reflects left atrial and filling pressure of the left ventricle. Often, a wide discrepancy exists between left and right atrial pressure when pulmonary disease, overwhelming sepsis, or cardiac lesions are present. To utilize the data effectively, continuous measurements must be taken with a pressure transducer connected to a catheter accurately placed in the central venous system. Positive-pressure ventilation, pneumothorax, abdominal distention, or pericardial tamponade all elevate central venous pressure.

Pulmonary Artery Catheter

The pulmonary artery pressure catheter has altered the care of the child with severe cardiopulmonary derangement by allowing direct measurement of cardiovascular variables at the bedside. The indications for pulmonary catheter placement are listed in Table 1-6. With this catheter, it is possible to monitor central venous pressure, pulmonary artery pressure, pulmonary wedge pressure, and cardiac output. A 4-French, double-lumen catheter and a 5- to 8-French, triple-lumen catheter are available. The catheter is usually placed by percutaneous methods (as in the adult) except in the smallest pediatric patient, in whom a cutdown is sometimes required.

Table 1-6 Indications for Pulmonary Artery Catheter Placement

Indications
Inadequate systemic perfusion in the presence of elevated central venous pressure
Fluid management in noncardiogenic pulmonary edema
Evaluation of therapeutic interventions, such as changes in positive end-expiratory pressure, use of vasoactive drugs, or assisted circulation
Hemodynamic evaluation in children with pulmonary hypertension
Severe pulmonary disease with profound hypoxemia

Adapted from Perkin RM: Invasive monitoring in the pediatric intensive care unit. In Nussbaum E (ed): Pediatric Intensive Care, 2nd ed. Mt. Kisco, NY, Futura Publishing, 1989, p 259.

When the tip of the catheter is in a distal pulmonary artery and the balloon is inflated, the resulting pressure is generally an accurate reflection of left atrial pressure because the pulmonary veins have no valves. This pulmonary "wedge" pressure represents left ventricular filling pressure, which is used as a reflection of preload. The monitors display phasic pressures, but treatment decisions are made based on the electronically derived mean central venous pressure. A low pulmonary wedge pressure suggests that blood volume must be expanded. A high or normal pulmonary wedge pressure in the presence of continued signs of shock suggests left ventricular dysfunction.

Cardiac output is usually measured in liters per minute. When related to body surface area, the output is represented as the *cardiac index*, which is simply the cardiac output divided by the body surface area. The normalized cardiac index allows the evaluation of cardiac performance without regard to body size. The usual resting value for cardiac index is between 3.5 and 4.5 $L/min/m^2$. The determination of cardiac output by the thermodilution technique, which is possible with a Swan-Ganz pulmonary artery catheter, is widely used and has a good correlation with other methods. Accurate cardiac output determination depends on rapid injection, accurate measurement of injectant temperature and volume, and absence of shunting. Because ventilation affects the flow into and out of the right ventricle, three injections should be made at a consistent point in the ventilatory cycle, typically at end expiration.

Doppler measurement of aortic flow velocity allows measurement of cardiac output by the following formula:

$$\text{Cardiac output (mL/min)} = \text{Mean aortic blood flow velocity (cm/sec)} \times \text{Aortic cross-sectional area (cm}^2) \times 60$$

Aortic cross-sectional area is determined by standard ultrasonographic techniques. Using this cross-sectional measurement, pulsed Doppler aortic flow velocity is measured by a transducer placed at the suprasternal notch, in the esophagus, or in the trachea to derive cardiac output. Studies are underway to determine if cardiac output measured by this technique correlates well with thermodilution or the Fick method in critically ill pediatric patients. Previous studies have shown that cardiac output measured by intermittent Doppler measurement at the suprasternal notch was not of sufficient reliability to be employed for hemodynamic monitoring in critically ill children.[51]

Impedance cardiography (bioimpedance) is another noninvasive technique that measures stroke volume on a beat-by-beat basis.[52] Bioimpedance employs a low-level current applied to the thorax, where changes in the volume and velocity of blood flow in the thoracic aorta result in detectable changes in thoracic conductivity. Previous application of this technique in critically ill patients met with only limited success.[53] Late refinements in electrode configuration, algorithms, and microprocessors have produced more acceptable results. Studies in pigs demonstrated a good correlation of bioimpedance-derived cardiac output with thermodilutional cardiac output over a wide hemodynamic range.[54,55] These techniques have yet to be validated or proved effective in children.

Another study concluded that using right-sided heart catheters in treating critically ill adult patients resulted in an increased mortality.[56] However, a consensus committee report documents the continued safety and efficacy of right-sided heart catheters in the care of critically ill children.[57]

Venous Oximetry

Mixed venous oxygen saturation ($S\bar{v}O_2$) is an indicator of the adequacy of oxygen supply and demand in perfused tissues. Oxygen consumption is defined as the amount of oxygen consumed by the tissue as calculated by the Fick equation:

$$O_2\text{ Consumption} = \text{Cardiac output} \times \text{Arterial} - \text{venous oxygen content difference}$$

Reflectance spectrophotometry is currently used for continuous venous oximetry. Multiple wavelengths of light are transmitted at a known intensity by means of fiberoptic bundles in a special pulmonary artery or right atrial catheter. The light is reflected by red blood cells flowing past the tip of the catheter. The wavelengths of light are chosen so that both oxyhemoglobin and deoxyhemoglobin are measured to determine the fraction of hemoglobin saturated with oxygen. The system requires either in-vitro calibration by reflecting light from a standardized target that represents a known oxygen saturation or in-vivo calibration by withdrawing blood from the pulmonary artery catheter and measuring the saturation by laboratory co-oximetry.

Mixed venous oxygen saturation values within the normal range (68%-77%) indicate a normal balance between oxygen supply and demand, provided that vasoregulation is intact and distribution of peripheral blood flow is normal. Values greater than 77% are most commonly associated with syndromes of vasoderegulation, such as sepsis. Uncompensated changes in O_2 saturation, hemoglobin level, or cardiac output lead to a decrease in $S\bar{v}O_2$. A sustained decrease in $S\bar{v}O_2$ greater than 10% should lead to measuring Sao_2, hemoglobin level, and cardiac output to determine the cause of the decline.[58] The most common sources of error in measuring $S\bar{v}O_2$ are calibration and catheter malposition. The most important concept in $S\bar{v}O_2$ monitoring is the advantage of continuous monitoring, which allows early warning of a developing problem.[59]

Although most clinical experience has been with pulmonary artery catheters, right atrial catheters are more easily placed and may thus provide better information to detect hemodynamic deterioration earlier and permit more rapid treatment of physiologic derangements.[60] A study has shown that when oxygen consumption was monitored and maintained at a consistent level, the right atrial venous saturation was thought to be an excellent measure.[61]

SHOCK

Shock is a state in which the cardiac output is insufficient to deliver adequate oxygen to meet metabolic demands of the tissues. Cardiovascular function is determined by preload, cardiac contractility, heart rate, and afterload. Shock may be classified broadly as hypovolemic, cardiogenic, or septic.

Hypovolemic Shock

Preload is a function of the volume of blood presented to the ventricles. Because of the impracticality of measuring volume, preload is commonly monitored by atrial pressure measurements. In most clinical situations, right atrial pressure or central venous pressure is the index of cardiac preload. In situations in which left ventricular or right ventricular compliance is abnormal, or in certain forms of congenital heart disease, right atrial pressure may not correlate well with left atrial pressure. In infants and children, most shock situations are the result of reduced preload secondary to fluid loss, such as from diarrhea, vomiting, or trauma.

Virtually all forms of pediatric shock have significant intravascular and functional interstitial fluid deficits. Hypovolemia results in decreased venous return to the heart. Preload is reduced, cardiac output falls, and the overall result is a decrease in tissue perfusion. Invasive infection and hypovolemia are the most common causes of shock in both children and adults. The first step in treating all forms of shock is to correct existing fluid deficits. Inotropic drugs should not be initiated until adequate intravascular fluid volume has been established. The speed and volume of the infusate are determined by the patient's responses, particularly changes in blood pressure, pulse rate, urine output, and central venous pressure. Shock resulting from acute hemorrhage is initially treated with the administration of 10 to 20 mL/kg of Ringer's lactate solution or normal saline as fluid boluses. If the patient does not respond, a second bolus of crystalloid is given. Type-specific or crossmatched blood is given as needed.

The choice of resuscitation fluid in shock that results from sepsis or from loss of extracellular fluid (from conditions such as peritonitis, intestinal obstruction, and pancreatitis) is less clear. Our initial resuscitation fluids include Ringer's lactate or normal saline in older infants and children and half-strength Ringer's or 0.5 normal saline in the newborn. Despite our reluctance to use colloid-containing solutions for shock, we make an exception in the desperately ill newborn or premature infant with septicemia. To correct the reduced serum factors, for example in those children with a coagulopathy, we use fresh frozen plasma or specific factors as the resuscitation fluid.

The rate and volume of resuscitation fluid given is adjusted based on data obtained from monitoring the effects of the initial resuscitation. After the initial bolus is given, the adequacy of the replacement is assessed by monitoring urine output, urine concentration, plasma acidosis, oxygenation, arterial pressure, central venous pressure, and pulmonary wedge pressure, if indicated. When cardiac failure is present, continued vigorous delivery of large volumes of fluid may cause a further increase in preload to the failing myocardium and accelerate the downhill course. In this setting, as outlined previously, inotropic agents are given while monitoring cardiac and pulmonary function.

Cardiogenic Shock

Myocardial contractility is usually expressed as the ejection fraction, which is the proportion of ventricular volume that is pumped. Myocardial contractility is reduced with hypoxemia and acidosis. Inotropic drugs increase cardiac contractility but have their best effect when hypoxemia and acidosis are corrected.

Adrenergic receptors are important in regulating calcium flux, which, in turn, is important in controlling myocardial contractility. The α- and β-adrenergic receptors are proteins present in the sarcolemma of myocardial and vascular smooth muscle cells. β_1 receptors are predominantly in the heart and, when stimulated, result in increased contractility of myocardium. β_2 receptors are predominantly in respiratory and vascular smooth muscle. When stimulated, these receptors result in bronchodilation and vasodilation. α_1-Adrenergic receptors are located on vascular smooth muscle and result in vascular constriction when stimulated. α_2-Adrenergic receptors are found mainly on prejunctional sympathetic nerve terminals. The concept of dopaminergic receptors has also been used to account for the cardiovascular effects of dopamine not mediated through α or β receptors. Activation of dopaminergic receptors results in decreased renal and mesenteric vascular resistance and, usually, increased blood flow. The most commonly used inotropic drugs are listed in Table 1-7.

Epinephrine

Epinephrine is an endogenous catecholamine with α- and β-adrenergic effects. At low doses, the β-adrenergic effect predominates. These effects include an increase in heart rate, cardiac contractility, cardiac output, and bronchiolar dilation. Blood pressure rises, in part, not only due to increased cardiac output but also due to increased peripheral vascular resistance, which is noted with higher doses at which α-adrenergic effects become predominant. Renal blood flow may increase slightly, remain unchanged, or decrease depending on the balance between greater cardiac output and the changes in peripheral vascular resistance, which lead to regional redistribution of blood flow. Cardiac arrhythmias can be seen with epinephrine, especially with higher doses. Dosages for treating compromised cardiovascular function range from 0.05 to 1.0 μg/kg/min. Excessive doses of epinephrine can cause worsening cardiac ischemia and dysfunction from increased myocardial oxygen demand.

Isoproterenol

Isoproterenol is a β-adrenergic agonist. It increases cardiac contractility and heart rate, with little change in systemic vascular resistance. The peripheral vascular β-adrenergic effect and lack of a peripheral vascular α-adrenergic effect may allow reduction of left ventricular afterload. Isoproterenol's intense chronotropic effect produces tachycardia, which can limit its usefulness. Isoproterenol is administered intravenously at a dosage of 0.1 to 0.3 μg/kg/min.

Dopamine

Dopamine is an endogenous catecholamine with β-adrenergic, α-adrenergic, and dopaminergic effects. It is both a direct and an indirect β-adrenergic agonist. Dopamine elicits positive inotropic and chronotropic responses by direct interaction with the β receptor (direct effect) and by stimulating the release of norepinephrine from the sympathetic nerve endings, which interacts with the β receptor (indirect effect). At low dosages (<3 μg/kg/min), the dopaminergic effect of the drug predominates, resulting in reduced renal and mesenteric vascular resistance and improved blood flow to these organs. The β-adrenergic effects become more prominent at intermediate dosages (3 to 10 μg/kg/min), producing a higher cardiac output. At relatively high dosages (>15 to 20 μg/kg/min), the α-adrenergic effects become prominent with peripheral vasoconstriction.

Experience with the use of dopamine in pediatric patients suggests that it is effective in increasing blood pressure in neonates, infants, and children. The precise dosages for these desired hemodynamic effects are not known. The effects of low dosages of dopamine on blood pressure, heart rate, and renal function were studied in 18 hypotensive, preterm infants.[62] The blood pressure and diuretic effects were observed at 2, 4, and 8 μg/kg/min. Elevations in heart rate were seen only

Table 1-7 Vasoactive Medications Commonly Used in the Newborn

Vasoactive Agent	Principal Modes of Action	Major Hemodynamic Effects	Administration and Dosage	Indications
Epinephrine	α and β agonist	Increases heart rate and myocardial contractility by activating β_1 receptors	0.1 mL/kg of 1:10,000 solution given IV intracardial, *or* endotracheal 0.05-1.0 μg/kg/min IV	Cardiac resuscitation; short-term use when severe heart failure resistant to other drugs
Dopamine, low dose	Stimulates dopamine receptors	Decrease in vascular resistance in splanchnic, renal, and cerebral vessels	<2 μg/kg/min IV	Useful in managing cardiogenic or hypovolemic shock or after cardiac surgery
Dopamine, intermediate dose	Stimulates β_1 receptors; myocardial	Inotropic response	2=10 μg/kg/min IV	Blood pressure unresponsive to low dose
Dopamine, high dose	Stimulates α receptors	Increased peripheral and renal vascular resistance	>10 μg/kg/min IV	Septic shock with low systemic vascular resistance
Dobutamine	Synthetic β_1 agonist in low doses; α and β_2 effects in higher doses	Increased cardiac output, increased arterial pressure; less increase in heart rate than with dopamine	1-15 μg/kg/min IV	Useful alternative to dopamine if increase in heart rate undesirable
Isoproterenol	β_1 and β_2 agonist	Increased cardiac output by positive inotropic and chronotropic action and increase in venous return; systemic vascular resistance generally reduced; pulmonary vascular resistance generally reduced	0.1-0.3 μg/kg/min IV	Useful in low-output situations, especially when heart rate is slow
Sodium nitroprusside	Direct-acting vasodilator that relaxes arteriolar and venous smooth muscle	Afterload reduction; reduced arterial pressure	1-10 μg/kg/min IV (for up to 10 min); 0.5-2.0 μg/kg/min IV	Hypertensive crisis; vasodilator therapy
Milrinone	Phosphodiesterase inhibitor relaxes arteriolar and venous smooth muscle via calcium/cyclic adenosine monophosphate	Increased cardiac output, slight decreased blood presure, increased oxygen delivery	75 μg/kg bolus IV, then 0.75-1.0 μg/k g/min IV	Useful as an alternative or in addition to dopamine (may act synergistically) if increased heart rate undesirable

Adapted from Lees MH, King DH: Cardiogenic shock in the neonate. Pediatr Rev 9:263, 1988.

at 8 μg/kg/min. Further work is needed to better characterize the pharmacokinetics and pharmacodynamics of dopamine in children, especially in newborns.

Recent clinical evidence has demonstrated some beneficial effects from orally administered levodopa for treating cardiac failure in pediatric patients. Because enteral medications for heart failure are currently limited to digoxin and diuretics, using levodopa may improve our ability to treat heart failure without using parenteral ionotropes.[63]

Dobutamine

Dobutamine, a synthetic catecholamine, has predominantly β-adrenergic effects with minimal α-adrenergic effects. The hemodynamic effect of dobutamine in infants and children with shock has been studied.[64] Dobutamine infusion significantly increased cardiac index, stroke index, and pulmonary capillary wedge pressure, and it decreased systemic vascular resistance. The drug appears more efficacious in treating cardiogenic shock than septic shock. The advantage of dobutamine over isoproterenol is its lesser chronotropic effect and its tendency to maintain systemic pressure. The advantage over dopamine is dobutamine's lesser peripheral vasoconstrictor effect. The usual range of dosages for dobutamine is 2 to 15 μg/kg/min. One study found dobutamine significantly increased systemic blood flow in preterm infants when compared with dopamine. However, it did not demonstrate differences in outcomes.[65,66] The combination of dopamine and dobutamine has been increasingly used. However, little information regarding their combined advantages or effectiveness in pediatric patients has been published.

Milrinone

Milrinone, a phosphodiesterase inhibitor, is a potent positive inotrope and vasodilator that has been shown to improve cardiac function in infants and children.[67-69]

The proposed action is due, in part, to an increase in intracellular cyclic adenosine monophosphate and calcium transport secondary to inhibition of cardiac phosphodiesterase. This effect is independent of β-agonist stimulation and, in fact, may act synergistically with a β agonist to improve cardiac performance. Milrinone increases cardiac index and oxygen delivery without affecting heart rate, blood pressure, or pulmonary wedge pressure. Milrinone is administered as a 75-μg/kg bolus followed by infusion of 0.75 to 1.0 μg/kg/min.

Septic Shock

Afterload represents the force against which the left ventricle must contract to eject blood. It is related to systemic vascular resistance and myocardial wall stress. Systemic vascular resistance is defined as the systemic mean arterial blood pressure minus right arterial pressure divided by cardiac output. Cardiac contractility is affected by systemic vascular resistance and afterload. In general, increases in afterload reduce cardiac contractility and decreases in afterload increase cardiac contractility.

Septic shock is a distributive form of shock that differs from other forms of shock. Cardiogenic and hypovolemic shock lead to increased systemic vascular resistance and decreased cardiac output. Septic shock results from a severe decrease in systemic vascular resistance and a generalized maldistribution of blood and leads to a hyperdynamic state.[70] The pathophysiology of septic shock begins with a nidus of infection. Organisms may invade the bloodstream, or they may proliferate at the infected site and release various mediators into the bloodstream. Evidence now supports the finding that substances produced by the microorganism, such as lipopolysaccharide, endotoxin, exotoxin, lipid moieties, and other products, can induce septic shock by stimulating host cells to release cytokines, leukotrienes, and endorphins.

Endotoxin is a lipopolysaccharide found in the outer membrane of gram-negative bacteria. Functionally, the molecule is divided into three parts: (1) the highly variable O-specific polysaccharide side chain (conveys serotypic specificity to bacteria and can activate the alternate pathway of complement); (2) the R-core region (less variable among different gram-negative bacteria; antibodies to this region could be cross protective); and (3) lipid-A (responsible for most of the toxicity of endotoxin). Endotoxin stimulates tumor necrosis factor (TNF) and can directly activate the classic complement pathway in the absence of antibody. Endotoxin has been implicated as an important factor in the pathogenesis of human septic shock and gram-negative sepsis.[71] Therapy has focused on developing antibodies to endotoxin to treat septic shock. Antibodies to endotoxin have been used in clinical trials of sepsis with variable results.[72-74]

Cytokines, especially TNF, play a dominant role in the host's response. Endotoxin and exotoxin both induce TNF release in vivo and produce many other toxic effects via this endogenous mediator.[75-77] TNF is released primarily from monocytes and macrophages; however, it is also released from natural killer cells, mast cells, and some activated T lymphocytes. Other stimuli for its release include viruses, fungi, parasites, and interleukin-1 (IL-1). In sepsis, the effects of TNF release may include cardiac dysfunction, disseminated intravascular coagulation, and cardiovascular collapse. TNF release also causes the release of granulocyte-macrophage colony-stimulating factor (GM-CSF), interferon alfa, and IL-1. Antibodies against TNF protect animals from exotoxin and bacterial challenge.[78,79]

Previously known as the endogenous pyrogen, IL-1 is produced primarily by macrophages and monocytes and plays a central role in stimulating a variety of host responses, including fever production, lymphocyte activation, and endothelial cell stimulation to produce procoagulant activity and to increase adhesiveness. IL-1 also causes the induction of the inhibitor of tissue plasminogen activator and the production of GM-CSF. These effects are balanced by the release of platelet-activating factor and arachidonic metabolites.

IL-2, also known as T-cell growth factor, is produced by activated T lymphocytes and strengthens the immune response by stimulating cell proliferation. Its clinically apparent side effects include capillary leak syndrome, tachycardia, hypotension, increased cardiac index, decreased systemic vascular resistance, and decreased left ventricular ejection fraction.[80,81]

Studies done on dogs have suggested that, in immature animals, septic shock is more lethal and has different mechanisms of tissue injury.[82] These include more dramatic aberrations in blood pressure (more constant decline), heart rate (progressive, persistent tachycardia), blood sugar level (severe, progressive hypoglycemia), acid-base status (severe acidosis), and oxygenation (severe hypoxemia). These changes are significantly different from those seen in the adult animals that also experience improved survival of almost 600% (18.5 vs. 3.1 hours) compared with the premature animal.

The neonate's host defense can usually respond successfully to ordinary microbial challenge. However, defense against major challenges appears limited and provides an explanation for the high mortality rate with major neonatal sepsis. As in adults, the immune system consists of four major components: cell-mediated immunity (T cells), complement system, antibody-mediated immunity (B cells), and macrophage-neutrophil phagocytic system. The two most important deficits in newborn host defenses that seem to increase the risk of bacterial sepsis are the quantitative and qualitative changes in the phagocytic system and the defects in antibody-mediated immunity.

The proliferative rate of the granulocyte-macrophage precursor has been reported to be at near-maximal capacity in the neonate. However, the neutrophil storage pool is markedly reduced in the newborn compared with the adult. After bacterial challenge, newborns fail to increase stem cell proliferation and soon deplete their already reduced neutrophil storage pool. Numerous in-vitro abnormalities have been demonstrated in neonatal polymorphonuclear neutrophils, especially in times of stress or infection.[83] These abnormalities include decreased deformability, chemotaxis, phagocytosis, C3b receptor expression, adherence, bacterial killing, and depressed oxidative metabolism. Chemotaxis is impaired in neonatal neutrophils in response to various bacterial organisms and antigen-antibody complexes.[84] Granulocytes are activated by their interaction with endothelial cells followed by entry into secondary lymphoid tissues via the endothelial venules. Initial adhesion of granulocytes is dependent on their expression of L-selectin, a cell adhesion molecule expressed on the granulocyte cell surface. Evaluation of cord blood has demonstrated a significantly lower expression of L-selectin on granulocyte surfaces when compared with older newborn (5 days old) and adult samples, indicating a depressed level of interaction with vascular endothelial cells at the initial stage of adhesion.[85] Although phagocytosis has additionally been demonstrated to be abnormal in neonatal phagocytes, it appears that this phenomenon is most likely secondary to decreased opsonic activity rather than an intrinsic defect of the neonatal polymorphonuclear neutrophils.[86,87] Currently, there is inconclusive evidence to support or refute the routine use of granulocyte transfusions in the prevention or treatment of sepsis in the neonate.[88]

Preterm and term newborns have poor responses to various antigenic stimuli, reduced gamma globulin levels at birth, and reduced maternal immunoglobulin supply from placental transport. Almost 33% of infants with a birth weight less than 1500 g develop substantial hypogammaglobulinemia.[89] IgA and IgM are also low due to the inability of these two immunoglobulins to cross the placenta. Neonates, therefore, are usually more susceptible to pyogenic bacterial infections because most of the antibodies that opsonize pyogenic bacterial capsular antigens are IgG and IgM. In addition, neonates do not produce type-specific antibodies, which appears to be secondary to a defect in the differentiation of B lymphocytes into immunoglobulin-secreting plasma cells and T lymphocyte–mediated facilitation of antibody synthesis. In the term infant, total hemolytic complement activity, which measures the classic complement pathway, constitutes approximately 50% of adult activity.[90] Owing to lower levels of factor B, the activity of the alternative complement pathway is also decreased in the neonate.[91] Fibronectin, a plasma protein that promotes reticuloendothelial clearance of invading microorganisms, is deficient in neonatal cord plasma.[92]

Using intravenous immunoglobulins (IVIGs) for the prophylaxis and treatment of sepsis in the newborn, especially the preterm, low birth weight infant, has been studied in numerous trials with varied outcomes. In one study, a group of infants weighing 1500 g was treated with 500 mg/kg of IVIG each week for 4 weeks and compared with infants who were not treated with IVIG.[93] The mortality rate was 16% in the IVIG-treated group compared with 32% in the untreated group. Another recent analysis examined the role of IVIG to prevent and treat neonatal sepsis.[94] A significant benefit was noted from the prophylactic use of IVIG to prevent sepsis in low birth weight premature infants. However, using IVIG to treat neonatal sepsis produced a greater than 6% decrease in the mortality rate.

A review of 19 randomized controlled trials found a 3% decrease in the incidence of neonatal sepsis in preterm infants without a significant difference in all-cause and infection-related mortality when prophylactic IVIG was administered. Based on the marginal reduction of neonatal sepsis without a reduction in mortality, routine use of prophylactic IVIG cannot be recommended.[95]

Colony-stimulating factors are a family of glycoproteins that stimulate proliferation and differentiation of hematopoietic cells of various lineages. GM-CSF and granulocyte colony-stimulating factor (G-CSF) have similar physiologic actions. Both stimulate the proliferation of bone marrow myeloid progenitor cells, induce the release of bone marrow neutrophil storage pools, and enhance mature neutrophil effect or function.[94,96] Preliminary studies of GM-CSF in neonatal animals demonstrate enhancement of neutrophil oxidative metabolism, as well as priming of neonatal neutrophils for enhanced chemotaxis and bacterial killing. Both GM-CSF and G-CSF induce peripheral neutrophilia within 2 to 6 hours of intraperitoneal administration. This enhanced affinity for neutrophils returns to normal baseline level by 24 hours.[97] Recent studies confirm the efficacy and safety of G-CSF therapy for neonatal sepsis and neutropenia.[98] Other studies have demonstrated no long-term adverse hematologic, immunologic, or developmental effects from G-CSF therapy in the septic neonate. Prolonged prophylactic treatment in the very low birth weight neonate with recombinant GM-CSF has been shown to be well tolerated and have a significant decrease in the rate of nosocomial infections.[99,100] Confirmatory studies are currently being performed. The current recommended daily pediatric dose is 5 μg/kg/dose given subcutaneously.

Unique to the newborn in septic shock is the persistence of fetal circulation and resultant pulmonary hypertension.[101] In fact, the rapid administration of fluid can further exacerbate this issue by causing left-to-right shunting through a patent ductus arteriosus and subsequent congestive heart failure from ventricular overload. Infants in septic shock with a new heart murmur should receive indomethacin and undergo a cardiac echocardiogram to evaluate the heart. A single institution randomized trial demonstrated an improved outcome from ventricular overload with pentoxifylline in extremely premature infants.[102]

The critical care of a patient in septic shock can be challenging. Septic shock has a distinctive clinical presentation and is characterized by an early compensated stage where one can see a decreased systemic vascular resistance, an increase in cardiac output, tachycardia, warm extremities, and an adequate urine output. Later in the clinical presentation, septic shock is characterized by an uncompensated phase in which the patient develops a decrease in intravascular volume, myocardial depression, high vascular resistance, and a decreasing cardiac output.[103] Care of these patients is based on the principles of source control, antibiotics, and supportive care. Patients with severe septic shock often do not respond to conventional forms of volume loading and cardiovascular supportive medications. Recently, the administration of arginine vasopressin has been shown to decrease mortality in adult patients with recalcitrant septic shock.[104-106] Vasopressin, also known as antidiuretic hormone, is made in the posterior pituitary and plays a primary role in water regulation by the kidneys. The U.S. Food and Drug Administration (FDA)-approved uses of vasopressin and its derivatives are for diabetes. Other non–FDA-approved uses for vasopressin include gastrointestinal hemorrhage and in bleeding disorders such as type I von Willebrand's disease.[106] In septic shock, vasopressin has profound effects on increasing blood pressure in intravascular depleted states. The mechanisms behind this observation appear to be mediated by the ability of vasopressin to potentiate the catecholamine effects on blood vessels. Several observational and nonrandomized prospective studies have demonstrated the efficacy of terlipressin, an arginine vasopressin analog, to be effective as rescue therapy in catecholamine-resistant shock in children and neonates.[107,108] A single randomized, double-blinded, placebo-controlled study has been conducted that demonstrated a beneficial effect of vasopressin in recalcitrant septic shock.[109]

chapter 2

NUTRITIONAL SUPPORT OF THE PEDIATRIC PATIENT

Nilesh Mehta, MD, DCH • Tom Jaksic, MD, PhD

Despite advances in the field of nutritional support, the prevalence of malnutrition among hospitalized patients, especially those with a protracted clinical course, has remained largely unchanged over the past 2 decades.[1] The provision of optimal nutritional therapy requires a careful assessment of energy needs and the provision of macronutrients and micronutrients via the most suitable feeding route. The profound and stereotypic metabolic response to injury places unique demands on the hospitalized child. Standard equations available for estimating energy needs have proved to be unreliable in this population.[2,3] In addition, children with critical illness have marked net protein catabolism and often lack adequate nutritional support.[4] Ultimately, an individualized nutritional regimen should be tailored for each child and reviewed regularly during the course of illness. An understanding of the metabolic events that accompany illness and surgery in the child is the first step in implementing appropriate nutritional support.

THE METABOLIC RESPONSE TO STRESS

The metabolic response to illness due to stressors such as trauma, surgery, or inflammation has been well described. Cuthbertson was the first investigator to realize the primary role that whole-body protein catabolism plays in the systemic response to injury.[5] Based on his work, the metabolic stress response has been conceptually divided into two phases. The initial brief ebb phase is characterized by decreased enzymatic activity, reduced oxygen consumption, low cardiac output, and a core temperature that may be subnormal. This is followed by the hypermetabolic flow phase, characterized by increased cardiac output, oxygen consumption, and glucose production. During this phase, fat and protein mobilization is manifested by increased urinary nitrogen excretion and weight loss. This catabolic phase is mediated by a surge in cytokines and the characteristic endocrine response to trauma or surgery that results in an increased availability of substrates essential for healing and enhanced glucose production.

Neonates and children share similar qualitative metabolic responses to illness as adults, albeit with significant quantitative differences. The metabolic stress response is beneficial in the short term, but the consequences of sustained catabolism are significant because the child has limited tissue stores and substantial nutrient requirements for growth. Thus, the prompt institution of nutritional support is a priority in sick neonates and children. The goal of nutrition in this setting is to augment the short-term benefits of the pediatric metabolic response to injury while minimizing any long-term consequences. In general, the metabolic stress response is characterized by an increase in net muscle protein degradation and enhanced movement of free amino acids through the circulation (Fig. 2-1). These amino acids serve as the building blocks for the rapid synthesis of proteins that act as mediators for the inflammatory response and structural components for tissue repair. Remaining amino acids not used in this way are channeled through the liver where their carbon skeletons are utilized to create glucose through gluconeogenesis. The provision of additional dietary protein may slow the rate of net protein loss but does not eliminate the overall negative protein balance associated with injury.[6]

Carbohydrate and lipid turnover is also increased severalfold during the pediatric metabolic response. Although these metabolic alterations would be expected to increase overall energy requirements, data show that such an increase is quantitatively variable, modest, and evanescent. Overall, the energy needs of the critically ill or injured child are governed by the severity and persistence of the underlying illness or injury. Accurate assessment of energy requirements in individual patients allows optimal caloric supplementation and avoids the deleterious effects of both underfeeding and overfeeding. Children with critical illness demonstrate a unique hormonal and cytokine profile characterized by an elevation in serum levels

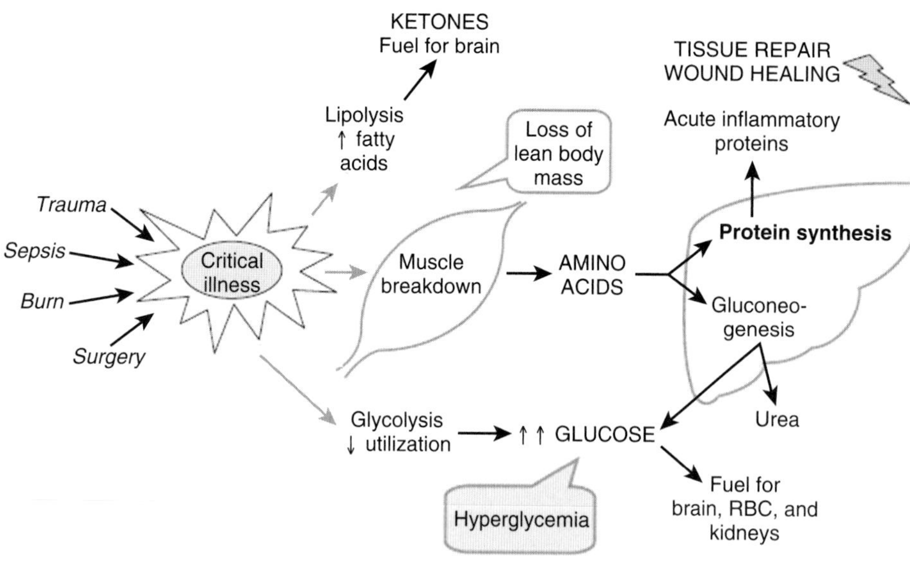

Figure 2-1. The metabolic changes associated with the pediatric stress response to critical illness and injury are illustrated. In general, net protein catabolism predominates and amino acids are transported from muscle stores to the liver, where they are converted to inflammatory proteins and glucose through the process of gluconeogenesis.

of insulin, the catabolic hormones (glucagon, cortisol, catecholamines), and specific cytokines known to interact with the inflammatory process.[7] Novel ways to manipulate these hormonal and cytokine alterations with an aim to minimize the deleterious consequences induced by the stress response are the focus of significant research.

BODY COMPOSITION AND NUTRIENT RESERVES

The body composition of the young child contrasts to that of the adult in several ways that significantly affect nutritional requirements. Table 2-1 lists the macronutrient stores of the neonate, child, and adult as a percentage of total body weight.[8,9] Carbohydrate stores are limited in all age groups and provide only a short-term supply of glucose when utilized. Despite this fact, neonates have a high demand for glucose and have shown elevated rates of glucose turnover when compared with those of the adult.[10] This is thought to be related to the neonate's increased brain-to-body mass ratio because glucose is the primary energy source for the central nervous system. Neonatal glycogen stores are even more limited in the early postpartum period, especially in the preterm infant.[11] Short periods of fasting can predispose the newborn to hypoglycemia. Thus, when infants are burdened with illness or injury, they must rapidly turn to the breakdown of protein stores to generate glucose through the process of gluconeogenesis. Lipid reserves are low in the neonate, gradually increasing with age. Premature infants have the lowest proportion of lipid stores because the majority of polyunsaturated fatty acids accumulate in the third trimester.[12] This renders lipid less useful as a potential fuel source in the young child.[13]

Table 2-1 The Body Composition of Neonates, Children, and Adults as a Percentage of Total Body Weight

Age	Protein (%)	Fat (%)	Carbohydrate (%)
Neonates	11	14	0.4
Children (age 10 yr)	15	17	0.4
Adults	18	19	0.4

The most dramatic difference between adult and pediatric patients is in the relative quantity of stored protein. The protein reserve of the adult is nearly twofold that of the neonate. Thus, infants cannot afford to lose significant amounts of protein during the course of protracted illness or injury. An important feature of the metabolic stress response, unlike in starvation, is that the provision of dietary glucose does not halt gluconeogenesis. Consequently, the catabolism of muscle protein to produce glucose continues unabated.[14] Neonates and children also share much higher baseline energy requirements. Studies have demonstrated that the resting energy expenditure for neonates is two to three times that of adults when standardized for body weight.[13,15,16] Clearly, the child's need for rapid growth and development is a large component of this increase in energy requirement. Moreover, the relatively large body surface area of the young child may increase heat loss and further contributes to elevations in energy expenditure.

The basic requirements for protein and energy in the healthy neonate, child, and adult, based on recent recommendations by the National Academy of Sciences, are listed in Table 2-2.[17] As illustrated, the recommended protein provision for the neonate is almost three times that of the adult. In premature infants, a minimum protein allotment of 2.8 g/kg/day is required to maintain in-utero growth rates.[18] The increased metabolic demand and limited nutrient reserves of the infant mandates early nutritional support in times of traumatic injury and critical illness in order to avoid untoward nutritional consequences.

Accurate assessment of body composition is necessary for planning nutritional intake, monitoring dynamic changes in the body compartments (e.g., the

Table 2-2 Estimated Requirements for Energy and Protein in Healthy Humans of Different Age Groups

Age	Protein (g/kg/day)	Energy (kcal/kg/day)
Neonates	2.2	120
Children (age 10 yr)	1.0	70
Adults	0.8	35

loss of lean body mass), and assessing the adequacy of nutritional supportive regimens during critical illness. Ongoing loss of lean body mass is an indicator of inadequate dietary supplementation and may have clinical implications in the hospitalized child. However, current methods of body composition analysis (e.g., anthropometry, weight, and biochemical parameters) are either impractical for clinical use or inaccurate in a subgroup of hospitalized children with critical illness. One of the principal problems in critically ill children is the presence of capillary leak, which is manifested as edema and large fluid shifts. These make anthropometric measurements invalid, and other bedside techniques have not been validated.

ENERGY EXPENDITURE DURING ILLNESS

For children with illness or undergoing operative intervention, knowledge of energy requirements is important for the design of appropriate nutritional strategies. Dietary regimens that both underestimate and overestimate energy needs are associated with injurious consequences. Owing to the high individual variability in energy expenditure, particularly in the most critically ill patients, the actual measurement of resting energy expenditure (REE) is recommended.

The components of total energy expenditure (TEE) for a child, in order of magnitude are (1) REE, (2) energy expended during physical activity, and (3) diet-induced thermogenesis (the heat generated by the consumption of food products). The sum of these components determines the energy requirement for an individual. In general, REE rates decline with age from infancy to young adulthood, at which time the rate becomes stable. In children with critical illness, the remaining factors in the determination of TEE are of reduced significance, because physical activity is low and diet-induced thermogenesis may not be significant.

REE can be measured using direct or indirect methods. The direct calorimetric method measures the heat released by a subject at rest and is based on the principle that all energy is eventually converted to heat. In practice, the patient is placed in a thermally isolated chamber and the heat dissipated is measured for a given period of time.[19] This method is the true gold standard for measured energy expenditure. Direct calorimetry is not practical for most hospitalized children, and REE is often estimated using standard equations. Unfortunately, REE estimates using standardized World Health Organization (WHO) predictive equations are unreliable, particularly in underweight subjects.[19-21]

REE estimation is difficult in critically ill or postoperative children. Their energy requirements show individual variation and are dependent on severity of injury. For instance, an infant with respiratory distress on pressure support is likely to have a high energy requirement owing to increased work of breathing. The same patient, when started on mechanical ventilation with muscle relaxants, is unlikely to have sustained high energy requirements. Infants with congenital diaphragmatic hernia on extracorporeal membrane oxygenation (ECMO) support have been shown to have energy expenditures of approximately 90 kcal/kg/day. After extubation, the same patients may have energy requirements as high as 140 kcal/kg/day. Although stress factors ranging from 1.0 to 2.7 have been applied to correct for these variations, calculated standardized energy expenditure equations have not been satisfactorily validated in critically ill children.[22-25]

Indirect calorimetry measures VO_2 (the volume of oxygen consumed) and VCO_2 (the volume of CO_2 produced) and uses a correlation factor based on urinary nitrogen excretion to calculate the overall rate of energy production.[26] The measurement of energy needs is "indirect" because it does not use direct temperature changes to determine energy needs. Indirect calorimetry, usually with the aid of a "metabolic cart," provides a measurement of the overall respiratory quotient (RQ), defined as the ratio of CO_2 produced to O_2 consumed (VCO_2/VO_2), for a given patient. Oxidation of carbohydrate yields an RQ of 1.0, whereas fatty acid oxidation gives an RQ of 0.7. However, the role of the RQ as a marker of substrate use and as an indicator of underfeeding or overfeeding is limited. The body's ability to metabolize substrate may be impaired during illness, making assumptions of RQ values and substrate oxidation invalid. Although RQ is not a sensitive marker for the adequacy of feeding in individual cases, RQ values greater than 1.0 are generally associated with lipogenesis secondary to overfeeding.[27,28] A recent study has suggested the utility of extremes of RQ in monitoring feeding adequacy.[29] An RQ higher than 0.85 reliably indicates the absence of underfeeding, and an RQ higher than 1.0 reliably indicates the presence of overfeeding. However, numerous factors, related and unrelated to feeding, can alter the value of a measured RQ in critically ill patients. Some of these factors include hyperventilation, acidosis effects of cardiotonic agents and neuromuscular blocking agents, and an individual response to a given substrate load, injury, or disease.[30] Furthermore, in the setting of wide diurnal and day-to-day variability of REE in critically ill individuals, the extrapolation of short-term calorimetric REE measurements to 24-hour REE may introduce errors. The use of steady-state measurements may decrease these errors. *Steady state* is defined by change in VO_2 and VCO_2 of less than 10% over a period of 5 consecutive minutes. The values for the mean REE from this steady-state period may be used as an accurate representation of the 24-hour TEE in patients with low levels of physical activity.[31] In a patient who fails to achieve steady state and is metabolically unstable, more prolonged testing is required (minimum of 60 minutes), and 24-hour indirect calorimetry should be considered. With the advent of newer technology, the application of indirect calorimetry at the bedside for continuous monitoring shows promise.

Indirect calorimetry is not accurate in the setting of air leaks around the endotracheal tube, the ventilator circuit, or through a chest tube, or in patients on ECMO support. High, inspired oxygen fraction ($FIO_2 >$ 0.6) will also affect indirect calorimetry. Indirect calorimetry is difficult to use in infants on ECMO because a large proportion of the patient's oxygenation and ventilation is performed through the membrane oxygenator. The use of indirect calorimetry for assessment and monitoring of nutrition intake requires attention to its limitations as well as expertise in the interpretation. Nonetheless, its application in children at high risk for underfeeding and overfeeding appears to be warranted.[32,33]

Nonradioactive stable isotope techniques have been used to measure REE in the pediatric patient. Stable isotope technology has been available for many years and was first applied for energy expenditure measurement in humans in 1982.[34,35] Both ^{13}C-labeled bicarbonate and doubly labeled water ($^2H_2{}^{18}O$) have been used to measure TEE in pediatric surgical patients[32,35] and have been shown to correlate well with indirect calorimetry.[36] The ^{13}C-labeled bicarbonate method allows the calculation of REE solely on the basis of infusion rate and the ratio of labeled to unlabeled CO_2 in expired breath samples.[36] Orally administered stable isotopes of water (^2H_2O and $H_2{}^{18}O$) mix with the body water, and the ^{18}O is lost from the body as both water and CO_2, while the ^2H is lost from the body only as water. The difference in the rates of loss of the isotopes ^{18}O and ^2H from the body reflects the rate of CO_2 production, which can be used to calculate the TEE.[37,38] However, the doubly labeled water method has its limitations in children with active capillary leak, decreased urine output, fluid overload, and diuretic use.[37]

In general, any increase in energy expenditure during illness or after surgery is variable. Recent studies suggest that the increase is far less than originally hypothesized. In children with severe burns, the initial REE during the flow phase of injury is increased by 50% but then returns to normal during convalescence.[39] In neonates with bronchopulmonary dysplasia in which the illness increases the patient's work of breathing, a 25% elevation in energy requirement is evident.[40] Newborns undergoing major surgery have only a transient 20% increase in energy expenditure that returns to baseline values within 12 hours postoperatively, provided that no major complications develop.[41,42] Stable, extubated neonates 5 days after surgery have been shown to have REE comparable to normal infants.[43] Effective anesthetic and analgesic management may play a significant role in muting the stress response of the neonate. Studies have demonstrated no discernable increase in REE in neonates undergoing patent ductus arteriosus ligation who received intraoperative fentanyl anesthesia and postoperative intravenous analgesic regimens.[42] A retrospective stratification of surgical infants into low- and high-stress cohorts based on the severity of underlying illness found that high-stress infants undergo moderate short-term elevations in energy expenditure after surgical intervention.[44] Low-stress infants do not manifest any increase in energy expenditures during the course of illness. Finally, by using stable isotopic methods, it has been found that the mean energy expenditures of critically ill neonates on ECMO are nearly identical to age- and diet-matched nonstressed controls.[45]

These studies suggest that critically ill neonates have only a small and usually short-term increase in energy expenditure. Although children have increased energy requirements from increased metabolic turnover during illness, their caloric needs may be lower than previously considered owing to possible halted or slow growth[46] and the use of sedation and muscle paralysis.[47] This could result in overfeeding when energy intake is based on presumed or estimated energy expenditure with stress factors. On the other hand, unrecognized hypermetabolism in select individuals results in underfeeding with nutritional consequences.[32] The variability in energy requirements may result in cumulative energy imbalances in the intensive care unit (ICU) over a period of time.[33] A direct relation has been reported between cumulative caloric imbalance and mortality rate in critically ill surgical patients.[48]

For practical purposes, the recommended dietary caloric intake for healthy children may represent a reasonable starting point for the upper limit of caloric allotment in the hospitalized child.[17] However, as discussed earlier, energy requirement estimates in select groups of patients remain variable and possibly overestimated, mandating an accurate estimation using measured energy expenditure where available. Regular anthropometric measurements plotted on a growth chart to assess the adequacy of caloric provision will allow relatively prompt detection of underfeeding or overfeeding in most cases. However, some critically ill children may be too sick for regular weights or have changes in body water that make anthropometric measurements unreliable.

MACRONUTRIENT INTAKE

Review of Protein Metabolism and Requirement during Illness

Amino acids are the key building blocks required for growth and tissue repair. The vast majority (98%) are found in existing proteins, and the remainder reside in the free amino acid pool. Proteins are continually degraded into their constituent amino acids and resynthesized through the process of protein turnover. The reutilization of amino acids released by protein breakdown is extensive. Synthesis of proteins from the recycling of amino acids is more than two times greater than that from dietary protein intake. An advantage of high protein turnover is that a continuous flow of amino acids is available for the synthesis of new proteins. This allows the body tremendous flexibility in meeting ever-changing physiologic needs. However, the process of protein turnover requires the input of energy to power both protein degradation and synthesis. At baseline, infants are known to have higher rates of protein turnover than adults. Healthy newborns have a protein turnover rate of 6 to 12 g/kg/day compared with 3.5 g/kg/day in adults.[49] Even greater rates of protein turnover have been measured in premature and low birth weight infants.[50] For example, it has been demonstrated that extremely low birth weight infants receiving no dietary protein can lose in excess of 1.2 g/kg/day of endogenous protein.[51] At the same time, infants must maintain a positive protein balance to attain normal growth and development, whereas the healthy adult can subsist with a neutral protein balance.

In the metabolically stressed patient, such as the child with severe burn injury or cardiorespiratory failure requiring ECMO, protein turnover is doubled when compared with that in normal subjects.[35,49] A study of critically ill infants and children found an 80% increase in protein turnover, which correlated with the duration of the critical illness.[52] This process redistributes amino acids from skeletal muscle to the liver, wound site, and tissues taking part in the inflammatory response. The factors required for the inflammatory response—acutely needed enzymes, serum proteins, and glucose—are thereby synthesized from degraded body protein stores. The well-established increase in hepatically derived acute phase proteins (including C-reactive protein, fibrinogen, transferrin, and α_1-acid glycoprotein), along with the concomitant decrease in transport proteins (albumin and retinol-binding protein) is evidence of this protein redistribution. As substrate turnover is increased during the stress response, rates of both whole-body protein degradation and whole-body protein synthesis are accelerated. However, protein breakdown predominates, thereby leading to a hypercatabolic state with ensuing net negative protein and nitrogen balance.[27] Protein loss is evident in elevated levels of excreted urinary nitrogen during critical illness. For example, infants with sepsis demonstrate a severalfold increase in the loss of urinary nitrogen that directly correlates with the degree of illness.[53] Clinically, severe protein loss can be manifested by skeletal muscle wasting, weight loss, delayed wound healing, and immune dysfunction.[54] In addition to the reprioritization of protein for tissue repair, healing and inflammation, the body appears to have an increased need for glucose production during times of metabolic stress.[55] The accelerated rate of gluconeogenesis during illness and injury is seen in both children and adults, and this process appears to be accentuated in infants with low body weight.[13,54] The increased production of glucose during illness is necessary, because glucose represents a versatile energy source for tissues taking part in the inflammatory response. For example, it has been shown that glucose utilization by leukocytes is significantly increased in inflammatory conditions.[56] Unfortunately, the provision of additional dietary glucose does not suppress the body's need for increased glucose production. Therefore, net protein breakdown continues to predominate.[14,57,58]

Specific amino acids are transported from muscle to the liver to facilitate hepatic glucose production. The initial step of amino acid catabolism involves removal of the toxic amino group (NH_3). Through transamination, the amino group is transferred to α-ketoglutarate, thereby producing glutamate. The addition of another amino group converts glutamate to glutamine, which is subsequently transported to the liver. Here, the amino groups are removed from glutamine and detoxified to urea through the urea cycle. The amino acid carbon skeleton can then enter the gluconeogenesis pathway. Alternatively, in skeletal muscle, the amino group can be transferred to pyruvate, thereby forming the amino acid alanine. When alanine is transported to the liver and detoxified, pyruvate is re-formed and can be converted to glucose through gluconeogenesis. The transport of alanine and pyruvate between peripheral muscle tissue and the liver is termed the *glucose-alanine cycle*.[59] Hence the transport amino acid systems involving glutamine and alanine provide carbon backbones for gluconeogenesis while facilitating the hepatic detoxification of ammonia by the urea cycle.

Increased muscle protein catabolism is a successful short-term adaptation during critical illness but is limited and ultimately harmful to the pediatric patient with reduced protein stores and elevated protein demands. Without elimination of the inciting stress, the progressive breakdown of diaphragmatic, cardiac, and skeletal muscle can lead to respiratory compromise, fatal arrhythmia, and loss of lean body mass. Moreover, a prolonged negative protein balance may have a significant impact on the child's growth and development. Healthy, nonstressed neonates require a positive protein balance of nearly 2 g/kg/day.[48,60] In contrast, critically ill, premature neonates requiring mechanical ventilation have a negative protein balance of −1 g/kg/day.[62,63] Critically ill neonates who require ECMO have exceedingly high rates of protein loss, with a net negative protein balance of −2.3 g/kg/day.[61] It has been well established that the extent of protein catabolism correlates with the ultimate morbidity and mortality of the surgical patient.

Fortunately, amino acid supplementation tends to promote increased nitrogen retention and positive protein balance in critically ill patients.[59,62] The mechanism appears to be an increase in protein synthesis while rates of protein degradation remain constant.[60,63] Therefore, the provision of dietary protein sufficient to optimize protein synthesis, facilitate wound healing and the inflammatory process, and preserve skeletal muscle mass is the single most important nutritional intervention in critically ill children. The quantity of protein needed to enhance protein accrual is greater in hospitalized sick children than in healthy children. Table 2-3 lists recommended quantities of dietary protein provision for hospitalized children. Extreme cases of physiologic stress, including the child with extensive burns or the neonate on ECMO, may

Table 2-3 Recommended Protein Requirements for Critically Ill Infants and Children

Age (yr)	Estimated Protein Requirement (g/kg/day)
0-2	2.0-3.0
2-13	1.5-2.0
13-18	1.5

necessitate additional protein supplementation to meet metabolic demands. It should be noted that toxicity from excessive protein administration has been reported, particularly in children with impaired renal and hepatic function. The provision of protein at levels greater than 3 g/kg/day is rarely indicated and is often associated with azotemia. In premature neonates, the possible beneficial effects of protein allotments of 3.0 to 3.5 g/kg/day are being actively investigated in an effort to replicate intrauterine growth rates. Studies using protein provisions of 6 g/kg/day in children have demonstrated significant morbidity, including azotemia, pyrexia, strabismus, and lower IQ scores.[62,64]

Protein Quality

In addition to the sufficient quantity of dietary protein, an increased focus has been placed on the quality of protein in nutritional feeding. The specific amino acid formulation that is best to increase whole-body protein balance has yet to be fully determined, although numerous clinical and basic science research projects are actively researching this topic. It is known that infants have an increased requirement per kilogram for the essential amino acids compared with the adult.[65] In particular, neonates have immature biosynthetic pathways that may temporarily alter their ability to synthesize specific amino acids. One example is the amino acid histidine, which has been shown to be a conditionally essential amino acid in infants up to age 6 months. Recent data suggest that cysteine, taurine, and proline also may be of limited capacity in the premature neonate.[66-69] Interest has also been expressed in the use of arginine as an "immunonutrient" to enhance the function of the immune system in critically ill patients. Although preliminary studies show that arginine supplementation may reduce the risk of infectious complications, its safety and efficacy in the pediatric population has yet to be established.[70]

The restricted availability of the amino acid cysteine may have clinical relevance in the critically ill child. Cysteine is a required substrate for the production of glutathione, the body's major antioxidant. In critically ill children, cysteine turnover is increased significantly. At the same time, rates of glutathione synthesis are decreased by 60%. In this way, cysteine may become a conditionally essential amino acid in the sick child. Recent experiments have demonstrated that the enteral feeding of cysteine in small quantities to rats dependent on total parenteral nutrition (TPN) significantly increases the hepatic concentration of glutathione.[71] The enteral supplementation of cysteine in a pediatric nutritional regimen warrants further investigation.

Glutamine is another amino acid that has been studied extensively in both pediatric and adult patients in the ICU. Glutamine is an important amino acid source for gluconeogenesis, intestinal energy production, and ammonia detoxification. In healthy subjects, glutamine is a nonessential amino acid, although it has been hypothesized that glutamine may become conditionally essential in critically ill patients. Because it is difficult to keep glutamine soluble in solution, standard TPN formulations do not include glutamine in the amino acid mixture. Although the preliminary data on glutamine supplementation in the clinical setting are encouraging, numerous problems with study methodology have been noted.[72] Additional prospective, randomized trials are needed to define its utility fully in both the adult and pediatric population.

In summary, during illness and recovery from trauma or surgery, there is increased protein catabolism. The short-term adaptive benefit of this response is, in time, outweighed by the loss of protein in critical organs and the consequent morbidity seen after the exhaustion of limited protein reserves. This sustained protein breakdown cannot be stopped by increasing caloric provision alone (as is the case in starvation), but protein balance may be restored by optimal (probably individual and disease specific) quantities of protein intake during this state. Future studies may also elucidate if specific amino acid mixtures may be of benefit to select subpopulations.

Modulating Protein Metabolism

The dramatic increase in protein breakdown during critical illness, coupled with the known association between protein loss and patient mortality and morbidity, has stimulated a wide array of research efforts. The measurement of whole-body nitrogen balance through urine and stool was once the only way to investigate changes in protein metabolism. New and validated stable isotope tracer techniques now exist to measure the precise rates of protein turnover, breakdown, and synthesis.[73] However, the modulation of protein metabolism in critically ill patients has proved difficult. Dietary supplementation of amino acids does increase protein synthesis but appears to have no effect on protein-breakdown rates. Thus, investigators have recently focused on the use of alternative anabolic agents to decrease protein catabolism. Studies have used various pharmacologic tools to achieve this goal, including growth hormone, insulin-derived growth factor I (IGF-I), and testosterone, with varying degrees of success.[74-76] One of the more promising agents, however, may be the anabolic hormone insulin. Multiple studies have used insulin to reduce protein breakdown in healthy volunteers and adult burn patients.[50,77] In children with extensive burns, intravenous insulin has been shown to increase lean body mass and mitigate peripheral muscle catabolism.[78] A recent prospective, randomized trial of more than

1500 adult postoperative patients in the ICU demonstrated significant reductions in mortality and morbidity with the use of intravenous insulin.[79] Preliminary stable isotopic studies demonstrate that an intravenous insulin infusion may reduce protein breakdown by over 30% in critically ill neonates on ECMO.[80] The use of intensive insulin therapy for critically ill children and adults continues to be another active area of clinical investigation. More recent studies examining the role of insulin for tight glycemic control in critically ill patients have been less encouraging and are discussed in the next section.

A Review of Carbohydrate Metabolism and Requirement during Illness

Glucose production and availability are a priority in the pediatric metabolic stress response. Glucose is the primary energy source for the brain, erythrocyte, and renal medulla and also is used extensively in the inflammatory response. Injured and septic adults demonstrate a threefold increase in glucose turnover, glucose oxidation, and gluconeogenesis.[16] This increase is of particular concern in neonates who have an elevated glucose turnover at baseline.[10] Moreover, glycogen stores provide only a limited endogenous supply of glucose in adults and an even smaller reserve in the neonate. Thus, the critically ill neonate has a greater glucose demand and reduced glucose stores. During illness, the administration of exogenous glucose does not halt the elevated rates of gluconeogenesis. Thus, net protein catabolism continues unabated.[14] It is clear, however, that a combination of dietary glucose and amino acids can effectively improve protein balance during critical illness, primarily through an augmentation of protein synthesis.

In the past, nutritional support regimens for critically ill patients used large amounts of glucose in an attempt to reduce endogenous glucose production. Unfortunately, excess glucose increases CO_2 production, engenders fatty liver, and results in no reduction in endogenous glucose turnover.[81] Therefore, a surplus of carbohydrate may increase the ventilatory burden on the critically ill patient. Adult patients in the ICU fed with high-glucose TPN demonstrate a 30% increase in oxygen consumption, a 57% increase in CO_2 production, and a 71% elevation in minute ventilation.[82] In critically ill infants, the conversion of excess glucose to fat has also been correlated with increased CO_2 production and higher respiratory rates.[83] In addition, excessive carbohydrate provision may play a role in the genesis of TPN-associated cholestatic liver injury. Finally, some data in critically ill neonates have shown that excess caloric allotments of carbohydrate are paradoxically associated with an increased rate of net protein breakdown.[84]

When designing a nutritional regimen for the critically ill child, excessive carbohydrate calories should be avoided. A mixed fuel system, with both glucose and lipid substrates, should be used to meet the patient's caloric requirements. When the postoperative neonate is fed a high-glucose diet, the corresponding RQ is approximately 1.0, and may be higher than 1.0 in selected patients, signifying increased lipogenesis.[85] A mixed dietary regimen of glucose and lipid (at 2 to 4 g/kg/day) lowers the effective RQ in neonates to 0.83.[86] This approach will provide the child with full nutritional supplementation while alleviating an increased ventilatory burden and difficulties with hyperglycemia.

Administration of high caloric (glucose load) diets in the early phase of critical illness may exacerbate hyperglycemia, increase CO_2 generation with increased load on the respiratory system, promote hyperlipidemia resulting from increased lipogenesis, and result in a hyperosmolar state. Recent reports have linked hyperglycemia with increased mortality and established the role of insulin-assisted tight glycemic control in improving outcomes in the critically ill adults.[79,87,88] A remarkable 43% reduction in mortality was reported in post–cardiac surgery patients in an adult ICU by implementing strict glycemic control (arterial blood glucose levels below 110 mg/dL) using insulin infusion in the treatment group compared with patients in the control group (average blood glucose level of 150-160 mg/dL).[79] The precise mechanism(s) responsible for this beneficial effect of tight glycemic control with insulin protocol remains unanswered. A recent meta-analysis of studies examining the role of tight glycemic control in adult ICUs has shown a high incidence of hypoglycemia in the treatment group and less impressive benefit.[89] Although the incidence of hyperglycemia in the pediatric population is high and may be associated with increased mortality and length of stay,[90] no data exist currently for similar benefits of tight glycemic control in the pediatric age group. Studies examining the role of tight glycemic control strategy (its benefits and risks) in the pediatric population are currently underway. Although it is prudent to avoid prolonged hyperglycemia in the pediatric ICU patients, in the absence of definitive data, aggressive glycemic control cannot yet be recommended in the critically ill children outside of a clinical trial setting.

A Review of Lipid Metabolism and Requirement during Illness

Along with protein and carbohydrate metabolism, the turnover of lipid is generally increased by critical illness, major surgery, and trauma in the pediatric patient.[91] During the early ebb phase, triglyceride levels may initially increase as the rate of lipid metabolism decreases. However, this process reverses itself in the predominant flow phase. During this time, critically ill adult patients have demonstrated twofold to fourfold increases in lipid turnover.[92] Recently it was shown that critically ill children on mechanical ventilation have increased rates of fatty acid oxidation.[93] The increased lipid metabolism is thought to be proportional to the overall degree of illness. The process of lipid turnover involves the conversion of free fatty acids and their glycerol backbone into, and hydrolytic cleavage from, triglycerides. Thirty to 40 percent of free fatty acids are oxidized for energy. RQ values may decline during illness, reflecting an increased utilization of fat as an energy source.[94] This suggests that fatty acids are a prime source of energy in metabolically stressed pediatric patients. In addition to the rich energy supply from lipid substrate, the glycerol moiety released from triglycerides may be converted to pyruvate and used to manufacture glucose. As seen with the other catabolic changes associated with illness and trauma, the provision of dietary glucose does not decrease fatty acid turnover in times of illness. The increased demand for lipid utilization in critical illness coupled with the limited lipid stores in the neonate puts the metabolically stressed child at high risk for the development of essential fatty acid deficiency.[95,96]

Preterm infants have been shown to develop biochemical evidence of essential fatty acid deficiency 2 days after the initiation of a fat-free nutritional regimen.[97] In the human, the polyunsaturated fatty acids linoleic and linolenic acid are considered essential fatty acids because the body cannot manufacture them by desaturating other fatty acids. Linoleic acid is used by the body to synthesize arachidonic acid, an important intermediary in prostaglandin synthesis. The prostaglandin family includes the leukotrienes and thromboxanes, all of which serve as mediators in such wide-ranging processes as vascular permeability, smooth muscle reactivity, and platelet aggregation. If an individual lacks dietary linoleic acid, the formation of arachidonic acid (a tetraene, with four double bonds) cannot occur and eicosatrienoic acid (a triene, with three double bonds) accumulates in its place. Clinically, a fatty acid profile can be performed on human serum. An elevated triene-to-tetraene ratio greater than 0.4 is characteristic of biochemical essential fatty acid deficiency, although this value is somewhat variable and dependent on the specific laboratory assay utilized. Signs of fatty acid deficiencies include dermatitis, alopecia, thrombocytopenia, increased susceptibility to infection, and overall failure to thrive. To avoid essential fatty acid deficiency in neonates, the allotment of linoleic and linolenic acid is recommended at concentrations of 4.5% and 0.5% of total calories, respectively. In addition, some evidence exists that the long-chain fatty acid docosahexaenoic acid (DHA), a derivative of linolenic acid, also may be deficient in preterm and formula-fed infants. At present, clinical trials are actively seeking to determine whether supplementation with long-chain polyunsaturated fatty acids will be of clinical benefit in this population.

Parenterally delivered lipid solutions also limit the need for excessive glucose provision. These lipid emulsions provide a higher quantity of energy per gram than does glucose (9 kcal/g vs. 4 kcal/g). This reduces the overall rate of CO_2 production, the RQ value, and the incidence of hepatic steatosis.[98] Some risks must be considered when starting a patient on intravenous lipid administration. These include hypertriglyceridemia, a possible increased risk of infection, and decreased alveolar oxygen-diffusion capacity.[99-101] Most institutions, therefore, initiate lipid provisions in children at 0.5 to 1.0 g/kg/day and advance over a period of days to 2 to 4 g/kg/day. During this time, triglyceride levels are monitored closely. Lipid administration is generally restricted to 30% to 40% of total caloric intake in ill children in an effort to obviate immune dysfunction, although this practice has not been validated in a formal clinical trial.

In settings of prolonged fasting or uncontrolled diabetes mellitus, the accelerated production of glucose depletes the hepatocyte of needed intermediaries in the citric acid cycle. When this occurs, the acetyl-coenzyme A (CoA) generated from the breakdown of fatty acids cannot enter the citric acid cycle. Instead, it forms the ketone bodies acetoacetate and β-hydroxybutyrate. These ketone bodies are released by the liver to extrahepatic tissues, in particular, skeletal muscle and the brain, where they can be used for energy production in place of glucose. During surgical illness, however, ketone formation is relatively inhibited secondary to elevated serum insulin levels.[102] Therefore, in surgical patients, ketone bodies do not significantly supplant the need for glucose and do not play a major role in the metabolic management of the pediatric stress response.

In addition to their nutritional role, fatty acids profoundly influence inflammatory and immune events by changing lipid mediators and inflammatory protein and coagulation protein expression. After ingestion, omega-6 and omega-3 fats are metabolized by an alternating series of desaturase and elongase enzymes that transform them into the membrane-associated lipids arachidonic acid, eicosapentaenoic (EPA), and docosahexaenoic (DHA) acids, respectively (Figs. 2-2 and 2-3).[103] Substitution of the intralipid component of TPN (rich in proinflammatory omega-6 fatty acids) with fish oil (a source of omega-3 fatty acids) may alleviate some of the toxic effects of long-term parenteral nutrition on the liver.[104] The beneficial effects of omega-3 fatty acids have been shown in animal and human models. Omega-3 fatty acids have an anti-inflammatory effect, with decreased cytokine production shown in some models.[103] More recently, a commercially available omega-3 fatty acid for parenteral administration has been used in children with exciting results. In a cohort of TPN-dependent children with TPN-associated hyperbilirubinemia, Omegaven (Fresenius Kabi, Hamburg, Germany), at a low lipid allocation of 1 g/kg/day, was associated with a normalization of bilirubin levels.[105] A clinical trial to test the relative benefits of Omegaven versus reduced omega-6 lipid allotments alone is underway in surgical neonates.

ROUTES OF NUTRITIONAL PROVISION

Enteral Nutrition

After the estimation of energy expenditure and macronutrient requirement in the hospitalized child, the next challenge is to facilitate the provision of this nutritional support. In most pediatric patients with a functioning gastrointestinal tract, the enteral route

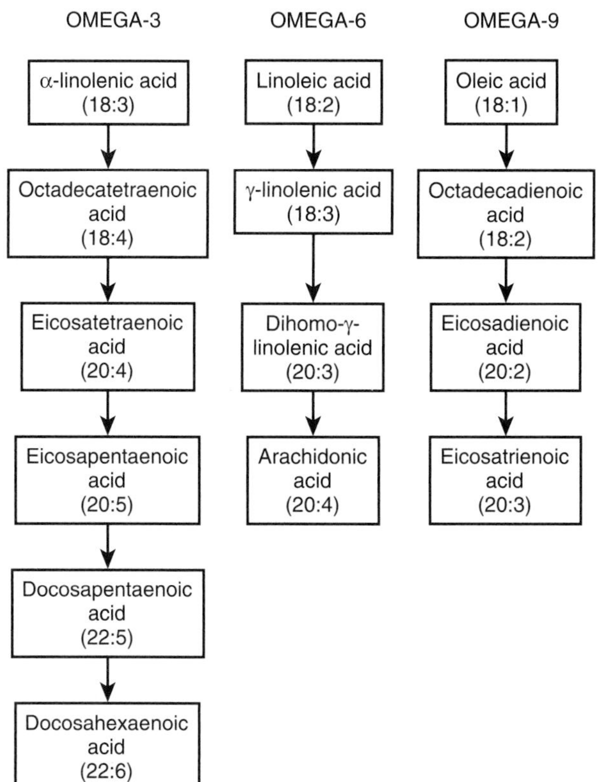

Figure 2-2. Fatty acid synthesis from omega-3, omega-6, and omega-9 fats. (From Lee S, Gura KM, Kim S, et al: Current clinical applications of omega-6 and omega-3 fatty acids. Nutr Clin Pract 21:323-341, 2006.)

of nutrient administration is preferable to parenteral nutrition. Enteral nutrition is physiologic and has been shown to be more cost effective without the added risk of nosocomial infection inherent in TPN. Early enteral nutrition has been shown to decrease infectious episodes and decrease the length of hospitalization in critically ill patients.[106] Based on level 1 and level 2 evidence in adult critical care literature, the Canadian Clinical Practice Guidelines for Nutrition Support have strongly recommended the use of early enteral feeding (within 24-48 hours after ICU admission).[107] The optimal route of nutrient delivery has not been systematically studied in children. In the absence of a randomized controlled trial comparing the effects of enteral versus parenteral nutrition, many centers have adopted institutional guidelines. Current practice includes the initiation of gastric or postpyloric enteral feeding within 48 to 72 hours after admission. Parenteral nutrition is being used to supplement or replace enteral nutrition in those patients in whom enteral nutrition alone is unable to meet their nutritional goals.

In children on enteral nutrition, there are insufficient data to make recommendations regarding the site of enteral feeding (gastric vs. postpyloric). Both enteral routes have been successfully used for nutritional support of the critically ill child.[108-110] In a study examining the role of small bowel feeding in 74 critically ill children randomized to receive either gastric or postpyloric feeds, no significant difference was observed in microaspiration, tube displacement, and feeding intolerance between the two groups.[111] The study was not powered to detect differences in mortality and enteral feedings were interrupted in a large number of subjects in this study. Moreover, caloric goals were met in only a small percentage of the population studied. A higher percentage of subjects in the small bowel group achieved their daily caloric goal when compared with the gastric fed group. Critically ill children receiving early (<24 hours after ICU admission) postpyloric feedings have been shown to have better feeding tolerance (decreased incidence of abdominal distention) compared with those in whom postpyloric

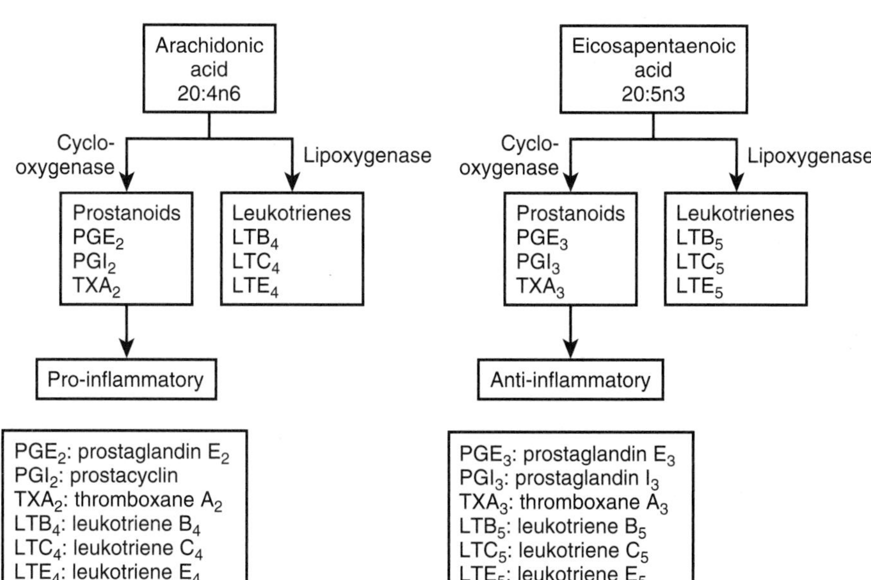

Figure 2-3. The pro- and anti-inflammatory products that are generated from the metabolism of arachidonic acid and eicosapentaenoic acid. (From Lee S, Gura KM, Kim S, et al: Current clinical applications of omega-6 and omega-3 fatty acids. Nutr Clin Pract 21:323-341, 2006.)

feeding was initiated late.[112] It may be prudent to consider postpyloric alimentation in patients who do not tolerate gastric feeding or those who are at a high risk of aspiration. Intolerance to enteral feeds may be a limiting factor, and supplementation with parenteral nutrition in this group of patients allows for improved nutritional intake.[113]

Prospective cohort studies and retrospective chart reviews have reported the inability to achieve daily caloric goal in many critically ill children.[4,114] The most common reasons for suboptimal enteral nutrient delivery in these studies are fluid restriction, procedures interrupting feeds, and feeding intolerance. In a study examining the endocrine and metabolic response of children with meningococcal sepsis, goal nutrition was achieved in only 25% of the cases.[7] Similar observations have been made in a group of 95 children in a pediatric ICU where patients received a median of 58.8% (range 0-277%) of their estimated energy requirements. In this review, enteral feedings were interrupted on 264 occasions to allow clinical procedures. In another review of nutritional intake in 42 patients in a tertiary-level pediatric ICU over 458 days, actual energy intake was compared with estimated energy requirement.[4] Only 50% of patients were reported to have received full estimated energy requirements after a median of 7 days in the ICU. Prolonged fluid resuscitation was a major factor hindering the achievement of estimated energy requirements despite maximizing the energy content of feeds.

Feeding protocols for transpyloric feeding tubes and changing from bolus to continuous feeds during brief periods of intolerance are strategies that may help achieve estimated energy goals in this population. Consistently underachieved enteral nutrition goals are thought to be one of the reasons for the absence of beneficial effect in multiple studies and meta-analyses on the efficacy of immunonutrition in preventing infection.[115] Addressing preventable interruptions in enteral feeding in critically ill children is essential to attaining goal feedings. At this time, there is not enough evidence to recommend the use of prokinetic medications, motility agents (for feeding intolerance or to facilitate enteral tube placement), prebiotics, probiotics, or synbiotics in critically ill children. Randomized studies comparing enteral feeds administered by bolus or continuously are also lacking.

In summary, enteral nutrition must be initiated early in hospitalized children with established peristalsis. Postpyloric enteral nutrition may be utilized in children with a high risk of aspiration or when gastric feeding is either contraindicated or has failed. Enterally administered feeds meet nutritional requirements in critically ill children with a functional gastrointestinal system and have the advantages of low cost, manageability, safety, and preservation of hepatic and other gastrointestinal function. Early introduction of enteral feeding in critically ill patients helps to achieve positive protein and energy balance and restores nitrogen balance during the acute state of illness. It maintains gut integrity and elicits release of growth factors and hormones that maintain gut integrity and function.[116] Despite its perceived benefits, current practice in ICUs shows a significant proportion of eligible patients deprived of enteral feeds.[117] Figure 2-4 offers an algorithm for initiating and advancing enteral nutrition in children admitted to the multidisciplinary ICU at Children's Hospital, Boston.

PARENTERAL NUTRITION

TPN bypasses the gut and provides intravenous administration of macronutrients and micronutrients to meet the nutritional requirements. TPN is indicated in children who are unable to tolerate enteral feeding for a prolonged period of time. Intravenous feeding may supplement enteral feeding or replace it entirely. Although widespread in its application, TPN is associated with mechanical, infectious, and metabolic complications and hence should only be used in carefully selected patients. In the setting of intact intestinal function, TPN is not indicated if enteral feeds alone can maintain nutrition.

The decision to initiate TPN is based on the anticipated length of fasting, the underlying nutritional status of the individual, and a careful examination of the risks associated with TPN use in relation to the consequences of poor nutritional intake. If the expected period during which there will be minimal or no enteral nutrition is longer than 5 days, the use of TPN is probably beneficial. In children with underlying malnutrition, prematurity, or conditions associated with hypermetabolism, TPN can be initiated earlier. The main limiting factor for provision of full nutritional support in the form of TPN is the availability of central access. Administration of full TPN requires a central venous catheter with its tip placed at the junction of the superior vena cava and right atrium. If a lower extremity central line is utilized, the tip of the catheter should be positioned at the junction of the inferior vena cava and right atrium. The large vessel diameter and maximal blood flow rate at these sites allows for the safe administration of the hypertonic TPN. To avoid the complications associated with malpositioned tips of central venous catheters, the practice at our institution is to document the location of the central venous catheter tip and the entry site before its use. Peripheral administration of TPN in the absence of an ideally located central venous catheter requires dilution (maximum 900 mOsm/L with 10% dextrose and 2% amino acids) to avoid the risks of phlebitis and sclerosis. The osmolarity of the TPN solution can be calculated using available on-line calculators or simple equations such as $\{(\text{dextrose [g/L]} \times 5) + (\text{protein [g/L]} \times 10) + (\text{lipid [g/L]} \times 1.5) + [(\text{mEq/L of } Na^+ + K^+ + Ca^{2+} + Mg^{2+}) \times 5]\}$.

The fluid and electrolytes status will guide the initial TPN prescription. The patient's hydration, size, age, and underlying disease will dictate the amount of the fluid to be administered. Fluid requirements in the pediatric age group are routinely estimated based on the Holliday-Segar method (Table 2-4). TPN should not routinely be used for replacing ongoing losses.

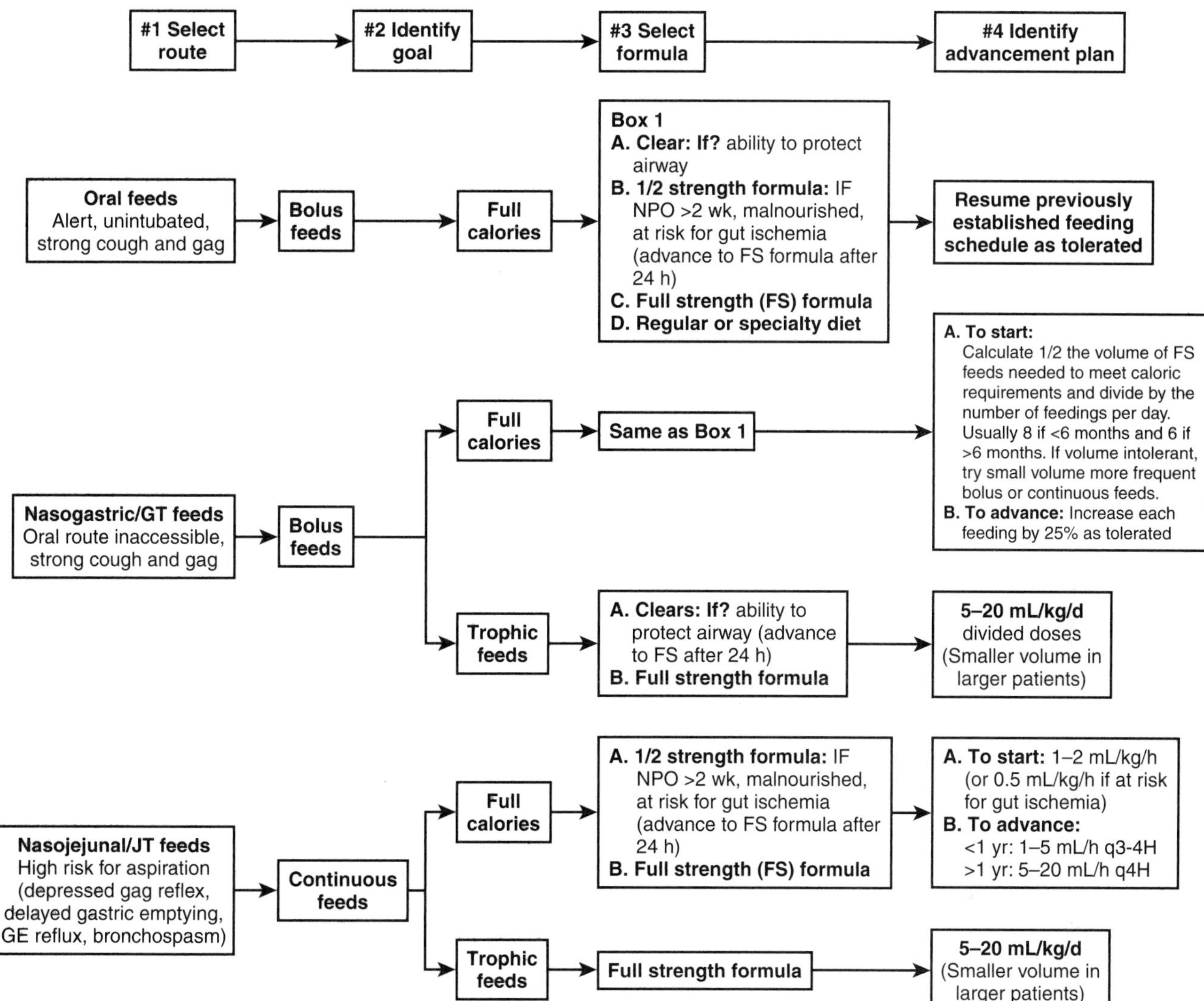

Figure 2-4. Example of an algorithm for a feeding regimen and route for patients admitted to a multidisciplinary intensive care unit. (Courtesy of Children's Hospital, Boston.)

Table 2-4 Daily Fluid Requirement for Infants and Children

Body Weight	Maintenance Daily Fluid Requirement
0-10 kg	100 mL/kg
10-20 kg	1000 mL + 50 mL/kg > 10 kg
> 20 kg	1500 mL + 20 mL/kg > 20 kg

Fluid shifts, increased insensible losses, drainage of bodily secretions, and renal failure can complicate electrolyte management in these patients. Parenteral nutrition should be ordered daily after reviewing the basic electrolytes (Na^+, K^+, Cl^-, HCO_3^-, Ca^{2+}) and blood sugar to allow adjustments in the macronutrient and micronutrient composition. In sick patients with significant gastrointestinal fluid loss (gastric, pancreatic, small intestinal, or bile), the actual measurement of electrolytes from the drained fluid is recommended. However, urgent changes in serum electrolytes should not be managed by changes in TPN infusion rate or composition because these represent imprecise methods to treat a potentially serious electrolyte abnormality. In addition, careful attention to phosphate and magnesium levels is also important. Hypophosphatemia may lead to hemolytic anemia, respiratory muscle dysfunction, and cardiac failure. A significant decrease in serum phosphate also may be seen with the re-feeding syndrome. In contrast, renal failure can result in the retention of phosphate and potassium and nutritional allotments must be reduced accordingly. Deficiency of magnesium can cause a fatal cardiac arrhythmia in both children and adults. Abnormalities of acid-base physiology also can influence the nutritional regimen of the hospitalized child. If a metabolic alkalosis develops from active diuresis or gastric suction, chloride administration should be used to correct the alkalosis. Severe, untreated alkalemia may inhibit the patient's respiratory drive, shift potassium intracellularly, decrease ionized calcium concentrations by increasing the affinity of albumin for calcium, and promote refractory cardiac arrhythmias. Metabolic acidosis is often seen in critically ill children and may be associated with hypotension, ischemia, or renal failure. In this case, the provision of acetate instead of chloride in the parenteral nutrition regimen may be useful.[118]

The three main macronutrients in TPN are carbohydrate, lipid, and protein. Lipid and dextrose are the principal sources of energy in TPN, whereas protein is utilized for lean body accretion. Protein is administered in the form of crystalline amino acids starting at 0.5 g/kg/day in preterm neonates and 1 g/kg/day in others. The protein intake is advanced daily in increments of 1 g/kg/day until the goal intake is achieved. Table 2-3 lists recommended quantities of dietary protein for hospitalized children. Dextrose provides the main source of energy in TPN and is initiated at a rate of 5 mg/kg/min using a 5% to 10% concentration. The glucose infusion rate in milligrams per kilogram per minute can be calculated with the help of the equation: [(% dextrose) × (1 dL/100 mL) × (1000 mg/1 g) (hourly rate in mL/hr) × (1 hr/60 min) × (1/weight in kg]. Infusion rates higher than 12 mg/kg/min are infrequently required. Moreover, overfeeding with carbohydrate is associated with lipogenesis (RQ > 1.0), hepatic steatosis, hyperglycemia, and osmotic diuresis. Three to 5 percent of the energy needs must be met using intravenous lipids, which are usually initiated at a rate of 1 g/kg/day and advanced in increments to reach a maximum of 3 g/kg/day, or 50% of the total energy intake. Intravenous lipids prevent essential fatty acid deficiency and are a concentrated and isotonic source of energy. Triglyceride levels should be monitored, and the intralipid infusion rate is lowered when hypertriglyceridemia is found. As noted previously, available evidence suggests that limiting lipids to 1 g/kg/day may be indicated in patients with intestinal failure–associated parenteral nutrition cholestasis or in those susceptible patients (i.e., neonates) who are likely to require a protracted course of TPN.[119]

The vitamin and micronutrient (trace element) needs of healthy children and neonates are relatively well defined in the literature.[17] In the neonate and child, required vitamins include the fat-soluble vitamins (A, D, E, and K) as well as the water-soluble vitamins (ascorbic acid, thiamine, riboflavin, pyridoxine, niacin, pantothenate, biotin, folate, and vitamin B_{12}). Because vitamins are not consumed stoichiometrically in biochemical reactions but instead act as catalysts, the administration of large vitamin supplements in metabolically stressed states is not logical from a nutritional standpoint. The trace elements required for normal growth and development include zinc, iron, copper, selenium, manganese, iodide, molybdenum, and chromium. Trace elements are usually used in the synthesis of the active sites of a ubiquitous and extraordinarily important class of enzymes called metalloenzymes. More than 200 zinc metalloenzymes alone exist. Both DNA and RNA polymerase are included in this group. As with vitamins, the role of metalloenzymes is to act as catalytic agents. Unless specific mineral losses occur, such as enhanced zinc loss with severe diarrhea, large nutritional requirements would not be anticipated during critical illness. Selenium and carnitine may be added after 30 days of exclusive TPN administration. The addition of copper and manganese in TPN of children with cholestasis is controversial. Usually, the dose is halved due to their biliary excretion. The pharmacologic use of vitamins and trace minerals in pediatric illness has not been adequately studied. Reviews of both vitamin and trace mineral toxicity clearly demonstrate that excessive dosage is a health risk.[120,121]

Careful biochemical monitoring is mandatory to prevent acute and long-term complications from TPN therapy. A TPN profile is recommended at initiation of therapy and then weekly. The profile includes serum levels of sodium, potassium, chloride, glucose, carbon dioxide, blood urine nitrogen, creatinine, albumin, magnesium, phosphate, total and direct bilirubin, and transaminases. For children requiring TPN longer than 30 days, selenium, iron, zinc, copper, and carnitine levels should be checked. It is essential to monitor daily vital statistics and routine anthropometry to ensure adequate growth and development. Critical care units benefit from the expertise of a dedicated nutritionist who should be consulted on a regular basis to guide optimal nutritional intake of patients.

Immune-Enhancing Diets

Immunomodulation is thought to play a significant role in the response to infectious insult and impacts outcome in children with sepsis. In 1997, Bone and colleagues outlined the role of the compensatory anti-inflammatory response that follows the initial proinflammatory response engendered by trauma or infection.[122] Therapies aimed at modulating or stimulating the immune response have been a focus of recent nutritional studies.

Unfortunately, investigations examining the role of immune enhancing diets in critically ill patients are marred by heterogeneous clinical populations, methodologic flaws, and the use of nutritional formulations that often contain multiple potentially active components. Thus, studies and meta-analyses often offer conflicting conclusions.[69,114,121-123] Furthermore, there are no published studies specifically evaluating the role of immunonutrition in critically ill children. Potentially promising, but unproven, additives include arginine, glutamine, cysteine, nucleic acids, and omega-3 fatty acids.

chapter 3

ANESTHETIC CONSIDERATIONS

Kathy M. Perryman, MD • Adam J. Schow, MD • Robert E. Binda, Jr., MD

Anesthetizing children is an increasingly safe undertaking. When discussing the risks and benefits of a surgical intervention with a child and his or her family, surgeons should feel confident that their pediatric anesthesiology colleagues can provide an anesthetic conducive to the demands of the surgery while safeguarding the child's health. As such, whether it is a question of appropriateness for outpatient surgery or how to manage a difficult clinical problem, surgeons and anesthesiologists should collaborate. This chapter is designed to inform surgeons of the considerations important to anesthesiologists. It is hoped that with better understanding between surgical and anesthesiology services, efficiency of case planning and operative patient care will improve.

PREANESTHETIC CONSIDERATIONS

Risk

In an effort to reduce patient complications, anesthesiologists have carefully analyzed their specialty over the past generation. The Pediatric Perioperative Cardiac Arrest (POCA) Registry, the Anesthesiology Patient Safety Foundation (APSF), and the American Society of Anesthesiologists (ASA) Closed Claims Project are among the important initiatives that have resulted in significant reductions in risk to patients undergoing anesthesia. Whereas anesthesia was historically considered a dangerous adventure, serious complications are now relatively rare. The reasons for this improvement include advances in pharmacology, improved monitoring technology and standards, increased rigor of subspecialty training, and the ability to target problems with the aforementioned risk analysis strategy.

Quantifying risk in pediatric anesthesia is fraught with difficulty owing to the inherent vagaries of determining just what complications are attributable to an anesthetic and to what degree. The risk of cardiac arrest for children undergoing anesthesia has been estimated at 1:10,000.[1,2] However, this number is hardly applicable universally because it does not discriminate based on patient co-morbidity or surgical disease. The risk of a healthy child suffering arrest during myringotomy tube placement would be dramatically smaller than the likelihood of a child with complex cardiac disease succumbing during a prolonged cardiac repair.[3]

A recent review of cardiac arrests in anesthetized children compared 193 events from 1998-2004 to 150 events from 1994-1997.[4] Medication-caused arrests decreased from 37% to 18%, which was attributed to a corresponding fall in halothane use and its attendant myocardial depression. It is interesting to note the dramatic reduction in unrecognized esophageal intubation as a leading cause of arrest, due in large part to the advent of pulse oximetry and an increased awareness of the problem. Another notable finding was the predominance of arrests due to inadequate response to hypovolemia or hyperkalemia associated with transfusion, frequently in spinal and craniofacial surgery. These events highlight the preventable nature of the most common arrests, with adequate vascular access and early recognition of bleeding as key to their avoidance.

Anesthesia Consultation

In some centers, all children are evaluated by an anesthesiologist prior to the day of surgery. In others, only selected patients are referred for anesthesia consultation. Any child with an ASA classification (Table 3-1) of 3 or greater should be seen by an anesthesiologist in consultation before the day of surgery. This may be modified in cases of hardship due to travel or when the patient is well known to the anesthesia service and the child's health is unchanged. Certain medical conditions are of particular interest to the anesthesiologist. Although this list is by no means exhaustive, such diseases would include any family history of malignant hyperthermia, abnormal airways, cardiac defects, pulmonary disease, neuromuscular disorders, or any other hypotonic condition. That being stated, whenever an organ system is moderately dysfunctional, consultation is desirable. Open consultation policies reduce frustration and delay on the day of surgery by resolving problems and concerns ahead of time.

At the time of consultation, selected laboratory studies may be ordered, but routine laboratory work is not

Table 3-1 ASA Physical Status Classification

ASA Classification	Patient Status
1	A normal healthy patient
2	A patient with mild systemic disease
3	A patient with severe systemic disease
4	A patient with severe systemic disease that is a constant threat to life
5	A moribund patient who is not expected to survive without the operation
6	A declared brain-dead patient whose organs are being removed for donor purposes
E	An emergency modifier for any ASA classification when failure to immediately correct a medical condition poses risk to life or organ viability

indicated. Medications should be individually assessed as to whether their schedule needs to be altered. In general, seizure medications, cardiac medications, and pulmonary medications should be continued even while NPO (nothing per os). Exceptions may include angiotensin-converting enzyme (ACE) inhibitors and diuretics; the latter may also require blood chemistries. Insulin-dependent diabetics have a particular urgency to be carefully evaluated before elective surgery. Their history of glucose control along with the length of NPO time and surgical stress require careful planning.

Upper Respiratory Tract Infections

Upper respiratory tract infections (URIs) deserve special mention. It is not uncommon for some patients to spend much of their childhood contracting, suffering from, or recovering from a URI. Historically, such patients' surgeries were cancelled due to concern over severe postoperative pulmonary morbidity.[5] Modern studies indicate that such morbidity is rare,[6,7] although transient complications are possible. These typically include postoperative stridor, laryngospasm, hypoxia, and coughing. While potentially worrisome, the vast majority of such complications are readily treatable and can be expected to resolve in the first postoperative day.

The decision to cancel or postpone a scheduled surgery (usually a delay of 4-6 weeks given concern for prolonged hyperreactivity of the bronchi) should not be made lightly. Families have often sacrificed time away from work, taken children out of school, arranged child care for other children, or have planned vacation around the surgical timing, and these social considerations deserve respectful attention. In one study, cases were more likely cancelled by anesthesia staff with more than 10 years of practice experience.[8] Factors to be considered include severity of illness, with intractable or productive cough, malaise, fever, or hypoxia by pulse oximetry. All these factors weigh toward cancellation. Also, a smaller child is exponentially more likely to struggle with bronchospasm because airway resistance is inversely proportional to the fourth power of the radius of the airway.

In contrast, clear rhinorrhea with a simple cough is not usually sufficient grounds for cancellation, provided the family understands the small chance of the need for postoperative supplemental oxygen and bronchodilator therapy. These complications may lead to delay in discharge or require inpatient admission for overnight observation. When the decision to cancel is uncertain, the best general guideline is probably to ask whether the child is in his or her usual state of health. If not, is the child reasonably likely to be better if surgery is postponed? Together with consultation with the surgeon, the answer to that question must in turn be weighed with the urgency of the surgery.

To summarize, some decisions are easy: a child with fever, malaise, hypoxia, or a severe cough should have elective surgery postponed. Similarly, a child with only clear rhinorrhea or a dry, intermittent cough can usually proceed to the operating room. Special attention should be paid to a child with a history of reactive airway disease when the absence of optimal management is more likely to lead to cancellation. For the patients who fall into the gray spectrum, surgeon, anesthesiologist, and parents must consider the urgency of the surgery, the likelihood of improvement of symptoms if the procedure is rescheduled, and the family's ability to accommodate a cancellation.

NPO

The most common cause for surgical delay or cancellation is a violation of NPO guidelines. These rules stipulate preoperative fasting for 6 hours from all oral intake (except breast milk for 4 hours and clear liquids for 2 hours). The rigidity of this rule can be a source of frustration to all. While the risk of aspiration is generally small, it is a real risk of severe morbidity or death. At this time, while some would wish to liberalize fasting guidelines, there are no data to support such changes and the difficulty in obtaining such data is likely prohibitive.

Mitigating circumstances for NPO rules are limited to emergent surgical intervention. In some cases, NPO carries a risk of morbidity from dehydration. One example would include children with single-ventricle cardiac physiology for whom prolonged fasting in the setting of hypotension with an inhalational induction could be fatal. When in question, NPO fasting should be compensated with intravenous hydration. Insulin-dependent diabetics and infants are among those requiring careful planning so that NPO times are not extended. They should be scheduled as the first case of the day when possible.

OUTPATIENT ANESTHESIA

Criteria for Ambulatory Surgery

Ambulatory surgery comprises 70% or more of the case load in most pediatric centers. Multiple factors should be considered when evaluating whether a child is suitable for outpatient surgery. In most cases, the child should be free of severe systemic disease (ASA class 1 or 2). Other factors that may determine the suitability of a child for outpatient surgery are family and social dynamics. For instance, will this child be cared for by a responsible and capable adult? Is the child to be cared for by a single parent who must work? How far must the child travel to receive appropriate medical attention, if needed?

Well-controlled systemic illnesses do not necessarily preclude outpatient surgery, but these questions must be answered in advance in a cooperative fashion between surgical and anesthesia services. If a child has a moderate degree of impairment but the disease is stable and the surgical procedure is of minimal insult, outpatient surgery may be acceptable. However, ASA class 3 children who present for surgery without prior evaluation run the risk of delaying the turnover of cases where efficiency is often at a premium.

The Former Preterm Infant

The potential dangers in performing outpatient surgery on former premature infants were first published in 1982.[9] The most life-threatening hazard is apnea after the surgical procedure, normally within the first 12 to 18 hours. Factors that contribute to the increased risk are not completely understood but may include immature neurologic development, particularly in the brain stem respiratory center, and less developed diaphragmatic musculature that leads to easier fatigability.[10] The age after birth at which this increased risk of apnea disappears is still being debated, despite numerous studies of this issue. A meta-analysis of pertinent studies was reported in 1995.[11] The results of this analysis indicated that a significant reduction occurred in the incidence of apnea at 52 to 54 weeks' postconceptual age, depending on the gestational age. A hematocrit less than 30% was identified as a risk factor, and it was recommended that infants with this degree of anemia be hospitalized postoperatively for observation no matter what the age. However, conclusions drawn from meta-analyses have been challenged for their validity. Moreover, the sample size of this study may not have been large enough to draw valid conclusions.[12]

No anesthetic technique appears to be clearly superior to other techniques, although some evidence has suggested an advantage to spinal anesthesia.[13] By far, general anesthesia is still the preferred anesthetic in most institutions.[14] Likewise, no medications can predictably prevent apnea, although caffeine may hold some promise.[15] Until more patients are systematically studied, the choice of when former preterm infants can undergo operation as outpatients is up to the discretion and personal bias of the anesthesiologist and surgeon. Institutional policies most commonly mention ages of 44 to 46 weeks, 50 weeks, or 60 weeks postconceptual age. Whereas the risk of postanesthesia apnea for preterm children varies widely depending on the degree of prematurity, the postconceptual age at presentation, and the significance of co-morbidities, one blanket rule for postoperative observation and monitoring is usually applied. Indeed, a recent survey of surgical practices showed that approximately one third of the surgeons chose to wait until 50 weeks' postconceptual age and that one third waited until 60 weeks if possible.[15] Legal issues direct such practices in some institutions, but regardless of the postconceptual age at time of surgery, an infant should be hospitalized if any safety concerns arise during the operative or recovery period.

INTRAOPERATIVE MANAGEMENT

Monitoring

Standard monitoring in pediatric anesthesia follows the ASA "Standards for Basic Anesthetic Monitoring."[16] The requirements are to continually evaluate the patient's oxygenation, ventilation, circulation, and temperature. This can be accomplished by the use of oximetry, capnography, electrocardiography, and blood pressure measurement. Temperature monitoring is indicated in most pediatric anesthetics.

Oxygenation is measured indirectly by pulse oximetry with an audible and variable pitch tone and low threshold alarm, which is also audible to the anesthesiologist. Adequate illumination and exposure of the patient to allow assessment of color is recommended. Measurement of inspired oxygen concentration is standard with the use of an anesthesia machine.

Besides traditional methods of ventilation assessment, such as chest rise, movement of the reservoir breathing bag, and auscultation of breath sounds, continual monitoring of expired carbon dioxide (CO_2) is required, unless there are special circumstances. A disconnect alarm device must be used in conjunction with mechanical ventilators.

Precordial or esophageal stethoscopes have been used for many years during all phases of general anesthesia as well as during transport of anesthetized children. Continuous auscultation provides the anesthesiologist with immediate detection of changes in heart rate and character and breath sounds. The precordial stethoscope is placed on the left anterior chest, enabling detection of changes in breath sounds that may indicate a change in endotracheal tube position (e.g., a right main-stem bronchus intubation) or critical changes in hemodynamics.[17,18]

The Difficult Pediatric Airway

As demonstrated in the POCA registry, many cardiac arrests result from respiratory complications. The difficult pediatric airway is implicated as an important cause in a significant number of these cases. Most difficult airways in the pediatric age group can be anticipated; and, unlike in adults, it is rare to encounter an unanticipated difficult airway in a normal-appearing child.

Another major difference between adult and pediatric difficult airways is that awake intubations are rarely feasible in children. Special equipment in multiple sizes is needed, and each anesthesiologist must be proficient in several techniques.[19] The ASA developed practice guidelines for management of the difficult airway along with the ASA Difficult Airway Algorithm. This guideline and the algorithm are continually updated and well known to anesthesiologists.[20,21] These references emphasize the importance of having a clear primary plan with multiple back-up contingency plans.

Many congenital syndromes are associated with difficult airway management, including Beckwith-Wiedemann, trisomy 21, Pierre Robin sequence, Treacher Collins, Goldenhar's, Apert, Freeman-Shelden, Klippel-Feil, Crouzon, and others.[19] Most difficult pediatric airways involve obstruction or lack of mobility of the airway above the glottis, with difficulty ventilating the patient due to the upper airway obstruction after the induction of anesthesia. Preservation of spontaneous ventilation and the use of continued positive airway pressure (CPAP) by mask are tools commonly used by pediatric anesthesiologists in the anesthetic management of these patients.

There are many useful techniques available to secure the airway: the lighted stylet, the fiberoptic intubating stylet, the flexible fiberoptic bronchoscope, direct laryngoscopy with intubating stylet, fiberoptic rigid laryngoscopy, digital intubation, the Bullard scope, an anterior commissure scope, the laryngeal mask airway (LMA), retrograde wire techniques, cricothyrotomy, and surgical tracheostomy. When a difficult airway is anticipated, it is important to have all necessary airway equipment present in the operating room before induction of anesthesia. Equally important, it is essential to have an individual experienced in pediatric bronchoscopy and difficult airway management and a second individual who is skilled in cricothyrotomy and/or tracheostomy. Indirect intubation methods should be utilized rather than repeated attempts at direct laryngoscopy because airway edema and bleeding increase with each attempt, decreasing the likelihood of success with subsequent indirect methods.[19]

Anesthetic Management of Anterior Mediastinal Masses

It has been recognized for many years that the anesthetic management of the child with an anterior mediastinal mass is very challenging and fraught with the risk of sudden airway and cardiovascular collapse. Signs and symptoms of airway compression and cardiovascular dysfunction may or may not be present, but the absence of signs and symptoms does not preclude the possibility of life-threatening collapse of the airway or cardiovascular obstruction.[22-24]

The inherent conflict between the need to obtain an accurate and timely tissue diagnosis and the very real concern regarding the safe conduct of the anesthetic requires an open dialogue between the consultants and the oncologists to reach an agreement on strategies to achieve these goals. Many experts recommend the development and utilization of an algorithm for anesthetic management of the child with an anterior mediastinal mass (Fig. 3-1). The algorithms address assessment of signs and symptoms, evaluation of cardiopulmonary compromise, and treatment options.[25-27]

Common symptoms of tracheal compression and tracheomalacia include cough, dyspnea, chest pain, dysphagia, orthopnea, and recurrent pulmonary infections. Cardiovascular symptoms may result from infiltration of the pericardium and myocardium or compression of the pulmonary artery or superior vena cava. Tumor-associated superior vena cava syndrome develops rapidly and is poorly tolerated. Emergency radiation therapy is the treatment of choice for this life-threatening condition.[26]

The diagnostic evaluation includes posteroanterior and lateral chest radiographs and computed tomography (CT) scans. Echocardiography is also an essential investigative tool to assess pericardial status, myocardial contractility, and compression of the cardiac chambers and major vessels, such as the pulmonary artery. Flow-volume loops and fiberoptic bronchoscopy can provide a dynamic assessment of airway compression that other tests cannot assess.

Local anesthesia for biopsy is recommended for patients with airway and/or cardiovascular obstruction (orthopnea or superior vena cava syndrome), abnormal echocardiogram, tracheal cross-sectional area less than 50% predicted and peak expiratory flow rate less than 50% predicted, or symptoms of stridor or wheezing (Fig. 3-2). If biopsy under local anesthesia is not feasible for a patient with any of these abnormalities, radiation therapy or steroid pulse therapy is recommended to reduce the tumor burden.[22,26,27]

The anesthetic plan depends on the age of the patient, possible peripheral tissue and fluid accessibility, severity of symptoms, and the presence or absence of cardiopulmonary compromise demonstrated on the diagnostic tests. The anesthetic choices include local anesthesia, sedation, and general anesthesia. Most children will require general anesthetics for invasive procedures. Children who present with symptoms should be considered strongly for preoperative treatment of the tumor to reduce its size and improve cardiopulmonary compromise. Premedication is inadvisable in most circumstances because any loss of airway muscle tone may upset the balance between negative intrathoracic pressure and gravity, resulting in airway collapse. Once the decision is made to sedate or anesthetize a child, the recommended plan includes maintenance of spontaneous respiration regardless of induction technique, which may be intravenous, inhalational, or a combination of these. It is essential to avoid the use of muscle relaxants because the resultant airway collapse can be fatal. Depending on the surgical procedure and the stability of the airway, the child may be intubated or a laryngeal mask airway may be used.

Positioning of the child is an important part of the anesthetic plan. The sitting position favors gravitational pull of the tumor toward the abdomen rather than allowing gravity to pull the tumor posteriorly onto the airway and major vessels in the supine position.

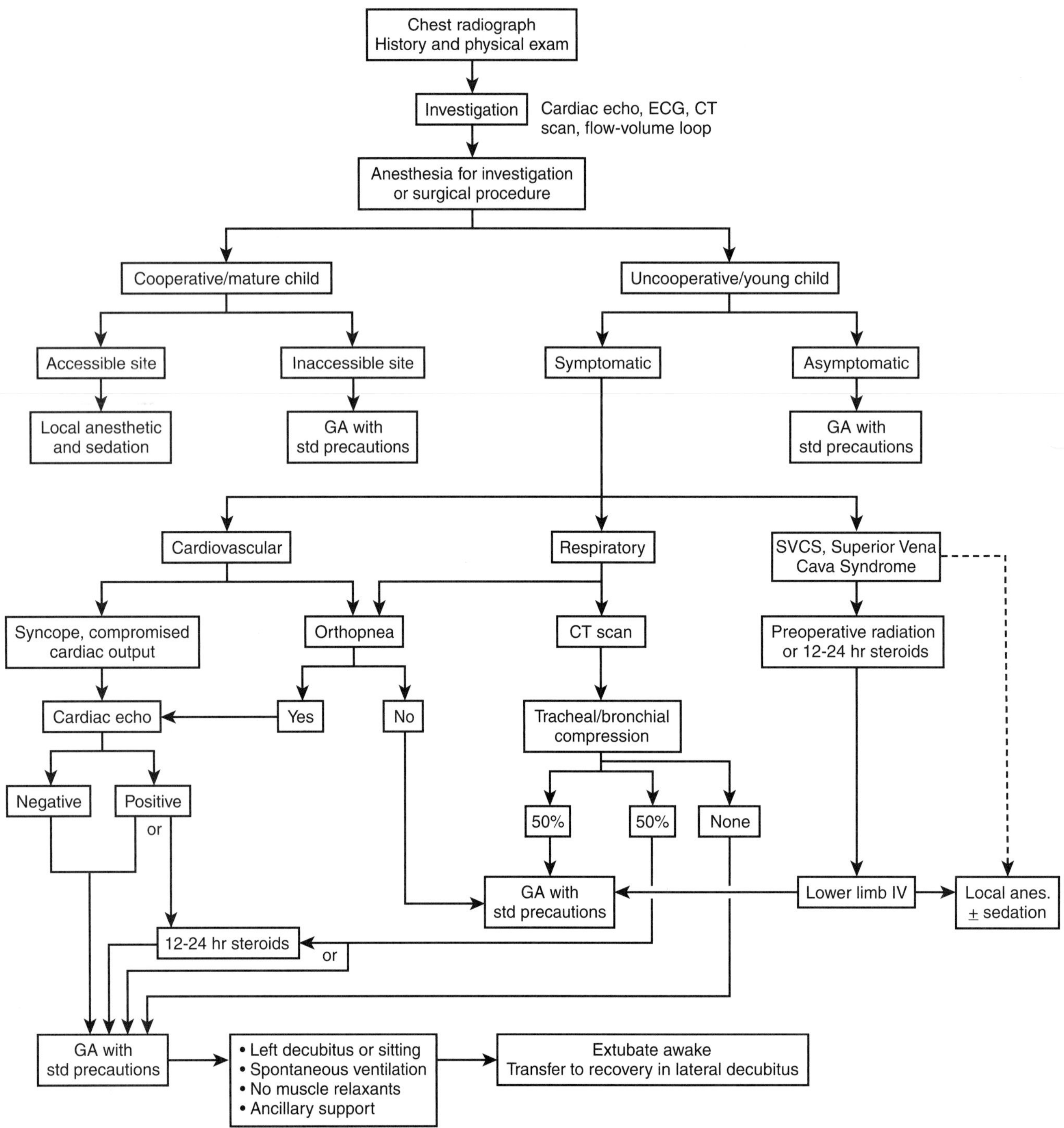

Figure 3-1. This algorithm describes management of the patient with a large anterior mediastinal mass. GA, general anesthesia. SVCS, superior vena cava syndrome. (Adapted from Cheung S, Lerman J: Mediastinal masses and anesthesia in children. In Riazi J [ed]: The Difficult Pediatric Airway. Anesthesiol Clin North Am 16:893-910, 1998.)

However, this position makes intubation challenging. Positioning the child in the lateral decubitus position is recommended even before induction for those who are symptomatic. Turning the child prone and lifting the sternum have been successful maneuvers to alleviate acute deterioration in ventilatory parameters or cardiovascular collapse secondary to tumor compression.[26] A rigid bronchoscope may also be used to relieve tracheal obstruction. Performing a median sternotomy and placing the child on cardiopulmonary bypass has been reported as an emergency measure but does not seem to be a practical alternative considering the time constraints of performing this procedure in the face of extreme hypoxia and hypotension. It is extremely important that the anesthesia, surgery, and the nursing teams be prepared with contingency plans to intervene emergently with alternative positioning and airway interventions.

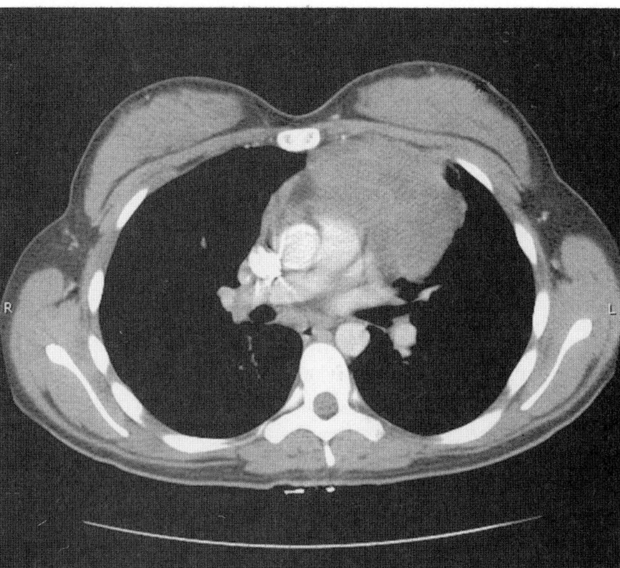

Figure 3-2. A 13-year-old girl presented with dyspnea and cervical adenopathy. As part of the evaluation, the CT scan showed this relatively large anterior mediastinal mass. The anesthesiologist did not believe that the child should undergo general endotracheal anesthesia because of concerns about tracheal compression from the mass. Therefore, she underwent cervical lymph node biopsy in the sitting position under local anesthesia.

Laparoscopic Surgery in Pediatric Patients

The successful application of minimally invasive surgical techniques in adults is commonplace now in the pediatric population. The cardiopulmonary effects of laparoscopic insufflation have been studied and published in adults and infants and deserve discussion here.

Laparoscopic fundoplication has gained in popularity in infants and children compared with open fundoplication because laparoscopic operations have been shown to reduce both short-term postoperative morbidity and long-term complications such as intestinal obstruction. In a comparison study of these two techniques in 212 children over 5 years, the laparoscopic operative time was longer, but the average hospital stay was reduced from 8.1 days to 3.5 days compared with the open approach.[28] Additional advantages are reduced discomfort and better cosmetic outcome.[29] It may be important to note that in spite of the many advantages of minimally invasive procedures, the systemic stress response is the same as for open surgeries.[30] Additionally, a recent study measured respiratory gas exchange intraoperatively in 19 open and 20 laparoscopic procedures and found a steady increase in oxygen consumption and core temperature in the laparoscopic group. This hypermetabolic response was more pronounced in younger children.[31]

An appreciation of the physiologic cardiocirculatory and pulmonary consequences during and after a laparoscopic operation is an important part of careful patient selection (Table 3-2). The widely varying nature of coexistent disease mandates close inspection of the potential impact of these laparoscopic-induced physiologic changes on each patient.

Table 3-2 Physiologic Effects of Creation of a Pneumoperitoneum
↑ Systemic vascular resistance
↑ Pulmonary vascular resistance
↓ Stroke volume
↓ Cardiac index
↑ P_{CO_2}
↓ Functional residual capacity
↓ pH
↓ P_{O_2}
↓ Venous return (head up)

Two critical factors create unique considerations for the anesthetic management of infants and children undergoing laparoscopic procedures: (1) the creation of a pneumoperitoneum with the resulting elevation of intra-abdominal pressure, and (2) the extremes of patient positioning that may be required for optimal exposure of intra-abdominal structures.[32]

Carbon dioxide remains the gas of choice because, unlike air, nitrous oxide, and oxygen, it does not promote combustion. In addition, CO_2 is also cleared more rapidly than the other choices. The cardiovascular consequences of intravascular gas embolism are relatively less risky than an insoluble gas such as helium. CO_2 uptake may be significantly greater in children, owing to the greater absorptive area of the peritoneum in relation to body weight and the smaller distance between capillaries and peritoneum. Hypercarbia has been demonstrated in adult and pediatric studies during CO_2 insufflation for laparoscopy.[33] Increases in minute ventilation by as much as 60% may be required to maintain baseline end-tidal CO_2 (ET_{CO_2}). Potentially deleterious consequences of hypercarbia are sympathetic nervous system activation with resultant increases in blood pressure and heart rate, along with increases in myocardial contractility and oxygen consumption. Hypercarbia sensitizes the myocardium to catecholamines and can predispose to cardiac arrhythmias.[32] ET_{CO_2} is not a reliable estimator of arterial CO_2 in children during laparoscopic surgery,[34] underestimating the value in as many as 30% of pediatric patients, so it is important to take this into consideration when planning for high-risk patients and include intra-arterial monitoring of blood gases in their management.

Some physiologic responses to hypercarbia are uniquely hazardous to infants, particularly neonates. Hypercarbia is a potent cerebrovascular dilator that, coupled with increased venous pressure due to increased intra-abdominal pressure, can result in increased intracranial pressure.[30,32] This presents the risk of intracranial hemorrhage in infants. Newborns are also at risk for reactive pulmonary hypertension when exposed to the stress of surgery, hypoxia, or hypercarbia. Infants with many forms of congenital heart disease are particularly vulnerable to the development of pulmonary hypertension.

Patients with preexisting ventriculoperitoneal shunts have been shown to develop acute intracranial pressure increases with concurrent decreases in cerebral perfusion pressure with an intra-abdominal pressure of 10 mm Hg or less.[35] This was ameliorated by monitored removal of cerebrospinal fluid. It is important to monitor intracranial pressure intraoperatively in patients with ventriculoperitoneal shunts, to avoid Trendelenburg positioning, and to use as low as possible intra-abdominal pressure to prevent neurosurgical complications.[34] In normal young children, creation of pneumoperitoneum results in an increase in middle cerebral artery blood flow velocity independent from hypercapnia, and CO_2 reactivity is maintained in the normal range.[36]

The increase in intra-abdominal pressure seen with laparoscopy results in well-documented cardiorespiratory changes. Respiratory derangements occur due to cephalad displacement of the diaphragm. This results in reduction in lung volume, ventilation-perfusion mismatch, and altered gas exchange. Bozkurt and coworkers demonstrated statistically significant decreases in pH and PaO_2 and increased $PaCO_2$ after 30 minutes of pneumoperitoneum.[30] Also, a 20% reduction in functional residual capacity occurs with induction of general anesthesia with an additional 20% decrease in functional residual capacity during laparoscopic surgery in adults.[30] The magnitude of the pulmonary effects correlates directly with intraperitoneal pressures.[37] Pediatric patients have a lower functional residual capacity relative to oxygen consumption and a higher closing volume than adults. Accordingly, infants have a smaller margin of safety and are less likely to tolerate the adverse respiratory effects of increased intra-abdominal pressure.

Significant cardiovascular changes have been demonstrated in response to increased intra-abdominal pressure and patient position. In the supine or Trendelenburg position, the venous return is augmented when the intra-abdominal pressure is kept below 15 mm Hg. The position preferred for upper abdominal procedures is reverse-Trendelenburg or supine. The head-up position reduces venous return and cardiac output.[38] Several pediatric studies have utilized echocardiography (supine),[39] impedance cardiography (15-degree head-down),[40] and continuous esophageal aortic blood flow echo-Doppler (supine)[41] to assess hemodynamic changes during laparoscopic surgery. These studies demonstrated significant reductions of stroke volume and cardiac index along with a significant increase in systemic vascular resistance. Pneumoperitoneum was found to be associated with significant increases in left ventricular end-diastolic volume, left ventricular end-systolic volume, and left ventricular end-systolic meridional wall stress.[39] All three studies demonstrated a decrease in cardiac performance and an increase in vascular resistance in healthy patients undergoing laparoscopy for lower abdominal procedures. The cardiovascular changes seen with pneumoperitoneum occur immediately with the creation of the pneumoperitoneum and resolve on exsufflation. However, a study of laparoscopic Nissen fundoplication in a pig model also showed a significant decrease in cardiac output that remained after the release of the pneumoperitoneum.[42] This study demonstrated a concomitant increase in mediastinal and pleural pressures thought to be due to dissection around the gastroesophageal junction. These parameters have not been studied in infants and children during upper abdominal procedures. However, the cardiopulmonary effects of low pressure pneumoperitoneum have been evaluated. Thirteen children, aged 6 to 36 months, undergoing laparoscopic fundoplication were studied in the 10-degree head-up position by noninvasive thoracic electrical bioimpedance looking at cardiac index, stroke volume, heart rate, mean arterial pressure, and peak inspiratory pressure at an intra-abdominal pressure of 5 mm Hg. The authors concluded that low-pressure pneumoperitoneum with intra-abdominal pressures not greater than 5 mm Hg does not decrease cardiac index in infants and children.[43]

In a study of cardiorespiratory function in 25 children undergoing laparoscopic Nissen fundoplication, 6 children developed postoperative hypoxemia, defined as an oxygen saturation of less than 95%. This desaturation has not been seen after laparoscopic surgery for inguinal hernia repair, leading the authors to conclude that interference with diaphragmatic function due to the surgical dissection may be the cause of the impaired oxygenation. Several of the children in the study had preexisting respiratory disease, presumably secondary to aspiration, which could also account for the desaturations.[44]

In summary, studies of the cardiopulmonary consequences of pneumoperitoneum for laparoscopic surgery have demonstrated a consistent and significant decrease in cardiac index, and an increase in systemic and pulmonary vascular resistance, unless low-pressure pneumoperitoneum is used. The reverse Trendelenburg position results in further reductions in preload and cardiac index. Postoperative diaphragmatic dysfunction may be a result of surgical dissection around the esophageal hiatus. Healthy infants and children without significant co-morbid conditions tolerate the cardiopulmonary effects of pneumoperitoneum well. Infants and children with significant cardiopulmonary disease require advanced planning and may need invasive monitoring during prolonged insufflation. Close monitoring of intra-abdominal pressure to ensure the use of minimally effective intra-abdominal pressure can minimize the adverse cardiopulmonary effects of pneumoperitoneum.

Anesthesia for Pediatric Thoracoscopy

Video-assisted thoracic surgery in pediatric patients has advantages over open thoracotomy, including reducing postoperative pain, decreasing hospitalization, improving cosmetic results, and decreasing the incidence of chest wall deformity.[45,46] Challenges for the anesthesiologist are numerous, making a thorough knowledge of the physiologic consequences of thoracoscopy and technical requirements in the ventilatory

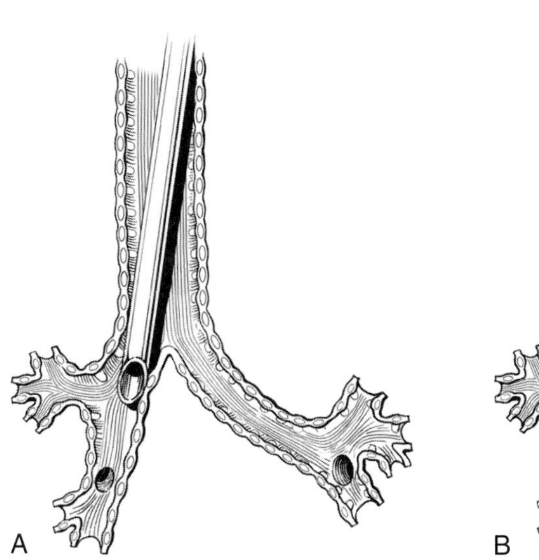

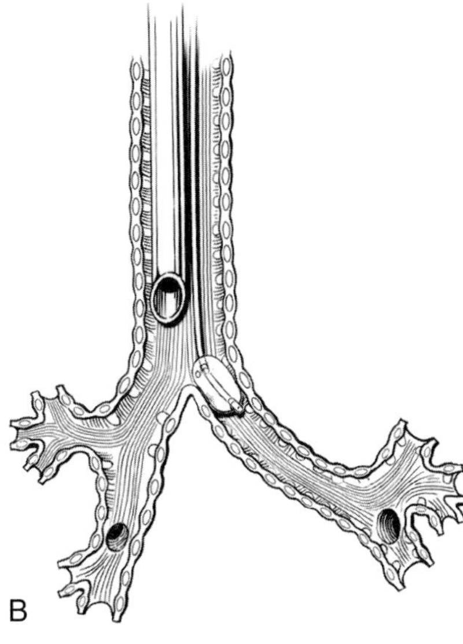

Figure 3-3. There are several methods available for single-lung ventilation in infants and children. The most common method is to use a conventional single-lumen endotracheal tube to intubate a main-stem bronchus (**A**). Another technique is to position the endotracheal tube in the trachea followed by insertion of a balloon-tipped bronchial blocker that is passed along the endotracheal tube and occludes the ipsilateral main-stem bronchus (**B**). The position of the bronchial blocker is usually confirmed using fiberoptic bronchoscopy.

management essential. An optimal anesthetic plan considers respiratory derangements due to positioning, lung exclusion, CO_2 insufflation into the pleural cavity, and methods of airway management for each age group in the pediatric population. Anesthesiologists must take into consideration the ventilation-perfusion mismatch that is induced by the lateral decubitus position in the anesthetized patient, single-lung ventilation, and CO_2 insufflation. In addition, much like laparoscopic insufflation, there are major hemodynamic implications during CO_2 insufflation of the chest cavity that compromises preload, stroke volume, cardiac index, and mean arterial pressure.[46]

In a recently published study of 50 pediatric patients undergoing thoracoscopy for a variety of surgical procedures, systolic and diastolic blood pressure was significantly lower and $ETCO_2$ was significantly higher during thoracoscopy. There was a statistically significant increase in $ETCO_2$ during single-lung ventilation compared with two-lung ventilation with intrapleural insufflation. Two-lung ventilation with insufflation was associated with a lower blood pressure than one-lung ventilation. The length of the thoracoscopy statistically significantly increased the $ETCO_2$.[46] These factors should be considered along with preoperative respiratory or cardiovascular compromise in planning the surgical procedure and anesthetic management. The magnitude of the physiologic changes induced by either one-lung or two-lung ventilation with insufflation is impacted by the patient's age, underlying co-morbid conditions, and the anesthetic agents utilized.

Multiple methods for single-lung ventilation have been described for infants and children. The most common and easiest method is to use a conventional single-lumen endotracheal tube (ETT) to intubate a main-stem bronchus (Fig. 3-3A). Fiberoptic bronchoscopy, in addition to clinical examination, is utilized to confirm proper placement. It is important to avoid obstruction of the right upper lobe bronchus or protrusion into the trachea from overinflation of the cuff (Fig. 3-4). A disadvantage of this technique is inadequate seal in the main-stem bronchus, causing problems with poor lung collapse on the operative side. Advantages of this technique are its simplicity and availability, because it can be performed in neonates.

Balloon-tipped bronchial blockers can be passed in or along the ETT and their position can be confirmed in the same manner as described earlier

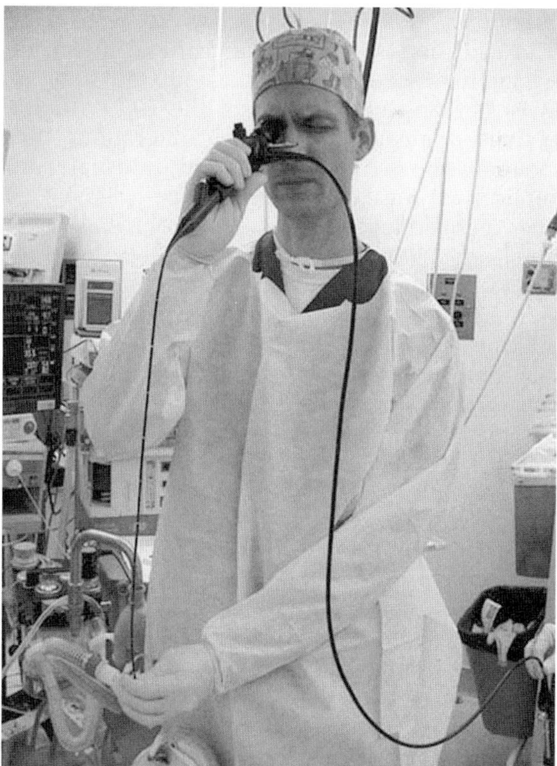

Figure 3-4. This photograph shows the anesthesiologist performing fiberoptic bronchoscopy to confirm proper placement of the bronchial blocker, which has been placed into the left main-stem bronchus in this young child.

(see Fig. 3-3B). Complications of this technique include obstruction of the trachea by dislodgement of the blocker balloon proximally, damage or rupture of the airway, and the inability to provide CPAP to the operated lung when needed. An Arndt wire–guided endobronchial blocker is now frequently used in pediatrics. This device utilizes the fiberoptic bronchoscope to guide the blocker into the desired position by attaching the blocker to the bronchoscope with a releasable wire. It is then locked into place proximally to stabilize its position. An additional advantage is its low-pressure and high-volume balloon, which should decrease the risk of mucosal injury.[47]

A Univent tube is a specially designed ETT with a second lumen containing a balloon-tipped bronchial blocker that can be advanced distally into the operative main-stem bronchus. This also requires a fiberoptic bronchoscope for placement. The smallest size available has a 3.5-mm internal diameter.

Double-lumen ETTs (DLTs) are available in right and left sides and consist of a longer bronchial tube fused with a shorter tracheal tube and two cuffs, one on each tube. Left-sided DLTs are used much more commonly than right-sided DLTs owing to the risk of obstructing the right upper lobe bronchus lumen. Limitations of these devices are related to the larger dimensions of the ETT, making its use restricted to patients 8 years and older. Advantages of DLTs are their relative ease of insertion and the ability to suction both lumens and provide oxygenated CPAP to the operative lung. Damage to the airway is possible with these rigid ETTs, as is true with all methods of single-lung ventilation.[46,48]

Complications related to anesthetic management are usually related to mechanical factors, such as airway injury and malposition of the ETTs. Additional problems related to physiologic alterations include hypoxemia and hypercapnia. An unusual surgical complication was reported in which a 3.5-kg infant with a congenital cystic adenomatoid malformation underwent attempted thoracoscopic resection of the lung cyst.[49] During CO_2 insufflation there was a sharp rise in $ETCO_2$ accompanied by severe hypoxemia and bradycardia due to occlusion of the ETT by blood. The procedure was immediately converted to an open thoracotomy, and it was discovered that there had been direct insufflation into the cyst and that the cyst communicated directly with the tracheobronchial tree. Another factor to consider is that $ETCO_2$ may be inaccurate during thoracoscopy, especially in small infants, because of alteration in dead space and shunt fraction, so there is usually a larger than usual gradient between $ETCO_2$ and arterial CO_2. In this unusual case, the abrupt rise in $ETCO_2$ was distinctly abnormal.

Risks associated with hypercarbia, especially in neonates, have been discussed earlier in this chapter. Therefore, it is important to try to maintain a reasonable range of increased CO_2 in neonates undergoing thoracoscopic procedures. The use of the high-frequency oscillating ventilator in neonates undergoing thoracoscopic repair of tracheoesophageal fistula has been described.[50] It is postulated that this ventilation method may allow better CO_2 elimination while optimizing the visualization for the surgeons. This technique has been used successfully at our institution recently as well and shows promise as a safe anesthetic management approach in these neonates.

Robotic Surgery

Minimal access surgery, despite its popularity, has some limitations that robot-assisted surgery is attempting to address. Robots can stabilize long instruments without tremor and overcome some of the technical challenges associated with the small workspace and two-dimensional visibility. One type of robot, AESOP (Automatic Endoscopic System for Optimal Positioning, Intuitive Surgical, Inc., Sunnyvale, CA), provides voice control of the telescope that is attached and stabilized by the robotic arm. This device is attached to the operating room table and does not impede access to the patient.[51]

AESOP has been used extensively and does not present any unique anesthetic management challenges. The da Vinci Robot (Intuitive Surgical, Inc., Sunnyvale, CA) is different and presents special challenges and limitations to patient access, which require advance preparation. Recently, a case report of a 2-month-old, 4.1-kg infant undergoing a Kasai procedure utilizing the da Vinci system described the hazards of minimal access.[52] The authors recommended practicing the crisis scenario of removing the robotic equipment and gaining access to the patient rapidly so that an emergency could be handled quickly. In the case of an airway emergency or cardiac arrest, the robotic instruments must be disengaged before backing the cart away from the operating table. This was performed in less than 1 minute in a practice run. Other recommendations were to use a left-sided precordial stethoscope to monitor for inadvertent right main-stem bronchus intubation and to consider fluoroscopy after patient positioning to confirm proper ETT depth. The precordial stethoscope is a low-tech, real-time method to check for left lung breath sounds. Intra-arterial blood pressure monitoring with interval blood gas sampling is also recommended, as well as urine output monitoring, because these procedures increase the setup and operative times currently. It is anticipated that operative times will decrease with experience.

Anesthetic Management of the Pediatric Congenital Heart Disease Patient Undergoing Noncardiac Surgery

Life expectancy of children with congenital heart disease (CHD) has continued to increase with the advancement of medical and surgical knowledge and expertise. Infants and children with complex congenital heart lesions are presenting more often for management of serious medical problems that may require surgical intervention before and between staged palliative cardiac procedures.

The diversity of anatomic and physiologic abnormalities encountered in children with CHD makes development of a generic anesthetic plan impossible. The main considerations for planning the anesthetic are the degree and type of cardiovascular and pulmonary impairment and the cardiopulmonary effects of the planned surgical procedure.[53,54] Unlike in adults, the estimation of risk in pediatric CHD patients undergoing noncardiac surgery has not been defined. We can, however, use the New York Heart Association (NYHA) functional classification as a guide for the need for further preoperative assessment. The potential deleterious physiologic consequences of anesthetics and surgery, such as laparoscopy, must be carefully examined in relation to the individual child's heart defect and associated hematologic and cardiopulmonary status.

Because cardiopulmonary dynamics are altered abruptly and significantly during procedures such as laparoscopy and thoracoscopy, preoperative assessment of cardiopulmonary reserve is vital. Evaluation for the presence of baseline hypoxemia, abnormalities of cardiac function, pulmonary abnormalities, and history of arrhythmias is essential.

Hypoxemia

Hypoxemic children should be evaluated for symptoms of hyperviscosity, such as headache, faintness, depressed mentation, fatigue, and muscle weakness. Preoperative phlebotomy is indicated for patients with a hematocrit greater than 65% and symptomatic hyperviscosity syndrome. Evidence of abnormal hemostasis, particularly prolongation of the prothrombin time or the partial thromboplastin time, occurs in up to 20% of patients with CHD. Reduction of red cell mass by preoperative phlebotomy has been reported to correct these abnormalities in some patients.[54] Prevention of dehydration with the intravenous use of fluids helps to reduce the hematocrit and optimizes preload. Children with hypoxemia due to CHD fall into two categories: (1) those with limited pulmonary blood flow with right-to-left shunting of blood and (2) those with unrestricted pulmonary blood flow with significant mixing of pulmonary and systemic venous blood. Anesthetic management is distinctly different in these two situations.[54]

When pulmonary blood flow is restricted, it is important to maintain adequate hydration and systemic arterial blood pressure to prevent worsening of the right-to-left shunt, which would further decrease pulmonary blood flow. Avoidance of additional increases in resistance to pulmonary blood flow would include careful adjustment of positive-pressure ventilation to prevent severe hypercarbia and high peak inspiratory pressure, both of which can diminish pulmonary blood flow. Unfortunately, even mild hyperventilation may be difficult to achieve during pneumoperitoneum with CO_2 without requiring high peak ventilatory pressures.[54] This may be particularly problematic in children with venous-dependent pulmonary blood flow, such as single ventricle physiology with Glenn or Fontan palliation.

The presence of unrestricted pulmonary blood flow mandates the preservation of ventricular function and the pulmonary to systemic blood flow (Qp:Qs) ratio at unity.[54] The choice of sevoflurane for induction, and either sevoflurane or isoflurane for maintenance, will minimize the myocardial depressant effect of the volatile anesthetic when kept below 1 MAC (mean alveolar concentration). Inotropic agents may be necessary to restore myocardial function during the anesthetic, especially in neonates.

Another important consideration in chronically hypoxemic patients is the development of myocardial fibrosis, reducing ventricular diastolic compliance and contractility. Myocardial cellular changes also occur, such as β-receptor downregulation. The chemoreceptor response to hypoxia is blunted, predisposing these patients to developing profound hypoxia in the postoperative period.[54]

Cardiac Failure

Patients with borderline cardiac function are at risk for intraoperative cardiac failure because of the negative inotropic effects of some anesthetic agents. Additional risks for cardiac failure occur during laparoscopy because of the acute decrease in preload and increase in systemic vascular resistance due to creation of the pneumoperitoneum. A case report by Tobias and Holcomb described the successful anesthetic management of two pediatric patients with dilated cardiomyopathy undergoing laparoscopic cholecystectomy.[55] Their anesthetic and surgical techniques were altered by avoiding anesthetic agents with negative inotropic effects, maintenance of the supine position, increasing ventilation to maintain normocarbia, slow insufflation with a pressure limit of 15 mm Hg, and use of intra-arterial monitoring of blood pressure and blood gases. Preoperative echocardiographic assessment of function and evaluation of exercise tolerance aids in decisions about the need for intraoperative monitoring and anesthetic drug and technique choices. Prophylactic management with inotropic infusions intraoperatively may be advisable.

Airway and Pulmonary Abnormalities

Abnormal airway anatomy is frequently seen in conjunction with CHD.[54] A short trachea is of particular significance in patients undergoing laparoscopic surgery due to the cephalad displacement of the diaphragm during pneumoperitoneum. Intraoperative main-stem bronchus intubation has been seen after insufflation in patients with normal tracheal length, so a high index of suspicion should be maintained, coupled with physical examination to prevent unrecognized main-stem bronchus intubation.[44] Use of a left anterior chest wall precordial stethoscope can be invaluable in the prompt detection of this potentially serious complication. Large and small airway obstruction due to CHD is also not uncommon. Airways can be compressed and/or obstructed by vascular rings, enlarged cardiac chambers, pulmonary artery, aorta, or artificial conduits. Small airway obstruction can result from bronchiolar smooth muscle hyperplasia in infants with pulmonary hypertension.[54]

Dead space is increased in children with decreased pulmonary blood flow. Positive-pressure ventilation and hypovolemia increase dead space further.[54] Anesthetic management of these children should emphasize maintenance of intravascular volume and ventricular function.

Excessive pulmonary blood flow leads to a progressive increase in pulmonary vascular resistance and airway obstruction. Children who have hypertrophied pulmonary vascular smooth musculature are susceptible to acute life-threatening pulmonary hypertensive episodes. Infants in this category include neonates, infants, and children with large ventricular septal defects or large patent ductus arteriosus. Particularly susceptible infants are those with complete atrioventricular canal and truncus arteriosus. Chronic exposure to excessive pulmonary blood flow results in irreversible pulmonary hypertension and right-to-left shunt. The anesthetic risk to symptomatic patients with this physiology (the Eisenmenger syndrome) appears to be considerable. These patients are usually NYHA functional class III or IV.[54] One case report describing the successful anesthetic management of an adult with Eisenmenger's syndrome presenting for laparoscopic cholecystectomy utilizing a technique consisting of general endotracheal anesthesia with infusion of norepinephrine to maintain systemic vascular resistance. This patient's history was consistent with NYHA functional class II. She had also tolerated a full-term pregnancy and vaginal delivery in the past.[56] Anesthetics that decrease systemic vascular resistance significantly, such as propofol, should be used only with extreme caution in patients with pulmonary hypertension or any cardiac defect in which a decrease in systemic vascular resistance is inadvisable.[18]

Neonates with or without CHD are at risk for reactive pulmonary hypertension due to the immaturity of the pulmonary vascular tree. Hypercarbia, hypoxemia, and stress can all trigger an acute pulmonary hypertensive crisis in this population. Neonates are also at risk for congestive heart failure when challenged with acute volume or pressure loads due to the immaturity of the neonatal myocyte. The Frank-Starling relationship is altered by the noncompliance of the neonatal ventricle so that the heart fails at a much lower pressure and volume. In neonates with CHD, the high risk of precipitating pulmonary hypertension and acute heart failure must be considered when selecting appropriate patients for minimally invasive surgery. In addition, infants with unrepaired CHD such as large ventricular septal defect, large patent ductus arteriosus, complete atrioventricular canal, truncus arteriosus, and single ventricle physiology are at high risk of death in the event of an acute pulmonary hypertensive crisis. The choice of surgical approach should take these factors into account. There is one published study of five infants with palliated hypoplastic left heart syndrome who underwent laparoscopic Nissen fundoplication and gastrostomy after modified Norwood procedures.[57] In the Norwood procedure, the right ventricle functions as the systemic ventricle and pulmonary blood flow is provided by a Blalock-Taussig shunt. In the modified Norwood procedure, the pulmonary blood flow is provided by a right ventricle to pulmonary artery conduit. All of the patients were monitored with arterial lines and blood gases were checked at regular intervals. Two patients received inotropic support prophylactically, and all five remained hemodynamically stable. Ventilation was meticulously managed to avoid high peak airway pressures and to maintain normocarbia. Pneumoperitoneum was limited to 12 mm Hg. $ETCO_2$ monitoring correlates poorly with $PaCO_2$ during peritoneal insufflation so frequent measurement of $PaCO_2$ was utilized for ventilation management. This is especially true in infants with cyanotic heart disease.[58] Decreases in cardiac index due to the systemic vascular resistance caused by pneumoperitoneum could decrease shunt flow, resulting in desaturation and acidosis. These patients had better preservation of diastolic blood pressure because of the right ventricle to pulmonary conduit modification of the Norwood procedure.[57]

Children who rely on passive venous return to the pulmonary circulation, such as those who have had Glenn or Fontan procedures, require special attention to ventilatory and fluid management during general anesthesia. The cardiac output in this population may be adversely affected by positive-pressure ventilation.

Residual defects in myocardial contractility and the ejection fraction predispose patients to acute heart failure when challenged by abrupt increases in afterload. Cyanotic patients should be considered to be at risk for decompensation when faced with increased afterload because of the known association of myocardial fibrosis with chronic cyanosis.[54]

Infants and children with intracardiac communications are at increased risk for shunting of blood and gas. The risk of gas embolism during laparoscopy is small, but should it occur in the presence of intracardiac communication, gas emboli could gain access to the systemic circulation. This could result in stroke or myocardial ischemia. Utilizing CO_2 as the insufflating gas decreases the likelihood of sustained arterial obstruction by a gas bubble because CO_2 would be absorbed more quickly than air or helium.

Children with repaired heart defects with little or no residual dysfunction tolerate anesthetics well. Subacute bacterial endocarditis prophylaxis recommendations should be utilized as indicated. A preoperative history revealing NYHA functional class I or II in conjunction with a recent echocardiogram demonstrating good function and no other serious concerns is valuable information in assessment of these children.

Recommendations for the anesthetic management of patients with CHD are seen in Table 3-3.

POSTANESTHESIA CARE

Pain Management

The incidence of postoperative pain in the pediatric population, although difficult to evaluate objectively, is probably similar to that in the adult population.

Table 3-3 Recommendations for the Anesthetic Management of Patients with Congenital Heart Disease

1. Preoperative medication with an anxiolytic, such as oral midazolam, should be considered to prevent agitation and increased oxygen consumption.
2. Preoperative intravenous fluids should be considered in patients at risk for hyperviscosity. Children with passive pulmonary blood flow should not be allowed to become dehydrated.
3. Prophylaxis for subacute bacterial endocarditis should be done as recommended by the American Heart Association.
4. Intraoperative monitoring with intra-arterial catheter and central venous pressure would be helpful in guiding fluid management and vasoactive drug therapy. Blood gas analysis can also be used to monitor arterial to end-tidal CO_2 and acid-base status.
5. Intraoperative transesophageal echocardiography could be helpful in aiding the intraoperative diagnosis of heart failure or air embolism in any patient with borderline or reduced cardiac function, intracardiac shunt, or passive pulmonary blood flow.
6. Induction with agents that have less negative inotropic effects, such as etomidate, ketamine, or sevoflurane, seems prudent. The use of an anticholinergic drug to prevent vagal reflexes and bradycardia during peritoneal insufflation is recommended in neonates whose cardiac output is heart rate dependent.
7. Maintenance of anesthesia with isoflurane should have minimal negative inotropic effect and may decrease systemic vascular resistance. A nondepolarizing muscle relaxant is required for optimal abdominal relaxation. Propofol should be used sparingly in any patient with pulmonary hypertension, if at all, because it reduces systemic vascular resistance and can result in sudden hypotension and cardiovascular collapse.
8. For laparoscopic procedures, slow insufflation and maintenance of the supine position are recommended to prevent sudden changes in cardiovascular parameters. It may not be possible to achieve adequate surgical exposure for upper abdominal procedures without some reverse Trendelenburg positioning. When a change in position is necessary, this should be done independently, rather than concurrently with insufflation. Hemodynamics should be allowed to equilibrate after each change before adding another variable.
9. Limiting insufflation pressure to 10-12 mm Hg to minimize cardiopulmonary alterations is recommended.
10. Postoperative analgesia is usually facilitated by the injection of local anesthetic into the small incisions by the surgeon at the end of the procedure. Additional analgesia can be provided by ketorolac and small doses of narcotic in the recovery room. If conversion to an open procedure is required because the patient does not tolerate the decrease in cardiac index and increase in systemic vascular resistance, a regional technique for postoperative analgesia may be considered. A normal coagulation profile is necessary to consider this option. The use of epidural analgesia for upper abdominal incisions has been shown to improve pulmonary function postoperatively and shorten the postoperative hospitalization.

It is reasonable, therefore, to assume that about 75% of children will report significant pain on the first postoperative day.[59] The ineffective treatment of postoperative discomfort in children is most often the result of four factors:

1. Individuals involved in the care of children are working with an evolving knowledge of the mechanisms of pain and its transmission in children. Attitudes toward the management of pain in children have often been biased by several observations made on newborns. It has been known for many years that newborns may cry for relatively short periods after experiencing noxious stimuli and then settle down and sleep without the use of analgesics.[60] In addition, microscopic examination of thalamocortical tracts in the newborn has shown a lack of myelin, leading investigators and clinicians to postulate that the pain perception of neonates is immature and rudimentary.[61] Finally, higher concentrations of endogenous opioids are present in the plasma and cerebrospinal fluid of neonates when compared with those of older children.[62] This type of information has led to the erroneous conclusion that neonates do not have a normal sensation of pain and therefore do not require postoperative pain therapy. Evidence indicates that neonates do experience pain in a manner similar to that of adults. Sophisticated observations of cry patterns, facial expressions, movements, and cardiovascular variables allow reproducible documentation of painful experiences in these smallest of patients.
2. Misconceptions remain regarding the pharmacokinetics of pain medications in children. Clearly, the neonate presents differences from older children and adults that must be taken into account. For instance, neonates appear to have a greater sensitivity to the respiratory depressant effects of narcotics. This may be explained by the fact that relatively fewer α_1 narcotic receptors (mediating analgesia) exist relative to the α_2 receptors (mediating respiratory depression) in neonates when compared with older individuals.[63] Evidence also suggests that for some narcotics the volume of distribution is larger and the elimination half-life is prolonged in premature infants. For example, the elimination half-life of fentanyl is 129 minutes in an adult and 230 minutes in a neonate. As a result, higher levels of narcotics persist in the cerebrospinal fluid of neonates for longer periods. Some have asserted that narcotics should be used in infants younger than 6 months only when observation in an intensive care setting is possible or postoperative ventilation is planned.[64]
3. The management of pain in the pediatric population is hampered by the difficulty that exists in assessing pain. Many children may respond to pain by emotionally withdrawing from their surroundings, and this may be misinterpreted by the medical and nursing staffs as evidence that they have no pain. In addition, when questioned as to their degree of pain, children may not volunteer useful information for fear of painful interventions. To circumvent these difficulties, several

visual and verbal scales have been developed for quantifying painful sensations or describing typical painful behaviors. These have met with varying degrees of success because they are difficult to implement, are time consuming to use, and still rely on patient comprehension and cooperation.

4. Individual biases exist in medical professionals caring for children. These biases run from the belief that pain is a natural consequence of surgery to the beliefs that the risks of respiratory depression and narcotic addiction outweigh the benefits that are associated with aggressive pain management.

The mainstay in pain control remains the use of narcotics. Not only is a bewildering array of narcotics available, but the methods of their administration also are changing. Dose-dependent respiratory depression is common to all narcotics and goes hand in hand with their analgesic properties. Other side effects that vary from drug to drug and patient to patient are somnolence, nausea and vomiting, pruritus, constipation, and urinary retention. Given time, patients develop tolerance to most, if not all, of these side effects while they continue to experience their analgesic properties. The side effects may be treated symptomatically while tolerance is developing, thereby making the patient much more comfortable and manageable. Changing the narcotics will often reduce or eliminate the side effects.

Morphine remains the standard by which most pain therapy is measured. Some pharmacologic differences between morphine and other analgesics must be appreciated to use this narcotic well. Although morphine has roughly the same plasma elimination half-life as other narcotics, its effect and duration of action may have considerable variability because of the drug's low lipid solubility.

Because a poor correlation exists between the plasma concentration of morphine and its desired analgesic effect—a fourfold variation has been measured in the plasma concentration of morphine at which patients medicate themselves for pain—many clinicians believe that morphine is best administered in a patient-controlled device (patient-controlled analgesia [PCA]). As the patient experiences changes in the level of morphine in the central nervous system, he or she is able to administer supplemental doses.

PCA dosing recommendations for morphine include a loading dose ranging from 0.04 to 0.06 mg/kg followed by intermittent PCA doses of 0.01 to 0.03 mg/kg. A lockout interval of 6 to 15 minutes and 0.2 to 0.4 mg/kg every 4 hours is the limit generally used.

When PCA devices are not used, the intermittent administration of morphine to opioid-naive children should be started at 0.05 to 0.1 mg/kg every 2 to 4 hours. If the treatment of pain is undertaken in a recovery room or intensive care setting, similar doses may be administered every 5 to 10 minutes until the child is comfortable. A background infusion approximately equivalent to one PCA dose per hour may be appropriate for patients with moderate to severe pain. Patients with a background infusion should be continuously monitored for cardiorespiratory depression by telemetry and pulse oximetry.

Fentanyl is a synthetic narcotic that usually has a relatively short duration of action as a result of rapid distribution into fat and muscle because of its high lipid solubility. With repeated dosing, the duration of action appears to increase.[65] When compared with morphine, fentanyl is about 100 times more potent. (Fentanyl dosages are calculated in micrograms rather than milligrams.) In controlled comparisons with equipotent dosages, morphine is generally found to provide better analgesia than fentanyl but with more side effects such as pruritus, hypotension, nausea, and vomiting.[66-68] Fentanyl may also demonstrate much more rapid tolerance to its analgesic effects than morphine or hydromorphone.

When using fentanyl for procedures, incremental dosing of 0.25 to 0.5 μg/kg every 5 minutes is safe. All of the respiratory depression from a single dose of fentanyl is evident within 5 minutes because of its rapid equilibration across the blood-brain barrier. The elimination rate of a single dose of fentanyl is reported to be about 1 μg/kg/hr.[69] A safe cumulative dose for procedures is 2 to 5 μg/kg.[70]

Other formulations of fentanyl have clinical applications in pain management. Although not approved for pediatrics at present, transdermal fentanyl, in doses of 25 to 100 μg/hr, has proved more effective in the treating of chronic pain than some traditional modalities.[71]

Hydromorphone is a well-tolerated alternative to morphine and fentanyl and is associated with less pruritus and sedation than morphine. Moreover, it has a longer duration of action than fentanyl. It is five to seven times more potent than morphine. The dosing schedule for PCA hydromorphone uses a loading dose of 5 to 15 μg/kg, a lockout of 6 to 15 minutes, supplemental PCA doses of 3 to 5 μg/kg, and a 4-hour limit of 100 μg/kg.

As more and more pediatric surgery is being performed on an outpatient basis, significant interest has developed in the role of non-narcotic analgesics for the management of postoperative pain. Many physicians have questioned the efficacy of acetaminophen for significant pain relief, although this may be more a question of the dosage used with recent investigators challenging established dosing recommendations for rectal administration.[72,73] Dosages for analgesia were based on recommendations for fever control (10 to 20 mg/kg), but these doses failed to produce serum levels shown to be effective even in reducing temperature. To achieve adequate serum levels for analgesia, doses of 30 to 40 mg/kg rectally are required. A dose of 30 mg/kg of acetaminophen rectally has proved to have analgesic properties similar to 1 mg/kg of ketorolac.[74]

Ketorolac is an oral and parenteral nonsteroidal anti-inflammatory drug shown to have excellent pain-control characteristics. Dosage recommendations are 0.5 mg/kg intravenously every 6 to 8 hours for 48 hours. Doses greater than 15 mg may yield diminishing analgesic return with increasing side effect profiles. Doses greater than 30 mg are generally not recommended. One of the drawbacks associated with ketorolac is its inhibition of platelet aggregation, which has been associated with increased bleeding after tonsillectomy.[75] Attention must also be paid to patients with renal impairment, risk for gastric ulcers, and the question of poor union of extensive orthopedic repairs.

Clonidine has gained favor as an adjunct in regional anesthesia. A centrally acting α_2 agonist with a sedative effect, clonidine confers an analgesic benefit. It has been shown to increase the analgesic duration of caudal blocks by as much as 18 hours.[76] Clonidine has also been used effectively in epidural infusions. In adults, clonidine may carry a risk of hypotension, but this side effect is not prominent in children. Moreover, clonidine is not beset by problems of nausea and pruritus. For this reason, it has compared favorably as a substitute for neuraxial opioids, long the standard adjuvant to local anesthetics.

Regional anesthetic techniques used concomitantly with general anesthesia have had a resurgence in both adult and pediatric patients. These techniques include local infiltration of the wound, peripheral nerve blocks, and caudal, epidural, or spinal blocks. Part of the intent of these techniques is to prevent sensitization of the peripheral and central nervous systems, which could result in prolonged or excessive postoperative pain. This approach is often referred to as preemptive analgesia. Whether preemptive analgesia exists in children is still unresolved.[77] Anecdotal reports of improved, prolonged analgesia during the postoperative period when regional anesthetic techniques are used preemptively still await scientific validation.

In selected cases, peripheral nerve blocks appear to be a superior pain control modality. They offer the benefit of absent central side effects (nausea, pruritus, sedation, urinary retention) and can allow for faster recovery. It is increasingly common for these blocks to be performed under ultrasound guidance, which may, in some cases, confer increased accuracy and reduced time consumption.

Whether undergoing an operation on an inpatient or an outpatient basis, infants and children should be afforded maximal pain relief. Recent developments in and understanding of pain-relieving techniques place this goal within the reach of all clinicians caring for children during the postoperative period.

Recovery and Criteria for Discharge

The recovery period for infants and children may be more crucial than for adult patients. Although the risks of intraoperative problems are similar in adults and children, 3% to 4% of infants and children have major complications in the recovery period, whereas only 0.5% of adults experience these complications. In general, children should be comfortable, awake, stable, off supplemental oxygen, have normal vital signs, and be able to take oral fluids before discharge from outpatient surgery. These variables have been quantified with the Modified Aldrete Score (Table 3-4), which lists the important factors taken into consideration for discharge.

Table 3-4 Modified Aldrete Score

Variable*	Score
Able to move, voluntarily or on command	
• Four extremities	2
• Two extremities	1
• No extremities	0
Respiration	
• Able to breathe deeply and cough freely	2
• Tachypnea, shallow or limited breathing	1
• Apnea	0
Circulation	
• Blood pressure within 20 mm Hg of preoperative level	2
• Blood pressure within 20-50 mm Hg of preoperative level	1
• Blood pressure ± 50 mm Hg of preoperative level	0
Consciousness	
• Fully awake	2
• Arousable to voice	1
• Unresponsive	0
Oxygen saturation	
• > 92% on room air	2
• > 90% with oxygen	1
• < 90% with oxygen	0

*These variables are taken into consideration for discharge from outpatient surgery.

Common impediments to discharge include pain, emergence delirium, nausea, laryngospasm or croup, and hypoxia. Because general anesthesia is nearly universal in children, regional anesthesia is less common than in adults. However, pediatric outpatients are excellent candidates for a host of regional blocks.[78] Some blocks require specialized equipment like a nerve stimulator or ultrasound, but others such as an ilioinguinal block can be performed by landmarks alone. Local infiltration by the surgeon is encouraged when a neuraxial or peripheral block is not performed.

Emergence delirium is a vexing problem characterized by agitation in a child without apparent physiologic cause. The child is disoriented and often does not recognize his or her own parents. While not intrinsically dangerous, the problem is disturbing to parents and caregivers alike, poses a risk of self-injury, delays discharge, and invariably consumes recovery room resources. It is possible that sevoflurane, with its rapid elimination half-life, is more likely to be associated with emergence delirium.[79] However, other published data show no difference in emergence delirium relative to isoflurane.[80]

Postoperative nausea and vomiting (PONV) is most effectively managed with a combination of steroids (dexamethasone, 0.05-0.5 mg/kg) and serotonin antagonists as first-line therapy.[81] Adequate hydration and avoidance of nitrous oxide, volatile anesthetics (in favor of propofol), and neostigmine all are validated as reducing PONV. Metoclopramide, a commonly prescribed promotility drug, while possibly having a salutary effect on intraoperative hiccups, bestows little benefit for PONV. Perhaps the most cost-effective perioperative antiemetic is droperidol. Unfortunately, its use has been dramatically curtailed due to a black box warning from the U.S. Food and Drug Administration regarding possible QT prolongation associated with its use. There is much disagreement about the data behind this warning.[82]

Respiratory complications are the most serious of the common problems seen after outpatient surgery. Laryngospasm, while possibly life threatening, is almost always transient and treatable by continuous positive mask pressure with a small dose of propofol (1-2 mg/kg) as an immediate backup. Rescue with succinylcholine is indicated at the first sign of relative bradycardia, which is often audible before it is visualized on an electrocardiogram. Postoperative croup is usually treatable with nebulized racemic epinephrine, and bronchospasm is managed with nebulized β agonists such as albuterol.

Intraoperative Awareness

Intraoperative awareness is a rare condition in which surgical patients can recall their surroundings or an event and sometimes even pain related to their surgery while they were under general anesthesia. The definition of intraoperative awareness is becoming conscious during a procedure performed under general anesthesia and subsequently having recall of these events. Recall is explicit memory of specific events that took place during the general anesthesia. A Sentinel Event Alert was issued by the Joint Commission (JC) regarding the prevention and management of intraoperative awareness in October 2004. The ASA published a Practice Advisory for Intraoperative Awareness and Brain Functioning Monitoring in April 2006.[83]

The incidence of intraoperative awareness in adults has been reported to be 0.1% to 0.9% in older studies[84] and 0.0068% or 1 per 14,560 patients in a 2007 report of 87,361 patients. Most experts estimate the true incidence in adults to be 0.1% to 0.2%. There is a dearth of literature about intraoperative awareness in infants and children, but there is a 2005 study of 864 children in which there was a reported incidence of 0.8%.[85] Some of these data may be confounded by the memory of entering the operating room after administration of the preoperative sedation or a memory of emergence. Certainly, the likelihood of a clear memory of a painful surgery is a much rarer event than the generic incidence commonly reported. There are multiple adverse effects related to intraoperative awareness including post-traumatic stress disorder in adults and children and medical-legal implications. Therefore, it is important to understand the risk factors, preventive measures that can be taken, and management of the condition when it occurs.

Surgical and anesthetic risk factors for intraoperative awareness include cardiac surgery, cesarean section, trauma surgery, emergency surgery, the use of muscle relaxants with reduced anesthetic dosage, and the use of nitrous oxide/opioid anesthetics. Known patient risk factors are substance use or abuse, previous intraoperative awareness, a history of difficult intubation or anticipated difficult intubation, and patients with opioid tolerance, such as chronic pain patients on high doses of opioid. Additionally, ASA class 4 or 5 patients and any patient with limited hemodynamic reserve are at risk for intraoperative awareness.

Preventive measures include conventional monitoring, equipment checklists, and verification of proper functioning of intravenous access, infusion pumps, and connections. Benzodiazepine prophylaxis should be selected on a case-by-case basis depending on the patient and surgical risk factors. The common use of volatile anesthetics in pediatrics should decrease the risk of intraoperative awareness. Detection of signs and symptoms of possible awareness intraoperatively may include hypertension, tachycardia, movement, lacrimation, sweating, and decreased lung compliance.

Brain function monitors have been suggested as a method of prevention, and the ASA practice advisory and the JC alert addressed this methodology in their reports. These monitors measure spontaneous electrical activity and convert a single channel of frontal electroencephalograph into an index of hypnotic level. The consensus of the ASA task force found that a specific numerical value may not correlate with a specific anesthetic depth and that the values do not have uniform sensitivity across different anesthetic drugs or types of patients. There is insufficient evidence to recommend the routine use of brain function monitors to either reduce the frequency of intraoperative awareness or monitor the depth of anesthesia. Both the ASA and the JC recommend case-by-case decision by the anesthesiologist for selected patients.[83]

These advisories recommend that the anesthesiologist may consider discussing the risk of intraoperative awareness with patients in substantially increased risk groups preoperatively. The patient can be reassured of the measures that will be taken to prevent intraoperative awareness and that if it occurs it is rarely associated with pain. If intraoperative awareness does occur, the anesthesiologist should discuss the episode with the patient to obtain details and discuss possible reasons for the event. Counseling or other psychological support should be offered.

It is important to remember that intraoperative awareness is a rare occurrence and usually not associated with pain. It is more likely to occur in high-risk surgery because of the need to maintain hemodynamic stability. Parental and patient questions should be referred to the anesthesiologist as soon as possible so that early intervention and counseling can be offered to lessen the resulting trauma.

SEDATION

Twenty-five years ago, the American Academy of Pediatrics (AAP) asked the Section on Anesthesiology to develop guidelines for monitoring children undergoing sedation by non-anesthesiologists. That year, three children died in sedation disasters in a single

Table 3-5 Current Definitions of Sedation Levels

Analgesia	Relief of pain without intentionally producing sedation
Minimal sedation/ anxiolysis	A drug-induced state during which the patient responds normally to verbal commands. Ventilatory and cardiovascular functions are unaffected.
Moderate sedation/ analgesia	A drug-induced state during which the patient responds purposefully to verbal commands and/or light touch. Airway and adequate ventilation are maintained without intervention and cardiovascular function is maintained.
Deep sedation/ analgesia	A drug-induced depression of consciousness during which the patient cannot be easily aroused but responds purposefully to noxious stimulation (reflex withdrawal). Assistance may be required to maintain airway and adequate ventilation. Cardiovascular function is usually maintained.
General anesthesia	A drug-induced loss of consciousness during which the patient is not arousable, even by painful stimulation (no reflex withdrawal). Assistance to maintain airway is often required, and positive-pressure ventilation may be required to maintain adequate ventilation. Cardiovascular function may be impaired.

dental office in California. At that time, an analysis of pediatric sedation by non-anesthesiologists revealed a disturbingly high morbidity and mortality rate. In the ensuing years, the AAP, the ASA, the American Academy of Pediatric Dentists (AAPD), and the American College of Emergency Physicians (ACEP) have worked independently and collectively to evaluate the problem, develop guidelines, and institute standardized practices. This has improved the safety of pediatric sedation in practices where these guidelines are followed.

A multidisciplinary review of over 600 adverse drug reports was undertaken and reviewed independently by two pediatric anesthesiologists, one pediatric emergency medicine specialist, and one pediatric critical care specialist, who then debated each case.[86] An epidemiologist/statistician then guided the group through the analysis of these events. The results demonstrated no relationship between adverse outcomes (death/neurologic injury) and route of drug administration (intravenous, nasal, rectal, intramuscular, oral, inhalation [nitrous oxide plus other sedatives]), or drug class. Failure to rescue the patient and inadequate cardiopulmonary resuscitation skills were the major contributing factors. Most of these patients presented with some form of respiratory depression. Other contributory causes were drug overdoses, drug-drug interactions, inadequate monitoring, inadequate recovery, prescription/transcription errors, drug administration without medical supervision, drug administration by a technician, inadequate equipment, and premature discharge from recovery or inadequate recovery procedures.

The major goals of procedural sedation are to provide anxiety relief, pain control, and reasonable movement control.[87,88] Inadequate sedation causes psychological trauma and difficulty completing a high-quality diagnostic or therapeutic procedure and results in excessively high cancellation rates for radiologic procedures.[87,88] In 2002 the AAP, ASA, and the JC all began to use the same sedation terminology, which recognizes the fact that "conscious sedation" is not realistic in children and that children younger than age 6 are considered to be deeply sedated from the beginning of the sedation process. Levels of sedation occur on a continuum, and it is difficult to predict every patient's response. For this reason, it is agreed by all groups that the practitioner must be able to rescue the patient from the next deeper level of sedation than the one targeted.[89,90] The current definitions of sedation levels are found in Table 3-5.

The JC mandates standardization for sedation outside the operating room with processes similar to those utilized for monitored anesthesia care delivered by qualified anesthesia providers in the operating room.[89] The JC also requires that sedation practices throughout the hospital be "monitored and evaluated by the Department of Anesthesia." In response to regulatory guidelines and in recognition of the need to institute a safe, systematic approach to sedation of children, many children's hospitals have developed dedicated sedation services using experts (anesthesiologists or other highly trained individuals) to perform sedation rather than a variety of providers with a range of training. The benefits of this are many, including optimizing patient safety, reducing sedation failure rates to 0%, and meeting regulatory and administrative requirements.[87,88]

The principles outlined in the *2006 Guidelines for Monitoring and Management of Pediatric Patients During and After Sedation for Diagnostic and Therapeutic Procedures: An Update* are seen in Table 3-6.[91] Appropriate monitoring of patients includes visual observation, pulse oximetry, and measurement of vital signs by an appropriately credentialed health care professional who is not performing the procedure. Capnography (noninvasive measurement of expired CO_2) is mandated during general anesthesia and is now being encouraged during deep sedation by the JC and the AAP.[92] Several published studies have now demonstrated that the use of nasal or nasal/oral cannulas for continuous CO_2 analysis provides early detection of inadequate ventilation and prompts faster intervention.[93-95] This has been shown to decrease the number of episodes of oxygen desaturation.[95]

Credentialing and privileging practitioners for sedation requires adherence to federal, state, and local laws as well as governing bodies' requirements for physicians, dentists, and nurses. Medical staff bylaws define credentialing requirements, which are also significantly influenced by the JC recognition that moderate and deep sedation are high-risk activities. Therefore,

Table 3-6 The 2006 Guidelines for Monitoring and Management of Pediatric Patients during and after Sedation for Diagnostic and Therapeutic Procedures: An Update

- No administration of sedating medication without the safety net of medical supervision
- Pre-sedation evaluation of underlying medical or surgical conditions by the practitioner ordering the medication (JC requirement)
- Appropriate fasting for elective procedures, balancing the depth of sedation and risk for urgent procedures
- Focused airway examination for airway obstruction potential, such as large tonsils or anatomic airway abnormalities
- A clear understanding by the ordering practitioner of the pharmacokinetic and pharmacodynamic effects of the sedative medications, as well as an appreciation of drug interactions
- Appropriate training and skills in airway management to allow rescue of the patient
- Age- and size-appropriate equipment for airway management and venous access
- Appropriate medications and reversal agents
- Sufficient numbers of care providers to carry out the procedure and monitor the patient
- Appropriate monitoring during and after the procedure
- A properly equipped and staffed recovery area
- Recovery to pre-sedation level of consciousness before discharge from medical supervision
- Appropriate discharge instructions

From Coté CJ, Karl HW, Notterman DA, et al: Adverse sedation events in pediatrics: Analysis of medications used for sedations. Pediatrics 106: 633-644, 2000.

individuals seeking privileges for procedural sedation must meet threshold criteria.[96] Each practitioner must be a qualified, licensed professional with documented competency-based education, training, and experience in evaluating patients before sedation and performing moderate or deep sedation, including the ability to rescue patients who progress into a deeper-than-desired level of sedation. The individual must possess airway skills capable of managing a compromised airway and maintaining oxygenation and ventilation to qualify for moderate sedation privileges. For deep sedation privileges, the practitioner must be able to rescue the patient from general anesthesia and be able to manage an unstable cardiovascular system in addition to a compromised airway.[96] Each medical facility develops criteria based on these principles. For JC accreditation, the institution must be able to document that its system is safe and effective, with consistent quality improvement activities across the institution. In addition, the institution must be able to document that all patients sedated by non-anesthesiologists are comparably assessed, monitored, discharged, and have similar sedation outcomes.[89]

CONCLUSION

Many children who present for surgery are frightened and uncomfortable; it is the anesthesiologist's privilege to help calm and comfort these children. Guiding the child through an operation safely, amnestically, and under conditions amenable to the surgery are goals shared by both the anesthesiologist and surgeon alike. These shared goals are most likely to be met when surgical and anesthesia services communicate openly at the time of surgical scheduling, preoperatively, intraoperatively, and postoperatively. When such an understanding exists, the prospect of a child's operation proceeding safely, efficiently, and with a desired outcome is optimized.

chapter 4

RENAL IMPAIRMENT

Uri S. Alon, MD • Bradley A. Warady, MD

BODY FLUID REGULATION

Effective kidney function maintains the normal volume and composition of body fluids. Although there is a wide variation in dietary intake and nonrenal expenditures of water and solute, water and electrolyte balance is maintained by the excretion of urine, with the volume and composition defined by physiologic needs. Fluid balance is accomplished by glomerular ultrafiltration of plasma coupled with modification of the ultrafiltrate by tubular reabsorption and secretion.[1,2] The excreted urine, the modified glomerular filtrate, is the small residuum of the large volume of nonselective ultrafiltrate modified by transport processes operating along the nephron. The glomerular capillaries permit free passage of water and solutes of low molecular weight while restraining formed elements and macromolecules. The glomerular capillary wall functions as a barrier to the filtration of macromolecules based on their size, shape, and charge characteristics. The glomerular filtrate is modified during passage through the tubules by the active and passive transport of certain solutes into and out of the luminal fluid and the permeability characteristics of specific nephron segments. The transport systems in renal epithelial cells serve to maintain global water, salt, and acid-base homeostasis rather than to regulate local cellular processes, such as volume and metabolic substrate uptake, that occur in nonrenal epithelial cells.

An adequate volume of glomerular filtrate is essential for the kidney to regulate water and solute balance effectively. Blood flow to the kidneys accounts for 20% to 30% of cardiac output. Of the total renal plasma flow, 92% passes through the functioning excretory tissue and is known as the effective renal plasma flow. The glomerular filtration rate (GFR) is usually about one fifth of the effective renal plasma flow, giving a filtration fraction of about 0.2.

The rate of ultrafiltration across the glomerular capillaries is determined by the same forces that allow the transmural movement of fluid in other capillary networks.[3] These forces are the transcapillary hydraulic and osmotic pressure gradients and the characteristics of capillary wall permeability. A renal autoregulatory mechanism enables the kidney to maintain relative constancy of blood flow in the presence of changing systemic arterial and renal perfusion pressures.[1] This intrinsic renal autoregulatory mechanism appears to be mediated in individual nephrons by tubuloglomerular feedback involving the macula densa (a region in the early distal tubule that juxtaposes the glomerulus) and the afferent and efferent arterioles. A decrease in arteriolar resistance in the afferent arteriole, with maintenance of the resistance in the efferent arteriole, sustains glomerular hydraulic pressure despite a decrease in systemic and renal arterial pressures.

Under normal conditions, the reabsorption of water and the reabsorption and secretion of solute during passage of the glomerular filtrate through the nephron are subservient to the maintenance of body fluid, electrolytes, and acid-base homeostasis. In the healthy, nongrowing individual, the intake and the expenditure of water and solute are equal and the hydrogen-ion balance is zero. Renal function may be impaired by systemic or renal disease and by medications such as vasoactive drugs, nonsteroidal anti-inflammatory drugs, diuretics, and antibiotics. Hypoxia and renal hypoperfusion appear to be the events most commonly associated with postoperative renal dysfunction.

RENAL FUNCTION EVALUATION

The evaluation of kidney function begins with the history, physical examination, and laboratory studies. Persistent oliguria or significant impairment in renal concentrating capacity should be evident from the history. Examination of the urinary sediment may provide evidence of renal disease if proteinuria and/or cellular casts are present. Normal serum concentrations of sodium, potassium, chloride, total CO_2, calcium, and phosphorus indicate appropriate renal regulation of the concentration of electrolytes in body fluids. The serum creatinine concentration is the usual parameter for GFR. Important limitations and caveats must be observed when using creatinine to estimate GFR.

Urinary creatinine excretion reflects both filtered and secreted creatinine because creatinine is not only filtered by the glomerular capillaries but also secreted by renal tubular cells. As a consequence, creatinine clearance, which is calculated by using serum creatinine concentration and the urinary excretion of creatinine, overestimates true GFR measured by using inulin clearance by 10% to 40%.[4] Serum creatinine concentration and the rate of urinary creatinine excretion are affected by diet. The ingestion of meat, fish, or fowl, which are substances containing preformed creatinine and creatinine precursors, causes an increase in serum creatinine concentration and in urinary creatinine excretion.[5] The overestimation of GFR by creatinine clearance increases as kidney function deteriorates owing to the relative increase in the tubular component of urine creatinine.

During the past 10 years, the serum concentration of cystatin C, a nonglycosylated 13.3-kD basic protein, has been shown to correlate with GFR as well as or better than serum creatinine.[6-9] From about age 12 months and up until age 50 years, normal serum cystatin C concentrations are similar in children and adults (0.70 to 1.38 mg/L). Beginning at about age 50 years, serum cystatin C concentration increases, related to the decline in GFR associated with age. Serum cystatin C concentration is not affected by gender, inflammatory conditions, or diet. Accurate automated systems allow the measurement of cystatin C.[10] At this time, the measurement of cystatin C has not been incorporated into routine clinical practice. However, in the near future, it may become a new tool in the assessment of GFR.

Urine Volume

The appropriate urine volume in any situation depends on the status of body fluids, fluid intake, extrarenal losses, obligatory renal solute load, and renal concentrating and diluting capacity. Patients with impaired renal concentrating capacity require a larger minimal urinary volume for excretion of the obligatory renal solute load than do those with normal renal concentrating ability. Patients with elevated levels of antidiuretic hormone retain water out of proportion to solute and are prone to hyponatremia. Increased levels of antidiuretic hormone may occur because of physiologic factors such as hypertonicity of body fluids or decrease in the effective circulatory volume (as encountered with low levels of serum albumin or with generalized vasodilatation as in the sepsis syndrome).

Table 4-1 Usual Maintenance Water Requirements

Weight Range (kg)	Maintenance Water
2.5-10	100 mL/kg
10-20	1000 mL + 50 mL/kg > 10 kg
20	1500 mL + 20 mL/kg > 20 kg

Recently, some authors have expressed concern that "usual maintenance fluids" (Table 4-1), providing 2 to 3 mEq/L of sodium, potassium, and chloride per 100 calories metabolized, may contribute to the development of hyponatremia in children hospitalized with conditions likely to be associated with antidiuretic hormone excess.[11] The children at risk are those with nonosmotic stimuli for antidiuretic hormone release, such as central nervous system disorders, the postoperative state, pain, stress, nausea, and emesis. It has been proposed in patients prone to develop the syndrome of inappropriate secretion of antidiuretic hormone that isotonic 0.9% normal saline might be a better choice for maintenance fluid therapy.[12]

The urinary volume making the diagnosis of oliguric renal failure likely is based on an estimate of the minimal volume needed to excrete the obligatory renal solute load. The reference base for the calculation of urine volume is per 100 mL of maintenance water, not per kilogram of body weight.[13] The minimal urinary volume for excretion of the obligatory renal solute load is derived by using the following assumptions:

1. Approximately 30 mOsm of obligatory renal solute/100 mL of usual maintenance water is taken as the obligatory renal solute load in children aged 2 months and older.[13]
2. Urinary concentrating capacity increases rapidly during the first year of life and reaches the adult level of 1200 to 1400 mOsm/L at about the second year.[14,15] The maximum urinary concentrating capacity of the term infant from 1 week to 2 months of age is about 800 mOsm/L; from 2 months to 3 years, about 1000 mOsm/L; and beyond that age, about 1200 mOsm/L. Table 4-2 provides an estimate of the minimal urinary volumes that permit excretion of the obligatory renal solute load, assuming an appropriate physiologic response to renal hypoperfusion. The minimal urinary volumes have been calculated by dividing the expected obligatory renal solute load by the

Table 4-2 Minimal Urinary Volumes for Excretion of Obligatory Renal Solute

	Assumptions		Urinary Volume	
Age	*Renal Solute Load (mOsm/100 cal)*	*Maximum Urine Concentration (mOsm/kg)*	*Urine (mL) per 100 mL (per 24 hr)*	*Maintenance Water (per hr)*
1 wk to 2 mo	25 (?)	800	31.3	1.3
2 mo to 2 yr	30 (?)	1000	25.0	1.0
2 yr	30	1200	20.8	1.0

maximal urinary concentrating capacity. Significantly lower urinary volumes are present among patients with oliguric acute renal failure (ARF). Noteworthy is the recent re-characterization of ARF as acute kidney injury (AKI) to better describe the renal dysfunction that has occurred.[16,17]

3. The presence of oliguric renal failure, based on urine volume, can be diagnosed only in the hydrated patient who has adequate blood pressure for renal perfusion and has no urinary tract obstruction. Oliguric AKI is probably not present in a newborn as old as 2 months with a urinary volume equal to or greater than 1.3 mL/hr/100 mL maintenance water or in an older patient with a urinary volume equal to or greater than 1.0 mL/hr/100 mL of maintenance water. Urine output less than these levels requires further evaluation for oliguric AKI.
4. Nonoliguric AKI occurs about as frequently as oliguric AKI. It is diagnosed when an adequately hydrated patient with normal blood pressure and urine volume has elevated serum creatinine and urea nitrogen concentrations. Some of the infants and children with nonoliguric AKI also have decreased serum bicarbonate and calcium concentrations and increased serum potassium and phosphorus concentrations.

Glomerular Filtration Rate

GFR is the most useful index of renal function because it reflects the volume of plasma ultrafiltrate presented to the renal tubules. Decline in GFR is the principal functional abnormality in both acute and chronic renal failure. Assessment of GFR is important not only for evaluating the patient with respect to kidney function but also for guiding the administration of antibiotics and other drugs. Inulin clearance, which is the accepted standard for measurement of GFR, is too time consuming and inconvenient to be used in the clinical evaluation of most patients. Serum urea nitrogen concentration shows so much variation with dietary intake of nitrogen-containing foods that it is not a satisfactory index of GFR. Serum creatinine concentration and creatinine clearance have become the usual clinical measures for estimation of GFR. However, precautions should be taken when creatinine alone is used for estimation of GFR because of the effect of diet as well as common medications on serum creatinine concentration and excretion rate. Ingestion of a meal containing a large quantity of animal protein increases serum creatinine levels about 0.25 mg/dL in 2 hours and increases creatinine excretion rate about 75% over the next 3- to 4-hour period.[5] Serum creatinine concentrations are increased by ingestion of commonly used medications such as salicylate and trimethoprim.[18,19] These agents compete with creatinine for tubular secretion through a base-secreting pathway. They do not alter GFR but do elevate the serum creatinine concentration.

Because of the difficulties in timed urine collection, several equations have been developed to estimate GFR. The most commonly used is the one developed by Schwartz[20] and is based on serum creatinine value and the child's height:

$$\text{GFR (mL/min/1.73m}^2\text{)} = \\ k \times \text{Ht (cm)/serum creatinine (mg/dL)}$$

where k for low birth weight infants is 0.33, full-term infants, 0.45; males 2 to 12 and females 2 to 21 years old, 0.55; and males 13 to 21 years old, 0.70.

However, k value changes with creatinine analysis methodology (see later). Improvement in the precision of this formula can be achieved by formulas containing additional endogenous markers such as urea and cystatin C.[20]

Creatinine is formed by the nonenzymatic dehydration of muscle creatine, at a rate of 50 mg creatinine/kg muscle.[4] The serum creatinine concentration in the neonate reflects the maternal level for the first 3 to 4 days of life and somewhat longer in the premature infant. After this time, the serum creatinine concentration should decrease. From age 2 weeks to 2 years, the value averages about 0.4 ± 0.04 mg/dL (35 ± 3.5 μM).[21] The serum creatinine concentration is relatively constant during this period of growth because the increase in endogenous creatinine production, which is directly correlated with muscle mass, is matched by the increase in GFR. During the first 2 years of life, GFR increases from 35 to 45 mL/min/1.73 m^2 to the normal adult range of 90 to 170 mL/min/1.73 m^2. The normal range for serum creatinine concentration increases from 2 years through puberty, although the GFR remains essentially constant when expressed per unit of surface area. This occurs because growth during childhood is associated with increased muscle mass and, therefore, increased creatinine production, which is greater than the increased GFR per unit of body weight.[21] Table 4-3 shows the mean values and ranges for plasma or serum creatinine levels at different ages.[22] Normative data of serum creatinine may differ from one laboratory to another, based in large part on whether the Jaffe kinetic method or the enzymatic method is used for the creatinine determination, because the latter method provides lower values.[23] At present, most laboratories provide their normative range for age concomitantly with the reported result.

Fractional Excretion of Substances

Fractional excretions are indexes of renal function that are helpful in evaluating specific clinical conditions. Conceptually, a fractional excretion is the fraction of the filtered substance that is excreted in the urine. Fractional excretions are calculated by using creatinine clearance to estimate GFR and the serum and urine concentrations of the substance studied.

Fractional Excretion of Sodium (FENa)

The normal FENa is usually less than 1% but may be elevated with high salt intake, adaptation to chronic renal failure, and diuretic administration.[24] When a decrease in renal perfusion pressure occurs, which is

Table 4-3 Plasma Creatinine Levels at Different Ages

Age	Height (cm)	True Plasma Creatinine* (mg/dL)	
		Mean	Range (±2 SD)
Fetal cord blood		0.75	0.15-0.99
0-2 wk	50	0.50	0.34-0.66
2-26 wk	60	0.39	0.23-0.55
26 wk-1 yr	70	0.32	0.18-0.46
2 yr	87	0.32	0.20-0.44
4 yr	101	0.37	0.25-0.49
6 yr	114	0.43	0.27-0.59
8 yr	126	0.48	0.31-0.65
10 yr	137	0.52	0.34-0.70
12 yr	147	0.59	0.41-0.78
Adult male	174	0.97	0.72-1.22
Adult female	163	0.77	0.53-1.01

*Conversion factor: mmol/L = mg/dL × 88.4
Adapted from Changler C, Barratt TM: Laboratory evaluation. In Holiday MA (ed): Pediatric Nephrology, 2nd ed. Baltimore, Williams & Wilkins, 1987, pp 282-299.

common in intravascular volume depletion or congestive heart failure, the normal renal response results in a marked increase in the tubular resorption of sodium and water and in the excretion of a small volume of concentrated urine containing a small amount of sodium. This physiologic response to decreased renal perfusion is an FENa less than 1%. The FENa is usually greater than 2% in ischemic AKI (also known as acute tubular necrosis), reflecting the impaired ability of the tubules to reabsorb sodium.

When using FENa to aid in differentiating prerenal azotemia from AKI, it is essential that no recent diuretic therapy has been given. Another caveat is in the patient with a decrease in renal perfusion superimposed on chronic renal failure, in which case the tubules will not be able to preserve sodium in spite of the dehydration. However, with fluid and electrolyte replenishment, kidney function will improve to some extent. The FENa, as well as the other diagnostic indices used to help differentiate prerenal azotemia from ischemic AKI, are not pathognomonic for either disorder. Furthermore, the FENa is often less than 1% in cases of acute kidney injury due to a glomerular disease, in which tubular function remains intact. However, FENa provides helpful information when integrated into the overall clinical evaluation.

Fractional Excretion of Bicarbonate (FEHCO_3^-)

Renal tubular acidosis (RTA) describes a group of disorders in which metabolic acidosis occurs as a result of an impairment in the reclamation of filtered HCO_3^- or as a result of a defect in the renal hydrogen ion excretion, in the absence of a significant reduction in GFR.[25] RTA is considered in the differential diagnosis of the patient with metabolic acidosis, a normal serum anion gap (hyperchloremic metabolic acidosis), and a urinary pH above 6.0. However, a patient with proximal RTA, due to the decreased reclamation of filtered HCO_3^-, may have a urinary pH below 6.0 when the plasma HCO_3^- concentration is below the lowered renal threshold for HCO_3^- reabsorption. Another exception, with respect to the presence of an elevated urinary pH in RTA, occurs in type IV RTA, a form of distal RTA in which the normal serum anion gap metabolic acidosis is associated with hyperkalemia. Also, under certain conditions, these patients might be able to lower their urine pH (see later).

Besides several genetic disorders such as cystinosis, proximal tubular damage is often seen in children receiving chemotherapy. The diagnosis of a defect in proximal tubular reabsorption of HCO_3^- is made by showing that the FEHCO_3^- is greater than 15% when the plasma HCO_3^- concentration is normalized by sufficient alkalinization. This results in flooding of the distal nephron with HCO_3^-, so the urine becomes highly alkaline. The FEHCO_3^- is calculated just as is the FENa, but with serum and urine HCO_3^- substituted for sodium. A normal individual ingesting a usual diet reabsorbs all the filtered HCO_3^-, and the FEHCO_3^- is zero. A urinary pH of 6.2 or less indicates that urinary HCO_3^- excretion is negligible.

Urinary P_{CO_2} or Urine Minus Blood P_{CO_2}

Classic distal RTA is caused by a defect in the secretion of H^+ by the cells of the distal nephron. It is characterized by hyperchloremic metabolic acidosis, urine with a pH greater than 6.0 at normal as well as at low serum HCO_3^- concentrations, and an FEHCO_3^- less than 5% when serum HCO_3^- is normal.[25,26] Normally, the cells of the distal nephron secrete H^+ into the lumen where, in the presence of filtered HCO_3^-, carbonic acid (H_2CO_3) is formed. Slow dehydration of the H_2CO_3

into $CO_2 + H_2O$ in the medullary collecting ducts, renal pelvis, and urinary bladder results in urinary PCO_2 greater than 80 mm Hg or urine minus blood (U-B) PCO_2 greater than 30 mm Hg. Urinary PCO_2 is evaluated after administering a single dose of sodium bicarbonate ($NaHCO_3^-$) (2 to 3 mEq/kg) or acetazolamide (17 ± 2 mg/kg) to flood the distal nephron with HCO_3^-.[27] Rather than acetazolamide, $NaHCO_3^-$ should be used in a patient with significantly reduced serum HCO_3^- levels at the time of the test. Urinary PCO_2 should be measured only after urinary pH exceeds 7.4 or urinary HCO_3^- concentration exceeds 40 mEq/L or both. A defect in distal nephron secretion of H^+ is diagnosed if U-B PCO_2 is less than 20 mm Hg or urine PCO_2 is below 60 mm Hg.

As noted earlier, type IV RTA, a form of distal RTA associated with low urinary pH (<6.0) and hyperkalemia, is a result of decreased H^+ and K^+ secretion in the distal tubule and is related to a failure to reabsorb sodium.[25,26] Type IV RTA is probably the most commonly recognized type of RTA in both adults and children. The hyperkalemia inhibits ammonia synthesis, resulting in decreased ammonia to serve as a urinary buffer. Therefore, a low urinary pH occurs despite decreased H^+ secretion ($NH_3 + H^+ = NH_4^+$). Type IV RTA is physiologically equivalent to aldosterone deficiency, which is one cause of the disorder. In children, it may reflect true hypoaldosteronism but it is much more common as a consequence of renal parenchymal damage, especially that due to obstructive uropathy. In pediatric patients, the physiologic impairment of type IV RTA resolves in a few weeks to months after relief of an obstructive disorder.[2,8]

MEDICAL ASPECTS OF MANAGING THE CHILD WITH POSTOPERATIVE IMPAIRMENT OF RENAL FUNCTION

Pathophysiology of Acute Kidney Injury

Acute kidney injury is characterized by an abrupt decrease in kidney function. Because AKI is caused by a decrease in the GFR, the initial clinical manifestations are elevations in serum urea nitrogen and creatinine concentrations and, frequently, reduction in urine output. Among pediatric surgical patients, an impairment in kidney function is most common in those who are undergoing cardiopulmonary procedures.[29,30] In recent years, research has focused on the identification of biomarkers that indicate imminent kidney failure, even before a rise in serum creatinine is noted.[31]

The most important factor in the pathogenesis of postoperative kidney failure is decreased renal perfusion. In the early phase, the reduction in renal blood flow results in a decline in GFR. Intact tubular function results in enhanced resorption of sodium and water. This clinical condition is recognized as prerenal azotemia. Analysis of the patient's urine reveals a high urinary osmolality of greater than 350 mOsm/kg H_2O and a urine sodium concentration less than 10 mEq/L (20 mEq/L in the neonate).[32] The most useful index of the tubular response to renal hypoperfusion with intact tubular function is FENa. The FENa test is invalid if the patient received diuretics before giving the urine sample. When kidney function is intact in the hypoperfused state, FENa is less than 1% in term infants and children and below 2.5% in premature infants.[33] In most patients with prerenal azotemia, intravascular volume depletion is clinically evident. However, in patients with diminished cardiac output (pump failure), clinical appreciation of reduced renal perfusion can be obscured because body weight and central venous pressure may suggest fluid overload. Similarly, assessment of volume status is difficult in patients with burns, edema, ascites, anasarca, or hypoalbuminemia. The reduced effective intra-arterial volume might be evident from the reduced systemic blood pressure, tachycardia, and prolonged capillary refill time.

Prerenal azotemia can be alleviated by improving renal perfusion either by repleting the intravascular fluid volume or by improving the cardiac output. The improved kidney function is recognized by increased urine output and normalization of serum urea nitrogen and creatinine concentrations. However, if renal hypoperfusion persists for a significant period or if other nephrotoxic factors are present, parenchymal kidney failure can result. Factors that may predispose the patient to AKI include preexisting congenital urinary anomalies or impaired kidney functions, septicemia, hypoxemia, hemolysis, rhabdomyolysis, hyperuricemia, drug toxicity, and use of radiocontrast agents. On rare occasions, abdominal compartmental syndrome causing tense ascites may impair renal perfusion. In that setting, kidney failure may be alleviated by abdominal decompression.[34]

Medical Management

The child with postoperative oliguria and an elevated serum creatinine concentration should be assessed for possible prerenal azotemia. If the child is found to be hypovolemic, an intravenous fluid challenge of 20 mL/kg of isotonic saline or plasma is commonly infused. In most instances, however, it may be physiologically advantageous to provide a solution in which bicarbonate accounts for 25 to 40 mEq/L of the anions in the fluid bolus (0.5 isotonic NaCl in 5% glucose, to which is added 25 to 40 mEq/L of 1 M $NaHCO_3$ and additional NaCl or $NaHCO_3$ to bring the solution to isotonicity). If no response is observed and the child is still dehydrated, the dose can be repeated. When the urine output is satisfactory after fluid replenishment, the child should receive appropriate maintenance and replacement fluids and should be monitored. Body weight, urinary volume, and serum concentrations of urea nitrogen, creatinine, and electrolytes also should be monitored.

If urinary output is inadequate after the fluid challenge, an intravenous infusion of furosemide, 1 mg/kg, may be given in a bolus. Patients with kidney failure may require higher doses, up to 5 mg/kg. If no response occurs after the initial infusion of furosemide, a second, higher dose can be repeated after 1 hour. Some patients may require furosemide every 4 to 8 hours to maintain satisfactory urinary volume. A protocol with constant furosemide infusion has been successfully used in oliguric children after cardiac surgery.[35] Furosemide is infused at 0.1 mg/kg/hr, with the dose increased by 0.1 mg after 2 hours if the urinary volume remains less than 1 mL/kg/hr. The maximum dose is 0.4 mg/kg/hr. At times, urine output can be increased by the use of vasoactive agents such as dopamine. However, their efficacy in otherwise altering the course of AKI is not well established.[36-39] It is of utmost importance to maintain adequate blood pressure and effective renal plasma flow.

Careful monitoring of the patient's fluid and electrolyte status is essential. Those children who fail to respond to furosemide are at risk for fluid overload. Overzealous fluid administration during anesthesia and surgery and for the management of persistent hypoperfusion, along with decreased urinary output, can result in hypervolemia, hypertension, heart failure, and pulmonary edema. In extreme cases, fluid administration must be decreased to the minimum necessary to deliver essential medications. In less severe instances, and in euvolemic patients with impaired kidney function, total fluid intake should equal insensible water loss, urine volume, and any significant extrarenal fluid losses. Urine output must be monitored hourly, and fluid management must be re-evaluated every 4 to 12 hours, as clinically indicated. Valuable information about the patient's overall fluid status can be obtained by carefully monitoring blood pressure, pulse, and body weight. The preoperative values of these parameters help serve as a baseline for postoperative evaluation. Ideally, the patient's hemodynamic status should be assessed continuously by using central venous pressure monitoring. In patients with complicated cardiac problems, a Swan-Ganz catheter that monitors pulmonary wedge pressure should be used.

Fluid overload can lead to hyponatremia. In most cases, because total body sodium remains normal or high, the best way to normalize serum sodium concentration is by restriction of fluid intake and enhancement of urinary volume.[40] In patients with acute symptomatic hyponatremia, careful infusion of NaCl 3% solution (512 mEq Na/L or 0.5 mEq/mL) may be given to correct hyponatremia. Rapid correction at a rate of 1 to 2 mEq/hr over a 2- to 3-hour period, with an increase of serum sodium level by 4 to 6 mEq/L, is usually well tolerated and adequate. Infusion of 6 mL/kg of 3% NaCl increases serum sodium concentration by about 5 mEq/L. Hyponatremia present for more than 24 to 48 hours should not be corrected at a rate more rapid than 0.5 mEq/L/hr.

In children with AKI, hyperkalemia often develops. The early sign of potassium cardiotoxicity is peaked T waves on the electrocardiogram. Higher levels of serum potassium can cause ventricular fibrillation and cardiac asystole. The treatment of hyperkalemia is shown in Table 4-4. Emergency treatment of hyperkalemia is indicated when the serum potassium concentration reaches 7.0 mEq/L or when electrocardiographic changes are noted.

Table 4-4 Treatment of Hyperkalemia

Cardiac Protection
Calcium gluconate, 10%, 0.5-1.0 mL/kg body weight injected intravenously and slowly over 5-10 min, with continuous monitoring of heart rate
Shift of Potassium into the Intracellular Compartment
Sodium bicarbonate, 1-2 mEq/kg body weight intravenously over 10-20 min, provided that salt and water overload is not a problem
Glucose, 1g/kg body weight, and insulin, 1 unit per every 4 g of glucose, intravenously over 20-30 min
Stimulants of β_2-adrenergic receptors, such as salbutamol, intravenously or by inhalation
Elimination of Excess Potassium
Furosemide 1mg/kg, or higher in the face of decreased GFR
Cation exchange resin, sodium polystyrene sulfonate, 1 g/kg body weight, administered orally or rectally in 20% to 30% sorbitol or 10% glucose, 1 g resin/4 mL. Additional 70% sorbitol syrup may be given if constipation occurs
Dialysis

In children with AKI, metabolic acidosis rapidly develops. Owing to decreased kidney function, fewer hydrogen ions are excreted. Organic acids accumulate in the body, causing a reduction in the serum HCO_3^- concentration. Although a child with uncompromised ventilatory capacity is able to hyperventilate and achieve partial compensation, a child with compromised pulmonary function or a hypercatabolic state is at risk for profound acidosis. Metabolic acidosis is usually treated by administering $NaHCO_3^-$. However, attention should be directed toward the excess sodium load associated with this mode of therapy. Because hypocalcemia develops in many patients with AKI, treatment with alkali should be done with care to protect them from hypocalcemic tetany due to a shift of ionized calcium from free to albumin bound. It is not necessary to correct the metabolic acidosis completely to prevent the untoward effects of acidemia. Increasing the serum HCO_3^- concentration to 15 mEq/L is usually satisfactory.[41]

Dialysis

The inability to control medically the fluid and electrolyte or acid-base disorders caused by renal failure necessitates the initiation of dialysis therapy. The indications for urgent dialysis are persistent oligoanuria, hyperkalemia, metabolic acidosis, fluid overload, severe electrolyte and mineral disturbances, and uremic syndrome.

The most common indication for postoperative dialysis in a child is hypervolemia caused by repeated attempts at fluid resuscitation, administration of medications, and total parenteral nutrition.[42] Repeated intravenous catheter flushes and endotracheal tube

Table 4-5 Characteristics of Dialysis Modalities

Variable	CRRT	PD	HD
Continuous therapy	Yes	Yes	No
Hemodynamic stability	Yes	Yes	No
Fluid balance achieved	Yes, pump controlled	Yes/no, variable	Yes, intermittent
Easy to perform	No	Yes	No
Metabolic control	Yes	Yes	Yes, intermittent
Optimal nutrition	Yes	No	No
Continuous toxin removal	Yes	No/yes, depends on the nature of the toxin—larger molecules not well cleared	No
Anticoagulation	Yes, requires continuous anticoagulation	No, anticoagulation not required	Yes/no, intermittent anticoagulation
Rapid poison removal	Yes/no, depending on patient size and dose	No	Yes
Stable intracranial pressure	Yes	Yes/no, less predictable than CRRT	Yes/no, less predictable than CRRT
ICU nursing support	Yes, high level of support	Yes/no, moderate level of support (if frequent, manual cycling can be labor intensive)	No, low level of support
Dialysis nursing support	Yes/no, institution dependent	Yes/no, institution dependent	Yes
Patient mobility	No	Yes, if intermittent PD used	No†
Cost	High	Low/moderate. Increases with increased dialysis fluid used	High/moderate
Vascular access required	Yes	No	Yes
Recent abdominal surgery*	Yes	No	Yes
Ventriculoperitoneal shunt	Yes	Yes/no, relative contraindication	Yes
Prune belly syndrome	Yes	Yes/no, relative contraindication	Yes
Ultrafiltration control	Yes	Yes/no, variable	Yes, intermittent
PD catheter leakage	No	Yes	No
Infection potential	Yes	Yes	Yes
Use in acute kidney injury–associated inborn errors of metabolism	Yes	No	Yes
Use in acute kidney injury–associated ingestions	Yes	No	Yes

*Omphalocele, gastroschisis, frequent or extensive abdominal surgery.
†Varies, depending on the location of the hemodialysis catheter.
CRRT, continuous renal replacement therapy; PD, peritoneal dialysis; HD, hemodialysis.

lavages can add a significant amount of water and solute to the total intake. Fluid overload in the postoperative patient can cause pulmonary edema and hypertension.

Dialysis Therapy

The three modes of dialysis therapy include hemodialysis (HD), peritoneal dialysis (PD), and continuous renal replacement therapy (CRRT). Although PD has historically been used most often in children, more recent data have revealed an increased use of CRRT in those centers where the expertise and resources are available.[42,43] Recognition of the needs of the patient, the resources of the treating facility, and the advantages and disadvantages of each dialytic technique dictate which modality is best (Table 4-5).[42]

The intrinsic factors that affect the efficacy of PD include peritoneal blood flow, peritoneal vascular permeability, and peritoneal surface area.[44] Although removal of up to 50% of the peritoneal surface area does not seem to interfere with dialysis efficacy,[45] hypoperfusion of the peritoneal membrane vasculature renders dialysis ineffective.[46] PD is feasible in the postoperative patient even in the presence of peritonitis or immediately after major abdominal procedures.[47-49] However, it is contraindicated in the presence of a diaphragmatic defect. Increased intra-abdominal pressure caused by the intraperitoneal administration of dialysis fluid can cause respiratory embarrassment and contribute to fluid leakage from the sites of surgical incisions and the entrance of the peritoneal catheter. Under such circumstances, the smallest effective dialysis fluid volume is used. It can be gradually increased over time. Common complications associated with PD are peritonitis, exit-site infection, dialysate leakage, catheter obstruction from omentum or fibrin, and abdominal wall hernia. The provision of antibiotics at the time of catheter placement may decrease the risk of peritonitis.[50] The use of fibrin glue at the site of catheter entry into the peritoneum has been associated with a decreased incidence of dialysate leakage during the immediate postoperative period.[51] A rare complication is abdominal organ perforation, seen most commonly with the use of stiff dialysis catheters.[52] A study in 2000 showed placement of a Tenckhoff catheter to be superior to use of the stiffer Cook catheter (Cook Medical, Bloomington, IN) in terms of complication-free survival.[53] More recently, there is evidence for equal outcomes with the Cook Multipurpose Drainage catheter, a flexible catheter that is placed at the bedside, in contrast to the Tenckhoff catheter, which typically requires surgical placement.[54]

PD is performed with dialysis solutions that contain a 1.5%, 2.5%, or 4.25% glucose concentration. Dialysate with a 1.5% glucose concentration has an osmolality of 350 mOsm/kg H_2O, which is moderately hypertonic to normal plasma (280 to 295 mOsm/kg H_2O). With increased glucose concentration, the tonicity of the solution increases, reaching 490 mOsm/kg H_2O with 4.25% glucose, the highest concentration commercially available. Other factors being equal, the higher the tonicity of the dialysate, the greater the ultrafiltrate (fluid removed from the body). Owing to the rapid movement of water and glucose across the peritoneal membrane, the effect of PD on fluid removal is maximal when short dialysis cycles of 20 to 30 minutes are used. When solutions containing glucose concentrations higher than 1.5% are used, close monitoring of the patient's serum glucose concentration is necessary. If hyperglycemia with a blood glucose concentration of greater than 200 mg/dL develops, it can be controlled by the addition of insulin to the dialysate solution or by intravenous insulin drip. The volume of fluid removed by dialysis in a 24-hour period should generally be limited to 500 mL in the neonate, ranges from 500 to 1000 mL in infants and 1000 to 1500 mL in young children, and should be limited to 3000 mL in children weighing more than 30 kg.[55] The effect of dialysis on the removal of solutes depends mainly on the length of the dwell time of the dialysate within the peritoneal cavity and the molecular weight of the solute. The following are the relative rates of diffusion of common substances: urea > potassium > sodium > creatinine > phosphate > uric acid > calcium > magnesium. Standard dialysate solutions do not contain potassium.[56] Therefore, hyperkalemia may be controlled with a few hours of effective PD.

Hemodialysis has the advantage of more rapid ultrafiltration and solute removal than either PD or CRRT. It is technically more difficult to perform than PD and thus requires particular expertise of the personnel conducting the procedure. Adequate vascular access is the most important requirement, and a variety of temporary pediatric catheters are available.[57] Ideally, placement of the dialysis catheter in the subclavian vein should be discouraged because of the potential development of subclavian stenosis and the subsequent inability to create a dialysis fistula in the ipsilateral arm of those patients who go on to develop end-stage renal disease. The intermittent nature of HD requires that fluid restriction be instituted in the patient who is anuric to help prevent the development of hypervolemia. Fluid removal can also be problematic in the patient who is hypotensive and receiving HD because of poor patient tolerance and is better accomplished by either PD or CRRT in this clinical setting.

The types of CRRT consist of continuous venovenous hemodialysis (CVVHD), continuous venovenous hemofiltration (CVVH), and continuous venovenous hemodiafiltration (CVVHDF). Although the complexity and cost of CRRT precludes its potential for global utilization, it is now widely practiced in many tertiary pediatric centers because of the safety and efficacy of the procedure in even the sickest patients. The choice of one method of CRRT over another depends on whether one chooses to make use of the diffusive (CVVHD) or convective (CVVH) method or a combination of the two (CVVHDF) properties of the technique. As in HD, a well-functioning vascular access is crucial to the performance of CRRT. Recent data suggest that the optimal access is the one with the largest diameter, preferably located within the internal jugular vein.[58] Likewise, large extracorporeal blood volumes are necessary for the CRRT (and HD) circuit and require the use of blood products in the small patient in whom the circuit volume exceeds 10% of the patient's blood volume. Particular attention must be paid to the possible development of hemofilter-related reactions that might occur with the initiation of therapy.[59,60] The predictability and efficiency of ultrafiltration and solute removal make CRRT an ideal dialytic technique for hemodynamically unstable patients. The capability of removing fluid in a well-controlled, continuous manner also makes adequate nutritional delivery possible. In children at risk for hemorrhage, a protocol using citrate instead of heparin as the anticoagulant has been developed.[61,62] Finally, although it is well recognized that the institution of dialysis is indicated for the control of solute and fluid removal, new information has provided direction regarding the preferred timing of dialysis initiation. Fluid overload itself appears to be a significant risk factor for mortality, and its early and aggressive management with dialysis may prove particularly beneficial.[63]

ACUTE KIDNEY INJURY IN THE NEONATE

Acute kidney injury occurs in as many as 24% of all patients admitted to the neonatal intensive care unit.[39,64,65] The definition of AKI in a term neonate is most often considered to be a serum creatinine level above 1.5 mg/dL for more than 24 hours in the setting of normal maternal renal function.[66] On occasion, it may be diagnosed in the term infant with a serum creatinine value less than 1.5 mg/dL when it fails to decrease in a normal manner over the initial days/weeks of life.[67-69] The limited availability of cystatin C data from the neonatal population currently precludes its routine use to define AKI.[70,71]

AKI is of the oliguric variety when the elevated serum creatinine concentration is accompanied by a urine output below 1 mL/kg/hr after the initial 24 hours of life and when urine output fails to improve in response to a fluid challenge.[68,72] In contrast, in some neonates, solute retention develops, as evidenced by an elevated serum creatinine level, with a normal (>1.0 mL/kg/hr) urine flow rate. These neonates are diagnosed as having nonoliguric AKI.[73] The nonoliguric form is particularly common in neonates with AKI secondary to perinatal asphyxia and appears to be associated with a better prognosis than does the oliguric form.[69,73] The diagnosis of nonoliguric AKI can be missed if patients at risk for developing renal insufficiency are monitored solely by the evaluation of urine output without repeated assessments of the serum creatinine concentration.

The causes of AKI traditionally have been divided into three categories: prerenal, intrinsic, and postrenal (Table 4-6). This division, based on the site of the lesion, has important implications because the evaluation, treatment, and prognosis of the three groups can be quite different.

Prerenal Acute Kidney Injury

Impairment of renal perfusion is the cause of 70% of AKI during the neonatal period.[39,64,65,67-69] Prerenal AKI may occur in any patient with hypoperfusion of an otherwise normal kidney. Although prompt correction of the low perfusion state usually reverses kidney function impairment, delay in fluid resuscitation may result in renal parenchymal damage.

Intrinsic Acute Kidney Injury

Intrinsic AKI occurs in 6% to 8% of admissions to the neonatal intensive care unit and implies the presence of renal cellular damage associated with impaired kidney function.[67] Intrinsic AKI usually falls into one of the following categories: ischemic (acute tubular necrosis), nephrotoxic (aminoglycoside antibiotics, indomethacin), congenital renal anomalies (autosomal recessive polycystic kidney disease), and vascular lesions (renal artery or vein thrombosis, especially with a solitary kidney).[74]

Postrenal Acute Kidney Injury

Postrenal AKI results from obstruction of urine flow from both kidneys or from a solitary kidney. The most common causes of postrenal AKI in neonates are posterior urethral valves, bilateral ureteropelvic junction obstruction, and bilateral ureterovesical junction obstruction.[75,76] Although these types of obstructions are characteristically reversible, neonates with long-standing intrauterine obstruction have varying degrees of permanent impairment of renal function.[77,78] This impairment may be due not only to the presence of renal dysplasia but also to cellular damage secondary to AKI.

Clinical Presentation

Clinical presentation of the neonate with AKI often reflects the condition that has precipitated development of the renal insufficiency. Accordingly, sepsis, shock, dehydration, severe respiratory distress syndrome, and other related conditions may be present. Nonspecific symptoms related to uremia, such as poor feeding, lethargy, emesis, seizures, hypertension, and anemia, also are frequently present.

Table 4-6 Major Causes of Acute Renal Failure in the Newborn

Prerenal Failure

- Systemic hypovolemia: fetal hemorrhage, neonatal hemorrhage, septic shock, necrotizing enterocolitis, dehydration
- Renal hypoperfusion: perinatal asphyxia, congestive heart failure, cardiac surgery, cardiopulmonary bypass/extracorporeal membrane oxygenation, respiratory distress syndrome, pharmacologic (tolazoline, captopril, enalapril, indomethacin)

Intrinsic Renal Failure

- Acute tubular necrosis
- Congenital malformations: bilateral agenesis, renal dysplasia, polycystic kidney disease
- Infection: congenital (syphilis, toxoplasmosis), pyelonephritis
- Renal vascular: renal artery thrombosis, renal venous thrombosis, disseminated intravascular coagulation
- Nephrotoxins: aminoglycosides, indomethacin, amphotericin B, contrast media, captopril, enalapril, vancomycin
- Intrarenal obstruction: uric acid nephropathy, myoglobinuria, hemoglobinuria

Postrenal (Obstructive) Renal Failure

- Congenital malformations: imperforate prepuce, urethral stricture, posterior urethral valves, urethral diverticulum, primary vesicoureteral reflux, ureterocele, megacystis megaureter, Eagle-Barrett syndrome, ureteropelvic junction obstruction, ureterovesical obstruction
- Extrinsic compression: sacrococcygeal teratoma, hematocolpos
- Intrinsic obstruction: renal calculi, fungus balls
- Neurogenic bladder

Adapted from Karlowicz MG, Adelman RD: Acute renal failure in the neonate. Clin Perinatol 19:139-158, 1992.

Diagnostic Evaluation

Evaluation of the neonate with AKI should include a thorough patient and family history and a physical examination. Suspected prerenal causes of acute oliguria are usually addressed diagnostically and therapeutically by volume expansion, with or without furosemide. If this approach does not result in increased urine output, a more extensive evaluation of kidney function is indicated.

Laboratory studies are an important component of the evaluation and should include the following measures: complete blood cell count and determination of serum concentrations of urea nitrogen, creatinine, electrolytes, uric acid, calcium, glucose, and phosphorus. The serum creatinine value during the first several days of life is a reflection of the maternal value. In term infants, a value of 0.4 to 0.5 mg/dL is expected after the first week of life. In contrast, the expected value in preterm infants is related to their gestational age, with an initial increase followed by a gradual decrease.[79,80] In all cases, a urinalysis should be obtained to check for the presence of red blood cells, protein, and casts suggestive of intrinsic renal disease.

Urine indices can help distinguish intrinsic renal failure from prerenal azotemia in the oliguric patient.[36-38] As mentioned previously, the index usually found to be most useful is the FENa. This factor is based on the assumption that the renal tubules of the poorly perfused kidney reabsorb sodium avidly, whereas the kidney with intrinsic renal disease and tubular damage is unable to do so. Accordingly, in most cases of neonatal oliguric renal failure secondary to intrinsic disease, the FENa is greater than 2.5% to 3.0%, a value that is different from that of the older child.[39,65,72,81] The FENa should be measured before administering furosemide. In addition, the results should be interpreted with caution in the very premature infant who normally has an even higher (i.e., > 5%) FENa.[66,81,82]

Ultrasonography commonly is the initial imaging study performed.[83] The urinary tract should be evaluated for the presence of one or two kidneys and for their size, shape, and location. Dilation of the collecting system and the size and appearance of the urinary bladder should be evident. A voiding cystourethrogram (VCUG) may also be necessary, specifically when the diagnosis of posterior urethral valves or vesicoureteral reflux is entertained. In most cases, a VCUG is deemed preferable to radionuclide cystography in this setting because of its superior ability to provide reliable anatomic information about the grading of vesicoureteral reflux or the appearance of the urethra.[84] Antegrade pyelography or diuretic renography with either ^{99m}Tc-dimercaptosuccinic acid (DMSA) or ^{99m}Tc-mercaptoacetyltriglycine (MAG_3) as the radiopharmaceutical agent may be needed to evaluate for ureteral obstruction. Finally, radiologic assessment of the differential kidney function may be performed with radioisotope scanning as well.

Management

The treatment of neonatal AKI should proceed simultaneously with the diagnostic workup. Bladder catheter placement is a good immediate therapy for posterior urethral valves, whereas high surgical drainage may be needed for other obstructive lesions in the neonate. The fluid challenge for the neonate should consist of 20 mL/kg of an isotonic solution containing 25 mEq/L of $NaHCO_3^-$ infused over a 1- to 2-hour period. In the absence of a prompt diuresis of 2 mL or more of urine per kilogram during 1 to 2 hours, intravenous furosemide at 1 to 3 mg/kg may be helpful. As noted previously, the potential role of low-dose (0.5 to 3.0 µg/kg/min) dopamine continues to be debated.[37,38] The failure to achieve increased urinary output after volume expansion in the neonate with an adequate cardiac output (i.e., renal perfusion) and an unobstructed urinary tract indicates the presence of intrinsic kidney disease and the need to manage oliguric or anuric kidney failure appropriately.

Maintenance of normal fluid balance is of primary concern in the management of the patient with AKI. Daily fluid intake should equal insensible water loss, urine output, and fluid losses from nonrenal sources. In term infants, insensible water losses amount to 30 to 40 mL/kg/day, whereas premature infants may require as much as 50 to 100 mL/kg/day.[82,85] A frequent assessment of the neonate's body weight is essential for fluid management. The electrolyte content of the fluids administered should be guided by frequent laboratory studies. Insensible water losses are electrolyte free and should be replaced by using 5% dextrose in water.

Important systemic disturbances that may arise secondary to AKI include hyperkalemia, hyponatremia, hypertension, hypocalcemia, hyperphosphatemia, and metabolic acidosis. All exogenous sources of potassium should be discontinued in patients with AKI. Despite this restriction, elevated serum potassium levels develop in many neonates and must be treated aggressively owing to the potential for cardiac toxicity.[33,68] Treatment should be initiated by correction of metabolic acidosis with $NaHCO_3^-$. One to 2 mEq/kg should be given intravenously over a 10- to 20-minute period, provided that salt and water balance is not problematic. The quantity of $NaHCO_3^-$ to be prescribed also can be calculated in the following manner: (0.3 × body weight [kg] × base deficit [mM]).[68] Associated hypocalcemia should be treated with the intravenous administration of 10% calcium gluconate at a dose of 0.5 to 1.0 mL/kg injected slowly over a 5- to 15-minute period with continuous monitoring of the heart rate. If a progressive increase in the serum potassium concentration is noted, additional treatment measures may include the use of a sodium-potassium exchange resin (sodium polystyrene sulfonate in 20% to 30% sorbitol, 1 g/kg by enema), with recognition of its frequent ineffectiveness and/or associated complications when used in low birth weight infants.[86] The use of glucose (0.5 to 1.0 g/kg) followed by insulin (0.1 to 0.2 unit regular insulin per gram glucose over a 1-hour period) may be the preferred approach. Either intravenous salbutamol or inhaled albuterol is an additional therapeutic option.[87-89] Dialysis should be considered if these measures prove unsuccessful.[89]

Hyponatremia and systemic hypertension are most often related to overhydration in the infant with oliguria. These problems should be treated initially with fluid restriction or water removal with dialysis, if necessary. The addition of high-dose intravenous furosemide (5 mg/kg) may be beneficial. Serum sodium levels below 125 mEq/L can be associated with seizures, and levels below 120 mEq/L should be corrected rapidly to at least 125 mEq/L by calculating the amount of sodium required in the following manner:

$$Na^+ \text{ (mEq)} = ([Na^+] \text{ Desired} - [Na^+] \text{ Actual}) \times \text{Weight (kg)} \times 0.8$$

When serum sodium levels are less than 120 mEq/L and are associated with symptoms (e.g., seizures), prompt treatment with hypertonic (3%) saline is indicated. The provision of 10 to 12 mL/kg of 3% saline is generally therapeutic.

The treatment of persistent hypertension may include parenterally administered hydralazine (0.1 to 0.6 mg/kg/dose), labetalol (0.20 to 1.0 mg/kg/dose or 0.4 to 3.0 mg/kg/hr infusion), or enalaprilat (5.0 to 10 μg/kg/dose). Orally administered amlodipine (0.06 to 0.6 mg/kg/day) can be prescribed for the patient who is without symptoms. Treatment of the patient with marked or refractory hypertension can include intravenous sodium nitroprusside (0.5 to 10 μg/kg/min infusion), nicardipine (0.5 to 3 μg/kg/min infusion), or labetalol.[90] Caution should be exercised when initiating therapy with captopril (initial oral dose, 0.01 to 0.05 mg/kg/dose), owing to the profound hypotension that can occur in neonates in association with higher doses.[68,91,92]

In the infant in whom AKI does not fully resolve and becomes chronic renal failure, hyperphosphatemia (serum phosphorus level > 7 mg/dL) necessitates the use of a low phosphorus infant formula and calcium carbonate (50 to 100 mg/kg/day) as a phosphate binder.[93] The use of aluminum hydroxide as a binder is contraindicated, owing to its association with aluminum toxicity in infants and children with renal insufficiency.[94] No experience has been published about the use of newer phosphate-binding agents, such as sevelamer, in the neonatal population.[95-97]

Hypocalcemia, as reflected by a low total serum calcium level, often occurs in AKI in association with hypoalbuminemia. Less commonly, the ionized calcium level is low and the patient is symptomatic. In these cases, intravenous 10% calcium gluconate, 0.5 to 1.0 mL/kg, over a 5-minute period with cardiac monitoring should be given until the ionized calcium level is restored to the normal range.[68] It is important to remember that permanent correction of a low serum calcium level can be achieved only by oral supplementation of calcium and active vitamin D metabolites.

Metabolic acidosis may arise as a result of retention of hydrogen ions and may require $NaHCO_3^-$ for correction. The dose of $NaHCO_3^-$ to be given can be calculated as follows:

$$NaHCO_3^- \text{ (mEq)} = (\text{Desired bicarbonate} - \text{Observed bicarbonate}) \times \text{Weight (kg)} \times 0.5$$

This dose may be given orally or added to parenteral fluids and infused during several hours.

Adequate nutrition should be provided, with the goal of 100 to 120 calories and 1 to 2 g of protein/kg/day, provided intravenously or orally. For neonates who can tolerate oral fluids, a formula containing low levels of phosphorus and aluminum, such as Similac PM 60/40 (Abbott Labs, Abbott Park, IL), is recommended. An aggressive approach to nutrition may well contribute to kidney recovery by providing necessary energy at the cellular level.[33]

Although most neonates with AKI can be managed conservatively, occasional patients require PD or CRRT for the treatment of the metabolic complications and fluid overload.[55,98-100] The mortality rate in this group of patients commonly exceeds 60%. Twenty-three patients who received PD at Children's Mercy Hospital during the neonatal period had a mortality rate of 35% at 1 year.[101] The somewhat lower mortality rate in our center probably reflects the improved outcome of neonates with renal structural abnormalities leading to AKI (17% mortality rate) compared with those infants with multisystem disease. In a report of 12 neonates in whom AKI developed after cardiac surgery and who received CVVH, 7 (59%) of the infants survived and no complications were noted related to the hemofiltration procedure.[102] In another report, on the use of CRRT in 85 children weighing less than 10 kg, 16 weighed less than 3 kg.[100] In these patients, the procedure was well tolerated, other than for the need of pressor support, with survival rates of 25% and 41% for those weighing less than 3 kg and from 3 to 10 kg, respectively. When CRRT is used with infants receiving extracorporeal membrane oxygenation, excessive hemolysis has been documented on occasion.[103]

OBSTRUCTIVE UROPATHY

Obstructive uropathy in the neonate is the most common renal abnormality diagnosed prenatally and is most often the result of ureteropelvic junction obstruction, posterior urethral valves, or ureterovesical junction obstruction.[75] Obstruction also represents a significant cause of end-stage renal disease in children, accounting for 13% of all cases, and is the underlying cause of end-stage renal disease in nearly 90% of affected boys younger than age 4 years.[104-106] Accordingly, early recognition and treatment of these lesions are desirable because of the adverse effects obstruction can have on kidney function.[40,41,77,78,107] Regardless, after surgical intervention and relief of obstruction, alterations of GFR, renal blood flow, and renal tubular function may occur.[78,107,108] Specifically, injury to the renal tubule may result in an impaired capacity to reabsorb sodium, to concentrate urine, and to secrete potassium and hydrogen, all of which may have profound clinical implications. The resorption of other solutes, such as magnesium, calcium, and phosphorus, may also be affected.[78,108]

The ability of the renal tubule to reabsorb salt and water after relief of the obstruction typically depends on whether the obstruction is unilateral or bilateral. In unilateral obstruction, the proximal tubules of the juxtamedullary nephrons are unable to reabsorb salt and water maximally, whereas the fractional reabsorption of salt and water is increased in the superficial nephrons.[108] However, the amount of sodium excreted by the previously obstructed kidney is not different from that of the contralateral kidney, because tubuloglomerular balance is maintained. In contrast, relief of bilateral obstruction or, on occasion, unilateral obstruction in neonates results in a postobstructive diuresis characterized by a marked elevation in the absolute amount of sodium and water lost.[109] In part, these changes are a result of an osmotic diuresis secondary to retained solutes, such as urea.[109,110] Some contribution may also occur from atrial natriuretic factor, the plasma level of which is elevated during obstruction, as well as from enhanced synthesis of prostaglandins.[108,111] Decreased renal medullary tonicity and decreased hydraulic water permeability of the collecting duct in response to antidiuretic hormone, the latter a result of reduced aquaporin channels, contribute to the impaired concentrating ability of the kidney.[35,107,112]

The clinical conditions associated with prolonged salt wasting are severe volume contraction and circulatory impairment. Conditions associated with the concentrating abnormalities are secondary nephrogenic diabetes insipidus and hypernatremic dehydration. Accordingly, management must ensure the provision of adequate amounts of fluid and salt. Sodium intake should be monitored by serum and urine electrolyte determinations. Fluid intake should equal insensible losses, urine output, and nonrenal losses and should be guided by frequent assessments of body weight.

Ureteral obstruction also can result in the impairment of hydrogen and potassium secretion and the syndrome of hyperkalemic, hyperchloremic metabolic acidosis, or type IV RTA.[113-115] This clinical situation appears to be the result of the impaired turnover of the sodium-potassium pump or a decreased responsiveness of the distal renal tubule to the actions of aldosterone. In a portion of the patients with this presentation, the FE_{Na} is normal and the FE_K is inappropriately low, relative to the elevated serum level. Treatment is directed toward correcting the underlying obstructive abnormality with surgery as well as providing $NaHCO_3^-$ to alleviate the metabolic acidosis and hyperkalemia.

Finally, the outcome of obstructive uropathy in the neonate in terms of preservation of GFR is, in part, related to how promptly surgical intervention and relief of obstruction take place. In these patients, the serum creatinine value obtained at age 12 months has been shown to be predictive of long-term kidney function.[40,41,78,107]

chapter 5

COAGULOPATHIES AND SICKLE CELL DISEASE

Kathleen A. Neville, MD, MS • Brian M. Wicklund, MD, CM, MPH • Gerald M. Woods, MD

The pediatric surgeon will encounter patients with various hematologic disorders, including children with hemophilia and sickle cell disease (SCD), who represent the largest populations that have been followed by hematologists for an extended period. We discuss these two conditions because of the unique surgical challenges that these patients provide to the pediatric surgeon, pediatric hematologist, and other physicians involved.

BIOCHEMISTRY AND PHYSIOLOGY OF HEMOSTASIS

The hemostatic system functions to arrest bleeding from injured blood vessels and to prevent the loss of blood from intact vessels. It also maintains a delicate balance that prevents unwanted clots from forming and dissolves blood clots that previously formed. This system, which is comprised of both thrombotic and thrombolytic proteins, platelets, and cells lining blood vessels, maintains hemostasis. Pathologic defects in this regulatory system result in either bleeding or thrombosis when too little or too much clot is formed or when dissolution of a clot is not properly regulated.

Obtaining a complete patient and family history is essential to effectively anticipate hemostatic disorders. Preoperative preparations can be made only if a good history is taken so that medications that interfere with coagulation or platelet function can be discontinued. Laboratory studies help identify and characterize the problems that are uncovered by the history. However, consideration and workup of potential genetic bleeding and platelet disorders largely depends on a meticulous bleeding history for both the patient and family members and on a detailed physical examination.

Three distinct structures are involved in the process of hemostasis: blood vessels, platelets, and circulating hemostatic proteins. Together, these components form the coagulation system, the naturally occurring anticoagulation system, and the fibrinolytic system. Coagulation must act rapidly to stop the loss of blood from an injured vessel, but the clot that is formed must remain localized so that it does not interfere with the passage of blood through the intact circulation. The anticoagulation system prevents the extension of the clot beyond the site of injury. The fibrinolytic system removes excess hemostatic material that has been released into the circulation and slowly lyses the clot once it is no longer needed.

The stimulus that initially causes clot formation occurs as a consequence of disruption of endothelial cells. This leads to exposure of collagen and subendothelial tissues. The hemostatic response to tissue injury consists of four stages. First, vasoconstriction by the contraction of smooth muscle in the injured vessel wall reduces blood flow. Second, platelets adhere to the exposed endothelium, aggregate, and release their granular contents. This activity stimulates further vasoconstriction and recruits more platelets. This action results in "primary hemostasis" that occludes the gap in the blood vessel and stops blood loss through the vessel. Third, the extrinsic and intrinsic coagulation systems are activated to form fibrin, which stabilizes the platelets and prevents disaggregation. Fourth, fibrinolysis results from the release of plasminogen activators from the injured vessel wall. These activators limit the coagulation process. Once healing has taken place, they begin dissolution of formed clot so that vascular patency can be restored.[1]

Endothelial Cells

Endothelial cells line the lumen of all blood vessels. They maintain the integrity of the blood vessel and prevent extravasation of blood into the surrounding tissue.[1] When the vessel is intact, it provides a thromboresistant surface that prevents the activation of the coagulation system. Passive thromboresistance is provided by endothelial proteoglycans, primarily endogenous heparin sulfate. Heparin is an anticoagulant compound that acts as a co-factor in converting antithrombin to a potent inhibitor of activated clotting factors. Active thromboresistance is achieved through several mechanisms, including the synthesis and release of prostacyclin (PGI_2), a potent vasodilator and an inhibitor of platelet adhesion and aggregation.[1,2]

When the endothelium is injured, tissue factor (thromboplastin) is produced and rapidly promotes local thrombin formation.[3] Tissue factor binds factor VII and converts it to factor VIIa (Fig. 5-1). The production of factor VIIa is the first step in activation of the extrinsic coagulation pathway, which begins the activation of the common pathway. It also activates factor IX, which is the major activator of the common pathway, resulting in the formation of fibrin.[4] The contribution that these processes make to the control of bleeding depends on the size of the interrupted vessel. Capillaries seal with little dependence on the hemostatic system, but arterioles and venules require the presence of platelets to form an occluding plug. In arteries and veins, hemostasis depends on both vascular contraction and clot formation around an occluding primary hemostatic plug.[5]

Platelets

In the resting state, platelets circulate as disk-shaped, anuclear cells that have been released from megakaryocytes in the bone marrow. They are 2 to 3 μm in size and remain in circulation for approximately 10 days unless they participate in coagulation reactions or are removed by the spleen. Normal blood contains 150,000 to 400,000 platelets per microliter.[5] In the resting state, platelets do not bind to intact endothelium.

Platelet Adhesion

Once platelets bind to injured tissue and are activated, their discoid shape changes. They spread on the subendothelial connective tissue and degranulate. Degranulation occurs when platelets internally contract and extrude storage granule contents into the open canalicular system. Dense granules release serotonin, adenosine diphosphate (ADP), calcium, and adenosine triphosphate (ATP). Alpha granules release factor V, fibrinogen, von Willebrand factor (FVIII:vWF), fibronectin, platelet factor 4, β-thromboglobulin, and platelet-derived growth factor.[6,7] Lysosomal vesicles also

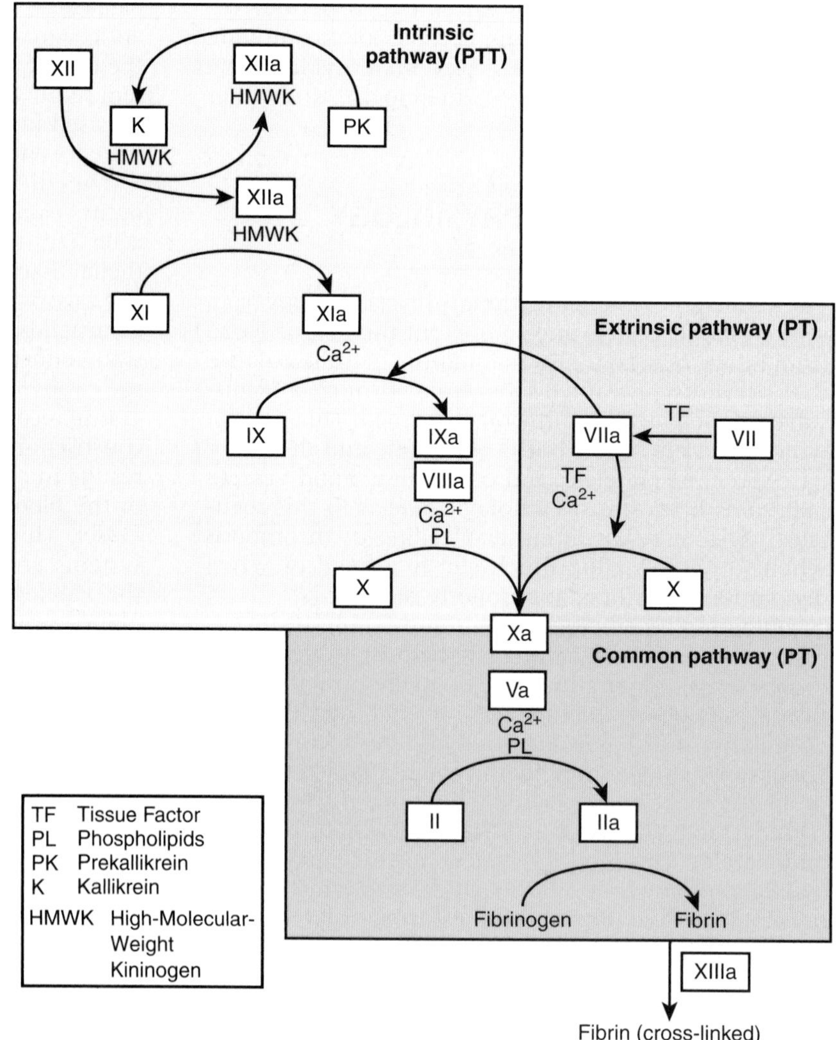

Figure 5-1. The coagulation cascade.

are present within platelets. The material released from the granules recruits and aggregates more platelets from the circulation onto the already adherent platelets.[7]

When a vessel is disrupted, platelet adhesion occurs through the binding of collagen and vWF (found in the subendothelium) to the platelet membrane. For platelet adhesion to occur, platelets must express specific glycoprotein Ib receptors on their surface to bind the vWF complex. If this specific glycoprotein is missing, platelets are unable to adhere to areas of injury.[8] Platelets in Bernard-Soulier syndrome lack glycoprotein Ib and are unable to adhere and form the initial hemostatic plug.[9] If the vWF is defective or deficient in amount, platelets do not adhere to sites of vascular injury. The result is von Willebrand's disease, of which several specific types and subtypes have been defined.[10-12] If an operation is performed on a patient with either Bernard-Soulier syndrome or von Willebrand's disease without the transfusion of normal amounts and types of platelets or vWF, respectively, serious bleeding can result because of the inability to form an initial hemostatic platelet plug. Very high concentrations of PGI_2 also can inhibit platelet adhesion to exposed subendothelium.[5]

After platelet adhesion has occurred, in addition to degranulation and an increased local concentration of ADP, small amounts of thrombin are formed, and platelet membrane phospholipase is activated to generate thromboxane A_2. Thromboxane A_2 and serotonin released from the dense granules stimulate vasoconstriction and induce the exposure of membrane receptors for fibrinogen (glycoproteins IIb/IIIa). Fibrinogen binding to stimulated platelets then induces aggregation.[7]

Platelet Aggregation

Aggregation is a complex reaction that involves platelet granule release, cleavage of membrane phospholipids by phospholipases A_2 and C, alterations in intracellular cyclic adenosine monophosphate (cAMP) levels, mobilization of intracellular calcium, and the expression of fibrinogen receptors on the platelet surface. If fibrinogen receptors (glycoproteins IIb and IIIa) or fibrinogen are missing, platelets do not aggregate.[13] Glanzmann's thrombasthenia is a deficiency of glycoproteins IIb and IIIa in which platelets adhere normally but do not aggregate. These patients have a serious, life-long bleeding disorder.[6]

After aggregation, platelets function to enhance thrombin formation. The platelet membrane provides specific binding sites for factors Xa and V. The result is an efficient site for the assembly of the prothrombinase complex, which converts prothrombin into thrombin.[7] Thrombin formation results in the formation of a stable hemostatic plug of adherent platelets surrounded by a network of fibrin strands.

Generation of Thrombin

Tissue injury induces activation of the plasma-based coagulation system, resulting in the generation of thrombin from prothrombin. Thrombin is the enzyme responsible for transforming liquid blood into a fibrin gel. The initial activation of factor VII by tissue factor results in the production of thrombin by the extrinsic system. Tissue factor is released after injury to the endothelial cells but is not expressed on the surface of the cells.

The majority of thrombin production results from the activation of the intrinsic coagulation system, not the extrinsic system. Exposed subendothelium converts factor XII to factor XIIa and thereby activates the intrinsic pathway, although it is interesting to note that deficits in factor XII do not cause a bleeding disorder. Activation of factors XI and IX follows, and activated factor IX in combination with factor VIII, calcium, and platelet phospholipid activates factor X. Activated factor VII, complexed with tissue factor, activates factor IX. Factor Xa with factor V then cleaves prothrombin into the active molecule thrombin, which can convert fibrinogen into fibrin.[4,14]

Formation of Fibrin

When thrombin acts on fibrinogen, fibrin monomers result after the proteolytic release of fibrinopeptides A and B. The monomeric fibrin then polymerizes into a gel.[4,14] With additional stabilization of the fibrin gel provided by factor XIII, fibrin surrounds and stabilizes the platelet plug. This process makes the multimeric fibrin more resistant to plasmin digestion and completes the formation and stabilization of the blood clot.[15]

Several regulatory proteins serve to localize thrombin formation to the surface of the blood vessel. Endothelial cells have receptors for protein C, an anticoagulant protein. Protein C from the plasma binds to these receptors. Protein S is a co-factor for the activation of protein C. Thrombomodulin is an endothelial surface protein that acts in combination with thrombin to activate the bound protein C. Activated protein C then degrades factors Va and VIIIa, which inhibit thrombin formation.[16]

Heparin-like anticoagulant molecules are present on endothelial cells. They act in combination with antithrombin III to inhibit factors XIIa, XIa, IXa, and Xa and thrombin. Inhibition of these factors prevents the spread of clot to uninjured adjacent vessels and the blockage of large vessels by excessive clot formation.[14,16] Endothelial cells, as mentioned previously, produce PGI_2, a potent vasodilator and inhibitor of platelet aggregation and adhesion.

Fibrinolysis

The regulatory process that dissolves fibrin and preserves vessel patency is called fibrinolysis. Circulating plasminogen is converted into plasmin by tissue plasminogen activators. These activators are released from the vessel walls at the site of blood clotting. They bind to the fibrin clot and convert plasminogen to plasmin. Plasmin enzymatically degrades fibrin, fibrinogen, and other plasma proteins, and this process results in the dissolution of formed clot.[14,16]

CLINICAL EVALUATION

Currently, no screening test to evaluate hemostasis is completely reliable in the preoperative evaluation of patients. A careful history, including a full family history, is still the best means of uncovering mild bleeding problems, including von Willebrand's disease or qualitative platelet abnormalities.[17] These disorders may easily escape standard laboratory screening procedures, such as prothrombin time (PT), activated partial thromboplastin time (aPTT), platelet count, and bleeding time. aPTT screening yields many false-positive results caused by both analytical problems and detection of clinically insignificant disorders. In addition, a normal aPTT may lead to a false sense of safety because it does not exclude all serious bleeding disorders. Therefore, it is imperative to identify patients at risk who need laboratory evaluation by obtaining a thorough history. Because no method can reliably predict all bleeding complications, postoperative monitoring remains mandatory for all patients.[18] Likewise, patients with mild disorders who have not previously undergone surgical procedures may have no history of bleeding problems and might be identified preoperatively only if screening tests are performed.[17] It is important to consider the history as the most important component of a diagnostic strategy and to investigate thoroughly any story of unusual bleeding, even if the screening tests are normal.[19] Conversely, studies examining the utility of a screening preoperative PT and aPTT in patients undergoing tonsillectomy and adenoidectomy concluded that routine screening with a PT and aPTT for all patients regardless of history cannot be recommended.[18,20] In obtaining a history from the patient and parents, positive answers to the questions posed in Table 5-1 indicate the need for further evaluation.[17,21-23]

If there is a history of abnormal bleeding, the following points must be established. The type of bleeding (i.e., petechiae, purpura, ecchymosis, and single or generalized bleeding sites) can give an indication of the underlying defect. Petechiae and purpura are most frequently associated with platelet abnormalities, either of function or of numbers. Von Willebrand's disease is most frequently associated with mucosal bleeding, including epistaxis, whereas hemophilia is most often associated with bleeding into joints or soft tissue ecchymosis, or both. Bleeding when the umbilical cord separates is most often associated with a deficiency in factor XIII, as is unexplained bleeding of the central nervous system.[15,24] A single bleeding site, such as repetitive epistaxis from the same nostril, is frequently indicative of a localized, anatomic problem and not a system-wide coagulation defect.

The course or pattern of the bleeding (i.e., spontaneous or after trauma) and its frequency, duration of problems, and severity can provide clues to whether a bleeding disorder is present. A family history of bleeding is important to define, and the pattern of inheritance (i.e., X-linked or autosomal; recessive or dominant) can help narrow the differential diagnosis (e.g., hemophilia A and B are X-linked recessive diseases, whereas von Willebrand's disease is autosomal dominant).

Table 5-1 Questions to Ask about Potential Bleeding Problems

1. Is there any history of easy bruising, bleeding problems, or an established bleeding disorder in the patient or any family members?
2. Has excessive bleeding occurred after any previous surgical procedure or dental work? Have the parents or any siblings had excessive bleeding after any surgical or dental procedures, specifically tonsillectomy or adenoidectomy?
3. Have frequent nosebleeds occurred, and has nasal packing or cautery been needed? Has bleeding without trauma occurred into any joint or muscle?
4. Does excessive bleeding or bruising occur after aspirin ingestion?
5. Does significant gingival bleeding occur after tooth brushing?
6. Has there been any significant postpartum hemorrhage?
7. Has the patient been taking any medication that might affect platelets or the coagulation system?
8. If the patient is male and was circumcised, were any problems noted with prolonged oozing after the circumcision?
9. If the patient is a child, do the parents remember any bleeding problems when the umbilical cord separated?
10. If the patient is menstruating, does she have profuse menstruation?
11. Has the patient ever received any transfusions of blood or blood products? If so, what was the reason for the transfusion?

Any previous or current drug therapy must be fully documented, and a search is made for any over-the-counter medications that the patient might be taking but does not consider "medicine" and has therefore not mentioned. Aspirin, ibuprofen, cough medications containing guaifenesin, and antihistamines can lead to platelet dysfunction or uncover a previously undiagnosed bleeding disorder such as von Willebrand's disease.[25,26] The presence of other medical problems including renal failure with uremia, hepatic failure, malignancies, gastrointestinal malabsorption, vascular malformations, cardiac anomalies with or without repair, and autoimmune disorders is essential to elicit because these may have associated coagulopathies.

The physical examination is used to help narrow the differential diagnosis and guide the laboratory investigation of hemostatic disorders. Certain physical findings may be associated with specific coagulation abnormalities, whereas others may be indicative of underlying systemic disease with an associated coagulopathy. Petechiae and purpuric bleeding occur with platelet and vascular abnormalities. Mucocutaneous bleeding suggests a platelet disorder and includes petechiae, ecchymoses, epistaxis, and genitourinary and gastrointestinal bleeding. Bleeding into potential spaces such as joints, fascial planes, and the retroperitoneum is instead suggestive of a coagulation factor deficiency. Bleeding from multiple sites in an ill patient can be seen with disseminated intravascular coagulation (DIC) or thrombotic thrombocytopenic purpura (TTP). Hemophilia patients often have palpable purpura and deep muscle bleeding that is painful but may be difficult to detect. Findings compatible with a collagen disorder include the body habitus of Marfan syndrome; blue sclerae; skeletal deformities; hyperextensible joints and skin; and nodular, spider-like, or pinpoint telangiectasia. Other signs may be indicative of systemic disease. For example, hepatosplenomegaly and lymphadenopathy may suggest an underlying malignancy, whereas jaundice and hepatomegaly may be indicative of hepatic dysfunction.

LABORATORY EVALUATION

When the bleeding history and/or family history suggest the possibility of a bleeding disorder, or if it is impossible to obtain a history due to family or social circumstances, it is customary to proceed with a series of laboratory investigations to look for a possible bleeding diagnosis. Generally, screening tests are performed first and can include a blood cell count, PT, and aPTT (Fig. 5-2).[19] Additional tests can be done to measure fibrinogen levels, assess the thrombin time, screen for inhibitors of specific coagulation factors, measure specific factor levels, and test for platelet function and von Willebrand's disease.[19,27] Patients also can be evaluated for evidence of DIC by using multiple assays to test for the presence of various fibrinopeptides and products from the breakdown of fibrin or fibrinogen.

Platelet Count

The platelet count measures the adequacy of platelet numbers to provide initial hemostasis. Thrombocytopenia (a platelet count of < 150,000/µL) is one of the most common problems that occur in hospitalized patients. As stated previously, typical manifestations include bruising, menorrhagia, and gastrointestinal or urinary tract bleeding. The risk of bleeding is inversely proportional to the platelet count. When the platelet count is less than 50,000/µL, minor bleeding occurs easily and the risk of major bleeding increases. Counts between 20,000 and 50,000/µL predispose to bleeding with trauma, even minor trauma; with counts less than 20,000/µL, spontaneous bleeding may occur; with counts less than 5,000/µL, severe spontaneous bleeding is more likely. However, patients with counts less than 10,000/µL may be asymptomatic for years.[28] Surgical bleeding does not usually occur until the platelet count is less than 50,000 platelets/µL.[29] A platelet count of less than 50,000/µL is considered a cutoff criterion for transfusions, and the prophylactic use of platelet transfusion is indicated for any invasive procedure. Patients with thrombocytopenia and significant bleeding should also receive transfusion of platelets.[29]

Bleeding Time and the PFA-100 Analyzer

The bleeding time is defined as the length of time required for a standardized incision to stop oozing blood that can be absorbed onto filter paper. A variety of procedures have been used, but all have variable sensitivity and have been difficult to reproduce accurately, leading many centers to drop the bleeding time from the list of approved laboratory tests.[30] The PFA-100 Analyzer (Siemans Healthcare Diagnostics, Deerfield, IL) is now widely used as a replacement for the

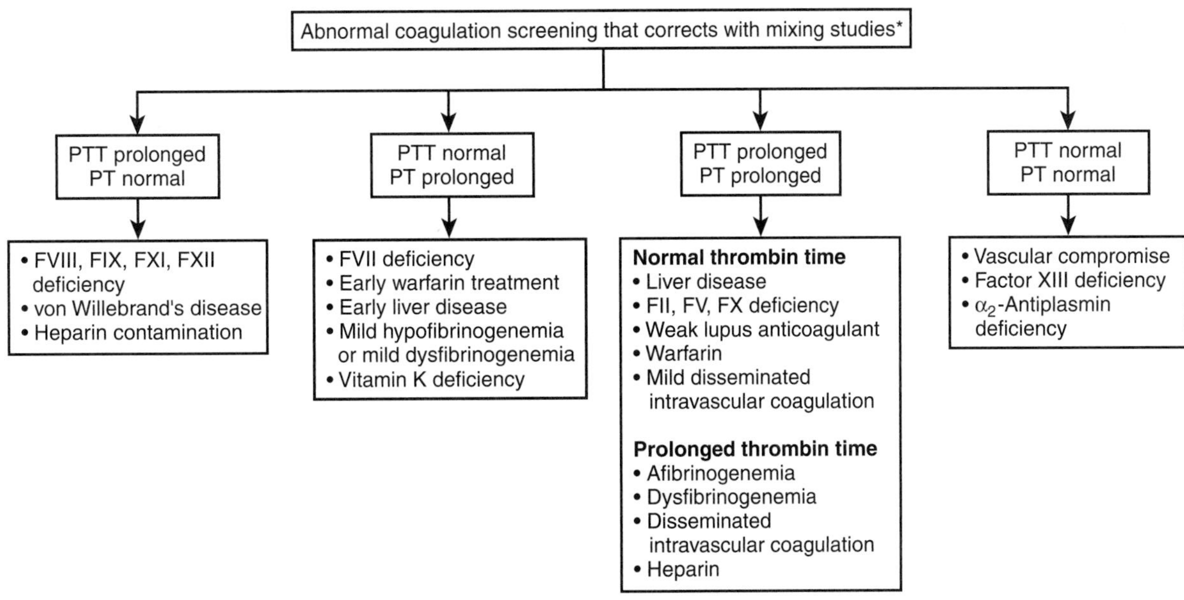

*Repeating an abnormal coagulation screening with a mixture of 1 part patient plasma and 1 part normal plasma ("mixing studies") will normalize the test if a factor deficiency is present, but the screening test will remain abnormal if an anticoagulant is present. These anticoagulants rarely are a cause of thromboembolic disease and even more rarely cause bleeding.

Figure 5-2. Screening tests for abnormal coagulation.

bleeding time. It creates an in-vitro high shear stress condition that results in the activation of platelet-dependent and vWF-dependent attachment and aggregation of platelets to a collagen-ADP or collagen-epinephrine surface. In most cases, the PFA-100 closure time is superior to the bleeding time in the detection of von Willebrand's disease, aspirin effect, or platelet dysfunction.[30] However, test results can be influenced by the sample's hematocrit. Although the PFA-100 does not detect all platelet dysfunctions or cases of von Willebrand's disease, when used in conjunction with a standardized questionnaire, it will likely detect impaired hemostasis in most cases.[30,31]

Prothrombin Time

The PT is a measure of the function of the extrinsic and common coagulation pathways. It represents the time (in seconds) for the patient's plasma to clot after the addition of calcium and thromboplastin (an activator of the extrinsic pathway).[32,33] Isolated prolongation of the PT is seen most commonly in patients who are deficient in vitamin K due to previous antibiotic treatment. It also occurs with factor VII deficiency, mild hypofibrinogenemia, dysfibrinogenemia, and warfarin treatment. The PT may also be prolonged when significant liver dysfunction occurs.[32,33]

Partial Thromboplastin Time

The aPTT measures the function of the intrinsic and common coagulation pathways. The aPTT represents the time (in seconds) for the patient's plasma to clot after the addition of phospholipid, calcium and an intrinsic pathway activator. The aPTT detects deficiencies in factors XII, XI, IX, and VIII and in the common pathway, but mild factor deficiencies may be missed. The aPTT also is used to monitor anticoagulation with heparin.[32,33]

Several inherited disorders of coagulation are not detected by the preceding tests. Results from standard hemostatic screening tests such as the aPTT and international normalized ratio (INR) assessments are normal in factor XIII (FXIII) deficiency. Therefore, assessment of clot stability is the most common screening test used for FXIII deficiency with a quantitative assay required to confirm the diagnosis of FXIII deficiency.[34] Von Willebrand's disease patients may have normal or prolonged aPTTs, and patients with a deficiency in α_2-antiplasmin have a normal aPTT. Both the PT and aPTT are prolonged in patients with deficiencies of factors X and V, prothrombin, and fibrinogen and in patients with DIC or severe liver disease.[32,33]

Fibrinogen

The standard method for fibrinogen determination measures clottable fibrinogen by using a kinetic assay. Normal levels of fibrinogen are 150 to 350 mg/dL. Because fibrinogen is the substrate for the final reaction in the formation of a clot, and all plasma-based screening tests depend on the formation of a clot as the end point of the reaction, fibrinogen levels below 80 mg/dL prolong the PT, aPTT, and thrombin time and therefore make the results uninterpretable. Large amounts of fibrin degradation products interfere with the formation of fibrin and cause an artificially low level of measured fibrinogen. Partially clotted samples also cause a low level of fibrinogen to be assayed. An immunologic-based assay for fibrinogen is used to measure both clottable and nonclottable fibrinogen. This test is most often used in identifying patients with a dysfibrinogenemia in whom the functional level of fibrinogen is low and the immunologic level is normal.[33,35]

Inhibitor Screening Tests

Repeating the PT or aPTT by using a 1:1 mix of patient plasma with normal plasma is a useful procedure for investigating a prolonged PT or aPTT. Normal plasma has, by definition, 100% levels of all factors. When mixed with an equal volume of patient plasma, a minimum of 50% of any given factor is present, which should normalize the PT or aPTT. Correction of the clotting time suggests the presence of a factor deficiency, whereas lack of normalization suggests the presence of an inhibitor that interferes with either thrombin or fibrin formation.[32,33]

Two types of acquired inhibitors prolong the aPTT. One blocks or inactivates one of the intrinsic factors, whereas the other is a lupus-like inhibitor that interferes with phospholipid-based clotting reactions. The first type of inhibitor occurs in 10% to 15% of hemophilia A patients and can occur spontaneously, but it is extremely rare in nonhemophiliac children.[36] The lupus-like inhibitor is associated not with bleeding problems but rather with an increased risk of thrombotic problems in adults. Lupus-like inhibitors are mentioned because they commonly cause prolongations of the aPTT.[37] Specific investigation of either of these situations should be referred to a coagulation reference laboratory.

Platelet Function Studies

Platelet function studies measure in-vitro platelet aggregation. In this procedure, platelet-rich plasma is incubated with an agonist and then changes in the amount of light transmitted through the platelet suspension are recorded. Agonists used to induce platelet aggregation include collagen, epinephrine, ADP, thrombin, and ristocetin. Three distinct phases are seen in the reaction. The first is an initial change in the shape of the platelets, leading to a temporary decrease in light transmission. Next is the first wave of aggregation, which is a reversible platelet-platelet interaction. With additional stimulation, the final phase—the second wave of aggregation—occurs and produces irreversible platelet aggregation. The second wave of aggregation is due to the release reaction of the platelet granules and thromboxane A_2 synthesis. The release reaction is extinguished by aspirin and is absent in patients with an inherited storage pool defect, congenital deficiency in thromboxane A_2 synthesis, or cyclooxygenase deficiency.[7] The PFA-100 has become the test of choice to replace the bleeding time and is used to screen for a variety of disorders, but full characterization of platelet function requires traditional platelet aggregation studies in a specialized laboratory.

Specific Factor Assays

Specific factor assays are available for all known coagulation, fibrinolysis, and anticoagulation factors to quantify their levels in plasma. These tests are not indicated unless a screening test result is abnormal. The only exception involves the patient with a history that is suggestive of von Willebrand's disease, factor XIII deficiency, or dysfibrinogenemia. In these cases, the aPTT may not be sensitive enough to detect the disorder. Further testing may be justified by clinical suspicion based on the patient's history.[32,33] For von Willebrand's disease, the workup consists of measuring factor VIII levels, vWF antigen levels, ristocetin co-factor activity, and ristocetin-induced platelet aggregation. Analysis of the distribution of vWF multimers can be useful to the hematologist in identifying the specific type of von Willebrand's disease.[10-12]

Tests for Disseminated Intravascular Coagulation

The tests that are available in most hospital laboratories for identification of DIC are semiquantitative fibrin or fibrinogen degradation product assays, which involve a slide agglutination procedure or a D-dimer assay. An increased amount of these degradation products suggests that either plasmin has circulated to lyse fibrin and fibrinogen or the patient's hepatic function is insufficient to clear the small amounts of regularly produced degradation products. The D-dimer test is a slide agglutination procedure that tests for the presence of two D subunits of fibrin that are cross-linked by factor XIII. This test provides specific evidence that plasmin has digested fibrin clot and not fibrinogen. It is positive in patients with DIC, in patients with resolving large intravascular clots, and in patients with hepatic insufficiency. Specific assays to demonstrate the presence of soluble fibrin monomer complexes or fibrinopeptides produced by the conversion of prothrombin to thrombin also are useful in some situations and available in specialized laboratories.[33,38]

HEMOPHILIA A AND B

Hemophilia A and B are X-linked recessive bleeding disorders caused by decreased levels of functional procoagulant factors VIII and IX, respectively. Approximately 80% of all hemophilia patients have factor VIII deficiency, which is classic hemophilia. The remaining 20% have factor IX deficiency, which is called Christmas disease. These are rare disorders, with a prevalence of only 13.4/100,000 males.[39] Until 1964, the treatment of hemophilia was limited by volume restrictions imposed by the use of whole blood or fresh frozen plasma. At that time, the factor VIII–rich fraction of fresh frozen plasma called cryoprecipitate was discovered.[40] Specific lyophilized factor VIII concentrates have since been developed, as have prothrombin-complex concentrates containing factors II, VII, IX, and X. Also, concentrates containing only factor IX for the treatment of hemophilia B patients and factor VIII/vWF concentrates for the treatment of von Willebrand's disease have been developed.[41,42] The lyophilized factor concentrates have allowed storage of the clotting factor using standard refrigeration and have permitted the outpatient treatment of bleeding episodes plus the development of home self-infusion programs.[43] This treatment, combined with the development of comprehensive hemophilia treatment centers, has produced a remarkable change in the outlook for these patients who previously developed significant joint deformities in their teens to 20s and were frequently wheelchair bound in adult life. Home therapy has decreased the damage caused by hemarthroses, with hemophiliac children born since the mid 1970s having far fewer joint deformities than do older hemophiliacs. These factor concentrates have allowed surgical procedures to be performed with much less risk, even to the point that orthopedic procedures can be readily accomplished.[44] Moreover, the comprehensive hemophilia treatment system has shown a 40% reduction in mortality for hemophilia patients.[45]

Viral infections transmitted by cryoprecipitate and factor concentrates were the major problem faced by hemophilia patients in the late 1970s to mid 1980s. Approximately 60% of all hemophilia patients became human immunodeficiency virus (HIV) positive in the 1980s, but there have not been any HIV infections from clotting factor concentrates since 1987.[46] Hepatitis C is the other major viral infection that was transmitted by plasma-derived factor concentrates used to treat hemophilia. Estimates from the mid 1980s are that more than 90% of multiply transfused hemophiliacs were positive for non-A, non-B hepatitis and that more than 95% had been infected with hepatitis B.[47] A different study shows that 75% of HIV-negative hemophiliacs, treated with earlier plasma-derived factor concentrates, have evidence of hepatitis C infection.[48] Again, no documented cases of hepatitis C transmission by clotting factor concentrates after 1987 are known.[46] Since 1993, recombinant produced factor VIII concentrates have been available. At present, only recombinant factor VIII and IX concentrates are used for the treatment of patients with newly diagnosed hemophilia A and B.[49]

Hemophilia patients are classified into three categories based on their level of circulating procoagulant. Those with factor levels below 1% are severe hemophiliacs, have a high risk of bleeding, and usually require replacement therapy two to four times per month.[39,50] Bleeding occurs in areas subject to minor trauma. Hemarthroses, hematomas, and ecchymoses are common. Recurrent hemarthroses can cause pseudotumors of the bone, whereas hematomas can cause compression damage to tissue or nerves and even ischemic compartment syndromes. Bleeding episodes in severe hemophiliacs can be irregularly spaced, with periods of recurrent hemarthrosis requiring frequent replacement doses of factor concentrate, interspersed with periods during which little or no concentrate is used.[39] In moderate hemophiliacs, who have procoagulant levels of 1% to 5%, spontaneous hemorrhage occurs infrequently but relatively minor trauma can cause bleeding into joints or soft tissues.

Mild hemophiliacs, with levels greater than 5%, rarely have bleeding problems and typically have problems only with major trauma or surgical procedures.[36,39] Some mild hemophilias may not be diagnosed until late childhood or adulthood. Therefore, a history may not be present to alert the pediatric surgeon to the risk of bleeding. Moreover, because one third of all cases of hemophilia are caused by new mutations, there may not be a family history to arouse suspicion of a bleeding problem.[36] Preoperative laboratory testing may provide the only point at which mild hemophilia is diagnosed.

The indications for surgical intervention in hemophiliacs are the same as those for patients with a normal clotting system, but they most frequently center on areas of damage secondary to bleeding episodes. In 1985, the results of a review of 350 consecutive operations performed at the Orthopedic Hospital in Los Angeles were published.[51] Because the study represented patients from before the start of home therapy and comprehensive care, the group was expected to have significant orthopedic problems secondary to multiple hemarthroses. Of the 350 procedures reviewed, 312 were characterized as serious and 38 of lesser intensity; 318 operations were on hemophiliacs with moderate and severe hemophilia and 30 on patients with mild hemophilia. As expected, musculoskeletal procedures made up two thirds of all operations on moderate and severe hemophiliacs and half of all operations on mild hemophiliacs. One death occurred in a child with a massive intracranial hemorrhage who did not survive an emergency craniotomy.[51] Bleeding problems during operation were not observed, but 23% of all serious operations were complicated by postoperative hemorrhages. Only operations on the knee had significantly more postoperative hemorrhages (40%). Operations on other joints and soft tissue areas had similar rates of complications (15%). Most of the postoperative hemorrhages occurred with plasma factor levels greater than 30%, which is the minimum level that is considered hemostatic. The authors also noted that the incidence of postoperative hemorrhage decreased after postoperative day 11, although other studies have found that vigorous physical therapy may cause postoperative hemorrhage and have therefore recommended the continuation of factor replacement throughout the period of physical therapy.[51,52]

The management of the hemophilic patient requires close cooperation among surgeons, hematologists, and personnel in the hemophilia center, the coagulation laboratory, and the pharmacy or blood bank. Careful preoperative planning is essential to the success of the procedure, and an adequate supply of clotting factor concentrate must be available to cover the patient's needs before the patient is admitted. The patient also must be screened for the presence of an inhibitor to either factor VIII or IX during the 2 to 4 weeks before the operation. If an inhibitor is present, management of the patient becomes much more complex and depends on the strength of the inhibitor. A low-titer inhibitor may be overcome with increased doses of human clotting factor, but high-titer inhibitors may require the use of activated prothrombin complex concentrate (FEIBA) or recombinant activated factor VII (NovoSeven) to "bypass" the effect of the antibody against either factor VIII or IX. These patients have been desensitized with daily doses of human factor concentrate over a period of months to years, restoring their response to regular infusions of factor VIII or IX.[44,53,54]

At our institution, the hemophilia patient is seen in the hematology clinic on the morning of the scheduled operation. After a bolus dose of factor (usually 50 units/kg of factor VIII in hemophilia A patients), a continuous infusion of 4 to 8 units/kg/hr of factor VIII (for the hemophilia A patient) is started to maintain a factor level greater than 80% for the next 1 to 2 days.[55] The factor level is checked immediately before the operation and is the final screen for the presence of an inhibitor. The infusion is maintained throughout the procedure and is then reduced on the second or third postoperative day to allow the plasma levels to decrease to 50%. Replacement is continued for a full 10 to 14 days after the operation. Daily measurement of factor levels is necessary to ensure maintenance of appropriate levels. For neurosurgical or orthopedic procedures, much longer periods of factor coverage–even 4 to 6 weeks–are needed, especially if significant physical therapy is planned.[39,44]

Many hemophiliacs do their own factor infusions at home and are supported by home care pharmacies. With the advent of home nursing services, patients are being discharged home with prolonged periods of factor coverage. Hemophilia center personnel must be closely involved in the planning of these discharges to ensure that sufficient clotting factor is available at home and that close follow-up is maintained during periods of scheduled home therapy. Hemophilia patients should not receive any compounds that contain aspirin or ibuprofen. Any minor procedures that would require factor correction should be combined with the major procedure, if possible, to save on the use of factor concentrate.

Previously, the hemophilia B patient undergoing a surgical procedure had specific problems because of the thrombogenic risk inherent in the use of older factor IX concentrates. Since the advent of newer, more purified factor IX concentrates, surgical procedures in hemophilia B patients have been performed without excess thrombotic problems. Now, with high purity plasma-derived and recombinant-produced factor IX concentrates, there are no excess thrombosis risks.[56,57]

CLOTTING FACTOR DOSING

Factor VIII is dosed differently from factor IX, based on their half-lives. Factor VIII has an 8- to 12-hour half-life, and the infusion of 1 unit of factor per kilogram of body weight increases the plasma level by 2%. If a severe hemophilia A patient weighs 50 kg, an infusion of 25 units/kg, or 1250 units, of factor VIII will raise his factor level to 50%. Factor IX has a half-life of 24 hours and must be infused in larger amounts than factor VIII to raise the plasma level. Infusion of 1 unit/kg of factor IX will raise the plasma level only by 1%. Continuous infusion of highly purified factor IX, as well as factor VIII, has been shown to prevent excessive peaks and troughs of factor levels, is simpler to manage, and decreases the cost by decreasing the overall amount of factor used. It has not shown to cause any problems with excess thrombosis.[58] Recombinant factor IX has a marked variability in dose response to infusions, and individual recovery studies may be needed before it is used for surgical hemostasis. Often, a 20% increase in dose is needed to give the same factor levels as obtained by use of plasma-derived factor IX.[59]

NEONATAL HEMOSTASIS

The newborn's coagulation system is not fully mature until 6 months after birth. The lower levels of procoagulant, fibrinolytic, and anticoagulant proteins in neonatal patients complicate both surgical procedures and the care of sick and preterm infants. Platelet counts are within the usual adult normal ranges of 150,000 to 450,000/mL in healthy term and preterm infants. These platelets have a lower function than those of adults, but they function properly in hemostasis and produce a normal bleeding time.[59] Circulating coagulation factors do not cross the placenta, and infants with inherited deficiencies of clotting factors, fibrinolytic proteins, or natural anticoagulants may initially be seen in the neonatal period. Levels of fibrinogen, factor V, factor VIII, and vWF are within the adult normal range at birth.[60] All other procoagulants are at reduced levels, depending on gestational age. Vitamin K–dependent factors may become further depressed in infants who are breast fed and not given vitamin K at birth.[59]

Of more concern are the low levels of anticoagulant and fibrinolytic proteins. Very low levels of protein C have been associated with purpura fulminans in newborns. In sick infants, levels of antithrombin III and plasminogen may be inadequate to deal with increased levels of clot-promoting activity in the blood. Sick infants with indwelling catheters are at significant risk of thrombotic complications.[61]

DISSEMINATED INTRAVASCULAR COAGULATION

DIC is the inappropriate activation of both thrombin and fibrin. It may follow sepsis, hypotension, hypoxemia, trauma, malignancy, burns, and extracorporeal circulation. Hemorrhage due to the depletion of clotting factors as well as thrombosis due to the excess formation of clot are seen, and the end-organ damage caused by ischemia and impairment of blood flow causes irreversible disease and death.[62]

Acute DIC is associated with the consumption of factors II, V, VIII, X, and XIII, as well as fibrinogen, antithrombin III, plasminogen, and platelets. Review of the peripheral smear usually shows a microangiopathic hemolytic anemia. The PT and aPTT may both be prolonged, and the fibrinogen level may be initially elevated as an acute-phase reactant but ultimately decreases as the DIC worsens. The presence of D-dimers indicates the circulation of plasmin digesting formed fibrin and may indicate the presence of DIC, but it may also be elevated due to thrombus or hepatic dysfunction. Antithrombin III levels may be low, and the use of antithrombin III concentrates in septic shock may play a role in the future treatment of DIC. However, adult studies have not shown any improvement in mortality for patients with septicemia treated with antithrombin III.[63] At present, the major therapy for DIC is correction of the underlying disorder, with fresh frozen plasma and platelet transfusions as indicated to support hemostasis. Low-dose heparin infusions have been used to stop the ongoing consumption of clotting factors before starting replacement therapy but have not been shown to appreciably improve the outcome.[62,64]

MANAGEMENT OF QUANTITATIVE AND QUALITATIVE PLATELET DISORDERS

Thrombocytopenias are caused by either inadequate production of platelets by the bone marrow or by increased destruction or sequestration of the platelets in the circulation. The history and physical examination may be suggestive of a diagnosis that can be confirmed by laboratory testing. Medication use, a family history of blood disorders, a history of recent viral infection, short stature, absent thumbs or radii, or a congenital malformation may indicate a defect in platelet production. The destruction may be immunologic, as in immune thrombocytopenic purpura; mechanical, as in septicemia; or drug induced, as in patients with sensitivity to heparin or cimetidine. Establishing the cause of the thrombocytopenia determines the therapy needed to restore the platelet count in preparing the patient for operation. A bone marrow aspirate or biopsy, or both, can establish the number and morphology of the megakaryocytes and also rule out malignancy. The clinical response to therapeutic modalities, such as a platelet transfusion, also can be an important test and can help direct further investigations to define the diagnosis. In patients with immune-based platelet consumptions such as immune thrombocytopenic purpura, usually no response is found to platelet transfusion. Moreover, only a very short response may be seen in patients with other causes of increased consumption. Management of the patient is then aimed at reducing the consumption and should involve consultation with a hematologist about the use of corticosteroids, the use of intravenous immunoglobulin or anti-D immunoglobulin (WinRho), the discontinuation of medications, and other treatment modalities.[65]

If the thrombocytopenia is caused by a lack of production of platelets, due to either aplastic anemia, malignancy, or chemotherapy, transfusion with platelet concentrate to increase the platelet count above a minimum of 50,000/µL will allow minor surgical procedures to be performed safely. Most surgeons and anesthesiologists prefer for the platelet count to be greater than 100,000/µL before undertaking major surgery. Continued monitoring of platelet counts is vital because further transfusions may be needed to keep the platelet count above 50,000/µL for 3 to 5 days after operations.[66]

Qualitative platelet defects can be caused by rare congenital defects such as Bernard-Soulier syndrome, Glanzmann's thrombasthenia, or platelet storage pool disease. Alternatively, they can be caused by drug ingestions such as an aspirin-induced cyclooxygenase deficiency. In these situations, transfusion of normal donor platelets provides adequate hemostasis for the surgical procedure. Discontinuation of all aspirin-containing products 1 week before operation permits correction of the cyclooxygenase deficiency as new platelets are produced.[6,67]

DISORDERS OF THROMBIN GENERATION AND FIBRIN FORMATION

Patients with rare deficiencies of other clotting factors, such as factors XI, X, VII, V, prothrombin, and fibrinogen, can have clinical bleeding depending on the level of deficiency. Most of these disorders are inherited in an autosomal recessive manner and can therefore affect both male and female patients. Replacement therapy with fresh frozen plasma or, in certain situations, with prothrombin complex concentrates corrects the deficiency and should be conducted under the direction of a hematologist.[44,68]

Vitamin K deficiency, both in the neonatal period and due to malabsorption, can cause deficiencies of factors II, VII, IX, and X. Treatment with 1 to 2 mg of intravenous vitamin K may begin to correct the deficiencies within 4 to 6 hours. However, if a surgical procedure is contemplated, fresh frozen plasma (15 mL/kg) should be given with the vitamin K, and prothrombin times monitored for correction of the coagulopathy before the operation. Laboratory monitoring should be maintained during the postoperative period to ensure continuation of the appropriate factor levels. Repeated doses of fresh frozen plasma and vitamin K may be needed.[5]

Patients with factor XIII deficiency usually are initially seen with delayed bleeding from the umbilical cord, rebleeding from wounds that have stopped bleeding, intracranial hemorrhage, and poor wound healing. These problems may be treated with relatively small amounts of fresh frozen plasma (5 to 10 mL/kg). Because factor XIII has a half-life of 6 days, this treatment is usually needed only once to stop bleeding or at the time of operation.[15,44] Patients with dysfibrinogenemia or afibrinogenemia may be treated with fresh frozen plasma or cryoprecipitate.[44]

FIBRINOLYTIC AND THROMBOTIC DISORDERS

Failure to control excess fibrinolysis can result in a bleeding disorder, and deficiencies of the naturally occurring anticoagulants may result in excess clot formation. A severe hemorrhagic disorder due to a deficiency of α_2-antiplasmin has responded to treatment with aminocaproic acid or tranexamic acid, both antifibrinolytic agents.[36] Congenital antithrombin III, protein S, and protein C deficiencies are associated with recurrent thrombosis and are usually controlled with oral anticoagulants.[36] Factor V Leiden, prothrombin G20210A, and other activated protein C–resistance gene mutations will cause or add additional risk for thrombotic tendency in proportion to their homozygous or heterozygous states.[69-71] Operation requires discontinuation of the anticoagulation, and the patients will require replacement therapy during the procedure and in the postoperative healing period until anticoagulation can be restarted. Depending on the deficiency, antithrombin III concentrates or fresh frozen plasma can be used for replacement therapy, which should be conducted under the guidance of a hematologist with ready access to a full coagulation laboratory.

RECOMBINANT ACTIVATED FACTOR VII

Recombinant activated factor VII (rFVIIa) was developed for the treatment of bleeding in patients with hemophilia A or B who had inhibitors and was approved by the U.S. Food and Drug Administration (FDA) for this indication in 1999.[72-74] Good hemostasis with few side effects was seen in patients with intracranial hemorrhage, post-laparotomy and postpartum hemorrhage, and hemorrhage into the gluteal muscles (as a complication after cholecystectomy) and for surgical prophylaxis for major and minor procedures.[75-77] Home treatment programs for some patients who are hemophiliacs with inhibitors now use rFVIIa as frontline therapy for bleeding.[78] Children have a more rapid rate of clearance (elimination mean half-life, 1.32 hours in children vs. 2.74 hours in adults).[79] They also seem to have fewer side effects with this treatment.[74,80] Although various dosages and schedules have been studied, initial recommended therapy in hemophilia A or B with inhibitors is 90 mg/kg intravenously every 2 hours until the bleeding is controlled.[81]

The off-label use of rFVIIa has been reported in therapy-resistant severe bleeding from other conditions such as congenital factor VII deficiency, chronic liver disease, and inherited platelet disorders.[82-84]

Successes in patients without a known bleeding disorder who have trauma or postoperative hemorrhage also are described.[80,82,85,86] These reports should be interpreted with caution, because rFVIIa is currently not the standard of care in any of these off-label uses and exceptional circumstances impelled its use. It is highly recommended that rFVIIa be administered under the supervision of a physician experienced in its use who can anticipate the risks and respond to the complications, particularly risks of thrombosis, which are reported in 1% to 3% of patients.[72,87,88] rFVIIa shows great promise in the emergency treatment of uncontrolled hemorrhage for many situations and is becoming the standard of care for the treatment of intracranial hemorrage.[89]

SICKLE CELL DISEASE

General Principles

Sickle cell disease (SCD) is the most common disorder identified by neonatal blood screening, with approximately 2000 affected infants born in the United States each year. Overall, the incidence of SCD exceeds that of most other serious genetic disorders, including cystic fibrosis and hemophilia.[90,91] SCD is caused by a genetic mutation that results in an amino acid change in the β-globin and the production of sickle hemoglobin (Hb S) instead of normal hemoglobin (Hb A). The sickle cell gene, in combination with any other abnormal β-globin gene, results in SCD. There are many types of SCD. The most common include sickle cell anemia (Hb SS), the sickle β-thalassemias (Hb Sβ^0 and Hb Sβ^+), hemoglobin SC disease (Hb SC) and sickle cell/hereditary persistence of fetal hemoglobin (S/HPFH). Sickle cell anemia is the most common and, in general, the most severe form of SCD. Sickle β^0-thalassemia patients have clinical manifestations similar to those in patients with Hb SS disease. Sickle-C disease is the second most common form of SCD and generally has a more benign clinical course than does Hb SS or sickle β^0-thalassemia. Sickle β^+-thalassemia and S/HPFH patients also generally have a more benign clinical course. Patients with Hb SS disease and sickle β^0-thalassemia generally have lower hemoglobin levels and present a greater risk under general anesthesia than do patients with Hb SC disease and sickle β^+-thalassemia. Patients with S/HPFH may actually have hemoglobin levels that approach or are normal.

The red cell membrane is abnormal in patients with SCD, and the red cell life span is shortened by hemolysis. Intermittent episodes of vascular occlusion cause tissue ischemia, which results in acute and chronic organ dysfunction.[92] Consequently, patients with SCD require special considerations to prevent perioperative complications.

Because of the nature of the complications of SCD, people with this disorder are more likely to undergo surgery than the general population during their lifetime.[93] According to one study, the most common procedures were cholecystectomy; ear, nose, and throat procedures; orthopedic procedures; splenectomy; or herniorrhaphy.[94] Cholecystectomy, splenectomy, and orthopedic procedures are often required to treat complications of SCD.

Children with SCD can require surgical evaluation and treatment either because of complications of their SCD or unrelated processes. Moreover, symptoms associated with vaso-occlusive episodes, such as abdominal pain and bone pain with fever, may be difficult to distinguish from other pathologic processes, such as cholecystitis and osteomyelitis.

The differential diagnosis for acute abdominal pain in a patient with SCD includes uncomplicated sickle cell acute pain episode ("crisis"), cholelithiasis, appendicitis, pancreatitis, ulcer, constipation, pneumonia, pericarditis, and splenic sequestration. Whereas 50% of painful episodes include abdominal pain, they are usually associated with pain in the chest, back, and joints. However, whereas previous episodes of pain that are similar in character suggest an acute painful episode, and this population may have the usual problems that can present as abdominal pain, the incidence of gallstones with cholecystitis, peptic ulcer disease, and pyelonephritis is increased. Complications such as splenic or hepatic sequestration are almost unique problems in patients with this disease. Abdominal pain as a solitary symptom, especially when accompanied by fever, leukocytosis, and localized abdominal tenderness, is suggestive of pathology other than that which occurs with a sickle cell acute painful episode. A study that reviewed the presentation and management of acute abdominal conditions in adults with SCD suggested that a surgical condition is more likely if the pain does not resemble previous painful episodes and if no precipitating event is found.[95] Acute painful episodes were relieved within 48 hours with hydration and oxygen in 97% of patients, whereas no patient with a surgical disease achieved pain relief over the same period with these modalities. The leukocyte count and serum bilirubin were not helpful in establishing the correct diagnosis.

Vaso-occlusive episodes can also produce bone pain and fever, symptoms that are difficult to differentiate from those of osteomyelitis. The majority of bone pain in SCD is due to vaso-occlusion, but osteomyelitis secondary to *Salmonella* species or *Staphylococcus aureus* is not infrequent.[96,97] The presence of an immature white blood cell count or elevation of the sedimentation rate, C-reactive protein, or leukocyte alkaline phosphatase is suggestive of a bone infection and may be an indication for aspiration of the bone lesion. Radiographic studies including simple plain films, bone scan, or magnetic resonance imaging are generally less helpful but may be useful in arriving at the proper diagnosis when positive and combined with the appropriate clinical findings.[97]

Preoperative Assessment and Management

An optimal surgical outcome requires careful preoperative, intraoperative, and postoperative management by a team consisting of a surgeon, anesthesiologist, and hematologist. Potential sickle cell–related complications include acute chest syndrome, pain episodes, hyperhemolytic crisis, aplastic crisis, alloimmunization with delayed transfusion reactions, and infections. The outcome of children with SCD requiring a surgical procedure is improved by careful attention to the cardiorespiratory, hemodynamic, hydration, infectious, neurologic, and nutritional status of the child.[93,98-100] If possible, procedures should be performed when the child is in his or her usual state of health with regard to the SCD. Attention should be directed toward chronic manifestations of disease because predictors of a poor postoperative outcome include increased age, recent exacerbations of the disease, and preexisting infection and pregnancy.[101] Particular attention should be directed toward any recent history of acute chest syndrome, pneumonia, wheezing, and alloimmunization. Special efforts must be made to avoid perioperative hypoxia, hypothermia, acidosis, and dehydration because any of these events can result in serious morbidity.

Many centers perform preoperative transfusions with the aim of reducing the complications of surgery and anesthesia.[102] The largest study to examine the role of transfusion in the preoperative management of sickle cell anemia was a randomized study that compared exchange transfusion (with a goal of achieving an Hb value of > 10 g/dL and Hb S value of < 30%) versus simple transfusion (to achieve an Hb value of > 10 g/dL).[94,102] This study concluded that not only was simple transfusion as effective as exchange transfusion in preventing perioperative complications but it also provided a significantly lower rate of transfusion-related complications.[94] The question of which procedures are safe to perform in children with SCD without preoperative transfusion remains controversial because there is a lack of randomized controlled trials to answer this question. However, simple transfusion to increase the Hb level to 10 g/dL for major procedures and blood replacement for both profound anemia of less than 5 g/dL and intraoperative hemorrhage appear appropriate.[103] Several studies suggest that minor procedures can possibly be safely undertaken without transfusion.[93,102,104] Alloimmunization can be minimized by giving antigen-matched blood (matched for K, C, E, S, Fy, and Jk antigens).[100] Regardless of transfusion status, strong multidisciplinary collaboration is vital throughout the perioperative period.

Intraoperative Management

Anesthetic considerations are based more on the type of surgical procedure planned than on the presence of SCD because no single anesthetic technique has been shown to be the gold standard. However, regional anesthetic techniques may allow for opioid sparing in the postoperative period.[101] The goals of anesthetic management are to avoid factors that predispose the patient to sickling (e.g., hypoxemia, hypothermia, dehydration, and acidosis). Careful monitoring for hypoxia, hypothermia, acidosis, and dehydration is essential. Monitoring should include arterial blood gases, digital oxygen saturation, end-tidal carbon dioxide, temperature, electrocardiogram, blood pressure, and urine output.[101,105]

Postoperative Management

As with the preoperative and intraoperative periods, it is essential to prevent hypothermia, hypoxia, and hypotension throughout the postoperative period. Before extubation, the patient should be awake and oxygenating well. Once extubated, the patient must be carefully monitored with a digital oxygen saturation monitor and the pulmonary status critically assessed on a continuing basis. Continuous pulse oximetry should be provided in the early postoperative period. Assessment of fluid status should continue until the patient has resumed adequate oral intake and is able to maintain hydration without intravenous supplementation. All patients should receive incentive spirometry, as well as adequate hydration and oxygenation.

Appropriate levels of analgesia (preferably by a continuous intravenous line and patient-controlled analgesia, if appropriate) should be provided so the patient is comfortable enough to cooperate with ambulation and maintain pulmonary toilet without oversedation. Experienced respiratory therapists should administer a vigorous program for pulmonary toilet. The patient must be monitored closely for the occurrence of pulmonary edema or atelectasis that can progress to acute chest syndrome.[106]

SPECIFIC SURGICAL CONDITIONS

Adenotonsillectomy

Adenotonsillectomy is a fairly common procedure in children with SCD. Adenotonsillary hypertrophy, which may be associated with early functional hyposplenism and obstructive sleep apnea secondary to enlarged adenoids, occurs somewhat frequently.[93,107,108] As with other types of surgery, preoperative transfusions should be performed before surgery.[109] Clinicians should be aware that postoperative complications may be greater if obstructive sleep apnea is present and that a younger age may influence the likelihood of postoperative complications.[93,110]

Cholelithiasis and Cholecystectomy

Abdominal operations such as cholecystectomy and splenectomy are the most frequent type of surgery performed in patients with SCD.[93,103] At present, no clear consensus exists regarding the appropriate therapy for SCD children who have cholelithiasis. The reported prevalence of cholelithiasis varies from 4% to 55%.[111,112] This wide variation is dependent on the ages of the study population and the diagnostic modalities used.[113] We routinely screen symptomatic children with ultrasonography and laboratory studies (e.g., total and direct bilirubin, serum glutamic-oxaloacetic transaminase, serum glutamate-pyruvate transaminase, alkaline phosphatase, and γ-glutamyltranspeptidase). It is our practice to screen all SCD children for gallstones by no later than age 12 years.

A child with SCD and symptomatic cholelithiasis should undergo cholecystectomy after appropriate preoperative preparation to avoid the increased morbidity of an emergency operation on an unprepared patient.[113-118] If indicated, intraoperative cholangiography can be performed to assess for common duct stones.[119]

The utility of laparoscopic cholecystectomy in SCD was first reported in 1990.[120] Since that time, laparoscopic cholecystectomy has been performed with increasing frequency in children with SCD.[113,121-124] The advantages of laparoscopic cholecystectomy over open cholecystectomy are decreased pain, earlier feeding, earlier discharge, earlier return to school, and improved cosmesis. The presence of common duct stones at times complicates the laparoscopic approach and may require conversion to an open operation for removal. At present, the role of extracorporeal shock wave lithotripsy as a palliative therapeutic modality is uncertain.

Splenic Sequestration and Splenectomy

Before the advent of routine newborn screening for hemoglobinopathies, acute splenic sequestration was the second most common cause of mortality in children younger than age 5 years with sickle cell anemia.[125] Splenic sequestration classically was first seen with the acute onset of pallor and listlessness, a precipitate decrease in hemoglobin, thrombocytopenia, and massive splenomegaly.[126] It now appears that parental education along with earlier recognition and immediate treatment with volume support (including red blood cell transfusions) has resulted in significantly decreased mortality for this condition. It is rare for an otherwise uncomplicated patient with Hb SS disease who is older than 6 years of age to develop an acute splenic sequestration syndrome. However, patients with Hb SC and sickle β^+-thalassemia disease can experience splenic sequestration at an older age.[127]

The management of the SCD child with splenic sequestration is a clinical dilemma. The rate of recurrent splenic sequestration is high and greatly influences subsequent management, which may be divided into observation only, chronic transfusion, and splenectomy. Indications for these approaches are not clearly defined.[100] The benefit of splenectomy must be balanced with the increased risk of overwhelming bacterial sepsis in the younger asplenic SCD patient.[100,128] Partial splenectomy[129,130] and especially laparoscopic splenectomy[131] are being performed more commonly as the number of experienced practitioners grows.

CONCLUSION

Children with SCD may require various surgical procedures for which the principles outlined in this chapter should be utilized. As a consequence of their disease, school-aged and adolescent patients are at higher risk for other medical complications that may require surgical intervention. For example, patients with priapism that is refractory to medical management may require operative management.[132] The physician should make sure the operating and anesthesia teams are aware of the diagnosis of sickle cell syndrome and the need for special attention. In patients with Hb SS and Hb $S\beta^0$-thalassemia, simple transfusion to a hemoglobin level of 10 g/dL should be performed before all but the lowest-risk procedures. Alloimmunization should be minimized by giving antigen-matched blood (matched K, C, E, S, Fy, and Jk antigens). Patients with sickle cell disease, regardless of genotype, should all receive careful attention, with preoperative monitoring of intake and output, hematocrit, peripheral perfusion, and oxygenation status. Intraoperative monitoring of blood pressure, cardiac rhythm and rate, and oxygenation should be conducted for all surgical procedures. Postoperative care should include meticulous attention to hydration, oxygen administration with careful monitoring, and respiratory therapy.[100]

chapter 6

EXTRACORPOREAL MEMBRANE OXYGENATION

Jason S. Frischer, MD • Charles J. H. Stolar, MD

Extracorporeal membrane oxygenation (ECMO) is a lifesaving technology that employs partial heart/lung bypass for extended periods. It is not a therapeutic modality but rather a supportive tool that provides sufficient gas exchange and perfusion for patients with acute, *reversible* cardiac or respiratory failure. This affords the patient's cardiopulmonary system a time to "rest," at which point the patient is spared the deleterious effects of high airway pressure, high FIO_2, traumatic mechanical ventilation, and perfusion impairment. Since the early anecdotal reports of neonatal and pediatric ECMO, the Extracorporeal Life Support Organization (ELSO) has registered approximately 35,000 neonatal and pediatric patients treated with ECMO for a variety of cardiopulmonary disorders. The number of centers providing extracorporeal support and reporting to ELSO continues to increase along with the total number of cases.[1]

HISTORY

The initial effort to develop extracorporeal bypass was first led by cardiac surgeons. Their goal was to repair intracardiac lesions under direct visualization and, therefore, they needed to arrest the heart, divert and oxygenate the blood, and perfuse the patient so that repair could be performed. The first cardiopulmonary bypass circuits used in the operating room involved direct cross circulation between the patient and another subject (usually the patient's mother or father) acting as both the pump and the oxygenator.[2]

The first attempts at establishing cardiopulmonary bypass by complete artificial circuitry and oxygenation were constructed with disk-and-bubble oxygenators and were limited because of hemolysis encountered by direct mixing of oxygen and blood. The discovery of heparin and the development of semipermeable membranes (silicone rubber) capable of supporting gas exchange by diffusion were major advancements toward the development of ECMO.[3] During the 1960s and early 1970s, the silicone membrane was configured into a number of oxygenator models by a number of investigators.[4-7]

In 1972, the first successful use of prolonged cardiopulmonary bypass was reported.[8] The patient sustained a ruptured aorta following a motorcycle accident. Venoarterial extracorporeal bypass support was maintained for 3 days. A multicenter prospective randomized trial sponsored by the National Heart, Lung, and Blood Institute (a branch of the National Institutes of Health) studied the efficacy of ECMO for adult respiratory distress syndrome. In 1979, they concluded that the use of ECMO had no advantage over that of conventional mechanical ventilation in this study, and the trial was stopped early.[9] However, Bartlett and colleagues[10] noted that all of the patients in the study had irreversible pulmonary fibrosis before the initiation of ECMO. In 1976, they reported the first series of infants treated with long-term ECMO, with a significant number of survivors. Six (43%) of 14 patients with respiratory distress syndrome survived. Many of these patients were premature and weighed less than 2 kg. Also, 22 patients with meconium aspiration syndrome had a 70% survival. These neonates tended to be larger.

Since then, despite study design issues, three randomized controlled trials and a number of retrospective published reports have reported the efficacy of ECMO versus conventional mechanical ventilation.[11-18] Other centers started to employ ECMO. By 1996, 113 centers were maintaining ECMO programs registered with ELSO.[1] Over the next 2 decades, improvements in technology, a better understanding of the pathophysiology of pulmonary failure, and a greater experience in using ECMO have contributed to improved outcomes for infants with respiratory failure. In 2003, the University of Michigan reported an association between ECMO volume and an observed reduction in neonatal mortality seen in that state between 1980 through 1999.[19]

ELSO, formed in 1989, is a collaboration of physicians and scientists with an interest in ECMO. The organization provides the medical community with guidelines, training manuals and courses, and a forum in which these individuals can meet and discuss the future of extracorporeal life support. The group also provides a registry to investigators for the collection of data from almost all centers that maintain an ECMO program throughout the world. This database provides valuable information for analysis of this lifesaving biotechnology.[20,21]

CLINICAL APPLICATIONS

Neonates are the patients who benefit most from ECMO. Cardiopulmonary failure in this population secondary to meconium aspiration syndrome, congenital diaphragmatic hernia (CDH), persistent pulmonary hypertension of the newborn (PPHN), and congenital cardiac disease are the most common pathophysiologic processes requiring ECMO. For the pediatric population, the most common disorders treated with ECMO are viral and bacterial pneumonia, acute respiratory failure (non-acute respiratory distress syndrome [ARDS]), ARDS, sepsis, and cardiac disease. The experience with cardiac ECMO has been increasing over the past decade. Treatment of patients who are unweanable from bypass after cardiac surgery and as a bridge to heart transplantation in patients with postsurgical or end-stage ventricular failure are areas in which ECMO use is increasing.[1,22,23] Some less frequently used indications for ECMO include respiratory failure secondary to smoke inhalation,[24] severe asthma,[25] rewarming of hypercoagulopathic/hypothermic trauma patients,[26] and maintenance of an organ donor pending liver allograft harvest and transplantation.[27]

PATHOPHYSIOLOGY OF NEWBORN PULMONARY HYPERTENSION

Pulmonary vascular resistance (PVR) is the hallmark and driving force of fetal circulation. Normal fetal circulation is characterized by PVR that exceeds systemic pressures, resulting in higher right-sided heart pressures and, therefore, preferential right-to-left blood flow. The fetal umbilical vein carries oxygenated blood from the placenta to the inferior vena cava via the ductus venosus. Because of the high PVR, the majority of the blood that reaches the right atrium from the inferior vena cava is directed to the left atrium through the foramen ovale. The superior vena cava delivers deoxygenated blood to the right atrium that is preferentially directed to the right ventricle and pulmonary artery. This blood then takes the path of least resistance and shunts from the main pulmonary artery directly to the descending aorta via the ductus arteriosus, bypassing the pulmonary vascular bed and the left side of the heart. Therefore, as a consequence of these anatomic right-to-left shunts, the lungs are almost completely bypassed by the fetal circulation.

At birth, with the infant's initial breath, the alveoli distend and begin to fill with air. This is paralleled by relaxation of the muscular arterioles of the pulmonary circulation and the expansion of the pulmonary vascular bed. This causes a rapid drop in PVR to below systemic levels. This activity causes the left atrial pressure to become higher than the right atrial pressure, leading to closure of the foramen ovale, resulting in all venous blood flowing from the right atrium to the right ventricle and into the pulmonary artery. The ductus arteriosus also closes at this time. Therefore, all fetal right-to-left circulation ceases, completing separation of the pulmonary and systemic circulations. Anatomic closure of these structures takes several days to weeks. Thus, maintaining the pressure gradient of systemic pressure greater than the pulmonary circulation is vital to sustaining normal circulation.

Failure of the transition from fetal circulation to newborn circulation is described as PPHN or persistent fetal circulation.[28] Clinically, PPHN is characterized by hypoxemia out of proportion to pulmonary parenchymal or anatomic disease. Normally, in fetal and term neonates, the pulmonary arterioles are muscular only as far as the terminal bronchioles. In hypoxic fetuses and infants, the proliferation of smooth muscle on the arterioles may extend far beyond the terminal bronchioles, resulting in thickened and more reactive vessels. In response to hypoxic conditions, these vessels undergo significant self-perpetuating vasoconstriction. Although sometimes idiopathic, PPHN can occur secondary to a number of disease processes, such as meconium aspiration syndrome, CDH, polycythemia, and sepsis.

Treatment for PPHN is directed at decreasing right-to-left shunts and increasing pulmonary blood flow. Previously, most patients were treated with hyperventilation, induction of alkalosis, neuromuscular blockade, and sedation. Unfortunately, these therapies have not reduced morbidity, mortality, or the need for ECMO in the neonatal population. ECMO allows for the interruption of the hypoxia-induced negative cycle of increased smooth muscle tone and vasoconstriction. ECMO provides richly oxygenated blood and allows the pulmonary blood pressure to return to normal subsystemic values without the iatrogenic complications encumbered by overly aggressive "conventional" therapy. Recently, data recommending gentle ventilation and the use of inhaled nitric oxide for these children have been reported. Hyperventilation and neuromuscular blockade were not part of the treatment strategy.[29] The infants were allowed to breathe spontaneously. This strategy has decreased morbidity, mortality, and the need of ECMO.

PATIENT SELECTION CRITERIA

The selection of patients as potential ECMO candidates continues to remain controversial. The selection criteria are based on data from multiple institutions,

Table 6-1 Recommended Pre-ECMO Studies

Recommended Pre-ECMO Studies
Head ultrasonography
Cardiac echocardiography
Chest radiography
Complete blood cell count, with platelets
Type and crossmatch of blood
Electrolytes, calcium
Coagulation studies (prothrombin time, partial thromboplastin time, fibrinogen, fibrin degradation products)
Serial arterial blood gas analysis

patient safety, and mechanical limitations related to the equipment. The risk of performing an invasive procedure that requires heparinization of a critically ill child must be weighed against the estimated mortality of the patient with conventional therapy alone. A predictive mortality of greater than 80% after exhausting all conventional therapies is the criterion most institutions follow to select patients for ECMO. Obviously, these criteria are subjective and will vary between facilities, based on local clinical experience and available technologies. All ECMO centers must develop their own criteria and continually evaluate their patient selection based on ongoing outcomes data.

Recommended pre-ECMO studies are listed in Table 6-1. Indications for neonatal, cardiac, and pediatric ECMO all have their own modifiers. The definition of "conventional therapy" also is anything but consistent in any category. Nevertheless, ECMO is indicated when (1) there is a reversible disease process, (2) the ventilator treatment is causing more harm than good, and (3) tissue oxygenation requirements are not being met. A discussion of generally accepted selection criteria for using neonatal ECMO follows.

Reversible Cardiopulmonary Disorders

The underlying principle of ECMO relies on the premise that the patient has a reversible disease process that can be corrected with either therapy (including the possibility of organ transplantation) or "rest" and that this reversal will occur in a relatively short period of time. Prolonged exposure to high-pressure mechanical ventilation with high concentrations of oxygen can have a traumatic effect on the newborn's lungs and frequently leads to the development of bronchopulmonary dysplasia (BPD).[30] It has been suggested that BPD can result from high levels of ventilatory support for as little as 4 days or less.[31] The pulmonary dysfunction that follows barotrauma and oxygen toxicity associated with mechanical ventilation typically requires weeks to months to resolve. Therefore, patients who have been ventilated for a long time and in whom lung injury has developed are not amenable to a short course of therapy with ECMO. Most ECMO centers will not accept patients who have had more than 10 to 14 days of mechanical ventilation as candidates for ECMO, owing to the high probability of established, irreversible pulmonary dysfunction.

Echocardiography should be performed on every patient being considered for ECMO to determine cardiac anatomy and function. Treatable conditions such as total anomalous pulmonary venous return and transposition of the great vessels, which may masquerade initially as pulmonary failure, can be surgically corrected but may require ECMO resuscitation initially. Infants with correctable cardiac disease should be considered on an individual basis. ECMO also provides an excellent bridge to cardiac transplantation. ECMO as a bridge to lung transplantation is controversial because the time to receive a lung donor generally far exceeds the period of time one can be maintained on bypass.

Coexisting Anomalies

Every effort should be made to establish a clear diagnosis before the initiation of ECMO. Infants with anomalies incompatible with life do not benefit from ECMO. ECMO is not a resource that is intended to delay an inevitable death. Many lethal pulmonary conditions such as overwhelming pulmonary hypoplasia, congenital alveolar proteinosis, and alveolar capillary dysplasia may present as reversible conditions but are considered lethal.[32]

Gestational Age

The gestational age of an ECMO patient should be at least 34 to 35 weeks. In the early experience with ECMO, significant morbidity and mortality related to intracranial hemorrhage (ICH) was associated with premature infants (<34 weeks' gestation).[33] Despite modification of the ECMO technique over the past 2 decades, premature infants continue to be at risk for ICH. In preterm infants, ependymal cells within the brain are not fully developed, thus making these infants susceptible to hemorrhage. Systemic heparinization necessary to maintain a thrombus-free circuit adds to the risk of hemorrhagic complications.

Birth Weight

Technical considerations and limitation of cannula size restrict ECMO candidates to infants weighing at least 2000 g. The smallest single-lumen ECMO cannula is 8 French, and flow through a tube is proportional to the fourth power of the radius. Small veins permit only small cannulas, resulting in flow that will be reduced by a power of 4. Neonates who weigh less than 2 kg provide technical challenges in cannulation and in maintaining adequate blood flow through the small catheters.

Bleeding Complications

Infants with ongoing, uncontrollable bleeding or an uncorrectable bleeding diathesis pose a relative contraindication to ECMO.[20] Any correctable coagulopathy should be corrected before initiating ECMO because the need for continuous systemic heparinization adds an unacceptable risk of bleeding.

Intracranial Hemorrhage

Candidates for ECMO should not, as a rule, have had an ICH. A preexisting ICH may be exacerbated by the use of heparin and the unavoidable alterations in cerebral blood flow while receiving ECMO. Patients with small interventricular hemorrhages (grade I) or small intraparenchymal hemorrhage can be successfully treated on ECMO by maintaining a lower than optimal activated clotting time in the range of 180 to 200 seconds. These patients should be closely observed for extension of the intracranial bleeding. Patients posing a particularly high risk for ICH are those with a previous ICH, cerebral infarct, prematurity, coagulopathy, ischemic central nervous system injury, or sepsis. Consideration of these patients for ECMO should be individualized.[32]

Failure of Medical Management

ECMO candidates are expected to have a reversible cardiopulmonary disease process, with a predictive mortality of greater than 80% to 90% with all available modalities short of ECMO. Because different institutions have varying technical capabilities, opinions, and expertise, "optimal" medical management is a subjective term that varies widely. Vasoconstrictive agents, inotropic agents, pulmonary vascular smooth muscle relaxants, sedatives, and analgesics are all pharmacologic agents that are part of the medical management. Ventilatory management usually begins with conventional support but may also include the administration of surfactant, nitric oxide, inverse inspiration/expiration (I:E) ratios, or high-frequency ventilation. Ventilator and respiratory care strategies that incur significant barotrauma and other morbidity should be rigorously avoided.

ECMO use has been obviated in patients who otherwise meet ECMO criteria because of recent innovations in medical management. These innovations include the use of permissive hypercapnia with spontaneous ventilation, avoidance of muscle paralysis, and the avoidance of chest tubes. In 1978, the Children's Hospital of New York reported a nontraditional approach to the management of patients with PPHN, which has been successfully extended to infants with CDH.[34] Hyperventilation, hyperoxia, and muscle relaxants were not used, and permissive hypercapnia in conjunction with spontaneous ventilation was emphasized. Low-pressure ventilator settings were used and persistent $Paco_2$ of 50 to 80 mm Hg and a Pao_2 of 40 mm Hg were allowed. With careful attention to maintaining a *preductal* oxygen saturation greater than 90% or Pao_2 of 60 mm Hg or greater, 15 infants who met ECMO criteria with PPHN and in severe respiratory failure were initially treated with this approach and survived without ECMO.

Risk Assessment

Because of the invasive nature of ECMO, and the potentially life-threatening complications, investigators have worked to develop an objective set of criteria to predict which infants have an 80% mortality without ECMO. The two most commonly used measurements for neonatal respiratory failure are the alveolar-arterial oxygen gradient ($[A\text{-}a]Do_2$) and the oxygenation index (OI), which are calculated as follows:

$$(A\text{-}a)Do_2 = (Patm - 47)(Fio_2) - [(Paco_2)/0.8] - Pao_2$$

where Patm is the atmospheric pressure and Fio_2 is the inspired concentration of oxygen.

$$OI = \frac{MAP \times Fio_2 \times 100}{Pao_2}$$

where MAP is the mean airway pressure.

Although criteria for ECMO varies from institution and by diagnosis, it is generally accepted that, in the setting of optimal management, an $(A\text{-}a)Do_2$ greater than 625 mm Hg for more than 4 hours, or an $(A\text{-}a)Do_2$ greater than 600 mm Hg for more than 12 hours, or an OI of greater than 40 establishes both a relatively sensitive and specific predictor of mortality. Other criteria used by many institutions include a preductal Pao_2 less than 35 to 50 mm Hg for 2 to 12 hours or a pH of less than 7.25 for at least 2 hours with intractable hypotension. These are sustained values measured over a period of time and are not accurate predictors of mortality.[14,20,35-37] Patients with CDH are in their own category, and criteria for this situation are discussed later in this chapter.

Older infants and children do not have as well-defined criteria for high mortality risk. The ventilation index is determined by the following:

$$\frac{\text{Respiratory rate} \times Paco_2 \times \text{Peak inspiratory pressure}}{1000}$$

The combination of a ventilation index greater than 40 and an OI more than 40 correlates with a 77% mortality. A mortality of 81% is associated with an $(A\text{-}a)Do_2$ greater than 580 mm Hg and a peak inspiratory pressure of 40 cm H_2O. Indications for support in patients with cardiac pathology are based on clinical signs such as hypotension despite the administration of inotropes or volume resuscitation, oliguria (urine output < 0.5 mL/kg/hr), and decreased peripheral perfusion.

Congenital Diaphragmatic Hernia

Of most interest to surgeons are neonates with abdominal viscera in the thoracic cavity due to a CDH. These patients are plagued with pulmonary hypertension and have pulmonary hypoplasia both on the ipsilateral and contralateral lungs with regard to the hernia. Often, pulmonary insufficiency ensues and a vicious cycle of hypoxia, hypercarbia, and acidosis quickly ravages the child's well-being. This process must be interrupted by medical management, which has vastly improved over the past 2 decades with the use of permissive hypercapnia/spontaneous respiration, pharmacologic therapy, and delayed elective repair.

High-frequency oscillation may have its major role in forestalling respiratory failure when used as a "front end" strategy rather than as a "rescue therapy."[38] Surfactant plays no more than an anecdotal role. Nitric oxide is an important vasodilator in the treatment of pulmonary hypertension in these patients. Other pulmonary vasculature vasodilators such as epoprostenol, sildenafil, and iloprost are starting to demonstrate a significant efficacy in this patient population. The primary indicator for ECMO in the patient with CDH is when tissue oxygen requirements are not being met, as evidenced by progressive metabolic acidosis, mixed venous oxygen desaturation, and multiple organ failure. The other indicator is mounting iatrogenic pulmonary injury.

Permissive hypercapnia with spontaneous respiration is initiated with intermittent mandatory ventilation (IMV), 30 to 40 breaths per minute, equal I/E time, inspiratory gas flow of 5 to 7 L/min, peak inspiratory pressure (PIP) of 20 to 22 cm H_2O, and positive end-expiratory pressure (PEEP) of 5 cm H_2O. The FIO_2 is selected to maintain preductal SaO_2 greater than 90%. If this mode is not sufficient, as demonstrated by severe paradoxical chest movement, severe retractions, tachypnea, inadequate or labile oxygenation (preductal O_2 saturations < 80%), or $PaCO_2$ greater than 60 mm Hg, then a new mode of ventilation is needed.

High-frequency ventilation would be the next mode of therapy to be considered. It is delivered by setting the ventilator to IMV mode with a rate of 100, inspiratory time of 0.3, an inspiratory gas flow of 10 to 12 L, a PIP of 20, and a PEEP of 0 (due to auto-PEEP). The PIP is adjusted as needed based on chest excursion, with attempts to maintain PIP at less than 25 mm Hg.

High-frequency oscillation can be instituted if the high-frequency ventilation is refractory to improving the hypoxia and hypercarbia using the same parameters as just mentioned, but improvement may be no more than temporary. The goal is to maintain preductal oxygen saturations between 90% and 95%. Spontaneous breathing is preserved by rigorously avoiding muscle relaxants. Sedation is used only as needed. Meticulous attention to maintaining a clear airway and the well-being of the infant is obvious but critical.[39,40]

Before ECMO is initiated for an infant with CDH, the infant must first demonstrate some evidence of adequate lung parenchyma. Some programs use radiographic parameters to determine adequate lung volumes. The lung-to-head ratio (LHR) is measured by prenatal ultrasonography.[41] It is defined as the product of the orthogonal diameters of the right lung divided by the head circumference. Severe pulmonary hypoplasia is considered when the LHR is less than 1.0 and intermediate hypoplasia lies between 1.0 and 1.4.[42] The LHR is operator dependent and can only be obtained in a narrow gestational window and therefore leads to poor reproducibility across different centers.

In the past decade there has been a great advance in fetal magnetic resonance imaging (MRI), and this technology has recently been applied to CDH. Studies are starting to demonstrate that a percentage of the predicted lung volume (PPLV) can accurately predict disease severity in CDH. A group of investigators in Boston published a report that stated that a value less than 15 is associated with significantly higher risks, meaning prolonged support and/or death in this population.[43]

Many centers believe the best method to evaluate pulmonary hypoplasia and predict outcome is to evaluate the patient clinically. This is assessed by having a recorded best $PaCO_2$ less than 50 mm Hg and a preductal oxygen saturation greater than 90% for a sustained period of at least 1 hour at any time in their clinical course. With these criteria, successful ECMO should yield an overall survival rate of 75% or better. If patients with lethal anomalies, overwhelming pulmonary hypoplasia, or neurologic complications are not included, survival can approach 85%.[39,40,44]

Extracorporeal Cardiopulmonary Resuscitation

Studies demonstrate that 1% to 4% of pediatric intensive care unit admissions have a cardiac arrest. Survival to discharge for a patient who had an arrest in the pediatric intensive care unit ranges from 14% to 42%. The ELSO data demonstrate that approximately 73% of extracorporeal cardiopulmonary resuscitation (ECPR) was used for patients with primary cardiac disease. Overall survival to discharge in this population reached 38%. The American Heart Association recommends ECPR for in-hospital cardiac arrest refractory to initial resuscitation, secondary to a process that is reversible or amenable to heart transplantation. Conventional CPR must have failed, no more than several minutes should have elapsed, and ECMO must be readily available. ECPR is at its infancy, and this method of acute resuscitation needs to be explored further. Future research needs to analyze which patients will benefit the most with as little morbidity as possible.[45]

Second Course of ECMO

Approximately 3% of patients that are treated with ECMO will require a second course. The survival rates for patients in this cohort are comparable to the first course. Negative prognostic indicators for second-course ECMO patients include renal compromise patients, higher number of first-course complications, age older than 3 years old, or a prolonged second course.[46]

METHODS OF EXTRACORPOREAL SUPPORT

The goal of ECMO support is to provide an alternate means for oxygen delivery. Three different extracorporeal configurations are used clinically: venoarterial (VA), venovenous (VV), and double-lumen single cannula venovenous (DLVV) bypass. The inception of ECMO and its early days were characterized by VA

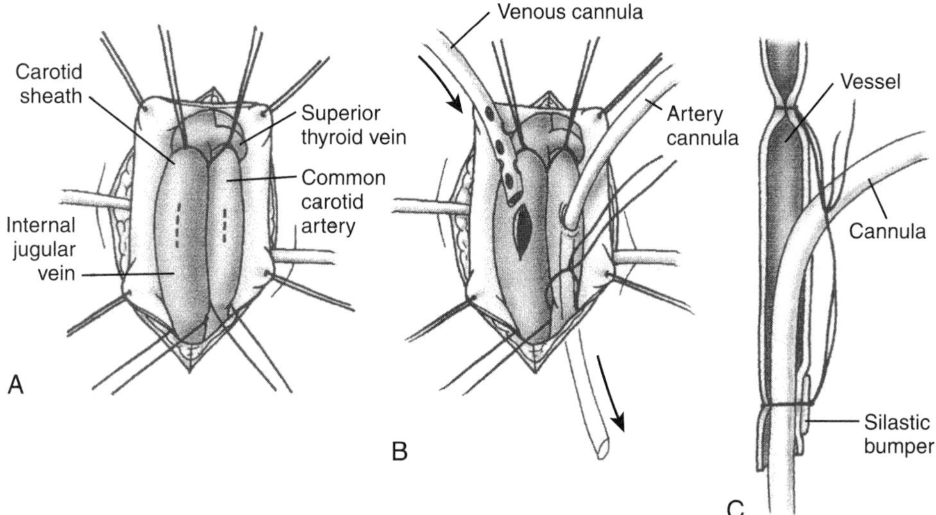

Figure 6-1. Details of the cannulation procedure. **A,** The carotid sheath is exposed, the sternocleidomastoid muscle is retracted laterally, and the common carotid artery and the internal jugular vein are dissected free. **B,** The patient is anticoagulated after the vessels are dissected and ligated cephalad. The arterial cannula is passed into the junction of the innominate artery and the aorta. The venous catheter is passed into the right atrium. **C,** A polymeric silicone (Silastic) bumper is used to facilitate ligation of the cannulas. The two ligatures on each vessel are then tied together.

ECMO because it offered the ability to replace both cardiac and pulmonary function. Venous blood is drained from the right atrium through the right internal jugular vein, and oxygenated blood is returned via the right common carotid artery to the aorta.

There are potential disadvantages with VA ECMO. A major artery must be cannulated and sacrificed. The risk of gas and particulate emboli into the systemic circulation is substantial, pulmonary perfusion is reduced, and decreased preload and increased afterload may reduce cardiac output, resulting in nonpulsatile flow. Finally, the coronary arteries are perfused by left ventricular blood, which is relatively hypoxic.

VV and DLVV avoid these disadvantages and provide pulmonary support but do not provide cardiac support. VV bypass is established by drainage from the right atrium via the right internal jugular vein with reinfusion into a femoral vein. DLVV is accomplished by means of a double-lumen catheter inserted into the right atrium via the right internal jugular vein. A major limitation of VV or DLVV ECMO is that a fraction of the infused, oxygenated blood reenters the pump and, at high flows, may limit oxygen delivery (recirculation). A limitation specific to DLVV is catheter size, which confines use of this method of support to larger neonates, infants, and smaller pediatric patients. VV and DLVV bypass have become the preferred method of extracorporeal support for all appropriate patients who do not require cardiac support.[20]

Cannulation

Cannulation can be performed in the neonatal or pediatric intensive care unit under adequate sedation and intravenous anesthesia, with proper monitoring. The infant is positioned supine with the head at the foot of the bed and the head and neck hyperextended over a shoulder roll and turned to the left. Local anesthesia is administered over the proposed incision site. A transverse cervical incision is made along the anterior border of the sternomastoid muscle, one finger-breadth above the right clavicle. The platysma muscle is divided, and dissection is carried down with the sternomastoid muscle retracted to expose the carotid sheath. The sheath is opened, and the internal jugular vein, common carotid artery, and vagus nerve are identified (Fig. 6-1A). The vein is exposed first and encircled with proximal and distal ligatures. Occasionally it is necessary to ligate the inferior thyroid vein. The common carotid artery lies medial and posterior, contains no branches, and is mobilized in a similar fashion. The vagus nerve should be identified and protected from injury.

If time permits, an activated clotting time (ACT) should be checked before heparinization. The patient is then systemically heparinized with 50 to 100 U/kg of heparin, which is allowed to circulate for 2 to 3 minutes, which should produce an ACT of more than 300 seconds. The arterial cannula (usually 10 Fr for newborns) is measured so that the tip will lie at the junction of the brachiocephalic artery and the aorta (2.5 to 3 cm or approximately one third the distance between the sternal notch and the xiphoid). The venous cannula (12-14 Fr for neonates) is measured so that its tip lies in the distal right atrium (6 to 8 cm or approximately half the distance between the suprasternal notch and the xiphoid process). The arterial cannula is usually inserted first with VA bypass. The carotid artery is ligated cephalad. Proximal control is obtained, and a transverse arteriotomy is made near the cephalad ligature (see Fig. 6-1B). To help prevent intimal dissection, stay sutures (of fine Prolene) are placed around the arteriotomy and used for retraction when placing the arterial cannula. The saline-filled cannula is inserted to its premeasured position and secured in the vessel with two silk ligatures (2-0 or 3-0). A small piece of vessel loop (bumper) may be placed under the ligatures on the anterior aspect of the carotid to protect the vessel from injury during decannulation (see Fig. 6-1C).

In preparation for the venous cannulation, the patient is given succinylcholine to prevent spontaneous respiration. The proximal jugular vein is then ligated cephalad to the site selected for the venotomy. Gentle traction on this ligature helps during the venous catheter insertion. A venotomy is made close to the ligature. The saline-filled venous catheter is passed to the level of the right atrium and secured in a manner similar to that used for the arterial catheter. Any bubbles are removed from the cannulas as they are connected to the ECMO circuit. Bypass is initiated. The cannulas are then secured to the skin above the incision. The incision is closed in layers, ensuring that hemostasis is meticulous.

For VV and DLVV bypass, the procedure is exactly as just described, including dissection of the artery, which is surrounded with a vessel loop to facilitate conversion to VA ECMO should that become necessary. The venous catheter tip should be in the mid-right atrium (5 cm in the neonate) with the arterial portion of the DLVV catheter oriented medially (pointed toward the ear) to direct the oxygenated blood flow toward the tricuspid valve.

The cannula positions for VA ECMO are confirmed by chest radiograph and transthoracic echocardiogram. The venous catheter should be located in the inferior aspect of the right atrium, and the arterial catheter at the ostium of the innominate artery and the aorta. With a double-lumen venous catheter, the tip should be in the mid-right atrium with return oxygenated blood flow toward the tricuspid valve.[47]

A challenging situation can arise when one attempts to cannulate a newborn with a right-sided CDH. Anatomic distortion can lead to cannulation of the azygos vein, which will then fail to provide adequate ECMO support. This can usually be detected by poor pump function and echocardiography, which will not be able to demonstrate the cannula in the superior vena cava or right atrium. In this situation, attempting cannula manipulation is often wrought with failure, and one should consider other avenues for venous drainage, including central cannulation.[48]

The small pediatric population (ages 2-12 years of age) presents a difficult and controversial scenario with regard to cannulation. Some centers continue to perform arterial cannulation via the carotid artery. The long-term outcome is unknown in this population after sacrificing the artery. Due to this concern, some centers will cannulate these patients via femoral access. The arterial cannula is large and often either partially or completely obstructs antegrade flow. This has the potential morbidity of distal limb ischemia, which can lead to sensory or motor deficits, tissue loss, or even limb loss. One potential way to avoid this morbidity is to provide antegrade flow via a percutaneously placed distal perfusion catheter (Fig. 6-2).[49]

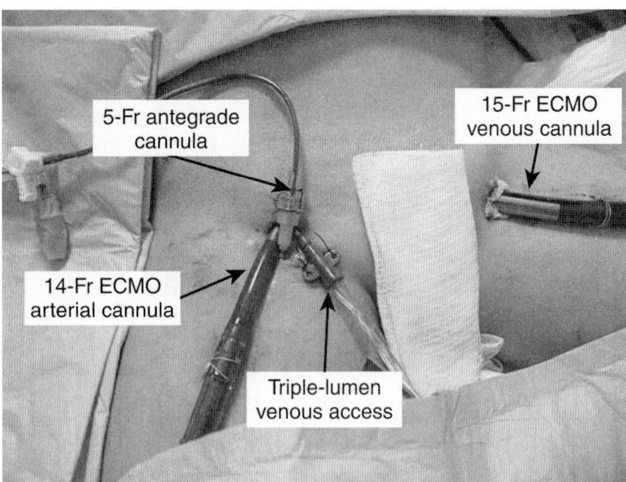

Figure 6-2. This infant has been cannulated for ECMO using the femoral artery and vein. To prevent possible distal limb ischemia, antegrade flow has been provided via a percutaneously placed distal perfusion catheter.

ECMO Circuit

Venous blood is drained from the infant by gravity through the cannula that is in the right atrium via the right internal jugular vein into a small reservoir or bladder (Fig. 6-3). An in-line oxymetric probe is located between the venous-return cannula and the bladder. This continuously monitors blood pH, Pao_2, Pco_2, and O_2 saturation. The monitor provides the information equivalent to the mixed venous blood gas (excluding any recirculation in VV or DLVV ECMO) and is extremely useful in monitoring the patient's status. The bladder is a 30- to 50-mL reservoir that acts as a safety valve. In the event that venous drainage does not keep up with arterial flow from the pump, the bladder volume will be depleted, sounding an alarm and automatically shutting off the pump. The blood flow through the circuit ceases to prevent gas bubbles forming from solution or drawing air into the circuit. Hypovolemia is one of the most common causes of decreased venous inflow into the circuit, but kinking and occlusion of the venous line should be suspected first. Raising the height of the patient's bed can improve venous drainage by gravity. An algorithm for managing pump failure due to inadequate venous return is shown in Figure 6-4.

A displacement roller pump pushes blood through the membrane oxygenator. The roller pumps are designed with microprocessors that allow for calculation of the blood flow based on roller-head speed and tubing diameter of the circuit. The pumps are connected to continuous pressure monitoring throughout the circuit and are servoregulated if pressures within the circuit exceed preset parameters. Another safety device, the bubble detector (not depicted in Fig. 6-3), is interposed between the pump and the membrane oxygenator that halts perfusion to the patient if air is detected within the circuit. The oxygenator consists of a long, two-compartment chamber composed of a spiral-wound silicone membrane and a polycarbonate

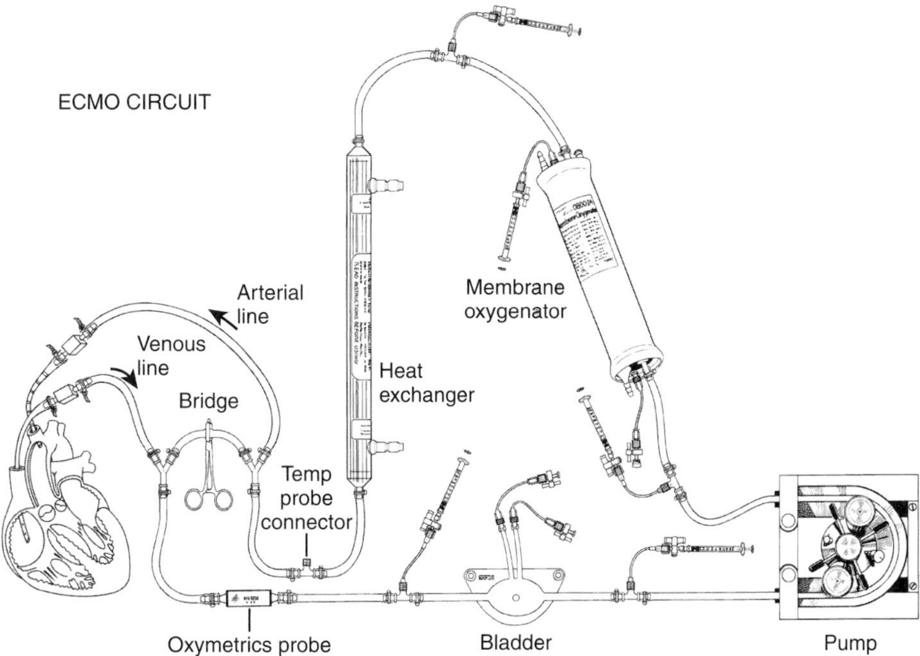
ECMO CIRCUIT
Arterial line
Venous line
Bridge
Membrane oxygenator
Heat exchanger
Temp probe connector
Oxymetrics probe
Bladder
Pump

Figure 6-3. Diagram of venoarterial extracorporeal membrane oxygenation circuit.

core, with blood flow in one direction and oxygen flow in the opposite direction. Oxygen diffuses through the membrane into the blood circuit, and carbon dioxide and water vapor diffuse from blood into the sweep gas. The size (surface area) of the oxygenator is based on the patient's size. Another oxymetric probe is located in the arterial return line distal to the oxygenator to provide information about the blood returning to the patient. The blood emerges from the upper end of the oxygenator and passes through the countercurrent heat exchanger and returns at body temperature to the aortic arch via the right common carotid artery.

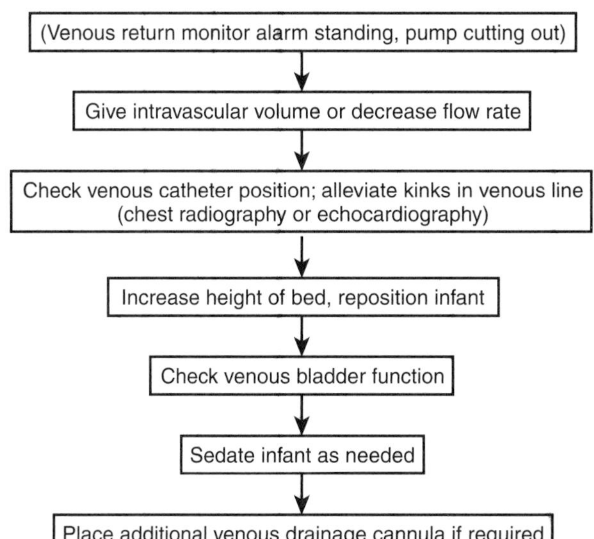
INADEQUATE VENOUS RETURN
(Venous return monitor alarm standing, pump cutting out)
Give intravascular volume or decrease flow rate
Check venous catheter position; alleviate kinks in venous line (chest radiography or echocardiography)
Increase height of bed, reposition infant
Check venous bladder function
Sedate infant as needed
Place additional venous drainage cannula if required

Figure 6-4. Suggested algorithm for the management of inadequate venous return during extracorporeal membrane oxygenation. (Adapted from DeBerry BB, Lynch J, Chung DH, Zwischenberger JB: Emergencies during ECLS and their management. In Van Meurs K, Lally KP, Peek G, Zwischenberger JB (eds): ECMO: Extracorporeal Cardiopulmonary Support in Critical Care, 3rd ed. Ann Arbor, MI, Extracorporeal Life Support Organization, 2005, pp 133-156.)

PATIENT MANAGEMENT ON ECMO

Once the cannulas are connected to the circuit, bypass is initiated, and the flow is slowly increased to 100 to 150 mL/kg/min. Continuous in-line monitoring of the (pre-pump) $S\bar{v}O_2$ and arterial (post-pump) PaO_2 as well as pulse oximetry is vital. The goal of VA ECMO is to maintain an $S\bar{v}O_2$ of 37 to 40 mm Hg and saturation of 65% to 70%. VV ECMO is more difficult to monitor because of recirculation, which may produce a falsely elevated $S\bar{v}O_2$. Inadequate oxygenation and perfusion are indicated by metabolic acidosis, oliguria, hypotension, elevated liver function test results, and seizures. Arterial blood gases should be monitored closely, with PaO_2 and $PaCO_2$ maintained at as close to normal levels as possible. The oxygen level of the blood returning to the patient should be maintained fully saturated. To increase a patient's oxygen level on ECMO, one can either increase the ECMO flow rate (~ cardiac output) or the hemoglobin must be increased to maintain hemoglobin at 15 g/dL (~ oxygen content). CO_2 elimination is extremely efficient with the membrane, and it is important to adjust the sweep (gas mixing) to maintain a $PaCO_2$ in the range of 40 to 45 mm Hg. This is important, especially during weaning, because a low $PaCO_2$ inhibits the infant's spontaneous respiratory drive. Vigilant monitoring allows timely adjustments. In addition to continuous blood gas monitoring, the arterial blood gas

Table 6-2 General Studies Obtained during ECMO

Laboratory Study	General Frequency and Comments
Chest radiography	Daily
Cranial ultrasonography	Only for neonates, the first 3 days and then as needed
Activated clotting time	Every 1 hr, more often if outside of parameters
Preoxygenator blood gas	Every 4 hr
Postoxygenator blood gas	Every 4 hr
Patient blood gas	Every 6 hr
Glucose monitoring test	Every 4 hr
Complete blood cell count with platelets	Every 6 hr; include a differential daily
Chem-7	Every 6 hr, including magnesium, calcium, and phosphorus daily
Fibrinogen	Daily and after infusion of cryoprecipitate and fresh frozen plasma; may also include prothrombin time and D-dimer

is directly measured every 4 hours. As soon as these parameters are met, all vasoactive drugs are weaned and ventilator levels are adjusted to "rest" settings. Gastrointestinal prophylaxis (H_2 antagonists or proton pump inhibitors) is initiated, and mild sedation and analgesia are provided, usually with fentanyl and midazolam. Paralyzing agents are avoided. Ampicillin and either gentamicin or cefotaxime are administered for antimicrobial prophylaxis. Routine blood, urine, and tracheal cultures should be obtained.[20,47] A daily chest radiograph is performed. Opacification or "white out" is often noted during the early ECMO course. The reasons for this are multifactorial and include decreased ventilatory pressures (both PIP and PEEP), reperfusion of the injured lung, and exposure of the blood to a foreign surface, causing an inflammatory response with the release of cytokines. A list of typical diagnostic tests is shown in Table 6-2.

Heparin is administered (30-60 mg/kg/hr) throughout the ECMO course to preserve a thrombus-free circuit. ACTs should be monitored hourly and maintained at 180 to 220 seconds. A complete blood cell count should be obtained every 6 hours and coagulation profiles obtained daily. To prevent a coagulopathy, platelets are transfused to maintain a platelet count greater than 100,000/mm^3. The use of fibrinogen and other clotting factors is controversial. The hematocrit should remain above 40% by using red blood cell transfusions so that oxygen delivery is maximized.[20]

Volume management of patients on ECMO is extremely important and very difficult. It is imperative that all inputs and outputs be diligently recorded and electrolytes monitored every 6 hours. All fluid losses should be repleted and electrolyte abnormalities corrected. All patients should receive maintenance fluids as well as adequate nutrition by using parenteral hyperalimentation. The first 48 to 72 hours of ECMO typically involve fluid extravasation into the soft tissues. The patient becomes edematous and often requires volume replacement (crystalloid, colloid, or blood products) to maintain adequate intravascular and bypass flows, appropriate hemodynamics, and urine output greater than 1 mL/kg/hr. By the third day of bypass, diuresis of the excess extracellular fluid begins and can be facilitated with the use of diuretics and, if necessary, an in-line hemofilter.[20,47]

Operative Procedure on ECMO

Surgical procedures, such as CDH repair, may be performed while the child remains on bypass, but one must account for the need for continued postoperative anticoagulation. Hemorrhagic complications are a frequent morbidity associated with this situation, and these complications increase mortality. To try to avoid these problems before the procedure, the platelet count should be greater than 150,000/mm^3, the ACT can be reduced to 180 to 200 seconds, and ECMO flow is increased to full support. Moreover, it is imperative that meticulous hemostasis is obtained throughout the operation. The fibrinolysis inhibitor aminocaproic acid (100 mg/kg) is administered just prior to incision, followed by a continuous infusion (30 mg/kg/hr) until evidence of bleeding ceases.[20,47]

Weaning and Decannulation

As the patient improves, less blood flow is required to pass through the ECMO circuit and the flow may be weaned at a rate of 10 to 20 mL/hr as long as the patient maintains good oxygenation and perfusion. The most important guide to VA ECMO weaning is the $S\bar{v}O_2$. For VV ECMO, it is the Sao_2. Flows should be decreased to 30 to 50 mL/kg/min, and the ACT should be at a higher level (200-220 seconds) to prevent thrombosis. Moderate conventional ventilator settings are used, but higher settings can be used if the patient needs to be weaned from ECMO urgently. If the child tolerates the low flow, all medications and fluids should be switched to vascular access on the patient and the cannulas may be clamped, with the circuit bypassing the patient via the bridge. If the possibility remains that the child may need to be placed back on bypass, then the cannulas should be flushed with heparin (2 U/mL). The patient is then observed for 2 to 4 hours. If this is tolerated, decannulation can be accomplished.

Decannulation is performed in a near-identical manner as cannulation. This should be executed under sterile conditions with the patient in the Trendelenburg position and with the use of a muscle relaxant to prevent air aspiration into the vein. Ventilator settings should be increased with the use of the muscle relaxant. The venous catheter is typically removed first to allow for better exposure, and the vessel is ligated. Repair of the carotid artery is controversial. Short-term results demonstrate acceptable patency rates and an equivalent short-term neurodevelopmental outcome when compared with children undergoing carotid artery ligation.[50,51] However, long-term follow-up of ECMO survivors is necessary to determine whether carotid artery repair is important. The incision should be irrigated and closed over a small drain, which is removed 24 hours later.[20,47]

COMPLICATIONS

Mechanical Complications

Membrane Failure

Failure of the membrane oxygenator is demonstrated by a decrease in oxygenation or retention of CO_2. The cause of such complications include either fibrin clot formation or water condensation, both of which diminish the membrane's ability to transfer oxygen and CO_2. An incidence of oxygenator failure or clot in the oxygenator is reported in 21.6% of respiratory ECMO runs in the neonatal and pediatric population.[1] This is potentially a serious complication and deserves due attention. The membrane should not be subject to high pressures, which should be continuously monitored. Pressure limits are specific for different manufacturers of membranes and for the size of the membrane. Signs of clot formation within the membrane can be detected by direct visualization of the top or bottom of the membrane, but the extent of the clot cannot be determined. The progressive consumption of coagulation factors, such as platelets and fibrinogen, also indicates that the membrane may be progressively building clot, and the need to change the oxygenator should be considered. Another sign of impending membrane failure is the formation of water vapor exiting the exhaust port of the oxygenator, along with rising CO_2 levels. The oxygenator can easily be exchanged without coming off bypass if the circuit was built with a double-diamond tubing arrangement with dual connectors both before and after the membrane. Such an arrangement allows parallel placement of a new oxygenator without having to come off bypass.

Raceway Tubing Rupture

Tubing rupture has become a much less frequent event with the introduction of Super Tygon (Norton Performance Plastics, Inc., Akron, OH) tubing. Extra tubing between the bladder and the oxygen membrane should be part of the initial circuit construction so that it can be used to rotate or "walk the raceway" tubing within the roller pump. This should be performed every 5 to 7 days and requires coming off pump for a matter of seconds. The tubing should be inspected repeatedly and all connections secured properly and replaced if defective. When a raceway rupture does occur, the pump must be turned off immediately, and the patient must be ventilated and perfused by conventional methods (increased ventilator pressures and oxygen, and CPR performed, if necessary). The raceway tubing should be replaced and the flow recalibrated.

Accidental Decannulation

Securing the cannulas properly and taping the tubing in place to the bed with some motion of the patient's head still possible will help prevent accidental decannulation. Unexpected decannulation is a surgical emergency, and immediate pressure should be applied to the cannula site along with discontinuation of bypass. Conventional ventilator settings should be increased simultaneously. The neck incision must be immediately re-explored to prevent further hemorrhage and the cannulas replaced if continued bypass is needed.

Patient Complications

Air Embolism

The ECMO circuit has several potential sources for entry of air. The initial cannulation procedure can be a source of air embolism. Thus, all visible air bubbles should be removed by using heparinized saline. Other entry points throughout the circuit include all of the connectors, the stopcocks, and the membrane oxygenator. Therefore, the circuit must be continually inspected. Air on the arterial side requires the patient to be taken off bypass immediately. The air should be aspirated from a port and the blood recirculated through the bridge until all air has been removed. Air on the venous side is not as urgent a problem, and the air can often be "walked" into the bladder where it can be aspirated without coming off bypass.

In the event that an air embolism reaches the patient, he or she should be immediately taken off ECMO and conventional ventilator settings adjusted to best meet the child's needs. The patient should be placed in the Trendelenburg position to prevent air from entering the cerebral circulation. Next, an attempt should be made to aspirate any accessible air out of the arterial cannula. If air enters the coronary circulation, inotropic support may be necessary. Before reinstituting ECMO, identifying and repairing the cause of the embolus is essential. Prevention of air embolism is vital. When setting up the circuit, all air must be removed and all connections made tight and thoroughly inspected before initiating bypass.

Neurologic Complications

For respiratory ECMO in neonates and pediatric patients, neurologic complications have an overall incidence of 26.3%.[1] ICH, infarct, and seizure carry significant mortality when encountered in ECMO patients. Frequent neurologic examinations should be performed and the use of paralytic agents avoided. The examination should include evaluation of alertness and interaction, spontaneous movements, eye findings, the presence of seizures, fullness of the fontanelles, tone, and reflexes. Cranial ultrasonography should be performed on all neonates before initiating ECMO to identify those patients in whom significant ICH already exists. A retrospective analysis revealed that birth weight and gestational age were the most significant correlating factors with ICH for neonates on ECMO.[33] Once the patient goes on ECMO, ultrasonography is repeated during the first 3 days when indicated by clinical condition. If the examination reveals a new moderate (grade II) hemorrhage or an expanding ICH, ECMO is usually discontinued and reversal of anticoagulation is advisable.

In the event that an ICH is suspected or detected on cranial ultrasonography and deemed to be small in size, it is reasonable to maintain a low ACT (180-200 seconds) with a platelet count greater than 125,000 to 150,000/mm^3. Serial head ultrasound imaging should be performed to monitor the progression of the hemorrhage.[20]

Cannula Site or Bleeding at Other Sites

The ECMO registry reports an 8.4% incidence of cannulation site bleeding and a 13% incidence of other surgical site bleeding.[1] Contact of blood with the foreign surface of the circuit activates the coagulation cascade. The number of platelets and their function are also affected. In conjunction with anticoagulation, the risk of bleeding while undergoing an operation on ECMO is considerable. To reduce this risk, meticulous hemostasis should be maintained during the procedure and before closure. If necessary, the surgeon should employ topical hemostatic agents. Lowering the ACT parameters to 180 to 200 seconds and maintaining a platelet count of at least 125,000/mm^3 can assist in obtaining hemostasis. If bleeding from the cannula incision is greater than 10 mL/hr for 2 hours despite conservative treatment strategies, it should be explored.[20]

Bleeding into the site of previous surgical interventions occurs frequently and must be handled aggressively. Constant monitoring for bleeding by observing a decreasing hematocrit, an increasing heart rate, a decline in the blood pressure, or an inadequate venous return are signs of hemorrhage. Treatment includes replenishing lost blood products, including coagulation factors, if necessary. ACT parameters should be decreased to 180 to 200 seconds and platelet count maintained at least greater than 125,000/mm^3. The use of agents that inhibit fibrinolysis, such as aminocaproic acid, also can help prevent bleeding. The use of recombinant activated factor VII (NovoSeven, Novo Nordisk, Inc., Princeton, NJ) has been described in the management of bleeding unresponsive to conventional methods. This is an off-label use of this agent, and thrombosis is a significant morbidity that has been described.[52] Often, one must evacuate the hematoma and explore for surgical bleeding, if necessary, as is the case in the postcardiac surgery patient left with an open chest and central cannulation. If bleeding is not quickly controlled, decannulation and removing the obligatory anticoagulation must be strongly considered.

Coagulation Abnormalities

ECMO patients have a coagulopathy secondary to consumption by the circuit. The treatment for this coagulopathy is removal of the source, and a circuit change is a logical approach. Disseminated intravascular coagulation (DIC) occurs in approximately 2.4% of ECMO cases.[1] DIC is characterized by the consumption of plasma clotting factors and platelets, resulting in deposition of fibrin thrombi in the microvasculature. Once the factor levels and platelet count decrease below certain levels, bleeding will occur. Sepsis, acidosis, hypoxia, and hypotension are the most common causes, which is why ECMO patients are at risk for developing DIC. The most common cause of coagulopathy is consumption of clotting factors by the circuit and only seldom is it due to sepsis or DIC.

Patent Ductus Arteriosus

The dramatic decrease in pulmonary hypertension seen usually in the first 48 hours of an ECMO run causes dramatic changes in the neonate's circulation. A left-to-right shunt through the patent ductus arteriosus (PDA) develops and causes less-efficient oxygenation, pulmonary edema, and poor peripheral perfusion. As a rule, the PDA closes spontaneously with the use of fluid restriction and diuresis. The use of indomethacin should be avoided because of its effects on platelet function. Rarely is PDA ligation required or indicated while on ECMO.

Renal Failure

Oliguria is common in ECMO patients and is often seen during the first 24 to 48 hours. The capillary leak that is seen after placing a child on ECMO may cause decreased renal perfusion, or it may be due to the nonpulsatile nature of blood flow that occurs with VA ECMO. Once the patient is considered to be adequately volume resuscitated, and fluid shifts have stabilized, the use of furosemide (1 to 2 mg/kg) can be used to improve urine output. If the creatinine level continues to rise, then renal ultrasonography is recommended. The use of continuous hemofiltration, which is easily added in-line to the ECMO circuit, is another mechanism to assist in managing the fluid shifts, hyperkalemia, and azotemia. Hemofiltration removes plasma water and dissolved solutes while retaining proteins and cellular components of the intravascular space.[20,53]

Hypertension

The reported incidence of hypertension on ECMO varies from 28% to as high as 92%.[54] According to the ELSO registry, 13.1% of respiratory ECMO patients require pharmacologic intervention. One group reported that detectable ICH occurred in 44% of their hypertensive patients and clinically significant ICH developed in 27%.[55] The patient should initially be assessed for reversible causes of hypertension, such as pain, hypercarbia, and hypoxia. Embolic renal infarction is another important cause of hypertension. Medical management includes the use of hydralazine, nitroglycerin, and captopril.

Infection

The incidence of nosocomial infections during ECMO has been reported as high as 30%. Associated risk factors include the duration of the ECMO run, the length of hospitalization, and surgical procedures performed before the initiation of ECMO or during the run.[56] The ELSO registry data from July 2008 states an 8.5% culture-proven infection rate in ECMO neonates and pediatric patients.[1] This is remarkably low, considering the large surface area of the circuit, the duration of bypass, and the frequency of access to the circuit. Fungal infections carry a significantly higher hospital mortality rate, and the onset of sepsis carries a higher morbidity and mortality rate in neonates, as would be expected.[57,58] Because of the large volume of blood products often transfused into ECMO patients, the risk of developing a bloodborne infectious disease is significant. One study reported that approximately 8% of a group of children who were treated with ECMO as neonates were seropositive for antibodies to hepatitis C virus.[59] With more stringent screening techniques, this number has probably decreased since its initial publication.

RESULTS

ECMO is a prime example of the evolution from an experimental technique to a commonly used therapeutic approach. The ELSO registry has accumulated data since the early 1980s from all registered centers throughout the world, allowing analysis of this management. The number of registered centers continues to rise, as does the number of ECMO cases. In 1992, over 1500 ECMO cannulations for neonatal respiratory disease were performed. In 2007, only 808 cases were reported. In contrast, the number of cardiac cases has steadily increased over the past 20 years with the exception of 2007. The decline in case volume is likely due to improvements in ventilation management strategies and the addition of new agents to our armamentarium for respiratory failure (inhaled nitric oxide, smooth muscle relaxants, and high-frequency oscillation).[1,20]

Overall survival to discharge for neonates and pediatric patients is 64.9% for all diagnoses.[1] Higher survival rates are seen in neonates with respiratory diseases (76%) versus pediatric patients with respiratory failure (55%), but the pediatric population (45%) fairs better than neonates (38%) with cardiac failure as the reason for ECMO (Table 6-3).[1] According to the 2007 ELSO Registry data, newborns with meconium aspiration syndrome who require ECMO have the best survival rate at 94%, whereas ECMO survival for infants with CDH is 51% (Table 6-4).[1]

The pediatric population of ECMO patients represents a diverse group with regard to patient age as well as diagnoses. Almost an equal number of respiratory cases (3854) and cardiac cases (4181) have been reported. This is in stark contrast to the neonatal population in which there is an almost 7:1 ratio of a primary respiratory to a primary cardiac diagnosis.[1] A higher complication rate exists with the pediatric patients, reflecting the longer duration of bypass required for reversal of the respiratory failure.

Table 6-3 ECMO Cases by Patient Group (ELSO Registry, 1980-2007)

Indication	No. Cases	Survival to Discharge (%)
Neonatal respiratory failure	22,429	76
Neonatal cardiac failure	3,416	38
Pediatric respiratory failure	3,854	55
Pediatric cardiac failure	4,181	45

ELSO, Extracorporeal Life Support Organization.[1]

Feeding and Growth Sequelae

Approximately one third of ECMO-treated infants have feeding problems.[60-62] The possible causes for the poor feeding are numerous and include interference from tachypnea, generalized central nervous system depression, poor hunger drive, soreness in the neck from the surgical procedure, manipulation or compression of the vagus nerve during the cannulation, sore throat from prolonged intubation, and poor oral-motor coordination.[63,64] Newborns with CDH have a higher incidence of feeding difficulties as compared to those with meconium aspiration syndrome. CDH children often have foregut dysmotility, which leads to significant gastroesophageal reflux, delayed gastric emptying, and obvious feeding difficulties. Respiratory compromise and chronic lung disease add to the problem.[63-65]

Normal growth is most commonly reported in ECMO-treated patients, yet these children are more likely to experience problems with growth than are normal controls. Head circumference below the fifth percentile occurs in 10% of ECMO-treated children.[66] Growth problems are most commonly associated with ECMO children who had CDH or residual lung disease.[64]

Table 6-4 Neonatal Respiratory ECMO Cases (ELSO Registry, 1980-2007)

Indication	No. Cases	Survival to Discharge (%)
Meconium aspiration syndrome	7,354	94
Respiratory distress syndrome	1,461	84
PPHN/PFC	3,630	78
Sepsis	2,561	75
Congenital diaphragmatic hernia	5,582	51

ELSO, Extracorporeal Life Support Organization[1]; PPHN, persistent pulmonary hypertension of the newborn; PFC, persistent fetal circulation.

Respiratory Sequelae

Respiratory morbidity is more likely to be iatrogenic than a consequence of congenital lung disease. Nevertheless, approximately 15% of infants require supplemental oxygen at 4 weeks of age in some series. At age 5 years, ECMO children were twice as likely to have reported cases of pneumonia as compared with controls (25% vs. 13%). These children with pneumonia are more likely to require hospitalization, and the pneumonia occurs at a younger age (half of the pneumonias were diagnosed before 1 year of life).[67,68] CDH infants have been found to have severe lung disease after ECMO and often require supplemental oxygen at the time of discharge.[64,68-71]

Neurodevelopmental Sequelae

Probably the most serious post-ECMO morbidity is neuromotor handicap. The total rate of handicap from 540 patients at 12 institutions is 6%, with a range from 2% to 18%.[66,72-84] Nine percent of ECMO survivors have significant developmental delay, ranging from none to 21%. This is comparable to other critically ill, non-ECMO–treated neonates.[85] A single center study using multivariate analysis identified ventilator time as the only independent predictor of motor problems at age 1 in CDH patients.[86] Auditory defects are reported in more than one fourth of ECMO neonates at discharge.[87] The deficits are detected by brain-stem auditory evoked response (BAER) testing, are considered mild to moderate, and generally resolve over time. The cause of the auditory defects also may be iatrogenic, caused by induced alkalosis, diuretics, or gentamicin ototoxicity. As a result, all patients should have a hearing screening at the time of neonatal intensive care unit discharge. Visual deficits are uncommon in ECMO neonates who weigh more than 2 kg.[88]

Seizures are widely reported among ECMO neonates, ranging from 20% to 70%.[89-92] However, by age 5 years, only 2% had a diagnosis of epilepsy. Seizures in the neonatal population are associated with neurologic disease and poorer outcomes, including cerebral palsy and epilepsy.[93] Severe nonambulatory cerebral palsy has an incidence of less than 5% and is usually accompanied by significant developmental delay.[66,72,77] Milder cases of cerebral palsy are seen in up to 20% of ECMO survivors. Overall, ECMO-treated neonates function within the normal range and the rate of handicap appears to be stable across studies with an average of 11%, ranging from 2% to 18%.[66,72,74-84] Again, this morbidity reflects how desperately ill these children are and is not a direct effect of ECMO.

chapter 7

MECHANICAL VENTILATION IN PEDIATRIC SURGICAL DISEASE

Samir Gadepalli, MD • Ronald B. Hirschl, MD

Amazingly, ventilation via tracheal cannulation was performed as early as 1543 when Vesalius demonstrated the ability to maintain the beating heart in animals with open chests.[1] This technique was first applied to humans in 1780, but there was little progress in positive-pressure ventilation until the development of the Fell-O'Dwyer apparatus. This device provided translaryngeal ventilation using bellows and was first used in 1887 (Fig. 7-1).[2,3] The Drinker-Shaw iron lung, which allowed piston-pump cyclic ventilation of a metal cylinder and associated negative-pressure ventilation, became available in 1928 and was followed by a simplified version built by Emerson in 1931.[4] Such machines were the mainstays in the ventilation of victims of poliomyelitis in the 1930s through the 1950s.

In the 1920s, the technique of tracheal intubation was refined by Magill and Rowbotham.[5,6] In World War II, the Bennett valve, which allowed cyclic application of high pressure, was devised to allow pilots to tolerate high-altitude bombing missions.[7] Concomitantly, the use of translaryngeal intubation and mechanical ventilation became common in the operating room as well as in the treatment of respiratory insufficiency. However, application of mechanical ventilation to newborns, both in the operating room and in the intensive care unit, lagged behind that for children and adults.

The use of positive-pressure mechanical ventilation in the management of respiratory distress syndrome (RDS) was described in 1962.[8] It was the unfortunate death of Patrick Bouvier Kennedy at 32 weeks of gestation in 1963 that resulted in additional National Institutes of Health (NIH) funding for research in the management of newborns with respiratory failure.[9] The discovery of surfactant deficiency as the etiology of RDS in 1959, the ability to provide positive-pressure ventilation in newborns with respiratory insufficiency in 1965, and demonstration of the effectiveness of continuous positive airway pressure in enhancing lung volume and ventilation in patients with RDS in 1971 set the stage for the development of continuous-flow ventilators specifically designed for neonates.[10-12] The development of neonatal intensive care units, hyperalimentation, and neonatal invasive and noninvasive monitoring enhanced the care of newborns with respiratory failure and increased survival in preterm newborns from 50% in the early 1970s to more than 90% today.[13]

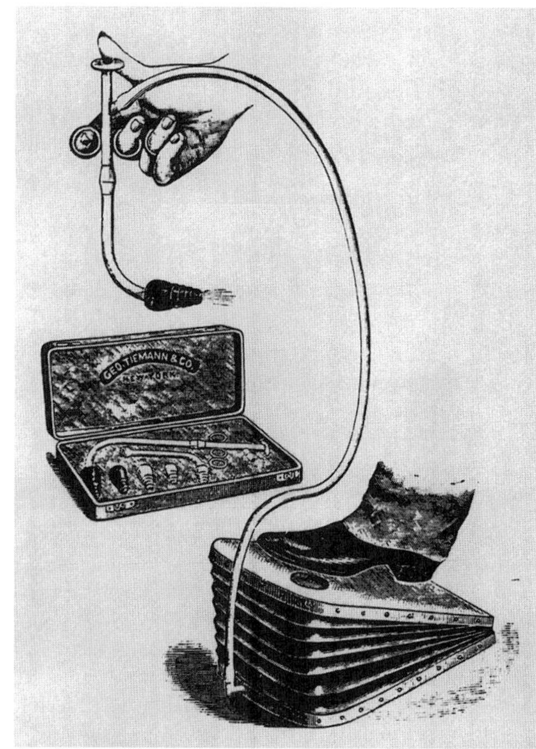

Figure 7-1. The Fell-O'Dwyer apparatus that was first used to perform positive-pressure ventilation in newborns. (Reprinted from Matas R: Intralaryngeal insufflation. JAMA 34:1468-1473, 1900.)

PHYSIOLOGY OF GAS EXCHANGE DURING MECHANICAL VENTILATION

The approach to mechanical ventilation is best understood if the two variables of oxygenation and carbon dioxide (CO_2) elimination are considered separately.[14]

Carbon Dioxide Elimination

The primary purpose of ventilation is to eliminate CO_2, which is accomplished by delivering tidal volume (VT) breaths at a designated rate. The product (VT· rate) determines the minute volume ventilation ($\dot{V}$E). Although CO_2 elimination is proportional to $\dot{V}$E, it is, in fact, directly related to the volume of gas ventilating the alveoli because part of the $\dot{V}$E resides in the conducting airways or in nonperfused alveoli. As such, the portion of the ventilation that does not participate in CO_2 exchange is termed the dead space (VD).[15] In a patient with healthy lungs, this dead space is fixed or "anatomic" and consists of about one third of the tidal volume (VD/VT = 0.33). In a setting of respiratory insufficiency, the proportion of dead space (VD/VT) may be augmented by the presence of nonperfused alveoli and a reduction in VT. Furthermore, dead space can unwittingly be increased through the presence of extensions of the trachea such as the endotracheal tube, a pneumotachometer to measure tidal volume, an end-tidal CO_2 monitor, or an extension of the ventilator tubing beyond the "Y." It is critical, therefore, that endotracheal tubes are shortened to a reasonable length and other safeguards are applied to ensure that the VD is minimized.

Tidal volume is a function of the applied ventilator pressure and the volume/pressure relationship (compliance), which describes the ability of the lung and chest wall to distend. At the functional residual capacity (FRC), the static point of end expiration, the tendency for the lung to collapse (elastic recoil) is in balance with the forces that promote chest wall expansion (Fig. 7-2).[15] As each breath develops, however, the elastic recoil of both the lung and chest wall work in concert to oppose lung inflation. Therefore, pulmonary compliance is a function of both the lung elastic recoil (lung compliance) and that of the rib cage and diaphragm (chest wall compliance).

The compliance can be determined in a dynamic or static mode. Figure 7-3 demonstrates the dynamic volume/pressure relationship for a normal patient. Note that application of 25 cm H_2O of inflating pressure (ΔP) above static FRC at positive end-expiratory pressure (PEEP) of 5 cm H_2O generates a VT of 40 mL/kg. The lung, at an inflating pressure of 30 cm H_2O when compared with ambient (transpulmonary) pressure, is considered to be at total lung capacity (TLC) (Table 7-1). Note that the loop observed during both inspiration and expiration is curvilinear. This is due to the resistance that is present in the airways and describes the work required to overcome air flow resistance. As a result, at any given point of active flow, the

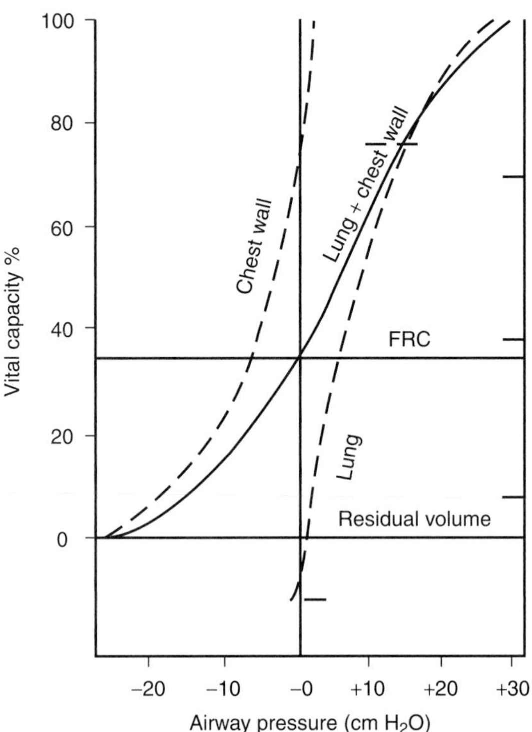

Figure 7-2. **Pulmonary function as a function of chest wall and lung compliance in healthy patients. At functional residual capacity, the tendency for the chest wall to expand and the lung to collapse is balanced.** (Adapted from West JB: Respiratory Physiology: The Essentials. Baltimore, Williams & Wilkins, 1985.)

measured pressure in the airways is higher during inspiration and lower during expiration than at the same volume under zero-flow conditions. Pulmonary compliance measurements, as well as alveolar pressure measurements, can be effectively performed only when no flow is present in the airways (zero flow),

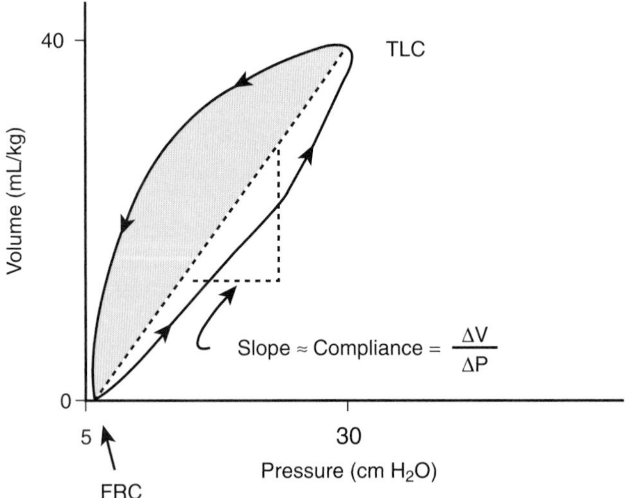

Figure 7-3. **Dynamic pressure/volume relation and effective pulmonary compliance (Ceff) in the normal lung. The volume at 30 cm H_2O is considered total lung capacity (TLC). Ceff is calculated by $\Delta V/\Delta P$.** (Adapted from Bhutani VK, Sivieri EM: Physiological principles for bedside assessment of pulmonary graphics. In Donn SM [ed]: Neonatal and Pediatric Pulmonary Graphics: Principles and Applications. Armonk, NY, Futura Publishing, 1998.)

Table 7-1 Definitions and Normal Values for Respiratory Physiologic Parameters

Variable	Definition	Normal Value
TLC	Total lung capacity	80 mL/kg
FRC	Functional residual capacity	40 mL/kg
IC	Inspiratory capacity	40 mL/kg
ERV	Expiratory reserve volume	30 mL/kg
RV	Residual volume	10 mL/kg
VT	Tidal volume	5 mL/kg
$\dot{V}_E$	Minute volume ventilation	100 mL/kg/min
$\dot{V}_E$	Alveolar ventilation	60 mL/kg/hr
VD	Dead space	mL = wt in lbs
VD/VT	% Dead space	0.33
CSt	Static compliance	2 mL/cm H_2O/kg
Ceff	Effective compliance	1 mL/cm H_2O/kg

which occurs at FRC and TLC. The change observed is a volume of 40 mL/kg and pressure of 25 cm H_2O pressure or 1.6 mL/kg/cm H_2O. This is termed *effective* compliance because it is calculated only between the two arbitrary points of end inspiration and end expiration.

As can be seen from Figure 7-4, the volume/pressure relationship is not linear over the range of most inflating pressures when a static compliance curve is developed. Such static compliance assessments are most commonly performed via a large syringe in which aliquots of 1 to 2 mL/kg of oxygen, up to a total of 15 to 20 mL/kg, are instilled sequentially with 3- to 5-second pauses. At the end of each pause, zero-flow pressures are measured. By plotting the data, a static compliance curve can be generated. This curve demonstrates how the calculated compliance can change depending on the arbitrary points used for assessment of the effective compliance (Ceff).[16]

Alternatively, the pulmonary pressure/volume relationship can be assessed by administration of a slow constant flow of gas into the lungs with simultaneous determination of airway pressure.[17,18] A curve may be fit to the data points to determine the optimal compliance and FRC.[19] The compliance will change as the FRC or end-expiratory lung volume (EELV) increases or decreases. For instance, as can be seen in Figure 7-4, at low FRC (point A), atelectasis is present. A given ΔP will not optimally inflate alveoli. Likewise, at a high FRC (point C), because of air trapping or application of high PEEP, the lung is already distended. Application of the same ΔP will result only in overdistention and potential lung injury with little benefit in terms of added VT. Thus, optimal compliance is provided when the pressure/volume range is on the linear portion of the static compliance curve (point B). Clinically, the compliance at a variety of FRC or PEEP values can be monitored to establish optimal FRC.[20]

Finally, it is important to recognize that a portion of the VT generated by the ventilator is actually compression of gas within both the ventilator tubing and the airways (Fig. 7-5). The ratio of gas compressed in the ventilator tubing to that entering the lungs is a function of the compliance of the ventilator tubing and the lung. The compliance of the ventilator tubing is 0.3 to 4.5 mL/cm H_2O.[21] A change in pressure of 15 cm H_2O in a 3-kg newborn with respiratory insufficiency and a pulmonary compliance of 0.4 mL/cm H_2O/kg would result in a lung VT of 18 mL and an impressive ventilator tubing/gas compression volume of 15 mL if the tubing compliance were 1.0 mL/cm H_2O. The relative ventilator tubing/gas compression volume would not be as striking in an adult. The ventilator tubing compliance is characterized for all current ventilators and should be factored when considering VT data. The software in many ventilators corrects for ventilator tubing compliance when displaying VT values.

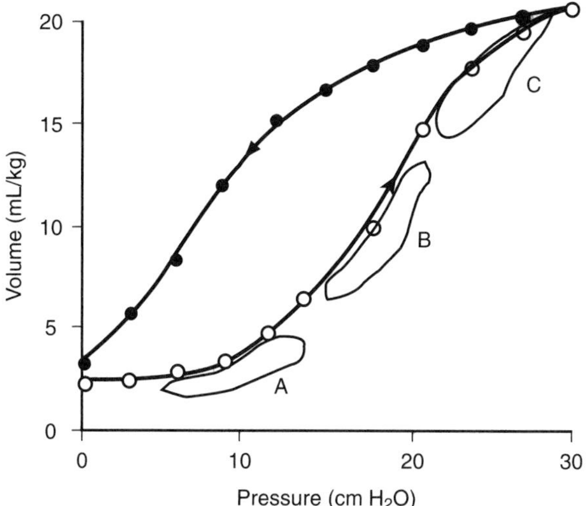

Figure 7-4. Static lung compliance curve in a normal lung. Effective compliance would be altered depending on whether FRC were to be at a level resulting in lung atelectasis (A) or overdistention (C). Optimal lung mechanics are observed when FRC is set on the steepest portion of the curve (B). (Adapted from West JB: Respiratory Physiology. Baltimore, Williams & Wilkins, 1985.)

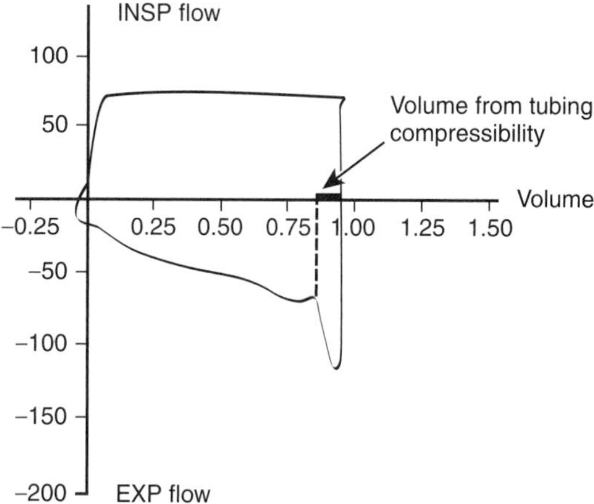

Figure 7-5. Flow/volume loops demonstrating the effect of ventilator tubing/gas compression volume in the ventilator tubing of a patient with respiratory insufficiency. The high flow during expiration results from gas decompressing from the ventilator tubing. (Adapted from Pilbeam SP: Mechanical Ventilation: Physiological and Clinical Applications. St. Louis, CV Mosby, 1998.)

Typical ventilator rate requirements in patients with healthy lungs range from 10 breaths/min in an adult to 30 breaths/min in a newborn. The VT is maintained at 5 to 10 mL/kg, resulting in a $\dot{V}E$ of about 100 mL/kg/min in adults and 150 mL/kg/min in newborns. In healthy lungs, these settings should provide sufficient ventilation to maintain normal $PaCO_2$ levels of approximately 40 mm Hg and should generate peak inspiratory pressures of between 15 and 20 cm H_2O above an applied PEEP of 5 cm H_2O. Clinical assessment by observing chest wall movement, auscultation, and evaluation of gas exchange determines the appropriate VT in a given patient.

Oxygenation

In contrast to CO_2 determination, oxygenation is determined by the fraction of inspired oxygen (FIO_2) and the degree of lung distention or alveolar recruitment, determined by the level of PEEP and the mean airway pressure (Paw) during each ventilator cycle. If CO_2 was not a competing gas at the alveolar level, oxygen within pulmonary capillary blood would simply be replaced by that provided at the airway, as long as alveolar distention was maintained. Such apneic oxygenation has been used in conjunction with extracorporeal carbon dioxide removal ($ECCO_2R$) or arteriovenous CO_2 removal ($AVCO_2R$), in which oxygen is delivered at the carina, whereas lung distention is maintained through application of PEEP.[22,23] Under normal circumstances, however, alveolar ventilation serves to remove carbon dioxide from the alveolus and to replenish the PO_2, thereby maintaining the alveolar/pulmonary capillary blood oxygen gradient.

Rather than depending on the degree of alveolar ventilation, oxygenation predominantly is a function of the appropriate matching of pulmonary blood flow to inflated alveoli (ventilation/perfusion matching [$\dot{V}/\dot{Q}$]).[15] In normal lungs, the PEEP should be maintained at 5 cm H_2O, a pressure that allows maintenance of alveolar inflation at end expiration, balancing the lung/chest wall recoil. An FIO_2 of 0.50 should be administered initially. However, one should be able to wean the FIO_2 rapidly in a patient with healthy lungs and normal $\dot{V}/\dot{Q}$ matching. Areas of ventilation but no perfusion (high $\dot{V}/\dot{Q}$), such as in the setting of pulmonary embolus, do not contribute to oxygenation. Therefore, hypoxemia supervenes in this situation once the average residence time of blood in the remaining perfused pulmonary capillaries exceeds that necessary for complete oxygenation. Normal residence time is threefold that required for full oxygenation of pulmonary capillary blood.

The common pathophysiology observed in the setting of respiratory insufficiency, however, is that of minimal or no ventilation, with persistent perfusion (low $\dot{V}/\dot{Q}$), resulting in right-to-left shunting and hypoxemia. Patients with the acute respiratory distress syndrome (ARDS) have collapse of the posterior, or dependent, regions of the lungs when supine.[24,25] Because the majority of blood flow is distributed to these dependent regions, one can easily imagine the limited oxygen transfer and large shunt secondary to $\dot{V}/\dot{Q}$ mismatch and the resulting hypoxemia that occurs in patients with ARDS. Attempts to inflate the alveoli in these regions, such as with the application of increased PEEP, can reduce $\dot{V}/\dot{Q}$ mismatch and enhance oxygenation.

Just as partial pressure of carbon dioxide in the artery ($PaCO_2$) is used to evaluate ventilation, partial pressure of oxygen in arterial blood (PaO_2) and arterial oxygen saturation (SaO_2) levels are the measures most frequently used to evaluate oxygenation. Lung oxygenation capabilities are also frequently assessed as a function of the difference between the ideal alveolar and the measured systemic arterial oxygen levels (A-a gradient), the ratio of the PaO_2 to the FIO_2 (P/F ratio), the physiologic shunt ($\dot{Q}ps/\dot{Q}t$), and the oxygen index (OI).

$$\text{A-a gradient} = (FIO_2 \cdot [PB - PH_2O] - PaCO_2/RQ) - PaO_2$$

where FIO_2 is the fraction of inspired oxygen, PB is the barometric pressure, PH_2O is the partial pressure of water, and RQ is the respiratory quotient or the ratio of CO_2 production (VCO_2) to oxygen consumption (VO_2).

$$\dot{Q}ps/\dot{Q}t = (CIO_2 - CaO_2)/(CIO_2 - CvO_2)$$

where $CvO_2/CaO_2/CIO_2$ are the oxygen contents of venous, arterial, and expected pulmonary capillary blood, respectively.

$$OI = (Paw \cdot FIO_2 \cdot 100)/PaO_2$$

where Paw represents the mean airway pressure.[15]

The overall therapeutic goal of optimizing parameters of oxygenation is to maintain oxygen delivery (DO_2) to the tissues. Three variables ascertain DO_2: cardiac output (Q), hemoglobin concentration (Hgb), and arterial blood oxygen saturation (SaO_2). The product of these three variables determines DO_2 by the relation:

$$\begin{aligned} DO_2 &= Q \cdot CaO_2 \\ \text{where } CaO_2 &= (1.36 \cdot Hgb \cdot [SaO_2/100]) \\ &\quad + (0.0031 \cdot PaO_2) \end{aligned}$$

Note that the contribution of the PaO_2 to DO_2 is minimal and, therefore, may be disregarded in most circumstances. If the hemoglobin concentration of the blood is normal (15 g/dL) and the hemoglobin is fully saturated with oxygen, the amount of oxygen bound to hemoglobin is 20.4 mL/dL (Fig. 7-6). In addition, approximately 0.3 mL of oxygen is physically dissolved in each deciliter of plasma, which makes the oxygen content of normal arterial blood equal to approximately 20.7 mL O_2/dL. Similar calculations reveal that the normal venous blood oxygen content is approximately 15 mL/O_2/dL.

Typically DO_2 is four to five times greater than the associated oxygen consumption (VO_2). As DO_2 increases or VO_2 decreases, more oxygen remains in the venous blood. The result is an increase in the oxygen hemoglobin saturation in the mixed venous pulmonary artery

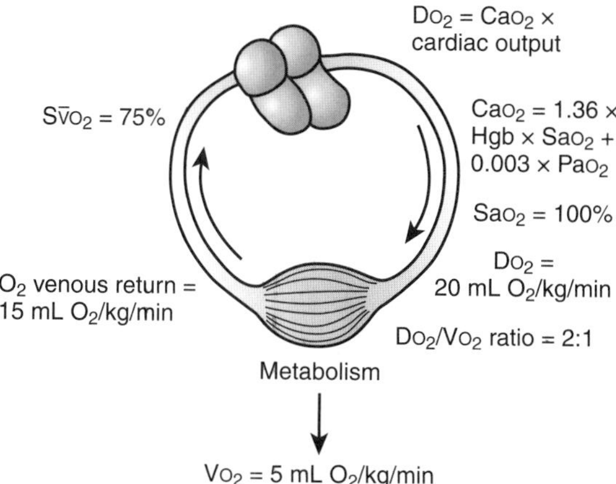

Figure 7-6. Oxygen consumption (Vo_2) and delivery (Do_2) relations. (Adapted with permission from Hirschl RB: Oxygen delivery in the pediatric surgical patients. Opin Pediatr 6:341-347, 1994.)

blood ($S\bar{V}O_2$). In contrast, if the Do_2 decreases or Vo_2 increases, relatively more oxygen is extracted from the blood, and therefore less oxygen remains in the venous blood. A decrease in $S\bar{V}O_2$ is the result. In general, the $S\bar{V}O_2$ serves as an excellent monitor of oxygen kinetics because it specifically assesses the adequacy of Do_2 in relation to Vo_2 (Do_2/Vo_2 ratio; Fig. 7-7).[26] Many pulmonary arterial catheters contain fiberoptic bundles that provide continuous mixed venous oximetry data. Such monitoring provides a means for assessing the adequacy of Do_2, rapid assessment of the response to interventions such as mechanical ventilation, and cost savings due to a diminished need for sequential blood

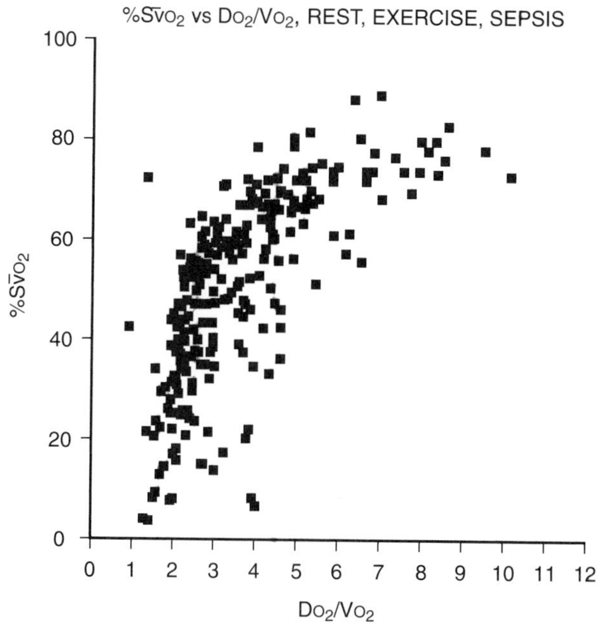

Figure 7-7. The relation of the mixed venous oxygen saturation ($S\bar{V}o_2$) and the ratio of oxygen delivery to oxygen consumption (Do_2/Vo_2) in normal eumetabolic, hypermetabolic septic, and hypermetabolic exercising canines. (Reprinted from Hirschl RB: Cardiopulmonary Critical Care and Shock: Surgery of Infants and Children: Scientific Principles and Practice. Philadelphia, Lippincott-Raven, 1997.)

gas monitoring.[26,27] If a pulmonary artery catheter is unavailable, the central venous oxygen saturation ($ScVO_2$) may serve as a surrogate of the $S\bar{V}O_2$.[28]

Four factors are manipulated in an attempt to improve the Do_2/Vo_2 ratio: cardiac output, hemoglobin concentration, Sao_2, and Vo_2. The result of various interventions designed to increase cardiac output, such as volume administration, infusion of inotropic agents, administration of afterload-reducing drugs, and correction of acid/base abnormalities, may be assessed by the effect on the $S\bar{V}O_2$ (Fig. 7-8). One of the most efficient ways to enhance Do_2 is to increase the oxygen-carrying capacity of the blood. For instance, an increase in hemoglobin from 7.5 to 15 g/dL will be associated with a twofold increase in Do_2 at constant cardiac output. However, blood viscosity is increased with blood transfusion, which may result in a reduction in cardiac output.[29] The Sao_2 can often be enhanced through application of supplemental oxygen and mechanical ventilation.

Assessment of the "best PEEP" identifies the level at which Do_2 and $S\bar{V}O_2$ are optimal without compromising compliance.[30,31] Evaluation of the best PEEP should be performed in any patient requiring an Fio_2 greater than 0.60 and may be determined by continuous monitoring of the $S\bar{V}O_2$ as the PEEP is sequentially increased from 5 to 15 cm H_2O over a short period. The point at which the $S\bar{V}O_2$ is maximal indicates optimal Do_2. The use of PEEP with mechanical ventilation is limited, however, by the adverse effects observed on cardiac output, the incidence of barotrauma, and the risk for ventilator-induced lung injury with application of peak inspiratory pressures greater than 30 to 40 cm H_2O.[32,33] Furthermore, oxygen consumption may be elevated secondary to sepsis, burns, agitation, seizures, hyperthermia, hyperthyroidism, and increased catecholamine production or infusion. A number of interventions may be applied to reduce Vo_2, such as sedation and mechanical ventilation. Paralysis may enhance the effectiveness of mechanical ventilation while simultaneously reducing Vo_2.[34,35] In the appropriate setting, hypothermia may be induced with an associated reduction of 7% in Vo_2 with each 1°C decrease in core temperature.[36]

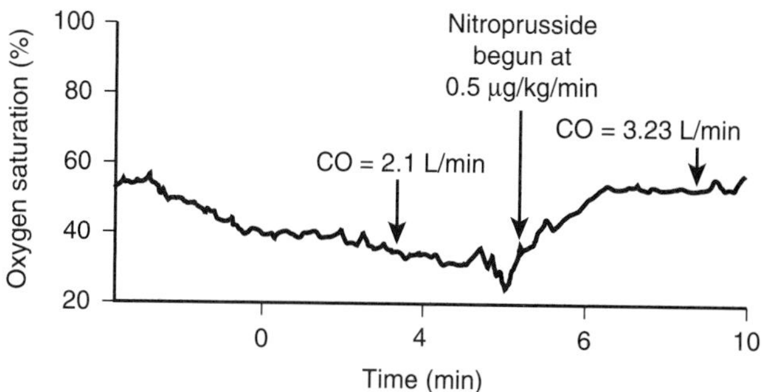

Figure 7-8. Alterations in $S\bar{V}o_2$ are shown as sodium nitroprusside is administered to reduce left ventricular afterload in the setting of cardiac insufficiency. (Reprinted from Hirschl RB: Cardiopulmonary Critical Care and Shock: Surgery of Infants and Children: Scientific Principles and Practice. Philadelphia, Lippincott-Raven, 1997.)

MECHANICAL VENTILATION

As discussed earlier, failure of gas exchange (CO_2 elimination or oxygenation) can be indications for mechanical ventilation. The ventilator can also be used to reduce the work of breathing and decrease oxygen consumption. Finally, mechanical ventilation is used in patients who are unable to breathe independently for neurologic reasons (primary hypoventilation, traumatic brain injury, inability to protect airway).

The Mechanical Ventilator and Its Components

The ventilator must overcome the pressure generated by the elastic recoil of the lung at end inspiration plus the resistance to flow at the airway. To do so, most ventilators in the intensive care unit are pneumatically powered by gas pressurized at 50 pounds per square inch. Microprocessor controls allow accurate management of proportional solenoid-driven valves, which carefully control infusion of a blend of air or oxygen into the ventilator circuit while simultaneously opening and closing an expiratory valve.[37] Additional components of a ventilator include a bacterial filter, a pneumotachometer, a humidifier, a heater/thermostat, an oxygen analyzer, and a pressure manometer. A chamber for nebulizing drugs is usually incorporated into the inspiratory circuit. The VT is not usually measured directly. Rather, flow is assessed as a function of time, thereby allowing calculation of VT. The modes of ventilation are characterized by three variables that affect patient and ventilator synchrony or interaction: the parameter used to initiate or "trigger" a breath, the parameter used to "limit" the size of the breath, and the parameter used to terminate inspiration or "cycle" the breath (Fig. 7-9).[38]

Gas flow in most ventilators is triggered either by time (controlled breath) or by patient effort (assisted breath). Controlled ventilation modes are time triggered: the inspiratory phase is concluded once a desired volume, pressure, or flow is attained, but the expiratory time will form the difference between the inspiratory time and the preset respiratory cycle time. In the assist mode, the ventilator is pressure or flow triggered. With the former, a pressure generated by the patient of approximately −1 cm H_2O will trigger the initiation of a breath. The sensitivity of the triggering device can be adjusted so that patient work is minimized. Other ventilators detect the reduction in constant ventilator tubing gas flow that is associated with patient initiation of a breath. Detection of this decrease in flow results in initiation of a positive-pressure breath.

The magnitude of the breath is controlled or limited by one of three variables: pressure, volume, or flow. When a breath is volume, pressure, or flow "controlled," it indicates that inspiration concludes once the limiting variable is reached. Pressure-controlled or pressure-limited modes are the most popular for all age groups, although volume-control ventilation may be of advantage in preterm newborns.[39,40] In the pressure modes, the respiratory rate, the inspiratory gas flow, the PEEP level, the inspiratory/expiratory (I/E) ratio, and the Paw are determined. The ventilator infuses gas until the desired peak inspiratory pressure (PIP) is provided. Zero-flow conditions are realized at end-inspiration during pressure-limited ventilation. Therefore, in this mode, PIP is frequently equivalent to end-inspiratory pressure (EIP) or plateau pressure. In many ventilators, the gas flow rate is fixed, although some ventilators allow manipulation of the flow rate and therefore the rate of positive-pressure development. Those with rapid flow rates will provide rapid ascent of pressure to the preset maximum, where it will remain for the duration of the inspiratory phase. This "square wave" pressure pattern results in decelerating flow during inspiration (Fig. 7-10). Airway pressure is "front loaded," which increases Paw, alveolar volume, and oxygenation without increasing PIP.[41] However, one of the biggest advantages of pressure-controlled

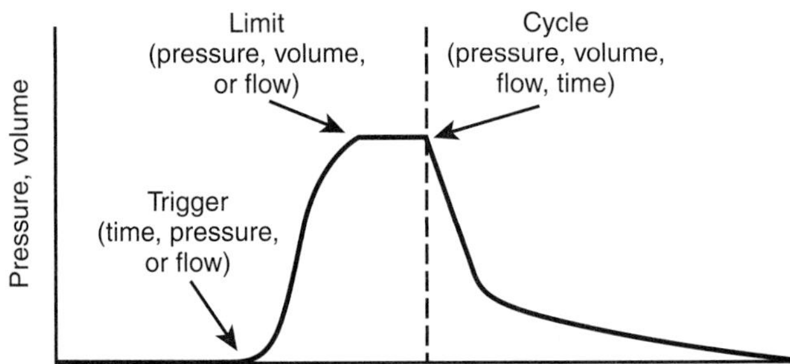

Figure 7-9. Variables that characterize the mode of mechanical ventilation.

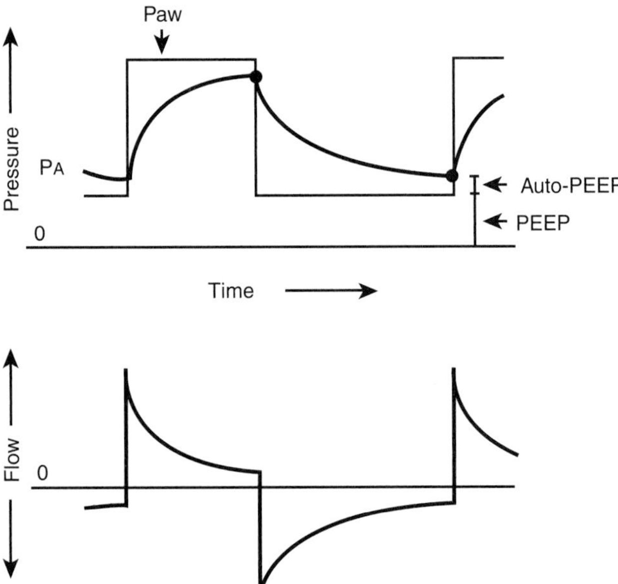

Figure 7-10. Pressure and flow waveforms during pressure-limited, time-cycled ventilation. Decelerating flow is applied, which "front loads" the pressure during inspiration. Auto-positive end-expiratory pressure is present when the expiratory time is inadequate for complete expiration. (Reprinted from Marini JJ: New options for the ventilatory management of acute lung injury. New Horizons 1:489-503, 1993.)

or pressure-limited ventilation is the ability to avoid lung overdistention and barotrauma/volutrauma (discussed later). The disadvantage of pressure-controlled or pressure-limited ventilation is that delivered volume varies with airway resistance and pulmonary compliance and may be reduced when short inspiratory times are applied (Fig. 7-11).[42] For this reason, both $\dot{V}_T$ and $\dot{V}_E$ must be monitored carefully.

Volume-controlled or volume-limited ventilation requires delineation of the VT, respiratory rate, and inspiratory gas flow. Gas will be inspired until the preset VT is attained. The volume will remain constant despite changes in pulmonary mechanics, although the resulting EIP and PIP may be altered. Flow-controlled or flow-limited ventilation is similar in many respects to volume-controlled or volume-limited ventilation. A flow pattern is predetermined, which effectively results in a fixed volume as the limiting component of inspiration.

The ventilator breath is concluded based on one of four variables: volume, time, pressure, or flow. With volume-cycled ventilation, inspiration is terminated when a prescribed volume is obtained. Likewise, with time-, pressure-, or flow-cycled ventilation, expiration begins after a certain period has passed, the airway pressure reaches a certain value, or when the flow has decreased to a predetermined level, respectively.

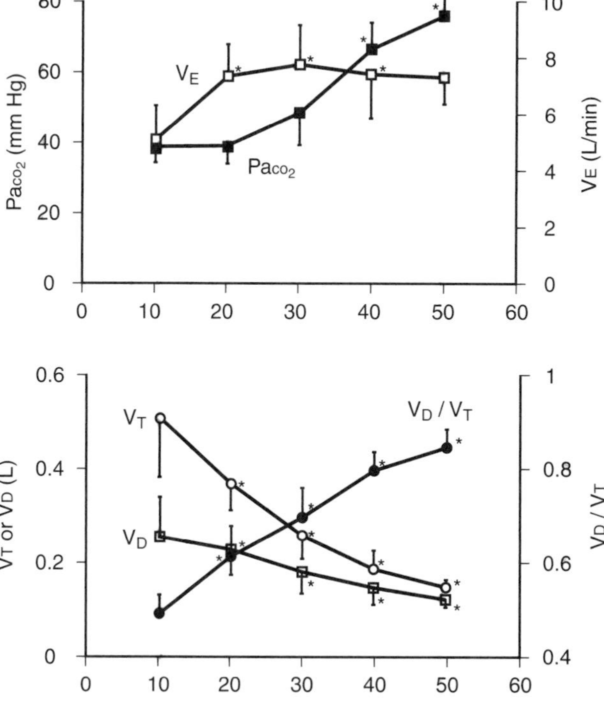

Figure 7-11. Effect of rate on tidal volume (VD/VT) and minute ventilation ($\dot{V}_E$) during pressure-limited ventilation. Note that $\dot{V}_E$ remains unchanged above 20 breaths/min. Simultaneously, VD/VT and $Paco_2$ increase, despite an increase in respiratory rate. (Reprinted from Nahum A, Burke WC, Ravenscraft SA: Lung mechanics and gas exchange during pressure-control ventilation in dogs: Augmentation of CO_2 elimination by an intratracheal catheter. Am Rev Respir Dis 146:965-973, 1992.)

A factor that limits inspiration suggests that the chosen value limits the level of the variable during inspiration, but the inspiratory phase does not necessarily conclude once this value is attained. For instance, during "pressure-limited" ventilation, gas flow continues until a given pressure limit is attained. However, the inspiratory phase may continue beyond that point. The limitation only controls the magnitude of the breath but does not always determine the length of the inspiratory phase. In contrast, during pressure-controlled ventilation, both gas flow and the inspiratory phase terminate once the preset pressure is reached because pressure is used to limit the magnitude of the breath and the gas flow.

Modes of Ventilation (Table 7-2)

Controlled Mechanical Ventilation

Controlled mechanical ventilation (CMV) is time triggered, flow limited, and volume or pressure cycled. Spontaneous breaths may be taken between the mandatory breaths. However, no additional gas is provided during spontaneous breaths. Therefore, the work of breathing is markedly increased in the spontaneously breathing patient. This mode of ventilation is no longer used.

Intermittent Mandatory Ventilation

Intermittent mandatory ventilation (IMV) is time triggered, volume or pressure limited, and either time, volume, or pressure cycled. A rate is set, as is a volume or pressure parameter. Additional inspired gas is provided by the ventilator to support spontaneous breathing when additional breaths are desired. The difference between CMV and IMV is that, in the latter, inspired gases are provided to the patient during spontaneous breaths.[43] IMV is useful in patients who do not have respiratory drive, for example, in those who are neurologically impaired or pharmacologically paralyzed. Work of breathing is still elevated in this mode in the awake and spontaneously breathing patient.

Synchronized Intermittent Mandatory Ventilation

In the SIMV mode, the ventilator synchronizes IMV breaths with the patient's spontaneous breaths (Fig. 7-12). Small, patient-initiated negative deflections in airway pressure (pressure triggered) or decreases in the constant ventilator gas flow (bias flow) passing through the exhalation valve (flow triggered) provide a signal to the ventilator that a patient breath has been initiated. Ventilated breaths are timed with the patient's spontaneous respiration, but the number of supported breaths each minute is predetermined and remains constant. Additional constant inspired gas flow is provided for use during any other spontaneous breaths. Advances in neonatal ventilators have provided the means for detecting small alterations in bias flow. As such, flow-triggered SIMV can be applied

Table 7-2 Modes of Ventilation

Mode	Trigger	Limit	Cycle	Comment
CMV	Time	Flow	Pressure/Volume	No longer used
IMV	Time	Volume/Pressure	Time Volume/Pressure	For no respiratory drive (neurologically impaired or paralyzed) Work of breathing elevated in spontaneously breathing patient
SIMV*	Pressure/Flow	Volume/Pressure	Time Volume/Pressure	Supports limited number of breaths
ACV*	Pressure/Flow	Volume/Pressure	Time Volume/Pressure	Supports all patient breaths Similar to IMV but patient controls breaths Sedation for hyperventilation and backup rate for apnea
PSV*	Pressure/Flow	Pressure	Flow Time	Supports all patient breaths Usually partially supported to allow for weaning Time cycled when termination-sensitivity for flow is off
VSV*	Pressure/Flow	Volume	Flow Time	Similar to PSV but volume used for partial support
VAPSV	Pressure/Flow	Pressure	Flow Time	Maintains a desired tidal volume using both VSV and PSV Dynamically maintains tidal volume
PAV*	Patient	Pressure	Patient	Size of the breath is determined by patient effort

*Patient-controlled rate.

to newborns, which appears to enhance ventilatory patterns and allows ventilation with reduced airway pressures and F_{IO_2}.[44,45] SIMV may be associated with a reduction in the duration of ventilation and the incidence of air leak in newborns in general, as well as in those premature infants with bronchopulmonary dysplasia and intraventricular hemorrhage.[46,47]

Assist-Control Ventilation

In the spontaneously breathing patient, brain stem reflexes dependent on cerebrospinal fluid levels of CO_2 and pH can be harnessed to determine the appropriate breathing rate.[15] As in SIMV, with ACV the assisted breaths can be either pressure triggered or flow triggered. The triggering-mechanism sensitivity can be set in most ventilators. In contrast to SIMV, the ventilator supports all patient-initiated breaths. This mode is similar to IMV but allows the patient inherently to control the ventilation needs and minimizes patient work of breathing in adults and neonates.[48,49] Occasionally, patients may hyperventilate, such as when they are agitated or have neurologic injury. Heavy sedation may be required if agitation is present. A minimal ventilator rate below the patient's assist rate should be established in case of apnea.

Pressure Support Ventilation

Pressure support ventilation (PSV) is a pressure- or flow-triggered, pressure-limited, and flow-cycled mode of ventilation. It is similar in concept to ACV, in that mechanical support is provided for each spontaneous breath and the patient determines the ventilator rate. During each breath, inspiratory flow is applied until a predetermined pressure is attained.[50] As the end of inspiration approaches, flow decreases to a level below a specified value (2 to 6 L/min) or a percentage of peak inspiratory flow (at 25%). At this point, inspiration terminates. Although it may apply full support, PSV is frequently used to support the patient partially by assigning a pressure limit for each breath that is less than that required for full support.[51] For example, in the spontaneously breathing patient, PSV can be sequentially decreased from full support to a PSV 5 to 10 cm H_2O above PEEP, allowing weaning while providing partial support with each breath.[52,53] Thus, V_T during PSV may be dependent on patient effort. PSV provides two advantages during ventilation of spontaneously breathing patients: (1) it provides excellent support and decreases the work of breathing associated with ventilation, and (2) it lowers PIP and Paw while higher V_T and cardiac output levels may be observed.[50,54,55]

Pressure-triggered SIMV and PSV may be applied to newborns. Inspiration is terminated when the peak airway flow decreases to a set percentage between 5% and 25%. This flow cutoff for inspiration, known as the termination sensitivity, may be adjusted. The higher the termination sensitivity value, the shorter is the inspiratory time. The termination sensitivity function also may be disabled, at which point ventilation is time cycled instead of flow cycled. Studies have demonstrated a reduction in work of breathing and sedation requirements when SIMV with pressure support is applied to newborns.

Volume Support Ventilation

Volume support ventilation (VSV) is similar to PSV except that a volume, rather than a pressure, is assigned to provide partial support. Automation with

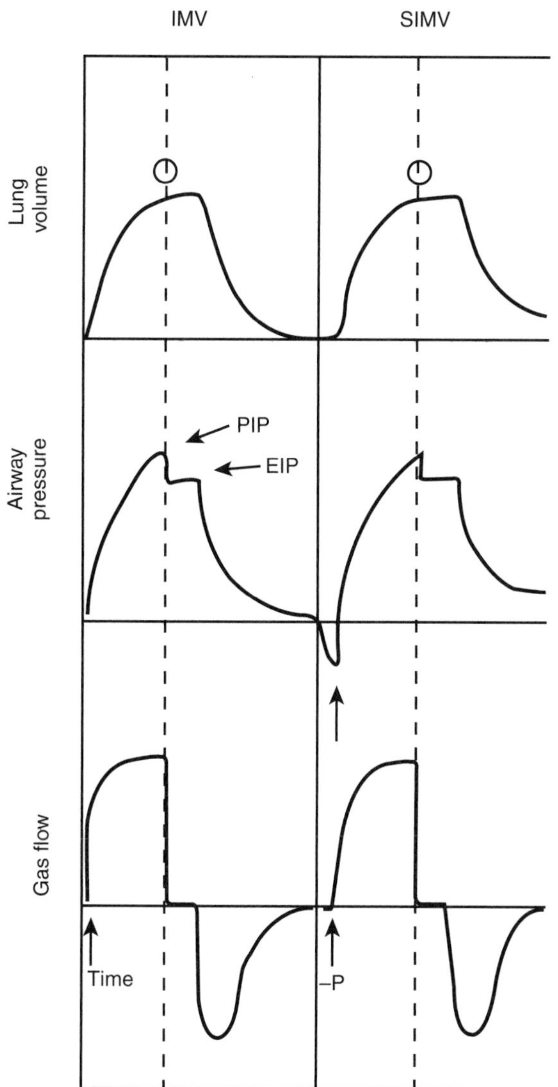

Figure 7-12. Pressure, volume, and flow waveforms observed during intermittent mandatory ventilation (IMV) and synchronized IMV (SIMV). In this case, an end-inspiratory pause has been added. Note the difference between peak (PIP) and end-inspiratory (EIP) or plateau pressure. *Arrows*, triggering variables; *open circles*, cycling variables. (Adapted from Bartlett RH: Use of the Mechanical Ventilator: Surgery. New York, Scientific American, 1988.)

VSV is enhanced because less need occurs for manual changes to maintain stable tidal and minute volume during weaning.[56] Both VSV and PSV are equally effective at weaning infants and children from the ventilator.[57]

Volume-Assured Pressure Support Ventilation

Volume-assured pressure support ventilation (VAPSV) attempts to combine volume- and pressure-controlled ventilation to ensure a desired VT within the constraints of the pressure limit. It has the advantage of maintaining inflation to a point below an injurious PIP level while maintaining VT constant in the face of changing pulmonary mechanics. Work of breathing may be markedly decreased while Ceff is increased during VAPSV.[58]

Proportional Assist Ventilation

Proportional assist ventilation (PAV) is an intriguing approach to the support of the spontaneously breathing patient. It relies on the concept that the combined pressure generated by the ventilator (Paw) and respiratory muscles (Pmus) is equivalent to that required to overcome the resistance to flow of the endotracheal tube/airways (Pres) and the tendency for the inflated lungs to collapse.[59]

With PAV, airway pressure generation by the ventilator is proportional at any instant to the respiratory effort (Pmus) generated by the patient. Small efforts, therefore, result in small breaths, whereas greater patient effort results in development of a greater VT. Inspiration is patient triggered and terminates with discontinuation of patient effort. Rate, VT, and inspiratory time are entirely patient controlled. The predominant variable to be set on the ventilator is the proportional response between Pmus and the applied ventilator pressure. This proportional assist (Paw/Pmus) can be increased until nearly all patient effort is provided by the ventilator.[60] Patient work of breathing, dyspnea, and PIP are reduced.[61,62] Elastance and resistance are set, as is applied PEEP. VT is variable, and risk of atelectasis may be present. PAV produces similar gas exchange with lower airway pressures when compared with conventional ventilation in infants.[63] Compared with preterm newborns being ventilated with the assist-control mode and with IMV, preterm newborns managed with PAV maintained gas exchange with lower airway pressures and a decrease in the oxygenation index by 28%.[64] Chest wall dynamics also are enhanced.[65] PAV represents an exciting first step in servoregulating ventilators to patient requirements.

Continuous Positive Airway Pressure

During continuous positive airway pressure (CPAP), pressures greater than those of ambient pressure are continuously applied to the airways to enhance alveolar distention and oxygenation.[66] Both airway resistance and work of breathing may be substantially reduced. However, because no support of ventilation is provided, this mode requires that the patient provide all of the work of breathing. This mode should be avoided in patients with hypovolemia, untreated pneumothorax, lung hyperinflation, or elevated intracranial pressure and in infants with nasal obstruction, cleft palate, tracheoesophageal fistula, or untreated congenital diaphragmatic hernia. CPAP is frequently applied via nasal prongs, although it can be delivered in adult patients with a nasal mask.

Inverse Ratio Ventilation

In the setting of respiratory failure, it would be helpful to enhance alveolar distention to reduce hypoxemia and shunt. One means to accomplish this is to maintain the inspiratory plateau pressure for a longer proportion of the breath.[67] The inspiratory time may be prolonged to the point at which the I/E ratio may be as high as 4:1.[68] In most circumstances, however, the I/E ratio is maintained at approximately 2:1. Inverse ratio ventilation (IRV) is usually performed during pressure-controlled ventilation (PC-IRV), although prolonged inspiratory times can be applied during volume-controlled ventilation by adding a decelerating flow pattern or an end-inspiratory pause to the volume-controlled ventilator breath.[69] One advantage of IRV is the ability to recruit alveoli that are associated with high-resistance airways that inflate only with prolonged application of positive pressure.[70] Unfortunately, IRV is associated with a profound sense of dyspnea in patients who are awake and spontaneously breathing. Therefore, heavy sedation and pharmacologic paralysis is required during this ventilator mode.

Because ET is reduced, the risk for incomplete expiration, identified by the failure to achieve zero-flow conditions at end expiration, is increased. This results in "auto-PEEP" or a total PEEP greater than that of the preset or applied PEEP. Care should be taken to recognize the presence of auto-PEEP and to incorporate it into the ventilation strategy to avoid barotrauma.[71] IRV also may negatively affect cardiac output and, therefore, decrease DO_2.[72] Some studies using IRV revealed an increase in Paw and oxygenation while protecting the lungs by reducing PIP.[73-76] Likewise, others suggest that early implementation of IRV in severe ARDS enhances oxygenation and allows reduction in FIO_2, PEEP, and PIP.[77] On the contrary, a number of studies have failed to demonstrate enhanced gas exchange with this mode of ventilation. Some series have suggested that IRV is less effective at enhancing gas exchange than is application of PEEP to maintain the same mean airway pressure.[78] Overall, it appears that oxygenation is determined primarily by the mean airway pressure rather than specifically by the application of IRV. As such, the usefulness of IRV remains in question.[79] Continuous monitoring of the $S\bar{V}O_2$ may aid in determining whether the addition of IRV has enhanced DO_2.

Airway Pressure Release Ventilation

Airway pressure release ventilation (APRV) is a unique approach to ventilation in which CPAP at high levels is used to enhance mean alveolar volume while intermittent reductions in pressure to a "release" level provide a period of expiration (Fig. 7-13). Re-establishment of CPAP results in inspiration and return of lung volume back to the baseline level. The advantage of APRV is a reduction in PIP of approximately 50% in adult patients with ARDS when compared with other more conventional modes of mechanical ventilation.[80,81] Spontaneous ventilation also is allowed throughout the cycle, which may enhance cardiac function and renal blood flow.[82,83] Some data suggest that $\dot{V}/\dot{Q}$ matching may be improved and dead space reduced.[84,85] In performing APRV, tidal volume is altered by adjusting the release pressure. Conceptually, ventilator management during APRV is the inverse of other modes of positive-pressure

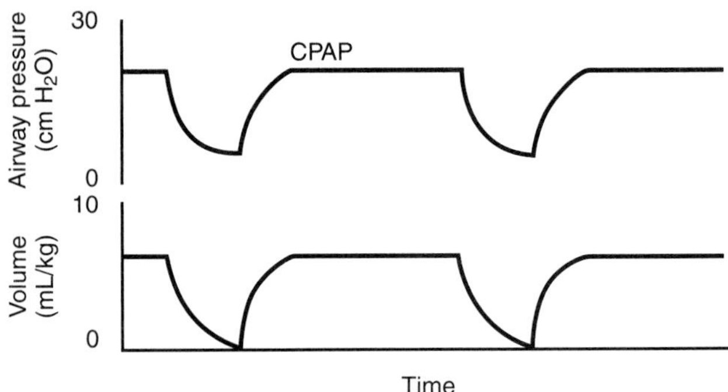

Figure 7-13. Typical pressure and volume waveforms observed during airway pressure release ventilation (APRV).

ventilation in that the PIP, or CPAP, determines oxygenation, while the expiratory pressure (release pressure) is used to adjust VT and CO_2 elimination. APRV is very similar to modes of ventilation, such as IRV, that use prolonged I/E ratios. However, APRV appears to be better tolerated when compared with IRV in patients with acute lung injury/ARDS, as demonstrated by a reduced need for paralysis and sedation, increased cardiac performance, decreased pressor use, and decreased PIP requirements.[86] The clinical experience with APRV is limited in the pediatric population.[87,88]

Bilevel Control of Positive Airway Pressure (BiPAP)

Although sometimes used in the setting of acute lung injury, BiPAP is frequently used for home respiratory support by varying airway pressure between one of two settings: the inspiratory positive airway pressure (IPAP) and the expiratory positive airway pressure (EPAP).[89,90] With patient effort, a change in flow is detected, and the IPAP pressure level is developed. With reduced flow at end expiration, EPAP is re-established. This device, therefore, provides both ventilatory support and airway distention during the expiratory phase. However, BiPAP ventilators should be used only to support the patient who is spontaneously breathing.

Monitoring during Mechanical Ventilation

Current mechanical ventilators incorporate highly accurate solid-state pressure transducers that provide data on a variety of pressures and gas flows. Volume is not measured directly. Instead, flow is integrated over time in the determination of volume. Ventilators can also calculate and display a variety of pressure/volume, flow/volume, or volume/pressure waveforms as well as demonstrate volume, flow, and pressure over time. Low-pressure alarms are present to detect disconnection and leaks and are set at approximately 10 cm H_2O below the anticipated PIP. High-pressure alarms are set approximately 10 cm H_2O above PIP to avoid incidental application of excessive pressure to the lungs. Apnea alarms typically are triggered if VT is not delivered for more than 10 seconds. Alarms for numerous other parameters such as PEEP, low VT, low and high rate, and low and high FIO_2 may be adjusted on various ventilators. Most ventilators also have an indicator that notifies the operator if the ventilator settings result in an I/E ratio that is greater than 1:1.

In the setting of respiratory insufficiency, mechanical ventilation should be used in conjunction with invasive monitoring such as systemic arterial, central venous, and pulmonary arterial catheters, as well as pulse oximetry and end-tidal CO_2 monitoring. Technology that allows frequent blood gas sampling without blood loss is now available for newborns and infants. It is likely that ventilators in the future will incorporate $S\bar{V}O_2$ or $Sc\bar{V}O_2$, SaO_2, and oxygen consumption data in determining online cardiac output and DO_2 values to help guide management.[91] As online blood gas monitoring becomes more accurate, FIO_2, rate, PIP, and PEEP will be servoregulated on the basis of SaO_2, $S\bar{V}O_2$, and $PaCO_2$ values.

Management of the Mechanical Ventilator

IMV and SIMV may suffice for patients with normal lungs, such as when needed after an operation.[92] If a patient is spontaneously breathing and is to be ventilated for more than a brief period, a flow- or pressure-triggered assist mode, pressure support, or PAV will result in maximal support and minimal work of breathing.[48,49] Ventilator modes that allow adjustment of specific details of pressure, flow, and volume are required in the patient with severe respiratory failure. With all these modes, the ventilator rate, VT or PIP, PEEP, and either inspiratory time alone or I/E ratio (if ventilation is pressure limited) must be assigned. Other secondary controls such as the flow rate, the flow pattern, the trigger sensitivity for assisted breaths, the inspiratory hold, the termination sensitivity, and the safety pressure limit also are set on individual ventilators. The normal $\dot{V}E$ is 100 to 150 mL/kg/min. The FIO_2 is usually initiated at 0.50 and decreased based on pulse oximetry. All efforts should be made to maintain the FIO_2 less than 0.60 to avoid alveolar nitrogen depletion and the development of atelectasis.[93,94] Oxygen toxicity likely is a result of this phenomenon, although free oxygen radical formation may play a role when an FIO_2 greater than 0.40 is applied for prolonged periods.[95] A short inspiratory phase with a low I/E ratio favors the expiratory phase and CO_2 elimination, whereas longer I/E ratios enhance oxygenation. In the normal lung, I/E ratios of 1:3 and inspiratory time of 0.5 to 1 second are typical.

Strategies in Respiratory Failure

Preventing Ventilator- Induced Lung Injury

A decrease in pulmonary compliance and FRC is seen in the patient with acute lung injury (PaO_2/FIO_2 ratio, 200-300) or ARDS (PaO_2/FIO_2 ratio, < 200). This is secondary to alveolar collapse and a decrease in the volume of lung available for ventilation and, in turn, to decreased pulmonary compliance. As a result, higher ventilator pressures are necessary to maintain VT and $\dot{V}E$. However, any attempt to ventilate the patient with respiratory insufficiency due to parenchymal disease with higher pressures can result in compromise of cardiopulmonary function and the development of ventilator-induced lung injury.[96]

The concept of ventilator-induced lung injury was first demonstrated in 1974 by demonstrating the detrimental effects of ventilation at PIP of 45 cm H_2O in rats.[97] Electron microscopy has been used to document an increased incidence of alveolar stress fractures in ex-vivo, perfused rabbit lungs exposed to transalveolar pressures more than 30 cm H_2O (Fig. 7-14).[98] Other studies have demonstrated increases in albumin leak, elevation of the capillary leak coefficient, enhanced wet-to-dry lung weight, deterioration in gas exchange, and augmented diffuse alveolar damage on histology with application of increased airway pressure (45 to 50 cm H_2O) in otherwise normal rats and sheep over a 1- to 24-hour period.[31,99,100] Pulmonary exposure to high pressures may potentially worsen nascent respiratory insufficiency and, ultimately, lead to the development of pulmonary fibrosis.

Such injury may be prevented during application of high PIPs by strapping the chest, thereby preventing lung overdistention, suggesting that alveolar distention or "volutrauma" is the injurious element, rather than application of high pressures or "barotrauma."[101] A low-VT (6 mL/kg) approach to mechanical ventilation in rabbits with *Pseudomonas aeruginosa*-induced acute lung injury appears to be associated with enhancement in oxygenation, increase in pH, increase in arterial blood pressure, and decrease in extravascular lung water when compared with a high-VT group (15 mL/kg).[102] A relation may also exist between ventilator gas flow rate and the development of lung injury.[103] Positive blood cultures have been seen in five of six animals exposed to high end-inspiratory pressure but rarely in those with low end-inspiratory pressure.[104]

Together, these data suggest that the method of ventilation has an effect on lung function and gas exchange as well as a systemic effect, which may include translocation of bacteria from the lungs. As such, avoidance of high PIPs and lung overdistention should be a primary goal of mechanical ventilation. Although the animal data would suggest that high PIPs and volumes may be deleterious, two multicenter studies have attempted to randomize patients with ARDS to high and low peak pressure or volume strategies. The first failed to demonstrate a difference in mortality or duration of mechanical ventilation in patients randomized to either the low-volume (7.2 ± 0.8 mL/kg) or the high-volume (10.8 ± 1.0 mL) strategy, although the applied PIP was not elevated to what would commonly be considered injurious levels in either group (low, 23.6 ± 5.8 cm H_2O; high, 34.0 ± 11.0 cm H_2O).[105] Another study revealed similar results but had similar design limitations.[106] A survival increase from 38% to 71% at 28 days, a higher

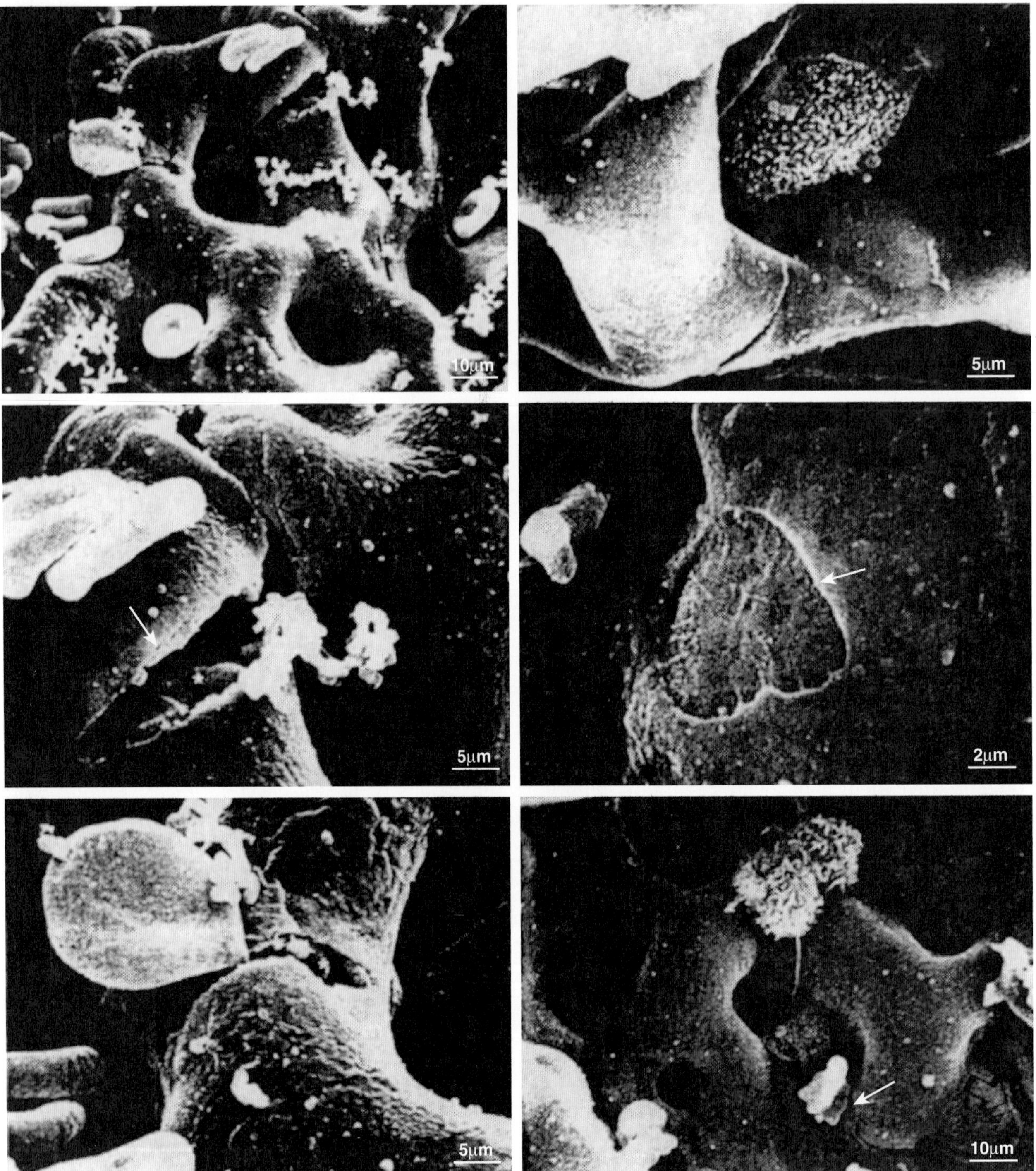

Figure 7-14. Scanning electron micrographs demonstrating disruptions in the blood-gas barriers (*arrows*) in rabbit lungs subjected to 20 cm H_2O airway pressure and 75 cm H_2O pulmonary arterial pressure. (Reprinted with permission from Fu Z, Costello ML, Tsukimoto K, et al: High lung volume increases stress failure in pulmonary capillaries. J Appl Physiol 73:123-133, 1992.)

rate of weaning from mechanical ventilation, and a lower rate of barotrauma has been demonstrated in patients in whom a lung-protective ventilator strategy was used. This strategy consisted of lung distention to a level that prevented alveolar collapse during expiration (see later) and avoidance of high distending pressures.[107] One study identified a significant reduction over time in bronchoalveolar lavage concentrations of polymorphonuclear cells ($P < .001$), interleukin (IL)-1β ($P < .05$), tumor necrosis factor (TNF)-α ($P < .001$), interleukin (IL)-8 ($P < .001$), and IL-6 ($P < .005$) and in plasma concentration of IL-6 ($P < .002$) among 44 patients randomized to receive a lung-protective strategy rather than a conventional approach.[108] The mean number of ventilator-free days at 28 days in the lung-protective strategy group was higher than in the control group (12 ± 11 vs. 4 ± 8 days, respectively; $P < .01$). Mortality rates at 28 days from

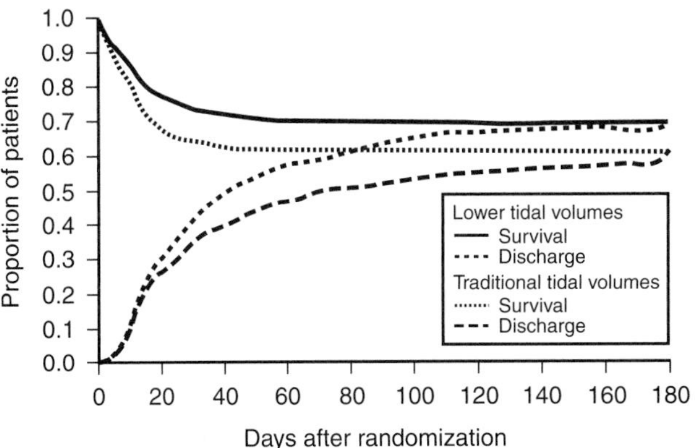

Figure 7-15. Probability of survival and of being discharged home and breathing without assistance during the first 180 days after randomization in patients with acute lung injury and the acute respiratory distress syndrome. The status at 180 days or at the end of the study was known for all but nine patients. (From The Acute Respiratory Distress Network: Ventilation with lower tidal volumes as compared with traditional tidal volumes for acute lung injury and the acute respiratory distress syndrome. N Engl J Med 342:1301-1308, 2000.)

admission were 38% and 58% in the lung-protective strategy and control groups, respectively (P = .19).

The NIH's Acute Respiratory Distress Network convincingly demonstrated that mortality was reduced with the use of a low-volume (6 mL/kg, mortality of 31%) when compared with a high-volume (12 mL/kg, mortality of 39%; P = 0.005) ventilator approach (Fig. 7-15).[109] Interestingly, no difference was found in gas exchange or pulmonary mechanics between groups to account for the difference in mortality. However, IL-6 levels and the incidence of organ failure were increased in the high-volume group when compared with the low-volume group. Similarly, multisystem organ failure scores increased significantly 72 hours after admission only in patients who were ventilated with a conventional rather than a lung-protective strategy, with renal failure being the most prevalent organ dysfunction.[110] Statistically significant correlations were noted between changes in overall multisystem organ failure score and changes in plasma concentration of inflammatory mediators, including IL-6, TNF-α, IL-1β, and IL-8. A significant correlation was also seen between the IL-6 level and the number of failing organs. Exposure of neutrophils (PMNs) to bronchoalveolar lavage fluid from a control group of ARDS patients resulted in increased PMN activation as compared with those exposed to bronchoalveolar lavage fluid from a group of patients managed with a lung-protective strategy.[111] The majority of clinicians are now convinced that avoidance of high PIP and support of lung recruitment, through the application of appropriate levels of PEEP (see later), should be a primary goal of any mechanical ventilatory program.

Permissive Hypercapnia

To avoid ventilator-induced lung injury, practitioners have applied the concept of permissive hypercapnia. With this approach, $Paco_2$ is allowed to increase to levels as high as 120 mm Hg as long as the blood pH is maintained in the 7.1 to 7.2 range by administration of buffers.[112] Mortality was reduced to 26% when compared with that expected (53%; $P < .004$) based on Acute Physiology and Chronic Health Evaluation II (APACHE II) scores when low-volume, pressure-limited ventilation with permissive hypercapnia was applied in the setting of ARDS in adults.[113] For burned children, the mortality rate was only 3.7% despite a high degree of inhalation injury when a ventilator strategy used a PIP of 40 cm H_2O and accepted an elevated $Paco_2$ as long as the arterial pH was greater than 7.20.[114] Other studies suggested that a strategy of high-frequency (40 to 120 breaths/min) ventilation with a low VT, low PIP, high PEEP (7 to 30 cm H_2O), and mild hypercapnia ($Paco_2$ from 45 to 60 mm Hg) enhances the survival rate in children with severe ARDS.[115]

Using Protective Effects of PEEP

Although application of high, overdistending airway pressures appears to be associated with the development of lung injury, a number of studies have demonstrated that application of PEEP or high-frequency oscillatory ventilation (HFOV) may allow avoidance of lung injury by the following mechanisms: (1) recruitment of collapsed alveoli, which reduces the risk for overdistention of healthy units; (2) resolution of alveolar collapse, which in and of itself is injurious; and (3) avoidance of the shear forces associated with the opening and closing of alveoli.[116,117] In the older child with injured lungs, a pressure of 8 to 12 cm H_2O is required to open alveoli and to begin VT generation.[107,118,119] Alveoli will subsequently close unless the end-expiratory pressure is maintained at such pressures, and cyclic opening and closing is thought to be particularly injurious because of application of large shear forces.[118] One way to avoid this process is through the application of PEEP to a point above the inflection pressure (Pflex), such that alveolar distention is maintained throughout the ventilatory cycle (Fig. 7-16).[120,121] In addition, as mentioned previously, it has been demonstrated that the distribution of infiltrates and atelectasis in the supine patient with ARDS is predominantly in the dependent regions of the lung.[122] This is likely the result of compression due to the increased weight of the overlying edematous lung. It has been shown that when the superimposed gravitational pressure from the weight of the overlying lung exceeded the PEEP applied to a given region of the lung, end-expiratory lung collapse increased, resulting in de-recruitment.[123] Thus, application of PEEP may result in recruitment of these atelectatic lung regions, simultaneously enhancing pulmonary compliance and oxygenation. PEEP and prone positioning (see later) are more effective if the need for ventilation is of extrapulmonary etiology rather than pulmonary etiology.[124]

As a result of these new data and concepts, the approach to mechanical ventilation in the patient with respiratory failure has changed drastically over

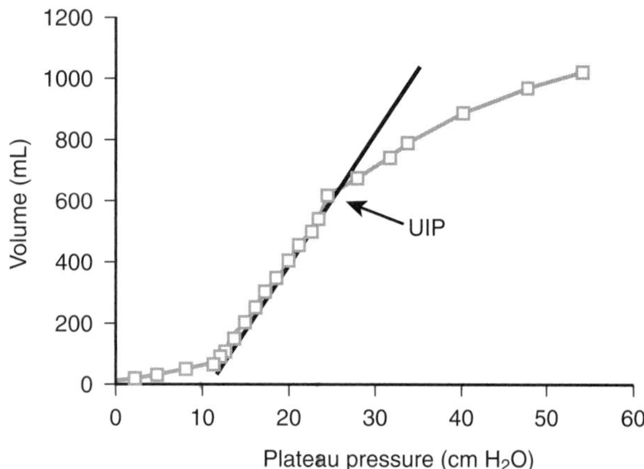

Figure 7-16. Static pressure/volume curve demonstrating the Pflex point in a patient with acute respiratory distress syndrome. Positive end-expiratory pressure should be maintained approximately 2 cm H_2O above that point. The upper inflection point (UIP) indicates the point at which lung overdistention is beginning to occur. Ventilation to points above the UIP should be avoided in most circumstances. (Reprinted from Roupie E, Dambrosio M, Servillo G: Titration of tidal volume and induced hypercapnia in acute respiratory distress syndrome. Am J Respir Crit Care Med 152:121-128, 1995.)

the past few years (Table 7-3). Time-cycled, pressure-controlled ventilation has become favored because of the ability to limit EIP to noninjurious levels at a maximum of 35 cm H_2O.[119] In infants and newborns, this EIP limit is set lower at 30 cm H_2O. The VT should be maintained in the range of 6 mL/kg.[109] A lung-protective approach also incorporates lung distention and prevention of alveolar closure. Pressure/volume curves should be developed on each patient at least daily, so that the Pflex can be identified and the PEEP maintained above Pflex. If a pressure/volume curve cannot be determined, then Pflex can be assumed to be in the 7- to 12-cm H_2O range, and PEEP, at that level or up to 2 cm H_2O higher, can be applied.[119,125,126] Recruitment maneuvers that use intermittent sustained

Table 7-3	Current Favored Approaches to the Treatment of ARDS
Pressure-limited ventilation	
VT ≈ 6 mL/kg	
IRV	
EIP < 35 cm H_2O	
PEEP > Pflex or > 12 cm H_2O	
Permissive hypercapnia	
$FIO_2 \le 0.06$	
$S\bar{v}O_2 \ge 65\%$	
$SaO_2 \ge$ 80%-85%	
Transfusion to hemoglobin > 13 g/dL	
Diuresis to dry weight	
Prone positioning	
Extracorporeal support	

ARDS, acute respiratory distress syndrome; VT, tidal volume; IRV, inverse ratio ventilation; EIP, end-inspiratory pressure.

inflations of approximately 40 cm H_2O for up to 40 seconds often can be beneficial by initially inflating collapsed lung regions.[127] The inflation obtained with the recruitment maneuver is then sustained by maintaining PEEP greater than Pflex.

As both PIP and PEEP are increased, enhancements in compliance and reductions in VD/VT and shunt are to be expected. If they are not observed, then one should suspect the presence of overdistention of currently inflated alveoli instead of the desired recruitment of collapsed lung units. Application of increased levels of PEEP also may result in a decrease in venous return and cardiac output. In addition, West's zone I physiology, which predicts diminished or absent pulmonary capillary flow in the nondependent regions of the lungs at end inspiration, may be exacerbated with application of higher airway pressures. This may be especially detrimental, because it is the nondependent regions that are best inflated and to which one would wish to direct as much pulmonary blood flow as possible.[15] As a result, parameters of DO_2 should be carefully monitored during application of increased PEEP.[128] One approach for monitoring delivery is by applying close attention to the $S\bar{v}O_2$ whenever the PEEP is increased to more than 5 cm H_2O. As mentioned, increasing the PEEP gradually in increments of 2.5 cm H_2O can be done until the desired level of oxygenation or lung protection is achieved or a decrease in $S\bar{v}O_2$ to below the maximum is observed. Effective lung compliance also should be monitored to ensure that alveolar recruitment is being achieved.

If oxygenation remains inadequate with application of higher levels of PEEP, FIO_2 should be increased to maintain SaO_2 greater than 90%, although levels as low as 80% may be acceptable in patients with adequate DO_2. As mentioned previously, one of the most effective ways to enhance DO_2 is with transfusion. All attempts should be made to avoid the atelectasis and oxygen toxicity associated with FIO_2 levels greater than 0.60.[93] Extending FIO_2 to levels more than 0.60 often has little effect on oxygenation, because severe respiratory failure is frequently associated with a large transpulmonary shunt. If inadequate DO_2 persists, a trial increase in PEEP level should be performed or institution of extracorporeal support considered.[129] Inflation of the lungs also can be enhanced by prolonging the inspiratory time by PC-IRV. Pharmacologic paralysis and sedation are required during performance of PC-IRV, although paralysis may have the additional benefit of decreasing oxygen consumption and enhancing ventilator efficiency.[35] PaO_2 may improve with application of PC-IRV.[130,131] Monitoring the effect on DO_2 and $S\bar{v}O_2$ is critical, however, to ensure the benefit of this intervention. The advantages of the alveolar inflation associated with a decelerating flow waveform during pressure-limited modes of ventilation also should be used.[41]

Prone Positioning

Altering the patient from the supine to the prone position appears to enhance gas exchange (Fig. 7-17).[132,133] Enhanced blood flow to the better-inflated

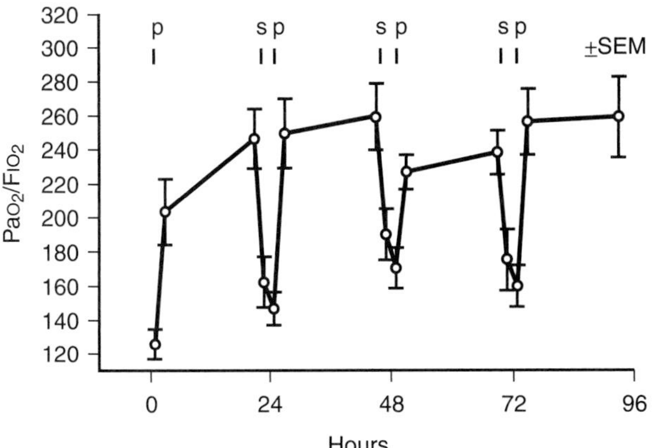

Figure 7-17. Pao_2 during supine (s) and prone (p) positioning. Note the increase in oxygenation when trauma patients with acute respiratory distress syndrome are in the prone position and a general trend toward increased Pao_2 with each return to the supine position. (Reprinted from Fridrich P, Krafft P, Hochleuthner H, Mauritz W: The effects of long-term prone positioning in patients with trauma-induced acute respiratory distress syndrome. Anesth Analg 83:1206-1211, 1996.)

anterior lung regions with the prone position would logically appear to account for the increase in oxygenation. However, data in oleic acid lung-injured sheep suggest that the enhancement in gas exchange may be due predominantly to more homogeneous distribution of ventilation, rather than to redistribution of pulmonary blood flow, because lung distention is more uniform in the prone position.[134-136] This effect may be reversed after a number of hours. Enhanced posterior region lung inflation frequently accounts for persistent increases in oxygenation when the patient is returned to the supine position. Therefore, benefit may be seen when the prone and supine positions are alternated, usually every 4 to 6 hours.[122] A randomized, controlled, multicenter trial evaluating the effectiveness of the prone position in the treatment of patients with ARDS was recently completed.[137] The prone group was placed in the prone position for 6 or more hours daily for 10 days while the control group remained in the supine position. Although the Pao_2/Fio_2 ratio was greater in the prone when compared with the supine group (prone, 63.0 + 66.8, vs. supine, 44.6 + 68.2; $P = 0.02$), no difference in mortality was noted between groups. It is clear that some patients will not respond to altered positioning, in which case this adjunct should be discontinued. Meticulous attention to careful patient padding and avoidance of dislodgement of tubes and catheters is of the utmost importance in successful implementation of this approach.

Adjunctive Maneuvers

Another means for enhancing oxygenation may be through administration of diuretics and the associated reduction of left atrial and pulmonary capillary hydrostatic pressure.[138] Diuresis results in a decrease in lung interstitial edema. In addition, reduction of lung edema decreases compression of the underlying dependent lung.[139] Collapsed dependent lung regions are thereby recruited. Although this treatment approach has not been proved in randomized clinical trials, reduction in total body fluid in adult patients with ARDS appears to be associated with an increase in survival.[140] One must be cognizant of the risks of hypoperfusion and organ system failure, especially renal insufficiency, if overly aggressive diuresis is performed. Overall, however, a strategy of fluid restriction and diuresis should be pursued in the setting of ARDS, while monitoring organ perfusion and renal function.[141] In a randomized trial, a conservative fluid management strategy improved the oxygenation index, the lung injury score, the ventilator-free days, and the number of days spent out of the intensive care unit while the prevalence of shock and dialysis use did not increase.[142] Although the study was limited to 60 days, the results further support keeping a patient with acute lung injury in a state of fluid balance.

Applying noninjurious PIPs and enhancing PEEP levels limits the ΔP (the amplitude between the PIP and the PEEP) and VT and compromises CO_2 elimination. Therefore, the concept of permissive hypercapnia, which was discussed previously, is integral to the successful application of lung-protective strategies. $Paco_2$ levels greater than 100 mm Hg have been allowed with this approach, although most practitioners prefer to maintain the $Paco_2$ at less than 60 to 70 mm Hg.[113] Bicarbonate or tris(hydroxymethyl)aminomethane (THAM) may be used to induce a metabolic alkalosis to maintain the pH at greater than 7.20. Few significant physiologic effects are observed with elevated $Paco_2$ levels as long as the pH is maintained at reasonable levels.[143] If adequate CO_2 elimination cannot be achieved while limiting EIP to noninjurious levels, then initiation of extracorporeal life support (ECLS) should be considered.

The one situation in which it may be acceptable to increase EIP to levels greater than 35 cm H_2O (30 cm H_2O in the infant and newborn) is in the patient with reduced chest wall compliance and relatively normal pulmonary compliance. Because pulmonary compliance is a combination of lung compliance and chest wall compliance, a decrease in chest wall compliance, such as due to abdominal distention, obesity, or chest wall edema, can markedly reduce pulmonary compliance despite reasonable lung compliance. This situation is analogous to studies discussed previously in which the lungs remain uninjured despite application of high airway pressures because the chest is strapped to prevent lung overdistention.[101] This is a frequent problem in secondary respiratory failure due to trauma, sepsis, and other frequent disease processes observed among surgical patients, including tightly placed dressings. A cautious increase in EIP in such patients may be warranted. Finally, a simple intervention, such as raising the head of the bed, may have marked effects on FRC and gas exchange in such patients.

Weaning from Mechanical Ventilation

Once a patient is spontaneously breathing and able to protect the airway, consideration should be given to weaning from ventilator support. Weaning in the majority of children should take 2 days or less.[144] The FIO_2 should be decreased to less than 0.40 before extubation. Simultaneously, PEEP should be lowered to 5 cm H_2O. The pressure support mode of ventilation is an efficient means for weaning because the preset inspiratory pressure can be gradually decreased while partial support is provided for each breath.[145] Adequate gas exchange with a pressure support of 7 to 10 cm H_2O above PEEP in adults and newborns is predictive of successful extubation.[146] Another study in adults demonstrated that simple transition from full ventilator support to a "T-piece," in which oxygen flow-by is provided, is as effective at weaning as is gradual reduction in rate during IMV or pressure during PSV.[147] In all circumstances, brief trials of spontaneous breathing before extubation should be performed with flow-by oxygen and CPAP. Prophylactic dexamethasone administration does not appear to increase the odds of a successful trial in infants, except in "high risk" patients who receive multiple doses starting at least 4 hours before extubation.[148,149] Parameters during a T-piece trial that indicate readiness for extubation include the following: (1) maintenance of the pretrial respiratory and heart rates; (2) inspiratory force greater than 20 cm H_2O; (3) $\dot{V}E$ less than 100 mL/kg/min; and (4) SaO_2 greater than 95%. If the patient's status is in question, transcutaneous CO_2 monitoring, along with arterial blood gas analysis ($PaCO_2 < 40$ mm Hg; $PaO_2 > 60$ mm Hg), may help to ascertain whether extubation is appropriate. The weaning trial should be brief. Under no circumstances should it last longer than 1 hour, because the narrow endotracheal tube provides substantial resistance to spontaneous ventilation. In most cases, the patient who tolerates spontaneous breathing through an endotracheal tube for only a few minutes will demonstrate enhanced capabilities once the tube is removed.

Frequent causes of failed extubation include persistent pulmonary parenchymal disease, interstitial fibrosis, and reduced breathing endurance. Pressure support ventilation is ideal for use in the difficult-to-wean patient because it allows gradual application of spontaneous support to enhance respiratory strength and conditioning (Table 7-4).[145] Enteral and parenteral nutrition should be adjusted to maintain the total caloric intake to no more than 10% above the estimated caloric needs of the patient. Excess calories will be converted to fat, with a high respiratory quotient and increased CO_2 production. Nutritional support high in glucose will have a similar effect.[149] Manipulation of feedings along with treatment of sepsis may reduce VCO_2 and enhance weaning. Pulmonary edema should be treated with diuretics. Some patients will benefit from a tracheostomy to avoid ongoing upper airway contamination, to decrease dead space and airway resistance, and to provide airway access for evacuation of secretions during the weaning process. In addition, the issue of "extubating" the patient is removed by tracheostomy tube placement. Spontaneous breathing trials, therefore, are easy to perform, and the transition from the mechanical ventilator is a much smoother and efficient process.[150] Tracheostomy in older patients can be performed by percutaneous means at the bedside.[151] Long-term complications are fairly minimal in older patients. However, in newborns and infants, the rate of development of stenoses and granulation tissue may be significant.[152,153]

Table 7-4	Management of the Patient for Whom Extubation Attempts Have Failed
Frequent spontaneous breathing trials	
Pressure support ventilation	
Caloric intake ≤10% above expenditure	
Minimize carbohydrate calories	
Diuresis to dry weight	
Treat infection	
Tracheostomy	

NONCONVENTIONAL MODES AND ADJUNCTS TO MECHANICAL VENTILATION

High-Frequency Ventilation

The concept of high-frequency jet ventilation (HFJV) was developed in the early 1970s to provide gas exchange during procedures performed on the trachea. HFJV uses small bursts of gas through a small "jet port" in the endotracheal tube typically at a rate of 420 breaths/min, with the range being 240 to 660 breaths/min.[154] The expiratory phase is passive.[155] The VT is adjusted by controlling the PIP, which is usually initiated at 90% of conventional PIP. CO_2 removal is most affected by the ΔP. Therefore, an increase in the PIP or a decrease in the PEEP will result in enhanced CO_2 elimination. Adjusting the Paw, PEEP, and FIO_2 alters oxygenation. HFJV is typically superimposed on background conventional VT mechanical ventilation.

The utilization of HFJV has decreased in favor of high-frequency oscillatory ventilation (HFOV), which uses a piston pump–driven diaphragm and delivers small volumes at frequencies between 3 and 15 Hz.[154] Both inspiration and expiration are active. Oxygenation is manipulated by adjusting Paw, which controls lung inflation similar to the role of PEEP in conventional mechanical ventilation. CO_2 elimination is controlled by manipulating the tidal volume, also known as the amplitude or power. In short, only four variables are adjusted during HFOV:

1. Mean airway pressure (Paw) is typically initiated at a level 1 to 2 cm H_2O higher in premature newborns and 2 to 4 cm H_2O higher in term newborns and children than that used during conventional mechanical ventilation.[155] For most disease processes, Paw is adjusted thereafter to maintain the right hemidiaphragm at the rib 8 to 9 level on the anteroposterior chest radiograph.
2. Frequency (Hz) is usually set at 12 Hz in premature newborns and 10 Hz in term patients. Lowering the frequency tends to result in an increase in VT and a decrease in $PaCO_2$.

3. Inspiratory time, which may be increased to enhance tidal volume, is usually set at 33%.
4. Amplitude or power (ΔP) is set to achieve good chest wall movement and adequate CO_2 elimination.

Gas exchange during high-frequency ventilation is thought to occur by convection involving those alveoli located close to airways. For the remaining alveoli, gas exchange occurs by streaming, a phenomenon in which inspiratory gas, which has a parabolic profile, tends to flow down the center of the airways whereas the expiratory flow, which has a square profile, takes place at the periphery (Fig. 7-18).[157] Other effects may play a role: (1) pendelluft, in which gas exchange takes place between lung units with different time constants, as some are filling while others are emptying; (2) the movement of the heart itself may enhance mixing of gases in distal airways; (3) Taylor dispersion, in which convective flow and diffusion together function to enhance distribution of gas; and (4) local diffusion.[158]

High-frequency ventilation should be applied to the newborn and pediatric patient for whom conventional ventilation is failing, because of either parameters of oxygenation or CO_2 elimination. The advantage of high-frequency ventilation lies in the alveolar distention and recruitment that is provided while limiting exposure to potentially injurious high ventilator pressures.[159] Thus, the approach during high-frequency ventilation should be to apply a mean airway pressure that will effectively recruit alveoli and maintain oxygenation while limiting the ΔP to that which will provide chest wall movement and adequate CO_2 elimination. CO_2 elimination at lower peak inspiratory pressures may be a specific advantage in patients with air leak, especially those with bronchopleural fistulas.[160] Once again, the effect on DO_2, rather than simply PaO_2, should be considered.

Although some studies with HFOV in preterm newborns suggested that the incidence of bronchopulmonary dysplasia was similar to that in the conventional ventilation group and that adverse effects were noted on intraventricular hemorrhage and periventricular leukomalacia, other trials noted an increase in the rescue rate and a reduction in bronchopulmonary dysplasia in this population.[161-165] One multicenter, randomized trial revealed that 56% of preterm newborns managed with HFOV were alive without the need for supplemental oxygen at 36 weeks postmenstrual age as compared with 47% of those receiving conventional ventilation ($P = .046$).[166] In an additional pilot study, those preterm infants managed with HFOV were extubated earlier and had decreased supplemental oxygen requirements.[167] Thus, although mixed, the data would suggest a reduction in pulmonary morbidity with the use of HFOV when compared with conventional ventilation.

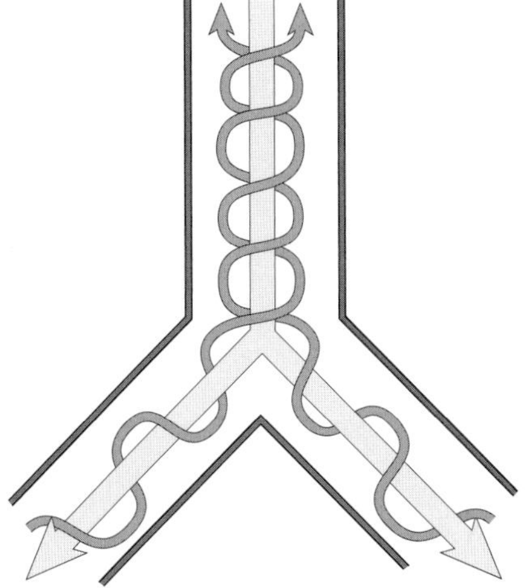

Figure 7-18. Streaming as a mechanism of gas exchange during high-frequency ventilation. Note that the parabolic wavefront of the inspiratory gas induces central flow in the airways, whereas expiratory gas flows at the periphery.

In term newborns and pediatric patients with respiratory insufficiency, studies suggest that the rescue rate and survival in those treated with HFOV is significantly increased when compared with conventional mechanical ventilation.[168-170] In a randomized controlled trial of HFOV and inspired (inhaled) nitrous oxide (iNO) in pediatric ARDS, HFOV with or without iNO resulted in greater improvement in the PAO_2/FIO_2 ratio than did conventional mechanical ventilation.[171] However, in contrast, one randomized controlled trial in term newborns failed to identify a significant difference in outcome between these treatment modalities.[172] In fact, a Cochrane Database review of randomized clinical trials comparing the use of HFOV versus conventional ventilation failed to show any clear advantage in the elective use of HFOV as a primary modality in the treatment of premature infants with acute pulmonary dysfunction.[173] Reductions in oxygenation index and FIO_2 were observed during HFOV in 17 adult patients with ARDS.[174] A multicenter, randomized, controlled trial of HFOV for adults with ARDS demonstrated a nonsignificant trend toward improved 30-day mortality in the HFOV group when compared with the conventional ventilation group (37% vs. 52%, respectively; $P = .102$).[175]

Intratracheal Pulmonary Ventilation or Tracheal Gas Insufflation

Intratracheal pulmonary ventilation (ITPV) involves infusion of fresh gas (oxygen) into the trachea via a cannula placed at the tip of the endotracheal tube. This gas flow effectively replaces the central airway dead space with fresh oxygen during the expiratory phase of the ventilatory cycle and functions to reduce dead space, which augments CO_2 elimination. For this purpose, a special "reverse thruster catheter" (RTC) was developed for gas insufflation that reverses the flow of gas at the tip such that it follows a retrograde path up the endotracheal tube (Fig. 7-19).[176] The catheter, which entrains gas, produces a Venturi effect and provides for more effective dead space reduction during expiration. ITPV has been shown to maintain reasonable levels of ventilation in normal animals at PIPs one half to one third of those required during conventional mechanical ventilation.

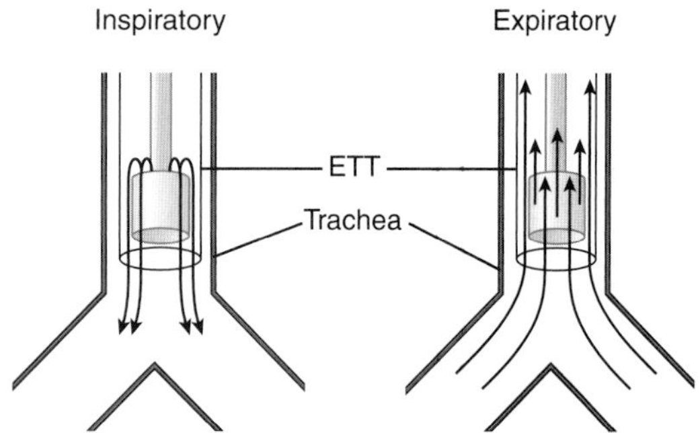

Figure 7-19. The reverse-thruster catheter used in performance of intratracheal pulmonary ventilation (ITPV). During inspiration, the exhalation valve on the ventilator closes, and gas flows prograde, filling the lung with a tidal volume of oxygen gas. During expiration, the gas flows retrograde, entraining and replacing the gas in the airways, thereby reducing dead space and $Paco_2$. (Reprinted with permission from Wilson JM, Thompson JR, Schnitzer JJ, et al: Intratracheal pulmonary ventilation and congenital diaphragmatic hernia: A review of two cases. J Pediatr Surg 28:484-487, 1993.)

This same group also demonstrated the ability to maintain adequate levels of CO_2 during ITPV, but not during CMV, in lambs in whom only 12.5% of the lung parenchyma remained available for gas exchange.[177] Others have demonstrated that PIPs could be reduced from 28.3 cm H_2O on CMV to 10.3 cm H_2O during ITPV (P = .028) in term lambs while maintaining gas exchange.[178] In the same study, initiation of ITPV in lambs resulted in a decrease in PIP from 44 to 32 cm H_2O (P = .002), with a simultaneous decrease in $Paco_2$ from 52.2 to 31.9 mm Hg (P = .029). This same group also demonstrated that initiation of ITPV in newborn lambs with congenital diaphragmatic hernia led to a decrease in $Paco_2$ from 110 ± 21 to 52 ± 24 (P = .0014).[179] The concept of reducing dead space by replacing upper airway gas during the expiratory phase also was applied by using a simple catheter, rather than the RTC, and has been termed *tracheal gas insufflation*.[42,180]

Clinical studies have demonstrated the ability of ITPV to reduce airway dead space and therefore the ventilator pressures required to achieve equivalent rates of CO_2 elimination when compared with those observed during conventional mechanical ventilation in adult patients with ARDS, pediatric patients on venoarterial ECLS, and newborns with congenital diaphragmatic hernia after ECLS.[181-183] Tracheal gas insufflation was compared with conventional ventilation in a randomized, controlled trial in preterm newborns: PIP and PEEP were lower, while generating the same $Paco_2$, and the time to extubation also was reduced.[184] In adult patients with ARDS, tracheal gas insufflation allowed a reduction in PIP without an increase in $Paco_2$.[185]

Inhaled Nitric Oxide Administration

Nitric oxide (NO) is an endogenous mediator that serves to stimulate guanylate cyclase in the endothelial cell to produce cyclic guanosine monophosphate (cGMP), which results in relaxation of vascular smooth muscle (Fig. 7-20).[186] NO is rapidly scavenged by heme moieties. Therefore, inhaled nitric oxide (iNO) serves as a selective vasodilator of the pulmonary circulation but is inactivated before reaching the systemic circulation. Diluted in nitrogen and then mixed with blended oxygen and air, iNO is administered in doses of 1 to 80 parts per million (ppm).

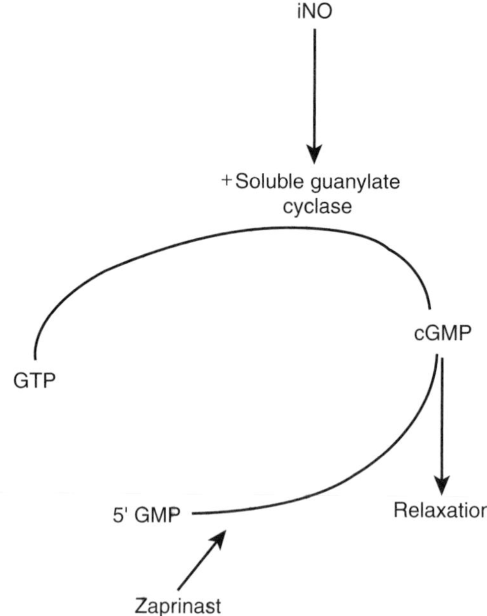

Figure 7-20. Mechanism of action of inhaled nitrous oxide (iNO) in inducing vascular smooth muscle relaxation. Zaprinast is a phosphodiesterase inhibitor that may increase the potency and duration of the effect of iNO. GTP, guanosine triphosphate; cGMP, cyclic guanosine monophosphate. (Reprinted from Hirschl RB: Innovative therapies in the management of newborns with congenital diaphragmatic hernia. Semin Pediatr Surg 5:255-265, 1996.)

Initial studies in adults with ARDS who were treated with iNO demonstrated a decrease in pulmonary vascular resistance and an increase in Pao_2, without change in systemic arterial pressure. In addition, a prospective, multicenter randomized trial of iNO in 177 adults with ARDS demonstrated a significant improvement in oxygenation compared with placebo over the first 4 hours of treatment (Pao_2 increase = 20%: iNO, 60%; CMV, 24%; P = .00002).[187-189] The initial increase in oxygenation translated to a reduction in Fio_2 over the first day and in the intensity of mechanical ventilation over the first 4 days of treatment. However, no differences were observed between the pooled iNO groups and placebo groups with respect to mortality rate and number of days alive and off mechanical ventilation. A subgroup of patients who received iNO at a dose of 5 ppm showed an improvement in the number of patients alive and off mechanical ventilation at day 28 (62% vs. 44%; P < .05). In another randomized, controlled trial in adults, iNO increased Pao_2/Fio_2 at 1 hour and 12 hours.[190] Beyond 24 hours, the two groups demonstrated an equivalent improvement in Pao_2/Fio_2. Pediatric patients with respiratory failure demonstrate increases in Pao_2 with iNO at 20 ppm.[191]

Unfortunately, a prospective, randomized, controlled trial investigating the effects of iNO therapy in children with respiratory failure revealed that although pulmonary vascular resistance and systemic oxygenation were acutely improved at 1 hour by administration of 10 ppm iNO, a sustained improvement at 24 hours was not identified.[192]

Only 40% of the iNO-treated term infants with pulmonary hypertension required ECLS when compared with 71% of the control subjects.[193] These results were corroborated by demonstrating a reduction in the need for ECLS in control newborns (ECLS, 64%) when compared with iNO-treated newborns (ECLS, 38%; $P = 0.001$).[194] The incidence of chronic lung disease was decreased in newborns managed with iNO (7% vs. 20%). Similar results were noted for infants with persistent pulmonary hypertension of the newborn (PPHN) who were on HFOV. The need for ECLS was decreased from 55% in the control HFOV group to 14% in the combined iNO and HFOV group ($P = .007$).[195] In a clinical trial conducted by the Neonatal Inhaled Nitric Oxide Study (NINOS) Group, neonates born at 34 weeks or older gestational age with hypoxic respiratory failure were randomized to receive 20 ppm iNO or 100% oxygen as a control.[196] If a complete response, defined as an increase in PaO_2 of more than 20 mm Hg within 30 minutes after gas initiation, was not observed, then iNO at 80 ppm was administered. Sixty-four percent of the control group and 46% of the iNO group died within 120 days or were treated with ECLS ($P = .006$). No difference in death was found between the two groups (iNO, 14% vs. control, 17%), but significantly fewer neonates in the iNO group required ECLS (39% vs. 54%). Follow-up at age 18 to 24 months failed to demonstrate a difference in the incidence of cerebral palsy, rate of sensorineural hearing loss, and mental developmental index scores between the control and iNO patients.[197] Other studies have similarly failed to identify a difference in pulmonary, neurologic, cognitive, or behavioral outcomes between survivors managed with iNO and those in the conventional group.[198]

An associated, but separate, trial demonstrated no difference in death rates and a significant increase in the need for ECLS when neonates with congenital disphragmatic hernia (CDH) were treated with 20 or 80 ppm of iNO versus 100% oxygen as control.[199] It should be noted, however, that some investigators have suggested that the efficacy of iNO in patients with CDH may be more substantial after surfactant administration or at the point at which recurrent pulmonary hypertension occurs.[200] iNO administration also may be helpful in the moribund CDH patient until ECLS can be initiated.

Some concern has been expressed for the development of intracranial hemorrhage in premature newborns treated with iNO. More than a 25% increase in the arterial/alveolar oxygen ratio (PaO_2/PAO_2) was observed in 10 of 11 premature newborns, with a mean gestational age of 29.8 weeks and severe RDS, in response to administration of 1 to 20 ppm iNO. However, in 7 of these 11 newborns, intracranial hemorrhage developed during their hospitalization.[201] Also, a meta-analysis of the three completed studies evaluating the efficacy of iNO in premature newborns suggests no significant difference in survival, incidence of chronic lung disease, or rate of development of intracranial hemorrhage between iNO and control patients.[202]

NO is associated with the production of potentially toxic metabolites. When combined with O_2, iNO produces peroxynitrates, which can be damaging to epithelial cells and also can inhibit surfactant function.[203,204] Nitrogen dioxide, which is toxic, also can be produced, and hemoglobin may be oxidized to methemoglobin. Additional concerns exist about the immunosuppressive effects and the potential for platelet dysfunction.

Surfactant Replacement Therapy

The use of exogenous surfactant has been responsible for a 30% to 40% reduction in the odds of death among very low birth weight newborns with RDS (Fig. 7-21).[205,206] In addition, in those premature neonates with birth weight more than 1250 g, mortality in a controlled, randomized, blinded study decreased from 7% to 4%.[207] Two general forms of surfactant are available: synthetic surfactant (e.g., Exosurf; Burroughs Wellcome, Raleigh-Durham, NC), which is made of dipalmytoyl phosphatidylcholine and is protein free; and natural surfactant (e.g., Survanta; Ross Laboratories, Columbus, OH; or Infasurf; ONY, Inc., Amherst, NY), which contains bovine surfactant extracts and associated proteins. Studies reveal

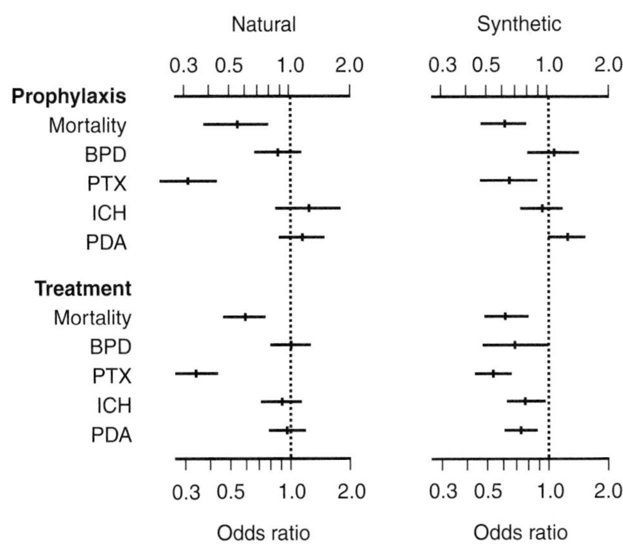

Figure 7-21. A meta-analysis of studies evaluating the outcome and complications of the prophylactic use and treatment approach to exogenous natural and synthetic surfactant administration in preterm newborns. BPD, bronchopulmonary dysplasia; PTX, pneumothorax; ICH, intracranial hemorrhage; PDA, patent ductus arteriosus. (Adapted from Jobe AH: Pulmonary surfactant therapy. N Engl J Med 328:861-868, 1993.)

a significantly lower risk of chronic lung disease in Survanta (27%), when compared with Exosurf (34%) infants with birth weights of 1001 to 1500 g.[208] Compared with Exosurf, Infasurf treatment results in a 62% decrease in the incidence of RDS (Infasurf, 16%, vs. Exosurf, 42%) and a 70% decrease in death due to RDS (Infasurf, 1.7%, vs. Exosurf, 5.4%).[209] On the other hand, intraventricular hemorrhage occurs more frequently in Infasurf-treated infants (Infasurf, 39.0%, vs. Exosurf, 29.9%). Another natural surfactant, porcine-derived poractant alfa (Curosurf; Chiesi Farmaceutici, Italy) has been shown to improve oxygenation more rapidly when compared with beractant (Survanta).[210]

A randomized, prospective, controlled trial in term newborns with respiratory insufficiency demonstrated that the need for extracorporeal membrane oxygenation (ECMO) was significantly reduced in those managed with surfactant when compared with placebo.[211] The benefit of surfactant was greatest in those with a lower oxygenation index (< 23). Another controlled, randomized study demonstrated the utility of surfactant in term newborns with the meconium aspiration syndrome.[212] The oxygen index minimally decreased with the initial dose but markedly decreased with the second and third doses of surfactant from a baseline of 23.7 to 5.9 (Fig. 7-22). After three doses of surfactant, PPHN had resolved in all but one of the infants in the study group versus none of the infants in the control group. The incidence of air leaks and need for ECLS were markedly reduced in the surfactant group compared with the control patients.

Studies have concluded that surfactant phospholipid concentration, synthesis, and kinetics are not significantly deranged in infants with CDH compared with controls, although surfactant protein A concentrations may be reduced in CDH newborns on ECMO.[213-215] Animal and human studies have suggested that surfactant administration before the first breath is associated with enhancement in Pao_2 and pulmonary mechanics.[216,217] However, among CDH patients on ECLS, no difference between those randomized to receive surfactant (n = 9) and those control patients receiving air (n = 8) was noted in terms of lung compliance, time to extubation, period of oxygen requirement, and the total number of hospital days.[213]

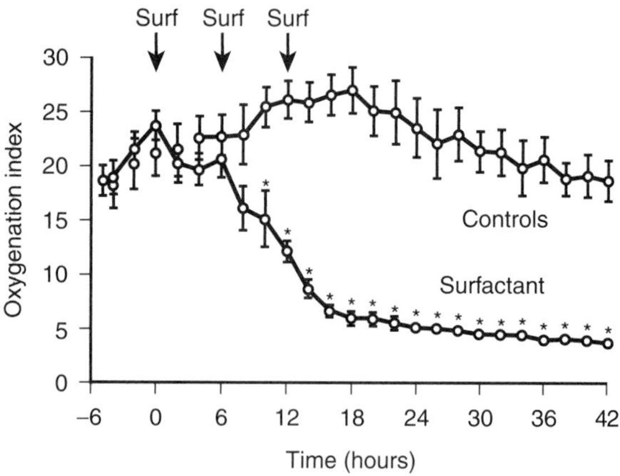

Figure 7-22. The effect of exogenous surfactant administration on oxygen index in term newborns with meconium-aspiration syndrome. (Reprinted from Findlay RD, Taeusch HW, Walther FJ: Surfactant replacement therapy for meconium aspiration syndrome. Pediatrics 97:48-52, 1996.)

Liquid Ventilation with Perfluorocarbon

Perfluorocarbons are clear, colorless, odorless, relatively dense fluids (1.9 g/mL) with relatively low surface tension (19 din/cm) that carry large amounts of oxygen (50 mL O_2/dL) and carbon dioxide (210 mL CO_2/dL).[218] Liquid ventilation has been performed by one of two methods[219]: (1) total liquid ventilation (TLV), in which the lungs are filled with perfluorocarbon to a volume equivalent of FRC, on which a device is used to generate tidal volumes of perfluorocarbon in the perfluorocarbon-filled lung[220]; and (2) administration of intratracheal perfluorocarbon to a volume equivalent of FRC followed by standard gas mechanical ventilation of the perfluorocarbon-filled lung, otherwise known as partial liquid ventilation (PLV).[221] The former technique appears to be somewhat more effective at enhancing gas exchange, whereas the latter technique is more easily generalized to critical care clinicians managing patients with severe respiratory insufficiency.

A number of studies have demonstrated the efficacy of PLV in enhancing gas exchange in animal models of respiratory insufficiency.[222-225] It appears that intratracheal administration of perfluorocarbon acts as a surrogate surfactant, recruits atelectatic lung regions, and redistributes pulmonary blood flow toward the better-ventilated, nondependent regions of the lungs in the patient with ARDS.[226] Of great interest is the demonstration of enhanced gas exchange with aerosolized perfluorocarbon in saline-lavaged, surfactant-depleted piglets. Pao_2 was higher and $Paco_2$ lower in the PLV and aerosolized perfluorocarbon group compared with that in the standard mechanical-ventilation animals.[227] The response was sustained even after discontinuation of aerosolization but not standard PLV. A number of phase I and II clinical studies have demonstrated the efficacy of PLV in enhancing oxygenation and pulmonary mechanics in adults, children, and newborns with respiratory insufficiency, including those with CDH and those who are premature.[228-231] Studies in pediatric and adult patients have demonstrated decreases in the (A-a)Do_2 from approximately 450 to 250 mm Hg within the first 48 hours after initiation of PLV.[232] Prospective, controlled, randomized pilot studies evaluating the safety and efficacy of PLV in adult and pediatric patients with respiratory insufficiency have shown no differences between the PLV and CMV groups since a surprisingly low mortality of 20% among the pediatric patients with isolated respiratory failure prohibited successful completion of the study, which was subsequently discontinued. Among adult patients with acute lung injury or ARDS, no differences in ventilatory pulmonary mechanics, gas-exchange parameters, or survival were noted between the PLV (n = 65) and CMV (n = 25) patients.[233] In May 2001, the results of a multicenter, prospective randomized study comparing PLV and CMV in adults with ARDS revealed no significant difference in mortality or 28-day ventilator-free days in the PLV compared with the CMV group.[234] Although PLV may be further evaluated in subgroups of adult and pediatric patients with respiratory failure, it is unlikely that PLV will play a general role in the treatment of adult or pediatric ARDS.

Premature newborns in whom surfactant therapy fails demonstrate a twofold increase in mean pulmonary compliance and a decrease in mean oxygen index from approximately 50 to 10 over the 24-hour period after initiation of PLV, although a pilot randomized study failed to reveal increased survival in the PLV compared with the CMV group.[235] Likewise, a prospective, randomized, controlled pilot trial evaluating PLV in term newborns with respiratory failure did not demonstrate an increase in survival in the PLV group compared with the CMV patients.

Studies have demonstrated the ability of in-utero tracheal ligation to correct the structural and physiologic effects of pulmonary hypoplasia in the sheep fetus with CDH.[236,237] The ability to induce lung growth has been demonstrated by distention of the isolated right upper lobe in newborn sheep with perflubron (LiquiVent; Alliance Pharmaceutical Corp., San Diego, CA) to a pressure of 7 to 10 mm Hg.[238] An increase in size and alveolar number in the right upper lobe was noted, while maintaining the air-space fraction and the protein/DNA ratio. The alveolar/arterial ratio was unchanged compared with that in the nondistended control animals. This technique of perfluorocarbon-induced lung growth (PILG) would apply to patients with CDH who required ECLS. The use of PILG demonstrated radiologic evidence of an increase in ipsilateral lung size in those patients managed with PILG (Fig. 7-23).[239] A randomized, prospective, controlled pilot study demonstrated encouraging survival rates in six (75%) of eight PILG-treated CDH patients on ECLS compared with two (40%) of five conventionally treated patients on ECLS.[240]

In 1989, the first report of the use of TLV in humans was published.[238,241] Three moribund, preterm newborns, for whom surfactant therapy had failed, were managed with TLV. Pulmonary compliance increased during the period of TLV. However, the gas-exchange response was variable, though for the first time the ability to sustain gas exchange during TLV in humans was demonstrated. A multicenter study of TLV in pediatric models of ARDS demonstrated increased oxygenation and pulmonary function with enhancement in cardiac output and decrease in histologic parameters of lung injury in the TLV group.[242] Although not yet effectively tested in the clinical setting, these data suggest that TLV may play a significant role in lavaging, re-inflating, and ventilating injured lungs.

VENTILATOR-ASSOCIATED PNEUMONIA

Ventilator- associated pneumonia (VAP), diagnosed at 48 hours or later on mechanical ventilation, is the second most common hospital-acquired infection in the neonatal (NICU) and pediatric (PICU) intensive care units. Occurring in 3% to 10% of all ventilated PICU patients and 6% to 32% of NICU patients, VAP results in higher mean lengths of ICU stay, increased mortality rates, and increased hospital costs.[243,244] Controversies exist on the definition, treatment, and prevention of VAP. Finally, many studies do not incorporate the pediatric population and therefore cannot be blindly applied to all patients.

Definitions for VAP differ for infants 1 year or younger (Table 7-5), children between 1 and 12 years old (Table 7-6), and those older than 12 years of age (Table 7-7). In all patients, mechanical ventilation must be present for more than 48 hours.[243,245] Microbial confirmation is not necessary for the NNIS/CDC criteria defined in the tables, and the use of quantitative cultures for diagnosis in children and neonates is variable. The technique of fiberoptic bronchoalveolar lavage (BAL) has been described in children but is not routinely used. Blind BAL findings of a bacterial index (defined as the $\log_{10}$ of the colony-forming units of microorganisms per milliliter of BAL fluid) greater than 5 are the most reliable method for diagnosing VAP in mechanically ventilated children and should be used most often.[246]

Investigations on the treatment of VAP focus on empirical use of antibiotics and duration of therapy. Broad-spectrum, early empirical antibiotics, when appropriately chosen, have been shown to decrease mortality in adults, but overuse can increase antibiotic resistance.[247,248] Risk factors for multidrug-resistant pathogens in pediatric patients include younger age, increasing pediatric risk of mortality score, previous PICU admissions, exposure to household contacts hospitalized over the past year, intravenous antibiotic use in the past 12 months, and exposure to chronic care facilities.[249,250] Once final cultures are available, it is important to de-escalate therapy to prevent overuse of antibiotics and the breeding of multidrug-resistant organisms. The question of optimal duration of therapy in adults was addressed using a multicenter, randomized, controlled trial comparing 8 days of antibiotic therapy versus 15 days. There was no difference in the mortality rates. Patients infected with nonfermenting gram-negative bacilli, however, benefited from the longer duration of therapy with a reduced relapse rate. Finally, patients treated for 8 days also had a reduced incidence of multidrug-resistant pathogens on relapse when compared with those treated for 15 days.[251]

Guidelines for the prevention of VAP have been established based on current evidence by the VAP Guidelines Committee and the Canadian Critical Care Trials Group.[244] Recommended therapeutic interventions include orotracheal route of intubation, a

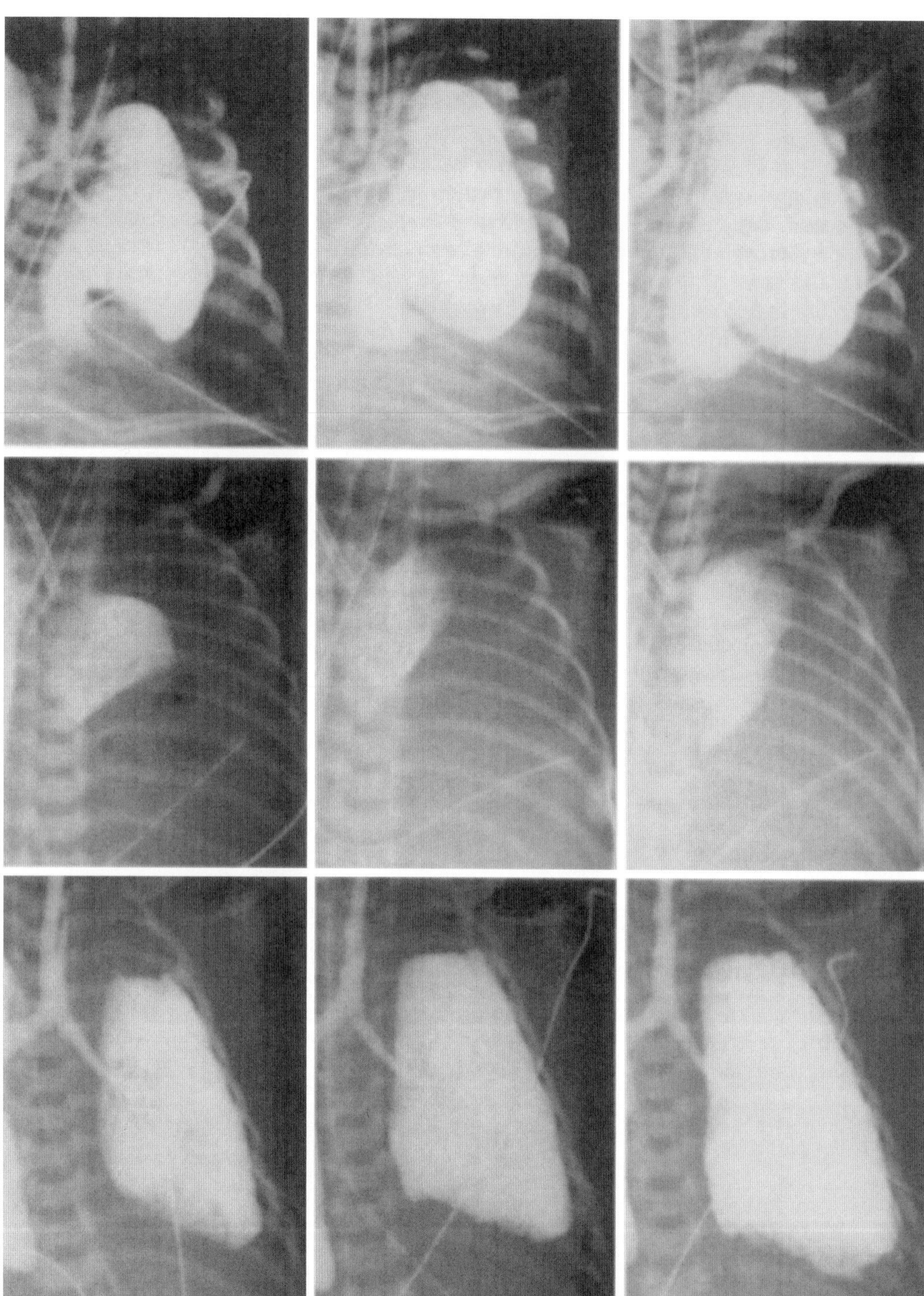

Figure 7-23. Progression of the distended lungs ipsilateral to the hernia with time (the perfluorocarbon is radiopaque) in the three patients who received 7 days of pulmonary distention with perfluorocarbon. Notice the evident increase in lung size, which was not observed in the contralateral lungs. (Reprinted with permission from Fauza DO, Hirschl RB, Wilson JM: Continuous intrapulmonary distension with perfluorocarbon accelerates lung growth in infants with congenital diaphragmatic hernia: Initial experience. J Pediatr Surg 36:1237-1240, 2001.)

Table 7-5 NNIS/CDC Criteria for Diagnosis of Ventilator-Associated Pneumonia in Infants 1 Year or Younger

Worsening gas exchange (oxygen desaturations, increased oxygen requirements, or increased ventilator demand) and three of the following:
Temperature instability with no other recognized cause
New onset of purulent sputum, change in character of sputum, increased respiratory secretions, or increased suctioning requirements
Apnea, tachypnea, nasal flaring with retraction of chest wall, or grunting
Wheezing, rales, or rhonchi
Cough
Bradycardia (< 100 beats/min) or tachycardia (> 170 beats/min)

From NNIS/CDC—National Nosocomial Infections Surveillance System/Centers for Disease Control.

Table 7-6 NNIS/CDC Criteria for Diagnosis of Ventilator-Associated Pneumonia in Children between Ages 1 and 12 Years

Three of the following:
Fever (>38.4°C) or hypothermia (<37°C) with no other recognized cause
Leukopenia (<4,000 white blood cells/mm^3) or leukocytosis (≥15,000 white blood cells/mm^3)
New onset of purulent sputum, change in character of sputum, increased respiratory secretions, or increased suctioning requirements
Rales or bronchial breath sounds
Worsening gas exchange (O_2 desaturations [pulse oximetry < 94%], increased oxygen requirements, or increased ventilation demand)

From NNIS/CDC—National Nosocomial Infections Surveillance System/Centers for Disease Control.

Table 7-7 NNIS/CDC Criteria for Diagnosis of Ventilator-Associated Pneumonia in Children Older Than 12 Years

One of the following:
Fever (>38°C) with no other recognized cause
Leukopenia (<4,000 white blood cells/mm^3) or leukocytosis (≥12,000 white blood cells/mm^3)
Two of the following:
New onset of purulent sputum, change in character of sputum, increased respiratory secretions, or increased suctioning requirements
New onset of worsening cough, dyspnea, or tachypnea
Rales or bronchial breath sounds
Worsening gas exchange ($PaO_2/FIO_2 \leq 240$, increased oxygen requirements, or increased ventilation demand)
Two or more abnormal chest radiographs (can be one if no pulmonary or cardiac disease) with one of the following:
New or progressive and persistent infiltrate
Consolidation
Cavitation
Pneumatoceles (in infants ≤1 year)

From NNIS/CDC—National Nosocomial Infections Surveillance System/Centers for Disease Control.

ventilator circuit specific for each patient, circuit changes if soiled or damaged but no scheduled changes, change of heat and moisture exchangers every 5 to 7 days or as indicated, use of closed endotracheal suctioning system changed for each patient and as clinically indicated, subglottic secretion drainage in patients expected to be mechanically ventilated for more than 72 hours, and the head of bed elevated at 45 degrees when possible. Consideration should be given to the use of rotating beds and oral antiseptic rinses.[252] Finally, in adult patients, a team approach and implementation of a VAP bundle encompassing all the evidence-based guidelines has successfully improved outcomes.[253]

chapter 8

VASCULAR ACCESS

Ravindra K. Vegunta, MBBS

One of the well-recognized challenges in providing medical care for infants and children is access to the vascular system. Pediatric surgeons are frequently called to provide vascular access in various settings and for a variety of indications. The most commonly used device for venous access in children is a peripheral intravenous (PIV) cannula. In adults, achieving venous access is often accomplished with minimal distress. However, in children, placement of an intravenous catheter can be quite traumatic to the child, the parents, and the attendant health care providers. In some situations it can be a fairly frustrating and time-consuming procedure.[1] In an emergency, alternative means of vascular access should be sought relatively quickly. Particular circumstances of each child may demand specific solutions for vascular access, namely, the choice of device and site chosen for its placement (see Table 8-1 for indications for vascular access and the respective device choices). It is imperative that one is aware of the limitations and potential adverse effects of the various vascular access devices (VADs) that are available. Unfortunately, practitioners often persist with a PIV cannula for a long time instead of committing to a higher level of access early. This reluctance is seen in all clinical settings, such as the emergency department, operating room, neonatal intensive care unit (NICU), and other patient care units. For example, a child may stay on low osmolar and inadequate intravenous nutrition through a PIV cannula instead of total parenteral nutrition (TPN) through a central vascular device. In an emergency, one should move on to other options promptly after a few failed attempts at PIV cannula placement. In the past, the options were a venous cutdown or an emergency central venous catheter (CVC) placement. These methods take considerable time and frequently require the availability of a pediatric surgeon. Over the past several years, intraosseous (IO) needle placement has become the most common contingency method of emergency vascular access in children (Fig. 8-1). The newer mechanical devices have allowed easier training of emergency medical personnel and improved the success rate of IO placement in the prehospital setting. In fact, with appropriate training, an IO needle can be placed more quickly than a PIV cannula.[2] Umbilical vessels are frequently used in sick neonates but can only be used for a finite period—maximum of 5 days for an umbilical artery catheter (UAC) and 14 days for an umbilical venous catheter (UVC).[3] Early placement of a peripherally introduced central venous catheter (PICC) is preferable in these infants. Persistence with using PIV cannulas leads to higher complication rates and reduces the number of future PICC placement sites. Local availability and policies of home health care personnel should be considered in deciding if a CVC or PICC would be more appropriate for home antibiotic therapy or home parenteral nutrition therapy that is indicated for a medium term (a few weeks). In choosing the appropriate VAD for an oncology patient, the requirements of the oncologist, the patient's age, expected activity level, expected chance of cure, number of previous VADs placed, and patency of the central veins all should be considered. The number of lumens, size of the catheter, type of catheter, and its location can all be tailored to the specific patient. Long-term maintenance of central venous access in patients suffering from intestinal malabsorption is particularly challenging. Once the six conventional sites of central venous access—bilateral internal jugular, subclavian, and femoral veins—are exhausted, one must become more creative in gaining central access.

Complications that are common to all types of VADs are extravasation of infusate, hemorrhage, phlebitis, septicemia, thrombosis, and thromboembolism. Prevention is the best way to manage these complications. Careful placement, with the use of ultrasound and/or fluoroscopic guidance as appropriate, can save time and reduce injury to adjacent structures. Maximal sterile barrier precautions are recommended during placement of the lines to reduce colonization and bloodstream infection rates.[4,5] Good stabilization will prevent dislodgement of the catheters and/or flipping of subcutaneous ports. Use of heparin-bonded catheters and heparin infusion have reduced the incidence of thrombosis of the veins while antibacterial-coated catheters are recommended for infection prevention.[4]

Table 8-1 Indications for Vascular Access in Infants and Children and the Recommended Devices

				CVC		
Indications	**PIV**	**PICC**	**IO**	*Non-tunneled*	*Tunneled*	*Subcutaneous Port*
Emergency venous access	X		X	X		
Short-term venous access	X			X		
Medium-term venous access	X	X		X		
Long-term venous access		X			X	X

PIV, peripheral intravenous catheter; PICC, peripherally introduced central venous catheter; IO, intraosseous needle; CVC, central venous catheter.

PERIPHERAL VENOUS ACCESS

As previously described, peripheral intravenous catheter placement is the most frequently used method of accessing the vascular compartment. Devices designed for this purpose are universally available, and the expertise needed for their placement is widely dispersed. Training new health care providers in these techniques is relatively straightforward. Nonetheless, obtaining PIV access in children in an emergency and in children who have had multiple previous intravenous catheters is particularly challenging.

In infants and children, PIV access is usually achieved by using the veins on the dorsum of the hand, forearm, dorsum of the foot, medial aspect of the ankle, and the scalp. In infants, the median vein tributaries on the ventral aspect of the distal forearm and wrist and the lateral tributaries of the dorsal venous arch on the dorsum of the foot may be available but typically admit only the finest-diameter catheters. The position of the distal long saphenous vein, anterior to the medial malleolus, is fairly constant and is frequently palpable, making it one of the most popular veins used for PIV access, particularly in infants. It allows a larger size catheter, and it is also possible to stabilize the catheter well. Several techniques have been shown to be beneficial in cannulating a peripheral vein, namely, warming the extremity, transillumination, and epidermal vasodilators.[6] Ultrasound guidance has been used to obtain access to basilic and brachial veins in the emergency department.[7] VeinViewer (Luminetx Corporation, Memphis, TN) is a device that is slowly gaining popularity based on near-infrared imaging and digital light processing technology.[8,9] It projects a real-time image of all the patent subcutaneous veins on the overlying skin. Unlike ultrasonography, there is no physical contact with the overlying skin and hence there is no compression or distortion of the veins. Scalp veins can be readily visible and accessible but tend to be difficult to maintain access for any length of time. Similarly, external jugular vein catheters tend to get dislodged promptly in a moving patient and may only be useful for a short time. Significant complications associated with PIV catheters include phlebitis, thrombosis, and extravasation with chemical burn or necrosis of surrounding soft tissue.

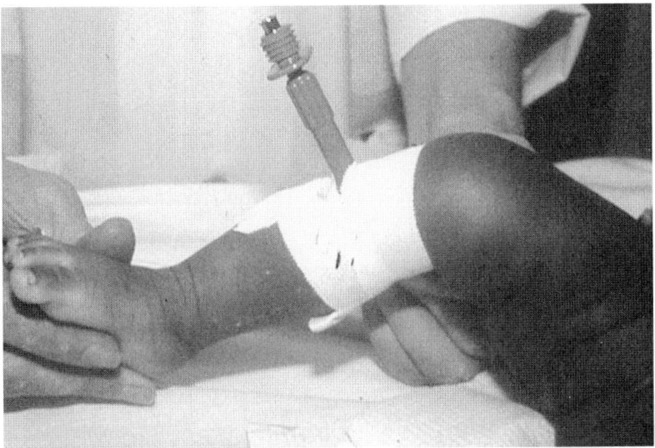

Figure 8-1. An intraosseous line has been inserted into the tibia of a young child for vascular access.

UMBILICAL VEIN AND ARTERY ACCESS

Sick neonates are often managed with catheters placed either in the umbilical vein (UVC) and/or one of the umbilical arteries (UAC). They are used for monitoring central venous or arterial pressure, blood sampling, fluid resuscitation, medication administration, and TPN. To minimize infectious complications, the UVCs are usually removed after a maximum of 14 days.[10] These catheters are typically placed by neonatal nurse practitioners or neonatologists by dissecting the umbilical cord stump within a few hours of birth. It is possible for the pediatric surgeon to cannulate the umbilical vessels after the umbilical stump has undergone early desiccation. A small vertical skin incision is made above or below the umbilical stump to access the umbilical vein or artery, respectively. Once the fascia is incised, the appropriate vessel is identified, isolated, and cannulated. The tip of the UVC is placed at the junction of the inferior vena cava (IVC) and the right atrium (RA).[11] The catheter is cut to reach the xiphisternum from the insertion site to locate the tip correctly. On the chest radiograph, the tip of the UVC should be above or at the level of the diaphragm. The tip of the UAC is positioned between the sixth and tenth thoracic vertebrae, cranial to the celiac axis (Fig. 8-2). Various calculations have been proposed to estimate the correct length of the catheter before insertion,

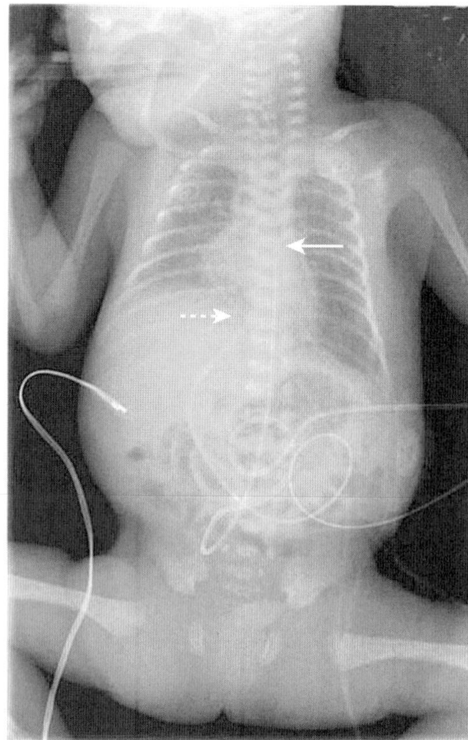

Figure 8-2. This abdominal and chest film in this newborn shows the UAC catheter at the level of the seventh vertebral body (*solid arrow*) and the umbilical venous catheter (*dotted arrow*) above the level of the diaphragm. These are the recommended positions for these catheters.

based on weight and other biometric measures of the infant.[12,13] The long-standing argument about the safety of a "high" versus "low" position for the UAC tip[14] has been laid to rest; the "high" position just described has been shown to be associated with a low incidence of clinically significant aortic thrombosis without any increase in other adverse sequelae.[15] Whereas the umbilical vessel catheters, without doubt, have saved many lives, they have also been associated with various complications. In addition to tip migration, sepsis, and thrombosis that are common to both, UVCs are associated with perforation of the IVC, extravasation of infusate into the peritoneal cavity, and portal vein thrombosis.[16] UACs are associated with aortic injuries, thromboembolism of aortic branches, aneurysms of the iliac artery and/or the aorta, paraplegia, and gluteal ischemia with possible necrosis.[11] Pooled rates of bloodstream infections associated with umbilical and CVCs in NICUs is reported to be 11.6 per 1000 catheter-days for premature infants with birth weight of less than 1000 g, 7.0 for infants weighing 1000 to 1500 g, and 4.0 for those weighing more than 2500 g.[17]

PERIPHERALLY INTRODUCED CENTRAL CATHETER

PICC lines provide a reliable central venous access in neonates and older children of all sizes without a need for directly accessing the central veins. Hence the potential for morbidity is low. PICC lines are suitable for infusion of fluids, medications, TPN, and blood products. They can be placed by specially trained registered nurses, advanced practice nurses, interventional radiologists, intensivists, and surgeons. Many institutions caring for sick children on a routine basis have developed special teams and protocols for placement of PICC lines to reduce variations in practice and increase availability.[18] Broadly, two techniques are used in the placement of PICC lines. The traditional technique involves placement of a relatively large cannula (about 19 gauge) in the vein of choice, through which the PICC is introduced. The technique that is currently most popular is the modified Seldinger technique. A regular small peripheral intravenous catheter (about 24 gauge) is first placed in a suitable extremity vein such as the basilic, cephalic, or long saphenous vein. A fine guide wire is advanced through this, the initial catheter is removed, the track is dilated, and the peel-away PICC introducer cannula is advanced over the guide wire. The guide wire is then removed, and the PICC line is introduced through the introducer (Fig. 8-3).[19] The tip of the PICC should be placed at the superior vena cava (SVC)/RA junction or the IVC/RA junction. Locations other than these are considered non-central and are associated with higher complications.[20] Lack of visible or palpable peripheral veins may necessitate use of ultrasound guidance to access a deeper vein such as the brachial vein. Accumulating evidence suggests that early placement of a PICC line is beneficial to the neonates compared with management with several peripheral venous catheters.[21,22] Delayed attempts

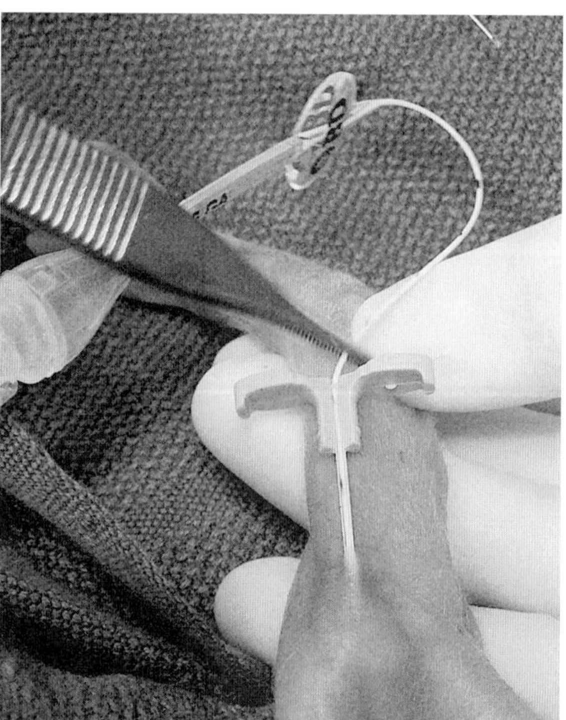

Figure 8-3. Placement of a PICC using the modified Seldinger technique described in the text. The axillary vein is being accessed in this premature infant.

at placement of a PICC line in these sick neonates may preclude its success because of lack of a suitable patent peripheral vein.[19] PICC lines are also eminently suitable for short- to medium-term (weeks) home intravenous therapy of antibiotic or parenteral nutrition.[23] The most common complications associated with PICC lines are infections, occlusion, and dislodgement of the catheter.[24] Symptomatic upper extremity venous thrombosis is seen as often as 7% in adults receiving chemotherapy through PICC lines versus 1% in those receiving no chemotherapy.[25]

CENTRAL VENOUS CATHETERS

Until recently, CVCs have been the mainstay of reliable central vascular access in children. With the development of PICC teams[18] and the increasing use of PICC lines, there has been a decline in the use of CVCs in neonates and older children. Non-tunneled CVCs are used for short- and medium-term indications, whereas surgically placed tunneled CVCs are used for medium- and long-term indications. In premature neonates, if PICC placement is not successful, tunneled CVCs are preferentially used because of their smaller size and durability as opposed to non-tunneled CVCs. The central veins accessed for placement of CVCs are the bilateral internal jugular veins, subclavian veins, and femoral veins. In older children and full-term neonates, the percutaneous Seldinger technique is used. In premature neonates and occasionally in older children, the relevant central vein or one of its tributaries, common facial vein[26] or external jugular vein in the neck, cephalic vein in the deltopectoral groove, or the long saphenous vein at the groin (Fig. 8-4)[27,28], is exposed surgically and cannulated directly. In the emergency situation, percutaneous femoral vein access is preferred because this area is away from all the other activity centered around the head, neck, and chest. Despite accumulating evidence, familiarity continues to dictate the choices made by pediatric surgeons in choosing the site of placement of CVCs.[28,29] In a recent, unpublished survey of 282 practicing North American pediatric surgeons, 84% preferred placing tunneled CVCs in NICU infants around the neck with the left subclavian, right internal jugular, and right external jugular veins being the vessels of choice (in that order), citing familiarity as the main reason. The tip of a CVC placed from the lower body should be positioned at the junction of the IVC and RA. The xiphoid process is a good surface landmark to estimate the length of catheter needed. On a radiographic image, the tip should project just above the diaphragm. Placing the tip high will ensure prompt dilution of the infusate and is likely to be associated with lower chance of thrombosis. If the tip is placed close to the IVC bifurcation or in the iliac veins, it cannot be considered truly "central," and hyperosmolar infusions should be avoided. A CVC placed through an upper body vein should be positioned such that the tip is at the junction of the SVC and RA. Surface landmarks for this location are less reliable. A point about 1 cm caudal to the manubriosternal junction, at the right sternal border, gives a close estimate to the SVC/RA junction in toddlers and older children. The lower margin of the third right costosternal junction has been shown to be the best surface landmark in adults for placement of the CVC tip at the SVC/RA junction.[30] Length recommendations have been made based on a child's weight for placement of right internal jugular and right subclavian CVCs.[31] On a chest radiograph, the tip of the catheter should project about two vertebral bodies caudal to the carina. The tunneled, surgically placed CVC can be left in for several months to years. The Broviac and Hickman catheters (Bard Access Systems, Salt Lake City, UT) are made of silicone and are available in various sizes, the smallest being a 2.7-Fr single-lumen catheter. These catheters have a Dacron cuff that allows tissue ingrowth, resulting in anchoring of the catheter within the subcutaneous tunnel. The cuff can be placed close to the exit site of the catheter to facilitate easier removal by dissection through the exit site itself. Placement of the Dacron cuff midway between the venotomy site and the exit site has the advantage of reduced chance of unintended removal of the catheter.

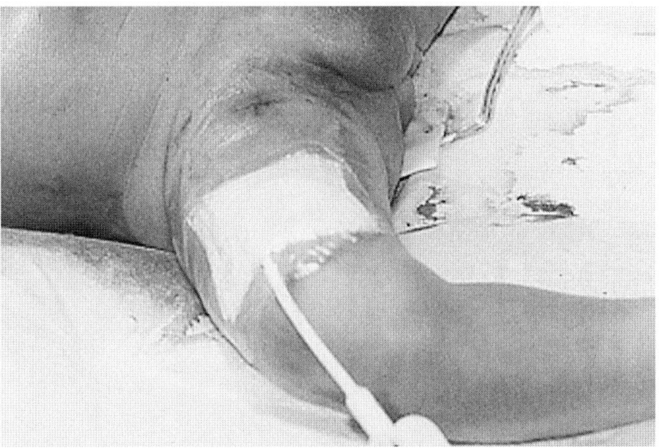

Figure 8-4. This broviac catheter was placed through a cutdown at the groin to access the long saphenous vein close to the saphenofemoral junction. The catheter is positioned in a subcutaneous tunnel in the thigh to exit just above the knee on the anteromedial aspect.

There is mounting evidence demonstrating the virtue of ultrasound guidance for percutaneous central venous access. Two devices developed for this purpose have been well studied: SiteRite (Bard Access Systems, Salt Lake City, UT) and SonoSite (SonoSite Inc, Bothel, WA). Real-time 2D ultrasound guidance is now recommended as the preferred method when placing a CVC into the internal jugular vein in adults and children in elective situations.[32,33] In a randomized controlled trial, real-time ultrasound guidance has been shown to be beneficial in internal jugular vein catheterization in infants weighing less than 7.5 kg when compared with an ultrasound image–based skin surface marking.[34] The benefits of ultrasound guidance include higher success rate,

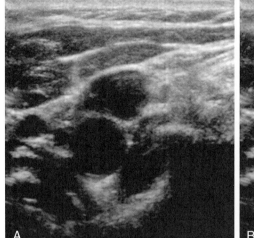

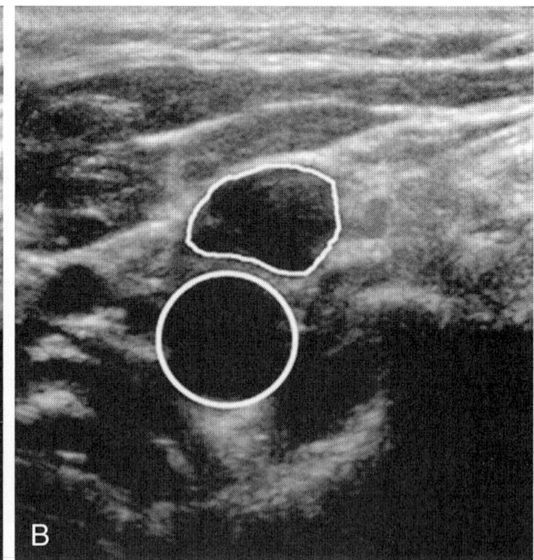

Figure 8-5. **A,** Representative ultrasound image of the right internal jugular vein and carotid artery as seen from the cranial end of an adult. **B,** The *circle* outlines the artery. The vein is just anterior and lateral to the artery and is shown by the *irregular ellipse*. The sternomastoid muscle is seen just anterior to the vein.

faster access, fewer needle passes, and fewer arterial punctures.[32-36] The ultrasound transducer is wrapped in a sterile sleeve, and sterile gel is used to obtain real-time images of the vessel being accessed. Either a short-axis view–across the diameter of the vessel (Fig. 8-5)–or the long axis view–along the length of the vessel–is used to visualize the needle approaching and entering the vessel. A guide wire is then passed into the vessel, followed by the routine Seldinger technique for placement of the CVC.[33,35] Because of the proximity of the clavicle, visualization of the subclavian vein is poor with ultrasound. Infraclavicular axillary vein cannulation has been performed with 96% success with ultrasound guidance for tunneled CVC placement into the subclavian vein.[37] There is limited evidence suggesting ultrasound guidance is helpful for subclavian vein and femoral vein cannulation in adults.[32]

The majority of bloodstream infections in children are associated with the use of a vascular access device. The pooled rate of catheter-associated bloodstream infections in pediatric intensive care units (PICUs) is reported to be 7.7 per 1000 catheter-days.[17] The incidence of umbilical catheter- and CVC-associated bloodstream infections in neonates is 4 to 11.3 per 1000 catheter-days. Tunneled CVCs placed in neonates in the NICU at the neck have been associated with a higher rate of complications than those placed in the groin; infection rates were 5.8 versus 0.7 per 1000 catheter-days.[28] Acute CVCs placed in 289 pediatric burn care unit patients also resulted in higher infection rates associated with subclavian and internal jugular CVCs compared with the femoral CVCs: 10 and 13.6 versus 8.2 per 1000 catheter-days.[29] This is thought to be due to the higher nursing and respiratory therapy activity at the head and neck in these patients who require intensive care. Although prophylactic antibiotics reduced the rate of CVC-associated septicemia in neonates, they are not recommended because no reduction in mortality was shown. Moreover, there is a potential risk for selection of resistant organisms.[38]

TOTALLY IMPLANTED CENTRAL VENOUS CATHETERS

Totally implantable intravascular devices (ports) are subcutaneous reservoirs attached to CVCs. The reservoirs are made with a metal or hard plastic shell and a silicone septum that is penetrated for access. They provide a reliable, long-lasting solution for patients who need intermittent access to their central veins. They are ideal for patients who desire to be involved in aquatic sports and other physical activities. They are most useful for patients with malignancies, coagulopathies, hemolytic syndromes, and renal failure, requiring recurrent vascular access. Ports are available with a low profile and as small as 5-Fr catheters for infants, with progressively larger ones for older children. Larger ports are available with dual lumens. More recently, some high-flow ports have been introduced (PowerPort-Bard Access Systems, Salt Lake City, UT) that allow high-pressure injection of intravenous contrast for radiologic imaging. Ports require special noncoring needles to keep the septum from leaking. Regular hypodermic needles should not be used with ports because they tend to cut out small cores of the silicone septum with each penetration. The cutting edge of the noncoring needle is in line with the needle, keeping it from cutting a core of the septum. The reservoir should be implanted in a subcutaneous pocket, over a firm base such as the chest wall. Placing the port in the abdominal wall is not acceptable because penetration of the skin and septum against a soft base is difficult, if not impossible. Preferred sites for port placement include the pectoral area, parasternal area, above and medial to the areola, and the subclavicular area, medial to the anterior axillary fold. In patients with a concern for cosmesis, the low pre-sternum area and the lateral chest wall are two locations that hide the scar when the port is eventually removed. In determining port placement, consideration should be given to the age of the patient, the intended activities, as well as the convenience of the caregivers. Placing a lateral chest wall port will make it difficult for an infant to be picked up under the axillae. Subclavicular placement will make it easy to access the port with minimal disrobing; in obese girls and young women, it is less likely to get displaced by the highly mobile breast tissue. However, the resultant scar is very difficult to hide. The presternal location will provide a very stable foundation for the port, even in the obese child. When placed over the lower sternum, it can be accessed with opening the front of a button-down top or shirt. Once the port is removed, the scar can be hidden nicely. Complications that are unique to a port are inability to access the port, disconnection of the catheter from the reservoir with extravasation, flipping of the port, fracture and embolization of the catheter, and breakdown of the overlying skin.[39] Unlike silicone catheters, polyurethane catheters have a tendency to adhere to the vein if left in place for more than 20 months.[40]

INTRAOSSEOUS ACCESS

Several studies have been published over the past 60 years establishing the safety and effectiveness of IO access for infusion of fluids and medications in children. Safety and efficacy of IO access in neonates has been specifically addressed in some recent studies.[41,42] IO access has also been shown to be faster than access with a PIV[2] and safer than an emergency CVC.

Bone marrow consists of rich lattice network of vessels. Whereas the peripheral veins collapse in patients in shock, the vascular spaces in the bone marrow do not.[43] The bioavailability of resuscitative drugs administered through IO access has been well established[44] and shown to be better than that of those administered through an endotracheal tube.[45] The current Pediatric Advanced Life Support (PALS) recommendation is to establish IO access promptly if PIV access cannot be attained rapidly in neonates and children of all ages who need intravenous drugs or fluids urgently.[46] Training in the technique of IO access placement is included in the PALS and the Advanced Trauma Life Support (ATLS) provider courses.[47] In children, the long bones of the lower extremities are used preferentially for IO placement. The proximal tibia is the most common site used, with the distal femur being the next most common. With full sterile precautions, a needle designed for bone marrow aspiration is advanced through the cortical bone to access the bone marrow. In an infant, a spinal needle may be used,[48] but in an older child, a generic bone marrow needle or a purposely designed IO needle such as the widely used Jamshidi needle (Cardinal Health, McGraw Park, IL) is used (see Fig. 8-1).[45] In the case of the proximal tibia, the subcutaneous, anteromedial flat surface of the tibia, 1 to 3 cm distal to the tibial tuberosity, is chosen. A small skin incision is made using the tip of a pointed scalpel or a large-bore hypodermic needle. The IO needle is positioned pointing posteriorly and angled slightly caudad. It is then advanced through the cortical bone using a screwing and unscrewing motion with constant pressure. Once the needle penetrates the outer cortex, a sudden "give" is felt. The needle is held in this position and the obturator is removed. A syringe is attached and bone marrow is aspirated to confirm correct placement. The IO needle is stabilized with a dressing. The femoral location is accessed by placing the needle 1 to 3 cm cephalad to the patella, angled slightly cranial to avoid the growth plate. Contraindications for IO placement include injury or suspected injury to the bone or soft tissue overlying the placement site. Recently introduced mechanical devices such as the Bone Injection Gun (BIG, Wasimed, Caesarea, Israel), FAST1 System (Pyng Medical Corporation, Vancouver, Canada), and EZ-IO (Vidacare, San Antonio, TX)[2,45] have helped to expand the use of IO access. The first two are spring-loaded devices. The FAST1 System is designed for sternal use in adults. The EZ-IO is a power drill–assisted device that makes IO placement easier in older children and adults.

Early concerns about potential adverse effects on the growth plates of long bones used for IO access have been allayed by animal studies.[48] The overall complication rate is estimated to be about 1%.[45] Extravasation of fluid is the most common adverse event. Compartment syndrome, osteomyelitis, skin and soft tissue infection, bone fractures, and fat embolism, although rare, have also been reported.[45]

VENOUS CUTDOWN

Although the advent and eventual broader acceptance of IO infusion has almost eliminated the need for venous cutdown and reduced the role of emergency placement of CVCs,[6] pediatric surgeons should maintain the knowledge and skills required to perform this procedure. The vessel of choice is the long saphenous vein near the medial malleolus. The vein is superficial and is of satisfactory size and there is minimal subcutaneous fat in this location. A transverse incision is made anterior and cephalad to the medial malleolus. The vein is readily identified by dissecting through the thin subcutaneous tissue and is stabilized by placing proximal and distal stay ligatures. The vein is then directly cannulated using a venous catheter of appropriate size relative to the vein. The catheter is anchored to the adjacent skin.

ALTERNATE ROUTES FOR CENTRAL VENOUS ACCESS

Patients who have had multiple previous CVCs can have unrecognized thrombosis or stenosis of the central veins that precludes the successful placement of a new catheter. Doppler ultrasonography or magnetic resonance angiography should be used to survey the central veins, including the brachiocephalic vein, the SVC, and the IVC.[49] Percutaneous access can be gained via a patent IVC by interventional radiologists either by a translumbar or a transhepatic approach.[50] A tunneled catheter can then be placed to reach the IVC/RA junction. The translumbar IVC catheters are quite durable, but the transhepatic ones tend to get withdrawn from the vascular space owing to the constant respiratory excursions of the diaphragm. The brachiocephalic vein, if patent, can similarly be accessed by interventional radiologists through a suprasternal route. In the absence of these options, the azygos vein may be accessed through one of the intercostal veins percutaneously[51] or surgically through a thoracotomy[52] or with thoracoscopic assistance.[53] Direct right atrial access has been used to manage patients with intestinal failure and occluded central veins[54] for long periods and in cardiac patients in an acute situation.

ARTERIAL CATHETER

Intra-arterial catheters allow continuous hemodynamic monitoring and blood sampling. Radial arteries at the wrist are most commonly used for intra-arterial access because of good collateral circulation. Dorsalis pedis and posterior tibial arteries are the other peripheral sites that are sometimes used. Femoral arteries are frequently used by cardiologists for catheter-based cardiac interventions and occasionally for monitoring. However, in general, it is advisable not to use the main artery of an extremity for chronic arterial catheter placement to avoid thromboembolic and ischemic complications. The adequacy of collateral arterial supply through the ulnar artery should be confirmed before placement of a radial arterial line by using the Allen test.[55-57] The right radial artery allows preductal monitoring and sampling. Percutaneous cannulation is often successful. If not, an arterial cutdown may be performed. Vasospasm is common and is self-limiting, reversing within a few hours. Thromboembolism can result in limb loss if the axillary, brachial, or femoral artery is catheterized. Digital ischemia can result from radial artery catheters. Local infections can occur when the catheters are left for several days. A pseudoaneurysm can result from injury to the adjacent vein during placement.

HEMODIALYSIS CATHETERS

The current recommendation is to use an autologous arteriovenous fistula (AVF) as the route of choice for hemodialysis.[58] AVFs permit high flow rates that facilitate effective dialysis. They also are reliable, are durable, and, once established, have low complication rates. Because patients are often referred late and AVFs take time to mature, there is frequently a need for CVCs for immediate dialysis. Temporary and tunneled long-term double-lumen hemodialysis catheters are placed preferentially through the right internal jugular vein, either percutaneously or by cutdown. The larger size of the vein and the straight internal path of the catheter allow a larger catheter to be placed safely through the right internal jugular vein. The long-term, cuffed hemodialysis catheters are precurved to allow right internal jugular placement with tunneling to the pectoral area. Flow rates achieved through hemodialysis catheters tend to be lower and they last a relatively short time. Totally implanted subcutaneous hemodialysis access systems are being developed.[59]

chapter 9

SURGICAL INFECTIOUS DISEASE

Bethany J. Slater, MD • Thomas M. Krummel, MD

Despite improvements in antimicrobial therapy, surgical technique, and postoperative intensive care, infection continues to be a significant source of mortality and morbidity for the pediatric patient. Widespread antibiotic use has brought with it the complication of resistant organisms,[1] and antibiotic selection has become increasingly complex as newer antibiotics are continually developed.[2] In addition, infections with uncommon organisms are becoming more common with diminished host resistance from immunosuppressive states such as immaturity, cancer, systemic diseases, and medications after transplant procedures. Surgical infections generally require some surgical intervention, such as drainage of an abscess or removal of necrotic tissue, as opposed to being treated solely with antibiotics.

Two broad classes of infectious disease processes affect a surgical practice: those infectious conditions brought to the pediatric surgeon for treatment and cure and those that arise in the postoperative period as a complication of surgical intervention.[3]

COMPONENTS OF INFECTION

The pathogenesis of infection involves a complex interaction between the host and pathogens. Four components are important: virulence of the organism, size of inoculum, presence of nutrient source for the organism, and a breakdown in the host's defense.

The virulence of any microorganism depends on its ability to cause damage to the host. Exotoxins, such as streptococcal hyaluronidase, are digestive enzymes released locally that allow the spread of infection by breaking down host extracellular matrix proteins. Endotoxins, such as lipopolysaccharides, are components of gram-negative cell walls that are released only after bacterial cell death. Once systemically absorbed, endotoxins trigger a severe and rapid systemic inflammatory response by releasing various endogenous mediators such as cytokines, bradykinin, and prostaglandins.[4] Surgical infections are often polymicrobial, involving various interactions among the species of microorganisms.

The size of the inoculum is the second component of an infection. The number of colonies of microorganisms per gram of tissue is a key determinant. The smallest number of bacteria required to cause clinical infection varies from species to species. Predictably, any decrease in host resistance decreases the absolute number of colonies necessary to cause clinical disease. In general, if the bacterial population in a wound exceeds 100,000 organisms per gram of tissue, invasive infection is present.[5]

For any inoculum, the ability of the organisms to find suitable nutrients is essential for their survival and comprises the third component of any clinical infection. Accumulation of necrotic tissue, hematoma, or other environmental contamination offers nutrient medium for continued organism growth and spread. Of special importance to the surgeon is the concept of necrotic tissue and infection. This tissue is recognized as a nutrient source for invading microorganisms.[6] Also, complement proteins and neutrophils accumulate in necrotic tissue that diverts them from the invading microorganisms.[7]

Finally, for a clinical infection to arise, the body's defenses must be broken. Even highly virulent organisms can be eradicated before clinical infection occurs if resistance is intact. Evolution has equipped humans with numerous mechanisms of defense, both anatomic and systemic.

DEFENSE AGAINST INFECTION

Anatomic Barriers

Intact skin and mucous membranes provide an effective surface barrier to infection.[8] These tissues are not merely a mechanical obstacle. The physiologic aspects of skin and mucous membranes provide additional protection. In the skin, the constant turnover of keratinocytes, temperature of the skin, and acid secretion from sebaceous glands inhibits bacterial cell growth. The mucosal surfaces also have developed advanced defense mechanisms to prevent and combat microbial invasion. Specialized epithelial layers provide resistance to infection. In addition, mechanisms such as the mucociliary transport system in the respiratory tract and normal colonic flora in the gastrointestinal tract prevent invasion of organisms. Any pathologic situation affecting the normal function of these anatomic barriers increases the host's susceptibility to infection. A skin injury or a burn provides open access to the soft tissues, and antibiotic use disrupts normal colonic flora. Such breakdowns in surface barriers are dealt with by the second line of defenses, the immune system.[9]

Immune Response

The immune system involves complex pathways and many specialized effector responses. The first line of defense is the more primitive and nonspecific innate system, which consists primarily of phagocytic cells and the complement system. The neutrophil is able to rapidly migrate to the source of the infection and engulf and destroy the infecting organisms by phagocytosis. Cytokines, low molecular weight proteins including tumor necrosis factor (TNF), and many interleukins attract and activate neutrophils and play a significant role in mediating the inflammatory response. In addition, the complement system, when activated, initiates a sequential cascade that also enhances phagocytosis, stimulates inflammation, and leads to lysis of pathogens. Neonates, in particular premature infants, have an immature immune system and must rely solely on the innate immune system and the protective agents in human breast milk.[10] The more specialized, adaptive immune system involves a highly specific response to antigens as well as the eventual production of a variety of humoral mediators.[11]

Humoral and Cell-Mediated Immunity

Specific, adaptive immunity has two major components. The humoral mechanism (B-cell system) is based on bursa cell lymphocytes and plasma cells. The cellular mechanism (T-cell system) consists of the thymic-dependent lymphocytes.[12] The adaptive immune system is an antigen-specific system that is regulated by the lymphocytes. A myriad of receptors on the T cells that are matched to particular individual antigens create these specific responses. Furthermore, antibody production from B cells enhances the antigen-specific interaction. The receptors of the T cells are produced by genes that undergo rearrangements, accounting for the enormous diversity of the unique receptors.[11]

Immunity provided by the B-cell system consists primarily of specific antibodies. Human antibodies are classified into five basic types of immunoglobulins. The first exposure of an antigen leads to the production of IgM antibodies, whereas subsequent exposure to the same antigen results in rapid production of IgG antibodies. Humoral antibodies may neutralize toxins, tag foreign matter to aid phagocytosis (opsonization), or lyse invading cellular pathogens. Plasma cells and non-thymic-dependent lymphocytes that reside in the bone marrow and in the germinal centers and medullary cords of lymph nodes produce the reactive components of this humoral system. These agents account for most of the human immunity against extracellular bacterial species.

The cellular or T-cell component of immunity is based on sensitized lymphocytes located in the subcortical regions of lymph nodes and in the periarterial spaces of the spleen. These lymphocytes form a part of the recirculating lymphocyte pool. The T cells are specifically responsible for immunity to viruses, most fungi, and intracellular bacteria. They produce a variety of lymphokines, such as transfer factors, that further activate lymphocytes, chemotactic factors, leukotrienes, and interferons.

Immunodeficiencies

Susceptibility to infection is increased when some component of the host defense mechanism is absent, reduced in absolute numbers, or significantly curtailed in function. Some of these derangements may have a congenital basis, although the majority are acquired as a direct result of drugs, radiation, endocrine disease, surgical ablation, tumors, or bacterial toxins. Immunodeficiencies from any cause significantly increase the risk of surgical infections both in hospitalized and postoperative patients. In addition, mycotic infections are an increasing problem in immunocompromised pediatric patients.[13]

Systemic diseases lead to diminished host resistance. For example, in diabetes mellitus, leukocytes often fail to respond normally to chemotaxis. Therefore, more severe and unusual infections often occur in diabetic patients.[14] In addition, tumors and other conditions that impair hematopoiesis lead to derangements in phagocytosis, resulting in an increased predilection for infection. Human immunodeficiency virus (HIV) infection in children is another major source of immunodeficiency. Vertical transmission from mother to child is the dominant mode of HIV acquisition among infants and children. Most of this transmission is thought to occur late in pregnancy or postnatally through breast feeding. Finally, poor nutritional status has adverse effects on immune function owing to a wide variety of negative influences on specific defense mechanisms, including decreased production of antibodies and phagocytic function.[15]

In patients with a primary immune defect, susceptibility to a specific infection is based on whether the defect is humoral, cellular, or a combination. Primary immunodeficiencies are rare but important because prompt recognition can lead to lifesaving treatment or significant improvement in the quality of life.[16] B-cell deficiencies are associated with sepsis from encapsulated bacteria, especially pneumococcus, *Haemophilus influenzae,* and meningococcus. Often a fulminating course rapidly ends in death, despite timely therapeutic measures. Although congenital agammaglobulinemia or dysgammaglobulinemia has been widely recognized, other causes of humoral defects include radiation, corticosteroid and antimetabolite therapy, sepsis, splenectomy, and starvation. Chronic granulomatous disease is caused by a deficiency in the respiratory burst action of phagocytes that leads to severe and recurrent bacterial and fungal infections in early childhood. Children with chronic granulomatous disease are prone to develop hepatic abscesses as well as suppurative adenitis of a single node or multiple nodes, both of which may require surgical drainage or excision.[17]

T-cell deficiencies are responsible for many viral, fungal, and bacterial infections. Cutaneous candidiasis is a good example of a common infection seen with a T-cell deficiency. DiGeorge syndrome is a developmental anomaly in which both the thymus and the parathyroid glands are deficient, thus increasing the risk for infection and hypocalcemic tetany during infancy. Bacterial toxins, immunosuppressive drugs, malnutrition, and radiation also can produce defects in cellular immunity.[18]

ANTIBIOTICS

The several classes of antibiotics are based on their molecular structure and site of action. The varying classes of antibiotics may be divided into bacteriostatic, which inhibit bacterial growth, and bactericidal, which destroy bacteria. The early initiation and correct choice of antibiotics is essential for timely and successful treatment of infections. In addition, it is important to have knowledge of the specific susceptibility patterns in a particular hospital or intensive care unit (ICU) to direct initial empirical antibiotic therapy. Finally, awareness of interactions and adverse reactions in pediatric patients of commonly utilized medications is critical.

The pharmacokinetics and monitoring of drug dosages in children is also important when treating patients with antibiotics. The efficacy and safety of many drugs have not been established in the pediatric patient, especially in the newborn.[19] Dosages based on pediatric pharmacokinetic data offer the most rational approach. The assumption that a child is a miniature adult as the basis for extrapolation of adult dosages to children is not ideal. Dosage requirements constantly change as a function of age and body weight. Furthermore, the volume of distribution and half-life of many drugs are often increased in neonates and children compared with adults for a variety of reasons.[20,21] Knowledge of a drug's pharmacokinetic profile allows manipulation of the dose to achieve and maintain a given plasma concentration. The body surface area (BSA) method of calculating drug dosages (Child's BSA [determined using nomogram)]/1.7 × Adult dose) approximates the pediatric dose of many drugs but does not always accurately determine dosage requirements in the premature and term newborn.

Newborns usually have extremely skewed drug-distribution patterns. The entire body mass can be considered as if it were a single compartment for purposes of dose calculations. For the majority of drugs, dose adjustments can be based on plasma drug concentration. Administering a loading dose is advisable when rapid onset of drug action is required. For many drugs, loading doses (milligrams per kilogram) are generally greater in neonates and young infants than in older children or adults.[22] However, prolonged elimination of drugs in the neonate requires lower maintenance doses, given at longer intervals, to prevent toxicity. Monitoring serum drug concentrations is useful if the desired effect is not attained or if adverse reactions occur. In the sick premature newborn, almost all medications are administered intravenously because gastrointestinal function and drug absorption are unreliable.

The neonate undergoing extracorporeal membrane oxygenation (ECMO) presents a special challenge to drug delivery and elimination. Because the ECMO circuit may bind or inactivate drugs and make them unavailable to the patient, dosing of drugs requires careful attention to drug response and serum levels. The pharmacokinetics under these conditions generally include a larger volume of distribution and prolonged elimination, with a return to baseline after decannulation.[23]

PREVENTION OF INFECTIONS

The most effective way to deal with surgical infectious complications is to prevent their occurrence. The clinician must recognize the variables that increase the risk of infection and attempt to decrease or eliminate them. A summary of the category 1 recommendations published by the Hospital Infection Control Practices Advisory Committee (HICPAC) of the Centers for Disease Control and Prevention that can be implemented by the surgical team is listed in Table 9-1.

Patient Characteristics

In the adult surgical population, patient characteristics and co-morbidities such as diabetes, liver failure, systemic corticosteroid use, obesity, extremes of age, and poor nutritional status are associated with an increased risk of surgical site infection. However, these chronic disease states are infrequently encountered in children. A prospective multicenter study of surgical wound infections in the pediatric surgical population found that postoperative wound infections were related to factors at the operation rather than to patient characteristics.[24] In this study of more than 800 pediatric patients, the only factors associated with increased surgical site infection were contamination at the time of operation and the duration of the procedure. In contrast, the presence of co-existing disease or anomalies, concurrent distant site infection, or American Society of Anesthesiologists (ASA) perioperative assessment score were not found to be associated with an increase in wound infection. Other investigators have similarly found that local factors at the time of operation, such as degree of contamination, tissue perfusion, and operative technique, play a more important role in initiation of a pediatric surgical site infection than the general condition of the patient.[25]

Table 9-1 Guidelines for Prevention of Surgical Site Infections

- Treat remote infections before elective surgery.
- Do not remove hair preoperatively unless it will interfere with operation.
- Adequately control serum blood glucose levels perioperatively.
- Require patients to shower or bathe with an antiseptic agent before the operative day.
- Use an appropriate antiseptic agent for skin preparation.
- Perform a surgical scrub for at least 2 to 5 minutes using an appropriate antiseptic.
- Administer a prophylactic antimicrobial agent only when indicated.
- Administer an antimicrobial agent such that bactericidal concentration of the drug is established in serum and tissues when the incision is made and maintained throughout the operation.
- Sterilize all surgical instruments.
- Wear a surgical mask.*
- Wear a cap or hood to fully cover hair on head and face.*
- Wear sterile gloves.*
- Use sterile gowns and drapes that are effective barriers when wet.
- Handle tissue gently, maintain effective hemostasis, minimize devitalized tissue and foreign bodies, and eradicate dead space at the surgical site.
- If drainage is necessary, use closed suction drain.
- Protect with a sterile dressing for 24 to 48 hours postoperatively an incision that has been closed primarily.

*Required by OSHA regulations.

From Mangram AJ, Horan TC, Pearson ML, et al. Guideline for Prevention of Surgical Site Infection, 1999. Centers for Disease Control and Prevention (CDC) Hospital Infection Control Practices Advisory Committee. Am J Infect Control 27:97-132, 1999.

Surgical Preparation

Preoperative preparation of the operative site and the sterility of the surgical team are very important in reducing the risk of postoperative infection. Hand scrubbing remains the most important proactive mechanism to reduce infection by reducing the number of microorganisms present on the skin during the surgical procedure. In the United States, the conventional method for scrubbing consists of a 5-minute first scrub followed by subsequent 2- or 3-minute scrubs for subsequent cases with either 5% povidone-iodine or 4% chlorhexidine gluconate. These scrubbing protocols can achieve a 95% decrease in skin flora.[26,27] Newer alcohol-based antiseptic cleaners with shorter applications, usually 30 seconds, have been developed and have been shown to be as effective as or even more effective than hand washing in decreasing bacterial contamination.[28-30] In addition, these solutions increase compliance and are less drying to the surgeon's skin. Preoperative showering with an antiseptic can reduce colony counts up to ninefold. Despite reducing the colony counts, no definitive data suggest that this actually reduces the risk of infection.[31] A similar reduction in the patient's skin flora can be achieved with aggressive preoperative cleansing and sterile draping.

Shaving the operative field, if necessary, should be done just before prepping the skin, and preferably with electric clippers or depilatory creams.[31-34] Preoperative shaving the night before has been shown to increase rates of infection.[32,33,35]

Normothermia has also been suggested as a means to decrease the incidence of surgical wound infections. Pediatric patients are at particular risk for experiencing hypothermia during surgery due to an increased area-to-body weight ratio leading to greater heat loss.[36] Intraoperative hypothermia can potentially lead to serious complications, including coagulopathy, surgical site infections, and cardiac complications. A prospective randomized trial of 200 adult patients undergoing colorectal surgery showed that intraoperative hypothermia caused delayed wound healing and a greater incidence of infections.[37] A number of techniques are available to warm infants and children during surgery, including warming intravenous fluids or using a warming mattress. In addition, supplemental oxygen given during the perioperative period in adult patients has been shown to decrease the rate of wound infection by as much as 40% to 50%.[38, 39] Finally, adequate control of glucose levels perioperatively has also been demonstrated to decrease morbidity and mortality in both adult and pediatric surgical patients, particularly in those patients undergoing cardiac surgery.[40,41]

Antibiotic Prophylaxis

Operative procedures can be classified into one of four types, as outlined in Table 9-2. In adults, several well-designed prospective trials have documented a decreased infection rate for all types of operative procedures with established antibiotic recommendations.[42] Important points for surgical antibiotic prophylaxis include using agents that cover the most

Table 9-2 Wound Classification

Class	Definition
Clean	An uninfected operative wound in which no inflammation is encountered and the respiratory, alimentary, genital, or infected urinary tract is not entered. In addition, clean wounds are closed primarily and, if necessary, drained with closed drainage.
Clean-contaminated	An operative wound in which the respiratory, alimentary, genital, or urinary tract is entered under controlled conditions and without unusual contamination
Contaminated	Open, fresh, accidental wounds. This includes operations with major breaks in sterile technique or gross spillage from the gastrointestinal tract and incisions in which acute, nonpurulent inflammation is encountered.
Dirty	Old traumatic wounds with retained devitalized tissue and those that involve existing clinical infection or perforated viscera

probable intraoperative contaminants for the operation, optimal timing for the initial dose of antibiotic so that bactericidal concentrations are reached at the time of incision, and maintaining the contribution levels throughout the operation.[31] Timing of the perioperative antibiotic coverage is crucial. The first dose is generally given 30 minutes to 1 hour before the start of the operation. In operations that take more than the half-life of the administered drug, a second dose of prophylactic antibiotics is indicated to re-achieve adequate serum levels.[43]

Prophylaxis accounts for nearly 75% of antibiotic use on pediatric surgical services. Additionally, prophylaxis is the major cause of the inappropriate use of antimicrobials in children. In one study of children younger than 6 years of age undergoing surgical procedures, prophylactic antibiotics were administered inappropriately to 42% of children receiving preoperative antibiotics, 67% of children receiving intraoperative antibiotics, and 55% of those receiving postoperative antibiotics.[44] In pediatric surgery, it is clear that antibiotic coverage is required during clean-contaminated, contaminated, or dirty cases. However, some disagreement exists concerning antimicrobial prophylaxis in clean operations. Antibiotic prophylaxis in a clean case in the pediatric population is now at the discretion of the operating surgeon.

Bowel Preparation

The efficacy of bowel preparation before an elective colon operation is well documented.[45,46] Bowel preparation includes mechanical irrigation and flushing of the colon to remove stool, oral antibiotics against colonic aerobes and anaerobes, and preoperative intravenous antibiotics that cover both common skin and colonic flora.[47] The preparation can be started on an outpatient basis the day before the operation, and the parenteral drugs are added to the regimen just before the procedure. Recently, there has been debate in the adult literature regarding the necessity of mechanical bowel preparation. In infants and children, protocols for bowel preparation have largely been extrapolated from the adult colorectal literature. It appears that the majority of pediatric surgeons use bowel preparations for elective colorectal surgery in an attempt to reduce surgical site infections.[48] Recently, others have proposed that omitting mechanical bowel preparation carries no increased risk of infectious or anastomotic complications.[49] If bowel preparation is used in the pediatric population, care must be taken to avoid dehydration.

Drains and Irrigation

The use of drains varies widely. Drains are indicated in those surgical procedures in which one expects an accumulation of blood, serum, exudate from the wound, and potential dead space.[50] Drains also are indicated when closure of a hollow viscous is imperfect. When a drain is used, a closed drainage system brought out through a separate stab incision away from the operative incision is preferable. Drains should be removed as soon as possible because they are foreign bodies that can impede wound healing and because bacteria can colonize the wound via a drain or its exit site.[51]

Irrigating the operative field is an important component in preventing postoperative infectious complications.[52] Irrigation with copious amounts of sterile saline mechanically removes loose debris, necrotic tissue, serum, and excess clot. Use of various types of irrigation solution have been used such as antibiotic or dilute povidone-iodine solutions.[53,54]

TYPES OF INFECTION

Postoperative Surgical Site Infection

Despite meticulous technique, perioperative antibiotics, and the proper use of drains and irrigation, surgical infectious complications still occur. Postoperative soft tissue infections can be divided into confined local lesions and invasive, spreading ones. Early diagnosis and prompt intervention help to avoid morbidity and occasional mortality. Erythema, fever, leukocytosis, tenderness, crepitus, and suppuration are diagnostic signs but are not always present. When confronted with one or more of these signs, clinical judgment must be made. Treatment should be suited to the extent of the infection and may include oral or intravenous antibiotics, simple incision and drainage, or extensive surgical debridement. Fortunately, soft tissue infections are uncommon in the pediatric surgical population, ranging from 2% to 20%.[25,55] The incidence of wound infection depends on the type of operative classification, varying from 1% to 11% in clean wounds and from 6% to 20% in contaminated wounds.

An abscess is a localized collection of pus in a cavity formed by an expanding infectious process. The pus is a combination of leukocytes, necrotic material, bacteria, and extracellular fluid. The usual cause is the staphylococcal species in combination with one or more organisms. The treatment is incision and drainage with packing to allow healing by secondary intention, followed by antibiotic therapy if associated with localized cellulitis or an immunocompromised patient. Drainage must be complete, or the abscess will reform. A phlegmon is an area of diffuse inflammation with little pus and some necrotic tissue. A phlegmon can often be treated with antibiotics, although it can progress to an abscess.

Streptococcal soft tissue infections are probably the most virulent and can arise within a few hours after surgical procedures. High fever, delirium, leukocytosis, and severe pain are hallmarks of the patient's presentation. Penicillin in high doses is the appropriate initial management for streptococcal infections, followed by operative debridement of necrotic tissue. *Bacillus* infections are the next most virulent infections. Inspection of the wound will show dark, mottled areas, as opposed to the bright pink of a streptococcal cellulitis.

Less than half of the patients with *Bacillus* infections have detectable gas crepitation. Severe pain is the most telling clinical symptom of this type of infection. High doses of penicillin (500,000 to 800,000 U/kg/day) are the hallmarks of treatment for these patients.

Nosocomial Infection

Nosocomial infections are defined as those infections that are hospital acquired.[56] As such, they are a potential threat to all hospitalized patients and increase morbidity and mortality significantly. Their incidence appears to be increasing as surgical care becomes more advanced and patients survive longer from previously fatal conditions. One report describing 676 operative procedures in 608 pediatric patients showed a nosocomial infection rate of 6.2%.[57] Fifty-three infectious complications were tabulated: wound, 17 (2.5%); septicemia, 14 (2.1%); pulmonary, 10 (1.5%); urinary tract, 5 (0.7%); abdominal, 5 (0.7%); and diarrhea, 2 (0.3%). The highest overall occurrence of infection was in the infant group (1 month to 1 year; 13 [8.1%] of 161). The probability of septicemia was highest in neonates (4.2%) compared with infants (3.1%) and older children (1.2%) ($P < .05$). The most common isolates were *Staphylococcus epidermidis* (10 of 17) from septic patients and gram-negative enteric bacteria (27 of 50) from organ and wound infections. Infection was associated with impaired nutrition, multiple disease processes, and multiple operations. In another study, ECMO use correlated with an increased incidence of nosocomial infection.[58] Two other factors that have been found to increase the risk of nosocomial infection in pediatric patients in ICUs are the length of the preoperative stay and exposure to invasive medical devices.[59]

Pneumonia can be a lethal nosocomial infection, with mortality ranging from 20% to 70% and accounting for 10% to 15% of all pediatric hospital-acquired infections.[60] The mortality rate is dependent on the causative organism. The risk factors for nosocomial pneumonia in the pediatric population include serious underlying illness, immunosuppression, length of time on a ventilator, and nasopharyngeal floral changes with prolonged hospitalization.[61] An increased risk has been found in patients with gastric alkalinization because the use of antacids in the ICU to prevent stress ulceration increases bacterial counts in the stomach and may potentially predispose the patient to increased bacterial translocation.[62]

Clostridium difficile is a well-recognized cause of infectious diarrhea that develops after antibiotic therapy in many patients, although it likely only accounts for 20% of antibiotic-associated diarrhea. It is a very common cause of nosocomial infection, and its incidence is increasing in frequency with associated increasing mortality.[63,64] The best method of prevention is the judicious and appropriate use of antibiotics. Prolonged antibiotic use has an association with increased rates of *C. difficile* colitis. Some studies have suggested the use of probiotics for the prevention and treatment of antibiotic-associated diarrhea.[65,66] The rationale for their use is that probiotics modify the makeup of colonic microflora. Some of the reports on the efficacy of probiotics in children are conflicting. However, a number of randomized controlled studies have demonstrated only a moderate beneficial effect of some strains of bacteria in preventing antibiotic-associated diarrhea. Until better evidence is available, the best method of prevention is the judicious and appropriate use of antibiotics.[67]

To decrease nosocomial infections in hospitals, the Centers for Medicare and Medicaid Services (CMS) released a proposal in 2008 to expand the list of hospital-acquired conditions (HAC) that would not be reimbursed by Medicare. These have been termed "Never Events" and include surgical site infections after specific elective surgeries, extreme glycemic aberrancies, ventilator-associated pneumonia, and *C. difficile*–associated diseases among others. Under this proposal, CMS will not reimburse hospitals for treatment (medical or surgical treatment) of these nosocomial entities.

Catheter Infections

Central venous catheters (CVCs) are essential in managing critically ill pediatric patients. The use of CVCs in pediatric patients has increased as prolonged vascular access has become increasingly necessary to provide parenteral nutrition, chemotherapy, antimicrobial therapy, and hemodynamic monitoring to an increasing number of children. However, the complication of catheter-related infection is common, despite considerable effort to reduce its occurrence. It is important to recognize the difference between colonization of the catheter and CVC infection. Colonization is defined as the presence of a positive culture without signs and symptoms of clinical infection. Infection is manifested as erythema at the site of insertion, tachycardia, and/or leukocytosis. Rates of infection are influenced by patient-related factors, by type and severity of illness, and by catheter-related parameters (catheter type, purpose, and conditions under which it was placed).[68] Coagulase-negative staphylococci, followed by enterococci, were the most frequently isolated causes of hospital-acquired bloodstream infections reported from National Nosocomial Infections Surveillance System report.[69] A number of factors are associated with the development of catheter-related infections, including the sterility of the insertion technique, type of solution being administered through the line, care of the catheter once inserted, proximity of the catheter to another wound, and the presence of another infection elsewhere.

The location of the catheter, such as the subclavian, internal jugular, or femoral veins, may be correlated with the risk of infection. Studies in pediatric patients have shown that femoral lines have an equivalent rate of infection to that of non-femoral lines.[68] For catheters that will remain for a long time, tunneling the catheter has been shown to significantly reduce the risk of catheter-related infection.[70,71]

Absolute sterile techniques should be maintained in all instances of line insertion whenever possible.

Emergency situations may necessitate less-than-sterile technique. The use of maximal sterile barriers, including sterile gown and gloves and a large sterile sheet, has been shown in adults to greatly reduce the risk of catheter-related infection.[72,73] Povidone-iodine has long been the standard for cleansing of the skin before catheter insertion. However, recent studies suggest that chlorhexidine significantly reduces the incidence of microbial colonization compared with povidone-iodine.[74]

The skin and catheter hub are the most common sources of colonization and infection. Thus, various methods have been tried to combat these risks. Silver ions have broad antimicrobial activity, and the use of silver-impregnated cuffs have been proposed as a preventive measure.[75,76] In addition, antimicrobial and antiseptic catheters and cuffs may decrease the incidence of catheter-related infections and potentially decrease hospital costs associated with these infections.[77,78] Catheters have been coated with chlorhexidine/silver sulfadiazine as well as minocycline/rifampin along with other agents. The use of these catheters in children is still under investigation but they have been approved by the U.S. Food and Drug Administration for use in patients weighing more than 3 kg. It is likely that these catheters become less effective in reducing infection risks after being in place for longer than 3 weeks because of a decrease in their antimicrobial activity.[78] Of note, no studies in adults have demonstrated a benefit for systemic antibiotic prophylaxis after insertion of a CVC. Studies in high-risk neonates and children have demonstrated conflicting results, although a few studies have found that vancomycin led to a reduction in catheter infections in select patient populations. However, concern exists for the emergence of resistance with the routine use of antimicrobial prophylaxis.[79,80]

Other Infections Requiring Surgical Care and Treatment

Although the infections discussed previously are possibly preventable and occur after surgical procedures or hospitalization, some infections are seen by the pediatric surgeon for treatment and cure for the first time.

Necrotizing Soft Tissue Infection

Necrotizing fasciitis is a rapidly progressing infection of the fascial tissues and overlying skin. Although it can occur as a postoperative complication or as a primary infection, necrotizing fasciitis is more likely in immunocompromised patients.[81] However, in the pediatric population, necrotizing fasciitis often affects previously healthy children.[82] Because the diagnosis is often not obvious, the clinician must look for clinical clues such as edema beyond the area of erythema, crepitus, skin vesicles, or cellulitis refractory to intravenous antibiotics. Skin necrosis is generally a late sign and is indicative of thrombosis of vessels in the subcutaneous tissue. Pediatric necrotizing fasciitis often occurs in the truncal region, as opposed to the extremities as is most common in adults (Figs. 9-1 and 9-2).[83] Although infections with a single organism often occur in adults with necrotizing fasciitis, polymicrobial infections predominate in children.[84] Prompt surgical intervention, including wide excision of all necrotic and infected tissue, along with the institution of antibiotics including penicillin, is mandatory to avoid progression and mortality. Necrotizing fasciitis can also occur as a complication of chickenpox.[85] Extensive debridement and antibiotic therapy initiated early are necessary to decrease the mortality from this rare complication of varicella lesions.

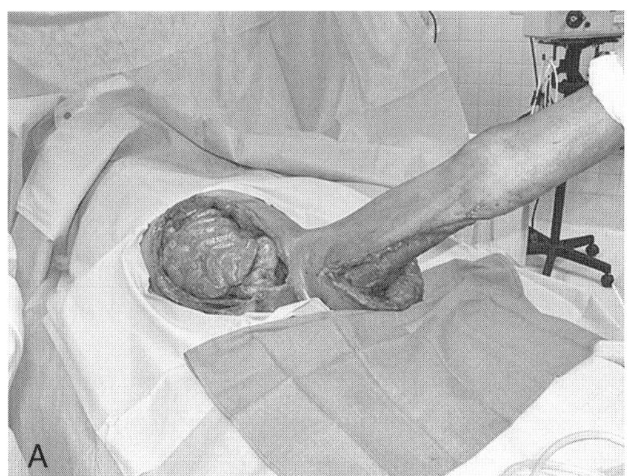

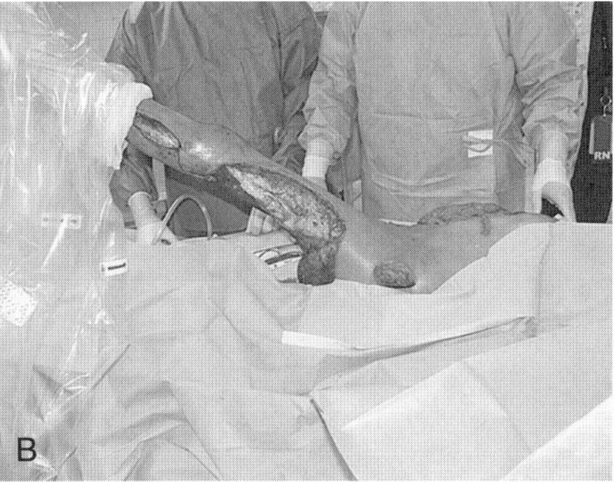

Figure 9-1. This 15-year-old was sick for 2 weeks with perforated appendicitis and presented in shock. After a midline incision for exploration for a rigid abdomen, his appendix was removed. The peritoneal cavity was extensively and copiously irrigated and the abdominal incision was left open. He returned to the operating room 2 days later for evaluation and was found to have necrotizing fasciitis of the rectus abdominis muscles bilaterally. Eventually, despite aggressive surgical debridement, this process spread to the retroperitoneum and down the left inguinal canal through a patent processus vaginalis. One week postoperatively, he was found to have edema and erythema of the left leg that prompted exploration. The necrotizing fasciitis had progressed down all compartments of the left thigh and the lateral compartment of the left lower leg. In the upper thigh, the semimembranosus and semitendinosus muscles had to be excised due to necrotic musculature. These photographs were taken on his ninth postoperative day. In **A**, the abdomen is seen to be open and the medial aspect of the left thigh is visualized. In **B**, the incisions in the left buttock area, the left lateral thigh, and the left lateral lower leg are seen.

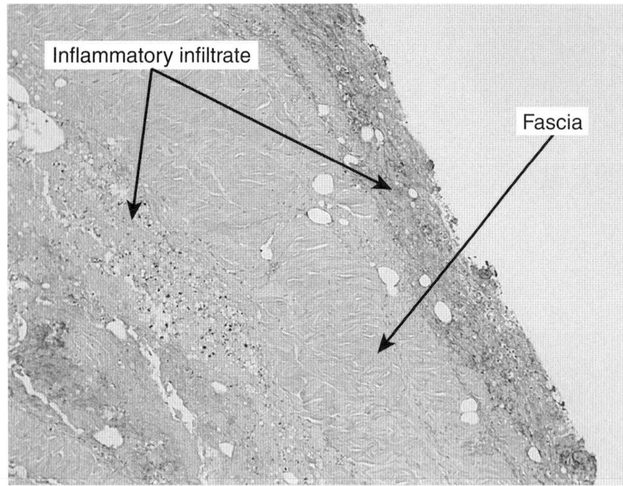

Figure 9-2. This photomicrograph depicts the histologic findings of necrotizing fasciitis in the patient shown in Figure 9-1. Note the inflammatory infiltrate on both sides of the fascia. The fascial cultures grew *Escherichia coli.*

Sepsis

Sepsis, by contemporary definition, distinguishes the systemic derangements that are caused by the infectious organisms and their byproducts from those that are caused by the host-systemic inflammatory response. In 1992, the Society of Critical Care Medicine published the results of a consensus conference to define accurately the terms regarding sepsis and the inflammatory response to injury and infection.[86] These definitions were updated in the 2001 Consensus Conference.[87] Although there has been a significant decrease in the mortality rate among children with sepsis, severe sepsis remains one of the leading causes of death in the pediatric population. In 2002, a group of experts gathered to focus specifically on pediatric sepsis.[88] Systemic inflammatory response syndrome (SIRS) has previously been defined in adults as the nonspecific inflammatory process after a variety of insults with sepsis specifically occurring from infection.[89] The main pediatric modifications for the definitions of SIRS and sepsis include the inclusion of temperature or leukocyte abnormalities in addition to tachycardia and tachypnea because these last two indices are common in many pediatric disease processes. Another difference was that hypotension is not necessary for the diagnosis of septic shock but rather cardiovascular dysfunction must be present. SIRS may progress to multiorgan dysfunction and death. Gram-negative organisms possess a lipopolysaccharide moiety on the cell wall that has been shown to incite most, if not all, of the toxic effects of end-organ failure.

Neonatal sepsis is defined as a generalized bacterial infection accompanied by a positive blood culture within the first month of life.[90] Neonatal sepsis occurring during the first week of life is caused primarily by maternal organisms transferred during delivery. Maternal contamination of the neonate can be transmitted through the placenta, via the birth canal, or by direct contamination of the amniotic fluid. The mortality of this early-onset variety approaches 50%. Late-onset neonatal sepsis is primarily nosocomial and is most often secondary to indwelling catheters or bacterial translocation from the gut. In the surgical neonate, three factors promote bacterial translocation and sepsis: (1) intestinal bacterial colonization and overgrowth, (2) compromised host defenses, and (3) disruption of the mucosal epithelial barrier.[91] The mortality of late-onset sepsis approaches 20%. The clinician must be alert for the subtle signs and symptoms of neonatal sepsis, which include lethargy, irritability, temperature instability, and a change in respiratory or feeding pattern. Neonates may not demonstrate leukocytosis. Empirical triple-antibiotic coverage may be started, pending the results of blood and other cultures.

Peritonitis

Peritonitis is defined as inflammation of the peritoneum.[92] It is divided into primary, secondary, and tertiary, depending on the cause. Spontaneous primary peritonitis is a bacterial infection without enteric perforation. Primary peritonitis is usually caused by a single organism. An infant with primary peritonitis usually does not exhibit signs of peritonitis but may have poor feeding, lethargy, distention, vomiting, and mild to severe abdominal tenderness. Definitive treatment may require only a course of broad-spectrum antibiotics. Secondary peritonitis is associated with gastrointestinal tract disruption. This can be caused directly by intestinal perforation, bowel-wall necrosis, or trauma or postoperatively as a result of iatrogenic injury or an anastomotic leak. In addition, secondary peritonitis also may result from an indwelling dialysis catheter or ventriculoperitoneal shunt.[93] These infections are generally polymicrobial. Treatment of secondary peritonitis is a combination of surgical intervention, removal of any prosthetic device, and antibiotics. Tertiary peritonitis, also called recurrent peritonitis, is characterized by organ dysfunction and systemic inflammation in association with recurrent infection. The mortality rate is very high, and treatment is very difficult.[94] Treatment consists of broad-spectrum antibiotics because the infection often includes nosocomial organisms and multidrug-resistant bacteria.

CONCLUSION

Infectious diseases can lead to significant morbidity and mortality for the pediatric surgical patient. Surgical infectious diseases may be encountered both as a complication of surgery post-operatively or as the primary reason for surgical intervention. The immune system has developed as a complex defense mechanism against infections. However, patients are particularly vulnerable to developing certain infections when their immune system is compromised by various immunodeficiencies. Given the substantial morbidity from infectious complications, pediatric surgeons have devoted much attention to the prevention of surgical infectious diseases by implementing measures such as antibiotic prophylaxis before skin incision, scrubbing, and sterile barriers. Early diagnoses and execution of effective treatment for surgical infectious diseases can decrease the morbidity and mortality in the pediatric population.

chapter 10

FETAL THERAPY

Shinjiro Hirose, MD • Michael R. Harrison, MD

New advances in imaging modalities have allowed clinicians to make early and accurate diagnoses of fetal anomalies. Most of these anomalies are best treated expectantly, with definitive therapy performed after birth. A subset of conditions can be treated by early delivery if the abnormality poses a threat to the fetus and if the fetus has reached a viable gestational age. An even smaller group of patients may have progression of their condition that can be corrected with in-utero treatment. Certain anomalies have been studied for the past 25 years and their natural history has been delineated. This time frame has allowed the development of potential strategies for ameliorating the derangement in pathophysiology associated with the condition. While advances in radiology have led to an earlier diagnosis of these abnormalities, techniques have also been developed to allow fetal intervention. These techniques, including maternal hysterotomy, minimal access fetoscopy, and percutaneous fetal access, were initially tested and validated in animal models. Further validation in humans was stringent because the mother's safety is of utmost importance in fetal surgery. In this chapter, we present an overview of the current state of fetal surgery, review specific fetal problems, and outline current management strategies.

GENERAL PRINCIPLES

Fetal intervention is complicated by both the risk to the unborn patient and to the mother. The mother has nothing to gain in terms of health benefits from any fetal intervention, yet she is at a significant risk for morbidity and even potential mortality with fetal surgery. To date, there have been no reported maternal deaths from fetal surgery, although significant short-term maternal morbidity is known. Complications can arise from endotracheal intubation, blood transfusion, premature rupture of membranes, chorioamniotic separation, chorioamnionitis, and placental abruption. Therefore, fetal surgery should be considered only if there is a severe, life-threatening or debilitating anomaly in the fetus that has been thoroughly investigated in animal models and has been shown to be improved by in-utero intervention.

Initial fetal surgical experiments were carried out in a variety of animal models (e.g., rat, rabbit, sheep, and nonhuman primates). These studies showed it was that in utero surgery could be performed safely and it was subsequently attempted in humans. The first open fetal surgical procedure was performed at the University of California, San Francisco (UCSF), and was reported in 1982.[1] Since that report, more than 380 fetal interventions have been performed at UCSF over the past 27 years with no maternal mortality. The primary morbidity after fetal surgery has been, and remains, preterm labor, resulting in premature delivery at 25 to 35 gestational weeks. Notably, in reviewing our experience, subsequent fertility after fetal intervention has been good.[2]

A crucial component contributing to the success of a fetal treatment program is a multidisciplinary approach, utilizing the skills of various specialists working in concert. At UCSF, all fetal referrals are presented at an open weekly meeting involving a multidisciplinary group consisting of perinatologists, anesthesiologists, neonatologists, cardiologists, radiologists, geneticists, and pediatric surgeons. In addition, specific subspecialists are involved for certain cases, such as pediatric neurosurgeons for fetal myelomeningocele (MMC) repair. The weekly discussion not only covers the medical and surgical aspects of the patient's care, but also includes the ethical and social concerns with each case. Finally, a special institutional fetal treatment oversight committee reviews all fetal interventions on a monthly basis. This group serves as a quality control mechanism as well as an ethical review board.

FETAL ACCESS

There are three general methods for accessing the fetus: (1) percutaneously, with ultrasound guidance; (2) minimally invasive fetoscopy; and (3) open hysterotomy. In all of these approaches, preoperative and intraoperative ultrasonography is crucial for defining the anomaly or anomalies, delineating the placental anatomy, determining the position of the fetus, detecting the location of the maternal blood vessels, and monitoring the fetal heart rate during the procedure. With percutaneous and fetoscopic procedures, ultrasonography is particularly important owing to the lack of direct exposure to the fetus and uterus during the procedure.

The mother is usually positioned supine with her left side down to minimize compression of her vena cava by the gravid uterus. Maternal anesthesia can be either spinal or general, depending on the nature and duration of the intervention. In addition, fetal anesthesia is needed when operating on the fetus. An intramuscular injection of an opiate and a nondepolarizing neuromuscular blocking agent are usually utilized.

Ultrasound-guided percutaneous procedures are performed through small skin incisions in the mother's skin. During these procedures, real-time ultrasonography is needed because the only visualization of the fetal and maternal anatomy is through these images.[3] Through ultrasound visualization, catheters and shunts can be inserted into the fetus for draining cystic masses, ascites, or pleural fluid into the amniotic space. In addition, radiofrequency ablation (RFA) probes can be deployed into the amniotic space to treat various twin gestational anomalies. The needles used to place these catheters, as well as the RFA device, are 1.5 to 2 mm in diameter, resulting in minimal morbidity to the mother.[4,5]

Fetoscopic procedures are generally performed using a 3-mm fetoscope and instruments or, sometimes, standard 5-mm laparoscopic telescopes and instruments. For many fetoscopic procedures, the 3-mm fetoscope with its 1-mm working channel is sufficient. It is important to identify a "window" in the uterus that is devoid of the placenta to reduce the risk of maternal bleeding, placental abruption, and fetal morbidity. When multiple ports and standard laparoscopic instruments are needed, we prefer a maternal laparotomy and direct uterine closure of the port sites. Occasionally, the amniotic fluid is not clear enough for adequate visualization. In such cases, we perform amnionic fluid exchange, using warmed crystalloid solutions to provide a clear operative view.

Open fetal procedures require general anesthesia and a combination of preoperative indomethacin and inhalational agents with a high mean alveolar concentration to maintain uterine relaxation.[6-8] The maternal incision is low and transverse with a vertical or transverse fascial incision, depending on the exposure needed. Preoperative and intraoperative ultrasonography is again crucial to avoid injury to the placenta. Uterine staplers with absorbable staples have been developed specifically for fetal surgery and allow a hemostatic hysterotomy with minimal blood loss. The fetus is monitored using ultrasonography and continuous pulse oximetry. The uterus is stabilized within the maternal abdomen. It is important to prevent herniation of the uterus, which would increase the tension on the uterine blood vessels. Also, fetal exposure is limited to the specific body part in question. Most of the fetus is left inside the uterus, and great care is taken not to handle or stretch the umbilical cord because this can cause fetal ischemia from injury or vasospasm. After the fetal procedure is completed, the fetus is returned to the uterus, the amniotic fluid is replaced, and the uterus is closed in multiple layers using absorbable sutures. Postoperatively, the mother and fetus are monitored continuously for uterine contractions and heart rate, respectively. Often, the uterus is irritable and contractions require control with tocolytic regimens. Also, open fetal surgery requires lifelong cesarean section for future pregnancies owing to the potential for uterine rupture with subsequent births.

Complications can occur after all types of fetal intervention. Bleeding can originate from the fetus, the placenta, the uterine wall, or the maternal abdominal wall. The uterine vessels are identified with ultrasonography and specifically avoided to prevent injury and minimize bleeding. Premature rupture of membranes and preterm labor remain problems after fetal surgery and are often the result of inadequate membrane closure, chorioamnionitis, chorioamniotic separation, and uterine contractions.

ANOMALIES AMENABLE TO FETAL SURGERY

Congenital Diaphragmatic Hernia

Despite significant advances in neonatal respiratory support, survival for children born with congenital diaphragmatic hernia (CDH) remains only 60% to 70% throughout the United States. Additionally, survival for all fetuses diagnosed with CDH may be as low as 20% to 27% owing to in-utero demise or death of infants with unrecognized CDH.[9-11] We have studied fetal lung development extensively and theorized that in-utero intervention may allow increased antenatal lung growth, pulmonary function, and survival postnatally.[12,13] In a fetal lamb model, compression of the lungs during the last trimester, either with an intrathoracic balloon or by creation of a diaphragmatic hernia, results in fatal pulmonary hypoplasia. In addition, removal of the compressing lesion allows the lung to grow and develop sufficiently to permit survival at birth.[14]

Initial attempts at fetal surgery for CDH involved in utero diaphragmatic hernia repair. Analysis of this initial group of patients revealed that open fetal surgery for CDH was feasible but did not show a survival advantage.[15] Fetuses with severe lung hypoplasia continue to have a poor prognosis and are identifiable prenatally by ultrasonography and magnetic resonance imaging. The factors associated with a poor outcome that can be assessed prenatally by ultrasonography are the presence of liver herniation into the chest and a low lung-to-head ratio (LHR). In our experience, survival has been 100% in fetuses with CDH without liver herniation on prenatal ultrasonography and 56% in fetuses with CDH and liver herniation into the chest.

The LHR is calculated as the area of the contralateral lung at the level of the cardiac atria divided by the head circumference. This value has been shown to correlate with survival: 100% survival with an LHR greater than 1.35, 61% survival with an LHR between 0.6 and 1.35, and 0% survival with an LHR less than 0.6.[16] Ultrasonography is critical in identifying other anomalies associated with CDH, particularly cardiac anomalies, because those portend an extremely poor prognosis. Magnetic resonance volumetric imaging of the lung for CDH is a promising modality for prognostic purposes.[17]

Over the past 20 years, we have been able to stratify the risk for fetuses with CDH. Over this same time period, extensive animal studies and observation in human fetuses born with congenital high airway obstruction have shown that lung growth may be driven by tracheal obstruction or occlusion, leading to pressurized fluid accumulating in the airway.[18-20] These reports led to the hypothesis that lung growth, resulting from the tracheal occlusion, may reduce the postnatal sequelae of CDH. Thus, our group has focused on in-utero tracheal occlusion as a method of augmenting lung growth in fetuses with CDH. Our preliminary efforts looked at the effect of in-utero extrinsic tracheal occlusion by placing an obstructing clip across the trachea using both an open and fetoscopic approach.[21] In a small number of patients, we found that survival was increased in the fetoscopic, but not the open, group, as compared with the control group, which consisted of patients undergoing standard postnatal care. This led to a National Institutes of Health (NIH)-funded trial comparing in-utero fetoscopic tracheal occlusion with standard postnatal care for fetuses diagnosed with severe left-sided CDH and no other detectable anomalies. Results of the trial showed a 75% overall survival with no difference between the tracheal occlusion group and the standard postnatal care group.[22] Interestingly and unexpectedly, the survival in the postnatal care group was considerably greater when compared with historical controls. Although this study did not demonstrate a difference in survival between the prenatal intervention group and the postnatal group, the results of this trial demonstrate the tremendous importance of proper randomized controlled trials for novel fetal surgical procedures.

Tracheal occlusion techniques have progressed from tracheal clipping to percutaneous, fetoscopic placement of a detachable, intratracheal balloon (Fig. 10-1). Animal studies have demonstrated complete tracheal occlusion with this approach, and it has now become the current method of choice for fetal tracheal occlusion in human fetuses.[23] Further data regarding tracheal occlusion have suggested that temporary, short-term reversible tracheal occlusion may be preferable to a longer duration of occlusion. Animal models of tracheal occlusion have demonstrated that long-term tracheal occlusion can be deleterious to type II pneumocytes (the cells that secret surfactant) and that this effect is not seen with a shorter duration of tracheal occlusion.[24] Other studies have also demonstrated the efficacy of short-term, reversible tracheal occlusion on lung growth in animals. A recent report demonstrated improved lung volumes after temporary balloon tracheal occlusion in human fetuses.[25] In 36 of 40 patients, the tracheal balloon was removed prenatally, limiting the duration of occlusion. In this group of patients, improved lung growth was associated with improved postnatal survival. Although reversal of the tracheal occlusion requires a second maternal and fetal intervention for the removal of the fetal intratracheal balloon, it obviates the need for an ex-utero intrapartum treatment (EXIT) approach at birth.[26,27] The EXIT procedure was initially developed to reverse the tracheal occlusion in this cohort of patients (Fig. 10-2). Therefore, with in-utero removal of the tracheal balloon, the EXIT procedure is no longer needed.

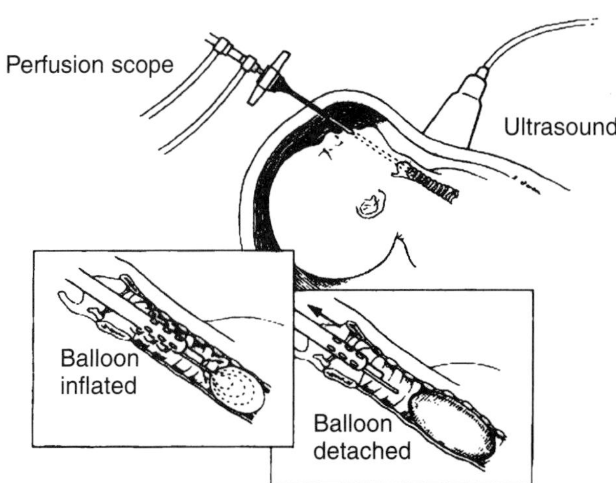

Figure 10-1. This schematic diagram shows the method of fetoscopic tracheal occlusion. A fetoscope is placed into the fetal mouth, the airway is identified, and a balloon is inserted into the trachea by using both fetoscopic and ultrasonographic visualization.

Based on these data, as part of a U.S. Food and Drug Administration (FDA)-sponsored trial, our group is currently offering reversible, fetal tracheal occlusion for fetuses with liver herniation in the chest and an LHR of less than 1.0, because these infants, as a group, continue to have greater than a 60% mortality.[28] In this study, we occlude the trachea at between 24 and 26 weeks' gestation and remove the balloon at between 32 and 34 weeks' gestation.

Tumors

Fortunately, fetal tumors are rare. When they do occur, most are benign. However, when they become large enough to impede the venous return to the heart or create high-output heart failure via arteriovenous shunts, they can cause nonimmune hydrops in the fetus. Hydropic changes include polyhydramnios, placentomegaly, fetal skin and scalp edema, and pleural, pericardial, and peritoneal fluid accumulation. If left untreated, fetal hydrops is nearly always fatal.[29,30] The two most common prenatally diagnosed tumors that cause nonimmune hydrops are congenital pulmonary

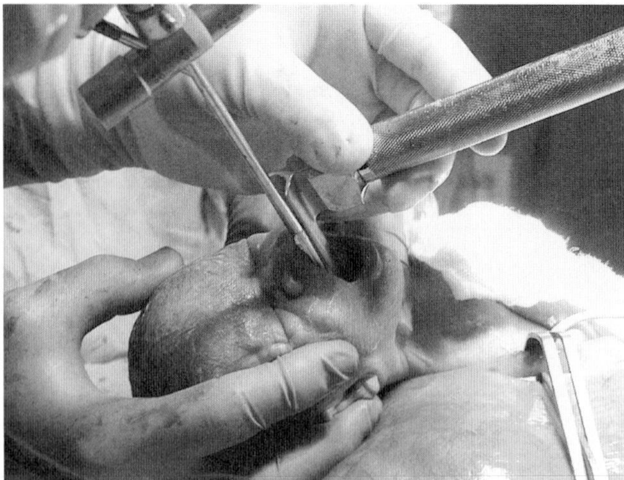

Figure 10-2. The EXIT procedure was initially developed as a means to reverse the in-utero tracheal occlusion in infants with a significant congenital diaphragmatic hernia. In the photograph, this infant is undergoing bronchoscopy as an EXIT procedure to remove the intratracheal balloon.

airway malformations (CPAMs) and sacrococcygeal teratoma (SCT).

Congenital Pulmonary Airway Malformations

CPAMs are pulmonary lesions with a broad range of clinical presentations. This new terminology includes congenital cystic adenomatoid malformations (CCAMs) and pulmonary sequestrations. CCAMs are much more likely than sequestrations to cause nonimmune hydrops in the fetus. CCAMs are characterized by an overgrowth of respiratory bronchioles with the formation of cysts of various sizes. Classification of CCAMs has historically been based on the size of the cysts.[31-34] Most fetuses diagnosed with a CCAM in utero develop normally and can be monitored with serial ultrasound studies. These asymptomatic patients can then undergo standard, postnatal resection. A small percentage of patients with the prenatal diagnosis of CCAM will develop nonimmune hydrops.[33,34] Various measurements have been developed to predict which fetuses are at risk for developing hydrops. The most accepted measurement is the CCAM volume ratio (CVR), defined as the product of the three longest cyst measurements on ultrasonography, multiplied by the constant 0.52, and then divided by the head circumference. In a recent paper, Crombleholme and colleagues identified a CVR of 1.6 as a cutoff for an increased likelihood of developing hydrops.[35]

Interestingly, CCAMs that are predominantly microcystic have a more predictable course than those that are macrocystic. Microcystic CCAMs undergo steady growth and tend to plateau at 26 to 28 weeks' gestation. In contrast, macrocystic CCAMs can have abrupt enlargements in size owing to rapid fluid accumulation in a large cyst. For these reasons, patients with microcystic CCAMs can be followed closely up to 26 to 28 weeks' gestation. At that point, the interval between ultrasound examinations can be lengthened. On the other hand, macrocystic CCAMs require close follow-up throughout the duration of the pregnancy.[32,36]

Once the fetus with hydrops reaches a viable gestational age, early delivery should be considered. In fetuses who are not yet viable outside the uterus and have one dominant macrocystic lesion, a thoracoamniotic shunt may reverse the hydrops fetalis.[37] Needle drainage has not proved to be an effective option because rapid reaccumulation of fluid occurs. Fetal thoracotomy with CCAM resection is an option in the pre-viable fetus with a microcystic CCAM or one without the presence of a dominant cyst. The fetal thoracic space is exposed through a fifth intercostal space thoracotomy after maternal hysterotomy (Fig. 10-3). The lobe containing the CCAM is identified and exteriorized through the incision. The pulmonary hilar structures are then mass ligated using an endoloop or endoscopic stapler. The thoracotomy is closed in layers.[38,39]

The experience with CCAM at UCSF and the Children's Hospital of Philadelphia has been published.[40] One hundred and thirty-four women pregnant with fetuses with CCAM were evaluated. Of this group, 120 elected to continue their pregnancies. Seventy-nine fetuses had no evidence of hydrops. Of these, 76 were followed and all survived. Three fetuses without evidence of hydrops and with large dominant cysts underwent thoracoamniotic shunt placement. All three fetuses survived. Twenty-five hydropic fetuses were followed with no intervention. All mothers delivered prematurely, and all fetuses died perinatally. Sixteen fetuses with hydrops underwent intervention: 13 underwent open fetal surgery while 3 underwent thoracoamniotic shunt placement. Two of the 3 survived in the group that underwent shunt placement, and 8 of 13 survived in the open fetal surgery group.

Recently, it has been shown that fetuses with large CCAMs and hydrops can be treated with maternal corticosteroids. This finding was discovered serendipitously at UCSF during the preparation of several hydropic fetuses for fetal surgery.[41] In these cases, maternal corticosteroids were administered to enhance fetal lung maturity. Subsequent ultrasound surveys showed resolution of the hydrops. These findings were later identified in similar patients at Children's Hospital of Philadelphia.[42] A multicenter, prospective trial is now underway to investigate the role of corticosteroids in the treatment and management of hydrops in fetuses with a large fetal CCAM.

Sacrococcygeal Teratoma

Sacrococcygeal teratoma is a rare tumor that is being diagnosed with increasing frequency in utero, allowing for observation of the prenatal natural history of the disease and appropriate perinatal management. As with CCAM, fetuses with SCT are susceptible to in-utero demise. SCTs can grow to a tremendous size in relation to the fetus and can cause high-output cardiac

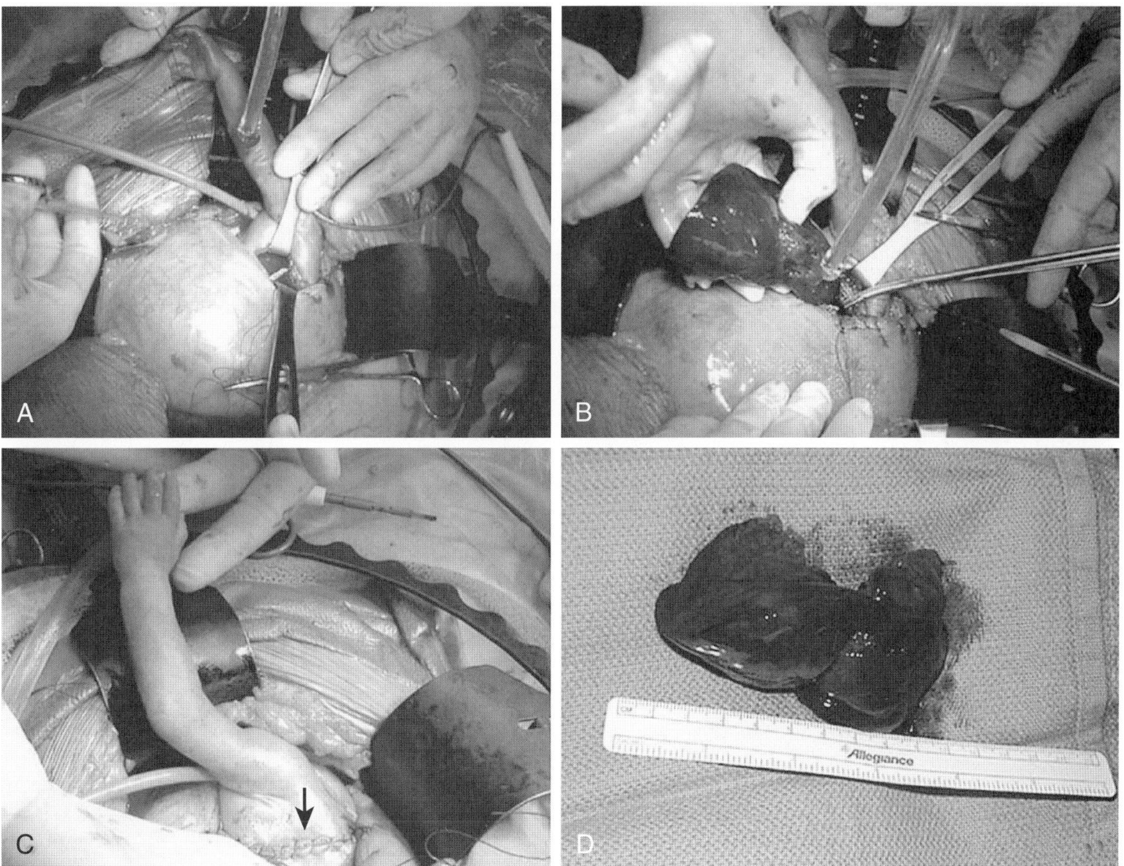

Figure 10-3. These photographs depict an infant with a large left upper lobe CCAM undergoing in-utero left lobectomy. **A,** The infant's left arm is visualized. Note the maternal hysterotomy and the left fetal thoracotomy (with retractors inserted) through the fifth intercostal space. **B,** The left upper lobe containing the CCAM has been identified and exteriorized through the thoracotomy incision. The pulmonary hilar structures were mass ligated using an endoloop. **C,** The fetal thoracotomy incision (*arrow*) has been closed. **D,** The left upper lobe specimen containing the CCAM is seen.

failure and nonimmune hydrops through vascular shunting. Rarely, tumors can hemorrhage internally or externally, resulting in fetal anemia and hypovolemia. Other potential problems with a fetus with a large SCT are dystocia and preterm labor. Delivery can be particularly difficult when the diagnosis has not been made prenatally. A traumatic delivery may result in hemorrhage or tumor rupture. Most clinicians favor cesarean delivery for fetuses with large SCTs. Thus, prenatal diagnosis and careful obstetric planning are critical in the appropriate management of such fetuses.

We have reported our initial experience with 17 fetuses and mothers with a prenatally diagnosed SCT.[43] Of the 17 fetuses, 12 developed hydrops. All 5 of the nonhydropic fetuses were delivered near term and survived. Of the 12 hydropic fetuses, 7 underwent fetal intervention with 3 survivors. Five hydropic fetuses were followed without fetal intervention, and none in this group survived. Other groups have also found an exceedingly high rate of fetal demise in fetuses with an SCT and hydrops. The group at Children's Hospital of Philadelphia recently published their experience with 30 fetuses with SCT.[44] There were 14 survivors, and four pregnancies were terminated. Fifteen fetuses had solid tumors. Of those, 4 developed signs of hydrops and underwent fetal debulking operations. Three of the 4 survived.

The most common approach for fetal intervention for an SCT is a maternal hysterotomy with resection or debulking of the tumor (Fig. 10-4). A predominantly cystic lesion may be amenable to percutaneous drainage or placement of a shunt. Also, tumor debulking using percutaneous coagulation techniques, such as with RFA or laser coagulation to decrease the vascular shunt, are minimally invasive alternatives to open resection that warrant further investigation.[30,45]

Abnormalities of Twin Gestations

Twin-Twin Transfusion Syndrome

Twin-twin transfusion syndrome (TTTS) is the most common complication (10%) of monochorionic twin pregnancies.[46] In monochorionic twin pregnancies, the two fetuses share one placenta and there are normal vascular connections between the fetuses. TTTS occurs when there is net flow from one twin to the other. As a result of the transfusion of blood from the donor twin to the recipient twin, hemodynamic

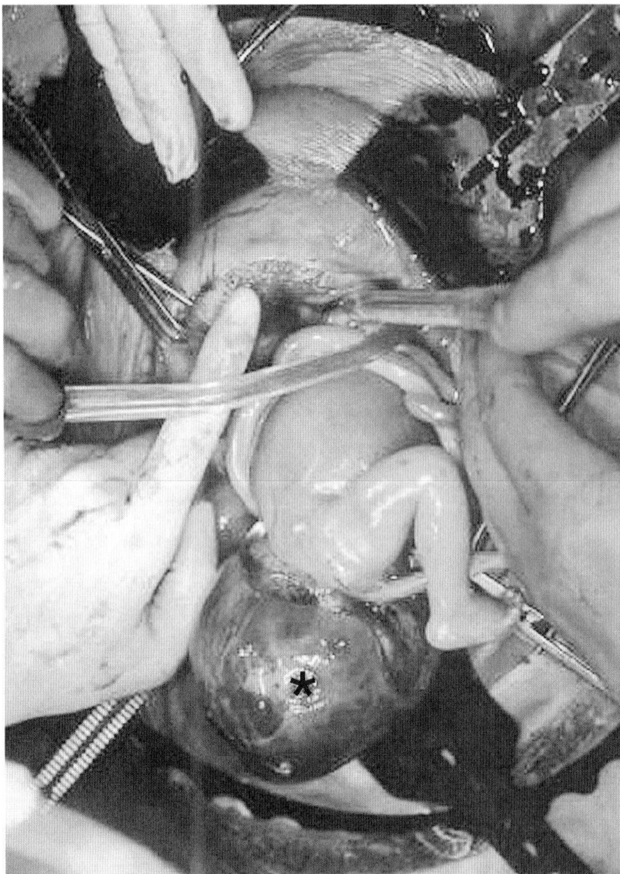

Figure 10-4. The sacrococcygeal teratoma (*asterisk*) was exposed after maternal laparotomy and excised in standard fashion.

compromise can occur in either, or both, twins. The donor twin suffers from a low flow state with resulting ischemia to the brain and kidneys. Conversely, the recipient twin has fluid overload and may develop congestive heart failure and hydrops. The hallmark of TTTS is oligohydramnios in the donor twin and polyhydramnios in the recipient. In addition, often there is a size discordance between the twins, with the donor being smaller than the recipient. Advanced disease is evidenced by progressive discordance in fluid volumes, with the donor becoming "stuck" in the amniotic sac owing to a lack of amniotic fluid. Moreover, worsening cardiac changes in the recipient twin portend a grave prognosis. If left untreated, TTTS carries an 80% to 90% mortality for both twins. In addition, in monochorionic twins, if one twin dies, the other is at risk for neurologic injury owing to a sump phenomenon in the placenta and demised fetus, and also for embolism.[47-49]

Clinicians have attempted a variety of treatments aimed at achieving improved outcome in one or both twins. The most commonly used approach is high-volume amnioreduction of the fluid in the polydramniotic sac. Because polyhydramnios may incite labor, the initial aim of amnioreduction is to reduce uterine volume to decrease the risk of preterm labor. In the International Amnioreduction Registry, high-volume amnioreduction has resulted in a survival rate of almost 60%.[50]

Several groups have used fetoscopic guidance to laser ablate the intertwin vascular connections. This can be done either nonselectively by ablating all intertwin connections or selectively by ablating only arteriovenous connections with flow in the causative direction. Fetoscopic laser ablation can be performed either percutaneously (using 1- or 2-mm endoscopes) or by maternal laparotomy (with 3- or 5-mm endoscopes). If the larger scopes are used, a maternal laparotomy is favored to close the uterine defect created by insertion of these larger ports. The telescopes are introduced through cannulas that have side channels for irrigation and for insertion of a laser. Recently, two large prospective trials have been published comparing amnioreduction to laser ablation of intertwin vessels.[51,52] The European trial enrolled 70 women in the amnioreduction arm and 72 women in the laser ablation arm. The trial was stopped early after interim analysis showed a clear survival advantage to laser therapy: 76% vs. 51% single survivor and 36% vs. 26% for dual survivors.[51] The North American trial also was stopped early after randomizing 42 mothers: 20 in the amnioreduction arm and 22 in the laser ablation one.[52] There was no survival benefit to either intervention, but the study was underpowered due to the early termination of the trial. This trial was complicated by the reluctance of referring physicians to send their patients to the various centers for randomization.

Twin Reversed Arterial Perfusion

Twin reversed arterial perfusion sequence (TRAP) is a rare disease of monochorionic twins that occurs when one normal twin acts as a "pump" for an acardiac, acephalic twin. The normal twin is put at risk for high-output heart failure and hydrops because of the need to maintain blood flow throughout the entire placenta as well as to the acardiac twin. The vascular flow in the acardiac twin is characteristically reversed. Thus, the acronym TRAP was coined to describe this anomaly. The natural history of TRAP is greater than a 50% mortality in the pump twin due to hydrops.[53,54] The risk of hydrops increases as the mass of the acardiac twin increases relative to the normal twin. Generally, intervention is needed when there is evidence of hydrops in the pump twin or when the estimated fetal weight of the acardiac twin is 50% or more relative to the twin functioning as the pump.

Multiple techniques have been used to separate the vascular connections in TRAP pregnancies. These include open hysterotomy and delivery, fetoscopic ligation, bipolar cautery, harmonic scalpel division, thermal coagulation, and laser coagulation. At UCSF, RFA is used to coagulate the umbilical cord insertion site on the acardiac twin's abdomen.[55-57] RFA was originally designed for ablation of solid tumors, but its small size and effective coagulation has been ideal for this application.[58] We have published our results with RFA for TRAP in 29 patients who underwent RFA between

18 and 24 weeks' gestation.[5] Survival was 86% percent overall, with 92% survival in monochorionic, diamniotic pregnancies.

Myelomeningocele

Myelomeningocele, or spina bifida, is characterized by an open neural tube and exposed spinal canal elements. MMC can occur anywhere along the spine, but most commonly occurs in the lumbar or cervical vertebral levels. Complications include neurologic deficits with motor and somatosensory abnormalities that correspond to the level of the spinal defect. In addition, autonomic function is also commonly deranged with an inability to control bladder or bowel function. Also, nearly all patients with MMC develop the Arnold-Chiari type II malformation of the hindbrain, and most will require ventriculoperitoneal shunting for hydrocephalus. Unlike patients who have been considered for fetal intervention, fetuses with MMC are generally born alive and healthy. However, the attendant morbidity from the neurologic abnormalities is severe, as up to 30% of patients die before reaching adulthood owing to respiratory, urinary, or central nervous system complications. Standard current therapy for MMC is postnatal repair of the spinal defect and extensive rehabilitation.[59]

The rationale for fetal intervention in MMC is the "two-hit" hypothesis, in which the first hit is the original neural tube defect that results in an open spinal canal. The second hit is postulated to be due to direct trauma to the exposed neural elements while the fetus is in utero.[60,61] It is this second hit that could potentially be ameliorated by fetal intervention.[62] Various animal models for fetal MMC have been created in rats, lambs, rabbits, and nonhuman primates to test this hypothesis. The data from these animal studies showed improved distal neurologic function, as well as correction of the Arnold-Chiari type II malformation, after in utero repair.[61,63]

Based on these animal data, two pilot studies in human fetuses have utilized MMC repair via an open hysterotomy (Fig. 10-5) and fetoscopy, with primary repair or skin allografts.[64-67] Preliminary results did not show improvement in lower extremity neurologic function, but did show improvement in the Arnold-Chiari type II malformation with reduced hindbrain herniation.[68-70] In addition, a possible decrease in the need for ventriculoperitoneal shunting was found when compared with historical controls.

MMC is unique in that it is the first nonlethal anomaly for which fetal surgery has been undertaken. However, it is associated with significant morbidity. Refinement in operative technique has minimized as much as possible the risk to the mother during these open fetal operations. Based on these data, the NIH has sponsored a prospective, multicenter, randomized controlled trial to investigate the efficacy of fetal surgery for MMC.[71] The results from this trial should be known in the near future.

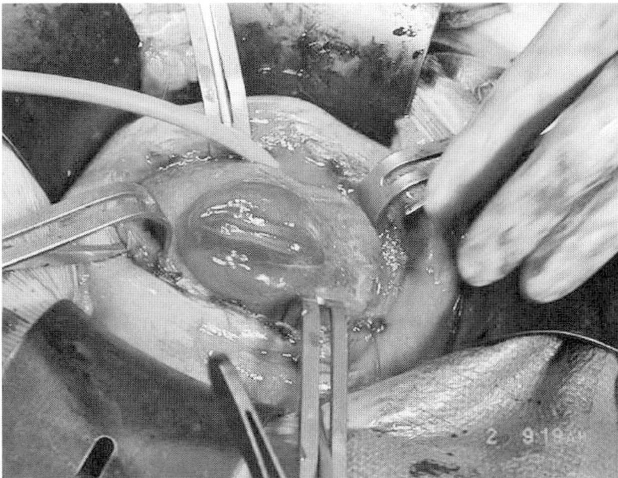

Figure 10-5. The myelomeningocele is exposed after maternal hysterectomy. The defect is closed by pediatric neurosurgeons using an operating microscope.

STEM CELLS AND GENE THERAPY

Gene therapy for prenatally identifiable diseases is being actively pursued for specific disorders. However, it is currently experimental. The rationale behind in-utero therapy with stem cells and/or virally directed genes includes avoiding the progression of disease in the fetus during gestation, as well as taking advantage of the developing immune system of the fetus, thus potentially negating postnatal problems of tolerance, rejection, and graft-versus-host disease.[72]

Specific issues for in-utero treatment of genetic diseases include the timing of diagnosis and therapy, how to deliver the stem cells or genes, the sources of the stem cells, and the longevity of treatment. With the advent of chorionic villus sampling, genetic diseases can now be identified in the first trimester. Timing of potential treatments is crucial to take advantage of the possible "pre-immune" status of the fetus, making fetuses potentially more receptive to exogenous genes or cells. Several investigators have utilized hematopoietic stem cells as a vector in an attempt to induce chimerism to treat the diseases.[73-75] Others have investigated the use of retroviral vectors to insert genetic material into the fetus.[76,77] This approach reduces the problem of obtaining the large numbers of stem cells needed to create even a modest amount of chimerism. Other approaches include using maternal stem cells or genetic material because studies have demonstrated early cross-trafficking of maternal cells in the fetus. Diseases that are a candidate for this approach include hematologic, immunologic, metabolic, and neurologic abnormalities (Table 10-1). To date, there have been over 30 reports of in-utero therapy with hematopoietic stem cells. However, the only durable treatment has been in patients with preexisting immunologic defects.[78,79] Currently, in-utero gene therapy and stem cell therapy are in their infancy but remain an active topic of research and investigation.

Table 10-1	Diseases for Which In Utero Stem Cell or Gene Therapy May Be Applicable
Hematologic	
α-Thalassemia Fanconi's anemia Chronic granulomatous disease Hemophilia A	
Immunologic	
Severe combined immunodeficiency (SCID) syndrome Wiskott-Aldrich syndrome	
Metabolic	
Wolman's disease	
Type II Gaucher's disease Pompe's disease Osteogenesis imperfecta Cystic fibrosis	
Neurologic	
Lesch-Nyhan syndrome Tay-Sachs disease Sandhoff's disease Niemann-Pick disease Leukodystrophies Generalized gangliosidosis Leigh disease	

SUMMARY

Fetal surgery has progressed from an investigational therapy to an accepted mode of therapy for selected fetal diseases. Multidisciplinary teams are critical for the success of any fetal treatment program. Regular, weekly meetings are necessary to keep all members of the team abreast of developments and new patients. Some diseases that historically have had a high perinatal mortality rate have shown improved survival with fetal surgery. NIH-funded, prospective trials have been performed for CDH and TTTS. Current clinical trials include evaluations for the efficacy of fetal intervention for MMC, hydrops, and CCAM, and reversible tracheal occlusion for CDH. In order to maximize the benefit to the fetus while minimizing the risk to the mother, fetal interventions were initially reserved for fetuses with lethal anomalies. MMC represents the first nonlethal anomaly that has been evaluated.

As minimal access techniques improve, and the maternal risks are further reduced, indications for fetal intervention may continue to broaden. New areas of investigation include tissue engineering, and stem cell and gene therapy. Maternal safety must remain paramount, and the risk to the mother should be minimized at all times. The study of these emerging techniques should occur initially with animal models and then in humans under the rubric of prospective, clinical trials.

section 2

TRAUMA

chapter 11

FOREIGN BODIES

Joseph L. Lelli Jr., MD

Infants and young children are naturally curious about their environment. It is this childhood inclination for exploration that results in the serious problems of aspiration, insertion, and ingestion of foreign bodies (FBs). The complications of FBs in the upper and lower airway, the gastrointestinal tract, and the ears carry a signification morbidity and mortality.

FB aspiration has been the cause of 160 annual deaths in children younger than the age of 14 years in the United States.[1] In 2007, the Annual Report of the American Association of Poison Control Centers noted 127,777 cases of ingestion of an FB by a minor. More than 70% of these cases (95,754) involved a child younger than age 6 years.[2] The Centers for Disease Control and Prevention (CDC) reported an estimated 15,653 children, 14 years of age or younger, who were treated in emergency departments in 2007 for choking-related episodes.[3] Although many of these events are benign, significant complications arise from FB entrapment, including but not limited to infection, obstruction, corrosion, fistula formation, hemorrhage, and nerve injury. FBs may be a secondary sign of underlying disorders such as pica, otalgia, rhinitis, neurologic dysfunction, and even child abuse. Despite significant advances in prevention, first aid, and intervention, FBs in the pediatric patient will remain a problem as long as children remain naturally curious.

Other factors contribute to ingestion and aspiration of FBs besides age. Contributing factors include the male gender, immature coordination of swallowing, lack of molars before age 4 years, neurologic impairment, seizure disorders, anatomic or functional esophageal disorders, immature laryngeal sphincter control, and an unsafe environment.[4,5] Children who are neglected or abused have been found to have an increased risk for FB indigestion or aspiration. The suspicion of child abuse should be raised if a very young child has a history of multiple previous episodes or is found to have multiple FBs on evaluation.[6,7]

Prior to 1930, the mortality rate associated with FBs was 24%. Owing in large part to the work of Chevalier Jackson,[8] the mortality rate was reduced to 2%. Jackson has been credited with the development of appropriate preparation of the patient and optimal positioning, as well as the equipment that made endoscopic removal of the FBs safe and successful.[9] In 1968, Harold Hopkins made the next significant evolution in endoscopy.[10,11] The Hopkins rod-lens telescope was added to the endoscope, bringing vastly improved illumination and visualization. As extraction devices evolved, the visualization during removal improved. Also, the incidence of complications began to decrease.[12]

Food items compose 50% to 80% of FBs removed by endoscopy from children's aerodigestive tracts.[13-16] In the 2007 CDC annual report, 60% of choking episodes treated in emergency departments were due to food substances, with 30% due to a nonfood substance.[3] Sixty-five percent of food-based choking episodes were due to candy or gum. The list of foods causing choking injury was similar in many published reports: hot dogs, nuts, seeds, and vegetable or fruit pieces.[14-17] Coins account for a significant portion of nonfood substances causing choking events in children.[1,16,18,19] Sixty-eight percent of the deaths in children younger than age 14 years reported to the Consumer Product and Safety Commission (CPSC) between 1972 and 1992 were due to nonfood items.[16] The cause of fatal choking was often balloons, balls, and other toys intended for children's use. The remaining 32% of causes of fatal choking episodes were household items. Two deaths in the CPSC database were due to choking on latex examination gloves given to children in clinicians' offices. The majority of choking deaths occurred in children 3 years of age and older with balloons and other conforming objects.[16]

The diagnosis of an FB in the aerodigestive tract may be challenging because of the difficulty in obtaining a reliable history from the child. The timely recognition of aspiration or ingestion relies heavily on clinical suspicion. Symptoms are mild or even absent in 40% to 60% of patients. Eighty percent of the asymptomatic patients have normal findings on physical examination. Twenty to 25 percent of FB events are not witnessed.[18,20,21] In one report, 15% of children evaluated by an emergency medicine physician for choking were not recognized as FB victims.[21] FBs persisted undetected in these children for 7 or more days, not suspected by caretakers, parents, or the physician. The clinician has a limited amount of data available when evaluating these patients. Therefore, a high index of suspicion for FB ingestion and aspiration must always be maintained.

AIRWAY FOREIGN BODIES

Approximately 75% of FB aspiration events in the pediatric age group occur in children younger than age 3 years. Boys are affected twice as frequently as girls. There are a number of factors that make young children more susceptible to aspiration. Children younger than age 3 years often cry, shout, and run with objects in their mouths and have immature coordination of swallowing and airway protection. They are also at an oral exploration stage of development when everything they hold tends to go into their mouths. These factors combine to make the child younger than age 3 years susceptible to FB aspiration (Table 11-1).

Most FBs are small enough to pass through the larynx and enter the trachea. The narrowest point in the child's airway is the cricoid ring. The 1% to 7% of airway FBs that become lodged in the laryngeal inlet are mostly seen in infants younger than 1 year of age (Fig. 11-1). Because the trachea is relatively large compared with the cricoid, FBs that lodge within it account for only an additional 3% to 12% of cases. These usually occur in cases of tracheomalacia, in the patient who has poor respiratory effort, or when previous postoperative stricture has occurred. In the majority of cases, the FB will pass easily through the trachea and lodge in the primary or secondary bronchi. A predominance of right bronchial involvement is somewhat dependent on age (Fig. 11-2). The prevalence for right-sided FBs is due to the greater diameter of the right bronchus, a smaller angle of divergence from the tracheal axis, greater air flow to the right lung, and the position of the carina to the left of the midline. In one anatomic study, the position of the carina was believed to be the only determining factor in the distribution of the FB.[22] The angle of the left bronchus and, therefore, the position of the carina is determined by the development of the aortic knob. The aortic knob reaches adult size by the age of 15 years, at which time it displaces the left main-stem bronchus downward. This creates a more obtuse angle at the carina, changing the more symmetric bronchial angles in young children. This may explain the increased propensity for right bronchus FBs in young children compared with those in older children and adults.

Table 11-1	Factors that Make Young Children Susceptible to Aspiration
Age younger than 3 years	
Male gender	
Often cry, shout, run, and play with objects in their mouths	
Do not have molars to chew certain foods adequately	
Immature coordination of swallowing and airway protection	
Oral exploration of their environment	
Immature laryngeal sphincter control	

The type of airway FB varies from generation to generation and country to country. For instance, in the United States, as diapers became disposable, the incidence of aspirated safety pins declined dramatically. Fifty years ago, a safety pin, usually opened, was an extremely common FB, but now it accounts for less than 5% in most reports. Small plastic products are now significant items in childhood FB aspiration. The CPSC mandates federal choking prevention standards. The standards use a small parts cylinder to determine if the small part on a toy is a choking hazard. When reviewing airway injuries and fatalities from FBs, 23% of fatalities were from toys with small parts that met the CPSC guidelines for size and 90% of all FBs found in the airway met the standard for being considered "safe." Nevertheless, food matter is still the most commonly aspirated FB for all generations and nations (Table 11-2).

The most important factor in evaluating a child who possibly aspirated an FB is an accurate history. The common signs and symptoms will be present in 50% to 90% of children who aspirate an FB. In a series of 100 FB aspiration cases, a choking crisis occurred in 95% and was the most sensitive clinical parameter.[23] FBs that lodge in the larynx and trachea can be completely obstructive, causing sudden death. Partial obstruction by an FB can lead to a sufficient inflammatory reaction in the surrounding tissue to produce total, or near total, obstruction. A history of choking without initial physical findings of reduced air exchange requires a high degree of suspicion if a timely diagnosis is to be made.[24] The larynx, trachea, and bronchi can initially accommodate FBs with minimal physical findings. This may account for the fact that 20% to 50% of FBs are detected more than 1 week after aspiration.[25]

The complications that develop as a result of aspiration are obstruction due to granulation tissue formation

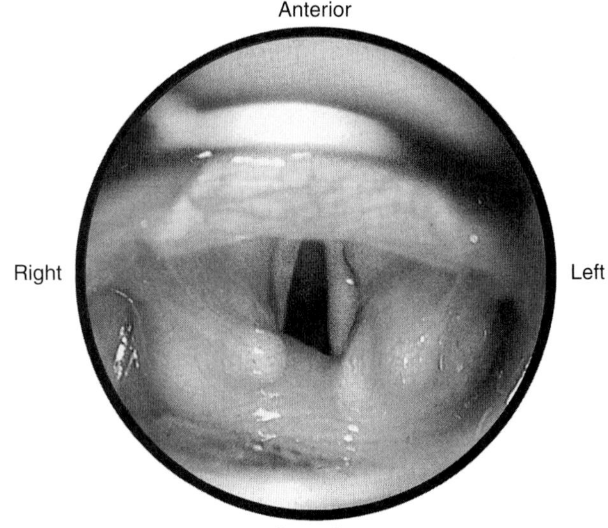

Figure 11-1. In this young infant, a coin became lodged anteriorly between the tongue and epiglottis in the vallecula.

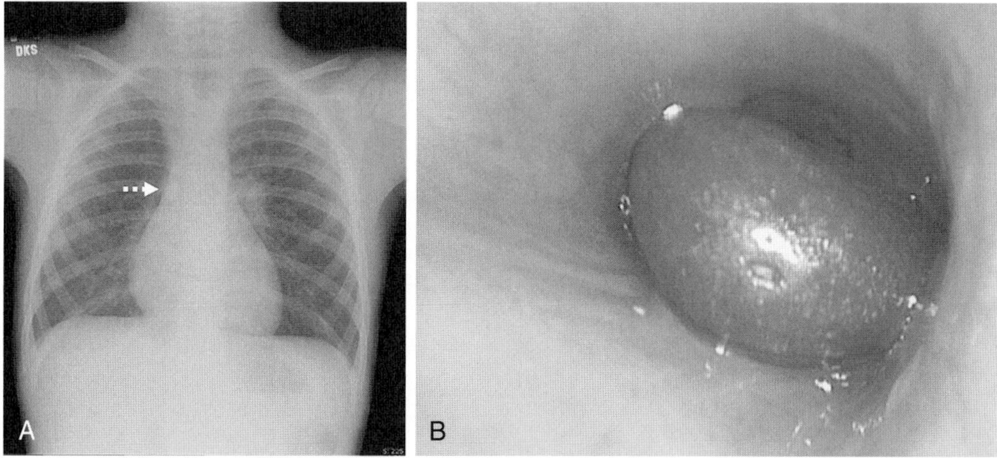

Figure 11-2. This 6-year-hold had a rock in his mouth, tripped, and aspirated the rock. **A,** On the chest radiograph, it is lodged in the right main-stem bronchus (*arrow*). **B,** The rock is seen at bronchoscopy. It was difficult to remove this rock because it was quite large, but it was able to be wedged between a Fogarty catheter and the bronchoscope and retrieved in this manner.

Table 11-2 Commonly Aspirated Foreign Bodies

Food Products	Nonfood Products
Candy/gum	Coins
Peanuts and other nuts	Toy parts
Seeds	Crayons
Popcorn	Pen tops
Hot dogs	Tacks, nails, needles, pins
Vegetable matter	Beads
Meat matter	Screws
Fish bones	

or strictures, atelectasis, bronchiectasis, pneumonia, empyema, lung abscess, perforation with pneumothorax, and systemic sepsis. Clinical findings that develop in a previously asymptomatic patient include croup, persistent cough, hemoptysis, fever, malaise, and respiratory compromise.[21,25,26] Because an unwitnessed choking event may not produce initial symptoms or physical findings, radiographic evaluation is essential for timely diagnosis and treatment.

Radiographic examination consists of anteroposterior and lateral views of the extended neck and chest. Chest radiographs in inspiration and expiration are beneficial in demonstrating unilateral air trapping that is present in up to 62% of patients when the bronchial FB acts as a one-way valve.[27] Air moves past the FB as the bronchus expands during inhalation, but the air is trapped, producing obstructive emphysema. Hyperinflation of the obstructed lobe or lung produces mediastinal shift to the contralateral or unobstructed side. For evaluation in the young patient who cannot cooperate with inspiration and expiration radiograms, left and right lateral decubitus radiographs may be helpful because the obstructed lung will not deflate while in the dependent position (Fig. 11-3). Although 56% of patients will have a normal chest radiograph within 24 hours of aspiration, others will demonstrate mediastinal shift (55%), consolidation (47%), pneumonia (26%), atelectasis (18%), or a radiopaque object (3%).[28] FBs that are present for a long time will develop complete obstruction and atelectasis secondary to a local inflammatory reaction.

A radiolucent FB is often evident only because of the ball-valve effect. The benefit of the radiographic assessment is dependent on the location of the FB. Laryngotracheal FBs can be evaluated radiographically with about a 90% yield. In cases of bronchial FBs, chest radiography is less diagnostic, with a sensitivity and specificity of 65% to 75%.[14,26-29] Radiographic evaluation is helpful in evaluating the patient with a choking history, but the definitive diagnostic assessment remains bronchoscopy.

General anesthesia provides a controlled environment for removal of most airway FBs. Only in the small group of patients with laryngeal FBs can removal be accomplished at times without anesthesia. Spontaneous ventilation, with the patients generating their own negative intrathoracic pressure, is the preferred technique. Positive-pressure ventilation is avoided because it can force the FB farther into the airway or may produce complete occlusion. However, assisted ventilation may be necessary for either oxygen desaturation or inadequate depth of anesthesia for the procedure. As in any standard operation, induction is performed with precautions taken to minimize secretions, laryngospasm, and hypoxia. After induction, the patient's head is extended and placed in the "sniffing" position. A laryngoscope is used to expose the larynx for insertion of the bronchoscope and to ensure that the FB is not within easy grasp of a McGill forceps. When the laryngeal inlet is deemed clear, the endoscopy is performed.

Endoscopic extraction of FBs from children requires a gentle, experienced hand. Great care is taken to protect the eyes, lips, teeth, tongue, and other laryngeal structures with insertion of the bronchoscope. The tongue is always swept to the left side with the laryngoscope to expose the glottis. The bronchoscope is inserted into the upper trachea and ventilation is

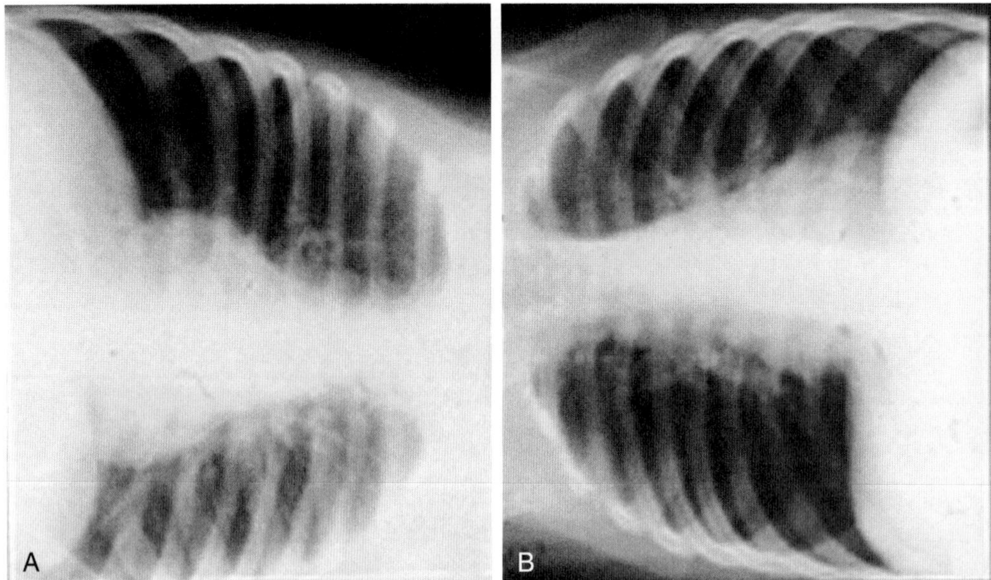

Figure 11-3. Radiographic evaluation in the young patient with a suspected foreign body aspiration can be difficult because inspiratory/expiratory chest radiographs may not be possible. Therefore, left and right lateral, decubitus films may be helpful because the obstructed lung will not deflate while in the dependent position. **A,** Radiograph with the child in a left lateral decubitus position. Note that the dependent left lung deflates appropriately. **B,** In the right lateral decubitus position, the right lung does not deflate, indicating a possible foreign body in the right main-stem bronchus. This was confirmed at bronchoscopy.

performed through the side arm. The tracheobronchial tree is then completely inspected, and the FB is removed.

The rigid bronchoscope is the primary instrument for evaluating the tracheobronchial tree for an FB. The instruments most commonly used are the Doesel-Huzly bronchoscope with Hopkins rod-lens telescope (Karl Storz Endoscopy, Tuttlingen, Germany) and the Holinger ventilating fiber-illuminated bronchoscope (Pilling Weck, Inc., Markham, ON). Both have the benefit of good exposure and the ability to shield FBs within the tube during extraction. The rigid instruments also allow the use of a diverse number of forceps. The length and diameter of the endoscope is dictated by the patient's age and size. In general, one should use the largest scope possible that will not cause trauma. The forceps used in most pediatric surgery practices are the positive-action, "center-action," or the passive-action forceps. The combination optical/illumination system with the forceps allows the greatest visibility.

Standard flexible bronchoscopy is being performed with increasing frequency in children older than age 12 years utilizing conscious sedation.[30] Older children can tolerate a larger and more versatile bronchoscope owing to their larger trachea. Additionally, the utilization of laryngeal mask anesthesia with a flexible bronchoscope passed through a side port in the mask has been used in younger as well as older children.

The primary causes of unsuccessful FB removal are inexperience, an impacted FB obscured by granulation tissue, and inadequate equipment. Many endoscopists describe the use of a Fogarty catheter for extraction of FBs inaccessible to grasping instruments. Removal may be limited by poor visualization associated with bleeding, granulation tissue, and edema. In cases with significant granulation tissue and bleeding or multiple FB fragments that migrate distally and become impacted, a second endoscopy may be required. Post-instrumentation laryngeal edema may require respiratory therapy intervention before the second procedure. The post-instrumentation edema responds well to inhaled epinephrine and intravenous corticosteroid treatment.[31,32] The second procedure may include repeated endoscopy or thoracotomy with bronchotomy, segmentectomy, or lobectomy as required.

In an attempt to minimize the complications associated with a delay in diagnosis of FB aspiration in young children, bronchoscopy based on a history of choking alone has been advocated.[12,14,17,21,25] A negative bronchoscopy rate of 10% to 15% has been deemed acceptable to prevent the morbidity associated with delayed diagnosis.[33] Individual patient circumstances, including access to expert care, will enter into decisions for this more aggressive approach.

ESOPHAGEAL FOREIGN BODIES

The esophagus is a muscular tube that has two shallow curves as it descends through the diaphragm to its termination at the gastric cardia. It is the narrowest portion of the alimentary tract and is protected at its upper end by the cricopharyngeus muscle where many ingested FBs lodge. The esophagus is narrowed somewhat at the aortic arch, left main-stem bronchus, and the diaphragm, areas where FBs will be trapped (Table 11-3).

Once they pass the cricopharyngeus, most swallowed objects will pass into the stomach. Congenital and acquired esophageal anomalies may contribute

Table 11-3	Level of Retention of Aspirated Esophageal Foreign Bodies
Cricopharyngeus muscle	63%–84%
Aortic crossover mid-esophagus	10%–17%
Lower esophagus sphincter	5%–20%

From Stack LB, Munter DW. Foreign bodies in the gastrointestinal tract. Emerg Med Clin North Am 14:493, 1996.

to FB obstruction of the esophagus. The middle and lower esophageal motility is abnormal in patients born with esophageal atresia. Also, it is relatively common for young children to swallow soft, rubbery foods and have them lodge firmly near the area of the esophageal anastomosis. FB obstruction may be seen in patients with an unsuspected vascular ring, ectopic salivary glands, cartilaginous rests, middle mediastinal mass, an esophageal stricture, achalasia, or duplication cyst. Twenty-two percent of patients older than age 5 years with esophageal FBs were noted to have anatomic abnormalities.[34,35] In a series of patients with an impacted esophageal food bolus, up to 70% had esophageal abnormalities.[36] In most cases in which the level is reported, ingested FBs lodge at the normal anatomic narrowing of the cricopharyngeus muscle or the level of the aortic arch (see Table 11-3).

Coins and smooth blunt objects are the most commonly ingested items in large pediatric series. The patients are most commonly between 18 and 48 months of age.[37] In one review of almost 200 patients, 89% of FBs were coins.[38] There is a well-documented cultural and geographic difference in the types of FBs ingested. In a review of 343 Chinese children, 42% had ingested fish bones and only 39% had ingested coins.[35] In a report from Belgium, only 89 (27%) of 325 patients were found to have ingested coins, but 16% had ingested sharp objects, a significantly higher percentage when compared with other nations. In older children, food boluses and school supplies–parts of pencils and pens–are most common.

The ingestion of an FB is often unrecognized and asymptomatic, as the FB passes uneventfully through the gut. Although swallowed FBs are not considered as dangerous as aspirated FBs, up to 1500 deaths per year have been documented from esophageal FB ingestion.[39] Clinical symptoms of a patient with an FB that obstructs the esophagus include the sudden onset of acute and severe coughing, pain in the pharyngeal or retrosternal region, gagging, poor feeding, and drooling, among others. Periesophageal inflammation from an unsuspected esophageal FB can cause airway symptoms such as wheezing, stridor, and coughing. Significant respiratory symptoms can be seen with an esophageal FB as the esophageal dilation can result in airway impingement.

The ingestion of small batteries creates a different set of serious problems. Batteries have been found in less than 2% of esophageal FBs historically but are being increasingly seen with the rise of small batteries in children's toys.[40] A 7-year review reported 2320 cases of battery ingestion, but only 9.9% of these patients

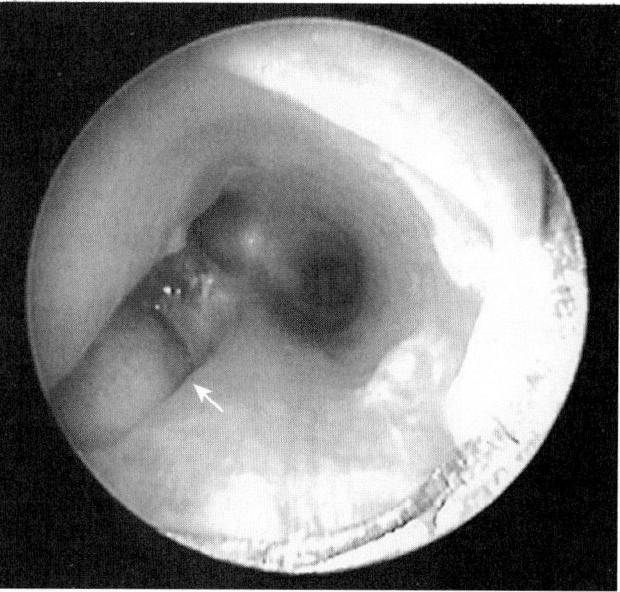

Figure 11-4. This infant accidentally swallowed a lithium battery. The battery was removed within a few hours of its ingestion. However, 1 week later, the patient developed respiratory distress and bronchoscopy revealed this tracheoesophageal fistula (*arrow*).

were symptomatic.[41] Batteries can cause unique injuries not seen with other FBs. These include direct caustic injury, pressure necrosis, tissue necrosis from electrical discharge, and toxin release (mercury poisoning). The main chemical ingredients of disc batteries include alkaline corrosive agents or heavy metals. Battery size and type may affect management and outcome. Disc batteries can cause corrosive injury to the esophagus within 4 hours.[42] Lithium batteries cause more adverse effects due to their greater size and voltage. A review of reported cases showed that batteries less than 15 mm almost never become lodged in the esophagus, whereas those that are larger than 20 mm account for most of the reported esophageal injuries.[43] A 3-volt lithium battery is enough to cause cellular electrolyte flux, releasing intracellular potassium, and can result in cell death and tissue necrosis. Complications caused by esophageal impaction of button batteries include tracheoesophageal fistula (Fig. 11-4), esophageal burn with and without perforation, aortoesophageal fistula, esophageal stricture, and death. Emergency endoscopy must be performed for batteries retained in the esophagus because of the high propensity of early mucosal injury.[44]

Radiologic evaluation for possible FB ingestion must include a lateral view and an anteroposterior view of both the neck and chest (Fig. 11-5). The radiologic evaluation of a child with a history of possibly swallowing a coin or a radiopaque object is highly sensitive and specific. In a review of the preoperative radiographs of 182 children with a history of FB ingestion (primarily coins), 96.7% had a positive radiographic finding confirmed by endoscopy.[37] Objects that are only faintly radiopaque such as bones or small items of aluminum are often seen on lateral views because

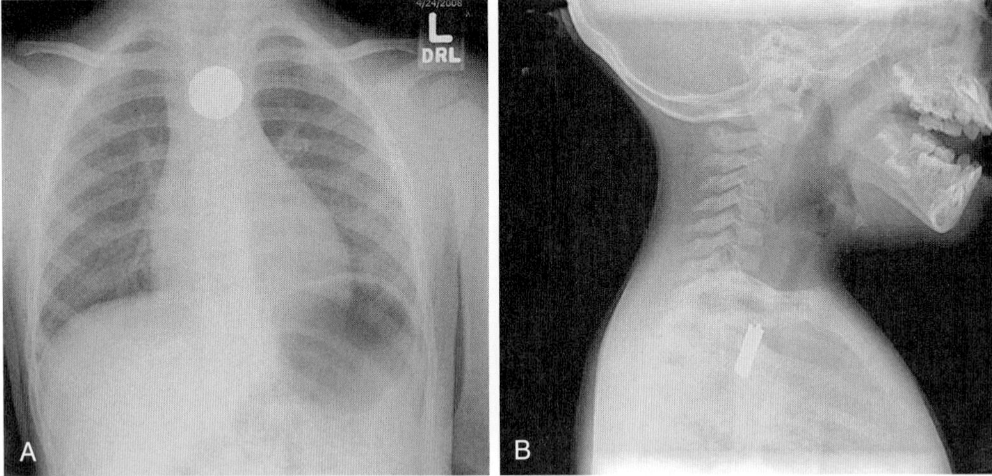

Figure 11-5. This infant was seen in the emergency department for swallowing difficulty and drooling. **A,** Anteroposterior radiograph shows a coin in the upper esophagus. **B,** However, on the lateral view, there are actually four coins superimposed on one another. The lateral view is very helpful for the purpose of determining whether more than one coin has been ingested.

the "end-on" view increases their radiodensity. Totally radiolucent FBs such as plastic beads or toys present a much more difficult radiographic challenge. In these cases, suspicion must be high enough to use contrast studies for the diagnosis. An esophagogram may demonstrate a radiolucent FB as a filling defect and may also reveal anomalies as compression by a vascular ring or an intrinsic stricture. Even though preoperative radiographic evaluation is accurate in demonstrating an FB in a child, the clinical situation should dictate the decision to perform esophagoscopy. Small coins, for example, lodged at the gastroesophageal junction, are likely to pass if given a chance. In an attempt to minimize the complications associated with the delay in diagnosis, endoscopy for suspicious cases with or without radiologic confirmation has been advocated. A negative esophagoscopy rate of 6.2% has been quoted as acceptable to prevent the morbidity associated with the missed diagnosis of an esophageal FB.[37]

Rapid diagnosis and treatment of FBs in the esophagus will decrease morbidity. Studies have been performed, however, to evaluate "watchful waiting" of asymptomatic esophageal coins. In a prospective randomized study, up to 30% of coins passed spontaneously within 8 to 16 hours of observation. Spontaneous passage appears to be associated with increasing age of the patient.[45,46] Watchful waiting, however, failed 70% of the time and was associated with an increased length of hospitalization.[46] Attempts at using glucagon to stimulate passage have proven to be ineffective.[47]

Three common techniques for FB removal from the esophagus are Foley catheter extraction, bougienage to push the FB into the stomach, and endoscopic retrieval. Foley catheter retrieval is generally easy and successful for removing smooth objects in the upper two thirds of the esophagus. The procedure is cost efficient and can be performed without anesthesia and usually under fluoroscopic guidance (Fig. 11-6). The risks of the procedure are potential airway compromise, esophageal injury, inability to visualize the esophageal reaction to the FB, and the discomfort of the awake

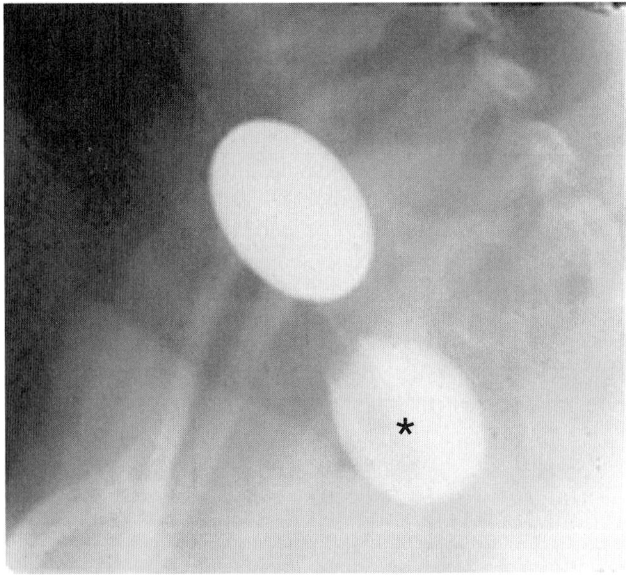

Figure 11-6. This radiograph shows the Foley catheter technique for removing a coin lodged in the upper esophagus. Under fluoroscopy, the Foley catheter is advanced past the coin and the balloon is filled with barium (*asterisk*). Under fluoroscopy, the catheter is then removed, bringing the coin with it. Care must be taken to ensure the patient does not aspirate the coin during its removal. This is a very cost-efficient way to remove coins in the upper esophagus in young children.

child. The success rate of 84% to 96% with Foley catheter extraction is less than with endoscopy.[48-51] Objects that have been retained in the esophagus for longer than 24 hours may have produced significant tissue reaction that significantly increases the risk of catheter extraction as well as the risk of failure for retrieving the FB. On occasion, the Foley catheter insertion itself has resulted in pushing FBs into the stomach.

Bougienage has been shown to be successful in selected cases. The patient has usually ingested a single coin within 24 hours of presentation, is stable, and has

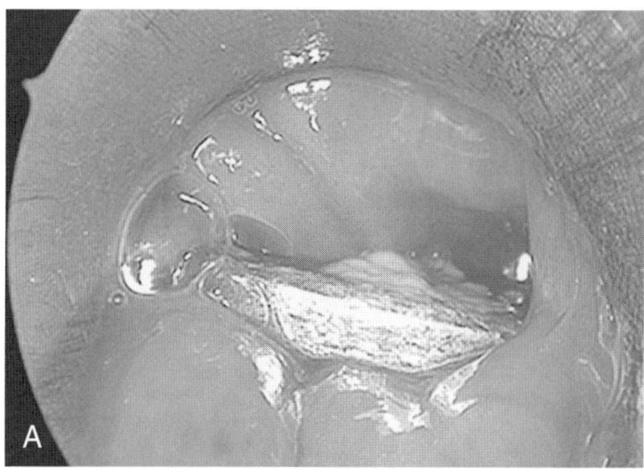

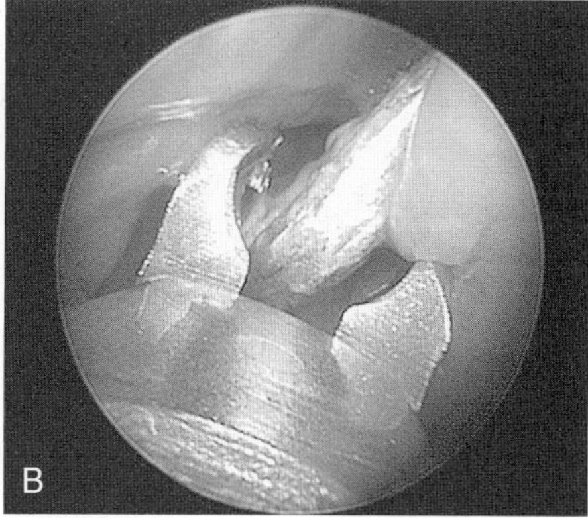

Figure 11-7. This coin was lodged in the esophagus of a 2-year-old child. It was unclear how long the coin had been in the esophagus. Therefore, rigid esophagoscopy was performed. **A,** The coin is seen through the esophagoscope. **B,** The optical graspers are being used to grasp the coin and remove it. The safety and success rate for rigid esophagoscopy and coin removal approaches 100% with minimal complications. This is usually a safe and successful way to remove a coin in the esophagus of children in whom the Foley catheter technique is not appropriate.

no history of esophageal abnormalities or FB aspiration. Blunt-tipped, weighted esophageal bougies are introduced to advance the coin or other smooth object into the stomach with the expectation the object will be passed per rectum. Roughly 90% to 95% of these objects will be evacuated spontaneously.[52] The concern with bougienage is that the nonevacuated FBs can lead to obstruction or perforation of the small intestine, requiring more difficult endoscopic retrieval or surgical exploration.

Rigid endoscopy is the most reliable and successful method used in retrieval of esophageal FBs (Fig. 11-7). The safety and success rate with rigid endoscopy has approached 100% with minimal complications. The procedure is performed in a controlled environment with the same precautions that apply to the use of the rigid bronchoscope. The patient is placed in the supine position with the head in the neutral sniffing position. The cervical spine is straight, allowing for passage of the endoscope over the cervical kyphosis. Esophagoscopes differ from the bronchoscopes in that they have a smooth, flared leading edge. This difference allows the endoscopist to lift the larynx with minimal trauma to expose and open the cricopharyngeus "sphincter." The appropriate size is the largest that can be accommodated without forcing the esophagoscope.

GASTROINTESTINAL FOREIGN BODIES

The vast majority of FBs that are ingested by children are not retained in the esophagus. In one study, 60% of patients who were evaluated for FB ingestion were found to have the FB in their stomach at the time of evaluation.[53] With the exception of sharp objects and batteries, most gastric FBs do not have to be removed because they are eliminated spontaneously.[44,54,55] In a study of 1481 children, 97% of ingested FBs that passed through the esophagus on radiographic study were spontaneously evacuated. The incidence of operative retrieval of ingested FBs found initially to be in the stomach is 1%, whereas the rate for ingested sharp objects is 15% to 30%. Some surgeons recommend early endoscopic retrieval of sharp FBs.[56] Commonly ingested sharp FBs include bones, nails, safety pins, needles, sharp toys, and toothpicks. Toothpick and bones are the most commonly ingested objects that require retrieval. If either of these objects becomes impacted in the intestinal mucosa, erosion may develop, which then can lead to perforation and peritonitis. Objects larger than 2 cm or longer than 3 cm that are swallowed by infants have been shown to have difficulty traversing the pyloric channel. In older children and adults, objects thicker than 2 cm and longer than 5 cm tend to have difficulty passing through the duodenal loop, causing functional gastric outlet obstruction. These objects also warrant endoscopic retrieval. Rarely, FBs become lodged distal to the ligament of Treitz. Although the ileocecal valve is the only natural narrowing in the lower intestinal tract, it is rarely the site for FB retention. Disc battery ingestion requires removal if lodged in the esophagus. Once the battery is in the stomach, it can be managed conservatively with spontaneous passage expected without complications.[57]

Ingestion of multiple magnets usually causes minimal initial physical findings. Late complications, however, include bowel perforation, volvulus, ischemia, and enteroenteral fistulas. Removal of magnets is recommended when there are more than one and while they are still in the stomach. Once they are distal to the stomach, observation is necessary to ensure that they all pass per the rectum.[58]

Bezoars are FBs that have accumulated over time in the alimentary tract. These can cause obstructive symptoms, bleeding, failure to thrive, weight loss due to early satiety, abdominal pain, anorexia, halitosis, and nausea. Common concentrations include plant and vegetable matter (phytobezoar), hair (trichobezoar), persimmons (disopyrobezoar), and neonatal casein curd (proteinacous) aggregations.

Trichobezoars can extend a long tail from the stomach down through the entire intestinal tract to or even beyond the ileocecal valve where they then cause an

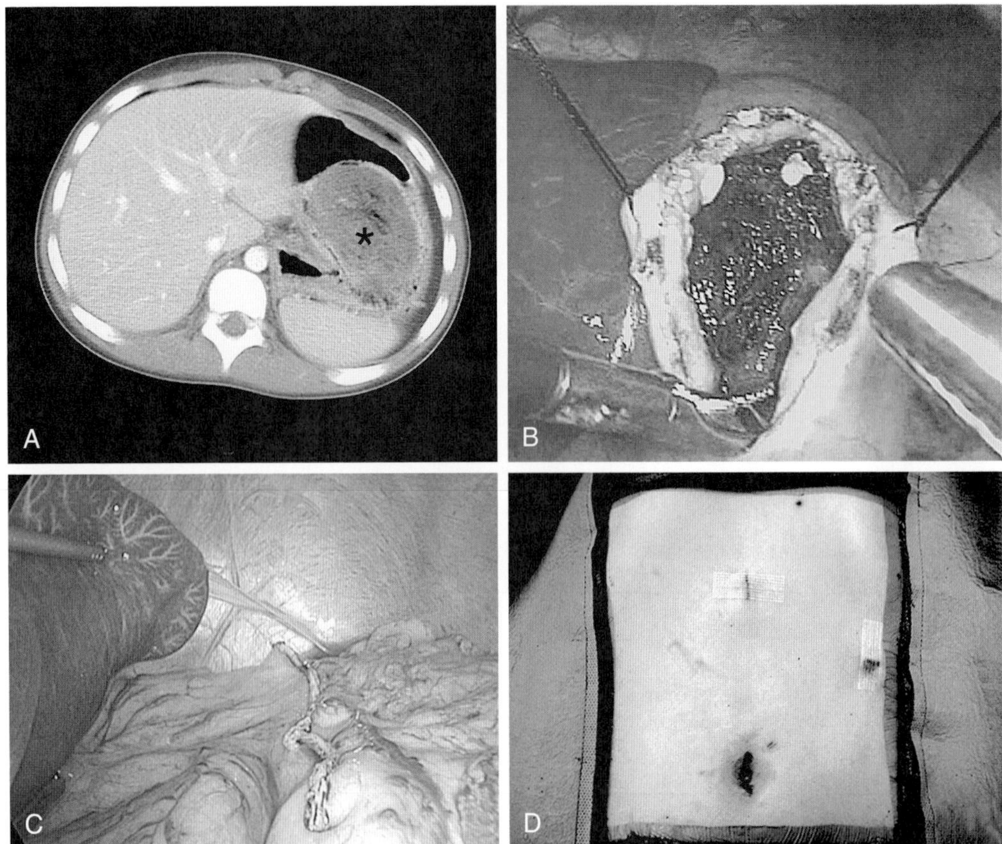

Figure 11-8. A 10-year-old girl was admitted to the hospital with decreasing oral intake, vomiting, and weight loss. **A,** An abdominal CT scan was performed that showed a large gastric bezoar (*asterisk*) in the stomach. Laparoscopic extraction of the trichobezoar was performed. **B,** The stomach was opened and the bezoar was visualized. The trichobezoar was extracted and placed in a bag which was then exteriorized through the umbilical incision. **C,** After extraction of the bezoar, the gastrotomy was closed with the endoscopic stapler. **D,** The incisions used for laparoscopic removal of the trichobezoar are seen in the postoperative photograph.

obstruction. Children with extensive trichobezoars causing this type of obstruction are referred to as having the Rapunzel syndrome.[59] Trichotillomania is a psychosomatic entity in which there is a desire to pull out one's hair and ingest it. Patients suffering from this disorder feel instant release of tension, a sense of relief, and security. This process can lead to the formation of trichobezoars.[60] Most cases of trichotillomania in children are considered "habit disorders" that are amenable to psychotherapy. Bezoars may be retrieved endoscopically or eliminated by enzymatic fragmentation. Laparotomy or laparoscopy may be warranted with large obstructing bezoars such as in the Rapunzel syndrome (Fig. 11-8).

EAR AND NOSE FOREIGN BODIES

FBs may be the cause of mouth breathing and rhinorrhea in children. Identification and removal require appropriate suspicion and adequate instrumentation. Although most FBs recently inserted are easily removed from the nose, those of long standing may not be as simple to remove. Nasal mucosal reaction with edema and granulation tissue develops rather quickly. The mucosal lining of the nose is a dynamic surface that requires uninterrupted mucociliary flow to remain free of crusting and inflammation. Interruption of the flow patterns by an FB readily produces inflammation and infection. FBs placed in the anterior nares can be inert or reactive. Common objects placed in the nares are dried beans, plastic objects, buttons, metals, food, erasers, nuts, seeds, and button batteries. Presenting signs and symptoms with nasal FBs include rhinorrhea, crusting, air flow obstruction, rhinitis, sinusitis, lymphadenopathy, epistaxis, otitis media, and adenoiditis.

Otitis media is a potential sequela of a posterior nasal reaction from an FB, causing eustachian tube obstruction. Plastic and other inert materials may be tolerated for long intervals, but granulation tissue develops to produce an obstruction. Button batteries may lead to septal perforation and destruction of cartilage, leading to a saddle-nose deformity. The site of maximal damage from button batteries has been shown to correspond to the negative pole of the battery.

Successful removal of a nasal FB in a child requires visualization and appropriate instrumentation. Usually this is a simple bedside procedure. The primary or emergency physician using tweezers, cerumen curet, or a cotton-tipped applicator can remove most FBs. Long-standing objects may be more complicated, requiring assistance from a surgical specialist. Tools that can be helpful in visualizing the object are the Frazier tip suction, the optic headlight, and the nasal speculum. The Hartmann forceps, wire loop, flexible cerumen curet, alligator forceps, and a right-angled hook are tools that increase the likelihood of recovering the FB. It is beneficial to place the instrument alongside or behind the object for successful removal. Great care must be taken not to impact the FB or to push it through the nose and risk aspiration.

The external ear canal is another orifice of interest to the curious child. The child can place a multitude of FBs in the ear canal. Symptoms may vary depending on the nature of the FB, the size of the FB, and the duration that the FB has been present. Local trauma can occur with bleeding and difficulty with hearing. The child may describe a fullness sensation. Complications can arise with inflammatory changes. Secondary infection may cause canal wall skin to bleed and slough, producing otorrhea and severe granulation tissue formation. The presence of a secondarily infected ear canal from an FB may mimic a chronic mastoid infection that will not respond to antibiotics. Disc batteries, as in the nose and gastrointestinal tract, are extremely caustic and can cause extensive damage to the external auditory canal, tympanic membrane, and middle ear. The removal of an FB requires that the patient be extremely cooperative. Therefore, the use of general anesthesia may be necessary to minimize iatrogenic injury.

chapter 12

BITES

Gary S. Wasserman, DO • Jennifer Lowry, MD • D. Adam Algren, MD

A wide variety of bites are seen in children. It is estimated that more than 1 million children are treated annually for bites (Table 12-1).[1] In this chapter we concentrate on bites of interest to the surgeon. The reader is referred elsewhere for discussions of management of venomous stings and injuries from marine life and general details of wound management.

TETANUS

The gram-positive anaerobic organism *Clostridium tetani* is the causative agent for tetanus, a severe and often fatal disease. According to the 2006 report of the Department of Health and Human Services Centers for Disease Control and Prevention (CDC), there were a total of 41 cases (27 females) reported in the United States.[2] Only two cases were reported in the age group younger than 15 years old, with six cases in the 15- to 24-year age group. No neonatal cases were described.

There has been a low incidence of tetanus since a peak of 102 cases in 1975. Mortality from tetanus is associated with co-morbid conditions such as diabetes and intravenous drug usage and occurs in the elderly, especially when vaccination status is unknown. Infection can occur weeks after a break in the skin, even after a wound has seemed to heal. The ideal anaerobic surroundings allow spores to germinate into mature organisms producing two neurotoxins: tetanolysin and tetanospasmin.[3] The latter is able to enter peripheral nerves and travel to the brain, causing the clinical manifestations of uncontrolled muscle spasms and autonomic instability. The incubation period varies from as short as 2 days to as long as months, with most cases occurring within 14 days.[4] In general, the shorter the incubation period, the more severe the disease and the higher the fatality risk.

Initially, the diagnosis must be made clinically because wound cultures are often negative and serum antitoxin antibodies have a long turn-around time. So-called "dirty" wounds—lacerations treated after 24 hours, abscesses, ulcers, gangrene, and wounds with nonviable tissue—are the most common injuries that become infected. However, a history of acute trauma is not necessary.

All wounds should be cleaned and debrided. Symptomatic and supportive care includes medications, such as benzodiazepines, to control tetanic spasms and antimicrobials for infections. Metronidazole (oral

Table 12-1 "Bites and Envenomations" to Humans—Calls to Poison Centers in 2006

Animal	Total Calls	Age < 6 yr	Age 6-19 yr	All Ages Treated at Facility	Severe Outcome/Death
Bat	647	84	135	392	0/0
Cat	797	97	136	452	0/0
Dog	1,718	330	577	1,217	6/0
Fox	20	0	2	18	0/0
Human	47	11	9	15	0/0
Other	959	118	262	463	1/0
Raccoon	118	10	17	71	0/0
Rodent/lagomorph	1,728	385	489	462	0/0
Skunks	251	43	51	10	0/0
Snakes	3,229	146	600	2,841	185/4
Spiders	14,613	1,469	2,284	3,509	51/1

n = 2,403,539 total human poisoning calls; n = 82,133 in the category of bites and envenomations.
Data from Bronstein AC, Spyker DA, Cantilena LR, et al (eds): 2006 Annual Report of the American Association of Poison Control Centers' National Poison Data System (NPDS). Clin Toxicol 45:815-917, 2007.

Table 12-2 Wound Tetanus Prophylaxis Guideline

Vaccination History (Td)	Clean/Minor Wounds	All Other Wounds
? or < 3 doses	Td or Tdap—No TIG	Td or Tdap—TIG
≥ 3 doses	Td or Tdap—No TIG if ≥ 10 yr since last dose	Td or Tdap—No TIG if ≥ 5 yr since last dose

Td, adult type diphtheria and tetanus toxoids vaccine; TIG, tetanus immune globulin (human); Tdap, booster tetanus toxoid, reduced diphtheria toxoid, and cellular pertussis.
From American Academy of Pediatrics: Tetanus (lockjaw), bite wounds. In Pickering LK, Baker CJ, Long SS, McMillan JA (eds): Redbook: 2006 Report of the Committee on Infectious Diseases, 27th ed. Elk Grove Village, IL, American Academy of Pediatrics, 2006, pp 191-195, 648-653.

or intravenous, 30 mg/kg/day, divided into four daily doses, maximum 4 g/day) is the antibiotic of choice because it decreases the number of vegetative forms of *C. tetani*.[5] An alternate choice is parenteral treatment with penicillin G (100,000 U/kg/day every 4 to 6 hours, not to exceed 12 million units/day) for 10 to 14 days. Human tetanus immune globulin (TIG) is administered to adults and adolescents as a one-time dose of 3000 to 6000 units intramuscularly. Some experts recommend that children receive 250 to 500 units to decrease discomfort from injection.[5] Infiltrating part of the dose locally is controversial.

Prevention in a potentially exposed patient depends on the nature of the wound and history of immunization with tetanus toxoid as recommended by the CDC. One should consult an infectious disease expert for the most updated therapy or the CDC's website: *www.cdc.gov/vaccines/*(Table 12-2).[5]

CAT, DOG, HUMAN, AND OTHER MAMMALIAN BITES

Children are frequent victims of mammalian bites. The most common complication from bites is infection: cats, 16% to 50%; dogs, 1% to 30%, and humans, 9% to 18%.[6] When the bite is from a cat, dog, or other mammal, the most common infectious organisms to consider include (but are not limited to) *Streptococcus, Staphylococcus, Actinomycetes, Pasteurella* species, *Capnocytophaga* species, *Moraxella* species, *Corynebacterium* species, *Neisseria* species, *Eikenella corrodens, Haemophilus* species, anaerobes, *Fusobacterium nucleatum,* and *Prevotella melaninogenica*.[5,7,8] Human bites are a potential source not only for bacterial contamination but also for hepatitis B and, possibly, human immunodeficiency virus (HIV) infection.[9]

Recommendations for bite wound management are presented in Table 12-3. Evidence-based medicine studies concerning the closure of bite wounds are not conclusive. Distal extremity wounds, especially hand/fist to teeth, are at higher risk for infection. Whether minimal risk wounds require prophylactic antimicrobial therapy is controversial. Antibiotics started within 8 to 12 hours of the bite and continued for 2 to 3 days may decrease infection rate.[5] The oral drug of choice is amoxicillin clavulanate. For penicillin-allergic patients, an extended-spectrum cephalosporin (5%-15% of penicillin-allergic people are also hypersensitive to cephalosporins) or trimethoprim-sulfamethoxazole plus clindamycin should be given.[5]

RABIES AND POSTEXPOSURE PROPHYLAXIS

Rabies is a viral disease usually transmitted through the saliva of a sick mammal (i.e., dogs, cats, ferrets, raccoons, skunks, foxes, bats, and most other carnivores). Most reported cases in the United States are caused by raccoons, skunks, foxes, mongooses, and bats.[2] Small rodents such as rats, mice, squirrels, chipmunks, hamsters, guinea pigs, and gerbils (also lagomorphs such as rabbits and hares) are almost never infected with rabies. Over the past decade, cats have been the most common domestic animal with rabies. In 2006, there were three cases of human rabies identified in the United States and all were fatal. This was a decline from a peak of seven cases in 2004 (with records dating back to 1975).[2] The rabies virus enters the central nervous system and causes an acute, progressive encephalomyelitis from which survival is extremely unlikely. The human host has a wide range for the incubation period from days to years (most commonly weeks to months).

Prophylactic treatment for humans potentially exposed to rabies includes immediate and thorough wound cleansing followed by passive vaccination with human rabies immune globulin (HRIG) and cell culture rabies vaccines, either human diploid (HDCV) or purified chick embryo (PCECV).[10-12] (Consult *www.cdc.gov/vaccines/* for the most up-to-date information.)

Table 12-3 Components of Bite Wound Management

- Obtain detailed history of injury.
- Evaluate injury and re-examine in 24-48 hours.
  - Check for foreign bodies and possible deep structure injury in small children.
- Evaluate for risk of tetanus, rabies, hepatitis B, human immunodeficiency virus.
- Perform meticulous cleansing and irrigation.
  - Irrigation of puncture wounds is controversial.
- Obtain wound culture as indicated.
  - Culture is recommended if wound appears infected or is of late presentation.
- Debride necrotic tissue or contaminants not removed by irrigation.
- Perform exploratory surgery as indicated.
- Primary closure is sometimes performed for dog bites but not recommended for human or cat bites.
- Consider antimicrobial therapy.

Many factors help determine the risk assessment in deciding which patient benefits from postexposure prophylaxis and which regimen should be given. The risk of infection depends on the type of exposure, surveillance, epidemiology of animal rabies in the region of contact, species of animal, animal behavior causing it to bite, and availability of the animal for observation or laboratory testing for rabies virus. The final decision for treatment with vaccines is complex. Therefore local, state, or CDC experts are available for assistance.

SPIDER BITES

There are about 40,000 species of spiders that have been named and placed in about 3000 genera and 105 families.[13] Families with over 100 genera are Salticidae (jumping spiders), Linyphiidae (dwarf or money spiders, sheet web weavers), Araneidae (common orb spiders), Theridiidae (cobweb weavers), Lycosidae (wolf spiders), Gnaphosidae (ground spiders), and Thomisidae (crab spiders). New species are constantly being discovered while others are becoming extinct. In regard to medically relevant spiders, few are known to cause significant clinical effects. In 2006, over 14,000 calls were made to U.S. Poison Control Centers (PCC) regarding spider bites.[1] Although PCC data are biased with over 85% of calls originating from the general public (see Table 12-1), one third of these cases were evaluated in a health care facility with 51 cases having a severe outcome with one death. Although it is unknown if surgical intervention was required in these cases, it is rare that a spider bite requires surgical care. Few spiders have been shown to have the ability to bite humans because their fangs cannot pierce our skin. The two most medically important spiders in the United States are Sicariidae (brown spiders) and Latrodectus (widow spiders).

Brown Spiders

Loxoscelism is a form of cutaneous-visceral (necrotic-systemic) arachnidism found throughout the world with predilection for North and South America.[14] There are four species of brown spiders within the United States that are known to cause necrotic skin lesions (*Loxosceles deserta, L. arizonica, L. rufescens,* and *L. reclusa*). *L. deserta* and *L. arizonica* can be found in the southwestern United States. *L. rufescens* is found sporadically all over the United States in very circumscribed infestations (typically one building). *L. reclusa* can usually be found in the South central United States, especially Missouri, Kansas, Oklahoma, Arkansas, Tennessee, and Kentucky.[15] Spiders can be transported out of their natural habitat but very rarely cause arachnidism in nonendemic areas. *L. reclusa* is tan to brown with a characteristic dark, violin-shaped marking on its dorsal cephalothorax, giving it the nickname "fiddleback spider." The spider can measure up to 1 cm in total body length with a 3 cm or longer leg span (Fig. 12-1) and only three pairs of eyes.

The incidence of *L. reclusa* bites predominantly occurs from April through October in the United States. The venom of the brown recluse spider contains at least 11 protein components. Most are enzymes with cytotoxic activity.[16] Sphingomyelinase D is believed to be the enzyme responsible for dermonecrosis and activity on red blood cell membranes.[17-19] In addition to the local effects, the venom has activity against neutrophils and the complement pathway that induces an immunologic response.[19-21] The resulting effect is a necrotic dermal lesion with the possibility of a systemic response that can be life threatening.

The prevalence of brown recluse spider envenomations is unknown. The victim may not feel the bite or may only feel a mild pinprick sensation. Many victims are bitten while they sleep and may be unaware of the

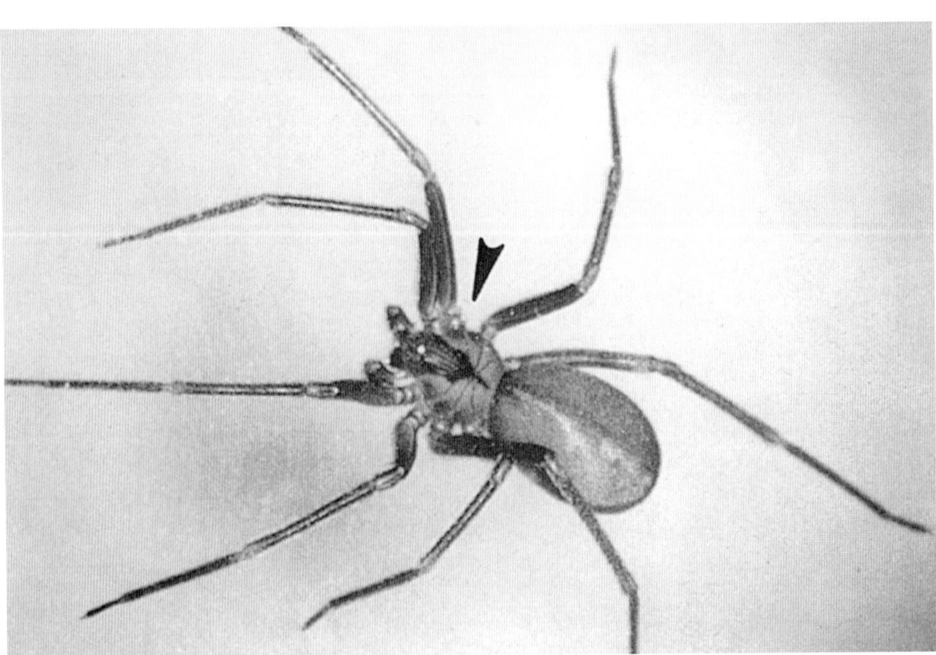

Figure 12-1. *Loxosceles reclusa* (brown recluse, "fiddleback") spider showing the classic violin-shaped marking on the back (dorsal side) of the cephalothorax. Note the long slender legs and oval body segment with short hairs. The *arrow* is pointing toward the classic violin marking. (From Ford M, Delaney K, Ling L, Erickson T: Clinical Toxicology. Philadelphia, Elsevier, 2001.)

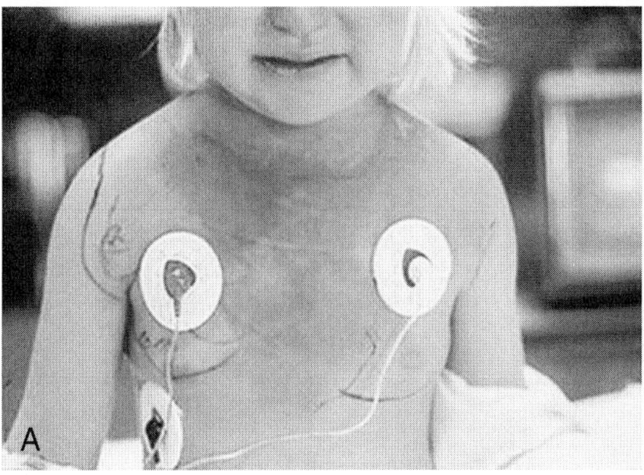

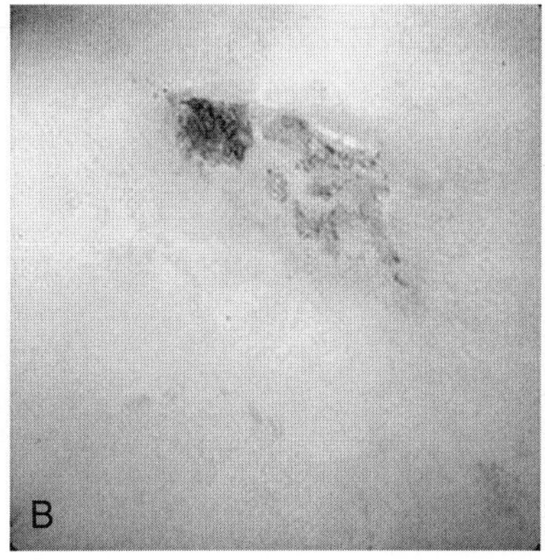

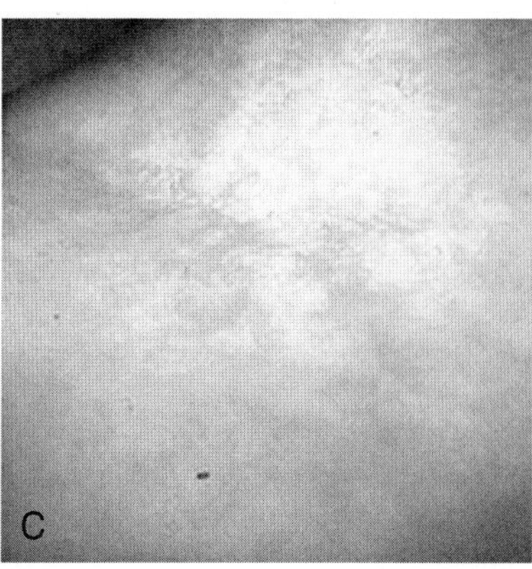

Figure 12-2. **A,** A 3-year-old girl hospitalized on the third day after a brown recluse spider bite for severe hemolytic anemia, hemoglobinuria, and ecchymosis (note the vast expansion of the ecchymosis secondary to hyaluronidase "spreading factor" in the venom). There is no necrosis or ischemia, but a small bleb/blister is present over the right clavicle that, although not pathognomonic, is often present early in lesion progression. Also note that the cutaneous lesion is mild in comparison with this patient's systemic presentation. **B,** On the 15th day after envenomation, the lesion measures 5 × 2 cm. Multiple small areas of necrosis have become apparent in the past week. The largest area indicates the original bite size. The lesion's edges have begun to involute with healing, and the ischemia is fading. **C,** Nine months after the bite, the necrotic wound has healed with no significant scarring.

envenomation until a wound develops. The majority of victims do not see the spider at the time of the bite.[22] Typically, the bite progressively begins to itch, tingle, and become ecchymotic, indurated, and edematous within several hours.[23] Often within hours, a characteristic bleb or bullae will form. The tissue under a blister is more likely to become necrotic, but the extent of necrosis is not predictable. As the wound ischemia and inflammation progresses, it becomes painful and may blanch or become erythematous, forming a "target" or "halo" design. Inflammation, ischemia, and pain increase over the first few days of the bite as enzymes spread. Over hours to weeks, an eschar forms at the site of the bite. Eventually, this eschar sloughs, revealing an underlying ulcer that may require months to heal, usually by secondary intention (Fig. 12-2). On very rare occasions, the ulcer does not heal and may require surgical intervention.

The need for hospitalization occurs if the patient develops systemic symptoms. Two studies documented that 14% to more than 50% of patients developed systemic symptoms, with fever being the most common symptom.[10] Other common symptoms include a maculopapular rash, nausea and vomiting, headache, malaise,

Table 12-4	Differential Diagnosis of Brown Recluse Spider Envenomations

- Acquired hemolytic anemias
- Bites from other creatures (e.g., snakes, spiders, insects) that can result in cutaneous lesions
- Dermatologic conditions (e.g., pyoderma gangrenosum)
- Hereditary hemolytic anemias
- Infectious causes (e.g., Lyme disease, infection with *Streptococcus, Staphylococcus,* or *Clostridium* species)
- Medical conditions causing necrotic lesions:
  - Emboli
  - Frostbite or thermal injuries
  - Ischemic injuries
  - Neoplastic wounds (e.g., ecthyma gangrenosum)
  - Trauma

muscle/joint pain, hepatitis, pancreatitis, and other organ toxicity. Life-threatening systemic effects include hemolysis (intravascular and/or extravascular), coagulopathy, and multiple organ system failure. Secondary effects include sepsis, necrotizing fasciitis, and shock.[24-26] Hemolysis usually manifests within the first 96 hours. However, late presentations can occur. When hemolysis does develop, it can take 4 to 7 days (or longer) to resolve. Complications such as cardiac dysrhythmias, coma, respiratory compromise, pulmonary edema, congestive heart failure, renal failure, and seizures can occur.

The diagnosis of a brown recluse spider envenomation is largely one of exclusion as it is rare to see or identify the spider. While the wound can look classic for an envenomation, other etiologies must be considered (Table 12-4). Certain laboratory findings can be consistent with a brown recluse spider envenomation but are not specific in making the diagnosis (Table 12-5).

Controversy surrounds the treatment of dermal and systemic symptoms of loxoscelism. Medications such as dapsone, nitroglycerin, and tetracycline have been used. Also, hyperbaric oxygen (HBO) therapy has been advocated as has surgical excision of the necrotic wound. However, none of these has shown consistently to be effective in treating or preventing the ulcer development. In South America, an antivenom has been developed and used in the treatment of *Loxosceles* envenomations. Unfortunately, the usual long delay in seeking medical care often leads to ineffective use of antivenom.[27] An antivenom is not available in North America.

Use of dapsone, a leukocyte inhibitor, has been advocated in case reports and animal studies.[28-30] However, other animal studies have shown no benefit from this treatment. In an animal study,[31] piglets received venom and were randomized to receive one of four treatments: no treatment, HBO, dapsone, or dapsone with HBO. Neither dapsone, HBO, nor the combination treatment reduced necrosis compared with controls. A second study compared the use of HBO, dapsone, or cyproheptadine against no treatment in decreasing

Table 12-5	Laboratory Findings Consistent with Systemic Effects of *Loxosceles* Envenomations
Hemoglobinemia	
Hemoglobinuria or hematuria	
Elevated plasma free hemoglobin or decreased free haptoglobin	
Leukocytosis	
Anemia	
Thrombocytopenia	
Coagulopathy (elevated prothrombin time, decreased fibrinogen, elevated D-dimer, decreased antithrombin III)	
Inflammatory markers (elevated C-reactive protein, elevated erythrocyte sedimentation rate, elevated liver and/or pancreatic enzymes)	
Immunology (positive antiglobulin tests: direct or indirect Coombs; decreased total serum complement or components; interference with blood screening or crossmatching)	

the necrotic wound after envenomation with *L. deserta* venom. No statistical difference was seen with respect to lesion size, ulcer size, or histopathologic ranking.[32] In addition, the use of dapsone is not without risk, especially hypersensitivity reactions.[33] Therapeutic doses of dapsone are associated with hemolytic anemia, methemoglobinemia, and other hematologic effects in patients with and without glucose-6-phosphate dehydrogenase deficiency and may complicate the clinical picture in treating these patients.

Topically applied nitroglycerin as a vasodilator had been advocated but is not effective in preventing necrosis. A randomized, blinded, controlled study was performed on rabbits envenomated with *Loxosceles* venom and showed that skin necrosis developed in all animals.[34] In addition, there was no difference in regard to the area of necrosis, amount of edema, and increase in creatinine phosphokinase (CPK) concentration. Alternatively, rabbits were inoculated with *Loxosceles* venom and randomized to receive topical doxycycline, topical tetracycline, or placebo.[35] Those who received topical tetracycline had reduced progression of the dermal lesion. However, treatment was started early at 6 hours after envenomation, which may not be realistic after a human bite. In addition, the agents used for this research study are not commercially available in the United States. Further studies need to be performed before topical tetracycline can be recommended.

As previously mentioned, HBO has been advocated for wound treatment to prevent progression of the necrotic wound. The initial use of HBO was based on the belief that tissue hypoxia was partially responsible for the subsequent necrosis seen after a bite. As mentioned previously, no statistical differences were noted in animal studies that compared dapsone and HBO.[31,32] Similar results have been seen in animal studies assessing the effect of HBO alone.[36,37] However, a randomized, controlled trial of HBO in a rabbit model in which standard HBO was used showed a significantly reduced wound diameter at 10 days.[38] No significant change in blood flow at the wound center or 1 to 2 cm from the wound center was seen. HBO is expensive and not without complications. At the present time, much of the literature contradicts the benefit of HBO for brown recluse spider envenomations. As such, it is not currently recommended as a first-line therapy for these bites but may be helpful in patients with underlying/preexisting vascular compromise such as sickle cell anemia or diabetes.

Early surgical intervention is not helpful because the venom diffuses rapidly throughout the soft tissues surrounding a bite.[39] In addition, patients may be more at risk for delayed wound healing and objectional scarring if surgery occurs within the first 72 hours of the bite.[40,41] Debridement of enlarging blebs is proposed with the theory that toxins exist within the blister fluid. However, necrosis almost always occurs beneath the blisters.[42] The question is whether surgical intervention should be advocated late after envenomation. The wound from the brown recluse spider may take 2 to 3 months to heal. Thus, skin grafting of a nonhealing necrotic area should be delayed up to 12 weeks to allow for neovascularization of the demarcated area.[43] Imaging studies of soft tissue areas are incorrectly interpreted as being "cellulitis" because of the noninfected inflammatory reaction within the tissue layers. This is especially noted in the head and neck regions as well as extremities.

Treatment of systemic signs and symptoms are largely symptomatic and involve supportive care. Patients should be monitored closely for hemolysis (and children hospitalized) if systemic symptoms such as fever and rash develop. Systemic corticosteroids seem to suppress hemolysis and may be needed for 5 to 10 days with a subsequent tapering dose.[43] Methylprednisolone can be administered as a 1.0- to 2.0-mg/kg intravenous loading dose (no maximum) followed by a 0.5 to 1.0 mg/kg maintenance dose every 6 hours. Hydration, to maintain good urine output, is required to prevent acute renal tubular necrosis if hemolysis or hematuria occurs. Antibiotics are not generally required early in the care of these patients because the spider does not inoculate humans with bacteria. However, secondary infections can occur and lead to sepsis, toxic shock syndrome, and necrotizing fasciitis. These complications require close observation and antibiotic therapy to cover anaerobic, staphylococcal, and streptococcal infections.

Black Widow Spider

The black widow spider (*Latrodectus mactans*) is found throughout North America except for areas of extreme cold.[44] They can usually be found outdoors in warm, dark places or in a garage or basement. They are web-making spiders and usually strike when their web is disturbed. The female spider is readily recognized as she is a black spider with a red marking on her abdomen in the shape of an hourglass. Widow spiders have a neurotoxic venom that is responsible for clinical effects. The venom, α-latrotoxin, acts on the neuromuscular junction to cause depletion of acetylcholine at motor endings and catecholamines at the postganglionic sympathetic synaptic sites followed by complete blockade of the neuromediator release.[45] Because the venom does not have cytotoxic properties, dermal effects including significant local pain are not seen.

In the majority of cases, a pinprick sensation may be felt at the time of a bite. A "halo" lesion may be present, but this tends to disappear within 12 hours of envenomation. Significant symptoms may present within 1 to 12 hours after the bite. Within several hours, tenderness may be felt in the regional lymph nodes and the affected extremity or surrounding tissues. Depending on where the bite occurs, pain migrates to large muscle groups in the thigh, buttock, and abdomen or to the chest. The most common presenting complaint to emergency departments is intractable abdominal, chest, back, or leg pain, depending on the site of the bite.[46] Board-like rigidity of the abdomen, shoulders, and back may develop that may lead to misdiagnosis of surgical abdomen or other etiology. The pain generally peaks at 2 to 3 hours but can last up to 72 hours.

Because the venom affects the autonomic nervous system, patients may present with symptoms of dysautonomia that include hypertension (sometimes severe), tachycardia, weakness, ptosis, eyelid edema, pruritus, nausea and vomiting, diaphoresis, hyperreflexia, difficulty breathing, and excessive salivation. Fatalities are rare but have been reported. Children are more at risk to develop systemic symptoms.

Treatment is largely symptomatic and supportive. For the most part, treatment is focused on analgesia. For those with mild pain, oral medications are appropriate. Patients may present with severe pain requiring opioids and benzodiazepines as adjunctive therapy. Calcium gluconate has been advocated in the past. However, it is not recommended because of lack of consistent effects in alleviating the symptoms. Antivenom is available and generally reserved for patients who have life-threatening symptoms or pain that is not relieved by opioids and benzodiazepines. Because it is an equine product, it has increased risk for anaphylaxis and serum sickness and it is not readily available in most hospital settings.

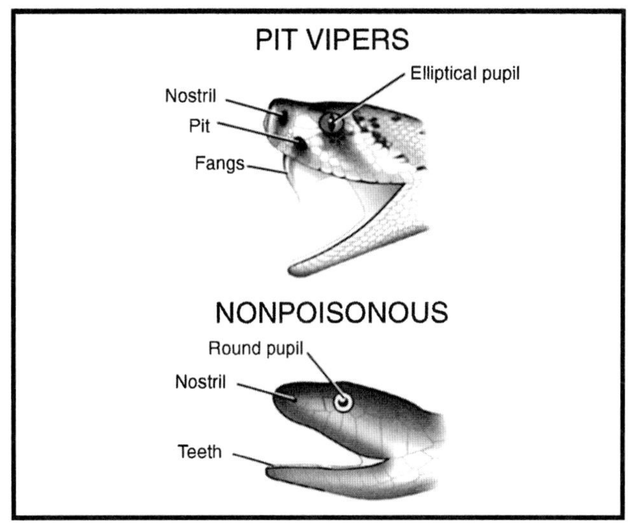

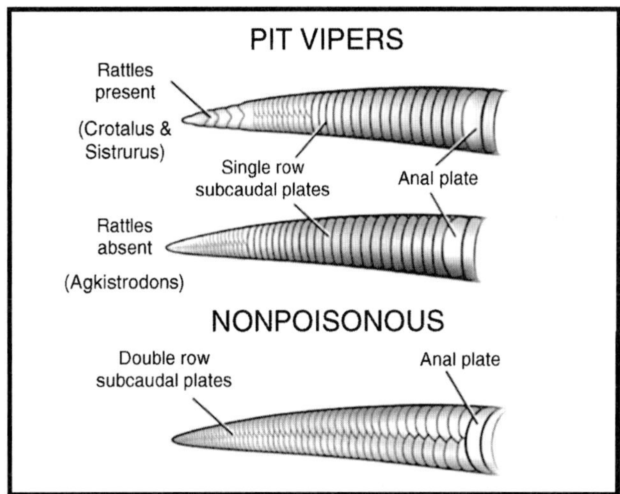

Figure 12-3. Identifying characteristics of pit vipers and nonpoisonous snakes. The presence or absence of a single row of subcaudal plates may be the only identifying feature in a decapitated snake. (From Ford M, Delaney K, Ling L, Erickson T: Clinical Toxicology. Philadelphia, Elsevier, 2001.)

CROTALID SNAKE ENVENOMATIONS

In the United States, there are two major classes of poisonous snakes: crotalids and elapids. Crotalids, otherwise known as pit vipers, are indigenous to almost every state and account for the vast majority of poisonous snakebites in the United States annually. Most snakebites occur during the warm summer months when both snakes and humans are more active and thus more likely to come into contact with each other. It is generally thought up to 20% of snakebites are "dry bites" and do not result in envenomation.[47]

Crotalids can be classified into three major groups: rattlesnakes, cottonmouths (water moccasins), and copperheads. Copperheads are responsible for the majority of crotalid envenomations. In general, these bites are less severe and rarely result in systemic toxicity.[48,49] Rattlesnake envenomations more commonly produce coagulopathy and systemic toxicity.

Crotalids have several physical features that can help distinguish them from nonpoisonous snakes (Fig. 12-3). Crotalids have triangular heads and elliptical pupils. Nonpoisonous snakes have round heads and pupils. Crotalids have a single row of subcaudal plates/scales distal to the anal plate, whereas nonpoisonous snakes have a double row of subcaudal plates. Most importantly, crotalids have two retractable fangs and the characteristic heat-seeking pit located between the nostril and the eye. Nonpoisonous snakes have short, pointy teeth but no fangs.

Crotalid Venom Pharmacology/Pathophysiology

Crotalid venom is a complex mixture of proteins, including metalloproteinases, collagenase, hyaluronidase, and phospholipase.[50] These enzymes act to destroy tissue at the site of envenomation. Damage to the vascular endothelium and basement membranes leads to edema, ecchymosis, and bullae formation. Concurrently with local tissue destruction, venom is absorbed systemically and can result in shock and coagulopathy. The potency of venom varies with the species of the snake, age, diet, and time of year.[47] Even within the same snake the composition and potency of venom can vary substantially based on these factors.

Clinical Effects

In questioning the patient, one should ascertain the circumstance and timing of the bite as well as any first aid methods that were used. Knowing what prehospital measures were instituted can be extremely helpful. Certain therapies such as incision, excision, and suction may result in significant local trauma and act to confound the assessment of local injury. The clinician should determine if the patient has previously received antivenom because sensitization can occur, thereby placing the patient at higher risk for an allergic reaction. Health care providers should be cautious regarding the reliability of victim identification of the offending snake. It is often assumed that rattlesnakes will rattle their tails before biting. However, this is not always the case. Also, rattles may be absent from rattlesnakes due to shedding or trauma. Victims occasionally trap or kill the snake and bring it to the emergency department. Vigilance is necessary when examining these snakes because they are capable of biting again. Even dead snakes have been known to bite reflexively for up to an hour after they are killed.[47]

Envenomations can result in significant local pain and swelling. The patient typically has two fang marks at the location of the bite. Often, there is mild bleeding or oozing from the wound. Swelling typically develops within 1 to 2 hours, and ecchymosis or bullae (some hemorrhagic) formation may appear. Several different models have been developed to grade the severity of snakebites.[47,51] The minimal, moderate, severe model is a simple tool that can help assess severity and determine the need for antivenom (Table 12-6).

Serial measurements of the extremity are required to detect any progression of swelling. Local effects have traditionally been documented by drawing a line demarcating the progression of the swelling. This technique requires subjective interpretation. Measurement of the limb circumference is more objective and can be easily repeated to determine any progression (Fig. 12-4). These measurements should be recorded every 15 minutes for the first 2 hours and then less frequently (every 30-60 minutes). In addition to measuring the limb circumference, serial neurovascular examinations can identify any ischemia or evidence of compartment syndrome.

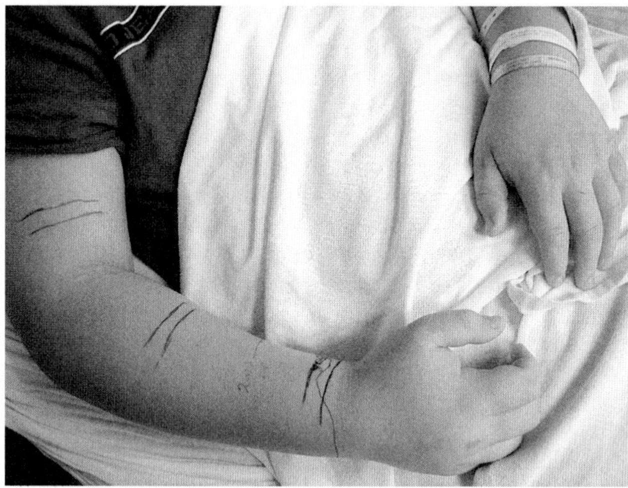

Figure 12-4. A 15-year-old boy was bitten on his right hand by a timber rattlesnake. Note the significant swelling of the arm. Serial limb circumference measurements documented progression of the swelling. The patient did well after treatment with Fab antivenom.

Table 12-6	Grading of Snake Envenomations
Minimal	Mild local swelling without progression; no systemic or hematologic toxicity
Moderate	Local swelling with proximal progression and/or mildly abnormal laboratory parameters (e.g., decreased platelets, prolonged coagulation studies)
Severe	Marked swelling with progression and/or significant systemic toxicity (shock, compartment syndrome) or laboratory abnormalities (severe thrombocytopenia/coagulopathy)

Adapted from Gold BS, Dart RC, Barish RA: Bite of Venomous Snakes. N Engl J Med 347:347-356, 2002.

Compartment syndrome is rare (<1%-2%) after snake envenomation because it is unusual for a snake's fangs to penetrate the muscle fascia. The true incidence is difficult to ascertain from the literature because many of the older case series report the use of prophylactic fasciotomies without measuring the compartment pressure.[52,53] Although swelling may be severe, it is almost always localized to the subcutaneous tissue. If there is concern for compartment syndrome in the setting of severe pain and swelling, measurement of compartment pressures is necessary. Even if elevated compartment pressures are found, treatment with antivenom is usually sufficient to alleviate the elevated pressures and reverse the compartment syndrome.[52-55] Given the efficacy and safety of the newer crotalid antivenom routine, prophylactic fasciotomies are not indicated in the setting of an envenomation.[56] Recent evidence has shown that prophylactic fasciotomies worsen local effects and do not improve clinical outcomes.[57,58] If compartment pressures are elevated, they should be re-measured after antivenom administration and repeat antivenom can be given, if required. If the pressures remain elevated for more than 4 hours despite antivenom, then fasciotomy is indicated (Fig. 12-5). Measurement of finger compartment pressures is not possible. If significant concern exists about the viability of the finger, a digit dermotomy is indicated.[58]

Systemic manifestations present in a variable fashion after envenomation. Nonspecific symptoms and

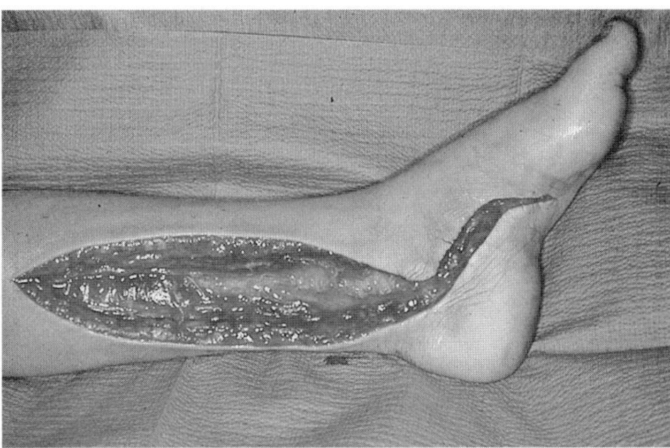

Figure 12-5. The need for fasciotomy for compartment syndrome may be suggested by excessive swelling in the soft tissue, but compartment pressures are rarely elevated significantly. Prophylactic fasciotomy is based on the belief that it protects against compartment syndrome. Such practices are unnecessary and can be catastrophic in venom-defibrinated patients. (From Brent J, Wallace K, Burkhart K, et al: Critical Care Toxicology: Diagnosis and Management of the Critically Poisoned Patient. Philadelphia, Elsevier, 2005.)

signs include nausea, vomiting, diaphoresis, and metallic taste. Hypotension and shock can occur in severe cases. Severe rattlesnake envenomations often develop coagulopathy with a disseminated intravascular coagulation-like syndrome. Thrombocytopenia has been noted to be severe and prolonged after timber rattlesnake envenomations.[59] Canebrake rattlesnake envenomations have been associated with significant rhabdomyolysis.[60] It should be noted that although crotalid envenomations have characteristic findings, there is one exception. The Mojave rattlesnake, native to California and Arizona, is able to produce neurologic symptoms, including weakness and respiratory failure. Its venom has evolved and contains a neurotoxin that inhibits the release of acetylcholine from the presynaptic neuron in the neuromuscular junction.

Management

After a crotalid bite, the victim should avoid exertion and have the involved extremity immobilized. These actions may act to decrease venom absorption into the systemic circulation. Rings, jewelry, and other constrictive clothing should be removed. Most importantly, the victim should be rapidly transported to the nearest emergency department.

Historically, different procedures and therapies have been advocated in the prehospital and in-hospital management of snakebites. Treatments such as cryotherapy and electric shock are associated with significant complications and are not recommended.[61] It is commonly thought that tourniquets should be applied to the affected extremity. However, their use has not been found to improve outcomes and evidence suggests they may worsen local toxicity.[62-64] Therefore, their use should be discouraged. Given the short transport times of most patients, the morbidity associated with tourniquet application (limb ischemia) outweighs any potential benefit. In those situations in which the victim is in a remote location that is hours away from an emergency department, the use of a constriction band can be considered. There are limited data to suggest that constriction bands decrease the rate of systemic venom absorption.[62] Constriction bands differ from venous tourniquets in that they serve to impede lymphatic return rather than blood flow. When placed correctly, two fingers should easily slip under a constriction band.

Pressure immobilization is another modality commonly recommended for snakebites worldwide. It involves wrapping the entire limb in an elastic compression bandage and then immobilizing the limb in extension with a splint. Although likely effective in cases of elapid envenomations,[65] their use in cases of crotalid envenomation should be discouraged. An animal model of crotalid envenomation demonstrated pressure immobilization slightly prolonged the time to death but was associated with a significant increase in extremity compartment pressures.[66]

Suction therapy with an extractor device has been previously suggested. A commercially available device is widely obtainable from sporting goods retailers. The general assertion is that when applied shortly after a bite occurs, the suction generated by the device would pull the venom out of the wound. However, it has been demonstrated that these devices are not efficacious and remove less than 1% of injected venom.[67] These devices may actually increase the amount of local tissue destruction.[68] Therefore, use of extractor devices in the prehospital or hospital setting is not recommended.

Incision therapy, often combined with suction, gained favor in the early 20th century. This procedure entailed making several parallel incisions longitudinally along the affected extremity. While early animal models demonstrated some survival improvement, subsequent human studies have failed to show any change in clinical outcomes.[69] Incising the wound also risks injury to underlying tendons, nerves, and blood vessels and increases infection rates.[69-71]

In-hospital management should initially focus on assessing and supporting the airway, breathing, and circulation. Anaphylactic reactions have been reported after envenomation.[72] The initial evaluation should assess the patient for evidence of shock and hypoperfusion. Hypotension mandates aggressive resuscitation with crystalloid fluid, antivenom (see later), and vasopressors, if required. If the patient arrives in the emergency department with a tourniquet in place, it should be slowly loosened and removed over 20 to 30 minutes. Rapid removal of a tourniquet could result in delivery of a venom bolus to the central circulation, resulting in decompensation of the patient.[62] Intravenous access should be obtained in the noninjured extremity, with placement of a second access line in those with significant envenomation. Opioids are often required for management of pain. The patient's tetanus should be updated, if needed. Prophylactic antibiotics are not warranted because the risk of infection resulting from snakebites is less than 5%.[73] Although snakes do carry pathogenic bacteria in their mouths, a majority of infections are secondary to the victim's normal skin flora.

The antivenom supplies of the hospital should be assessed in all cases of snakebites, even those cases in which antivenom administration does not appear to be indicated. This is prudent because the patient's clinical condition can change rapidly in the first several hours after envenomation. It is important for the clinician to arrange for procurement of antivenom or hospital transfer while the patient is stable and not in immediate need of antivenom. A complete blood cell count, chemistries, coagulation studies, fibrinogen, and creatine kinase are indicated in all cases of snakebites to assess systemic toxicity. Medical toxicologists and regional poison centers (1-800-222-1222) can serve as valuable resources to clinicians who are unfamiliar with the management of snake envenomations.

Antivenom is indicated for envenomations displaying more than minimal local effects (Table 12-7). The older Wyeth (Collegeville, PA) polyvalent antivenom that was introduced in the United States in 1954 is no longer manufactured. This product was a crudely purified, equine-derived IgG antibody directed against the venom of several crotalids. Because it contained foreign proteins and the highly immunogenic Fc portion of the antibody, the incidence of immediate hypersensitivity reactions was high. Approximately 50% of recipients developed urticaria or signs of anaphylactic shock.[74] This mandated that patients be observed in a critical care setting and have an epinephrine infusion at the bedside. Serum sickness, a delayed immunologic reaction to the foreign proteins, is another adverse effect associated with antivenom. This reaction typically occurs 1 to 3 weeks after antivenom administration and manifests clinically as a fever, rash, arthralgias, myalgias, and occasionally glomerulonephritis and pericarditis. It is generally self-limited and can be treated with corticosteroids and antihistamines. Serum sickness was common after polyvalent antivenom use, with an incidence of more than 50% if more than 5 vials were administered.[74]

Fortunately, a new polyvalent immune Fab antivenom (CroFab, Protherics, Inc., Brentwood, TN) is available that is much safer and associated with significantly fewer adverse reactions. It is a highly purified product that contains the Fab fragments of IgG antibodies. The product is sheep derived and is effective against all North American crotalid species. The incidence of immediate hypersensitivity reactions is less than 5% to 10%.[75-79] Many of the hypersensitivity reactions are mild (urticaria) and do not prevent further antivenom administration. Anaphylaxis is uncommon. Likewise, the incidence of serum sickness is also less than 5%.[78,79] The dosing of polyvalent immune Fab is based on the clinical severity and response of the patient to the antivenom (Fig. 12-6). The dosing is not weight based. Therefore, the dosing in children is the same as in adults. Skin testing is not required. Clinical trials have demonstrated improved outcomes when regular follow-up doses of antivenom were given for recurrence (see later) of local and systemic toxicity in those who received a single dose of antivenom. This resulted in the development of the currently recommended dosing schedule. Multiple studies have demonstrated that the polyvalent immune Fab antivenom is efficacious in ameliorating the local and systemic venom toxicity. Recent analysis of pediatric data also demonstrates excellent efficacy and safety in treating children as young as 18 months of age. There were no cases of anaphylaxis in pediatric patients (>100 cases) reported in five case series.[80-84] Liberal use should be considered for bites involving the hands or feet because these envenomations are associated with significant morbidity and prolonged recovery.[85]

Table 12-7	Indications for Crotalid Antivenom
Shock	
Coagulopathy and/or thrombocytopenia	
Compartment syndrome	
Significant swelling/progression of local effects	
Neurotoxicity (Mojave rattlesnake)	

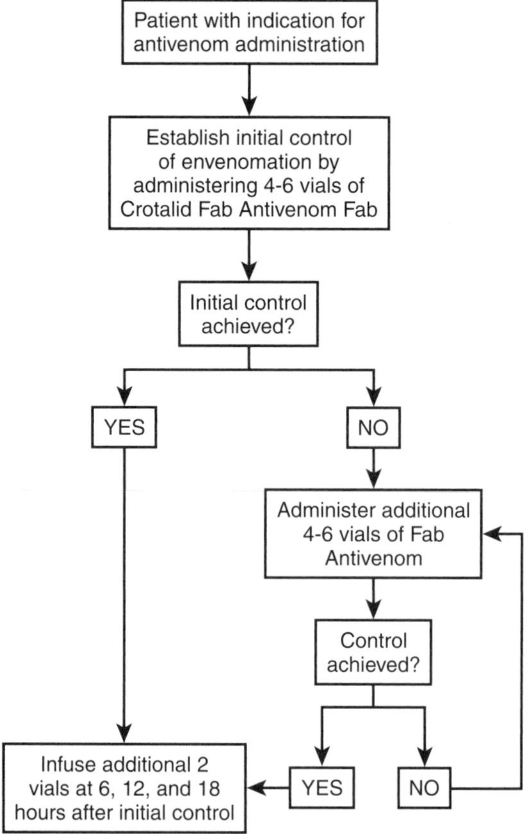

Figure 12-6. This schematic depicts management of the patient who needs crotalid polyvalent immune Fab antivenom.

Recurrence is defined as worsening of local and/or systemic toxicity after a period of improvement with antivenom therapy. This results from the pharmacokinetic differences between the antivenom and venom.[86] The Fab components have a low molecular weight and are small enough to be freely filtered by the kidney. This results in an elimination half-life of Fab antivenom of about 15 to 20 hours versus venom that has a half-life of approximately 40 hours.[86,87] Multiple reports have documented progression of swelling or worsening hematologic toxicity after antivenom therapy.[75,78,88] Those patients who develop hematologic toxicity during initial treatment are at highest risk for recurrence. Administration of antivenom is usually effective in treating further local progression. Although hematologic toxicity does not typically result in clinically significant bleeding, further antivenom administration is not effective in completely normalizing hematologic abnormalities.[78,89] Close monitoring is indicated, and treatment can be resumed in those with bleeding or markedly abnormal laboratory parameters.[89] A new Fab_2 immune antivenom (Anavip, Pharmasil, Inc., Columbia, MD) is currently in premarketing trials in the United States with the hope that it will have improved pharmacokinetics, thus potentially decreasing the incidence and severity of recurrence.

The disposition of patients who are bitten is dependent on the severity of the envenomation. Discharge after a 6- to 8-hour observation can be considered in those circumstances in which it is thought that no significant envenomation occurred (dry bite). There should be no appreciable local swelling, and results of initial laboratory studies and repeat laboratory studies before discharge should be normal. All patients with significant local swelling or evidence of systemic toxicity should be admitted for further evaluation and management. Rattlesnake bite victims from those areas in which the Mojave rattlesnake is endemic should be monitored for neurotoxicity.

CORAL SNAKE ENVENOMATION

The coral snake is the only poisonous elapid snake native to the United States. While there are several species of coral snakes in the United States, the species of greatest concern is found only in Florida and southern Georgia. These snakes are brightly colored and have bands in a distinctive pattern (black, yellow, red). This order gives rise to the common phrases, "red on yellow, kill a fellow" and "red on black, venom lack," that can help to differentiate a coral snake from the nonpoisonous king snake. Unlike crotalids, coral snakes have round heads and pupils. Instead of fangs they have short teeth. It has been described that these snakes have to be removed from the victim similar to removing Velcro. Up to 25% of bites do not result in significant envenomation.[90]

Unlike crotalids that produce local tissue destruction and coagulopathy, venom from elapids is associated with neurotoxicity. The resulting toxicity is likely related to an acetylcholinesterase present in the venom. After a bite, local effects tend to be mild. Of greater concern is the risk of progressive weakness and resulting respiratory failure. Neurologic symptoms (cranial nerve palsies, weakness) typically develop within 2 hours but may be delayed up to 13 hours.[90] Given the lack of significant local effects, surgical management is not indicated.

All patients with suspected coral snake bites should be admitted for observation. Treatment is supportive with close monitoring for respiratory compromise and antivenom administration. Coral snake antivenom is an equine-derived IgG. It should be administered in all cases of suspected coral snake bites, even if the victim is asymptomatic. This is recommended because antivenom only prevents progression of symptoms and does not reverse any neurologic signs that have occurred. The recommended dose is 3 to 5 vials in asymptomatic patients, followed by another 5 vials in those who develop symptoms. In the largest series of U.S. coral snake envenomations, immediate hypersensitivity reactions occurred in 15% of patients, whereas serum sickness was reported in 10%.[90]

chapter 13

BURNS

Dai H. Chung, MD • David N. Herndon, MD

For the past several decades, there have been major advances in the care of burns, resulting in significant improvement in the survival for patients with extensive burn injury. The development of the Lund and Browder burn diagram in 1944[1] allowed for assessment of the percent of the total body surface area (TBSA) burned. Other advances such as the determination of appropriate fluid resuscitation to treat burn shock and the introduction of topical antimicrobials (silver nitrate, mafenide acetate, silver sulfadiazine) have made significant impact as well. More recently, a better understanding of and further refinements in the areas of fluid resuscitation, infection control, support of the hypermetabolic response, treatment of inhalation injury, and early surgical excision and grafting of deep burn injuries have all contributed to a 50% decline in burn-related deaths and hospital admissions in the United States.[2,3]

Nearly 2 million burn injuries occur each year in the United States, with about half of these injuries occurring in children. Although a significant percentage of burn injuries are minor, approximately 50,000 patients suffer moderate to severe burns requiring hospitalization for treatment. Of these cases, approximately half are in children younger than 15 years of age. Children younger than the age of 5 account for 12% of burn-related hospital admissions. Moreover, nearly 40% of hospital admissions involve burns that affect more than 10% TBSA. The current mortality rate for burn patients is 5.6%, with burn injuries responsible for nearly 2500 deaths in children each year.[4]

Scald burns remain the most common cause of burn injury in children younger than 5 years of age. The majority of scald burns in infants and toddlers are from hot foods and liquids. Hot grease spills are notorious for causing deep burns to the involved areas. Hot tap water burns, which can easily be prevented by installing special faucet valves so that water does not leave the tap at a temperature above 120°F, frequently result in burns of larger areas to children. Children also frequently suffer product-related contact burns to their hands and faces from curling irons, ovens, steam irons, and fireworks. Contact with electrical outlets and electric cords also causes a significant percentage of electrical injuries.

Child abuse also represents a significant cause of burns in children. Burns with a bilaterally symmetric distribution, a stocking-glove distribution, burns to the dorsum of hands, and delay in seeking medical attention should all raise the suspicion for possible child abuse. In the adolescent age group, flame burns are more common, frequently occurring as a result of experimenting with fire and volatile agents.

PATHOPHYSIOLOGY

As the largest organ of the body, the skin guards against harmful environmental insults, prevents entry of microorganisms, and maintains fluid and electrolyte homeostasis. Skin is also important for thermoregulation, metabolism of vitamin D, and processing neurosensory inputs. The surface area of skin ranges from 0.2 to 0.3 m^2 in an average newborn to 1.5 to 2.0 m^2 in an adult. The epidermis is composed primarily of epithelial cells, specifically keratinocytes. The cells from the basal layer of keratinocytes (the stratum germinativum) divide and migrate outward to the strata spinosum, granulosum, lucidum, and eventually the stratum corneum. These cells then eventually desquamate. This entire process of epidermal maturation from the basal layer to desquamation generally takes 2 to 4 weeks. The basement membrane at the dermoepidermal junction is composed of mucopolysaccharides rich in fibronectin and functions as a barrier to the passage of macromolecules. The dermis is made up of fibroblasts producing collagen and elastin and is subdivided into a superficial papillary dermis and a deep reticular dermis. The papillary and reticular dermis are separated by a plexus of nerves and blood vessels. The reticular dermis and fatty layer contain skin appendages such as hair follicles, sweat glands, and sebaceous glands.

Thermal injury produces coagulation necrosis of the epidermis and a varying depth of injury to the underlying tissue. The extent of burn injury depends on the temperature, duration of exposure, skin thickness, tissue conductance, and specific heat of the causative agent. For example, the specific heat of lipid is higher than that of water. Therefore, grease burns often result in much deeper burns than a scald burn from water with the same temperature and duration of exposure. Thermal energy is easily transferred from high-energy molecules to those of lower energy during contact through the process of heat conduction. The skin generally provides a barrier to the transfer of energy to the deeper tissues. Therefore, much of the burn injury is confined to this layer. However, local tissue response to the zone of initial burn injury can lead to progression of the burn injury to surrounding tissue.

The area of cutaneous burn injury is divided into three zones: coagulation, stasis, and hyperemia (Fig. 13-1). The *zone of coagulation* comprises the initial burn eschar where cells become irreversibly damaged at the time of injury. The area immediately surrounding the necrotic area is called the *zone of stasis.* In this zone, most cells are initially viable but tissue perfusion becomes progressively impaired from the local release of inflammatory mediators, such as thromboxane A_2, arachidonic acid, oxidants, and cytokines.[5] Their influence on the microcirculation results in the formation of platelet thrombus, neutrophil adherence, fibrin deposition, and vasoconstriction, all of which lead to cell necrosis. Thromboxane A_2 inhibitors can significantly improve the dermal blood flow to decrease the zone of stasis.[6] Antioxidants as well as bradykinin antagonists also improve local blood flow.[7,8] Inhibition of neutrophil adherence to endothelium with anti-CD18 or anti-intercellular monoclonal antibodies improves tissue perfusion in animal models.[9,10] The *zone of hyperemia* is characterized by vasodilation with increased blood flow as part of the inflammatory response. This zone lies peripheral to the zone of stasis.

The burn-induced inflammatory response is not limited to the local burn wound. A massive systemic release of thromboxane A_2, along with other inflammatory mediators (bradykinin, leukotrienes, catecholamines, activated complements, and vasoactive amines) induces a significant physiologic burden on the cardiopulmonary, renal, and gastrointestinal organ systems.[11] Decreased plasma volume due to increased capillary permeability and subsequent plasma leak into the interstitial space can lead to depressed cardiac function. As a result of low cardiac output, renal blood flow can decrease, leading to a diminished glomerular filtration rate. Activation of other stress-induced hormones and mediators, such as angiotensin, aldosterone, and vasopressin, can further compromise renal blood flow, resulting in oliguria.[12] If not promptly recognized and treated, this condition can progress to acute tubular necrosis and subsequent renal failure, which contribute to poor outcome for burn patients.[13]

Burn injury can also affect remote organ systems such as the gastrointestinal tract. A rapid onset of atrophy of the small bowel mucosa occurs as a result of increased epithelial apoptosis and decreased epithelial proliferation.[14-16] Intestinal permeability to macromolecules, which are normally repelled by an intact mucosal barrier, increases after burns.[17] Transient mesenteric ischemia is thought to be an important contributing factor to an increase in intestinal permeability. This results in bacterial translocation and subsequent endotoxemia. Burn injury also causes a global depression of immune function. Macrophage production is decreased. Neutrophils are impaired in terms of diapedesis, chemotaxis, and phagocytosis; and cytotoxic T lymphocyte activity is decreased. These impaired functions of neutrophils, macrophages, and T lymphocytes contribute to an increased risk for infectious complications after burns.[18,19]

INITIAL MANAGEMENT

The burned patient must be immediately removed from the thermal source of injury, obviously including burning clothes and metal jewelry. Immediate cooling, such as pouring cold water on the wound, can minimize the depth of burn injury, but it must be used with extreme caution only in a small BSA because it can result in systemic hypothermia. In case of chemical burns, victims should be quickly removed from the continued exposure to the causative chemical agent(s) and the wounds irrigated with copious amounts of water, taking care not to spread the responsible chemical agent(s) to adjacent uninvolved skin areas. Attempts to neutralize causative chemicals are contraindicated because this process may produce additional heat and further add insult to the initial burn injury.

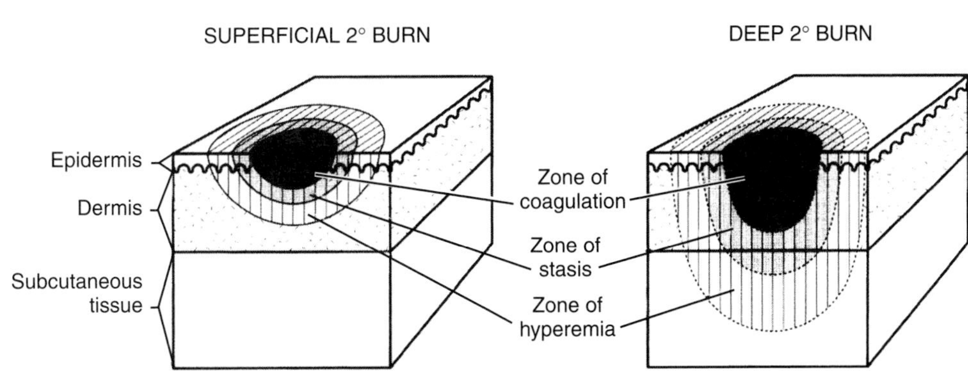

Figure 13-1. Three zones of burn injury: coagulation, stasis, and hyperemia.

As with any trauma patient, burn patients are quickly assessed through primary and secondary surveys. Airway, breathing, and circulation status are assessed, and any potential life-threatening conditions should be promptly identified and intervention initiated. Respiratory symptoms such as wheezing, tachypnea, and hoarseness should alert impending major airway problems. Therefore, the airway should be rapidly secured with 100% oxygen support. Oxygen saturation is monitored using pulse oximetry, and chest expansion is observed to ensure adequate and equal air entry. Circumferential full-thickness burns to the chest can significantly impair respiratory functions by constricting the chest wall and preventing adequate chest expansion. If necessary, escharotomy should be performed to allow better chest expansion and subsequent ventilation. Blood pressure may be difficult to obtain in burned patients with charred extremities. A change in the pulse rate is a sensitive indicator for intravascular volume status. The presence of tachycardia should prompt aggressive fluid resuscitation.

The burn depth is categorized according to the depth of the injury: epidermis, papillary dermis, reticular dermis, subcutaneous fat, and underlying structures. *First-degree* burns are confined to the epidermis. The epidermis appears intact and erythematous and is painful to touch. Therapy is targeted toward symptomatic relief. This typically involves application of a topical ointment containing aloe vera along with a nonsteroidal anti-inflammatory agent. First-degree burns (e.g., sunburn) heal spontaneously without scarring in 7 to 10 days. *Second-degree* burns are divided into superficial and deep, based on the depth of dermal involvement. Superficial second-degree burns are defined as burn injury limited to the papillary dermis and are typically erythematous and painful with blister formation. Superficial second-degree burns also heal spontaneously with the re-epithelialization process taking place in 10 to 14 days. Slight skin pigment discoloration is usually the only significant sequela. Deep second-degree burns extend into the reticular layer of the dermis. The deep epidermal appendages allow some of these wounds to slowly heal over several weeks, usually with significant scarring. However, in general, deep second-degree burn injury requires surgical debridement and skin grafting for more rapid recovery and shorter hospitalization. *Third-degree* burns involve full-thickness injury and result in complete destruction of the epidermis, dermis, and dermal appendages. These burns are characterized by a dry, leathery eschar that is insensate to any stimuli. Without any residual epidermal or dermal appendages, burn wounds can heal by re-epithelialization from the burn wound edges. However, this process is slow, requiring prolonged hospitalization with the risk for burn wound infection. *Fourth-degree* burns involve organs beneath the layers of the skin, such as muscle and bone.

Accurate and rapid determination of burn depth is vital to the proper management of the injury. In particular, the distinction between superficial and deep dermal burns is critical because this dictates whether the burns can be managed with or without excision and grafting. Evaluation by an experienced burn surgeon as to whether an apparent deep dermal burn will heal in 3 weeks is only about 50% accurate. Early excision and grafting provides better results than nonoperative therapy for such "indeterminate" burns. More precise objective methods to determine the burn depth include techniques such as using a multisensor heatable laser Doppler flowmeter and fluorescein to determine blood flow, ultrasonography to detect denatured collagen, and light reflectance of the wound.[20,21] Ultimately, burn wound biopsy seems to be the most precise diagnostic tool.[22] However, it is not clinically practical because it is invasive and provides only a static evaluation of the burn wound. It also requires an experienced pathologist to interpret the histologic findings. Although clinical examination by an experienced burn surgeon remains the most reliable method of determining the burn depth, other diagnostic tools such as laser Doppler imaging and videomicroscopy (visualizing intact dermal capillaries) are gaining popularity for routine clinical use.[23]

Full-thickness circumferential burns to the extremities produce constricting eschar, which can result in vascular compromise to the distal tissues. Accumulation of tissue edema beneath the nonelastic eschar impedes venous outflow first and eventually affects arterial flow. When distal pulses are absent by palpation or on Doppler imaging, escharotomies should be performed to avoid vascular compromise of the limb tissues. With the use of either the scalpel or electrocautery unit, escharotomies can be performed at the bedside along the lateral and medial aspects of the involved extremities (Fig. 13-2). When the hands are involved, incisions are carried down onto the thenar and hypothenar eminences and along the dorsolateral aspects of the digits. Because of the full-thickness burn depth, minimal bleeding is encountered. With

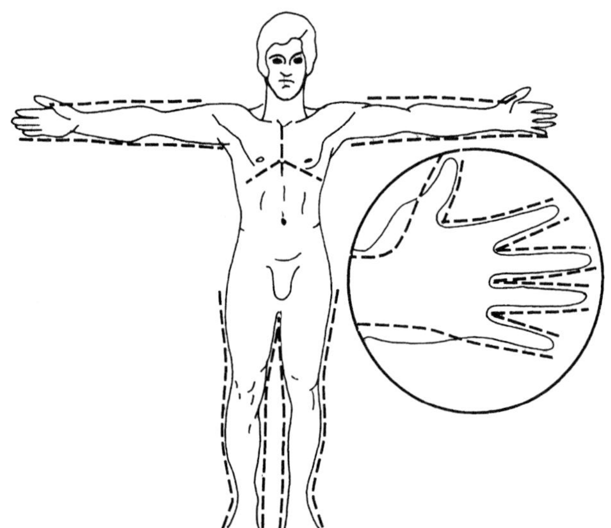

Figure 13-2. Escharotomies. The incisions are made on the medial and lateral aspects of the extremity. Hand escharotomies are performed on the medial and lateral digits and on the dorsum of the hand. (From Eichelberger MR [ed]: Pediatric Trauma: Prevention, Acute Care, Rehabilitation. St. Louis, Mosby, 1993.)

prolonged tissue vascular compromise, reperfusion after an escharotomy may cause reactive hyperemia and further edema formation in the muscle compartments. Ischemia-reperfusion injury also releases free oxygen radicals, resulting in transient hypotension. If increased compartment pressures are noted, fasciotomy should be performed immediately to avoid permanent ischemic injuries to the nerves, muscles, and other soft tissues.

Intravenous access should be established immediately to deliver lactated Ringer's solution according to the resuscitation guidelines. Peripheral intravenous access is preferred, but femoral venous access is an ideal alternative in patients with massive burns, particularly involving extremities. When achieving vascular access is problematic in small children (<6 years of age) with burned extremities, intraosseous access is an alternative route of fluid and medication administration. However, proper technique must be used to avoid potential injury to bone growth plate. A nasogastric tube is introduced in all patients with major burns in anticipation of a gastric ileus and potential vomiting. In addition, almost immediate implementation of enteral nutrition via a transpyloric feeding tube can effectively eliminate burn-induced small bowel ileus. A urinary catheter should be inserted to accurately monitor urine output as a measure of end-organ perfusion. Admission laboratory tests should include complete blood cell count, type and crossmatch, chemistry profile, urinalysis, coagulation profile, and chest radiograph. Whenever inhalation injury is suspected, arterial blood gas analysis with carboxyhemoglobin level should also be obtained.

The size of the burn is generally assessed by the "rule of nines" in adolescents and adults. Each upper extremity and head represent 9% of the TBSA and the lower extremities and the anterior and posterior trunks are 18% each. The perineum, genitalia, and neck each measures 1% of the TBSA. A quick rough estimate of the burn size can also be assessed by the use of the patient's palm, which represents 1% TBSA. However, the general use of this rule can be misleading in children because of different body proportions. Children have a relatively larger portion of their BSA in the head and neck and a smaller surface area in the lower extremities. For example, an infant's head constitutes 19% of TBSA compared with 9% in an adult. Thus, the modified "rule of nines" based on the anthropomorphic difference of infancy and childhood is generally used to assess pediatric burn size (Fig. 13-3).

Fluid Resuscitation

Appropriate fluid resuscitation should begin immediately after securing intravenous access. Peripheral intravenous access is sufficient in the majority of small to moderate size burns. Saphenous vein cutdowns are useful in cases of difficult intravenous access in larger patients. In children, percutaneous femoral central venous access may be easier and more reliable when dealing with a difficult peripheral intravenous access situation. Many guidelines exist as fluid resuscitation

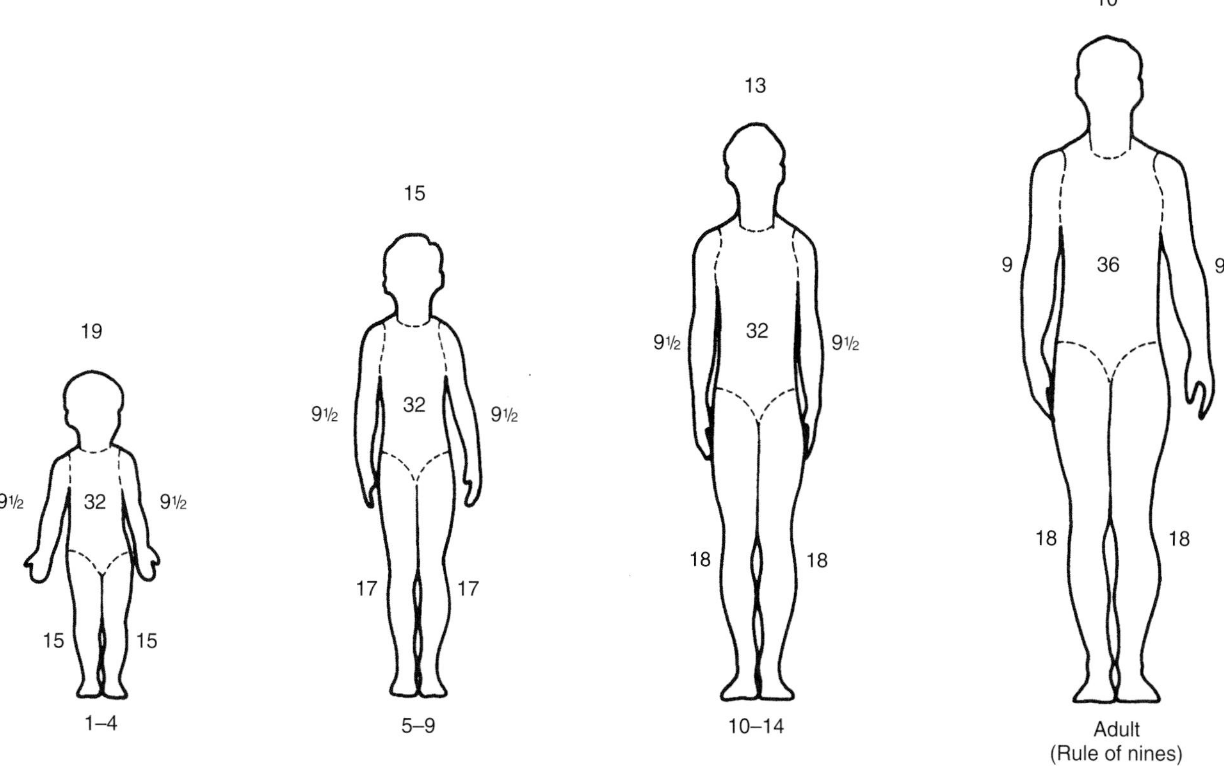

Figure 13-3. Modified "rule of nines" for pediatric burn patients. (Adapted from Lee J, Herndon DN: The pediatric burned patient. In Herndon DN [ed]: Total Burn Care, 3rd ed. Philadelphia, WB Saunders, 2007, p 487.)

Table 13-1	Formulas for Body Surface Area (BSA)
Dubois Formula	BSA (m^2) = height (cm)$^{0.725}$ × weight (kg)$^{0.425}$ × 0.007184
Jacobson Formula	BSA (m^2) = [height (cm) + weight (kg) − 60]/100

formulas, delivering various concentrations of colloid and crystalloid solutions. The Parkland formula (4 mL of lactated Ringer's per kilogram of body weight per percentage of TBSA burned) is most widely used, but the child's fluid resuscitation formula should be based on his or her BSA because of the disparity of BSA to weight. Children have greater BSA relative to their body weight. As a result, weight-based formulas can under-resuscitate children with minor burns and may grossly over-resuscitate children with extensive burns.[24] TBSA can also be assessed from height and weight using standard nomograms or calculated using formulas (Table 13-1). The Shriners-Galveston formula utilizes 5000 mL/m^2 BSA burn plus 2000 mL/m^2 BSA of lactated Ringer's solution given over the first 24 hours after burn injury. Half of this volume is administered during the first 8 hours and the remaining half over the following 16 hours (Table 13-2).

The primary goal of fluid resuscitation is to achieve adequate organ and tissue perfusion regardless of which guidelines are used. Fluid administration should be titrated to maintain a urine output of 1 mL/kg/hr. Approximately 50% of administered fluid is sequestered in nonburned tissues in 50% TBSA burn patients due to increased capillary permeability that occurs particularly in the first 6 to 8 hours after injury.[25] During this period, large molecules leak into the interstitial space to increase the extravascular colloid osmotic pressure. Therefore, to maintain adequate intravascular osmotic pressure, albumin is added 12 hours after the injury. After the first 24 hours, 3750 mL/m^2 BSA burn is given to replace evaporative fluid loss plus 1500 mL/m^2 BSA per 24 hours for maintenance. Dextrose-containing solutions, such as 5% dextrose with 0.25 to 0.5 normal saline, are used as the primary solution. Children younger than 2 years of age are susceptible to hypoglycemia due to limited glycogen stores. Therefore, lactated Ringer's solution with 5% dextrose is given during the first 24 hours in these patients.

Table 13-2	Burn Resuscitation Formulas	
Formula	**First 24 Hours**	**Fluid Solution**
Parkland	4 mL/kg per %TBSA burn	Lactated Ringer's (LR)
Brooke	1.5 mL/kg per %TBSA burn	LR + colloid 0.5 mL/kg per %TBSA burn
Shriners-Galveston	5000 mL/m^2 burned + 2000 mL/m^2 total	LR + 12.5 g albumin

TBSA, total body surface area.

Children often do not exhibit clinical signs of hypovolemia until more than 25% of their circulating volume is depleted and complete cardiovascular collapse is imminent. Tachycardia reflects a compensatory response to hypovolemia, but caution should be used not to overinterpret this finding, because a reflex tachycardia owing to postinjury catecholamine response is also common. A lethargic child with decreased capillary refill and cool, clammy extremities needs prompt attention. Measurement of the arterial pH and base deficit can help interpret the adequacy of fluid resuscitation. Hyponatremia is also a frequent complication in pediatric burn patients after aggressive fluid resuscitation. Frequent monitoring of serum chemistry with appropriate correction is required to avoid severe electrolyte imbalance. A serious complication such as central pontine myelinolysis can occur as a result of rapid correction of hypernatremia.[26]

Hypertonic saline resuscitation can be beneficial in treating burn-induced shock.[27] This hypertonic fluid maintains intravascular volume more effectively by removing fluid from the interstitial space by osmosis, resulting in a decrease in generalized tissue edema. However, it is not widely used because of its potential risks for hypernatremia, hyperosmolarity, renal failure, and alkalosis.[11] Some favor the use of a modified hypertonic solution by adding one ampule of sodium bicarbonate to each liter of lactated Ringer's solution during the first 24 hours of resuscitation.[28] Burn units with experienced multidisciplinary team members are best prepared to handle major burns. Patients who sustain a major burn injury (Table 13-3) should be transferred promptly to a nearby burn center for their care.

The ideal target for fluid resuscitation should be to maintain adequate visceral organ perfusion while minimizing soft tissue edema as a result of the diffuse capillary leak. Over-resuscitation during the first 24 hours post burn has been shown to be associated with an increased incidence of pneumonia, bloodstream infection, acute respiratory distress syndrome, multiple-organ failure, and death.[29] "Permissive hypovolemia" during burn fluid resuscitation has been shown to improve multiple-organ dysfunction scores,[30] further suggesting that this is a safe and beneficial approach during acute burn resuscitation.

Table 13-3	Major Burn Injury Criteria (American Burn Association)
Second-degree burns > 10% TBSA in patients younger than 10 yr	
Third-degree burns > 5% TBSA	
Burns involving the face, hands, feet, genitalia, perineum, and major joints	
Chemical burns	
Electrical burns including lightning injury	
Inhalation injury	
Burns with significant concomitant trauma	
Burns with significant preexisting medical disorders	

TBSA, total body surface area.

INHALATION INJURY

Inhalation injury remains the major contributor to mortality in burn patients. The mortality rate of children with isolated cutaneous burns is 1% to 2%, but this significantly increases to approximately 40% in the presence of inhalation injury.[31] Inhalation injury is caused primarily by inhaled toxins such as fumes, gases, and mists. Although the supraglottic region can be injured by both thermal and chemical insults, tracheobronchial and lung parenchymal injuries rarely occur as a result of direct thermal damage because the heat disperses so rapidly in the larynx. Hypoxia, increased airway resistance, decreased pulmonary compliance, increased alveolar epithelial permeability, and increased pulmonary vascular resistance can be triggered by the release of vasoactive substances (thromboxanes A_2, C_{3a}, and C_{5a}) from the damaged epithelium.[32] Neutrophil activation plays a critical role in this process. Pulmonary function has been shown to improve with the use of a ligand binding to E-selectins (inhibiting neutrophil adhesion) and anti-interleukin-8 (inhibiting neutrophil chemotaxis). Another significant respiratory tract pathology is sloughing of ciliated epithelial cells from the basement membrane, resulting in exudate formation. These exudates, consisting of lymph proteins, coalesce to form fibrin casts. These fibrin casts are frequently resistant to routine pulmonary toilet and can create a "ball-valve" effect in localized areas of lung. This eventually causes barotrauma.

The diagnosis is usually made on clinical history and physical findings at the initial evaluation. Victims trapped in a house fire with excessive smoke and fumes are likely to have sustained severe inhalation injury. Facial burns with singed hair and carbonaceous sputum suggest inhalation injury. Hoarseness and stridor should alert significant airway obstruction and the airway should immediately be secured with endotracheal intubation. Patients who present with disorientation and obtundation are likely to have an elevated carbon monoxide level (carboxyhemoglobin > 10%). Fiberoptic bronchoscopy remains the gold standard for diagnosing the presence of inhalation injury. It can demonstrate inflammatory changes in the tracheal mucosa such as edema, hyperemia, mucosal ulceration, and sloughing. A ventilation scan with xenon-133 can also identify regions of inhalation injury by assessing respiratory exchange and excretion of xenon by the lungs.[33] The use of these complementary diagnostic tools, bronchoscopy and xenon-133 scanning, is over 90% accurate in the diagnosis of inhalation injury. However, bronchoscopic examination of the airway at the bedside, without having to transport critically ill burn patients to nuclear medicine, is frequently sufficient to confirm the diagnosis of inhalation injury.

The treatment of inhalation injury begins at the scene of the burn accident. The administration of 100% oxygen rapidly decreases the half-life of carbon monoxide. The airway must be secured with intubation in patients with signs and symptoms of imminent respiratory failure. In the intensive care unit, inhalation treatment protocols have been effective in improving the clearance of tracheobronchial secretions and decreasing bronchospasm (Table 13-4). Aggressive pulmonary toilet with physiotherapy and frequent suctioning is important to prevent serious respiratory complications. The patient is frequently turned side to side along with chest physiotherapy every 2 hours. When physiologically stable, the patient is positioned out of bed in a chair as well as assisted to ambulate. Humidified air is delivered at high flow, and bronchodilators and racemic epinephrine are used to treat bronchospasm. Intravenous heparin has been shown to reduce tracheobronchial cast formation, minute ventilation, and peak inspiratory pressures after smoke inhalation. Inhalation treatments such as 20% acetylcysteine nebulized solution along with nebulized heparin is effective in improving the clearance of tracheobronchial secretions and minimizing bronchospasm and significantly improving reintubation rates and mortality.[34]

Table 13-4 Inhalation Injury Treatment Protocol

Treatment	Interval/Dosage
Suction and lavage	Every 2 hours
Bronchodilators (Albuterol)	Every 2 hours
Nebulized heparin	5000-10,000 units with 3 mL NS every 4 hours
Nebulized acetylcysteine	20%, 3 mL q4h
Hypertonic saline	Induces effective coughing
Racemic epinephrine	Reduces mucosal edema

NS, normal saline.

The presence of inhalation injury generally requires an increased amount of fluid resuscitation, up to 2 mL/kg/% TBSA burn more than would be required for an equal size burn without an inhalation injury. In fact, pulmonary edema that is associated with inhalation injury is not prevented by fluid restriction. Rather, inadequate resuscitation may increase the severity of pulmonary injury by sequestering neutrophils.[35] Corticosteroids have not been shown to be beneficial in inhalation injury. Prophylactic intravenous antibiotics are not indicated but are started with the clinical suspicion of pneumonia. Early pneumonia is usually the result of gram-positive organisms such as methicillin-resistant *Staphylococcus aureus*. Later infection is usually caused by gram-negative organisms, such as *Pseudomonas*. Antibiotic therapy should be guided by serially monitored sputum cultures and bronchial washings.

A recent report suggests that there is a distinct cytokine profile in pediatric burn patients with inhalation injury as an early predictor for high mortality.[36] Early alterations in serum levels of interleukin (IL)-6, IL-7, and IL-10 were found to be useful markers of high mortality in burned children with inhalation injury. Increased IL-6 and IL-10 as well as decreased IL-7 serum levels were associated with a greater risk for mortality, thus suggesting a valuable role for these diagnostic tools in the evaluation of severe pediatric burn patients with concomitant inhalation injury.

WOUND CARE

The appropriate wound care is generally determined by an accurate assessment of the burn depth and size (Table 13-5). First-degree burns require no particular dressing, but the involved areas should be kept out of exposure to direct sunlight. They are generally treated with topical ointments for symptomatic pain relief. Superficial second-degree burns are treated with daily dressing changes with topical antimicrobial agents. They can also be treated with simple application of petroleum gauze or synthetic dressings to allow for rapid spontaneous re-epithelialization. Deep second- and third-degree burn wounds eventually require excision of the eschar with skin grafting.

Antimicrobial Agents

Various topical antimicrobial agents have been used for management of burn wounds. None of these agents effectively prevent colonization of organisms that commonly harbor in the eschar, but they serve a purpose of maintaining bacterial quantity at less than 10^2 to 10^5 colonies/g of tissue. Routine punch quantitative wound biopsies of burned areas can document impending burn wound sepsis.

Silver sulfadiazine (Silvadene, Monarch Pharmaceuticals, Inc., Bristol, TN) is the most commonly used topical antimicrobial agent for burn wound dressings. Although it does not penetrate eschar, it has a broad spectrum of efficacy and soothes the pain associated

Table 13-5 Burn Wound Dressings

Dressings	Advantages	Disadvantages
Antimicrobial Salves		
Silver sulfadiazine (Silvadene)	Painless; broad-spectrum; rare sensitivity	Leukopenia; some gram-negative resistance; mild inhibition of epithelialization
Mafenide acetate (Sulfamylon)	Broad-spectrum; penetrates eschar; effective against *Pseudomonas*	Painful; metabolic acidosis; mild inhibition of epithelialization
Bacitracin/Neomycin/Polymyxin B	Ease of application, painless, useful on face	Limited antimicrobial property
Nystatin	Effective in inhibiting fungal growth; use in combination with Silvadene, Bacitracin	Cannot use in combination with mafenide acetate
Mupirocin (Bactroban)	Effective against *Staphylococcus,* including MRSA	Cost; poor eschar penetration
Antimicrobial Soaks		
0.5% Silver nitrate	Painless; broad-spectrum; rare sensitivity	No eschar penetration; discolors contacted areas; electrolyte imbalance; methemoglobinemia
Povidone-iodine (Betadine)	Broad-spectrum antimicrobial	Painful; potential systemic absorption; hypersensitivity
5% Mafenide acetate	Broad-spectrum antimicrobial	Painful; no fungal coverage; metabolic acidosis
0.025% Sodium hypochlorite (Dakin's solution)	Effective against most organisms	Mildly inhibits epithelialization
0.25% Acetic acid	Effective against most organisms	Mildly inhibits epithelialization
Silver-impregnated		
Aquacel, Acticoat	Broad-spectrum antimicrobial; no dressing changes	Cost
Synthetic Dressings		
Biobrane	Provides wound barrier; minimizes pain; useful for outpatient burns, hands (gloves)	Exudate accumulation risks invasive wound infection; no antimicrobial property
OpSite, Tegaderm	Provides moisture barrier; minimizes pain; useful for outpatient burns; inexpensive	Exudate accumulation risks invasive wound infection; no antimicrobial property
Transcyte	Provides wound barrier; accelerates wound healing	Exudate accumulation risks invasive wound infection; no antimicrobial property
Integra, Alloderm	Complete wound closure, including dermal substitute	No antimicrobial property; expensive; requires training, experience
Biologic Dressings		
Allograft (cadaver skin), Xenograft (pig skin)	Temporary biologic dressings	Requires access to skin bank; cost
Amniotic membrane	Minimizes dressing changes	Not widely used

MRSA, methicillin-resistant *S. aureus.*

with second-degree burns. Silver sulfadiazine on fine mesh gauze can be used separately or in combination with other antimicrobial agents, such as nystatin (Teva Pharmaceutical Industries, USA). The combination of Silvadene with nystatin has significantly reduced the incidence of *Candida* infection in burned patients.[37] The most common side effect is leukopenia. However, this is generally caused by margination of white blood cells and is usually transient.[38] When the leukocyte count falls below 3000 cells/mm^3, changing to another topical antimicrobial agent typically resolves this side effect.

Mafenide acetate (Sulfamylon, UDC Laboratories, Inc., Rockford, IL) is more effective in penetrating eschar and is frequently used in third-degree burns. Fine-mesh gauze impregnated with Sulfamylon (10% water-soluble cream) can be applied directly onto the burn wound. Sulfamylon has a much broader spectrum of efficacy, including *Pseudomonas* and *Enterococcus*. It is also available in a 5% solution to soak burn wounds, eliminating the need to perform frequent dressing changes. Sulfamylon is a potent carbonic anhydrase inhibitor and can therefore cause metabolic acidosis. This side effect can usually be avoided by limiting the use of Sulfamylon to only 20% TBSA at any given time and rotating application sites every several hours with another topical antimicrobial agent. In addition, the application of Sulfamylon can be painful, which limits its practical use in an outpatient setting, especially in children.

In addition to 5% Sulfamylon solution, other agents are available as a soak solution. These include 0.5% silver nitrate and 0.025% sodium hypochlorite (Dakin's solution). These soak solutions are generally poured onto the gauze dressings, avoiding frequent dressing changes with potential loss of grafts or healing cells. Silver nitrate is painless on application and has broad coverage, but its side effects include electrolyte imbalance (hyponatremia, hypochloremia) and dark gray or black stains. A new commercially available dressing containing biologically active silver ions (Aquacel, ConvaTec Ltd., UK; Acticoat, Smith & Nephew, London, UK) holds promise for retaining the effectiveness of silver nitrate but without its side effects. Dakin's (0.025%) solution is effective against most microbes, including *Pseudomonas*. However, it requires frequent dosing because of the inactivation of hypochlorite on contact with protein. Moreover, it can also retard healing.[39] Petroleum-based antimicrobial ointments, such as polymyxin B and bacitracin (Polysporin), are painless and transparent, allowing easier monitoring of the burn wounds. These agents are mostly effective against gram-positive organisms. Their use is limited to facial burns, small areas of partial-thickness burns, and healing donor sites. As with Silvadene, these petroleum-based agents can also be used in combination with nystatin to suppress skin *Candida* colonization.

The use of silver-impregnated antimicrobial dressings (Aquacel, Acticoat) has gained popularity in recent years. Aquacel Ag is a silver-impregnated hydrocolloid dressing that becomes adherent to the wound within 24 hours after application and can be left on for up to 2 weeks without change. The antimicrobial activity is equivalent to other silver-containing compounds.[40] A recent report demonstrated a shorter length of hospitalization as a result of reducing the complexity and number of dressing changes in pediatric burn patients when compared with treatment with silver sulfadiazine.[41]

The use of perioperative intravenous antibiotics has significantly contributed to an overall improvement in the survival of major burn patients during the past 2 decades. Bacteria colonized in the burn eschar can potentially shed systemically at the time of eschar excision and contribute to sepsis. It is our general practice to administer intravenous antibiotics against *Streptococcus*, *S. aureus*, and *Pseudomonas* perioperatively until quantitative cultures of the excised eschar are finalized. The antibiotic regimen should be guided by culture results and used appropriately for indicated clinical conditions.

Burn Wound Dressings

Superficial second-degree burns can be managed using various methods. A topical antimicrobial dressing using Silvadene is most commonly used, but synthetic dressings, such as Biobrane (UDL Laboratories, Rockford, IL) and OpSite (Smith & Nephew, London, UK), offer unique advantages of eliminating frequent painful dressing changes and potential tissue fluid loss. The general principle behind these synthetic products is to provide sterile coverage of superficial second-degree burn wounds to allow rapid spontaneous re-epithelialization of the involved areas.

Biobrane is a bilaminate thin membrane composed of thin semipermeable silicone bonded to a layer of nylon fabric mesh that is coated with a monomolecular layer of type I collagen of porcine origin. This dressing provides a hydrophilic coating for fibrin ingrowth that promotes wound adherence. It is supplied in simple sheets or preshaped gloves for easy application (Fig. 13-4).[42] After being placed onto clean fresh superficial second-degree burn wounds using Steri-strips and bandages, the Biobrane dressing dries and becomes well adherent to burn wounds within 24 to 48 hours. Once adherent, the covered areas are kept open to air and examined closely for the first few days to detect any signs or symptoms of infection. As the

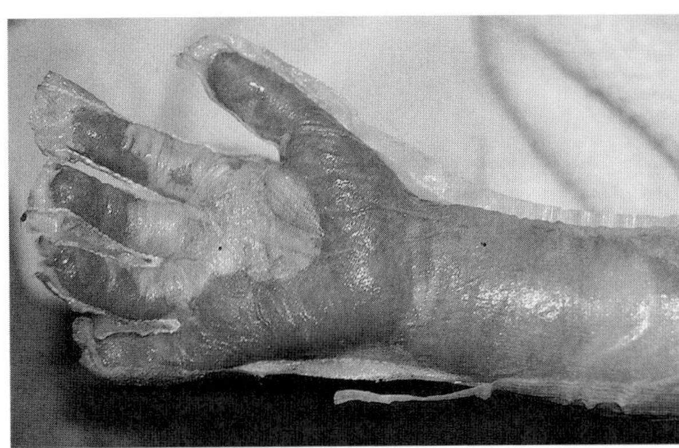

Figure 13-4. This burned right forearm and hand have been placed in a biobrane glove.

epithelialization occurs beneath the Biobrane sheet, it is easily peeled off the wound. Sterile aspiration of serous fluid underneath the Biobrane can preserve its use. However, if a foul-smelling exudate is detected, it should be removed and a topical antimicrobial dressing applied. The use of Biobrane has become widespread in the management of superficial second-degree burns because it has been shown to reduce pain and fluid and electrolyte loss, thereby allowing for application in an outpatient setting. Alternatively, OpSite or Tegaderm (3M Pharmaceuticals, St. Paul, MN) can also be used to cover superficial second-degree burn wounds. Commonly used as a postoperative dressing, it is easy to apply and provides an impervious barrier to the environment. It is also relatively inexpensive, and its transparent nature allows for easier monitoring of second-degree burn wounds. Despite lacking any special biologic factors (collagen and growth factors) to enhance wound healing, it promotes spontaneous re-epithelialization. Biobrane and OpSite are preferred to topical antimicrobial dressings when dealing with small superficial second-degree burn wounds, especially in the outpatient setting.

Synthetic and biologic dressings are also available for coverage of full-thickness burn wounds. Integra (Integra LifeSciences Corp., Plainsboro, NJ) consists of an inner layer made of a porous matrix of bovine collagen and the glycosaminoglycan chrondroitin-6-sulfate, which facilitates fibrovascular ingrowth.[43] The outer layer is polysiloxane polymer with vapor transmission characteristics similar to normal epithelium. Integra serves as a matrix for the infiltration of fibroblasts, macrophages, lymphocytes, and capillaries derived from the wound bed and promotes the rapid neodermis formation for the treatment of full-thickness burn wounds (Fig. 13-5). After the collagen matrix engrafts into the wound in approximately 2 weeks, the outer silicone layer is replaced with epidermal autografts. Epidermal donor sites heal rapidly without significant morbidity. Moreover, Integra-covered wounds have less scarring. However, they are also susceptible to wound infection and must be monitored carefully. The use of Integra for children with large TBSA burns was recently evaluated for short- and long-term follow-up.[44] Burned children treated with Integra demonstrated significantly decreased resting energy expenditure as well as increased bone mineral content and density, along with improved scarring at 24 months after burn injury, thus validating the use of this dermal substitute in the management of pediatric burned patients. Interestingly, Integra has also been successfully used as a dermal matrix host for the dispersal of keratinocytes as a novel skin-grafting technique.[45]

Alloderm (LifeCell Corp., Branchburg, NJ) is another dermal substitute with decellularized preserved cadaver dermis. This synthetic dermal substitute has a tremendous potential for minimizing scar contractures and improving the cosmetic and functional outcome. Biological dressings, such as xenografts from swine and allografts from cadaver donors, can also be used to cover full-thickness burn wounds as a temporary dressing. Particularly useful when dealing with large TBSA burns, biological dressings can provide immunologic and barrier functions of normal skin. The areas of xenograft and allograft are eventually rejected by the immune system and sloughed off, leaving healthy recipient beds for subsequent autografts. Although extremely rare, the transmission of viral diseases from the allograft is a potential concern.

Human amniotic membranes can also be used as an alternative burn wound dressing. Amnion has been used in the past for the treatment of burns. A recent prospective study compared the use of amnion as a biological dressing for pediatric facial burn patients to standard topical treatment.[46] Although patients in the amnion group had significantly fewer dressing changes, the overall time to healing, length of stay, and hypertrophic scarring were not different between the two treatment groups. Importantly, the use of amnion was not associated with an increased risk of infection, thus indicating the safe use of amnion as an alternative dressing for superficial second-degree burns.

Excision and Grafting

Early excision with skin grafting has been shown to decrease operative blood loss and length of hospitalization and ultimately to improve overall survival of

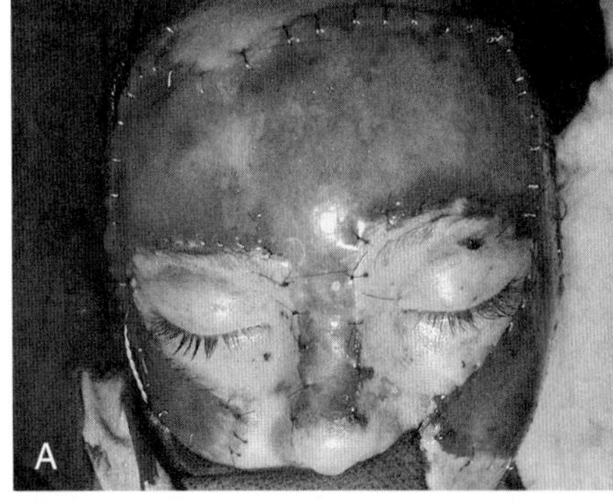

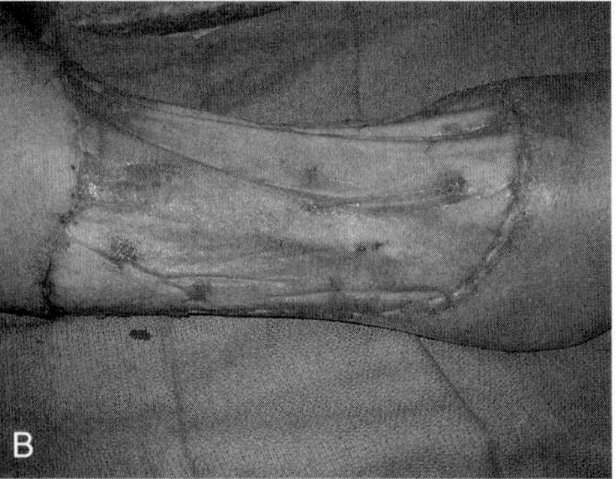

Figure 13-5. Synthetic and biological dressings are available for coverage of full-thickness burn wounds. When left on for 2 weeks, Integra serves as a matrix for neovascularization in the treatment of full-thickness burns. It can be used on the face **(A)** or in other locations **(B)**. At 2 weeks, a nonmeshed epidermal split-thickness skin graft (.006 to .008 inch) can be applied with good cosmetic results.

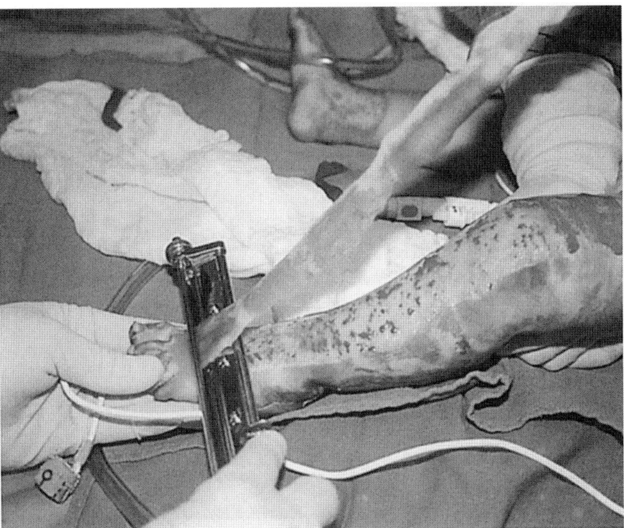

Figure 13-6. Tangential excision of eschar. The excision of eschar is performed to the depth of a viable, bleeding tissue plane. (From Herndon DN [ed]: Total Burn Care, 2nd ed. Philadelphia, WB Saunders, 2002, plate 2.)

burn patients.[3,47] Typically, tangential excision of the full-thickness burn wound is performed 1 to 3 days after burn injury when relative hemodynamic stability has occurred. Eschar is sequentially shaved using a powered dermatome and/or knife blades until a viable tissue plane is achieved (Fig. 13-6). Early excision of eschar (usually < 24 hours after burns) generally decreases operative blood loss due to the vasoconstrictive substances, such as thromboxane and catecholamines, in the burn wounds. Once the burn wounds become hyperemic 48 hours after burns, bleeding at the time of excision of the eschar can be excessive. Tourniquet and subcutaneous injections of epinephrine-containing solution can lessen the blood loss, but these techniques can potentially hinder the surgeon's ability to differentiate viable from nonviable tissues.[48] Topical hemostatic agents such as thrombin can also be used, but they are expensive and not very effective in preventing excessive bleeding from open wounds. In patients with deep full-thickness burns, electrocautery is useful to rapidly excise eschar with minimal blood loss. More importantly, the earlier the excision, the less blood loss occurs in burns greater than 30% TBSA.[49] However, scald burns are more difficult to assess the exact burn depth initially. Therefore, these burns require a more conservative approach with delayed excision. A recent innovative technique, Versajet hydrosurgery (Smith & Nephew, London, UK), utilizes streaming of water for tissue excision. This technique could eliminate significant bleeding associated with "traditional" tangential excision. In a prospective randomized trial, the Versajet technique was shown to produce a more precise and faster excision of burn wounds.[50]

Ideally, the excised burn wound is covered with autograft. Burn wounds less than 20% to 30% TBSA can be covered at one operation with split-thickness autografts. Split-thickness autografts are harvested and the donor sites are dressed with petroleum-based gauze, such as Xeroform (Kendall Healthcare, Miami, FL) or Scarlet-red (Tyco Healthcare, Mansfield, MA). OpSite can also be used to cover donor sites. It is preferable to use sheet autografts for better long-term aesthetic outcome, but narrowly meshed autografts (1:1 or 2:1) have the advantages of limiting the total surface area of donor harvest and allowing better drainage of fluid at the grafted sites. With massive burns, the closure of burn wounds is achieved by a combination of widely meshed autografts (4:1 to 6:1) with allograft (2:1) overlay (Fig. 13-7). Repeat grafting is required for large burns with sequential harvesting of split-thickness autograft from limited donor sites until the entire burn wound is covered. As the meshed autografts heal, the allografts slough. However, the formation of significant scar remains the major disadvantage of this technique. Therefore, the use of widely meshed graft is avoided on the face and functionally important areas. Full-thickness grafts that include both dermal and epidermal components provide the best outcome for wound coverage with diminished contracture and better pigment match. However, its use is generally limited to small areas owing to the lack of abundant full-thickness donor skin.

The limitation of donor sites in patients with burns over massive areas is partially addressed with the use of systemic recombinant human growth hormone (rHGH). Administration of rHGH has resulted in accelerated donor site healing, allowing more frequent donor site harvest in a given period of time.[51,52] Use of rHGH decreased donor site healing time by an average of 2 days, which ultimately improved the overall length of hospitalization from 0.8 to 0.54 days per percentage of TBSA burned.[51] These effects from rHGH are thought to be due to stimulation of insulin-like growth factor (IGF)-1 release and induction of IGF-1 receptors in the burn wound.[52] Given alone, insulin has been shown to decrease donor site healing time from 6.5 to 4.7 days.[53] The decrease in donor site healing by 1 day between each harvest can significantly impact overall length of hospital stay in patients with massive burns who require multiple grafting procedures. The administration of rHGH in burned children was associated with a 23% reduction in total cost of hospital care for a typical 80% TBSA burn.[51]

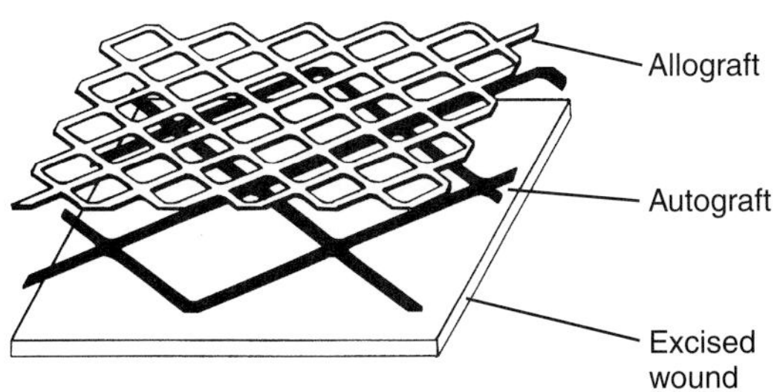

Figure 13-7. Schematic diagram of wound covering with 4:1 meshed autograft with 2:1 meshed allograft overlay. (From Eichelberg MR [ed]: Pediatric Trauma: Prevention, Acute Care, Rehabilitation. St. Louis, Mosby, 1993, p 581.)

The use of cultured keratinocytes from the patient's own skin has generated considerable interest as a potential solution for massively burned patients with limited donor sites.[54,55] This concept of using cultured skin to provide complete coverage is appealing, but there are several problems to overcome. First, cultures of keratinocytes grow slowly. Once grafted, they are very susceptible to mechanical trauma, with successful results in only 50% to 70%. Also, a significantly longer hospital stay has been reported with the use of cultured epithelial grafts in patients with burns of more than 80% TBSA.[56] However, this technology may hold promise in treating massive burns in the near future. Recently, the ReCell technique,[57] a new process of skin grafting that separates keratinocytes from small split-thickness skin grafts and disperses them for spraying onto the excised wound, has gained considerable interest. This technique results in the need for smaller donor sites and is associated with less pain.

HYPERMETABOLIC RESPONSE

Burn injury produces a hypermetabolic response that generally increases with increasing burn size and reaches a plateau at a 40% TBSA burn.[58] This response is characterized by increased energy expenditure, oxygen consumption, proteolysis, lipolysis, and nitrogen losses. These physiologic changes are induced by upregulation of catabolic agents such as cortisol, catecholamines, and glucagon, which act synergistically to increase the production of glucose, a principal fuel during acute inflammation.[59] Cortisol stimulates gluconeogenesis and proteolysis and sensitizes adipocytes to lipolytic hormones. Catecholamines stimulate the rate of glucose production through hepatic gluconeogenesis and glycogenolysis and also promotes lipolysis and peripheral insulin resistance. Thus, serum insulin levels are elevated but the cells are resistant.[60] This increase in glucagon, which is stimulated by catecholamines, further promotes gluconeogenesis.

A significant protein catabolism occurs in severe burns. Cortisol is catabolic and is partially responsible for the loss of tissue protein and a negative nitrogen balance. In addition, burn injury is associated with decreased levels of anabolic hormones such as growth hormone and IGF-1, which contributes significantly to net protein loss. The synthesis of protein, which is essential for the production of collagen for wound healing and antibodies and leukocytes for the immune response, requires a net positive nitrogen balance. Exogenous administration of rHGH, which increases protein synthesis, has been shown to improve nitrogen balance, preserve lean muscle mass, and increase the rate of wound healing.[52] However, the use of rHGH is associated with hyperglycemia along with increased free fatty acids and triglycerides, which limit its clinical applicability.

Excessive catecholamines in post-burn patients also contribute to persistent tachycardia and lipolysis. The consequences of these physiologic changes are cardiac failure and fatty infiltration of the liver. Propranolol lowers resting heart rate and left ventricular work and decreases peripheral lipolysis without adversely affecting cardiac output or the ability to respond to cold stress.[61-63] Therefore, a combination use of rHGH and propranolol appears ideal. A recent prospective randomized controlled trial showed efficacy in rHGH and propranolol treatment in attenuating hypermetabolism and inflammation in severely burned children.[64] In this study, patients receiving rHGH (0.2 mg/kg/day) and propranolol (to decrease heart rate by 15%) for more than 15 days demonstrated significantly decreased percent predicted resting energy expenditure, C-reactive protein, cortisone, aspartate aminotransferase, alanine aminotransferase, free fatty acid, IL-6, IL-8, and macrophage inflammatory protein-1β when compared with controls. Other markers, such as serum IGF-1, IGF-binding protein-3, growth hormone, prealbumin, and IL-7 increased in rHGH/propranolol-treated burned patients. These findings further validate the beneficial role of combination treatment with rHGH and a β blocker in pediatric burn patients.

Another anabolic agent of recent interest in the management of severe burns has been oxandrolone. Oxandrolone (Upsher-Smith Laboratories, Inc., Minneapolis, MN), an oral synthetic derivative of testosterone with a lower androgenic/anabolic ratio, has been safely used to improve lean body mass and weight gain in severely burned adults and children.[65] A large prospective double-blind randomized study involving 235 severely burned children (TBSA > 40%) showed that oxandrolone treatment significantly increased lean body mass along with serum total protein, prealbumin levels, and mean muscle strength.[66] Interestingly, the oxandrolone-treated group also had a shorter hospital stay.

NUTRITION

The metabolic rate of patients with burns significantly increases (1.5 × normal rate in a patient with 25% TBSA burns to 2 × in 40% TBSA burns).[67] Children are particularly vulnerable for protein-calorie malnutrition because of their proportionally less body fat and smaller muscle mass in addition to increased metabolic demands. This malnutrition is associated with dysfunction in various organ systems, including the immune system, and delayed wound healing. Feeding tubes are generally positioned in the duodenum under fluoroscopy immediately after the initial burn evaluation and enteral nutrition is started within hours after the injury. Early enteral feedings have been shown to decrease the level of catabolic hormones, improve nitrogen balance, maintain gut mucosal integrity, and decrease the incidence of sepsis and overall hospitalization.[68-70] Hyperalimentation in burn patients has clearly been shown to be associated with deleterious effects on the immune function, small bowel mucosal atrophy with an increased incidence of bacterial translocation, and a decrease in survival.[71,72]

Several formulas are used to calculate caloric requirement in burn patients. Both the Curreri

Table 13-6 Nutritional Requirements for Burned Children (Shriners Burn Hospital–Galveston)

Age Group	Daily Caloric Requirements
Infant and toddler	2100 kcal/m² total + 1000 kcal/m² burn
Child	1800 kcal/m² total + 1300 kcal/m² burn
Adolescent	1500 kcal/m² total + 1500 kcal/m² burn

(25 kcal/kg plus 40 kcal/% TBSA burned) and modified Harris-Benedict (calculated or measured resting metabolic rate times injury factor) formulas use the principle of providing maintenance caloric needs plus the additional caloric needs related to the burn size. Similar to fluid resuscitation formulas, a caloric requirement formula based on total and burned BSA is more appropriate for pediatric burn patients (Table 13-6).[73-75] The exact nutrient requirements of burn patients are not clear, but it is generally accepted that maintenance of energy requirement and replacement of protein losses are vital. The recommended enteral tube feedings should have 20% to 40% of the calories as protein, 10% to 20% as fat, and 40% to 70% as carbohydrates. Milk is one of the least expensive and best tolerated nutritional substances, but sodium supplement may be needed when milk is used in a large quantity to avoid dilutional hyponatremia. There are also numerous commercially available enteral formulas, such as Vivonex (Nestle-Nutrition, Switzerland) or PediaSure (Abbott Laboratories, Abbott Park, IL).

One recent report evaluated the efficacy of an anti-inflammatory, pulmonary enteral formula in the treatment of pediatric burn patients with respiratory failure.[76] Based on evidence that the inclusion of dietary lipids (e.g., omega-3 fatty acid, eicosapentaenoic acid) known to modulate the inflammatory response and the addition of antioxidants may improve cardiopulmonary function and respiratory gas exchange, this study evaluated the role of a specialized pulmonary enteral formula (SPEF) containing anti-inflammatory and antioxidant-enhanced components in pediatric burn patients. The use of SPEF was shown to be safe in pediatric patients and resulted in an improvement in oxygenation and pulmonary compliance in burn patients with acute respiratory distress syndrome (ARDS).

PAIN MANAGEMENT

Burn wound treatment and rehabilitation therapy produce pain for patients of all age groups. Infants and children do not express their pain in the same way as adults and may display pain through behaviors of fear, anxiety, agitation, tantrums, depression, and withdrawals. In older children, allowing the child to participate in providing wound care can help the child to have some control and alleviate fear and pain. Various combinations of analgesics with antianxiety medications are used effectively during procedures and wound dressing changes. Successful pain management of burned children requires understanding by the entire burn team members of how the pain is associated with burn depth and the phase of wound healing. Pain management protocols should be tailored to control background pain as well as specific procedure-related painful stimuli such as dressing changes, vascular access placement, and physical therapy. Scheduled administration of acetaminophen can often address background pain. Morphine sulfate or fentanyl is frequently used to manage postoperative pain. The intravenous use of ketamine (0.5-2.0 mg/kg) is quite effective and ideal for short procedures, such as dressing changes and vascular access placements. For burned children requiring deeper sedation and analgesia, a combination strategy with propofol and ketamine has also been shown to be effective.[77] Advanced pain management protocols can be administered safely by those experienced with the use of conscious sedation. Physical therapy, which is vital to optimize good functional outcome, can more effectively be employed if there is appropriate pain control. However, caution must be exercised to prevent any potential injury due to overmedication at the time of exercise therapy. Burn injury is extremely traumatic for affected children as well as their families.

NONTHERMAL INJURIES

Chemical Burns

Children accidentally come in contact with various household cleaning products. Treatment of chemical burns involves the immediate removal of the causative agent and lavage with copious amounts of water with caution for potential hypothermia. Fluid resuscitation is started, and care should be taken to ensure that the effluent does not contact uninjured areas. After completion of the lavage, the wounds should be covered with a topical antimicrobial dressing and appropriate surgical plans made. The rapid recognition of the offending chemical agent is crucial for proper management.[78] When there is doubt, the local poison control center should be contacted for identification of the product's chemical composition. The common offending chemical agents can be classified as alkali or acid. Alkalis, such as lime, potassium hydroxide, sodium hydroxide, and bleach, are among the most common agents involved in chemical injury. Mechanisms of alkali-induced burns are saponification of fat resulting in increased cell damage from heat, extraction of intracellular water, and formation of alkaline proteinates with hydroxyl ions. These ions induce further chemical reaction into the deeper tissues. Attempts to neutralize alkali are not recommended because the chemical reaction can generate more heat and add to the injury. Acid burns are not as common. Acids induce protein breakdown by hydrolysis and result in eschar formation. Therefore, these burns do not penetrate as deeply as the alkaline burns. Formic acid injuries are rare but can result in multiple systemic organ failures such as metabolic acidosis, renal failure, intravascular hemolysis, and ARDS. In general, hydrofluoric acid burns are managed differently from other acid burns.[79] After copious local irrigation with water, fluoride ion must be neutralized with topical application of 2.5% calcium gluconate gel. If not appropriately treated, free fluoride ion causes liquefaction necrosis of the affected soft tissues, including bones. Because of potential hypocalcemia, patients should be closely monitored for prolonged QT intervals.

Electrical Burns

Three to 5 percent of all admitted burn patients are injured from electrical contact. Fortunately, electrical burns are rare in children. Electrical burns are categorized into high- and low-voltage injuries. High-voltage injuries are characterized by a varying degree of local burns with destruction of deep tissues.[80] The electrical current enters part of the body and travels through tissues with the lowest resistance (nerves, blood vessels, and muscles). Heat generated by the transfer of the current damages deep tissues. This damage may not be easily visualized. Skin is mostly spared due to the high resistance to electrical current. Primary and secondary surveys, including electrocardiography, should be completed. If the initial electrocardiogram is normal, no further monitoring is necessary. However, any abnormal findings require continued monitoring for 48 hours and appropriate treatment of dysrhythmias when detected.[81] The key to managing electrical burns lies in the early detection and proper treatment of injuries to deep organs and tissues. Edema formation and subsequent vascular compromise is common to extremities. Fasciotomies are frequently necessary to avoid potential limb loss. If myoglobinuria develops, vigorous hydration with sodium bicarbonate and mannitol is indicated. Low-voltage injury is similar to thermal injury without transmission of the electrical current to deep tissues and usually only requires local wound care.

OUTPATIENT BURN CARE

The majority of all pediatric burns are minor, often resulting from scald accidents and affecting less than 10% TBSA, or from thermal injuries isolated to the hands from touching hot curling irons. Such injuries are usually limited to partial thickness of the skin and can be treated as an outpatient. After an initial assessment, the burn wound is gently washed with water and a mild bland soap with appropriate measures taken for pain control. Blisters are left intact, especially on the palms of the hand, because they can provide a natural barrier against the environment and help to avoid the need for daily dressing changes. Spontaneous resorption of the fluid occurs in approximately 1 week with the re-epithelialization process. Larger areas of blisters should be debrided and topical antimicrobial dressings applied. Silvadene is most commonly used with the fewest side effects. However, because silver sulfadiazine can impede epithelialization, its use should be discontinued when healing partial-thickness wounds are devoid of necrotic tissue and evidence of re-epithelialization is noted. Alternatively, antimicrobial dressings with triple antibiotic ointment (neomycin, bacitracin, and polymyxin B sulfate) and Polysporin are commonly used. Neither has any negative effects on epithelialization. For small superficial partial-thickness burns, nonmedical white petrolatum–impregnated fine mesh or porous mesh gauze (Adaptic, Johnson & Johnson Gateway, LLC, Piscataway, NJ) or fine mesh absorbent gauze impregnated with 3% bismuth tribromophenate in a nonmedicinal petrolatum blend (Xeroform) is usually sufficient without the need for topical antimicrobial agents.

Superficial burns to the face can be treated by applying triple antibiotic ointment only without any dressings. The frequency of dressing change varies from twice daily to once a week, depending on the size, depth of burns, and drainage. Those who advocate twice-daily dressing changes base their care on the use of topical antimicrobial agents whose half-life is 8 to 12 hours. Others who use petrolatum-based or bismuth-impregnated gauze recommend less frequent dressing changes of once every 3 to 5 days. The use of synthetic wound dressings (e.g., Biobrane) is also ideal for the treatment of superficial partial-thickness burns on an outpatient basis (see Fig. 13-4).[82] Although daily dressing changes are eliminated, Biobrane-covered wounds should still be monitored closely for signs of infection.

REHABILITATION

Rehabilitation therapy is a vital part of burn care. During the acute phase of burn care, splints are used to prevent joint deformities and contractures. By using thermoplastic materials, which are amendable to heat manipulation, splints can be fitted individually to each patient. Application of splints at all times, except during the exercise period, can potentially prevent severe contractures that occur in large burns. Patients are mobilized out of bed immediately after graft take, and aggressive physical therapy is encouraged. After the acute phase, hypertrophic scar formation is a major concern. Burn depth, patient's age, and genetic factors all play an important role in hypertrophic scar formation. In general, deep second-degree burns, requiring 3 weeks or more to heal, will produce hypertrophic scarring. Children are more prone to hypertrophic scar formation than adults, probably because of the high rate of cell mitosis associated with growth. Constant pressure, 24 hours per day, is the most effective way to decrease the incidence of hypertrophic scar formation. Pressure garments should be worn until scars mature. Scar maturation usually occurs 6 to 18 months after injury. In younger patients, scars mature at a much slower rate. In addition to splints and pressure garments, exercise therapy is a crucial component of rehabilitation therapy. Families should be thoroughly instructed on a program of range of motion exercises and muscle strengthening.

chapter 14

EARLY ASSESSMENT AND MANAGEMENT OF TRAUMA

Arthur Cooper, MD, MS

Trauma is the leading cause of mortality and morbidity in children from ages 1 to 14 years. It results in more death and disability than all other childhood diseases combined.[1] It is defined as forceful disruption of bodily homeostasis. Moreover, this term encompasses those injuries whose severity poses a demonstrable threat to life, which corresponds to an Injury Severity Score (ISS) of 10 or higher in children or a Pediatric Trauma Score (PTS) of 8 or lower.[2]

The term *first trauma* refers to the anatomic and physiologic disruption that results from acute injury. The term *second trauma*, defined and described by the American Trauma Society, refers to the social and familial dislocation associated with first trauma, which is often considerable in pediatric patients. Pediatric trauma remains a major public health problem in the United States, killing more than 10,000 pediatric patients annually nationwide[1] and causing some 10% of all pediatric hospitalizations,[3] about 15% of all pediatric intensive care unit admissions,[4] approximately 25% of pediatric emergency department visits,[5] and 50% or more of all pediatric ambulance runs.[6] Moreover, it also represents nearly 20% of all hospitalizations for serious injury among all age groups.[7]

TRAUMA EPIDEMIOLOGY

The incidence of serious traumatic injury, with hospitalization as the indicator of injury severity, is approximately 420/100,000.[8] Although the hospital-based fatality rate is 2.4/100,000, the population-based mortality rate is 11.8/100,000, indicating that 78% of lethally injured children die before hospital admission and demonstrating the need for effective injury prevention and prehospital care. The population-based mortality rate for pediatric injuries serious enough to require hospitalization is 3.2%.[7] Intracranial injuries are the cause of most pediatric trauma deaths because of the untoward effects of traumatic coma on airway patency, breathing control, and cerebral perfusion. Conversely, intrathoracic and intra-abdominal injuries are the cause of few pediatric trauma deaths, because they are infrequently associated with hypotensive shock.[9]

Most blunt trauma in childhood is sustained unintentionally (during the course of family, play, or sports activities), but 7% of serious injuries are due to intentional physical assault (of which nearly half, or 3%, are due to physical abuse).[10] Blunt injuries outnumber penetrating injuries in children by a ratio of 12:1, a ratio that has decreased significantly in recent years. While blunt injuries are more common, penetrating injuries are more lethal. Still, the leading killer of children is the motor vehicle, responsible for approximately 75% of all childhood deaths, which are evenly split between those resulting from pedestrian trauma and those resulting from occupant injuries (Table 14-1).

INJURY RISKS

Lack of adequate or appropriate supervision of children during play involving possible injury hazards is recognized by all caretakers as a major risk factor for unintentional injury in pediatric patients, but drug and alcohol use, obesity, poverty, and race also influence injury rates. Toxicology screens are reportedly positive in 10% to 40% of injured adolescents, while obese children and adolescents, despite less severe head injuries, appear to have more complications and require longer stays in the intensive care unit.[11-14] For reasons poorly understood, race and ethnicity may also affect injury risk independent of socioeconomic status, particularly among African-American children, whose rate of death from preventable injuries, head injuries, and child abuse is three to six times higher than that of white children.[15-17] Improper use of motor vehicle restraints may contribute to the increased fatality rates of African-American children, who are only one half as likely to be restrained as white children involved in motor vehicle accidents and only one third as likely to be placed in car seats during such events.[18]

Table 14-1 Incidence and Mortality of Pediatric Trauma

By Injury Mechanism	Incidence (%)	Mortality (%)
Blunt	92.0	3
Fall	27.2	0.4
Motor vehicle injury: occupant	21.2	4.2
Motor vehicle injury: pedestrian	11.9	4.8
Bicycle	8.6	1.9
Sport	7.5	0.7
Struck	4.2	2.9*
Beating	3.2	9.0
Animal bite	2.8	2.9*
All terrain/ recreational vehicle	2.0	2.5†
Motorcycle	1.2	2.5†
Machine	1.0	2.9*
Caught	0.7	2.9*
Penetrating	7.7	5
Gunshot wound	2.3	10.2
Stabbing	2.8	2.9*
Crush	0.1	2.9*
Other	3.2	2.9*
By Body Region	**Incidence (%)**	**Mortality (%)**
Multiple	46.3	5
Extremities	21.9	0
Head and neck	14.5	5
External	10.2	0
Abdomen	3.6	1
Face	1.8	0
Thorax	0.7	3
By Anatomic Diagnosis	**Incidence (%)**	**Mortality (%)**
Head injury	25.8	10
Fracture	25.9	4
Abrasion/contusion	19.6	3
Open wound	14.2	3
Thoracic/abdominal injury	9.1	14
Spine injury	2.0	9
Other	3.6	9

*Collective mortality of these seven categories.
†Collective mortality of these two categories.
From Discala C: National Pediatric Trauma Registry Annual Report. Boston, Tufts University Rehabilitation and Childhood Trauma Research and Training Center, 2002, with permission.

Analysis of the Crash Injury Research Engineering Network (CIREN) database has recently yielded valuable information about the pattern of childhood injuries after motor vehicle accidents: (1) child victims of frontal crashes were more likely to suffer severe spine and musculoskeletal injuries; (2) those of lateral crashes were more likely to suffer head and chest injuries; (3) those in front seats sustained more injuries to the chest, abdomen, pelvis, and axial skeleton than those in the rear seats; (4) seat belts were especially protective against pelvic and musculoskeletal injuries; (5) children involved in high-severity, lateral-impact crashes typically sustained injuries characterized by higher Injury Severity Scores (ISSs) and lower Glasgow Coma Scale (GCS) scores.[19,20] Special attention has also been directed toward appreciation of injuries suffered by seat belt-restrained, rear-seat child passengers. A "concussion cluster" is sustained by about 10%, an "abdominal/spine cluster" by about 55%, and a "mixture cluster" by the remainder.[21] Restraint devices have also been subjected to careful analysis in recent years: (1) they do not appear to protect young victims of motor vehicle accidents as well as older victims; (2) car seats may not significantly affect injury outcome; (3) improper application may predispose to abdominal injuries, even in low-severity crashes; (4) the presence of abdominal wall bruising in restrained children, although rare, is strongly indicative of intra-abdominal injury.[22-25] Direct impact from a bicycle handlebar remains highly predictive of the need for operation.[26]

INJURY OUTCOMES

In recent years, much effort has been devoted to outcomes research in pediatric trauma with the hope that benchmarking of treatment results may lead to better care for injured children. Both historical studies and contemporary investigations indicate that children survive more frequently and recover more fully in hospitals that specialize in pediatric trauma than in other hospitals. The availability of pediatric subspecialty and nursing support, as well as pediatric equipment, resources, and facilities, appears to matter far more than whether care is (1) provided in a children's hospital or a general hospital committed to treatment of injured children or (2) directed by a pediatric surgeon or an adult surgeon with a special interest in pediatric trauma care.[27-44] No less important than survival outcome is functional outcome, for which several studies now indicate improved outcomes in hospitals that specialize in pediatric trauma care. However, they also suggest that whereas children may recover from injury more quickly than adults, physical function may not fully normalize.[33-45] Even so, self-perceived long-term quality of life among seriously injured children may not be adversely affected, justifying an aggressive approach to pediatric trauma resuscitation.[46]

Perhaps the most important recent development for outcomes research in pediatric trauma has been the expansion of the National Trauma Data Bank™ (NTDB™) of the American College of Surgeons to fully embrace children. The NTDB™ annual report is based on the most recent 5 years of case records submitted to the NTDB™, which approximates 250,000 total pediatric reports (http://www.ntdb.org).[47] Although currently designed as a simple case repository, efforts are underway to develop a representative national sample from the NTDB™ to provide population estimates of severe pediatric injury, as well as benchmarks for quality of pediatric trauma care. Preliminary data suggest that such benchmarks perform as well as existing measures.[48]

INJURY PREVENTION

Injuries are not accidents but rather are predictable events that respond to risk- and harm-reduction strategies similar to those applied to other diseases. The Haddon Factor Phase Matrix neatly depicts these in graphic form (Fig. 14-1).[49] It demonstrates how strategies to lessen the burden of injury can be applied to the host, agent, and environment before, during, and after the traumatic event using enforcement, engineering, education, and economics as techniques to minimize the adverse impact of each factor.

Effective injury-prevention programs are community based and require extensive collaboration with civic leaders, governmental agencies, and neighborhood coalitions. Programs such as the National Safe Kids Campaign (http://www.safekids.org) and the Injury Free Coalition for Kids (http://www.injuryfree.org) have proven highly successful in reducing the burden of childhood injury in many communities.[50,51] Such programs require ongoing collaboration between trauma programs and local public health entities so the incidence of injury can be tracked by locality and specific plans made to target high-frequency risks, which can be precisely quantified using tools such as the Injury Prevention Priority Score (IPPS).[52,53]

INJURY MECHANISMS

The effects of injury on the pediatric patient are related to the laws of physics and biomechanics. The kinetic energy transferred is equal to one half of the mass of the impacting object times its velocity squared. However, because the child's body is smaller, it is compacted into a smaller space. In blunt trauma, the forces of impact are dependent on factors such as the size and speed of the vehicle or the vertical displacement after a fall. These impact forces can be mitigated through use of design elements such as roll bars and crumple zones in automobiles; active and passive restraint devices such as lap belts, shoulder harnesses, air bags, and age-specific and properly fitted infant car seats or child booster seats for young passengers; helmets for bicycle riders; safety surfaces beneath playground equipment; and window guards in medium- and high-rise buildings. In penetrating trauma, the forces of violation are dependent on the weapon used (specifically, the size of the missile it discharges and the muzzle velocity with which it is delivered).

Injury mechanism is the main predictor of injury pattern. Motor vehicle pedestrain trauma results in the Waddell triad of injuries to the head, torso, and lower extremity: pelvis, femur, or tibia (Fig. 14-2). Motor vechile occupant injuries may cause head, face, and neck injuries in unrestrained passengers. Cervical spine injuries, bowel disruption or hematoma, and Chance fractures occur in restrained passengers (Fig. 14-3). Bicycle trauma results in head injury in unhelmeted riders as well as upper extremity and upper abdominal injuries, the latter the result of contact with the handlebar (Fig. 14-4). Low falls, the most common cause of childhood injury, rarely produce significant trauma, but high falls from the second story or higher are associated with serious head injuries, with the addition of fractures of long bones if falling from the third story. Intrathoracic and intra-abdominal injuries result from falls from the fifth story (the height from which 50% of children can be expected to die after a high fall) (Table 14-2).[54]

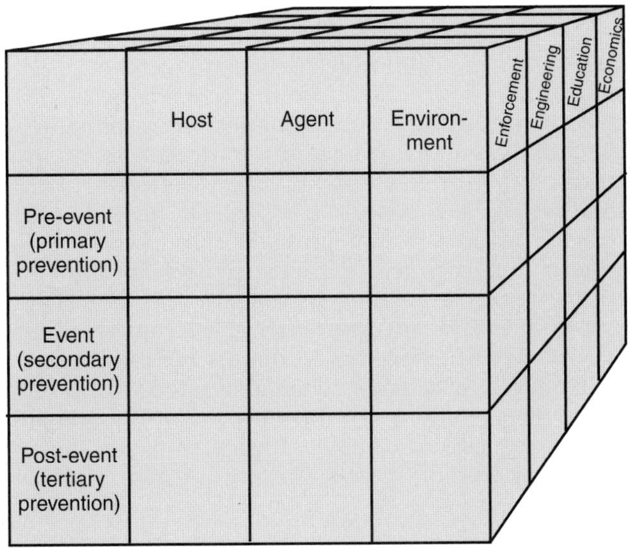

Figure 14-1. The Haddon Factor Phase Matrix, as modified and refined to include a third strategic dimension, integrates all phases of injury control into a single system. (Adapted from Haddon W: Advances in the epidemiology of injuries as a basis for public policy. Public Health Rep 95:411-421, 1980; and Runyan CW: Using the Haddon Matrix: Introducing the third dimension. Inj Prev 4:302-307, 1998).

INJURY PATTERNS

The injured child is subject to different mechanisms of injury than the adult. The body regions most frequently injured in major childhood trauma are the lower extremities, head and neck, and abdomen. In minor childhood injury, soft tissue and upper extremity injuries predominate. Because most pediatric trauma is blunt trauma involving the head, it is primarily a disease of airway and breathing rather than of circulation, bleeding, and shock. Even so, although neuroventilatory derangements (abnormalities in GCS score and respiratory rate) are five times more common than hemodynamic derangements, the latter are twice as lethal as the former.[9]

Injuries to specific body regions give rise to specific anatomic diagnoses (see Table 14-1). Because multiple injuries usually involve the head and neck, brain injury constitutes a major cause of injury mortality in childhood. Precise estimates of injury mortality by anatomic diagnosis cannot presently be calculated, owing to lack of population-based databases and the inability to determine with accuracy the relative contribution of individual diagnoses to injury mortality in multisystem trauma. Despite these constraints, brain injuries are directly (primary tissue injury) or indirectly (secondary

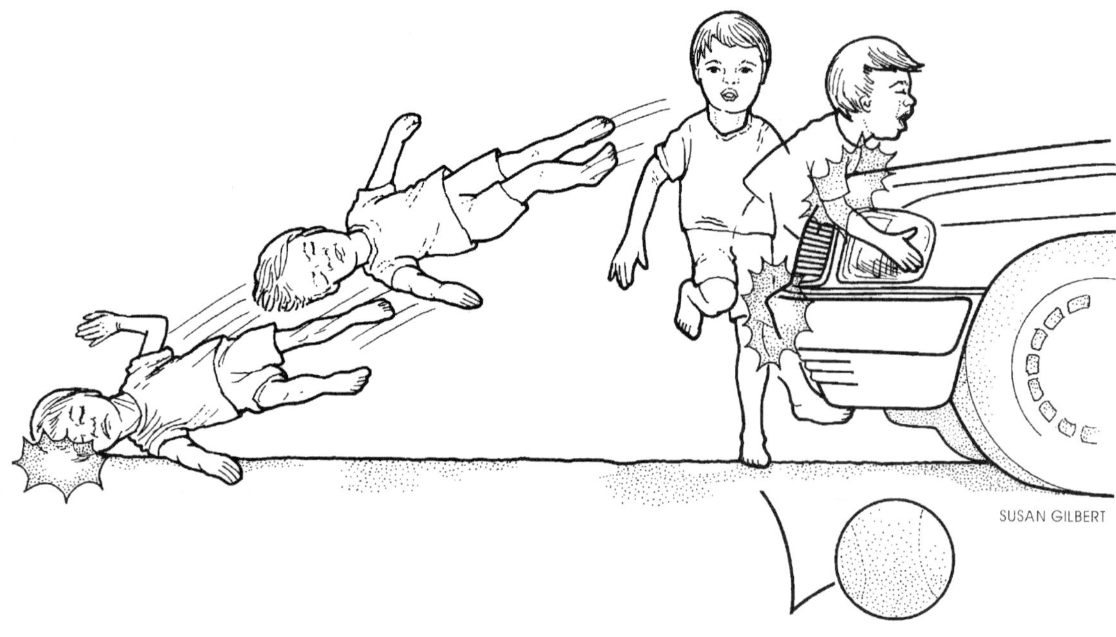

Figure 14-2. The Waddell triad of injuries to head, torso, and lower extremity is depicted. (From Foltin G, Tunik M, Cooper A, et al [eds]: Teaching Resource for Instructors of Prehospital Pediatrics. New York, Center for Pediatric Emergency Medicine, 1998. Accessed at http://www.cpem.org.)

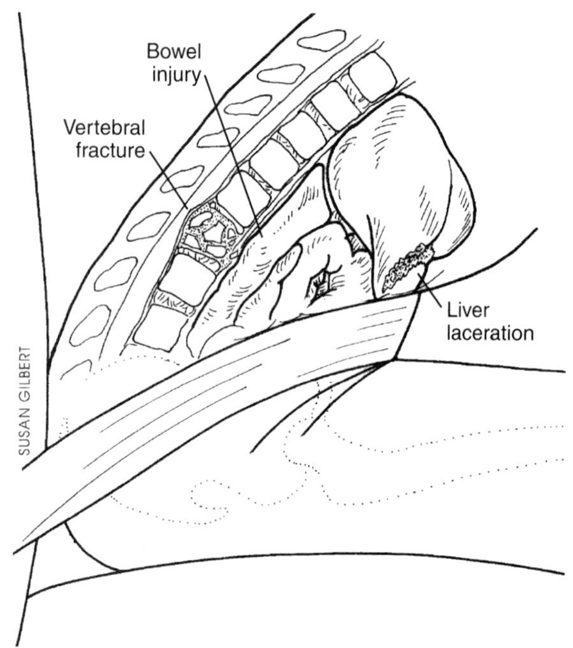

Figure 14-3. The mechanism for the development of intestinal and vertebral injuries from lap belts is shown. (From Foltin G, Tunik M, Cooper A, et al [eds]: Teaching Resource for Instructors of Prehospital Pediatrics. New York, Center for Pediatric Emergency Medicine, 1998. Accessed at http://www.cpem.org.)

hypoxic injury due to respiratory failure and shock) responsible for 75% of childhood trauma deaths.[55-57]

Head

Head injuries are potentially more dangerous in children than in adults for several reasons. First, developing neural tissue is delicate. The softer bones of the skull allow impacting forces to be transmitted directly to the underlying brain, especially at points of bony contact. Second, intracranial bleeding in infants in whom the fontanelles and sutures remain open may, on rare occasions, be severe enough to cause hypotensive shock. Third, the proportionately larger size of the head, when coupled with the injury mechanisms commonly observed in children, virtually guarantees that most serious blunt trauma in childhood will involve the brain and produce loss of consciousness. As a consequence, the voluntary muscles of the neck lose their tone, promoting development of soft tissue obstruction in the upper airway (which leads to hypoxia). It follows that diffuse brain injuries, particularly cerebral swelling (which results chiefly from cerebral hypoxia, loss of cerebral pressure autoregulation, and subsequent cerebral hyperemia, instead of vasogenic edema), are more common in childhood than in later years. Focal areas of cerebral contusion or laceration may occur adjacent to bony prominences in a coup-contrecoup pattern (typically in the frontal and temporal lobes), but major intracranial hemorrhage is uncommon and usually does not warrant surgical evacuation. Bilateral subdural hematomas in infants are indicative of child abuse (particularly when associated with retinal hemorrhages) and result from tearing of the bridging meningeal veins associated with the whiplash shaken impact syndrome.

Neck

Cervical spine injury is an uncommon event in pediatric trauma, occurring at a rate of 1.8/100,000 population, in contrast to closed-head injury, which occurs at a rate of 185/100,000 population.[58] When such injury does occur, it is more frequent at levels (C2, C1, and

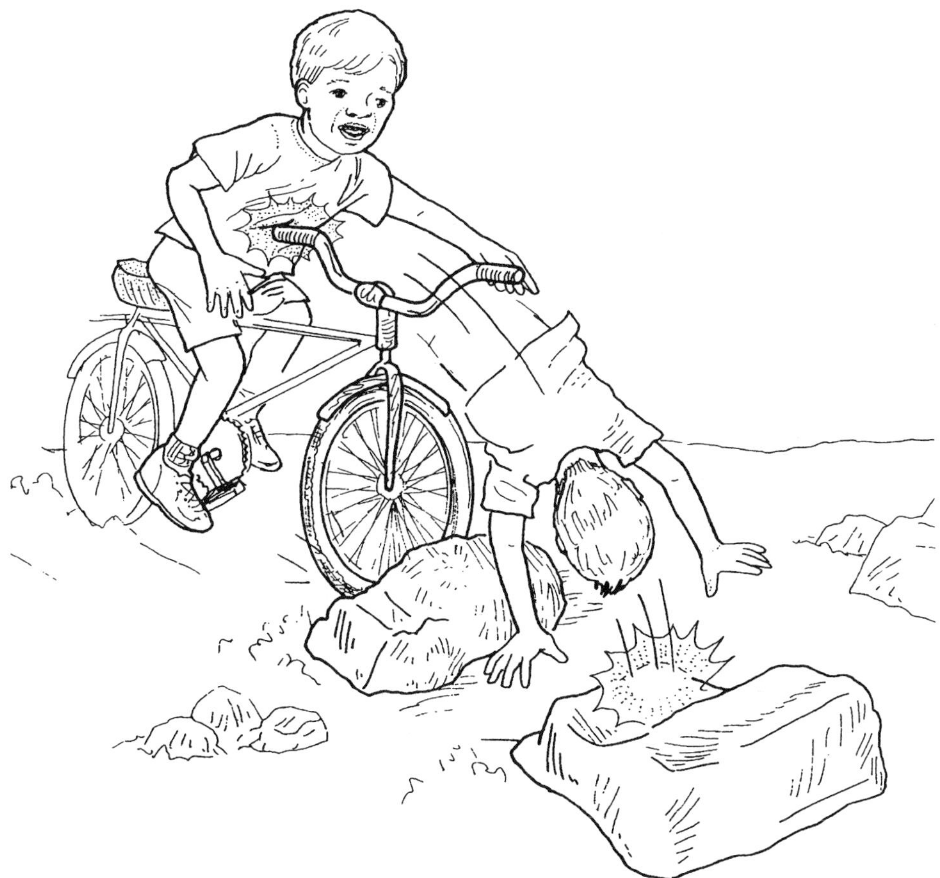

Figure 14-4. Children riding bicycles can sustain blunt abdominal trauma after contact with handlebars or head trauma from falling off the bicycle. (From Foltin G, Tunik M, Cooper A, et al [eds]: Teaching Resource for Instructors of Prehospital Pediatrics. New York, Center for Pediatric Emergency Medicine, 1998.)

the occipitoatlantal junction) above those whose nerve roots give rise to diaphragmatic innervation (C4), predisposing the child to respiratory arrest as well as muscular paralysis. The increased angular momentum produced by movement of the proportionately larger head, the greater elasticity of the interspinous ligaments, and the more horizontal apposition of the cervical vertebrae are responsible for this spectrum of injuries. Subluxation without dislocation causes spinal cord injury without radiographic abnormality (SCIWORA), from lateral shearing or axial stretching, despite the fact the stability of the cervical spine does not appear to be so affected as to warrant bracing. SCIWORA accounts for up to 20% of pediatric spinal cord injuries as well as a number of prehospital deaths previously attributed to head trauma.[59-61]

The greater elasticity of the interspinous ligaments also gives rise to a normal anatomic variant known as pseudosubluxation, which affects up to 40% of children younger than age 7 years. The most common finding is a short (2 to 3 mm) anterior displacement of C2 on C3, although anterior displacement of C3 on C4 also may be seen. The condition is accentuated when the pediatric patient is placed in a supine position, which forces the cervical spine of the young child into mild flexion because of the forward displacement of the head by the more prominent occiput. The greater elasticity of the interspinous ligaments also is responsible for the increased distance between the dens and the anterior arch of C1 that is found in up to 20% of children.

Chest

Serious intrathoracic injuries occur in 6% of pediatric blunt trauma victims[62] and require thoracostomy in about 50%. Thoracotomy is seldom needed. Lung injuries (52%), pneumothorax and hemothorax (42%), and rib and sternal fractures (32%) occur most frequently (Table 14-3). Injuries to the heart (6%), diaphragm (4%), great vessels (2%), bronchi (<1%), and esophagus (<1%) occur least frequently. Because blunt trauma is nearly 10 times more deadly when associated with major intrathoracic injury, this condition serves as a marker of injury severity, even though it is the proximate cause of death in less than 1% of all pediatric blunt trauma.[63]

The child compensates poorly for respiratory derangements associated with serious thoracic injury because of (1) a larger oxygen consumption but smaller functional reserve capacity (which makes the child more susceptible to hypoxia), (2) lesser pulmonary compliance yet greater chest wall compliance (which dictate chiefly a tachypneic response to hypoxia), and

Table 14-2 Common Injury Mechanisms and Corresponding Injury Patterns in Childhood Trauma

Injury Mechanism		Injury Pattern
Motor vehicle injury: occupant	Unrestrained	Head/neck injuries
		Scalp/facial lacerations
	Restrained	Internal abdomen injuries
		Lower spine fractures
Motor vehicle injury: pedestrian	Single	Lower extremity fractures
	Multiple	Head/neck injuries
		Internal chest/abdomen injuries
		Lower extremity fractures
Fall from height	Low	Upper extremity fractures
	Medium	Head/neck injuries
		Scalp/facial lacerations
		Upper extremity fractures
	High	Head/neck injuries
		Scalp/facial lacerations
		Internal chest/abdomen injuries
		Upper/lower extremity fractures
Fall from bicycle	Unhelmeted	Head/neck injuries
		Scalp/facial lacerations
		Upper extremity fractures
	Helmeted	Upper extremity fractures
	Handlebar	Internal abdomen injuries

From American College of Surgeons Committee on Trauma: Advanced Trauma Life Support for Doctors Student Manual, 8th ed. Chicago, American College of Surgeons, 2008.

Table 14-3 Incidence and Mortality of Injuries to Thoracic and Abdominal Organs

	Incidence (%)	Mortality (%)
Thoracic Organ		
Lung	52	18
Pneumothorax/hemothorax	42	17
Ribs/sternum	32	11
Heart	6	40
Diaphragm	4	16
Great vessels	2	51
Bronchi	<1	20
Esophagus	<1	43
Abdominal Organ		
Liver	27	13
Spleen	27	11
Kidneys	25	13
Gastrointestinal tract	21	11
Great vessels	5	47
Genitourinary tract	5	3
Pancreas	4	7
Pelvis	<1	7

From Cooper A, Barlow B, DiScala C, et al: Mortality and truncal injury: The pediatric perspective. J Pediatric Surg 29:33-38, 1994.

(3) horizontally aligned ribs and rudimentary intercostal musculature (which make the small child a diaphragmatic breather). The thorax of the child usually escapes major harm because the pliable nature of the cartilaginous ribs allows the kinetic energy associated with forceful impacts to be absorbed without significant injury, either to the chest wall itself or to underlying structures. Pulmonary contusions are the typical result but seldom are life threatening. Pneumothorax and hemothorax, due to lacerations of the lung parenchyma and intercostal vessels, occur less commonly but place the child in grave danger of sudden, marked ventilatory and circulatory compromise as the mediastinum shifts.

Abdomen

Serious intra-abdominal injuries occur in 8% of pediatric blunt trauma victims[62] and are caused by crushing the solid upper abdominal viscera against the vertebral column, sudden compression and bursting of hollow upper abdominal viscera against the vertebral column, or shearing of the posterior attachments or vascular supply of the upper abdominal viscera after rapid deceleration (see Table 14-3).[64] Injuries to the liver (27%), spleen (27%), kidneys (25%), and gastrointestinal tract (21%) occur most frequently and account for most of the deaths from intra-abdominal injury. Injuries to the great vessels (5%), genitourinary tract (5%), pancreas (4%), and pelvis (<1%) occur less frequently and account for few of the deaths that result from intra-abdominal injury. Most solid visceral injuries are successfully treated nonoperatively, especially those involving kidneys (98%), spleen (95%), and liver (90%).[65-67]

The abdomen of the child is vulnerable to injury for several reasons. Flexible ribs cover only the uppermost portion of the abdomen. Thin layers of muscle, fat, and fascia provide little protection to the large solid viscera. Also, the pelvis is shallow, lifting the bladder into the abdomen. Moreover, the overall small size of the abdomen predisposes the child to multiple rather than single injuries as energy is dissipated from the impacting force. Finally, gastric dilatation due to air swallowing (which often confounds abdominal examination by simulating peritonitis) leads to ventilatory and circulatory compromise by (1) limiting diaphragmatic motion, (2) increasing the risk of aspiration, and (3) causing vagally mediated dampening of the normal tachycardic response to hypovolemia.

Skeleton

Although they are the leading cause of disability, fractures are rarely an immediate cause of death in blunt trauma. They are reported to occur in 26% of serious blunt-injury cases and constitute the principal anatomic diagnosis in 22%.[10] Upper extremity fractures outnumber lower extremity fractures by 7:1, although, in serious blunt trauma, this ratio is 2:3. The most common long-bone fractures sustained during childhood pedestrian/motor vehicle accidents are fractures of the femur and tibia. Falls typically are associated with both upper and lower extremity fractures if the fall height is significant (from the window of a high-rise dwelling or the top of a bunk bed, but not from falls from standard beds or down stairs).[54,68-70] Because isolated long-bone and pelvic fractures are rarely associated with significant hemorrhage,[71] a diligent search must be made for another source of bleeding if signs of hypotensive shock are observed. This source is usually found in the abdomen.

The pediatric skeleton is susceptible to fractures because cortical bone in childhood is highly porous, whereas the periosteum is more resilient, elastic, and vascular. This results in higher percentages both of incomplete (torus and greenstick) fractures and complete but nondisplaced fractures. Long-term growth disturbances also may complicate childhood fractures. Diaphyseal fractures of the long bones cause significant overgrowth, whereas physeal (growth plate) fractures can cause significant undergrowth.

PREHOSPITAL CARE

Basic life support of the pediatric trauma patient consists of oxygen administration, airway adjuncts, bleeding control, and spine stabilization, providing assisted ventilation and fracture immobilization as needed. Spinal immobilization requires both neutral positioning (which cannot be achieved without placing a thin layer of padding beneath the torso from shoulders to hips)[72] and careful strapping (because forced vital capacity may be decreased by 4% to 59%).[73] One study suggested that cervical spine immobilization can be safely avoided in most pediatric trauma patients with minor injuries, but caution was urged in view of the known risks of SCIWORA and atlantoaxial instability.[74] Advanced life support of the pediatric trauma patient theoretically adds endotracheal intubation and volume resuscitation to this armamentarium, but neither intervention appears to improve outcome.[75-79]

Field triage of pediatric trauma patients to pediatric trauma centers is now well established. Regional protocols should direct ambulance transports to such centers where available. Although both the PTS[80] and the Revised Trauma Score (RTS)[81] reliably predict the need for pediatric trauma care, neither is optimally sensitive nor specific (Table 14-4). Good results also have been achieved by using checklists to identify anatomic, physiologic, and mechanistic criteria rather than calculated scores (Table 14-5).

Table 14-4 Trauma Scores Commonly Used in Children

	PEDIATRIC TRAUMA SCORE		
	+2	+1	-1
Size (kg)	>20	10-20	<10
Airway	Normal	Maintained	Unmaintained
Systolic blood pressure (mm Hg)	>90	50-90	<50
Central nervous system	Awake	Obtunded	Coma
Open wound	None	Minor	Major
Skeletal trauma	None	Closed	Open-multiple
	REVISED TRAUMA SCORE		
Glasgow Coma Scale	**Systolic Blood Pressure (mm Hg)**	**Respiratory Rate (breaths/min)**	**Code Value**
13-15	>89	10-29	4
9-12	76-89	>29	3
6-8	50-75	6-9	2
4-5	1-49	1-5	1
3	0	0	0

From Tepas JJ, Mollitt DL, Talbert JL, et al: The pediatric trauma score as a predictor of trauma severity in the injured child. J Pediatr Surg 22:14-18, 1987; and Champion HR, Sacco WJ, Copes WS, et al: A revison of the trauma score. J Trauma 29:623-629, 1989.

Table 14-5 Possible Indications for Transfer to a Pediatric Trauma Center

History of Injury
Patient thrown from a moving vehicle
Falls from >15 feet
Extrication time >20 min
Passenger cabin invaded >12 inches
Death of another passenger
Accident in a hostile environment (heat, cold water, etc.)
Anatomic Injuries
Combined system injury
Penetrating injury of the groin or neck
Three or more long-bone fractures
Fractures of the axial skeleton
Amputation (other than digits)
Persistent hypotension
Severe head trauma
Maxillofacial or upper airway injury
Central nervous system injury with prolonged loss of consciousness, posturing, or paralysis
Spinal cord injury with neurologic deficit
Unstable chest injury
Blunt or penetrating trauma to the chest or abdomen
Burns, flame, or inhalation
System Considerations
Necessary service or specialist not available
No beds available
Need for admission to pediatric intensive care unit
Multiple casualties
Family request
Paramedic judgment
Severity scores: Trauma Score ≤12; or
Revised Trauma Score ≤11; or
Pediatric Trauma Score ≤8

CNS, central nervous system; ICU, intensive care unit.
From Harris BH, Barlow BA, Ballantine TV, et al: American Pediatric Surgical Association: Principles of pediatric trauma care. J Pediatr Surg 27:423-426, 1992.

Table 14-6	Primary Survey, Resuscitation, and Secondary Survey
Primary Survey	
Airway: clear and maintain, protect cervical spine Breathing: ventilate and oxygenate, fix chest wall Circulation: control bleeding, restore volume Disability: GCS and pupils, call the neurosurgeon Exposure: disrobe, logroll, avoid hypothermia Foley catheter unless contraindicated* Gastric tube unless contraindicated†	
Secondary Survey	
History and physical: SAMPLE history, complete examination Imaging studies: plain radiographs,‡ special studies§	

*Meatal blood, scrotal hematoma, high-riding prostate.
†CSF oto-rhinorrhea, basilar skull fracture, midface instability.
‡Chest, pelvis, lateral cervical spine; others as indicated.
§FAST, CT as indicated.
GCS, Glasgow Coma Scale; CSF, cerebrospinal fluid; FAST, focused assessment by sonography in trauma; CT, computed tomography.
Adapted from American College of Surgeons Committee on Trauma: Advanced Trauma Life Support® for Doctors Student Manual, 8th ed. Chicago, American College of Surgeons, 2008.

EMERGENCY CARE

Primary Survey

Early management of childhood trauma begins in the field and continues in the emergency department.[82,83] Attention is first directed to the ABCDEs of trauma care: a "primary survey" of the Airway, Breathing, Circulation, and neurologic Disabilities, the purpose of which is to identify and correct deficits in ventilation, oxygenation, perfusion, and mentation, as well as conditions of the thorax and abdomen (e.g., tension pneumothorax and gastric dilatation) that pose an immediate threat to life (Table 14-6). The primary survey continues with complete Exposure of the patient to ensure that no injuries are missed, taking care to avoid hypothermia (through the use of blankets, over bed radiant warmers, and warmed intravenous fluids). It concludes with placement of adjuncts, such as a urinary and gastric catheter (unless contraindicated, respectively, by evidence of pelvic, or basilar skull or oromaxillofacial fractures). Together with other adjuncts (e.g., pulse oximetry and the trauma series of plain chest, pelvic, and lateral cervical spine radiographs that is obtained for all seriously injured patients), these steps facilitate the early recognition and treatment of immediate threats to vital functions.

Resuscitation

Resuscitation of the child trauma victim is conducted concurrent with the primary survey in a continuous cycle of assessment, intervention, and reassessment. An airway obstructed by soft tissues and secretions is opened while taking proper cervical spine precautions, then cleared (by using a large-bore Yankauer-type suction device) before its patency can be confirmed and assessment can proceed to the next step (Table 14-7).

Table 14-7	Airway/Cervical Spine
Open: jaw thrust/spinal stabilization Clear: suction/remove particulate matter Support: oropharyngeal/nasopharyngeal airway Establish: orotracheal/nasotracheal intubation* Maintain: primary/secondary confirmation† Bypass: needle/surgical cricothyroidotomy	

*Rapid sequential intubation technique: etomidate, then succinylcholine.
†1°, chest rise, air entry; 2°, exhaled CO2 detector, esophageal detector device, end tidal capnography; watch for DOPE: Dislodgement, Obstruction, Pneumothorax, Equipment failure.
Adapted from American College of Surgeons Committee on Trauma: Advanced Trauma Life Support® for Doctors Student Manual, 8th ed. Chicago, American College of Surgeons, 2008.

Abnormalities of breathing (ventilation and oxygenation) are next addressed with supplemental oxygen or assisted ventilation, if needed. Finally, the integrity of the circulation is assured through control of bleeding and administration of fluid.

Any child initially seen with major trauma should receive breathing support with high-concentration oxygen by the most appropriate means (Table 14-8). For the child with simple respiratory distress (increased work of breathing), a non-rebreather mask normally will suffice, provided the airway is open and breathing is spontaneous. For the child with frank respiratory failure (labored or inadequate work of breathing), assisted ventilation via face mask or an endotracheal tube attached to a bag-valve device should be initiated in preparation for endotracheal intubation. Orotracheal intubation with rapid-sequence induction techniques (etomidate and succinylcholine are now the preferred pharmacologic agents) and uncuffed endotracheal tubes (equivalent in diameter to the size of the naris or tip of the small finger, selected by using either a length-based resuscitation tape[84] or the formula 4 + age in years/4) is mandatory for all cases of respiratory failure.

The first step in management of the circulation is hemorrhage control. Direct pressure using sterile dressings is therefore applied to all actively bleeding external wounds. Blind clamping is avoided, owing to the potential risk of injury to neurovascular bundles.

Table 14-8	Breathing/Chest Wall
Ventilation: chest rise/air entry/effort/rate Oxygenation: central color/pulse oximetry Support: respiratory distress—NRB mask/respiratory failure—BVM ventilation Chest wall: ensure integrity/expand lungs Tension pneumothorax: needle decompression, chest tube* Open pneumothorax: occlusive dressing, chest tube Massive hemothorax: volume resuscitation, chest tube	

*Do not wait for confirmatory chest radiograph!
NRB, non-rebreather mask; BVM, bag valve mask.
Adapted from American College of Surgeons Committee on Trauma: Advanced Trauma Life Support® for Doctors Student Manual, 8th ed. Chicago, American College of Surgeons, 2008.

Table 14-9 Circulation/External Bleeding

Stop bleeding: direct pressure, avoid clamps; consider arterial tourniquets, topical hemostats
Shock evaluation: pulse, skin CRT, LOC
Blood pressure: avoid over/undercorrection
  Infant/child: low normal, 70 + (age x 2) mm Hg
  Adolescent: low normal, 90 mm Hg
Volume resuscitation: Ringer's lactate (RL), then packed cells
  Infant/child: 20 mL/kg RL, repeat x 1-2 with 10 mL/PRBCs
  Adolescent: 1-2 L, repeat x 1-2 with 1-2 units PRBCs

CRT, capillary refill time; LOC, level of consciousness; PRBCs, packed red blood cells. Consider obstructive and neurogenic as well as hypovolemic shock: exclude tension pneumothorax, cardiac tamponade, spinal shock.
Adapted from American College of Surgeons Committee on Trauma: Advanced Trauma Life Support® for Doctors Student Manual, 8th ed. Chicago, American College of Surgeons, 2008.

Military experience suggests that commercial arterial tourniquets, and topical hemostatic agents such as chitosan granules or powder, zeolite granules, and kaolin clay, are effective respectively, in stopping major arterial hemorrhage, and massive arteriolar, venular, and capillary oozing from large open wounds. However, because no results of their use in children have been reported to date, no recommendation can be made regarding their use in children.

The child with major trauma will require volume resuscitation if signs of hypovolemic shock are present (Table 14-9). This is best carried out by means of large-bore peripheral catheters placed percutaneously in the median cubital veins at the elbow or saphenous veins at the ankle or by cutdown in the saphenous veins at the ankle or groin. Intraosseous access may be necessary if intravenous access is not rapidly obtained. Simple hypovolemia usually responds to 20 to 40 mL/kg of warmed lactated Ringer's solution. However, frank hypotension (clinically defined by a systolic blood pressure less than 70 mm Hg plus twice the age in years) typically requires 40 to 60 mL/kg of warmed

Table 14-10 Disability/Mental Status

Pupils: symmetry, reaction
LOC: GCS
  Track and trend as a vital sign
  Significant change, 2 points
  Intubate for coma, GCS ≤8
Motor: strength, symmetry
Abnormality/deterioration: call neurosurgeon

Traumatic Brain Injury

Mild (GCS 13-15): observe, consider CT for history of LOC
Moderate (GCS 9-12): admit, obtain CT, repeat CT 12-24 hr
Severe (GCS 3-8): intubate, ventilate, obtain CT, repeat CT 12-24 hr

LOC, loss of consciousness; GCS, Glasgow Coma Scale; CT, computed tomography.
Adatped from American College of Surgeons Committee on Trauma: Advanced Trauma Life Support® for Doctors Student Manual, 8th ed. Chicago, American College of Surgeons, 2008.

Table 14-11 Exposure and Environment

Disrobe: Cut off clothes
Logroll: Requires four people
Screening examination: Front and back
Avoid hypothermia: Keep patient warm!

Adapted from American College of Surgeons Committee on Trauma: Advanced Trauma Life Support® for Doctors Student Manual, 8th ed. Chicago, American College of Surgeons, 2008.

lactated Ringer's solution followed by 10 to 20 mL/kg warmed packed red blood cells. Insertion of central venous catheters, except in rare cases in which venous access cannot otherwise be obtained, is not indicated. Urinary output should be measured in all seriously injured children as an indication of tissue perfusion.

Because of the ability of a child's blood vessels to compensate vigorously for hypovolemia by intense vasoconstriction, frank hypotension is a late sign of shock and may not develop until 30% to 35% of circulating blood volume is lost.[85] Thus, any child who cannot be stabilized after infusion of 40 to 60 mL/kg of lactated Ringer's solution and 10 to 20 mL/kg of packed red blood cells likely has internal bleeding and needs an emergency operation. If a child initially is in shock, has no signs of intrathoracic, intra-abdominal, or intrapelvic bleeding, but fails to improve despite seemingly adequate volume resuscitation, other forms of shock (obstructive, cardiogenic, neurogenic) should be considered: (1) tension pneumothorax or cardiac tamponade, (2) myocardial contusion, or (3) spinal cord injury. Yet, it must be emphasized that most children in hypotensive shock are victims of unrecognized hemorrhage that can be reversed only if promptly recognized and appropriately treated by means of rapid blood transfusion and immediate surgical intervention, particularly if major intrathoracic or intra-abdominal vessels are injured.[86-89]

Assessment of disability (neurologic status) relies on use of the GCS score (for level of consciousness) and evaluation of bilateral pupillary responses (to exclude mass lesions), and serves as a critical indicator of core organ function (Table 14-10). Traumatic coma (GCS score, 8) and pupillary asymmetry mandate immediate involvement of neurosurgical consultants. Further resuscitation is guided by findings on complete exposure of the patient (Table 14-11). The resuscitation phase concludes with use of adjuncts selected expressly to warn of conditions likely to affect the integrity of the airway, breathing, and circulation (Table 14-12).

Table 14-12 Primary Survey Adjuncts

Vital signs/pulse oximetry
Chest/pelvis/lateral cervical spine radiographs
Foley catheter/gastric tube
FAST/DPL

FAST, focused assessment by sonography in trauma; DPL, diagnostic peritoneal lavage.
Adapted from American College of Surgeons Committee on Trauma: Advanced Trauma Life Support® for Doctors Student Manual, 8th ed. Chicago, American College of Surgeons, 2008.

Secondary Survey

Once the primary survey has been performed, a secondary survey is undertaken for definitive evaluation of the injured child. This consists of a "SAMPLE" history (Symptoms, Allergies, Medications, Past illnesses, Last meal, Events, and Environment) and a complete head-to-toe examination, addressing all body regions and organ systems. The examination should be targeted particularly to the head and neck (for any history of blunt injury above the clavicles, alteration in level of consciousness, or neck pain or swelling) and to the chest (for any history of chest pain, noisy or rapid breathing, respiratory insufficiency, or hemoptysis, or if associated with severe deceleration injuries, such as high-speed motor vehicle accidents, which may suggest thoracic aortic injury). Finally, attention is turned to the abdomen (for any history of abdominal pain, tenderness, distention, or vomiting, especially if the emesis is stained with blood or bile, and, most important, abdominal bruising from seat belts, especially when associated with severe deceleration injuries, such as high-speed motor vehicle accidents, which may suggest abdominal aortic injury).[25,89] In examining the child, the physician's first responsibility is to identify life-threatening injuries that may have been overlooked during the primary survey, such as tension pneumothorax and gastric dilatation.

Drainage from the nose or ears, or any evidence of midface instability, suggests the presence of a basilar skull fracture (which precludes passage of a nasogastric tube) or an oromaxillofacial fracture (which may threaten the airway). Evidence of neck tenderness, swelling, torticollis, or spasm suggests the presence of a cervical spine fracture (which may not be detected on lateral cervical spine films in patients with SCIWORA). On chest examination, point tenderness, palpable bony deformity, crepitus or subcutaneous emphysema on inspection or palpation, or inadequate chest rise or air entry on auscultation or percussion suggests the presence of a rib fracture. Air or blood in the hemithorax indicates the need to search for an associated or subclinical pneumothorax or hemothorax. An abdomen that remains distended after gastric decompression suggests the presence of intra-abdominal bleeding (most often from the spleen or liver) or a disrupted hollow viscus (especially if fever, tenderness, or guarding are found together with abdominal distention or nasogastric aspirate stained with blood or bile).

All skeletal components should be palpated for evidence of instability or discontinuity, especially bony prominences such as the anterior superior iliac spines, which commonly are injured in major blunt trauma. In the absence of obvious deformities, fractures should be suspected if bony point tenderness, hematoma, spasm of overlying muscles, an unstable pelvic girdle, or perineal swelling or discoloration is found. The integrity of the pelvic ring may be tested in two ways: (1) by auscultating over one anterior superior iliac spine, while gently tapping over the other, to see if bone conduction is preserved, which will be the case only if the ring is intact; and (2) by compressing simultaneously, posteriorly, on the anterior superior iliac spines to see if the pelvic wings "spring" apart because of separation of the pubic symphysis, after first compressing simultaneously, medially, on the iliac crests to preclude further rift in a potential "open book" fracture. This is the compression-distraction test. Most long-bone fractures will be self-evident, but such injuries are occasionally missed during the secondary survey, which emphasizes the (1) assumption that a fracture is present on the basis of history alone (even if no obvious deformity is seen) until proven otherwise and (2) performance of ongoing evaluation of all injured extremities for evidence of pain, pallor, pulselessness, paresthesias, and paralysis (the classic signs of associated neurovascular trauma).

Laboratory evaluation is an integral part of the secondary survey. Arterial blood gases are of paramount importance in determining the adequacy of ventilation ($Paco_2$), oxygenation (Pao_2), and perfusion (base deficit).[90,91] However, the critically important determinant of blood oxygen content, hence tissue oxygen delivery (assuming the Pao_2 exceeds 60 mm Hg), is the blood hemoglobin concentration. Serial hemoglobin values better reflect the extent of blood loss than does the initial value. Elevations in serum levels of transaminases or amylase and lipase suggest injury to the liver or pancreas, but the infrequency of pancreatic injury makes the latter cost ineffective versus the former.[92,93] Urine that is grossly bloody or is positive for blood by dipstick or microscopy (> 50 red blood cells per high-power field) suggests kidney trauma. Damage to adjacent organs due to the high incidence of associated injuries should be suspected.[94]

Radiologic evaluation is another important part of the secondary survey. Arrangements should be made, before additional plain films are ordered beyond those already obtained during the primary survey, to obtain computed tomography (CT) of the head (without contrast) and abdomen (double contrast), as indicated. Other imaging studies may also be needed.

CT of the head should be performed whenever loss of consciousness has occurred, or in accordance with evidence-based decision rules that demonstrate abnormal mental status, clinical signs of skull fracture, history of vomiting, scalp hematoma, and headache to be associated with less-than-minimal risk of traumatic brain injury.[95] CT of the chest adds little to what is already known from the chest radiograph obtained during the primary survey, since the incidental pulmonary contusions identified by CT of the chest do not correlate with increased fatality. CT of the abdomen should be obtained (1) in intubated patients; (2) with signs of internal bleeding (abdominal tenderness, distention, bruising, or gross hematuria), a history of hypotensive shock (which has responded to volume resuscitation), or a hematocrit less than 30%; (3) if a femur fracture is evident; (4) if serum transaminase levels are elevated; (5) if significant microscopic hematuria is present, or (6) if the mechanism of injury is deemed significant.[96-99] Focused assessment with sonography for trauma (FAST) may be useful in detecting intra-abdominal blood. However, it is not sufficiently reliable to exclude blunt abdominal injury in hemodynamically stable children, although it does have the advantage that such injuries can be detected by repeated examination.[100-107] Therefore, like diagnostic peritoneal lavage, which it has largely supplanted, FAST adds comparatively little to the management of pediatric abdominal trauma. Unstable patients with suspected intra-abdominal injuries are candidates for immediate operation, whereas stable patients are managed nonoperatively without regard to the presence of intra-abdominal blood.[108-112] However, FAST has been successfully used in screening for intra-abdominal injuries.[113]

Critical Care

Definitive management of childhood trauma begins once the primary survey and resuscitation phases have concluded. This care is the responsibility not of a single individual or specialty but of a multidisciplinary team of professionals specializing in pediatric health care led by a surgeon with experience in the care of both trauma and children. It begins with the secondary survey and re-evaluation of vital functions and progresses through the tertiary survey (a scrupulous repetition of the primary and secondary surveys conducted by the admitting team once the patient is transferred to definitive care) to ensure no injuries were missed. It persists throughout the duration of hospitalization and concludes with rehabilitation, fully encompassing the operative, critical, acute, and convalescent phases of care. Avoidance of secondary injury (injury due to persistent or recurrent hypoxia or hypoperfusion) is a major goal of definitive management and mandates reliance on continuous monitoring of vital signs, GCS score, oxygen saturation, urinary output, and, when necessary, arterial and central venous pressure.

Definitive management of childhood trauma also depends on the type, extent, and severity of the injuries sustained. Any child requiring resuscitation should be admitted to the hospital under the care of a surgeon experienced in the management of childhood injuries. Such a child should initially not receive oral intake (because of the temporary paralytic ileus that often accompanies major blunt abdominal trauma and because general anesthesia may later be required) but intravenous fluid at a maintenance rate (assuming both normal hydration at the time of the injury and normalization of both vital signs and perfusion status after resuscitation). Soft tissue injuries also should receive proper attention, including wound closure and tetanus prophylaxis. Intravenous lines inserted under substerile circumstances should be replaced to prevent the development of thrombophlebitis.

Brain

The overall mortality and morbidity of major pediatric trauma are closely linked with the functional outcome of the brain injury that typically occurs after significant blunt impact. The results of treatment of severe closed-head trauma are somewhat better in children age 3 to 12 years than in adults, an advantage that is ablated in the presence of hypotension. Conversely, outcomes are worse in children younger than 3 years. Although the general principles of definitive management of traumatic brain injury are similar in children and adults, nonoperative management predominates because diffuse brain injuries are more common than focal injuries in pediatric patients. Surgically remediable causes of intracranial hypertension must be treated if found, but medically remediable causes are addressed aggressively. The goal of treatment is to optimize cerebral blood flow through the maintenance of cerebral perfusion pressure and avoidance of prolonged hyperventilation, which causes cerebral ischemia.

Current management of traumatic brain injury in children should adhere to evidence-based consensus guidelines (see Chapter 17).[114] Conservative treatment, including discharge to home care under the supervision of responsible adult caretakers who have been instructed to return if signs of increased intracranial pressure (nausea, vomiting, increasing lethargy) develop, suffices for management of mild head injury (GCS score, 13 to 15). At the same time, noncontrast CT is indicated for all patients who have a documented loss of consciousness or are amnestic, in accordance with evidence-based decision rules.[95] Expectant management, consisting of hospital admission, CT, and continuous neurologic observation, is used for all patients with moderate head injury (GCS score, 9 to 12).

Controlled ventilation is initiated after endotracheal intubation via rapid-sequence technique for all patients with severe head injury (GCS score, 3 to 8, or a rapid deterioration in GCS score of ≥ 2 points). Hyperventilation ($Paco_2$, 25 to 30 mm Hg) and mannitol (0.5 mg/kg) are reserved for patients with evidence of transtentorial (pupillary asymmetry, neurologic posturing) or cerebellar (ataxic breathing) herniation.

Immediate operation is necessary for all acute collections of intracranial (epidural, subdural, intracerebral) blood of sufficient size to cause a mass effect, for all open skull fractures, and for all depressed skull fractures that invade the intracranial vault by more than the thickness of the adjacent skull. Intravenous antibiotics are used only for patients with open skull fractures. Anticonvulsants (phenytoin preceded by diazepam, as needed) are indicated for all patients with active seizures, impact seizures, or moderate or severe brain injury but should be discontinued after 2 weeks of therapy because no benefit accrues after this treatment interval.[115] Therapy with corticosteroids is not advantageous in traumatic brain injury.[116] Moreover, nitrogen losses may be accelerated.[117]

Acute complications of severe traumatic brain injury include hyperglycemia, diabetes insipidus, the syndrome of inappropriate antidiuretic hormone secretion, and brain death. The first three are managed, respectively, through the use of insulin, desmopressin, and water restriction. Brain death results from uncontrolled intracranial hypertension and is manifested in a normothermic patient by the total absence of brain stem function on neurologic examination, a positive apnea test, isoelectric activity on the electroencephalogram on two successive occasions (preferably 24 hours apart), or complete absence of cerebral perfusion on nuclear scan or cerebral arteriography.

Due consideration should be given to organ preservation and donation under such circumstances.

Spine

The cervical region is often injured. High-dose methylprednisolone was previously thought efficacious in mitigating the effects of spinal cord injury. Currently, it is now believed to add little, if any, benefit to the management of patients with spinal cord injury.[118,119] Early care with volume resuscitation followed by vasopressor agents as needed should focus on management of neurogenic shock and immobilization of associated fractures (extrication collar and backboard followed by skeletal traction with Gardner-Wells tongs), realizing that SCIWORA is more common in children than in adults. Later care addresses repair of associated vertebral fractures through the use of halo traction with or without surgical fusion.

The critical care of patients with spinal cord injury is chiefly supportive. Alternating-pressure or air-fluidizing mattresses should be used whenever available to prevent the development of decubitus ulcers. Indwelling urinary catheterization, followed by intermittent clean catheterization, should be used to prevent the development of urinary stasis and subsequent infection. Aggressive pulmonary toilet, including bronchoscopy, should be used to prevent the development of pulmonary infections, especially in patients with intercostal or diaphragmatic muscle paralysis.

Chest

Most life-threatening chest injuries can be managed expectantly, or by tube thoracostomy inserted via the fifth intercostal space in the midaxillary line (Table 14-13). Indications for resuscitative thoracotomy are limited to patients with physical or electrocardiographic signs

Table 14-13 Early Assessment and Management of Chest Injuries in Childhood

	Clinical Signs	Emergency Treatment
Immediate Threats		
Upper airway obstruction	Incomplete: noisy breathing Snoring (soft tissue collapse) Gurgling (secretions, blood) Stridor (edema, foreign body) Hoarseness (larnygeal fracture)	Incomplete: clear obstruction Jaw thrust, oral airway Oropharyngeal suction Foreign body retrieval Tracheostomy and repair
	Complete: rocking chest-wall motions unrelieved by simple measures	Complete: needle or surgical cricothyroidotomy
Tension pneumothorax	Ipsilaterally decreased breath sounds, contralaterally shifted trachea, hyper-resonance to percussion	Needle decompression without waiting for chest radiograph followed by urgent tube thoracostomy
Open pneumothorax	Chest-wall defect, sucking chest wound	Occlusive dressing followed by urgent tube thoracostomy
Massive hemothorax	Ipsilaterally decreased breath sounds, midline trachea, dullness to percussion	Volume resuscitation together with urgent tube thoracostomy
Cardiac tamponade	Muffled heart tones, distended neck veins, narrowed pulse pressure, Focused Assessment by Sonography in Trauma (FAST)	Pericardiocentesis followed by urgent operative repair
Flail chest	Paradoxical chest-wall motions, bony crepitus	Endotracheal intubation for respiratory failure
Potential Threats		
Pulmonary contusion	Rales, rhonchi	Supplemental oxygen
Myocardial contusion	Cardiac arrhythmias	Monitoring, antiarrhythmics
Diaphragmatic rupture	Elevated hemidiaphragm, nasogastric tube in hemithorax	Urgent operative repair
Aortic rupture	Murmur radiating to back, widened mediastinum	Urgent operative repair
Bronchial disruption	Persistent large air leak, persistent pneumothorax despite thoracostomy	Urgent operative repair
Esophageal disruption	Food or saliva draining from thoracostomy, pneumomediastinum	Urgent operative repair
Possible Threats		
Simple pneumothorax	Ipsilaterally decreased breath sounds, midline trachea, hyper-resonance to percussion	Urgent tube thoracostomy
Simple hemothorax	Ipsilaterally decreased breath sounds, midline trachea, dullness to percussion	Urgent tube thoracostomy
Rib fractures	Bony crepitus	Analgesics
Traumatic asphyxia	Multiple petechiae of head and neck	Supportive and expectant

of life in the field or emergency department after penetrating chest trauma. The universally dismal results preclude its use in blunt chest or abdominal trauma,[120] even though cardiopulmonary resuscitation by itself is associated with a 23.5% survival rate.[121] Emergency thoracotomy is reserved for injured patients with massive hemothorax (20 mL/kg) and ongoing hemorrhage (2 to 4 mL/kg/hr), massive air leak, and food or salivary drainage from the chest tube. Severe pulmonary contusions, if complicated by aspiration, overhydration, or infection, can predispose the patient to development of acute respiratory distress syndrome (ARDS) or post-traumatic pulmonary insufficiency. These complications require aggressive ventilatory support and, occasionally, extracorporeal membrane oxygenation. Traumatic asphyxia, characterized by facial and conjunctival petechiae, requires no specific treatment but serves to indicate the considerable severity of the impacting force.

Critical care of the respiratory insufficiency that accompanies severe chest injury also is expectant. To avoid both oxygen toxicity and resorption atelectasis, it is best to use the least amount of artificial respiratory support necessary to maintain the PaO_2 at 70 to 80 mm Hg (hence the SpO_2 at 90% to 100%) and the $PaCO_2$ (or the $PETCO_2$) at 35 to 45 mm Hg. Continuous positive airway pressure (CPAP) or positive end-expiratory pressure (PEEP) should be used for maintenance of functional residual capacity whenever the FIO_2 exceeds 40%, but adverse effects on the circulation should be avoided. Peak inspiratory pressure should be kept below 20 to 25 cm H_2O whenever positive-pressure ventilation is required, especially if pneumothoraces, or fresh bronchial or pulmonary suture lines, are present. Pulmonary contusions uncomplicated by aspiration, overhydration, or infection can be expected to resolve in 7 to 10 days. Thus, the judicious use of pulmonary toilet, crystalloid fluid, loop diuretics, and therapeutic (not prophylactic) antibiotics to preclude the development of ARDS or post-traumatic pulmonary insufficiency is required.

Abdomen

Immediate management of intra-abdominal and genitourinary injuries in children is chiefly nonoperative, although not necessarily nonsurgical, as mature surgical judgment is needed to determine whether, or when, operation is needed. Bleeding from renal, splenic, and hepatic injuries is mostly self-limited and resolves spontaneously in most cases, unless the patient is in hypotensive shock or the transfusion requirement exceeds 40 mL/kg of body weight (half the circulating blood volume) within 24 hours of injury.[65-67] Laparotomy for management of renal, pancreatic, gastrointestinal, and genitourinary injuries is performed as indicated, including damage-control methods for patients in extremis and staged closure for patients with abdominal compartment syndrome (Table 14-14).[122] A pancreatic pseudocyst is heralded by the development of a tender epigastric mass 3 to 5 days after upper abdominal trauma and is likely to respond to nonoperative management composed of 4 to 6 weeks of bowel rest and total parenteral nutrition. However, the presence of a high-grade pancreatic injury on CT of the abdomen suggests that nonoperative management may fail and that either an internal drainage procedure or, in selected cases, endoscopic retrograde cholangiopancreatography with pancreatic ductal stenting, may ultimately be required.[123-125]

Table 14-14 Indications for Early Operation in Abdominal Trauma in Childhood

Blunt
Hemodynamic instability despite adequate volume resuscitation
Transfusion requirement >50% of estimated blood volume
Physical signs of peritonitis
Endoscopic evidence of rectal tear
Radiologic evidence of intraperitoneal or retroperitoneal gas
Radiologic evidence of gastrointestinal perforation
Radiologic evidence of renovascular pedicle injury
Radiologic evidence of pancreatic transection
Bile, bacteria, stool, or >500 WBC/mm³ on peritoneal lavage
Penetrating
All gunshot wounds
All stab wounds associated with evisceration; blood in stomach, urine, or rectum; physical signs of shock or peritonitis; radiologic evidence of intraperitoneal or retroperitoneal gas
All suspected thoracoabdominal injuries (unless excluded by thoracoscopy or laparoscopy)
Bile, bacteria, stool, or >500 WBC/mm³ on peritoneal lavage

WBCs, white blood cells.

Skeleton

Because fractures of the long bones are rarely life threatening unless associated with major bleeding (bilateral femur fractures, unstable pelvic fractures), the general care of the injured patient takes precedence over orthopedic care. At the same time, early stabilization will serve both to decrease patient discomfort and to limit the amount of hemorrhage. Closed treatment predominates for fractures of the clavicle, upper extremity, tibia, and femur (infants and preschoolers), although fractures of the femur increasingly involve the use of external fixation and intramedullary rods (school-age children and adolescents). Operative treatment is required for open fractures, displaced supracondylar fractures (because of their association with ischemic vascular injury), and major or displaced physeal fractures (which must be reduced anatomically). Owing to the ability of most long-bone fractures to remodel, reductions need not be perfectly anatomic. However, remodeling is limited in torus and greenstick fractures as the hyperemia typical of complete fractures is unlikely to occur.

Critical care of skeletal injuries consists of careful immobilization, with emphasis on the avoidance of immobilization-related complications (e.g., friction burns and bed sores) through the use of supportive and assistive devices (e.g., egg-crate or similar mattresses and a trapeze to permit limited freedom of movement). Fracture-associated arterial insufficiency is recognized by the presence of a pulse deficit on serial observation. Detection of compartment syndrome may require measurement of compartment pressure, which mandates fasciotomy when greater than 40 cm H_2O. Traumatic fat embolism, after long-bone fracture, and rhabdomyolysis, after severe crush injury, are rare but require aggressive respiratory support and crystalloid diuresis. Early rehabilitation is vital to optimal recovery and mandates routine physiatric consultation on admission.

Physical Support

The care of children with major traumatic injury also involves assessment and treatment of somatic pain, for quantification of which two scales have now been validated, although neither correlates with injury severity.[126] In patients who are not eating, nutritional support and anti-acid therapies with both topical and systemic agents to avoid gastric stress ulcer bleeding are recommended.[127] In children with hematomas of the liver, spleen, or pelvis, low-grade fever may develop as these are resorbed, but high spiking fevers should prompt investigation for a source such as infected hematomas, effusions, or pelvic osteomyelitis. In children with large retroperitoneal hematomas, hypertension may develop on rare occasions, presumably owing to pressure on the renal vessels. The temporary use of antihypertensive agents may be required, but the hematomas usually resolve without the need for surgical decompression. Children with chest tubes or long-term indwelling urinary catheters are at risk for systemic infection and should receive prophylactic or suppressive antibiotics as long as the tube is required.

Emotional Support

Efforts must be made to attend to the emotional needs of the child and family, especially for those families facing the death of a child or a sibling.[128] In addition to the loss of control over their child's destiny, parents of seriously injured children also may feel enormous guilt, whether or not these feelings are warranted. The responsible surgeon should attempt to create as normal an environment as possible for the child and allow the parents to participate meaningfully in postinjury care. In so doing, treatment interventions will be facilitated as the child perceives that parents and staff are working together to ensure an optimal recovery.

SPECIAL CONSIDERATIONS

Child Abuse

Child abuse is the underlying cause of 3% of major traumatic injuries in childhood.[10] A detailed review of the mechanisms, patterns, presentations, and findings of physical abuse is beyond the scope of this chapter, but child abuse may be suspected when (1) an unexplained delay occurs in obtaining treatment, although this occasionally occurs with unintentional injury as well, (2) the history is vague or otherwise incompatible with the observed physical findings, (3) the caretaker blames siblings or playmates or other third parties, or (4) the caretaker protects other adults rather than the child.[129,130] Although the recognition and sociomedicolegal management of suspected cases of child abuse require a special approach, assessment and medical treatment of physical injuries is no different from that for any other mechanism of injury. Most important, confrontation and accusation hinder treatment and rehabilitation and have no place in the surgical management of any pediatric patient, regardless of the nature of the injury (although reports of suspected child abuse must be filed with local child protective services in every state and territory).

Penetrating Injuries

Early involvement of social services, psychiatric support, pastoral care, and responsible law enforcement and child protective agencies is mandatory, especially in cases of nonaccidental injury for which the initial history is rarely accurate and the potential for recidivism is significant. All penetrating wounds are contaminated and must be treated as infected. Accessible missile fragments should be removed (once swelling has subsided) to prevent the development of lead poisoning (especially those in contact with bone or joint fluid).[131] Thoracotomy is usually not required except for massive hemothorax (20 mL/kg) or ongoing hemorrhage (2 to 4 mL/kg/hr) from the chest tube, persistent massive air leak, or food or salivary drainage from the chest tube. Laparotomy is always required for gunshot wounds as well as stab wounds associated with hemorrhagic shock, peritonitis, or evisceration. Thoracoabdominal injury should be suspected whenever the torso is penetrated between the nipple line and the costal margin, if peritoneal irritation develops after thoracic penetration, if food or chyle is recovered from the chest tube, or if injury-trajectory or imaging studies suggest the possibility of diaphragmatic penetration. Tube thoracostomy, followed by laparotomy or laparoscopy for repair of the diaphragm and/or damaged organs, is mandated with such signs.[132]

Systems Issues

Pediatric patients, at high risk of death from multiple and severe injuries, are best served by a fully inclusive trauma system (each component of which experienced in pediatric care) that incorporates all appropriate health care facilities and personnel to the level of their resources and capabilities.[133,134] Moreover, collaboration with local public health agencies (in programs for injury prevention and control), as well as local public health, public safety, and emergency-management agencies (in regional disaster-planning efforts) is necessary.[133,134] Although the regional trauma center is at the hub of the system (and ideally also is the regional pediatric trauma center), area trauma centers may be needed in localities distant from the regional trauma center. All trauma centers, whether adult or pediatric, must be capable of the initial surgical management of pediatric trauma. This requires the immediate availability of a resuscitation team trained and credentialed for the management of pediatric trauma. All other hospitals in the region should participate as they are able but must be fully capable of initial resuscitation, stabilization, and transfer of pediatric trauma patients. Finally, a regional trauma advisory committee should include pediatric representation that has the authority to develop and implement guidelines for triage of pediatric trauma within the system to verified pediatric-capable trauma centers, since participation in the trauma center verification process has been shown to result in better survival outcomes.[135,136] Mature systems should expect that seriously injured pediatric patients will be preferentially transported to pediatric trauma centers.[137]

Transport Issues

Pediatric victims of multisystem trauma should undergo direct primary transport from the injury scene to a pediatric-capable trauma center.[27-44] If this is not possible, additional secondary transport from the initial trauma receiving hospital to the pediatric trauma center is needed. Transport providers must be capable of critical pediatric assessment and monitoring and skilled in the techniques of endotracheal intubation and vascular access, as well as drug and fluid administration in children.[138,139] Specialized pediatric-transport teams, staffed by physicians and nurses with advanced training in pediatric trauma and critical care treatment and transport, should be used whenever possible because complications related to endotracheal intubation and vascular access are the leading causes of adverse events during transport. These adverse events occur at twice the rate of those in the pediatric intensive care unit and 10 times more frequently when specialized teams are not used.[140,141]

Hospital Preparedness

Regional pediatric trauma centers should be located in trauma hospitals with comprehensive pediatric services (e.g., a full-service general, university, or children's hospital) that demonstrates an institutional commitment to pediatric trauma care, including child abuse.[27-36,133] Adult trauma centers can achieve results comparable to those of pediatric trauma centers if pediatric subspecialty support (pediatric emergency and critical care medicine) is available.[37-44,133] Finally, an organized pediatric trauma service must be available within the regional pediatric trauma center that, in addition to exemplary patient care, supports education and research in pediatric trauma and provides leadership in pediatric trauma system coordination.

Emergency Preparedness

Recent literature describing pediatric disaster management has focused on multiple casualty incidents involving children that resulted from motorized transport crashes, natural disasters, and terrorist incidents, underscoring the need for meaningful involvement of pediatric trauma surgeons and pediatric trauma hospitals in regional disaster-planning efforts for pediatric patients. Airplane crashes predominantly cause severe traumatic brain injuries, severe intrathoracic hemorrhage, and femur fractures, whereas bus crashes predominantly cause closed-head injuries, soft tissue damage, and superficial lacerations.[142,143] Injuries sustained during major hurricanes appear to result chiefly in open wounds, gastroenteritis, skin infections, and, to a lesser extent, hydrocarbon and bleach ingestions, whereas those from earthquakes appear to result chiefly in orthopedic and soft tissue injuries as well as burns.[144-146] Building collapses after massive bomb explosions are associated with high fatality rates (due chiefly to lethal head and torso injuries, as well as traumatic amputations).[147] In the aftermath of the April 19, 1995, bombing of the Murrah Federal Building in Oklahoma City, Oklahoma, and the September 11, 2001, suicide airliner attacks on the World Trade Center in New York and the Pentagon near Washington, DC, thoughtful approaches to pediatric disaster planning as well as dissemination of policy guidelines from key professional organizations and experts in pediatric emergency and disaster medicine have evolved.[148-156]

chapter 15

THORACIC TRAUMA

Devin P. Puapong, MD • David W. Tuggle, MD

Thoracic trauma is an important cause of morbidity and mortality in children. Although it accounts for a small minority of pediatric trauma injuries (4%-25%), it is associated with a 20-fold increase in mortality when compared with pediatric trauma patients without thoracic trauma.[1-10] Moreover, the mortality rate of head and abdominal trauma in association with thoracic trauma in children increases to 25%. Children with neurosurgical trauma, thoracic trauma, and abdominal trauma may have a mortality rate that approaches 40%. Isolated thoracic trauma in a child is associated with a mortality rate of approximately 5%, which is largely due to penetrating trauma.[1]

Epidemiologic studies have reported a twofold to threefold higher incidence of thoracic trauma in boys as compared with girls.[9-15] Most injuries (80%-95%) are the result of blunt trauma, typically resulting from a traffic accident in which the child involved is a passenger or pedestrian.[2,10] Not surprisingly, many children will have involvement of other organ systems with a high Injury Severity Score (ISS). When penetrating trauma does occur, older children and adolescents are more likely to be the victims. This is associated with a higher mortality rate.[5]

Contusion or laceration of the pulmonary parenchyma is the most common injury and may be associated with rib fractures and pneumothorax or hemothorax. Injuries to other organs such as the tracheobronchial tree (<1%), esophagus (<1%), aorta (<1%), diaphragm (4%), and heart (6%) are uncommon but not insignificant.[12]

ANATOMY AND PHYSIOLOGY

Children have unique anatomic and physiologic properties that are salient to the diagnosis and management of thoracic trauma. As in any trauma patient, sequential management of the airway, breathing, and circulation is of primary importance. The pediatric airway may be complicated by numerous factors. The head of an infant is proportionally much larger than that of an adult, thus predisposing to neck flexion and occlusion of the airway in the supine position. The larger tongue and soft palate, as well as the more anterior glottis, can make the airway difficult to visualize. The child's trachea is shorter relative to body size, narrower, and more easily compressed compared with the adult. The subglottic region is the narrowest part of the airway in children. Because of its small cross-sectional diameter, the pediatric airway is more susceptible to plugging with mucus and to small amounts of airway edema.

With regard to breathing, the chest wall is more compliant in children, with less muscle mass for soft tissue protection. This allows a greater transmission of energy to underlying organs when injury occurs. The thinner chest wall also allows for easier transmission of breath sounds, which may obscure the diagnosis of a hemothorax or pneumothorax. Children are also at an increased risk for hypoxia owing to their higher oxygen consumption per unit body mass and their lower functional residual capacity to total lung volume ratio.

When assessing circulation, it is important to note that the mediastinum is more mobile than in older patients, and this is particularly true in young children. Unilateral changes in thoracic pressure, such as with a pneumothorax, can lead to a tension pneumothorax. This can shift the mediastinum to the extent that venous return is markedly reduced. The pathophysiologic effect is similar to hypovolemic shock. This response is more pronounced than is typically seen in an adult.

Children compensate for a decrease in cardiac output by increasing their heart rate. In the infant, improvement in stroke volume provides little in the way of compensation in the hypotensive child. Pediatric patients also have a higher body surface area to weight ratio than the adult, which predisposes them to hypothermia. This, in turn, may complicate the assessment of perfusion.

SPECIFIC INJURIES AND MANAGEMENT

Thoracic injuries in children can be categorized by location:

I. Chest Wall
   a. Flail chest
   b. Open pneumothorax

c. Rib fracture
d. Traumatic asphyxia

II. Pleural Cavity/Pulmonary Parenchyma
a. Tension pneumothorax
b. Hemothorax
c. Simple pneumothorax
d. Pulmonary contusion/laceration
e. Diaphragmatic injury

III. Mediastinum
a. Pericardial tamponade
b. Aortic/great vessel injury
c. Tracheobronchial injury
d. Cardiac contusion
e. Esophageal injury

Chest Wall

Rib Fractures

Young children have a compliant thorax and begin to resemble adults around 8 to 10 years of age. As a consequence, rib fractures are relatively uncommon in young children and occur more frequently in adolescents. Rib fractures are often suspected with physical examination and are identified on a chest radiograph (CXR) during the initial assessment. By themselves, rib fractures are infrequently a cause of major morbidity or mortality, but they are indicators of significant energy transfer.[16] If a rib fracture is found in a child younger than 3 years of age, child abuse should be considered.[17,18] Bone scans and bone surveys are useful in diagnosing remote fractures of the bony thorax in abused children, and follow-up studies improve identification of these injuries.[19] In older children, rib fractures should draw attention to the risk of an associated underlying injury. Fractures and dislocations of the bony thorax and joints may cause significant long-term pain. In addition to pneumothorax and hemothorax, children with first rib fractures may have fractures of the clavicle, central nervous system injury, facial fractures, pelvic fractures, extremity injuries, and major vascular trauma.[20,21] When children present with multiple rib fractures, mortality has been reported to be as high as 42%.[21] A careful survey of the child must be performed to look for significant injuries in other regions of the body.

The management of rib fractures is typically supportive. Good pain relief will prevent atelectasis and pneumonia. Because rib fractures can be associated with a hemothorax or pneumothorax, immediate drainage of fluid and blood collections or air with a tube thoracostomy is appropriate.

Flail Chest

Because of the increased pliability of the chest wall, multiple rib fractures in series (flail chest) are not commonly seen in younger children.[22] However, when flail chest does occur, respiratory effort can be depressed with a paradoxical motion of the flail segment. The large force required to produce this injury invariably results in injury to the underlying lung, which contributes to the respiratory compromise. Treatment of the pediatric flail chest includes good pain relief, adjusted to avoid respiratory depression. Nonsteroidal anti-inflammatory medications are useful to treat the pain from rib fractures after the acute phase. Occasionally, positive-pressure ventilation may be required in children with a flail chest and respiratory insufficiency. In the case of a severe flail chest there is some evidence to suggest that operative fracture stabilization of a flail chest will decrease morbidity and improve outcome in selected cases.[23]

Open Pneumothorax

Open pneumothorax (sucking chest wound) occurs when there is a gaping defect in the chest wall typically caused by blast injury, severe avulsion injuries, or impalement (Fig. 15-1). This is not commonly seen in children but may be acutely life threatening when present. The negative pressure in the pleural cavity sucks air into the thorax. Air trapping results in collapse of the ipsilateral lung and mediastinal shift as with a tension pneumothorax. Treatment requires placement of an occlusive dressing to prevent further air from entering the chest cavity as well as chest tube insertion to drain any hemo/pneumothorax that may have accumulated.

Traumatic Asphyxia

Traumatic asphyxia is typically caused by a large compressive force on the chest combined with deep inspiration against a closed glottis (Valsalva maneuver). The increased thoracic pressure compresses the right atrium, precluding blood return from the superior vena cava, and resulting in rupture of venules and capillaries of the face and head.[24] Patients will exhibit conjunctival hemorrhages, facial swelling, and petechial hemorrhages on the face and upper chest. Although severe cases may result in loss of vision or

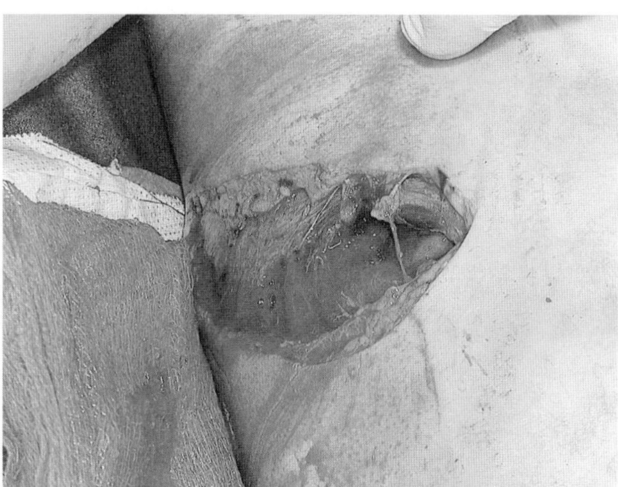

Figure 15-1. Open pneumothorax (sucking chest wound) in a child who was impaled by a door handle along his right lateral chest wall.

other permanent neurologic sequelae, the morbidity and mortality associated with traumatic asphyxia is generally related to associated injuries. The majority of children who survive exhibit good outcomes.[25,26]

Pleural Cavity and Pulmonary Parenchyma

Pneumothorax—Pulmonary Lacerations

Pneumothorax may occur with penetrating injury to the chest wall or air leak into the pleural space from a pulmonary laceration or disruption of the airway more proximally. It is a relatively common finding in children with blunt and penetrating thoracic trauma. An air leak from the injury may dissect under the pleura to cause pneumomediastinum and subcutaneous emphysema. A simple pneumothorax is often asymptomatic because the lack of increased intrathoracic pressure limits the recognition of symptoms. For this reason, a screening CXR is an important component of the evaluation of pediatric thoracic injury. Air within the pleural cavity can layer anteriorly, posteriorly, or in the subpulmonic space, and a simple pneumothorax can be easily missed on chest film but can be identified on a subsequent computed tomographic (CT) scan.[27] However, a recent study analyzing the utility of CT scan as a screening modality to replace initial CXR concluded that although a CT scan is highly sensitive, it should not be used as a primary imaging tool given its cost and the acceptable sensitivity of routine CXR.[28] Ultrasonography is another diagnostic modality that has been shown to be nearly as sensitive as CT in determining the presence of an occult pneumothorax and has gained wide acceptance as a screening tool for traumatic pneumothorax.[29,30]

The need for intervention in the presence of a simple pneumothorax will depend on the degree of pneumothorax and the patient's clinical condition (Fig. 15-2). Some authors have suggested that if the volume of the pneumothorax is greater than 20% of the pleural space, then drainage is indicated.[31] Although insertion of a chest tube can be considered appropriate in almost every circumstance of traumatic pneumothorax, there are alternatives to conventional chest tubes, such as pigtail catheters.[32] Additionally, there may be a benefit in treating with supplemental oxygen alone. The rationale for this therapy is that atmospheric gas (78% nitrogen) comprises the majority of the entrapped air collection. If the nitrogen level in the blood is "washed out" by increased inspired oxygen, a nitrogen gradient will be created that will cause accelerated absorption of the air collection. Oxygen can be delivered by way of nasal cannula, a hood, or a mask. Treatment with supplemental oxygen is usually only required for 24 to 48 hours.

In contrast, tension pneumothorax is a life-threatening condition that requires expeditious decompression of the involved hemithorax. A tension pneumothorax likely causes symptoms due initially to hypoxemia[33] and later to increased intrapleural pressure with subsequent decreased venous return and cardiovascular collapse. If the clinician suspects a tension pneumothorax in a patient with appropriate signs and symptoms, it is reasonable to proceed with needle decompression of the pneumothorax without waiting for a CXR to confirm the clinical suspicion. If rapid drainage of intrapleural air cannot be accomplished with a needle, insertion of a pigtail catheter or a chest tube should be performed. A tension pneumothorax treated initially with needle decompression will usually require placement of a chest tube due to the continuing collection of air under pressure in the involved hemithorax. If one or both lungs have been under compression due to a prolonged tension pneumothorax, re-expansion pulmonary edema can occur.[34]

Systemic air embolism can occur with any pulmonary parenchymal injury and increased intrabronchial pressure, creating a bronchopulmonary venous fistula.[35] This is most often seen when positive-pressure

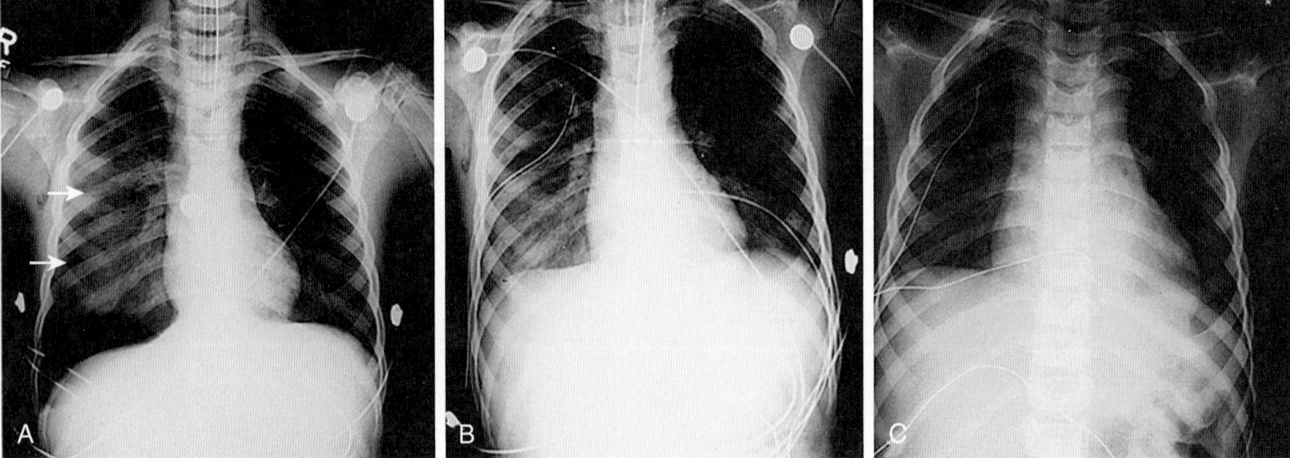

Figure 15-2. This 7-year-old was involved in a motor vehicle accident. The patient was not wearing restraints at the time of injury and had multiple other injuries. **A,** Multiple rib fractures and pneumothorax with collapsed right lung (*arrows*) are seen. **B,** A chest tube has been placed for initial management. **C,** Several days later there has been complete re-expansion of the lung and resolution of the right lower lobe pulmonary contusion.

ventilation is required to support the injured patient. Sudden neurologic findings or cardiovascular decompensation may be the initial sign that air has embolized to the coronary or cerebral vessels. If this complication is recognized, steps should be taken to prevent further air embolism. If possible, the removal of the intravascular air should be considered. Treatment options include tube thoracostomy, but more often an emergency thoracotomy will provide immediate reversal of the physiology promoting air embolism. The hilum of the lung should be occluded to prevent further escape of air into the venous system, and operative control of the bronchial-venous interface should be obtained. The mortality associated with this complication is high.

Hemothorax

Hemothorax can result from blunt or penetrating injury to any of the intrathoracic vessels, the chest wall vessels, the pleura, or the pulmonary parenchyma. Occasionally, a rib fracture may lacerate intercostal blood vessels or the lung. Rarely, the aorta or vena cava may be injured by pressure or shearing. Blood in the thorax may be asymptomatic unless the volume of blood is large. Smaller volumes may be more easily detected on CT scan, which also allows for measurement of Hounsfield density to aid in the diagnosis.[36] Each hemithorax can hold approximately 40% of a child's blood volume.[37] It is difficult to estimate the amount of blood loss on a CXR. Prompt chest tube placement allows for evacuation of blood from the pleural space and re-expansion of the lung. It also allows the surgeon to assess the volume of blood lost and whether the blood loss is ongoing.

There are instances in which an operation may be needed to stop ongoing intrathoracic blood loss. The immediate blood loss after tube thoracostomy of 15 mL/kg or ongoing losses of 2 to 3 mL/kg/hr for 3 or more hours are indicators for thoracic exploration in children to control bleeding.[38,39] If undrained, the hemothorax can become organized with the clot eventually replaced by a fibrothorax that can cause a restrictive lung defect. This predisposes to atelectasis, ventilation-perfusion mismatching, and pneumonia.

Residual blood is an excellent culture medium. Empyema and sepsis can result from infection of an undrained hemothorax. Tube thoracostomy may not adequately evacuate an organizing post-traumatic hemothorax in up to 12% of patients.[40] In this situation, thoracoscopy is indicated to evacuate the residual clot. Patients who undergo earlier thoracoscopy may experience less morbidity according to some authors.[41,42] However, there are also data to suggest that thrombolytic therapy with streptokinase or urokinase is equally effective at treating a retained hemothorax.[40]

Chylothorax

Chylothorax caused by injury to thoracic lymphatic channels is an uncommon complication of thoracic trauma. Chylothorax usually becomes evident 3 to 7 days after injury. The diagnosis is made by obtaining a sample of the pleural fluid and identifying the lymphatic and lipid content. Treatment includes tube thoracostomy and either enteral feedings with medium-chain triglycerides or parenteral nutrition.

Pulmonary Contusion

One of the most common thoracic injuries in children is a pulmonary contusion, which can occur with blunt or penetrating trauma.[1] The flexible chest wall of the child allows contusion of the lung without rib fracture, resulting in areas of lung consolidation and chest wall contusion. Microscopically, pulmonary contusions show alveolar hemorrhage, consolidation, and edema. The presence of a pulmonary contusion contributes to decreased pulmonary compliance, hypoxia, hypoventilation, and a ventilation-perfusion mismatch. A CXR taken during the initial assessment may demonstrate a pulmonary contusion. However, because this is invariably a supine film, it is sometimes difficult to differentiate fluid/blood in the pleural space from a lung contusion. To this end, a chest CT scan can show areas of pulmonary contusion not appreciated on the radiograph and can differentiate a parenchymal process (contusion) from free fluid.[43] When a contusion is seen on CXR, however, these children typically have a larger volume of lung that has been injured with a higher degree of impaired oxygenation.[44] Also, a significant percentage will require ventilatory support.[45] When a pulmonary contusion is seen only on CT, the morbidity of the injured child does not appear to be affected when compared with children with normal CT findings.[45] The overall injury severity, associated injuries, and outcomes in these patients are similar to those seen in adults.[43] Treatment includes appropriate fluid resuscitation, supplemental oxygen, pain management, and strategies to prevent atelectasis and pneumonia.

A significant percentage of patients may develop pneumonia or the acute respiratory distress syndrome (ARDS) after pulmonary contusion.[13] In an occasional patient, the pulmonary contusion may cause life-threatening hypoxia that cannot be supported with conventional ventilation, including high-frequency oscillation. Extracorporeal life support has been used in extreme circumstances to support patients with severe pulmonary contusions or ARDS.[46] Children with pulmonary contusions may have prolonged changes in respiratory function and radiographic abnormalities. These changes may persist for an extended period of time after resolution of the symptoms.[47] However, these children do not appear to suffer from any significant long-term sequelae.[15]

Diaphragmatic Injuries

Blunt diaphragmatic rupture is an uncommon occurrence. The left diaphragm is involved more often because of the protective effect of the right lobe of the liver. There have been occasional reports of bilateral injury (Fig. 15-3).[48,49] The frequency of associated

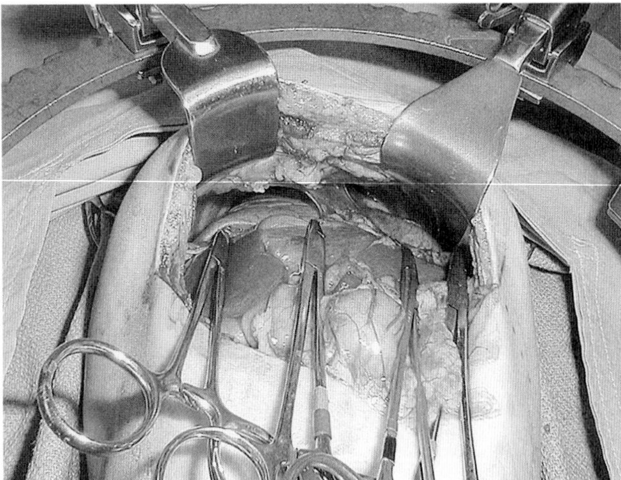

Figure 15-3. Bilateral diaphragmatic rupture after blunt abdominal trauma. The hemostats have been placed on the lower rim of the diaphragmatic rupture.

injuries, especially liver and spleen injuries, is very high.[49] Blunt injury to the diaphragm may have several manifestations. Children may have chest pain that radiates to the shoulder, shortness of breath, or abdominal pain. On physical examination, breath sounds may be diminished on the ipsilateral side and bowel sounds may be heard.[50]

On radiographic imaging, an abnormal diaphragm contour, a high-riding diaphragm, or a questionable overlap of abdominal visceral shadows may indicate injury. Visceral herniation or the abnormal placement of a nasogastric tube into the hemithorax should be considered diagnostic. Many diaphragmatic ruptures are not identified in the first few days after injury and may not be detected for a considerable period of time.[51] CXR findings may be obscured by associated contusion or atelectasis in the lung bases. In patients requiring intubation, herniation of abdominal viscera through the injury may not occur until after the patient is off positive-pressure ventilation.[52] CT has been used to establish this diagnosis, but the CT may appear normal in some patients. A heightened awareness of this injury should be present to avoid the late complications of visceral herniation or bowel complications. Repair of an acute diaphragmatic rupture is often best accomplished using an abdominal approach (see Fig. 15-3). If a late diagnosis of a diaphragmatic injury is made, a thoracic approach for repair is often considered to avoid the scarring and adhesions that might have formed.

When penetrating trauma is sustained below the nipple line, consideration should be given to the presence of a diaphragmatic injury. Imaging evaluation is unreliable in this setting. Therefore after determining whether other life-threatening injuries to the heart, lung, liver, spleen, or gastrointestinal tract exists, consideration should be given for operative exploration and repair.[50] If exploration is undertaken, laparoscopy, thoracoscopy, thoracotomy, or laparotomy have all been used with success.

Mediastinum

Airway Injury

Injuries to the tracheobronchial tree are infrequent in children. Airway disruption may occur with penetrating injury or with blunt injury such as high-energy acceleration or deceleration. Up to three fourths of these injuries are noted within 2 cm of the carina and almost half occur within the first 2 cm of the right main-stem bronchus.[53] Most patients with tracheal injuries have mediastinal air on CXR, although more distal injuries may rupture into the pleural space and present as a tension pneumothorax. Other findings associated with a major airway injury include a persistent large air leak from a chest tube, mediastinal air, cervical subcutaneous emphysema without pneumothorax, or florid respiratory compromise. Rarely, complete transection of a distal main-stem bronchus will appear on CXR with total lung collapse and mediastinal displacement.[54] Persistent pneumomediastinum and pneumothoraces on CXR after adequate tube thoracostomy should alert the clinician to consider an injury to the tracheobronchial tree (Fig. 15-4).

Once recognized, these injuries require prompt diagnosis and treatment. Pleural air or fluid collections should be drained until an accurate diagnosis of the airway injury is made. Mechanical ventilation may be necessary because of respiratory failure in this setting. Fiberoptic bronchoscopy allows for evaluation of the

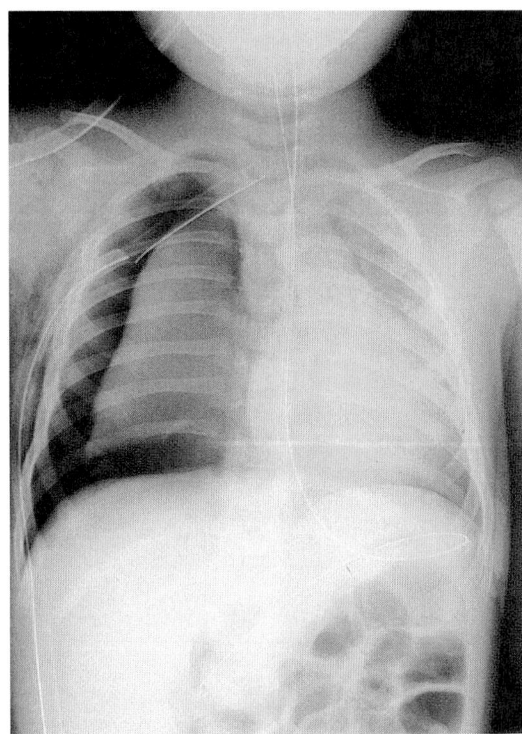

Figure 15-4. Chest radiograph of a 2-year-old patient who was run over by an automobile. Note the persistent large right pneumothorax despite the adequate placement of a chest tube. This patient was found to have a complete disruption of the right main-stem bronchus at the orifice of the right upper lobe bronchus

airway and may improve the probability of successful intubation. Many airway injuries are diagnosed by rigid or flexible bronchoscopy. Chest CT with a multiple-array scanner may have a role in visualizing tracheal or bronchial injuries especially if three-dimensional reconstructions of the airway are used (virtual bronchoscopy) (Fig. 15-5).[55,56]

A delay in diagnosis, however, is not uncommon in children. A retrospective review found that 75% of cases with a delayed diagnosis of tracheobronchial injury occurred in children younger than the age of 15.[57] This was thought to be related to the probability that incomplete tears in children cause minimal symptoms and the possibility that children involved in a severe accident with the loss of a family member may be reluctant to express physical complaints.

In general, when a tracheobronchial injury is identified, surgical repair is indicated. Repair may be delayed if the symptoms can be managed without morbidity. Repair of some bronchial injuries can be successful even a year after injury.[53] Occasionally, more distal bronchial injuries may heal with nonoperative management.[58] Distal bronchial injuries, both acute and chronic, are generally well managed by pulmonary resection, whereas more proximal airway trauma is best treated by surgical repair. Nonoperative management of a tracheobronchial injury may result in a high incidence of airway stenosis. When the diagnosis of a tracheobronchial injury is substantially delayed, scarring may obliterate the airway lumen and cause chronic collapse of the lung segment or lobe. The degree of injury may also play a role in determining whether a repair, as opposed to a resection, is needed. Complete transections are commonly associated with an obliterated distal bronchus, which may spare the pulmonary parenchyma from infection, thus making repair possible. Incomplete tears, on the other hand, form granulation tissue and scar that result in a patent, but narrowed lumen, predisposing the supplied lung to recurrent infection and retained secretions. This usually necessitates future resection. Three-dimensional reconstructions of the trachea and bronchi, taken from spiral CT images, have been found to be useful in planning surgical treatment. If the esophagus and the airway are injured near one another, a traumatic tracheoesophageal fistula can occur.[59]

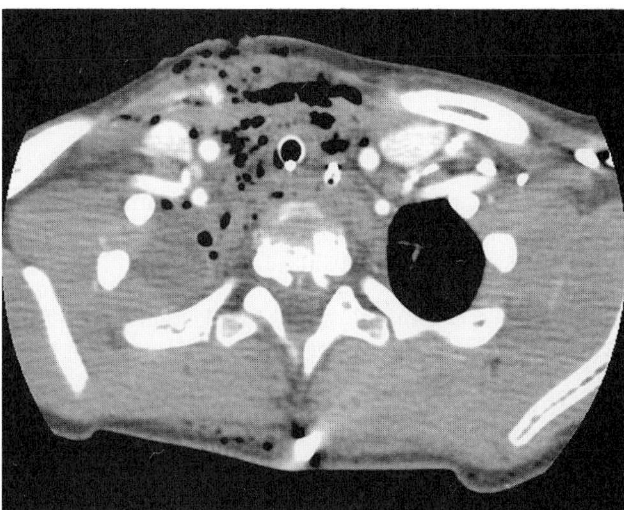

Figure 15-5. CT scan of the chest in a child who sustained penetrating trauma. This image was taken from the upper thoracic region. Note the air in the subcutaneous tissue and mediastinum. This child was found to have a tracheal and an esophageal injury.

Heart and Great Vessel Injuries

Injuries to the heart and great vessels of the thorax are rare in young children. The National Trauma Data Bank reports the incidence of blunt aortic injury to be 0.1% with a mortality rate of over 40%.[60] Traumatic thoracic aortic disruptions can occur in children as young as 4 years of age.[61,62] However, these injuries are more likely in the older child. Eighty percent of children who sustain a thoracic aortic tear will have significant associated injuries to the lung, heart, skeletal system, abdominal organs, or central nervous system.[63] Only one half of these patients will have external evidence of thoracic injury. Most aortic injuries in children are related to falls or motor vehicle collisions, especially when children are unrestrained.

The diagnosis of an aortic injury in a child can be difficult. Findings on a chest film may include a left apical cap, pulmonary contusion, mediastinal widening, a shift of the trachea to the right, downward depression of the left main-stem bronchus, and an indistinct aorta (Fig. 15-6A).[62] However, none of these findings is specific enough to make the diagnosis of aortic injury. A normal CXR, however, is highly predictive for the absence of an aortic injury.[64] A CT scan may reveal a mediastinal hematoma or an actual aortic injury. Transesophageal echocardiography has also been useful for diagnosing an aortic injury.[65] Whereas thoracic CT and transesophageal echocardiography can diagnose aortic injuries, aortic angiography gives excellent anatomic detail (see Fig. 15-6B). The most common finding with a traumatic aortic injury is a pseudoaneurysm located at the proximal descending aorta. This is thought to occur secondary to tethering of the aorta by the ligamentum arteriosum at the time of injury, resulting in a tear in the aortic intima and media.[66]

There is no large collective study of children with aortic injuries. However, of those who survive until diagnosis, more than 70% will live to discharge.[62,63] Spinal cord ischemia is a complication with thoracic aortic injury and may be associated with preoperative cardiovascular instability.[67] Although urgent operative repair is thought to be the best treatment in most patients, recent experience has demonstrated the ability to delay operative intervention by using β-adrenergic blockers while other injuries are managed.[61,67,68] Several pediatric patients have received aortic endostents to repair an aortic injury.[68-70] Although this experience is limited, in the future its risk-benefit ratio may be better than that of open operative intervention.[69]

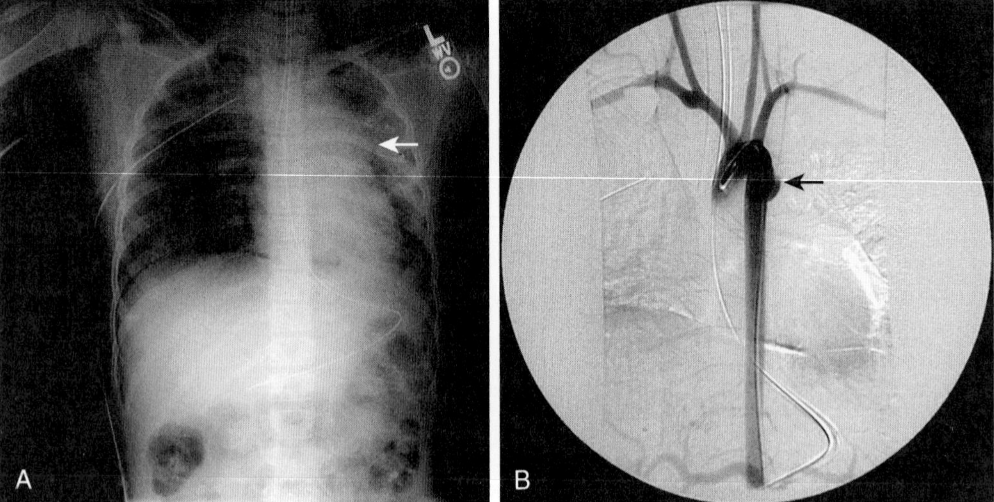

Figure 15-6. An 8-year-old patient presented with injuries from being an unrestrained passenger in a motor vehicle accident. **A,** On the chest radiograph, note the widened mediastinum and loss of definition of the aortic knob (*arrow*). There is also a right pneumothorax that was treated with tube thoracostomy. **B,** An aortogram shows a pseudoaneurysm (*arrow*) at the location of the ligamentum arteriosum just distal to the left subclavian artery, representing the partial transection of the descending aorta at this point.

Blunt cardiac injury such as myocardial contusion, cardiac laceration, or cardiac rupture is rare, occurring in less than 5% of children with blunt thoracic trauma.[71,72] Penetrating trauma is more often a cause of cardiac and aortic injury in this age group. Cardiac contusion accounts for 95% of blunt cardiac injuries in the child, followed by valvular dysfunction and ventricular septal defect.[72] Clinical manifestations of cardiac injury after blunt thoracic trauma include arrhythmia, new-onset murmur, and heart failure. These findings, however, may be absent in children, and CXR and electrocardiographic findings are generally nonspecific.[72]

The management of a cardiac contusion is supportive. Children with a cardiac contusion who are hemodynamically stable on presentation rarely have deterioration of their cardiac rhythm. Patients should be monitored with continuous electrocardiography and frequent blood pressure determinations. Echocardiography should be performed early in the evaluation of children with a significant cardiac contusion. In patients with a suspected cardiac contusion, serum cardiac troponin I levels may be useful to confirm the diagnosis.[73]

Inotropic agents are occasionally needed to provide cardiac support in the presence of a cardiac contusion. Whereas blunt cardiac injury with heart rupture and cardiac tamponade is very rare, only immediate diagnosis and treatment will be lifesaving, as is also true for penetrating cardiac trauma. A delayed diagnosis of cardiac rupture in children has been described.[74,75] Immediate ultrasonography in the emergency department may provide the clinical information necessary to identify this injury quickly.[76] Pericardiocentesis in this setting may provide a temporary solution while operative intervention is organized. If urgent pericardiocentesis is required in a child, it should be kept in mind that the distance from the skin to the pericardium is significantly reduced in younger patients relative to adults. Undercompensating or overcompensating for chest wall thickness may lead to inadequate decompression or iatrogenic cardiac injury. Once stabilized, children with a blunt cardiac injury should be followed closely and monitored for sequelae such as valvular insufficiency or ventricular septal defect.[72] Very rarely, extracorporeal life support may be needed to manage a child with a severe blunt cardiac injury.

Commotio cordis has become a widely recognized problem in pediatric thoracic trauma.[77] Typically, a young baseball player is struck in the chest with a hit or thrown ball and collapses suddenly. Commotio cordis is characterized by the absence of cardiac contusion, coronary artery abnormalities, structural abnormalities, or conduction system pathology. It is thought that a sudden blow to the chest will result in a disorganized cardiac rhythm followed by rapid cardiovascular collapse. Although chest protective devices seem useful, they do not provide total protection against asystole.[78] Automatic electrical defibrillators may have a place in treating this rare sports-related injury.

Esophagus

Pediatric esophageal injuries are uncommon, occurring in less than 1% of children sustaining either blunt or penetrating thoracic trauma.[79-81] The esophagus is a relatively elastic, mediastinal structure that is largely protected by the bony thorax. This elasticity allows the esophagus mobility so that when blunt force is applied it can move or decompress, which limits the likelihood of rupture. Penetrating injuries are more likely to cause esophageal trauma (see Fig. 15-5). Esophageal disruption may manifest as dyspnea, dysphagia, cyanosis, mediastinal air, subcutaneous emphysema, pleural effusion, chest or epigastric pain, fever, or sepsis.[82] Initial symptoms, however, may be vague and nonspecific. Esophagography with a water-soluble contrast agent and esophagoscopy are typically the studies that will identify an esophageal injury.

If the esophagus is ruptured or perforated, conventional treatment is operative repair. This is performed for the purpose of drainage and/or repair of the injured esophagus. Treatment is initiated with fluid resuscitation and parenteral antibiotics.[83] Operative repair consists of direct suture closure of the injury. If possible, pleural flap coverage and tube thoracostomy are performed. If an operation is undertaken early after the injury, this treatment, along with bowel rest and total parenteral nutrition has good success. If the perforation is not identified early, treatment becomes more difficult. If the perforation is more than 24 hours old, operative closure becomes technically much more difficult owing to the degree of inflammation and the amount of contamination. Techniques used in this circumstance include attempted repair, esophageal isolation, multiple drain placement, gastrostomy, and total parenteral nutrition.

In selected cases of esophageal perforation, nonoperative management may be successful.[82] This might be the case with certain types of blunt trauma and with iatrogenic injury such as a perforation at the time of endoscopy. Nonoperative management is based on the clinical status of the patient and the injury seen on imaging studies. For example, a patient might have a small leak identified, manifested by mediastinal air or pneumothorax. If there is no fever, no effusion, and the patient looks well, nonoperative treatment with total parenteral nutrition and intravenous antibiotics, along with serial examinations, may be reasonable.

chapter 16

ABDOMINAL AND RENAL TRAUMA

Steven Stylianos, MD • Barry A. Hicks, MD

The management of children with major abdominal injuries has changed significantly in the past 2 decades. An increased awareness of the anatomic patterns and physiologic responses characteristic of trauma in children has resulted in the successful nonoperative treatment of most abdominal solid organ injuries.[1] Our colleagues in adult trauma care have acknowledged this success and have applied many of the principles learned in pediatric trauma to their patients.[2,3] A recent review of the National Pediatric Trauma Registry (NPTR) indicates that 8% to 12% of children with blunt trauma have an abdominal injury.[4] Fortunately, more than 90% survive. Only 22% of the deaths in the NPTR were related to the abdominal injury. Although abdominal injuries are 30% more common than thoracic injuries, they are 40% less likely to be fatal.

Historically, adult trauma surgeons unfamiliar with the nonoperative management of solid organ injuries raised doubts about the wisdom of this approach. Their concerns included the potential for increased transfusion requirements, increased length of hospitalization, and missed associated injuries. Some even questioned the need for involvement of pediatric surgeons in pediatric trauma care. The clinical experience accumulated over the past 20 to 30 years, which has settled these concerns, is reviewed.

Few surgeons have extensive experience with massive abdominal solid organ injury requiring immediate surgery. It is imperative that surgeons familiarize themselves with current treatment algorithms for life-threatening abdominal trauma. Important contributions have been made in the diagnosis and treatment of children with abdominal injury by radiologists and endoscopists. The resolution and speed of computed tomography (CT), screening capabilities of focused assessment with sonography for trauma (FAST), and the percutaneous, angiographic, and endoscopic interventions of nonsurgeon members of the pediatric trauma team have all enhanced patient care and improved outcomes. Each section of this chapter focuses on the more common blunt injuries and unique aspects of their care in children.

DIAGNOSTIC MODALITIES

The initial evaluation of the acutely injured child is similar to that of the adult. Plain radiographs of the cervical spine, chest, and pelvis are obtained after the primary survey and evaluation of the airway, breathing, and circulation.[5] Plain abdominal radiographs offer little in the urgent evaluation of the pediatric trauma patient. The rapid availability and quality of imaging modalities has improved dramatically in recent years, both in the urban and in the rural settings. Prompt identification of potentially life-threatening intra-abdominal injuries with rapid resuscitation and therapeutic intervention is now possible in the overwhelming majority of children.

Computed Tomography

CT has become the standard of care in the evaluation of the pediatric trauma patient. Newer-generation CT scanners are now readily accessible in most health care facilities. CT is noninvasive, rapid, and highly accurate in identifying and qualifying the extent of abdominal injury. This has significantly reduced the incidence of nontherapeutic exploratory laparotomy.[6] A head CT, when indicated, should be performed without use of a contrast agent before abdominal CT to avoid having the contrast conceal a hemorrhagic brain injury. Intravenous contrast is then administered, and the vascular and parenchymal resolution is enhanced utilizing a "dynamic" scanning mode. The finding of a contrast "blush" on CT in children with blunt liver injury has been associated with larger transfusion requirements and a higher mortality rate.[7] A CT blush after significant hepatic or splenic injury should prompt the surgeon caring for the child to consider surgical or interventional radiologic control of the bleeding based on the hemodynamic status and stability of the child. Enteral contrast for enhancement of the gastrointestinal tract is generally not required in the acute trauma setting and can actually be detrimental secondary to aspiration of the contrast agent.[8]

Not all children with potential abdominal injuries are candidates for acute CT evaluation. Obvious

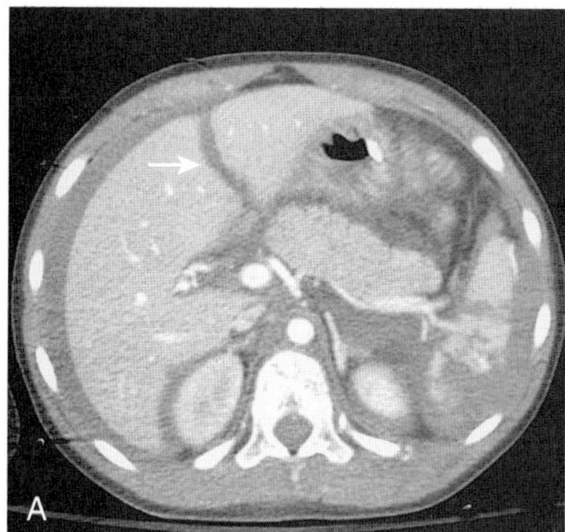
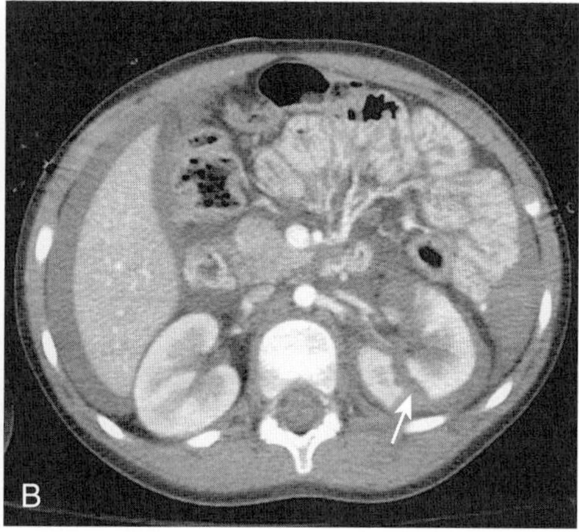

Figure 16-1. CT scans are highly accurate in demonstrating solid organ injuries. **A,** Hemoperitoneum with a liver laceration (*arrow*) and a shattered spleen is seen. **B,** Hemoperitoneum and a left renal laceration (*arrow*) is shown.

penetrating injury necessitates immediate operative intervention. Diagnostic laparoscopy may be very beneficial in determining if peritoneal penetration has occurred in the setting of an abdominal or flank stab wound.[9] The hemodynamically unstable child should never be taken from an appropriate resuscitation arena for a CT scan. These children may benefit from an alternative diagnostic study, such as diagnostic peritoneal lavage (DPL), FAST, or urgent operative intervention. Hemodynamically unstable patients with clinical evidence of abdominal trauma who are hypotensive and not responsive to resuscitative efforts should go immediately to the operating room without imaging.

Modern generation CT scanners are highly sensitive in the evaluation of possible solid organ (Fig. 16-1A) and retroperitoneal injuries (see Fig. 16-1B). The greatest limitation of abdominal CT in trauma is the lack of ability to reliably identify acute intestinal rupture.[10,11] Findings suggestive but not diagnostic of intestinal perforation are pneumoperitoneum, bowel wall thickening, free intraperitoneal fluid, bowel wall enhancement, and dilated bowel.[12] There must be a high index of suspicion for a hollow viscus injury in the child with free intraperitoneal fluid and no identifiable solid organ injury on CT (Fig. 16-2).[13]

Recent concerns about the risk of the radiation involved in CT have arisen, particularly in the pediatric population. Epidemiologic studies of populations exposed to radiation have shown that children are considerably more sensitive to radiation than adults. Because children have more rapidly dividing cells and have a longer life expectancy, the odds that children may develop cancers from x-ray radiation may be significantly higher than adults.[14] The actual lifetime risk from CT is not clearly known. Efforts to reduce the numbers of CT scans, unnecessary scans, and efforts to reduce the CT-related radiation dose in individual patients are important measures that should be kept in mind when caring for and evaluating the injured child.

Focused Abdominal Sonography for Trauma

Clinician-performed sonography for the early evaluation of the injured child has been shown to be useful in many situations but does have limitations. Examination of Morrison's pouch, the pouch of Douglas, the left flank to include the perisplenic region, and a subxiphoid view to visualize the pericardium is the standard four-view FAST examination. This bedside study may be useful as a rapid screening study, particularly in the patient too unstable to undergo an abdominal CT scan. Free intraperitoneal fluid seen on FAST examination in the unstable child not responding to resuscitative measures may support a decision to operate immediately. This modality is the study of choice for the evaluation of possible hemopericardium with tamponade.

A negative FAST exam (absence of hemoperitoneum) does not exclude a significant solid organ or hollow viscus injury.[15] There is at least a 15% false-negative rate for detecting hemoperitoneum with sonography. FAST may miss up to 25% of liver

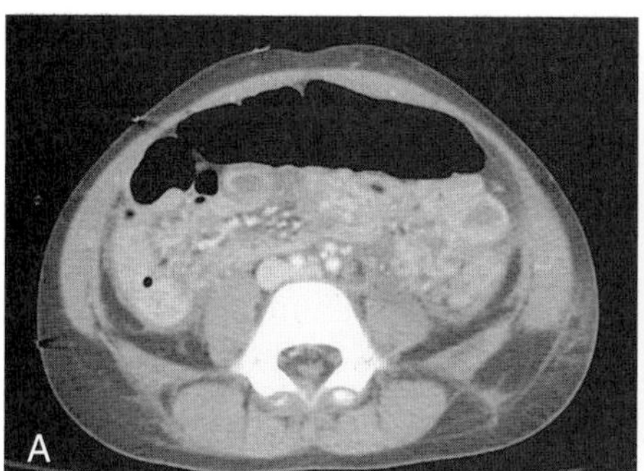
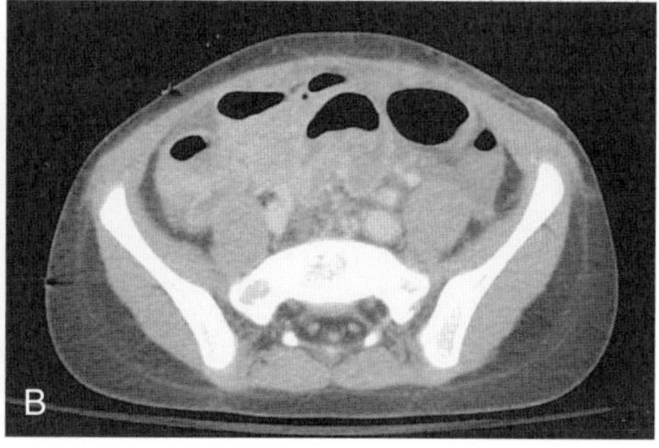

Figure 16-2. **A,** Bowel wall thickening and enhancement is seen on a CT scan of a patient with documented traumatic small bowel perforation. **B,** Free intra-loop fluid and bowel wall thickening are found on this CT scan in a patient with a small bowel perforation from a lap belt injury.

and spleen injuries, most acute renal injuries, retroperitoneal bleeding, and virtually all pancreatic, mesenteric, and bowel and bladder injuries.[16] Compared with CT, FAST is only about 63% sensitive for detecting moderate amounts of free intraperitoneal fluid in the trauma setting. Also, the documentation of free fluid in the abdomen does not necessarily indicate the need for surgical intervention. FAST may be very useful in decreasing the number of CT scans performed for "low-likelihood" injuries. The study may be repeated on a serial basis and results correlated with the clinical scenario.

Diagnostic Peritoneal Lavage

Since its description in 1965, the use of DPL has diminished significantly, especially in the pediatric population. The ready availability of high-resolution CT scanners and the nonoperative management of many pediatric injury patterns have increased, thus minimizing the utility of DPL. Although very accurate for identifying hemoperitoneum, retroperitoneal injuries may be missed with DPL. Incisional pain after a negative DPL may interfere with serial examinations in a child being managed nonoperatively. Also, a positive DPL may lead to a nontherapeutic laparotomy if based on hemoperitoneum alone. Because the majority of solid organ injuries do not require surgical intervention, intraperitoneal blood documented by DPL has little clinical significance. The need for operative management is determined by clinical instability, associated injuries, and the requirement for ongoing blood replacement.

There are clinical situations in which a DPL may prove to be very beneficial. The hemodynamically unstable child may have a rapid DPL to exclude the abdomen as a source of significant hemorrhage. Children with a lap belt injury pose a particular diagnostic challenge, particularly if concomitant neurologic injury is present. The initial abdominal CT is frequently normal in those with lap belt injuries, including acute hollow viscus perforations, but a DPL may document the presence of an occult visceral injury with the return of bile, bacteria, feculent matter, or an increased leukocyte count. Infusion of 10 mL/kg of normal saline into the peritoneal cavity is followed by allowing the infusate to drain. The criteria for a positive lavage are listed in Table 16-1.

Diagnostic and Therapeutic Laparoscopy

The use of laparoscopy for the injured child may have its place in the evaluation armamentarium of the hemodynamically stable patient. The sensitivity is comparable to that of DPL, but the specificity is higher, as would be expected by actually visualizing the injury.[17] A decrease in the number of nontherapeutic laparotomies has been demonstrated in adult series.[18] Studies also have shown that not only may the traumatic injury be identified with laparoscopy but the definitive repair also can be frequently performed (Fig. 16-3).[19,20]

Table 16-1	Positive Peritoneal Lavage Criteria
10 mL gross blood return with lavage catheter insertion	
>100,000 red blood cells/mm^3	
>500 white blood cells/mm^3	
Bile, bacteria, or vegetable matter on microscopic examination	
Amylase >175 IU/dL	

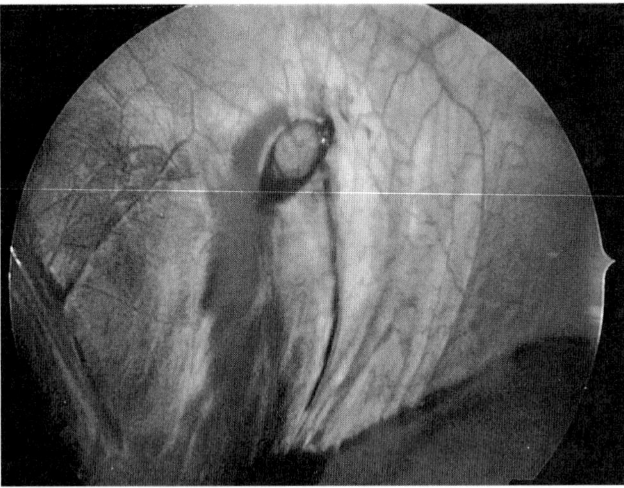

Figure 16-3. Diagnostic laparoscopy in a stable patient after a stab wound to the upper abdomen revealed this diaphragmatic injury. Repair was performed by using minimal access techniques.

Interventional Radiology in Pediatric Trauma

The role of the interventional radiologist in the evaluation and treatment of the injured child continues to expand as technology and indications prove to be safe and efficacious. Initially utilized solely for the assessment and identification of vascular injuries, the use of image-guided therapy is now an important part of the trauma team approach that leads to optimal care of the injured patient.[21] Endovascular transcatheter therapies, including placement of stents, embolotherapy, and thrombolysis, offer both primary and adjunctive modes of therapy for vascular injuries. Drainage of fluid collections, bile leaks, pancreatic pseudocysts, or loculated thoracic fluid or air collections can be very useful in the treatment of the injured child.

SOLID ORGAN INJURY

Spleen and Liver

The spleen and liver are the organs most commonly injured in blunt abdominal trauma, with each accounting for one third of the injuries. Nonoperative treatment of isolated splenic and hepatic injuries in stable children is now standard practice. Although nonoperative treatment of children with isolated, blunt spleen or liver injury has been universally successful,

Table 16-2 Resource Utilization and Activity Restriction in 832 Children with Isolated Spleen or Liver Injury

CT Grade	I	II	III	IV
Admitted to intensive care unit	55.0%	54.3%	72.3%	85.4%
No. hosp days (mean)	4.3 days	5.3 days	7.1 days	7.6 days
No. hosp days (range)	1-7 days	2-9 days	3-9 days	4-10 days
Transfused	1.8%	5.2%	10.1%*	26.6%*
Laparotomy	None	1.0%	2.7%†	12.6%†
Follow-up imaging	34.4%	46.3%	54.1%	51.8%
Activity restriction (mean)	5.1 wk	6.2 wk	7.5 wk	9.2 wk
Activity restriction (range)	2-6 wk	2-8 wk	4-12 wk	6-12 wk

*Grade III vs. grade IV, $P < .014$.
†Grade III vs. grade IV, $P < .0001$.
From Stylianos S and APSA Trauma Committee: Evidence-based guidelines for resource utilization in children with isolated spleen or liver injury. J Pediatr Surg 35:164-169, 2000.

great variation is seen in the management algorithms used by individual pediatric surgeons. Review of the NPTR and recent surveys of the American Pediatric Surgical Association (APSA) membership confirm the wide disparity in practice.[22,23] Controversy also exists regarding the utility of CT grading as a prediction of outcome in liver and spleen injury.[24-27] In 1999, the APSA Trauma Committee defined consensus guidelines for resource utilization in hemodynamically stable children with isolated liver or spleen injury. These guidelines are based on CT grading and were developed by analyzing a contemporary, multi-institution database of 832 children treated nonoperatively at 32 centers in North America from 1995 to 1997 (Table 16-2).[28] Consensus guidelines on the length of intensive care unit (ICU) stay, length of total hospitalization, use of follow-up imaging, and physical activity restriction for clinically stable children with isolated spleen or liver injuries (grades I to IV) were defined by analysis of this database (Table 16-3).

The guidelines were then applied prospectively to 312 children with liver or spleen injuries treated nonoperatively at 16 centers from 1998 to 2000.[29] (It is imperative to emphasize that these proposed guidelines assume hemodynamic stability.) Patients with other minor injuries such as nondisplaced, noncomminuted fractures or soft tissue injuries were included as long as the associated injuries did not influence the variables in this study. The patients were grouped by severity of injury and defined by CT grade. Compliance with the proposed guidelines was analyzed for age, organ injured, and injury grade. All patients were followed for 4 months after injury. The extremely low rates of transfusion and need for operation document the stability of the study patients.

Specific guideline compliance was 81% for criteria for ICU hospitalization, 82% for length of hospitalization, 87% for follow-up imaging, and 78% for activity restriction. A significant improvement in compliance was noted from year 1 to year 2 for ICU stay (77% vs. 88%; $P < .02$) and activity restriction (73% vs. 87%; $P < .01$). No differences in compliance were found by age, gender, or organ injured. Deviation from guidelines was the surgeon's choice in 90% and patient related in 10%. Six (1.9%) patients were readmitted, although none required operation. Compared with the previously studied 832 patients, the latter 312 patients managed prospectively under the proposed guidelines had a significant reduction in ICU stay ($P < .0001$), total hospitalization ($P < .0006$), follow-up imaging ($P < .0001$), and interval of physical activity restriction ($P < .04$) within each grade of injury.

From these data, it was concluded that prospective application of specific treatment guidelines based on injury severity resulted in conformity in patient management, improved utilization of resources, and validation of guideline safety. Significant reduction of ICU care, hospital stay, follow-up imaging, and

Table 16-3 Proposed Guidelines for Resource Utilization in Children with Isolated Spleen or Liver Injury

CT Grade	I	II	III	IV
Days in intensive care unit	None	None	None	1 day
Hospital stay	2 days	3 days	4 days	5 days
Predischarge imaging	None	None	None	None
Postdischarge imaging	None	None	None	None
Activity restriction*	3 wk	4 wk	5 wk	6 wk

*Return to full-contact, competitive sports (i.e., football, wrestling, hockey, lacrosse, mountain climbing) should be at the discretion of the individual pediatric trauma surgeon. The proposed guidelines for return to unrestricted activity include "normal" age-appropriate activities.
From Stylianos S, and APSA Trauma Committee: Evidence-based guidelines for resource utilization in children with isolated spleen or liver injury. J Pediatr Surg 35:164-169, 2000.

activity restriction was achieved without adverse sequelae when compared with the retrospective database. Recent single-institution studies have suggested that further reduction in resource utilization may be safe.[30,31] A large retrospective series showed that once hemodynamic stability was achieved and there was no evidence of ongoing bleeding, patients are unlikely to begin bleeding again.[30] This evidence challenges the assumption that bed rest is the key variable in treatment. In reality, bed rest is simply a period of observation, for which the current recommendations may be longer than necessary. Another institution has employed a management strategy based on the patient's hemodynamic status instead of injury grade and recorded a dramatic decrease in hospital stay compared with the current guidelines without an adverse event.[31] A prospective, multicenter trial is underway to delineate the safety of an abbreviated protocol.

The surgeon's decision to operate for spleen or liver injury is best based on evidence of continued blood loss such as hypotension, tachycardia, decreased urine output, and decreasing hematocrit unresponsive to crystalloid and blood transfusion. The rates of successful nonoperative treatment of isolated blunt splenic and hepatic injury now exceed 90% in most pediatric trauma centers or adult trauma centers with a strong pediatric commitment.[28-31] A recent study of more than 100 patients from the NPTR indicated that nonoperative treatment of spleen or liver injury is indicated even in the presence of associated head injury, if the patient is hemodynamically stable.[32] In this study, the rates of operative intervention for blunt spleen or liver injury were similar with or without an associated closed-head injury.

Surgeons unfamiliar with current treatment algorithms for blunt splenic injuries in children occasionally question the nonoperative approach. This is important because the majority of seriously injured children are treated outside dedicated pediatric trauma centers. Although several adult trauma services have reported excellent survival rates for pediatric trauma patients, analysis of treatment for spleen and liver injuries reveals an alarmingly high rate of operative treatment.[33-36] It is possible that adult trauma surgeons, influenced by their past experience with adult patients, are more likely to favor operative treatment than are their pediatric surgical colleagues. Adult trauma surgeons caring for injured children must consider the anatomic, immunologic, and physiologic differences between pediatric and adult trauma patients and incorporate these differences into their treatment protocols. The major concerns regarding nonoperative management are related to the potential risks of increased transfusion requirements, missed associated injuries, and increased length of hospital stay. Each of these concerns has been shown to be without merit.[23,37-42]

Outcomes in the Treatment of Blunt Spleen Injury

Many early attempts at comparing care in pediatric trauma focused on the treatment of blunt spleen injury. Hospital and physician expertise were used as the basis for comparison in the treatment of children with blunt splenic injury in seven studies between 1985 and 1998 (Table 16-4).[33,34,36,43-45]

In one study there was a marked difference in the incidence of operative treatment of a splenic injury within a single trauma center, depending on physician expertise (pediatric surgeon vs. nonpediatric surgeon).[36] The overall splenectomy rate was nearly twofold higher in children treated by adult surgeons (24% vs. 13%, $P < .05$). Transfusion requirements and hospital costs were lower for patients managed nonoperatively. A significant increase in the use of nonoperative treatment for pediatric spleen injury in Vermont between 1985 to 1995 was found after the institution of statewide educational programs.[34] The rate of nonoperative treatment of pediatric splenic injury at the state trauma center remained significantly higher (77% vs. 57%, $P < .001$) than at rural hospitals. In a report on the treatment of 126 children with splenic injury using the New Hampshire Uniform Hospital Discharge Data Sets, a large majority of patients (84%) were treated by adult surgeons at general hospitals.[33] Risk-adjusted operative rates were 10% at the children's hospital compared with 41% at general hospitals ($P < .005$). The authors concluded that the overwhelming majority of splenectomies and splenorrhaphies could have been avoided if general hospitals treated children with splenic injury in a manner similar to the treatment at the children's hospital. In a report from

Table 16-4 Studies (1985-1998) Comparing Operative Rates for Pediatric Blunt Spleen Injury

Authors	Study Period	No. Patients	Study Site	Rate of Operation	*P* Value
Keller et al.	1985-1991	41	Single center	17%-PS vs. 61%-NPS	<.01
Frumiento and Vane	1985-1990	127	State UHDDS	64.5%-TC vs. 92.3%-RH	< .001
Frumiento et al.	1990-1995	140	State UHDDS	23.1%-TC vs. 43.1%-RH	< .001
Mooney et al.	1991-1994	126	State UHDDS	10%-PTC vs. 41%-GH	< .005
Potoka et al.	1993-1997	772	State trauma outcome study	8.5%-PTC vs. 32%-ATC	< .001
Jacobs et al.	1992-1998	54	Single center	8%-PS vs. 23%-NPS	NS
Myers et al.	1993-1998	35	Single center	8%-NPTR vs. 11%-NPS	NS

PS, pediatric surgeon; NPS, nonpediatric surgeon; UHDDS, Uniform Hospital Discharge Data Set; TC, trauma center; PTC, pediatric trauma center; ATC, adult trauma center; GH, general hospital; RH, rural hospital; NPTR, National Pediatric Trauma Registry; NS, not significant.

the Pennsylvania Trauma Outcome Study, more than 13,000 injured children were treated from 1993 to 1997 at two regional pediatric trauma centers (PTCs) and 24 adult trauma centers (ATCs).[43] Significantly more children had successful nonoperative treatment for spleen (91.5% vs. 62.1%, $P < .001$) and liver injury (96.6% vs. 84.1%, $P < .05$) at a PTC compared with an ATC despite similar injury severity.

In contrast, two reports on children treated at single institutions during the mid to late 1990s found rates of nonoperative treatment for pediatric splenic injury by adult trauma surgeons similar to those of the just-referenced pediatric centers.[44,45] These two studies highlight the fact that dedicated trauma surgeons, familiar with contemporary processes of care advanced in pediatric centers, can achieve excellent results. They also implicate the potential importance of information dissemination and education efforts based on the benchmarks derived from examination of large public data sources. A statewide quality improvement initiative in Washington state was associated with a reduction in the rate of splenectomy in children in both pediatric and adult hospitals.[46]

Despite the two studies mentioned previously, several recent studies provide a basis for ongoing concern regarding the disparity of appropriate treatment in children with blunt spleen injury.[47-51] Using large nonselected databases and adjusting for risk, these studies indicate that the disparity in care between adult and children's hospitals is substantial and continuing on a regional and national basis (Table 16-5).

In an analysis from the Healthcare Cost and Utilization Project's National Inpatient Sample (HCUP-NIS), which contains a sample of discharges from 1300 hospitals in 28 states (representing 20% of all hospital discharges in the United States), children with splenic injury treated at rural hospitals had a risk-adjusted odds ratio for laparotomy of 1.64 (95% confidence interval [CI], 1.39-1.94) when compared with those treated at an urban teaching hospital.[47] The APSA Center on Outcomes compared the treatment of pediatric spleen injury using discharge datasets from four states.[48] The authors found a risk-adjusted odds ratio for laparotomy of 2.1 (95% CI, 1.4-3.1) when comparing treatment at nontrauma centers versus centers with trauma expertise. In a review of more than 2600 children with spleen injury from the New England Pediatric Trauma Database, the authors found that similarly injured patients treated by nonpediatric surgeons had a risk-adjusted odds ratio for laparotomy of 3.1 (95% CI, 2.3-4.4) when compared with those treated by pediatric surgeons.[49] The last two studies found even greater disparity when comparing the treatment of children with isolated spleen injury as contrasted to those with multiple injuries. Data from the Kids' Inpatient Database (KID2000) of the Healthcare Cost and Utilization Project, sponsored by the Agency for Healthcare Research and Quality, were recently reviewed.[50] This administrative database represents an 80% sample of non-newborn discharges from 2784 hospitals in 27 states (2.5 million pediatric discharges). The authors found a risk-adjusted odds ratio for laparotomy of 5.0 (95% CI, 2.2-11.4) when comparing treatment at general hospitals versus children's hospitals in pediatric patients with spleen injury. In a review of discharge data from 175 hospitals in Pennsylvania, the risk-adjusted odds ratio for laparotomy was 6.2 (95% CI, 4.4-8.6) when comparing treatment at adult trauma centers versus pediatric trauma centers.[51] Although all these studies suggest marked differences in the processes of care, administrative datasets do not readily allow risk adjustment for differences in physiologic status at presentation, a potential major limitation.

A recent report surveyed 281 surgeons (114 pediatric, 167 adult) regarding their treatment of children with solid organ injury.[52] For all clinical scenarios, adult surgeons were more likely to operate or pursue interventional radiologic procedures than their pediatric colleagues (relative risk [RR]: 8.6 with isolated solid organ injury, $P < .05$; 14.8 with multiple solid organ injuries, $P < .001$; 17.9 solid organ injury with intracranial hemorrhage, $P < .0001$). Adult surgeons were also more likely to consider any transfusion a failure (13.3% vs. 1.2%, $P < .01$) and had a much lower transfusion threshold.

The importance of these data is further amplified by the fact that the overwhelming majority

Table 16-5 Studies Comparing Operative Rates for Pediatric Blunt Spleen Injury: Adult vs. Children's Hospitals

Authors	Study Period	No. Patients	Database	Adjusted Odds Ratio (95% CI) for Operation	Ratio	*P* Value
Todd et al.	1998-2000	2569	HCUP-NIS	1.64 (1.39-1.94) RH vs. UTH	N/A	N/A
Stylianos et al.	2000-2002	3232	State UHDDS	2.1 (1.4-3.1) NTC vs. TC	34:66	< .0001
Mooney and Forbes	1990-1998	2631	NEPTD	3.1 (2.3-4.4) NPS vs. PS	68:32	< .0001
Bowman et al.	2000	2851	KID2000	5.0 (2.2-11.4) GH vs. CH	87:13	< .001
Davis et al.	1991-2000	3245	State UHDDS	6.2 (4.4-8.6) ATC vs. PTC	84:16	< .0001

HCUP-NIS, Healthcare Cost and Utilization Project's National Inpatient Sample (1300 hospitals in 28 states; 20% of all hospital discharges in United States); RH, rural hospital; UTH, urban teaching hospital; NEPTD, New England Pediatric Trauma Database; PS, pediatric surgeon; NPS, nonpediatric surgeon; UHDDS, Uniform Hospital Discharge Data Set; PTC, pediatric trauma center; ATC, adult trauma center; KID2000, Kids' Inpatient Database of the Healthcare Cost and Utilization Project, Agency for Healthcare Research and Quality (2784 hospitals in 27 states; 2.5 million pediatric discharges); CH, children's hospital; GH, general hospital; TC, trauma center; NTC, nontrauma center; CI, confidence interval.

Table 16-6 Operative Rate in Children with Spleen Injury

	Trauma Center	Nontrauma Center	*P* Value	APSA Benchmarks
Multiple injuries (n = 1299)	15.3%	19.3%	< .001	11%-17%
Isolated spleen injuries (n = 1933)	9.2%	18.5%	< .0001	0%-3%
Total (n = 3232)	12.1%	18.8%	< .0001	5%-11%

From Stylianos S, Egorova N, Guice KS, et al: Variation in treatment of pediatric spleen injury at trauma centers versus non-trauma centers: A call for dissemination of APSA benchmarks and guidelines. J Am Coll Surg 202:247-251, 2006.

(68%-87%) of pediatric patients are treated at hospitals or by physicians with the higher likelihood of operation.[49-51] However, in contrast, hospitals with trauma expertise had a significantly lower rate of operation for both multiply injured patients (15.3% vs. 19.3%, $P < .001$) and those with isolated injury (9.2% vs. 18.5%, $P < .0001$) when compared with nontrauma centers (Table 16-6).[48]

The operative rates at both trauma centers and nontrauma centers exceeded published APSA benchmarks (Table 16-7) for all children with spleen injury (3%-11%) and those with isolated spleen injury (0%-3%).[28,29,33,50,51,53] Thus, trauma centers and their corresponding state or regional trauma systems may represent rational targets for dissemination of current pediatric trauma guidelines and benchmarks. Broad application of existing APSA guidelines for spleen injury should encourage conformity of care and result in reduced rates of operative intervention and diminished resource utilization.[29]

Failure of nonoperative management can have serious consequences. Therefore, patient selection is important. Two recent multi-institutional reviews sought to evaluate the timeline and the characteristics of patients who fail nonoperative management.[54,55] One hundred twenty of 1813 (6.6%) children with solid organ injury underwent laparotomy in a median time of 2.4 hours, with 90% of the patients having surgery within 24 hours. Pediatric patients who sustained pancreatic injuries were more likely to fail nonoperative management (odds ratio [OR] 7.49; 95% CI, 3.74-15.01) compared with those who suffered other injuries. The patients who failed nonoperative management had a higher Injury Severity Score (28 ± 17) than those who were managed successfully nonoperatively (14 ± 10, $P < .001$). Severely head-injured patients (Glasgow Coma Scale score [GCS] = 8) had a higher failure rate for nonoperative management (OR 5.09; 95% CI, 3.04-8.52). Factors associated with an increased failure rate include a bicycle-related injury mechanism, isolated pancreatic injury, more than one solid organ injury, and an isolated grade 5 solid organ injury. The time to failure of nonoperative management peaked at 4 hours and then declined over 36 hours from admission. Thus, continued surgical evaluation and assessment during the entire hospitalization is required to limit morbidity and mortality.

Missed Associated Abdominal Injuries

Advocates of surgical intervention for splenic trauma cite their concern about missing associated abdominal injuries if an operation is not performed. One study reported successful nonoperative treatment in 110 (91%) of 120 children with blunt splenic trauma. In that report, 22 (18%) had associated abdominal injuries.[39] Only 3 (2.5%) of these 120 patients had gastrointestinal injuries, and each was found at early celiotomy performed for a specific indication. No morbidity occurred from missed injuries or delayed surgical intervention. Similarly, a review of the NPTR from 1988 through 1998 revealed 2977 patients with solid abdominal visceral injury. Only 96 (3.2%) had an associated hollow viscus injury.[40] Higher rates of hollow viscus injury were observed in assaulted patients and those with multiple solid visceral injury or pancreatic

Table 16-7 Pediatric Surgery Benchmarks for Operative Rate in Children with Spleen Injury

Authors	Database	Study Period	No. Patients	Operative Rate: Pediatric Surgeon and/or Children's Hospital/PTC	Spleen Injuries
Bowman et al.	KID 2000-AHRQ	2000	363	3%	All
Davis et al.	Pennsylvania Trauma Outcome Study-UHDDS	1991-2000	507	5%	All
Mooney et al.	New England Pediatric Trauma Database-UHDDS	1990-1998	866	11%	All
Stylianos	APSA Trauma Committee-Multicenter registry	1995-2000	652	3%	Isolated
Mooney and Forbes	Children's Hospital-Boston Trauma registry	1993-1999	82	0%	Isolated

KID2000, Kids' Inpatient Database of the Healthcare Cost and Utilization Project, Agency for Healthcare Research and Quality (2784 hospitals in 27 states; 2.5 million pediatric discharges); UHDDS, Uniform Hospital Discharge Data Sets; PTC, pediatric trauma center.

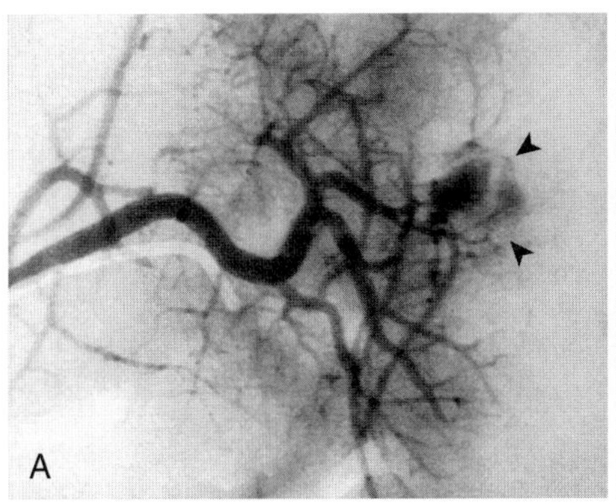

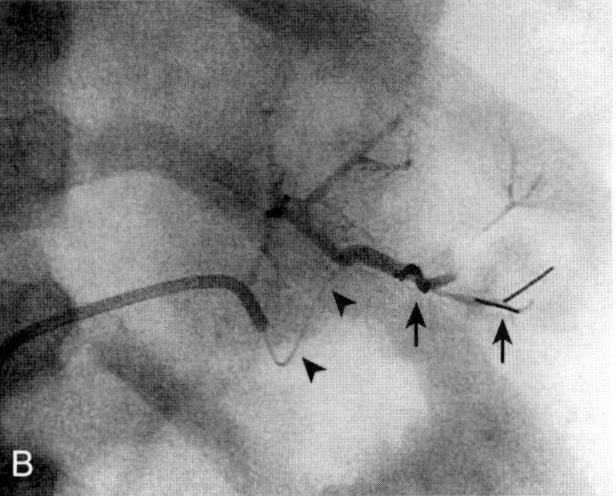

Figure 16-4. **A,** Splenic pseudoaneurysm (*arrowheads*) has developed after nonoperative treatment of blunt splenic injury. **B,** Successful angiographic embolization has been accomplished. The microcatheter used to deploy the coils is marked by the arrowheads and the embolic coils are marked by the arrows.

injury. Differences in mechanism of injury may account for the much lower incidence of associated abdominal injuries in children with splenic trauma. No justification exists for an exploratory celiotomy solely to avoid missing potential associated injuries in children.

Complications of Nonoperative Treatment

Nonoperative treatment protocols have been the standard for most children with blunt liver and spleen injury during the past 2 decades. The cumulative experience allows an evaluation of both the benefits and risks of the nonoperative approach. Fundamental to the success of the nonoperative strategy is the early, spontaneous cessation of hemorrhage. Transfusion rates for children with isolated spleen or liver injury have decreased to less than 10%, confirming the lack of continued blood loss in the majority of patients.[26-29,56] Despite these many favorable observations, obvious ongoing hemorrhage and hemodynamic instability require the presence of skilled surgeons, operating room staff, and blood bank capabilities. The role of angioembolization in adult trauma patients with splenic injury is expanding with variable success.[57,58] To date, most pediatric trauma centers have not utilized angioembolization in acutely bleeding patients with splenic injury.[59,60]

Isolated reports of significant delayed hemorrhage with adverse outcome continue to appear.[61-64] Two children with delayed hemorrhage 10 days after blunt liver injury have been reported.[63] Both children had persistent right upper quadrant (RUQ) and right shoulder pain despite having normal vital signs and stable hematocrits. The authors recommended continued in-house observation for injured patients until symptoms resolve. Recent reports described patients with significant bleeding 38 days after a grade II spleen injury and 24 days after a grade IV liver injury.[62,64] These rare occurrences create anxiety in identifying the minimal safe interval before resuming unrestricted activities.

Routine follow-up imaging studies have identified pseudocysts and pseudoaneurysms after splenic injury.[65-67] Splenic pseudoaneurysms are often asymptomatic and appear to resolve with time. The true incidence of self-limited, post-traumatic splenic pseudoaneurysms is unknown as routine follow-up imaging after successful nonoperative management has been largely abandoned. Once it is identified, the actual risk of splenic pseudoaneurysm rupture also is unclear. Angiographic embolization techniques can be used to treat these lesions successfully, obviating the need for operation and loss of splenic parenchyma (Fig. 16-4).[65]

Splenic pseudocysts may reach enormous size, leading to pain and gastrointestinal disturbance (Fig. 16-5). Simple percutaneous aspiration leads to a high recurrence rate. Laparoscopic excision and marsupialization is highly effective.

The immunocompetence of a shattered spleen that heals without surgery is debated, and vaccination practices in these children vary widely. Recent evidence using differential interference contrast microscopy in adult trauma patients indicates immunocompetence in patients with healed grade IV injuries.[68]

Sequelae of Damage Control Strategies

Even the most severe solid organ injuries can be treated nonoperatively if a prompt response to resuscitation occurs.[69] In patients who are hemodynamically unstable, despite fluid and packed red blood cell transfusion, emergency laparotomy is indicated. Most spleen and liver injuries requiring operation are amenable to simple methods of hemostasis,

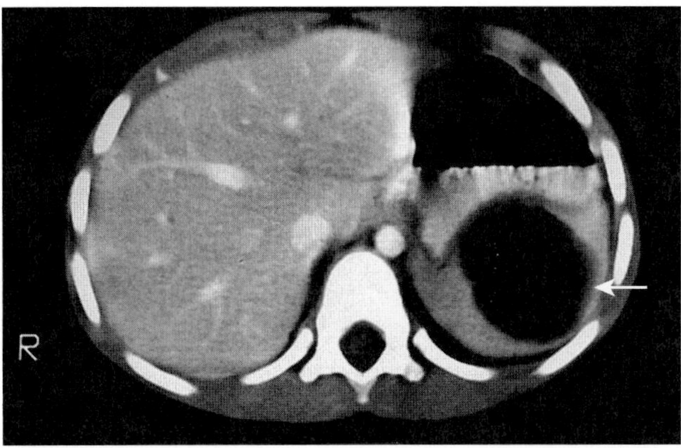

Figure 16-5. CT scan showing a post-traumatic splenic pseudocyst (*arrow*).

using a combination of manual compression, direct suture, and an increasing array of topical hemostatic agents.[70,71] In young children with significant hepatic injury, the sternum can be divided rapidly to expose the suprahepatic or intrapericardial inferior vena cava. Children will tolerate clamping of the inferior vena cava above the liver as long as their blood volume is replenished. With this exposure, the liver and major perihepatic veins can be isolated and the bleeding controlled to permit direct suture repair or ligation of the injured vessel.

The early morbidity and mortality of severe hepatic injuries are related to the effects of massive blood loss and replacement with large volumes of cold blood products. The consequences of prolonged operations with massive blood-product replacement include hypothermia, coagulopathy, and acidosis. Although the surgical team may keep pace with blood loss, serious physiologic and metabolic consequences are inevitable, and many of these critically ill patients are unlikely to survive. A multi-institutional review identified exsanguination as the cause of death in 82% of 537 intraoperative deaths at eight academic trauma centers.[72] The mean serum pH was 7.18, and the mean core temperature was 32°C before death. Survival in only 5 (40%) of 12 consecutive operative cases of retrohepatic vascular or severe parenchymal liver injury in children has been reported.[73]

Maintenance of physiologic stability during the struggle for surgical control of severe bleeding is a formidable challenge even for the most experienced operative team, particularly when hypothermia, coagulopathy, and acidosis occur. This triad creates a vicious cycle in which each derangement exacerbates the others. The physiologic and metabolic consequences of this triad often preclude completion of the procedure. Lethal coagulopathy from dilution, hypothermia, and acidosis can rapidly occur.[74]

Increased emphasis on physiologic and metabolic stability in emergency abdominal operations has led to the development of staged, multidisciplinary treatment plans, including abbreviated laparotomy, perihepatic packing, temporary abdominal closure, angiographic embolization, and endoscopic biliary stenting.[75-77] In a series of 22 patients with grade IV or V hepatic injuries treated between 1992 and 1997, mean blood loss was estimated at 4.6 L and mean packed red cell transfusion was 15 units.[78] Ten patients underwent packing of the hepatic injuries at the first operation. Fifteen patients had postoperative angiographic embolization in an attempt to control hemorrhage (Fig. 16-6). Survival was 92% in 13 grade IV patients and 78% in 9 grade V patients.

Abbreviated laparotomy with packing for hemostasis allowing resuscitation before planned reoperation is an alternative in unstable patients in whom further blood loss would be untenable. This "damage control" philosophy is a systematic, phased approach to the management of the exsanguinating trauma patient.[79-81] Packing of the retroperitoneum while avoiding entry into the abdomen in unstable patients with severe pelvic fractures has also gained popularity.[82] The three phases of damage control are detailed in Table 16-8. Although controversial, several resuscitative endpoints have been proposed beyond the conventional vital signs and urine output, including serum lactate, base deficit, mixed venous oxygen saturation, and gastric mucosal pH. Studies from recent military experience indicate that the optimal ratio of transfused packed red blood cells and fresh frozen plasma should approach 1:1 in massive transfusion scenarios.[83]

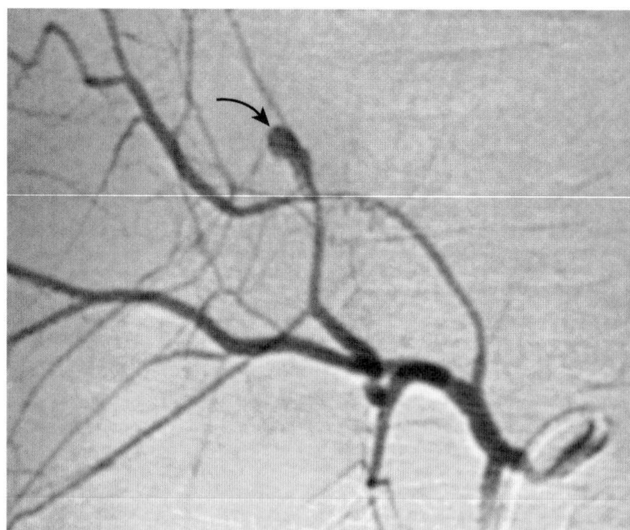

Figure 16-6. This hepatic artery angiogram was performed in a patient with persistent hemorrhage after initial damage-control laparotomy. The site of hemorrhage is identified (*arrow*), and embolization was successfully performed.

There has been increasing experimental and clinical evidence that recombinant activated factor VII (rFVIIa) may be a useful adjunctive therapy in injured patients with ongoing hemorrhage. In the laboratory, reduced clot formation due to hypothermia was reversed with rFVIIa.[84] Military experience indicates a survival advantage in injured soldiers requiring massive transfusion with early use of rFVIIa.[85] The use of rFVIIA has been described in eight children with blunt injuries to the spleen, liver, or kidney and signs of ongoing hemorrhage.[86] Bleeding was successfully controlled after a single dose of rFVIIa. Only three patients required transfusion, and there were

Table 16-8	"Damage Control" Strategy in the Exsanguinating Trauma Patient
Phase 1	Abbreviated laparotomy for exploration Control of hemorrhage and contamination Packing and temporary abdominal wall closure
Phase 2	Aggressive resuscitation in intensive care unit Core rewarming Optimize volume and oxygen delivery Correction of coagulopathy
Phase 3	Planned reoperation for packing change, evacuation, and definitive repair of injuries Abdominal wall closure

no thromboembolic events. The indications, optimal dosages and intervals, and risk profile still need to be developed before rFVIIa can be a mainstay in pediatric trauma care.

Once patients become normothermic, coagulation factors replaced, and oxygen delivery optimized, a second procedure is performed for pack removal and definitive repair of the injuries. A review of nearly 700 adult patients from several institutions who were treated with abdominal packing demonstrated hemostasis in 80%, survival of 32% to 73%, and abdominal abscess rates of 10% to 40%.[87,88]

Although abdominal packing with planned reoperation has been used with increasing frequency in adults during the past 2 decades, little published experience has been reported in children.[89-96] Nevertheless, this technique has a place in the management of children with massive intra-abdominal bleeding, especially after blunt trauma. A 3-year-old child required abdominal packing for a severe liver injury, making closure of the abdomen impossible.[90] A polymeric silicone "silo" was constructed to accommodate the bowel until the packing could be removed. The patient made a complete recovery.

The combined technique of abdominal packing and a "silo" allows time for correction of the hypothermia, acidosis, and coagulopathy without compromise of respiratory mechanics. A recent review reported 22 infants and children with refractory hemorrhage (ages 6 days to 20 years) who were treated with abdominal packing.[91] The anatomic site of hemorrhage was the liver and/or hepatic veins in 14, retroperitoneum and/or pelvis in 7, and the pancreatic bed in 1. Primary fascial closure was accomplished in 12 (55%) patients, and temporary skin closure or prosthetic material was used in the other 10. Abdominal packing controlled hemorrhage in 21 (95%) of the 22 patients. Removal of the packing was possible within 72 hours in 18 (82%) patients. No patient re-bled after removal of abdominal packing. However, 2 patients died with the packing still in place. In 7 (32%) patients, an abdominal or pelvic abscess developed. All were successfully drained by laparotomy (6 patients) or percutaneously (1 patient). Six of the 7 patients with abdominal sepsis survived. Overall, 18 (82%) patients survived. Two deaths were due to multisystem organ failure, 1 patient succumbed to cardiac failure from complex cardiac anomalies, and another died of exsanguination after blunt traumatic liver injury. No differences were noted in the volume of intraoperative blood transfusion, time to initiate abdominal packing, physiologic status, or type of abdominal closure between survivors and nonsurvivors.

Although the success of abdominal packing is encouraging, it may contribute to significant morbidity such as intra-abdominal sepsis, organ failure, and increased intra-abdominal pressure. Fluid samples taken from 28 patients with abdominal packing found peritoneal endotoxin and mediator accumulation even when cultures were sterile.[97] The assumption was that fluid accumulating after damage-control laparotomy can contribute to neutrophil dysfunction by enhancing neutrophil respiratory burst and inhibiting neutrophil responses to specific chemotactic mediators needed to fight infection. Thus, the known propensity of such patients for both intra-abdominal and systemic infection may be related to changes in neutrophil receptor status and effector function related to an accumulation of inflammatory mediators in the abdomen. Early washout, repetitive packing, and other efforts to minimize mediator accumulation deserve consideration.

It is essential to emphasize that the success of the abbreviated laparotomy and planned reoperation depends on a decision to use this strategy before irreversible shock. Abdominal packing, when used as a desperate, "last-ditch" effort after prolonged, failed attempts at hemostasis, has been uniformly unsuccessful. Indications for abdominal packing based on physiologic and anatomic criteria have been identified. Most have focused on intraoperative parameters including pH (~7.2), core temperature (<35°C), and coagulation values (prothrombin time >16 seconds) in the patient with profuse hemorrhage requiring large volumes of blood-product transfusion.

The optimal time for re-exploration is controversial because neither the physiologic endpoints of resuscitation nor the increased risk of infection with prolonged packing is well defined. The obvious benefits of hemostasis provided by packing also are balanced against the potential deleterious effects of increased intra-abdominal pressure on ventilation, cardiac output, renal function, mesenteric circulation, and intracranial pressure. Timely alleviation of the secondary "abdominal compartment syndrome" may be a critical salvage maneuver for patients. We recommend temporary abdominal wall expansion in all patients requiring packing until the hemostasis is obtained and visceral edema subsides.

A staged operative strategy for unstable trauma patients represents advanced surgical care and requires sound judgment. Intra-abdominal packing for control of exsanguinating hemorrhage is a lifesaving maneuver in highly selected patients in whom coagulopathy, hypothermia, and acidosis render further surgical procedures unduly hazardous. Early identification of patients likely to benefit from abbreviated laparotomy techniques is crucial for its success.

Abdominal Compartment Syndrome

Abdominal compartment syndrome is a term used to describe the deleterious effects of increased intra-abdominal pressure.[98] The "syndrome" includes respiratory insufficiency from worsening ventilation/perfusion mismatch, hemodynamic compromise from preload reduction due to inferior vena cava compression, impaired renal function from renal vein compression as well as decreased cardiac output, intracranial hypertension from increased ventilator pressures, splanchnic hypoperfusion, and abdominal wall overdistention. The causes of intra-abdominal hypertension in trauma patients include hemoperitoneum, retroperitoneal and/or bowel edema, use of abdominal/pelvic packing, and secondary to massive resuscitation of

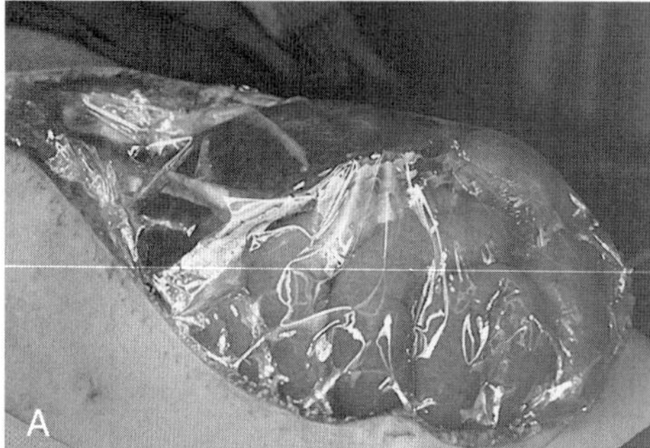

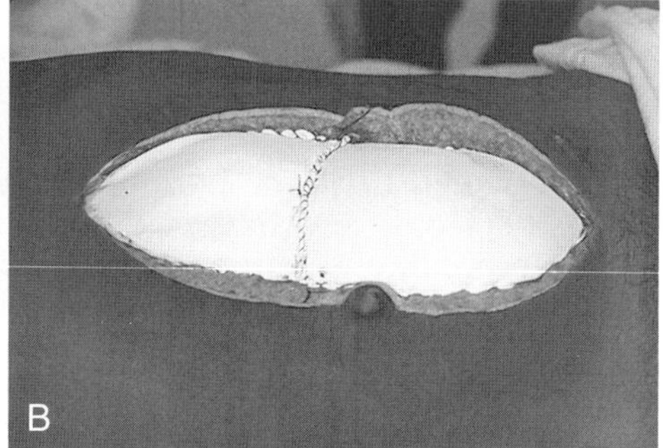

Figure 16-7. **A,** Abdominal wall expansion was performed in this patient with a bowel bag. **B,** Abdominal wall expansion in this patient was accomplished with a polytetrafluoroethylene patch.

non-abdominal trauma.[99] The combination of tissue injury and hemodynamic shock creates a cascade of events including capillary leak, ischemia-reperfusion, and release of vasoactive mediators and free radicals that combine to increase extracellular volume and tissue edema. Experimental evidence indicates significant alterations in cytokine levels in the presence of sustained intra-abdominal pressure elevation.[100,101] Once the combined effects of tissue edema and intra-abdominal fluid exceed a certain level, abdominal decompression must be considered.

The adverse effects of abdominal compartment syndrome have been acknowledged for decades. However, abdominal compartment syndrome has only recently been recognized as a life-threatening, yet potentially treatable entity.[76,102] The measurement of intra-abdominal pressure can be useful in determining the contribution of abdominal compartment syndrome to altered physiologic and metabolic parameters.[103-105] Intra-abdominal pressure can be determined by measuring bladder pressure. This involves instilling 1 mL/kg of saline into the urinary catheter and connecting it to a pressure transducer or manometer via a three-way stopcock. The symphysis pubis is used as the zero reference point, and the pressure is measured in centimeters of H_2O or millimeters of mercury. Intra-abdominal pressures in the range of 20 to 35 cm H_2O or 15 to 25 mm Hg have been identified as an indication to decompress the abdomen. Many surgeons prefer to intervene according to alterations in other physiologic and metabolic parameters rather than a specific pressure measurement. One series reported 11 adult trauma patients with abdominal compartment syndrome, measured by pulmonary artery catheters and gastric tonometry, had improved preload, pulmonary function, and visceral perfusion after abdominal decompression.[104]

Experience with abdominal decompression for abdominal compartment syndrome in children is limited.[91,102,105-107] Nonspecific abdominal CT findings in children with abdominal compartment syndrome include narrowing of the inferior vena cava, direct renal compression or displacement, bowel wall thickening with enhancement, and a rounded appearance of the abdomen.[106] One study reported the use of patch abdominoplasty in 23 infants and children, of whom only 3 were trauma patients.[107] These authors found that patch abdominoplasty for abdominal compartment syndrome effectively decreased airway pressures and oxygen requirements. Failure to respond with a decrease in airway pressures or FIO_2 was an ominous sign in their series. Several authors found that abdominal decompression resulted in decreased airway pressures, increased PO_2, and increased urine output in children with abdominal compartment syndrome.[102,105,107] Many materials have been suggested for use in temporary patch abdominoplasty, including Silastic sheeting, polytetrafluoroethylene (PTFE) sheeting, intravenous bags, cystoscopy bags, ostomy appliances, and various mesh materials (Fig. 16-7). The vacuum pack technique, used increasingly in adults, is applicable in pediatric patients and seems promising (Fig. 16-8).[80,96]

Bile Duct Injury

Nonoperative management of pediatric blunt liver injury is highly successful but is complicated by a 4% risk of persistent bile leakage.[108,109] The majority of patients with bile leaks sustained high grade (III-V) injuries.[110] Radionuclide scanning is recommended when biliary injury is suspected.[111] Delayed views may show a bile leak even if early views are normal. Endoscopic retrograde cholangiopancreatography (ERCP) can be performed with placement of

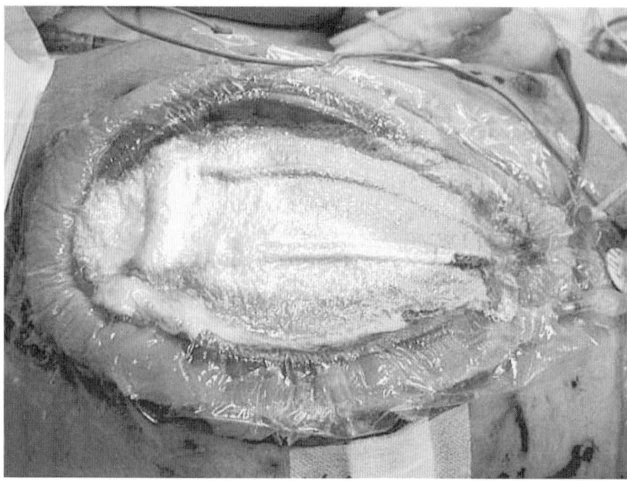

Figure 16-8. This photograph shows an open abdomen in a child treated with vacuum packing for hemostasis.

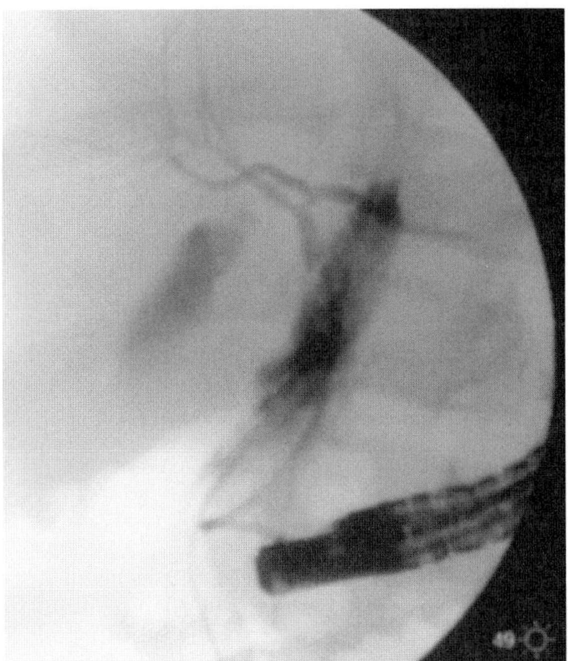

Figure 16-9. Endoscopic retrograde cholangiopancreatography demonstrates several areas of bile leaks after blunt liver injury.

transampullary biliary stents for biliary duct injury after blunt hepatic trauma. Although ERCP is invasive and requires conscious sedation, it can pinpoint the site of injury and allow treatment of the injured ducts without laparotomy (Fig. 16-9). Endoscopic transampullary biliary decompression is a recent addition to treatment for patients with persistent bile leakage. The addition of sphincterotomy during ERCP for persistent bile leakage after blunt liver injury has been advocated to decrease intrabiliary pressure and promote internal decompression.[112-115] Also, it is important to note that endoscopic biliary stents may migrate or clog.

Injury to the Pancreas

Blunt traumatic injury to the pancreas occurs infrequently in children and can be very difficult to diagnose. It is estimated that injuries to the pancreas compose 3% to 12% of intra-abdominal injuries in children sustaining blunt trauma.[116] The lack of surrounding fat planes and the small size of the retroperitoneal gland make it challenging to document even a major ductal injury by routine CT.[117] A dynamic CT pancreatogram, with multiple thin slices while infusing a contrast medium, gives much more detail than routine abdominal CT. Magnetic resonance cholangiopancreatography also is a useful diagnostic modality but is not appropriate in the acute resuscitative phase of the child with multiple injuries.[118] Elevations in serum amylase and lipase levels are very common in abdominal trauma but are not indicative of the extent of injury or need for surgical intervention. Hyperamylasemia also may occur with salivary gland injury, bowel perforation or obstruction, intracranial hemorrhage, or other nonspecific mesenteric injuries.[119] In contrast, ERCP is a very accurate technique in evaluating potential injury to the pancreatic ductal system.[120] It is not widely used in the early evaluation of the acutely injured child because of the highly specialized skills required, the need for general anesthesia, and the likelihood of significant need for treatment of associated head and thoracic injuries.

Nonoperative management of blunt injuries to the liver, spleen, and kidney in children is accepted as the standard of care in the majority of cases. Controversy exists when discussing management of the child with a significant pancreatic injury. Those with a pancreatic contusion without major ductal disruption will heal spontaneously. Successful nonoperative treatment of 28 children with pancreatic injuries ranging from contusions to complete transections by CT scan has been described.[121] Pseudocysts developed in 36% of patients and were treated with observation or percutaneous aspiration.

Direct visualization of the pancreas is very important when exploring a child's abdomen for a traumatic injury. The lesser sac is entered above the transverse colon, and the body and tail of the gland are carefully inspected. A Kocher maneuver is then used to inspect the duodenum and head of the pancreas. The posterior surface of the gland may be accessed by mobilization of the spleen along with the tail of the pancreas from a lateral to medial direction.

In the child with a major pancreatic ductal injury (Fig. 16-10), early operative intervention has been reported to shorten hospitalization and lessen dependence on total parenteral nutrition compared with those children who were initially managed nonoperatively.[122-125] Pseudocyst formation occurs in 45% to 100% of ductal injuries managed nonoperatively.[121,126] Of these, a significant number, up to 60%, may resolve with time. Percutaneous or cyst-enteric drainage procedures may be needed if resolution does not occur spontaneously. These children have an increased length of hospitalization as well as an increased dependence on total parenteral nutrition compared with those undergoing early distal pancreatectomy.

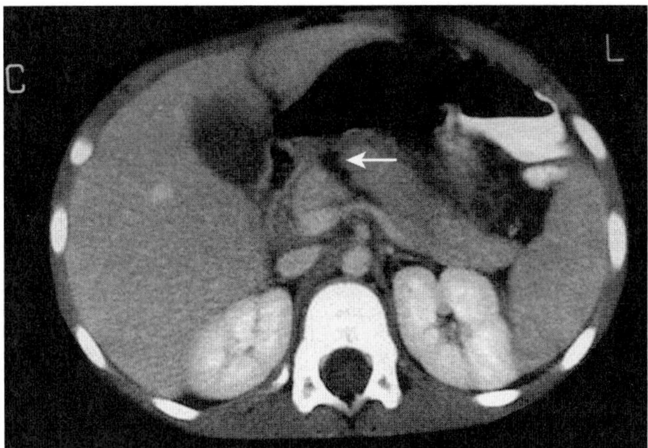

Figure 16-10. This abdominal CT scan demonstrates blunt transection of the pancreas (*arrow*).

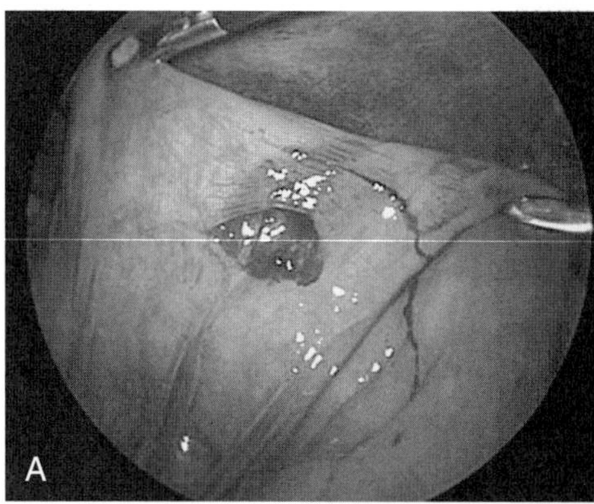

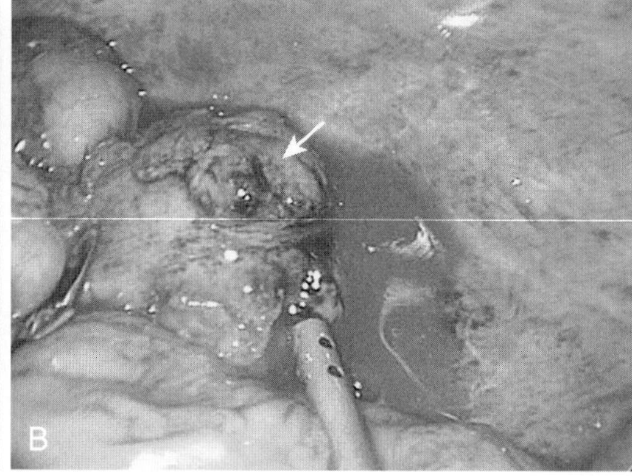

Figure 16-11. In some patients it is not always clear whether a significant intestinal injury has occurred from either blunt or penetrating trauma. Dingnostic laparoscopy is a useful technique in these patients. **A,** Perforation of the bowel from penetrating trauma is seen at laparoscopy. This was closed primarily. **B,** Full-thickness injury to the colon (*arrow*) in a patient with blunt trauma is shown. The laparoscopic approach was converted to an open operation for treatment of this injury.

ERCP as a diagnostic and therapeutic option has recently gained some favor in selected centers with pediatric ERCP expertise. Documentation of a ductal injury, sphincterotomy, and possible stenting of the injury are all maneuvers useful for healing.[120,127,128]

HOLLOW VISCUS INJURY

Gastrointestinal tract injuries in children may occur by either blunt or penetrating mechanisms. Penetrating injuries to the abdomen account for less than 10% of cases of abdominal trauma in most series. They require minimal diagnostic evaluation before operative management if penetration of the peritoneal cavity is evident, if the child has a clinical examination consistent with peritoneal irritation, or in the unstable child. Blunt intestinal injury may be seen with obvious indications for surgical intervention or may have a more subtle, insidious presentation. The mechanism may be from a compressive force (crush injury or child abuse), a deceleration shearing force (fall from a height), or a combination of the two (lap belt injury).

CT diagnosis of a bowel injury is often quite difficult. CT findings have been described in an effort to improve its diagnostic accuracy in victims of blunt abdominal trauma. Bowel wall thickening and enhancement, mesenteric stranding, and free intraperitoneal fluid in the absence of solid organ injury should alert the caregiver to a possible hollow viscus injury. Pneumoperitoneum often is not present, even with a full-thickness bowel wall disruption. Virtually all neurologically intact patients have findings or symptoms suggestive of peritoneal contamination from a perforated viscus, such as pain, tachycardia, rebound tenderness, or guarding.[129] Laparoscopy can be useful for diagnostic purposes in some patients (Fig. 16-11). The unconscious patient with multiple injuries presents a significant diagnostic challenge, and a high index of suspicion is needed.[130] These neurologically injured patients may benefit from DPL if the abdominal CT shows suspicious findings but laparotomy poses substantial risks due to associated injuries.

Children who have a visible contusion of the anterior abdominal wall from a seat-belt lap restraint have been documented to have an increased incidence of abdominal injuries (Fig. 16-12). These include both solid and hollow abdominal organs as well as associated fractures of the lower thoracic and lumbar spine. These children must have frequent in-hospital assessments, serial physical examination by the same surgeon, and diagnostic imaging to assess for abdominal and spinal injuries. Several series have documented 80% to 100% of children with major blunt intestinal injuries who had evidence of abdominal wall ecchymosis.[10,129] The presence of a visible contusion does not, in itself, mandate exploration but should prompt careful observation.

Injury to the Stomach

Injuries to the stomach due to penetrating mechanisms are variable in the amount of tissue destruction and are dependent primarily on the velocity of the offending missile or penetrating object. Blunt injury to the stomach, which is relatively infrequent, occurs when a compressive force causes a burst injury in a patient with a full stomach following a meal.

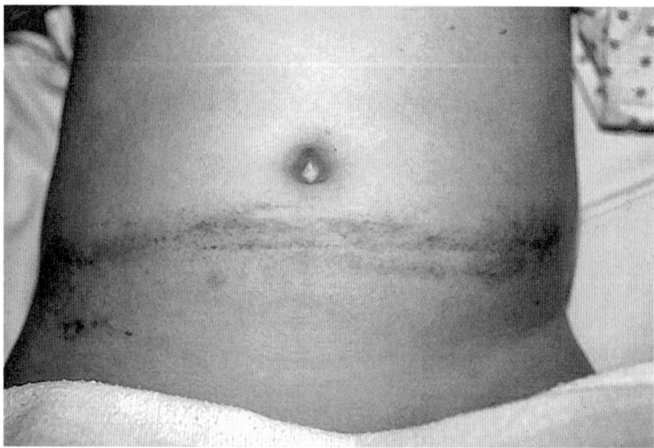

Figure 16-12. A lap belt sign is seen across this child's lower abdomen. This child had an underlying intestinal injury.

The diagnosis of a gastric injury from blunt force is often problematic. Free air may not be seen on the initial radiograph or CT scan. A nasogastric tube lying outside the stomach contour on a radiograph or CT scan is diagnostic. The child with abdominal wall ecchymosis, tenderness, and/or free fluid in the peritoneal cavity should prompt the suspicion of hollow viscus injury.

Surgical exploration for a suspected gastric injury is initiated with an upper midline laparotomy incision. The stomach and duodenum should be adequately mobilized, and hemorrhage should be controlled. Particular attention should be paid to the lesser curve and to the posterior stomach near the gastroesophageal junction, which are sites of possible missed injuries.[131] The lesser sac should always be opened to explore the posterior wall of the stomach adequately. Owing to the excellent blood supply of the stomach, repairs usually heal well.

Injury to the Duodenum

Duodenal injuries may be extremely difficult to manage because of the intimate association with the pancreas, extrahepatic biliary system, and intra-abdominal vascular systems. Thorough mobilization is key to identifying injuries, both blunt and penetrating. The technique used to repair a duodenal injury is dependent on the overall status of the patient, the location of the injury, and the amount of tissue destruction encountered. Extravasation of air or enteral CT contrast material into the paraduodenal, pararenal, or retroperitoneal space is the key finding in those patients with a duodenal perforation. This is not seen in patients sustaining a duodenal hematoma.[132]

An intramural duodenal hematoma due to blunt force applied to the epigastrium (kick, punch, handlebar) may be managed nonoperatively if the child has no evidence of full-thickness injury or peritonitis (Fig. 16-13).[133] The CT scans or upper gastrointestinal contrast studies typically reveal duodenal narrowing, spiraling, or partial obstruction of the duodenum. No contrast or air is seen outside the bowel lumen. When managed nonoperatively, nasogastric decompression and total parenteral nutrition may be required for an average of 1 to 3 weeks. If a duodenal hematoma is encountered during exploration for additional abdominal trauma, the serosa may be incised and the clot carefully evacuated, taking care not to enter the duodenal lumen.

Full-thickness duodenal injuries may be closed primarily if the amount of tissue destruction is not excessive and if the closure will not compromise the duodenal lumen or drainage of the biliary and pancreatic ductal system. Adequate surgical drainage of the paraduodenal area is important if a pancreatic injury or major duodenal tissue devitalization has occurred. Duodenal closure may be obtained with the aid of a Roux limb of jejunum sewn to the viable debrided duodenum. A duodenal drainage tube for decompression is left in place. Temporary pyloric exclusion with an absorbable suture via a gastrotomy also may be valuable in the management of a complex duodenal repair. This allows healing of the duodenum before spontaneous recanalization of the pyloric channel once the pyloric sutures resorb. A gastrostomy tube for decompression may also be utilized instead of a nasogastric tube. Placement of a feeding jejunostomy will be helpful for enteral nutritional support. Surgical drains placed near the injured tissue at the time of initial repair will control a fistula resulting from any enteric leak. Somatostatin analogs may be helpful in decreasing pancreatic and intestinal secretions and are useful in management of a fistula should one occur. Rarely is a pancreaticoduodenectomy required for blunt trauma in children.[134]

Small Bowel Injury

Penetrating injury to the abdomen frequently injures the small intestine. The small bowel must be carefully and systematically visualized for mesenteric and bowel wall injuries. Extensive injuries should be managed by resection and anastomosis. Isolated perforations and lacerations may be repaired with debridement and closure, with care to avoid luminal narrowing.

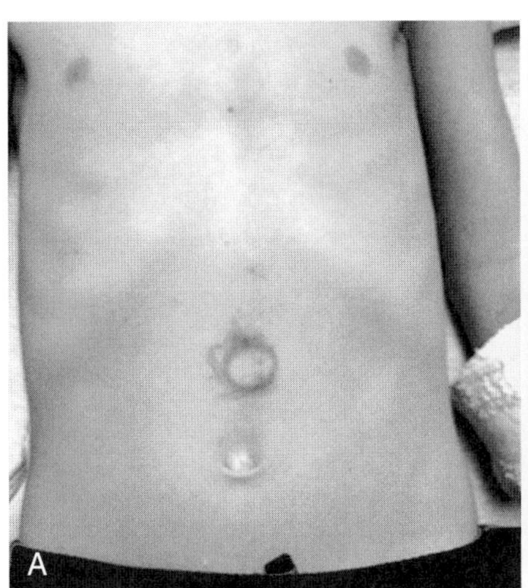

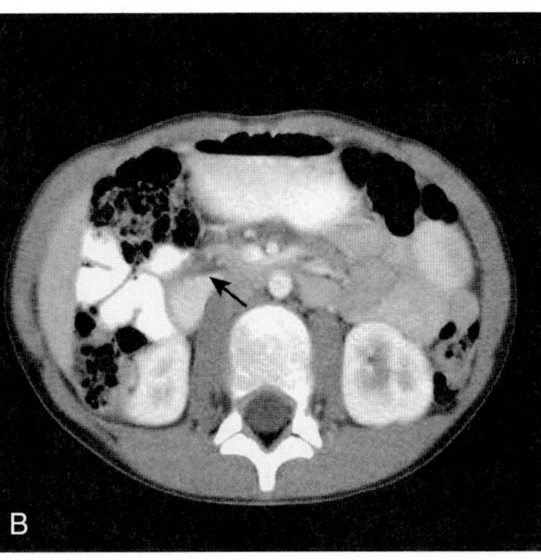

Figure 16-13. This child sustained a duodenal hematoma (**B**, *arrow*) from a handlebar injury to the epigastrium (**A**).

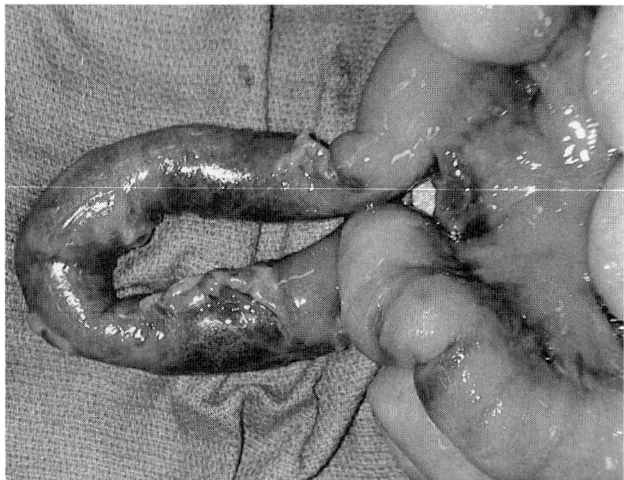

Figure 16-14. The small bowel mesentery has been avulsed, resulting in ischemic bowel.

Hematomas in the mesentery should be explored, and control of bleeding vessels should be meticulously performed. If a segment of bowel is in jeopardy because of a mesenteric injury, bowel resection and primary anastomosis should be performed to avoid stricture formation. Injuries to the superior mesenteric artery or vein should be repaired with a vein patch as needed to avoid stenosis of the affected vessel. Delayed diagnosis of injuries may also be seen with a delayed bowel infarction due to rapid deceleration injury with avulsion of the bowel from its mesentery (Fig. 16-14). A late sequela of blunt intestinal injury is intestinal stricture.[135] Crush injury to the bowel wall results in ischemic injury and resulting scarring and fibrosis. Intolerance of feeding, bilious emesis, and evidence of a bowel obstruction 1 to 6 weeks after blunt abdominal trauma is the most common presenting scenario.

Injury to the Colon

Injuries to the colon in children may occur by the same mechanisms as small bowel injuries, but the consequences may be more significant. Delayed diagnosis with peritoneal contamination may result in severe and life-threatening septic complications. If isolated colonic injuries are identified and repaired early in a hemodynamically stable child, a primary bowel anastomosis with appropriate perioperative antibiotic coverage is safe. This approach also avoids the potential complications of stomas and the need for reoperation for stoma closure. Once a colonic injury has been identified and controlled, multiple factors influence surgical management. In the absence of shock or delayed diagnosis with severe fecal contamination, many colon injuries may be safely repaired primarily. A diverting stoma may be necessary if extensive abdominal wall or perineal tissue devitalization is present, if the child is in shock, or if severe peritoneal soilage has occurred. Care must be taken in selecting the site for placement of the proximal diverting stoma to avoid ongoing wound contamination.

Rectal Injuries

The etiology of the majority of perineal and rectal injuries in children is either accidental falls in a straddle fashion onto sharp or blunt objects or sexual abuse. Typically, rectal perforations require proximal diversion with an end colostomy and drainage of the distal injured perirectal space. Identification of these injuries may be difficult. The ability to ascertain the extent of the injury will frequently require a formal examination under general anesthesia (Fig. 16-15). In the female, care is taken to carefully inspect the vaginal vault for evidence of a penetrating injury either through or into the vagina.[136] Proctosigmoidoscopy in a nonprepared colon may not clearly localize an obvious perforation, but the presence of endoluminal blood must be assumed to be evidence of injury. After proximal colostomy and presacral drainage has been performed, the distal rectum should be cleared of any remaining feces. Meticulous repair of the injured anal sphincter musculature must be performed. Any nonviable tissue should be debrided at this setting. Closure of the rectal injury or perforation may be accomplished transanally if the injury is low enough to permit this approach.

Urinary Bladder

The bladder can rupture either in an intraperitoneal or an extraperitoneal location. The young child's bladder is predominantly an intra-abdominal organ. Blunt trauma to a child with a full bladder is the mechanism in the vast majority of bladder injuries. Careful examination for possible pelvic fractures and associated intra-abdominal injuries must be performed. Gross hematuria is frequently, but not always, present as a presenting symptom. Plain cystography or CT cystography is the study of choice to evaluate a suspected bladder injury based on hematuria or an abnormal abdominal CT scan. Contrast extravasation from the bladder or a large amount of free intraperitoneal

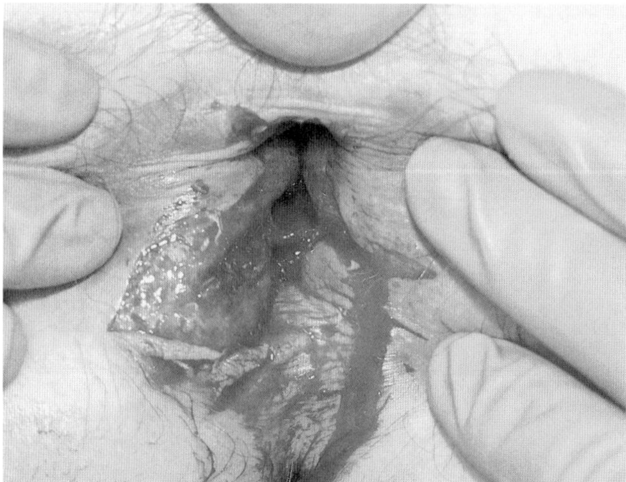

Figure 16-15. This teenager developed this full-thickness straddle rectal injury after falling off a trampoline. It was possible to close the injury over drains placed in the perirectal tissues. He has recovered uneventfully with full continence.

fluid not explained by solid organ injury in a child with hematuria should prompt a study to exclude bladder perforation. Extraperitoneal bladder rupture may be treated with bladder catheter drainage, which allows complete healing in most cases. Intraperitoneal rupture will require surgical repair after adequate debridement of devitalized tissue. One or two layered closure with absorbable suture material and adequate bladder decompression with transurethral or suprapubic drains are utilized. Careful inspection for associated concomitant injuries is essential to avoid preventable sequelae.

INJURY TO THE DIAPHRAGM

Traumatic injury to the diaphragm is infrequently observed, even at the largest pediatric trauma centers. The etiology may be either blunt or penetrating mechanisms. In most series, blunt traumatic rupture of the diaphragm after motor vehicle crashes accounts for 80% to 90% of cases. These injuries are caused by massive compressive forces to the abdomen, which create acceleration of abdominal contents cephalad, followed by rupture of the diaphragmatic muscle. The pressure gradient between the pleural and peritoneal cavities enables abdominal viscera to herniate into the thoracic cavity.

The diagnosis is frequently suggested by a plain chest radiograph as part of the secondary survey of the injured child. Other studies are occasionally helpful but may not aid in the diagnosis.[137] The plain radiographic findings include the following:

- Obscured hemidiaphragm
- Elevated hemidiaphragm
- Gas in herniated viscus above the diaphragm
- Tip of nasogastric tube in thorax
- Atypical pneumothorax
- Plate-like atelectasis adjacent to the diaphragm

Historically, it was believed that left-sided traumatic diaphragmatic hernias were much more common, accounting for 80% to 90% of reported cases. More recent series and autopsy studies have shown that actually the right- and left-sided ruptures occur with equal frequency.[138] It is likely that these traumatic hernias do occur equally, but the more severe injuries causing a right-sided rupture result in fewer survivors, resulting in fewer documented cases in trauma series.

Multiple-system and multiple-organ injury in this population is the rule rather than the exception. In the Toronto series of 16 pediatric patients with traumatic diaphragmatic rupture, 81% had multiple injuries, which included liver lacerations (47%), pelvic fractures (47%), major vascular injuries (40%), bowel perforations (33%), fractures of the long bones (20%), renal lacerations (20%), splenic lacerations (13%), and closed-head injuries (13%).[137] As would be expected, many complications in this group of severely injured patients were noted, with a significant risk of fatal injury.

Emergent operative exploration with minimal diagnostic testing is often necessary in patients with multiple abdominal injuries. Observation and careful palpation of both diaphragms must be a routine part of the abdominal exploration in this setting. Direct suture repair of the injury is usually possible after debridement of any devitalized tissue. Pledgeted sutures may aid in buttressing the repair made with mild tension without tearing the muscle. If the defect to be closed is too large to repair primarily without undue tension, a prosthetic patch of PTFE or an acellular collagen patch implant can be used in the manner of repairing congenital diaphragmatic hernias in the newborn. Successful laparoscopic or thoracoscopic repair of diaphragmatic injuries in hemodynamically stable children and in delayed repairs is technically feasible, with care being taken to search for additional associated injuries.[139,140] Renal avulsion into the chest through a traumatically ruptured diaphragm has been reported.[141,142] Because of the rarity of this injury, a high index of suspicion must be maintained when the mechanism and associated injuries suggests the possibility of this injury.[143] As always, a thorough and systematic exploration of the entire abdomen and palpation of the retroperitoneal structures is emphasized.

RENAL TRAUMA

The kidney is the most commonly injured organ in the urogenital system. Children appear to be more susceptible to major renal trauma than adults.[144] Several unique anatomic aspects contribute to this observation, including less cushioning from perirenal fat, weaker abdominal musculature, and a less well-ossified thoracic cage. The child's kidney also occupies a proportionately larger space in the retroperitoneum than does an adult's kidney. In addition, the pediatric kidney may retain fetal lobulations, permitting easier parenchymal disruption.

Renal trauma is broadly classified as being blunt or penetrating. Blunt trauma is more common, accounting for more than 90% of injuries in some series.[145] The kidney, which is relatively mobile within Gerota's fascia, can be crushed against the ribs or vertebral column, resulting in parenchymal lacerations or contusions. The kidney also can be lacerated by fractured ribs. Penetrating trauma accounts for only 10% to 20% of renal injuries, yet it is responsible for the majority of renal injuries that require operation.[146] Penetrating injuries to the chest, abdomen, flank, and lumbar regions should be assumed to have caused renal injury until proven otherwise.

Preexisting or congenital renal abnormalities, such as hydronephrosis, tumors, or abnormal position, make the kidney vulnerable to relatively mild traumatic forces. Historically, congenital abnormalities in injured kidneys have been reported to vary from 1% to 21%, although recent reviews have shown that the incidence rates are closer to 1% to 5%.[147,148] Renal abnormalities, particularly hydronephrosis, may be discovered as a result of minor blunt abdominal trauma. Rarely, the child may be seen with an acute abdomen secondary to intraperitoneal rupture of a hydronephrotic kidney.[149]

Major deceleration/flexion injuries may produce renal arterial or venous injuries due to stretching of a normally fixed vascular pedicle. This type of injury may be more common in children because of their increased flexibility and relatively increased renal mobility.[150-152] Post-traumatic thrombosis of the renal artery follows an intimal tear that occurs because the media and adventitia of the renal artery are more elastic than the intima. The intimal tear produces thrombosis that results in renal ischemia. A high index of suspicion must be maintained to identify these injuries in a timely fashion.

Diagnosis

Once the patient has been resuscitated and life-threatening injuries have been addressed, evaluation of the genitourinary system can be undertaken. After any blunt injury, the presence of hematuria (microscopic or gross), a palpable flank mass, or flank hematomas are indications for urologic evaluations. Most major blunt renal injuries occur in association with other major injuries of the head, chest, and abdomen. Urologic investigations should be undertaken when trauma to the lower chest is associated with rib, thoracic, or lumbar spine fractures. It also should be performed in all crush injuries to the abdomen or pelvis when the patient has sustained a severe deceleration injury. Because a renal pedicle injury or ureteropelvic junction disruption may not be associated with one of the classic signs of renal injury such as hematuria, radiologic evaluation to demonstrate bilateral renal function should always be considered in patients with a mechanism of injury that could potentially injure the upper urinary tract.

Gross hematuria is the most reliable indicator for serious urologic injury.[153] The need for imaging in the patient with blunt trauma and microscopic hematuria is not so clear. Moreover, the degree of hematuria does not always correlate with the degree of injury.[154] Renal vascular pedicle avulsion or acute thrombosis of segmental arteries can occur in the absence of hematuria, whereas mild renal contusions can appear with gross hematuria.[155] In adults, the vast majority of patients with blunt trauma with microscopic hematuria and no evidence of shock (systolic blood pressure < 90 mm Hg) have minor renal injuries and thus do not need to be studied radiographically.[155,156] Guidelines for evaluating the pediatric population are not so clearly defined. All children with any degree of microscopic hematuria after blunt trauma have traditionally undergone renal imaging. Recently, a meta-analysis of all reported series of children with hematuria and suspected renal injury revealed that only 11 (2%) of 548 patients with insignificant microscopic hematuria (<50 red blood cells/high-power field [RBCs/HPF]) had a significant renal injury.[157] However, all 11 of these patients were found to have multiple organ trauma and renal imaging would have been performed in the course of evaluation despite the relatively minor amount of microscopic hematuria. Detection of significant renal injury was found to increase to 8% with significant microhematuria (>50 RBCs/HPF) and to 32% in those with gross hematuria after blunt trauma. Thus, it seems reasonable to consider observation without renal imaging in children with microscopic hematuria of less than 50 RBCs/HPF who are stable, unless they have multiple organ system injuries.

Historically, excretory urography (intravenous pyelography [IVP]) has been the radiographic imaging study of choice in suspected renal trauma. The sensitivity has been reported as high as 90% in diagnosing renal injury. Unfortunately, IVP misses other intra-abdominal injuries and may miss or understage renal injury in children by 50% compared with CT.[158,159] CT is now used almost exclusively as the imaging study of choice for suspected renal trauma in hemodynamically stable adults and children.[160] CT is both sensitive and specific for demonstrating a parenchymal laceration or urinary extravasation, for delineating segmental parenchymal infarcts, for determining the size and location of the surrounding retroperitoneal hematoma, and/or for diagnosing associated intra-abdominal injury (Fig. 16-16). CT also allows accurate staging of the renal injury.

The most commonly used staging system for renal trauma is from the American Association for the Surgery of Trauma. This classification categorizes renal trauma into five grades that have predictive value in the subsequent management strategy of these injuries.[161] The ultimate goal of staging is to provide sufficient information for management that results in the preservation of renal parenchyma and the salvage of injured kidneys.

Ultrasonography also has been used to assess renal trauma. However, in comparison to CT, its sensitivity in demonstrating renal injury is only 25% to 70%. Also, it may miss associated intra-abdominal injuries. Unfortunately, FAST has been shown to have a low sensitivity for solid organ injury in children. It also provides little information concerning renal function or pedicle injuries. At present, renal ultrasonography is not currently recommended as a useful screening

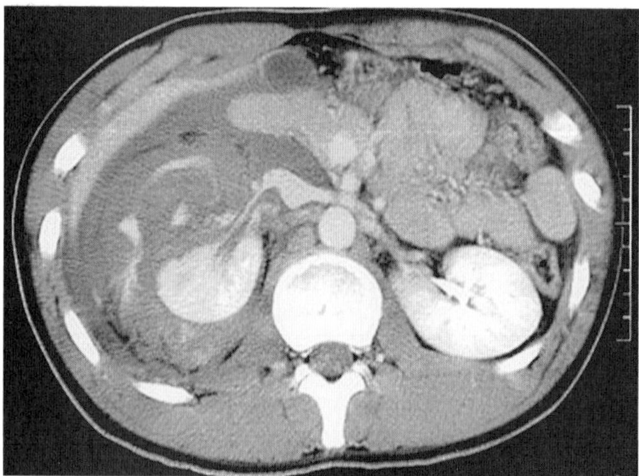

FIGURE 16-16. Severe right kidney disruption, resulting in a large perirenal hematoma, is seen on this CT scan after intravenous administration of a contrast agent.

tool for urologic evaluation in the setting of blunt renal trauma.[162]

It is imperative to acknowledge that major renal injuries such as ureteropelvic junction disruption or segmental arterial thrombosis may occur without the presence of hematuria or hypotension. Therefore, a high index of suspicion is necessary to diagnose these injuries. Nonvisualization of the injured kidney on IVP and failure of contrast uptake with a large associated perirenal hematoma on CT are hallmark findings for renal artery thrombosis. Ureteropelvic junction disruption is classically seen as perihilar extravasation of contrast agent with nonvisualization of the distal ureter.[163]

Treatment

In most patients, attempts should be made to manage all renal injuries nonoperatively.[164-166] Minor renal injuries constitute the majority of blunt renal injuries and usually resolve without incident.[167,168] The management of major renal parenchymal lacerations, although accounting for only 10% to 15% of all renal trauma patients, is currently controversial. Operative intervention is not always mandatory, and many major renal injuries due to blunt trauma can be managed without operation.[169-171] When necessary, the goals of surgical renal exploration are either to treat major renal injuries definitively with preservation of renal parenchyma when possible or to evaluate thoroughly a suspected renal injury. The need for surgical exploration is much higher in patients with penetrating trauma as opposed to blunt trauma.

The indications for renal exploration vary greatly between individual trauma centers. Most centers expectantly manage grade I to III injuries with bed rest and observation. Controversies arise in the management of grade IV to V injuries. The majority of blunt renal injuries sustained are minor contusions and lacerations. Even in the presence of gross hematuria, most blunt renal injuries will not require exploration and have excellent long-term outcomes.[171] Absolute indications for renal exploration include persistent life-threatening bleeding; an expanding, pulsatile, or uncontained retroperitoneal hematoma; or suspected renal pedicle avulsion. Relative indications for exploration include substantial devitalized renal parenchyma or urinary extravasation. Injuries with significant (>25%) nonviable renal tissue associated with parenchymal laceration that are managed nonoperatively have a complication rate of more than 75%.[172] When such renal injuries are associated with an intraperitoneal organ injury, the postinjury complication rate is much higher unless the kidney is surgically repaired. By surgically repairing such injuries, surgeons reduced the overall morbidity from 85% to 23%.

Urinary extravasation alone does not demand surgical exploration. In patients with major renal injury and urinary extravasation who are managed nonoperatively, urinary extravasation resolved spontaneously in 87%.[165] Extravasation persisted in 13% and was successfully managed endoscopically. Incomplete staging of the renal injury demands either further imaging or renal exploration and reconstruction. Most commonly, these patients undergo renal exploration because they are bleeding persistently or because they have an associated injury that requires laparotomy.

When the nonoperative approach is chosen, supportive care with bed rest, hydration, antibiotics, and serial hemoglobin and blood pressure monitoring is required. After the gross hematuria resolves, limited activity is advised for 2 to 4 weeks until microscopic hematuria ceases. Complications can occur during the period of observation within the first 4 weeks of injury and include delayed bleeding, abscess, sepsis, urinary fistula, urinary extravasation, urinoma, and hypertension. The greatest risk is life-threatening hemorrhage occurring within the first 2 weeks of injury. Immediate surgical exploration or angiographic embolization is indicated. Angiographic embolization is an alternative to exploration in a hemodynamically stable patient in whom persistent gross hematuria signifies persistent low-grade hemorrhage from the injured kidney. Persistent urinary extravasation has successfully been managed by percutaneous drainage. Hypertension in the early post-trauma period is uncommon. Hypertension may develop in the ensuing months and, in most instances, is treated medically.

Renal Exploration and Reconstruction

If operation is required, early control of the vessels increases the rate of renal salvage.[173] When proximal vascular control is initially achieved before any renal exploration, nephrectomy is required in fewer than 12% of cases.[174] When primary vascular control is not achieved and massive bleeding is encountered, in the rush to control bleeding, a kidney that could have been salvaged may need to be removed. The surgeon must carefully identify the kidney's relations with the posterior abdomen and the posterior parietal peritoneum. The colon is lifted from the abdomen and placed on the anterior chest to allow mobilization of the small bowel. The inferior mesenteric vein and the aorta are identified at this point, and the posterior peritoneum is incised medial to the inferior mesenteric vein. The aorta is dissected superiorly to the ligament of Treitz, where the left renal vein is found crossing anterior to the aorta. Retraction of the left renal vein exposes both renal arteries beneath it. These arteries may now be isolated and controlled with vessel loops. Once vessel isolation is complete, an incision is made in the peritoneum just lateral to the colon. The colon is reflected medially to expose the retroperitoneal hematoma in its entirety, and the kidney may be exposed. If significant bleeding is encountered, the ipsilateral renal vessels may be occluded. Warm ischemia time should not surpass 30 minutes.[174]

Renal vascular injuries must be addressed promptly. Major lacerations to the renal vein are repaired directly with venorrhaphy. Repair of renal arterial injuries may require a variety of techniques, including resection with end-to-end anastomosis, bypass graft with autogenous vein or a synthetic graft, and arteriorrhaphy.

Traumatic renal artery occlusion requires many of the same techniques for repair. However, this must be performed in the first 12 hours from the time of injury. Otherwise, the kidney is usually nonviable after this length of ischemia.

Single Kidney and Sports Participation

Physician opinions and practice patterns regarding the participation of children and adolescents with single, normal kidneys in contact/collision sports vary widely. A recent survey of the American Society of Pediatric Nephrology indicated that the majority (62%) of nephrologists do not permit contact/collision sports participation in patients with a solitary kidney.[175] Interestingly, only 5% barred cycling. These opinions are not supported by the literature because a sports-related kidney injury was found in 0.4 per million children per year from all sports, and cycling caused three times more kidney injuries than football.

chapter 17

PEDIATRIC HEAD TRAUMA

Kelly Tieves, DO

Traumatic brain injury (TBI) is an important cause of death and disability in children.[1] Among children from birth to 14 years, there are an estimated 2685 deaths, 37,000 hospitalizations, and 435,000 emergency department visits each year in the United States for TBI. An estimated 30,000 children and youth suffer permanent disability. The two highest-risk age groups are birth to 4-year-olds and 15- to 19-year-olds. Falls and abuse account for the majority of injury in the infants and small children, whereas motor vehicle crashes are the predominant mechanism of injury in teens and young adults.[2,3] In the entire American population, more than 1.4 million people sustain TBI each year, with over 50,000 deaths, 235,000 hospitalizations, and 1.1 million treated and released from an emergency department.[2] The economic burden of TBI totaled an estimated $60 billion in the United States in 2000.[4]

Although TBI is often referred to as the leading cause of death and disability in children, there are currently no population-based studies to estimate the actual personal and public health burden of TBI in children and youth. The number of mild injuries in children, including concussions, is estimated to be three to four times that of the more severe cases. Current studies, including longitudinal outcome studies in adults, often omit this population from study, producing underestimates of the burden of disease.[5]

Head trauma as a result of child abuse remains a significant concern.[6] In children younger than age 1 year, nonaccidental trauma secondary to abuse is the most common cause of fatal TBI.[7,8] Head trauma associated with abuse has a higher rate of subdural hematoma, subarachnoid hemorrhage, and retinal hemorrhages when compared with nonabusive head trauma. Public health campaigns have brought attention to the dangers of shaking a young child and provided resources to parents and caretakers who may be at risk of harming a child.[9]

Although the reasons are not entirely clear, there has been a general trend in improved outcome after severe TBI in children.[10] Declines in morbidity and mortality have been due to improved prehospital care, regionalization of pediatric trauma care, adherence to evidence-based practice guidelines, more aggressive care, such as intracranial pressure (ICP) monitoring and early surgical evacuation of mass lesions, improved diagnostic imaging (computed tomography [CT], magnetic resonance imaging [MRI]), and advances in intensive care. In July 2003, evidence-based practice guidelines were published for the acute medical management of severe TBI in infants, children, and adolescents.[11] These guidelines have provided a format to decrease variability in care across centers, but there is a striking lack of data from well-designed, randomized controlled trials.

BRAIN INJURY MECHANISMS

Nonpenetrating Cranial Trauma

Head injuries can be classified by their pathologic or morphologic descriptions. Blunt or nonpenetrating trauma occurs as the result of a direct impact on the brain and calvaria. These injuries often occur after a motor vehicle collision or fall and account for the vast majority of TBI in the United States. This type of injury typically results in focal damage to the underlying brain (*coup*). In some instances, *contrecoup* damage occurs from the rebound movement of the viscoelastic brain within its rigid encasement. The predominant contrecoup damage occurs on the side opposite the impact. This is commonly seen with subdural hemorrhages with associated cortical contusion when the brain rebounds off the skull, causing disruption of delicate surface vessels. The inner surface of the skull at its base is irregular, ridged, and restrictive at its anterior margins. As a result, the anterior and inferior portions of the temporal and frontal lobes are often injured by abrupt brain acceleration or deceleration in a sagittal plane.

Penetrating Trauma

Penetrating injury, caused by bladed weapons and projectiles, such as handguns and rifles, cause cerebral lacerations with deleterious effects on the underlying neurons, their functional interconnections, and the cerebral vasculature at the surface of the brain. Penetrating injuries also carry a risk of increased infection, especially if foreign material is introduced into the brain.

Axonal Shearing

Axonal injury or shearing occurs as the result of changes in the angular momentum of the head. Axonal injury or shear injury is often coupled with vascular injury. Axonal shearing may occur between white matter bundles and deeper subcortical neuronal structures such as the basal ganglia and thalamus and within the upper brain stem where the cerebrum rotates on its axis. This shearing injury coupled with vascular injury is classically observed as petechial hemorrhages in white matter and commonly referred to as diffuse axonal injury (DAI). Impact depolarization occurs at the time of severe impact injury, resulting in the release of the excitatory amino acid glutamate and with massive increases in extracellular potassium, which initiates excitotoxicity. This cascade plays a crucial role in secondary injury and is discussed later. The neurologic impact due to axonal shearing can present as a transient loss of consciousness or as profound and persistent neurologic deficits, even leading to death.

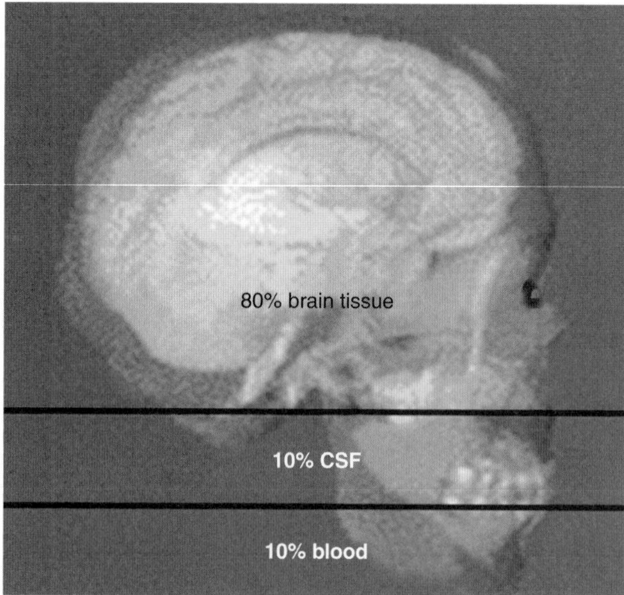

Figure 17-1. Monro-Kellie doctrine. The Monro-Kellie doctrine states that the cranial compartment is incompressible and that the volume inside the cranium is a fixed volume. The cranium and its constituents (blood, cerebrospinal fluid [CSF], and brain tissue) create a state of volume equilibrium such that any increase in volume of one of the cranial constituents must be compensated by a decrease in volume of another.

Concussion

The term *concussion* is often used to describe the constellation of symptoms that occur after mild to moderate TBI when no hematoma nor other intracranial pathologic process is identified. Classic symptoms include headache, nausea, vomiting, difficulty concentrating, retrograde and/or anterograde amnesia, and personality changes. These findings are the result of neuronal dysfunction and axonal injury that can occur even after a mild TBI. Complete recovery after concussion injury is common. However, long-term consequences have been described and include impaired attention and working memory and slowed processing speed.

PATHOPHYSIOLOGY

The intracranial contents include brain parenchymal tissue, cerebrospinal fluid (CSF), and blood. The brain parenchyma accounts for approximately 80% of the intracranial contents, with the remainder being evenly distributed between CSF and blood. The majority of the CSF is in the subarachnoid spaces, and the remainder is in the ventricles, with the postcapillary circulation containing most of the intracranial blood.

The Monro-Kellie doctrine is a simple, yet vitally important concept relating to the understanding of ICP dynamics (Fig. 17-1). Given that the cranium is a rigid, nonexpansile container, it states that the total volume of the intracranial contents must remain constant and any increase in the volume of one component must be at the expense of the others, assuming the intracranial volume remains constant. Thus, very early after injury, a mass such as an expanding hematoma may be enlarging while the ICP remains normal. Once the limit of displacement of CSF and intravascular blood has been reached, ICP rapidly increases (Fig. 17-2). In children with distensible skulls, there is controversy about the application of this principle. Some argue that the open fontanelle allows for expansion of the intracranial contents and therefore affords increased protection from elevation of ICP. However, studies have indicated that the smaller neural axis of infants and young children results in a less compliant pressure-volume relationship with an increased risk of intracranial hypertension.[12,13] Although this doctrine is important to understanding the dynamics of ICP, it uses a hydraulic approach to the cerebral circulation.

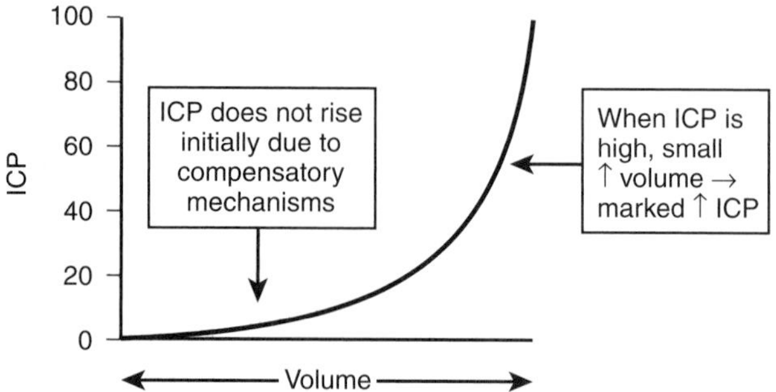

Figure 17-2. Intracranial pressure (ICP)-volume relationship. Small increases in brain volume do not lead to immediate increase in ICP because of the ability of the cerebrospinal fluid to be displaced into the spinal canal as well as the slight ability to stretch the falx cerebri between the hemispheres and the tentorium between the hemispheres and the cerebellum. However, once the ICP has reached around 25 mm Hg, small increases in brain volume can lead to marked elevations in ICP.

Subsequent work has shown that the relationship between ICP and cerebral blood flow (CBF) is much more complex and variable. Whereas simultaneous measurement of ICP and CBF would be most helpful in optimizing therapeutic strategies, the Monro-Kellie doctrine provides a reasonable basic explanation of intracranial dynamics.

CBF is defined as the velocity of blood through the cerebral circulation. In normal adults, CBF is 50 to 55 mL/100 g of brain tissue/min. In children, CBF may be much higher depending on their age. At 1 year of age it approximates adult levels, but at 5 years of age, normal CBF is approximately 90 mL/100 g/min and then gradually declines to adult levels by the mid to late teens. Flow is inversely related to vascular resistance, with resistance increasing as vessel diameter becomes smaller. CBF is proportional to the pressure gradient and, in accordance to Poiseuille's law, inversely proportional to blood viscosity. Brain injury severe enough to cause coma can cause a 50% reduction in CBF during the first 6 to 12 hours after injury.[14,15] It usually increases over the next 2 to 3 days, but for those patients who remain comatose, CBF remains below normal for days or weeks after injury. There is increasing evidence that such low levels of CBF are inadequate to meet the metabolic demands of the brain early after injury and that regional, if not global, cerebral ischemia is common.[16,17]

Cerebral perfusion pressure (CPP) is the differential pressure of arterial inflow and venous outflow to the brain. CPP is considered the transmural pressure gradient that is ultimately the driving force required for supplying cerebral metabolic needs. Intracranial venous pressure is usually slightly less than ICP and CSF pressure. As ICP increases from head injury, the difference between CPP and ICP narrows. At a CPP of 10 mm Hg, blood vessels collapse and blood flow ceases.

Current techniques available to measure CBF are still considered experimental in the management of severe TBI. Such techniques include transcranial Doppler and xenon-enhanced CT imaging. Because CPP is easily determined in the clinical situation in which ICP monitoring is done, it has become a critical parameter for defining treatment options. Studies have shown a good correlation between CPP and CBF in patients with intact cerebral autoregulation.[18] However, cerebral autoregulation is often disrupted after severe TBI and measures of cerebral vascular resistance may be more useful in guiding therapy.[19,20]

Historically, treatment protocols were principally directed toward reducing ICP. Hyperventilation and fluid restriction were important components in these older protocols. Current treatment strategies seek to optimize CPP while reducing ICP, with little reliance on hyperventilation or fluid restriction. Maintenance of a CPP of greater than 70 mm Hg was initially recommended in the adult TBI guidelines developed by the Brain Trauma Foundation. However, more recent studies have shown conflicting data regarding the optimal CPP and how best to achieve it. Current adult evidence-based guidelines recommend maintenance of a 50 to 70 mm Hg CPP. CPP is likely an age-related continuum, thus making problematic treatment protocols based on a single number for all age groups. To date, no study has demonstrated that active maintenance of CPP above any target threshold in pediatric TBI improves mortality or morbidity. However, there seems to be a threshold of less than 40 mm Hg that is associated with increased mortality. Guidelines for pediatric TBI suggest maintenance of CPP greater than 40 mm Hg and a CPP between 40 and 65 mm Hg may be optimal for an individual patient.[11]

Cerebral autoregulation refers to a homeostatic process that allows CBF to remain constant given a wide range of mean arterial pressures (MAP). Arterial vessels can dilate or constrict in response to various physiologic changes, including ICP and systemic arterial pressure to maintain normal flow and normal brain metabolism. In healthy adult patients, CBF remains constant with a MAP between 60 and 160 mm Hg or a CPP between 50 and 150 mm Hg.[21] Normally, reflexive vasoconstriction will occur in the presence of elevated systemic blood pressure to impede intracranial hypertension. In contrast, a moderate decrease in systemic blood pressure will paradoxically result in increased ICP because reflex vasodilatation will occur in compensation. When perfusion pressure falls below 50 mm Hg, cerebral ischemia occurs and compensatory cerebral arteriole vasodilatation is exhausted. When perfusion pressure exceeds 150 mm Hg, cerebral arteriolar impedance is overcome, the affected vessels passively dilate, and fluid is forced through a damaged endothelium into the brain, causing diffuse vasogenic edema. Impaired cerebral autoregulation after TBI and age-related changes in CBF make the immature brain susceptible to secondary injury both from diminished as well as excess CBF. Not only is diminished blood flow and cerebral ischemia associated with poor neurologic outcome, excess CBF, or hyperemia, it is also associated with impaired cerebral autoregulation and poor neurologic outcome.[22]

In addition to changes in CBF, the brain has some structural differences from its adult counterpart that may explain the different responses to injury often seen in children after TBI. The brain doubles in size in the first 6 months of life and reaches approximately 80% of adult size by age 2. The developing brain has a higher water content and incomplete neuronal synapse formation and arborization. In addition, incomplete myelinization and neurochemical changes result in neuronal plasticity after birth. The subarachnoid space is generally smaller and offers less protection than the mature brain, owing to less buoyancy, and thereby provides less protection to the brain parenchyma during changes in head momentum. This contributes to the higher incidence of diffuse cerebral edema and parenchymal injuries in children.

Primary Brain Injury

Primary injury occurs as a result of direct injury to the brain parenchyma due to shear forces at the time of impact. Both cortical disruption and axonal injury can occur, resulting in a cascade of events contributing to secondary brain injury (see later). Cortical disruption, if occurring within minutes to hours, is not likely to be amenable to resuscitative therapy.

Skull fractures occur commonly with head injury and are readily diagnosed with CT. In children, a skull fracture should prompt an evaluation of the underlying brain parenchyma given the significant impact it takes to injure the skull. Fractures of the skull vault can occur in either a linear or a stellate fashion. Fractures involving the skull base are typically associated with a greater force than simple cranial vault fractures. The classic signs of basilar skull fractures include Battle's sign (ecchymoses over the mastoid process associated with an ipsilateral skull fracture), raccoon eyes and CSF rhinorrhea (associated with a cribriform plate fracture), and otorrhea (associated with fracture of the mastoid air cells or temporal bone fracture). Meningitis associated with a basilar skull fracture occurs in 2% to 9%.[23] Despite the risk of infection, the routine use of prophylactic antibiotics is not recommended because this does not prevent meningitis from occurring and tends to select out for resistant organisms.[24,25] Vaccination against *Streptococcus pneumoniae* should be considered for all patients with a basilar skull fracture and CSF leak because of the increased risk of pneumococcal-associated meningitis.[26]

Post-traumatic intracranial hemorrhage includes epidural hematomas, subdural hematomas, and subarachnoid hemorrhages. Epidural hematomas usually occur in the middle fossa and are often associated with an injury to the middle meningeal artery, although they can occur in the anterior or posterior fossa. The classic CT description is a lenticular hematoma, bound by suture lines, because of the tightly bound dura (Fig. 17-3). Clot formation under the calvaria compresses the dura and can cause rapid neurologic deterioration as the brain becomes further displaced. Skull fractures overlying the epidural hematoma are common. The classic presentation of a patient with a lucid interval followed by clinical deterioration is rare in children. Only after the hematoma enlarges is clinical evidence of elevated ICP noted. Typical symptoms include headache, lethargy, emesis, irritability, confusion, and decreased level of consciousness. Progressive deterioration results in seizures, changes in vital signs with hypertension and respiratory instability, pupillary changes, posturing, and cardiovascular compromise. Prompt neurosurgical evacuation is imperative for patient survival and good outcome. Evacuation of extremely large clots (>40 mL) in children often results in very good long-term results, provided that surgical intervention is timely.

Subdural hemorrhages are classified as acute (<3 days old), subacute (3 to 10 days old), and chronic (>10 days old). Acute and subacute subdural hemorrhages are not infrequent in infants, often the result of birth injury or abuse (Fig. 17-4). They usually result from torn or bridging veins or from associated contusions hemorrhaging into the subdural space. The superficial cortical veins in small children lack any reinforcement from arachnoidal trabeculae and

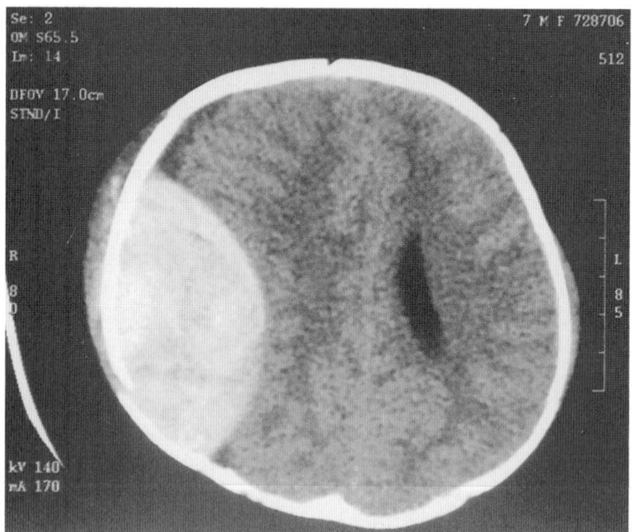

Figure 17-3. CT scan demonstrates a very large epidural hematoma that compresses the right hemisphere and causes midline shift. This 7-month-old patient reportedly fell and became obtunded. On examination, she had a fixed and dilated right pupil. She had a good recovery after immediate surgical evacuation of her epidural hemorrhage, with persistent partial third nerve and facial palsies on the side ipsilateral to the hemorrhage. (Courtesy of Dr. Lisa Lowe.)

are susceptible to inertial loading. Infants are particularly susceptible to the development of a subdural hemorrhage. Subdural hematomas tend to follow the convexities of the brain and cover the entire hemisphere. CT demonstrates hyperdense crescent-shaped

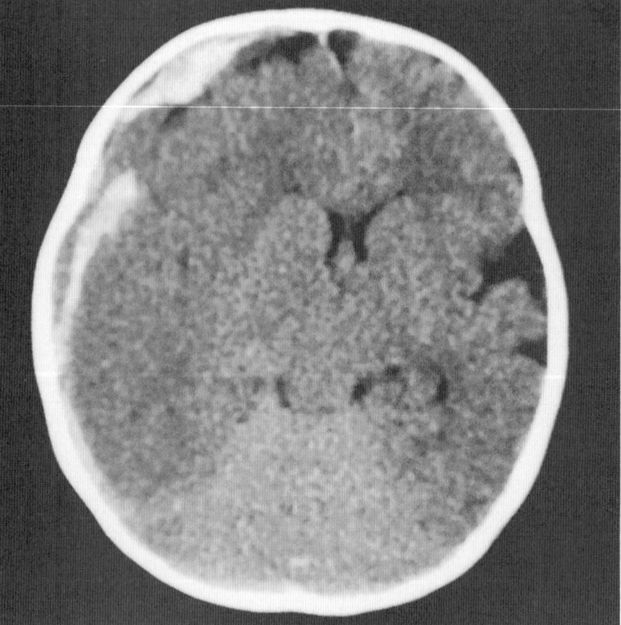

Figure 17-4. Hyperacute subdural bleeding is seen on the right side on this cranial CT scan. Compression of right-sided cerebral structures is found with no intraparenchymal bleeding. Despite immediate craniotomy and evacuation of the subdural blood, the patient had a prolonged convalescence. He is hemiparetic on the left side and has significant developmental and cognitive delay. (Courtesy of Dr. Lisa Lowe.)

blood collections at the surface of the brain, often associated with mass effect and cortical edema. On CT, particularly when anemia is present, acute subdural hematomas may have an isodense appearance that belies their actual hemorrhagic character later found at the time of operation. Surgical intervention is indicated when neurologic deterioration occurs as a result of the combined effect of subdural hemorrhage and parenchymal injury, either from the compressive effect of the subdural blood or from the combined effect of impact forces on the entire cerebrum and diffuse bleeding. In infants, it is possible to tap the subdural space at the level of the fontanelle and produce rapid decompression. Large subdural hematomas with significant mass effect require more extensive craniotomies. Acute subdural hemorrhages are usually associated with a worse prognosis than patients with an epidural hematoma, primarily related to the underlying brain damage.

Subacute subdural hematomas in the context of trauma are much less frequent in the pediatric population. However, they will be seen in emergency settings when they are a cause of neurologic problems and when they are considered a manifestation of previous or recurrent nonaccidental head trauma. As with acute hematomas, subacute subdural hematomas will have a nonspecific presentation. Affected children have both the symptoms of increased ICP (coma, irritability, lethargy, emesis, seizures) and the signs of elevated ICP (frontal bossing, enlarged heads, dilated scalp veins, sun-setting eyes, papilledema, and bulging fontanelles). The CT scan often shows isodense or hypodense fluid collections at the cerebral convexities. MRI studies are often valuable in making the diagnosis of these bleeding events. As with acute subdural hematomas, surgical intervention is often necessary.

Chronic subdural hematomas can cause pathologic elevation of the ICP and may require surgical intervention to control cranial growth and CSF pressure. Patients present with symptoms similar to those of a subacute subdural hematoma. Interventions include serial percutaneous drainage, limited craniotomies to drain and irrigate the subdural space, and subdural/peritoneal shunts.

Subarachnoid bleeding in acutely traumatized children is common and rarely the result of aneurysmal bleeding (Fig. 17-5). Bleeding occurs from disruption of the fragile pia-arachnoidal vasculature. Often this occurs over the convexities of the brain affected by coup type of injuries or the frontotemporal poles affected by contrecoup injuries. Subarachnoid hemorrhage from trauma can also occur in the interhemispheric fissure and in the basilar cisterns. If subarachnoid bleeding is an isolated finding resulting from minor trauma, no specific therapies are indicated except symptomatic amelioration of chemical meningitis, meningismus, and photophobia. Subarachnoid hemorrhage may result in hydrocephalus and may require ventricular shunting to relieve the increased ICP. In patients with severe TBI, subarachnoid hemorrhage is associated with a poor outcome and may be further associated with cerebral vasospasm. Techniques such as transcranial Doppler imaging can be utilized to identify vasospasm. Nimodipine, a calcium channel blocking agent, has been used in vasospasm occurring in the setting of postaneurysmal subarachnoid bleeding. Nimodipine is not often used in the context of TBI, in part because of its hypotensive effects. Moreover, in children, there are little data looking at its efficacy in the setting of post-TBI subarachnoidal bleeding.[27,28]

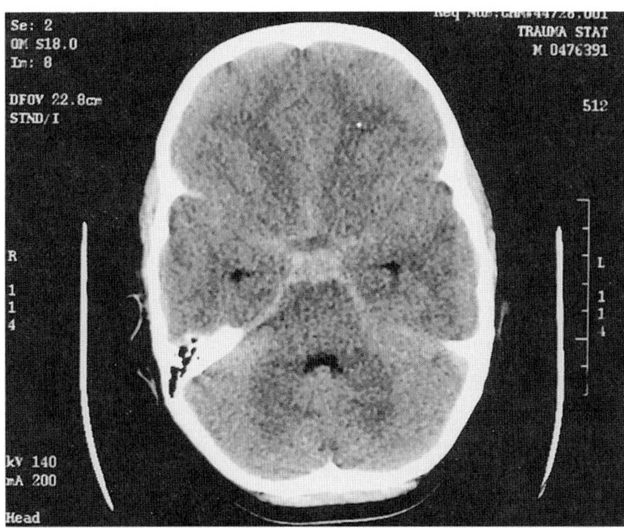

Figure 17-5. Subarachnoid hemorrhage secondary to trauma is present on this cranial CT scan without contrast. Blood is seen in the perimesencephalic, prepontine, and suprasellar cisterns. The patient was involved in a motor vehicle accident and complained of headache. He was neurologically normal. (Courtesy of Dr. Lisa Lowe.)

Secondary Brain Injury

The cornerstone of management of TBI is the prevention of secondary injuries. Secondary brain injury includes both the evolution of damage within the brain related to a cascade of macroscopic and microscopic events as described here and the effects of secondary insults, including hypoxia and hypotension. Endogenous secondary brain injury involves the macroscopic cascade of edema, ischemia, necrosis, elevated ICP, and inadequate CPP. The cellular changes after TBI have been the focus of much research, and several cellular mechanisms have been elucidated and are described later.

Brain swelling or edema traditionally has been described as either vasogenic or cytotoxic. Vasogenic edema results from the disruption of the blood-brain barrier. The blood-brain barrier is maintained by tight junctions between endothelial cells that line the vessels of the brain. Injury to these cells allows extravasation of fluid and proteins into the interstitial space of the brain parenchyma. Disruption of these cells may occur from the primary impact injury or result from free radical formation, cytokines, and other secondary mechanisms of brain injury. Cytotoxic edema is edema of the cells themselves, resulting from a failure of cellular ion homeostasis and membrane function. The time course of brain edema is variable. It is thought, however, that vasogenic edema occurs early after injury and cytotoxic edema occurs in a more delayed fashion.

Edema of the brain is an important marker for injury and is also a cause of secondary injury. In children, rapid formation of edema is commonly seen on serial CT scans after trauma. In early (<24 hours after injury), fatal closed-head injuries in children, CT scans often demonstrate little or no significant parenchymal bleeding. However, diffuse brain swelling is seen with obliteration of the ventricles and loss of the basilar cisterns and subarachnoid space. As edema progresses and the compensatory mechanisms of the brain are exhausted, ICP increases markedly with small changes in intracranial volume (see Fig. 17-2). Cerebral edema typically develops early after injury, typically peaking at 72 to 96 hours and then gradually resorbs over the course of a week in survivors.[29]

Sustained elevations in ICP above 20 mm Hg are poorly tolerated by the injured brain and have been associated with poor neurologic outcome and increased mortality in pediatric patients.[30] Sustained elevation in ICP may result in cerebral ischemia if cerebral perfusion is impaired and ultimately may result in cerebral herniation.

Studies in adults utilizing xenon CT have shown a reduction in CBF that occurs early after severe TBI.[14,31] This hypoperfusion may be further exacerbated by hypotension and hypoxia. It is clear that this early hypoperfusion or ischemia occurring after severe TBI is associated with poor outcome.[32,33] Proposed mediators involved in early post-traumatic ischemia include direct vascular disruption, production of endothelin-1 (a potent vasoconstrictor), loss of endogenous vasodilators (endogenous nitric oxide synthase), and likely many other complex, interrelated cellular and metabolic events.

The release of excitatory amino acids, such as glutamate, results in neuronal injury after TBI. Glutamate is the most studied and most abundant neurotransmitter in the brain. However, toxic levels cause neuronal cell death.[34,35] After TBI, glutamate and other excitatory amino acids are released, resulting in neuronal swelling. Glutamate works on a variety of receptors; the best demonstrated is the *N*-methyl-D-aspartate (NMDA) receptor, which results in large fluxes of calcium into the neuron. The resultant stimulation of enzymes leads to cell death with the breakdown of the cytoskeleton, free radical formation, alterations in gene expression and protein synthesis, and membrane dysfunction. Studies have failed to demonstrate efficacy of anti-excitotoxic therapies, perhaps owing to their application in all patients with TBI rather than those with excitotoxicity and because treatment may have been initiated too late.[36]

Oxidative stress with free radical formation is an important mechanism leading to secondary injury. Free radicals are molecules or atoms possessing an unpaired electron in the outer orbit, making them highly reactive. Free radicals damage endothelial cells and injure the brain parenchyma. This results in disruption of the blood-brain barrier and resultant vasogenic and cytotoxic edema. Free radical scavengers, such as vitamin E, ascorbic acid, and superoxide dismutase attempt to minimize injury by binding with the free radicals. However, these mechanisms often become overwhelmed and the process becomes self-perpetuating. Clinical studies are ongoing to identify pharmacologic free radical scavenging agents.

Apoptosis requires a cascade of intracellular events for completion of cell death and is thus termed *programmed cell death*. The signals for cell death have now been elucidated in vitro and are becoming more clearly understood in vivo. Calcium influx into the cell, oxidative stress, and energy depletion all appear to be important intracellular triggers of apoptosis. Knowledge of the mechanisms involved in cellular signaling of apoptosis is important in the development of new therapeutic approaches to the management of TBI. As our understanding of the complex biochemical, cellular, and molecular responses to TBI progresses, application of therapeutic strategies and agents may help halt the secondary injury processes.

INITIAL EVALUATION AND MANAGEMENT OF HEAD INJURY

The key principles of management after TBI rest on the foundation of the Monro-Kellie doctrine and the avoidance of secondary brain injury. Interventions that decrease CSF and hyperemia, while ensuring adequate oxygenation and blood flow, form the basis for all management strategies discussed here.

The initial management and resuscitation, as with any trauma management, begins with the assessment of airway, breathing, and circulation. Ensuring adequate oxygenation and ventilation and promptly addressing sources of ongoing blood loss serve as the basic principles in the management of persons suspected or confirmed to have head injury. Hypotension and hypoxia in the field are proven secondary injury insults that are associated with poor outcomes, with hypotension being considerably more detrimental than hypoxia.[32,37] There has been no documented advantage to endotracheal intubation over effective bag-valve-mask ventilation in the field.[38,39] Providers inexperienced in pediatric airway management should defer endotracheal intubation. Efforts should be made to control bleeding, including scalp lacerations, which may be a source of shock in the pediatric patient. The administration of isotonic crystalloid solution should be utilized to promptly restore the intravascular volume. The withholding of fluid because of concerns of concomitant head injury is unjustified and may contribute to secondary brain injury with ineffective CBF. Young children are prone to hypoglycemia; however, hypoglycemia occurring early after trauma is rare. Hyperglycemia may be detrimental during periods of cellular hypoxia owing to a shift to anaerobic metabolism and lactate production. Therefore, unless there is documented hypoglycemia, dextrose-containing fluids should be avoided in the early phases of resuscitation.

Current recommendations do not support ICP-directed measures in the field, even if the patient has focal or lateralizing signs, such as a decreased level of consciousness and an enlarging pupil, with the possible exception of hyperventilation and hyperosmolar therapy for signs of herniation.[11,40] Every effort should be made to transport the patient to a pediatric trauma center or to an adult center equipped to manage pediatric trauma patients. Careful attention should be paid to cervical spine immobilization because there is an increased risk of spinal cord injury with TBI.

On arrival in the emergency department, the Advanced Trauma Life Support (ATLS) protocol of the American College of Surgeons should be followed.[41] This provides a systematic approach to the traumatized patient and emphasizes evaluation and management of airway, breathing, and circulation first. Early hospital evaluation and management is the same as that described for the prehospital setting. Placement of a secure airway utilizing endotracheal intubation should be performed in the initial hospital management if not already performed in the prehospital setting. After initial stabilization and fluid resuscitation, a brief neurologic examination should be performed, preferably before the administration of sedation and neuromuscular blockade. Adjunctive diagnostic studies should be performed only after the initial resuscitation phase.

The severity of brain injury is often classified using the modified Glasgow Coma Scale (GCS) score.[42] Even with modifications, the GCS score has limitations in its use for infants and very young children (Table 17-1). In addition, the use of sedation and pharmacologic paralysis, orbital swelling making eye opening impossible, endotracheal intubation making verbal responses impossible, and preexisting conditions such as alterations in motor function further limit the use of the GCS score. Nonetheless, it is the best tool currently available to classify TBI and to share information between treating physicians.

Table 17-1 Modified Glasgow Coma Scale for Infants and Children

Child	Infant	Score
Eye Opening		
Spontaneous	Spontaneous	4
To verbal stimuli	To verbal stimuli	3
To pain only	To pain only	2
No response	No response	1
Verbal Response		
Oriented, appropriate	Coos and babbles	5
Confused	Irritable cries	4
Inappropriate words	Cries to pain	3
Incomprehensible words or nonspecific sounds	Moans to pain	2
No response	No response	1
Motor Response		
Obeys commands	Moves spontaneously and purposefully	6
Localizes painful stimulus	Withdraws to touch	5
Withdraws in response to pain	Withdraws in response to pain	4
Flexion in response to pain	Decorticate posturing (abnormal flexion) in response to pain	3
Extension in response to pain	Decerebrate posturing (abnormal extension) in response to pain	2
No response	No response	1

Mild TBI: GCS 14-15

Approximately 80% of patients presenting to the emergency department with brain injury are categorized as having a mild brain injury. These patients may have a brief loss of consciousness and be amnestic to the events surrounding the injury. Most patients with mild TBI recover fully. However, a small percentage of patients will experience deterioration, resulting in severe neurologic dysfunction unless prompt recognition and resuscitation is performed. All patients should have a general examination to exclude other injuries and a limited neurologic examination. Adjunctive studies such as cervical spine evaluation and other imaging studies should also be performed as needed. Although less common in younger children, alcohol or other intoxicants can confuse the findings and make examination results unreliable. Neuroimaging is essential in the evaluation in all but the completely asymptomatic and neurologically normal patient. Unenhanced, or noncontrast, CT is the initial and most reliable diagnostic tool, particularly for identifying bleeding.

Patients who are asymptomatic, fully awake and alert, and neurologically normal may be observed for several hours and safely discharged. It is imperative that they be discharged with a reliable caretaker and one who understands the signs and symptoms that should prompt emergent re-evaluation. Discharge instructions should be given in both written and verbal format. When appropriate, a follow-up visit should be scheduled with the patient's primary care provider. Admission to the hospital should be considered for patients with penetrating injuries, a history of loss of consciousness or a deteriorating level of consciousness, moderate to severe headache, intoxication, skull fracture, or lack of availability of CT. Additionally, all patients with a CSF leak or other significant associated injuries should be admitted for observation.

Moderate TBI: GCS 9-13

Approximately 10% of patients presenting with TBI will fall into the moderate category. They should undergo the same initial examination as those presenting with mild TBI but additionally will need laboratory studies and CT. All patients should be admitted to a facility with definitive neurosurgical care. Frequent re-evaluation of neurologic status is imperative. Approximately 90% of patients with moderate TBI will improve and will be discharged from the hospital. Ten percent experience deterioration of their condition and require management as described next for severe TBI. An emergent repeat CT should be performed in those whose condition deteriorates.

Severe TBI: GCS 3-8

The treatment of severe TBI begins with the fundamentals of resuscitation previously described including restoration of an adequate circulating blood volume, blood pressure support, appropriate ventilation, and adequate oxygenation. Patients with severe head injury often have multisystem injuries and require a multidisciplinary team to aggressively identify and treat all injuries. An evidence-based approach to resuscitation and treatment of patients with severe brain injury is presented in Figure 17-6.[11]

Respiratory Monitoring and Management

Ensuring adequate oxygenation to avoid worsening of neuronal ischemia is essential. If the patient did not have an endotracheal tube placed in the field, the airway should be secured, with special attention paid to avoidance of hypoxia, hypercarbia, or hypocarbia. Ventilation should be provided with a goal $Paco_2$ of 35 to 40 mm Hg. The cerebral vasculature is sensitive to changes in the $Paco_2$. In the head-injured patient, hypercapnia ($Paco_2$ > 45 mm Hg) can cause significant elevation in ICP because of CO_2-induced dilatation of the cerebral vasculature resulting in increased cerebral blood volume and flow. The immediate effect of hyperventilation is a reduction of ICP, although this response is neither universal nor sustained. Hyperventilation reduces ICP by causing cerebral vasoconstriction, with a subsequent reduction in CBF in reactive vascular beds. Hyperventilation should be reserved for those patients with obvious signs of brain stem herniation, often hallmarked by Cushing's triad (abnormal respiratory pattern, hypertension, and bradycardia) and nonreactive, dilated pupils.

Patient Positioning

The head of the bed should be elevated at 15 to 30 degrees and the head maintained in the midline position to facilitate venous drainage from the head, thus allowing maintenance of cerebral perfusion. Temperature management will be discussed in more detail later; however, avoidance of hyperthermia is important in early brain resuscitation.[43] Moreover, patients who are identified early in resuscitation to have isolated head trauma and have hypothermia should undergo passive rewarming.

Acute Surgical Management

A CT scan should be obtained promptly in all patients after initial resuscitation and stabilization. Patients with intracerebral hematomas causing a mass effect should undergo prompt neurosurgical evacuation. The traditional definition of a significant mass effect has been greater than 5 mm of midline shift. Midline shift is measured on axial views of the CT scan. A line is drawn at the midline of the skull in the sagittal plane and then a perpendicular line is extended to the septum pellucidum. The basilar cisterns are also evaluated for compression.

Sedation and Analgesia

Sedation and analgesia are commonly used in children with TBI. However, there is little clinical evidence guiding their use. Sedation and analgesia can help facilitate the care of the patient including maintenance of the airway and placement of invasive catheters or other monitoring devices. These measures can also facilitate the transport of the patient for diagnostic or therapeutic procedures. Sedation and analgesia may be useful in maintaining or decreasing ICP by decreasing the metabolic rate and thereby decreasing CBF. Studies have demonstrated a twofold to threefold increase in basal metabolic rate for oxygen accompanying painful or stressful stimuli. Noxious stimuli, such as suctioning, can increase ICP. Painful and noxious stimuli and stress can also increase sympathetic tone, resulting in hypertension and bleeding from operative sites.[44,45] However, these medications must be used with caution, because sedative or narcotic related vasodilatation may decrease CBF with resulting hypotension or conversely increase CBF by causing cerebral vasodilatation.

Intracranial Pressure Monitoring and Management

The use of ICP devices has become standard in this country in the treatment of severe head injury, even in the absence of prospective, randomized clinical trials to establish efficacy in improving outcome. There are two lines of evidence to support the use of ICP monitoring in the pediatric TBI patient. There is strong evidence that supports the association between intracranial hypertension and poor neurologic outcome.[46] Second, ICP monitoring and aggressive treatment of intracranial hypertension are associated with the best reported clinical outcomes.[47] The "Guidelines for the Acute Management of Severe Traumatic Brain Injury in Infants, Children, and Adolescents" recommend that ICP monitoring may be considered in patients with a GCS score less than 8.[11] The guidelines also state that the presence of open fontanelles and/or sutures in an infant does not preclude the development of intracranial hypertension or negate the utility of ICP monitoring. The treatment threshold for intracranial hypertension is typically defined as an ICP

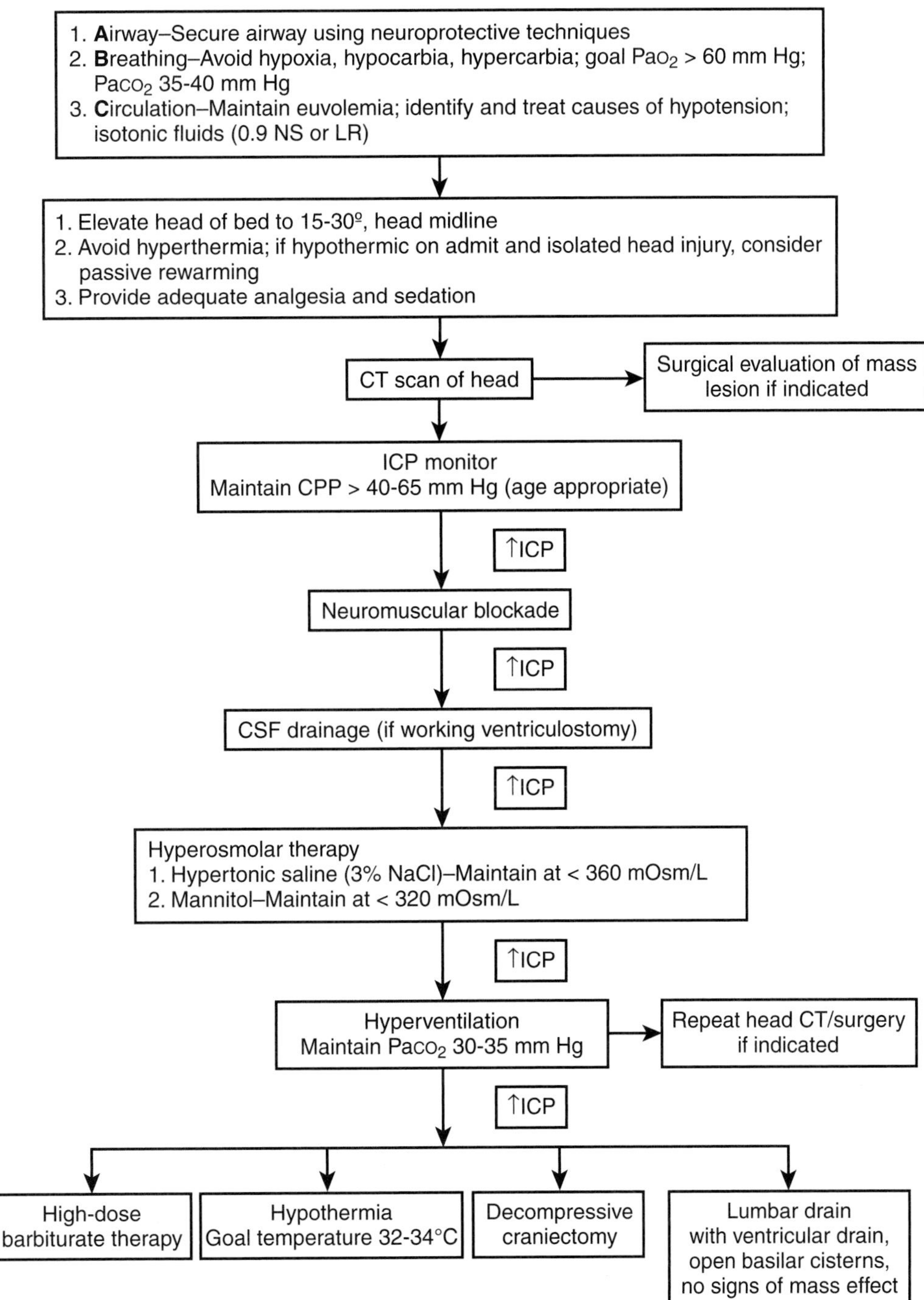

Figure 17-6. This algorithm provides an evidence-based approach for treatment of pediatric patients with severe head trauma. NS, normal saline; LR, lactated Ringer's; ICP, intracranial pressure; CSF, cerebrospinal fluid.

greater than 20 mm Hg. Age-specific and injury mechanism–specific ICP thresholds have yet to be defined. In more recent years, focus has switched from ICP-directed therapy to CPP-directed therapy and is discussed later.

Although there is no single ICP monitoring device that is superior to the others, intraventricular devices are effective monitors that allow CSF drainage as part of treatment of ICP. Ventricular CSF drainage may serve as a treatment option in the setting of refractory intracranial hypertension. However, if not placed early after injury, placement may be difficult when damaged brain and cerebral edema have effaced the normal ventricle. Intraparenchymal monitors have fiberoptic or strain-gauge transducers that provide continuous pressure readings and can be placed, with relative ease, in any region of the brain. Newer monitors can measure brain tissue oxygen levels and permit manipulations to optimize regional oxygenation, including adjustments in the fraction of inspired oxygen (FIO_2)

and blood transfusion. Coagulation abnormalities are a relative contraindication to the insertion of these devices. Therefore, prompt correction using plasma or activated factor VIIa should be considered before placement.[48]

The optimal CPP for a given individual is not clear. Global and/or regional cerebral ischemia commonly complicates brain injury. Studies have consistently shown that a CPP less than 40 mm Hg is associated with increased mortality.[46,49] A CPP between 40 and 65 mm Hg likely represents an age-related continuum with interindividual variability. Studies have suggested that avoidance of hypotension, rather than elevation of CPP, is beneficial.[46] Efforts to increase CPP in adults to a supernormal level with the use of fluids and vasoactive infusions are associated with significant risks, including pulmonary complications, fluid overload, pressor toxicity, and renal insufficiency. Furthermore, in cases of disrupted autoregulation, exacerbation of intracranial hypertension can result.

Neuromuscular Blockade

Neuromuscular blockade is commonly used as a treatment strategy for patients with increased ICP. Neuromuscular blocking agents should be used only in those patients with a secure airway, who are mechanically ventilated and adequately sedated. The proposed mechanisms of neuromuscular blocking agents in reducing ICP include a reduction in airway and intrathoracic pressure with facilitation of cerebral venous outflow and prevention of shivering, posturing, or breathing against the ventilator.[50] Neuromuscular blockade should be reserved for the patient with increased ICP who is unresponsive to sedation and analgesia because its use has been associated with prolonged ICU stays and increased risk of nosocomial infections.

Hyperosmolar Therapy

The use of hyperosmolar agents to decrease ICP was first described in the early 1900s. Hypertonic saline and mannitol were among the first agents used, and mannitol has become the mainstay of therapy over the past couple decades. The mechanism of action of mannitol has been well studied. However, its effect on survival and functional outcome after TBI has not been well demonstrated. Mannitol has two primary mechanisms. The first is an initial rheologic effect, resulting in a decrease in blood viscosity that occurs within minutes of administration. A resultant decrease in blood vessel diameter occurs as a result of autoregulation with reflex vasoconstriction that leads to a decrease in cerebral blood volume and ICP.[51] Second, mannitol acts as a potent osmotic diuretic, thus pulling fluid from the interstitial space into the intravascular space. Because of its diuretic effect, intravascular volume can be depleted with the risk of decreasing cerebral perfusion, resulting in secondary brain ischemia. Careful attention must be paid to promptly replenishing intravascular volume. Another reported risk of mannitol therapy is acute tubular necrosis. Monitoring of serum osmolarity is recommended when using mannitol, with osmolar levels greater than 320 mOsm/L to be avoided. Most of the reports showing the development of renal damage occurred in the era of dehydration therapy for cerebral edema. It is unclear whether the same osmolar thresholds are valid in the current era of maintaining normal intravascular volume. The beneficial effects of mannitol are best achieved with rapid bolus administration, with dosage ranges of 0.25 to 1.0 g/kg. Chronic administration of mannitol has been associated with a reverse osmotic shift resulting in rebound cerebral edema and disruption of the blood-brain barrier.

More recently, hypertonic saline has re-emerged as a hyperosmolar agent and is the preferred agent in the TBI patient with hypovolemia.[52,53] Hypertonic saline includes 3% to 23.4% saline, with 3% saline the most studied in pediatrics. There is no evidence that one concentration is more effective than another for reducing intracranial hypertension. Similar to mannitol, hypertonic saline requires the presence of an intact blood-brain barrier to exert its effect. Hypertonic saline is an osmolar agent and it pulls fluid from the interstitium into the intravascular space, without a strong diuretic effect, thus maintaining blood volume and resultant cerebral perfusion. Hypertonic saline can be used as a bolus (3 to 5 mL/kg) or continuous infusion (0.1 to 1.0 mL/kg/hr titrated to the minimum dose needed to achieve a reduction in ICP). In addition to the hyperosmolar effect, hypertonic saline has been reported to have several other potentially beneficial effects for the trauma patient, including vasoregulatory, hemodynamic, neurochemical, and immunologic properties. Serum osmolarity of 360 mOsm/L has been reported with the use of hypertonic saline and has been well tolerated in the pediatric patient with a head injury.[52] The primary theoretical concerns associated with the risk of hypertonic saline include the development of central pontine myelinolysis (rapid shrinking of the brain associated with mechanical tearing of bridging vessels leading to subarachnoid hemorrhage), renal failure, and rebound intracranial hypertension (Table 17-2).

Prophylactic administration of mannitol or other hyperosmolar therapy either in the field or in the hospital is no longer routinely recommended. Hyperosmolar therapy should be reserved for those patients with documented intracranial hypertension or those with signs of impending herniation to avoid potential secondary injury and complications associated with hyperosmolar therapy.

Anticonvulsant Prophylaxis

Anticonvulsants are often administered to patients with TBI. Current clinical evidence supports their use to prevent early post-traumatic seizures, which are typically defined as seizures occurring within the first 7 days after injury. Early post-traumatic seizures occur with a greater frequency in infants and children with severe TBI than adults. They may further increase brain metabolic demands, may increase ICP, and may

Table 17-2 A Comparison of Mannitol and Hypertonic Saline (for Hyperosmolar Therapy)

	Mannitol	3% Hypertonic Saline
Bolus dosing guidelines	0.25-1.0 g/kg rapid bolus	3-5 mL/kg
Infusion guidelines	None	0.1-1.0 mL/kg/hr
Effectiveness	May wane with repeated administration	Effective after repeated administration; effective when mannitol efficacy has waned
Augmentation of MAP	Moderate	Greater, more prolonged
Rheologic properties	Yes	Yes
Diuretic effect	Osmotic diuretic, may necessitate volume replacement to avoid hypovolemia	Diuresis through action of atrial natriuretic peptide
Maximum serum osmolarity	320 mOsm/L	360 mOsm/L
Adverse effects	Renal failure, hypotension, rebound elevation in ICP	Rebound elevation in ICP, central pontine myelinolysis, bleeding, electrolyte abnormal
Proposed beneficial effects	Antioxidant effects	Restoration of resting membrane potential and cell volume, inhibition of inflammation

MAP, mean arterial pressure; ICP, intracranial pressure.
From Knapp JM: Hyperosmolar therapy in the treatment of severe head injury in children: Mannitol and hypertonic saline. AACN Clin Issues 16: 199-211, 2005. Reprinted with permission.

lead to secondary brain injury. Prophylactic anticonvulsants do not prevent late (occurring > 7 days from injury) post-traumatic seizures.

Medically Refractory Intracranial Hypertension

It is estimated that 21% to 42% of children with severe TBI will develop refractory intracranial hypertension despite medical and surgical management.[11] In this population of children, therapies and interventions with higher risk profiles may need to be considered. Decompressive craniectomy, high-dose barbiturate therapy, hyperventilation, lumbar drain placement, and the use of moderate hypothermia should be considered in the patient with medically refractory intracranial hypertension.

Decompressive Craniectomy

Children are more likely than adults to have diffuse brain swelling after TBI and may be more amenable to a treatment strategy utilizing early decompressive craniectomy. Decompressive craniectomy should be considered in children with severe TBI and medically refractory intracranial hypertension in infants with abusive head trauma. The main goal of decompressive craniectomy is to control ICP, thereby maintaining CPP and cerebral oxygenation. Improved outcomes have been demonstrated in several small single-center studies, and it appears to be most effective when done early, before the development of extensive secondary brain injury.[54,55]

Barbiturate Therapy

High doses of barbiturates are known to reduce ICP and have been used in the management of increased ICP for decades. Their side effects limit their current use to those patients with injuries refractory to first-line therapies. Barbiturates are effective in lowering ICP by suppression of brain metabolism and altering vascular tone. In addition to the ICP-lowering benefits, barbiturates also inhibit free radical–mediated lipid peroxidation and have membrane-stabilizing effects. Small case series of children with severe TBI suggest that barbiturates may be effective in lowering ICP in the setting of refractory intracranial hypertension.[56,57] Their use is associated with myocardial depression, increased risk of hypotension, and the need for blood pressure support with intravascular fluids and inotropic infusions. It is important that barbiturates be used in the setting of systemic monitoring with the ability to rapidly detect hemodynamic instability.

Hyperventilation

Hyperventilation has been a mainstay in the management of severe TBI, but more recent concerns about its role in cerebral ischemia have lessened its use. As discussed previously, the cerebral vasculature is sensitive to changes in $Paco_2$, with hypocarbia producing cerebral vasoconstriction and a resultant decrease in CBF. Historically, hyperemia, or excessive CBF, was thought to be the primary mechanism resulting in cerebral edema after TBI, thus making hyperventilation a reasonable approach to the management of the patient with severe TBI. More recent pediatric studies have demonstrated that hyperemia is uncommon after severe TBI. Hyperventilation may decrease cerebral oxygenation, resulting in secondary brain ischemia.[58,59] Aggressive hyperventilation ($Paco_2 < 30$ mm Hg) may be considered for refractory intracranial hypertension. Monitoring of CBF, jugular venous oxygen saturation, or brain tissue oxygenation may help identify cerebral ischemia in this setting.

Lumbar Drain

Placement of a lumbar drain can be considered in patients with refractory intracranial hypertension that is unresponsive to the first-line therapies. It is recommended that the patient have a working ventriculostomy in place or documentation of open basilar cisterns on CT.

Therapeutic Hypothermia

The avoidance of hyperthermia and use of therapeutic hypothermia after TBI is based on the rationale that temperature plays an important role in mechanisms contributing to secondary brain injury (excitotoxicity, free radical formation). Despite evidence in animal models demonstrating efficacy of therapeutic moderate hypothermia (32°-34°C), large randomized clinical studies in both adults and children have been unable to prove the effectiveness of hypothermia on improved outcome after TBI.[60-65] Studies extrapolated from the adult literature indicate that hyperthermia adversely affects outcome, and it may be advisable to consider passive rewarming of the mild to moderately hypothermic trauma patient with isolated head injury.[43]

CONCLUSION

With continued advancements in medical care, more children are surviving TBI.[10] The highest mortality rates occur in children younger than 2 years of age and older than 15 years of age. Survivor outcomes range from full recovery to severe physical and/or mental disabilities. Generally, children and adolescents recover better than those older than 21 years. The immature brain is very susceptible to secondary brain injury, and an open fontanelle may mask signs until rapid decompensation occurs.

chapter 18

PEDIATRIC ORTHOPEDIC TRAUMA

Gregory A. Mencio, MD • Michael T. Rohmiller, MD • Neil E. Green, MD

Musculoskeletal trauma is the most common emergency condition in children.[1] In children ages 1 to 14, accidents are the leading cause of death.[2] However, most orthopedic injuries sustained by children are not life threatening. The chance of a child sustaining a fracture before age 16 is 42% for boys and 27% for girls.[3] It has been estimated that between 1% and 2% of children present with a fracture each year.[4] As participation in sporting and recreational activities increases, the number of fractures is likely to increase. A 2006 study looking at the impact of trauma on an urban pediatric orthopedic practice demonstrated that fracture treatment (both operative and nonoperative) accounted for approximately one third of the total work-related relative value units generated by this group.[5] The most common fractures seen were of the distal radius (23%), forearm (14%), tibia (13%), and elbow (10%). The most common fracture-related operations were performed on the elbow (23%), tibia (12%), femur (9.8%), forearm (5.5%), and the distal aspect of the radius (5%).

Patient gender, age, climate, time of day, and social situation in the home have been shown to impact the frequency of orthopedic injuries. In children, boys sustain fractures at 2.7 times the rate of girls.[6] However, as girls become more involved in athletic events, this margin may narrow. It has been shown that fracture location varies with chronologic age, a finding that is probably due to a combination of the anatomic maturation of the child and the age-specific activities of childhood.[3] Several authors have shown that fractures are more common during the summer months when children are out of school.[4,6,7] It has also been shown that there is a strong association between sunshine and fractures and a negative association between rain and fractures.[8] Likewise, two studies have documented that the afternoon is the most frequent time for fractures to occur.[9,10] This correlates with the time of peak activity for children. Injuries in the home during the late afternoon and evening account for more than 83% of all injuries to children.[11] Moreover, the overall incidence of fractures occurring at home increases with the age of the child.[4,12] In a Swedish study, the physical quality of the home environment did not correlate well with the fracture incidence.[13] The major correlation was with the degree of social handicaps such as welfare or alcoholism in the family. Similarly, a study from Manitoba elicited the social situation at home as a major influence of children's injuries.[14]

No discussion of pediatric orthopedic trauma is complete that does not include a discussion of nonaccidental trauma. The incidence of physical abuse to children is estimated to be 4.9 per 1000. Of those abused, 1 of every 1000 will ultimately die as a result.[15] Early recognition and reporting of nonaccidental trauma is essential because children who return home after hospitalization with unrecognized abuse have a 25% risk of serious injury and a 5% risk of death.[16] Children at highest risk for abuse are first-born children, premature infants, stepchildren, and handicapped children.[17] Most cases of child abuse involve children younger than 3 years of age. Any child presenting with fractures, particularly if they involve the long bones, should be viewed with circumspection as to the cause.[18]

PATHOPHYSIOLOGY

The major difference between children and adults is that children are constantly growing. In the immature skeleton, longitudinal and appositional growth takes place through the physes (growth plates) that are located at the ends of the long bones, in the end plates of the vertebral bodies, or at the periphery of the round bones in the feet and hands. Thus, the physis is essential for normal skeletal growth but is also the weakest portion of the bone in children. Consequently, fractures in children frequently involve this structure. It is estimated that in children approximately 30% of fractures of the long bones include an injury to the physis.[19-21] Most fractures that involve the growth plates heal without consequence. However, some injuries can result in permanent damage with significant sequelae such as angular deformity or complete cessation of growth.

The ends of every long bone consist of an epiphysis (near the joint), physis, and metaphysis (area of newly formed bone). At the time of skeletal maturity, the physis closes, which means there is no further longitudinal growth. Fracture healing in children is rapid and the potential for remodeling is great due to the growth potential and dynamism of the immature skeleton. These characteristics allow for nonoperative treatment of some fractures in children that demand operative treatment in skeletally mature patients. Remodeling of fractures predictably occurs in the plane of primary motion of the adjacent joint (usually flexion/extension), to a lesser degree in the coronal plane (varus and valgus deformities), and is virtually nonexistent in the transverse plane with rotational malalignment.[22]

Classification of fractures is done to predict outcome and guide treatment. Fractures in children are classified according to the pattern of involvement. Currently, most orthopedic surgeons use the Salter-Harris classification (Fig. 18-1).[23] Type I injuries involve the physis only and may be missed on radiographs if they are not displaced. Type II injuries start in the physis and exit the metaphysis. Type III injuries involve the physis and epiphysis, exiting into the joint, and type IV fractures involve both the epiphysis and metaphysis. Classic teaching states that type I and II injuries heal without growth abnormalities if reduced appropriately. More recent literature disputes some of this dogma.[24-26] Type III and IV injuries usually occur in older children and require anatomic realignment via open reduction to restore congruity of the joint to minimize the risk of arthritis. Also, it restores continuity of the physis to decrease the risk of growth disturbance. Type V injuries are crush injuries and are not usually recognized at presentation, but this pattern carries a high risk of growth arrest.[27]

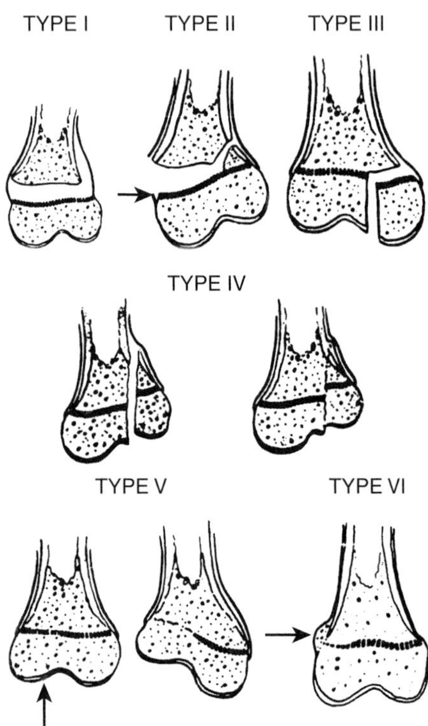

Figure 18-1. Salter-Harris classification of physeal injuries with Rang modification. (From Rang ML [ed]: The Growth Plate and Its Disorders. Edinburgh, E&S Livingstone, 1969, p 139.)

COMPLEX INJURIES

Children sustain injuries that are different from adults owing to their size and activities. A common example is a pedestrian struck by a car. An adult will frequently sustain an injury to the tibia or knee from the car's bumper. However, the same mechanism will result in a fracture of the femur or pelvis and a chest or head injury in a small child.[28] Motor vehicle accidents (MVAs) are the most common cause of multiple injuries to children, both as occupants and pedestrians.[28,29] Although not restricted to MVAs, spine trauma is frequently seen in the child with multiple injuries. Awareness of the possibility of cervical spine trauma is mandatory in any child who presents with facial injuries.[30,31] Likewise, ecchymosis in the lower abdomen consistent with the lap belt portion of the seat belt should alert the physician to the possibility of significant intra-abdominal and/or spine injury.[32-34] Frequently seen with the use of lap belts without shoulder restraint, the lap belt syndrome consists of flexion-distraction injuries to the lumbar spine (Chance fracture), hollow viscus rupture, and traumatic pancreatitis (Fig. 18-2).[35] This terminology has evolved to include a wider spectrum of intra-abdominal hollow viscus, solid organ, and vascular injuries that can occur in conjunction with a characteristic flexion-distraction injury to the spine. This injury occurs when a car lap belt restraint acts as a fulcrum over which the torso is violently flexed anteriorly and distracted posteriorly.

Open fractures are considered one of the true orthopedic emergencies in children.[36] These injuries usually result from high-energy mechanisms and are often seen in the setting of multiple trauma. Open fractures in children and adults are classified according to the system of Gustilo-Anderson (Table 18-1).[37-39] The four goals of treatment of open fractures are prevention of infection, bony union, prevention of malunion, and return to function of limb and patient.[36,40] To attain these goals, open fractures must be treated by early irrigation and débridement along with broad-spectrum antibiotic therapy.[37-39] Kindsfater and Jonassen found that early treatment of tibial shaft fractures in children resulted in fewer cases of osteomyelitis when compared with those treated later.[41] As a counterpoint, data from our institution demonstrated no difference in infection or nonunion rates in 390 open fractures of the lower extremities in adults.[42] However, there is no consensus on the effect of delaying surgical treatment of open fractures in regard to rates of infection and need for secondary surgical procedures to promote bone healing.[36,43-49]

FRACTURES OF THE LOWER EXTREMITY

Because of the high energy required, fractures of the pelvis and proximal femur are rare but serious injuries in children. Approximately two thirds of patients with pelvic fractures have associated injuries, and approximately one third have residual, long-term morbidity.[50,51] Pelvic fractures rank second to head

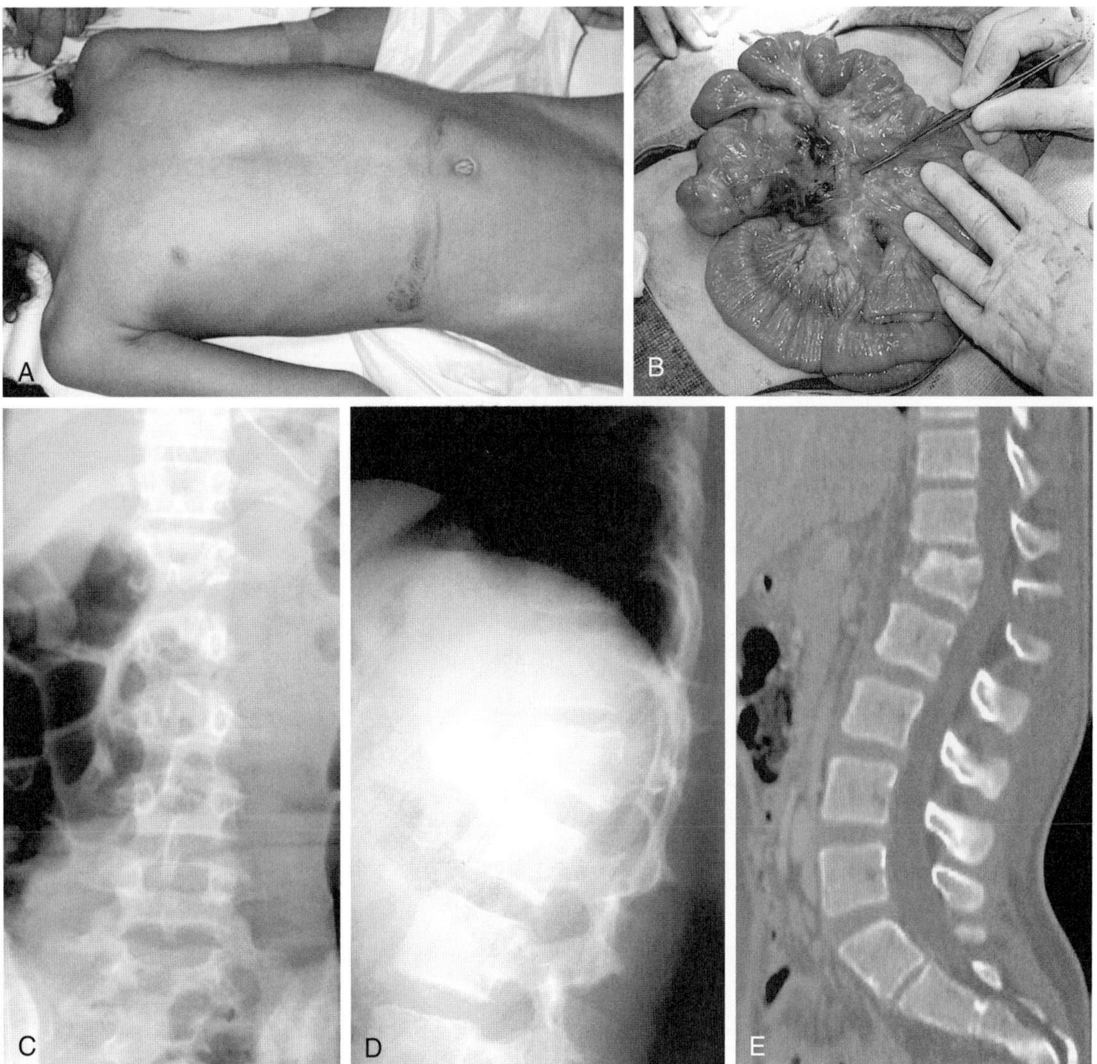

Figure 18-2. **A,** A 12-year-old girl was involved in a motor vehicle accident resulting in ecchymosis in the lower abdomen caused by the lap belt portion of a three-point restraint. This child had a laceration of the omentum discovered at laparotomy (**B**) and a flexion-distraction fracture of L1 with disruption of all three columns of the spine (**C-E**) that required surgical stabilization.

Table 18-1 Severity Classification for Open Fractures

Grade	Description
I	Wound < 1 cm
II	Transitional wound (1-10 cm)
III	Wound > 10 cm
IIIA	Extensive soft tissue injury
IIIB	Reconstructive soft tissue injury
IIIC	Vascular injury

From Gustilo RB, Mendoza RM, Williams DN: Problems in the management of type III (severe) open fractures: A new classification of type III open fractures. J Trauma 24:747-796, 1984; Gustilo RB, Anderson T: Prevention of infection in the treatment of 1025 open fractures of long bones: Retrospective and prospective analyses. J Bone Joint Surg Am 50:453-458, 1976.

injuries in terms of complications, including life-threatening visceral injuries. The mortality rate from pelvic fractures is between 9% and 18%, which is lower than in adults.[50] Children with multiple injuries should be checked carefully for fractures of the pelvis. Some common findings for pelvic fractures are the presence of a hematoma beneath the inguinal ligament (Desot's sign), decreased distance between the greater trochanter and anterior superior iliac spine on the affected side in lateral compression injuries (Roux's sign), and the presence of a bony prominence or hematoma on rectal examination (Earl's sign). An anteroposterior radiograph of the pelvis is usually sufficient as the initial screening study, although increasingly these injuries are diagnosed by spiral tomography that is performed as part of the initial trauma evaluation.[52] Most pediatric pelvic fractures, even those in which the pelvic ring is disrupted, can be treated nonoperatively with good outcomes.[51]

Fractures of the femoral neck are serious injuries that typically require operative treatment.[53-62] Osteonecrosis caused by disruption of the blood supply to the femoral epiphysis is a dreaded complication of this fracture that occurs in up to 75% of children after this injury.[53-58,62-65] The risk of developing osteonecrosis correlates with a higher anatomic location of the fracture in the femoral neck, extent of displacement, and delay in reducing the fracture. Accordingly, fractures and dislocations of the proximal femur are treated as orthopedic emergencies. They require immediate anatomic reduction, which may be achieved by closed or open techniques, and internal fixation (Fig. 18-3).[55,59,62,66-69]

Pediatric femoral shaft fractures are common injuries. The incidence and mechanism of pediatric femoral shaft fractures vary with patient age and gender. Child abuse accounts for up to 67% of femur fractures in children younger than age 1, but only 11% of fractures in children between ages 1 and 2 years old.[70-72] Classic teaching states that spiral fractures in preambulatory children are pathognomonic for abuse. However, other studies have demonstrated that any fracture pattern can occur as the result of abuse.[71]

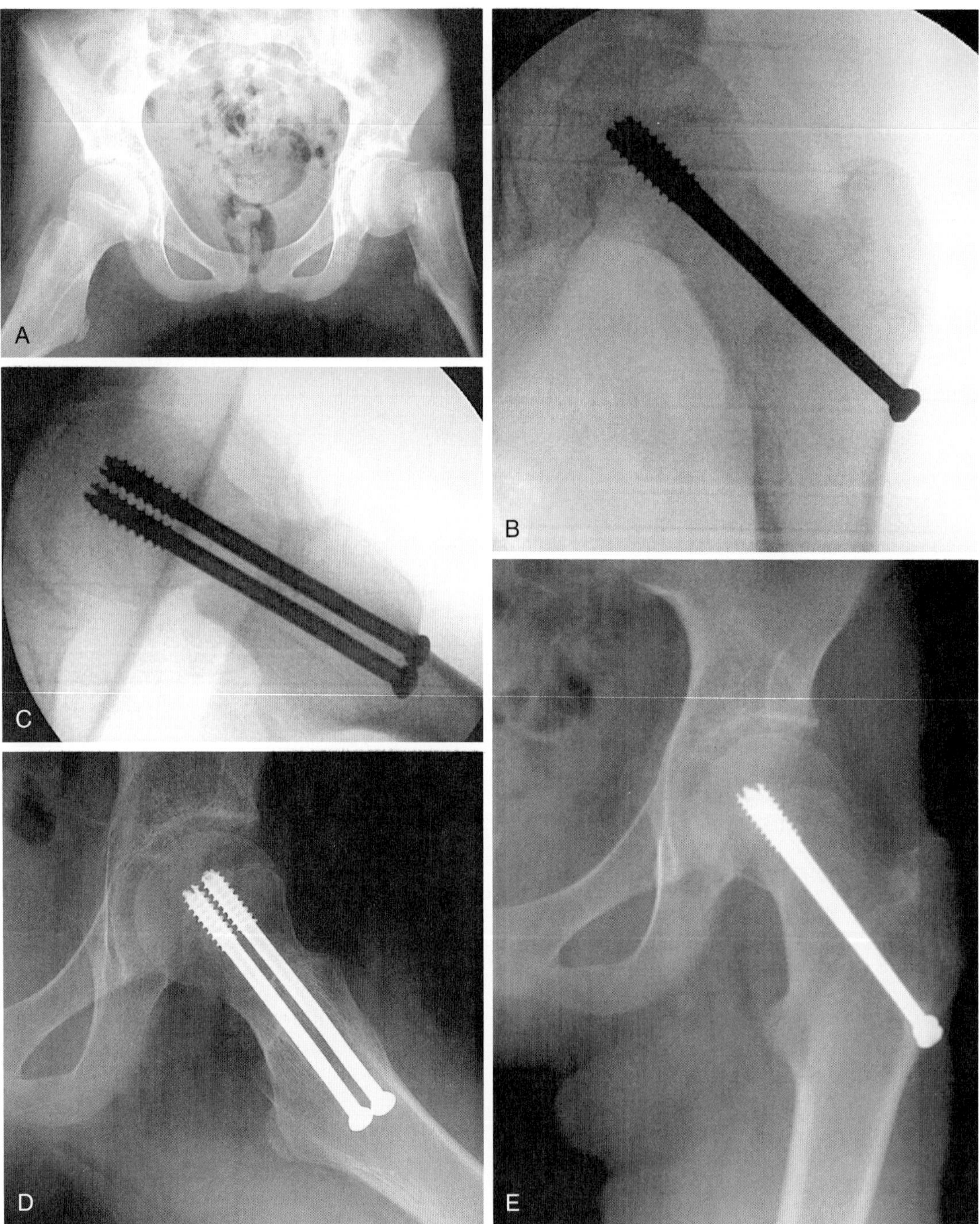

Figure 18-3. **A,** Anteroposterior radiograph of the pelvis of a 12-year-old girl injured as the result of a fall shows a displaced transcervical fracture of the left femoral neck. The fracture was treated as an emergency with closed reduction and internal fixation with two cannulated screws. **B** and **C,** Intraoperative fluoroscopic images demonstrate anatomic reduction of the fracture. **D** and **E,** Radiographs 1 year later show healing of the fracture and no evidence of osteonecrosis.

Falls are the leading cause of femur fractures in children aged 2 to 3 years, and MVAs are the most common cause in older children.[70] Although bleeding after a femur fracture can be fairly extensive, transfusion in isolated, closed injuries is rarely needed. Therefore, other causes of blood loss must be considered if there is hemodynamic instability or a falling hematocrit at 24 hours after injury in a patient with a femur fracture, especially in the setting of multiple trauma.[73]

Treatment of femur fractures also varies with age.[72] Younger children (<4-5 years) are usually treated nonoperatively by closed reduction and immediate spica cast immobilization.[74-77] Older children (4-10 years) are treated with flexible nails[78-85] or plates.[86-88] Adolescents (>10 years or >100 lbs) and teenagers may be treated as adults with solid, reamed, femoral nails, which should be introduced through the tip of the greater trochanter, rather than through the piriformis fossa, to avoid injury to the vascular supply to the femoral head. In contrast to adults, the timing of femur fracture stabilization in children, even in the setting of multiple trauma, does not appear to have an effect on the development of pulmonary complications.[89] The implications are that surgery can be deferred until the general medical condition of the child permits, with the caveat that expeditious stabilization of femur (as well as other long bone) fracture(s) will facilitate mobilization and nursing care in the overall management of the child.

Knee injuries in children differ from those in adults. In children, the cartilage of the physes, apophyses, menisci, and articular surface are weaker than the knee ligaments and are thus more prone to injury.[90] Therefore, fractures about the knee occur more commonly than ligamentous injuries in skeletally immature individuals.[91] The distal femoral physis is the largest and fastest growing physis. It is often injured as a result of a direct blow and is a common injury in American football players. Most fractures are Salter-Harris type I or II injuries. These fractures can usually be treated by closed reduction and percutaneous, cross-pin stabilization. Fractures extending into the articular surface (type III and IV injuries) require open reduction and internal fixation if displacement of the articular surface is greater than 2 mm. Because of the size of this growth plate, its complex, undulating anatomy, and the forces required for displacement, fractures of the distal femoral physis, even type I and II injuries, may result in permanent growth disturbance in up to 50% of cases.[92] All of these fractures should be followed for a minimum of 1 year to evaluate for sequelae of complete (limb-length inequality) or partial (angular deformity) growth arrest.

Proximal tibial physeal injuries are uncommon owing to the reinforcement provided by the knee joint capsular attachments and collateral ligaments. However, vascular compromise of the lower leg due to a popliteal artery injury is possible with displaced fractures of the proximal tibial physis, particularly with extension-type injuries in which the proximal portion of the tibial metaphysis is displaced posteriorly. Such injuries tent the popliteal artery at the level of the physis and proximal to the trifurcation, where it is relatively tethered by the peroneal branch as it courses through the fascia entering the anterior compartment of the leg (Fig. 18-4). Close attention to the vascular examination of the lower extremity is critical after injuries to the proximal tibia. Intra-articular injuries including patellar fractures, tibial spine/plateau fractures, osteochondral fractures, and ligamentous/meniscal injuries typically present as a hemarthrosis. These fractures are not typically emergencies and can be splinted initially and then treated definitively at a later time.

Nonphyseal fractures of the tibia and fibula are among the most common injuries involving the lower extremity in children.[93,94] Fortunately, most of these injuries are low energy and can be treated nonoperatively with good long-term results and few complications. However, one must always be cognizant of the possibility of compartment syndrome after closed or open fractures of the tibial shaft.[95] Indications for operative treatment of tibial shaft fractures include open fractures, fractures with neurovascular injury or impending compartment syndrome, those with unacceptable alignment after closed reduction, and fractures occurring in the setting of multiple trauma.

Foot and ankle fractures are typically caused by indirect, torsional forces. Injuries to the distal tibial and fibular physes account for 25% to 38% of all children's physeal injuries.[96,97] Sports injuries account for up to 58% of physeal fractures about the ankle.[98] Nonoperative treatment has historically been the treatment of choice except for intra-articular fractures and those unable to be adequately reduced by closed means. Recent data suggest improved results with open reduction of distal tibial physeal injuries.[24] Computed tomography (CT) is very useful in defining the pathoanatomy of fractures with intra-articular involvement or unusual patterns, and has proved to be very helpful in making management decisions as well as in preoperative planning.[99] Foot fractures are uncommon and infrequently cause problems for the child. Most foot fractures can be treated nonoperatively with immobilization and restricted weight bearing with good functional results. More complex problems that require operative intervention include fractures of the talar neck and calcaneus, fractures or dislocations of the tarsometatarsal (Lisfranc) joint, and open fractures and lawn mower injuries.[99]

SPINE INJURIES

Cervical Spine Injuries

Cervical spine injuries in children are relatively uncommon but potentially catastrophic. Accurate diagnosis requires an awareness of the injury patterns, anatomic characteristics, and radiographic variants of the immature cervical spine.[100] These injuries account for approximately 1% of all pediatric fractures and only 2% of all spine fractures.[101-103] Pediatric cervical spine injuries are fundamentally different from their adult counterparts owing to the anatomic characteristics of the immature spine and, to a lesser extent, the differences in the mechanisms of injury between adults and children.[104] The cervical spine in children is inherently

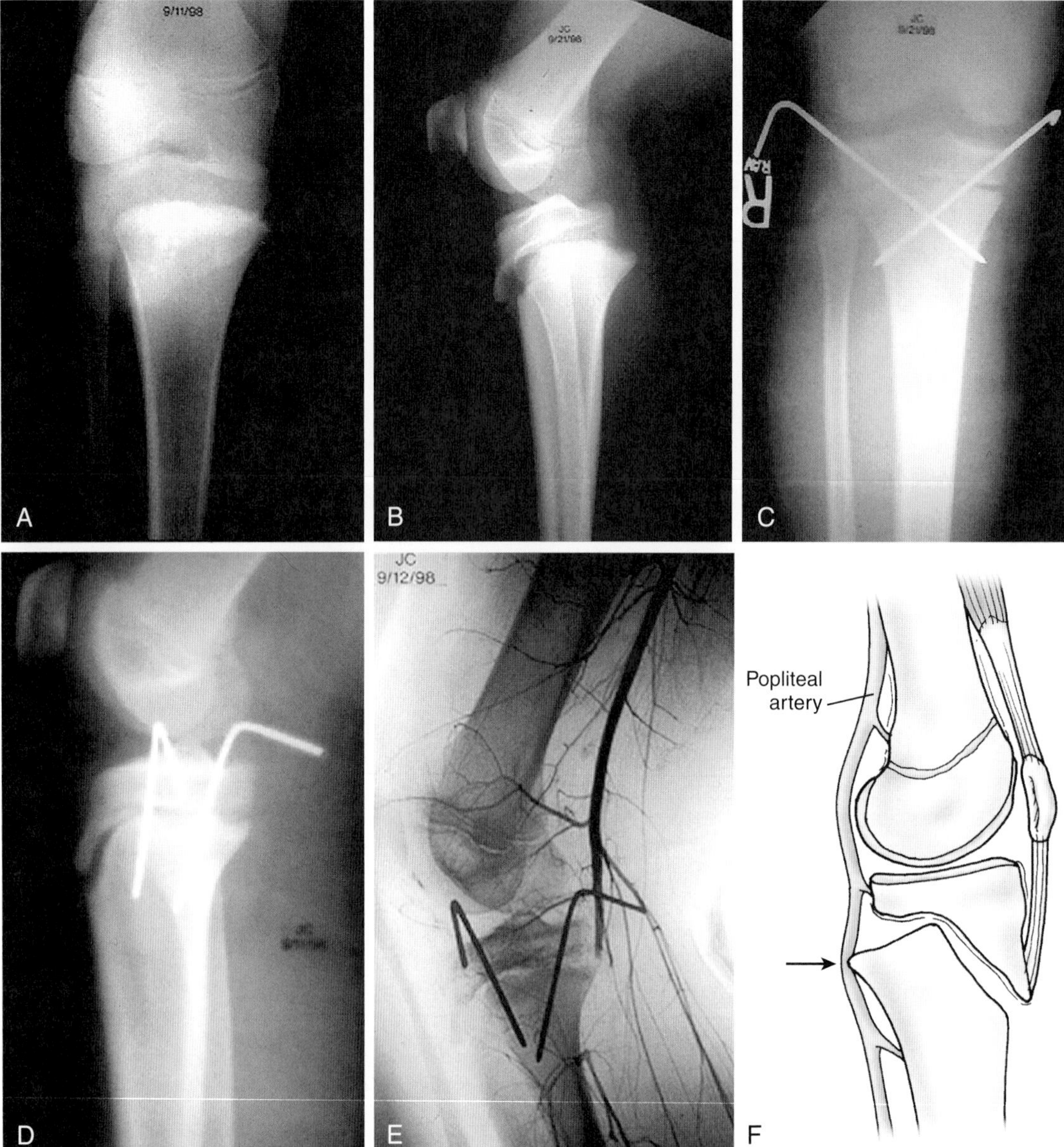

Figure 18-4. Anteroposterior (**A**) and lateral (**B**) radiographs of a 13-year-old boy showing a Salter-Harris type I fracture of the proximal tibial physis with posterior displacement of the distal fragment after an extension-type injury. **C** and **D,** Distal pulses were diminished before and after closed reduction and stabilization of the fracture. **E,** Arteriogram shows occlusion of the popliteal artery at the level of the fracture. Vascular repair with an interposition graft was performed successfully. **F,** Drawing shows the relation of the popliteal artery to the proximal tibial physis and the mechanism of vascular injury in this fracture. (From Green NE: Fractures and dislocations about the knee. In Green NE, Swiontkowski MF [eds]: Skeletal Trauma in Children. Philadelphia, WB Saunders, 2003.)

mobile because of a generalized laxity in the interspinous ligaments and joint capsules, underdeveloped neck musculature, thick cartilaginous end plates, incomplete vertebral ossification (wedge-shaped vertebral bodies), and shallow-angled facet joints, particularly in the upper segments (between the occiput and C4).[104]

In infants and young children, injuries to the upper cervical spine (above C3) predominate because the head is disproportionately large and creates a large bending moment in the upper cervical spine. In an 11-year experience with 122 pediatric neck injuries, none of the 21 patients age 8 years or younger had evidence of injury below C3.[105] Also, multiple-level spinal injuries are more common, occurring in approximately 25% of children with cervical spine fractures.[105-108] Spinal cord injury without radiographic abnormality (SCIWORA) occurs more frequently in children than in adults.[102,104] After age 8 to 10 years, the anatomic and biomechanical characteristics of the cervical spine are more like an adult and injuries to the cervical spine are much more likely to occur in the subaxial region (below C3). Evaluation and treatment of these injuries are essentially the same as in an adult.[100,102,104,109]

Mechanisms of injury vary somewhat with age. In neonates, birth trauma is the most common cause of cervical spine injury and occult spinal cord injury has been demonstrated at necropsy in 30% to 50% of stillborns. Excessive distraction and/or hyperextension of

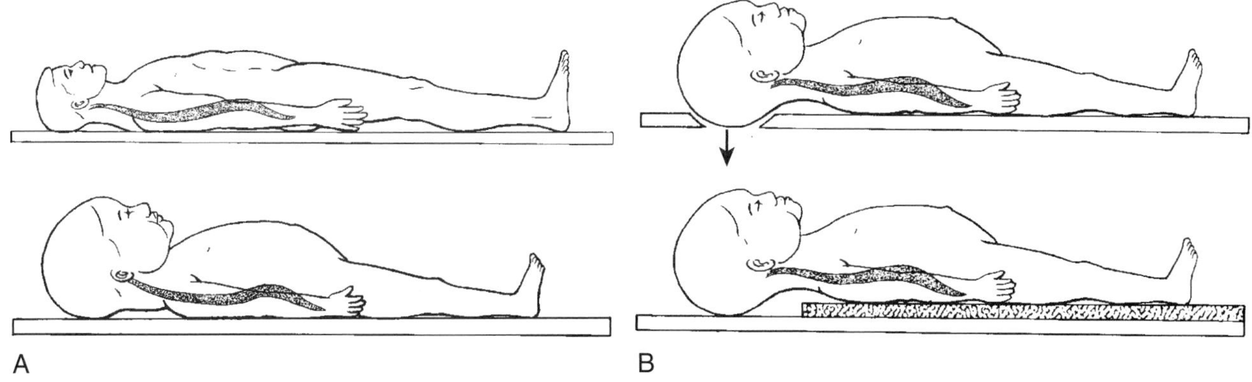

Figure 18-5. **A,** Drawings of an adult and a child on a normal spine board contrasting the differences in position of the head and neck during emergency transport. Because of the disproportionate head-to-body ratio in children, the child's cervical spine is flexed. **B,** Two methods of modifying the traditional spine board for pediatric patient transport are shown. In the upper illustration, a cutout in the board allows the occiput to be recessed. In the lower illustration, the area under the thorax is built up with padding. Both methods effectively allow the head to translate posteriorly, creating more normal alignment of the cervical spine. (Reprinted from Herzenberg JE, Hensiger RN, Dedrick DK: Emergency transport and positioning of young children who have an injury to the cervical spine. J Bone Joint Surg Am 71:15-21, 1989.)

the cervical spine are thought to be the most common mechanisms of injury and may be associated with abnormal intrauterine position (transverse lie) or a difficult cephalic or breech delivery.[110,111] In infants and young children, nonaccidental trauma is a significant cause of injury to the cervical spine. Avulsion fractures of the spinous processes, fractures of the pars or pedicles (most commonly C2), or compression fractures of multiple vertebral bodies are the most common patterns of injury and are thought to result from severe shaking or battering.[112,113] These injuries may be associated with other signs of nonaccidental trauma, including fractures of the skull, ribs, or long bones, and superficial ecchymoses. In older children (up to about age 10), the most common causes are pedestrian-MVAs and falls. In children older than 10 years of age, the most common causes are passenger-related MVAs, sports-related injuries, and diving accidents.

Appropriate methods of immobilizing children for transport and evaluating them clinically and radiographically are crucial to avoid detrimental outcomes. The goal of immobilization during transport of the injured child with potential spine trauma is to avoid excessive angulation of the spinal column so as to avoid causing or exacerbating spinal cord injury. Immobilization of children younger than 8 years of age on a standard spine board during emergency transportation has been shown to cause excessive flexion of the cervical spine due to the disproportionately large diameter of the head relative to the torso. It has been recommended that the child's spine board be modified by building up the area under the torso with padding to allow the head to fall back slightly or cutting out the area under the occiput to recess the skull (Fig. 18-5).[114] In addition to proper spine board immobilization, an appropriately fitting cervical collar is necessary to achieve neutral alignment of the cervical spine after injury.[115]

Clinical evaluation of a child suspected of having an injury to the cervical spine is often hampered by an inability to obtain an accurate history and the unreliability of the physical examination.[100,102,109,116-118] Historically, overt or occult injury to the cervical spine is more likely to occur as a result of falls from a height of more than 4 feet, pedestrian- or cyclist-MVAs, and unrestrained occupant-MVAs. Head or facial trauma, altered mental status, and/or loss of consciousness are also risk factors. Neck pain, guarding, and torticollis are the most reliable signs of an injury to the cervical spine in children. Extremity weakness, sensory changes (numbness or tingling), bowel and bladder dysfunction, and, less frequently, headaches, seizures, syncope, and respiratory distress are signs of injury to the spinal cord.[31,100,101,106,119-127] When these conditions are present, the cervical spine should be immobilized until imaging studies can be completed and the spine cleared (Table 18-2).[100]

Radiographic evaluation of the cervical spine in children is hampered by the presence of normal anatomic variants that can be mistaken for trauma. Synchondroses and incompletely ossified, wedge-shaped vertebral bodies can simulate fractures.[128-131] Anterior angulation of the odontoid is a normal variant in approximately 5% of children and may be mistaken for a Salter-Harris type I fracture of the dens. Physiologic subluxation of C2 on C3 or C3 on C4 of up to 3 mm is a normal variant (pseudosubluxation) in about 40% of children younger than age 8 years that is often misinterpreted as pathologic instability.[130,132] Focal kyphosis of the midcervical spine is a normal

Table 18-2	Risk Factors for Cervical Spine Injury
Mechanism of injury	
Pedestrian/ or cyclist/motor vehicle accident	
Unrestrained occupant/motor vehicle accident	
Fall > 4 feet	
Loss of consciousness	
Neck pain, limited range of motion, torticollis	
Abnormal neurologic examination	
Numbness, tingling	
Extremity weakness	
Head or facial trauma	

From Weiser ER, Mencio GA: Pediatric cervical spine injuries: Assessment and treatment. Semin Spine Surg 13:142-151, 2001.

variant in about 15% of children younger than age 16 years that can also be misinterpreted as pathologic.

Initial radiographic evaluation should include cross-table lateral and anteroposterior radiographs. On the lateral view, it is essential to see the C7-T1 disc space. Oblique films are additionally helpful in defining detail of the pedicles and facet joints.[128] Open-mouth odontoid images are technically difficult to perform and rarely helpful.[133] CT is a much better way to image the upper cervical spine and also provides excellent definition of known fractures, confirmation of suspicious areas, and excellent visualization of the cervicothoracic level, which can be difficult to adequately image with plain radiography. CT evaluation of the cervical spine has been shown to be more efficacious than conventional images in evaluating the cervical spine in adult and pediatric trauma and to lower institutional costs and complications in urban trauma centers.[126,134,135] Magnetic resonance imaging (MRI) is the preferred study to evaluate the spinal cord and soft tissue structures, including ligaments, cartilage, and intervertebral discs.

Once a cervical collar has been placed on a child or the neck immobilized, either at the scene of an accident or in the emergency department, formal clearance of the cervical spine is necessary before immobilization is discontinued.[117] In general, the cervical spine may be cleared based on clinical examination alone if the child is awake, alert, and cooperative; if there are no signs of cervical injury; and if the mechanism of injury is not consistent with cervical trauma.[100,117] For children younger than age 8 to 10 years who are obtunded or otherwise unable to be examined, and all those with a profile suggestive of injury to the cervical spine, clearance may be based on a five-view cervical spine radiographic series, consisting of anteroposterior, lateral, open-mouth odontoid, and two oblique views, and CT of the axial region of the spine, from the occiput to C2. In a study at our institution in which this protocol was followed, 8 of 112 children were diagnosed with cervical spine injuries. Two of 6 children with bony injuries (33%) were diagnosed only by the CT scan. No injuries were missed, and cervical immobilization was discontinued in a timely fashion.[136] The rationale for CT includes the predisposition for injuries to occur in the upper cervical region in children younger than 8 years old and the technical difficulty of imaging this area with plain radiographs.[100] In a subsequent study from our institution, helical CT was shown to have higher specificity, sensitivity, and negative predictive value than conventional radiographs in evaluating the cervical spine in children with blunt trauma.[135]

Others have advocated a definitive role for MRI as an adjunct to plain films and CT, particularly in identifying soft tissue injury.[137-139] In one study of 79 children, MRI revealed injuries in 15 patients with normal radiographs and excluded injuries suspected on plain radiographs and CT scans in 7 and 2 patients, respectively.[137] In 25 obtunded or uncooperative children, MRI demonstrated 3 with significant injuries.

Halo vest immobilization is being used with increasing frequency in children with cervical spine injuries. It affords superior immobilization to a rigid cervical collar and is easier to apply and more versatile than a Minerva cast. It permits access for skin and wound care while avoiding the skin problems (maceration, ulceration) typically associated with both hard collars and casts. However, complication rates associated with pediatric use of halo vest immobilization as high as 68% have been reported.[140] Pin site infections are the most common problems, but pin perforation, cerebrospinal fluid leaks, and brain abscesses have also been described.[109,140] In children younger than age 6 years, a CT scan of the skull to measure calvarial thickness can be helpful in determining optimal sites for pin placement.[141] In children older than age 6 years, the standard adult halo construct utilizing four pins (two anterolaterally, two posterolaterally) inserted at standard torques of 6 to 8 inch-pounds generally works well (Fig. 18-6A). In younger children, more pins (up to 12) placed with lower insertional torques (2-4 inch-pounds) have been advocated (see Fig. 18-6B).[140,141] Standard pediatric halo rings fit most children, but infants and toddlers usually require custom rings. Although standard pediatric halo vests are available, custom vests or body casts generally provide superior immobilization.[142]

The possibility of SCIWORA should be considered in children, particularly in those younger than 8 years old.[143-146] MRI may be diagnostic in demonstrating spinal cord edema or hemorrhage, soft tissue or ligamentous injury, or apophyseal or disc disruption but is completely

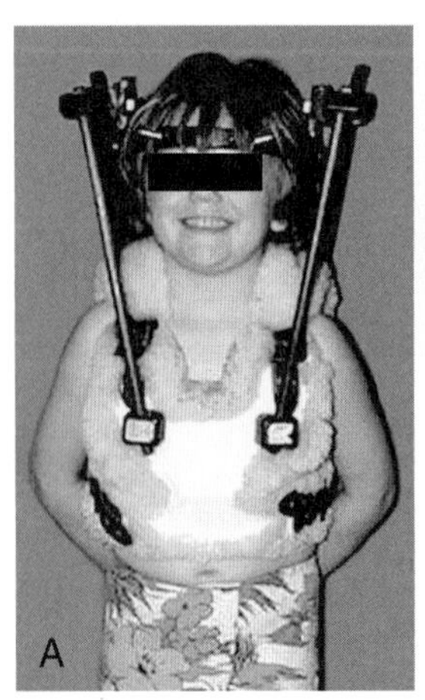

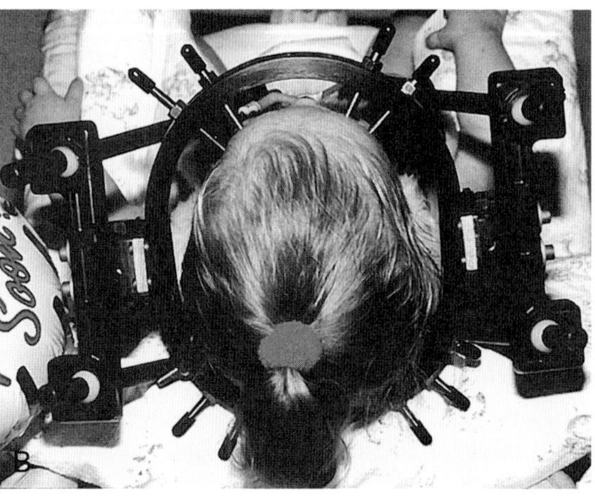

Figure 18-6. **A,** Six-year-old immobilized in standard halo construct with four pins (two anterolateral, two posterolateral) inserted at torques of 6 to 8 inch-pounds. **B,** Three-year-old child with halo ring with 10 pins inserted at low torque, in contrast to the usual four-pin configuration used in older children and adults. (From Weiser ER, Mencio GA: Pediatric cervical spine injuries: Assessment and treatment. Semin Spine Surg 13:142-151, 2001.)

normal in approximately 25% of cases. SCIWORA is the cause of paralysis in 20% to 30% of children with injuries of the spinal cord. Potential mechanisms of SCIWORA include hyperextension of the cervical spine, which can cause compression of the spinal cord by the ligamentum flavum, followed by flexion, which can cause longitudinal traction. Other mechanisms include transient subluxation without gross failure or unrecognized cartilaginous end plate failure (Salter-Harris type I fracture).

Regardless of the specific mechanism, injury to the spinal cord occurs because of the variable elasticity of the elements of the spinal column in children.[147] Experimentally, it has been shown that the bone, cartilage, and soft tissue in the spinal column can stretch about 2 inches without disruption but the spinal cord ruptures after one-fourth inch.[111,146,148] Spinal cord injury occurs when deformation of the musculoskeletal structures of the spinal column exceeds the physiologic limits of the spinal cord.[147] Injury may be complete or incomplete and may occur at more than one level.[149] Partial spinal cord syndromes reported in SCIWORA include Brown-Séquard and anterior and central cord syndromes as well as mixed patterns of injury.[143-145,147]

Prognosis after SCIWORA is correlated to MRI findings, if any are present, and to the severity of neurologic injury.[143-145] Effective management demands careful evaluation of the cervical spine to exclude osseous or cartilaginous injury or mechanical instability. In addition, stabilization of the spine is needed to prevent recurrent injury.[143-146] Immobilization with a rigid cervical collar for 2 to 3 months is usually adequate treatment for SCIWORA. There are no reports of recurrent spinal cord injury when the cervical spine has been immobilized in this manner. Surgery is occasionally necessary for unstable injury patterns. The prevalence of scoliosis after infantile quadriplegia is over 90%. Therefore, long-term follow-up is necessary to monitor for vertebral column deformity.

Administration of high-dose corticosteroids within the first 8 hours of spinal cord injury has been shown to improve the chances of neurologic recovery in adults.[150-153] According to guidelines from the third National Acute Spinal Cord Injury Study (NASCIS), when treatment is initiated within 3 hours of injury, methylprednisolone should be administered as an intravenous bolus of 30 mg/kg over 15 minutes followed by a continuous infusion of 5.4 mg/kg/hr over the next 23 hours. Also, if treatment cannot be started until more than 3 to 8 hours after injury, the corticosteroids should be given for 48 hours. After 8 hours, there is no benefit and corticosteroids should not be administered.[152,153] Although the effect on younger children (<13 years old) is not known, we universally initiate this protocol in all patients with spinal cord injuries at our institution.

Thoracic, Lumbar, and Sacral Spine Injuries

Thoracic, lumbar, and sacral fractures are also relatively uncommon in children. MVAs or falls cause the majority of these injuries. Child abuse can be a cause in younger children.[122,154-158] The most common injuries are compression fractures and flexion-distraction injuries. Compression fractures are caused by a combination of hyperflexion and axial compression. Because the disc in children is stronger than cancellous bone, the vertebral body is the first structure to fail. It is common for children to sustain multiple compression fractures. Compression rarely exceeds more than 20% of the vertebral body. In the multiply injured patient, helical CT is increasingly becoming the preferred imaging modality for diagnosing and characterizing these fractures.[52,159] These fractures are managed conservatively with rest, analgesics, and bracing.[158]

Flexion-distraction injuries (seat belt injuries) occur in the upper lumbar spine in children wearing a lap belt.[35,160-167] With sudden deceleration, the seat belt slides up on the abdomen where it provides an axis about which the spine rotates. As a result, the torso is forcibly flexed and the spinal column fails in tension, resulting primarily in disruption of the posterior column with variable patterns of extension into the middle and anterior columns. These injuries may be missed on axial CT because of the transverse plane of orientation of the fracture. A lateral radiograph showing widening of the interspinous distance (see Fig. 18-2D) and a CT with sagittal reconstruction (see Fig. 18-2E) are the most helpful studies in diagnosing this fracture. Approximately two thirds of patients have an injury to a hollow viscus, a solid organ injury, and even an injury to the abdominal aorta. These injuries often result in greater morbidity than the spine fracture and may be life threatening, particularly if unrecognized initially.[35,168,169] Fortunately, neurologic injury is unusual. Lap belt injuries with mostly bony involvement and kyphosis less than 20 degrees can be treated with hyperextension casting. Those with posterior ligamentous disruption and soft tissue injury require surgical stabilization with compression instrumentation and posterior arthrodesis.

Fracture-dislocations of the spine are unstable injuries that usually occur at the thoracolumbar junction and often are associated with neurologic deficits. They are rare injuries in children that require surgical stabilization and fusion. Burst fractures are also rare injuries in children that result from axial compression and typically occur at the thoracolumbar junction or in the lumbar spine.[170] The need for operative treatment is determined by the stability of the fracture and the presence of neurologic deficits. Fractures of the sacrum are usually associated with pelvic fractures. Fractures that involve the sacral foramina or central sacral canal are associated with neurologic deficits in 28% and 50% of patients, respectively. Decompression of the sacral nerve root(s) and stabilization of the sacral fracture may be necessary to improve neurologic function. In most instances, however, fractures of the sacrum can be treated nonoperatively.

FRACTURES OF THE UPPER EXTREMITY

Fractures of the clavicle are among the most common injuries in children. They are usually uncomplicated and require little, if any, treatment other than sling immobilization for comfort. Distal clavicular fractures in the immature child may mimic acromioclavicular separation. The trauma surgeon should be aware of this injury and not mistake it for a true acromioclavicular dislocation. The periosteal sleeve of the distal clavicle remains intact with the coracoclavicular ligaments attached.[21,171-173] The fracture heals very rapidly with an enormous amount of callus and requires no treatment other than sling immobilization for comfort. There will be complete remodeling of the bone.

Injuries to the medial end of the clavicle are somewhat rare but potentially problematic from the standpoint of recognition and neurovascular complications. The medial clavicle consists of the clavicle and its medial growth plate plus the ligaments of the sternoclavicular joint. The physis of the medial clavicle is the last one in the body to close, and frequently does not close until after age 21.[21,173,174] The so-called dislocation of the sternoclavicular joint in the teenager and young adult is almost always a type I physeal fracture. It is important to recognize this distinction because a true dislocation likely would be unstable, whereas a type I fracture of the physis is a stable injury once reduced.

Anterior or posterior displacement of the medial end of the clavicle may occur as a result of indirect trauma to the shoulder with a secondary force vector that determines the final resting position of the bone. Posterior displacement almost always occurs by a direct mechanism such as when one falls on something such as a football and others land on top of him. The medial portion of the clavicle is pushed posteriorly, resulting in an injury directly through the growth plate of the medial clavicle. The patient presents to the emergency department with pain and swelling about the sternoclavicular joint. The shoulder is usually held forward. There is no pain about the distal clavicle or the shoulder joint. Although uncommon, compression of the mediastinal structures is the most devastating complication of this injury.

Diagnosis of the injury requires awareness of the injury and a CT scan to confirm the diagnosis. Radiographs may show the posterior dislocation, but it is most clearly seen on CT scan with thin cuts through the medial clavicle and sternoclavicular joint (Fig. 18-7A). Treatment of this type I fracture of the medial clavicular growth plate is usually easily handled by closed reduction under general anesthesia (see Fig. 18-7B). Although open reduction is rarely necessary, internal fixation with a large, nonabsorbable suture placed through the thick periosteal sleeve is usually sufficient. Smooth pins should be avoided because of the risk of migration. Open reduction should be performed in conjunction with a general, vascular, or thoracic surgeon assisting or available in the event of unrecognized or iatrogenic injury to the great vessels. However, the most common problem associated with persistent posterior displacement is dysphagia.

Once the fracture (posterior dislocation) is reduced, alignment is maintained with a hard figure-of-eight bandage. This should be applied in the operating room with the patient still asleep using cast padding applied in a criss-crossing, figure-of-eight manner with the shoulders abducted. This bandage is then covered with fiberglass to keep the shoulders in that position. This injury should be stable enough within 3 to 4 weeks to discontinue the immobilization and begin gentle motion of the shoulder. Healing is rapid, and return of function is expected.

Fractures about the proximal humerus can usually be treated nonoperatively. In all age groups, the tremendous arc of motion in the shoulder joint allows a fairly large margin for fracture alignment. In the younger child, the rapid growth of the proximal humeral physis, which accounts for about 80% of the length of the bone, also contributes to rapid and predictable remodeling of all but the most angulated fractures. In these children, no treatment other than immobilization for comfort is necessary.[175,176] Markedly displaced fractures in the teenager, however, may not remodel because there is not sufficient remaining growth.[176-178] Most injuries in this age group are Salter-Harris type II fractures of the proximal humerus physis, which are usually not stable in addition to being significantly angulated and displaced. These fractures need to be reduced and usually require fixation. Generally these fractures can be stabilized with percutaneous Steinmann pins or cannulated screws inserted from the distal fragment into the proximal fragment using C-arm visualization.[179,180] Internal fixation should be supplemented with a sling and swathe. If pins are used, they should remain for 3 to 4 weeks after which gentle range of motion may begin. The fracture will heal very

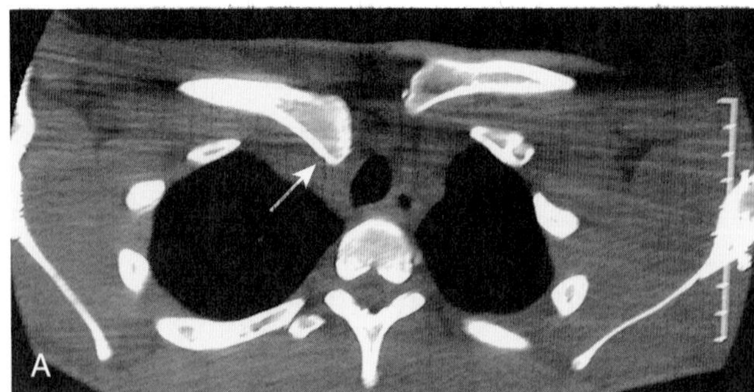

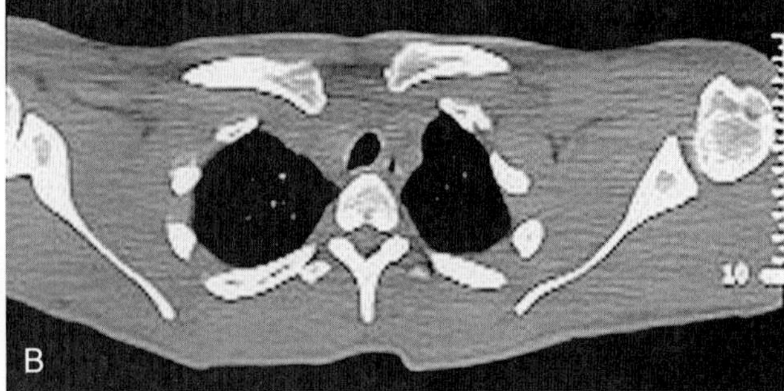

Figure 18-7. A 16-year-old boy injured his right clavicle when he was checked into the board while playing hockey. He complained of difficulty swallowing. Anteroposterior radiograph of the right clavicle appeared normal. **A,** CT scan with thin cuts through the sternoclavicular joint shows posterior displacement of the medial end of the clavicle (*arrow*). **B,** Note restoration of alignment after closed reduction.

quickly. Permanent injury to the growth plate is not an issue because this fracture generally occurs very close to the end of skeletal growth.

Fractures about the elbow in children can be difficult to diagnose because the anatomy of the immature elbow is confusing owing to the presence of numerous centers of ossification. Knowledge of the sequence of appearance and maturation of the secondary ossification centers is mandatory. A comparison radiograph of the contralateral elbow is often helpful in correctly identifying the nature of the injury.[181]

The most common fracture about the distal humerus in the child is a supracondylar fracture. These fractures are classified according to the amount of displacement. Type III fractures are the most severe, with both fragments completely displaced. The injury usually occurs from a fall on the outstretched hand. In children who are ligamentously lax, the elbow will hyperextend and shear off the distal portion of the humerus through the olecranon fossa.[182]

The major problems with this injury are swelling and nerve and/or vascular injury. In the past, it has been thought that this fracture should be treated immediately. However, we now recognize that this fracture does not need immediate operative stabilization unless there are other extenuating circumstances, such as vascular injury, compartment ischemia, or an open wound. Currently, the general policy is to delay treatment until the next day if the patient presents in the middle of the night and correct the fracture during the daylight hours with operating room personnel who are familiar with the procedures required. Initially, the elbow is splinted in less than 90 degrees of flexion with a loose bandage over a posterior splint.[183,184] These fractures can usually be reduced by closed manipulation and stabilized by percutaneous pins (Fig. 18-8). Occasionally, open reduction and pinning of this fracture is necessary if a perfect anatomic reduction is not possible, or if there are other extenuating circumstances such as an open fracture or a vascular injury that requires exploration.

There has long been a controversy as to the treatment of the pulseless extremity in patients who have sustained a supracondylar fracture. Absence of the pulse with this fracture is not uncommon. It is believed that the absence of the pulse may either be the result of vascular spasm and/or direct vascular injury. However, the collateral circulation about the elbow is so rich that the circulation to the forearm and hand usually remains normal. Treatment of the vascular injury has been debated for decades in the orthopedic and

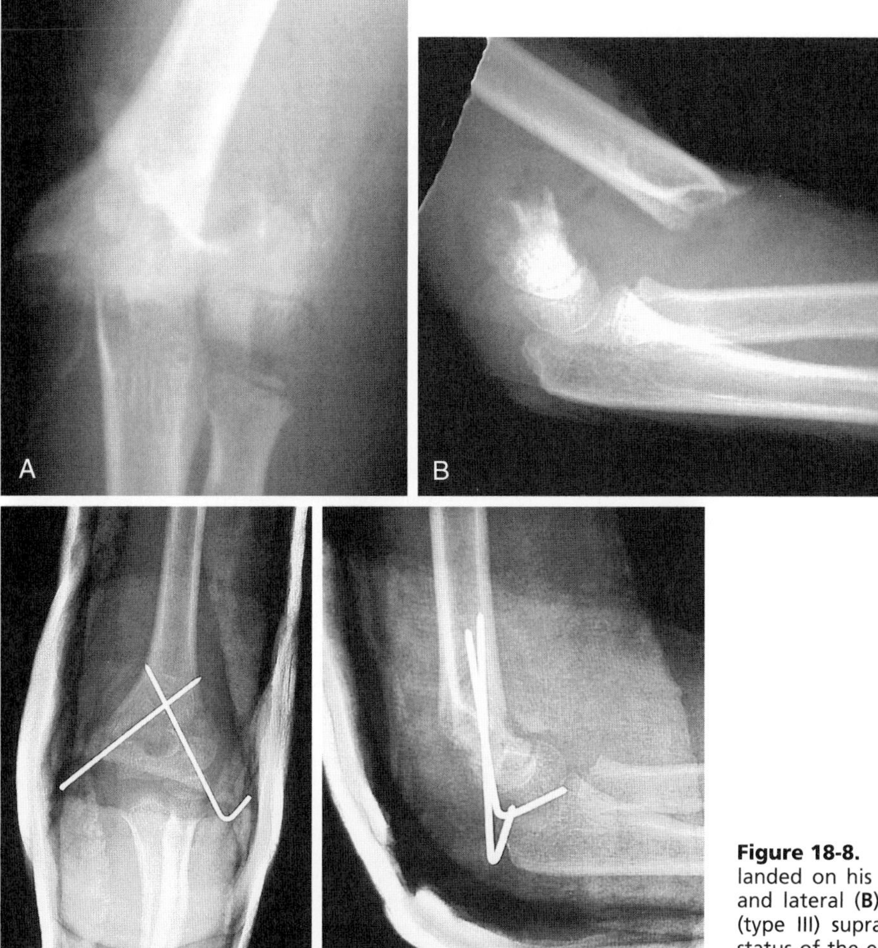

Figure 18-8. A 6-year-old fell while horseback riding and landed on his outstretched left arm. Anteroposterior **(A)** and lateral **(B)** radiographs show a completely displaced (type III) supracondylar humerus fracture. Neurovascular status of the extremity was intact. **C** and **D,** The child was treated with closed reduction and percutaneous fixation with smooth Steinmann pins.

vascular surgery literature. The current practice is observation as long as circulation to the hand and forearm is clinically normal.[182,183,185] It has been shown by follow-up studies that vein grafts for these vascular injuries will frequently clot because of the excellent collateral circulation about the elbow.[186] The only true indication for vascular exploration is the pulseless, ischemic extremity, which is a true surgical emergency. In this instance, the fracture should be reduced and stabilized with crossed pins before vascular repair.[187,188]

Compartment syndrome is a feared complication that is actually quite uncommon in the modern era of treatment. By stabilizing the fracture with internal fixation, the need to immobilize the elbow in hyperflexion, which has been shown to increase the risk of vascular compression and forearm compartment swelling, is avoided.[182]

The signs of compartment syndrome are well known, but the main one is pain that is out of proportion to the fracture itself. Once this fracture is stabilized, the child should be comfortable and not have significant pain. Passive extension of the fingers should be possible to a neutral position. If not, it suggests the need for investigation of a compartment syndrome by removal of the splint, palpation of the forearm compartment, and pressure measurements, if necessary. If the pressures are elevated, consistent with a forearm compartment syndrome, fasciotomy should be performed quickly.

Salter-Harris type I fractures of the distal humerus are less common than other injuries about the elbow. However, they are frequently misdiagnosed. For that reason alone, it is an important fracture to understand. Equally important is the recognition that in very young children this fracture often occurs as the result of nonaccidental trauma. Therefore, this injury should trigger investigation into the possibility of abuse as the mechanism of occurrence.[189] The differential diagnosis of this injury requires an understanding of the anatomy of the distal humerus and the pathology of the lesion itself. With a type I fracture of the distal humerus, the entire epiphysis moves away from the rest of the humeral shaft and is displaced in a medial (more typical) or lateral direction. This fracture usually occurs in very young children in whom only the capitellum is ossified. Radiographically, in the type I fracture, the capitellum appears displaced from its normal position relative to the distal humerus and is distinguished from dislocation of the elbow by the fact that the radius and ulna remain in line with the capitellum and all three structures are displaced relative to the distal humerus (Fig. 18-9). In an elbow dislocation, the radius and

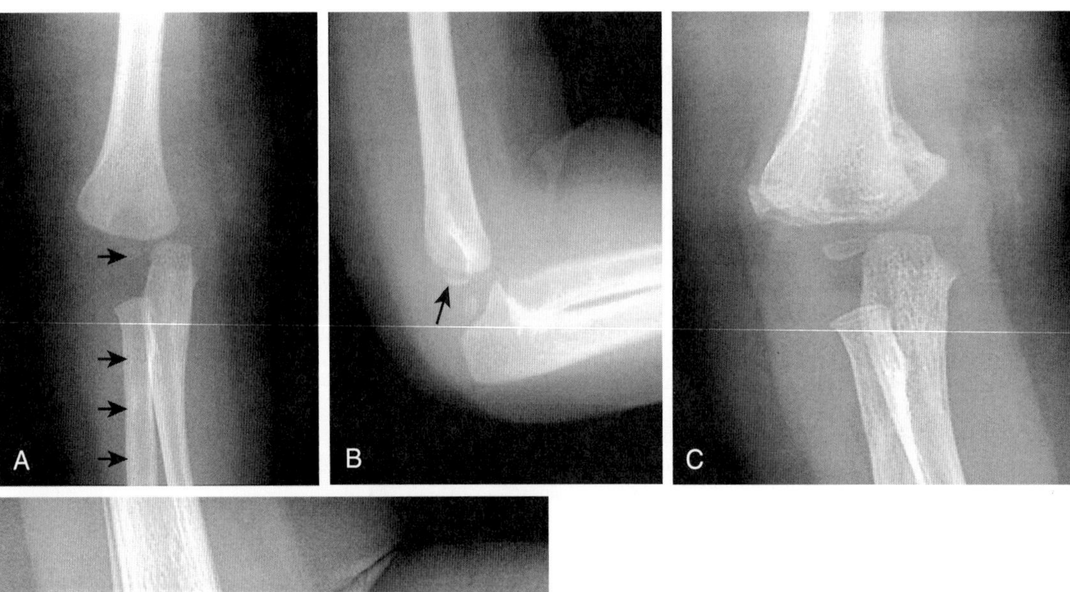

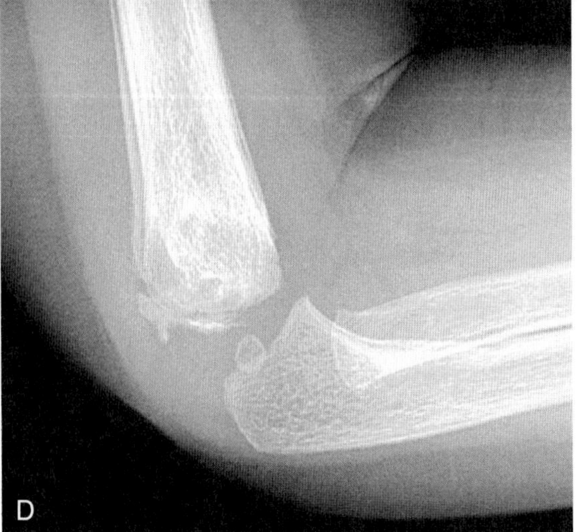

Figure 18-9. An 11-month-old infant, ultimately determined to have been the victim of abuse, presented with a swollen arm. **A,** On the anteroposterior radiograph of the elbow, the capitellum, the proximal radius, and the ulna are displaced from their normal positions relative to the distal humerus (*arrows*), consistent with a fracture-separation of the distal humeral epiphysis. In an elbow dislocation, the radius and ulna are displaced relative to the distal humerus but the capitellum is not displaced from its normal position in the distal humerus. **B,** The lateral radiograph of the elbow shows a small metaphyseal fragment (*arrow*), also consistent with a fracture of the distal humeral physis and not with dislocation of the elbow. This fracture was treated with cast immobilization. **C** and **D,** Note the exuberant fracture callus 3 weeks after the injury.

ulna are displaced relative to the distal humerus and are not in line with the capitellum. Also, the capitellum is not displaced from its normal position in the distal humerus.[182]

This fracture may also occur in newborns as a result of birth trauma. In this instance, the fracture is usually stable, will heal in a few days, and requires only splint immobilization for comfort. In the child, this fracture may require closed manipulation and pinning if the fracture is expediently diagnosed before some healing has occurred. Unfortunately, especially in instances of nonaccidental trauma, the child is usually seen well after this injury has already begun to heal and manipulation of the fracture is either not possible or ill advised.

Fractures of the lateral condyle of the humerus must also be distinguished from the Salter-Harris type I fractures of the distal humeral physis. With fractures of the lateral condyle, the radius and ulna remain aligned with the humerus but the capitellum is displaced from its normal position (Fig. 18-10). If the condylar fracture is displaced at all, it requires open reduction and pin fixation because the risk of nonunion is high when it is treated nonoperatively. Nonunion will result in a progressive valgus deformity of the elbow with an ulnar nerve palsy.[190-192]

Forearm fractures have traditionally been treated with closed manipulation and casting. In most instances, especially with distal fractures, this treatment is highly successful and results in normal function of the extremity. Our preference is to perform closed reduction of these fractures in the emergency department using intravenous ketamine (2 mg/kg) or other methods of conscious sedation. Ketamine has proved to be an excellent drug for sedation in the ambulatory management of these and other fractures because it has a fast onset of action, particularly after intravenous administration, has a very short half-life, and does not cause respiratory depression or suppression of the gag reflex. The child is monitored with electrocardiography and pulse oximetry by a nurse or physician who is not involved in the management of the fracture according to the guidelines for conscious sedation from the American Academy of Pediatrics. Midazolam (Versed) is also frequently used to prevent emergence reactions that are sometimes seen with ketamine, especially in the older child.[193,194]

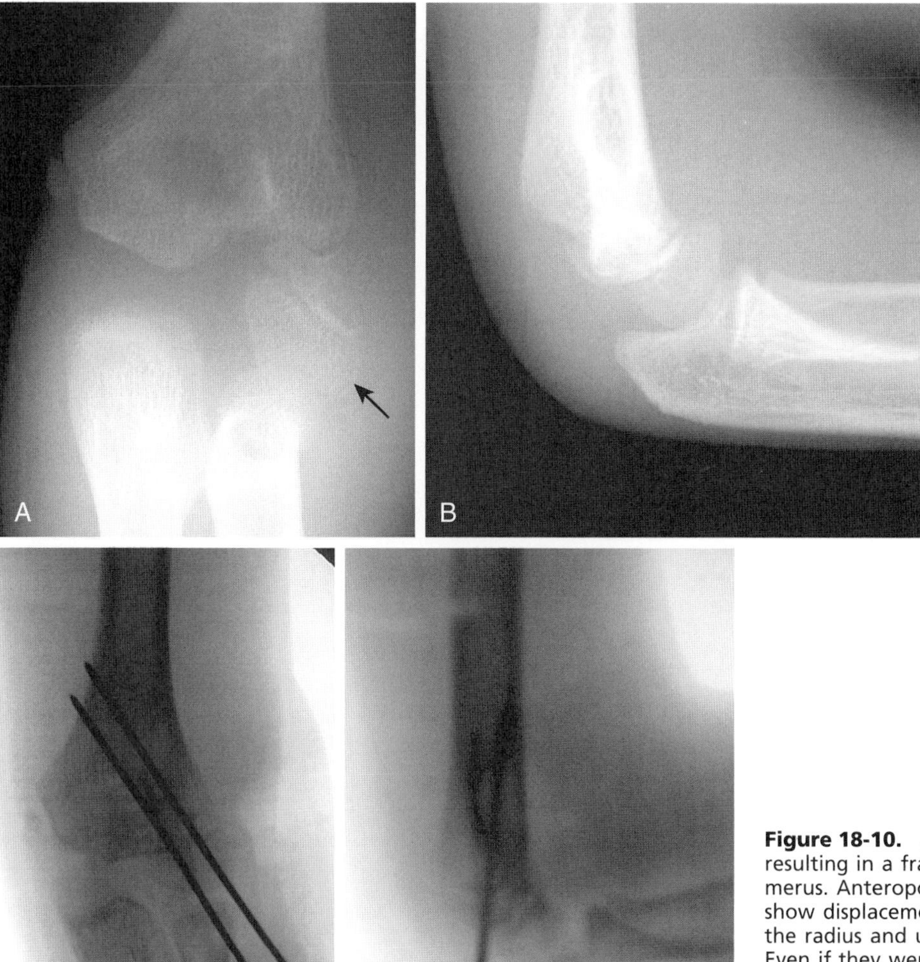

Figure 18-10. A 7-year-old child fell from a bunk bed, resulting in a fracture of the lateral condyle of the humerus. Anteroposterior (**A**) and lateral (**B**) radiographs show displacement of the capitellum (*arrow*), whereas the radius and ulna remain aligned with the humerus. Even if they were minimally displaced, the risk of joint incongruity and nonunion is high after nonoperative treatment of this fracture. Anteroposterior (**C**) and lateral (**D**) radiographs of the elbow after open reduction and pin fixation show anatomic alignment.

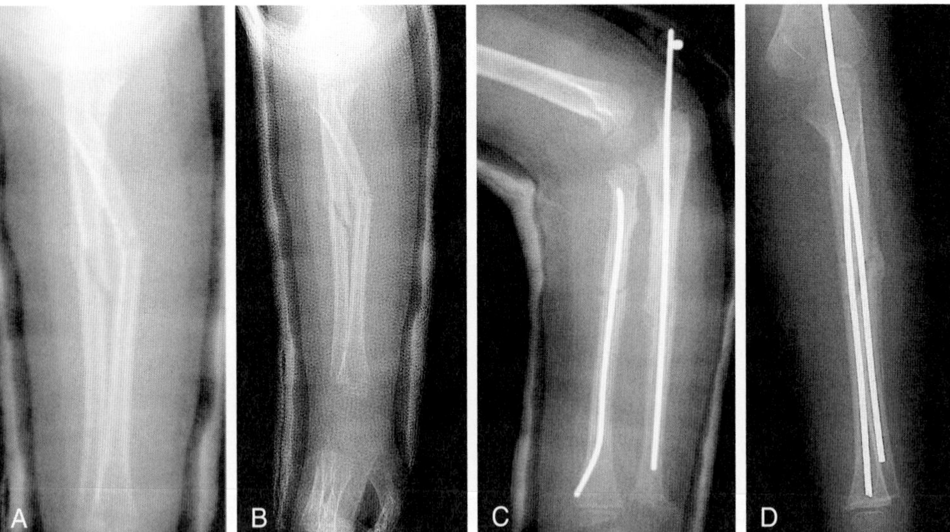

Figure 18-11. Anteroposterior (**A**) and lateral (**B**) radiographs show diaphyseal fractures of the radius and ulna in a 6-year-old, with angulation after closed treatment. **C** and **D,** Fractures were treated with internal fixation by using flexible titanium nails inserted via 1-cm incisions, distally in the radius and proximally in the ulna, and advanced across the fracture under fluoroscopic visualization.

The use of a portable fluoroscopy unit is essential in treating pediatric forearm fractures, both to guide reduction of the fracture and to confirm alignment after immobilization. After manipulation of the fracture, the extremity is immobilized in a sugar tong splint that will allow for swelling. When swelling is no longer a concern, the sugar tong splint is incorporated into a long-arm, fiberglass cast. After 3 weeks, a short-arm cast is applied for another 3 weeks, after which progressive use and motion is started.

Fractures of the shaft of both bones of the forearm, especially from the midportion of the forearm proximally, are poorly treated with cast immobilization alone, especially in children older than the age of 8 or 9 years. It is difficult to maintain reduction of these fractures in a cast or splint. Also, angulation or malrotation in the diaphysis of either the radius or ulna will result in loss of rotation in the forearm (Fig. 18-11). For this reason, fractures of the shafts of the radius and ulna are being treated by internal fixation using flexible titanium nails with increasing frequency.[195-203] These fractures can usually be reduced by closed manipulation (although open reduction may occasionally be required) and by percutaneous insertion of titanium or stainless steel intramedullary nails.

chapter 19

NEUROSURGICAL CONDITIONS

Gregory W. Hornig, MD • Clarence Greene, Jr., MD

BRAIN TUMORS

Brain tumors are rare in the first year of life, with an incidence of 1 per 100,000 infants.[1] This incidence increases with age. By the age of 2 years, central nervous system (CNS) tumors occur in 2 to 5/100,000 children. Brain tumors represent the most common solid tumors in the pediatric population.[2]

In the group of brain tumors considered congenital, the most common are teratomas (37%), followed by primitive neuroectodermal tumors (PNETs) (12%), astrocytomas (10%-15%), and choroid plexus tumors (8%).[3] In a slightly older population of children, teratomas become less frequent and other neoplasms become relatively more common, including astrocytomas (34% of brain tumors in children younger than 24 months of age), PNETs (23%), and ependymomas (11%). There is also a group of tumors that are sometimes considered non-neoplastic. These include developmental tumors, which derive from aberrant proliferative growth during embryonic brain development and include craniopharyngiomas, lipomas, dermoids, and colloid cysts.[4]

Cerebellar Astrocytomas

Low-grade astrocytomas occur throughout the CNS and constitute a fourth of all pediatric brain tumors. Cerebellar astrocytomas are common (12%-17% of pediatric CNS tumors), and their treatment has the most favorable outcome of all intra-axial neoplasms in the CNS.[5] Most of these tumors are found in children younger than the age of 10 years. The symptoms of cerebellar astrocytomas include headache (80%), vomiting (80%), gait disturbance, and decreased level of consciousness. Signs include ataxia in 80%, papilledema, cranial nerve palsies (including blindness and diplopia), and dysmetria. The rapid progression of signs and symptoms is often a function of cerebrospinal fluid (CSF) obstruction because the tumor occupies the fourth ventricle or the aqueduct and causes hydrocephalus. Treatment of the hydrocephalus is often required urgently in very sick children. Temporary diversion of CSF via external ventriculostomies or shunts often precedes removal of the tumor.

Many of the signs and symptoms of posterior fossa neoplasms have an indolent progression. It is not unusual for headache and vomiting and ataxia to continue for many months in patients who are treated for otitis, viral syndromes, gastrointestinal disorders, or failure to thrive. It is the experience of many neurosurgeons that nearly all brain tumors in young children are misdiagnosed initially, sometimes for long periods of time. The relentlessness and progression of symptomatology is the decisive factor that leads to diagnostic studies.

Surgical removal of these tumors is often possible, but new neurologic deficits can occur in 30% of patients, although at least half of these new deficits are transient.[6] Neurologic trauma during surgery occurs because of the proximity of vital brain stem and delicate cranial nerve structures to the tumor, which is often large and firm. Postoperative pseudomeningoceles (the bulging of skin at the occipital incision site) and hydrocephalus are not uncommon (10%-26%) and require additional treatment. Temporary continuation of postoperative CSF diversion via external ventriculostomy is favored by many surgeons to reduce the likelihood of permanent ventriculoperitoneal shunts.

The unambiguous goal of surgical therapy for low-grade tumors remains complete removal. When total resection of these tumors is confirmed, the long-term survival without recurrence occurs in about 90% of cases but much depends on the biologic aggressiveness of the tumor. Some histologic features such as mitosis, endothelial proliferation, and necrosis suggest a high-grade lesion with a much poorer prognosis. In cases of "low grade" astrocytomas with unanticipated rapid recurrence, additional treatment can be attempted, including further surgery and adjunctive chemotherapy and/or radiotherapy. Frequent follow-up scans continue for at least 5 years after the operation.

Ependymomas

Ependymomas represent about 10% of pediatric brain tumors and are slightly less common than PNETs and astrocytomas. More than two thirds of ependymomas in children occur in the posterior fossa (Fig. 19-1) and the symptoms they cause are similar to posterior fossa or cerebellar astrocytomas: headache, vomiting, lethargy, and ataxia. These symptoms result from a combination of compression along the dorsal brain stem and hydrocephalus. Many extend from the obex (in the inferior aspect of the fourth ventricle) and then extrude through the lateral opening of this ventricle (foramen of Luschka) into the cerebellopontine angle. Here they invade and compress cranial nerves with resulting facial weakness, diplopia, swallowing dysfunction, and hearing loss. When large, they often extend beyond the foramen magnum and can compress the cervical cord. In regard to their cell of origin, they are not limited to the ependymal layer of the ventricle but can arise from cerebellar, cerebral, or spinal cord parenchyma.

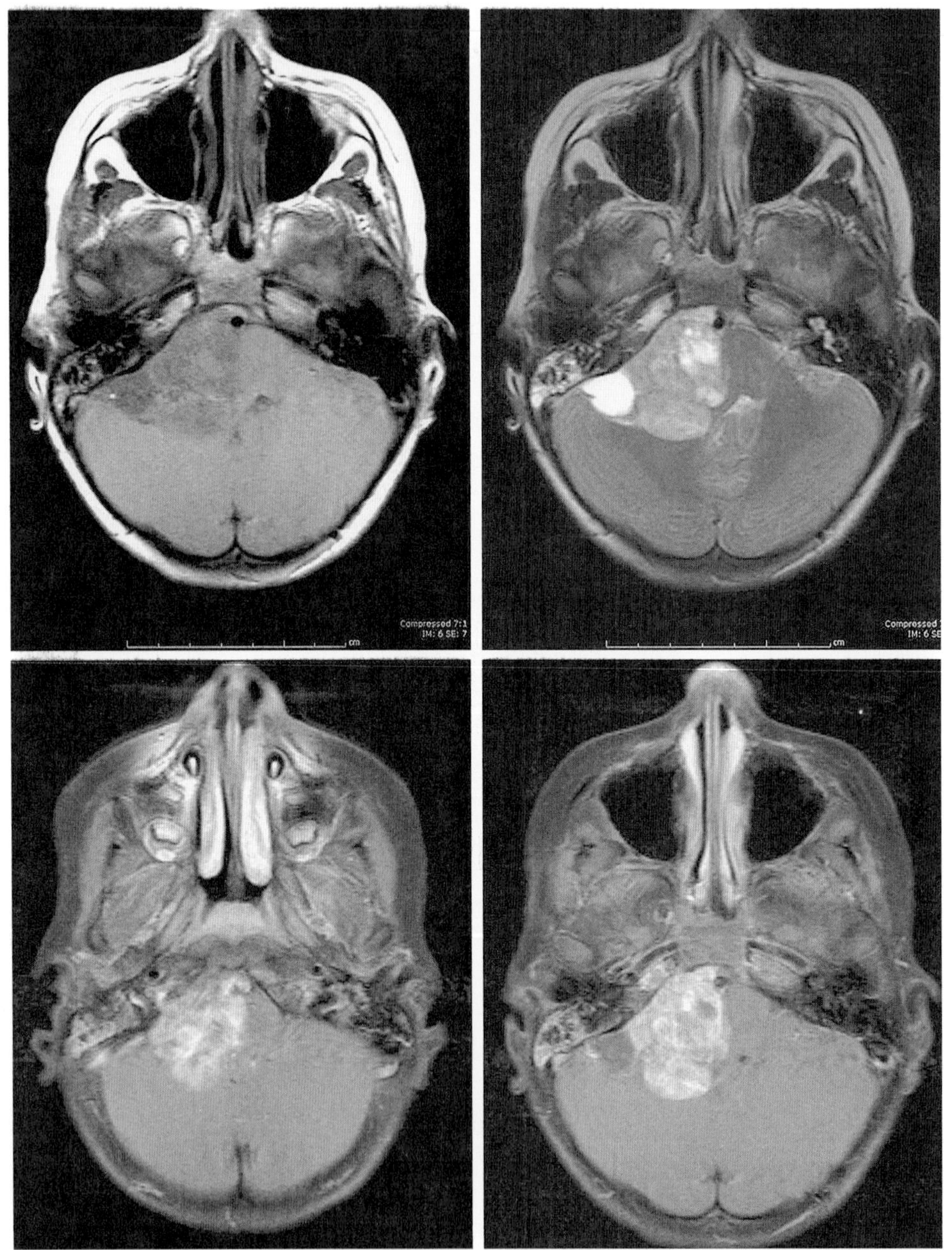

Figure 19-1. MR image of a posterior fossa ependymoma. The tumor involves the lateral aspect of the posterior fossa and contains calcifications typical of ependymomas. The brain stem is severely distorted by the mass effect of the tumor. The tumor also compresses cranial nerves on the right side, making complete tumor removal problematic. This patient had right facial weakness, diplopia, and mild left hemiparesis postoperatively.

Aggressive surgical resection has been the goal of neurosurgical treatment of these difficult tumors, but there is high probability of new or worsening neurologic deficits as a result of surgical trauma. Modern surgical results have clearly demonstrated a correlation between postoperative residual tumor and tumor recurrence and/or progression. In the 30% of children where the tumor is totally resected, there is still a 20% to 40% possibility of recurrence, even after conventional radiotherapy.[7] In cases of near-total resection, the rate of progression-free survival falls to 30%.[8] Most of the recurrences are local and radiation therapy has become the mainstay of treatment, even with complete resection. Very small children, usually younger than age 3 years, are faced with comparatively greater morbidity from conventional radiotherapy, and radiation therapy is often deferred. Chemotherapy has been used with some success in this group of patients. The role of chemotherapy without irradiation has generally not been favorable in other groups. Retrospective studies have failed to prove substantial benefit in survival when chemotherapy is added to surgery and radiation therapy for newly diagnosed ependymomas.

Treatment of ependymomas has remained problematic. Large, invasive tumors are clearly difficult to remove without significant risk to the patient, and residual tumors are largely refractory to chemotherapy and radiation. Some surgeons have suggested staged surgical attacks with an initial subtotal debulking followed by a second aggressive approach after chemotherapy. Whether this approach provides durable survival has not been established. Surveillance of treated patients with ependymomas must continue for many years, independent of histologic grading and extent of resection. Radiosurgery is also being used to treat focal areas of recurrent or unresectable tumor.

Medulloblastomas

Medulloblastomas are the most common malignant solid tumor in children and constitute 20% of pediatric brain tumors.[9] They are usually located in the posterior fossa and they are also referred to as primitive neuroectodermal tumors (PNETs) because they are histologically identical to tumors (pineoblastomas, neuroblastomas, and retinoblastomas) located in other locations that are believed to have derived from progenitor subependymal neuroepithelial cells undergoing malignant transformation. Nearly half of medulloblastomas have chromosomal abnormalities, particularly the deletion of 17p chromosome that contains the tumor suppressor gene *TP53*.[10]

Hydrocephalus often occurs with medulloblastomas because of their location within the cerebellar vermis (a midline structure), often filling the fourth ventricle (Fig. 19-2). Children with this tumor often have symptoms of elevated intracranial pressure (ICP) (obtundation, headache, nausea/vomiting, irritability) and have signs suggestive of posterior fossa compression (dysmetria, ataxia, diplopia, head tilt, and papilledema). Lumbar puncture should not be done after computed tomography (CT) or magnetic resonance imaging (MRI) has established the presence of a posterior fossa tumor and obstructive hydrocephalus. CSF diversion treatments (usually via an external drain) are usually done either before or in conjunction with craniotomy. Conversion of these temporary devices to permanent ventriculoperitoneal shunts is not uncommon in children with large tumors and marked preoperative ventriculomegaly.

Complete resection of medulloblastomas is often possible, although permanent postoperative deficits can occur in as many as 14% of patients with worsening of preoperative deficits after aggressive surgery.[6] The "posterior fossa syndrome" that can occur in up to 13% of children after surgery is characterized by mutism, drooling and swallowing difficulties, ocular palsies, and increasing ataxia.[11] These problems resolve entirely in most patients after several months. Improvement is thought to occur with resolution of swelling within the inferior vermis.

Staging is important with medulloblastomas because patients have a predictable outcome depending on age, metastases, pathology, and extent of surgical resection. Poor survival is correlated with age younger than 4 years, residual tumor measuring more than 1.5 cm,[2] and tumor dissemination, particularly "drop" metastasis along the spinal column. After craniospinal radiation in eligible patients, survival occurs in 50% to 70% of patients with standard or low-risk medulloblastomas. Newer treatment protocols include chemotherapy first, which is followed by radiotherapy consisting of lowered cumulative craniospinal doses (24 to 36 Gy to the entire brain) with hyperfractionated delivery, usually 1 Gy twice daily. Survival in these "good risk" patients is nearly 90% after 5 years. Survival in high-risk patients is 60% to 65% with current multimodality therapy, with the worst outcomes in affected infants. Children younger than 3 years of age are usually treated first with chemotherapy, with irradiation deferred for 1 to 2 years. Radiation is sometimes avoided altogether in the 40% with progression-free survival.[12]

Recurrent medulloblastoma after surgery and radiotherapy is not amenable to cure, but a combination of aggressive therapies can allow remission of disease. These treatments include reoperation, radiosurgery, and high-dose chemotherapy with autologous stem cell rescue. Each of these treatments carries significant morbidity, including loss of cognitive skills, growth retardation, endocrine problems, and the risk of second tumors and vascular malformations in previously irradiated areas.

Supratentorial Nonglial and Glial Neoplasms

There are multiple nonglial tumors involving the cerebral hemisphere. Supratentorial tumors are fairly common, and the majority of these are glial in origin, usually designated in ascending order of malignancy as astrocytomas, anaplastic astrocytomas, or glioblastoma multiforme. Nonastrocytic tumors include

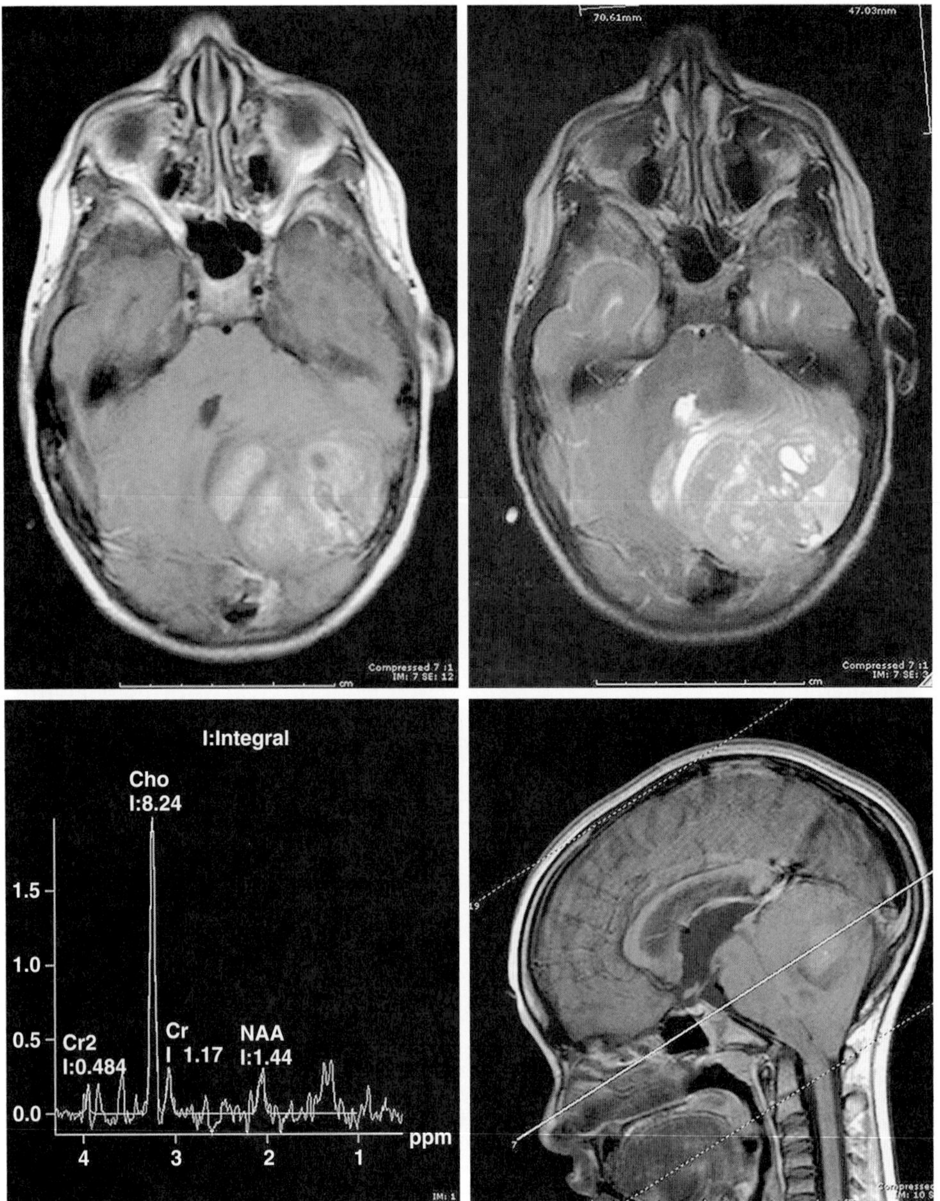

Figure 19-2. MRI and MRS (magnetic resonance spectroscopy) of a posterior fossa medulloblastoma, with compression of fourth ventricle. The MRS profile (*bottom left*) shows a choline peak with depression of *N*-acetyl aspartate (NAA) typical of aggressive tumors.

PNETs (including cerebral neuroblastomas), choroid plexus tumors (papillomas and carcinomas), teratomas (including dysembryoplastic neuroepithelial tumors [DNETs], germinomas, oligodendrogliomas, meningiomas, and gangliogliomas. In this latter grouping, operative resection is the requisite initial treatment. In the last three tumors, adjunctive therapies are not recommended after gross total resection if the tumor is relatively benign.

Seizures are much more common with supratentorial tumors because they affect the eloquent neocortex, particularly tumors in the medial or lateral temporal cortex. Older individuals are afflicted with these tumors and can present with personality changes, cognitive difficulties, headache, and growth deficits.

Germ cell tumors are composed of germinomas and teratomas and arise in pineal and suprasellar regions predominantly. Germ cells tumors often metastasize and cannot be surgically cured. Therefore, they are often best treated with radiation and chemotherapy. This combination of therapies is often quite successful with the majority of germ cell neoplasms.

Ependymomas that occur in the cerebral hemispheres remain problematic in terms of treatment, although hemispheric tumors generally have comparatively better outcomes. Incomplete resection (often because of diffuse involvement within critical brain regions) and leptomeningeal spread are significant adverse risk factors. Age is also a factor. Children younger than 3 years of age have significantly diminished progression-free survival (10%-15%) compared with older children.[13]

As with medulloblastoma, glial and nonglial tumors often have genetic abnormalities, with chromosomal abnormalities and gene mutations. Many low-grade lesions progress to become more malignant. The pathway to this malignant progression is complex. Chromosomal translocations and mutations occur as initiating events before the amplification of deleterious genes that support tumor progression. In medulloblastomas, the loss of regulation of the Sonic hedgehog developmental signaling pathway causes inactivation of the retinoblastoma tumor-suppressor gene and thereby induces the proto-oncogene *MYCN*.[14] *MYCN* is a key transcription factor that leads to proliferation of neuronal progenitor cells, and its overexpression is common in medulloblastomas. In 50% to 60% of malignant gliomas, mutations of the *TP53* suppressor gene on chromosome 17 result in malignant differentiation of glial cells and the loss of normal apoptosis. Multiple cells in the adult brain, including neural stem cells and glial progenitor cells, are self-renewing and have robust proliferative potential. As such, even small numbers of these cells can undergo malignant transformation and lead to the development of gliomas. Additionally, aberrant regulation of gene transcription can independently lead to tumor progression, either by amplification or loss of inhibition of genes involved in cell division. Extracellular growth factor activation such as vascular endothelial growth factor (VEGF) can lead to malignant transformation by phosphorylation of tyrosine kinases that deregulate signaling pathways. The interaction of VEGF and its receptor leads not only to increased endothelial proliferation but also to cell migration, cell proliferation, vascular permeability, and the loss of apoptosis.[15]

There is a growing appreciation of the myriad causes of neoplastic growth, often by agents that do not directly alter DNA but cause subtle changes in gene expression. For example, hypermethylation (adding a methyl group to cytosines that precede guanines) of promoter regions of tumor-suppressor genes or DNA repair genes can lead to transcriptional silencing of regulatory regions in glioma cells, leading to tumor development.[16] Even microRNA genes, composed of 21-23 nucleotides, are important regulators of gene expression and can function as oncogenes when they downregulate tumor suppressor genes. The precise regulation of cell-cycle control is disrupted in all instances of glial tumorigenesis. The highly complex causes of this loss of regulation remain an enigma.

For surgical treatment of brain tumors there exists a strong association between resection extent and outcome. From the neurosurgical viewpoint, maximal resection should be attempted without inordinate surgical morbidity. The advent of frameless stereotaxy for precise tumor localization, "functional" localization with intraoperative monitoring (e.g., somatosensory evoked potential mapping to determine the location of the motor cortex), presurgical functional MRI to determine location of speech areas, and intraoperative scanning (via real-time ultrasonography, CT, or MRI) have each added considerably to the safety of surgery. Nonetheless, surgery can only achieve resection of targeted areas. Infiltrative tumors (which typically extend well beyond the target borders) cannot be ablated using current surgical technology. The roles of chemotherapy, molecular manipulation, and conformal radiation therapy remain essential to the goal of controlling high-grade brain neoplasms partially treated with surgery. Unfortunately, high-grade brain lesions remain stubbornly resistant to the intensive multimodality treatments that follow surgical resection. Survival curves for highly malignant brain lesions have not changed substantially in the past several decades.

Radiotherapy for Pediatric CNS Tumors

The target for radiation therapy is cellular DNA. Ionizing radiation damages double-stranded DNA, leading to cell death. Unlike normal cells, which have a preserved ability to repair radiation damage, neoplastic cells often are replicating at abnormally high rates and radiation interferes with their mitotic or proliferative ability. With slowly growing tumors such as craniopharyngiomas, the response to radiation is subtle and such tumors may take many months to show a clinical response. The critical sublethal dose required to preserve normal tissue but damage brain tumors, the so-called therapeutic window, is quite well understood and depends on a number of factors, including vulnerability of affected tissue (which can depend on the age of the patient and locale of the target; optic nerve radiation, as an example, is poorly tolerated), tumor vulnerability, volume irradiated, total dose, fraction size, and interfraction interval. As total volume of irradiation increases, the cumulative radiation dose must necessarily decrease to reduce the morbidity of treatment. The conventional cumulative radiation dose for most pediatric CNS tumors is in the 50- to 60-Gy range, although some tumors (e.g., germinomas) are much more sensitive to radiation and can respond to treatment in the 30- to 50-Gy range.[17] Identification of tumor type is therefore an important determinant of radiation therapy, and biopsy is often a prerequisite for treatment.

Radiotherapy has enjoyed significant technologic advances with the advent of improved radiologic definition of tumors and sophisticated computer-assisted planning in three-dimensional systems. Stereotactic radiosurgery (SRS) has become routine in the United States, and single high-dose fractions can be delivered with great precision using high-energy photons produced either by linear accelerators or cobalt sources (gamma knife). Proton-beam therapy utilizes charged nuclear particles to deliver energy in discrete target points after the proton has nearly come to rest. As such, the proton can traverse normal brain without losing energy. As it comes to rest, it gives off most of its energy in less than 1 cm in the form of a Bragg "peak," providing a distinctively sharp rise in absorbed energy at the targeted tissue.

All these stereotactic methods are very precise and ideal for small targets, which are usually noninfiltrative lesions with well-delineated borders. The complications arising from targeting structures larger than 3.5 cm limit the radiosurgical approach. As such, the utility of treating small noninfiltrative tumors is optimal with single-fraction radiosurgery. For larger lesions in vulnerable areas of the brain (e.g., brain stem, retina, or cranial nerves), fractionation can be used with either repeat head fixation or localization systems to minimize complications of SRS therapy. In pediatric patients, SRS is mainly used as a boost to tumors that have recurred or persisted after conventional fractionated radiation therapy.

Stereotactic radiotherapy is distinct from radiosurgery in that it utilizes SRS techniques (usually with radiation from linear accelerators, with computer-assisted planning and delivery devices) using fractionation such as limited radiation of delivery of less than 200 cGy per day. The targets of this therapy are usually discrete and spare nearby normal structures (e.g., the optic nerve, the optic chiasm, the hypothalamus) that cannot tolerate the radiation delivered with single-dosing methods such as the gamma knife. This conformal radiation provides the radiobiologic advantages of fractionation along with the precision and control of SRS. Tumors typically treated in this manner are craniopharyngiomas, optic system tumors, and pituitary adenomas.

TREATMENT OF SPASTICITY AND MOVEMENT DISORDERS

Spasticity is defined as an abnormal response to passive muscle stretch. As the velocity of passive movement of a joint is increased, increased resistance develops. During examination of an affected extremity, there can be as little as a "catch" to passive movement or, in more severe cases, no movement at all. Spastic children often have muscle stiffness, fatigue, and pain. If the condition is severe and chronic, muscle contractures and joint dislocation can occur, particularly in the flexor muscles and internal rotator muscles. In children with spastic quadriparesis, the typical stance is one of flexed elbows and wrists, with standing and walking on toes, the knees and hips flexed, and the legs internally rotated.

Spasticity occurs because of an imbalance of excitatory Ia afferents from muscle spindles into the spinal cord and inhibitory descending impulses from the basal ganglia and cerebellum. In most children, the inhibitory impulses are diminished because of early CNS injury or injury to the spinal cord, which conducts the descending inhibitory impulses. Hence, treatment is directed toward either increasing the inhibitory neurotransmitters (usually γ-aminobutyric acid [GABA]) or reducing the afferent excitatory transmission from muscle spindles. Baclofen achieves the former, and dorsal rhizotomy (via cutting afferent nerve roots) interrupts the reflex transmission from muscle spindles.[18,19]

The children most susceptible to spasticity are those with low birth weight due to prematurity who have suffered a variety of cerebral insults, particularly hypoxic-ischemic encephalopathy with its predilection for causing periventricular white matter loss. Other affected infants have antepartum or intrapartum insults that lead to specific brain injuries that interrupt pyramidal pathways that mediate the inhibitory spinal pathways.

Treatment of spasticity should aim to improve function and facilitate care. Multidisciplinary clinics usually assess the potential candidate for surgical treatment. The best candidates for lumbosacral rhizotomy are motivated, older children (age 5-6 years) with spastic diplegia (affecting the legs predominantly) who lack severe contractures and have relatively good leg strength. Children with weak legs and spasticity can lose function with rhizotomy because they depend on their increased tone to maintain marginal ambulatory function. Rhizotomy can produce, to their detriment, a nonadjustable and permanent decrease in spasticity. Very young children are not good candidates for baclofen pumps because of the size of the device. Oral baclofen can be most useful in these very young children. Baclofen pumps are advantageous in children with severe spasticity that interferes with their care and in children with quadriplegia, often with a greater reduction of spasticity in the legs than the arms. The treatment is not permanent and nonablative, and the dosing is amenable to adjustments. It is particularly useful in children with spinal cord insult from trauma or inflammatory processes (transverse myelitis) and in patients with familial spastic paraparesis.

Botulinum toxin produces neuromuscular blockade and thereby reduces muscle contractions and spasticity. It is typically injected into spastic muscles and for a period of several months will decrease spasticity and increase range of motion. These injections are often used to extend the period of time until a definitive procedure can be done in very young children, often decreasing the risk of developing muscle contractures that are fixed deformities not amenable to any spasticity treatments.[20]

EPILEPSY SURGERY

Epilepsy affects about 1% of the population and starts commonly in the first decade of life. Surgical control of epilepsy is a well-established therapy when medical control of seizures cannot be achieved. Temporal lobectomy has been a mainstay of pediatric neurosurgical care for more than 40 years, and temporal resections constitute more than half of the epilepsy interventions currently performed in pediatric patients. The efficacy of surgery for temporal lobe epilepsy is well established. In a randomized, controlled trial of surgery versus medical therapy, 64% of patients were free of disabling seizures after surgery compared with only 8% of those in the medical arm.[21] Surgery additionally may curtail the cognitive and psychosocial disabilities that can occur with medically intractable seizures, particularly in remediable syndromes that begin in infancy, before the acquisition of language and social skills. The quality of life for patients with epilepsy is unambiguously related to the recurrence of seizures, and uncontrolled seizures carry a substantial risk of disability and death.

Drug-resistant epilepsy is thought to be reasonably predicted after only two antiepileptic medications have proven ineffective. After the failure of a third medication, the probability of being seizure free is less than 10%. Therefore, despite the invasiveness of surgery, it is highly reasonable to consider operative intervention 1 or 2 years after the onset of disabling epileptic seizures, particularly in the 30% of epileptic children who have complex partial seizures emanating (unilaterally) from the temporal area. Surgery requires comprehensive preoperative evaluation by epilepsy specialists, along with multiple imaging and monitoring studies. Invasive monitoring is fairly common in pediatric patients, who tend to have seizures that are multilobar. Newer noninvasive modalities such as magnetoencephalography are rapidly achieving success in determining the source of seizures.

The success of temporal lobe surgery has led to more aggressive approaches to control epilepsy originating elsewhere in the brain. The pathologic substrates of pediatric extratemporal epilepsies are quite diverse, including cortical dysplasia, developmental abnormalities of neuronal migration, gliosis, tumors, neurocutaneous disorders (e.g., Sturge-Weber syndrome, tuberous sclerosis), and inflammatory lesions. These entities are often intensely epileptogenic from an early age. In such lesions, the MRI abnormality does not strictly correlate with the source of seizures and the epileptogenic focus may, in fact, be relatively diffuse and involve eloquent cortex. Nonetheless, some series show excellent results in more than 50% of patients, particularly if there is complete resection of an epileptogenic focus, including the focal area of interictal abnormality.[22] Intelligence quotient scores tend to be stable or improved in the majority of children selected for surgery.

In some patients, seizures can be lateralized to one hemisphere by preoperative methods but not precisely localized. These patients can be considered for hemispherectomy if there is significant unilateral dysfunction. As radical as such operative resection would appear, the improvement of hemisphere disconnection procedures is in the 70% range for seizure freedom, with likely hemiparesis and hemianopia found postoperatively (although these deficits are often present before surgery). Newer techniques involve a disconnection of the hemisphere without anatomic removal of the affected hemisphere, thereby reducing some of the complications associated with volumetric removal of large portions of the brain.[23]

Corpus callosum sectioning is a palliative surgery in patients who have seizures without focal onset. In patients with drop attacks, division of all or part of the corpus callosum can result in improvement in about 60% of patients by reducing the severity of their seizure and decreasing the likelihood of severe injury from falling.[24]

Vagal nerve stimulation (VNS) is useful for the treatment of partial seizures, providing about a 50% reduction in seizure frequency in patients with intractable seizures who are not candidates for resection. The morbidity of implantation of the vagal nerve stimulator is extremely small, and the efficacy of the device rivals that of new antiepileptic medications. As opposed to medications, there is no toxicity and no issues of compliance.[25]

HYDROCEPHALUS

Other than trauma, hydrocephalus is the single most common entity pediatric neurosurgeons are called on to manage. This disorder of CSF circulation and absorption accounts for 0.6% of all pediatric hospital admissions, 1.8% of all pediatric hospital days, and 3.1% of all pediatric hospital charges.[26-29] The care of hydrocephalic patients is a major health care expenditure, hovering near $1 billion in the United States per year.[30] Although hydrocephalus can afflict individuals at any age, the range of causes and manifestations are larger and often more complex than in the adult population.

CSF is a clear fluid, which is primarily secreted within the ventricles of the brain by the choroid plexus. A considerable volume may be formed by interstitial fluid from the intercellular clefts in the brain and spinal cord.[31-33] The total production of CSF has been calculated at 0.31 mL/kg/hr.[34] The volume in the system turns over nearly four times per day.

The circulation of CSF is complex. CSF exits the brain through the fourth ventricle and has a pulsatile course through the subarachnoid space over the convexities of the brain, the basal cisterns, the spinal subarachnoid space, and ultimately back intracranially to the vertex of the brain. There, the CSF transits through midline arachnoid granulations into the venous system at the superior sagittal sinus. This transfer is passive from a higher-pressure system into a lower-pressure environment.

Escape of the CSF through alternative routes exist, although none is adequate to maintain normal nervous system function. Many mothers have observed that their children look puffy around the eyes when their shunt is malfunctioning. There is perhaps escape of CSF through the craniofacial lymphatics that might account for this observation. This transit of CSF has been confirmed in other mammals, and there is advancing evidence of this in humans.[35-37]

Congenital Hydrocephalus

Hydrocephalus may be an isolated development or be associated with many syndromes and brain maldevelopment conditions such as holoprosencephaly and schizencephaly.

The most common genetic hydrocephalus is X-linked hydrocephalus. It occurs in 1:30,000 male births and represents 2% to 5% of nonsyndromal cases of hydrocephalus. The aqueduct of Sylvius is narrowed, causing subsequent dilation of the third and lateral ventricles, sparing the fourth ventricle (Figs. 19-3 to 19-5). In its fullest expression, other neurologic abnormalities can occur. Twenty-five percent of males with clear aqueduct stenosis will have X-linked

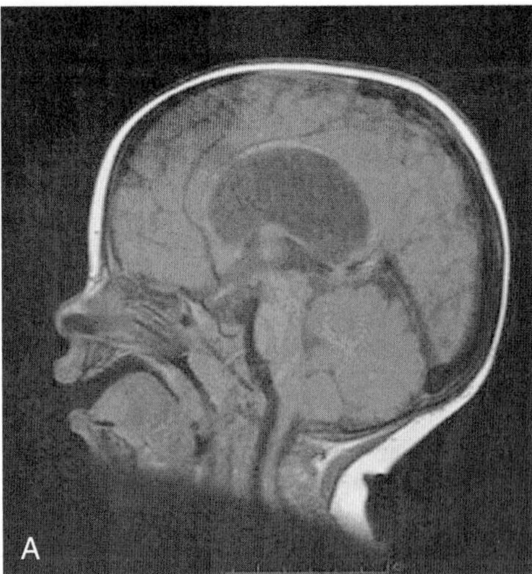

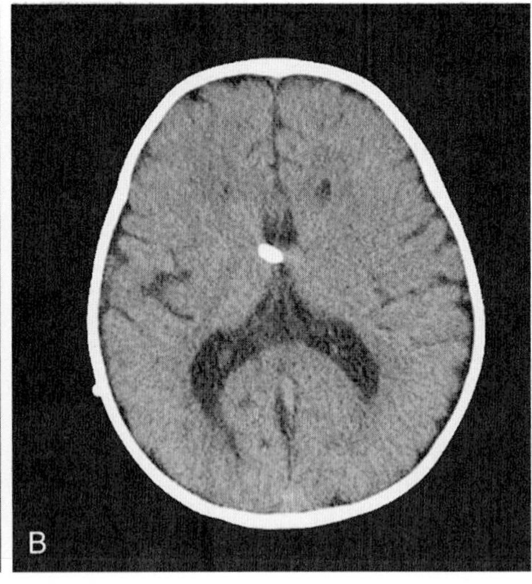

Figure 19-3. **A,** Sagittal MR image showing aqueduct stenosis and dilated third and lateral ventricles. **B,** Axial CT after ventriculoperitoneal shunt.

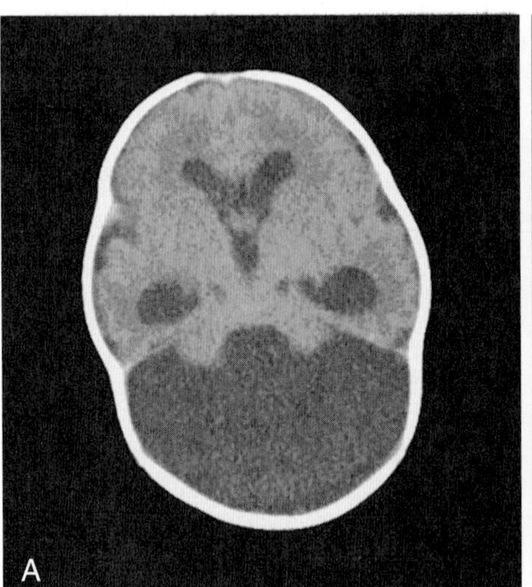

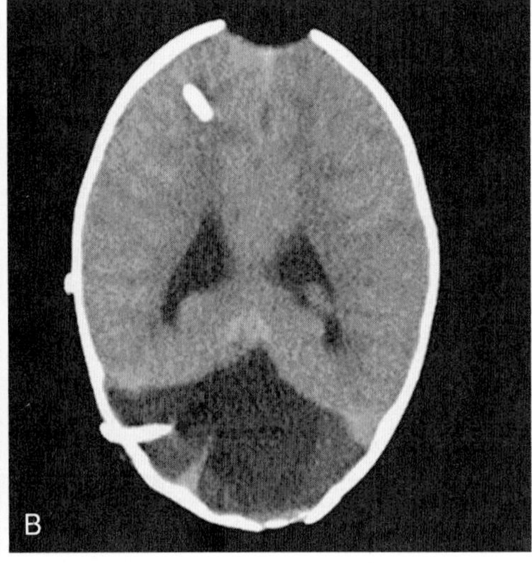

Figure 19-4. **A,** Axial CT scan of Dandy-Walker malformation. **B,** The axial CT scan shows supratentorial and posterior fossa shunt catheters. The posterior fossa shunt was required after the cyst continued to expand.

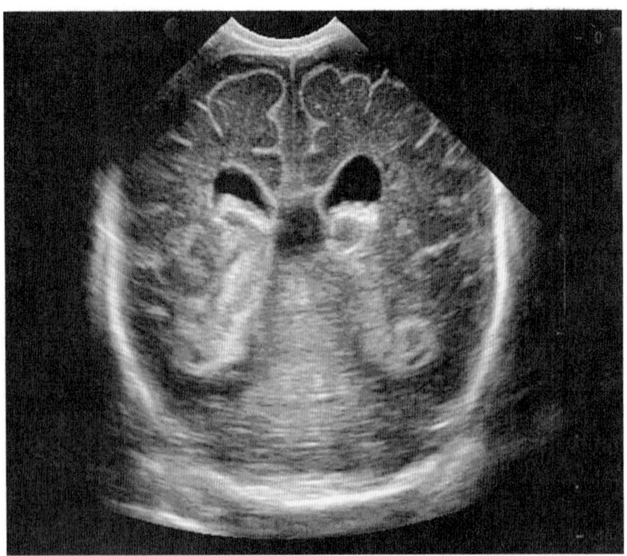

Figure 19-5. Ultrasound image shows a grade III bilateral intraventricular hemorrhage with ventricular dilation.

hydrocephalus, which is very important in advising couples about future pregnancies.[38] Other causes of aqueduct stenosis can be thickening of the tectum of the midbrain from hamartoma, glioma formation, or from intrauterine infections.[39]

The Chiari II malformation includes alternation in the size and shape of the posterior fossa, descent of the midline cerebellar tonsils through the foramen magnum, and straightening of the brain stem along with a beaking appearance of the tectum or dorsal midbrain. This is the next most common etiology of hydrocephalus and is always present to some degree in children who have the spinal dysraphism of myelomeningocele or meningocele. Chiari II malformation interrupts the egress of CSF from the fourth ventricle as well as disrupts the pulsatile flow of CSF around the confines of the posterior fossa. Children with untreated or undertreated hydrocephalus and Chiari malformation are at risk for the development of hydromyelia or syrinx.

The Dandy-Walker malformation is next in frequency for causing hydrocephalus. In the fullest expression of this anomaly, one finds a retrocerebellar cyst, which can be quite sizable with a cleft or defect in the vermis of the cerebellum, agenesis of the corpus callosum, and extracranial anomalies such as cardiac septal defects and syndactyly. These children are at higher risk for developmental delays and epilepsy.

In Dandy-Walker malformation, the hydrocephalus is due to an alternation in CSF flow at the exit of the fourth ventricle. Dandy-Walker malformation may be further complicated by a "double compartment" hydrocephalus. The cyst formation may block escape of the CSF at the distal end of the aqueduct of Sylvius with resultant dilation of the third and lateral ventricles. In addition, the choroid plexus within the fourth ventricle will create CSF with no access to the subarachnoid space and subsequent enlargement of the cyst. In infants, this may lead to an unsightly distortion of the cranium and signs and symptoms of hindbrain compression. Not infrequently, additional surgical attention must be directed to the cyst, usually a CSF shunt catheter, either joined with a ventriculoperitoneal shunt or a separate shunt entirely (see Figs. 19-3 and 19-4).[40,41]

Acquired Hydrocephalus

In the United States there are more than 50,000 very low birth weight infants born each year. Almost 20% of these neonates suffer some degree of intraventricular hemorrhage, most related to bleeding within the germinal matrix adjacent to the ventricles of the brain (see Fig. 19-5). These hemorrhages are graded on a I to IV scale (Table 19-1). Grade I is subependymal only, grade II shows extension into the ventricle, grade III has ventricular dilation, and grade IV includes clot in the parenchyma of the brain. At least 25% of these neonates will develop posthemorrhagic hydrocephalus.[42] Intraventricular blood is a powerful irritant to the ependymal lining of the ventricles as well as to the arachnoid membranes. The resultant inflammatory response and scarring can lead to obstruction of flow of CSF from the ventricle or, more commonly, an intense arachnoiditis with severe restriction of the CSF pathways at the base of the brain. Traumatic intracranial bleeding will manifest the same pathophysiology, leading to "posttraumatic" hydrocephalus. In the worst cases, the resultant inflammation will be both intraventricular and in the subarachnoid space. It can lead to multiple scar septations within the ventricles and "multiple compartment" hydrocephalus.[43]

Table 19-1 Grading System for Intraventricular Hemorrhage Based on Ultrasound Findings

Grade	Cranial Ultrasound Findings
I	Hemorrhage in germinal matrix only
II	Ventricular hemorrhage without ventricular dilation
III	Ventricular hemorrhage with ventricular dilation
IV	Brain parenchymal hemorrhage

By definition, meningitis is inflammation of the arachnoid. In severe cases, especially in the very young, hydrocephalus may be the consequence of compromised subarachnoid spaces. Fetal infection with toxoplasmosis, cytomegalovirus, and *Cryptococcus* are infrequently encountered but are devastating to the developing brain, and the concurrence of hydrocephalus is only more tragic to the infants. Finally, subdural emphysema and brain abscess may lead to altered CSF flow and subsequent hydrocephalus.

It is extremely rare to see a child with congenital hydrocephalus become shunt independent. Thus, such children need to be approached with caution in making such a diagnosis.[44,45]

Brain tumors frequently occur in the midline in children and cause CSF obstruction. In fact, it is often the signs and symptoms of hydrocephalus, not the tumor itself, that brings these children to medical attention. Fortunately, if the tumor can be excised, the hydrocephalus in the majority will resolve without additional surgical management.

There is one entity, congenital or acquired, that creates an overproduction of CSF. This condition is hyperplasia or a tumor of the choroid plexus. Choroid plexus papilloma or carcinomas (<1% of brain tumors) are not infrequently diagnosed in the neonatal period. The choroid plexus tumor is usually obvious on brain imaging studies for investigation of a large head or to delineate the type of hydrocephalus present. Hyperplasia of the plexus might not be as evident and may only become recognized when seeking why hydrocephalus treatment is not effective. CSF ascites, pleural effusion, or failure of an endoscopic third ventriculostomy are examples of treatment failure due to excessive CSF. Choroid plexus hyperplasia may generate hundreds of milliliters of CSF above normal and overwhelm the absorptive capacity of peritoneal, pleural, or other shunt termini.

Diagnosis

The brain imaging of communicating hydrocephalus typically demonstrates dilation of all the ventricles of the brain and infrequently the subarachnoid space. Patients with postmeningitic hydrocephalus are a typical example. The signs and symptoms of hydrocephalus are age dependent and often relate to the rapidity of the ventricular expansion. In the neonate and young infant, there are typically few symptoms. The child often feeds well and is attentive and happy, and the only clue may be an accelerated rate of head growth.

In older children with a firmer calvaria, hydrocephalus usually creates a more pronounced increase in ICP and the increased pressure will generate more symptoms. Most commonly, there is head pain or excessive irritability in the nonverbal child. Vomiting, detachment, or disinterest in play is common. Other common observations are poor school performance

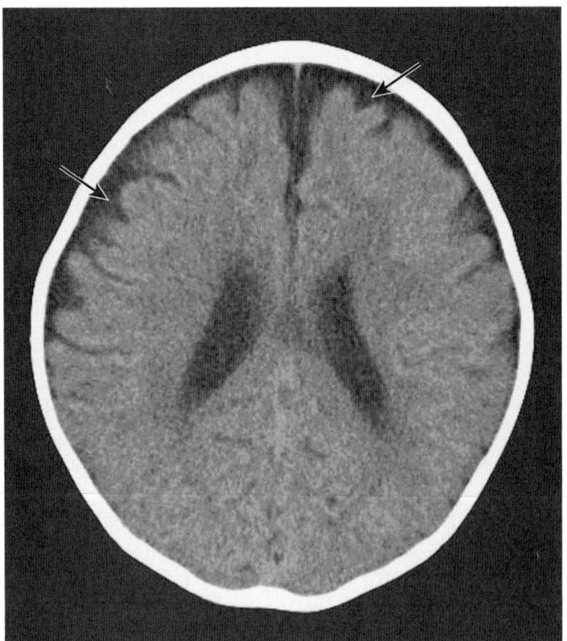

Figure 19-6. Axial CT scan shows mildly dilated lateral ventricles and a generous subarachnoid space in the frontal and frontoparietal areas (*arrows*).

and easy fatigability. Visual changes such as blurriness or change in color perception can be noted by older children. Recumbence increases ICP, and therefore typically the headaches and vomiting are more pronounced in the morning. Seizures may occur, but not usually as a presenting or solitary event.

Physical findings commonly include a large head, a full but not tense anterior fontanelle, and prominent scalp veins. Peculiar to infants is the "sunset" eye appearance. This downward and outward deviation of the eyes is a neuronal mediated response to pressure on the superior colliculi of the midbrain by a dilated third ventricle. After treatment, the extraocular disturbance regresses. Older children may demonstrate a Parinaud sign: the failure of upward gaze, the mature version of the sunset eyes phenomena. Papilledema and altered visual fields often are evident.

Suspicions are to be confirmed by brain imaging studies. Ultrasonography in infants with an open fontanelle is a good screening study, but even if hydrocephalus is diagnosed with that technique, MRI or CT is required to more fully understand the etiology (Fig. 19-6).

Treatment

The first reproducibly successful treatments for hydrocephalus of all types occurred in the early 1950s. Lumboureteral shunts had been successfully employed in patients with communicating hydrocephalus.[46] Success was then reported with ventricular to jugular vein shunts incorporating a miniaturized spring and ball valve.[47] As silicone replaced the earlier stiffer plastics, the ventriculoperitoneal shunt became and remains the mainstay of hydrocephalus therapy.[48]

Development of shunt hardware has matured. The quality of the silicone has improved, making the tubing more pliable and less hazardous to abdominal organs. Valves can be adjusted to various opening pressures with external magnets. Tubing that incorporates antibiotics within or coating it are available. With these mechanical advances, life expectancy of the shunt itself has improved and the complications have diminished, although only slightly. Realistically, there is little difference in the performance of one brand of shunt over another, despite the claims of the multiple vendors.[49]

Shunt occlusions and infections are still vexing in our efforts to have these children lead a normal life. Nearly half of all shunt operations are revisions for occlusion or removals for infections. Perioperative antibiotic usage, although not without controversy, has reduced the shunt infection rate to 8% or less in busy pediatric centers.[50] There is no consensus as to which antimicrobial agents or what dose is most efficacious.[51]

Alternatives to ventriculoperitoneal shunts are still useful, if not required in some complex cases. Lumboperitoneal shunts have regained some popularity among pediatric neurosurgeons in selected patients with free communication of CSF from the intracranial compartment to the spinal subarachnoid space. The development of a Chiari I malformation presumably from chronic CSF drainage that draws the cerebellar tonsils downward has given many neurosurgeons pause before considering this shunt in young patients.[52-54] When circumstances make the peritoneum inhospitable to CSF absorption, alternate termini for the tube include the venous system, pleural space, and even the gallbladder.[55]

An alternative to CSF shunting has re-emerged with the miniaturization of endoscopic equipment. Creating an opening in the floor of the third ventricle to look around an obstruction at the aqueduct or the outlet of the fourth ventricle is very appealing. The concept dates from 1922 but was a failure. New technology for minimally invasive surgery has given a rebirth to the idea and, today, most pediatric neurosurgeons are eager to use endoscopic third ventriculostomy (ETV) in lieu of CSF shunts (Fig. 19-7). When successful, the hydrocephalus is managed without the need for foreign body implant and without the inherent risks of infection or valve or catheter failure. This approach has been found to be successful in 60% of properly selected children.[56] The potential complications, such as uncontrollable hemorrhage, neuroendocrine dysfunction, and short-term memory loss, are severe, more so than with shunting. Nevertheless, there is great appeal in having hydrocephalus treated effectively without hardware in the body.

Shunt Malfunctions

Despite the progress in shunt design and materials, shunts will fail, and at a surprisingly high rate. Forty percent fail within the first year of implant. At 15 years, there is an 80% likelihood of failure. Again, the signs and symptoms will be age dependent. Infants

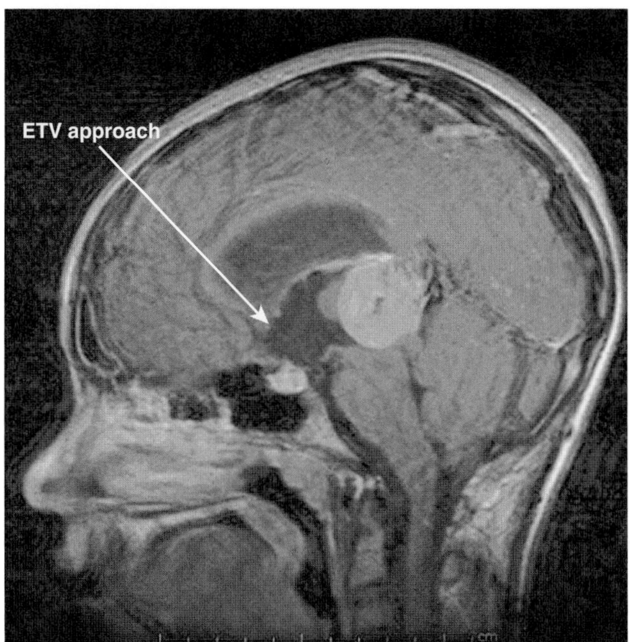

Figure 19-7. Sagittal MRI of patient with a large tumor in the posterior third ventricle causing aqueduct occlusion. The *arrow* depicts the approach for an endoscopic third ventriculostomy (ETV) to bypass the obstruction and relieve the hydrocephalus. At the same operation, the tumor was sampled.

may have minimal symptoms because of the expandable cranium, whereas older children may quickly become dreadfully ill as the ICP increases. Headache, vomiting, and altered mental status predominate as symptoms. The clinical assessment typically includes a brain imaging study, a shunt survey (plain films of the shunt) to look for a fracture of the tube, a shortened end, or a migration. Although a change in the ventricular size noted on imaging is a strong clue to the diagnosis, normal ventricular size can often be a falsely reassuring sign. It is not uncommon for symptomatic children to have no dilation of their ventricles, presumably related to loss of brain compliance.[57,58] Often a percutaneous needle tap of the shunt reservoir or valve will be needed to measure pressure. Some surgeons use radioisotope or contrast flow studies. When in doubt, surgical exploration of the shunt is the best option.[59]

SPINAL DYSRAPHISM

There are multiple types of spinal dysraphism, or neural tube defects, in children. The most common are myelomeningocele, lipomyelomeningocele, and meningocele.

Myelomeningocele

Myelomeningocele is the most frequently encountered spinal neural tube defect. In the United States, the incidence is 0.3 per 1000 live births, a decrease of nearly 50% since the widespread use of folic acid in women planning pregnancy or begun in the first trimester.[60] It is rarely a diagnostic problem and is now frequently discovered with fetal ultrasonography. Diagnostic confirmation with ultrasonography and amniocentesis has presented the opportunity for pediatric neurosurgeons to councel couples as to the ramifications of the disorder and allow them to make an informed decision about continuing the pregnancy.

Essentially, these are defects in the skin, fascia, posterior elements of the spine, and the conus medullaris of the cord, along with a failure in neurulation during the 26th to 28th weeks of gestation. Myelomeningocele is most frequent in the lumbar and lumbosacral area (Fig. 19-8). Often of considerable size, it might be confused with a sacral teratoma. The neonatal assessment may require MRI of the entire spinal canal to exclude concurrent anomalies. Cranial ultrasonography is usually sufficient to evaluate for hydrocephalus. The surgical challenge is not so much in closing the exposed nervous system but in obtaining a tension-free cutaneous closure. The initial surgery is directed at freeing the exposed end of the incompletely fused spinal cord from the cutaneous attachments and closing a pseudo-dural layer to protect it. Not infrequently, the skin closure is the more complex segment of the operation, and plastic surgical techniques (relaxing flank incisions, skin grafts, rotational flaps) may be required to accomplish this closure.

The more rostral the defect, the more severe the neurologic deficit, and the more severe the challenges presented to the patient throughout his or her lifetime. To some degree, all of these children have a concurrent Chiari II malformation, which will lead to hydrocephalus in most patients.

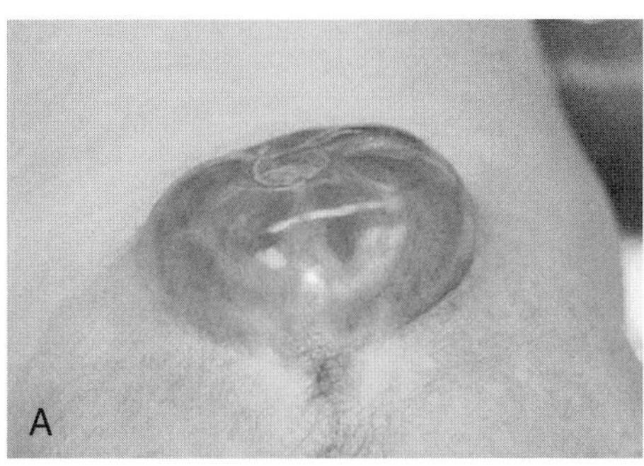

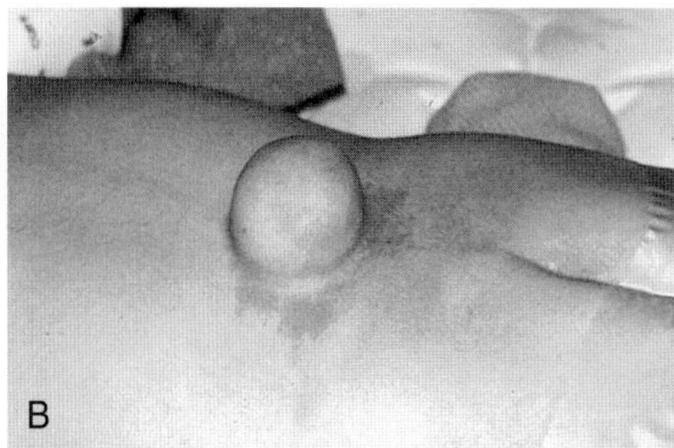

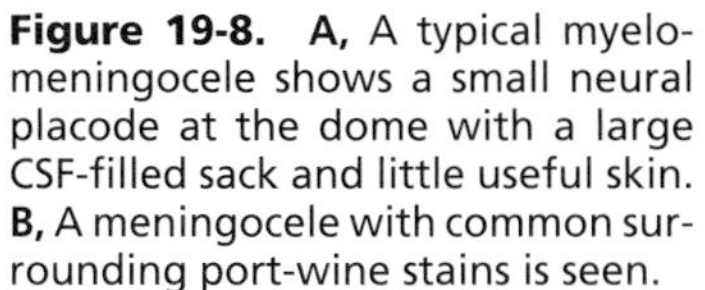

Figure 19-8. **A,** A typical myelomeningocele shows a small neural placode at the dome with a large CSF-filled sack and little useful skin. **B,** A meningocele with common surrounding port-wine stains is seen.

Lipomyelomeningocele

Lipomyelomeningocele is a complex anomaly that consists of a subcutaneous meningocele, fascia and bony defects, and a lipoma interfacing with the spinal cord, which is located dorsally, dorsolateral, or terminally. Externally, these lesions appear in the midline and can range from tiny subtle fatty lumps to large masses often accompanied by skin tags, port-wine stains, and an altered intragluteal fold (Fig. 19-9). Before the availability of CT, the connection with the spinal canal was often missed and cosmetic removal of the subcutaneous fat was performed, often with significant negative sequelae. These lesions often require tedious microdissection with release of any tethering effect on the spinal cord to prevent neurologic (weakness, sensory loss), urologic (neurogenic bladder), or orthopedic (scoliosis, leg-length discrepancies) consequences. These children do not have Chiari malformation, sparing them the burden of hydrocephalus.

Operative correction of the asymptomatic infant with a lipomyelomeningocele is not without controversy. Unfortunately, the natural history of these anomalies is unknown. The rationale for early operation in these patients is to release any tethering on the spinal cord and prevent neurologic, urologic, or orthopedic consequences of spinal cord injury. However, a significant number of patients have suffered the same deficits postoperatively that the surgery was planned to prevent. Some children progress despite surgery, which may be related more to a dysfunctional conus than to tethering effects. The absolute correct approach to this lesion remains elusive.[61,62]

Meningocele

The least common of the neural tube defects is the simplest one. A meningocele consists of a defect in the skin, fascia, posterior spine, and meninges but not the nervous system. When this anomaly occurs, it has a predilection for the lumbosacral area, although it can develop anywhere along the neural axis. Unlike the myelomeningocele, these lesions are almost always covered by nearly normal skin. Therefore, there is no CSF leak. Because the spinal cord and nerve roots are not involved, the children do not have neurologic, urologic, or orthopedic symptomatology. A Chiari II malformation is prevalent in these patients. Therefore, hydrocephalus and the other maladies discussed earlier are possible.

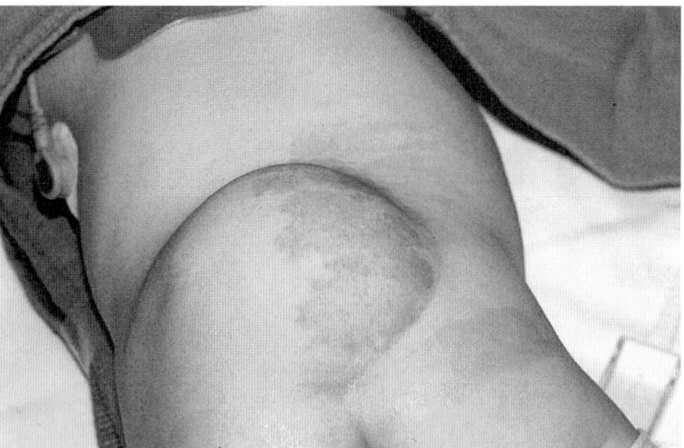

Figure 19-9. A sizable lipomyelomeningocele is seen with cutaneous port-wine stains.

Tethered Spinal Cord Syndrome

With any of the spinal dysraphisms, there is a high probability the conus medullaris lies below the L2 disc space and is deemed to be "tethered" by radiographic imaging. The spinal cord moves slightly rostrad and caudad with ambulation. When constricted from free excursion, stretching of the neurons and microvascular ischemia will lead to neurologic dysfunction. This chronic injury leads to a plethora of signs and symptoms, most commonly neurogenic bladder, motor weakness or increasing tone in the lower extremities, sensory loss, and skeletal growth anomalies, including scoliosis. Operative exploration for lysis of adhesions or division of whatever structure is impeding the tethered cord is required. Unfortunately, the process may be recurrent throughout the child's growing years. All children with spinal dysraphism are at risk for tethered cord syndrome, and long-term follow-up is essential.

section 3

THORACIC

chapter 20

CONGENITAL CHEST WALL DEFORMITIES

Donald Nuss, MB, ChB • Robert E. Kelly, Jr., MD

Congenital chest wall deformities fall into two groups: those with overgrowth of the cartilages causing either a depression or protuberance and those with varying degrees of either aplasia or dysplasia.

Pectus excavatum, also known as an "excavated, sunken, or funnel chest," is the most common chest wall anomaly, constituting about 88% of deformities (Table 20-1). Pectus carinatum, a chest wall protuberance, comprises approximately 5% of chest wall deformities, whereas combined excavatum/carinatum deformities constitute 6%. Jeune's syndrome, or asphyxiating chondrodystrophy, is an extreme form of mixed pectus excavatum/carinatum and is very rare. Poland's syndrome (0.8%) and bifid sternum represent different forms of aplasia of the anterior chest wall. Poland's syndrome consists of varying degrees of dysplasia of the breast, the pectoralis muscles, and ribs. In bifid sternum, partial or complete failure of the midline fusion of the sternum is seen. This may result in ectopia cordis or varying degrees of sternal dysplasia and deficiencies of associated structures such as the heart, pericardium, diaphragm, and anterior abdominal wall (pentalogy of Cantrell).

Many of these deformities are present at birth. Some cases, such as ectopia cordis, are incompatible with life and have rarely been successfully repaired. Chest wall deformities are frequently associated with a systemic weakness of the connective tissues and with poor muscular development of the abdominal region, thorax, and spine. Therefore, a markedly increased association with Marfan syndrome, Ehlers-Danlos syndrome, and scoliosis, as well as with omphalocele in the case of bifid sternum, has been identified, all of which complicate the management of these patients (see Table 20-1).

Table 20-1 Incidence and Etiology of Congenital Chest Wall Anomalies Seen at Children's Hospital of the King's Daughters

Total children evaluated	2141
Pectus excavatum only	1805
Mixed excavatum/carinatum	116
Carinatum only	208
Poland syndrome	12
Male-female ratio	4:1
Family history of pectus excavatum	36.2%
Incidence of scoliosis	21.7%
Incidence of Marfan syndrome diagnosed	1.7%
Marfanoid—presumed Marfan syndrome	12.0%
Patients with Ehlers-Danlos syndrome	0.7%

Data collected through 12/31/2007.

PECTUS EXCAVATUM

Pectus excavatum is a depression of the anterior chest wall of variable severity and can usually be characterized as mild, moderate, or severe. All variations in depth, symmetry, and breadth of the deformity can be seen. The deformity may be localized and deep ("cup-shaped"; Fig. 20-1A), or diffuse and shallow ("saucer-shaped"; see Fig. 20-1B), or asymmetric (see Fig. 20-1C). The depth and extent of the depression determine the degree of cardiac and pulmonary compression, which, in turn, determines the degree of physiologic effect.Only one third of patients referred from our own region had a deformity severe enough to require surgical correction. Even with referral of patients with a severe deformity from other centers, our ratio of surgical interventions has been only about 50% (Table 20-2).

The deformity may be noted at birth and progresses with growth. During rapid pubertal growth, the progression may become especially pronounced, a fact apparently unknown to many pediatricians, who mistakenly advise families of younger patients that the condition will resolve spontaneously. We have seen many families who were given this advice and missed the opportunity to have the deformity repaired before puberty while the chest was still soft and malleable and before it interfered with physical performance.

History

Pectus excavatum was recognized as early as the 16th century. Johan Schenck collected literature on the subject, as cited by Ebstein.[1] A classic article by Bauhinus

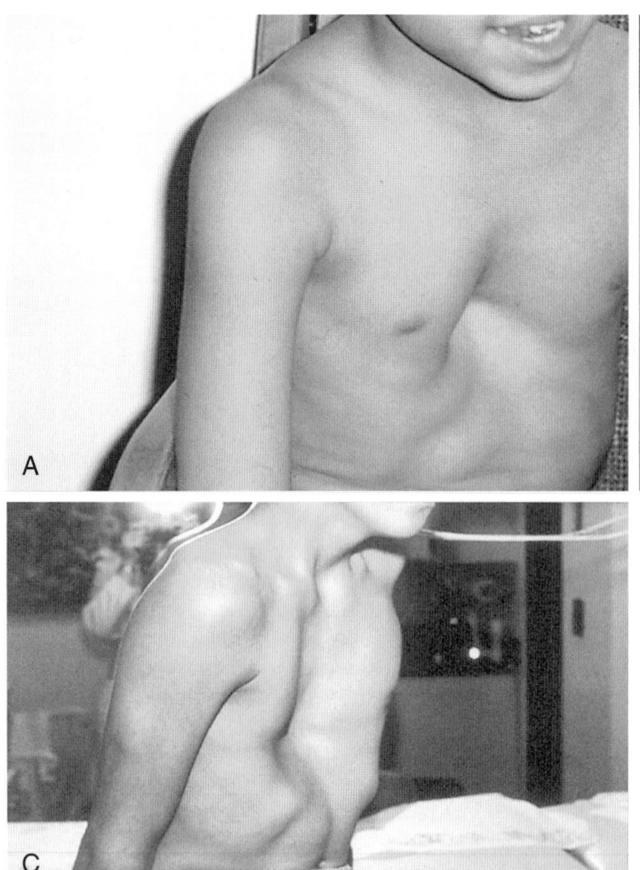

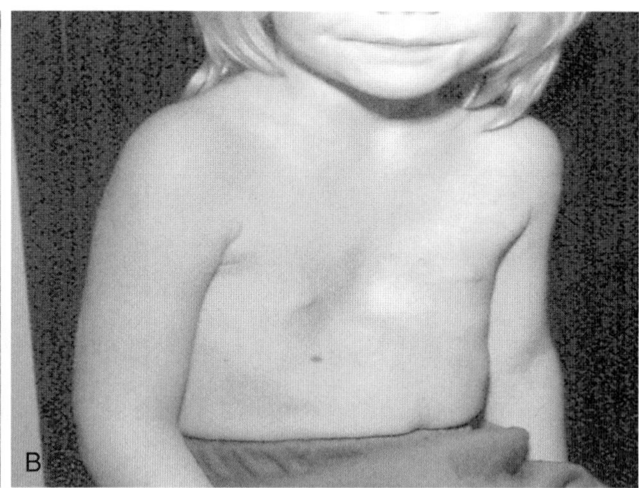

Figure 20-1. **A,** Localized or "cup-shaped" pectus excavatum. **B,** Diffuse or "saucer-shaped" deformity. **C,** Eccentric deformity.

in 1594 described the clinical features of pectus excavatum in a patient who had pulmonary compression with dyspnea and paroxysmal cough, attributed to a severe pectus excavatum.[2] The familial predisposition was first noted by Coulson in 1820,[3] who cited a family of three brothers with pectus excavatum, and Williams in 1872,[4] who described a 17-year-old patient who was born with a pectus excavatum and whose father and brother also had the condition.

Table 20-2	Presenting Symptoms in 1015 Patients Who Have Undergone Surgical Correction of Pectus Excavatum at Children's' Hospital of the King's Daughters
Shortness of breath, lack of endurance, exercise intolerance	89.2% (906)
Chest pain, with or without exercise	67.0% (680)
Frequent respiratory infections	23.9% (243)
Asthma/asthma-like symptoms	27.8% (282)
Cardiology Indicators	
Cardiac compression	89% (793/889)
Cardiac displacement by CT	88% (783/889)
Murmurs	29% (257/889)
Mitral valve prolapse	15% (132/889)
Pulmonary Indicators	
FVC < 80%	26%
FEV1% < 80%	32%
FEF25-75% < 80%	45%

Data collected through 12/31/2007.

Numerous other case reports appeared in the 19th century, including a five-case report by Ebstein in 1882 that covered the clinical spectrum of this condition.[5] Treatment at that time was limited to "fresh air, breathing exercises, aerobic activities and lateral pressure."[6,7]

Thoracic surgery remained "forbidden territory" until the early years of the 20th century. The first attempt at surgical correction was a tentative approach in 1911 by Meyer, who removed the second and third costal cartilages on the right side without improvement of the deformity.[8] Sauerbruch, one of the pioneers of thoracic surgery, used a more aggressive approach in 1913 by excising a section of the anterior chest wall, which included the left fifth to ninth costal cartilages as well as a segment of the adjacent sternum.[7] Before his operation, the patient was incapacitated by severe dyspnea and palpitations, even at rest, and was unable to work in his father's watch factory. After recovery, the heart could be seen to pulsate under the muscle flap, but the patient was able to work without dyspnea and was married 3 years later.

In the 1920s, Sauerbruch performed the first pectus repair that used the bilateral costal cartilage resection and sternal osteotomy technique later popularized by

Ravitch.[9] He also advocated external traction to hold the sternum in its corrected position for 6 postoperative weeks. His technique was soon adapted by others in Europe and rapidly gained popularity in the United States. In 1939, Ochsner and DeBakey published their experience with the procedure and reviewed the entire surgical literature on the subject.[10] Also in 1939, Lincoln Brown published his experience in two patients and reviewed the literature with particular reference to the etiology of pectus excavatum.[11] He was impressed with the theory that short diaphragmatic ligaments and the pull of the diaphragm on the posterior sternum were the causative factors.

Ravitch initially subscribed to the short ligament theory as well. As a result, he advocated even more radical mobilization of the sternum, with transection of all sternal attachments, including the intercostal bundles, rectus muscles, diaphragmatic attachments, and excision of the xiphisternum. In 1949, he published his experience with eight patients in which he used this radically extended modification of Sauerbruch's technique of bilateral cartilage resection and sternal osteotomy.[12] However, he did not utilize external traction.

The abolition of external traction may have led to an increased recurrence of the condition. As a result, Wallgren and Sulamaa introduced the concept of internal support in 1956 by using a slightly curved stainless steel bar that was pushed through the caudal end of the sternum from side to side and bridged the newly created gap between the sternum and ribs.[13,14] In 1961, Adkins and Blades modified internal bracing further by passing a straight stainless steel bar behind rather than through the sternum.[15] This technique was rapidly adapted for patients of all ages.

As early as 1958, Welch and Gross advocated a less radical approach than that of Ravitch.[16,17] Welch produced excellent results in 75 cases without dividing all the intercostal bundles or the rectus muscle attachments. However, he still advocated performing the procedure in young patients. Conversely, Pena was very disturbed by the idea of resecting the rib cartilages from very young patients and demonstrted that asphyxiating chondrodystrophy developed in baby rabbits after cartilage resection during their growth phase.[18] Later, Haller also reported the risk of acquired asphyxiating chondrodystrophy as well.[19] As a result, many surgeons stopped performing open pectus repair in young children and waited until they had reached puberty. They also decreased the amount of cartilage resected and spoke about a "modified Ravitch procedure," which effectively was the original Sauerbruch procedure.

In 1997, we published our 10-year experience with a minimally invasive technique that required no cartilage resection and no sternal osteotomy but instead relied on internal bracing made possible by the flexibility and malleability of the costal cartilages.[20]

The rationale for this technique was based on the three following observations:

1. *Malleability of the chest.* Children have a soft and malleable chest. In young children, the chest is so soft that even minor respiratory obstruction can cause severe sternal retraction. Trauma rarely causes rib fractures, flail chest, and so on, because the chest is so soft and malleable.[21-23] Thus, the American Heart Association recommends "using only two fingers" when performing cardiac resuscitation in young children and "only one hand in older children" for fear of crushing the heart.
2. *Chest reconfiguration.* In middle-aged and older adults, a barrel-shaped chest configuration develops in response to chronic obstructive respiratory diseases such as emphysema. If older adults are able to reconfigure the chest wall, children and teenagers should be able to remodel as well, especially with the increased malleability of their anterior chest wall.
3. *Bracing.* The role of braces and serial casting in successfully correcting skeletal anomalies such as scoliosis, clubfoot, and maxillomandibular malocclusion by orthopedic and orthodontic surgeons is well established. The anterior chest wall, being even more malleable than the previously mentioned skeletal structures, is therefore ideal for this type of correction.

Incidence and Etiology

Pectus excavatum occurs in approximately 1 in 1000 children and constitutes 88% of all chest wall deformities (see Table 20-1). However, this is not the case in all countries. In Argentina, pectus carinatum is more common than pectus excavatum.[24] Pectus excavatum also is rare in African-Americans. A genetic predisposition, already noted in the 19th century, was found in 36% of our patients. We have seen families with three siblings, as well as cousins and other family members, who had a pectus deformity severe enough to require correction. We also have seen patients whose fathers and grandfathers have the deformity. The male-to-female ratio of 4:1 in our series of pectus excavatum patients is similar to that of other large series.[25] Female patients have an increased risk of associated scoliosis. Inheritance is autosomal dominant, autosomal recessive, X-linked, and multifactorial in different families.[26]

The association with a connective tissue disorder is higher than in the normal population. The vast majority of our patients have an asthenic build and a definitive diagnosis of Marfan syndrome has been found in 1.7% of our patients. An additional 12% have had clinical features suggestive of Marfan syndrome. Ehlers-Danlos syndrome was present in another 0.7%. Mild scoliosis was noted in 21.7% of the patients. In our experience, severely asymmetric pectus excavatum tends to aggravate the postural abnormality of scoliosis. Early correction of the pectus excavatum has improved the mild scoliosis in some patients.

Clinical Features

Pectus excavatum is noted in infancy in approximately one third of patients[25] and usually progresses slowly as the child grows. Because young children have

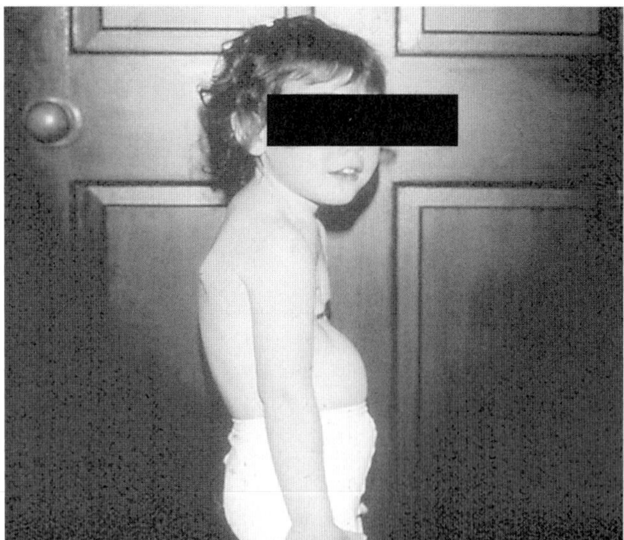

Figure 20-2. Classic pectus posture with thoracic kyphosis, forward sloping shoulders, and lumbar lordosis.

significant cardiac and pulmonary reserve and their chest wall is still very pliable, the majority of young children are asymptomatic. However, as they become older, the deformity becomes more severe and the chest wall becomes more rigid. Eventually, they find that they have difficulty keeping up with their peers when playing aerobic sports. A vicious cycle may develop as patients stop participating in aerobic activities because of their inability to keep up. Subsequently, their exercise capacity diminishes further. The downward spiral is given added impetus by the fact that these patients, already embarrassed by their deformity, will avoid situations in which they have to remove their shirts in front of other children, further inhibiting participation in school and team activities.

By withdrawing from participation in activities with their peers, they also become depressed, which may affect their schoolwork. Most pectus patients have a typical geriatric or "pectus posture" that includes thoracic kyphosis, forward-sloping shoulders, and a protuberant abdomen (Fig. 20-2). A sedentary "couch potato" lifestyle may aggravate this posture, and the poor posture depresses the sternum even farther. For this reason, we empirically recommend an aggressive pectus posture exercise and breathing program, both preoperatively and postoperatively.

Many patients have a relatively mild deformity during childhood. Because pediatricians are unaware of the potential for marked progression of the deformity with growth, they reassure the parents that it will resolve spontaneously or even improve. Although the deformity may not always deepen, it is unlikely that it will resolve spontaneously. When the patients grow rapidly during puberty, the deformity often suddenly accelerates. A mild deformity may become severe in as little as 6 to 12 months. These patients give a history that "my chest suddenly caved in." It is the rapid progression that alarms parents and induces them to seek surgical consultation despite their pediatrician's reassurance. Patients with a rapid progression of their deformity exhibit the most pronounced symptom-complex.

The earliest complaints are shortness of breath and lack of endurance with exercise. As the deformity progresses, chest pain and palpitations with exercise may occur, giving rise to exercise intolerance. Other symptoms include frequent and prolonged respiratory tract infections, which may lead to the development of asthma (see Table 20-2).

A recent study showed that these patients have a poor body image, which has a major impact on self-worth.[27] Therefore, it is important to correct the deformity before it affects their ability to function normally. One of our patients, a 35-year-old lawyer, confided that he had not married because he was too ashamed of his chest abnormality to have a serious relationship. A 16-year-old patient left a note for his parents, before attempting suicide, detailing the harassment and abuse that he had received from children at school. Just as one would not consider leaving a child with a cleft lip untreated, one should not leave a child with a severe pectus untreated. Both have a physiologic and psychological impact on the patient.

Cardiac and Pulmonary Effects of Pectus Excavatum

A great deal has been written about cardiopulmonary function in patients with pectus excavatum.[28] Some authors have shown significant compromise of cardiac or pulmonary function, or both.[29,30] Others have been unable to demonstrate significant variation from predicted values.[31] Several factors play a role when testing cardiopulmonary function. These include the severity of the deformity, the inherent physical fitness of the individual patient, the patient's age, associated conditions, whether the tests are done supine or erect, and whether they are done at rest or during exercise. Recently, a study has shown statistically significant and clinically meaningful improvements in stroke volume, cardiac output, and cardiac index after minimally invasive repair of pectus excavatum.[32] Also, an improvement in exercise cardiopulmonary function has been noted as well.

Cardiac effects fall into three categories: decreased cardiac output, mitral valve prolapse, and arrhythmias (see Table 20-2). Compression of the heart results in incomplete filling and decreased stroke volume, which in turn, results in decreased cardiac output.[29,30,33,34] Second, the cardiac compression interferes with normal valve function. Mitral valve prolapse was present in 17% of our patients and in up to 65% of those in other published series, compared with only 1% in the normal pediatric population.[35-37] Dysrhythmias, including first-degree heart block, right bundle branch block, Wolff-Parkinson-White syndrome, and so on, have been found in 16% of our patients.[38]

Pulmonary effects also fall into three categories: restrictive lung disease, atelectasis due to lung compression, and paradoxical respiration in severe cases. The result is varying degrees of pulmonary compromise, prolonged respiratory infections, and even the development of asthma (see Table 20-2). Children with a severe deformity from birth tend to compensate by increasing the diaphragmatic component of their respiration. This partly compensates for their deformity and is found in patients who, despite a severe deformity, are able to achieve low-normal pulmonary function studies at rest. However, they demonstrate a lack of endurance during exercise because they have little or no reserve. Stress testing has shown an increase in oxygen consumption for a given exercise when compared with that of normal patients.[39] This shows that the work of breathing is increased and explains why they lack endurance.

Evaluation and Indications for Operation

A complete history and physical examination is performed in all patients and includes documenting photographs. Patients with a mild to moderate deformity are treated with a posture and exercise program in an attempt to halt the progression and are followed at 6-month intervals (Fig. 20-3).

Patients with a severe deformity or those with a documented progression also are treated with the exercise and posture program. Additionally, they undergo objective studies to evaluate whether their condition is severe enough to warrant surgical correction. These studies include pulmonary function tests (FTP), a thoracic computed tomography (CT) scan, and a cardiac evaluation that includes an electrocardiogram (ECG) and an echocardiogram.

Pulmonary function tests are performed in all patients old enough to cooperate with testing. They are best done while the patient is exercising but also are helpful in the resting state. The cardiology evaluation includes an electrocardiogram, an echocardiogram, and an examination by a pediatric cardiologist to determine the presence of cardiac compression, murmurs, mitral valve prolapse, conduction abnormalities, or other structural abnormalities. CT scans are very helpful because they clearly show the degree of cardiac compression and displacement, the degree of pulmonary compression and atelectasis, asymmetry of the chest, sternal torsion, compensatory development of a barrel-chest deformity in long-standing deformities, and ossification of the cartilages in patients with previous repairs (Fig. 20-4A, B). They also are used to calculate the CT index, which gives an objective measurement for comparing the severity between different patients. The CT index is calculated by dividing the transverse diameter by the anteroposterior diameter (see Fig. 20-4C).[40]

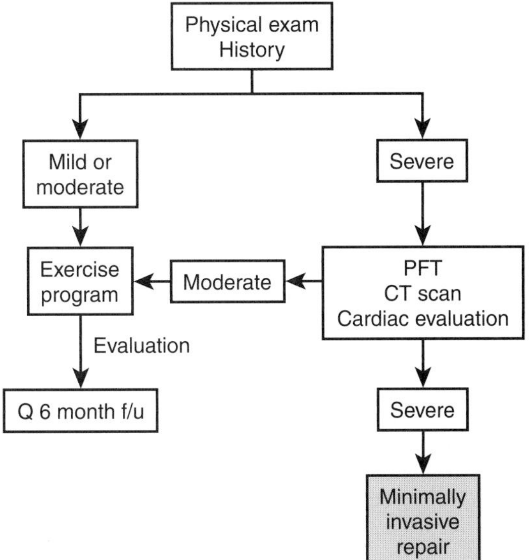

Figure 20-3. Algorithm for evaluation and treatment of patients with pectus deformities.

Determination of a severe pectus excavatum and the need for repair include two or more of the following criteria: (1) a CT index greater than 3.25; (2) pulmonary function studies that indicate restrictive or obstructive airway disease, or both; (3) a cardiology evaluation in which compression is causing murmurs, mitral valve prolapse, cardiac displacement, or conduction abnormalities on the echocardiogram or ECG tracings; (4) documentation of progression of the deformity with associated physical symptoms other than isolated concerns of body image; (5) a failed Ravitch procedure; or (6) a failed minimally invasive procedure. With these criteria, fewer than 50% of patients in our referral practice are found to have a deformity severe enough to warrant surgical correction.[20,41]

The age parameters for surgical correction depend on the type of procedure selected. Unlike the more invasive procedures (e.g., Ravitch procedure, sternal turnover), no interference with growth plates occurs with the minimally invasive procedure. Therefore, it can be done at any age, as evidenced by the fact that we have successfully operated on patients from ages 17 months to 31 years (Fig. 20-5). However, the concern with patients younger than 11 years is that if the procedure is done at too young an age, many years of subsequent growth remain during which the pectus excavatum may recur.

Our experience has shown that the optimal age for repair is 11 to 14 years. At this age, the patient is prepubertal, the chest is still soft and malleable, there is a quick recovery with a rapid return to normal activities, and results are excellent (Fig. 20-6). After puberty, the flexibility of the chest wall is decreased, sometimes requiring the insertion of two bars, which makes the procedure more difficult. It also takes patients longer to recover. However, all of our patients older than age 20 years have been extremely pleased with their results. Several other centers have reported success with patients up to age 44 years.[33,42,43]

Surgical Technique

Minimally Invasive Pectus Repair

The minimally invasive pectus repair (Fig. 20-7) involves making incisions on each side of the chest and creating a subcutaneous tunnel from the lateral thoracic incision to the top of the pectus ridge on each

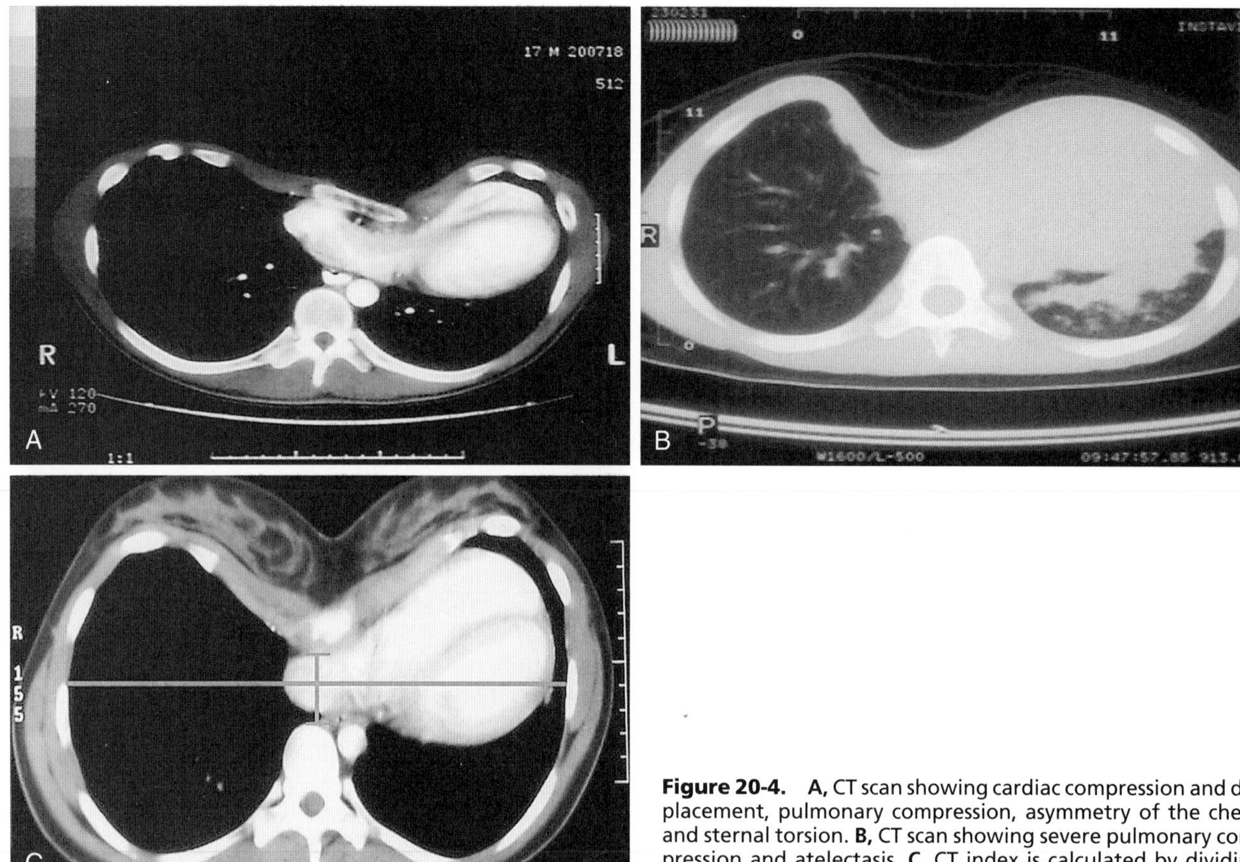

Figure 20-4. **A,** CT scan showing cardiac compression and displacement, pulmonary compression, asymmetry of the chest, and sternal torsion. **B,** CT scan showing severe pulmonary compression and atelectasis. **C,** CT index is calculated by dividing the transverse diameter by the anteroposterior diameter.

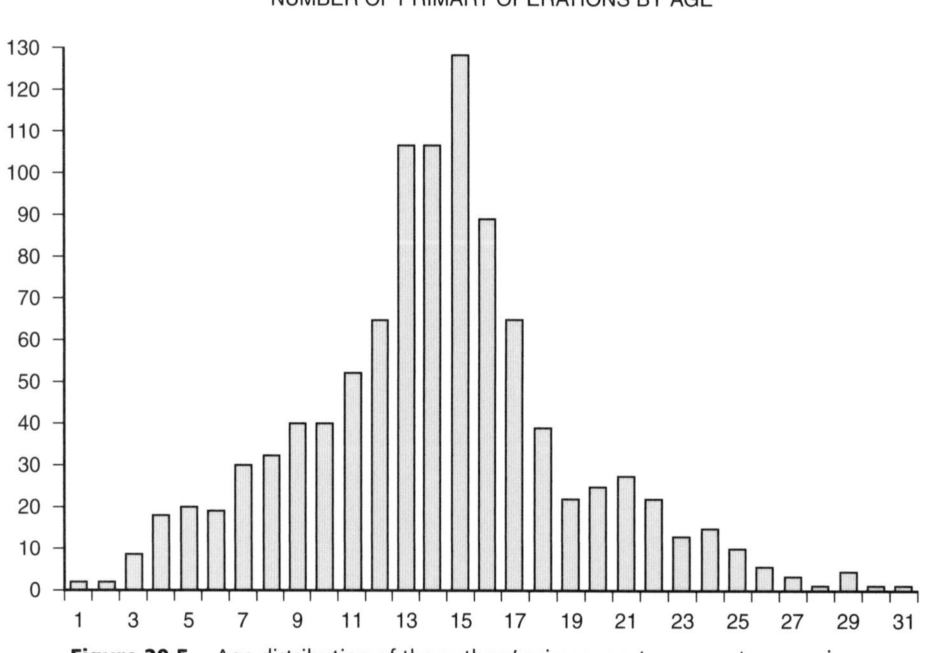

Figure 20-5. Age distribution of the authors' primary pectus excavatum repairs.

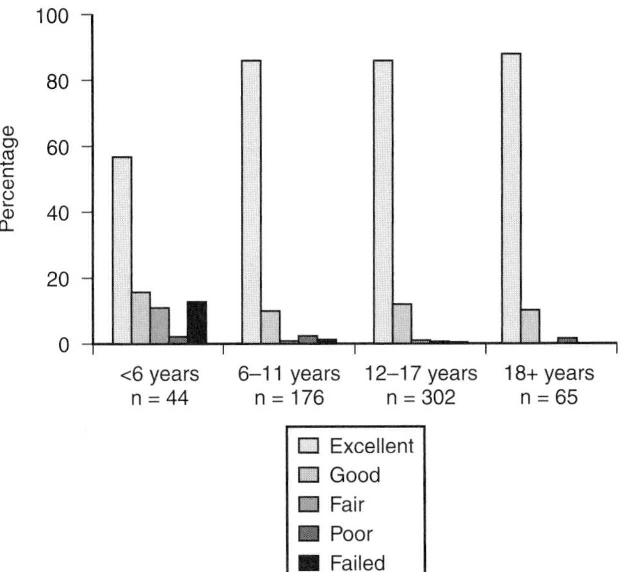

Figure 20-6. Long-term results of minimally invasive pectus repair by age groups.

side. At the top of the ridge, bilateral thoracostomy incisions are made and a large introducer is inserted into the chest cavity under thoracoscopic guidance. Very carefully, with the thoracoscope in place and under good vision, the pleura and pericardium are dissected off the undersurface of the sternum and the introducer is slowly advanced across the mediastinum and exteriorized through the thoracostomy incision on the contralateral side. When the introducer is in place, the sternum is lifted out of its depressed position by the introducer. Once the sternal depression has been corrected, an umbilical tape is attached to the introducer, and the introducer is slowly withdrawn from the chest. The pectus support bar is then attached to the umbilical tape and is slowly guided through the substernal tunnel, under thoracoscopic guidance, with its convexity facing posteriorly until it emerges on the contralateral side.

The length of the bar is determined by measuring the distance from midaxillary line to midaxillary line and subtracting 2.5 cm (1 inch). The bar is bent to the desired configuration using a bar bender. Once the bar is in position inside the chest with the convexity facing posteriorly, it is turned over by using specially designed bar flippers, resulting in correction of the pectus excavatum. The bar is secured using a stabilizer on one end of the bar and placing sutures around the bar and underlying ribs. Alternatively, stabilizers can be used on both sides to secure the bar in place. The sutures are usually placed with an autosuture needle under thoracoscopic control. It is essential that the bar be adequately stabilized or it will become displaced. Once the bar has been stabilized, the incisions are closed. The thoracoscope is removed, and the pneumothorax is evacuated by using a water-seal system. The patient is kept on a thoracic epidural analgesia for 3 postoperative days and is then discharged from the hospital, usually on the fourth or fifth day. Patients need to refrain from sports activities for 6 weeks after surgery. All patients are started on an exercise and posture program to facilitate chest expansion and to maintain a good posture.

Pain management for both the open and closed pectus repairs is the same and is designed to pre-empt the pain cascade. This is accomplished by the use of epidural analgesia and non-steroidal anti-inflammatory agents, which are started immediately before surgery and continued post-operatively for three days. In addition, narcotics and muscle relaxants are added post-operatively. When patients are discharged, they are given prescriptions for non-steriodal, anti-inflammatory medications, muscle relaxants, and narcotic medication. Patients less than 13 years of age are generally able to stop all pain medications after 7 to 10 days while patients 13 and over may require pain medication for 10 to 14 days post-operatively.

Open Technique

The preoperative preparation and evaluation are the same for the open approach for repair of pectus excavatum as for minimally invasive technique. However, because of the risk of interference with growth plates in young children and the development of asphyxiating chondrodystrophy, the procedure should be reserved for patients who have completed their growth.[18,19] The open procedure is best suited for the older patients, especially those who have asymmetric or eccentric deformities, and patients with mixed pectus carinatum/excavatum deformities.

The open technique involves making an anterior thoracic incision and elevating skin and muscle flaps until all the costal cartilages from T3 to T6 are exposed. The perichondrium is then incised longitudinally, and the deformed cartilages are either partially or completely removed. Most surgeons now advocate removing only a small section (1 to 2 cm) of the deformed cartilages, as was originally advocated by Sauerbruch and Gross.[9,17] An anterior table, wedge-shaped, sternal osteotomy is performed at the angle of Louis. The sternum is elevated, and the osteotomy is closed with nonabsorbable sutures. Some surgeons utilize a pectus strut that is inserted under the sternum to bridge the gap between the ribs and the sternum and to prevent the sternum from sinking back into the chest. The perichondrial "sleeves" are approximated with absorbable sutures, drains are inserted, the muscle flaps are sutured back into position, and the incisions are closed. Postoperative management is similar to that for the minimally invasive technique except that patients are required to refrain from contact sports for at least 3 months.

Results

The minimally invasive approach for the repair of pectus excavatum received rapid acceptance by the surgical community because the technique requires neither rib incision nor resection nor sternal osteotomy. The blood loss is minimal, the operating time is short, and the patient rapidly returns to regular activity.[43-50]

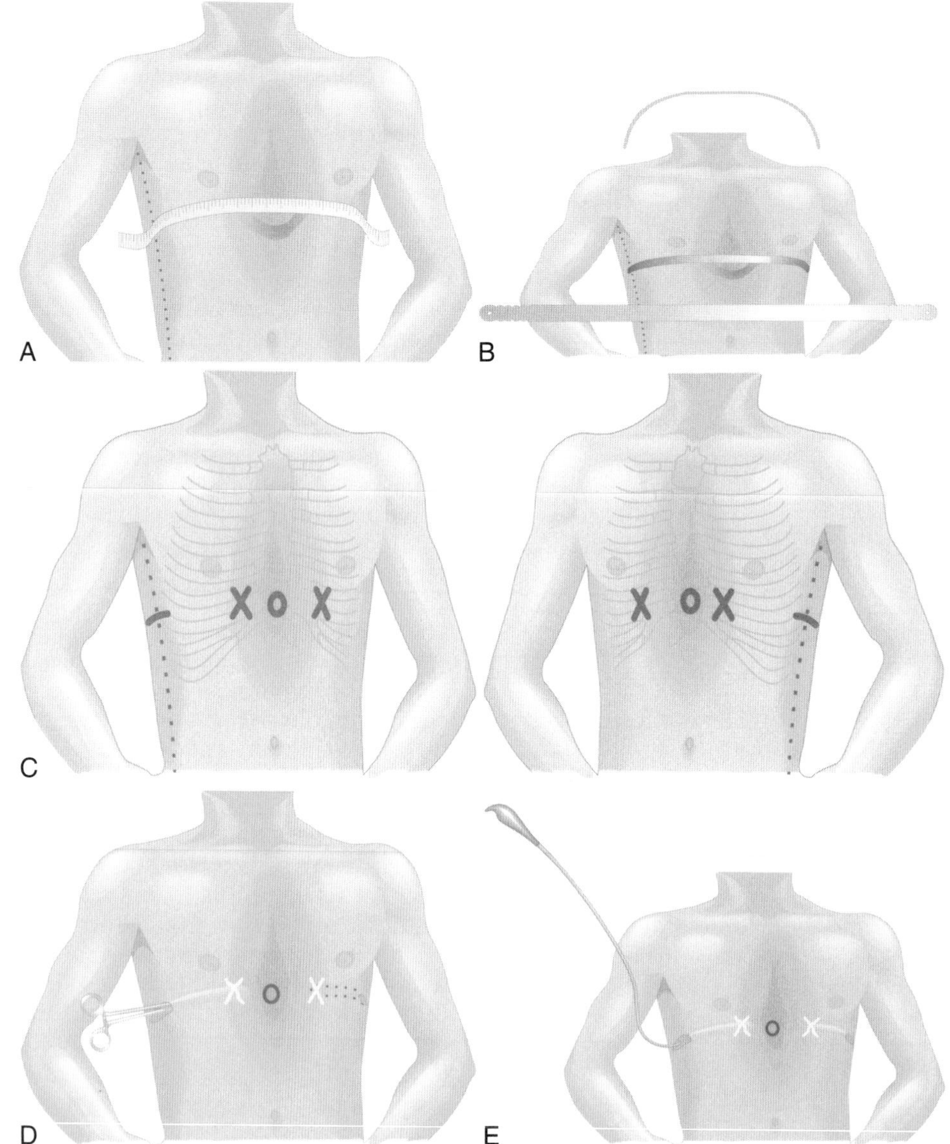

Figure 20-7. **A,** To calculate the length of the pectus bar, measure the distance from right to left midaxillary line and subtract 1 to 2 cm (1 inch). **B,** Bend the Lorenz pectus support bar to conform to the desired chest wall curvature. **C,** Mark the deepest point of the pectus excavatum with a circle by using a marking pen. If this point is inferior to the sternum, then move the circle superiorly to the lower end of the sternum just above the xiphoid. This point sets the horizontal plane bar for insertion. **D,** After confirming by thoracoscopy that the internal and external anatomy match up well, make lateral thoracic skin incisions and raise skin flaps anteriorly toward the "X" marked on the external skin at the top of the pectus ridge. **E,** Retract skin incision anteriorly to allow visualization of the intercostal space previously marked with an "X". Under thoracoscopic control, insert the appropriate-size Lorenz introducer through the right intercostal space at the top of the pectus ridge and at the previously marked "X."

Although our initial report in 1998 presented a 10-year experience, the numbers were limited (42 patients) and the long-term results were affected by the early learning experience of using a support bar that was too soft. Moreover, in some patients, the bar was removed too soon.[20] From 1988 through December 2007, 1015 patients have had their primary operation at our institution (Table 20-3). Six hundred and ninety patients have had their bars removed. Since the original presentation, numerous important modifications have been made, both to the surgical technique (e.g., routine use of thoracoscopy) and instruments, to minimize the risks of the procedure and facilitate insertion and stabilization of the support bar. These modifications have markedly reduced the risks and complications and have been previously reported.[41]

In our series of 1015 patients with pectus excavatum, only 7 (0.7%) had a mixed pectus excavatum and carinatum. One (0.1%) patient had associated Poland's syndrome, and one (0.1%) had an associated complex cardiac anomaly (atrioventricular canal). Marfan syndrome was confirmed or suspected in 13.7% of the patients, and Ehlers-Danlos syndrome was noted in 0.7% of the patients. The male-to-female ratio in patients undergoing repair was more than 4:1. The median age was 14.6 years, with a range from 19 months to 31 years. Preoperative evaluation included CT scan with a median CT index of 4.6 (range, 2.4 to

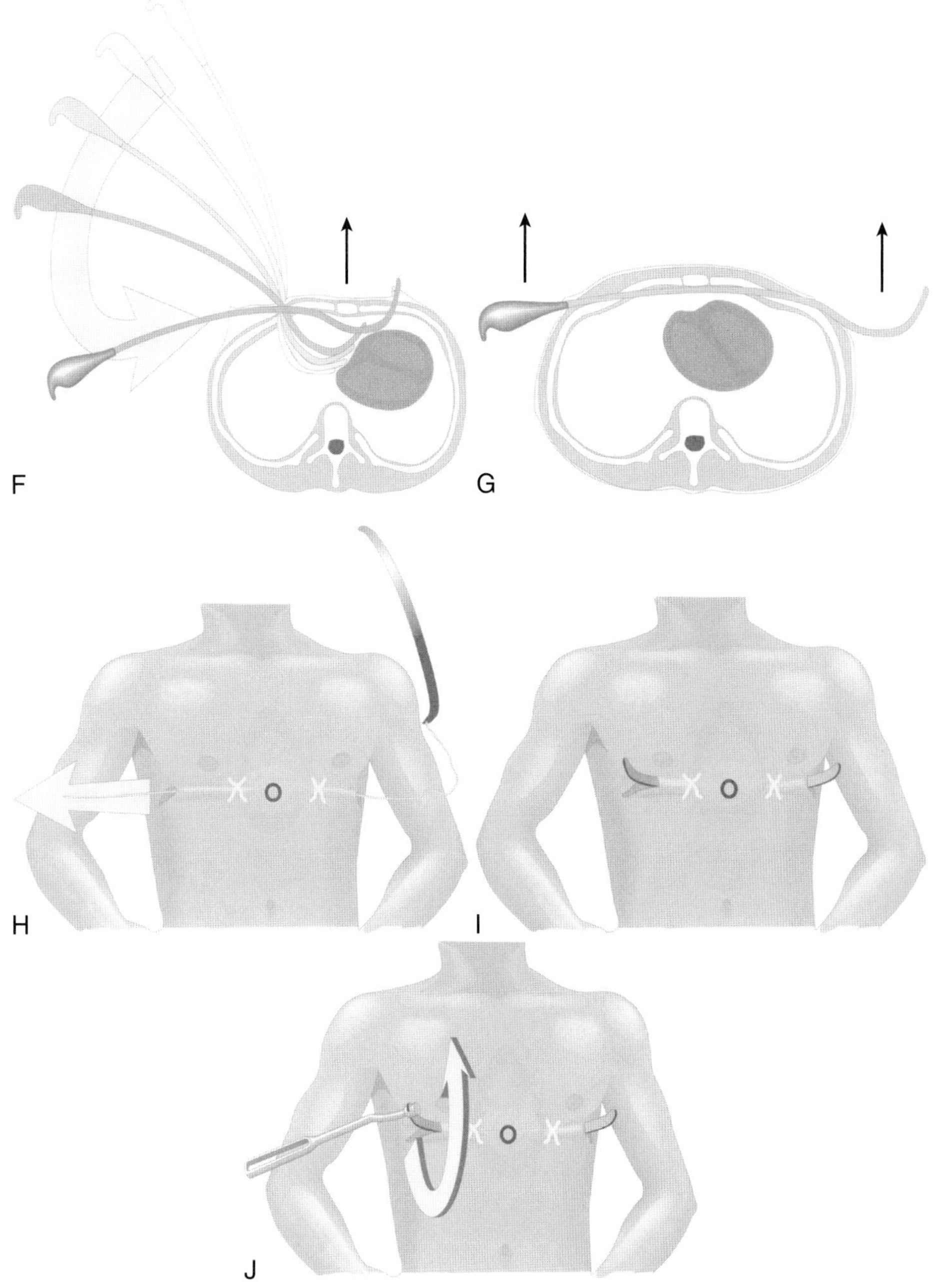

Figure 20-7—cont'd. F, When the substernal tunnel has been completed, gently push the tip of the introducer through the contralateral intercostal space at the previously marked "X," medial to the top of the pectus ridge on the left side. **G,** Use the introducer to elevate the sternum. The surgeon lifts on the right side, and the assistant lifts the left side of the introducer. **H,** Attach the previously prepared pectus bar to the umbilical tape and slowly guide the bar through the tunnel by using the umbilical tape for traction. **I,** The bar is inserted with the convexity facing posteriorly. **J,** When the bar is in position, use the specially designed Lorenz bar rotational instrument (bar flipper) to turn the bar over.

21). Cardiac compression was noted on echocardiography or CT scan, or both, in 793 of 889 patients (89%). Mitral valve prolapse was noted in 132 of 889 patients (15%). Resting pulmonary function tests were completed in 454 patients and demonstrated abnormalities in 43%.

In 730 (72%) patients, a single bar was inserted. Two bars were needed in 285 (28%) patients. Blood loss in most patients was minimal (±10 mL), with the exception of 4 patients in whom a hemothorax developed. Epidural analgesia was used for 3 days in the vast majority of patients. The median length of stay was 5 days.

Complications

Early Complications

No deaths or cardiac perforations occurred during the 1015 repairs at our institution. Pneumothorax requiring chest tube drainage occurred in 36 (3.6%) repairs,

Table 20-3 Results from Patients Undergoing Repair of Pectus Excavatum at Children's Hospital of The King's Daughters

Minimally Invasive Technique	*Materials and Methods*
2141 patients evaluated for chest wall deformity	
1101 patients had minimally invasive pectus repair	
1015 patients underwent primary operations	
86 patients have had re-do operations:	
41 failed Ravitch procedures	
43 failed Nuss procedures	
2 failed Leonard procedures	
Minimally Invasive Technique	***Operation and Length of Stay***
Single pectus bar	71.9%
Double pectus bar	27.7%
Triple pectus bar	0.4%
No stabilizers	12% (124/1015)
Stabilizers	88% (891/1015)
PDS sutures	48% (434/891)
Wired stabilizers	42% (372/891)
Not wired	10% (85/891)
Median age	14.64
Median Haller CT index	4.6
Median length of stay	5 days

and hemothorax occurred after 4 (0.4%) repairs. Four (0.4%) pleural effusions required treatment with either a chest tube or aspiration (Table 20-4).

Pericarditis requiring treatment with indomethacin occurred after 5 (0.5%) repairs. One patient required pericardiocentesis. Pneumonia occurred after 6 (0.6%) repairs, and medication reactions have occurred after 36 (3.6%) repairs. Wound infections occurred after 11 (1.1%) repairs. These resulted in bar infections and eventual early bar removal in 2 (0.02%) patients. One hundred seventy-nine patients had a transient Horner syndrome at varying times during the thoracic epidural administration.

Late Complications

Fifty-eight (5.8%) bars became displaced, and 43 (4.2%) required repositioning. In the 43 cases in which patients required repositioning of the bars, 16 occurred before stabilizers were available, a time period covering our first 105 repairs. After the introduction of stabilizers, the incidence of bar displacement decreased from 15.2% to 6.5%. When the bar and stabilizers were wired together, the incidence of bar displacement decreased to 4.3%. Since we combined placing a stabilizer on the left and polydioxanone (PDS, Ethicon, Inc., Somerville NJ) sutures around the bar and underlying rib on the right, the incidence of bar displacement has dropped to 1%.

In two patients, a late hemothorax developed secondary to trauma. Both underwent thoracoscopy with drainage of the hemothorax. At the time of thoracoscopy, no active bleeding was found. Therefore, an injury to an intercostal vessel was presumed. Whether hemothoraces would have developed in these patients as a result of their thoracic trauma if they had not had a pectus bar placed in situ is unknown. We do have several patients who were involved in major automobile accidents who sustained head and musculoskeletal trauma but no chest injuries.

Twenty-nine (2.9%) of 1015 patients have had unsuspected allergies to the metal in the bar. These allergies initially presented as rashes in the area of the bar or stabilizer and required revision to custom-made bars of other alloys. Mild overcorrection occurred in 32 (3.2%) patients. In 4 (0.4%), a true carinatum deformity developed. Of the patients in whom a true carinatum deformity developed, 3 had Marfan syndrome and the other had Ehlers-Danlos syndrome. No patient has developed thoracic chondrodystrophy.

Overall Results and Long-Term Follow-up

Patients are evaluated at 6 months after the operation and then yearly until the bar is removed. Long-term assessment has allowed classification of the results into excellent, good, fair, or failed categories.

An excellent repair indicates that the patient experienced complete repair of the pectus deformity and resolution of associated symptoms. A good repair is distinguished by a markedly improved but not completely normal chest wall appearance and resolution of associated symptoms. A fair result indicates a mild residual pectus excavatum without complete resolution of symptoms. A failed repair is defined as a recurrence of the pectus deformity and associated symptoms or the need for additional surgery (or both) after final removal of the bar.

In addition, patients with ECG conduction abnormalities or mitral valve prolapse had follow-up

Table 20-4 Early Complications after Initial Pectus Excavatum Repair at Children's Hospital of the King's Daughters

Complication	% (No.)
Pneumothorax w/spontaneous resolution	60.4% (613)
Pneumothorax w/chest tube	3.6% (36)
Horner's syndrome	17.7% (179)
Bar displacement	5.7% (58)
Drug reaction	3.6% (36)
Overcorrection	3.2% (32)
Bar allergy	2.9% (29)
Suture site infection	1.0% (10)
Pneumonia	0.6% (6)
Hemothorax	0.6% (6)
Hemothorax (post-traumatic)	0.2% (2)
Pericarditis	0.5% (5)
Pleural effusion (requiring drainage)	0.3% (3)
Death	0%
Cardiac perforation	0%

Data collected through 12/31/2007.

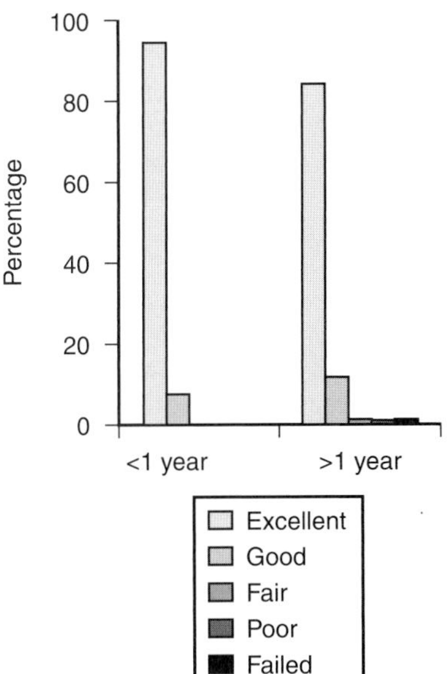

Figure 20-8. The authors' outcomes evaluated over time since bar removal.

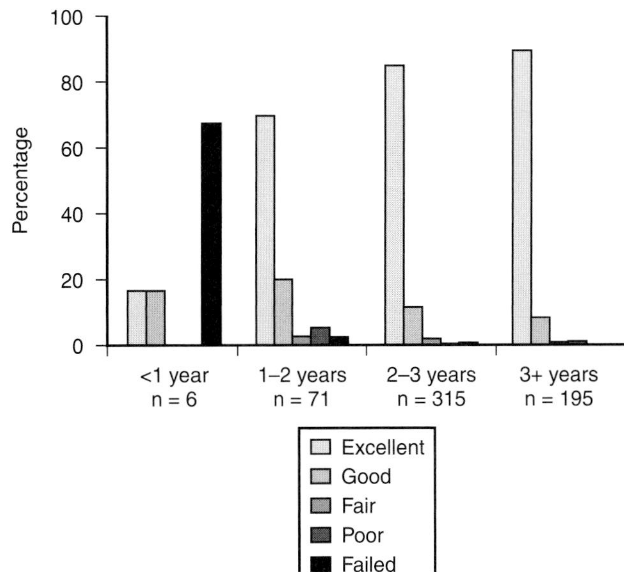

Figure 20-9. The authors' outcomes evaluated by the length of time the bar was left in situ.

assessments. Patients old enough to have pulmonary function studies preoperatively were reassessed with repeated studies.

It has been noted that patients who are sedentary and who do not perform the pectus breathing exercises tend to have mild recurrences over time. Therefore, we strongly emphasize the importance of aerobic activities and deep breathing exercises.

As of December 2007, there were 690 primary repair patients who had undergone bar removal. The cosmetic and functional results of the 587 patients who were more that 1 year post-bar removal were deemed excellent in 84%, good in 12%, fair in 1.5%, and failed in 2.5% (Fig. 20-8). The long-term results are affected by the length of time the bar was left in place (Fig. 20-9).

Bar Removal

We advise the pectus bar be left in place for 2 to 4 years, with 3 years being an optimal time. We evaluate patients on an annual basis and monitor their growth, activity level, and pulmonary function test results and encourage them to do their pectus exercises and participate in aerobic sports. Patients between the ages of 6 and 10 years often do not grow rapidly. Therefore, they tolerate the bar well for 3 or even 4 years. Conversely, we have had teenagers who have undergone a massive growth spurt, completely outgrowing the bar and requiring bar removal after 2 years. We consider the exercise programs to be as important as the surgical correction. Many children and adults lead sedentary lifestyles and never perform aerobic activities. Therefore, their lungs never expand beyond the resting tidal volume (approximately 10% of total lung capacity). Deep breathing with breath holding for 10 to 15 seconds and aerobic activities, such as running (e.g., soccer, basketball) and swimming, are vigorously encouraged. We have seen a mild recurrence over the long term in patients who do not follow our exercise protocol.

Pectus excavatum can be corrected with excellent long-term results without the need for costal cartilage incision, cartilage resection, or sternal osteotomy. A significant number of patients have been safely and effectively managed at long-term follow-up. Pectus excavatum repair without cartilage resection is a simpler operation with tolerable morbidity. As a result, it has received rapid acceptance by the surgical community.

PECTUS CARINATUM

Pectus carinatum, or protrusion deformity of the chest, occurs less frequently than does pectus excavatum. It comprises about 5% of patients with chest wall deformities.[51] The prominence may be in the upper manubrium of the sternum, which is called a chondromanubrial deformity.[52] The most common protrusion occurs in the lower or body of the sternum (the gladiolus) and is called chondrogladiolar. The protrusion may be unilateral, bilateral, or mixed.[53] About 80% of patients who develop pectus carinatum are boys. Although the etiology is unknown, a genetic component of causation is suggested by the approximately one fourth of patients with a family history of chest wall defect.[51,54] Pectus carinatum has been reported to occur after treatment for pectus excavatum.[55]

The natural history of the condition differs from that of pectus excavatum. Pectus carinatum is usually noted in adolescence and is seen most commonly around the time of a growth spurt, rather than at birth as is often seen with pectus excavatum. Symptoms of dyspnea, reduced endurance, or tachypnea with exertion were noted in all 260 patients in one study.[56]

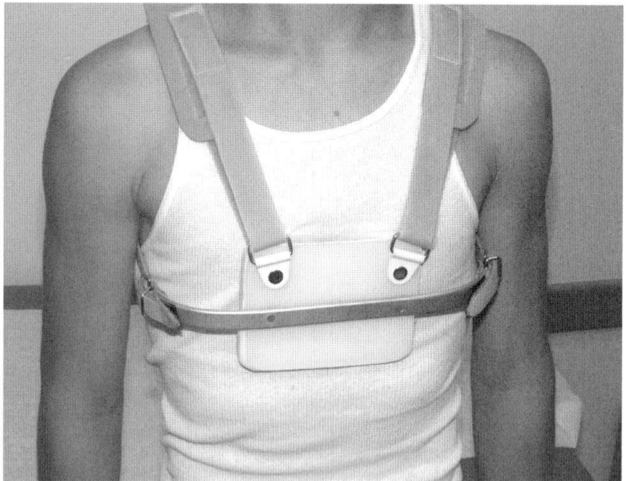

Figure 20-10. This photograph shows a patient who is being treated with bracing for a prominent pectus carinatum.

Associated mitral valve disease has been reported as well.[57,58] Other associations include Marfan syndrome and scoliosis (in 15%).[51]

Orthotic bracing has been applied successfully in some patients with pectus carinatum. Reports have described correction or improvement in this condition by means of a brace analogous to that used for treatment of scoliosis but that exerts pressure in the anteroposterior direction (Fig. 20-10).[24,59]

Our group has had limited success with bracing. Poor compliance contributes to failure of bracing in one third of cases. Surgical treatment consists of costochondral resection with sternotomy. Multiple studies emphasize the importance of performing bilateral cartilage resection, even with unilateral deformity of the cartilages, to prevent recurrence.[25,53,60,61] Recently, minimally invasive correction has been described.[62]

Postoperative complications are uncommon, and recurrence is reported to be rare in centers with a large experience.

POLAND'S SYNDROME

Poland's syndrome affects 1 in 30,000 live births and is sporadic in occurrence.[63] It is a constellation of anomalies that present in a variety of ways. Clinical manifestations can include any or all of the following: absence of the pectoralis major, pectoralis minor, serratus anterior, rectus abdominis, and latissimus dorsi muscles (Fig. 20-11). Athelia or amastia, nipple deformities, limb deformities (syndactyly, brachydactyly), absent axillary hair, and limited subcutaneous fat can also be found.

In 1841, Alfred Poland, an English medical student, published a partial description of the deformity.[64] However, the syndrome was initially described in the French and German literature in 1826 and 1839.[65,66]

Poland's syndrome does not appear to be genetic, although rare occurrences within families have been reported. The right side is more commonly affected and is present in boys 70% of the time.[63] Approximately 15% of patients with breast hypoplasia/aplasia have Poland's syndrome. The etiology is unclear, but theories include abnormal migration of the embryonic tissues forming the pectoralis muscles, hypoplasia of the subclavian artery, or in-utero injury.

No correlation has been identified between the extent of hand deformities and the chest wall deformities. Varying degrees of either can occur with mild hypoplasia to total aplasia of muscles, ribs, and cartilage. The latter can lead to major chest wall depression and paradoxical respiratory motion.

Surgical repair is rarely required, except in those patients with aplasia of the ribs or a major depression deformity.[67,68] When necessary, chest wall reconstruction with correction of contralateral carinatum-type protrusions can usually be performed at the same time (Fig. 20-12). Autologous rib grafts, or a variety of bioprosthetic agents, can be used with or without a latissimus dorsi flap. The use of custom-made chest wall prostheses has been associated with significant problems such as migration, erosion of local tissues, and adverse cosmesis. Chest wall reconstruction should take place before breast reconstruction in a girl with hypoplasia or aplasia of the breast.

STERNAL DEFECTS

Sternal defects are midline defects of the upper torso that range from the relatively benign sternal cleft (sternal defect without displacement of the heart) to the very rare and almost uniformly fatal thoracic ectopia cordis (the heart is out of the chest without a skin covering).

Cleft sternum (bifid sternum, partial ectopia cordis) is a rare malformation (0.15% of all chest wall malformations in some series) and is due to partial or total failure of sternal fusion at an early stage of embryonic development. Sternal clefts can be classified as either complete (the rarest form), superior, or inferior.[69]

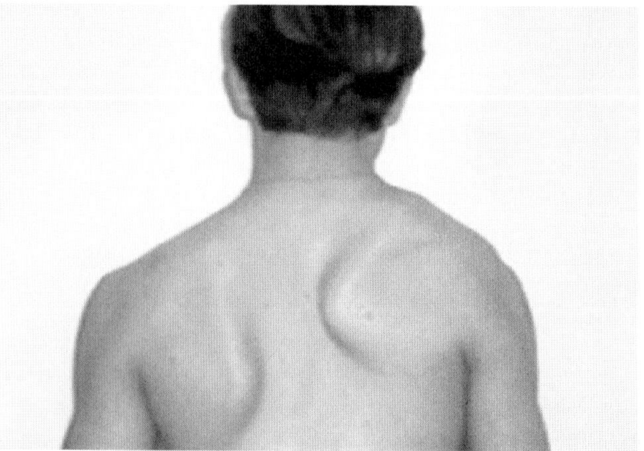

Figure 20-11. A 12-year-old boy with Poland's syndrome and absence of the serratus anterior muscles, leading to a winged scapula on the right.

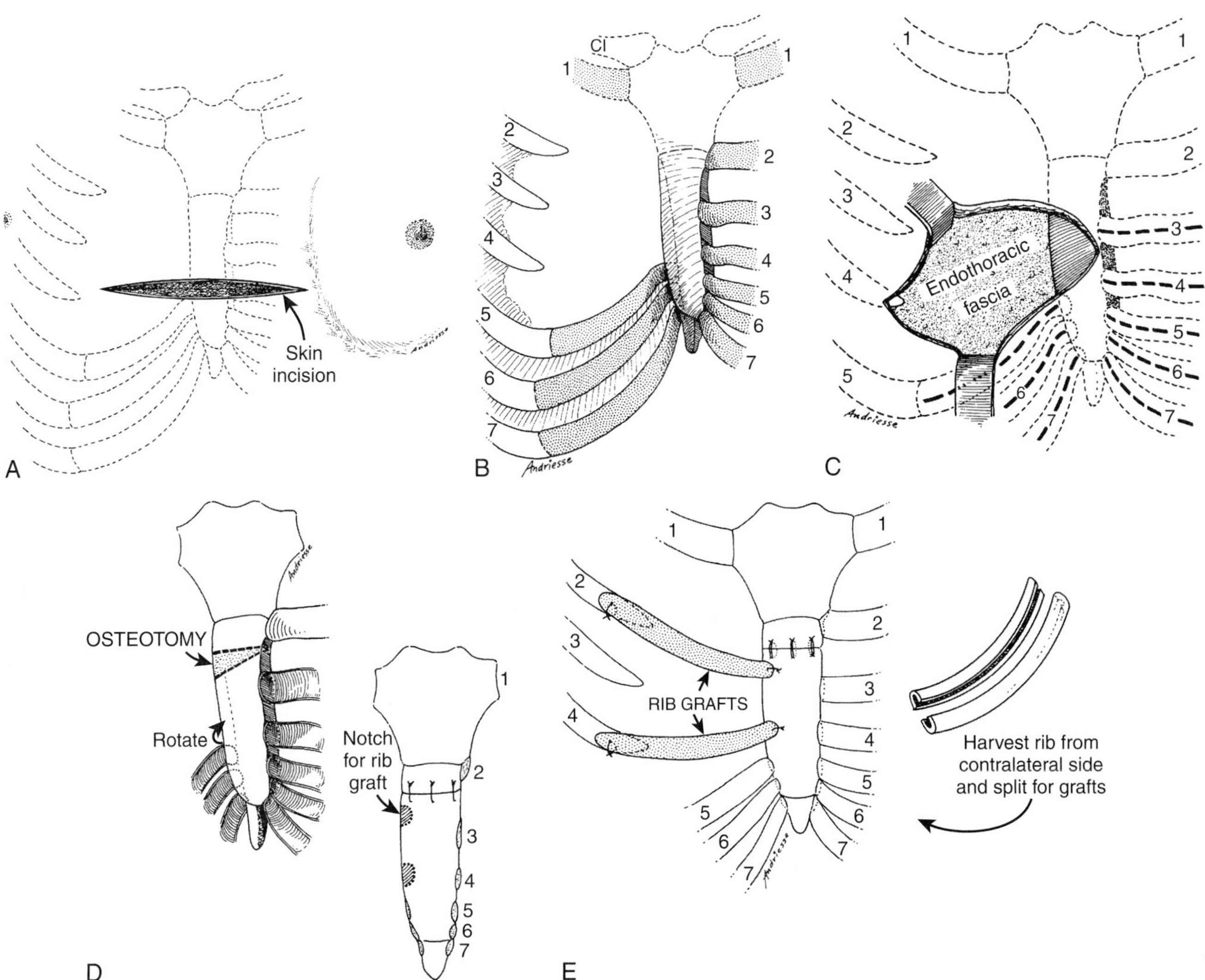

Figure 20-12. **A,** The transverse incision is placed below and within the nipples. In girls, it is placed in the future inframammary crease. **B,** A schematic depiction of the deformity with rotation of the sternum, depression of the cartilages of the involved side, and carinate protrusion of the contralateral side. **C,** In cases with aplasia of the ribs, the endothoracic fascia is encountered directly below the attenuated subcutaneous tissue and pectoral fascia. The pectoral muscle flap is elevated on the contralateral side, with the pectoral fascia, if present, on the involved side. Subperichondrial resection of the costal cartilages is carried out as shown (*dashed line*), preserving the costochondral junction. Rarely this resection must be carried to the level of the second costal cartilage. **D,** A transverse, offset, wedge-shaped sternal osteotomy is created below the second costal cartilage. Closure of this defect with heavy silk sutures or elevation of the sternum with a strut corrects both the posterior displacement and the rotation of the sternum. **E,** In cases with rib aplasia, rib grafts are harvested from the contralateral fifth or sixth ribs, split, and secured medially with wire sutures into notches created in the sternum and with wire to the native ribs laterally. Ribs are split as shown, along their short axes, to maintain maximal mechanical strength. (From Shamberger RC, Welch KJ, Upton J III: Surgical treatment of thoracic deformity in Poland's syndrome. J Pediatr Surg 24:760-766, 1989.)

Superior clefts are either U shaped (proximal to the fourth cartilage) or V shaped (reaching the xiphoid process). They are most often isolated, with only minor associated lesions. The heart is in a normal position, and cardiac anomalies are rare. Surgical repair, which is very successful, is warranted once the diagnosis is made and can be done electively. Optimally, it is performed in the neonatal age when the sternal bars can be approximated easily because of flexibility and minimal compression of mediastinal structures (Fig. 20-13). After age 1 year, primary repair is difficult and more extensive techniques may be needed, such as the use of autologous structures (costal cartilage, ribs) or prosthetic materials.[70,71]

Thoracic ectopia cordis (true ectopia cordis) is a lesion in which the heart has no overlying somatic structures. It is very rare and usually occurs with some form of an abdominal wall defect, with the heart sitting on the chest and the apex pointed toward the chin (Fig. 20-14). Intrinsic cardiac anomalies are frequent, especially tetralogy of Fallot, pulmonary artery stenosis, transposition of the great arteries, and ventricular septal defects.[72] Survival in patients with thoracic ectopia cordis is rare, with only three survivors being reported. Most patients die because of torsion of the great vessels and compression of the heart while attempting to reduce it back in the chest. The goals of therapy are to cover the heart, preserve cardiac output

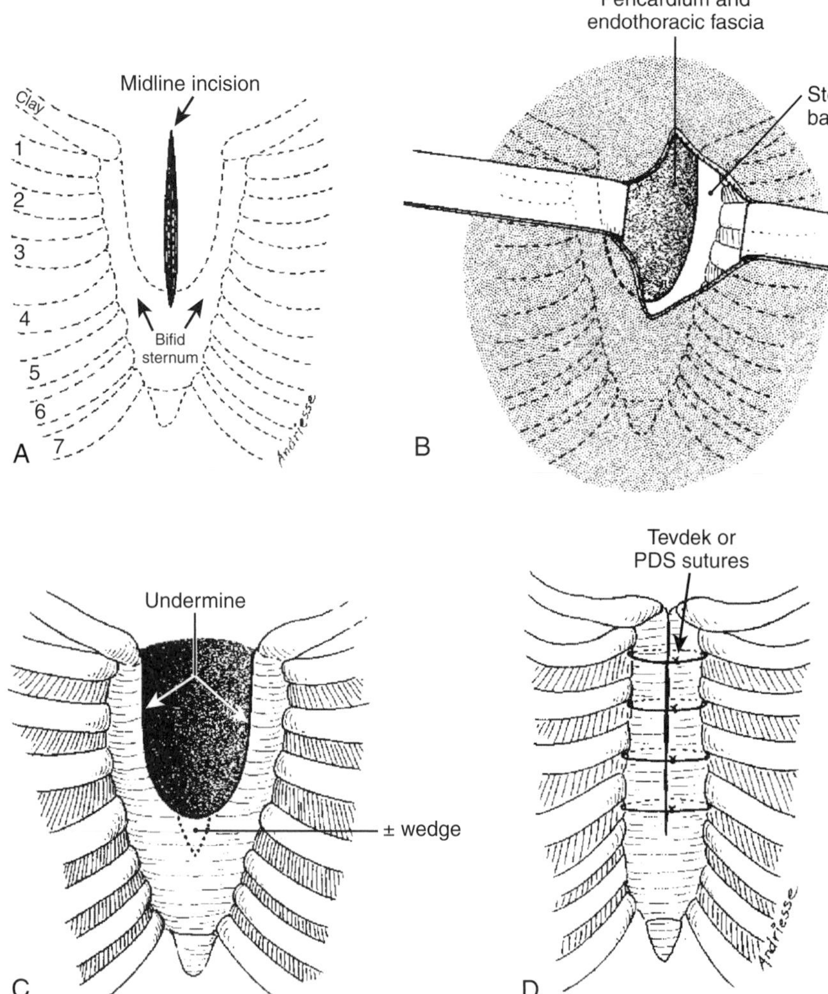

Figure 20-13. **A,** Repair of a bifid sternum is best performed through a longitudinal incision extending the length of the defect. These defects are characteristically cleft superiorly, as shown. **B,** Directly beneath the subcutaneous tissues, the sternal bars are encountered, with the origin of the pectoral muscles on the lateral aspect of the bars. The endothoracic fascia and pericardium are just below these structures. **C,** The endothoracic fascia is mobilized off the sternal bars posteriorly with blunt dissection to allow safe placement of the sutures. Approximation of the sternal bars may be facilitated by excising a wedge of cartilage inferiorly. Repair is best accomplished in the neonatal period because of the flexibility of the chest wall. **D,** Closure of the defect is achieved with 2-0 Tevdek or polydioxanone sutures. (From Shamberger RC, Welch KJ: Sternal defects. Pediatr Surg Int 5:156-164, 1990.)

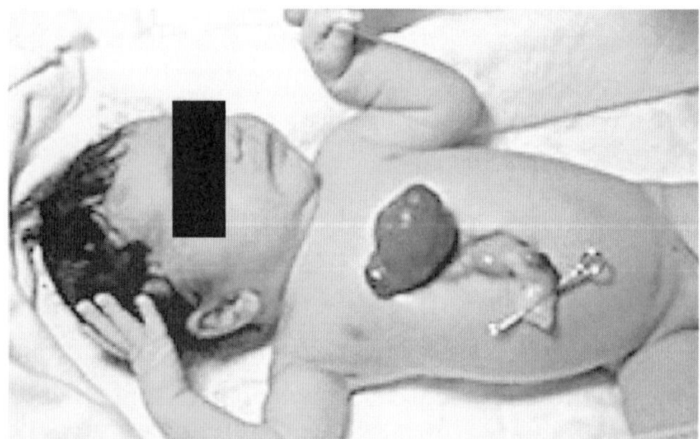

Figure 20-14. An infant with thoracic ectopia cordis with no significant abdominal wall defect present. Note the characteristic high insertion of the umbilicus and anterior projection of the apex of the heart.

by preventing kinking of the great vessels, repair the associated abdominal wall defect, and stabilize the thoracic cavity so that spontaneous ventilation can be effective.[72-74]

Thoracoabdominal ectopia cordis (Cantrell's pentalogy) involves lesions in which the heart is covered by an omphalocele-like membrane (Fig. 20-15).[74] Intrinsic cardiac anomalies also are common in these patients, with tetralogy of Fallot and ventricular septal defects being the most common. Cantrell's pentalogy consists of an inferior sternal cleft, ectopia cordis, midline abdominal wall defects or omphalocele, pericardial defects, and one or more cardiac defects. Repair in these patients is much more successful than in thoracic ectopia cordis. Initial surgical management addresses the lack of skin overlying the heart and abdominal cavity. After initial stabilization and echocardiogram, the goal of the initial operation is to provide coverage of the midline defects, separate the abdominal and pericardial compartments, and repair the diaphragm. Various techniques to gain closure include flap mobilization, skin closure only, and a variety of bioprosthetic agents. The congenital heart defect is repaired at a later date.

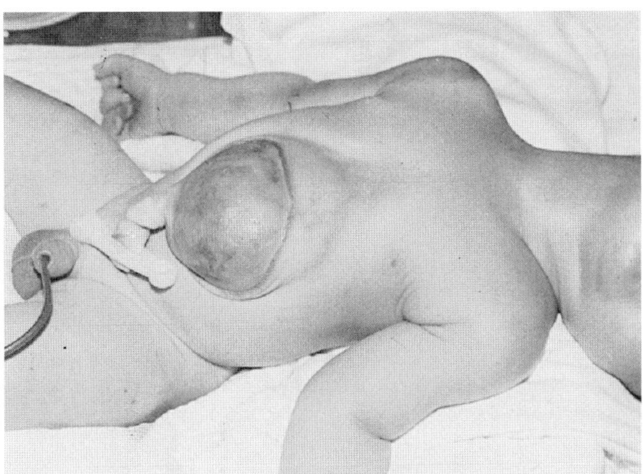

Figure 20-15. A newborn with the external features of Cantrell's pentalogy is seen. Flaring of the lower thoracic cavity is present, with a large epigastric omphalocele. The transverse septum of the diaphragm and the inferior portion of the pericardium are absent. The patient also has tetralogy of Fallot.

THORACIC INSUFFICIENCY SYNDROME ASSOCIATED WITH DIFFUSE SKELETAL DISORDERS

Thoracic insufficiency syndrome may be defined as any disorder that produces the inability of the thorax to support normal respiration or lung growth.[75] It includes a spectrum of disorders including asphyxiating thoracic dystrophy (Jeune's syndrome), acquired asphyxiating thoracic dystrophy (after open pectus excavatum repair), spondylothoracic dysplasia (Jarcho-Levin syndrome), congenital scoliosis with multiple vertebral anomalies and fused or absent ribs (jumbled spine), and severe kyphoscoliosis. These disorders have been viewed and treated as separate entities, with little coordinated effort between specialties. However, they are best addressed with a unified approach integrating pediatric general and orthopedic surgeons as well as pediatric pulmonologists.

Jeune's syndrome is an autosomal recessive inherited osteochondrodystrophy with variable expressions.[76] In mild forms, the chest may support adequate respiration. In more severe cases, the thorax is narrowed both transversely and vertically, with short, wide horizontal ribs and irregular costochondral junctions (Fig. 20-16). This chest wall configuration produces a rigid chest with very little intercostal excursion for normal respiration, leading to ventilatory dependence and death from respiratory failure.[77,78] Pathologic examination of pulmonary structures varies, with some findings of pulmonary hypertension. However, most patients have normal bronchial development with variable alveolar density.[79,80] This suggests that the extrinsic chest wall plays a significant role in the underlying hypoplasia. Other associated skeletal abnormalities in Jeune's syndrome include short stubby extremities, fixed elevated clavicles, hypoplastic iliac wings, and a high incidence of C1 spinal stenosis.[81-83] These patients also have varying degrees of renal dysplasia.[84]

Spondylothoracic dysplasia (Jarcho-Levin) syndrome occurs in two forms with different inheritance patterns. Type I is an autosomal recessive deformity characterized by multiple vertebral hemivertebrae and posterior rib fusions.[85] This produces a marked shortening of the thoracic spine and a crab-like appearance of the chest on a standard radiograph (Fig. 20-17).[86] Associated malformations are noted in 30% of patients and include cardiac and renal anomalies. The type I form is often fatal by age 15 months, and a high incidence is reported in Puerto Rican families.[87] Type II

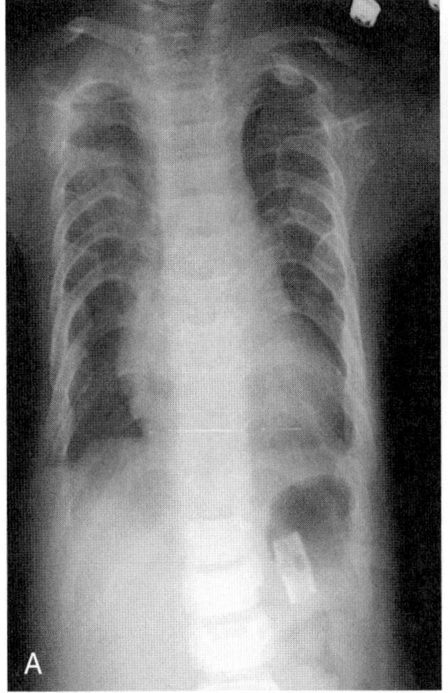

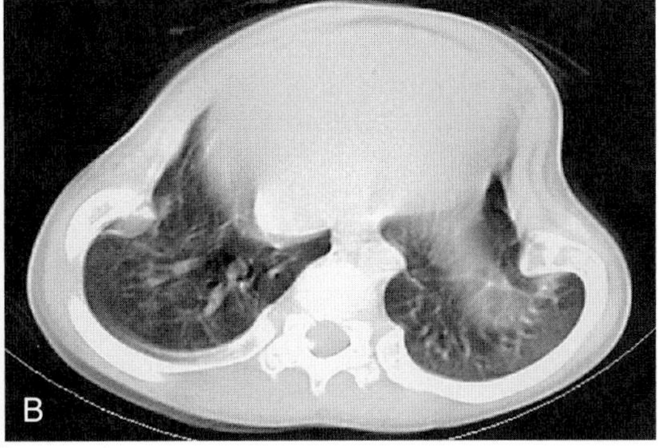

Figure 20-16. **A,** Chest radiograph of a patient with Jeune's syndrome (asphyxiating thoracic dystrophy). The thorax is narrow, and the ribs are short and wide. **B,** CT scan demonstrating Jeune's asphyxiating thoracic dystrophy.

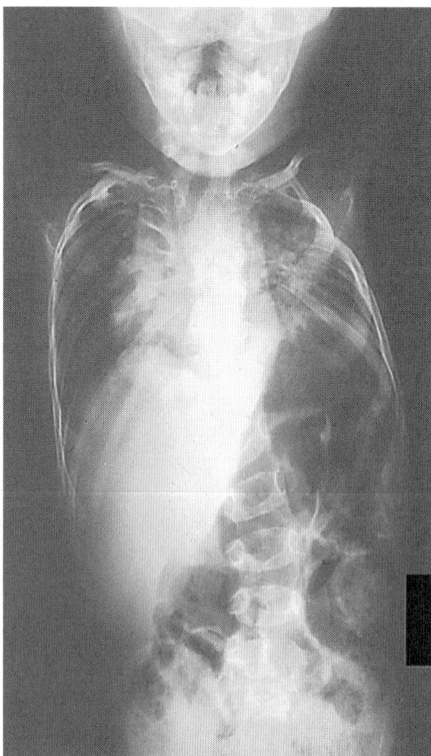

Figure 20-17. Chest radiograph of a patient with Jarcho-Levin syndrome with a markedly shortened thoracic spine producing a crab-like appearance.

spondylothoracic dysplasia has an autosomal dominant inheritance pattern and is associated with near-normal longevity. It is seen most commonly in white children.[87]

Thoracic insufficiency also may arise secondary to too early or too extensive pectus operations.[19] Complex spine anomalies producing the so-called jumbled spine, unilateral thoracic hypoplasia seen with the VACTERL association, and kyphoscoliosis may be a cause of thoracic insufficiency.[88-92]

Surgical techniques to correct the spectrum of these complex disorders have attempted to address the issue of thoracic volume by various approaches. In both congenital (Jeune's) and acquired (post-pectus) thoracic dystrophy, one approach has been an anterior longitudinal sternal split with widening of the sternum. This has been accomplished with methylmethacrylate, bone grafts or rib, and metal plates.[93-95] A staged approach with a methylmethacrylate plate followed by secondary removal of the plate and latissimus dorsi flaps to cover the created sternal cleft also has been described.[96] Sternal elevation has also been reported in cases of acquired thoracic dystrophy by both the open and the minimally invasive techniques used for standard pectus repair.[19,41] A lateral staged approach with staggered rib osteotomies, staggered division of the chest wall, intercostal muscles, and pleura, with transposition of alternating ribs by using metal plate fixation, also has been described.[97]

These approaches have had variable results because they are not easily revised to allow continued growth of the chest wall to allow lung expansion. The lateral thoracic expansion may also interfere with intercostal muscle function after division of multiple intercostal muscles and nerves. In regard to patients with Jarcho-Levin syndrome, jumbled spine, and kyphosis, pediatric general surgeons have done little to approach these problems that they considered either lethal or solely in the domain of the orthopedic surgeon.

A promising technique to address patients with the spectrum of causes for thoracic insufficiency syndrome rejoins the disciplines of pediatric general, thoracic, and orthopedic surgery. Expansion thoracoplasty and the use of a vertical expandable prosthetic titanium rib (VEPTR) developed by Campbell and Smith addresses many problems in the spectrum of these disorders. This technique allows serial expansion of the chest wall to allow continued growth of the thorax and spine until skeletal maturity is achieved.[98] More than 300 patients with various disorders have been treated with this approach. In Jeune's asphyxiating thoracic dystrophy, 14 patients have undergone staged bilateral expansions. Anterior rib osteotomies adjacent to the costochondral junction and posterior osteotomies adjacent to the transverse process of the spine in the 3rd to 9th ribs are performed. This creates a mobilized segment of chest wall that is distracted posterolaterally and anchored to a curved VEPTR that is attached to the 2nd and 10th ribs (Fig. 20-18). The segment is anchored to the VEPTR with 2-mm titanium rings, stabilizing the segment and allowing reossification of the multiple osteotomies (Fig. 20-19). The second stage is performed 3 months later, and then the devices are expanded every 6 months.

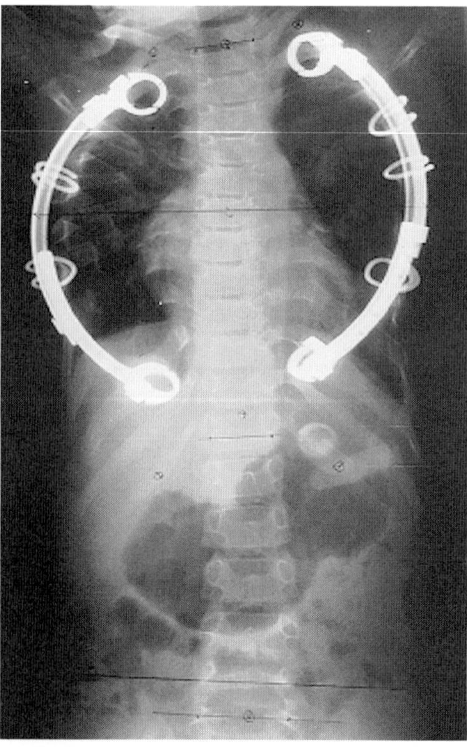

Figure 20-18. Bilateral vertical expandable prosthetic titanium rib (VEPTR) fixed with titanium rings to ribs of the patient with Jeune's asphyxiating thoracic dystrophy seen in Figure 20-16A.

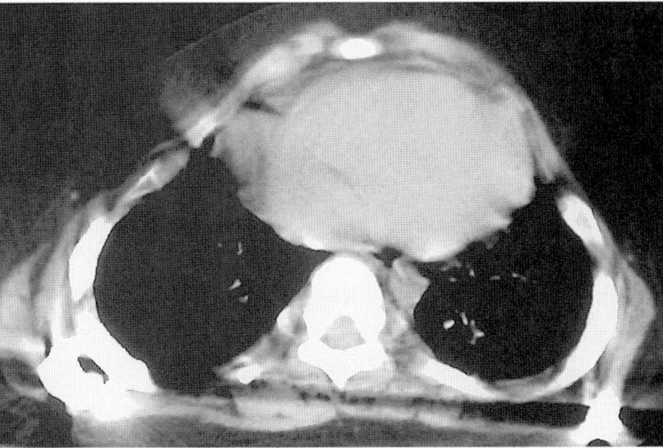

Figure 20-19. Postoperative CT scan of the patient from Figure 20-16B after VEPTR placement, demonstrating expansion of the thorax.

In patients with fused or absent ribs and scoliosis, a wedge thoracostomy through the fused segment of ribs not only allows expansion of the chest, but also correction of the scoliosis and the rotational spinal deformity (producing a windswept thorax).[92,99] It also stimulates increased spinal height in both congenital scoliosis and Jarcho-Levin syndrome, in which bilateral devices are placed (Fig. 20-20).

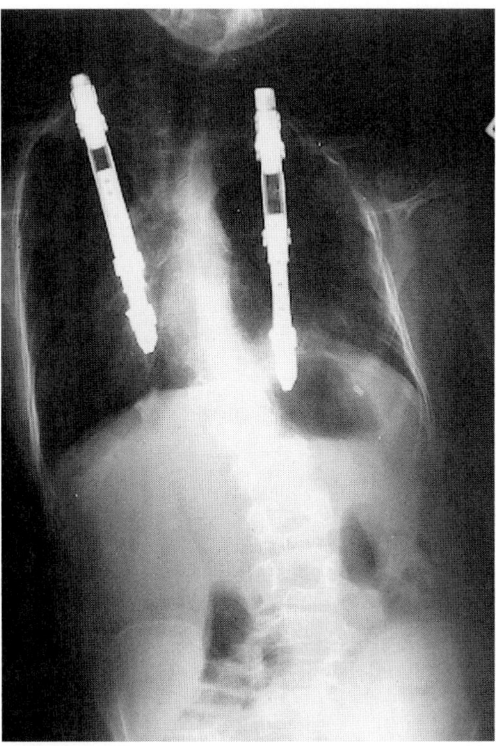

Figure 20-20. Bilateral VEPTRs were placed in the patient in Figure 20-17 with Jarcho-Levin syndrome.

chapter 21

TRACHEAL OBSTRUCTION AND REPAIR

H. Biemann Othersen, Jr., MD • André Hebra, MD

Pediatric surgeons are often involved in the management of acute or chronic airway obstruction. Moreover, iatrogenic injury of the pediatric airway occasionally occurs. The large number of operative techniques for the treatment of tracheal stenosis shows that no single procedure or technique is universally applicable and successful. Prevention of, or prompt therapy for, injury is all-important.[1,2]

PRACTICAL EMBRYOLOGY AND ANATOMY

A working knowledge of the embryonic development of mediastinal structures aids in understanding the etiology and associated anomalies of tracheal obstruction. Malformations of the great vessels (vascular rings) should be suspected and investigated when evaluating a child with complete tracheal rings. The most common vascular malformation associated with complete tracheal rings is a pulmonary vascular sling. This anomaly occurs when the left pulmonary artery arises to the right of the trachea, around which it curves and compresses just above the carina, and then passes between the trachea and esophagus before reaching the left lung (Fig. 21-1).[3] Other vascular ring malformations may produce varying degrees of tracheal, bronchial, and esophageal compression.

TRACHEAL MALFORMATIONS

Congenital Subglottic Stenosis

The anatomy of the pediatric airway has been compared to an inverted cone, with the trachea fitting telescopically into the cricoid above it, the cricoid into the thyroid cartilage, and then the thyroid into the hyoid space, as illustrated in Figure 21-2.[4] Congenital subglottic stenosis is the most common morphologic abnormality of the trachea and presents as a narrowing of the airway at the distal end of the larynx, just at the beginning of the trachea. This subglottic region lies at the junction of the cricoid cartilage and trachea and is the narrowest point of the child's airway. The cricoid cartilage is the only normally complete cartilaginous ring in the airway. Congenital abnormalities of this subglottic area consist of narrowing or malformation of the cricoid cartilage, the etiology of which is not truly known.

When compared with an adult, the anatomy of the trachea and larynx differs in several ways (Fig. 21-3). The child's epiglottis is short and small, and the valleculae are very shallow. Also, the larynx points posteriorly

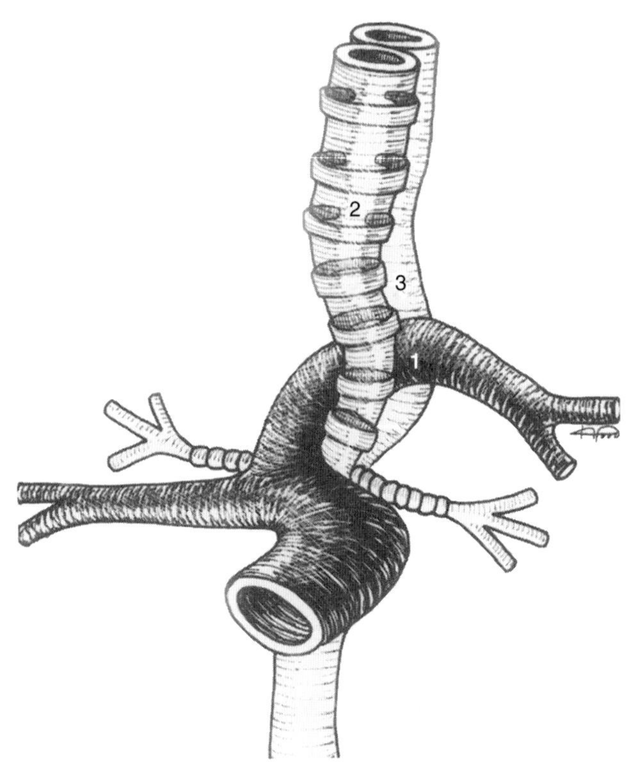

Figure 21-1. Complete tracheal rings in distal trachea and pulmonary vascular sling. 1, Left pulmonary artery; 2, trachea; 3, esophagus.

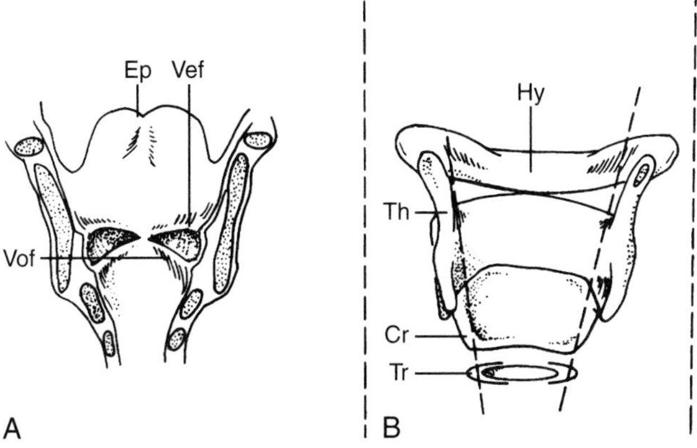

Figure 21-2. A, Ventral area of the larynx in the neonate viewed from behind. The ventricle, or "third cavity," is bounded above by the ventricular folds (Vef) and below by the vocal folds (Vof). Ep, epiglottis. **B,** Laryngeal cartilages (without arytenoids). Th, thyroid; Cr, cricoid; Tr, trachea; and Hy, hyoid viewed from behind. *Inner dashed lines* show telescopic configuration in the neonate as opposed to the rectangular shape in the adult (*outer dashed lines*). (From Othersen HB Jr [ed]: The Pediatric Airway. Philadelphia, WB Saunders, 1991.)

toward the nasopharynx, and the arytenoid apparatus is large in relation to the lumen of the larynx. Finally, the narrowest point of the normal pediatric airway is the cricotracheal junction. In the adult, it is the glottis. Cricoid stenosis is exceeded only by laryngomalacia and vocal cord paralysis in the frequency of congenital airway anomalies.

In the normal trachea, the cartilaginous rings are horseshoe shaped, with the posterior wall composed of connective tissue and muscle. Thus, the lumen may change as the trachea expands or contracts with respiration. Long stenotic segments in the trachea usually consist of tracheal rings that are complete. When the cartilaginous rings are complete, the lumen is rigid and usually much smaller than the normal trachea. If it does not produce early respiratory distress, complete cartilaginous rings may be detected when an inflammatory process within the trachea produces mucosal edema, which further compromises the rigid lumen and results in acute airway obstruction. Occasionally, tracheal intubation for an elective operative procedure may be impossible and the narrowed segment is discovered.

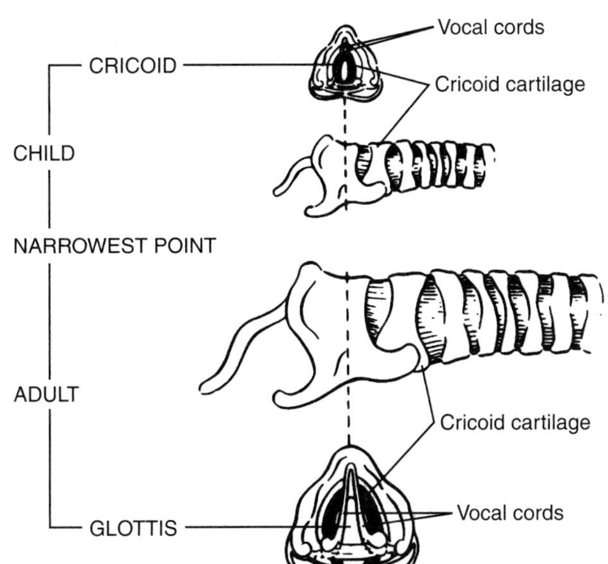

Figure 21-3. Difference between adult and pediatric airway. (From Othersen HB Jr: Intubation injuries of the trachea in children: Management and prevention. Ann Surg 189:601-606, 1979.)

Acquired Subglottic and Tracheal Stenosis

Acquired airway malformations usually result from intrinsic injury with subsequent inflammation, ulceration, and scarring, leading to severe subglottic or tracheal scarring and narrowing. Occasionally external trauma is the initiating event,[2] but an iatrogenic event can exacerbate an unstable situation. For example, a child with a congenitally small airway might be asymptomatic until an endotracheal tube is inserted. The tube may be of an appropriate size but, because of the congenital stenosis, it will fit tightly and can lead to ulceration and stricture. Particularly difficult to treat are those injuries that occur well below the subglottic region, usually produced by an endotracheal balloon that has caused compression and ulceration in the trachea. Frequently, these areas of injury are below the usual site for a tracheostomy. The cuff may even erode into overlying vessels (Fig. 21-4).

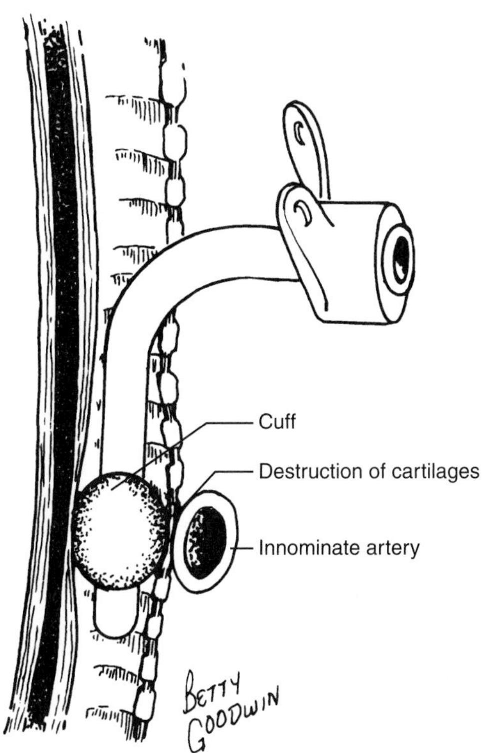

Figure 21-4. The inflated cuff of a tracheostomy tube may erode anteriorly into the innominate artery. (From Othersen HB Jr [ed]: The Pediatric Airway. Philadelphia, WB Saunders, 1991.)

VASCULAR COMPRESSIONS

Compression and partial obstruction of the trachea may be caused by abnormalities of the aortic arch that impinge on or encircle the trachea or esophagus or both.[5,6] When both the trachea and esophagus are compressed, swallowing frequently produces acute airway compression and respiratory distress. Vascular rings are often asymptomatic in neonates and infants, yet can lead to significant airway obstruction in a child.[7]

The physiologic impingement on the trachea by a vascular ring is similar to that seen in patients after repair of esophageal atresia. The persistently distended upper esophageal pouch can displace the trachea anteriorly, producing tracheomalacia, or softened tracheal rings (Fig. 21-5). Particularly with swallowing, the distended esophageal pouch may compress the trachea against the innominate artery (Figs. 21-6 and 21-7). This sequence of events is thought responsible for a condition called reflex apnea. Consequently, surgical correction of this problem consists of anterior mobilization and suspension of the innominate artery (Fig. 21-8).[8-12] The treatment of a pulmonary vascular sling usually requires not only relocation and reimplantation of the pulmonary artery but also tracheal repair for the stenotic distal trachea.[7,12,13]

Stridor and dyspnea are symptoms that may be produced by vascular impingement on the trachea. Patients with severe compression from a double aortic arch are usually symptomatic, but their manifestations are variable (Fig. 21-9). Some patients are initially seen with frequent coughing and stridor accompanied by dyspnea and cyanosis, whereas small infants may have

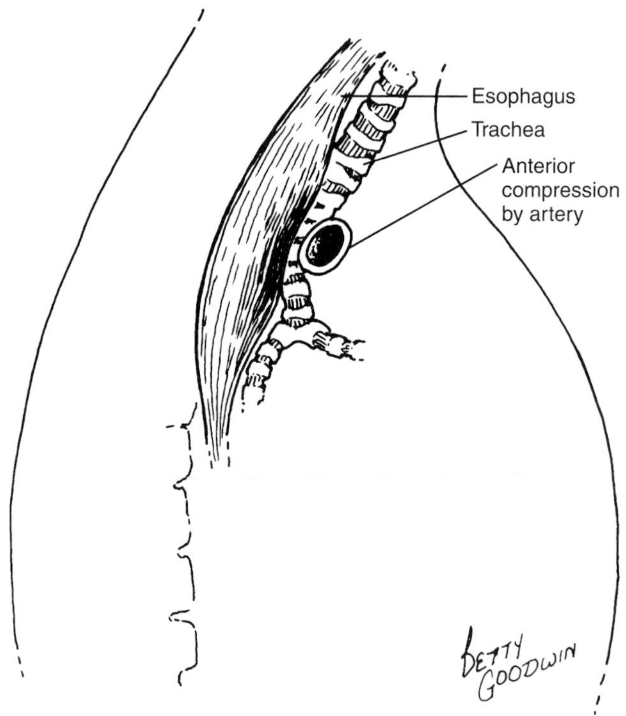

Figure 21-6. A lateral view shows how the dilated proximal esophagus displaces the trachea and compresses it against the overlying innominate artery. (From Othersen HB Jr [ed]: The Pediatric Airway. Philadelphia, WB Saunders, 1991.)

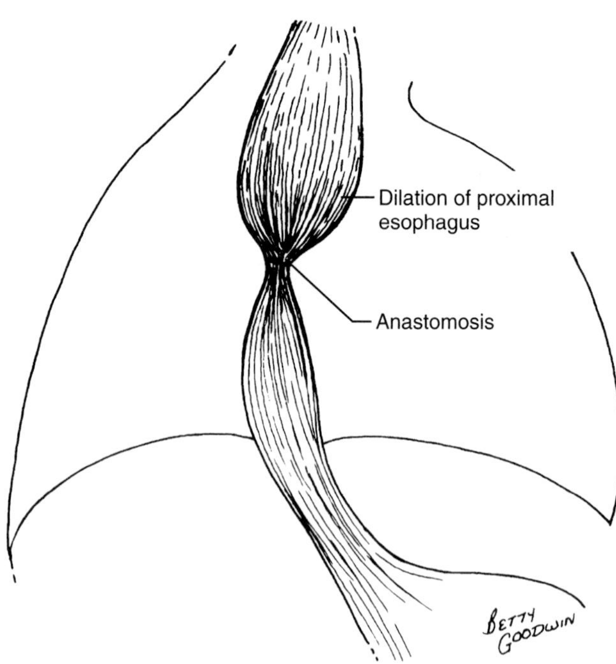

Figure 21-5. After repair of esophageal atresia, the proximal esophagus, which is already enlarged, is further dilated by an anastomotic stricture. (From Othersen HB Jr [ed]: The Pediatric Airway. Philadelphia, WB Saunders, 1991.)

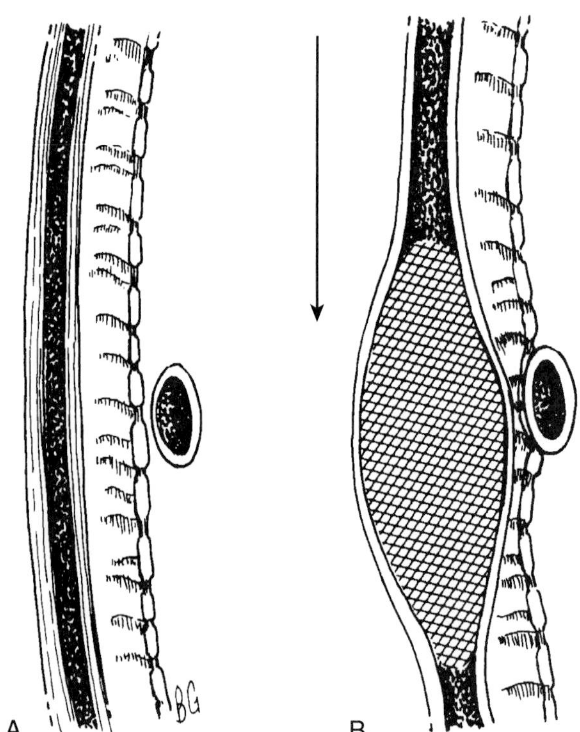

Figure 21-7. **A** and **B**, An enlarged diagram of Figure 21-6 illustrates how the compression is increased by ingestion of food. (From Othersen HB Jr [ed]: The Pediatric Airway. Philadelphia, WB Saunders, 1991.)

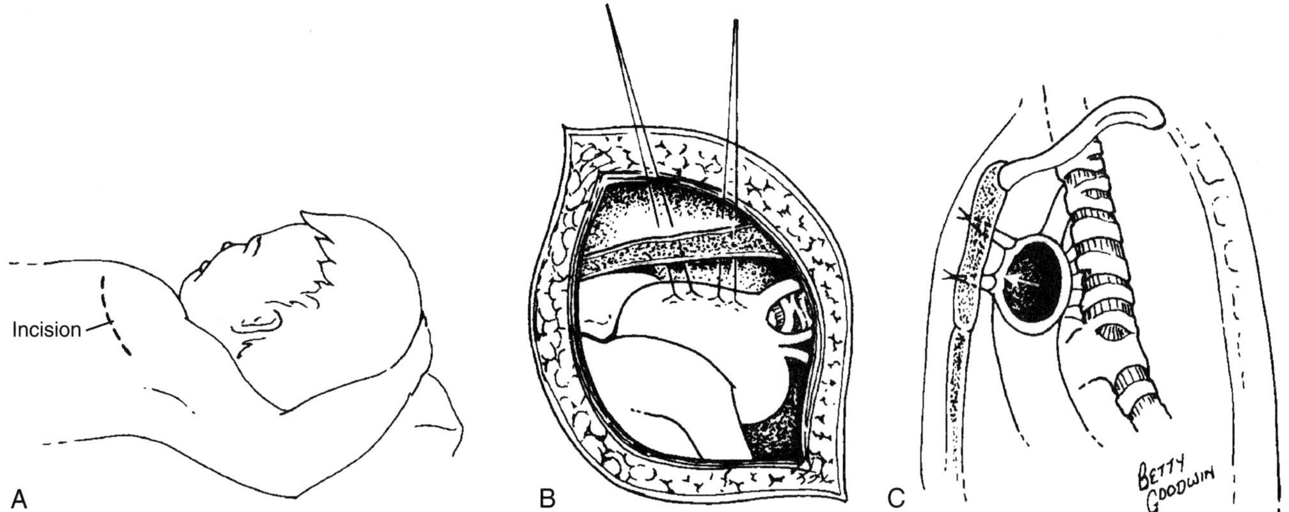

Figure 21-8. The operative technique for aortopexy. **A,** Anterior left thoracotomy in the third interspace. **B,** Sutures placed into the wall of the innominate artery and the aortic arch. **C,** Sutures passed through the sternum and tied to elevate the compressing vessels. Tracheal attachments pull the anterior wall of the trachea forward. (From Othersen HB Jr [ed]: The Pediatric Airway. Philadelphia, WB Saunders, 1991.)

reflex apnea. The symptoms of vascular impingement on the trachea are usually more dramatic than those of compression of the esophagus.

The diagnosis of vascular ring anomalies has classically been made or suspected from a barium esophagogram with indentations on the esophageal column of barium and a decrease in the tracheal air column. Offset of the axis of the barium column above and below the indentation is diagnostic of a double aortic arch. Newer imaging techniques with rapid computed tomographic (CT) scans allow a graphic reconstruction of the trachea and adjacent vessels (Fig. 21-10). Magnetic resonance imaging (MRI) enhanced with intravenous administration of a contrast agent allows excellent visualization of the trachea and vessels.

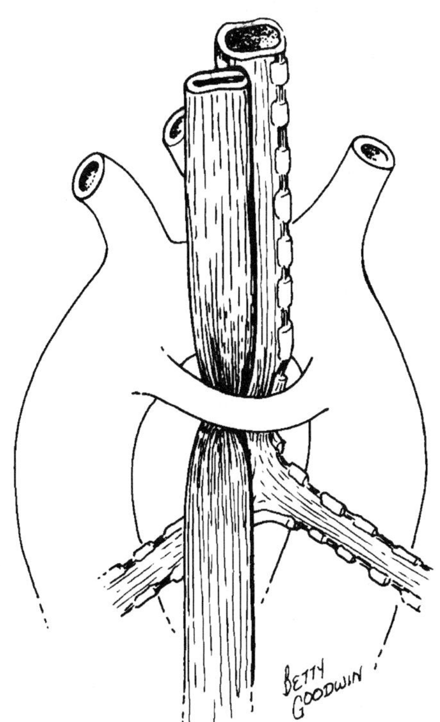

Figure 21-9. Both trachea and esophagus are compressed by a double aortic arch. (From Othersen HB Jr [ed]: The Pediatric Airway. Philadelphia, WB Saunders, 1991.)

Occasionally, a child will appear with acute airway obstruction or other medical problems requiring intensive care, during which endotracheal intubation and a concomitant nasogastric tube are inserted. The presence of tubes in both airway and esophagus makes detection of a vascular ring difficult and can generate complications. In a child who is already intubated, performance of contrast radiographic procedures may not be possible. Ultrasonography or CT and contrast-enhanced MRI may delineate the vascular abnormality. When both tracheal and esophageal intubations are necessary in a patient with a double aortic arch, the encircling vessels may sustain pressure necrosis. Erosion into the aortic arch produces an acute aortoesophageal fistula that may not be manifest until either the endotracheal or the esophageal tube is removed. A sentinel hemorrhage may occur before a massive, and often fatal, hemorrhage into the esophagus. The passage of a Sengstaken-Blakemore tube with inflation of the esophageal balloon can be lifesaving by tamponading the fistula.[14] Because no reliable diagnostic study is available to demonstrate an aortoesophageal fistula, the observation of a sentinel hemorrhage in such a patient with ultrasound confirmation of a double aortic arch is a clear indication for urgent cardiopulmonary bypass and repair.[14]

Vascular rings cause airway constriction and not vascular problems. Thus, simple division of the vascular ring is often not enough to relieve tracheal compression. Significant numbers of patients are now being treated by the thoracoscopic approach.[15] A vessel that continues to compress the airway must not be dissected away from the trachea but suspended anteriorly,

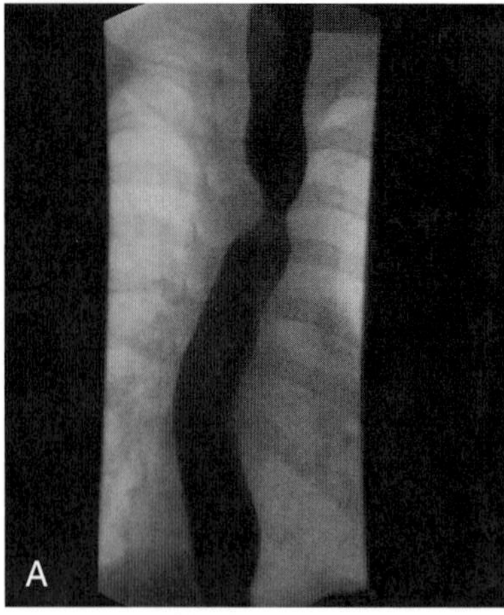

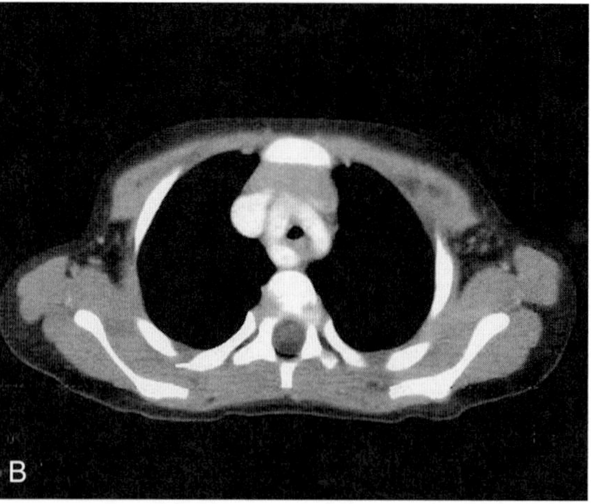

Figure 21-10. This infant presented with stridor. There was a suggestion of tracheal indentation on the chest radiograph. Therefore, a barium esophagogram was performed **(A)** and shows the double indentations diagnostic of a double aortic arch. On the right **(B)**, a CT scan shows contrast in the double arch that is encircling the trachea and esophagus (collapsed).

often to the back of the sternum, so that the vascular tracheal attachments will lift the anterior tracheal wall and enlarge the lumen (see Fig. 21-8). Regardless of the approach, from the right or from the left,[16] or other technical variations,[17] the recurrent laryngeal and phrenic nerves must be identified and protected. Flexible endoscopic observation of the trachea during these maneuvers can corroborate relief of the compression.[5]

TRACHEOMALACIA

Often tracheomalacia is produced by the constant pressure of a cardiovascular structure. Thus, it is almost always necessary to suspend the offending vessel and utilize its attachments to the trachea to expand the tracheal lumen. Occasionally, tracheomalacia can be primary in nature and there is no obvious compression. In these cases, suspension of the large mediastinal vessels may enlarge the tracheal lumen.[18-21] Interestingly in the United Kingdom (Scotland), guidelines have been promulgated for the use of thoracoscopic aortopexy to treat severe primary tracheomalacia.[22] The National Health Service believed that these guidelines were necessary because individual surgeons would operate infrequently on infants and children who are good candidates for operative correction.

INFLAMMATORY OBSTRUCTIONS

Viral laryngotracheitis (croup), bacterial or membranous tracheitis, and epiglottitis are inflammatory conditions that may require surgical intervention. The acute inflammatory airway process may progress rapidly to a life-threatening obstruction and require emergency tracheostomy. However, in all cases of inflammatory obstruction, endotracheal intubation before tracheostomy is advisable, if at all possible. It is important to distinguish croup and bacterial tracheitis from epiglottitis because the treatments are quite different (Table 21-1).

Children with epiglottitis characteristically tolerate endotracheal intubation without airway injury because the inflammation and edema are supraglottic and not circumferential. They do, however, present more risks of intubation failure because of the severe edema of the epiglottis. Some hospitals have strict protocols requiring diagnostic laryngoscopy in the operating room with anesthesia standby for suspected cases of epiglottitis because an emergency tracheostomy is occasionally necessary. Conversely, with viral or bacterial laryngotracheitis, the inflammatory process involves the entire circumference of the airway and prolonged intubation may lead to permanent scarring.[1,23]

Table 21-1 Characteristics of Laryngotracheobronchitis and Epiglottitis

Characteristic	Laryngotracheobronchitis	Epiglottitis
Incidence	Common	Uncommon
Etiology	Viral	*Haemophilus influenzae* type b
Age	6 months to 3 years	2-6 years
Clinical picture	Gradual onset, preceding upper respiratory tract infection, barking cough	Rapid onset, fever, drooling, dysphagia
Physical examination	Respiratory distress, inspiratory stridor, low-grade temperature	Anxious, muffled voice, chin forward, drooling, high temperature
Laboratory studies	WBC usually <10,000/mm^3 with lymphocytosis; radiograph shows narrowing of subglottic region	WBC often >10,000/mm^3 with band cells increased; radiograph shows swollen epiglottis

WBC, white blood cell count.
Adapted from McLain LG: Croup syndrome. Am Fam Physican 36:213, 1987.

Croup characteristically occurs during viral seasons in children age 3 months to 3 years. Children in whom the classic "croupy" cough develops frequently have a history of an antecedent respiratory infection, usually with a high fever.[24] Bacterial tracheitis, a nonviral infectious disease, is seen with fever and rapid development of upper airway obstruction, characterized by copious mucopurulent secretions. Epiglottitis typically affects children who are age 2 to 6 years and have sore throat and dysphagia. Consequently, speech may be slurred and drooling of saliva is prominent. Lateral radiographs of the neck may show an edematous epiglottis.[25]

Fortunately, most of these inflammatory processes are now controlled with antibiotics and respiratory care without surgical intervention. Treatment includes oxygen with increased humidification and inhalation of racemic epinephrine. Endotracheal intubation is well tolerated in epiglottitis and usually causes no further injury while antibiotic therapy produces resolution of the epiglottic edema. However, in cases of viral or bacterial tracheitis, even brief (24-48 hours) intubation may cause ulceration in a trachea that is already acutely inflamed and swollen. Therefore, it may be best to use endotracheal intubation to establish a definitive diagnosis. If resolution does not occur within 48 to 72 hours, a temporary tracheostomy may be advisable.

The decreasing incidence of epiglottitis is probably due to the increasing use of immunization against *Haemophilus influenzae* type b, the most common causative organism.[26] Other infectious organisms, however, may produce the typical epiglottic swelling. Intubation is usually not necessary for more than 24 to 48 hours until antibiotics can control the infection. Croup also is now more easily treated without intubation with racemic epinephrine inhalation combined with administration of dexamethasone, 0.6 mg/kg, either orally, intramuscularly, or intravenously.

Regardless of the cause of the inflammatory process, rapid obstruction of the airway can occur in a small child. The surgeon must be prepared to work with the anesthesiologist and pediatrician to establish an airway by endotracheal intubation, bronchoscopy, or tracheostomy.

INJURIES

Intrinsic Injuries

Most intrinsic laryngotracheal injuries are iatrogenic and produced by inappropriate introduction of an endotracheal tube or instrumentation of the airway. Benign laryngeal tumors, such as a subglottic hemangioma and lymphangioma, require repeated endoscopic treatments that can be injurious to the larynx. Thus, in such patients, it may be wise to consider a preliminary tracheostomy. Therapy consists of removal of the obstruction with CO_2 or KTP lasers. Laser therapy for these lymphovascular malformations can be painstaking and tedious, requiring multiple treatments.

Other techniques such as sclerotherapy have been applied to these same intrinsic airway lesions. Intralesional corticosteroid injection has been reported to promote rapid involution of a subglottic hemangioma.[27] OK-432 has shown promise when injected into lymphovascular lesions around the head and neck.[28,29] OK-432, derived from group A *Streptococcus pyogenes*, stimulates a local inflammatory reaction that leads to involution of the lymphovascular mass. This compound has been used extensively in Japan and Europe.[30] One such series of children with lymphangioma described a case of partial airway obstruction resulting from OK-432 injection and cautioned against use of this agent around the airway.[31] Controlling the depth of injection of this agent and others is difficult and may result in damage to the airway in an area where treatment is difficult.

Another intrinsic injury is a thermal burn of the trachea. The inhalation of hot gases, steam, and toxic smoke produces acute injury that can lead to inflammation and edema in addition to actual burn necrosis. These individuals require special considerations in their management.[32,33] Whenever an endotracheal tube is passed through an inflamed glottis and upper trachea, early tracheostomy should be considered. With more extensive involvement, prolonged stenting with a T-shaped tracheostomy or T-tube with open proximal and distal limbs may be required.[33] Also, the overaggressive use of lasers or cautery may produce direct tissue thermal injury or may lead to an airway fire.

Extrinsic Injuries

Extrinsic injury to the larynx and trachea may occur when an unrestrained child in an automobile strikes his or her neck on the dashboard or the back of the front seat (Fig. 21-11). A blow directly to the neck from

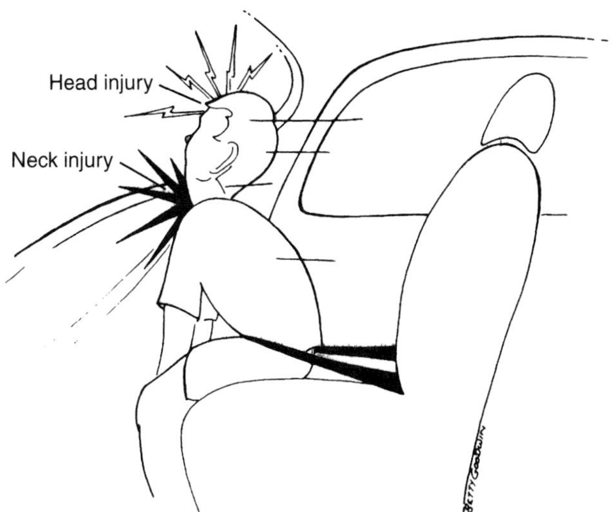

Figure 21-11. Mechanism of head injury. With a padded dashboard, external evidence of injury is minimal. (From Othersen HB Jr: Cardiothoracic injuries. In Touloukian RJ [ed]: Pediatric Trauma. New York, John Wiley & Sons, 1978.)

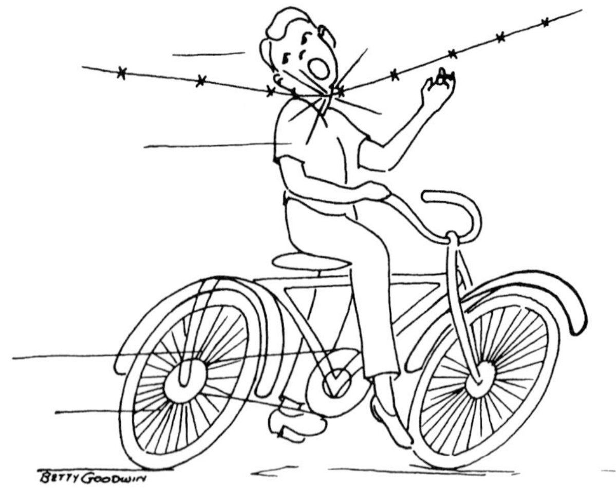

Figure 21-12. This neck injury may produce fracture or transection of the airway with little evidence of skin injury. (From Othersen HB Jr: Cardiothoracic injuries. In Touloukian RJ [ed]: Pediatric Trauma. New York, John Wiley & Sons, 1978.)

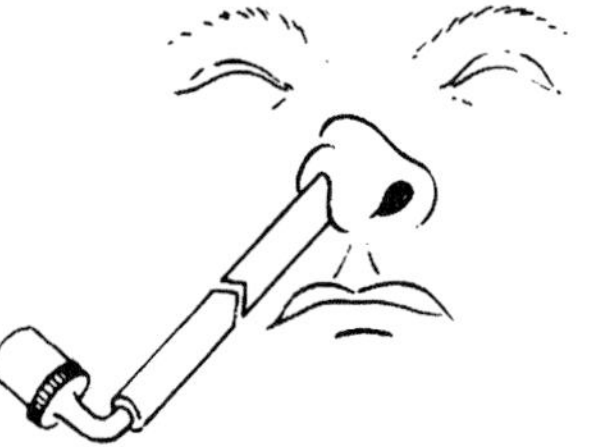

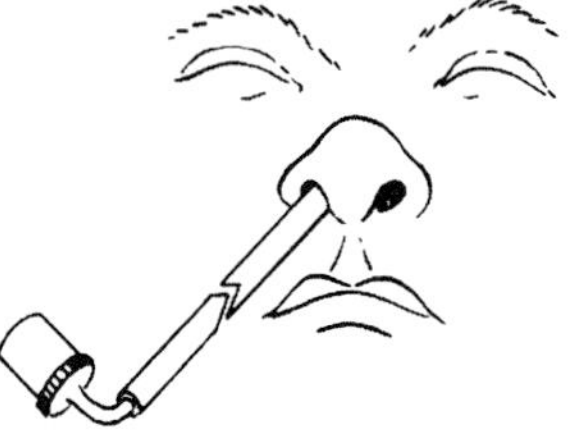

Endotracheal tube too large Endotracheal tube just right

Figure 21-13. An endotracheal tube should fit through the external naris without deforming it. (From Othersen HB Jr [ed]: The Pediatric Airway. Philadelphia, WB Saunders, 1991.)

a wire when falling or when riding a bicycle ("clothesline injury") (Fig. 21-12) may damage the larynx or trachea. Transection of both the trachea and esophagus can occur without visible external neck injuries beyond slight erythema. Crepitus may be present. A good history is essential in determining the mechanism of injury.[34] In these instances, and particularly in conjunction with severe craniofacial injuries, a tracheostomy performed under general anesthesia but without endotracheal intubation is usually advisable, because attempts at intubation may further compromise the tenuous airway. Penetrating injuries in children are infrequent, but the same general principles used for management in adults should be followed.[35]

ENDOTRACHEAL INTUBATION

Endotracheal intubation may be difficult in small children. The best laryngoscopic blade for children is a straight blade, such as the Miller or the Wis-Hipple. The latter is a straight blade with a design that allows passage of a bronchoscope or endotracheal tube through the blade. The child's head should be in the neutral position and not extended. Because the larynx is anterior in small infants, extension of the head draws the airway even farther anteriorly and makes visualization of the larynx difficult. With the infant's head in the neutral, or "sniffing," position and not extended, the laryngoscope blade is introduced and the tongue and floor of the mouth lifted to expose the epiglottis. Once the epiglottis is seen, extension or flexion of the head and neck may be required to improve visualization. Although many elect to stiffen the endotracheal tube with a curved stylet for all intubations, the use of a stylet may make introduction of the tube somewhat more difficult in a child because the stylet is usually curved slightly at the tip. When the tube is inserted through the glottis, the tip may impinge on the narrow anterior subglottic region. A tube without a stylet tends to follow the lumen more easily.

Usually an endotracheal tube that approximates the size of the child's external nares will be appropriate (Fig. 21-13). For pediatric patients, a commonly applied formula to determine the correct endotracheal tube size is (age + 16)/4 or age/4 + 4. If a child must be rapidly intubated with a tube that fits snugly and allows no air leak, this fact should be noted and documented. At the earliest possible opportunity, the snugly fitting tube should be changed to a smaller size. If intubation is required for a long period (usually > 2-3 weeks), tracheostomy should be considered. An air leak is generally an indication that the tube is not too snug.

Usually a cuffed endotracheal tube is not necessary in children because compensation for air leaks can be accomplished by increasing the volume of air delivered by a ventilator. However, with massive craniofacial injuries and bleeding or with severe gastroesophageal reflux, a cuff may be necessary to prevent aspiration of blood or gastric contents. Otherwise, it is best not to use a cuff for fear of damage to the trachea below the cricoid region. The mechanism for production of a tracheal injury by endotracheal tubes has been known for some time,[36] and steps for prevention have been suggested.[1,37] Although many surgeons elect to intubate the patient initially via the mouth, it is easier to overestimate the endotracheal tube size and produce a subglottic injury when compared with a nasally passed tube. Additionally, the conscious or unconscious movement of the tongue will produce a shearing injury to the glottis and subglottis with prolonged orotracheal intubation. The considerations for determining whether endotracheal intubation should be continued or tracheostomy performed are summarized in Table 21-2.

TRACHEOSTOMY

Our experience has been that tracheostomy with a linear tracheal incision through the second, third, and, possibly, fourth rings without excising any of the anterior wall of the trachea is the preferred technique in children (Fig. 21-14). Cruciate incisions should not be used because the flaps created may be inverted and narrow the lumen. However, some surgeons continue to espouse a technique called Starplasty.[38,39] Cruciate incisions in the skin and the anterior tracheal wall are sutured together to produce a permanent ostomy. This

Table 21-2 Indications for Endotracheal Intubation and Tracheostomy

Clinical Situation	Endotracheal Intubation	Tracheostomy
Emergencies	Always, except →	Severe craniofacial or head and neck injuries
Neonates and infants <6 months	Oral intubation unless no hope of extubation →	When long-term intubation is required or when there is difficulty in maintaining intubation because of activity
Infants >6 months and children	Maintain for 7-14 days and then →	When long-term intubation or ventilatory support is required for conditions such as severe head injuries
Epiglottitis	Until infection has cleared	Usually not necessary
Croup or other severe glottic inflammatory diseases	If does not respond to inhalations of racemic epinephrine or with airway obstruction as a temporary measure before →	When glottic edema and inflammation are severe

technique should be reserved for permanent tracheostomy because operative closure is necessary when a tracheostomy tube is no longer needed.

Tracheostomy is best performed with an endotracheal tube in place so that the airway is controlled. A transverse incision made in the lower neck is deepened to allow lateral retraction of the strap muscles after the midline is opened. This dissection is then carried down to the trachea. In small children, palpation of the ridges of the tracheal cartilages is frequently more valuable than visualization for determining the appropriate level of tracheotomy. The incision in the trachea is made below the thyroid isthmus, no higher than the second ring. The tracheostomy tube specifications are illustrated in Table 21-3. Traction sutures of polypropylene, left long and labeled "Left" and "Right," allow easier reintubation in the event of accidental dislodgement within the first week. If the tracheostomy has been in place for longer than 2 weeks, bronchoscopy can be helpful during decannulation.

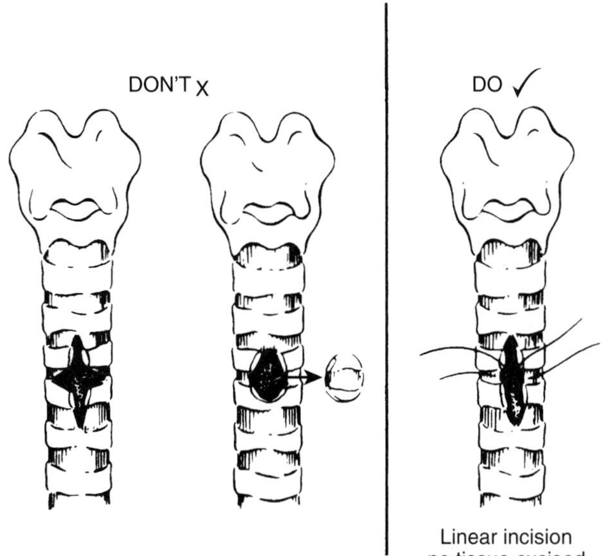

Figure 21-14. Two techniques of tracheostomy to be avoided in children and the preferred linear incision. (From Othersen HB Jr: Intubation injuries of the trachea in children: Management and prevention. Ann Surg 189:601-606, 1979.)

A large granuloma frequently develops at the superior rim of the tracheostomy stoma and may need endoscopic excision.

TRACHEAL REPAIR

Congenital Stenosis

Most congenital obstructions have a cartilaginous base but also have a fibrous tissue component. As mentioned earlier, many congenital stenotic lesions in the airway are asymptomatic until an acute event such as an injury, acute tracheal inflammation, or endotracheal intubation. At that point, the constriction of the airway becomes symptomatic. Complete tracheal rings may first be suspected when the child requires an anesthetic and an endotracheal tube meets a tracheal obstruction.[40]

For treatment of long-segment obstruction from complete tracheal rings, we have devised a procedure in which either the KTP or CO_2 laser is used to divide each complete cartilaginous ring in the posterior midline.[41] With an endoscopic balloon, the trachea is gradually dilated as the rigid bronchoscope is advanced. When all complete rings have been divided, a tube is inserted to serve as a stent. If long-term stenting is required, a T-tube is used (see later). If this procedure is done carefully without forceful dilation, no air leak should occur because the esophagus posteriorly fills the gap in the posterior tracheal wall. With a short segment of complete rings, resection and anastomosis has been accepted as effective therapy, but few surgeons have a large experience with this technique.[42] Other groups have used resection for long and short lesions but are now considering slide tracheoplasty.[43]

An improvement on standard resection procedures, slide tracheoplasty allows reconstruction without tension.[44] The narrowed segment is transected in its midportion, and the remaining stenotic segments are incised. One end of the trachea is opened in the posterior midline, and the other is incised in the anterior midline. Long-term evaluation has been satisfactory.[45] The diameter of the resulting anastomosis is broad enough to avoid airway narrowing.

Table 21-3 Tracheostomy Tube Specifications

Tube Type	French Size	ID	OD	Length (mm)
Shiley				
Neonatal	00			
	0	3.4	5.0	32
	1	3.7	5.5	34
Pediatric	00	3.1	4.5	39
	0	3.4	5.0	40
	1	3.7	5.5	41
	2	4.1	6.0	42
	3	4.8	7.0	44
	4	5.5	8.0	46
Argyle (Dover)	000	2.5	4.0	32
	00	3.0	4.7	34
	0	3.5	5.4	36
	1	4.0	6.0	36
	2	4.5	6.6	40
	3	5.0	7.3	46
	4	5.5	7.8	50
	5	6.0	8.5	54
Silastic	1	3.0	5.5	35
(Dow Corning)	3	4.0	7.0	40
	4½	5.0	8.0	43
	6	7.0	10.0	46

ID, inside diameter; OD, outside diameter.

Some surgeons have compared laryngotracheal reconstruction with cricotracheal resection and attempted to categorize the indications for each procedure.[46] The surgical therapy for these patients continues to evolve, as evidenced by a recent review of 50 patients treated for congenital tracheal stenosis at a single institution over an 18-year span (1982 - 2000).[47] Although the operation originally preferred was pericardial tracheoplasty,[48] four procedures were compared: pericardial-patch tracheoplasty (28 patients), tracheal autograft (12 patients), tracheal resection (8 patients), and slide tracheoplasty (2 patients). These authors concluded that their operation of choice for short segments would be resection. Resection with tracheal autograft was preferred for long-segment stenoses (more than eight rings).[49] In this latter procedure, the stenotic trachea is incised anteriorly and the midportion is excised. A primary anastomosis is made posteriorly, and the anterior defect is closed with a free autograft fashioned from the excised trachea. Others have used human cadaver tracheal allografts for reconstruction.[50,51] The ideal surgical treatment for congenital tracheal stenosis has not yet been devised.

Anterior cricoid split is a procedure that is useful in treating moderate subglottic stenosis in neonates and young infants.[52,53] Infants selected for the anterior cricoid split procedure should weigh more than 1500 g and require assisted ventilation or inspired oxygen of more than 35%. They should also not be in cardiac failure. This technique is illustrated in Figure 21-15.[54] Proper selection of patients for anterior cricoid split is crucial. After anterior cricoid split, those infants who can be successfully extubated have excellent long-term outcomes, whereas those who continue to need intubation will require tracheostomy.

Acquired Stenosis

When an endotracheal tube is removed, tracheal injury may be manifested by stridor or dyspnea. Prompt therapy may allow the trachea to heal without cicatricial stenosis. We treat the patients by introducing an endotracheal tube of a size that allows a slight air leak to serve as a temporary stent. A polyvinyl (Portex, Smiths Medical, St. Paul, MN) tube is pliable, softens at body temperature, and is preferred. This soft tube can be left in place while the patient is treated with high doses of systemic corticosteroids (0.8 to 1 mg dexamethasone/kg/day) in an attempt to soften the dense scar. Before insertion of the stent, the trachea may require gentle dilation by using balloon dilators. Rigid dilators may produce more injury, because even though they dilate they also impart a shearing force to the tracheal mucosa. Balloons dilate with only radial forces. Dexamethasone is continued in the dose of 0.8 to 1 mg/kg/day divided into four doses (0.2 to 0.25 mg/kg/dose) for at least 72 hours. Longer treatment may be necessary for more severe injuries. The corticosteroids are then rapidly tapered, and the endotracheal tube is removed once the patient is stable and spontaneously breathing without ventilatory assistance.

If a dense stenosis has already occurred, the previously described technique will not be effective. Acquired tracheal obstruction can be classified as granulomatous, inflammatory, fibrous, or calcific. Congenital obstructions are usually cartilaginous. With dense fibrous and calcific strictures, open resection and reconstruction is usually necessary. However, endoscopic laser incision with gradual and gentle balloon expansion of the lumen combined with insertion of an endotracheal stent may allow a functional airway to remodel over a period of time. Some authors advocate treatment of tracheal granulation tissue with mitomycin C.[55] Topical application of mitomycin C during endoscopic surgery helps reduce recurrence of granulation tissue. If stenosis recurs when the stent is removed, the stent can be reinserted and a balloon tracheoplasty performed with the stent in situ.

T-tubes have been used effectively as stents in the past for both children and adults.[33] Newer expandable metal stents are frequently used in adults. Some of these nickel-titanium (nitinol)-coated stents have been used in children in selected cases.[56] However, these stents may not be appropriate for children because the child will grow and the metal stent does not. Removal of the stent is then necessary and may be hazardous. Moreover, the ingrowth of granulation tissue through the interstices of the metal stent may produce obstruction in itself and lead to severe hemorrhage when removal is attempted. Finally, the medical conditions for which the stents are placed in children are different from those in adults. Stent use in adults is often due to neoplastic conditions that are associated with a short life expectancy. However, in children, a stent may be required for years.

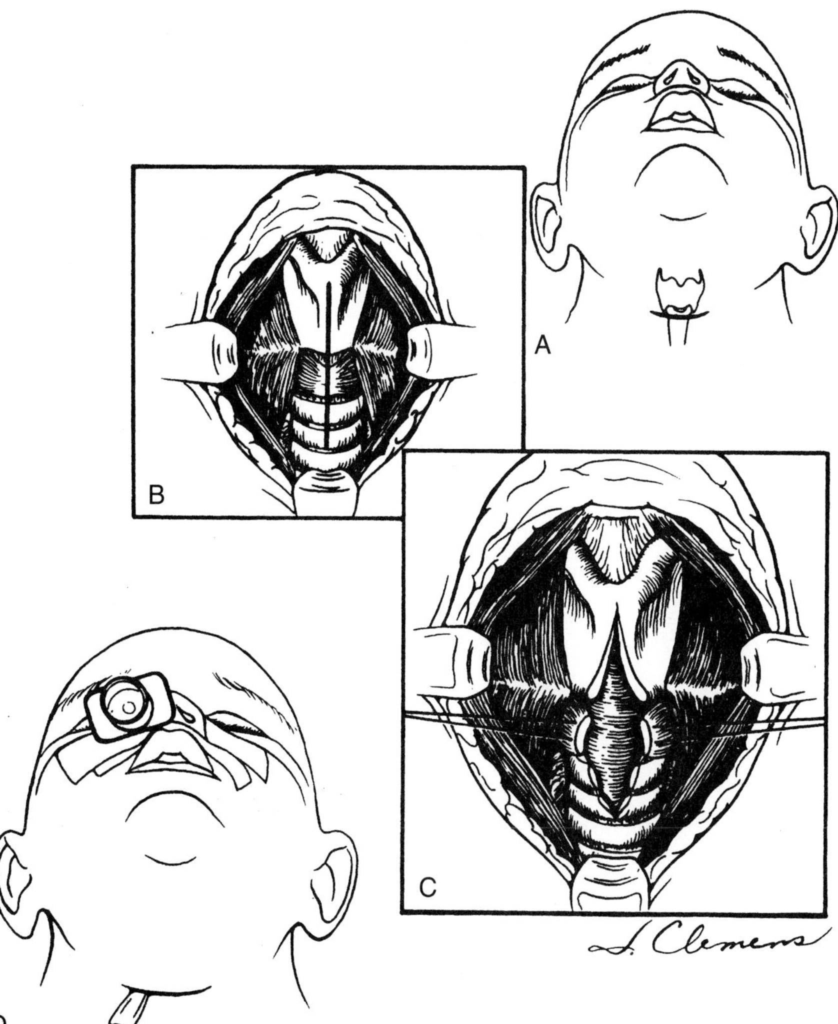

Figure 21-15. The anterior cricoid split procedure. **A,** Make a horizontal incision over the cricoid cartilage. **B,** Use a combination of sharp and blunt dissection to expose the larynx and upper trachea. **C,** Split the lower portion of the thyroid cartilage, the cricoid cartilage, and upper tracheal rings. **D,** Close the wound loosely over a drain with the airway stented by a nasotracheal tube. (From Othersen HB Jr [ed]: The Pediatric Airway. Philadelphia, WB Saunders, 1991.)

Straight tracheal stents of silicone rubber have been successfully used in adults, but fixation by projections from the circumference of the tube is necessary to prevent migration when it is not used as a T-tube.[57,58] The small diameter of a child's trachea makes these stents impractical. A T-shaped tube inserted through a tracheotomy with proximal and distal tracheal extensions can be readily inserted into a child's airway and will not migrate.

We prefer a modification of the Montgomery T-tubes for tracheal stents in children. These tubes are made of silicone rubber and are pliable yet rigid enough to serve as a stent. The tubes can be constructed to the exact dimensions necessary to fit the individual child's trachea. The proximal limb can be placed below the vocal cords, and the distal limb can be made as long as necessary for bridging the obstruction. Also, the cervical tube can be used for suctioning or for insufflation in an emergency. If these measures do not improve the airway obstruction, the T-tube can be removed by the parents and replaced with an endotracheal tube inserted through the cervical stoma. Finally, the modified T-tube allows normal laryngeal breathing and phonation when the side arm is plugged. Our technique for insertion of a T-tube is shown in Figure 21-16.

Open Laryngotracheoplasty

Many variations exist in the operative techniques of procedures available for tracheal reconstruction for a scarred and stenotic trachea.[59,60] First, an open procedure can be done with or without cardiopulmonary bypass.[61] Recently, there has been a tendency to avoid bypass and use only endotracheal anesthesia. Second, the repair can be performed with or without an augmentation graft. The grafts may include tracheal autografts, costal cartilage, cartilage from other sites such as thyroid or alar cartilage, autologous or allogeneic pericardium, skin, and tracheal allografts. Third, a stent may be used to maintain the lumen and can remain in place for hours, days, months, or years.

When open laryngotracheoplasty is performed without a cartilage graft, it is essentially a cricoid split or the expansion of the lumen with the use of a castellated

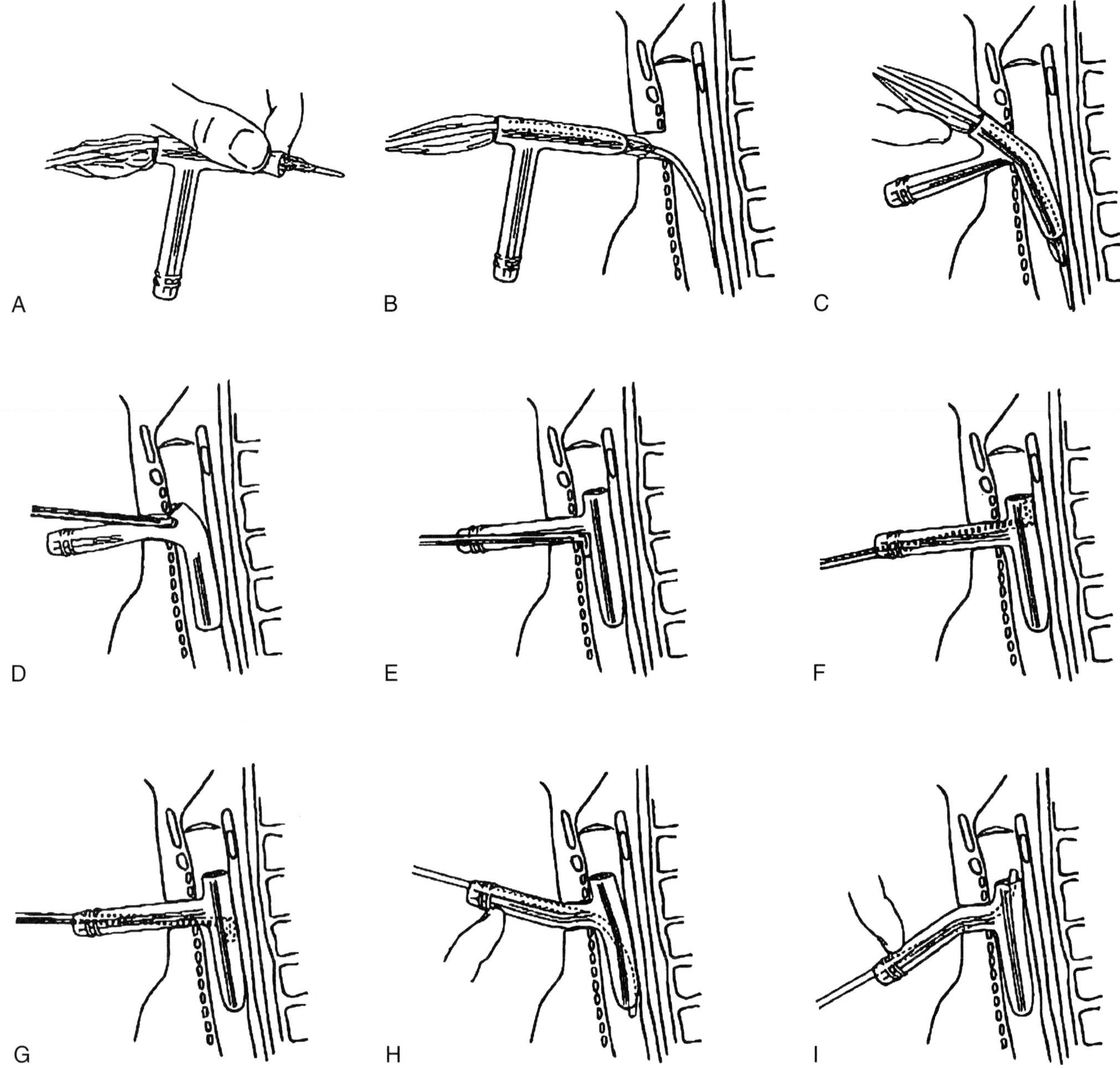

Figure 21-16. **A** to **I**, T-tube stent insertion with the aid of a dilating balloon to stiffen the T-tube during insertion.

incision.[62] These procedures are often performed with an internal stent.

The classic cartilage laryngotracheoplasty utilizes a cartilage graft (Fig. 21-17).[63,64] An omental flap may help a long cartilaginous graft survive.[65] The cartilage is inserted anteriorly after incising the stenotic segment.[46,66] Cartilage inserts also can be placed posteriorly and laterally in sites where the stenotic cricoid is incised. Ciliated mucosa has been found on the surface of a mature costal cartilage graft if the perichondrium faces the airway lumen.[67] Another option is resection and primary anastomosis. The stenotic portion of the trachea is excised, and an end-to-end anastomosis is performed.[68]

A slide tracheoplasty uses autologous trachea by dividing the trachea in the midportion of the stenotic segment. The upper and lower portions of the stenosis are incised in the midline, one anteriorly and the other posteriorly, and the anastomosis is then performed.[69,70]

Another option for repair of tracheal stenosis is by anterior incision and closure of the defect with pericardium. All pericardial patch operations are done on cardiopulmonary bypass.[47] However, experience at some centers has not been as good because of complications secondary to patch collapse.[71] The original proponents of pericardial patching have now reported improved results with a free tracheal autograft in which the excised stenotic segment is flattened and used as a free anterior autograft to expand the lumen at the anastomosis.[49]

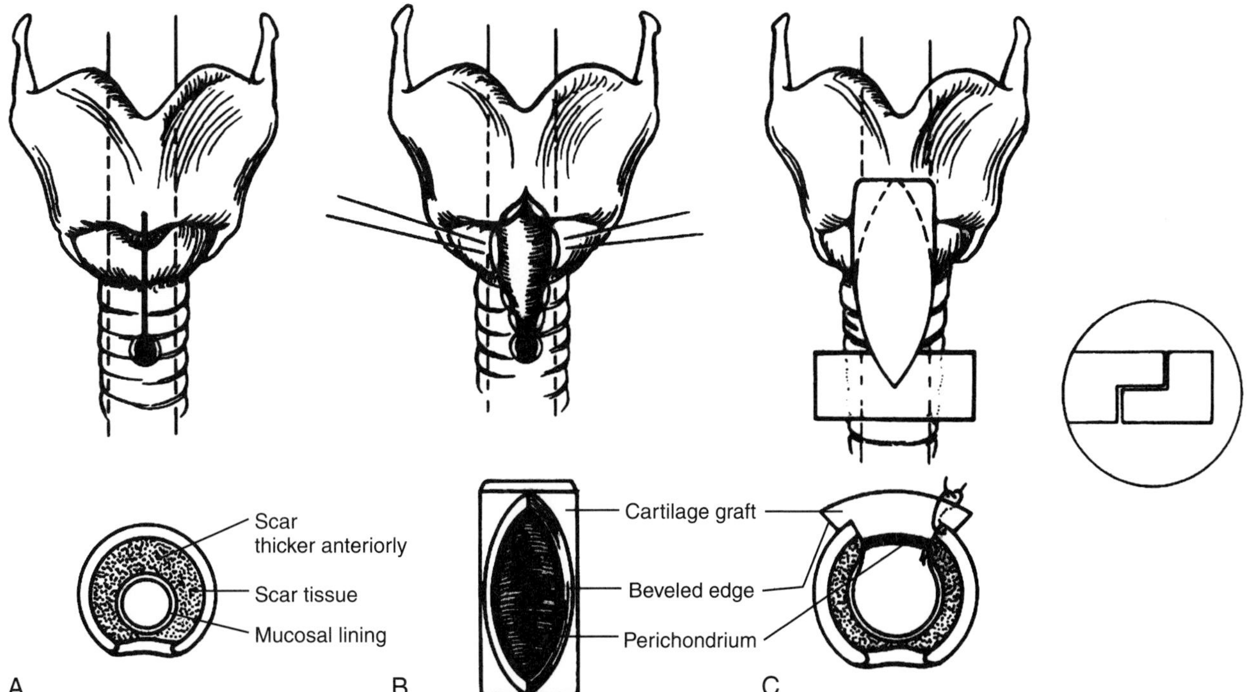

Figure 21-17. An autogenous costal cartilage graft reconstruction. **A,** Expose the larynx and upper trachea. **B,** Incise the aforementioned region, remaining superior to the tracheostomy stoma if the stenosis does not involve this site. **C,** Sew the costal cartilage to the incised edges of the larynx and trachea, placing the perichondrium internally. (From Othersen HB Jr [ed]: The Pediatric Airway. Philadelphia, WB Saunders, 1991.)

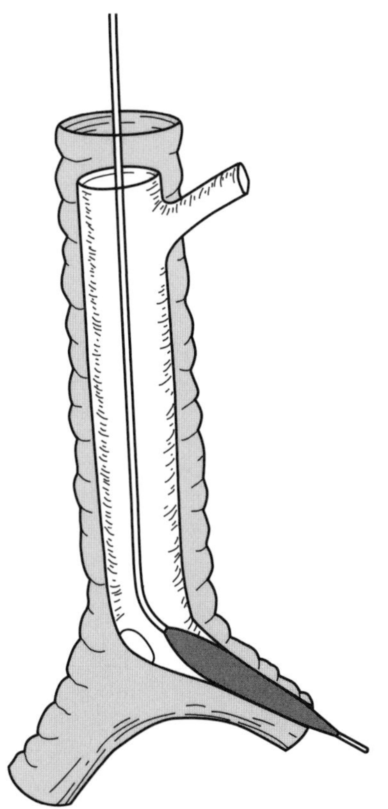

Figure 21-18. Diagram of a custom bifurcated T-tube with extension into the left main-stem bronchus and a hole for the right main-stem bronchus. A guide wire is placed with visualization by a flexible scope and a balloon catheter passed over it. With the balloon inflated, introduction of the stent is facilitated.

Silicone T-tubes are often used as internal stents to maintain the tracheal lumen and allow tracheal remodeling.[72] These tubes can be placed temporarily to allow for growth of the airway or to maintain the lumen while the airway heals after tracheoplasty. Alternatively, T-tubes can be effective as a permanent stent for the difficult pediatric airway or in cases of failed tracheoplasty. In very complicated and difficult cases, we have utilized custom-made T-tubes. One such custom T-tube is shown in Figure 21-18. This tube was necessary for treatment of tracheomalacia at the carina. A bifurcated Y-tube is difficult to insert. Thus, a bronchial arm extended into one bronchus and a hole allowed aeration of the other bronchus.[73]

CONCLUSION

One group has attempted to set up a foundation to develop a "disease-based and operation-specific model" to predict the outcome of airway reconstruction.[74] The operations for pediatric laryngotracheal reconstruction are challenging, and multiple procedures may be required. Therefore, prevention of tracheal stenosis or injury is extremely important.

Minimally invasive approaches by thoracoscopy will improve the techniques available for operative repair. However, the principles of surgical correction must be the same for the thoracoscopic or for the open approach.[15]

To summarize, the following principles are essential in treating the pediatric airway:

1. Be gentle. Endotracheal tube insertion should be atraumatic and of a size that allows an air leak.
2. If injury occurs and dilation is necessary, use balloon, not rigid, dilators.
3. Stents may aid in the healing process by maintaining the lumen.
4. Immediate high-dose and short-term corticosteroid therapy may be helpful in acute injuries, and their use may prevent dense cicatrix.
5. In all children with an endotracheal tube in place, document the size of the tube, presence or absence of an air leak, cuff inflation, and considerations regarding possible tracheostomy.

chapter 22

CONGENITAL BRONCHOPULMONARY MALFORMATIONS

Karl G. Sylvester, MD • Saif Ghole, MD • Craig T. Albanese, MD

A variety of developmental abnormalities of the tracheobronchial tree and pulmonary parenchyma are found in the newborn. Some of these have a genetic basis and produce widespread physiologic abnormalities. Many of these, such as surfactant protein deficiency, alveolar capillary dysplasia, and generalized pulmonary hypoplasia, are newly described and are not in the traditional scope of care of the pediatric surgeon. Thus, they are not addressed in this chapter. In this chapter, the more focal anatomic abnormalities of the foregut and its anlagen, traditionally termed *bronchopulmonary malformations* (BPMs), are covered. Although these lesions have been recognized for years and grouped as related for discussion purposes, no uniform pathologic or embryologic reason exists for this clustering. Rather, this grouping remains appropriate to facilitate an understanding of the common clinical presentation and management of BPMs.

With the advent of near-routine prenatal ultrasonography, a great deal has been learned about the natural history and pathophysiology of BPMs. Currently, ultrasound findings are altering many of the conventional beliefs and understanding of these lesions. Moreover, prenatal identification and a more accurate depiction of their natural history have given rise to advanced fetal interventions. The lessons learned from prenatal ultrasonography have also affected the postnatal management of cystic lung lesions, because previously unrecognized and likely clinically silent malformations are being detected with ever greater frequency. Still, despite these advances, BPMs defy a common embryologic classification and, as a whole, their pathophysiology remains varied.

EMBRYOLOGY AND CLASSIFICATION

The traditional understanding is that the tracheobronchial tree and proximal gastrointestinal tract arise from a common foregut anlagen.[1-3] At the end of the third week of gestation, the laryngotracheal groove or diverticulum can be seen in the caudal end of the embryonic foregut. This groove arises as a ventral enlargement of the foregut and then grows caudad to form the primordium of the trachea and lung bud. This outgrowth of endoderm is ventral and in parallel with the more dorsal portion of the foregut or future esophagus. Next, the lateral walls of the foregut, now called longitudinal ridges, begin to approximate in the midline, forming the tracheoesophageal septum. The separation of the dorsal esophagus and the more ventral tracheobronchial tree is thought to be caused by this tracheoesophageal septum and is complete by the sixth week of gestation. If this process fails or is incomplete, congenital defects affecting the trachea, conducting airways, or esophagus may result.

Some now question this traditional embryologic description.[4] Several lines of evidence tend to refute these long-held beliefs. With the use of scanning electronic microscopy at various stages of development, findings in chick embryos have described a paired caudal "lung bud" diverticulum with no identifiable tracheal primordium.[4] Even more elusive is the developmental program of the lung primordia after separation from the foregut anlagen, which occurs between 6 and 16 weeks' gestation. Current advances in molecular biologic techniques, including conditional mutants and transgenic mice, have allowed a more in-depth investigation and understanding of the molecular regulators of airway and pulmonary parenchymal development. In more generalized terms, the epithelium of the trachea, bronchi, and alveoli originate from endoderm, whereas muscle and cartilage originate from mesoderm.[2] Subsequent epithelial mesenchymal interactions result in the changes of branching morphogenesis and yield site-specific specialized epithelia for air conduction and gas exchange.[5,6] Studies in mice have established non-overlapping cell lineages of conducting airways (trachea and bronchi) as being distinct from those of peripheral airways (bronchioles, acini, and alveoli), well before formation of the definitive lung buds.[7,8] Similarly, studies in knockout mice and conditional mutants have revealed the involvement of many of the secreted protein morphogens involved in

Table 22-1 Bronchopulmonary Malformations: Classification by Site of Origin

Trachea and Bronchi	Pulmonary Parenchyma	Vascular
Agenesis	Congenital pulmonary airway malformations	Hemangioma
Atresia, stenosis	Bronchopulmonary sequestration	Arteriovenous malformation
Tracheal bronchus	Congenital lobar emphysema	Scimitar syndrome
Esophageal bronchus/lung (communicating bronchopulmonary malformation)	Agenesis	Congenital pulmonary lymphangiectasia
Bronchogenic cyst	Aplasia	Lymphangioma
Enteric duplication cyst	Hypoplasia	Congenital chylothorax
Neuroenteric cyst	Bronchiolar cysts (cystic bronchiectasis—multiple)	
Bronchial cysts (peripheral)	Lobulation anomalies	

organogenesis throughout mammalian development, such as members of the BMP, FGF, Hhh, and Wnt families.[8-11]

Knowledge of this embryology serves to elucidate the reasons for the frequent consideration of the close relation between anomalies of the proximal gastrointestinal tract and pulmonary system. Congenital BPMs comprise a broad spectrum of clinical lesions from both systems, including esophageal duplications, cystic lung lesions, and anomalies of solid pulmonary parenchyma with abnormal vascular supply. Classification of congenital BPMs therefore is not easy from either a morphologic or an embryologic standpoint. A simplified listing of BPMs by anatomic location becomes the most useful classification system for the clinician charged with managing the myriad presentations and diagnoses (Table 22-1).

PRENATAL DIAGNOSIS AND THERAPY

The widespread use of prenatal ultrasonography has expanded our understanding of the natural history and pathophysiology of some of the more common BPMs.[12] With ever-increasing sophistication in prenatal imaging, a wide range of lesions including bronchogenic and enteric cysts, mediastinal cystic teratomas, congenital lobar emphysema, bronchial atresia, and the cystic lung masses of congenital pulmonary airway malformations (CPAMs) and bronchopulmonary sequestrations (BPSs) are now identified with regularity.[13] Confusion still can occur, particularly in the fetus with a basilar cystic lung lesion in which the diagnosis of congenital diaphragmatic hernia (CDH) also is possible. More recently, ultrafast magnetic resonance imaging (MRI) of many of these same lesions has allowed an even more detailed distinction based on an assessment of their anatomic variability.[14] Overall, prenatal imaging of BPMs also has demonstrated the rarity of other associated anomalies, a fact of importance when therapeutic options are considered.[15]

The most commonly identified prenatal pulmonary anomaly remains the cystic lung lesion (Fig. 22-1).[12,16] An irregularity in the ultrasound echogenicity of lung parenchyma has become the initial diagnostic hallmark of the congenital cystic lung masses.[17] CPAMs, which are manifest histologically by an adenomatoid increase in terminal respiratory bronchioles, can be classified according to their prenatal ultrasound findings.[13,17,18] Microcystic lesions appear as a solid echodense mass.[17] Macrocystic lesions, which are composed of either a single dominant cyst or several daughter cysts measuring more than 5 mm in diameter, appear more echolucent and less dense.[15] In contrast to a CPAM, a BPS is defined by its morphologic characteristics of nonfunctioning lung parenchyma without communication to the tracheobronchial tree and with an anomalous systemic blood supply.[18] These characteristics are the clinically relevant diagnostic findings both grossly and by prenatal ultrasonography. A BPS appears, like some CPAMs, as an echodense homogeneous mass.[13,17] The finding on color Doppler imaging of a systemically derived feeding arterial vessel, as opposed to bronchial circulation, is pathognomonic of BPS.[12,17] Microcystic CPAMs and BPSs can have an otherwise identical sonographic appearance if the anomalous blood supply is not identified. Ultrafast fetal MRI can aid in the distinction between these two lesions.[13,14,19] However, in the majority of cases without definitive in-utero pathologic manifestations, the distinction is perhaps irrelevant.

Cystic fetal lung lesions may manifest several alternative outcomes. The overall prognosis of cystic lung masses relates to size, although with great

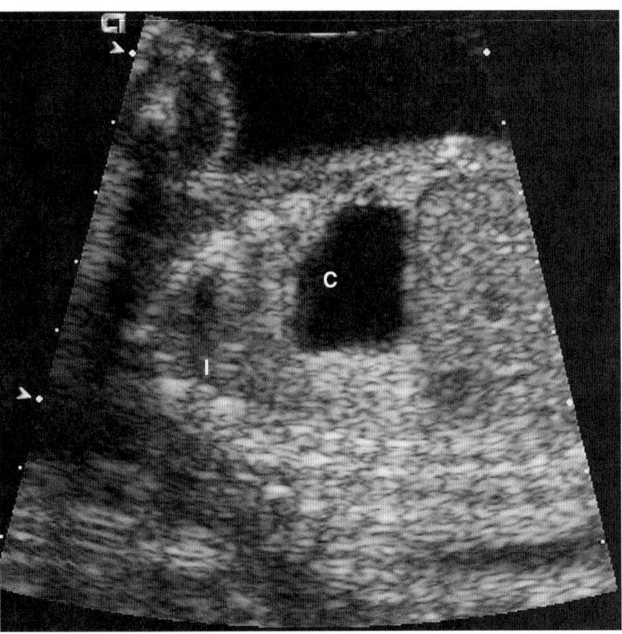

Figure 22-1. This fetal ultrasound image shows a large unilocular cystic lesion above the fetal liver in the chest. C, cystic lesion; I, inferior vena cava.

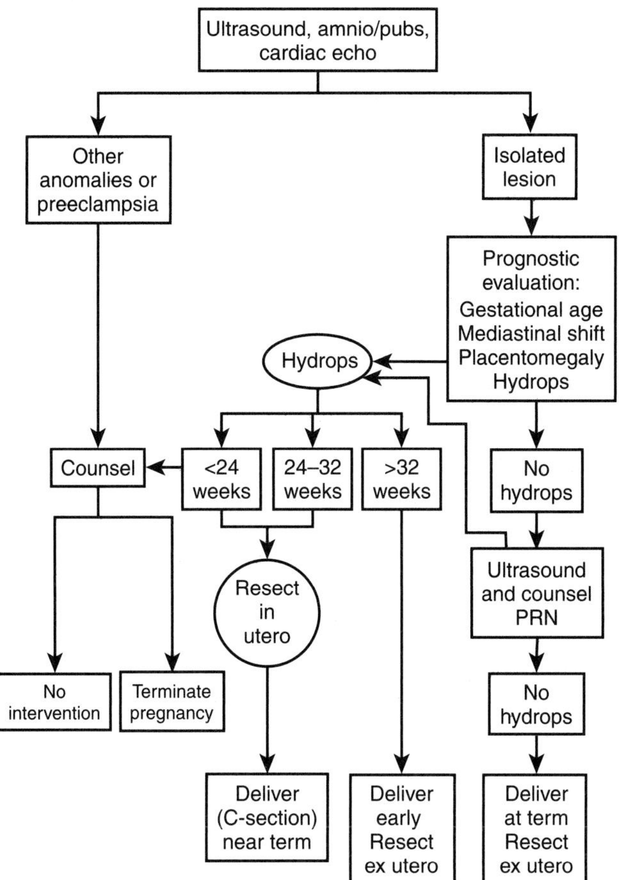

Figure 22-2. Proposed algorithm for the management of a fetus found by prenatal ultrasonography to have a thoracic mass. Pubs, percutaneoues umbilical blood sampling.

variability.[13,20] Small pulmonary masses as an incidental finding may be entirely asymptomatic both in utero and after birth. Very large masses can have reproducible physiologic effects on the developing fetus. Compression of the fetal esophagus may impede the normal swallowing of amniotic fluid and can result in polyhydramnios. Simple mass effect can displace normal or unaffected lung, producing pulmonary hypoplasia. Through a similar mechanism of extreme vena caval obstruction and cardiac compression, low-output cardiac failure and fetal hydrops can develop. Either polyhydramnios or hydrops can occur in isolation because they do not represent a continuum of pathophysiology. Hydrops is manifested by fetal ascites, pleural and pericardial effusions, and skin or scalp edema, or both. These findings have historically been viewed as a harbinger of fetal or neonatal death.[13,15] The ability to identify a lesion and witness its pathophysiologic evolution has produced a management scheme based on prognosis that now includes fetal intervention. This algorithm is outlined in Figure 22-2.

In 2003, an extensive 7-year experience with 350 prenatally diagnosed cystic fetal lung lesions was reported.[15] In this experience, 15% of CPAMs and 68% of BPS lesions were observed to decrease in size during gestation. Other groups have reported similar findings of involution of fetal cystic lung masses.[21-23] The mechanism by which these lesions involute remains unknown. Despite the strong association of hydrops due to a cystic lung mass and fetal death, a recent series of three cases of hydrops resolution with fetal survival was reported after the administration of prenatal corticosteroids.[21] Although the occasional case of fetal hydrops has been documented to resolve with spontaneous tumor shrinkage, it remains the collective experience that hydrops portends a poor either prenatal or postnatal outcome.[12,13,15,17,21-23] Overall, caution should be exercised when discussing the prognosis of the fetus because an understanding of which lesions will shrink remains unclear.

In an effort to derive a more objective prognostic tool, measurements of overall cyst size relative to the remainder of the fetus have been compared. The index of CPAM volume ratio (CVR) is obtained by dividing the CPAM volume by the fetal head circumference.[20] This index was found to be predictive of fetal hydrops when the ratio is greater than 1.6. Through these and similar serial ultrasound observations, it has been shown that most CPAMs do not increase in size relative to overall fetal size after 28 weeks' gestation. Based on these data, the authors' recommendations for fetuses less than 28 weeks' gestation are twice-weekly ultrasound examinations, given a CVR greater than 1.6, and weekly scans for those with smaller indices.[15,20]

The reproducible finding on prenatal ultrasonography that fetuses with very large cystic lung lesions and hydrops remain at risk has led to the development of fetal therapeutic options. Fetal thoracentesis and thoracoamniotic shunting have been performed with some success in fetuses with large, space-occupying pleural effusions, usually associated with BPS, or for the dominant cyst in a principally macrocystic CPAM.[15,24,25] Thoracentesis alone has proven ineffective because of the rapid reaccumulation of fluid and should therefore be considered as only a temporizing measure. Shunt placement for the continuous decompression of large single-cyst–predominant masses has resulted in the consistent resolution of hydrops in several centers.[24,25] In one report, nine fetuses were successfully treated for macrocystic CPAM with thoracoamniotic shunting, all with complete hydrops resolution, and with eight survivors.[15,26] Given an average time to delivery of 13 weeks, it seems that percutaneously placed shunts are well tolerated by the gravid uterus with respect to preterm labor after therapeutic fetal intervention. Of course, microcystic CPAMs associated with hydrops would not be amenable to shunting, based on knowledge of their microscopic anatomy and subsequent behavior. Somewhat paradoxically, the rare BPS with hydrops also has been treated successfully with shunting.[13] In BPS with hydrops, fluid accumulates in the pleural and peritoneal spaces and is believed to produce a tension hydrothorax from the obstructed flow of either fluid or lymph. All surviving fetuses should undergo more definitive postnatal resection after delivery and stabilization.

Numerous studies in the fetal lamb model that simulate a large thoracic mass with the mechanisms of compression, hydrops, and subsequent resolution, have been studied.[12,27-29] The techniques of fetal surgical resection, anesthetic, and tocolytic management were extensively investigated in nonhuman primates before the first clinical application of open fetal therapy.[12] Drawing on these collective experiences, guidelines based on the gestational age of the fetus, size of the lesion, maternal health and well-being, and the presence of hydrops have allowed selected fetuses with life-threatening lesions to be surgically approached (see Fig. 22-2). Open fetal surgery is offered at a few selected centers after a comprehensive multidisciplinary screening process.[16] Extensive prenatal ultrasonography and echocardiography is done to exclude associated anomalies.[12,16] In addition, amniocentesis or percutaneous umbilical blood sampling is performed to confirm a normal karyotype. With the knowledge that prenatal hydrops from mass effect is highly predictive of fetal death, massive multicystic or predominantly solid CPAMs associated with hydrops can be resected in utero before 32 weeks' gestation. The largest reported series to date described 22 cases, with 11 healthy survivors of procedures performed between 21 and 31 weeks' gestation.[15] Findings at operation in the original 22 cases necessitated 16 single lobectomies, 4 double lobectomies, and 2 pneumonectomies. In the 11 survivors, histologic confirmation of CPAM was acquired and all survivors had postresection resolution of hydrops within 1 to 2 weeks. In addition, compensatory fetal lung growth was noted as the mediastinum returned to a more anatomic configuration. In this same series, 11 failures were noted from a variety of causes. The same lessons of advanced fetal hydrops or maternal preeclampsia, also known as the maternal mirror syndrome, were causative in several cases. Mirror syndrome is a maternal hyperdynamic state that remains poorly understood.[30] It seems that there is a rationale for the belief that close ultrasound follow-up is warranted to identify fetuses before the complications of hydrops render the fetus unsalvageable. Preterm labor precipitated fetal delivery and death in several others. Thus, it seems that the lessons learned about the indications and limitations of the open operative fetal cases are reproducible.

For fetuses that have reached 32 weeks' gestation or more at the time of presentation, early elective delivery is recommended to effect ex-utero resection (see Fig. 22-2).[15,16] However, the outcome remains dismal for hydropic fetuses, even with advanced postnatal support, including extracorporeal membrane oxygenation (ECMO). The combined results and experience cited earlier have demonstrated that fetal CPAM resection is a viable option for selected fetuses with otherwise fatal BPMs and hydrops.

Table 22-2 Comparison of CPAM Classification Schemes

	Stocker (Classic)	Anatomic (Current)
Cyst Size	I (>2 cm)	Macrocystic (>5 mm)
	II (<2 cm)	Microcystic (<5 mm)
	III (solid)	
	II	Microcystic
Associated Anomalies		
Prognosis		
Favorable	I	Macrocystic
Unfavorable	III	Microcystic
Echogenicity		
Solid (echogenic)	III	Microcystic
Cystic (echolucent)	I, II	Macrocystic

POSTNATAL MANAGEMENT

Several fetal anomalies can be confused with CPAMs and BPSs.[3] Chief among these are CDHs, bronchogenic and enteric cysts, mediastinal cystic teratomas, congenital lobar emphysema (CLE), and bronchial atresia.[31-34] Smaller lesions may be asymptomatic at birth. Before the increased use of prenatal ultrasonography, many of these lesions went unnoticed, even on perinatal chest radiography. Current practice is to obtain computed tomography (CT) of the chest either before discharge or in the first several weeks of life. Planned elective resection of asymptomatic CPAMs and BPSs is recommended, given the accumulating evidence for the risks of either infection or occult malignant transformation.[3,35-38] However, this remains debatable and practice patterns are still evolving for the small asymptomatic lesions. Moderate-sized lesions may cause some respiratory embarrassment at birth, either from hyperinflation or from the secondary mass effects on normal lung. The traditional postnatal management of planned delivery with multidisciplinary neonatal evaluation, stabilization, and eventual excision has produced an excellent overall prognosis. On rare occasions when severe perinatal respiratory distress is anticipated, a strategy using ECMO has been described.[13,15]

CONGENITAL PULMONARY AIRWAY MALFORMATION

CPAM is traditionally described as a multicystic lung mass resulting from a proliferation of terminal bronchiolar structures with an associated suppression of alveolar growth. On histologic examination, these cysts are lined by cuboidal or columnar epithelium.[18] A pathologic classification system adopted by Stocker and colleagues[39] is important to note for historic purposes but does not currently represent a clinically helpful designation to predict the natural history.

The Stocker classification system subdivides cysts based on size into three major subtypes (Table 22-2).[39] Type I lesions have large multiple cysts of varying size, each measuring at least 2 cm and lined by a ciliated pseudostratified columnar epithelium. Type II cysts are also multilocular, yet they tend to be smaller, are

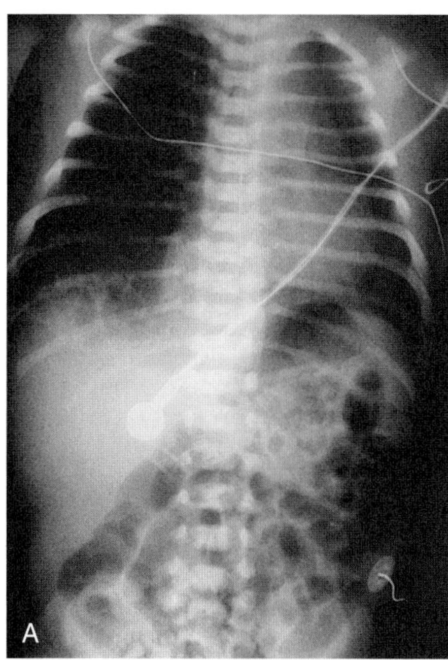

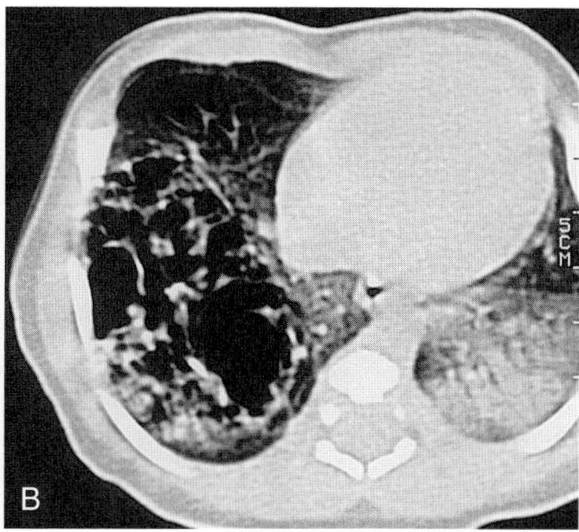

Figure 22-3. **A,** Chest radiograph of a neonate with mild respiratory distress and oxygen requirement. Note the small cystic appearance of the right lower lung field overlying the diaphragm and the shifting of the mediastinum to the left. **B,** Chest CT scan demonstrates multiple small and larger cysts suggestive of a congenital pulmonary airway malformation of the right lower lobe.

more uniform in size (daughter cysts are < 2 cm), and are lined by ciliated cuboidal to columnar epithelium. Type III lesions are macroscopically and microscopically solid, without cystic components. Many problems of overlap with hybrid lesions and atypical cysts that do not fit this classification system have subsequently been identified.[40,41] One published report documented a complex lesion with elements of a CPAM, BPS, and bronchogenic cyst, prompting speculation about a previously unidentified common ontogeny.[41]

Currently, a more generalized classification of cysts into macrocystic (>5 mm diameter) and microcystic (<5 mm diameter) subtypes is more commonly used and seems more clinically relevant (see Table 22-2).[42] The macrocystic lesions are not true cysts because they do communicate with the more proximal conducting airways. Therefore, these lesions typically are first seen in early infancy with progressive respiratory distress because air trapping leads to cystic expansion and compression of normal lung. These lesions are being identified prenatally with increasing frequency and are only infrequently associated with hydrops or pulmonary hypoplasia. Therefore, macrocystic lesions have a generally favorable prognosis and are frequently asymptomatic at birth.

Microcystic CPAM lesions can be distinguished from the macrocystic type radiographically, pathologically, and clinically.[16,42] These lesions appear more homogeneous and solid on imaging. Similar to the macrocystic lesions, they are not true cysts. The microcystic lesions, however, are currently believed to be more frequently associated with other developmental abnormalities. Therefore, these patients have a worse prognosis.[16,42] The small-cyst CPAMs may be seen in association with developmental airway obstruction due to bronchial atresia or stenosis. The pathologic features are consistent and demonstrate focal areas of increased bronchiolar proliferation, variable alveolar development, and regional displacement of unaffected lung parenchyma.

Macrocystic CPAMs most typically affect only one lobe and may have one or more dominant cyst-like structures with multiple smaller daughter cysts. While all cysts have some respiratory epithelial lining, some also contain mucigenic epithelium resembling stomach. In some series, at least 25% of these lesions have an associated systemic, nonpulmonary, arterial supply. Confusion between macrocystic and microcystic lesions may exist shortly after birth, with both appearing as solid on early imaging. The cystic nature of the macrocystic lesions becomes apparent within a few postnatal days as amniotic fluid is replaced by air (Fig. 22-3). When very large cystic changes occur on imaging, other diagnoses such as pulmonary interstitial emphysema, pneumatocele, pleuropulmonary blastoma, and intraparenchymal lymphangioma need to be considered.

BRONCHOPULMONARY SEQUESTRATION

Sequestrations should be distinguishable from CPAMs by their pathologic, radiologic, and clinical characteristics.[16] A pulmonary sequestration is classically described as a cystic mass of nonfunctioning lung parenchyma that lacks a demonstrable connection to the tracheobronchial tree. In addition, this sequestered mass of lung tissue receives its blood supply anomalously from the systemic circulation. However, as with many of these lesions, exceptions are common, with a wide variety of arterial supply and venous drainage combinations being described. Because of the anomalous blood supply, many believe the true embryologic

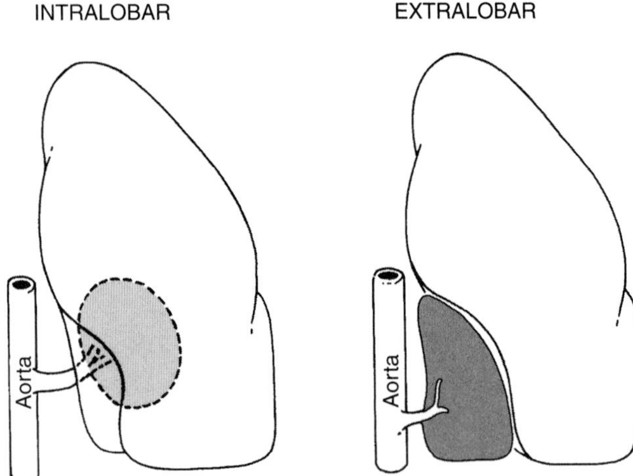

Figure 22-4. Locations for a pulmonary sequestration. These lesions occur either within the lung or outside the visceral pleura.

derivation of these lesions should classify them as vascular anomalies. However, because the majority of the clinical symptoms are respiratory, we continue to classify these as lung lesions. Sequestrations are largely solid lesions. Pathologically, these lesions demonstrate parenchymal maldevelopment, reflected as microcystic abnormalities similar to type II microcystic CPAMs.

Sequestrations are typically classified as either intralobar or extralobar (Fig. 22-4). If the lesion is contained within the same investing pleura as normal lung, it is intralobar. Extralobar lesions are found outside the investing parietal pleura of adjacent normal lung. Intralobar sequestrations are usually found in the lower lobe basilar segments and are more common in the patient's left hemithorax. Extralobar lesions have a more variable occurrence pattern. However, their typical location is also basilar, below the more normally formed lung (Fig. 22-5A). Extralobar lesions also have been found in the upper thorax, below the diaphragm in the upper abdomen (see Fig. 22-5B), throughout the mediastinum, and within the pericardium.[16,32,43-47]

Many sequestrations are asymptomatic. Given the lack of communication to the tracheobronchial tree, infectious complications most likely develop from hematogenous seeding. Extralobar sequestrations are frequently identified as an incidental finding, with approximately 15% occurring below the diaphragm and, not infrequently, in association with a left-sided CDH.[45] The radiographic findings for either intralobar or extralobar sequestrations are usually that of an opacified solid lung mass or a cystic parenchymal lesion with an air-fluid level secondary to infection. Intralobar BPS accounts for the majority of lesions overall, yet extralobar lesions are more likely to have other associated anomalies in as many as 50% to 65% of cases.[47,48] The most commonly recognized anomalies associated with BPS, in addition to CDH, include diaphragmatic eventration and other foregut malformations such as tracheoesophageal fistula and esophageal duplication.[43,44,48]

Historically, angiography was performed to confirm the anomalous systemic blood supply and to help in planning surgical management. Currently, the hallmark anomalous vascular supply can be identified by Doppler ultrasonography, CT, or MR angiography or a combination of these modalities. Typically, a single large feeding vessel arising from the abdominal aorta is found (Fig. 22-6). This vessel can be typically found within a pedicle or stalk. However, not infrequently, more than one major vessel is found to supply the sequestration. The venous anatomy may be even more variable, with systemic, bronchial, and azygous system involvement. If a bronchus is found within the pedicle, communication with the gastrointestinal tract should be sought.

SURGICAL MANAGEMENT OF CONGENITAL PULMONARY AIRWAY MALFORMATION AND BRONCHOPULMONARY SEQUESTRATION

Although somewhat debatable, the finding of a CPAM or BPS, regardless of symptoms, is an indication for resection, given the risk of either infection or malignant transformation. In an asymptomatic newborn,

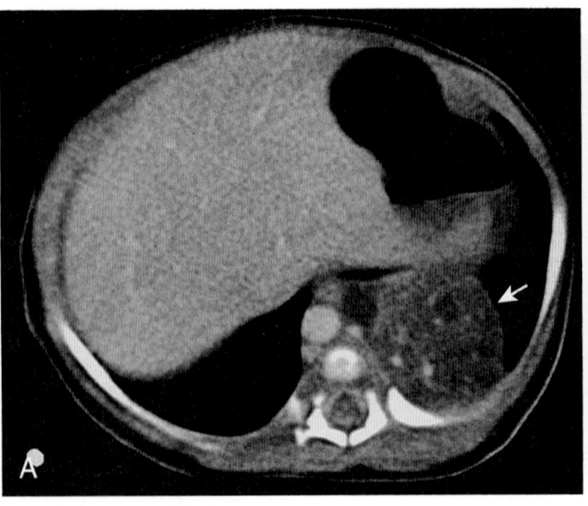

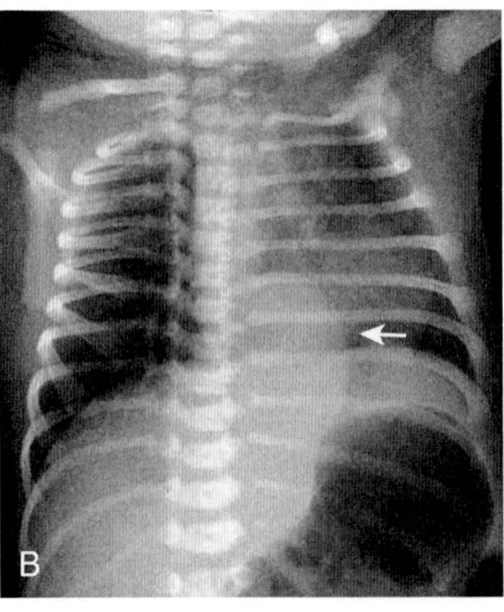

Figure 22-5. **A,** The CT scan demonstrates an extralobar sequestration in the typical basilar location of the left chest (*arrow*). **B,** In a different patient, the chest radiograph shows a large transdiaphragmatic extralobar sequestration (*arrow*).

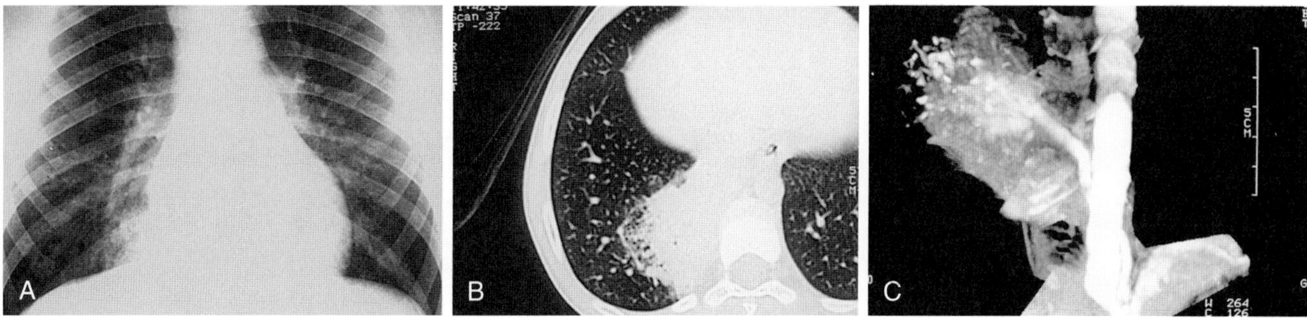

Figure 22-6. Systemic arterial feeding vessel from the infradiaphragmatic aorta to an intralobar sequestration. **A,** Chest radiograph. **B,** CT scan. **C,** Three-dimensional reconstruction of the CT scan.

the resection can be electively performed at 3 to 6 months of age. Both pleuropulmonary blastoma and bronchoalveolar carcinoma have been reported in infants, children, and adults with known CPAMs.[35-38] The preoperative chest CT can help in planning the operative approach. Traditionally, a lateral thoracotomy has been performed, depending on the location of the target lesion. Either a lobectomy, or less frequently, a segmentectomy allows complete removal of the majority of these lesions. For extralobar sequestrations, the preoperative imaging and localizing studies are even more important, given the possibility that some lesions are located below the diaphragm. Obviously, for extralobar lesions, a nonanatomic resection is possible and is facilitated by the stalk or pedicle-like nature of the feeding vessel.

Over the past decade, the thoracoscopic approach for resection of CPAMs and BPSs has been well described.[49-55] The advantages of this approach include a reduction in postoperative pain, decrease in hospital stay, improvement in cosmesis, and, importantly, the avoidance of morbidities (namely, musculoskeletal complications) associated with a thoracotomy.[54] The first large series of thoracoscopic pulmonary procedures in infants and children was reported in 2000.[51] The vast majority of the 113 cases reported were pulmonary biopsies and wedge resections. Lobectomies were performed with a hybrid technique of directed thoracoscopy and mini-thoracotomy. This report predated many of the instruments that are currently used for hemostasis and tissue sealing. The Ligasure (Tyco, Inc., Norwalk, CT), for example, also can be used to seal neonatal lung parenchyma when an incomplete fissure is encountered. Since this initial review, numerous reports attesting to the safety and efficacy of the thoracoscopic technique in the management of BPS and CPAM have been published.[49,50,52,53,55] In a recent report, 65 of the 97 patients underwent thoracoscopic resection for either CPAM or BPS.[53] All but 4 of the 97 lobectomies performed were completed thoracoscopically. Three postoperative complications were described (pneumothorax, pneumonia, and persistent air leak). Postoperative hospitalization averaged 2.4 days in patients who underwent successful thoracoscopic surgery. In 2007, a two-surgeon experience was published detailing a series of 144 consecutive pediatric lobectomies, 112 of which were performed for CPAM/sequestrations.[49] Lung abnormalities were diagnosed prenatally (by ultrasonography and/or MRI) and postnatally (by CT). The majority of these resections were lower lobectomies, which are technically less difficult than upper lobe resections. The median operating time was 125 minutes, and the median postoperative hospitalization was 2.8 days. Long-term follow-up (1-10 years) has not revealed any problems with musculoskeletal deformity or weakness.

In a 2008 study, thoracoscopic resection was compared with open resection in the treatment of 36 consecutive postnatally treated CPAMs over a 10-year period at UCSF Children's Hospital.[55] The 12 patients undergoing thoracoscopic resection were noted to have significantly shorter postoperative hospitalization (2 days vs. 5 days, $P = .0003$), a shorter time required for the chest tube (2 days vs. 3 days, $P = .047$), and a lower incidence of postoperative complications (16.7% vs. 58.3%, $P = .03$) than the 24 patients who underwent an open operation. However, the thoracoscopic resection group did experience a longer average operative time (164 minutes vs. 104 minutes, $P = .02$). The average hospital costs were noted to be similar in both groups, further validating the use of thoracoscopic techniques in the management of bronchopulmonary malformations. (See Chapter 28 for further information about the thoracoscopic approach.)

With further evolution in the thoracoscopic technique, a broader range of lesions, such as bilateral disease and very large lesions, can be approached. On the other hand, it may be best to stage bilateral cases to give the remaining normal lung a period of accommodation between elective resections. Currently, the main limiting factor for the thoracoscopic approach is the child whose condition is unstable because of the mass effect, because the large size may eliminate the effective working space needed for thoracoscopic resection. On occasion, intraoperative cyst rupture has provided the necessary working space for resection by minimal-access techniques. An exceedingly large lesion requiring pneumonectomy also will require additional plans for managing potential pulmonary hypertension or the temporary respiratory insufficiency that can result from pulmonary hypoplasia. ECMO may be useful as a temporizing measure in such cases.

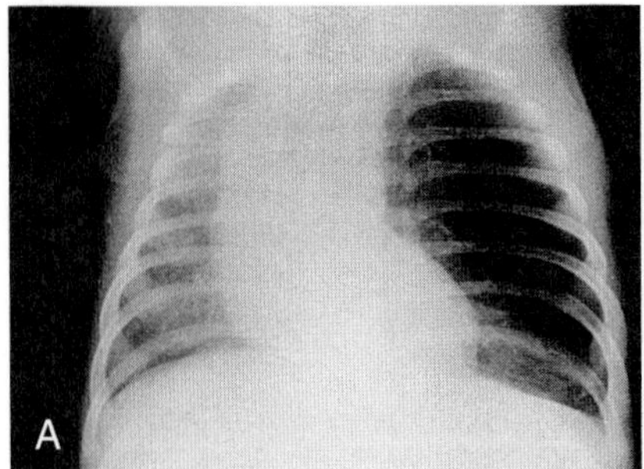

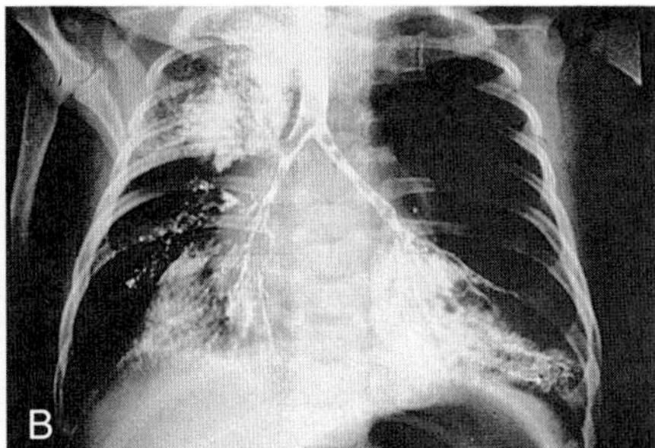

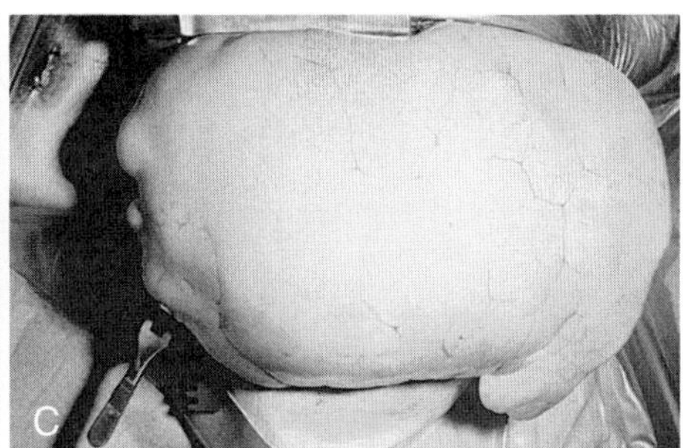

Figure 22-7. **A,** Chest radiograph demonstrates the characteristic changes in an infant with congenital lobar emphysema (CLE). Marked overdistention of the left upper lobe caused the mediastinal shift, flattening of the diaphragm, and likely subsequent respiratory distress. **B,** Bronchogram shows the absence or occlusion of the left upper lobe bronchus, producing the typical findings in CLE. **C,** Operative photograph demonstrates the dramatic herniation of an emphysematous lobe through the thoracotomy incision.

EMPHYSEMATOUS LESIONS

On occasion, CLE can be confused with a macrocystic CPAM.[31,34] Radiographically, CLE appears as overdistention involving one or more lobes (Fig. 22-7A). This is believed to be caused by a variant of bronchomalacia with a focal cartilaginous deficiency of the tracheobronchial tree, leading to regional airway collapse with expiration.[2,3] With postnatal air exchange, air trapping behind a structurally inadequate conducting airway leads to these emphysematous changes. Other rare causes include extrinsic compression from anomalous pulmonary vessels or by a very large ductus arteriosus (see Fig. 22-7B).[3,56] In the premature infant with significant respiratory distress syndrome, pulmonary interstitial emphysema, in its more chronic form, can evolve into a variant of CLE. One third of cases remain classified as idiopathic.[2,3,57]

The clinical presentation of CLE can be as varied as its numerous causes. With massive lobar overdistention (see Fig. 22-7C), compression of the normal lung and the mediastinum can cause respiratory and cardiovascular collapse. In these cases, emergency thoracotomy is necessary as a lifesaving maneuver. In less dramatic presentations, progressive tachypnea and expansion lead to assisted ventilation and radiographic identification of the offending lesion. Plain chest radiographs and CT scans have been used both for diagnosis and for determining the appropriateness of surgical resection and the boundaries of normal lung. In most cases, resection of the abnormal lung allows re-expansion and compensatory growth of the normal lung. Expectant management is acceptable for the largely asymptomatic lesion.[57] However, complete resolution of the radiographic findings is rare, and, for this reason, surgical resection is indicated.[57-59] The aforementioned concerns of retained secretions as a nidus for infection exist with CLE as for CPAMs.

The acquired forms of emphysematous pulmonary lesions generally are first seen in a more time-dependent fashion than are the lesions caused purely by congenital structural defects.[57-59] A history of chronic ventilation of a poorly compliant premature lung precedes the development of pulmonary interstitial emphysema and its sequelae of lobar emphysema or parenchymal cysts. Many of these lesions will resolve spontaneously. However, if the mass effect produces some of the same clinical symptoms of compression of the normal lung and mediastinum, then surgical intervention is indicated. In the most chronic forms of CLE, operative therapy for cystic pulmonary lesions from prolonged ventilator barotrauma can be quite difficult because little residual normal lung will be available for continued gas exchange.

LOBULATION ANOMALIES AND ISOMERISM

Significant variations of lung anatomy occur with respect to the pattern of lung lobulation. The most common variability is an absent or incomplete fissure separating the anatomic lobes. Absent fissures occur in 30% of individuals, whereas incomplete fissures can be seen in more than half of the general population.[2,3] However, these variations do not indicate disordered lobulation and, as such, have no clinical significance, other than to the operating surgeon. True lobulation and segmentation abnormalities can result in extra lobes such as a cardiac lobe (division of the left lower lobe into two separate lobes) or supersegmentation of the lower lobes.[2,3] The majority of these anomalies are without clinical relevance. Lobulation anomalies can occur with abnormal bronchial patterns as seen with accessory tracheal lobes with direct airway connection to the trachea.

The azygos lobe is a malformation usually of the right upper lobe that is caused by an aberrant azygos vein that is suspended by pleura and acts as a mesentery that produces the defect.[2] These lesions also most likely are clinically silent. Reports have mentioned esophageal lung, also termed *communicating bronchopulmonary foregut malformation,* in which a tract is preserved between the respiratory and alimentary systems.[60] These anomalies are almost always seen in association with esophageal atresia and tracheal stenosis or fistula.

Pulmonary isomerism is the mirror-image reversal of pulmonary lobar sidedness, in which the left lung has three lobes and the right has two.[2] This abnormality may or may not be associated with situs inversus but nearly always involves other organ system abnormalities, most notably congenital cardiac lesions. In addition, asplenia and polysplenia have been described with relative frequency. The associated cardiac lesions are usually responsible for the majority of the clinically relevant morbidity.

PULMONARY AGENESIS, APLASIA, AND HYPOPLASIA

Pulmonary agenesis is the complete failure of both airway and parenchymal development. Pulmonary aplasia is used to describe the incomplete development of lung parenchyma supplied by a rudimentary bronchus. Pulmonary hypoplasia is distinguished by a normal tracheobronchial tree and underdeveloped pulmonary parenchyma. Agenesis can occur either unilaterally or bilaterally. In the latter case this would be incompatible with life. In cases of unilateral agenesis, frequently other associated severe developmental abnormalities are also found.[2] Most commonly, these include the elements of the VACTERL syndrome. The etiology and embryonic pathophysiology of aplasia and agenesis remain largely unknown.

Pulmonary hypoplasia is the most commonly encountered anomaly of underdeveloped lung parenchyma. There are a variety of known causes. The compressive effects of lung, mediastinal, or cardiac masses or herniated abdominal viscera, as seen with CDH, can result in arrested pulmonary parenchymal development. Other causes include the abnormal mechanical effects of fetal diaphragmatic excursion or fetal lung and amniotic fluid volume. Specifically, abnormal or absent fetal breathing or oligohydramnios, with or without renal dysgenesis or obstructive uropathy, can be causative of pulmonary hypoplasia.[61]

The diagnosis and treatment of pulmonary hypoplasia is dependent on the underlying etiology.[61] For example, severe respiratory impairment can be seen with pulmonary hypoplasia from a CDH. In these cases, stabilization of the underlying physiologic impairment is the priority. In cases of aplasia or agenesis, the chest radiographs may demonstrate opacification of the ipsilateral hemithorax and an ipsilateral mediastinal shift with volume loss. In addition, asymmetry of the chest with obviously impaired respiratory movement of the affected side is seen. Treatment is initially directed at any associated anomalies, with particular focus on congenital cardiac lesions. If an operation is needed to remove a nonfunctioning lobe or lung, every effort is made to preserve functional parenchyma. In cases that render an empty hemithorax, consideration should be given to the intrathoracic placement of a tissue expander to prevent significant musculoskeletal disfigurement from the eventual mediastinal and skeletal shift toward the volume loss side (Fig. 22-8).

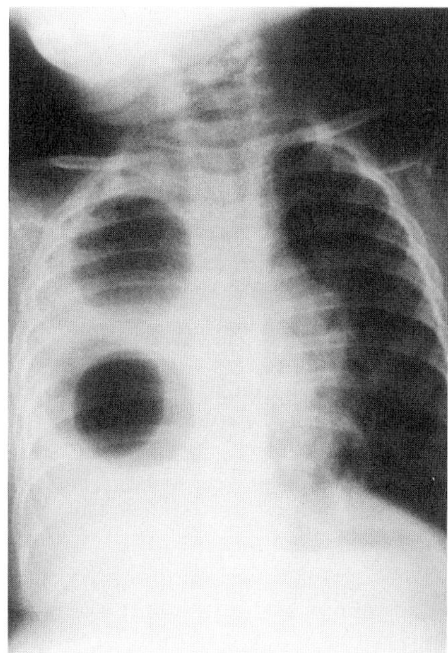

Figure 22-8. This chest radiograph was taken of a 3-year-old who underwent right pulmonary plumbage with insertion of three Ping-Pong balls 1 year earlier.

MEDIASTINAL CYSTS

As has been discussed, many of the commonly recognized congenital bronchial malformations, such as bronchial agenesis, atresia, or stenosis, produce parenchymal abnormalities that distinguish these lesions clinically. However, a subset of congenital malformations is unique to the bronchial tree and has been traditionally grouped under the nomenclature of bronchogenic cysts or foregut duplication cysts. As discussed earlier, the embryologic derivation of these from a common foregut anlagen, their occurrence in the chest, and their most frequent clinical symptoms make their inclusion appropriate in a discussion of BPMs. The nomenclature in common usage remains confusing. In general, the term *foregut duplication cyst* appropriately links these lesions embryologically as arising from a common developmental structure. When one considers their histologic architecture, these lesions can be divided into three subdivisions: (1) bronchogenic cysts, (2) enteric duplication cysts, and (3) neuroenteric cysts, all of which reveal their common endodermal origins.[62]

Bronchogenic cysts are lined by respiratory bronchial epithelium, are mucus filled, and may contain cartilage in their walls.[2,62] Enteric duplication cysts are lined by intestinal epithelium (either esophageal or gastric) and may contain smooth muscle. Most commonly, enteric cysts occur within the muscular wall of an otherwise intact esophagus without communication with the lumen. Neuroenteric cysts are the embryologic exception, arising from a failure of separation of notochord and foregut. These lesions contain gastrointestinal mucosa with well-developed smooth muscle walls and communicate with the central nervous

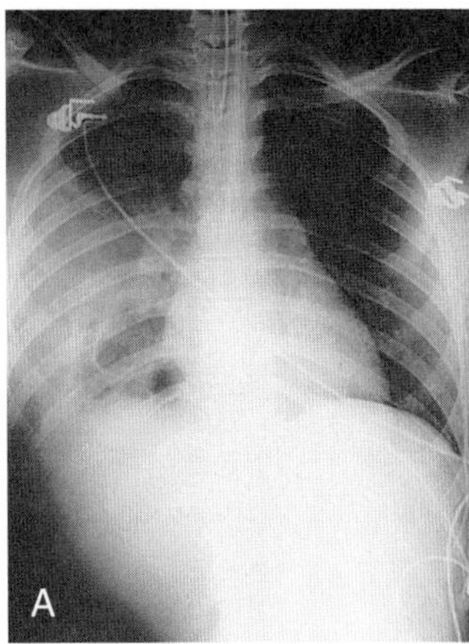

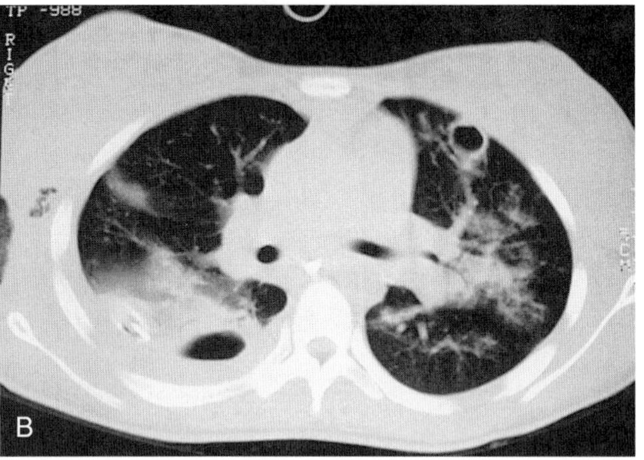

Figure 22-9. **A,** Chest radiograph in this 10-year-old child shows a right upper lobe infiltrate. **B,** Chest CT scan demonstrates a large bronchogenic cyst with an air-fluid level indicating bronchial communication.

system (CNS), spinal cord, and perhaps dura. This association explains their frequent coexistence with congenital vertebral defects, most commonly hemivertebrae.[63] Neuroenteric cysts are, however, much rarer than either bronchogenic or enteric cysts.

Foregut duplications must be considered in the differential diagnosis of a cystic mediastinal lesion (Fig. 22-9). Bronchogenic cysts can be diagnosed prenatally, perinatally, or in an older child. The lesion may be seen in the newborn with acute respiratory distress because a large lesion can compress adjacent normal lung tissue. They may be totally asymptomatic in an older child or may occur with infection in an occult lesion. Occasionally, the lesion is discovered incidentally on chest radiography performed for unrelated reasons. Further studies should include CT of the chest to identify the lesion and its relation to surrounding structures. Mediastinal cysts also have been identified on prenatal ultrasonography and are followed up perinatally with these same imaging modalities. Close scrutiny of the mediastinal structures is indicated because all bronchogenic cysts, whether symptomatic or not, should be excised, given their propensity for expansion, infection, and hemorrhage.[64] Because bronchogenic cysts are most commonly discrete lesions, they can be successfully approached thoracoscopically. Care must be taken to avoid injury to either the bronchial or esophageal wall, particularly when they share a common wall. The development of intracorporeal suturing techniques has enhanced our ability to excise these lesions endoscopically. Previous infection makes their removal more difficult by either the open or thoracoscopic approach, given the fibrovascular reaction that occurs surrounding infected lesions.

Bronchogenic cysts also may occur within the pulmonary parenchyma separate from the hilar structures. Peripheral bronchogenic cysts may be multiple, in which case they are more appropriately termed *bronchiolar cysts* or *cystic bronchiectasis*.[2] The more peripheral bronchogenic or pulmonary cysts are lined by ciliated respiratory epithelium and likely result from abnormalities during the latter portion of the pseudoglandular stage of lung development, as contrasted to the more central lesions that are true foregut abnormalities.[2] These lesions invariably communicate with the airway and often create obstruction of accompanying bronchi. Peripheral lesions may initially be seen early from the accumulation of mucus that leads to obstruction, or they may be seen later as infected peripheral lesions. They may be confused with necrotizing pneumonia. Diagnostic evaluation almost always includes CT. The treatment is surgical resection, given the natural history of persistence with recurring symptoms. (See Chapters 25, 28, and 40 for further information about bronchogenic cysts and esophageal duplications.)

VASCULAR ANOMALIES

Although the majority of pulmonary vascular anomalies are more appropriately discussed with congenital cardiac defects, several vascular malformations of the peripheral pulmonary parenchyma are within the scope of treatment for most pediatric surgeons. Pulmonary arteriovenous malformations (AVMs) typically are seen initially with a triad of symptoms, including dyspnea on exertion, cyanosis, and clubbing of the digits. The symptoms are produced because of the significant right-to-left shunting produced by these lesions. Radiographically, pulmonary AVMs appear as solid, frequently peripheral, lobulated masses of varying size. A CT scan reveals the tortuous nature of the involved vessels. Angiography may be needed to delineate the exact nature of the lesion. Complications of pulmonary AVMs include cardiac failure and, less commonly, rupture and hemorrhage, either into a neighboring bronchus or into the pleura. Treatment options include segmental surgical resection or catheter-directed embolization (which may be the preferred approach for the emergently bleeding AVM).

A rare entity known commonly as scimitar syndrome is a distinct variation of both BPS and the AVM anomalies. Also known as congenital venolobar syndrome, scimitar syndrome consists of a hypoplastic and malformed right lung with anomalous venous return directly to the vena cava.[2] Similarly, the arterial supply is variable and normally includes a hypoplastic right pulmonary artery and a systemic arterial branch from the aorta to the right lower lobe. Occasionally confused with BPS, this lesion always involves the right lung and maintains its bronchial connection to the airway. The syndrome takes its name from the scimitar appearance on a plain radiograph, arising as the lateral outline of the abnormal pulmonary venous connection with the vena cava (Fig. 22-10). This constellation of anatomic abnormalities produces a left-to-right shunt. Associated intracardiac anomalies frequently occur. Treatment options include redirecting the venous drainage to the left atrium or a right lower lobectomy.

Lymphatic malformations in the thorax are rare but, when present, can take one of two different forms. Congenital pulmonary lymphangiectasia is an anomaly with diffuse dysplasia and dilation of the pulmonary lymphatics. This can be seen in association with generalized lymphangiectasia. It may be secondary to pulmonary venous hypertension, or it can be seen as an isolated finding. With generalized lymphangiectasia, the treatment is supportive, whereas the less frequent focal abnormalities may be amenable to surgical excision.

Congenital chylothorax is the accumulation of chyle in the pleural space. In the newborn, this results either from a congenital abnormality of the thoracic duct or from birth trauma. Frequently, the exact etiology cannot be identified, rendering the label "idiopathic." For the majority of congenital chylothoraces, treatment is supportive with enteral diet modification or total parenteral nutrition. Serial thoracenteses or tube thoracostomy (or both) are the mainstays of therapeutic interventions that are largely temporizing and not curative. Recalcitrant cases may necessitate interventional radiology–guided attempts at embolization, thoracoscopic thoracic duct ligation, or placement of a thoracoabdominal shunt. These lesions can be fatal.

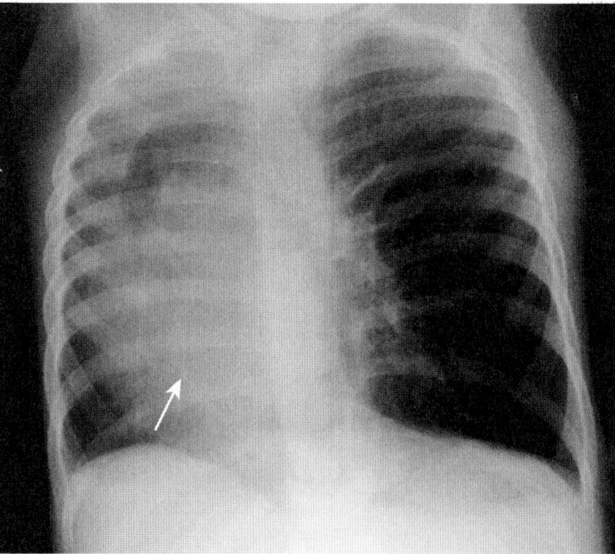

Figure 22-10. Chest radiograph shows the classic appearance of a patient with scimitar syndrome. The right lung is hypoplastic, and the anomalous pulmonary venous drainage to the inferior vena cava (IVC) is marked with the *arrow.* The outline of this vein gives the appearance of a scimitar. This vein probably drains into the supradiaphragmatic IVC. The vein is usually larger if it is partially obstructed or is draining into the IVC below the diaphragm. (Photo courtesy of Dr. Jim Brown, Children's Mercy Hospital.)

chapter 23

ACQUIRED LESIONS OF THE LUNG AND PLEURA

Bradley M. Rodgers, MD • Marc P. Michalsky, MD

Acquired pulmonary and pleural lesions in the pediatric age group continue to pose a significant challenge for the surgical community. Despite dramatic advances in antibiotic therapy and the implementation of widespread immunization protocols, the emergence of opportunistic infections and changes in disease patterns have led to increasing complexity with regard to the choice of treatment modalities. Furthermore, the widespread and often inappropriate use of antibiotics, along with increased numbers of immunocompromised children (as a result of better chemotherapeutic regimens and emergence of human immunodeficiency virus [HIV] infections) has led to increases in the prevalence of several acquired pulmonary and pleural processes previously regarded as uncommon. The treatment of these diseases poses a significant challenge and requires that the surgeon caring for such children is well versed in the varied and often complex therapeutic options.

EMPYEMA

Empyema is the accumulation of infected fluid within the thoracic cavity. In the pediatric population, this pathophysiologic process is typically associated with severe pneumonia and an associated parapneumonic effusion. Although pneumonia remains the leading cause of thoracic empyema in both the pediatric and adult populations, other potential sources of pleural infection include the extension of mediastinal, retropharyngeal, and/or paravertebral infectious processes. In addition, empyema may also develop as a complication of thoracic surgery or as a consequence of direct trauma to the thoracic cavity.[1] Although the incidence of this disease process is reported to be as low as 0.6% in hospitalized pediatric patients,[1] the associated mortality may be as high as 8%.[2-7]

Pathogenesis

In the early 1960s, the American Thoracic Society characterized three pathologic stages of empyema that remain pertinent today (Table 23-1).[8] Stage I, commonly referred to as the "exudative stage," generally consists of thin pleural fluid (with minimal cells) that moves freely within the thoracic cavity and is associated with mobile lung parenchyma. This phase, often referred to as a "parapneumonic effusion," occurs within the initial 24 to 72 hours and is typically amenable to a combination of simple drainage (thoracentesis or chest-tube placement) and broad-spectrum antibiotics. Stage II, or the "fibrinopurulent stage," lasts for 7 to 10 days and is marked by the presence of fibrinous debris and fluid laden with large numbers of polymorphonuclear cells. At this phase, the fluid is often acidic, in comparison with fluid collected during the exudative stage. A notable difference, compared with the earlier stage, is the fact that the fluid is often compartmentalized as a result of the formation of

Table 23-1 Characteristics of the Three Stages of Empyema

Stage	Time after Onset of Empyema	Fluid Characteristics	Treatment
I. Exudative	24-72 hours	Thin fluid, few cells	Drainage (needle or chest tube)
II. Fibrinopurulent	5-10 days	Fibrinous debris, many PMNs, loculated septations	Fibrinolysis (thoracoscopic debridement for failures)
III. Organizing	2-4 weeks	Thickened visceral and parietal pleura	Pleurectomy—open usually

PMNs, polymorphonuclear leukocytes.

multiple septations (Fig. 23-1). The presence of organized loculations makes effective tube drainage more difficult. With this limitation in mind, the use of computed tomography (CT) becomes an invaluable tool when planning the placement of chest tubes in the hopes of establishing adequate drainage of the thoracic cavity. Stage III, or the "organizing stage," typically occurs 2 to 4 weeks after the initial process has begun and is marked by thickening of the visceral and parietal pleura as a consequence of significant fibroblast ingrowth. The result is the establishment of an organized peel or rind (Fig. 23-2), which is intimately associated with the visceral pleura and which serves to entrap the underlying lung parenchyma.

The bacteriologic characteristics associated with thoracic empyemas have changed significantly over the past half-century. Although pneumococcal species were the predominant organisms associated with the development of thoracic empyemas in the mid-20th century, the introduction of penicillin and pneumococcal vaccine has resulted in *Staphylococcus aureus* now being the leading bacterial pathogen.[7,9] *S. aureus* has been reported to be cultured in the majority of pediatric patients and in approximately 50% of adult patients with documented empyema.[9]

Additional organisms include *Streptococcus pneumoniae, Haemophilus influenzae, Pseudomonas aeruginosa,* and several *Bacteroides* species. However, the effective treatment of *S. aureus* has resulted in the emergence of a variety of other species with a greater proportion of gram-negative organisms.[1] Recent series have shown the emergence of antibiotic-resistant organisms, including penicillin-resistant *S. pneumoniae* and methicillin-resistant *S. aureus.* Several contemporary series have demonstrated resistant organisms to comprise the majority of gram-positive cultures from pediatric empyemas.[7,9-11] Interestingly, some relatively recent series cite a re-emergence of *H. influenzae* and streptococcal species among pediatric patients,[12] although it has been speculated that the increasing use of vaccination against *H. influenzae* may further affect the current trends.

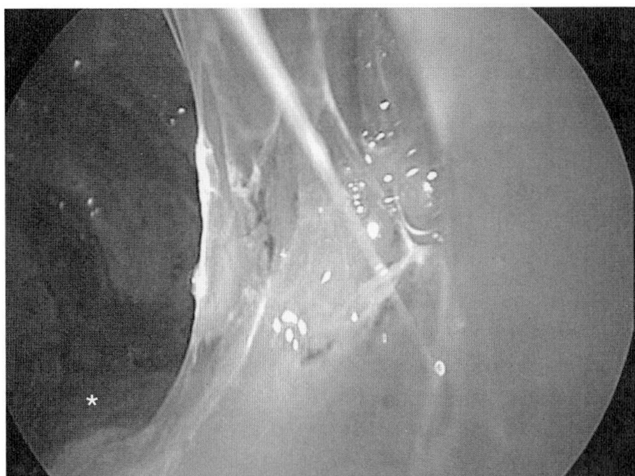

Figure 23-1. This thoracoscopic view shows the inflammatory septations that can develop after the development of an empyema. These septations often result in loculations of the fluid, which makes chest tube drainage alone ineffective. Note the collapsed lung (*asterisk*) as a result of this inflammatory material.

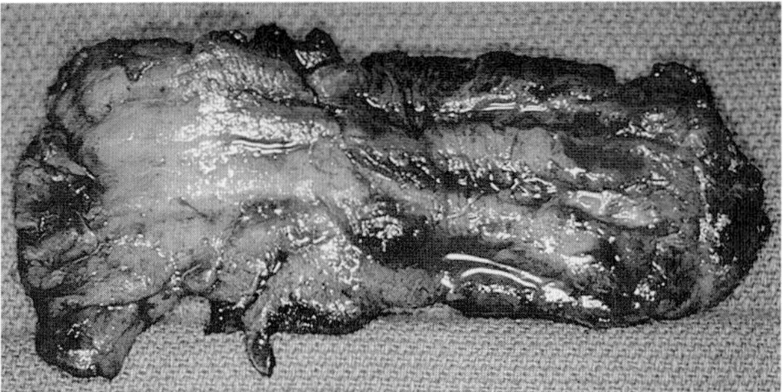

Figure 23-2. This gross specimen demonstrates significant pleural thickening encountered in the latter stages of thoracic empyema.

Clinical Presentation and Diagnosis

Because the usual cause of empyema in children is infection related to an underlying pneumonia, the typical clinical presentation consists of a recent history of upper respiratory tract symptoms with fever and cough. This clinical scenario often progresses to a state of respiratory distress, accompanied by malaise, persistent fever, and pleuritic chest pain.[4,7,12-14] The patient's typical appearance often includes lethargy with pronounced tachycardia, shallow and rapid breathing, and diminished breath sounds with dullness to percussion on the affected side. Dehydration requires aggressive resuscitation with intravenous fluids. A paralytic ileus is commonly encountered at the initial presentation.

A chest radiograph obtained at the time of presentation often reveals the presence of a moderate to large pleural effusion in conjunction with pleural thickening and underlying pneumonia (Fig. 23-3). The ability to differentiate between a simple parapneumonic effusion and a complicated effusion or empyema requires an analysis of the pleural fluid. Thoracentesis may reveal thick pleural fluid, with a purulent appearance, clearly indicating an empyema. Standard criteria for differentiating between a complicated effusion and an uncomplicated parapneumonic effusion include analysis of pleural fluid pH, glucose, and lactate dehydrogenase. A pH value less than 7.20, a glucose level less than 60 mg/dL, or a lactate dehydrogenase value greater than 1000 units/L suggests a complicated pleural effusion. Recently, one study has suggested the use of pleural tumor necrosis factor-α (TNF-α) for differentiating a complicated effusion.[15] These investigators have suggested that a TNF-α level greater than 80 pg/mL suggests a complicated effusion.

CT and/or ultrasonography of the chest are helpful during the initial evaluation of children with a pleural effusion (Fig. 23-4). These studies may help assess the condition of the underlying lung parenchyma during advanced stages of the disease process and allow identification of loculated fluid collections that have not been adequately drained. The identification of complex and undrained loculations suggests the need for more aggressive surgical management.

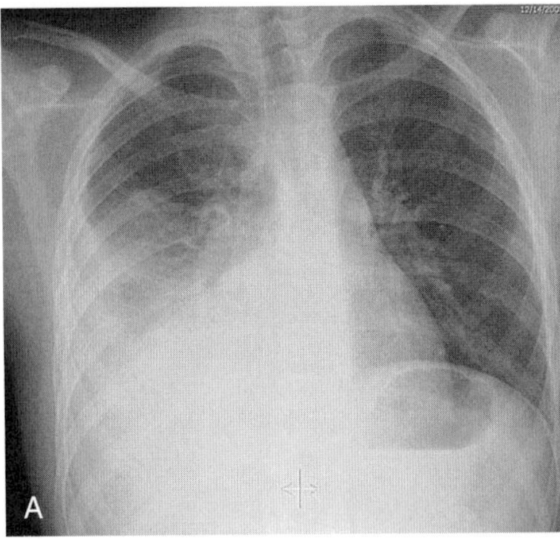

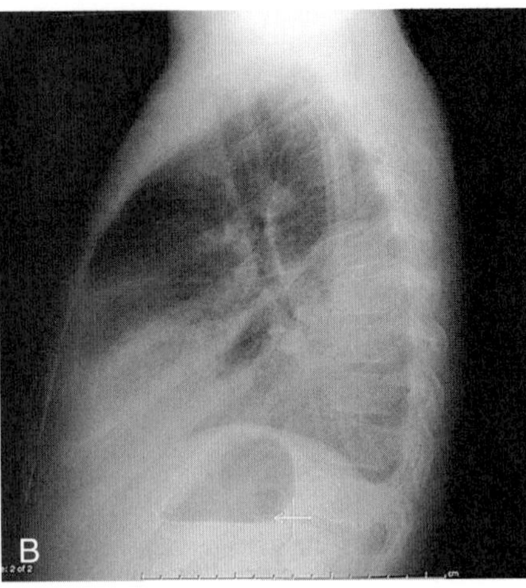

Figure 23-3. Anteroposterior (**A**) and lateral (**B**) chest radiographs show a large right thoracic empyema. The decubitus radiograph did not show any layering of the pleural fluid.

Therapy

The optimal course of therapy for children with empyema has been the topic of much debate over the past several decades. The treatment is dictated by the stage at which the individual patient is first seen (Fig. 23-5). Several authors have proposed treatment pathways encompassing several clinical and radiologic factors in an effort to help define optimal therapeutic management of this patient population.[6,11]

For patients initially seen during stage I disease, the fluid is usually thin and communicates freely throughout the thoracic cavity. The optimal treatment for empyema diagnosed in this stage consists of drainage of the infected fluid. This can be accomplished through the use of paracentesis or chest tube drainage.

The combination of drainage and antibiotics often results in rapid improvement in the clinical picture. The early clinical effects (24-48 hours) of closed chest tube drainage and antibiotic therapy are often quite dramatic with defervescence, decrease in the serum leukocyte count, and improved respiratory status. Failure to demonstrate rapid clinical improvement often indicates the presence of residual pleural fluid. A typical uncomplicated course involves removal of the chest tube(s) within 1 to 2 weeks' time and discharge from the hospital soon thereafter.

Although serial chest radiographs are often used to guide the effectiveness of therapy in patients with early disease, complete resolution of the radiologic findings may take weeks to months. The persistence of such radiographic abnormalities during the convalescent phase must be carefully followed. Specifically, when presented with a patient whose overall clinical picture continues to improve, one must consider the potential "lag time" encountered for resolution of the radiographic abnormalities and thereby avoid the mistake of misinterpreting such radiologic findings as being consistent with a diagnosis of chronic empyema.

Tube thoracostomy is rarely capable of completely evacuating the pleural space in a child who has progressed to an advanced disease stage (i.e., stages II and III). Most often, these patients require more invasive surgical techniques to ensure complete evacuation of the affected pleura. Advancement of the disease process to stage II is marked by a change in the consistency of the pleural fluid. During this stage, the fluid is often thick

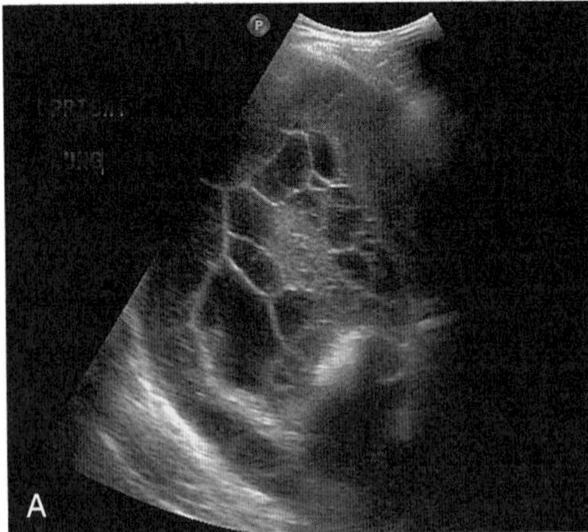

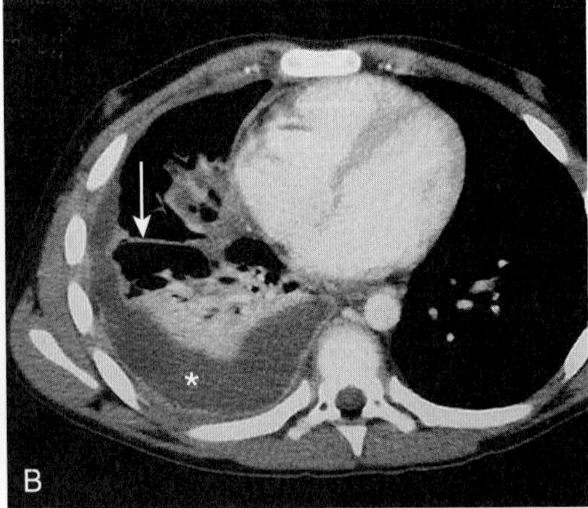

Figure 23-4. Ultrasonography and/or CT of the chest are helpful during the initial evaluation of children with a pleural effusion and possible empyema. **A,** In the ultrasound study, note the loculations identified in the pleural fluid. **B,** On the CT scan, a large pleural effusion (*asterisk*) is noted. Also there is collapse of the underlying lung parenchyma as well as septations (*arrow*).

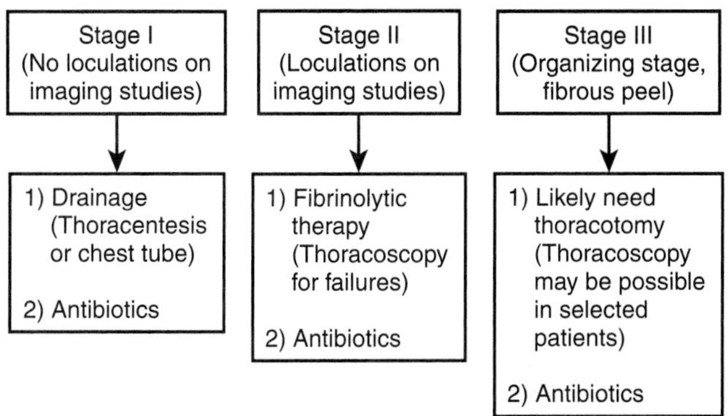

Figure 23-5. This schematic shows management of empyema depends on the stage. Simple drainage is usually possible for stage I disease. However, most patients present to the surgical service with stage II disease. Fortunately, stage III disease is not frequent today but was quite prevalent 30 years ago.

and turbid. In addition, free communication of the fluid, typically noted in the earlier disease process, is hindered by the presence of fibrinous strands within the fluid itself and frankly organized loculations (see Figs. 23-1 and 23-4). This results in the formation of multiple, non-communicating fluid compartments within the pleural space. When patients are encountered in the later stages of the disease process, or in those for whom initial therapy with chest tube drainage and intravenous antibiotics fails, more complicated therapy is needed.[7,9,16-32]

Historically, surgeons utilized formal thoracotomy for decortication as the treatment for children in these more advanced stages of the disease process. Over the past decade, most pediatric surgeons have employed thoracoscopy for this purpose (Fig. 23-6).[18-20] This minimally invasive technique allows complete evacuation, irrigation, and debridement of the involved pleural space during the fibropurulent stage (stage II) but is less effective during the more advanced, or organized, stage III. Nonetheless, thoracoscopy has replaced open thoracotomy for the surgical treatment of empyema in the vast majority of children who require operative intervention.

In the past several years, there have been a number of reports describing the effective use of fibrinolytic therapy to facilitate evacuation of the pleural space in children with empyema.[21-32] Initially, streptokinase and urokinase were used for this purpose. More recently, tissue plasminogen activator (tPA) has been the principal agent utilized. Recently, two prospective randomized trials comparing fibrinolytic therapy to thoracoscopic debridement and decortication have been completed.[31,32] The study designs for each of these two trials were very similar. The primary difference was that tPA was used for fibrinolysis in the Kansas City trial[31] and urokinase was used in the London trial.[32] In comparing the two treatment groups, there was no significant difference in length of hospitalization after initial intervention (fibrinolysis or thoracoscopy), days until the patient was afebrile, days of oxygen therapy, or the number of doses of analgesics. The primary difference was in the statistically significant higher cost involved with the thoracoscopy group. Interestingly, the excess cost was almost identical for each study. Failure of fibrinolysis occurred in 16% in both randomized trials. These patients then required thoracoscopic debridement.

Based on this level 1 evidence showing fibrinolytic therapy to be as effective and less costly than thoracoscopy, we have changed our treatment algorithm and have begun initially treating these patients with fibrinolytic therapy. In our own clinical experience, children in whom residual pleural fluid loculations are confirmed radiographically after placing a chest tube receive 3 days of intrapleural fibrinolytic therapy. Alteplase (Genentech Inc, San Francisco, CA) (0.1-0.2 mg/kg), a tPA produced by recombinant DNA technology, is mixed with 60 mL of saline and injected into the chest cavity through the chest tube. The tube is not clamped and is left open to underwater seal. If residual fluid remains at the completion of this 3-day trial of fibrinolytic therapy, these patients proceed to thoracoscopic debridement and decortication.

Outcomes

Despite the complex nature of this disease process, and the need to individualize patient care, the overall morbidity and mortality is relatively low. Patients

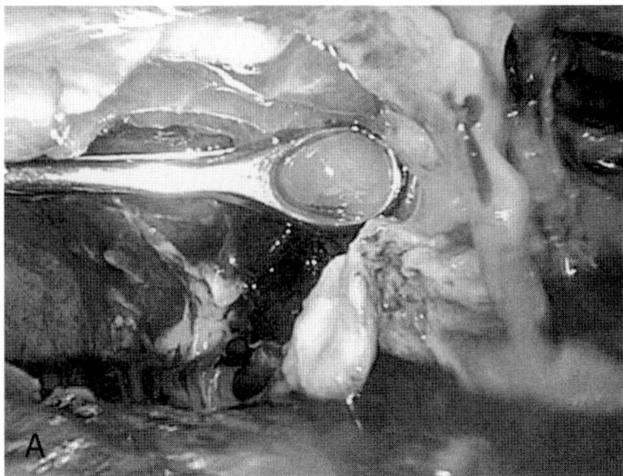

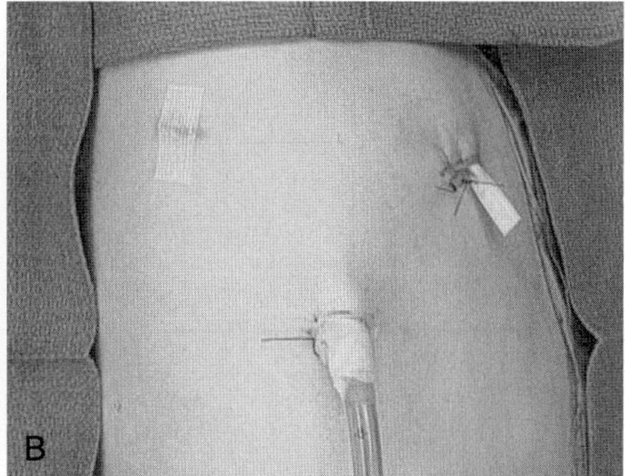

Figure 23-6. Over the past decade, most surgeons have utilized thoracoscopy for surgical management of empyema. **A,** Often, sponge forceps can be placed directly through the incisions to extract the inflammatory debris. **B,** In the postoperative photograph, three 8- to 10-mm incisions have been used for the thoracoscopic debridement. The chest tube is exteriorized through the most inferior incision. A small Penrose drain has been placed in one of the incisions because this was the site of a catheter that had been placed by the pediatric service for drainage of the empyema.

rarely have significant sequelae if treated successfully, although some reports indicate chronic pleural scarring and restrictive pulmonary pathophysiology as the result of a prior history of empyema.[2] The outcomes appear similar for initial fibrinolytic therapy as with thoracoscopy, but fibrinolytic therapy is more cost effective. However, 10% to 20% of patients initially treated with fibrinolysis will require thoracoscopic debridement.[31,32]

BRONCHIECTASIS

First described by Laënnec in 1819,[33] bronchiectasis is defined as a permanent dilatation of segmental airways and continues to be cited as the cause for a significant number of deaths due to respiratory insufficiency. In 1950, Reid described three pathologic forms of bronchiectasis: saccular, cylindrical, and fusiform (or varicose).[34] Saccular bronchiectasis tends to occur in third- and fourth-order bronchioles, whereas cylindrical bronchiectasis occurs in sixth- to seventh-order bronchioles. The fusiform variety has an intermediate type of pathology and involvement. Many forms of cylindrical bronchiectasis are largely reversible with control of the underlying infection and probably should best be referred to as "pseudobronchiectasis." As better treatment paradigms have been established, the frequency of bronchiectasis has decreased significantly in the industrialized world, although it continues to be a major problem in developing nations.

Pathogenesis

Bronchiectasis should not be thought of as a diagnostic entity in itself. Rather, the term refers to the morphologic abnormalities that represent the final common pathway of a variety of conditions causing long-standing pulmonary inflammation. The etiology of bronchiectasis can be divided into congenital or acquired, depending on the source and cause of the inflammation (Table 23-2). Most patients with congenital causes are found to have bilateral disease, whereas most patients with acquired bronchiectasis present with only unilateral disease. Although the disease process may involve any pulmonary segment, it is most commonly encountered in the left lower lobe or lingula or in the right middle lobe. A specific cause for the development of bronchiectasis is found in less than 40% of patients. Recent series indicate that about 50% of those patients in whom a specific cause is determined developed their first pulmonary insult before age 14 years.[35,36]

The bronchial dilatation develops after destruction of the elastic lamina and muscularis of the bronchial walls, secondary to recurrent infection. The pathologic process usually begins with impaired pulmonary clearance of mucus and bacteria and results in an increased endoluminal pressure. Migration of leukocytes into the bronchial lumen leads to degranulation and release of tissue-damaging oxidants, neutrophil elastase, and myeloperoxidases, in addition to the inflammatory cytokines TNF-α, Interleukin (IL)-8, and IL-6.[37] The ciliated epithelium is destroyed, leading to an increased propensity for recurrent infection. Repeated localized infection leads to replacement of the ciliated epithelium by squamous epithelium and loss of the supporting cartilage, allowing further bronchial inflammation and dilatation.

Table 23-2 Congenital and Acquired Conditions Associated with the Development of Bronchiectasis
Congenital
Cystic fibrosis Kartagener's syndrome Immunodeficiency states Ciliary dyskinesia states
Acquired
Pneumonia Repeated aspiration (gastroesophageal reflux disease) Sequestration Tuberculosis Airway foreign body Endobronchial tumor Smoking Human immunodeficiency virus infection

The overall incidence of bronchiectasis in the United States has declined progressively since the 1950s. This has been attributed to the widespread use of bacterial and viral immunizations in childhood and aggressive antibiotic treatment of pulmonary infection. The near elimination of tuberculosis in this country is also considered a factor in this decline. Conversely, there is a suggestion that the incidence of bronchiectasis is beginning to increase in children as fewer are uniformly vaccinated and resistant strains of tuberculosis are being encountered more frequently. An accelerated form of bronchiectasis has been described in patients with HIV infections.[38]

Clinical Presentation and Diagnosis

Children with active bronchiectasis initially appear with systemic signs of infection such as fever, fatigue, and anorexia. This presentation is often accompanied by a productive cough, pleuritic chest pain, and hemoptysis. Physical examination usually reveals coarse inspiratory crackles and expiratory wheezes. Because few specific signs of bronchiectasis exist, the diagnosis often is delayed. The initial diagnostic workup should include a chest radiograph. Although this is sensitive for the diagnosis of bronchiectasis in only 50% of patients, it may show focal increase and "crowding" of interstitial markings. In diffuse, long-standing disease, a coarse honeycomb appearance may be seen (Fig. 23-7). For many years, the specific diagnosis of bronchiectasis depended on the performance of bronchography, a relatively invasive test in children. In the past decade, high-resolution CT scans have replaced bronchography for this purpose. Modern thin-section CT scans have more than a 90% correlation with bronchographic findings.[39] The characteristic changes

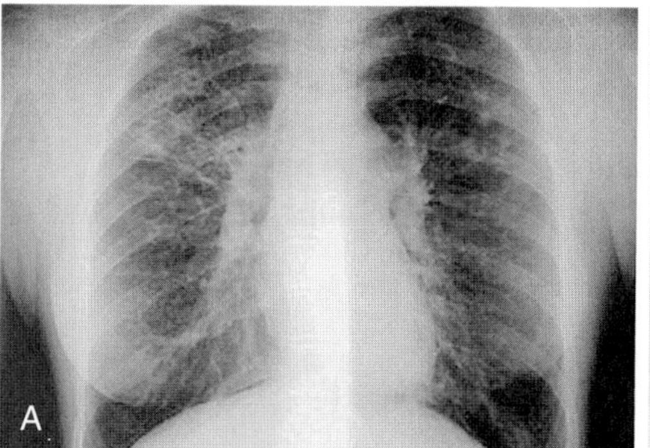

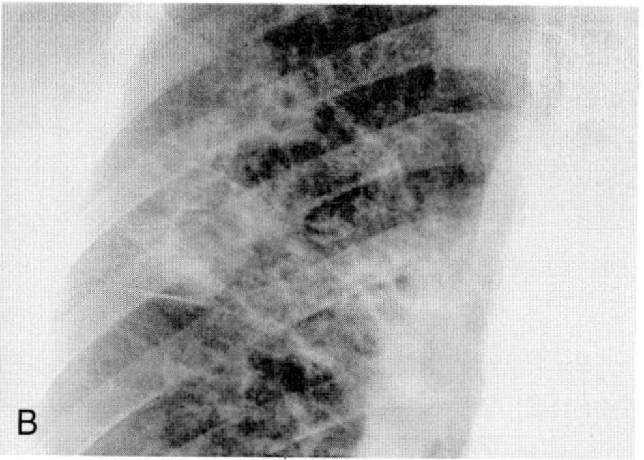

Figure 23-7. **A,** Chest radiograph demonstrating the classic appearance of bronchiectasis in a pediatric patient with cystic fibrosis. **B,** Magnified view of patient in **A** demonstrating honeycombed appearance.

on thin-section CT include focal regions of volume loss and vascular crowding, "ring shadows" of dilated bronchi sectioned on end, bronchoarteriolar ratios less than 1, loss of bronchial tapering, and visualization of bronchi within 1 cm of the pleural surface. Of these findings, the presence of bronchi within 1 cm of the pleural surface appears to correlate best with bronchographic findings.[40] Additional types of CT studies that may be useful in evaluating patients with bronchiectasis include inspiratory-expiratory CT, which can give insights into the pathophysiologic processes involved; spiral CT and virtual bronchoscopy, which may allow better visualization of peripheral bronchi; and CT angiography, which may demonstrate neovascularization of the chronically inflamed bronchi.

Therapy

The best therapy for bronchiectasis involves prevention of the disease by aggressively treating recurrent pulmonary infections. The development of bronchiectasis may be inevitable in children with congenial causes such as cystic fibrosis or ciliary dyskinesia, but the disease in those patients with acquired causes should, for the most part, be preventable. Aggressive treatment of children with recurrent pulmonary infections should be accomplished with targeted antibiotic therapy and pulmonary physical therapy. A high index of suspicion must be maintained for bronchial obstruction, either by foreign body or endobronchial tumors, and bronchoscopy plays an important role in the early management of these children.

Pulmonary resection is reserved for those children who have repeated localized involvement despite adequate medical therapy. The absence of vascular perfusion, as determined by either angiography or perfusion nuclear scans, is an indication for operation for end-stage disease.[40] Those patients will generally experience a good operative result. Patients with perfused segments may have reversible, cylindrical bronchiectases and should probably continue to receive medical management. Occasionally, massive hemoptysis will be the indication for surgical resection, although embolization of bronchial vessels using interventional radiology may eliminate resection as an emergency procedure.

The principles of surgical therapy should be to preserve uninvolved pulmonary tissue by the liberal use of segmental pulmonary resection.[41] On the other hand, resection of all diseased segments is critical for a successful operative result, including staged bilateral thoracotomy, if necessary. Care must be taken to avoid contamination of the dependent lung while the patient is in the lateral decubitus position. The use of bifurcated endotracheal tubes or cuffed tubes with main-stem bronchial blockers is recommended.[42] Haciibrahimoglu and colleagues described the operative results of pulmonary resection in 35 children with bronchiectases treated at their institution between 1985 and 2001.[43] Eleven percent of these children had pulmonary tuberculosis. The average age at thoracotomy was 10.6 years, and 68.5% of the patients had cylindrical bronchiectases. There was a single death in this series. Follow-up studies revealed that 64.7% of the children were asymptomatic and 23.5% were significantly improved clinically. About 12% had no clinical improvement. The authors stress the importance of careful selection of patients and complete resection of the disease. It is generally conceded that surgical outcomes are better in younger patients. Finally, thoracoscopic lobectomy for acquired disease is becoming more frequently utilized.

Outcomes

While resolution of bronchiectasis may be anticipated with effective treatment of the underlying infectious process, patients with chronic underlying pulmonary diseases, such as cystic fibrosis, are likely to experience less favorable outcomes. In addition, outcomes may also be influenced as a result of the specific infectious organisms and treatment regimens.[44] Most of these patients are found to have significant airway obstruction that progresses over time. Pulmonary function studies indicate intrathoracic airway obstruction of the medium to small airways associated with hyperinflation. Sophisticated studies indicate an increased residual volume and a reduced FEV_1 in these patients.[44]

LUNG ABSCESS

Lung abscess in the pediatric population is considered to be relatively rare and typically results from an infection with mixed aerobic and anaerobic flora.

The treatment of a lung abscess in an infant or child follows the same basic principles of postural drainage and pulmonary toilet used in adults, but it is more often ineffective, secondary to the small airway size.[45,46]

Pathogenesis

The etiologic conditions associated with formation of a primary pulmonary abscess are not clearly identified in many cases. Associated events include aspiration of gastric contents, operations involving the upper respiratory tract, foreign body aspiration, or prolonged unconsciousness.[47,48] In addition, formation of a lung abscess may be associated with a preceding necrotizing pneumonia characterized by a significant degree of necrosis.[46] The resulting inflammation leads to the formation of a cavity surrounded by a thick fibrous wall.

As in adults, the development of a lung abscess in a child is the result of contamination with a mixed spectrum of both aerobic and anaerobic organisms. Specifically, one or more species of anaerobic oral bacteria, along with *Staphylococcus*, *Streptococcus*, or gram-negative enteric organisms, are recovered from culture of the airway and/or abscess fluid. The most commonly recovered organisms include *S. aureus*, *Streptococcus viridans*, group A hemolytic *Streptococcus*, *S. pneumoniae*, and *H. influenzae*. Less commonly encountered species include *Escherichia coli*, *Pseudomonas*, *Klebsiella*, *Peptococcus*, and *Peptostreptococcus*.

Clinical Presentation and Diagnosis

The presentation of a pediatric patient with a lung abscess is characterized by tachycardia, fever, malaise, pleuritic chest pain, and a productive, often foul-smelling cough. Underlying disorders may include an immunocompromised state, severe neurologic impairment, chronic lung disease, or poor oral hygiene. When a lung abscess is encountered in infants, underlying conditions such as congenital cystic adenomatoid malformation, bronchogenic cysts, or airway foreign bodies should be suspected. In older children, an intralobar pulmonary sequestration should be evaluated as a potential etiologic factor.

Most primary lung abscesses are located in the posterior segment of the right upper lobe and the superior segments of the right and left lower lobes. In contrast, secondary and/or recurrent collections may be found in multiple locations with no specific anatomic predilection. Chest radiographs are often nondiagnostic during the early phase of development but can go on to reveal striking abnormalities, including cavitary lesions with or without associated air-fluid levels. In a recent study, the etiologic organisms were identified in most cases of lung abscess (82%) despite prior use of antibiotics.[49] Immunocompromised children developing lung abscesses often grow fungal organisms and require more aggressive therapy.[46]

Therapy

As with any abscess, the therapeutic goal is centered on establishing adequate drainage. Unlike in the adult patient, however, the use of postural drainage in the treatment of lung abscesses in infants and children, along with coughing and chest physiotherapy, is less effective. This observation is thought to be due to smaller airways and less effective patient-driven pulmonary toilet (i.e., purposeful coughing and incentive spirometry). In addition, bronchoscopy, with direct catheter suction and irrigation of the cavity, has been recommended as a diagnostic and therapeutic modality, often producing excellent results.[42] In concert with these maneuvers, a prolonged course (2 to 3 weeks) of broad-spectrum antibiotics is also needed.

Bacterial organisms recovered from most cases of lung abscesses have been susceptible to penicillin, although antibiotic-resistant organisms are being found more frequently. Improved results can usually be achieved by a combination of ampicillin and metronidazole or clindamycin. Although the typical antibiotic regimen is administered intravenously throughout the hospital stay, completion of the prescribed course in an outpatient setting with oral antibiotics is often successful and has not been shown to result in an increased incidence of recurrent disease.

In patients who fail medical therapy, more invasive surgical intervention may be required. The procedure of choice for a solitary abscess located directly beneath the parietal pleura is pneumonostomy. Alternatively, thoracotomy and pulmonary resection may be required for abscesses that are more centrally located.[46,47] Patients with fungal isolates and immunocompromised patients generally require early and aggressive pulmonary resection.

Outcomes

As described previously, successful management of a lung abscess is based on adequate drainage in combination with long-term antibiotic therapy. Resolution of the infectious and inflammatory processes can be seen over a period of several weeks. Although unusual, recurrence of a lung abscess at the site of the primary lesion can occur if the underlying cause persists (e.g., poorly treated gastroesophageal reflux in a nonambulatory patient). The mortality associated with primary lung abscess in immunocompetent children is very low. Increased complications and less favorable outcomes are seen, however, in immunocompromised individuals and in the neonatal population.

CHYLOTHORAX

Chylothorax, defined as an abnormal collection of lymphatic fluid within the pleural space, is rare and may be encountered at any age. First described as a clinical entity by Asellius in the 17th century,[50] chylothorax typically occurs during infancy and childhood and is seen less often in adults.

Pathogenesis

Although the exact course of events responsible for the development of many chylous effusions remains uncertain, related pathophysiologic factors are often subcategorized as being traumatic or nontraumatic in origin. Potential traumatic events include a multitude of potential iatrogenic causes secondary to thoracic surgical procedures, penetrating thoracic injuries or crush wounds, and injuries related to the birth process (presumably secondary to hyperextension of the spine). Nontraumatic causes associated with chylous effusions include various congenital abnormalities (i.e., lymphangiomatosis), venous thrombosis (which also may be associated with traumatic causes), and mediastinal and thoracic infections or malignancies.

During the neonatal period, the development of a chylous effusion has been commonly referred to as spontaneous and/or congenital. Although presentation during this early period has been associated with various dysmorphic syndromes, most cases have no identifiable etiology. In these patients, it is presumed that the formation of a chylous effusion is the result of a structural defect involving the lymphatic vessels.[51,52] Although reports of nontraumatic chylous effusions in the postneonatal period have been reported, traumatic causes, as described earlier, are far more common. Injury to the main thoracic duct as well as to major tributaries has been reported as a result of both blunt and penetrating thoracic trauma, with an incidence of as high as 0.9% after cardiac surgery in children.[53]

Clinical Presentation and Diagnosis

Chylothorax typically presents as significant respiratory distress. However, it may be encountered as an incidental finding during routine prenatal ultrasonography or while obtaining a thoracic imaging study for other indications. In the case of postoperative chylothorax, a seemingly unremarkable postoperative effusion may rapidly increase once enteral nutrition is resumed, raising the suspicion of an injury to the thoracic duct and/or the network of intrathoracic lymphatic vessels. In addition to the obvious respiratory embarrassment that can occur as a result of the accumulation of significant volumes of fluid within the thoracic cavity, prolonged loss of chyle results in severe nutritional deficiencies, immunologic disturbances, and electrolyte derangement.

The diagnosis of chylothorax is established by using fluid analysis. The gross appearance is typically described as "milky," although straw-colored fluid is often encountered in patients who are not being fed. Chylothorax should be considered if the pleural fluid is noted to contain a total fat content greater than 400 mg/dL, triglycerides greater than 200 mg/dL, or a specific gravity greater than 1.012. In addition, Gram stain analysis demonstrates the presence of more than 90% lymphocytes and Sudan red staining may reveal the presence of chylomicrons.[54]

The term *pseudochylothorax* refers to the circumstance of a prolonged (i.e., several weeks) pleural effusion, which may have a milky appearance, and elevated triglyceride levels. In the patient with no obvious risk factors for true chylothorax, this entity may be differentiated by using lipoprotein electrophoresis.[55]

Therapy

Treatment of chylothorax has traditionally been nonoperative. As many as 80% of patients respond to conservative management.[54] Most treatment algorithms are based on adequate drainage of the pleural fluid in combination with attempted trials of dietary modifications. Although no strict guidelines exist, many authors recommend several attempts at draining chylous fluid using thoracentesis. With persistent reaccumulation, however, formal chest tube drainage is needed.

The use of medium-chain triglyceride (MCT)–based formulas, with a high protein content, leads to spontaneous resolution in some patients. The success of this management is thought to be the result of effectively reducing the amount of chyle produced while still providing adequate nutrition. This is the result of preferential absorption of MCT into the portal venous system rather than into the intestinal lymphatic network. The resultant reduction in chyle formation is thought to improve the likelihood of achieving spontaneous resolution. In cases in which this therapeutic approach fails, many physicians use complete cessation of enteral feeds along with the concurrent administration of total parenteral nutrition (TPN).

Because considerable volumes of pleural fluid can be lost daily (representing large amounts of protein and lymphocytes), vigorous efforts to replenish these losses, typically with albumin, are needed to avoid the development of severe nutritional and hemodynamic derangements. In addition to drainage of the pleural space in combination with dietary interventions and/or TPN, recent literature supports the use of somatostatin in the treatment of ongoing chylous effusions.[56,57] Although the exact mechanism of action is not understood, these reports cite the reduced need for surgical intervention, the potential for early return to enteral feeding, and shorter overall hospitalization with minimal side effects. Although the majority of such reports cite the use of somatostatin analogs in the treatment of postsurgical chylous effusions, recent experience, including that of the authors, suggests a potential role for its use in the case of spontaneous chylothorax as well.[57-59]

If nonoperative therapy fails to stop the lymphatic drainage, several surgical options are available. The ideal timing of such operative interventions remains unclear. Most authors advocate a trial of nonoperative therapy for only 5 to 14 days before considering surgical intervention.[54] The principles of operative intervention focus on attempts to ligate the thoracic duct or obliterate areas of leakage either directly (if visualized) or by pleurodesis.[60] Moreover, they are dictated by the nature of the chylothorax (i.e., traumatic or nontraumatic). Many of these patients are now managed with thoracoscopy. Right thoracoscopy with occlusion of the thoracic duct as it crosses the

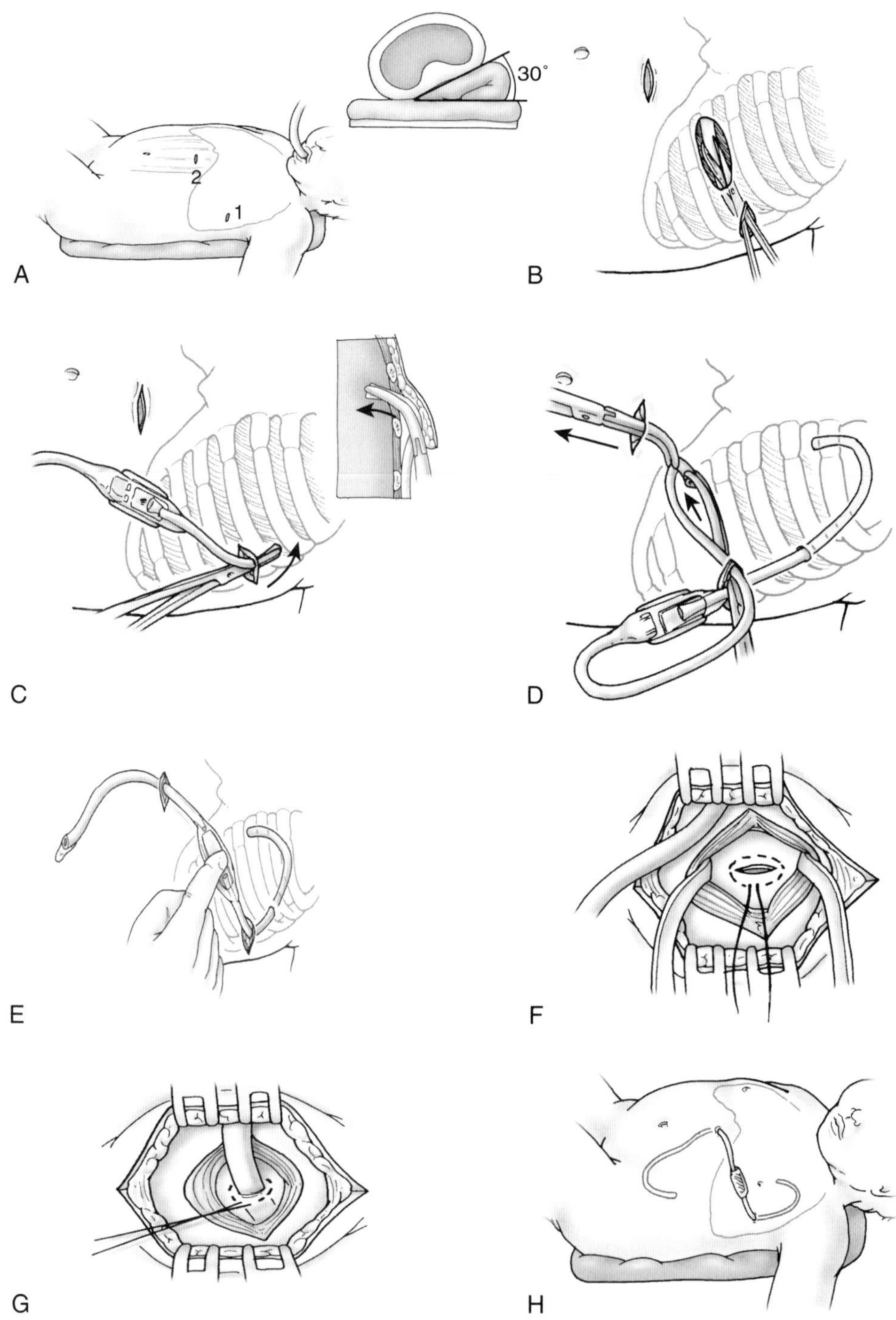

Figure 23-8. Insertion of pleuroperitoneal shunt. **A,** The affected hemithorax is elevated 30 degrees. The two incisions are planned to allow the pump chamber to rest on the costal margin. **B,** A small incision is made over the rib in the anterior axillary line, and a deep subcutaneous pocket is created inferiorly. **C,** Insertion of pleuroperitoneal shunt into the pleural space is done with a large curved clamp. The pleural catheter is tunneled 2 to 3 cm and bluntly passed through the intercostal space. The catheter must be carefully passed through the intercostal muscle at an angle to avoid kinking. **D,** A second small incision is made overlying the rectus muscle, and the peritoneal catheter is tunneled through this incision. The distal end of the shunt device is delivered to the second incision, as shown. The pumping chamber is drawn into the subcutaneous pocket by traction on the peritoneal catheter. **E,** The flow of chyle is confirmed before the distal catheter is inserted into the peritoneum. **F** and **G,** A purse-string suture is used to secure the peritoneal catheter at the level of the posterior rectus fascia. **H,** Both incisions should be closed with an absorbable suture, leaving a totally implanted system. (From Murphy M, Newman B, Rodgers B: Pleuroperitoneal shunts in the management of persistent chylothorax. Ann Thorac Surg 48:195-200, 1989.)

diaphragm has been shown to be a useful technique in patients with traumatic disruption of the thoracic duct after an operation.[61,62] Others have described direct suture of the area of chylous leak with the concurrent application of fibrin glue.[63] The use of a pleural-peritoneal shunt has been advocated as a less invasive technique to manage refractory chylothorax (Fig. 23-8). In these patients, pleural chyle is manually pumped into the peritoneal cavity where it is absorbed, presumably into the venous system.[64] These shunts are left for 3 to 4 months until the chylous leak seals. Recently, a technique of percutaneous injection of the cisterna chyli with platinum coil embolization of the thoracic duct has been utilized for adults with refractory chylous effusions. This technique has proven to be remarkably successful and probably would be applicable for use in adolescents but not infants. Cope has described a greater than 70% success rate with this technique in patients with high-output chylothorax in whom conservative therapy has not been successful.[65]

Outcomes

Because of the relatively small number of cases in the current literature, the natural course of childhood chylothorax and the exact success rate of nonsurgical therapy in the pediatric age group remain unclear. Despite this, however, most patients appear to be successfully treated with pleural drainage and a combination of dietary intervention and/or TPN and somatostatin. Most authors agree that a relatively short period of nonoperative therapy should be tried before an operation is considered.

TUBERCULOSIS

Tuberculosis (TB) is a virulent pulmonary infection caused by *Mycobacterium tuberculosis.* Primary pulmonary infection with atypical mycobacterial organisms is rare in children. After several decades of dramatic reduction in the frequency of pulmonary TB, particularly in the United States, a worldwide increase is now being seen. In 1993, the World Health Organization declared pulmonary tuberculosis "a global emergency."[66] In 1995, pulmonary TB caused more fatalities worldwide than any other infectious disease. It is currently estimated that about one third of the world's population is inoculated with TB.

The incidence of pulmonary TB in the United States has shown a progressive increase over the past 2 decades for a number of reasons, including immigration of individuals from countries with a high incidence of infection, increasing incidence of HIV infection, increasing intravenous drug abuse, and a general worsening of social conditions in many of the larger cities.[66] Children, particularly in the younger age groups, are at high risk, often living in close contact with infected adults. Pulmonary TB in young children is usually the primary form of the disease, whereas adolescents tend to have reinfection TB and lung cavitation.

Clinical Presentation and Diagnosis

The diagnosis of pulmonary tuberculosis in children can be quite difficult. The patient may remain asymptomatic throughout much of the early phase of the disease, and bacteriologic confirmation can be difficult. Adequate sputum collection in young children is difficult, and gastric washings demonstrate *M. tuberculosis* organisms in only about 30% of the cases. Primary diagnosis is highly dependent on abnormalities noted on chest radiographs and by surveying patients living in close contact with infected adults. Seventy-five to 90 percent of these patients will be noted to have pulmonary opacities due to parenchymal involvement that tend to be more heavily concentrated in the subpleural location.[67] Eighty-five to 90 percent of these children will be noted to have hilar or subcarinal lymphadenopathy on plain chest radiographs (Fig. 23-9).[68] Calcification of these nodes is rarely seen. Liberal use of CT scans may facilitate identification of these pathologic changes. Cavitary disease, so common in adult patients with pulmonary TB, is rarely seen in infected children in the first 5 years of life but becomes more common in adolescents, presumably from reinfection. Approximately 60% of adolescents with TB will be noted to have cavitary disease in one or the other of the upper lobes on a chest radiograph.[69] Bacterial confirmation of pulmonary TB also is easier in the adolescent. A suggestion of pulmonary TB on a chest radiograph should be supported by a skin test.

The incidence of pulmonary TB is greatest in patients with compromised immunity, such as bone marrow transplant patients, diabetics, and those with HIV infection.[70] Symptoms may be variable and radiologic changes more dramatic among the immunocompromised subpopulation. The mortality of HIV-infected patients with pulmonary TB approximates 70%.[71]

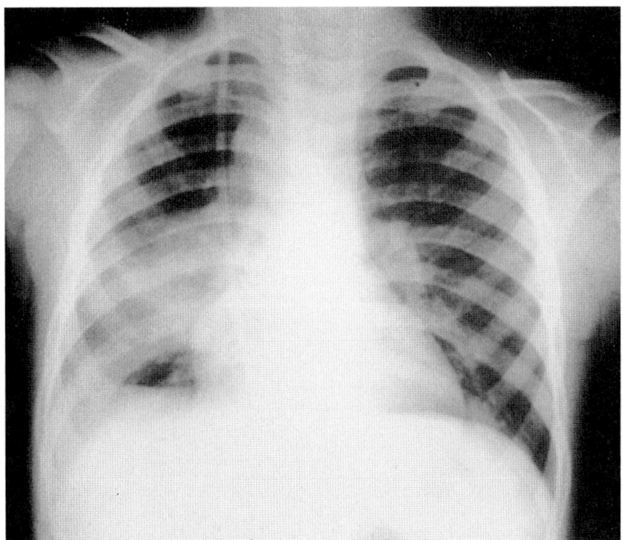

Figure 23-9. Chest radiograph of a 12-year-old girl with pulmonary tuberculosis demonstrates bilateral hilar infiltrates.

Therapy

First-line therapy for patients with pulmonary tuberculosis consists of multidrug antibiotic therapy. A 6-month course of isoniazid and rifampin forms the basis for most antibiotic regimens. This may be supplemented with 2 months of pyrazinamide. These drugs appear to have an acceptable toxicity spectrum in children. Isoniazid causes changes in liver enzymes in children much less commonly than in adults. In otherwise normal children who are compliant with this regimen, a 100% cure rate should be expected. Drug treatment should be initiated as soon as the diagnosis is confirmed because a delay in treatment has been linked to increased mortality.[71]

Surgery for pulmonary TB in children is generally indicated to treat complications and to reduce the bacillary load.[72,73] In younger patients, enlargement of hilar and subcarinal lymph nodes can cause bronchial obstruction with distal atelectasis. In these patients, in addition to adding a fourth antibiotic, usually streptomycin or ethambutol, a short course of prednisone (2 mg/kg/day) may be beneficial.[74] Serial chest CT scans can be used to monitor the progress of this disease and its response to therapy. These scans also identify those patients with endobronchial extension of the disease who may be helped by bronchoscopy. If corticosteroids and antibiotics fail to relieve the bronchial compression, these patients should have a thoracotomy/thoracoscopy with partial resection of the hilar and subcarinal nodes to relieve the airway compression.[74] Actual pulmonary resection should be avoided in these young children. Indications for surgical treatment in adolescents with cavitary disease include continued positive sputum cultures after 6 months of appropriate antibiotic therapy and massive hemoptysis. In all of these patients, operative management can be very challenging because of the degree of scarring from the chronic infection. Blood loss may be substantial.[75]

In the past decade, the emergence of antibiotic-resistant strains of *M. tuberculosis* organisms has become problematic. By definition, these organisms are resistant to isoniazid and rifampin, significantly limiting options for therapy. Currently, drug-resistant *M. tuberculosis* is the primary indication for TB surgery in the United States.[76] Although primary infection with drug-resistant organisms in young children has not yet been reported, such infection in adolescents has been encountered.

HISTOPLASMOSIS

The lung is the most commonly involved site of clinical infection from endemic fungal organisms in North America, which include *Histoplasma capsulatum, Blastomyces dermatitidis,* and *Coccidioides.*[77] Histoplasmosis, a thermal dimorphic fungus found in mold within the soil, has a nearly worldwide distribution, with endemic concentrations in the eastern half of the United States and a large proportion of Latin America.[77] The presence of a large concentration of bird and bat feces within the soil of these areas appears to be associated with endemic or hyperendemic rates of infection. Manipulation of this infected soil can result in airborne dissemination and infection of individuals with no other obvious source of exposure. Although outbreaks of histoplasmosis have been attributed to specific sources in the past, the fact that airborne spores can travel considerable distances is thought to be responsible for the majority of current cases having no obvious source of exposure.[78,79]

Pathogenesis

The majority of infections are mild or completely asymptomatic and associated with patchy infiltrates on chest radiographs. After being inhaled into the lungs, *H. capsulatum* spores germinate into yeast forms and result in an influx of macrophages, neutrophils, and T cells. T-cell immunity typically develops 10 to 14 days after the initial exposure and is responsible for the typically self-limiting process observed among immunocompetent individuals. Although primary infection and subsequent T-cell immunity does provide some degree of protection, reinfection and/or reactivation may occur.[77]

Clinical Presentation and Diagnosis

The incubation period ranges from 1 to 3 weeks and may result in an acute clinical infection. Alternatively, the patient may be completely asymptomatic. The majority of symptomatic patients have a "flu-like" illness consisting of general myalgia, malaise, a non-productive cough, headache, and fever. Progressive or diffuse disease is encountered in patients with some element of immune compromise. Chest radiographs during acute infection typically show diffuse, often bilateral, infiltrates. Cavitation and miliary processes may be observed as a result of chronic infection. As seen in Figures 23-10 and 23-11, hilar adenopathy may be observed in both acute and chronic disease states.

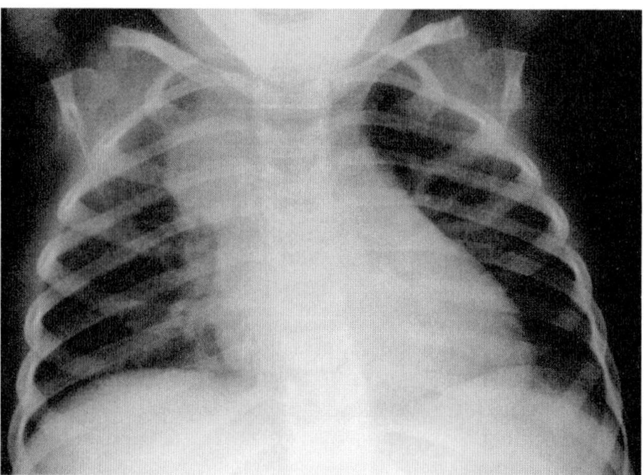

FIGURE 23-10. Chest radiograph of a child with histoplasmosis demonstrates hilar lymphadenopathy.

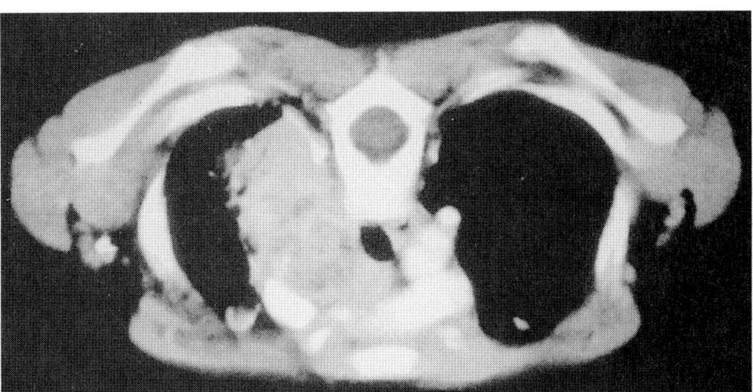

Figure 23-11. This CT scan of the chest demonstrates hilar lymphadenopathy secondary to pulmonary histoplasmosis.

Intraoperative specimens often appear to be firm and rubbery, making them grossly indistinguishable from lymphadenopathy secondary to other infectious and noninfectious causes. Less common manifestations include acute overwhelming pulmonary infections, fibrosing mediastinitis, pericarditis, and enlargement of mediastinal lymph nodes. These processes can result in dysphagia, pleuritic chest pain, airway obstruction, and superior vena caval syndrome. Surgical intervention in the cases of major vascular and airway obstruction is hazardous. It should be considered only in severe cases in which medical therapy has failed to improve the patient's condition.

Therapy

As previously mentioned, the majority of immunocompetent patients experience a self-limiting process and, therefore, require only supportive therapy. Treatment with antifungal agents is typically reserved for patients who have persistent symptoms (longer than 2 to 3 weeks) or demonstrate progressive disease based on serial radiologic examinations. Itraconazole has been used for treatment of mild persistent disease. Amphotericin B is strongly recommended for patients with more severe manifestations of histoplasmosis, followed by oral itraconazole or ketoconazole after achieving an adequate clinical response. Operative intervention may be required for constrictive pericarditis or to relieve obstructive airway and/or vascular complications from the disease process.

DIFFUSE INTERSTITIAL DISEASE

Chronic interstitial lung disease (ILD) may result from infectious as well as noninfectious processes (Table 23-3). It is characterized by restrictive lung physiology and abnormal gas exchange that produces considerable morbidity and mortality. The list of differential diagnoses to consider in the etiology of diffuse ILD comprises more than 100 separate conditions in both adults[80] and children.[81,82] The clinical disease patterns range from a chronic, slowly progressive picture in a relatively stable patient to one of acute pulmonary decompensation, requiring emergency lifesaving maneuvers. Sorting through the potential causes may delay treatment, and the ability to establish a specific diagnosis can be time consuming and difficult. It is not uncommon for pediatric surgeons to be involved in such cases to help establish the correct diagnosis with lung biopsy. Prompt diagnosis, especially in the case of immunocompromised or otherwise debilitated children, may require an urgent lung biopsy to guide further therapeutic interventions. The importance of such information cannot be overemphasized. In the case of an extremely unstable patient, the use of thoracoscopy and/or thoracotomy may be needed, even in the intensive care unit setting, to obtain the necessary tissue specimens. In addition, surgical intervention may be required to deal with respiratory failure. In severe cases of acute respiratory compromise, a pediatric surgeon may also be asked to insert the cannulas for extracorporeal membrane oxygenation. In addition, the need for long-term ventilatory and prolonged airway management may require the creation of a tracheostomy.

Table 23-3	Infectious and Noninfectious Processes Associated with the Development of Chronic Interstitial Lung Disease
Infectious	
Pneumocystis	
Cryptococcus	
Aspergillus	
Streptococcus	
Chlamydia	
Mycoplasma pneumoniae	
Rickettsia	
Adenovirus	
Parainfluenzavirus	
Respiratory syncytial virus	
Cytomegalovirus	
Varicella-zoster virus	
Herpes simplex virus	
Noninfectious	
Hypersensitivity pneumonitis	
Sarcoidosis	
Neoplasms	
Systemic lupus erythematosus	
Graft-vs.-host disease	
Radiation pneumonitis	
Adult respiratory distress syndrome	
Aspiration pneumonitis (gastroesophageal reflux disease)	
Chemotherapeutic agents	
Fat embolism	
Allergic alveolitis	
Pulmonary hemosiderosis	

Pathogenesis

Although the precise pathophysiology responsible for the development of ILD remains poorly understood, current evidence suggests that the processes responsible for its development are related to inflammation at the level of the interstitial and perialveolar tissues.

This common feature appears to explain the presence of similar histologic, radiologic, and clinical characteristics among a heterogeneous group of pulmonary disorders.[81] Histologic evidence suggests that the establishment and subsequent progression of the interstitial process involves injury to both epithelial and endothelial structures.[83] Furthermore, recent studies have focused on the potential of a genetic determination in ILD, hypothesizing the existence of an aberrant immunologic defect(s), which results in a failure of the normal immunomodulatory and mucociliary functions. This paradigm results in a predisposition for development of a pathologic interstitial pulmonary process.[84]

Clinical Presentation and Diagnosis

As discussed previously, the spectrum of ILD can be quite varied. Studies have attempted to correlate survival with associated symptoms and the physical examination. Determinants evaluated for correlation with survival include the patient's age, weight, duration of symptoms, presence of crackles on auscultation of the lung fields, clubbing of fingers, and severity-of-illness score (Table 23-4).[84]

The task of establishing the correct diagnosis relies on the combined results of several diagnostic modalities, such as radiologic studies, bronchoalveolar lavage, and lung biopsy. Although the use of plain chest radiographs can offer the ability to follow disease progression, chest films offer little specific diagnostic and/or prognostic information. One study of 39 adult patients with pulmonary fibrosis demonstrated a possible correlation between disease severity (as measured by standard pulmonary function testing) and high-resolution CT images.[85] Practical applications of such observations are less clear in the pediatric population.

The results of bronchoalveolar lavage are disappointing. In a prospective analysis of children with ILD undergoing bronchoalveolar lavage, a definitive primary diagnosis was made in only 5 (17%) of 29 patients. Although its use provided important information overall, its ability to determine the primary cause of diffuse ILD was limited.[86]

Several other invasive techniques have been outlined as useful for obtaining lung tissue in an effort to establish the diagnosis. These techniques are generally well tolerated and include percutaneous needle biopsy, transbronchial lung biopsy, open-lung biopsy, and thoracoscopy for biopsy. Although the use of lung biopsy has been considered the most definitive method for diagnosis, it has been found to be nondiagnostic in as many as 30% of patients.[86] In addition to the modalities described, more-focused diagnostic modalities such as radiologic evaluation for gastroesophageal reflux disease should always be considered in newly diagnosed cases because gastroesophageal reflux disease has been cited as an important contributory process that should not be overlooked in children.[87]

Table 23-4 Severity-of-Illness Score Correlates Degree of Illness with Overall Survival Rates among Patients with Diffuse Interstitial Lung Disease

Score	Severity of Illness
1	Asymptomatic
2	Symptomatic: room air oxygen saturation normal under all conditions
3	Symptomatic: room air oxygen saturation normal during resting but abnormal (<90%) with sleep or exercise
4	Symptomatic: abnormal resting room air oxygen saturation (<90%)
5	Symptomatic: pulmonary hypertension

Therapy

The therapy for chronic ILD is often challenging and necessitates a detailed and systematic review of all historic, physical, and environmental factors that may help lead to a specific diagnosis. Because pediatric ILD is relatively rare, controlled clinical studies addressing treatment algorithms do not presently exist. The paucity of reliable diagnostic guidelines often leaves the physician with little choice but to initiate a treatment regimen based on what appears to be the most likely diagnosis. Therapeutic interventions can range from simple expectant therapy for mild or self-limited cases to the initiation of complex rescue therapy requiring high-frequency oscillating ventilation and/or extracorporeal membrane oxygenation in the most severe cases. Pharmacologic therapy with various immunosuppressants, administered after confirming the absence of a responsible bacteriologic organism, also is a common practice. Corticosteroids are the most commonly used agents in noninfectious disease, followed by hydroxychloroquine. Less commonly used agents include chloroquine, cyclosporine, colchicines, and methotrexate.[86] In all cases, supportive measures in the form of nutritional and psychosocial support and environmental modification (i.e., avoiding identified irritants or allergens) are important elements in treatment.

Outcomes

The natural history of chronic ILD that is unresponsive to therapy appears to be progressive fibrosis and resultant failure of the normal gas exchange mechanisms. The morbidity and mortality as well as the long-term outcome associated with chronic ILD vary depending on the associated etiologic factors and existing comorbid conditions. Despite several attempts to identify reliable means with which to monitor the progression of the disease process and the clinical response to therapy, investigators have failed to offer a clear consensus regarding management and outcome issues.[87]

PNEUMATOCELE

Pneumatoceles are defined as thin-walled, air-filled, intraparenchymal pulmonary cysts and typically occur in association with underlying bacterial pneumonia or as a result of trauma. Although the formation of pneumatoceles is relatively infrequent and has been associated with a variety of underlying bacterial organisms, the majority appear to be the result of staphylococcal pneumonia.[88,89] Other pathogens that have been identified as being associated with pneumatocele formation include *Streptococcus, H. influenzae, Klebsiella, E. coli,* and *Pseudomonas.* In addition, pneumatoceles have been found in cases of pulmonary TB and measles.[90]

Pathogenesis

Although the exact pathologic mechanisms responsible for the formation of pneumatoceles are uncertain, the development of a severe inflammatory reaction and the subsequent destruction of the alveolar and interstitial architecture have been attributed to the release of bacterial exotoxins. The resulting air leak occasionally culminates in a phenomenon whereby continued accumulation within the thin-walled defect results in the formation of a tension pneumatocele. The development of a tension pneumatocele may potentially compress adjacent structures or rupture into the free pleural space, resulting in a tension pneumothorax. Additional complications associated with pneumatoceles include the establishment of secondary infections, empyema, and bronchopleural fistulas.[91]

Clinical Presentation and Diagnosis

The clinical presentation and symptoms seen in children with an identified pneumatocele are usually indistinguishable from those encountered in the case of bacterial pneumonia without associated pneumatoceles. The diagnosis of pneumatoceles is typically made by chest radiograph and/or CT scan. In addition, they have occasionally been confused with simple pulmonary cysts and congenital diaphragmatic hernias. Serial examination and the overall clinical course often help to differentiate pneumatoceles from other pathologic abnormalities.

Therapy

The majority of pneumatoceles appear to involute over time, requiring no specific therapy other than supportive care and appropriate antibiotic coverage. In the case of a rapidly enlarging and/or tension pneumatocele, resulting in respiratory compromise, urgent decompression may be required. In addition to closed-tube thoracostomy or cystostomy, percutaneous catheter drainage techniques, in combination with fluoroscopy and ultrasonography, have been reported to be an effective means of decompression in such patients.[92,93] Open drainage with decortication and oversewing of the cyst wall is rarely necessary.

Outcomes

The majority of pneumatoceles decrease in size and resolve over a period of several weeks to months, assuming that the underlying infectious cause is adequately treated. In uncomplicated cases, no residual pulmonary compromise or radiologic sequelae are likely.

chapter 24

CONGENITAL DIAPHRAGMATIC HERNIA AND EVENTRATION

KuoJen Tsao, MD • Kevin P. Lally, MD

The management and treatment of posterolateral congenital diaphragmatic hernia (CDH) remains a challenge for pediatric surgeons. Despite tremendous advances in prenatal diagnosis, surgical treatment, and neonatal critical care, CDH remains a significant cause of mortality and long-term disability. The clinical challenges lie in the broad spectrum of disease and the relative small volume of patients at individual institutions, resulting in a limited experience with the most severe CDH infants. Although some institutions have become leaders in the treatment, management, and research of CDH, the vast majority will treat fewer than 10 infants with CDH per year.[1] Thus, broad clinical experience is difficult to achieve.

In 1946, Gross reported the first successful repair of CDH in an infant younger than 24 hours old.[2] CDH was considered a surgical emergency, and immediate repair was the practice at that time, with excellent survival rates of greater than 90%.[3] Since then, it has become apparent that such survival rates only included infants who lived to have an operation and did not include those who died before birth or soon thereafter. Accounting for this "hidden mortality" of CDH,[4] actual survival may be closer to 50%.

Although surgical intervention is necessary to repair a CDH, the most recent advances have been in nonsurgical therapies. Lung-protective ventilator strategies, extracorporeal membrane oxygenation (ECMO), and preoperative stabilization before surgery have all led to a significant decrease in mortality. In addition, improved understanding of pulmonary hypoplasia and hypertension associated with CDH has led to innovative therapies.

EPIDEMIOLOGY

The incidence of CDH has been reported between 1 in 2000 to 5000 births.[5-7] In the United States, approximately 1000 infants are born with CDH with a prevalence of 2.4 per 10,000 live births.[8,9] The incidence in stillborn infants is less clear. An estimated one third of infants with CDH are stillborn and often have other associated congenital anomalies.[10] Presumed to have the most severe form of CDH, infants who die in utero contribute to the "hidden mortality" of the disorder.[11,12]

Isolated CDH infants are typically male with one third having a major congenital anomaly.[8] However, when stillbirths are included, females with CDH tend to be more prevalent than males.[5,13] Approximately 80% of CDHs are left sided. Bilateral defects are rare and are often associated with other major anomalies.[14] Although the exact cause remains unknown, mothers who are thin or underweight may have an increased risk of bearing an infant with CDH.[15]

GENETICS

Once thought to be only a sporadic isolated anomaly, it is becoming increasingly understood that genetics plays an important role in the development of CDH. A first-degree relative has an expected disease rate of approximately 2%.[16] Several structural chromosomal abnormalities including deletions, translocations, and trisomies have been identified.[17,18] Genetic abnormalities associated with CDH include both anomalies of chromosome number (Turner's syndrome; trisomies 13, 18, 21, 22, and 23) and conditions with specific chromosomal aberrations (i.e., 15q24-q26 deletions).[19] A gene distal to the 15q21 locus may be important for normal development of the diaphragm.[19,20] Several specific genes have been implicated in the development of CDH based on human and animal studies, including chick ovalbumin upstream promoter-transcription factor II (COUP-TFII), Wilms' tumor 1 gene (*WT1*), homolog of Drosophila slit 3 (*SLIT3*), and Friend of GATA2 (*FOG2*).[21]

CDH may present as an isolated defect or in association with other non–CDH-related anomalies. Several associated anomalies such as lung hypoplasia, intestinal malrotation, some cardiac malformations, and patent ductus arteriosus are considered to be sequelae of isolated CDH. Non–CDH-related defects involving the cardiovascular, central nervous, gastrointestinal, and genitourinary systems may be a consequence of an underlying field defect of unknown etiology. Non–hernia-related anomalies associated with CDH have been estimated to occur in 40% to 60% of cases.[22,23]

CDH has been associated with over 50 syndromes.[24] In some cases, the diaphragmatic malformation is the predominant defect as in Fryns and Donnai-Barrow syndromes, in which CDH occurs in a high proportion of these patients.[25,26] In other cases, diaphragmatic defects occur in a small percentage but are still greater than the general population as in Simpson-Golabi-Behmel and Beckwith-Wiedemann syndromes. The inheritance patterns for these syndromes include dominant and recessive as well as autosomal and X-linked varieties.[21] Identifying the patterns of non–hernia-related anomalies with CDH and recognizing genetic syndromes are vital in determining the prognosis, treatments, counseling, and outcomes for these infants and their families.[14,18] Other syndromic patterns have been described, including Brachmann-de Lange and Pallister-Killian syndromes.[27-29] If an antenatal diagnosis of CDH is made by fetal ultrasonography, amniocentesis with karyotype and chromosomal analysis is warranted.

ASSOCIATED ANOMALIES

The impact of associated anomalies with CDH on prognosis and outcome cannot be overstated. Ninety-five percent of stillborn infants with CDH have an associated major anomaly.[5] In addition, more than 60% of infants who do not survive the immediate neonatal period have associated anomalies.[30] Of those infants who survive preoperative stabilization and come to operative repair, less than 10% have additional anomalies.[30] Although the severity of pulmonary hypoplasia and hypertension are the major determinants of overall survival, infants with CDH with another major defect have a greater morbidity and mortality. The survival advantage for infants with isolated CDH is significant compared with those with associated non–hernia-related anomalies (43.7% vs. 7.1%).[22] Because of this dismal outcome, the emphasis on detailed and accurate prenatal diagnosis has influenced the management and treatment of CDH. Twenty percent of prenatally diagnosed CDH infants have a chromosomal anomaly, with 70% having an associated structural malformation. In contrast, only 35% of postnatally diagnosed CDH infants have an associated anomaly.[22]

Non–hernia-related anomalies have been associated with many different organ systems. Cardiac anomalies account for 63% of those identified.[31] Hypoplastic left ventricle with hypoplasia of the aortic arch is the most common cardiac anomaly. Often confused with hypoplastic left heart syndrome, this defect does not have the same impact as hypoplastic left heart syndrome but may exacerbate pulmonary hypertension, right-to-left shunting, and hemodynamic instability. In addition, other common cardiac defects include atrial septal defects, ventricular septal defects, and other outflow tract anomalies (transposition of the great vessels, tetralogy of Fallot, double-outlet right ventricle, and aortic coarctation).[30,32,33] In a review of 2636 infants with CDH, approximately 15% of infants had an associated cardiac defect.[34] After eliminating those lesions that were deemed hemodynamically insignificant (patent foramen ovale, atrial septal defects, patent ductus arteriosus), only 10.6% of the cohort had significant cardiac lesions in which overall survival was 41.1%, compared with the group with nonsignificant findings (70.2%). Defects within the tracheobronchial tree have been reported, including tracheal stenosis, trifurcated trachea, and tracheal bronchus.[35] Neural tube defects are the most common central nervous system anomaly.[36]

EMBRYOLOGY

Diaphragm Development

The embryologic development of the human diaphragm is a combination of complex, multicellular, multiple-tissue interactions that are poorly understood. Precursors to the diaphragm begin to form during the fourth week of gestation. Historically, the diaphragm has been thought to develop from the fusion of four embryonic components: anteriorly by the septum transversum, dorsolaterally by the pleuroperitoneal folds, dorsally by the crura of the esophageal mesentery, and posteriorly by the body wall mesoderm (Fig. 24-1).[37,38] As the embryo begins to develop, the septum transversum migrates dorsally and separates the pleuropericardial cavity from the peritoneal cavity. At this point there is still a communication between the pleural and peritoneal cavities but the pleural and pericardial cavities are separated. The septum transversum interacts with the pleuropericardial folds and mesodermal tissue surrounding the developing esophagus and other foregut structures, resulting in the formation of a primitive diaphragmatic structure known as the pleuroperitoneal fold (PPF). Bound by pericardial, pleural, and peritoneal folds, the paired PPFs separate the pleuropericardial and peritoneal cavities. Eventually, the septum transversum develops into the central tendon.[37-41] Phrenic axons and myogenic cells destined for neuromuscularization migrate to the PPF and form the mature diaphragm.[42]

However, the exact mechanism in which the diaphragm becomes muscularized remains poorly understood. As the PPF develops during the sixth week of gestation, the pleuroperitoneal membranes close concurrently and separate the pleural and abdominal cavities by the eighth week of gestation. Typically, the right side completes closure before the left. Historically, the primitive fetal diaphragm has been thought to become muscularized by the inner thoracic musculature as the diaphragm closes.[43] Some have suggested that the posthepatic mesenchymal tissue

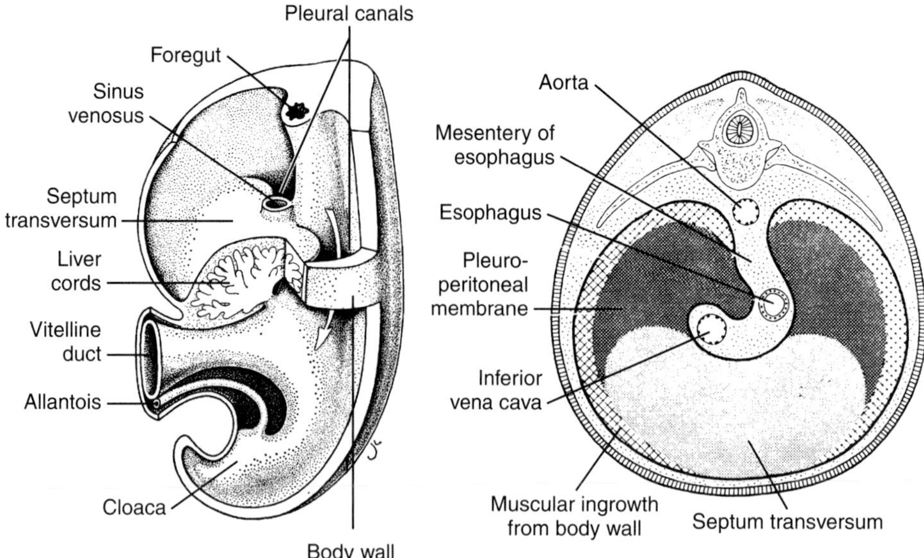

Figure 24-1. Historically, the diaphragm has been thought to develop from fusion of its four embryologic components. According to this theory, the septum transversum fuses posteriorly with the mediastinal mesenchyme. The pleuroperitoneal canals (*white arrow*) allow free communication between the pleural and peritoneal cavities. Closure of these canals is completed as the pleuroperitoneal membranes develop. The four embryologic components of the developing diaphragm are shown in cross section. (From Skandalakis IJ, Colborn GL, Skandalakis JE: In Nyhus LM, Baker RJ, Fischer JE [eds]: Mastery of Surgery, 3rd ed. Boston, Little, Brown, 1996.)

interacting with the PPF contributes to the diaphragmatic musculature development.[44] Others implicate a progressive development of the pleuroperitoneal membrane.[45]

An improved understanding of diaphragmatic muscularization has supported an alternative hypothesis for its embryogenesis. Inactivation of c-*met,* a tyrosine kinase receptor in mice, has demonstrated that the musculature of the diaphragm has a distinct origin other than the thoracic body wall.[46] C-*met* encodes for a receptor protein that is responsible for the delamination and migration of muscle cell precursors (MPCs) from somites.[47] The body wall theory of diaphragm muscularization is challenged by c-*met* null mutant mice that have an amuscular diaphragm and a normal body wall musculature. This hypothesis is further supported by the expression of *Lbx1* on diaphragmatic MPCs, a transcription factor only found on migrating MPCs and not seen on body wall myocytes.[48] Furthermore, immunologic staining of the diaphragm musculature revealed no MPCs from the body wall.[42] Thus, it appears that during the process of embryologic folding, a primitive diaphragmatic structure is formed, the PPF. Subsequently, the phrenic nerve and MPCs migrate from somatic origins, populate, and muscularize the newly formed PPF (Fig. 24-2). This process corresponds to week 10 of human gestation.

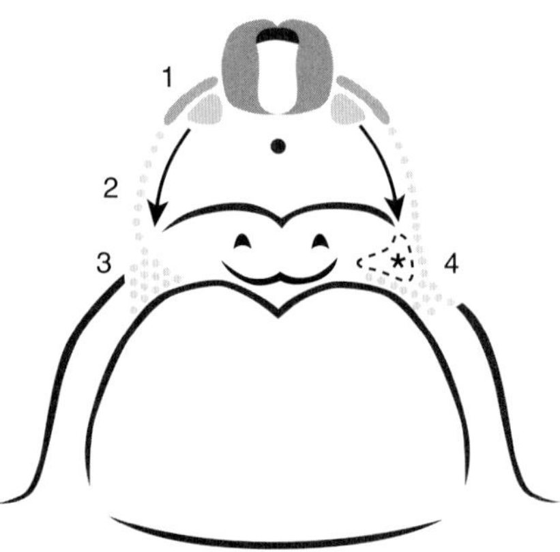

1. Muscle precursor cells delaminate from the lateral dermomyotomal lip.
2. Delaminated cells migrate through the lateral body wall.
3. MPCs arrive in the PPF, from which point they spread out to populate the growing diaphragm.
4. In CDH, the dorsolateral region of the PPF is missing (*) and MPCs are concentrated in the remaining tissue, ultimately leading to thickening of the diaphragm around the defect.

Figure 24-2. This schematic depicts a different embryologic pathway for diaphragmatic development and CDH formation than seen in Figure 24-1. On the left side (1-3) is the proposed normal pathway for diaphragm development. On the right side (4) is the pathway for CDH formation. MPC, muscle precursor cells; PPF, pleuroperitoneal fold. (From Clugston RD, Greer JJ: Diaphragm development and congenital diaphragmatic hernia. Semin Pediatr Surg 16:94-100, 2007.)

Lung Development

Fetal lung development is divided into five overlapping stages[49,50]:

1. The *embryonic stage* of lung development begins during the 3rd week of gestation as a diverticular formation of the caudal end of the laryngotracheal groove. The primary lung buds and trachea form from this diverticulum by the 4th week, and lobar structures are seen by the 6th week.
2. The *pseudoglandular stage* occurs between the 5th and 17th weeks of gestation with the formation of formal lung buds as well as the main and terminal bronchi.

3. The *canalicular stage* is highlighted by the development of pulmonary vessels, respiratory bronchioles, and alveolar ducts between weeks 16 and 25 of gestation. Type 1 pneumocytes begin to appear as well as the precursors for type 2 pneumocytes. At this stage, functional gas exchange is possible.
4. The *saccular stage* continues from 24 weeks' gestation to term with the maturation of alveolar sacs. Airway dimensions and surfactant synthesis capabilities continue to mature as well.
5. The *alveolar stage* begins right after birth with the appearance of mature alveoli. This stage extends well after birth with continued increase and development of functional alveoli.

Fetal pulmonary vascular development occurs in concordance with the associated lung development and follows the pattern of airway and alveolar maturation. A functional unit known as the acinus consists of the alveoli, alveolar ducts, and respiratory bronchioli. The pulmonary vasculature develops as these units multiply and evolve during the canalicular stage. The preacinar structure consists of the trachea, major bronchi, lobar bronchi, and terminal bronchioles. The pulmonary vascular development for the preacinus is typically completed by the end of the pseudoglandular stage.[51-53] In theory, any impedance to normal pulmonary development will concurrently hinder proper pulmonary vascular development.

Pulmonary development is recognized as a complex series of interlocking programmed events regulated by genetic signals, transcription factors, growth factors, and hormones. These events regulate the temporal and spatial interactions between epithelium and endothelium. Early transcription signals, such as thyroid transcription factor-1 and hepatocyte nuclear factor-3β, regulate pulmonary development from the primitive foregut mesenchyme. Other pathways of pulmonary development include Sonic hedgehog, transforming growth factor-β, Notch-delta pathway, and Wingless-Int.[21,54] In addition, glucocorticoids, thyroid hormone, and retinoic acid have all been shown to regulate pulmonary organogenesis.[55]

PATHOGENESIS

The development of CDH has been attributed to a defective fusion of the pleuroperitoneal membrane, to improper development of the PPF, or to a consequence of abnormal development of the posthepatic mesenchymal plate.[37,38,56] Others suggest that the muscular defect in CDH occurs before the complete closure of the canal as a result of abnormal formation of the diaphragm or PPFs.[39]

Traditionally, herniation of abdominal viscera through the diaphragmatic hernia was thought to impair lung development secondary to direct pulmonary compression resulting in pulmonary hypoplasia. Other evidence suggests that lung hypoplasia may occur early during embryogenesis before visceral herniation.[57-59] Still others have postulated a corollary theory that primary lung maldevelopment leads to the fetal diaphragmatic defect, although this is not widely accepted.[37] This latter theory has been refuted by the transgenic mice with the *Fgf10* gene.[60] Inactivated *Fgf10* null-mutant mice do not develop lung tissue but have normal diaphragms suggesting independent pathways to diaphragm and lung development. This phenomenon is also seen in humans where infants with lung agenesis have normal diaphragms.[61,62]

Pulmonary hypoplasia is characterized by a decrease in bronchial divisions, bronchioles, and alveoli. The alveoli and terminal saccules exhibit abnormal septations that impair the air-capillary interface and its ability for gas exchange.[57] At birth, the alveoli are thick walled with intra-alveolar septations. These immature alveoli have increased glycogen content leading to thickened secretions that further limit gas exchange. Animal models of CDH have demonstrated pulmonary hypoplasia with decreased levels of total lung DNA and total lung protein. In addition, the pulmonary vasculature appears to be less compliant with abnormally thick-walled arterioles.[63] Surfactant levels are also decreased that may result in immature functioning lungs.[64-66] Abnormalities in pulmonary development are not limited to the ipsilateral lung of the CDH. The contralateral lung also exhibits structural abnormalities of pulmonary hypoplasia. These sequelae are most profound in cases in which mediastinal shift leads to contralateral lung compression. This supports the theory that lung compression may be the major cause of pulmonary hypoplasia.

The understanding of abnormal pulmonary development in CDH has been widely aided by the nitrofen murine model.[67] Nitrofen (2,4-dichloro-phenyl-*p*-nitrophenyl ether) is an environmental teratogen that is relatively harmless to adult mice. However, if given during pregnancy, it can cause pulmonary, cardiac, skeletal, and diaphragmatic abnormalities.[68,69] Diaphragmatic defects resulting from the administration of nitrofen in mice are very similar to those seen in humans with regard to size, location, and herniation of abdominal viscera.[33,70,71] Depending on the time of exposure during gestation, resultant pups will develop either right or left CDH. In addition, the offspring will exhibit features of pulmonary hypoplasia, including reduced airway branching, surfactant deficiency, pulmonary vascular abnormalities, and respiratory failure at birth. These mutations are the result of many alterations in developmental pathways of embryonic mice.[55,72] The nitrofen model of CDH also suggests that not all of the pulmonary hypoplasia in CDH is due to lung compression. The effect of nitrofen in causing CDH is consistent with many theories that congenital anomalies are the result of environmental insults.

Other structurally similar teratogens to nitrofen have been shown to induce CDH in animal models. Bisdiamine (*N,N'-bis* [dichloroacetyl]-l,8-octamethylenediamine) is a spermatogenesis inhibitor. BPCA (4-biphenyl carboxylic acid) is a breakdown product of a thromboxane A_2 receptor antagonist. SB-210661 is a benzofuranyl urea derivative and 5-lipoxygenase inhibitor. All these agents cause similar diaphragmatic defects during the same embryologic periods in rodents. Although the exact etiology of CDH is unknown, all these compounds commonly affect the retinoic acid synthesis pathway by inhibiting retinol dehydrogenase-2 (RALDH2).[73] The direct correlation between nitrofen and the retinoic acid system is supported by studies using transgenic mice with a LacZ reporter linked to a retinoic acid response element (RARE). The expression of RARE is reduced with the administration of nitrofen.[74]

Although the etiology is not fully understood, an alternative hypothesis to traditional CDH formation has been suggested by the nitrofen model. The primary defect appears to affect only the development of the PPF.[39] In nitrofen-exposed fetuses, a defect is clearly seen in the posterolateral portions of the PPF.[75] This is further supported by observations of posterolateral-type CDH in vitamin A–deficient rats and mice with an inactivated *Wt1* gene.[75] In addition, nitrofen exposure does appear to affect muscularization of the PPF.[76] Studies in MPC migration and myoblast proliferation and differentiation suggest that muscularization continues and a thickened diaphragm is formed in the setting of an abnormal PPF (see Fig. 24-2).[42,76] This concept of abnormal PPF formation with intact muscularization as the primary etiology of CDH is in contrast to other theories that CDH is a result of failed closure of the pleuroperitoneal membranes or a defect in diaphragmatic muscularization.

Several clinical observations and molecular studies have supported the importance of the retinoic acid pathways in the development of CDH. Vitamin A–deficient rodents will produce offspring with CDH of variable severity.[77] Retinoic acid receptor knockout mice produce fetuses with CDH.[78] Lower plasma levels of retinoic acid and retinol binding protein have been found in infants with CDH compared with controls.[74] The conversion of retinoic acid to retinaldehyde has been prevented by inhibiting RALDH2 with nitrofen with the development of posterolateral diaphragmatic defects in rats.[73]

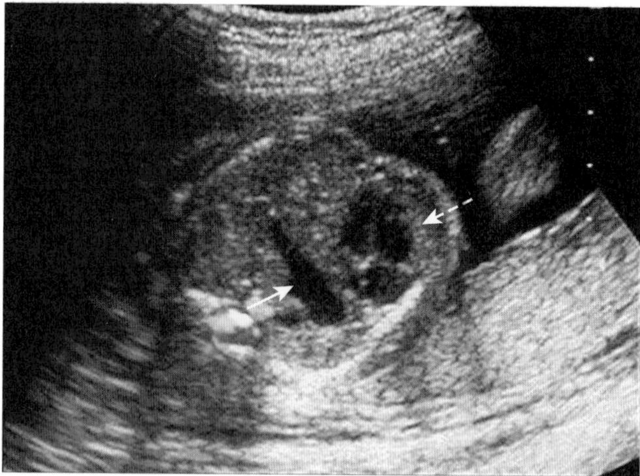

Figure 24-3. Fetal ultrasound image at the level of the four-chamber heart (*dotted arrow*). Gastric bubble (*solid arrow*) at the level of the four-chamber heart suggests CDH. This is the level used to calculate the lung-head ratio.

DIAGNOSIS

Prenatal Diagnosis

Owing to the wide discrepancy of disease severity and potential fetal therapies, accurate and timely prenatal diagnosis of CDH has become paramount. The diagnosis of CDH can be made by ultrasonography in 50% to 60% of pregnancies (Fig. 24-3).[44] Typically diagnosed at 24 weeks' gestation, CDH has been reported as early as 11 weeks' gestation.[79] In some tertiary medical centers, up to 93% of the neonates with CDH may have a prenatal diagnosis.[80] Fetal ultrasound findings include polyhydramnios, bowel loops within the chest, an echogenic chest mass, and an absent or intrathoracic gastric bubble. Severe or advanced CDH may exhibit intrathoracic "liver up," mediastinal shift, and hydrops fetalis.[81] Although most CDH can be detected during the second trimester, some sonographic features may not be exhibited until later in pregnancy.[82]

Independent sonographic features of CDH have not been shown to be accurate prognosticators for poor prognosis. However, two distinct features in combination have been utilized to risk stratify: (1) a low lung-to-head ratio (LHR) and (2) liver herniation into the chest. The LHR is calculated by the cross-sectional area of the contralateral lung at the level of the cardiac atria divided by the head circumference (see Fig. 24-2). Survival of CDH fetuses based on LHR has been statistically supported. In one series, there was 100% survival with LHR greater than 1.35, 61% with LHR between 1.35 and 0.6, and no survival with LHR less than 0.6.[83] Survival based on liver herniation alone is 56%, compared with 100% survival without liver herniation.[84] The combination of liver herniation and low LHR (LHR < 1.0) has a demonstrated 60% mortality for infants with prenatally diagnosed CDH.[85-87] Although fetal ultrasonography has been adopted as the most reliable prognostic test for CDH, its wide and inconsistent utilization has created variable results among centers. An LHR of 1.0 in one institution may be consistently different than the same results in another institution. Subsequently, LHR and liver herniation as prognosticators should be approached with some caution.[88]

Recently, fetal magnetic resonance imaging (MRI) of infants with CDH has been introduced as an adjunctive tool to evaluate fetal lung volume and liver location (Fig. 24-4). MRI-based fetal lung volume has been utilized in a manner similar to fetal ultrasonography. Several studies have touted the predictive value of fetal MRI in assessing risk. Lung volumes of CDH are calculated and compared with the predicted fetal lung volumes as a ratio. When the measured-to-expected fetal lung volumes ratio is less than 25%, there is a significant decrease in postnatal survival.[89] Fetal lung volumes predicting the need for ECMO or degree of severity are less precise.[90,91] Because of the nonstandardized approach to postnatal care for infants with CDH, conclusions regarding predictive outcomes using

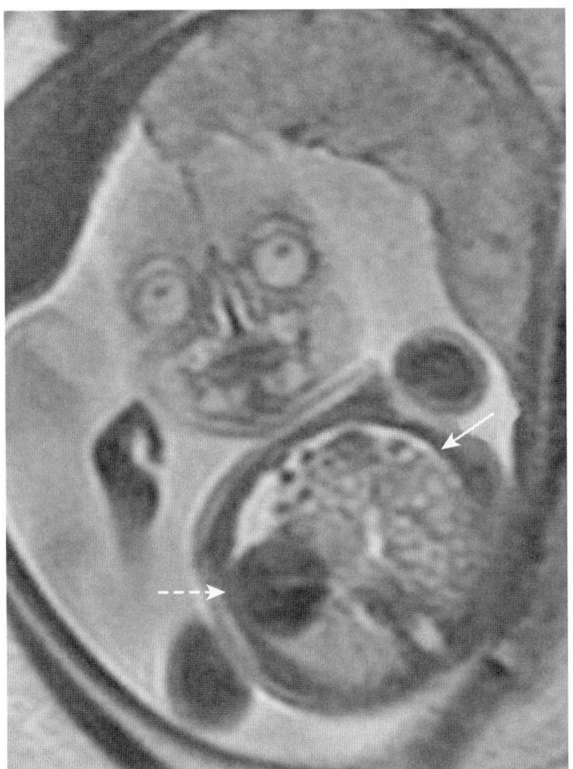

Figure 24-4. Fetal MR image of a left-sided CDH at 28 weeks' gestation. A large CDH with herniation of the small bowel and stomach is found within the left hemithorax (*solid arrow*). There is dextroposition of the fetal heart (*dotted arrow*). There is no evidence of liver herniation.

all prenatal imaging modalities should be used with caution. Nonetheless, prenatal assessment can clearly identify the most severe cases.

Prenatal diagnosis in early pregnancy provides an opportunity to optimize the prenatal and postnatal care of the fetus and mother by providing accurate prenatal counseling, discussion of possible fetal intervention, and/or termination of pregnancy. Although prenatal imaging provides valuable information, it does not consider the influences of postnatal care, especially in tertiary medical centers, on survival or overall outcome.

Clinical Presentation

Newborns with CDH typically present with respiratory distress. Clinical scenarios may range from immediate respiratory distress with associated low Apgar scores to an initial stable period and a delay in respiratory distress for 24 to 48 hours to late presentations that may occur years into life. Initial signs include tachypnea, chest wall retractions, grunting, cyanosis, and pallor. There may be clinical signs of ongoing fetal circulation and subsequent shunting. On physical examination, infants will often have a scaphoid abdomen and an increased chest diameter. The point of maximal cardiac impulse is often displaced (contralateral to the diaphragmatic defect), suggesting mediastinal shift. Bowel sounds may be auscultated within the chest cavity with a decrease in breath sounds bilaterally. Chest excursion may be low, suggesting a lower tidal volume.

The diagnosis of CDH is typically made by chest radiography demonstrating intestinal loops within the thorax (Fig. 24-5). The location of the gastric bubble should be determined with the placement of an orogastric tube. In rare circumstances, a contrast radiograph is necessary. The abdominal cavity may have minimal to no intestinal gas. Right-sided CDH may be more difficult to diagnose (Fig. 24-6). Salient features such as intestinal and gastric herniation may not occur. Rather, features of lobar compression may be the only radiographic sign and may be confused with congenital cystic adenomatoid malformations, pulmonary sequestrations, bronchopulmonary cysts, neurogenic cysts, or cystic teratomas.

Although most infants with CDH will be diagnosed within the first 24 hours, as many as 20% may present beyond the neonatal period.[92] These infants usually present with milder respiratory symptoms, chronic pulmonary infections, pleural effusions, pneumonias,

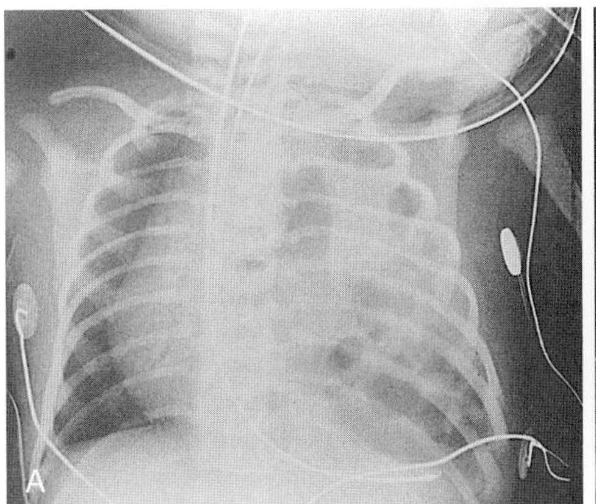

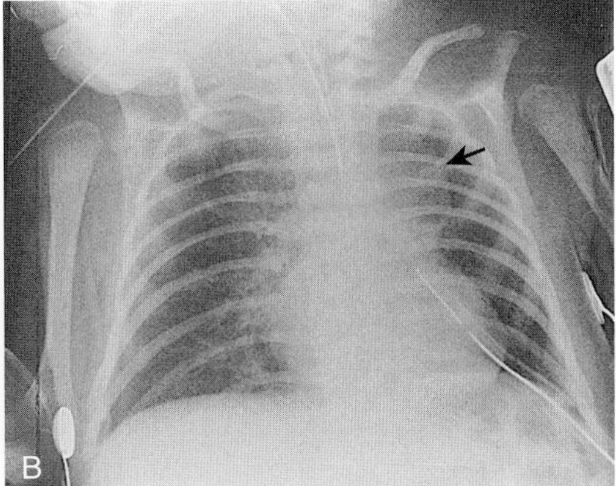

Figure 24-5. **A,** Anteroposterior chest radiograph in a neonate with a CDH demonstrating air-filled loops of bowel within the left chest. The heart and mediastinum are shifted to the right, and the hypoplastic left lung can be seen medially. **B,** Postoperative radiograph demonstrating hyperexpansion of the right lung with shift of the mediastinum to the left. The edge of the severely hypoplastic left lung is again easily visualized (*arrow*).

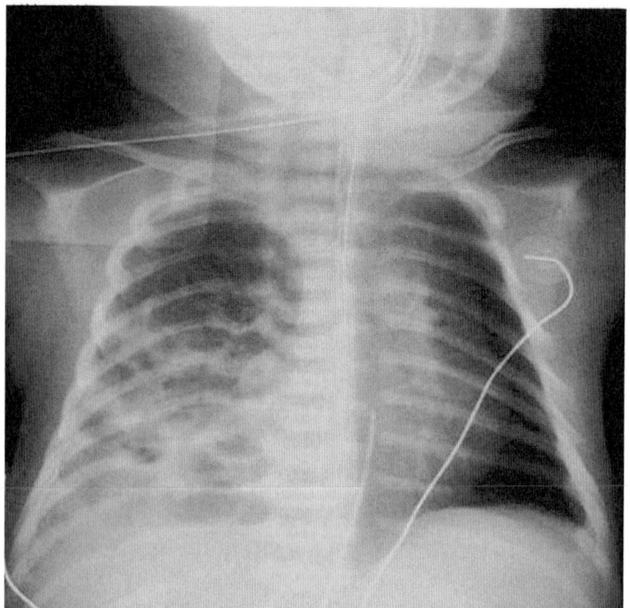

Figure 24-6. This infant presented with respiratory distress and a right CDH.

feeding intolerance, or gastric volvulus. Older children may present with symptoms of mediastinal compression due to acute gastric distention.[93] Because CDH invariably causes abnormal intestinal rotation and fixation, some children may present with intestinal obstruction or volvulus. Occasionally, CDH may be asymptomatic and discovered only incidentally.[67,94-97] Patients who present later in life have a much better prognosis due to milder or absent pulmonary hypoplasia and hypertension.

TREATMENT

Prenatal Care

The prenatal diagnosis of CDH has increased with the greater use of fetal ultrasound examinations. Advanced-level ultrasonography may be initiated after screening ultrasonography demonstrates discordant size and dates. A comprehensive sonographic evaluation should be made to diagnose associated anomalies (cardiovascular and neurologic) as well as signs of fetal compromise (i.e., hydrops fetalis). Once diagnosed, a karyotype should be obtained via amniocentesis or chorionic villus sampling. The mother and fetus should be referred to a tertiary perinatal center with advanced critical care capabilities such as ECMO, nitric oxide (NO) therapy, and oscillating ventilators.[98] A prenatal diagnosis of CDH allows the mother and family to be properly informed of treatment options and outcomes.

Some highly selective patients may be candidates for fetal intervention. Historically, open fetal repair of CDH was attempted but with dismal outcomes.[84] Based on clinical observations in infants with congenital tracheal atresia,[99] fetal intervention has shifted from direct repair of the diaphragm to lung expansion techniques. A fetoscopically placed endotracheal occlusive balloon for temporary tracheal occlusion has been introduced as a therapy for the most severe cases, LHR less than 1.0, and liver herniation.[100] However, the only National Institutes of Health (NIH)–sponsored, prospective, randomized trial comparing tracheal occlusion with conventional therapy did not demonstrate a survival or morbidity advantage with fetal intervention.[101] However, this study did suggest that a subgroup of the most severe patients (LHR < 0.9) may still benefit from tracheal occlusion. Thus, tracheal occlusion remains of great interest as potential fetal therapy but should only be performed in the setting of a clinical trial. Currently, there is no clinical evidence that supports temporary tracheal occlusion for the treatment of prenatally diagnosed CDH.

Resuscitation and Stabilization

After the confirmation of the diagnosis of CDH, initial postnatal therapy is targeted at resuscitation and stabilization of the infant in cardiopulmonary distress. Management should be targeted at the physiologic sequelae of pulmonary hypoplasia and hypertension. Immediately after delivery, a rapid overall assessment is necessary to determine hemodynamic stability and severity of disease. In severe cases, prompt endotracheal intubation is warranted without high-pressure bag ventilation to avoid gastric and intestinal distention. A nasogastric tube should be introduced along with placement of arterial and venous catheters to assist in resuscitative maneuvers. Acid-base balance and oxygenation-ventilation status should be carefully monitored.

Invasive monitoring with arterial and venous catheters is important for accurate assessment of overall perfusion of the infant and estimation of the significance of pulmonary hypertension and hypoplasia. Umbilical venous catheters may be used and should be placed across the liver into the right atrium to measure central venous pressures, but this may be difficult to achieve. In addition, oxygen content and/or saturation that reflects cerebral perfusion should be available from a preductal source by either a right radial arterial catheter or a transcutaneous saturation probe.

Initial mechanical ventilation should be utilized for stabilization. High airway pressures with a peak inspiratory pressure (PIP) greater than 25 cm H_2O should be avoided to prevent iatrogenic barotrauma. Positive-pressure ventilation should maintain the preductal arterial saturation (Sao_2) above 85% with a minimal amount of PIP. In order to maintain lower PIP, a moderate level of hypercarbia ($Paco_2$, 45 to 60 mm Hg) is accepted without a compensatory acidosis (pH > 7.2). Occasionally, higher levels of $Paco_2$ are tolerated.

Pulmonary hypertension and associated cardiac anomalies are evaluated with echocardiography. Clinically, pulmonary hypertension may be exhibited by differential preductal and postductal arterial saturations. However, echocardiography can better characterize the severity of disease and the degree of pulmonary hypertension. Sonographic findings of pulmonary hypertension include poor contractility of the right ventricle, flattening of the interventricular septum, enlarged right-sided heart chambers, and tricuspid valve regurgitation. There may be right-to-left or bidirectional shunting across the ductus arteriosus.

Preductal oxygen saturations less than 85% may impair adequate tissue perfusion. In general, a preductal $Pa{O_2}$ should be maintained above 60 mm Hg and a postductal $Pa{O_2}$ above 40 mm Hg. Failure to provide adequate tissue oxygenation may result in metabolic acidosis, which may exacerbate the pulmonary hypertension. Pulmonary vascular resistance is increased by hypoxia and acidosis, which all should be avoided or corrected. If severe ductal shunting develops, inhaled NO can be utilized, although pulmonary hypertension in association with CDH is less responsive than other causes of pulmonary hypertension. Despite its common utilization, NO as a rescue strategy in this setting has failed to demonstrate benefit in infants with CDH.[102,103]

Almost all infants with CDH and severe pulmonary hypertension will exhibit some left ventricular dysfunction. Vasopressor agents such as dopamine, dobutamine, and milrinone may be utilized in hemodynamically unstable patients. These inotropic agents may augment left ventricular output and increase systemic pressures to ameliorate the right-to-left ductal shunting.

Mechanical Ventilation

Mechanical ventilation is a critical component in the care of infants with respiratory failure secondary to CDH. The physiologic limits of the hypoplastic lung make mechanical ventilation a challenge. Hypoplastic lungs in CDH infants are characterized by a decreased number of airways and smaller airspaces. In conjunction, the pulmonary vasculature exhibits decreased vascular branching and increased adventitial and medial wall thickness.[104,105] This combination results in varying degrees of respiratory failure and pulmonary hypertension. Fortunately, pulmonary and vascular development continues after birth.[106,107] Because of this ongoing maturation, mechanical ventilation strategies have trended to less aggressive approaches with the goal of stabilizing ventilator therapy to maintain oxygenation while limiting the risks of ventilator-induced lung injury, a major contributor to mortality.[108]

The type of mechanical ventilator in infants with CDH is clinician preference, but most cases of CDH can be managed using a pressure-cycled mode. The initial fraction of inspired oxygen ($F{IO_2}$) of 1.0 is utilized to maintain adequate oxygen saturation. Typically, the utilization of higher rates and lower peak airway pressures (18 to 22 cm H_2O) while titrating the $F{IO_2}$ can maintain a preductal $Pa{O_2}$ greater than 60 mm Hg or better (a preductal $Sa{O_2} > 85\%$) and a $P{CO_2}$ less than 60 mm Hg. Maintaining an acceptable pH and $P{CO_2}$ is important in managing the pulmonary hypertension.[109,110] The ventilation strategy of induced respiratory alkalosis by hyperventilation to reduce ductal shunting has been abandoned by most centers.[111-114] Lung-protective ventilation strategies include pressure-limited ventilation rates between 30 and 60 breaths/min along with PIP less than 25 cm H_2O to minimize barotrauma.[111,115] Spontaneous respirations are maintained by avoiding neuromuscular paralysis and minimally set respiratory rates. This combination of spontaneous respiration and permissive hypercapnia has been a well-documented preoperative stabilization strategy with survival rates of almost 90% reported from some centers in patients with isolated CDH.[111-113]

If conventional ventilation fails to reverse hypercapnia and hypoxemia, high-frequency ventilation strategies may be employed. The role of high-frequency oscillatory ventilation (HFOV) in infants with CDH is based on its ability to avoid ventilatory-induced lung injury by preserving end-expiratory lung volume without overdistention. As the understanding of the CDH lungs continued to evolve, HFOV strategies also changed. Initially used in a high-pressure lung recruitment mode, this strategy demonstrated no benefit due to the nonrecruitable nature of the hypoplastic lungs.[116,117] High-frequency strategies as a rescue therapy for infants with profound hypoxia and refractory hypercapnia on conventional ventilators have been without much success.[118,119] As the concept of preoperative stabilization became better defined, HFOV began to be used as means to avoid barotrauma early in the treatment course before refractory respiratory failure, with some institutions using HFOV as primary therapy.[120-122] These strategies of preoperative stabilization regardless of ventilator modalities to prevent lung injury and delayed surgery have resulted in improved survival.[108,120-123]

To achieve lower peak airway pressures, HFOV should be maintained at a mean airway pressure less than 16 cm H_2O. HFOV should be considered when PIP exceeds 25 cm H_2O with conventional therapy. The $P{CO_2}$ should be maintained in the range of 40 to 55 mm Hg by adjusting the amplitude between 35 to 45 cm H_2O. Eight rib expansion of the contralateral hemithorax has been used as an initial guide to achieve optimal lung expansion without overdistention.[120,122] Tidal volumes are directly related to the amplitude and inversely related to frequency. Thus, significant increases in tidal volume can be seen when frequencies are below 10 Hz. This can result in hyperinflation, which in turn may adversely affect the pulmonary vasculature, including venous return. Constant assessment of acid-base status and end-organ perfusion is necessary as lung compliance changes, or as the CDH is repaired.

Surfactant

Several animal studies of CDH have shown altered surfactant levels and composition.[63,124-129] However, human data to support this have been controversial.[65] Experimentally, surfactant decreases pulmonary vascular resistance, improves pulmonary blood flow, and reduces ductal shunting.[130] In addition, surfactant administration has been shown to augment NO delivery and improve gas exchange.[131] These findings led clinicians to utilize exogenous surfactant empirically. However, clinical evidence in term and preterm infants with CDH has not shown benefit. In one study, it was suggested that surfactant therapy in term infants with CDH was associated with an increased use of ECMO, an increased incidence of chronic lung disease, and higher mortality.[128] Similar findings were found in preterm infants despite adjusting for Apgar scores and gestational age.[127] Even as a rescue therapy in CDH infants on ECMO, surfactant failed to demonstrate a survival advantage.[64,126] Despite the lack of proven efficacy, exogenous surfactant therapy continues to be used with unknown risk and unclear benefit. Proponents of this therapy argue that the clinical evidence is based on a heterogeneous population of disease severity and that failed therapy may be due to its use in the most severe CDH infants. Given the clinical data, surfactant therapy should only be used in a randomized, controlled fashion.

Nitric Oxide

Inhaled NO is a potent pulmonary vasodilator that has been shown to have tremendous benefit in the treatment of persistent pulmonary hypertension of the neonate (PPHN).[118,132-135] In clinical studies, NO improved oxygenation and decreased the need for ECMO in infants with respiratory failure secondary to PPHN.[135,136] However, the efficacy of NO for pulmonary hypertension secondary to CDH has not been as well supported. The need for ECMO or a reduction in mortality has not been shown with NO use in CDH infants.[137] In the Neonatal Inhaled Nitric Oxide Study Group trial, the CDH subgroup had a greater likelihood for ECMO or death.[102] The response to NO is variable and unpredictable in infants with CDH. Some may demonstrate a rebound pulmonary hypertension that is more difficult to control than the initial disease.[138] Furthermore, the effect appears to be transient and does not prevent progression toward ECMO use.[139,140] Thus, the role of inhaled NO has not been clearly defined and should not be routinely used. NO should be reserved for infants who persistently demonstrate suprasystemic pulmonary pressures in the setting of optimized pulmonary and cardiac function to reduce right ventricular pressures.[115,140]

Other pulmonary vasodilator agents have been utilized in the treatment of pulmonary hypertension in infants with CDH. Sildenafil is a 5-phosphodiesterase (5-PDE) inhibitor that has been utilized as a transitional medication to wean off NO for unresolving pulmonary hypertension. Widely used for PPHN and pulmonary hypertension secondary to congenital heart disease, sildenafil can be used in both oral or intravenous forms.[140,141] Epoprostenol (intravenous prostacyclin) and bosentan (a nonspecific endothelin-1 receptor inhibitor) have all been used in infants with CDH but the experience to date is limited.[142-144]

Extracorporeal Membrane Oxygenation

ECMO for infants with CDH was first introduced as a potential therapy for infants who likely had severe ventilator-associated lung injury.[145] Since then, ECMO strategies have evolved as understanding of CDH with its associated pulmonary hypoplasia and hypertension has improved. CDH accounts for approximately one fourth of all infants requiring ECMO for respiratory failure. Almost 30% of CDH infants will receive ECMO during their hospital course.[146-149] Prior to the era of preoperative stabilization, ECMO was associated with only a modest improvement in survival in high-risk CDH infants.[150-152]

Initially, strict criteria were established as indications for ECMO use in CDH. These included an oxygenation index greater than 40 and persistent alveolar-arterial gradient greater than 610 mm Hg.[148,153,154] Today, those criteria have been softened and the most common indication for ECMO is a "failure to respond" to therapy. In efforts to maintain lung-protective ventilation, clinicians have opted for ECMO rather than escalation of positive airway pressures. Relative contraindications include significant congenital anomalies, lethal chromosomal anomalies, intracranial hemorrhage, and gestational age less than 34 weeks. Ideally, ECMO candidates should have a birth weight greater than 2 kg owing to increased risk of intracranial hemorrhage, but some have reported benefit in infants weighing less than 2 kg.

ECMO was initially utilized as a postoperative rescue therapy, but its role has evolved.[155,156] In combination with other adjunctive modalities such as HFOV, ECMO is now routinely used as a component of preoperative stabilization. The strategy of stabilization with ECMO and delay in surgery has been shown to be beneficial, with a reported survival of 67% in high-risk patients.[10,157] These findings were further supported by the CDH study group that reported 85% of infants had ECMO before repair. Of those, 54% were repaired while still on ECMO and 29% repaired after ECMO with 16% never making it to repair. Infants who underwent repair while on ECMO had a 50% mortality, compared with 17% after ECMO.

The optimal timing of CDH repair is controversial and surgeon dependent. With more repairs of CDH on ECMO, bleeding became an increasingly recognized complication.[157,158] The introduction of aminocaproic acid, a fibrinolysis inhibitor, has significantly decreased bleeding complications.[147] Bleeding may also be reduced with early repair on ECMO before the development of coagulopathy and significant edema.[148] Some surgeons have recommended repair when pulmonary hypertension has resolved but prior to decannulation.[66] This allows reinstitution of ECMO if respiratory failure and/or pulmonary hypertension recurs. Others have requested that infants be decannulated and on conventional ventilation before repair. Although rare, recurrent pulmonary hypertension can occur after surgery, requiring a second run of ECMO.[159] Survival for second-run ECMO patients is approximately 50%.[160]

Today, ECMO is routinely used to stabilize patients before operation. Although results are dependent on patient selection and entry criteria, survival has been reported between 60% and 90%.[98,111,146,161,162] Without ECMO, the predicted mortality in the high-risk cohort reaches 80%.[146] Despite these data, ECMO for CDH is not universally accepted. Some authors report no survival advantage with ECMO.[163,164] Others cite an increased neurologic complication rate with ECMO use in CDH infants compared with other indications such as PPHN.[165,166] Some institutions report an 80% survival of infants with CDH without use of ECMO.[167,168] Nonetheless, in most centers ECMO remains a component in the armamentarium for treating CDH infants with refractory cardiopulmonary failure.

Surgery

The surgical approach to the repair of CDH has changed dramatically in the past 25 years. Historically, neonates with CDH were brought to the operating room almost immediately after birth to emergently relieve the compressed lung by reducing the intra-abdominal contents from the chest. Often, this maneuver was followed by a transient period of cardiopulmonary stability or improvement.[169,170] However, frequently, the infant would develop progressive respiratory failure, elevated pulmonary vascular pressures, right-to-left ductal shunting, unrecoverable hypoxemia, and eventually death. With improved understanding of the pathophysiology of CDH, repair of CDH is no longer considered a surgical emergency. Nonetheless, timing of the surgical repair of the diaphragm remains controversial.

The shift toward a delay in surgery after preoperative stabilization occurred after evidence was introduced that pulmonary compliance was actually worse after repair.[171] Several factors have been implicated, including increased intra-abdominal pressure and distortion of the repaired diaphragm. In addition, surgical repair has not been shown to improve gas exchange. Several studies have evaluated early versus delayed repair of CDH without demonstrating a difference in mortality or need for ECMO.[172-174] These include two randomized trials of early (<12 hours) versus delayed repair after 24 hours[174] and after 96 hours.[172] Since the adoption of the delayed repair strategy, several centers have reported improved survival rates.[111,174-177] Although modifications of surgical techniques and timing have contributed to this improvement, concomitant advances in neonatal critical care as well as a better understanding of the disease and outcomes have been the greater contributors to decreased mortality. Importantly, there has been no clinical evidence that specifically attributes a delay in surgery to improved outcomes over immediate repair.[178]

Timing of operation remains with clinical judgment and surgeon discretion. Some clinicians will opt for repair once the respiratory failure has stabilized (low peak airway pressures and inspired oxygen requirements) and after echocardiography demonstrates a resolution or stability of the pulmonary hypertension. This typically occurs 24 to 48 hours after clinical evidence of ductal shunting has resolved. Although CDH can be repaired on HFOV, most surgeons will wait until the infant is transitioned to a conventional mechanical ventilator.

The repair of a CDH may be as variable as the clinical management. A subcostal incision on the ipsilateral side of the hernia is the traditional approach. Less than 10% of surgeons prefer a thoracic approach.[179] The intra-abdominal contents should be reduced out of the thorax with careful attention to the spleen, which can be caught and torn on the rudimentary rim of diaphragm. A true hernia sac, which is only present less than 20% of the time, should be identified and excised.[180] The thoracic and abdominal cavities should be inspected for associated pulmonary sequestrations. The extent of the diaphragmatic hernia should be examined and assessed.

The type of repair is dependent on the size of the diaphragmatic defect. If the defect is small, a tension-free primary closure should be performed with nonabsorbable sutures with or without pledgets. If the defect is large, attempted primary closure may cause significant tension or flattening of the diaphragm, resulting in decreased pulmonary compliance. Alternatively, a diaphragmatic replacement may be employed to restore a tension-free, diaphragmatic shape (Fig. 24-7). Several types of prosthetic and biosynthetic patch materials have been utilized. Traditionally, a polytetrafluoroethylene (PTFE or Gore-Tex, W. L. Gore, Newark, DE) patch has been used.[179] With the use of a 1-mm thickness patch, the prosthesis is cut slightly larger than the diaphragmatic defect and is sewn to the residual diaphragm or surrounding tissue with nonabsorbable suture. The disadvantage of prosthetic material is the lack of material growth, resulting in a significant recurrence rate of nearly 50%.[181] To prevent this, the patch is tailored in a "cone shape" that may resemble the native diaphragm. This technique has demonstrated a reduction in recurrence rate from 26% to 9%.[182] Large defects with an adequate

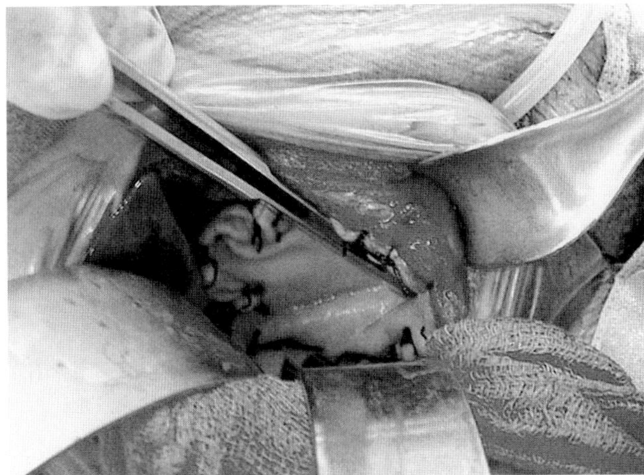

Figure 24-7. A large left posterolateral diaphragmatic hernia was approached through a subcostal incision. After reduction of the abdominal viscera, the large defect was closed using a biosynthetic patch (Alloderm).

posterior rim of diaphragm may require suturing the patch to the abdominal wall or encircling the ribs for adequate fixation.

Outcomes regarding the type of prosthetic patch material are mixed. Opponents of prosthetic patch material, such as PTFE, cite an unacceptable recurrence rate, chest wall deformity, and intra-abdominal complications, such as small bowel obstruction.[181,183-186] With a recurrence rate as high as 50%, alternative biosynthetic materials have been introduced to repair CDH. Currently, the most popular material is small intestine submucosa (Surgisis or SIS, Cook, Inc., Bloomington, IN) or human acellular dermal matrix (Alloderm, LifeCell, Branchburg, NJ). These bioactive patches may serve as a matrix for permanent tissue ingrowth.[187] Some institutions have adopted bioactive materials as the primary patch for repair of large diaphragmatic hernias. Proponents of biosynthetic patches claim the patch material is less adherent to small bowel and allows for tissue engraftment that grows with the patient. However, the largest series comparing SIS to Gore-Tex demonstrated similar recurrence rates and no difference in small bowel obstruction.[187] Long-term outcomes with biosynthetic patches for CDH remain to be seen. Certainly, the type of CDH patch material needs to be studied in a prospective fashion.

Recurrences after CDH repairs have prompted investigation into alternatives to prosthetic and biosynthetic materials. Some surgeons have utilized muscle flaps for primary and recurrence repairs. In small case series, an abdominal wall muscle flap using internal oblique and transversalis abdominal muscles has been described to cover very large primary or recurrent diaphragmatic defects.[188-191] Thoracic wall musculature has also been widely utilized. Latissimus dorsi and serratus anterior muscles have been described with isolated success.[33,188,192] Local advancement with a reversed latissimus dorsi flap with microneural anastomosis of the thoracodorsal nerve to the phrenic nerve has been described for recurrent herniations.[192] With this technique, the neodiaphragm was able to demonstrate nonparadoxical motion by fluoroscopy and ultrasonography. Muscle flaps may be advantageous in very large defects and in diaphragmatic agenesis.

Postoperative tube thoracostomy is not necessary and probably not indicated.[111,114] An exception may be CDH repair on ECMO because bleeding complications should be expected. The thoracic space will eventually fill with air and fluid, the lung will gradually grow, and the rib spaces may narrow to decrease the overall thoracic cavity. Tube thoracostomy is used only for postoperative chylothorax or accumulation of pleural fluid causing hemodynamic compromise.[193] If a chest tube is warranted, the tube is placed in the thoracic cavity before final closure of the diaphragm. Chest tubes should be placed to water seal rather than suction. Aggressive negative pressure can shift the mediastinum to the ipsilateral hemithorax creating overdistention of the contralateral lung. Symptomatic pleural fluid may be treated with repeated thoracentesis. If used, chest tubes should be removed early to avoid infection.

If the CDH is repaired via laparotomy, the abdominal domain may not be able to accommodate the reduction of the intestinal contents. Closure of the abdominal wall may result in an abdominal compartment syndrome. A "tight abdomen" may cause respiratory compromise in an already tenuous infant. Careful attention should be paid to the peak airway pressures as the abdominal fascia is closed. Respiratory compromise should prompt the abdomen to be left open. This scenario is more often seen with CDH infants on ECMO.[194] Temporary closure can be achieved with skin, prosthetic silo, or abdominoplasty.[195] Delayed closure, especially in those infants on ECMO, should be attempted after the general edema has resolved or the intra-abdominal domain has enlarged.[196]

Special operative considerations should be made for CDH infants on ECMO. In addition to the abdominal compartment issues, hemorrhagic complications are more likely due to the anticoagulation required for ECMO. Fibrin or thrombin sealants should be liberally used to reduce suture line hemorrhage. Aminocaproic acid should be given before operation and for 2 to 3 days postoperatively to prevent bleeding complications.

The therapeutic goals of postoperative ventilation should be similar to the preoperative goals, that is, to minimize barotrauma. Infants may experience a transient period of cardiopulmonary improvement that may allow clinicians to wean ventilatory support. However, rapid decreases in FIO_2 should be avoided to prevent triggering pulmonary vasospasm and recurrent pulmonary hypertension.

Advances in minimally invasive techniques have led to an increase in thoracoscopic and laparoscopic repairs of CDH (Fig. 24-8). Concerns regarding the minimally

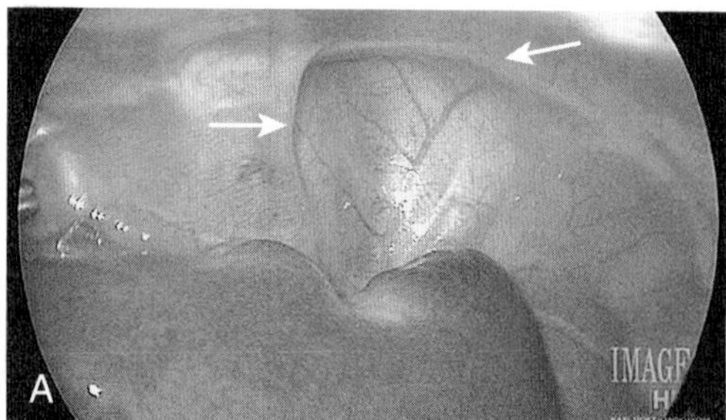

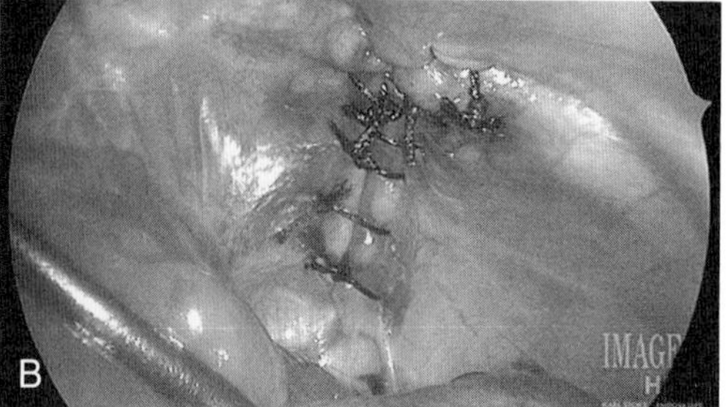

Figure 24-8. **A,** Laparoscopic view of a left-sided CDH in a 2-week-old with respiratory distress. The bowel and spleen have been reduced. The edges of the diaphragmatic defect are well seen (*arrows*). A very thin sac was present. **B,** The sac was removed and a primary closure was possible.

invasive approaches have centered around prolonged operations precipitating respiratory complications, triggering or exacerbating pulmonary hypertension, and resulting in an unnecessary increase in mortality. With careful patient selection, minimally invasive repairs have been successfully performed, both laparoscopically and thoracoscopically.[197-199] This approach has been utilized with primary repair as well as prosthetic patch closure of the CDH.[200] Laparoscopic and thoracoscopic operations are feasible without a demonstrable advantage to either. However, patient selection remains the main determinant of success. A preoperative patient selection criteria for thoracoscopic repair of CDH has been proposed.[199] Preoperative requirements included minimal ventilatory support (PIP < 24 mm Hg), no clinical or sonographic evidence of pulmonary hypertension, and an intra-abdominal stomach. In a small series of seven patients, results were similar to open CDH repairs. The long-term outcomes with minimally invasive approaches to CDH remain to be seen.

OUTCOMES

Clinical outcomes in regard to the treatment and management of infants with CDH have traditionally been difficult to interpret. Because the estimated incidence of CDH is low (1 in 2500 to 4000 live births), it has become evident that single institutions, regardless of their volume, would have difficulty in generating meaningful, evidence-based outcomes.[9,10] In addition, patient characteristics and clinical practices are very different and each institution's ability to offer state-of-the-art neonatal critical care is highly variable. Furthermore, data from a very heterogeneous disease population, such as CDH, are often pooled to generate single reports.

Congenital Diaphragmatic Hernia Registry (CDHR)

The Congenital Diaphragmatic Hernia Study Group (CDHSG) was established in 1995 as an international group of clinicians and researchers interested in developing a registry of all infants born with CDH. The CDHSG recognized the limitations of individual institutions in producing meaningful data on their own. As an observational database, the CDHR was created by a network of voluntary centers to ask specific clinical questions, recommend specific therapy as needed, and monitor outcomes of various management and treatment strategies. Since 1995, more than 90 centers from 10 countries have submitted data on more than 4000 infants with CDH. Participation among centers has varied, but currently there are over 50 active centers in the CDHSG with an average total submission of 340 infants per year.[1]

Data from the CDHR must be used with caution as with all outcome studies of CDH. There is a wide spectrum of patients within institutions and a wide spectrum of institutions within the CDHSG. Patients are only followed until hospital discharge or death. Thus, long-term follow-up outcomes are not available. Nonetheless, large international registries such as the CDHR offer some advantages. The CDHR is a vehicle to collect data from a large number of patients. The CDHR reflects changes in management and outcomes over time. Finally, individual institutions can compare their risk-adjusted outcomes to other institutions as a method of quality assurance.

Survival

As with all outcomes studies regarding CDH, survival analysis remains difficult to interpret due to the tremendous variations in patient disease, management strategies, and operative techniques. Unique to individual institutions are differences in ventilation strategies, availability and entry criteria for ECMO, and operative timing. One method to achieve better comparisons of outcomes is the development of risk stratification of patient disease. In 2001, the CDHSG published the first attempt at predicting outcome based on risk stratification.[201] The study examined 1054 infants with CDH by applying a risk assessment tool created by a logistical equation. Patients were categorized into low-, moderate-, and high-risk groups, which correlated with actual mortality. Overall survival was 64% in which birth weight and 5-minute Apgar scores had the strongest correlation. Survival rates for CDH among institutions are highly variable even when risk adjusted. Although the overall survival of liveborn infants has been reported around 60%, individual centers have varied from 25% to 83%.[9] This variation may be a reflection of the increasing prenatal diagnosis of CDH in which the most severe cases are transferred to tertiary care centers.

Pulmonary Outcomes

For many infants who survive the neonatal period with CDH, pulmonary function is excellent. Prior to the era of ECMO and lung-protective ventilation, long-term survivors were routinely reported as healthy children without respiratory disease.[53,202-204] However, with improved survival, more severe CDH infants are available for follow-up. Children with a history of CDH have demonstrated both functional and radiographic evidence of chronic lung disease.

Pulmonary function has been reported to be normal in 50% to 70% of CDH survivors.[53,202,205,206] The remainder exhibit some form of restrictive or obstructive respiratory symptoms. Approximately 25% of children beyond the age of 5 years have demonstrable signs of obstructive airway disease. One hundred consecutive CDH survivors were recently evaluated. ECMO and the need for patch repair were independent predictors of pulmonary outcome.[206] The use of ECMO significantly correlated with diuretic dependence at the time of discharge.[81] While only 16% required oxygen at discharge, 53% required at least transient usage of bronchodilators within the first year. Similarly, 41% were either dependent on or intermittently needing corticosteroids during the first year. Others have demonstrated similar pulmonary morbidities. In another study, chronic lung disease was found in 22% of surviving infants with CDH with a 2-year follow-up.[207] As with previous studies, ECMO and patch repair were the dominant factors of poor outcomes.

Respiratory infections appear to have a higher prevalence in children with CDH.[107,202,208-210] Viral bronchiolitis, such as respiratory syncytial virus (RSV), is the most common pathogen seen in children younger than 3 years of age, suggesting a need for RSV prophylaxis.[206] Recurrent pneumonias have been reported in 26% to 39% of CDH survivors with at least 10 years of follow-up.[107,209]

Obstructive pulmonary disease is commonly reported in children with CDH. Asthma and general symptoms of bronchospasm and wheezing are well documented.[155,210,211] Although the severity of these symptoms appear to improve with age, most children will still exhibit some combination of obstructive and restrictive pulmonary function and are more reactive to pharmacologic agents.[210-213] After correcting for lung size, lower functional volumes and not primary obstruction of the airways were the cause of abnormal pulmonary function tests in one study.[211]

Although lung development begins early in gestation, alveolar and pulmonary vascular maturation continue well after birth. In CDH, lung hypoplasia will affect both lungs with a reduction in airway and pulmonary artery divisions. As demonstrated in ventilation/perfusion ($\dot{V}/\dot{Q}$) radionuclide scans, pulmonary hypoplasia will persist despite continued lung growth.[211,212,214] $\dot{V}/\dot{Q}$ mismatches are predominantly due to abnormal lung perfusion. Follow-up $\dot{V}/\dot{Q}$ scans have demonstrated an increase in lung volume but not in lung perfusion. Because the pulmonary vasculature and alveoli grow concurrently, normalization or improvement in pulmonary function must be due to increased lung volume. This is further supported by increased alveolar size after neonatal repair of CDH.[215,216] Although $\dot{V}/\dot{Q}$ scans in children with CDH have provided valuable information, their predictive value for chronic lung disease in CDH survivors remains to be determined. In a review of 137 CDH infants, 61% had $\dot{V}/\dot{Q}$ mismatching at the time of their last scan. Patch repair and ECMO again had the strongest association, but definitive causation could not be established.[217]

Chest radiographs (CXR) are routinely abnormal and consistently demonstrate evidence of bronchopulmonary dysplasia.[202,206,213,218] Common features of chronic lung disease include hyperlucency, hyperinflation, persistent lung hypoplasia, decreased pulmonary vasculature, unknown opacities, persistent mediastinal shifts, and a chronic abnormal diaphragm position. In general, plain radiographs have no correlation with clinical symptoms in CDH with the exception of recurrent hernias. Approximately one third of CDH children will have an abnormal chest film.[213]

Neurologic Outcomes

As more infants with CDH are surviving, multidisciplinary follow-up has become as important as the in-hospital care. Although most patients may resolve their pulmonary or gastrointestinal issues, neurodevelopmental morbidities may be harder to detect. The lack of close follow-up and adequate simple tools to measure neurodevelopment may lead to undetected morbidity. Thus, close monitoring of neurodevelopment is imperative. Continued motor and language problems, even at 3 years of age, have been found.[219]

A significant percentage of CDH survivors will have neurodevelopmental sequelae, including developmental delay, motor and cognitive disabilities, and behavior disorder.[165,166,220-222] Several factors have been attributed to these outcomes, including ECMO use, disease severity with prolonged hypoxia, and prolonged hospitalizations. However, confounding evidence has made deciphering the root cause of neurodevelopmental sequelae from CDH difficult. In 1995, one study evaluated 82 CDH children at 1 year who had required ECMO use.[220] Developmental delay was significantly more prevalent when compared with children in whom ECMO was used for other indications. Another study demonstrated associated abnormal neuroimaging in children with neurodevelopmental delays in ECMO survivors of CDH.[165] However, other studies with large patient groups have not implicated ECMO. Stolar and colleagues reported on 51 ECMO survivors and concluded that ECMO was not a risk factor for neurologic deficits.[166] Another study found no differences in neurologic outcomes in 130 children who underwent ECMO for CDH compared with other diseases.[207] Other factors such as low socioeconomic status and prematurity have also been suggested as contributors.[166,221-223]

Sensorineural hearing loss (SNHL) is a common neurologic sequela of CDH. The prevalence of SNHL ranges from none in some series to 100% in others.[207,224] The etiology of SNHL remains difficult to decipher. SNHL is seen in patients with and without ECMO.[224-226] Several ototoxic medications are routinely used in the acute and chronic care of infants with CDH, such as diuretics, antibiotics, and muscle relaxants.[227] Even mechanical ventilation has been linked to SNHL.[228] Most likely, it is a combination of treatment and severity of disease. Stringent audiologic testing is warranted because SNHL may cause speech delays and further impair other aspects of neurodevelopment.

Gastrointestinal Outcomes

Gastroesophageal reflux disease (GERD) is a common gastrointestinal sequela of CDH. The cumulative incidence has been reported to be 40% of all CDH survivors. Approximately half require surgical intervention,[229] although individual centers have reported higher percentages.[230,231] The incidence among institutions is variable, depending on the mode of diagnosis: clinical symptoms, upper gastrointestinal contrast radiographs, pH monitoring, or impedance plethysmography. Although GERD can be self-limiting, several studies have reported long-term symptoms. One study reported that 63% of patients required GERD medications after 2 years.[232] Another report found a similar percentage (63%) in a long-term follow-up of 29 years.[231] A final study noted that 50% had symptomatic GERD after 1 year of age.[208]

Despite its high prevalence, the etiology of GERD in association with CDH is unclear. Certainly, anatomic changes with CDH may contribute to GERD. Esophageal ectasia may occur due to abnormal fetal development secondary to mediastinal shift, resulting in an abnormal lower esophageal sphincter.[233] The presence of an intrathoracic stomach due to herniation may cause the maldevelopment of the gastroesophageal junction.[234,235] The side of the CDH may cause a differential growth pattern and subsequent shortening of an intra-abdominal esophagus.[236] Distortion of the esophageal hiatus and increased intra-abdominal pressure from reduction of the viscera have also been implicated as postsurgical causes of GERD.[237] Owing to the frequency of symptomatic GERD, primary antireflux surgery has been recommended by some surgeons, especially for large defects.[207]

A significant number of CDH survivors demonstrate evidence of failure to thrive.[230,238] Many fall well below the 25th percentile in weight despite adequate caloric intake and aggressive feeding management (i.e., via gastrostomy). Symptomatic GERD may be a contributor, but an underestimation of the caloric needs may be the more significant reason. Survivors of CDH may have an increased metabolic demand due to chronic lung disease, resulting in increased respiratory work. These factors, in addition to oral aversion due to prolonged hospitalization, result in nutritional demands that may be underappreciated.

Gastrointestinal surgical issues are commonly seen in CDH children. Adhesive intestinal obstruction, intestinal ischemia, volvulus secondary to malrotation, and intestinal perforation are well documented. Intestinal obstruction occurs in up to 25% of patients.[229] Postoperative adhesions due to repair of the diaphragm or antireflux surgery have been reported, with the use of prosthetic patch material as a significant factor.[186] Other causes include malrotation, intestinal dysmotility, and recurrent hernia with incarceration. Recurrent CDH occurs in approximately 50% of patients within 3 years and is most commonly associated with a large defect size and subsequent use of prosthetic patch material.[225] Patients who underwent ECMO appear to have the highest risk of recurrence.[239] This is most likely due to the patients having the most severe disease secondary to the largest defects with the subsequent need for prosthetic patch repair.

Musculoskeletal Outcomes

The relationship between musculoskeletal development and CDH is evidenced by the frequency of chest wall deformities seen in children with CDH. The estimated incidence is between 21% and 48%.[225,231] Pectus deformities, chest asymmetry, and scoliosis are the most common. Scoliosis may be severe and continue to progress until adulthood. Some authors have suggested that the reason for progression is due to tension on the diaphragm, thoracotomies without muscle-sparing techniques, or a small hemithorax due to hypoplastic lungs.[12,231] Most patients are asymptomatic and do not require surgical intervention.

Follow-up Guidelines

Critically ill infants with CDH often require prolonged and intensive therapies such as ECMO during hospitalization. These result in long-term sequelae that require medical attention after discharge. Pulmonary, neurologic, gastrointestinal, and musculoskeletal complications necessitate a multidisciplinary team of surgical, medical, and developmental specialists. In 2008, the Section on Surgery and Committee on Fetus and Newborn for the American Academy of Pediatrics established a series of guidelines for the follow-up care of infants with CDH.[240] These recommendations begin before discharge and extend through age 16 years. The guidelines include a formal follow-up plan to facilitate the early recognition of co-morbidities (Table 24-1).

NOVEL INTERVENTIONS

Even with advances in neonatal critical care, the treatment of infants with CDH remains a challenge to pediatric surgeons, neonatologists, and intensivists. Despite increased survival rates in the past 25 years, many infants with CDH die or develop debilitating morbidities. Thus, researchers continue to investigate novel therapies for infants with CDH.

Fetal Intervention

The impetus for fetal therapy for CDH coincided with the advances in prenatal diagnosis. Improvements in fetal ultrasonography revealed the true natural history of CDH and the hidden mortality during gestation and soon after birth. These poor outcomes prompted the researchers at the University of California, San Francisco, to explore fetal surgery for CDH. Subsequently, fetal CDH intervention evolved from open fetal surgery to the current state of endoscopic endoluminal tracheal occlusion.

The prerequisite for any fetal intervention is the ability to accurately diagnose CDH and predict severity of disease and survival. The most widely accepted prenatal sonographic prognosticators have been liver herniation and LHR, which have been discussed previously. Liver herniation and an LHR less than 1.0 are recognized as fetal characteristics that portend the poorest outcomes.[241]

After years of unfavorable outcomes with open fetal repair of CDH, prenatal intervention evolved to tracheal occlusion. Based on clinical observations that tracheal atresia causes pulmonary hyperplasia, novel animal experiments of lung distention, and an improved understanding of fetal lung growth, therapeutic tracheal occlusion was introduced as a treatment for pulmonary hypoplasia secondary to CDH.[99,242-244] Current techniques involve endoscopic placement of an occlusive balloon without

Table 24-1 Recommended Schedule of Follow-up for Infants with CDH

	Before Discharge	1-3 mo after Birth	4-6 mo after Birth	9-12 mo after Birth	15-18 mo after Birth	Annual through 16 yr
Weight, length, occipital-frontal circumference	X	X	X	X	X	X
Chest radiograph	X	If patched	If patched	If patched	If patched	If patched
Pulmonary function tests			If patched		If patched	If patched
Childhood immunizations	Per childhood guidelines	X	X	X	X	X
RSV prophylaxis	RSV season during first 2 years after birth (if evidence of chronic lung disease)	X	X	X	X	X
Echocardiogram and cardiology follow-up	X	If previously abnormal or if on supplemental oxygen	If previously abnormal or if on supplemental oxygen	If previously abnormal or if on supplemental oxygen	If previously abnormal or if on supplemental oxygen	If previously abnormal or if on supplemental oxygen
Head CT or MRI	If (1) abnormal finding on head ultrasound examination; (2) seizures/abnormal neurologic findings; or (3) ECMO or patch repair	As indicated	As indicated	As indicated	As indicated	As indicated
Hearing evaluation	Auditory brain-stem evoked response or otoacoustic emissions screen	X	X	X	X	Every 6 mo to age 3 yr, then annually to age 5 yr
Developmental screening evaluation	X	X	X	X		Annually to age 5 yr
Neurodevelopmental evaluation	X			X		Annually to age 5 yr
Oral aversion screening	X	X	If oral feeding problems	If oral feeding problems	If oral feeding problems	If oral feeding problems
Upper gastrointestinal study, pH probe, and/or gastric scintiscan	Consider for all patients	If symptoms	If symptoms	Consider for all patients	If symptoms	If symptoms
Esophagoscopy		If symptoms	If symptoms	If symptoms or if abnormal gastrointestinal evaluations	If symptoms	If symptoms
Scoliosis and chest wall deformity screening (physical examination, chest radiograph, and/or CT of the chest)				X		X

RSV, respiratory syncytial virus; ECMO, extracorporeal membrane oxygenation.
Adapted from Lally KP, Engle W: Post-discharge follow-up of infants with congenital diaphragmatic hernia. Pediatrics 121:627-632, 2008.

maternal laparotomy or general anesthesia.[245] Tracheal balloons are placed between 24 and 28 weeks' gestation and deflated at 34 weeks. This strategy of temporary tracheal occlusion is based on avoiding the need for an ex-utero intrapartum treatment (EXIT) procedure at delivery. In addition, prolonged tracheal occlusion has been demonstrated to differentiate type II pneumocytes into type I pneumocytes, resulting in surfactant deficiency and necessitating the need for balloon removal.[246-248]

An NIH-sponsored randomized trial comparing fetal tracheal occlusion versus standard postnatal care was reported in 2003.[101] After 24 cases (11 by tracheal occlusion), the study was terminated early due to comparable survival outcomes (77% by postnatal care, 73% by tracheal occlusion) during interim analysis. The hazard ratio for mortality associated with tracheal occlusion, as compared with conventional therapy, was 1.2 (95% confidence interval [CI]: 0.29 to 4.67). However, when stratified based on LHR, survival was significantly better for LHR greater than 0.9. In fact, the hazard ratio for death with tracheal occlusion was 0.13 (95% CI: 0.03 to 0.64). This study recognized the wide spectrum of disease based on LHR and speculated that the patients with the most severe disease may still benefit from tracheal occlusion. Despite these results from the randomized trial, tracheal occlusion continues to be investigated owing to the significant mortality of infants with LHR less than 1.0 and liver herniation.

The FETO (Fetoscopic Tracheal Occlusion) task group, a European perinatology organization, created a multicenter prospective observational study.[100] In an attempt to select a more severe subset based on data from the NIH trial, the study included fetuses with liver herniation and LHR less than 1.0. In the initial 21 patients (15 left-sided CDH and 6 right-sided CDH), the investigators reported a survival of 48% for tracheal occlusion compared with 8% in the non-occlusion group. In addition to the survival advantage, the study also demonstrated an improvement in perinatal complications such as prematurity and premature rupture of membranes. The latest series reported overall survival of 57% for tracheal occlusion with survival greater than 62% for LHR between 0.6 and 1.0.[241] Although impressive, these results warrant further investigation in that the survival for LHR of 0.8 to 0.9 (78%) was higher than survival for LHR greater than 1.0 treated postnatally (65%). Furthermore, study limitations have prevented the widespread adoption of tracheal occlusion based on the European data. Control cases were taken from multiple centers that could not provide a standardized postnatal approach or reflect recent advances in postnatal care.

Long-term outcome with morbidity has yet to be reported for tracheal occlusion. However, one study examined pulmonary function in 20 patients (9 with conventional therapy and 11 with tracheal occlusions) from the NIH-sponsored randomized trial.[249] Infants were evaluated during the first 24 hours of life, before and after operative repair, and before elective extubation. The study demonstrated slight improvements in respiratory compliance and alveolar-arterial oxygenation gradients in patients who had undergone tracheal occlusion. However, other long-term outcomes remain to be seen. Based on the only randomized clinical trial, there appears to be no significant benefit from tracheal occlusion for the treatment of CDH. Although proponents of fetal intervention suggest that a subgroup of the most severe patients (liver herniation and LHR < 0.9) may still benefit from fetal intervention, the true efficacy of fetal tracheal occlusion for these severely affected infants will require a prospective randomized trial before its universal acceptance.

Prenatal Glucocorticoids

The hypoplastic lungs of CDH infants are structurally and functionally immature. Biochemical markers for lung maturity demonstrate decreased total lung DNA, total lung protein, and desaturated phosphatidylcholine in addition to deficiency of surfactant.[63] In animal models of CDH, prenatal administration of glucocorticoids has demonstrated a reduction in alveolar septal thickness, increased DNA synthesis, and increased total lung protein production.[250,251] Thus, antenatal administration of glucocorticoids has been used to improve lung function.[252,253] Initial results from small patient studies seemed promising. However, a prospective randomized trial conducted by the CDHSG failed to demonstrate any benefit to antenatal corticosteroid therapy for CDH.[254] In the multicenter trial, mothers received three weekly administrations of prenatal betamethasone. The study, which included 32 patients (15 on placebo and 17 on steroids), failed to show a difference in overall survival benefit, length of mechanical ventilation, length of hospitalization, or need for supplemental oxygen at 30 days. The study compared its results with a large cohort from the CDHR with comparable outcomes.

ANTERIOR HERNIAS OF MORGAGNI

Anterior diaphragmatic hernias of Morgagni account for less than 2% of all congenital diaphragmatic hernias. The foramen of Morgagni hernia results from the failure of the crural and sternal portions of the diaphragm to fuse. This can occur on either side at the junction of the septum transversum and thoracic wall where the superior epigastric artery (internal mammary artery, intrathoracically) traverses the diaphragm. Approximately 90% of unilateral hernias occur on the right.[255] Only 7% occur bilaterally.[256] Operatively, these may communicate in the midline and appear as a very large anterior hernia. Typically, a hernia sac is present with herniation of omentum, small intestine, and/or large intestine but may also contain liver and spleen. Malrotation may also be found. The majority of children with Morgagni hernia are asymptomatic and thus are rarely diagnosed during the neonatal period. When these hernias become symptomatic, pulmonary symptoms are usually not

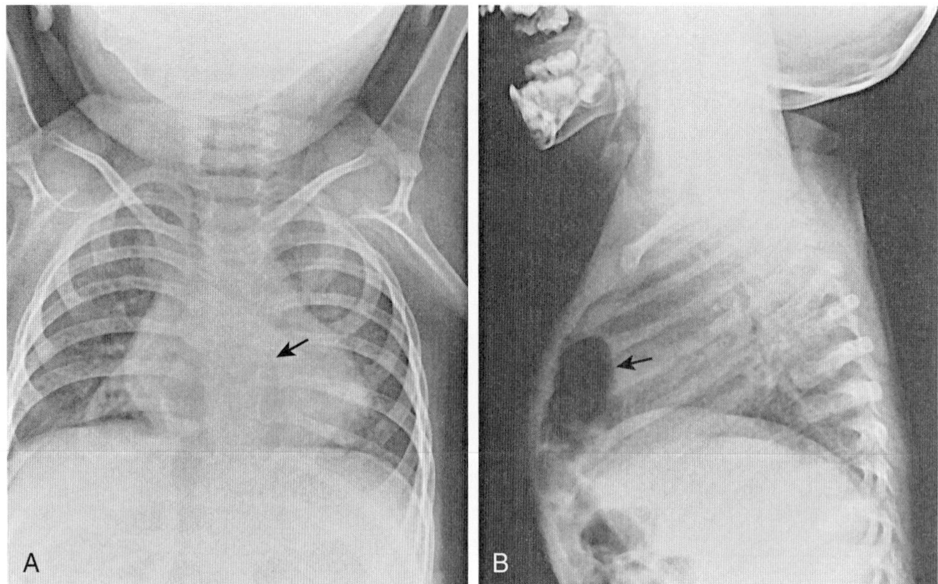

Figure 24-9. **A,** Chest radiograph in a neonate with a retrosternal hernia. Anteroposterior film demonstrates air-filled loops of bowel above the diaphragm and posterior to the sternum (*arrow*). **B,** Lateral projection confirms the retrosternal position of the herniated viscera (*arrow*).

the primary complaint. Children may have general epigastric discomfort such as vomiting and coughing due to intermittent obstruction.[255,257] Acute cases may present as intestinal ischemia with necrosis and perforation as well as gastric volvulus.[258,259] Herniation into the pericardium causing tamponade has been reported.[260]

Chest radiographs of Morgagni hernias may exhibit a well-defined air-fluid level in the midline of the chest. A lateral chest radiograph will demonstrate the hernia in the retrosternal space (Fig. 24-9). Small hernias may require a contrast radiograph or CT scan to confirm the diagnosis. Because of the risk of incarceration and strangulation, these hernias should be repaired relatively soon after diagnosis. Operative repair usually entails reduction of herniated viscera, excision of the hernia sac, and closure of the diaphragm to the posterior rectus sheath at the costal margin. Open procedures can be performed through an upper transabdominal incision. Laparoscopic techniques have been well documented (Fig. 24-10).[261,262] Although most defects can be repaired primarily, large defects may require patch repairs. The use of PTFE and biosynthetic (Surgisis, Cook Inc., Bloomington IN) patches has been described.[197,263] The long-term outcome regarding recurrence is yet to be defined.

An anterior diaphragmatic hernia may be found in association with a pentalogy of Cantrell due to a failure in the development of the septum transversum.[264] Pentalogy of Cantrell is a rare cluster of congenital anomalies that include omphalocele, cardiac defects, ectopic cordis, and an anterior diaphragmatic defect extending into the pericardium. The cardiac defect is the most severe problem and is the main cause of mortality.

DIAPHRAGMATIC EVENTRATION

Eventration is the abnormal elevation of the diaphragm resulting in a paradoxical motion during respiration that interferes with proper pulmonary mechanics and function.[265,266] Congenital eventration results from the incomplete development of the central tendon or muscular portion of the diaphragm. Most commonly left sided, bilateral congenital eventration has been reported.[267] The muscle is typically present but does not move in a coordinated fashion. The diaphragm is

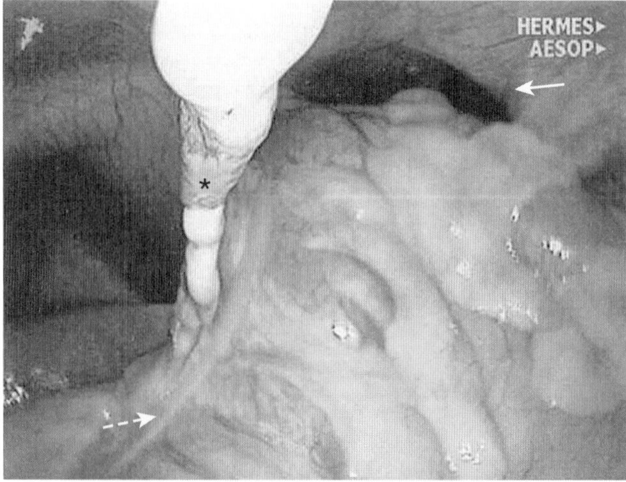

Figure 24-10. Laparoscopic view of a Morgagni hernia. This anterior hernia (*white arrow*) is to the left of the falciform ligament (*asterisk*) with a deep sac that was excised. The large bowel (*dotted arrow*) was reduced from the hernia defect, and the defect was closed with a biosynthetic patch. (From Holcomb GW III, Ostlie DJ, Miller KA: Laparoscopic patch repair of diaphragmatic hernias with Surgisis. J Pediatr Surg 40:e1-e5, 2005.)

thin, which may be indistinguishable from a hernia sac in CDH. Large eventrations may interfere with lung development due to the paradoxical motion, and the elevated diaphragm may decrease the thoracic space. Similar to CDH, congenital eventration can result in lung hypoplasia, although this is uncommon. Persistent fetal circulation and pulmonary hypertension are usually not seen with eventration. Diaphragmatic eventration may also be acquired due to paralysis of the phrenic nerve. This can occur secondary to mediastinal tumors, congenital heart surgery, or birth trauma. The incidence after congenital cardiac surgery has been reported to be approximately 5%, with the highest incidence after Fontan and Blalock-Taussig shunt procedures.[268,269]

Diaphragmatic eventration may be asymptomatic but typically presents acutely as respiratory distress and tachypnea in the newborn or more indolently with recurrent respiratory infections and wheezing. Neonates may have feeding intolerance due to discoordinated sucking and breathing. Older children may demonstrate exercise intolerance. Both lungs are usually affected by the paradoxical motion. On inspiration, the eventrated diaphragm rises, which causes the mediastinum to shift and compress the contralateral lung.

Eventration is typically suspected on a plain radiograph when an elevated hemidiaphragm is seen (Fig. 24-11). The diagnosis is subsequently confirmed by ultrasonography or fluoroscopy. Motion studies demonstrate a paradoxical movement of the diaphragm during respiration with a shift of the mediastinum.[270] Prenatal diagnosis of congenital eventration has been reported using fetal ultrasonography and MRI.[271,272] Occasionally, CT is required to distinguish eventration from pleural effusions, mediastinal tumors, bronchogenic cysts, and pulmonary sequestrations.

Small eventrations may be left untreated. Eventually, the child will overcome and compensate for the abnormal diaphragmatic dynamics. Initial treatment should include respiratory support, but mechanical ventilation is usually not necessary. However, larger defects that cause functional pulmonary impairment or promote recurrent infections should be repaired. Neonates with large eventrations benefit from early repair rather than a course of conservative treatment.[270,273] Acquired eventrations may require repair for the patient to be weaned from mechanical ventilation.

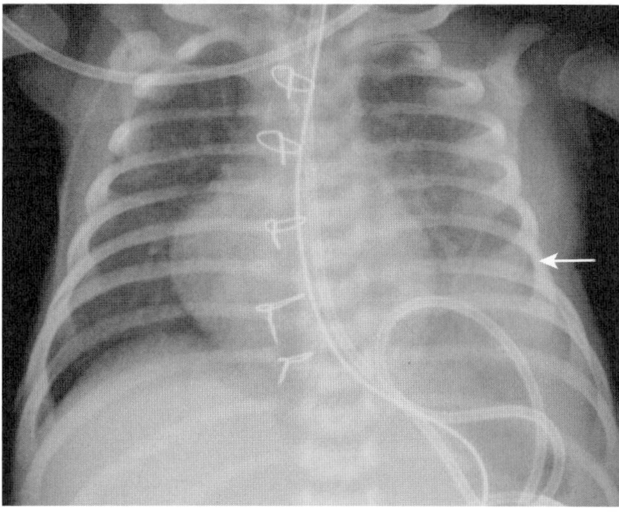

Figure 24-11. Anteroposterior chest radiograph of a 4-week-old male neonate demonstrates a left-sided diaphragmatic eventration (*arrow*) after repair of total anomalous pulmonary venous return. The abdominal viscera remain beneath an intact left hemidiaphragm.

Surgical repair can be accomplished through the chest or abdomen. The eventrated diaphragm is plicated with a series of nonabsorbable sutures. The sutures should imbricate generous amounts of the diaphragmatic tissue without injury to the phrenic nerve. Edges of the diaphragm should overlap until the plicated muscle is taut. Subsequently, the diaphragm becomes immobilized, resulting in an increased tidal volume and preventing mediastinal shift. Minimally invasive techniques have been well described using thoracoscopic and laparoscopic approaches.[274-276]

chapter 25

MEDIASTINAL TUMORS

Juan A. Tovar, MD, PhD

The mediastinum is the body compartment limited by the sternum, the spine, the diaphragm, and both lungs. For teaching purposes, it is divided into three parts: anterior, middle, and posterior (Fig. 25-1). The boundaries of the anterior mediastinum are the sternum anteriorly; the trachea, great vessels, and pericardium posteriorly; and the pleurae and the lungs laterally. This compartment contains the thymus, lymphoid structures, and nerves and vessels embedded into a mesenchymal and fatty environment. The middle mediastinum contains the trachea, main-stem bronchi, the heart and great vessels, as well as the hilar lymph nodes. The posterior mediastinum accommodates the aorta, the thoracic esophagus, and the sympathetic nerve chains.

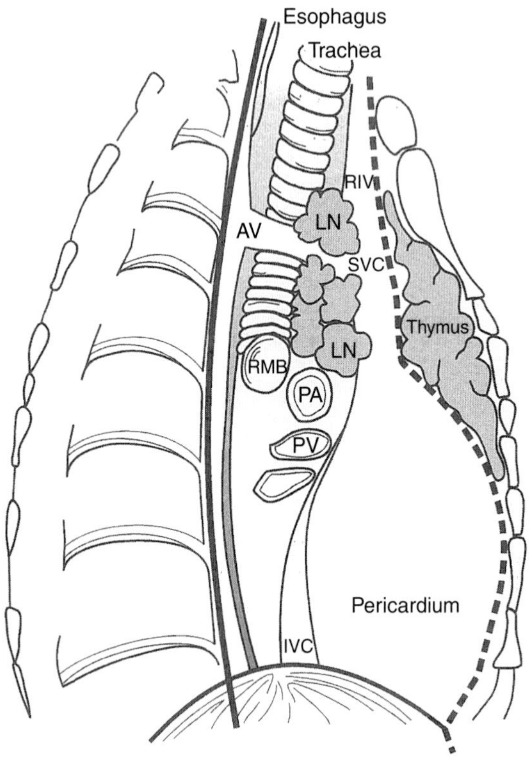

Developmentally, the foregut runs longitudinally in the middle of the embryonal mediastinum and differentiates to form the esophagus and trachea. The tracheobronchial tree and the lungs originate from a ventral bud from the foregut that subsequently grows and branches while interacting with the surrounding mesenchyme to produce the lungs. Neural crest cells migrate along the foregut axis to innervate the gastrointestinal tract and form the sympathetic chains. The anterior mediastinum is one of the regions through which embryonal germ cells migrate toward their final settlement in the gonads. The thymus is derived from paired primordia located in the third pharyngeal pouches that subsequently migrate into the anterior mediastinum where they fuse to form a single organ. All these events explain why tracheobronchial and esophageal malformations, neural crest and germ cell tumors, and thymic tumors and cysts are located in this compartment. Finally, the lymphaticovenous confluence and the vascular structures in the upper mediastinum account for the presence of some vascular tumors and malformations in this area. The most frequent location of the different mediastinal tumors is summarized in Table 25-1.

Figure 25-1. Anatomic division of the mediastinum: anterior compartment extends from the sternum to the *dotted line* anterior to the pericardium. Middle mediastinum extends posteriorly to the anterior border of the vertebrae (*solid line*). IVC, inferior vena cava; PV, pulmonary vein; PA, pulmonary artery; LN, lymph node; SVC, superior vena cava; AV, azygous vein; RMB, right main-stem bronchus; RIV, right internal jugular vein.

Table 25-1 Topographic Classification of Mediastinal Tumors in Children

Compartment	Benign	Malignant
Anterior	Teratoma Thymic hyperplasia Thymic cysts (rare)	Non-Hodgkin's lymphoma Hodgkin's lymphoma Thymic tumors (rare)
Middle	Lymphangioma Foregut cysts and duplications	Non-Hodgkin's lymphoma Hodgkin's lymphoma
Posterior	Ganglioneuroma	Neuroblastoma

CLINICAL FEATURES

Mediastinal tumors and cysts are occasionally diagnosed before birth and may even benefit from prenatal instrumentation.[1,2] Most mediastinal masses seen during infancy and childhood do not produce symptoms and are discovered with imaging performed for concurrent conditions. Respiratory embarrassment, orthopnea, stridor, wheezing, or even severe distress and/or superior vena cava syndrome are seen in some instances. Sternal bulging may appear in young infants with large anterior tumors. Recurrent laryngeal or phrenic nerve palsies or Horner syndrome may reveal the presence of the tumor when it involves the nerve trunks. Sudden paraplegia or paraparesia is occasionally observed in dumbbell-shaped tumors involving the spinal cord. Finally, secretion of catecholamines, α-fetoprotein, or gonadotropins may also uncover the tumor.

DIAGNOSTIC METHODS

Modern imaging allows accurate preoperative diagnosis in most cases. Plain radiographs of the thorax show widening of the superior mediastinal shadow or masses in either hemithorax. Ultrasonography may be useful as well.[3] Computed tomography (CT) helps to locate the tumor and to provide information about its cystic or solid nature, revealing calcifications, necrotic areas, and other details such as occasional widening of the spinal foramina in cases with intraspinal extension. Calcifications are suggestive of neuroblastoma or teratoma, but other tumors, such as lymphangiomas or some histiocytoses, may have calcified areas that should be taken into account upon diagnosis.[4-6] CT is also important for assessing the patency of the airway and the risks of anesthesia.[7] Magnetic resonance imaging (MRI) is used to better define the nature of the masses of vascular origin, but it may be very useful in other tumors as well, particularly for evaluating the intraspinal space.[8,9]

In some tumors, particularly those for which surgery is not the primary treatment, histology, cell markers, and molecular biology features must be ascertained before undertaking therapy. Cells can be obtained by biopsy of distant lymph nodes in the cervical or suprasternal notch areas, or by fine-needle aspiration (FNA) guided by ultrasonography or CT, or by pleural or pericardial fluid aspiration.[10-12] When this is not feasible, operative biopsy may be required. Thoracoscopy or anterior mini-thoracotomy through the bed of the second or third rib (the Chamberlain approach) may provide material for biopsy.[13-15] Mediastinoscopy is rarely needed in children.[16,17]

PRINCIPLES OF MANAGEMENT

It is vitally important for all involved in the care of a child with an anterior mediastinal mass to remember the possible respiratory collapse that may occur after induction and even before relaxation. Ventilation can be critically difficult, particularly in children with lymphoma in whom thorough preanesthetic assessment using CT sections of the upper chest and respiratory tests is necessary. The anesthetic risk is high if the cross-sectional surface of the tracheal lumen is decreased by 50% or more on the CT scan.[14] These patients also have marked reductions in the maximum expiratory flow rates, and special modalities of anesthesia (e.g., spontaneous ventilation, laryngeal mask, rigid tubes) may be required.[7]

Except for lymphomas that respond to chemotherapy and/or radiotherapy and in which surgery is usually adjuvant, all other mediastinal masses in children should be removed. Excision can be accomplished by median sternotomy, which is an excellent approach in terms of exposure and postoperative pain,[17] but thoracotomy on either side might be better depending on the anatomic extent of the mass. Thoracoscopy is an alternative in some cases, although it must be adapted to the principles of oncologic surgery and avoid spillage of tumor cells or fluids (particularly true for germ cell tumors).[17-19]

LYMPHOMA

Non-Hodgkin's Lymphoma

Non-Hodgkin's lymphoma (NHL) is one of the more frequent tumors of the mediastinum. It is a systemic disease in which there is massive proliferation of lymphoblasts in the lymph nodes. Lymphoblasts can ontogenically divide into B cells (related to tumoral immunity and produced in the bone marrow) and T cells (involved in cellular immunity that are processed in the thymus). In children, B cells cause undifferentiated Burkitt's or non-Burkitt's lymphomas, which constitute about 50% of all lymphomas. These lymphomas are found in the abdominal organs, whereas T cells cause lymphoblastic lymphomas (about 40% of all) and are generally located in the thymus and/or lymph nodes of the anterior mediastinum. Finally, the remaining 10% correspond to large cell lymphomas. These are similar to undifferentiated tumors but may be of T- or B-cell origin and appear on either side of the diaphragm.

Undifferentiated lymphomas express surface IgM and CD19 and CD20 antigens, whereas lymphoblastic lymphomas contain the enzyme TdT (terminal deoxynucleotidyl transferase) and express T-cell markers such as CD5 and CD7.[19] Burkitt-type lymphomas often have 8:14, and less often 8:22 or 2:8 translocations, involving the *MYCC* proto-oncogene, whereas T-cell lymphomas occasionally have 14q11 translocations.[20,21]

At the time of diagnosis, these tumors have usually spread beyond the original site and involve the regional nodes and distant organs such as the pleural or pericardial spaces or the bone marrow. (In this case, they are practically indistinguishable from acute lymphoblastic leukemia.) The liver and other abdominal organs and the central nervous system may occasionally be involved as well.

Rapid growth of mediastinal lymphomas may distort the airway, causing respiratory distress, wheezing, and orthopnea. The vena cava may be compressed, generating cervicofacial edema and jugular distention. Systemic symptoms are possible, and hematologic disturbances may appear when the bone marrow is invaded. Lymph nodes may be enlarged and palpable elsewhere, particularly in the neck, axillae, and supraclavicular or suprasternal regions.

Imaging depicts an enlargement of the mediastinum with or without involvement of the airway. Sometimes fluid can be seen in the pleural or pericardial spaces and obtained for cytologic analysis.[12,22] If neither peripheral lymph nodes nor fluids are available for biopsy or puncture, fine-needle aspiration under ultrasonography or CT is required for cytologic analysis. If this is still not diagnostic, biopsy by thoracoscopy or the anterior Chamberlain approach may be necessary. In both cases, the anesthetic risks and precautions should be emphasized.[23,24]

Staging of NHL takes into account the extent of the disease in terms of overall bulk of the tumoral tissue. The most used classification includes mediastinal cases as stage III except when the bone marrow and/or the central nervous system are involved (stage IV).[25] Standard imaging procedures and tissue and cell investigations allow proper staging, but other procedures such as gallium-67 isotopic scanning may be helpful as well.[26,27] The role of combined positron emission tomography (PET) and CT in children is still undefined.

Surgery is not a primary option in the treatment of mediastinal NHL because this disease responds well to chemotherapy and corticosteroids, limiting the contribution of the surgeon to providing adequate biopsy material for cytologic assessment. Chemotherapy based on acute lymphoblastic leukemia protocols leads to long-term survival in more than 80% of these children.[25,28]

Hodgkin's Lymphoma

Hodgkin's lymphoma is less frequent in this location and occurs more often in preadolescent and adolescent individuals. The main feature is the Reed-Sternberg cell, which is probably the malignant counterpart of the dendritic interdigitating cell that has a role in antigen presentation. These cells are embedded in lymph nodes in which the proportions of fibrous stroma, lymphocytes, and plasma cells are variable, allowing classification into the following types: lymphocyte predominant, lymphocyte depleted, mixed cellularity, and nodular sclerosis. Most children with Hodgkin's lymphoma have the nodular sclerosis type, but the youngest ones may have lymphocyte predominant or mixed cellularity varieties.[29]

Hodgkin's lymphoma originates in one group of lymph nodes but extends to contiguous or distant nodes after lymphatic pathways. Confirmation of the diagnosis and a detailed histology assessment require biopsies that are probably impossible from frozen section analysis alone. The extent of the disease determines the modality and the intensity of the treatment. Therefore, accurate staging is imperative before selection of the treatment protocol. The Ann Arbor classification of four stages with subgroups, according to the presence or absence of systemic symptoms, remains the most widely used system, but the mapping of the involved organs or lymph node groups requires refined imaging tools.

Hodgkin's lymphoma may be localized primarily in the anterior and middle mediastinum in children and may cause the same compressive effects as NHL (Fig. 25-2). Biopsies are sometimes possible from extrathoracic nodes. If not, the Chamberlain operation or thoracoscopy usually allow retrieval of enough tissue for diagnosis. The widespread preference for chemotherapy over radiotherapy in children, perhaps except in some adolescents, has limited the use of staging laparotomy. Staging laparotomy should be reserved for those cases with stage II thoracic involvement in which

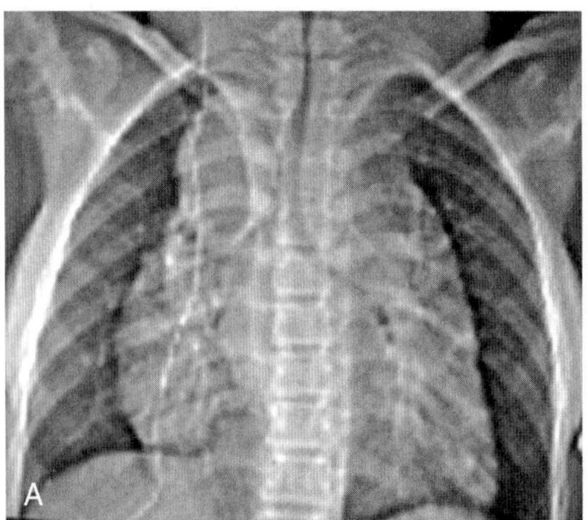

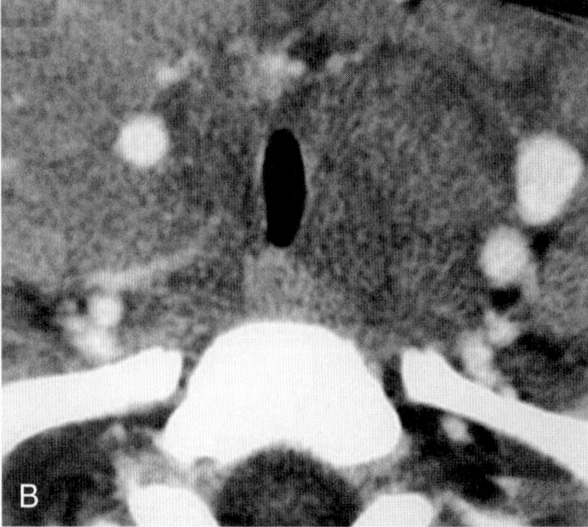

Figure 25-2. Imaging studies in an 11-year-old boy with Hodgkin's lymphoma. **A,** Widening of the mediastinum is accompanied by compression of the upper trachea that is seen on the chest radiograph. **B,** Transverse section on a CT scan of the upper mediastinum shows the extent of this tracheal compression by adenopathy that displaces the vessels laterally.

localized radiotherapy as the sole treatment requires excluding transdiaphragmatic involvement.[30] PET/CT seems promising as a noninvasive staging modality.[29]

Like NHL, surgery is not the primary treatment of Hodgkin's lymphoma, except in very localized cases. However, it may be occasionally performed in children in whom unusual imaging pictures, such as cystic spaces within the enlarged thymus, are suggestive of other diagnoses and lead to removal of the organ.[31]

GERM CELL TUMORS

The primitive germ cells may produce various types of tumors. Tumors from the gonadal germ cells (seminoma and dysgerminoma) and those of the totipotential cells may be either in the line of extraembryonic tissues (yolk sac tumors and choriocarcinoma) or in the line of embryonic tissues (teratomas). In fact, these different tissues can be found sometimes in the same tumor.

Teratomas

These tumors comprise only 8% to 16% of the tumors in this region at all ages and are uncommon in children.[32-35] They consist of solid or organoid masses containing tissues derived from all three blastodermic layers (ectoderm, endoderm, and mesoderm). Their histologic features are heterogeneous and may include cystic or solid areas as well as mature and immature components. Their incidence is higher in individuals with Klinefelter's syndrome.[36,37]

Mediastinal teratomas originate most often from the thymus or pericardium and are therefore located almost invariably in the anterior compartment of the mediastinum. They are as frequent in girls as in boys, in contrast to the situation in adults in whom there is a clear male predominance.[38-40] They develop relatively early in fetal life, and may cause hydrops and fetal demise.[2,41] These masses can be diagnosed prenatally. However, in most cases, they are detected after birth because of respiratory distress or later in life because of vague symptoms (thoracic or cervical pain, dyspnea) that are more frequent in children than in adults. The diagnosis is often an incidental finding from chest radiographs performed for other causes. Mediastinal teratomas should be suspected whenever a mass with or without calcifications is seen in the anterior mediastinal compartment. However, this diagnosis often is not made until the operation.

Most mediastinal teratomas are benign in children, but the prognosis is definitely worse if they contain elements of other germ cell tumors such as yolk sac, embryonal carcinoma, seminoma, germinoma, or choriocarcinoma.[35,37] Some of these lesions may induce precocious puberty or detectable pancreatic secretions.[37,42]

Surgical excision is the treatment of choice for mediastinal teratomas. Median sternotomy provides excellent exposure, but lateral thoracotomies may be preferred when the tumor extends into either hemithorax. Thoracoscopy has been described for removal of some benign mediastinal tumors.[43] Chemotherapy with carboplatin, bleomycin, and etoposide, which is very effective in malignant germ cell tumors, may allow secondary surgery after tumor shrinkage in cases that cannot be initially removed.[37] Although wide adherence to adjacent tissues usually makes a complete resection difficult, it is essential to avoid recurrence. In fact, these tumors have an excellent prognosis when resection is complete. α-Fetoprotein is a good tumor marker because it is usually elevated in malignant and immature tumors and very seldom in mature ones.[44]

Nonteratomatous Germ Cell Tumors

Very rarely, pure extraembryonal germ cell tumors (seminoma/dysgerminoma, embryonal carcinoma, yolk sac tumor, or choriocarcinoma) may appear in the anterior mediastinum. These are malignant and require complete removal and chemotherapy, as explained earlier for the malignant components of teratomas.[37,44]

TUMORS AND CYSTS OF THE THYMUS

During their migration, the thymic primordia leave behind thymopharyngeal ducts (not unlike the thyroglossal duct of the migrating thyroid gland) that progressively obliterate and disappear. Epithelial tumors and cysts are therefore possible in this organ along with lymphocytic and mesenchymal tumors.

Thymic Hyperplasia

The thymus plays an important role in the development of cellular immunity in infancy. Therefore, its size is larger at this age and regresses later in life. Sometimes real hyperplasia may suggest the development of a thymic mass. However, the absence of symptoms and clinical compromise of the mediastinal vessels as well as some radiologic features (e.g., the absence of compression of the airway or the "boat sail" shape of the inferior boundaries of the organ) rule out this suspicion. Treatment with corticosteroids is usually enough to make the enlarged thymus regress, and observation may be a better choice.

Thymic Cysts

Cysts derived from the thymopharyngeal ducts may appear in the anterior mediastinum and/or in the neck. They are lined by pharyngeal epithelium, which is often ciliated. They have secretory and thymic elements (Hassall's corpuscles) and may be inflamed or infected. When they reach a certain size, they are either palpable (in the neck) or detected on imaging of the mediastinum.[45,46] Also, they may cause respiratory symptoms by compression.[47] Thymic cysts can also be found in rare instances of malignant lymphoma and in patients with human immunodeficiency virus (HIV) infection in whom they can be multilocular.[31,48] These cysts require surgical excision through a cervical or transsternal approach.

Malignant Thymic Tumors

In contrast with adults, malignant neoplasia of the thymus is exceedingly rare in children. However, some instances of malignant thymoma without or with myasthenia gravis and thymic carcinoma have been reported.[33,49,50]

VASCULAR TUMORS AND ANOMALIES

Modern classifications of vascular anomalies and tumors have facilitated the understanding of their apparently unpredictable clinical course. It is currently accepted that the vascular tumors of congenital hemangioma with its two varieties (noninvoluting [NICH] and rapidly involuting [RICH]), hemangioma, kaposiform hemangioendothelioma, and the capillary, venous, arteriovenous, or lymphatic vascular malformations have very different clinical behaviors and require an individualized approach.[51] Although rare, these conditions may locate in the mediastinum where they may pose difficult therapeutic problems. Pathologic reviews of these mediastinal tumors at all ages illustrate the wide range of stable or regressive behavior.[52]

Vascular Tumors

Most hemangiomas located in the anterior mediastinum are in continuity with cervicofacial components. They may be asymptomatic or cause respiratory compromise when they extend into the airway. If they are asymptomatic, they should not be treated because they tend to regress over time. However, if airway compression is present, active anti-angiogenic treatment with corticosteroids and/or interferon-2α or vincristine must be promptly used. Interferon-2α has been found to cause severe neurologic complications.[51]

Kaposiform hemangioendothelioma is dangerous because when it is large, it may be accompanied by a Kasabach-Merritt syndrome in which there is massive platelet trapping with risks of hemorrhage. These tumors involve the thoracic wall and often the mediastinum. Full anti-angiogenic therapy together with close hematologic monitoring and eventually surgery are required. This tumor has a mortality rate close to 20%.[51]

Vascular Malformations

Venous and arteriovenous malformations are very rarely located in the mediastinum, and the vast majority are lymphangiomas. They may be located anywhere in the body but particularly near the confluences of large venous and lymphatic collections that are found in the mediastinum.[53,54] The tumor may extend into either hemithorax and eventually into the neck and the base of the mouth. Lymphangiomas are multicystic and infiltrate the anatomic structures (Fig. 25-3). Reaction to local infections may make the mass swell or even suppurate. Respiratory symptoms may arise in cases with airway compromise.[55] Modern imaging is very helpful for diagnosis, particularly MRI.

Mediastinal lymphangiomas do not tend to involute spontaneously. The treatment strategy must take into account that they are benign, that total removal is often impossible, and that a too radical operation may endanger nerve trunks or other structures.[56,57] Sclerosis with OK-432 or bleomycin is an alternative or a complement in cases in which incomplete removal has already reduced the volume of the tumor.[51] Only in cases of single, wide cysts is the result of sclerosing procedures generally satisfactory.[58] For masses with multiple infiltrating cysts of small size, partial debulking may be satisfactory to reduce symptoms.[56]

FOREGUT CYSTS AND DUPLICATIONS

Abnormal branching of the tracheobronchial anlage from the ventral face of the foregut may form closed spaces lined by either esophageal or bronchial mucosa. These cysts are located in the mediastinum in close contact with either the trachea and main-stem bronchi or the esophagus. The secreting mucosa progressively enlarges the cysts, which can then become symptomatic. In rare instances, the foregut malformation is more extensive and involves both the respiratory and digestive tracts and combine esophageal duplications with

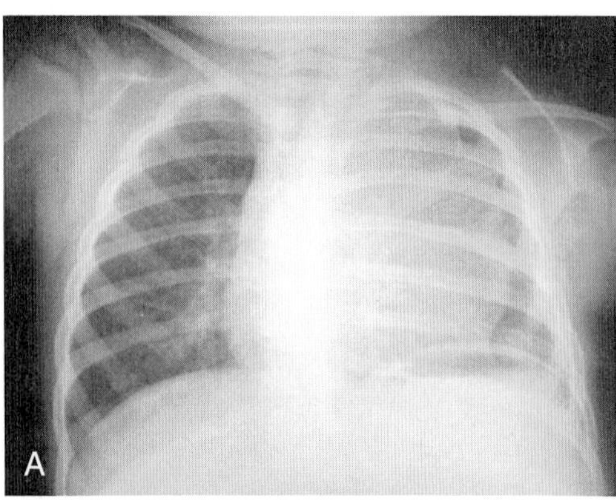

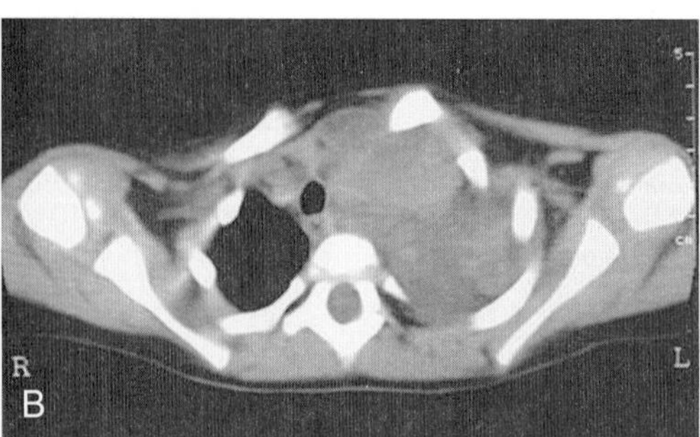

Figure 25-3. A 3-year-old girl presented with a left cervicomediastinal lymphangioma. **A,** Chest radiograph depicts the large mass. **B,** CT scan shows displacement of the trachea and other mediastinal structures by cysts of variable density.

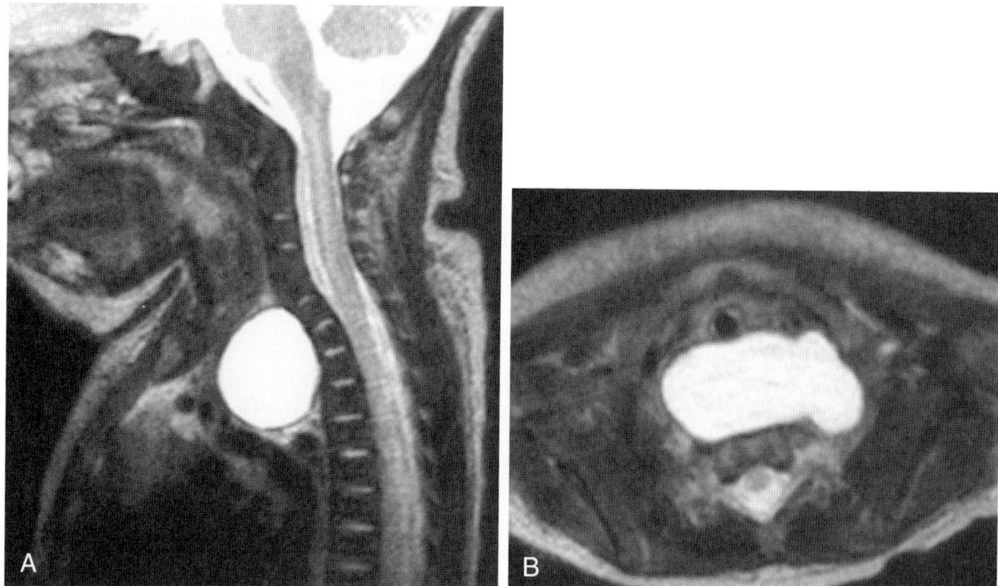

Figure 25-4. This newborn with the prenatal diagnosis of an upper mediastinal cyst had respiratory distress at birth. These T2-weighted MR images show a large prevertebral mucus cyst that displaces the trachea forward (**A**) and extends to both sides (**B**). In **A**, deformation of the anterior vertebral bodies due to prolonged prenatal compression can be seen. This bronchogenic cyst was successfully removed thoracoscopically.

airway malformations.[59,60] When the foregut cyst is due to a persistence of the embryonic neuroenteric communication, it involves both the foregut and the neural tube. It splits the notochord and, as a consequence, is accompanied by split vertebral bodies. This rare variety is termed a neuroenteric cyst.[61-63]

Prenatal diagnosis of mediastinal cysts is possible.[64] However, most cases are diagnosed because of symptoms of respiratory or gastrointestinal compression that become evident at birth (Fig. 25-4) or later in life, or are found during imaging for unrelated symptoms. Very seldom, these mediastinal cysts may bleed due to mucosal ulceration.

When the cysts are located close to the trachea and main-stem bronchi, they are usually lined by ciliated epithelium and are considered to be "bronchogenic cysts" (Fig. 25-5).[65,66] Those located in contact or within the wall of the esophagus are lined by esophageal or mixed epithelium and are known as "esophageal duplication cysts." Both types are filled with more or less mucoid fluid depending on the proportion of secretory glands in their lining.

Plain chest radiographs may show paramediastinal round opacities, and esophagograms depict esophageal compression from outside or intraluminal imprinting by the cyst. CT and/or MRI depict precisely the size and location of the cysts and the nature of their content. Endoscopy may be useful in cases in which the cyst is within the wall of the esophagus, and it can demonstrate external compression in other cases.

The treatment of foregut cysts and duplications should be surgical because of their secretory nature. Prenatal diagnosis may allow intrauterine treatment, which has been described.[67] Thoracoscopy has become

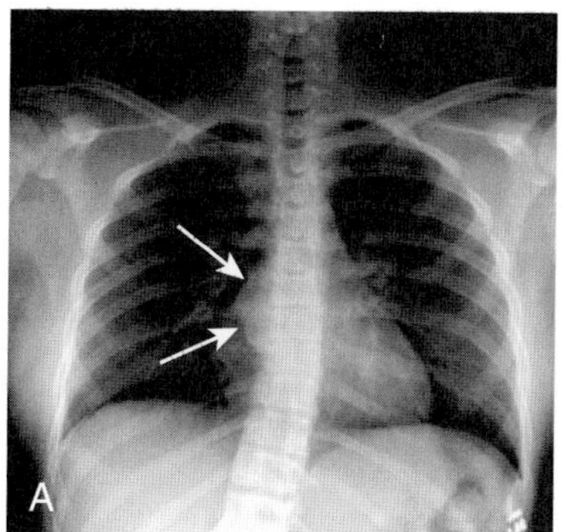

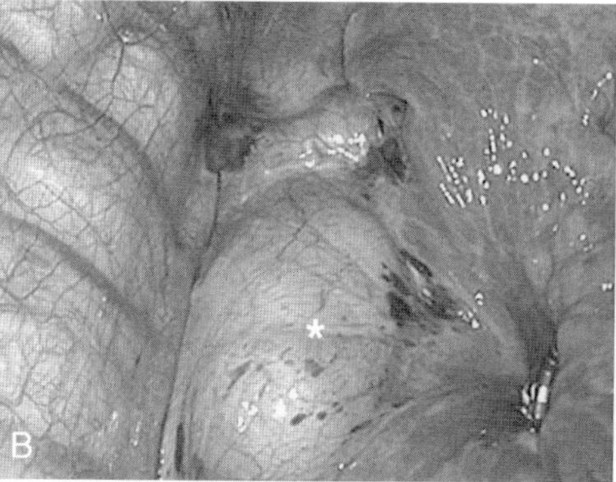

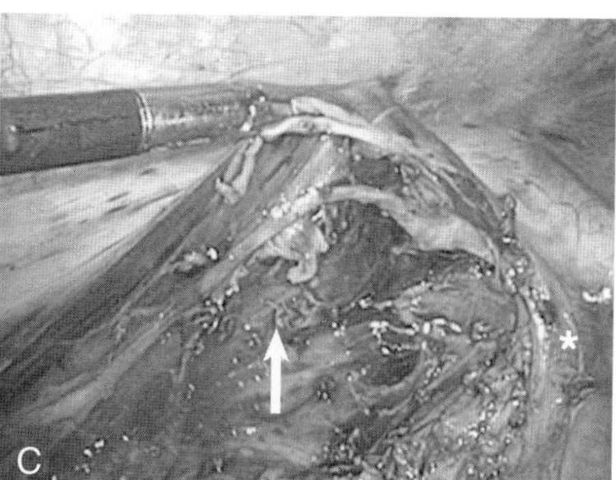

Figure 25-5. This 12-year-old developed some respiratory distress that prompted the chest radiograph (**A**), which shows a right bronchogenic cyst (*arrows*). **B,** The lesion (*asterisk*) is seen at thoracoscopy. **C,** After removal of the cyst, the esophagus (*arrow*) is seen to lie in the posterior bed of the resection. The cyst was intimately adherent to the right main-stem bronchus (*asterisk*).

the preferred approach in recent years.[68-72] Most esophageal duplications and bronchogenic cysts can be removed by this approach. Dissection from the esophageal wall may be delicate, but, because these cysts are generally not communicated with the esophageal lumen, they can be mobilized without damage to the mucosa. Intraoperative esophageal fiberoptic observation may be helpful.[73] As in other duplications, it is essential to completely remove the secreting mucosa to prevent recurrence or cancer later in adulthood.[65]

NEURAL TUMORS

These tumors originate from the sympathetic chains located on both sides of the spine and may exhibit different degrees of differentiation, ranging from malignant neuroblastomas to mature ganglioneuromas (Fig. 25-6). These two components may appear together in the same tumor. For unknown reasons, thoracic neural tumors are less malignant than those located in the abdomen.[74] Also, thoracic neuroblastomas tend to behave less aggressively. The proportion of INSS stages 1 and 2 and of favorable histologic pattern are definitely higher than in other locations. Moreover, these tumors are less likely to have biologic and molecular predictors of malignancy, such as *MYCN* amplification.[74-77]

The tumors involve the sympathetic trunks and a variable number of ganglia. Sometimes they may extend into the spinal canal through one or several foramina (dumbbell- or hourglass-shaped tumors).[78,79] The upper or apical tumors may extend to the neck and often involve the stellate ganglion. The lower ones may extend into the abdomen through the posterior diaphragmatic insertions and/or the aortic hiatus. The aorta and the esophagus on the left side and the azygos vein on the right may be in close contact with the tumor, which sometimes passes across the midline. Intercostal arteries and veins are often intratumoral.

Horner syndrome and/or heterochromia of the iris may lead to the diagnosis.[80,81] Paraplegia due to spinal cord compression may occur suddenly.[82] However, most cases are silent and are discovered by imaging procedures for concurrent conditions or vague symptoms. The proportion of secreting tumors in this location is low and paraneoplastic symptoms such as hypertension and diarrhea are rare. A limited number of malignant tumors spread from the primary site and metastasize to distant regions such as the bone marrow or the bones.[77]

Imaging reveals a round or fusiform mass with paraspinal extrapleural signs and sometimes hemorrhagic, necrotic, or calcified areas. The ribs and the spinal pedicles may be distorted, with the foramina enlarged. In hourglass-shaped tumors, the intraspinal component is better depicted by MRI (Fig. 25-7).[78]

All tests required for neuroblastoma workup (e.g., metaiodobenzylguanidine scan, catecholamine metabolite excretion) are routinely used for tumors in this location as well.

In cases with paraplegia, emergency laminectomy or laminotomy with removal of the intraspinal extension is generally preferred,[82,83] although some groups advise chemotherapy initially.[84] Except in very extensive tumors and in those with bone metastases in which chemotherapy should precede surgical removal, mediastinal neural tumors are primarily excised.[85] This operation may be difficult, particularly when the tumor extends beyond the midline or into the neck, the spinal canal, or below the diaphragm. Mobilization of the aorta with division of several intercostal vessels may be required. Clearance of the tumor should be as complete as possible, although in many cases minimal macroscopic residual disease is unavoidable. In cases of thoracoabdominal tumors, splitting the diaphragm and dissecting the retroperitoneal mass from above at the same operative setting is advantageous. Thoracoscopic excision is increasingly being utilized.[18,86,87]

Irrespective of their histology, the survival of patients with thoracic neuroblastoma is encouraging and always better than that of their abdominal counterparts. Some sequelae are unavoidable. Paraplegia may persist when the cord has been permanently damaged (this happens in tumors that cause prenatal compression).[88,89]

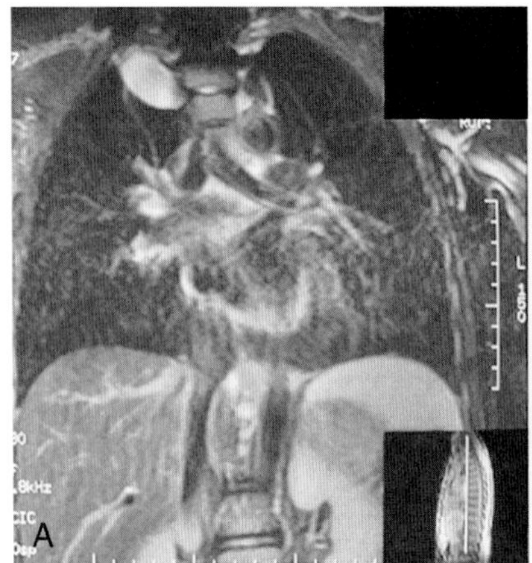

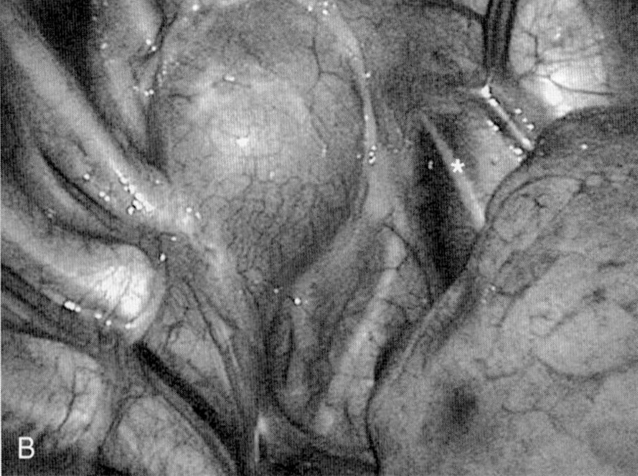

Figure 25-6. A 16-year-old presented with a Horner syndrome and was found to have a right superior mediastinal mass. **A,** MR image of the mass. **B,** At thoracoscopy, the mass can be visualized cephalad to the azygos vein and just lateral to the superior vena cava (*asterisk*). This ganglioneuroma was able to be removed thoracoscopically.

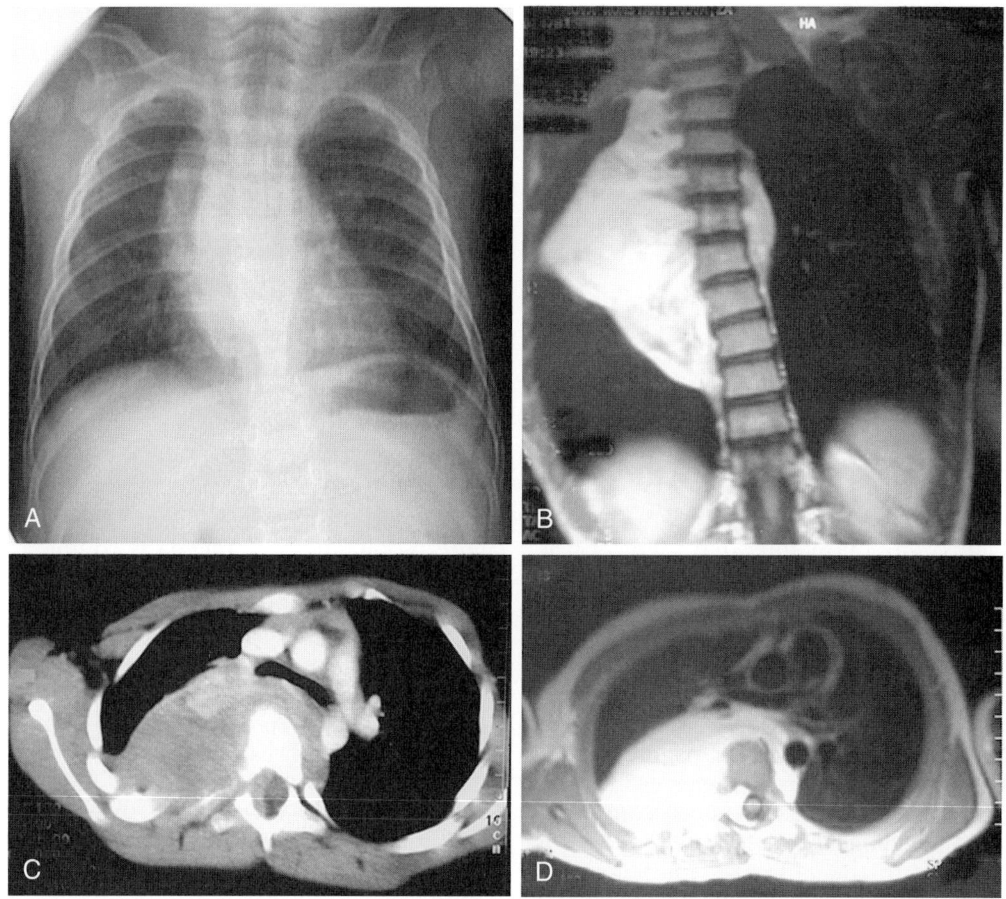

Figure 25-7. This 7-year-old patient had a long-standing history of neuroblastoma that was treated with chemotherapy but the lesion was not resected. The tumor is seen as a fusiform mass extending to both sides of the thorax on the plain radiograph (**A**) and MR image (**B**). **C,** CT scan shows rib and vertebral body deformations with widening of the foramina and displacement of the great vessels. **D,** MR image depicts the dumbbell-shaped nature of the tumor, which invaded the spinal canal, although without paraplegia. Combined spinal and right thoracotomy approaches allowed complete resection of the mass.

Permanent paraplegia may occasionally occur due to intraoperative spinal cord ischemia.[90] Division of the segmental vessels may cause localized paralysis of upper abdominal or thoracic muscles. Removal of the stellate ganglion usually leads to permanent Horner syndrome. Finally, scoliosis may ensue after laminectomies and should be avoided whenever possible.

OTHER RARE MEDIASTINAL TUMORS

Rarely, other mediastinal tumors have been reported in children. These include pseudoinflammatory tumor,[91] Langerhans' cell histiocytosis with calcification,[5,92] thymolipoma,[93] sarcoma,[94] and liposarcoma.[95]

chapter 26

THE ESOPHAGUS

Nicole Chandler, MD • Paul M. Colombani, MD

The esophagus is a hollow muscular tube consisting of mucosa, submucosa, and muscularis layers. The esophagus lacks a serosal layer. The upper one third of the esophagus is striated muscle under voluntary control, and the distal two thirds of the esophagus is composed of smooth muscle under autonomic control. Two sphincters control passage of contents into the gastrointestinal tract: an anatomic upper esophageal sphincter (UES) and a physiologic lower esophageal sphincter (LES). The UES consists of the cricopharyngeus and inferior pharyngeal constrictors. The LES is histologically similar to the muscular component of the esophagus.

The blood supply to the proximal esophagus is derived from the fourth brachial arch. The fourth brachial arch gives rise to the subclavian artery and its branches, including the inferior thyroid artery, which supplies the cervical esophagus. The thoracic esophagus is supplied directly from branches of the aorta. The excellent submucosal plexus of the proximal esophagus allows for extensive mobilization without compromise to the blood supply, whereas caution should be taken distally because of the segmental distal esophageal blood supply. The abdominal esophagus has a generous blood supply from the phrenic branches and gastric vessels.

Embryologically, the trachea and esophagus are intimately related. The trachea and esophagus both develop from the foregut as a median ventral diverticulum. Familiarity with the embryologic development of the esophagus and trachea is important to understand the congenital abnormalities that arise from these structures. The classic description of these malformations proposes an impaired process of septation of the trachea and esophagus.[1]

In humans, normal development of the foregut begins during the fourth week of gestation. At 22 days' gestation, the foregut endoderm differentiates into a ventral respiratory part and a dorsal esophageal part. The separation of the respiratory part from the esophageal part is achieved by the formation of lateral longitudinal tracheoesophageal folds. The trachea and esophagus elongate first distally and then proximally. At 6 to 7 weeks' gestation, the separation of the esophagus and trachea is complete. At birth, the esophagus is 8 to 10 cm in length.[2] This length will double in the first few years of life.

Lesions of the upper esophagus are best approached through the right chest to avoid problems with the aortic arch. The azygos vein should be ligated and divided where it crosses the esophagus. As long as the superior vena cava is patent, the azygos vein can be divided without consequence. Lesions of the lower esophagus can be explored through either the right or left chest. To expose the distal esophagus via the left chest, the inferior pulmonary ligament must be divided, taking care not to injure the inferior pulmonary vein that runs in the upper part of the pulmonary ligament.

The mucosa is the strongest layer of the esophageal wall. When the esophagus is divided, the mucosa will retract proximally and distally. Meticulous approximation of the esophageal mucosa is essential for a technically sound anastomosis.

ENDOSCOPY

In current pediatric practice, esophagoscopy is frequently used to evaluate dysphagia and gastroesophageal reflux as well as to dilate esophageal strictures, evaluate for trauma, and aid in sclerotherapy for bleeding esophageal varices and in the placement of gastrostomy tubes. Both rigid and flexible esophagoscopes are available for use in children of all ages.

Flexible endoscopy is the technique of choice for routine diagnostic esophagoscopy. The rigid esophagoscope is more versatile and provides a larger diameter that allows for better visualization and a larger channel for biopsies. It also does not require air insufflation of the esophagus, which is crucial in the setting of trauma because air will not be forced through a perforation into the mediastinum.

The main value of rigid esophagoscopy in current pediatric practice is for therapeutic procedures such as dilation of an esophageal stricture or removal of a foreign body. Rigid esophagoscopy requires general anesthesia with endotracheal intubation and muscle relaxation. The child is positioned supine with a roll under the shoulders to extend the neck. With care taken to protect the teeth, the esophagoscope, with its bevel up, is introduced into the oral cavity along the hard and soft palates to identify the cricopharyngeus muscle and enter the esophagus. Once the most distal aspect of evaluation is reached, it is easy to examine the esophagus fully when withdrawing the scope to identify any lesions or foreign bodies missed on insertion.

Flexible endoscopes are now available for upper endoscopy in premature infants all the way to adolescents in a reliable, safe, and efficient manner. Endoscopy with a flexible scope can be performed under sedation or general anesthesia. The endoscope is passed though the pharynx and cricopharynx into the upper esophagus. This is most safely done under direct vision. The scope should be advanced down the esophagus carefully, making sure to always maintain visualization of the esophageal lumen. The endoscope should never be advanced blindly. If the lumen is not apparent, the scope should be withdrawn slightly with gentle insufflation until the lumen is identified. Once the stomach is entered, it should be insufflated to allow inspection of the mucosa. In small infants, overdistention of the stomach may lead to respiratory distress.

Complications related to passage of a rigid or flexible endoscope are typically at the level of the cricopharyngeus muscle. Perforation of the cricopharyngeus occurs in about 0.03% with flexible endoscopy and 0.1% in rigid esophagoscopy.[3] Perforation during diagnostic esophagoscopy is exceedingly rare.

An emerging technique uses the natural orifices of the body, such as the mouth, anus, or vagina, to access the peritoneal cavity and pelvis. Natural orifice transluminal endoscopic surgery is expected to further reduce pain, scarring, and recovery time associated with intraperitoneal surgery. The size limitations imposed by existing technology will limit the applicability of these techniques in children.

A more thorough description of pediatric esophagoscopy and emerging therapeutic endoscopic techniques can be found elsewhere.[4-7]

FOREIGN BODY ESOPHAGEAL INJURY

Coins are the most frequently ingested foreign body.[8,9] When foreign bodies become lodged in the esophagus, they may cause serious complications. Ten to 20 percent of foreign bodies may lodge in the esophagus and place the patient at risk for developing complications such as aortoesophageal fistula,[10] esophageal perforation,[11] esophageal stricture,[12] tracheoesophageal fistula,[13] and respiratory distress.[14] There are four sites of physiologic narrowing in the esophagus: (1) the cricopharyngeus of the UES, (2) the aortic notch, (3) the left main-stem bronchus, and (4) the LES. The cricopharyngeus is the narrowest point in the gastrointestinal tract. Endoscopic removal has been the preferred approach in many referral centers and has been highly successful with low complication rates.

Key principles of endoscopic management of esophageal foreign bodies are to protect the airway, maintain control of the object during extraction, and avoid causing additional damage. Children are more likely than adults to be asymptomatic and have an increased frequency of respiratory symptoms. There should be a high suspicion of foreign body ingestion in infants with excessive drooling, refusal of food, and unexplained coughing or gagging. Anteroposterior and lateral chest radiographs are the best diagnostic tests for radiopaque objects. The flat surface of a coin is best seen on the anteroposterior view when it is lodged in the esophagus, whereas the lateral view will show the flat surface when it is lodged in the trachea (Fig. 26-1).

Rigid esophagoscopy has long been considered the gold standard for removal of retained foreign bodies. This procedure has been proven to be highly successful with low complication rates. Other approaches have been described to treat esophageal coins, including flexible endoscopy, bougienage, Foley balloon extraction under fluoroscopy, and brief observation trials.

A randomized, prospective study comparing limited observation versus immediate endoscopic retrieval found a 25% spontaneous passage of esophageal coins over a 16-hour observation time.[15] Children were considered for observation only if the patient was

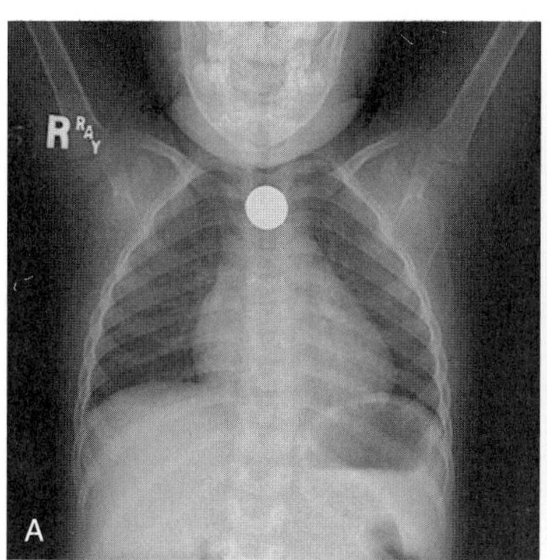

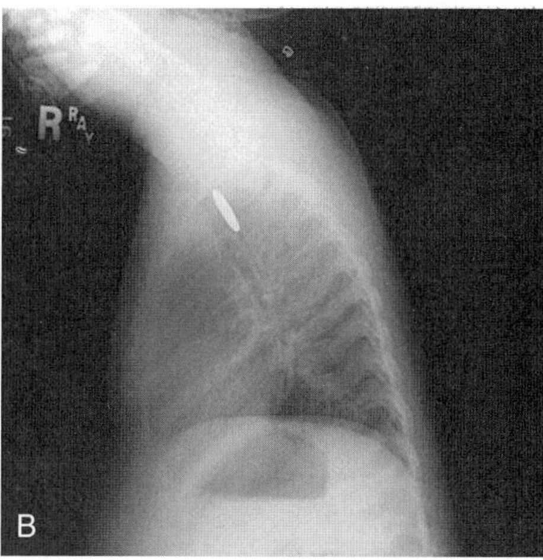

Figure 26-1. Anteroposterior (**A**) and lateral (**B**) radiographs demonstrate a coin lodged at the cricopharyngeus muscle. Note that coins will most often orient with the flat surface facing anteroposteriorly.

asymptomatic, the ingestion was less than 24 hours before presentation, and there was no intrinsic esophageal or tracheal abnormality. There were no complications related to observation. Spontaneous passage was found to be more likely in older children and coins lodged in the lower esophagus. The authors of the study concluded that a short observation period is safe and appropriate for selected patients.

In another study, patients who presented with asymptomatic, witnessed coin ingestion were prospectively enrolled to receive bougienage treatment.[16] This study reported a 90% success rate with a single pass of a weighted bougie dilator to push the coin into the stomach. No complications were reported. There was a significant decrease in hospital costs as well as time to discharge for patients treated with bougienage (2 hours vs. 8 hours, $P < .001$). These authors concluded bougienage is a safe, effective, and economically sound treatment for coins in the esophagus.

A decision analysis model was used to compare four strategies for managing coins in the esophagus in children: endoscopic removal under general anesthesia, esophageal bougienage, outpatient observation for 12 to 24 hours, or an inpatient observation period.[17] Esophageal bougienage resulted in no complications and the lowest total cost per patient of the four strategies. Both observation strategies resulted in a spontaneous passage rate of 23% and an overall complication rate of 4.2%. The endoscopic approach had the highest complication rate (5.8%) and cost. With nearly 25% of patients spontaneously passing ingested coins, a brief period of observation may reduce complications and cost compared with routine endoscopic removal of all esophageal coins.

A retrospective review looked at 555 patients with retained esophageal foreign bodies that were treated with balloon extraction under fluoroscopy (see Fig. 11-6).[8] Dysphagia (37%) and sialorrhea (31%) were the most common presenting symptoms of retained foreign bodies. The upper esophagus was the most common site of impaction in 73% of patients. Coins consisted of 88% of the retained foreign bodies. Other foreign bodies included round batteries, rings, keys, food particles/bones, washers, and pins. The procedure was performed by passing a 10-Fr to 12-Fr lubricated Foley balloon through the nares and advancing it beyond the foreign body. The balloon was inflated with 5 mL of diluted barium. Under fluoroscopy, the inflated balloon was withdrawn until the foreign body reached the posterior pharynx; then the patient was turned to a decubitus position to expel the foreign body. The foreign body was successfully removed in 80% of patients. In 8%, the foreign body was pushed into the stomach, for an overall success rate of 88%. There were no major complications or aspirations. Two patients had minor postprocedural epistaxis. The children in whom Foley balloon extraction was not successful underwent endoscopic retrieval of the foreign body. In infants younger than age 1 year, the failure rate of this procedure was 25%. Patients 1 to 2 years old had a 13% failure rate. Because patients did not require general anesthesia or an inpatient admission, a significant cost savings was demonstrated for patients undergoing balloon extraction.

In a meta-analysis, a total of 1706 coin removal attempts were reviewed with a 97.7% success rate and 2.1% complication rate.[18] The only reported failures were attempted Foley catheter retrievals. Of the 1005 endoscopic retrievals, 2.5% had complications and nearly all were airway related. No complications were reported with bougienage. There was a 1.8% complication rate with 658 attempted Foley catheter extractions. Epistaxis, vomiting, and transient respiratory distress were the most common complications.

There is much more concern for serious injury with the ingestion of button batteries. There are four mechanisms of injury caused by batteries: (1) the toxic effect due to absorption of substances, particularly batteries containing mercuric oxide; (2) electrical discharge and mucosal burn; (3) pressure necrosis; and (4) caustic injury from leakage. Severe esophageal damage may occur in as little as 4 hours after ingestion and perforation in as little as 6 hours after ingestion.[19] Emetics should not be given, owing to ineffectiveness and possible reflux of a battery back into the esophagus.

There have been 20 reported cases of esophageal injury from ingested button batteries from 1979 to 2004.[20] Complications from the ingestion of button batteries include death from vascular invasion and uncontrollable hemorrhage,[21] esophageal perforation,[22] tracheoesophageal fistula (see Fig. 11-4),[23,24] and bilateral vocal cord paralysis.[25]

A total of 2382 cases of battery ingestion was collected by a National Button Battery Ingestion Hotline.[19] As expected, children younger than 5 years of age were at greatest risk, accounting for 61.8% of ingestion cases. The most common batteries came from hearing aids, watches, games, and toys. Hospitalization for ingestion was infrequent. Endoscopic intervention was required in 2.1% of cases, and surgery was needed in 0.4% of cases. Two children had major morbidity from battery ingestion. In both cases, the battery became lodged in the esophagus and produced a burn injury to the esophageal mucosa, which required long-term dilations. Current management protocols call for emergent removal of all batteries lodged in the esophagus by endoscopy, because direct visualization of the mucosa is required to assess the degree of injury. Removal by the balloon technique or magnetic devices is not recommended at this time because esophageal injury cannot be assessed by these methods. Batteries that have passed beyond the esophagus need not be retrieved unless the patient shows signs of intestinal injury. However, outpatient follow-up is critical to ensure safe passage by inspection of stools and/or repeated radiographs to document clearance from the intestinal tract. Further information about esophageal foreign bodies can be found in Chapter 11.

CHEMICAL ESOPHAGEAL INJURIES

In 2004, the U.S. Poison Control Centers reported household ingestions and related deaths with nearly 125,000 ingestions in children younger than the age of 5.[26] Household bleaches and oven cleaners are the most frequently ingested substances. The mean age for ingestions was 3.7 years, and 60% of patients were male.[27]

The extent of injury is dependent on several factors, including the composition of the substance, volume, concentration, and duration of contact. Acidic injury results in immediate pain and coagulative necrosis with eschar formation and is more likely to result in gastric injury. Alkali ingestions more commonly result in esophageal injury. Alkalis combine with tissue proteins to cause liquefactive necrosis and saponification and generally penetrate deeper into tissues. Alkali absorption leads to vascular thrombosis, impeding blood flow to damaged tissues.

Alkali ingestions have three phases of injury: liquefactive necrosis, reparative phase, and scar retraction. In liquefactive necrosis, the injury rapidly penetrates the deep layers of the esophagus until the alkali is buffered by tissue fluids. Between 5 days and 2 weeks is considered the reparative phase. Sloughing of the necrotic debris is followed by development of granulation tissue and collagen deposition. The esophageal wall is thinnest during this subacute phase and at highest risk for perforation. Scar formation begins after 2 weeks. During this time, there is deposition of collagen, resulting in esophageal stricture.

Caustic injuries are classified similar to burn injuries (Table 26-1). The classification of injury is based on endoscopic evaluation and is used clinically to help predict subsequent clinical outcomes and course. First-degree injuries are superficial and will result in edema and erythema. The esophageal mucosa will slough, but no stricture will form. Second-degree injuries involve the mucosa, submucosa, and muscle layers. They result in deep ulceration and granulation tissue after which collagen deposition and contraction occur. If there is circumferential injury, a stricture may develop. Third-degree injuries are transmural with deep ulcerations that result in a black appearance to the lining of the esophagus. These injuries can result in perforation. Patients with grade 2b or 3 develop strictures in 70% to 100% of cases.[28] Grade 3b are the most severe injuries and carry a 65% mortality.[28] These patients may need emergent esophageal resection.

After ingestion, patients can be asymptomatic or may present with nausea, vomiting, dysphagia, odynophagia, drooling, abdominal pain, chest pain, or stridor. There have been no conclusive data to correlate laboratory values or symptoms with degree of injury. Initial management of these patients should focus on airway management and volume resuscitation. Direct laryngoscopy can be useful for identifying laryngeal edema. Inducing emesis should be discouraged because additional exposure to the substance can cause increased mucosal damage. A chest and abdominal radiograph should be obtained to look for signs of perforation. Computed tomography (CT) of the chest can also be used in selected cases.

Endoscopic evaluation should be carried out in the first 24 to 48 hours after ingestion. Contraindications to endoscopy include shock, respiratory distress, peritonitis, mediastinitis, or evidence of perforation. Endoscopy should not be performed after 5 days, once the reparative phase has begun, because the esophagus is at its thinnest and the risk of perforation is highest. Once the degree of injury is identified, further evaluation of the distal esophagus also increases the risk of perforation.

In addition to endoscopy, endoscopic ultrasonography has been used to delineate the depth of tissue injury and a separate grading system has been proposed.[29] Endoscopic ultrasonography may be able to identify deeper tissue injury over endoscopy alone but has not added prognostic value over endoscopy.[30] Further investigations need to be carried out to determine the usefulness of this technique in evaluating corrosive esophageal injuries.

Patients with grade 1 or 2a injury are allowed oral intake and are typically discharged soon after injury. Patients with grade 2b and 3 injuries should be observed for 24 to 48 hours and then may have their diets slowly advanced. With severe injuries, esophageal strictures are common, occurring in up to 70% of patients with grade 2b injuries and up to 100% in patients with grade 3 injuries. Because of the frequency with which strictures occur, patients with grade 2 or 3 injuries should have a barium swallow performed for early detection. A barium swallow on day 21 after injury is indicated to evaluate for strictures (Fig. 26-2). Once a stricture is identified, gradual dilations are performed. Strictures refractory to dilation may need surgical resection.

A systematic pooled analysis on the use of corticosteroids in second-degree caustic burns of the esophagus from 1956 to 2006 showed the overall percentages of strictures for corticosteroid therapy and nonsteroid therapy groups were 12.3% and 19%, respectively.[31] In this study, there was no statistical difference. Additionally, corticosteroid therapy posed additional complications, including perforation and infection. At this time, existing data fail to support the use of corticosteroids or antibiotics in the prevention of esophageal strictures in patients with caustic-induced grade 2 esophageal injuries.[32]

A 30-year report from a single institution with esophageal caustic injuries was recently reported.[33] Eighty patients were treated over this time period. The degree of injury was first or second degree in 58%, more extensive second degree in 26%, and third degree in 16%. Overall, 29% had medical complications, including chemical pneumonitis, atelectasis, aspiration pneumonia, dysphagia, and gastroesophageal

Table 26-1 Classification of Caustic Esophageal Injuries

Grade	Endoscopic Findings
1	Mucosal edema and erythema
2a	Friability, hemorrhage, blisters, erosions, erythema, white exudate
2b	Findings of grade 2a plus deep or circumferential ulceration
3a	Small and scattered area of necrosis
3b	Extensive necrosis

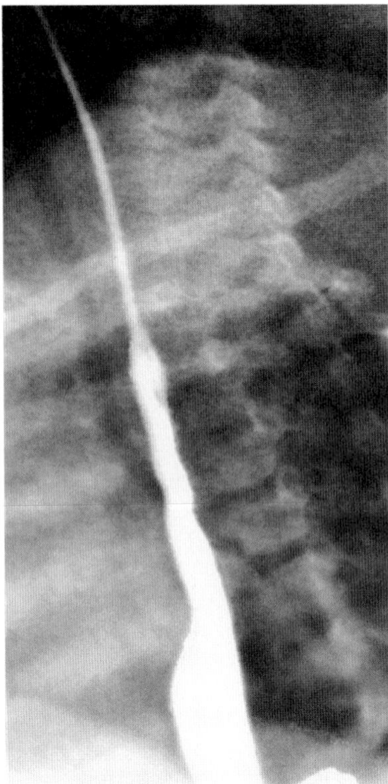

Figure 26-2. This barium swallow was performed 3 weeks after lye ingestion. Note the significant narrowing in the proximal two thirds of the esophagus.

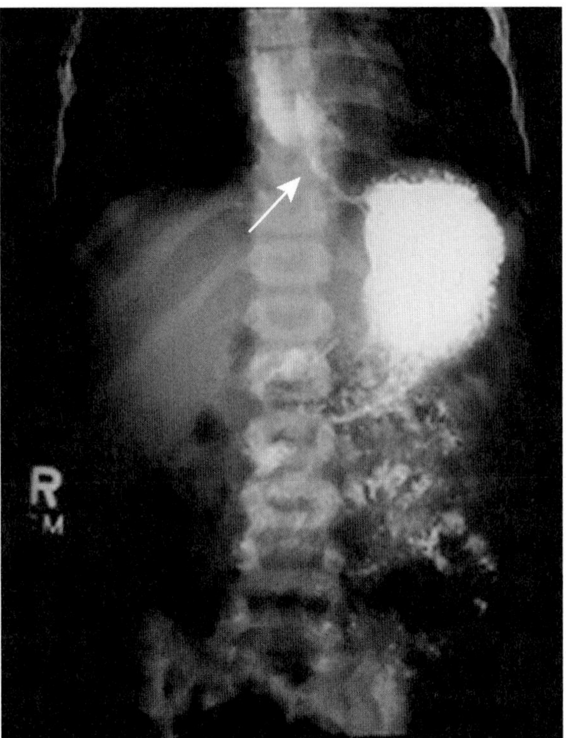

Figure 26-3. This barium study was performed in a child with dysphagia and pain. There is marked narrowing (*arrow*) of the distal esophagus secondary to gastroesophageal reflux and a peptic stricture.

reflux, and 20% developed severe esophageal strictures. Nearly 14% of patients required esophageal replacement, which consisted of gastric tube conduit reconstruction with anastomosis to the cervical esophagus. The time from initial injury to esophageal replacement ranged from 12 months to 14 years, with a mean of 5 years. Because of the heterogeneous nature of ingestions and the various substances, location, and degree of injury, the optimal management remains controversial.

Treatment modalities for esophageal strictures include bougienage, esophageal stent placement, intralesional corticosteroid injection, and endoscopic dilations after stricture formation. Once strictures have formed, patients require endoscopic balloon dilation or bougienage. Multiple dilations may be required for strictures to resolve. Surgical intervention may be necessary if these treatments fail, if malignant transformation occurs, or if lengthy or tight strictures develop.

ESOPHAGEAL STRICTURES

In general, esophageal strictures in children do not involve malignancies. The causes of benign esophageal strictures in childhood include reflux esophagitis, corrosive ingestion, and anastomotic scarring. Anastomotic and corrosive strictures may be aggravated by gastroesophageal reflux. The incidence of stricture in patients with gastroesophageal reflux approaches 15%.[34] Management includes relief of the obstruction as well as correction of the reflux. Anastomotic strictures are discrete and short, whereas corrosive strictures tend to be irregular and long. Peptic esophageal strictures are short and usually located in the lower third of the esophagus (Fig. 26-3).

Uncontrolled gastroesophageal reflux can result in esophageal stricture as a consequence of repeated insults to the esophageal mucosa. Vomiting and failure to thrive are present in nearly all patients with strictures resulting from gastroesophageal reflux. Many patients will also have concomitant pulmonary disease. The majority of strictures are located in the lower third of the esophagus and less frequently occur in the middle third. In addition, a hiatal hernia may also be present.

One group reported their success in treating these gastroesophageal reflux-associated strictures with preoperative dilations and antireflux procedures.[35] Twelve percent of all antireflux operations performed by this group were for gastroesophageal reflux with stricture formation. Preoperative management included oral antacids, prokinetic agents, histamine-2 (H_2) receptor blocker, maximal nutritional support, and optimization of respiratory compromise. Antireflux surgery was delayed until nutritional optimization was met and esophagitis resolved. A mean of 3.6 dilations per patient was required. Postoperative dilations were performed until the stricture was no longer present. They reported that most patients (88%) had complete resolution of the stricture and associated gastroesophageal reflux with this management protocol.

In another series, patients did not undergo preoperative dilation.[34] They were treated preoperatively with antacids and an H_2-receptor blocker to reduce the inflammation and edema related to esophagitis and were provided nutritional support. Operative management included intraoperative dilation, Nissen fundoplication, and guided dilations postoperatively. These patients required a mean of 3.4 postoperative dilations and achieved good results with a mean follow-up of 3 years.

Chronic esophagitis related to gastroesophageal reflux is the inciting event in the formation of strictures. Characteristically, esophageal strictures produce few early symptoms, which are initially insidious in onset. Correction of gastroesophageal reflux with concomitant dilation and continued postoperative dilations is sufficient in most cases to resolve symptoms of reflux and allow strictures to heal. By utilizing this treatment approach, more aggressive forms of surgical management of esophageal strictures are not usually required.

A recent retrospective study looked at the management of 125 patients who had corrosive ingestion and the outcomes of early prophylactic bougienage for stricture.[36] Of the 125 patients, 54 were found to have an esophageal burn injury on endoscopy and 32 required treatment for stricture. This group's management protocol was to perform early endoscopy if the ingested substance was strongly acidic, alkaline, or unknown and if symptoms were apparent within 24 to 48 hours. In this study, 27% had symptoms at the time of admission, most commonly dysphagia, and 57% of these symptomatic patients had a normal endoscopy. Overall, 25% of the patients with esophageal burns of all degrees developed a stricture. All patients with grade 3 injury developed severe esophageal strictures. Varying degrees of stricture developed in patients with grade 2b injury. Mild strictures developed in 4 of 15 patients with grade 2a injury. No patient with a grade 1 injury developed a stricture.

Patients with severe 2b or 3 injuries were treated with either early prophylactic dilations or dilations were initiated after the formation of stricture. In the first group, 20 patients underwent early bougienage beginning the first week after injury. In the second group, eight patients started dilations based on esophagograms showing stricture at 3 weeks after ingestion. In this retrospective study, in the group who had early dilations, the strictures resolved after 6 months of dilations, whereas the group who had dilations starting later required dilations for 1 year or longer.

Stenting for esophageal strictures is commonly utilized in adults but not widely used in children. Use of a retrievable and expandable nitinol stent was used successfully in eight children with corrosive esophageal strictures.[37] The stents were removed after a mean of 13 days. Two patients required dilations after the stent was removed for persistent stenosis. Placement of the stent was associated with mild symptoms of chest pains and vomiting that resolved after stent removal.

Bougienage dilation has traditionally been used in children. However, balloon catheter dilation is now being increasingly used for the treatment of esophageal strictures. One theoretical advantage of balloon catheter dilation is that the stricture is gradually dilated by a uniform radial force. In contrast, bougienage exerts an abrupt shearing axial force that may cause significant injury of the mucosa and may lead to further scarring and stricture. In one report, 77 children with mean age of 1.8 years underwent a total of 260 dilations (3.4 per patient) for treatment of an esophageal stricture for various causes, including achalasia, post-esophageal atresia repair, reflux esophagitis, post fundoplication, and caustic injury. An esophageal perforation occurred in 1.5%. Successful outcomes were seen in 97% over a 6-year follow-up period.[38]

ESOPHAGEAL PERFORATION

Iatrogenic esophageal perforation is a potentially life-threatening condition if not recognized and treated promptly. Pain, fever, dyspnea, and tachycardia are early symptoms of esophageal perforation after dilation for an esophageal stricture.[39] Clinical findings include pneumomediastinum, pleural effusion, subcutaneous emphysema, and pneumothorax. Proximal thoracic perforations lead to signs in the left thoracic cavity, whereas distal perforations usually show findings on the right side. Complications include mediastinitis, septicemia, empyema, and death.[39] Perforations can occur with both bougie dilators and balloon dilators. Most perforations can be recognized at the time of dilation, especially if endoscopy is used to inspect the esophagus after dilation. Conservative treatment including nasogastric decompression, broad-spectrum antibiotics, nutritional support, and drainage of the effusion or pneumothorax has been successful in the majority of patients (Fig. 26-4).

Perforation of the esophagus in children with caustic esophageal injury is difficult to manage and typically occurs during the first dilation of an esophageal stricture. In a report of 22 children treated for esophageal perforation that occurred secondary to a caustic esophageal stricture, 80% were successfully treated with conservative therapy.[40] However, although the esophageal perforations healed with conservative measures, most patients were left with a residual stricture.

Operative management is still considered the mainstay of therapy in adults with esophageal perforation. Many authors have reported successful nonoperative therapy in children with esophageal perforations. In contrast to nonoperative management of esophageal perforations, minimally invasive techniques offer the advantage of identifying the perforation, debriding the necrotic tissue, and draining the pleural cavity.[41]

CONGENITAL ESOPHAGEAL STENOSIS

Congenital esophageal stenosis is a rare childhood condition with an incidence of 1 in 25,000 to 50,000 live births.[42,43] It is associated with esophageal atresia

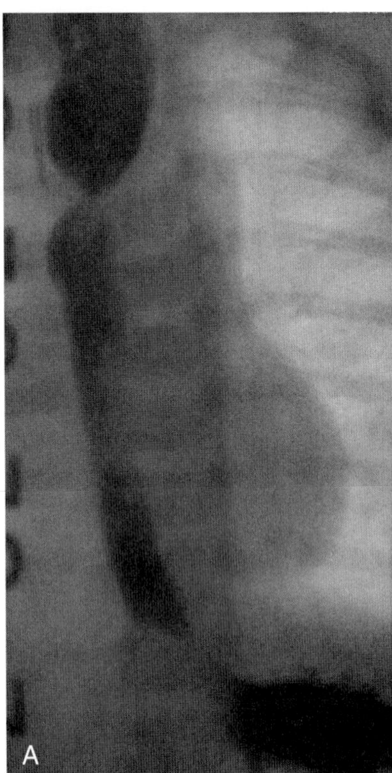

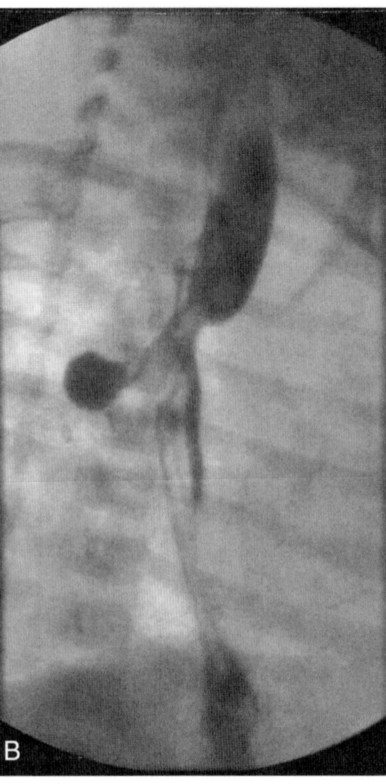

Figure 26-4. **A,** This infant developed a stricture at the anastomosis after esophageal atresia repair. Multiple balloon dilations were required. **B,** Unexpectedly, at the time of one of these dilations, an esophageal perforation developed. Note the contrast leak through the esophageal perforation. This child was managed nonoperatively, and the perforation eventually sealed without the need for operative intervention.

in one third of patients. The remaining are considered to be isolated cases.[44,45] Three histopathologic variants are seen: tracheobronchial remnants, membranous diaphragms or webs, and diffuse fibrosis of the muscularis and submucosa.[46] Most infants have normal physical findings at birth. As a result, congenital esophageal stenosis is rarely diagnosed in the neonatal period. The onset of symptoms, most commonly vomiting, dysphagia, and failure to thrive, typically develop with the introduction of solid food at ages 4 to 10 months. Respiratory symptoms are found in about 10% of patients.[47] An esophagogram may show an abrupt or tapered stenosis, commonly at the junction of the middle and distal third of the esophagus (Fig. 26-5). Additional workup, including pH probe and endoscopy, is necessary to exclude the more common diagnosis of gastroesophageal reflux-associated stricture and esophagitis. When associated with esophageal atresia, the stenosis is usually found in the distal one third of the esophagus.[47,48]

The absence of esophagitis will be confirmed on esophagoscopy. However, tracheobronchial remnants can be missed on biopsy specimens that are taken too superficially.[48] Endoscopic ultrasonography has been shown to be helpful in differentiating tracheobronchial remnants as the cause of the stenosis from stricture due to gastroesophageal reflux.[49,50]

Dilatation of a congenital esophageal stenosis does not provide long-term benefit. Case reports have described successful treatment with endoscopic electrocauterization and balloon dilation.[51] However, limited resection of the stenosis through the left chest (either open or thoracoscopically[45]) with primary end-to-end anastomosis is the treatment of choice for long-term relief.

ESOPHAGEAL DUPLICATION

Congenital esophageal duplication is a rare anomaly of the esophagus, with an incidence of 1 in 8000 births, accounting for 10% to 15% of all gastrointestinal duplications.[52] Histologic criteria for diagnosis include attachment to the esophagus, enclosure of the duplication by two muscle layers, and lining of the duplication by epithelium. Patients tend to present with respiratory symptoms, vomiting, regurgitation, and a possible neck mass. Diagnosis can be made by contrast esophagography. Because the duplication may increase in size with time and compress surrounding structures, operative resection is the treatment of choice. This can be approached via posterolateral thoracotomy or thoracoscopy. Operative guidelines include preserving the vagus and phrenic nerves and reconstructing the muscular wall of the esophagus. Air insufflation of the esophagus intraoperatively with endoscopy or with a nasogastric tube should be utilized to assess the integrity of the esophageal wall after resection. See Chapter 40 for further information about esophageal duplications.

ESOPHAGEAL ACHALASIA

Achalasia is an uncommon disorder with an incidence of 4 to 6 cases per million per year. Only 5% of cases occur in children younger than the age of 15 years.[53] In contrast to adults, the disease is more common in boys than girls (1.86:1) and is unusual during infancy. Achalasia is a primary esophageal motor disorder of unknown etiology, characterized by three findings: increased LES

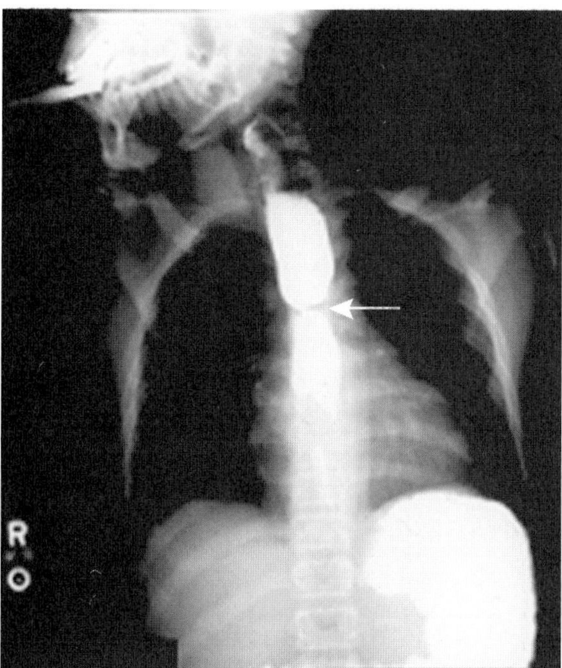

Figure 26-5. This child presented with significant dysphagia and weight loss. An esophagogram revealed marked narrowing of the midesophagus (*arrow*) due to congenital esophageal stenosis. This child underwent resection of the stenosis and primary repair of the esophagus.

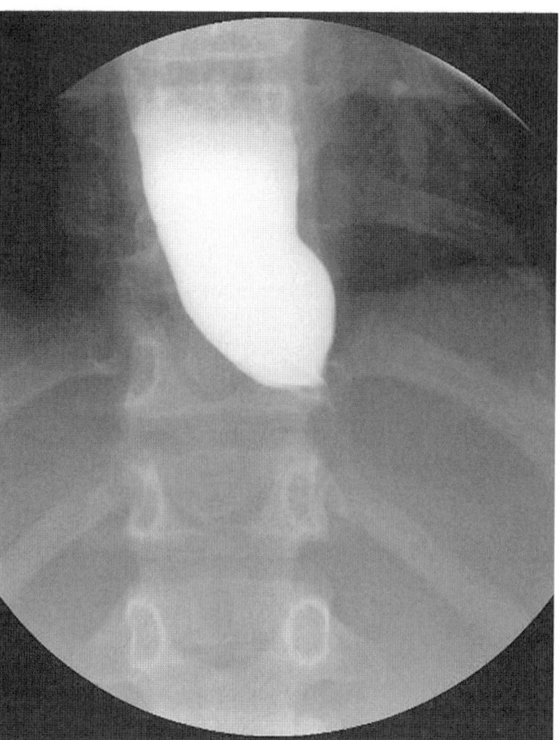

Figure 26-6. This barium swallow was performed in a 16-year-old patient with dysphagia secondary to achalasia. The classic "bird's beak" narrowing of the distal esophagus at the level of the spastic, contracted esophagus is seen. Also, note the dilated esophagus proximal to the lower esophageal sphincter.

resting pressures, absent esophageal body contraction, and impaired LES relaxation during swallowing. In children, this has been associated with various syndromes, including trisomy 21 and triple A syndrome (achalasia, alacrima, and ACTH insensitivity).

Presenting symptoms of achalasia are age dependent. Infants present with frequent regurgitation, choking, pneumonia, and failure to thrive. Symptoms in older children are similar to those seen in adults and include vomiting, regurgitation, and dysphagia. Esophagography and the clinical history are sufficient to make the diagnosis in most cases. A barium esophagogram will show the typical dilated esophagus and a narrowed distal segment, the "bird's beak" sign (Fig. 26-6). Decreased or absent peristalsis of the esophageal body can be noted at the time of fluoroscopy. Esophageal manometry will reveal an elevated LES pressure, failure of the sphincter to relax with swallowing, and low-amplitude, nonprogressive, or absent peristaltic contractions in the esophageal body.

The aims of therapy are to reduce the LES pressure to facilitate esophageal emptying, improve symptoms, and prevent stasis-related complications. Treatment has utilized several approaches: pharmacologic agents, dilatation, and esophagomyotomy.

Pharmacologic treatment with calcium channel blockers can result in a decrease in the LES pressure, but the response is short-lived. The need for long-term medicine limits its usefulness in children. Botulinum toxin (Botox) has become popular in recent years for the treatment of achalasia. It is a neurotoxin that binds to presynaptic cholinergic terminals in skeletal muscle, inhibiting the release of acetylcholine at the neuromuscular junction, which creates a chemical denervation. While initially effective, there is a high recurrence rate that also limits its applicability in children.

Treatment with Botox results in inflammation and fibrosis of the LES. This can result in a significantly more difficult operation at the time of esophagomyotomy.[54] Even though Botox effectively initiates the resolution of symptoms associated with achalasia in children, 50% of patients are expected to need an additional procedure within 7 months after one injection. A randomized controlled trial compared adult patients treated with either Botox or laparoscopic myotomy for the treatment of achalasia.[55] They found that laparoscopic myotomy is as safe as Botox treatment and should be the initial treatment for achalasia. Because the results are poor and may interfere with the ability to perform an esophagomyotomy, Botox has almost no role in the treatment of achalasia in children, except perhaps those who are not candidates for general anesthesia.

In 1994, a worldwide survey collected data on 175 cases of achalasia in children.[56] Only 6% were infants at diagnosis even though 18% reported onset of symptoms in the first year of life. The duration of symptoms was less than 3 years before diagnosis in most (80%) patients. Operative treatment was performed in 95%. Forceful dilatation of the distal esophagus was needed in 26%. Transabdominal myotomy was successful at alleviating symptoms in 73% of patients, and this increased to 91% with the addition of an antireflux procedure. Patients who had a transthoracic approach were less likely to have relief of symptoms, regardless of whether an antireflux procedure was performed. The apparent benefit of an antireflux procedure in this group of patients suggests some advantage to controlling post-myotomy gastroesophageal reflux in high-risk patients, although this conclusion has not been found in other reports.

The outcomes after esophagomyotomy are similar for both pediatric and adult patients, as reported in a recent retrospective review.[57] A total of 337 patients underwent laparoscopic myotomy with anterior fundoplication, 14 of whom were younger than 18 years of age. More than half the pediatric patients had frequent and severe dysphagia, choking, regurgitation, and chest pain. Both children and adults had similar duration of symptoms before diagnosis. A significant number of pediatric patients had initial nonoperative management consisting of Botox in 7%, dilatation in 14%, and both in 28%. Postoperatively, all patients underwent an early esophagogram to evaluate for a missed esophagotomy or gastrotomy. At median follow-up of 37 months, 77% of the pediatric patients' symptoms improved, compared with 88% improvement in adults.

A review over 21 years evaluated 19 pediatric patients who underwent a transthoracic modified anterior esophagomyotomy.[58] In each case, a longitudinal incision was carried down to the submucosa and the muscularis was freed laterally on each side until at least 50% of the esophageal circumference was mobilized. The esophagomyotomy began from the aortic arch and extended 1 cm onto the stomach. A minority of patients had concomitant antireflux procedures. All patients who underwent antireflux procedures required postoperative esophageal dilatations in the first postoperative year. Overall, 90% of patients had complete and permanent relief of their swallowing difficulties.

Another relatively large study reported the experience of 20 patients with achalasia who were treated with modified esophagomyotomy.[53] Seventy percent did not have an antireflux procedure. The incidence of postoperative gastroesophageal reflux was noted in 1 patient (5%), whereas postoperative dysphagia requiring dilation occurred in 5 patients. Complete relief of symptoms was achieved in 70%.

Esophagomyotomy is a proven intervention, but incomplete myotomy may lead to clinical failure. One study found that patients who had a myotomy without intraoperative manometry were more likely to experience recurrence of symptoms.[59] Performance of an adequate myotomy is a key feature to successful long-term relief of symptoms. The reasons for inadequate myotomy include a gastric component to the LES or an inadequate proximal myotomy, resulting in residual high-pressure zones.

It is the opinion of most authors that the treatment of choice for achalasia remains esophagomyotomy. The operation may be performed either through the chest or abdomen. Both laparoscopic and thoracoscopic approaches have been used with success. The transthoracic approach may provide better exposure to perform a long myotomy, which is necessary in patients with a long proximal area of involvement. On the other hand, the transabdominal approach may be better suited for when an antireflux procedure is also needed. In children, it is still controversial whether an antireflux should be performed at the same time as esophagomyotomy. In adults, 30% to 50% of patients develop significant gastroesophageal reflux after esophagomyotomy. Studies in children have shown a lower overall rate of postmyotomy reflux of 5% to 36%.[53,58] As a result, concomitant fundoplication may not be necessary for every child with achalasia.

ESOPHAGEAL REPLACEMENT

The most common indications in the pediatric population for esophageal replacement are esophageal atresia and strictures related to reflux or corrosive injury. The colon was the first conduit used as esophageal replacement and remains the most commonly used technique in practice today. Other alternatives have distinct advantages over colon interposition but require advance planning on the part of the surgeon. The alternatives include gastric tube, gastric transposition, and jejunal interposition graft. Which conduit is best for any given patient depends on multiple factors, including the location and length of the native esophagus that remains, the original diagnosis for the patient, the patient's size and age, and previous procedures on the esophagus, stomach, or colon.

Regardless of the conduit used, there are several principles that are important. First, the esophagus is the best conduit and should be preserved at all costs, provided it functions relatively normally and has no malignant potential (e.g., Barrett's esophagus). Second, a short straight tract is best because esophagoscopy and dilatations are frequently required. Almost all conduits function as passive tubes rather than by means of intrinsic peristaltic activity. A retrosternal tunnel is often the shortest and straightest route. Third, the prevention of reflux into any conduit is important. An interposition procedure that incorporates the distal normal esophagus with its gastroesophageal junction has an advantage. Fourth, persistence is exceedingly important. Anastomotic dilatations should not be necessary except during the healing phase. Strictures should be revised surgically (Fig. 26-7). Complex interpositions that do not function well should be revised to provide the straightest, lowest resistance conduit possible.

Colon Interposition

The right, transverse, or left colon on its vascular pedicle has been used as an esophageal replacement, either in an isoperistaltic or an antiperistaltic direction. It can be placed in a substernal position or a transthoracic posterior mediastinal location. The colon is pulled

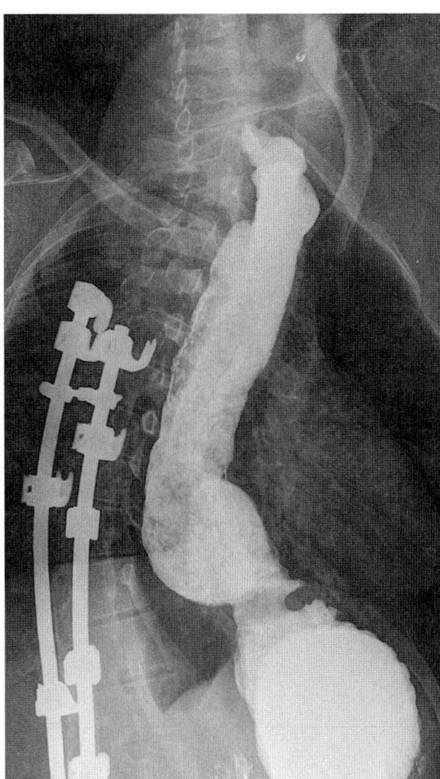

Figure 26-7. Barium swallow of a 28-year-old patient after successful left colon interposition for isolated esophageal atresia. The patient developed bleeding and dysphagia from peptic ulceration at the distal anastomosis, requiring revision.

up into the neck, and an end-to-side or end-to-end esophagocolic anastomosis is performed in the neck. The gastrocolic anastomosis is then performed, followed by an antireflux procedure and pyloroplasty. The steps involved with a right colon interposition for esophageal atresia are seen in Figure 26-8, and the operative steps for a left or transverse colon interposition are seen in Figure 26-9.

Colon interposition is a relatively straightforward procedure, and the colon is readily placed into the thorax without causing respiratory compromise. Disadvantages of this approach include the need for three anastomoses and an increased risk for anastomotic leak, strictures at the esophagocolic anastomosis, and tortuosity or redundancy of the graft over the long term.

In a study of 38 colon interpositions, 61% of surgeons utilized the right colon and 39% used the transverse left colon.[60] In addition, 63% were placed substernally and 37% were routed in a transthoracic posterior mediastinal location. Early complications included cervical anastomotic leaks in 29%, pneumonia, wound infection, pneumothorax/hemothorax, wound dehiscence, prolonged ventilation, and perforated graft secondary to ischemia. Late complications included significant proximal strictures, distal strictures, redundancy of the graft, intestinal obstruction, and dumping syndrome. Of significance, cervical anastomotic stricture development correlated strongly with leak at the cervical anastomosis. The overall graft failure rate, requiring graft replacement, was 18%. Although 45% of the patients required additional procedures, 80% of patients eventually had good functional results.

A recent report of 850 esophageal replacement procedures from one institution described a 30-year experience.[61] Gastric pull-up procedures were used in 75 cases, retrosternal colon interpositions in 550 cases, and posterior mediastinal colon interpositions in 225 cases. The posterior mediastinal colon interposition procedure has evolved as these authors' preferred procedure because it provides the most direct route and has a very low incidence of complications. Including the most recent 250 cases of substernal colon interpositions, the authors have had a 10% cervical anastomotic leak rate, 50% of whom developed an anastomotic stricture, and a 1% mortality rate. Only 0.6% of patients developed late graft stenosis. These remarkable statistics may reflect the value of experience rather than the intrinsic value of one procedure over another.

More intraoperative ischemic complications of colon interpositions have occurred with the right colon placed in the substernal position when compared with the left colon placed in the posterior mediastinum.[62] This may occur because up to 70% of patients have a right colon that lacks a marginal artery necessary to nourish the colon transplant.[63] Ischemia also may result from the angulation necessary for the substernal placement of the interposition. Several authors report an incidence of this complication of approximately 30%.[64-66] Leak at the esophagocolic anastomosis is probably caused by technical errors or minor degrees of ischemia, but stricture formation is almost undoubtedly caused by ischemia. Repeated dilatation is not often successful. Therefore, most anastomotic strictures that persist more than 6 months after the interposition procedure will ultimately require surgical revision. Both the management of an esophageal leak and the surgical management of an esophageal stricture are less difficult if the anastomosis is made in the neck.

Another consideration in the selection of an interposition route is the possibility of subsequent acquired heart disease, necessitating sternotomy. The approach to access the heart is difficult in patients who have had a colon interposition in a substernal location. Similarly, patients who previously had a sternotomy for cardiac surgery usually need an alternative route for an interposition.[67]

Timing of Colon Interposition

In those patients in whom esophageal atresia exists without a distal fistula and in whom attempts at stretching are successful, the colon can be interposed in the newborn period. Most pediatric surgeons, however, create a cervical esophageal fistula, place a gastrostomy, and carry out interposition when the patient is age 6 months or older. Both approaches have theoretical and practical advantages. Most

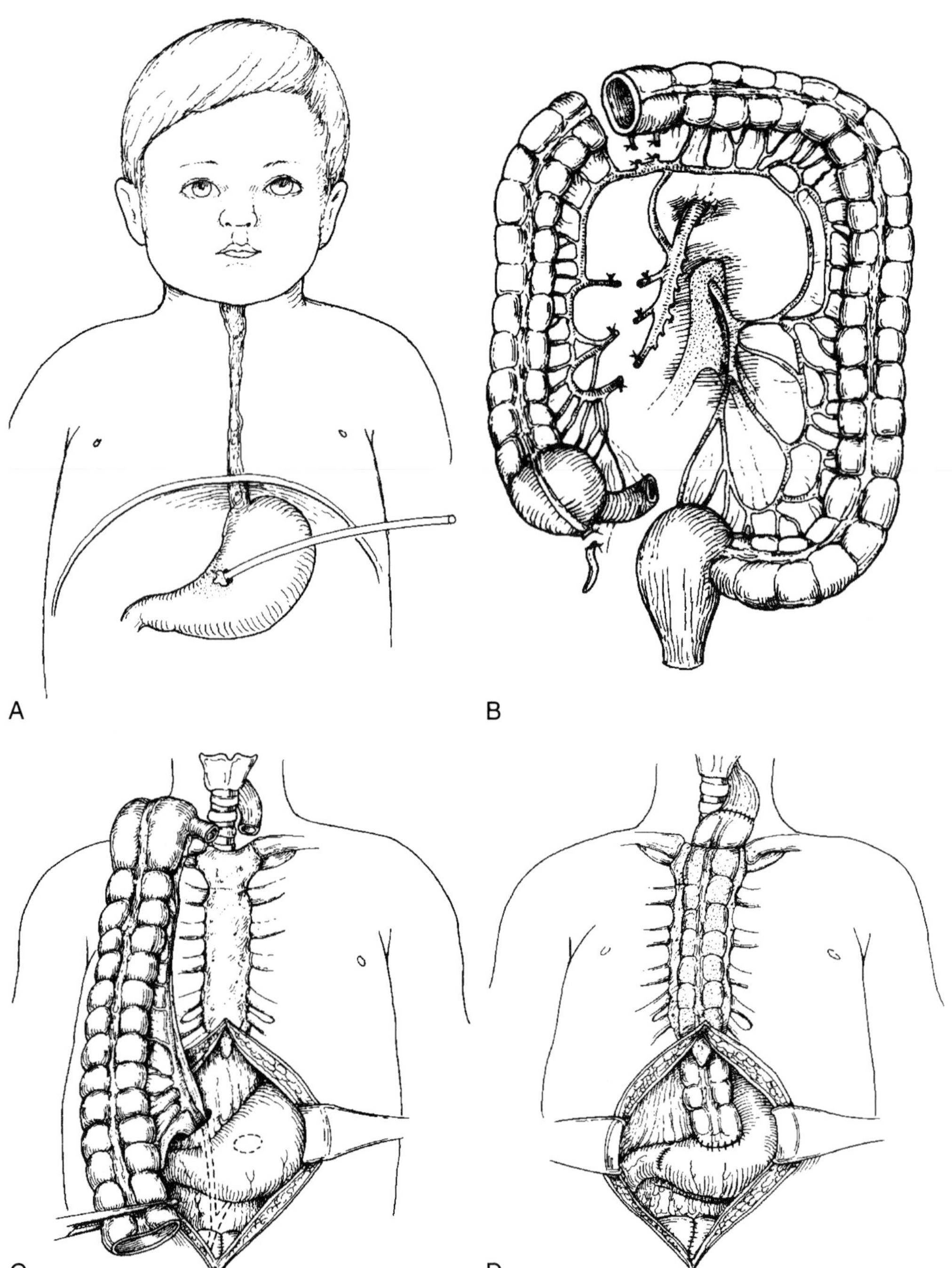

Figure 26-8. **A,** For any esophageal lesion in which a substitution procedure may be anticipated, the gastrotomy should be placed on the lesser curve at about the level of the incisura, so that a right or left colon or gastric tube interposition may be carried out without compromising the blood supply. **B,** The right colon and terminal ileum are isolated, based on blood supply from the arcades and from the middle colic artery. **C,** The colon on its pedicle is brought up through the lesser sac and positioned substernally in an isoperistaltic fashion. **D,** Most frequently, excision of the terminal ileum and cecum is accomplished. Careful tailoring of the distal end allows a straight conduit to be anastomosed to the antrum. Pyloroplasty may or may not be added to the procedure. The incidence of significant gastrocolic reflux is reduced by a drainage procedure.

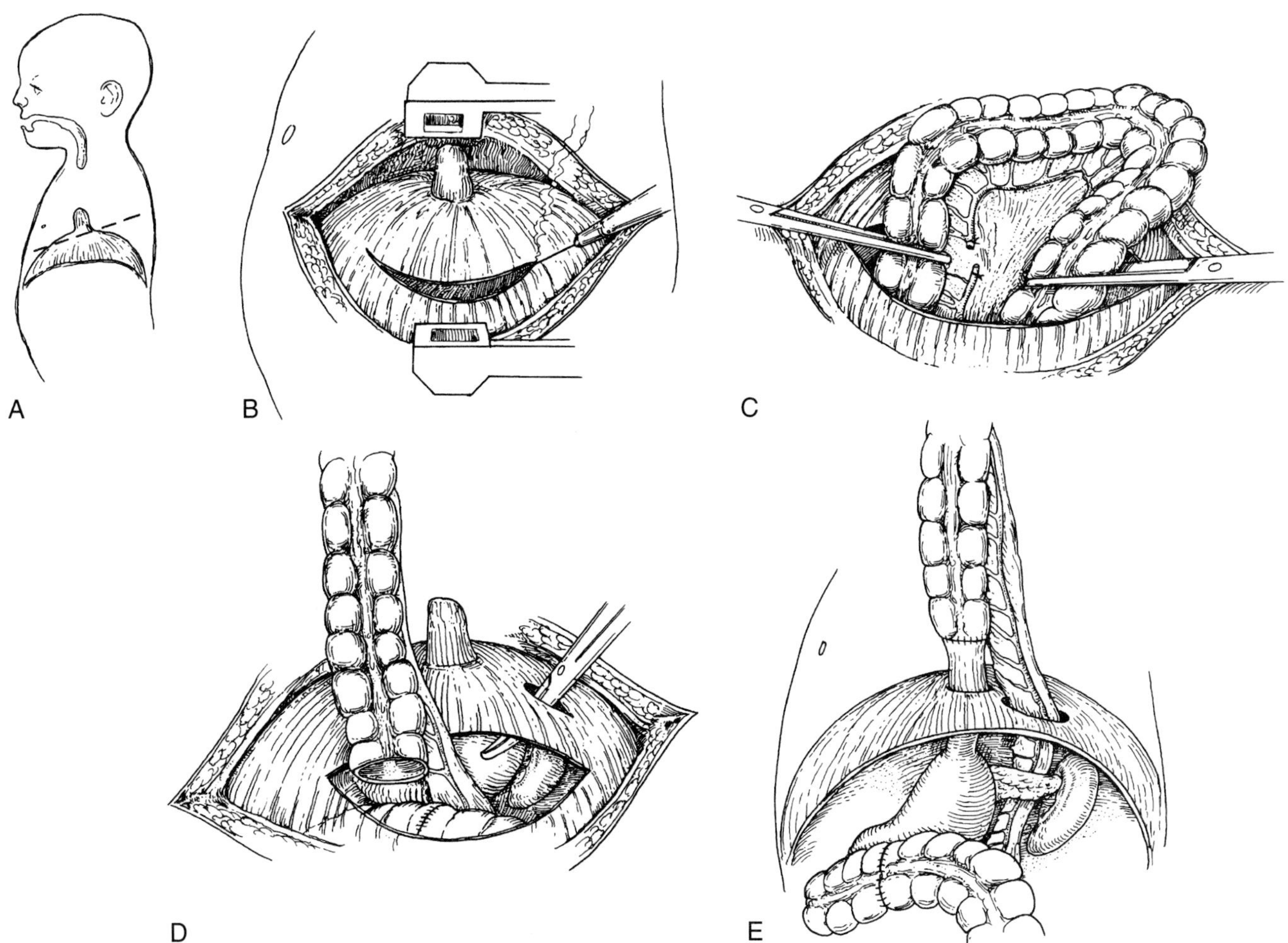

Figure 26-9. The left colon or transverse colon substitution described by Waterston is illustrated in this patient with isolated esophageal atresia. However, it works equally well for other lesions requiring esophageal replacement. **A,** A standard posterolateral left thoracotomy at about the sixth intercostal space. **B,** Incision of the diaphragm peripherally. **C,** A section of colon is isolated and its vascular pedicle is developed, usually based on the left colic artery. It may be necessary to base it on the middle colic artery, in which case, this interposed colon is placed in an antiperistaltic manner. **D,** The colon and its vascular pedicle are delivered behind the spleen and pancreas and through a separate posterior opening in the diaphragm, so that the abdominal viscera do not stretch or otherwise obstruct the blood supply to this colon segment. **E,** The distal anastomosis may be made to the remnant of distal esophagus or to the posterior aspect of the stomach.

(Continued)

reported experience has been in patients who are 12 to 18 months of age. However, if the patient has been without oral intake for many months, once an esophageal substitution has been created, the infant may not want to eat. Therefore, sham feedings by mouth should accompany gastrostomy feedings so that the patient associates a full stomach with swallowing.

Gastric Tube Esophageal Replacement

The reported experience with gastric tube esophagoplasty is much smaller than that with colon interposition, perhaps because the number of patients needing esophageal substitution has diminished in the developed world.

Gastric tubes have become popular because they can be constructed rapidly with a stapling device. The gastric tube is constructed from the greater curve of the stomach with the blood supply based on the left gastroepiploic artery. These tubes can be constructed from the antrum up, or from the fundus down, and can be constructed so that there is enough gastric tube to reach the neck (Fig. 26-10). The advantages of a gastric tube are its excellent and reliable blood supply, its resistance to ulceration from gastric acid reflux, and its ability to bridge long gaps. The tube is also resilient and does not become tortuous or dilated over time. Theoretical disadvantages are a long suture line, continued acid production by the tube, and reduced stomach capacity.

A series of 21 patients who underwent isoperistaltic gastric tube replacement over a 12-year period has been reported.[68] Two patients developed cervical anastomotic leaks, which healed with conservative treatment, and two other patients developed strictures that were treated with dilatations. There were two dilations of the intrathoracic gastric tube and two cases

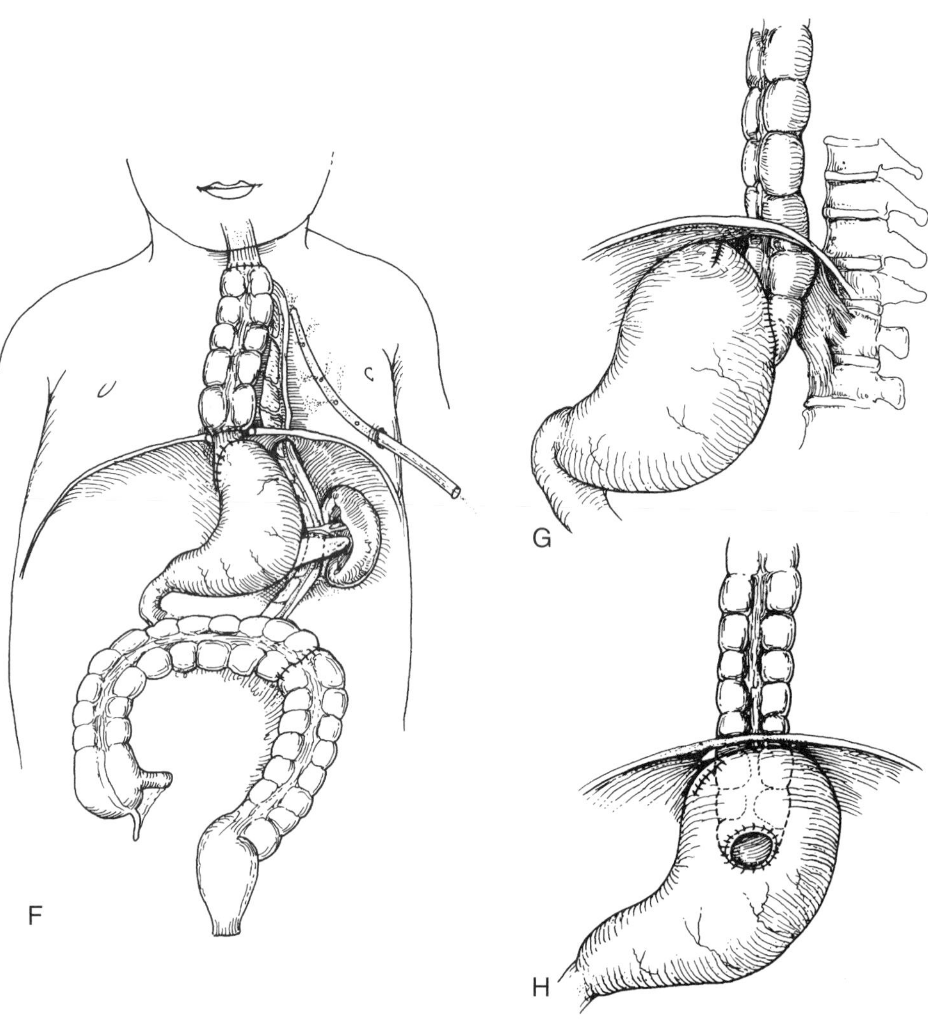

Figure 26-9—cont'd **F,** The upper anastomosis is made to the esophagus either within the mediastinum or within the neck. Adequate drainage of the pleura is necessary to prevent empyema. A fundoplication after the method of Thal also may be added to this procedure, if the distal esophagus is used. This technique reduces the amount of reflux that can interfere with the healing or that can produce ulcers in the colon. **G,** A lateral view of an alternative method of cologastrostomy with Waterston's procedure. **H,** The segment of colon is shown within the abdominal cavity, which will possibly reduce the incidence of gastrocolic reflux.

of dumping syndrome that resolved within 2 years of operation. In another two patients who required anastomosis to the pharynx, there was loss of graft function related to an intractable stricture or a "nonfunctioning" anastomosis.

In this study, pH monitoring was performed in a majority of these patients. All probes that were placed in the gastric tube showed continued acid production. In four cases, pH monitoring showed the presence of acid reflux in the native esophagus. Evaluation with endoscopy showed four patients with mild esophagitis above the anastomosis and two had Barrett's esophagus. At median follow-up of 2.5 years, 76% of the patients were sustained entirely on oral feedings and 50% had normal growth patterns.

Gastric Transposition

The gastric transposition (or pull-up procedure) is performed by mobilizing the entire stomach on a vascular pedicle, relocating the entire stomach into the mediastinum, and creating an anastomosis to the cervical esophagus in the neck. In addition, many surgeons will perform a routine pyloroplasty to prevent delayed gastric emptying. The advantages of this approach are the excellent blood supply to the stomach, that only a single anastomosis is needed, and that the entire esophagus can be replaced with a low risk of necrosis, leak, or stricture. Potential disadvantages are that the stomach acts as a space-occupying mass in the chest, leading to respiratory compromise. Figure 26-11 depicts a postoperative barium study after a gastric pull-up procedure for extensive strictures after lye ingestion.

A single institution recently reported its outcomes with 173 cases since 1981.[69] Their preference is locating the transposed stomach in a posterior mediastinal location without thoracotomy, using blunt dissection via the hiatus, and cervical incisions. An anastomotic leak occurred in 12%, and most sealed with conservative treatment. Anastomotic strictures developed in 19.6%, with all but three patients responding to endoscopic dilatations. The long-term outcome was considered good to excellent in 90%, although many patients preferred eating small frequent meals. There was no documented evidence of deterioration in the function of the gastric transposition in 72 patients who were observed for longer than 10 years.

In older patients who have had multiple procedures, the blood supply to the stomach may be compromised and a long gastric tube is not advised. These patients

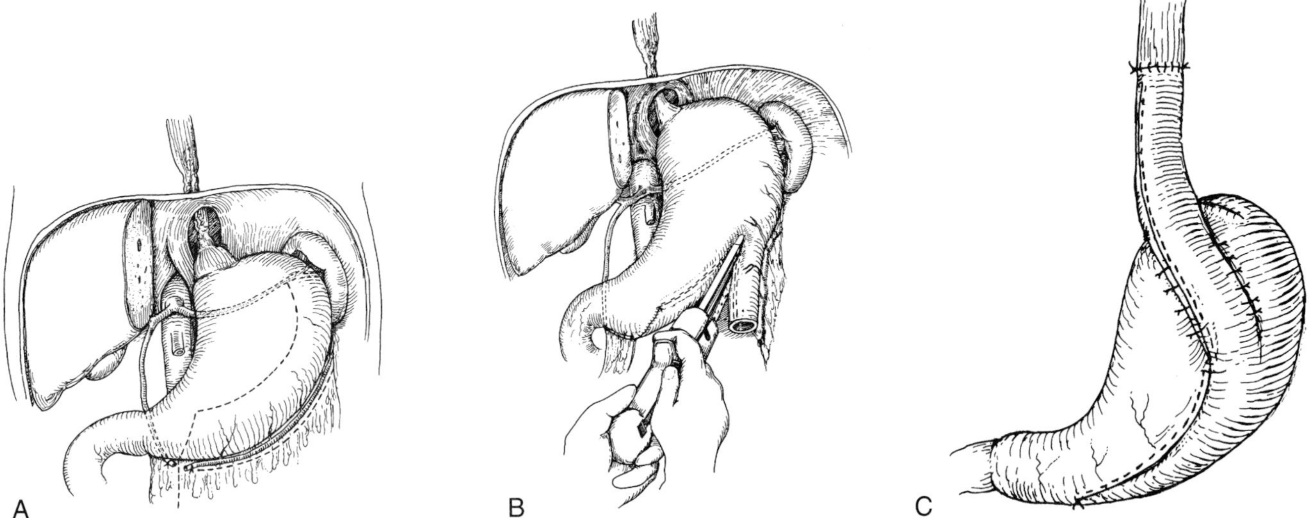

Figure 26-10. Graphic depiction of the technique to create a reversed gastric tube for esophageal replacement. **A,** Inspection of the blood supply to the stomach and preservation of the gastroepiploic artery for creating the tube. **B,** The use of a stapler to create the tube along the greater curvature of the stomach. **C,** The completed reversed tube is brought up to the chest for the esophageal anastomosis.

also may not have adequate stomach length to reach the cervical esophagus. In such patients, a gastric pull-up, combined with a short gastric tube, may be used to get the additional stomach length required to reach the neck.

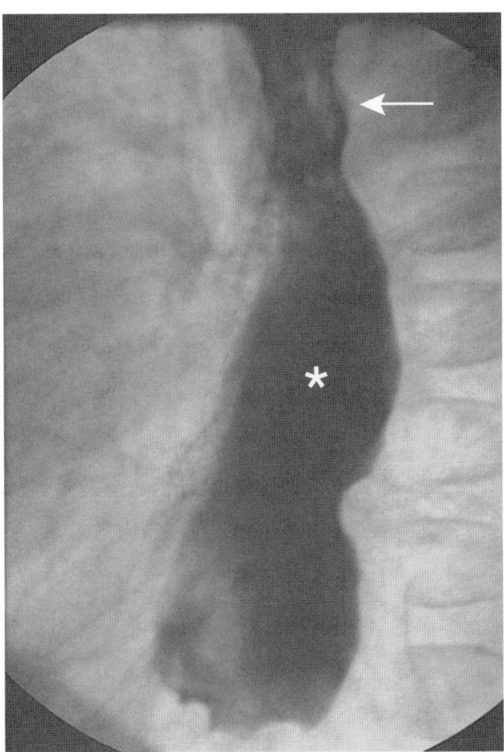

Figure 26-11. This infant underwent a gastric pull-up after a failed colonic interposition for isolated esophageal atresia. The native esophagus is identified by the *arrow,* and the gastric pull-up is marked with an *asterisk.*

Jejunal Substitution

The jejunum as an esophageal substitute has been used much more commonly in adults than in children. Advantages to using jejunum include a diameter that is similar to the esophagus and does not occupy much space in the thoracic cavity. Also, the jejunum retains its peristaltic activity. Significant disadvantages include the precarious vascular supply of a pedicled jejunal graft. Also, a tension-free anastomosis may be difficult to achieve.

A recent report of eight patients who underwent esophageal substitution with free and pedicled jejunal grafts resulted in significant perioperative morbidity, including three intraoperative repeat interpositions for immediate graft loss.[70] There were four upper anastomotic leaks and four late anastomotic strictures. Less than 50% of patients were able to achieve a completely oral diet without reliance on gastrostomy feeds. In spite of technically sound outcomes, these authors concluded that significant complications exist, including death, graft necrosis, ischemia, and strictures.

Complications of Esophageal Substitution

Regardless of the conduit used, substitution of the esophagus carries a number of predictable complications. The most serious one is vascular insufficiency with necrosis of the interposition. This complication is most commonly seen when using the colon and is recognized at the time of interposition as a blue, pulseless graft. Adjustment of the colon graft to relieve tension or twisting of the pedicle may be effective in improving the blood supply. Intraoperative hypotension may result in the colon graft taking on the appearance of vascular insufficiency. If the geometry

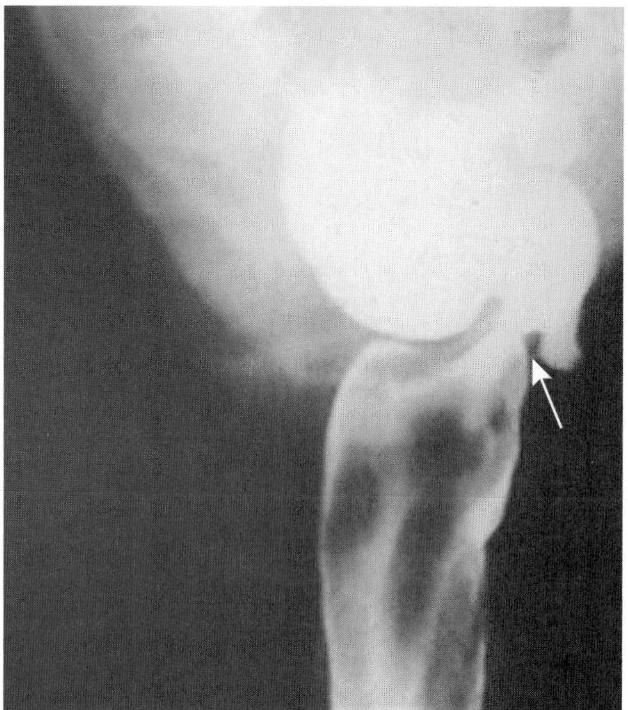

Figure 26-12. A stricture (*arrow*) developed at the esophagocolonic anastomosis after colon interposition for esophageal substitution. The likely cause was vascular insufficiency.

of the graft and the patient's blood pressure are both satisfactory, the graft must be abandoned because its vascularity will rarely improve after completion of the operation.

Interposition of a well-vascularized graft is sometimes followed several days later by fever, increased leukocytosis, and drainage from the proximal anastomosis. An anastomotic leak from tension or mild ischemia may be managed expectantly if the conduit appears viable. A contrast study, however, may demonstrate that the mucosal pattern of the interposed segment is ischemic. The interposition must be inspected and removed if it is necrotic. In this case, a cervical esophagostomy should be established and a different form of substitution planned. Many investigators have reported using the left colon after failure of the right colon. Others may not be inclined to sacrifice additional colon and would perform a gastric tube or gastric interposition.

Proximal strictures between the esophagus and the interposition usually are the result of insufficient blood supply to the interposition (Fig. 26-12). Anastomosis to a scarred esophagus also results in stricture. After a reasonable healing period, persistent strictures should be revised surgically rather than dilated repeatedly.

Ulceration in either a gastric tube or interposed colon is probably the result of reflux and stasis, which may be caused by kinks in the interposition or by delayed gastric emptying. The latter can be a complication of vagal injury either from the original caustic ingestion or from the surgical attempts at previous esophageal reconstruction. Whether a pyloroplasty or a drainage procedure is necessary in all interpositions is a matter of opinion. Certainly, the elimination of "sink-trap" kinks in the interposition is important to prevent ulceration. Revision of the lower end of the interposed colon to eliminate redundancy must be performed with great care to prevent damage to the vascular pedicle and loss of the entire graft. An excellent review of esophageal replacement in children was recently published.[71]

chapter 27

ESOPHAGEAL ATRESIA AND TRACHEOESOPHAGEAL MALFORMATIONS

Klaas Bax, MD, PhD

The first reports describing successful correction of esophageal atresia (EA) date to the early 1940s.[1-3] These described two different procedures: staged repair and primary anastomosis through a left-sided extrapleural approach. An extrapleural approach had already been reported in 1940 but the child died.[4] At that time, the mortality rate for this condition was nearly 100%, but it dropped rapidly in the years to come.[5-9]

CLASSIFICATION

EA and tracheoesophageal fistula (TEF) present in many forms. It is clear that EA should be thought of as a spectrum of anomalies (Fig. 27-1).[10] A simplified classification, believed needed for daily practice, was published in 1929[11] and modified in 1944[3] and again in 1953.[12] These classifications tend to be confusing, however, by naming the same subclasses differently. For clarity, it is much better to give descriptive names to the major subtypes.[13]

Esophageal Atresia with Distal Fistula (EA/TEF)

This is the most common subtype, accounting for about 85% of EA anomalies.[14,15] The very dilated proximal esophagus has a thickened wall and descends into the superior mediastinum usually to the third or fourth thoracic vertebrae. The distal esophagus is slender and has a thin wall. It enters the trachea posteriorly either at the level of the carina or 1 to 2 cm higher. The distance between the esophageal ends varies from very small to a quite wide gap. Very rarely, the distal fistula may be occluded, leading to the misdiagnosis of EA without distal fistula.[16]

Pure Esophageal Atresia

Pure EA has an incidence of about 7%.[15] The proximal and distal esophagus end blindly in the posterior mediastinum. The proximal end is dilated and has a thickened wall as in EA/TEF. If there is no concomitant proximal fistula, the upper esophagus ends at the level of the azygos vein. The distal esophagus is short and usually suspended by a fibrotic band. The distance between the two segments is considerable, usually precluding immediate anastomosis.

Esophageal Atresia with Proximal Fistula

The association of a proximal fistula in a patient with pure EA seems higher than is generally appreciated. In a recent series of 13 children without distal fistula, a proximal fistula was found in 7.[14] An upper esophageal fistula is usually not found at the end of the pouch.[3,11,12] This fistula is similar to the H-type starting proximally on the trachea and ending distally in the dilated proximal esophagus. It is located at the thoracic aperture or higher in the neck. Although limited in length, its diameter may vary from tiny to large. If not diagnosed preoperatively, it may be suspected during operative repair when gas leaks out upon opening the proximal esophagus.

Esophageal Atresia with Proximal and Distal Fistulas

The incidence of EA with proximal and distal fistulas is reported to be less than 1%.[15] EA with one distal fistula and two proximal fistulas has also been described.[17] Also reported is near-complete membranous obstruction of the esophagus in conjunction with a single TEF at the level of the membrane, communicating with both parts of the esophagus.[18]

H-type Fistula without Esophageal Atresia

H-type TEF without atresia is usually discussed together with EA because it may be part of the VACTERL association. It occurs with an incidence of about 4%.[15] The fistula starts from the membranous trachea and runs

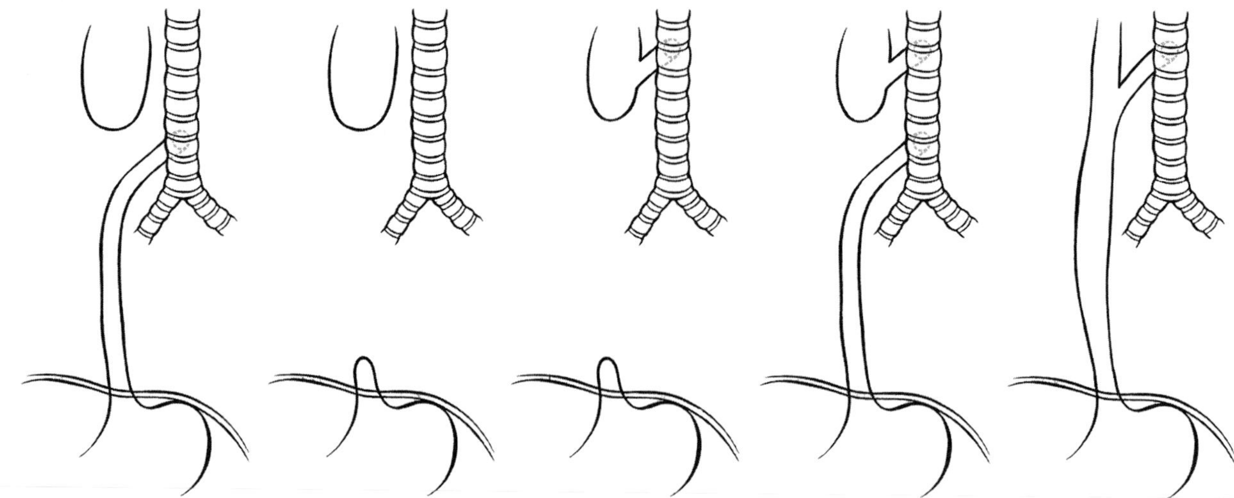

Figure 27-1. Classification of EA and/or TEF (*from left to right*):

Esophageal atresia with distal tracheoesophageal fistula:	Vogt IIIb, Ladd III, Gross C
Esophageal atresia without fistula:	Vogt II, Ladd I, Gross A
Esophageal atresia with proximal fistula:	Vogt IIIa, Ladd II, Gross B
Esophageal atresia with proximal and distal fistulas:	Vogt IIIc, Ladd V, Gross D
Tracheoesophageal fistula (H-type) without atresia:	Vogt IV, Gross E

caudad to enter the esophagus. Normally it is short, although the diameter may be variable. The fistula is usually situated at the thoracic aperture or higher in the neck.[19]

EMBRYOLOGY

The embryology of the foregut is still subject to controversy.[20] What is known, however, is that during the fourth week of gestation the foregut starts to differentiate into a ventral respiratory part and a dorsal esophageal part. The laryngotracheal diverticulum then evaginates ventrally into the mesenchyme. The traditional theory postulates that the ventral respiratory system separates from the esophagus by the formation of lateral tracheoesophageal folds that fuse in the midline and create the tracheoesophageal septum. At 6 to 7 weeks of gestation, the separation between trachea and esophagus is complete. Incomplete fusion of the folds would result in a defective tracheoesophageal septum and abnormal connection between the trachea and esophagus.

This theory of longitudinal tracheoesophageal folds merging to a septum has been challenged.[21-24] In chicken embryo studies, these folds could not be demonstrated. Instead, cranial and caudal folds were found in the region of tracheoesophageal separation. According to this theory, EA/TEF would then be due to an imbalance in the growth of these folds.[22,23] Furthermore, rat studies suggest that EA/TEF results from disturbances in either epithelial proliferation or apoptosis.[24]

The Adriamycin (doxorubicin) rat model has greatly helped with understanding the development of EA/TEF.[25] From this model, it appears the EA develops first, with the lung bud arising from the atretic foregut dividing into three rather than two branches.[26] The middle branch would be the distal esophagus eventually connecting with the stomach. This hypothesis, however, has not been substantiated.[23,27] Also, in the Adriamycin rat model, notochord abnormalities are observed in 90% of the animals.[28] Abnormal ventral branches from the notochord impinging on the foregut, midgut, dorsal aorta, and kidney are common. At the same time, an ectopic expression of Sonic hedgehog occurs in the tissues between the notochord and the gut. Knockout mice models have helped elucidate the functions of different genes in the development of the foregut and aberrations such as EA/TEF.[20]

EPIDEMIOLOGY

The total birth incidence of EA/TEF varies between 2.55 and 2.82 per 10,000 births.[29-31] EA is usually a sporadic occurrence. There is a slight male preponderance of 1.26. There is no evidence for a link between EA/TEF and maternal age when chromosomal cases are excluded.[32] The recurrence risk among parents of one affected child is 0.5% to 2%, increasing to 20% when more than one child is affected. The empirical risk of an affected child born to an affected person is 3% to 4%.[33] The relative risk for EA/TEF in twins is 2.56 when compared with singletons.[34] The concordance rate in twins is low, but the same gender rate is high.[30]

Environmental factors that have been implicated include the use of methimazole in early pregnancy,[35,36] prolonged use of contraceptive pills,[37] progesterone and estrogen exposure,[38] and maternal diabetes and thalidomide exposure.[39] EA is occasionally seen in the fetal alcohol syndrome[40] and in maternal phenylketonuria.[41]

Chromosomal anomalies are found in 6.6% to 10% of the cases.[29,30,42] The lower incidence was found in a study excluding births before 28 weeks of gestation. The total number of trisomy 18 cases exceeds the total number of trisomy 21 cases. Because the incidence of trisomy 18 is higher, this would seem to indicate that trisomy 18 is a greater risk for EA development.[32] Three separate genes have been associated with EA/TEF: *MYCN* haploinsufficiency in Feingold syndrome, *CHD7* in CHARGE syndrome, and *SOX2* in the anophthalmia-esophageal-genital (AEG) syndrome.[43-45]

EA may occasionally be part of the Opitz G/BB syndrome, Fanconi anemia, oculo-auriculo-vertebral syndrome, Bartsocas-Papas syndrome, or Frijns syndrome.[46]

ASSOCIATED ANOMALIES

Obviously, the factor or factors responsible for the early disturbance in organogenesis causing EA may affect the organogenesis of other organs or systems developing at the same time. EA can be divided clinically into isolated EA and syndromic EA, occurring at roughly the same rate.[46]

The most frequent associated malformations encountered in syndromic EA are:

- Cardiac (13%-34%)
- Vertebral (6%-21%)
- Limb (5%-19%)
- Anorectal (10%-16%)
- Renal (5%-14%)

Vertebral anomalies are confined mainly to the thoracic region. An earlier claim that the presence of 13 pairs of ribs is a good indicator of long-gap EA has not been substantiated.[47]

Nonrandom associations have been documented as well. Two of these are the VACTERL association (Vertebral, Anorectal, Cardiac, Tracheo-Esophageal, Renal, and Limb abnormalities) and the CHARGE association (Coloboma, Heart defects, Atresia of the choanae, developmental Retardation, Genital hypoplasia, and Ear deformities). In 1973, VACTERL was originally described as VATER, an acronym made up of Vertebral defects, Anal atresia, T-E fistula with esophageal atresia, and Radial dysplasia.[48] It was later extended with the C for cardiac anomalies and the L for limb anomalies.[38] In a cohort of 463 patients with EA, 107 (23%) had at least two additional VACTERL defects.[49] Seventeen of these patients had a chromosomal defect or a syndrome without a known genetic defect. Interestingly, as many as 70% of the remaining 90 patients had additional defects other than those of the VACTERL association.

The association of coloboma with multiple congenital anomalies was first described in 1961.[50] The name CHARGE association was first used in 1981.[51] EA has been observed occasionally in patients with CHARGE association.[52] These patients have high mortality and morbidity rates.

DIAGNOSIS

Antenatal Diagnosis

The prenatal diagnosis of EA/TEF relies, in principle, on two nonspecific signs: polyhydramnios and an absent or small stomach bubble. Polyhydramnios is associated with a wide range of fetal abnormalities. Most commonly, however, it pursues a benign course. Similarly, the ultrasonographic absence of a stomach bubble may point to a variety of fetal anomalies. The combination of a small stomach together with a dilated esophagus in the neck (the pouch sign) has been confirmed to be diagnostic for pure EA in a number of patients.[53-55] Nevertheless, it is encountered in only a few patients.[54] Depending on whether the pouch is confined to the neck or descends into the mediastinum, a longer or smaller gap may have to be bridged postnatally.[54,55] Current ultrasound technology does not allow for a definite diagnosis of EA/TEF. Therefore, counseling of the parents should be guarded.[56] The application of 3D power Doppler imaging seems promising, both antenatally and postnatally. Aortic arch anomalies, for example, have been diagnosed using this modality.[57,58]

Magnetic resonance imaging (MRI) has served to identify fetal thoracic lesions.[59,60] Furthermore, in a study involving 10 fetuses considered to be at risk for EA on the basis of the ultrasound findings, MRI proved 100% sensitive for the identification of the five cases of EA/TEF.[61] The MRI criterion for EA/TEF in this series was nonvisualization of the intrathoracic portion of the esophagus. In another study, however, fetal MRI for suspected chest lesions did not visualize the esophagus in 54 of 85 (64%) examinations.[59]

Postnatal Diagnosis

When pregnancy was complicated by polyhydramnios, free passage through the esophagus should be tested with a nasogastric tube. The same holds true when the child presents with anomalies that fit in the VACTERL association (e.g., radial aplasia).

As EA prevents the passage of saliva down the esophagus, saliva accumulates in the proximal esophagus and mouth. Salivation is obvious and the child exhales through the saliva so that bubbles are formed. Under such circumstances, feeding should be withheld and esophageal continuity tested. This is best done with a stiff, wide 10-Fr catheter inserted through the nose or, in case of choanal atresia, the mouth. In EA, the catheter will stop about 12 cm from the nostrils. A plain radiograph of the chest and abdomen will show the tip of the catheter arrested in the superior mediastinum (T2-T4) (Fig. 27-2). Often, the dilated upper esophageal pouch is well visualized by the air it contains. Gas in the stomach signifies the presence of a distal TEF. Note that the catheter must be a stiff one. Otherwise it may curl up in the upper esophagus and the findings be confused with those of EA. On the other hand, the diagnosis of EA should be questioned when the tip of the catheter passes beyond the carina. Traumatic perforation of the

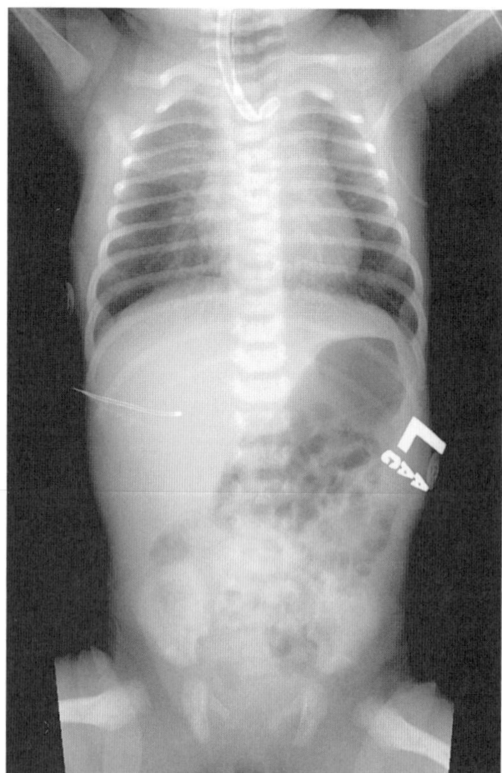

Figure 27-2. This plain radiograph depicts the classic features seen in an infant with EA and TEF. A nasoesophageal tube is seen in the upper pouch and has kinked a little at the end of the pouch. There is air in the stomach and bowel, which signifies the presence of a distal TEF.

esophagus, causing an esophageal pseudodiverticulum, may also lead to the misdiagnosis of EA.[62,63] Rarely, a catheter can descend through the trachea and distal fistula into the stomach.

Radiographs may reveal associated anomalies such as vertebral and rib anomalies or duodenal atresia (Fig. 27-3) . The absence of air in the stomach points to EA without distal fistula (see Fig. 27-3A). Mediastinal ultrasonography has been suggested as a helpful adjunct in the diagnosis of pure EA.[64]

Surprisingly, the length of the esophageal gap is usually not known preoperatively. Absence of air in the stomach has been linked with a long gap, but has also been described in association with a distal fistula occluded with mucus.[16] Even in true long-gap EA (atresia without distal fistula), the gap length varies. It can be measured radiologically, either with metal bougies or with a contrast agent at the time of the gastrostomy. Note that the amount of pressure on the metal bougies will affect the distance measurement. In one report, operative management was linked to the measured length of the gap: less than two vertebrae, then primary anastomosis; two to six vertebrae, then delayed primary anastomosis; more than six vertebrae, then esophageal replacement.[65] A long gap in EA/TEF has been associated with azygos vein anomalies and with the presence of 13 rib pairs.[47,66] Others have not substantiated these relationships.

In EA/TEF, a longer gap between the two esophageal ends should be expected when the distal fistula arises from the carina. The longest gaps in EA with distal fistula are seen in patients with the distal fistula originating from the carina in combination with a short proximal esophageal pouch. It is customary to push on the nasoesophageal catheter when the first chest film is made. However, this maneuver may lead to the wrong impression that a rather long proximal pouch is present. Using contrast radiographs to delineate the upper pouch is certainly more accurate but this can result in aspiration of contrast material. Even when the distance is relatively well assessed preoperatively by means of contrast imaging of the proximal pouch in combination with tracheoscopy for identification of the origin of the distal fistula, other factors may affect

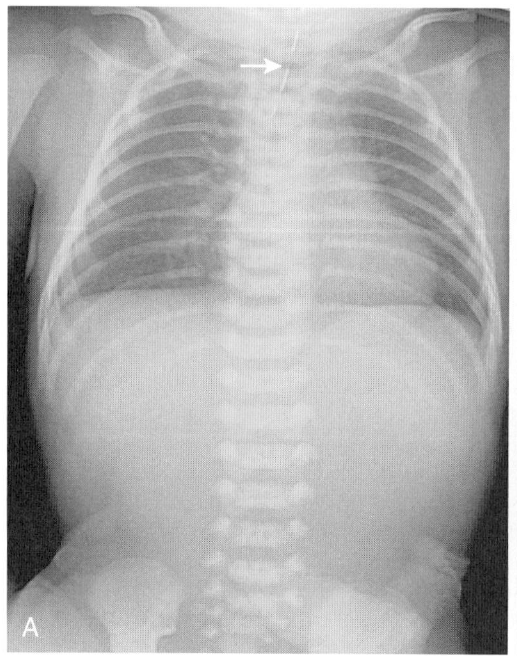

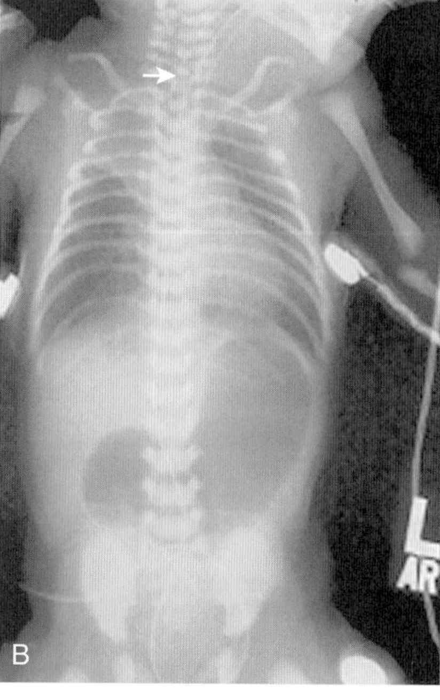

Figure 27-3. These two radiographs depict less common presentations of EA. **A,** Isolated EA. The nasoesophageal tube (*arrow*) is seen in the proximal pouch. There is no air in the gastrointestinal tract. **B,** This patient has EA with distal TEF and duodenal atresia and has been endotracheally intubated. A nasoesophageal catheter (*arrow*) sits in the upper esophageal pouch. An endotracheal tube is also seen. The stomach and bulbous duodenum are distended with air but no air is seen distal to the duodenum.

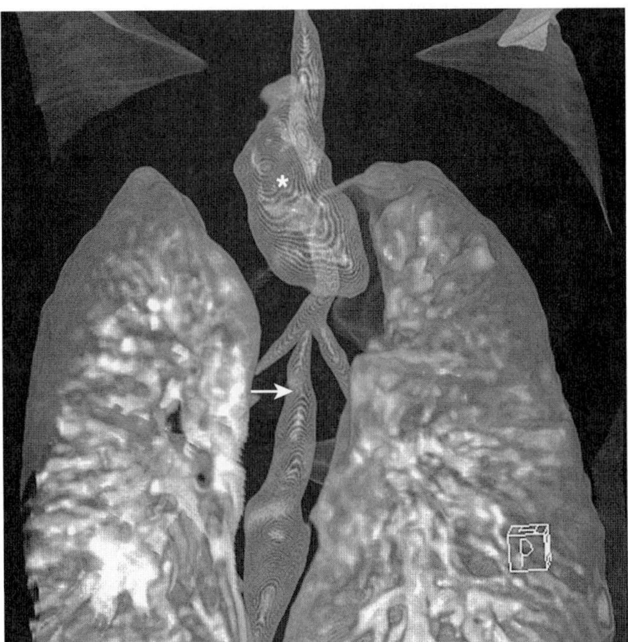

Figure 27-4. This preoperative CT scan reconstruction shows EA with a distal TEF. The distal TEF (*arrow*) originates at the carina. The upper esophageal pouch is very dilated (*asterisk*). The distance between the upper pouch and lower esophagus is relatively short.

the surgical plan. Ultrasonography may reveal cardiac and/or aortic arch anomalies. A right descending aorta, which occurs in about 2.5% of the cases, makes a left-sided thoracic approach preferable.[67,68] Renal ultrasound images and spine radiographs should be obtained as well. Because EA may be part of a syndrome, consultation by a geneticist is recommended.

There is little doubt that better preoperative imaging of the neck and chest would allow for better preoperative planning. At present, two imaging modalities are available: CT and MRI. Although MRI would certainly be preferable for its absence of radiation exposure, it requires general anesthesia. On the other hand, MRI is better for diagnosing cardiac and aortic arch anomalies,[69] CT has been done in children with EA/TEF (Fig. 27-4).[70-73]

MANAGEMENT

Preoperative Management

Once the diagnosis of EA has been established, the child is taken to a pediatric surgical center in a transport incubator. A double-lumen 10-Fr suction tube is placed in the upper esophagus and set to continuous suction.[74] The child is in a head-up position and on his or her side. Intravenous access is important, and the vital signs are monitored.

If the child is in respiratory distress, endotracheal intubation and ventilation may be needed. Forceful ventilation will overdistend the stomach, causing diaphragmatic splinting and even gastric rupture.[75,76] Gentle low-pressure ventilation is therefore essential. Alternatively, high-frequency ventilation should be attempted, but emergency ligation of the fistula may be lifesaving.[65,76,77] After ligation of the fistula only, a delayed primary anastomosis should not be postponed longer than 7 to 14 days because recanalization is likely to occur.[65,78,79]

Generally, the operative treatment of an EA/TEF is not regarded as an emergency procedure. Thus, there is time to confirm the diagnosis in the pediatric surgical center and to assess for associated anomalies.

OPERATIVE REPAIR

Esophageal Atresia with Distal Fistula

The operation can be performed through a thoracotomy or using a thoracoscopic approach. The side of entrance to the chest is opposite the turn of the aortic arch: right for a left descending aorta, left for a right descending aorta. If a right-sided aortic arch is not detected until surgery has begun, change to the left side is appropriate if the thoracoscopic approach has been chosen. If a thoracotomy has been performed, an anastomosis from the right should be attempted but has a higher morbidity in this setting.[67,68] The operation is performed with the patient under general anesthesia and with adequate venous access. A right radial artery arterial line is beneficial for monitoring the pH and blood gases, especially during a thoracoscopic approach under CO_2 pneumothorax.

Laryngotracheobronchoscopy

The value of routine preoperative laryngotracheobronchoscopy is much debated because the incidence of the combination of a proximal and distal fistula is less than 1%.[65] With the availability of small-diameter flexible fiberscopes, tracheobronchoscopy can now be performed after intubation through the endotracheal tube.[80,81] Forceful ventilation must be avoided, not only to prevent lung damage[82] but also to prevent gastric distention and perforation of the stomach by insufflation through the distal fistula.[75,76,83] Laryngotracheobronchoscopy may reveal abnormalities such as a laryngotracheoesophageal cleft, tracheal stenosis, or a tracheal bronchus to the right upper lobe. The entrance of the distal fistula is usually well seen (Fig. 27-5). Its distance to the carina provides a clue as to the gap between the esophageal segments: the closer the fistula is to the carina, the longer the distance. An indication of the severity of tracheomalacia is only possible when the child is breathing spontaneously. Even then, it remains difficult to predict the severity.

Positioning the Tip of the Endotracheal Tube

If possible, the tip of the endotracheal tube (ET) is positioned more distally than the origin of the TEF.[84-87] This is quite feasible when the distal fistula originates

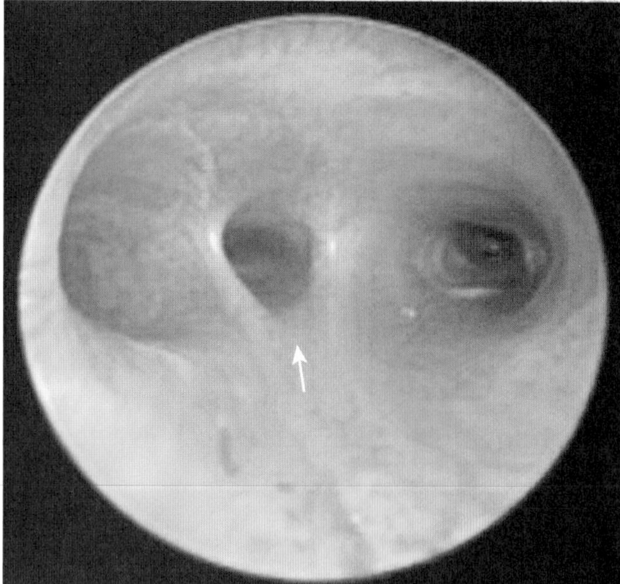

Figure 27-5. At bronchoscopy, the distal TEF (*arrow*) is seen at the carina. It is usually found between the midtrachea and carina.

at a distance well proximal to the carina. Still, in a series of 149 patients with EA/TEF, tracheobronchoscopy revealed that 2 of the 154 fistulas were bronchial, 15 carinal, 34 just 1 cm proximal to the carina, 91 halfway up the trachea, and 12 cervical.[88] On the other hand, when the fistula originates too close to the carina, the slightest movement may cause the ET tip to enter the distal fistula or one of the main-stem bronchi. Inadvertent entrance of the ET into the right main-stem bronchus is especially troublesome during a right thoracoscopic operation. An appropriate depth for the tip of the tube can be predicted by measurements taken during the laryngotracheobronchoscopy, if performed. Preoperative flexible bronchoscopy through the tube is ideal when the diameter of the ET allows passage of the flexible scope. However, identifying a proximal fistula is more difficult because the ET may be occluding it. Moreover, a proximal fistula with a distal fistula is rare. Nevertheless, there are several reports describing proximal fistulas that were missed and caused significant morbidity.[89,90]

Repair through Thoracotomy

In case of a left descending aorta, the child is placed in a true left lateral decubitus position close to the right edge of a shortened operating table. A small pad is placed underneath the chest to open the right-sided intercostal spaces. The surgeon stands to the right of the patient with the assistant opposite. In case of a right descending aorta, the child is placed in a right lateral decubitus position close to the left edge of the table. The surgeon then stands on the left with the assistant on the right of the table. In case the chest is opened on the right and a right descending aorta is encountered, the esophagus can be repaired to the right of the aortic arch. However, in this situation, there is a higher anastomotic leak rate.[67]

The patient's arm is positioned over the head (Fig. 27-6). Suction is removed from the Replogle tube, but the tube is left in place so that it can be advanced during the operation to make identification of the proximal pouch easier.

A slightly curved 4- to 5-cm long incision is made 1 cm below the inferior tip of the scapula. With the use of a muscle-sparing approach, the auscultatory triangle is opened and the muscles are retracted (i.e., the latissimus dorsi posteriorly and the serratus anterior anteriorly).[91] If the serratus muscle needs to be transected, this should be done as low as possible to preserve the long thoracic nerve. The fourth or fifth intercostal space is then entered.

An extrapleural approach has been suggested to protect the pleural space in case of an anastomotic leak, but there is no evidence that it is better than a transpleural one.[92,93] In the extrapleural approach, the pleura is gently pushed away from the endothoracic fascia, first in the middle of the incision so that an infant rib spreader can be inserted and opened (see Fig. 27-6B). With the rib spreader opened even farther, the pleura is carefully pushed away posteriorly until the posterior mediastinum is exposed.

The distal fistula may start from the trachea directly underneath the azygos vein, in which case the azygos vein is transected between 3-0 or 4-0 absorbable ligatures (Fig. 27-7). If the distal fistula originates more cephalad on the trachea, the vein can be left intact. Recently, a relationship between azygos vein transection and anastomotic leak has been suggested.[94,95] Rarely, there is an azygos lobe in which the azygos vein loops anteriorly and causes a fissure in the upper lung lobe. An extrapleural approach then becomes more difficult unless the anomaly is recognized and the vein divided.[96]

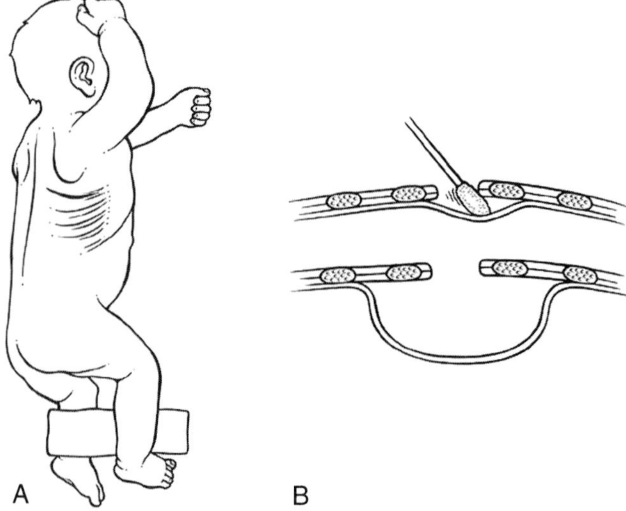

Figure 27-6. A, The infant is positioned for a right thoracotomy. The ipsilateral arm is positioned over the head of the patient. A 4- to 5-cm incision is made 1 cm below the tip of the scapula. **B,** This schematic depicts a peanut or sterile cotton swab being used to gently push the pleura away from the chest wall.

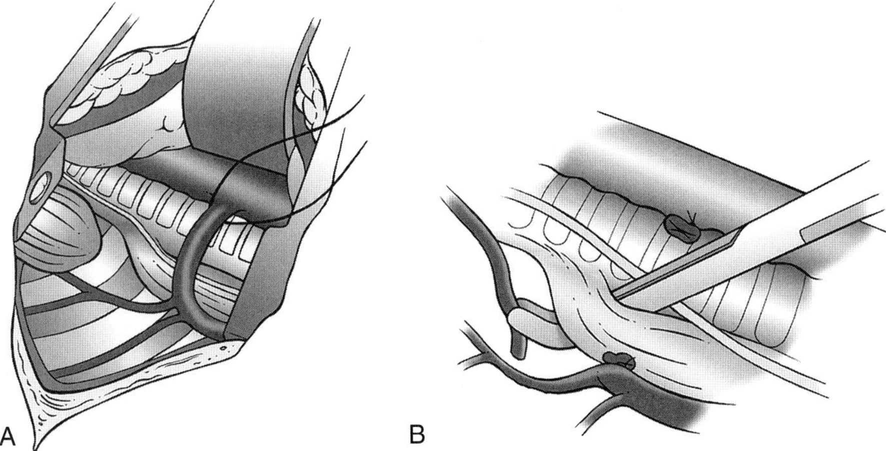

Figure 27-7. **A,** Ligation of the azygos vein. **B,** The distal fistula is being mobilized from its insertion in the trachea.

The distal esophagus is usually easily found because it looks fleshy with the glittering vagal nerve lying over it. The origin of the distal fistula is usually easy to find as the trachea and adjacent esophagus distend during each inspiration. The fistula should be dissected and mobilized close to the trachea, which will spare as many vagal nerve branches as possible (see Fig. 27-7B). The fistula can be encircled with a vessel loop. There are several ways of closing the fistula on the tracheal side. Ligation in continuity[97] can result in a higher recanalization rate.[78,79,98] To avoid slipping of the ligature on the tracheal side, a suture can be placed through the muscular layer of the upper corner of the fistula, after which the fistula is encircled, tied, and transected a few millimeters distally. This can be done with a 5-0 absorbable suture. Alternatively, the upper and lower corners of the fistula can be marked with a traction suture and the fistula is transected. The remaining hole in the trachea is then closed with interrupted 5-0 absorbable sutures. This closure can be checked by irrigating with warm water and applying a higher ventilation pressure to assess for an air leak.

The proximal esophagus is easily identified by asking the anesthesiologist to push on the Replogle tube. A traction suture, taking a good bite of the muscular wall, is placed in the most distal part of the proximal pouch (Fig. 27-8). The proximal pouch can easily be freed posteriorly and laterally by blunt dissection. Behind the trachea, however, the pouch may be strongly adherent. Usually, it is dissected sharply, staying on the esophageal side to avoid entrance into the trachea. Extensive dissection is not warranted, however, because this may damage the tracheal or esophageal walls and may interfere with innervation to the upper esophagus.[99] It has been documented that the recurrent laryngeal nerve gives motor branches to the upper esophagus. Extensive dissection of the proximal pouch searching for a proximal fistula should not be performed routinely because the incidence of a proximal fistula in combination with a distal one is only about 1%. If a proximal fistula is present, it is usually of the H-type. If missed at birth and diagnosed after repair of the atresia, it can be repaired through the neck at a later date. If the trachea is opened during the dissection of the proximal pouch, one should be wary that a proximal fistula may have been opened as well. There is no common wall between the trachea and esophagus.

The distal end of the proximal pouch is now opened by amputating the most distal muscular wall together with the traction suture so that the mucosa becomes visible. The mucosa is then opened.

An end-to-end anastomosis is performed with 5-0 absorbable sutures starting in the middle of the back wall of the two esophageal segments (Fig. 27-9). It is important to include both the mucosa and the muscular wall with each suture. The sutures in the back part of the anastomosis are tied on the inside. Then the front part of the anastomosis is performed with sutures tied on the outside. Before finishing the anastomosis, a 6-Fr nasogastric tube is passed into the stomach until the esophagus stretches. The tube is then withdrawn to

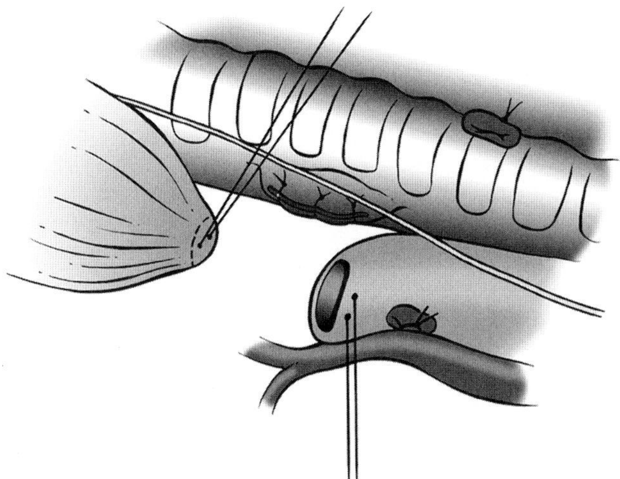

Figure 27-8. Dissection of the proximal esophageal pouch. A traction suture has been placed in the distal end of the upper pouch, which is freed posteriorly and laterally. Freeing of the upper esophageal pouch from the trachea should not be extensive because this is usually not needed. The distal tip of the upper esophagus containing the traction suture is then amputated. The distal TEF has been divided.

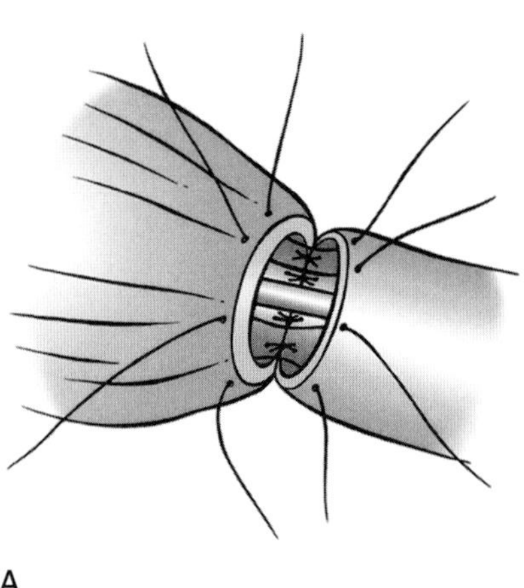

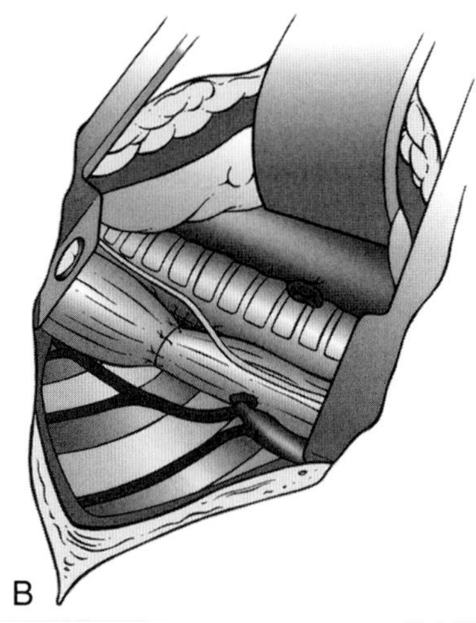

Figure 27-9. Esophageal anastomosis. **A,** The back wall of the anastomosis has been sutured from the inside, and a small nasogastric tube has been passed through the anastomosis. The front part of the anastomosis is being sutured with knots on the outside. **B,** Completed anastomosis.

release the esophageal tension. The stomach contents are aspirated. Care is taken not to accidentally withdraw the tube entirely.

A chest drain is not routinely utilized.[100,101] A small nasogastric tube is inserted until the very end of the closure of the chest, enabling the removal of residual air. When a trans-rib approach is used, the periosteum should be closed in layers with fine but strong absorbable sutures. If repaired properly, the ribs will heal nicely. When an intercostal approach has been used, the adjacent two ribs should be approximated with one 3-0 absorbable suture. These sutures should be tied gently so that the intercostal space is not obliterated. The subcutis can be co-apted with a few absorbable sutures, and the skin is closed with adhesive strips.

Thoracoscopic Repair

There are several retrospective reports describing experience with the thoracoscopic approach.[102-106] The child is positioned in a true left lateral decubitus position close to the left edge of a shortened operating table in an infant with a left descending aorta (Fig. 27-10). A pad is placed underneath the chest to widen the right-sided intercostal spaces. The table is turned 15 degrees reverse Trendelenburg and 15 degrees tilt to the left. Thus, the lung will fall caudad and inferiorly by gravity once CO_2 is insufflated. The right arm is positioned over the head. The Replogle tube is released but left in place for later identification of the upper pouch. The surgeon stands to the left of the table with the camera person to his or her left and the scrub nurse at the opposite lower side of the table. The screen is at the level of the infant's right shoulder. An infant with a right descending aorta is placed in a right lateral decubitus position close to the right edge of the table. The surgeon is then on the right of the table with the screen at the level of the left shoulder.

The first cannula is inserted 1 cm distal and anterior to the tip of the scapula (Fig. 27-11). This is performed with an open technique. A small incision is made in the direction of the skin folds. With a small clamp, a small opening is made parallel with the upper border of the rib. When loss of resistance is reached, a cannula with a blunt trocar is inserted. The sleeve of the cannula is sutured to the intercostal musculature. In infants larger than 2 kg, a 6-mm cannula with a 5-mm, 30-degree, 24-cm-long telescope is used. In infants smaller than 2 kg, a 3.8-mm cannula with a 3.3-mm, 30-degree, 24-cm-long telescope is used.

After creation of the working space, two 3.5-mm cannulas are inserted under endoscopic visualization, one more cephalad in the midaxilla and one more

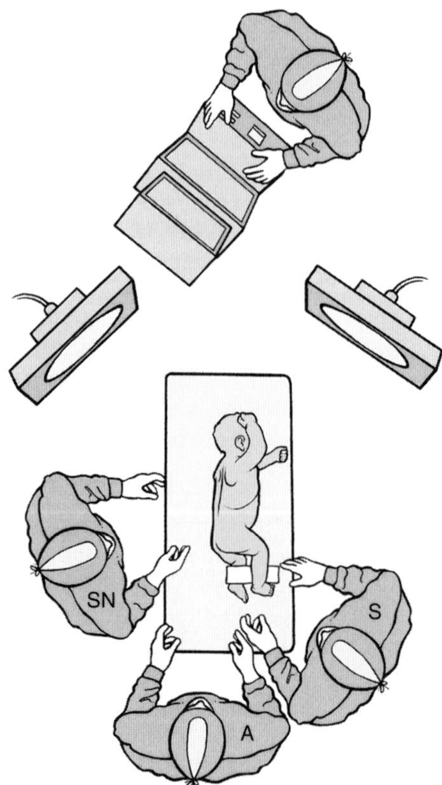

Figure 27-10. This infant is positioned for right thoracoscopic repair. The surgeon (S) stands on the left side of the operating table when the aortic arch turns to the left. The surgeon, operative field, and screen are in line. The assistant (A) is situated to the left of the surgeon when the surgeon is right-handed. The scrub nurse (SN) stands to the right of the operating table.

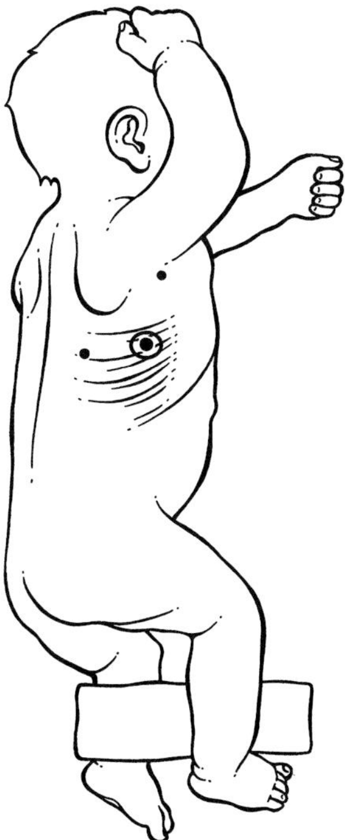

Figure 27-11. Cannula position for thoracoscopic repair. The cannulas are inserted in triangulation. The telescope cannula (*circle and dot*) is inserted 1 cm below the inferior angle of the scapula and slightly anterior. One working cannula is inserted in the midaxillary line in the axilla. The second working cannula is introduced at the level of the telescope cannula but more posteriorly on the chest wall.

posteriorly behind the scapula. Two 3-mm, 20-cm-long working instruments are introduced through these ports. A lung retractor is usually not needed.

One-lung ventilation in neonates can be achieved with the use of a bronchial blocker.[107-109] An alternative approach is midtracheal intubation in conjunction with CO_2 pneumothorax. After insertion of the first cannula and telescopic verification that the cannula is in the thorax, CO_2 insufflation is started with a flow of 0.1 L/min and a pressure of 5 mm Hg. Initial desaturation is the rule. CO_2 pneumothorax is then released but is restarted when the anesthesiologist agrees. Adaptation of the ventilator settings, especially increasing the ventilation rate, is usually effective in reaching a steady state. This usually occurs after 5 to 10 minutes. End-tidal CO_2 is not reliable, and arterial blood gases should be monitored regularly.[85,110-112] How much acidosis that can be accepted is not known. Nevertheless, case reports have demonstrated that EA repair is tolerated even in neonates with complex cardiac conditions.[113,114]

When the fistula departs from the trachea above the azygos vein, this area will distend with each ventilation. In this case there is no need to divide the azygos vein. The anesthesiologist is asked to push on the Replogle tube. Dissection is started by opening the pleura between the upper pouch and the spinal column in a longitudinal direction. The upper pouch is dissected posteriorly and laterally but not in front, as explained earlier (Fig. 27-12).

The fistula is now dissected close to its entrance in the trachea. A 10-cm-long, 5-0 Vicryl (Ethicon, Inc., Somerville, NJ) suture on a V18 needle is introduced through the axillary cannula and is placed through the upper muscular edge of the fistula. The suture is tied, brought around the fistula, and tied again (see Fig. 27-12B). The fistula is then transected a few millimeters distal to the tie. The distal end of the fistula will retract but can be easily found later. If the entrance of the fistula in the trachea is behind the azygos vein, the vein should be divided. This can easily be done between ligatures or monopolar hook coagulation. The vein is coagulated on both sides of the initial coagulation site and transected in the middle. The fistula is then mobilized as described for the open approach.

The Replogle tube is pushed down so that the lowest point of the pouch can be identified. This point is opened with hook diathermy. The defect is then opened farther with scissors. The hole should be large enough so as to prevent stenosis. A 10-cm-long, 5-0 Vicryl suture on a V18 needle is introduced, and the first suture is placed in the middle of the back wall of the upper esophageal pouch, starting from the inside. The needle is then placed in the middle of the back wall of the distal esophagus. If a considerable distance needs to be bridged, a tumbled flat knot is made and glided until both walls appose (see Fig. 27-12C). Further sutures are placed in the back wall of the upper and lower esophagus. The knots are tied on the inside. The front part of the anastomosis is performed with the knots on the outside. Before completing the anastomosis a 6-Fr nasogastric tube is inserted, as described earlier.

A drain is not usually left. The cannulas are removed and so is residual CO_2. The port sites do not need suturing, and adhesive tape for the skin will suffice.

Wide Gap Esophageal Atresia with Distal Fistula

In almost all cases of EA with distal fistula, an anastomosis can be made. Paralysis and ventilation for 5 days have been advocated if the anastomosis is very tense.[115-118] The effectiveness of this strategy should be questioned, however, because the tensile strength of an anastomosis at 5 days is low. When the fistula originates at the carina, the distance may occasionally be too long for making a simple anastomosis.[88,119] Likewise, a short upper esophageal pouch may preclude a primary anastomosis.[120] Various maneuvers have been described to overcome this problem (Table 27-1).

Esophageal Atresia without Distal Fistula

Initial Treatment

An airless abdomen is the signature of EA without distal fistula. Very rarely, a blocked distal fistula is responsible for the airlessness of the abdomen.[16] One should be aware that the incidence of a proximal fistula, in the absence of a distal fistula, is relatively high. In

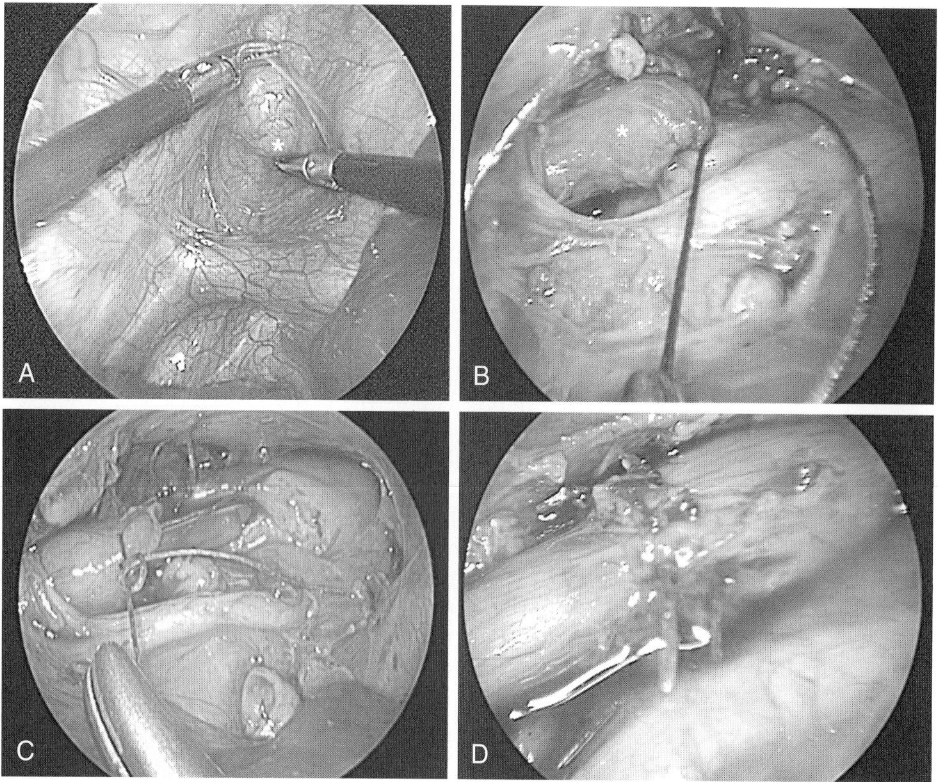

Figure 27-12. Thoracoscopic approach. **A,** Proximal pouch (*asterisk*) dissection is seen. **B,** The distal fistula (*asterisk*) has been isolated close to the trachea and is being suture ligated. **C,** The back wall of the esophageal anastomosis has been finished with interrupted sutures knotted on the inside. The front part of the anastomosis is being performed using a tumbled square knot. A nasogastric tube can be seen in this photograph. **D,** Completed anastomosis.

one series of EA without distal fistula, the incidence of an upper pouch fistula even exceeded 50%.[14] A proximal fistula in EA without distal fistula is of the H-type, running from a more cranial tracheal position to a more caudal esophageal position. It is usually located at the thoracic inlet.

The initial treatment is a gastrostomy with laryngotracheobronchoscopy during the same anesthesia, aimed at ruling out a proximal fistula and other associated anomalies. In EA without a distal fistula and in the absence of a duodenal obstruction, the stomach is usually small. It may be difficult to bring the anterior gastric wall against the abdominal wall. Sometimes, even the shortest distance to the anterior wall cannot be bridged. In this situation, part of the gastrostomy tube is allowed to traverse the peritoneal cavity.[121] A siliconized urinary catheter of appropriate size (8 or 10 Fr) is inserted through the abdominal wall and into the stomach through a small gastrotomy. The balloon is filled with 1 mL only. Initial feeding should be with small quantities. The gastrostomy balloon must not be placed too close to the pylorus because this may cause distal obstruction.

Esophageal Reconstruction

The first question that arises is the timing of the esophageal reconstruction. This moment will depend on the gap length to be bridged. A period of around 12 weeks is often suggested.[65,122,123]

During this waiting period, the proximal esophagus is emptied by continuous suction on a transnasally placed 10-Fr Replogle tube. The tube can get obstructed and should be replaced regularly. Moreover, insertion should be occasionally changed from the one nostril to the other to avoid damage. If the child shows persisting respiratory problems, a proximal fistula should be searched for again. If possible, the proximal fistula should be closed at the time of the esophageal reconstruction. Severe respiratory problems may be a reason, however, to perform the esophageal reconstruction, including division of the fistula, at an earlier time. An alternative is cervical esophagostomy, but this may jeopardize the ability to perform a primary anastomosis in the future. Traditionally, the cervical esophagostomy is done on the left, but there is no good reason why this could not be done from the right. Home care during the waiting period has been advocated, but most of the reported patients have required a long time in the hospital before they were sent home for further observation.[124,125]

The gap between esophageal segments is usually expressed in terms of the number of vertebral bodies, thus taking the child's length into account. The residual gap to be bridged should be periodically measured. This can be done with a simultaneous contrast study of the upper and lower esophagus or by simultaneous insertion of a metal bougie transorally into the upper esophagus and through the gastrostomy into the lower esophagus. The metal bougie ends should overlap before attempting a primary anastomosis.

If an attempt at reconstruction is planned at 3 months of age, the surgeon should proceed according to the preoperative estimation of the feasibility of performing a primary anastomosis. Several techniques to lengthen the native esophagus have been described, such as esophageal myotomy or extensive mobilization

Table 27-1 Maneuvers for Lengthening the Esophagus in Long-Gap Esophageal Atresia*

***Nonoperative Maneuvers* (in combination with delayed primary anastomosis)**
Spontaneous growth[122]
Bougienage
Proximal[227,228]
Proximal and distal[229]
Magnetic[230]
Operative Measures
Using the native esophagus
Upper pouch mobilization
Myotomy of the upper pouch[231]
Flap lengthening of the upper pouch[232,233]
Multistaged extrathoracic elongation of the proximal pouch[234]
Using thoracoscopy[235]
Lower pouch mobilization[236,237]
Myotomy of the lower pouch[238]
Myotomy of the upper and lower pouch[239]
Traction sutures[240,241]
Thoracoscopic placement[126]
Transluminal thread with olives[242,243]
Thoracoscopic assistance[235]
Lower pouch hydrostatic distention[244]
Elongation of the lesser curvature[245,246]
Using esophageal replacement
Colon[247]
Stomach
Tube[248,249]
Transposition[250]
Laparoscopic assistance[251]
Jejunum
Pedicle graft[252,253]
Free graft[254]
Ileum[255]

*See references for further information.

of the proximal and even distal esophagus (see Table 27-1). There is little doubt that all these maneuvers damage the esophagus and that their long-term results may be less than optimal. If a delayed primary anastomosis with or without lengthening is not feasible, an alternative procedure is indicated, such as a gastric pull-up or a jejunal, ileal, or colonic interposition (see Table 27-1).

Thoracoscopy is ideal to have a look at the gap length to be bridged (Fig. 27-13). Moreover, the ends can be dissected and mobilized thoracoscopically. An anastomosis can be performed thoracoscopically as well. Also, a thoracoscopic Foker procedure can be accomplished.[126]

Postoperative Management

Mechanical ventilation with muscle relaxation for 5 days has been advocated after an anastomosis is performed under considerable tension.[115-118] Again, evidence for the effectiveness of this approach is lacking.[127] A chest drain is needed only when there is considerable doubt regarding the quality of the anastomosis.[101] Feeding can be started early through the nasogastric tube, which is the main reason for leaving such a tube. When sialorrhea ceases, oral feeding can be started. The child can then be fed ad libitum. If the child is doing well, there is no need for a routine imaging study of the esophagus postoperatively.[128]

COMPLICATIONS

Anastomotic Leaks

An overall leak rate of 17% has been reported by several authors.[9,128,129] Major leaks occur much less frequently—3.5% in the first study[128] and 4.5% in the more recent one,[129] which confirms the statement that most leaks are minor. Two series reported a much lower leak rate of, respectively, 6% and 7%.[5,8] In the largest thoracoscopic report, the leak rate was 7.6%.[104] Published reports often include all types of EA and do not always mention whether the leak was detected at routine esophagography only.

Anastomotic Stricture

As with anastomotic leaks, no uniform definition is used for anastomotic stricture. It has been defined as a narrowing of more than 50% of the lumen[130] or as a narrowing detected on a contrast study or at esophagoscopy in combination with symptoms.[131] Reported incidences range from 17%,[128] 36%,[8] 40%,[132] 41%,[133] to 59%.[5] Four of 104 patients (3.8%) undergoing thoracoscopic repair developed a stricture, which was defined on the initial esophagogram.[104] Routine dilatation is certainly not indicated because many patients never require dilatation.[133] Anastomotic tension, anastomotic leakage, and gastroesophageal reflux[134-137] have been implicated as risk factors. Strictures usually respond well to dilation. Resection of the stricture is rarely required. Balloon dilatation seems superior, but there is no hard evidence.[130]

Recurrent Tracheoesophageal Fistula

The reported incidence of recurrent TEF varies between 3% and 15%. In one study, the 10% incidence in the period 1986 to 1995 had dropped to 5% in the period 1996 to 2005.[5] In another study, it had dropped from 17% before 1980 to 3% in the period 1990 to 1999.[8] Yet another study reported a similar recurrence incidence of 3%.[128] In the 104 patients in one thoracoscopic series, 2 (1.9%) developed recurrent TEFs.[104]

A recurrent fistula is suspected when the child starts to cough during feeding, has apneic or cyanotic episodes, or has repeat respiratory infections. Often the abdomen is distended with air. On a chest film there may be signs of pneumonia. Sometimes, an air-filled esophagus is seen. The diagnosis can sometimes be made by video-esophagography using a water-soluble contrast medium (Fig. 27-14). Bronchoscopy confirms

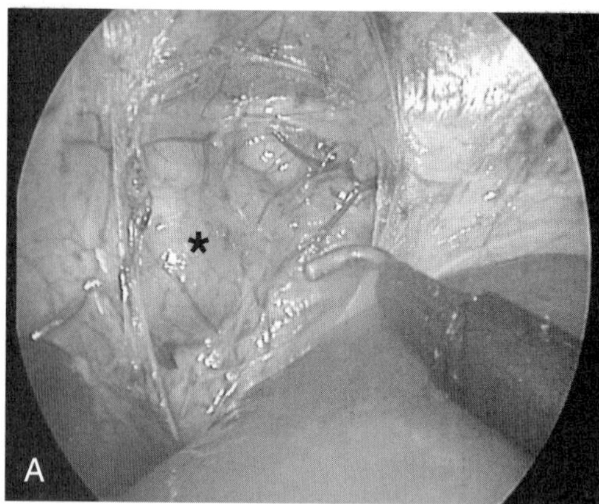

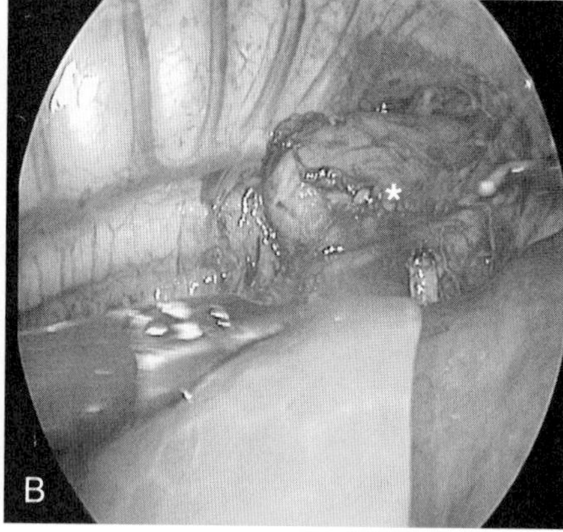

Figure 27-13. Thoracoscopic view of esophageal atresia without fistula in a 3-month old neonate. **A,** The short distal esophageal segment (*asterisk*) is seen in the inferior portion of the mediastinum. **B,** The proximal pouch (*asterisk*) reaches to the azygos vein, which has been coagulated and transected.

the diagnosis. While pressing on the stomach, the fistula may open and become clearly visible. Alternatively, a small catheter may be fed into it. Several tracheoscopic treatment possibilities have been tried, such as electrocoagulation of the trajectory and injection of TissueCol (Baxter, Deerfield, IL)[138] or plugging of the fistula with Surgisis (Cook, Inc., Bloomington, IN) (Fig. 27-15).[139] Use of a laser, in combination with TissueCol, is another option.[140] Should these attempts fail, surgery should be considered, either with an open or thoracoscopic approach.

Prevention of a recurrent TEF can be difficult. Interposition of tissue between the tracheal closure and esophageal anastomosis has been advocated for this purpose. Native tissue such as pleura or pericardium can be used. Recently, a report described interposing Surgisis between the trachea and esophagus to help prevent a recurrent TEF (Fig. 27-16).[141]

Tracheomalacia

Tracheomalacia is defined as a generalized or localized weakness of the trachea that allows the anterior and posterior walls to come together during expiration or coughing.[15] The area of collapse is usually restricted to the region of the fistula. In one series, autopsy revealed structural abnormalities of the trachea in 75% of infants with EA/TEF.[142] The cartilage of the rings is softened, and the length of the transverse muscle is increased. As a result, the airway collapses during expiration, which produces expiratory stridor varying from a hoarse barking cough to acute life-threatening incidents of cyanosis or apnea.[143] In EA without fistula, tracheomalacia does not seem to occur very often,[144] which questions whether upper esophagus dilatation is really a causative factor. Tracheomalacia is implicated in the pathogenesis of reactive airway disease in patients with EA/TEF.

Symptoms vary from mild to life-threatening apneic spells. Severe symptoms usually appear when the child

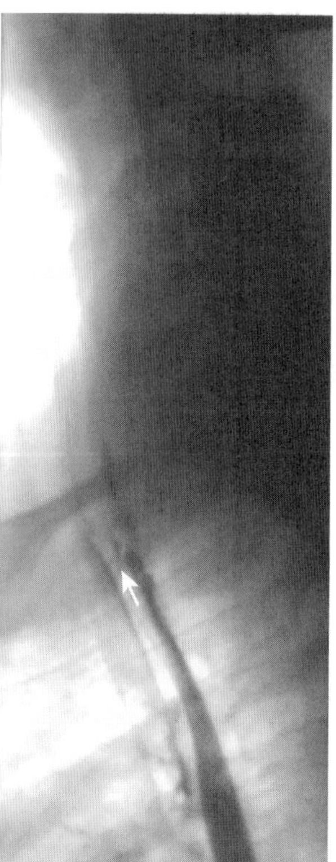

Figure 27-14. On this water-soluble contrast study, a recurrent TEF (*arrow*) is seen.

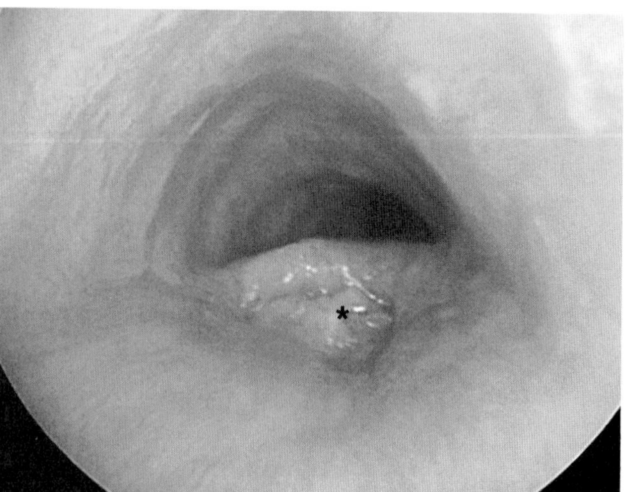

Figure 27-15. This bronchoscopic view shows Surgisis (*asterisk*) placed into a recurrent TEF. In this patient, the fistula was successfully occluded using this technique.

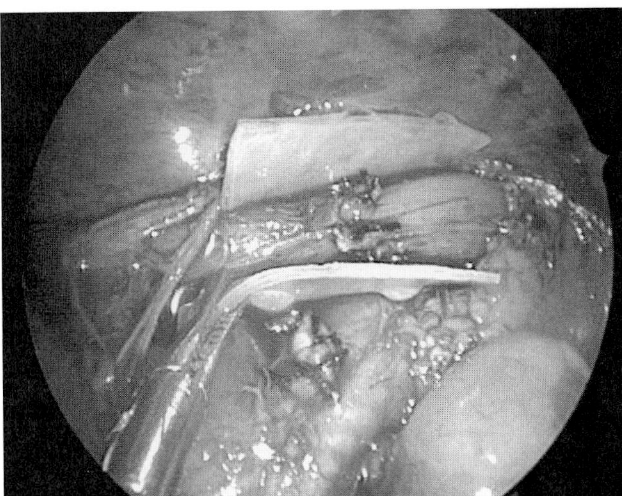

Figure 27-16. After thoracoscopic repair of esophageal atresia and distal fistula in this infant, Surgisis was interposed between the tracheal closure and esophageal anastomosis to help prevent a recurrent TEF. (From St. Peter SD, Calkins CM, Holcomb GW III: The use of biosynthetic mesh to separate the anastomoses during the thoracoscopic repair of esophageal atresia and tracheoesophageal fistula. J Laparoendosc Adv Surg Tech 17:380-382, 2007. Reprinted with permission.)

is a few months old. The diagnosis is confirmed by tracheobronchoscopy. In patients with EA/TEF, it is often difficult to clinically distinguish these symptoms from those of a recurrent fistula, an anastomotic stricture, or gastroesophageal reflux.[145]

Treatment is required in the severely symptomatic form of tracheomalacia. The therapy of choice is aortopexy.[143,146,147] The principle behind this operation is that the ascending aorta and arch are suspended against the posterior surface of the sternum. By doing so, the anterior wall of the trachea, which is loosely attached to the aorta, is suspended as well. This aortic suspension opens the tracheal lumen.[143] If the anterior aorta cannot reach the posterior sternum, a pericardial flap based at the aortic root can be fashioned.[148,149] Aortopexy is classically performed through a left anterolateral thoracotomy or median sternotomy[147,150] but can also be performed through a low cervical incision and partial sternal split[151] or thoracoscopically either from the left[152,153] or from the right.[154] It is best to check the effect of the suspension during the operation by simultaneous tracheoscopy.

Disordered Peristalsis/ Gastroesophageal Reflux

Disturbed motility of the esophagus in EA patients has been recognized for a long time.[155-157] Many adolescents and adults, operated on at birth for an EA with distal fistula and who considered themselves healthy, show symptoms of esophageal dysfunction, including dysphagia, episodes of foreign body impaction, heartburn, vomiting, and various respiratory disorders.[158] Similar findings were reported in another study as well.[159] Foreign body obstruction has been reported with an incidence of 13% in this study population.[160]

The oral phase of swallowing is normal, but the pharyngeal and esophageal phases are abnormal in all patients, both at video-fluoroscopy[161,162] and with manometry.[163-165] It is doubtful there are patients with normal peristalsis.

Whether the cause of these disturbed motility problems is congenital or acquired has been a long-standing debate. Preoperative simultaneous manometry in the upper and lower pouch in two children with EA without fistula revealed coordinated contractions in both the upper and lower esophagus on swallowing and a reflex relaxation of the lower esophageal sphincter.[166] Postoperatively, it revealed simultaneous, instead of coordinated, contractions in the repaired esophagus with only partial relaxation of the lower esophageal sphincter. These findings seem to favor the hypothesis that the motility disturbance is caused by surgical damage. Subsequently, the same authors confirmed their observations experimentally in a dog model.[166,167] A dissection study on autopsy material of EA patients also supports the hypothesis of surgical damage.[99] In the Adriamycin-induced EA rat model, however, a deficient extrinsic and intrinsic nerve plexus in the lower esophagus is present.[168,169] Achalasia-like dysmotility in EA has also been reported.[170]

Whatever the cause for the disturbed motility in patients with corrected EA, it brings several problems, not the least of which is gastroesophageal reflux (GER). Whereas GER in otherwise normal children has a tendency to improve during the first year of life, it does not improve in individuals with corrected EA, not even after several decades.[158] The incidence of significant reflux in patients with EA has been stated to be 40%, and about half will require antireflux surgery.[65] In one center, the incidence of significant GER rose from 39% in the period 1975 to 1984 to 63% in the period 1985 to 1988.[171] In another study, it rose from 25% in 1958 to 72% in 1982.[8,172] A progressive rise in significant reflux was seen up to the age of 5 years.[173] A considerable number of patients with repaired EA have complaints in adult life pointing toward GER as the etiology.[159,174] Early normal pH values in the esophagus do not exclude significant reflux on follow-up.[175] Antireflux medication including gastric acid suppression is successful in only about half of the cases.[121] Antireflux operations in patients with repaired EA have a high failure rate,[176] but there seems to be no other alternative. In view of the motility disturbances, partial wraps have been advocated,[177] but hard evidence for their superiority is lacking. The question remains whether patients with repaired EA should be screened as adults. However, there is no correlation between subjective and objective findings, there are no reports of treatment of Barrett's esophagus, and the incidence of cancer in EA patients seems not to be increased.[159,178]

Respiratory Morbidity

Respiratory morbidity in patients with repaired EA is high. In a series of 334 patients aged 1 to 37, just under half were subsequently hospitalized with a respiratory illness.[179] Two thirds of the admissions were before 5 years of age. Even a high proportion of the adult patients reported respiratory symptoms.[180] These symptoms can be attributed to tracheomalacia and GER. Aortopexy is effective in preventing further life-threatening spells but does not prevent the increased susceptibility to respiratory infections.[181]

Thoracotomy-Related Morbidity

Thoracotomy, especially in the newborn, may lead to significant morbidity, such as winged scapula, elevation or fixation of the shoulder, asymmetry of the chest wall, rib fusion, scoliosis, and breast and pectoral muscle maldevelopment.[182-189] Moreover, chronic pain after thoracic surgery is a serious problem, at least in adults, and has been reported in more than 50% of patients.[190,191] The negative consequences of a thoracotomy can certainly be alleviated by choosing the thoracoscopic approach.[104]

OUTCOME

Short-Term Outcome

The classification system for assessing short-term outcome was first proposed by Waterston in 1962 (Table 27-2).[192] In later years, factors such as earlier diagnosis and referral, improvements in perioperative care (including anesthesia), and improvements in the diagnosis and treatment of associated anomalies considerably improved the outcomes. Thus, using the original Waterston classification and applying it to the cohort of patients treated at Great Ormond Street in London from 1980 to 1992, there was a 99% survival in group A, 75% in group B, and 71% in group C.[6] The authors then developed a new classification system based on birth weight and the presence of congenital cardiac anomalies (Table 27-3).[6] Another classification system from Montreal takes into account only life-threatening anomalies or major associated anomalies together with ventilator dependence.[193] Finally, two studies on gap length as a prognostic factor found significant differences in prognosis.[194,195]

Table 27-2 Waterston Classification for Short-Term Outcomes after Repair of EA/TEF

Group	Birth Characteristics	Survival
A	> 5½ lb body weight and well	95%
B	1. Birth weight: 4 to 5½ lb and well 2. Higher birth weight, moderate pneumonia, and congenital anomaly	68%
C	1. Birth weight < 4 lb 2. Higher birth weight, severe pneumonia, and severe congenital anomaly	6%

Data from Waterston DJ, Carter RE, Aberdeen E: Oesophageal atresia: Tracheo-oesophageal fistula: A study of survival in 218 infants. Lancet 1:819-822, 1962.

Table 27-3 New Classification System for Short-Term Outcomes after Repair of EA/TEF Based on Birth Weight and Cardiac Status

Group	Birth Characteristics	Survival*
I	Birth weight > 1500 g with no major cardiac anomaly	97% (283/293)
II	Birth weight < 1500 g or major cardiac anomaly	59% (41/70)
III	Birth weight < 1500 g and major congenital anomaly	22% (2/9)

*Survival found in 357 infants with EA and 15 infants with an H-type TEF treated at Great Ormond Street Hospital, London, 1980-1992.
Data from Spitz L, Kiely EM, Morecroft JA, et al: Oesophageal atresia: At-risk groups for the 1990s. J Pediatr Surg 29:723-725, 1994.

Long-Term Outcome

As described previously, EA is associated with high morbidity.[174,189,196,197] Interestingly, young adult patients with a history of EA score well on the Course of Life Questionnaire.[198] It seems they have learned to live with their inconveniences.

ISOLATED TRACHEOESOPHAGEAL FISTULA

Incidence and Associated Malformations

The incidence of isolated TEF is about 4% in series taking EA and TEF together.[14,15] Isolated TEF is associated with the same anomalies as seen in EA, although at lower incidences.[199]

Pathology

The fistula runs from the trachea downward to the esophagus, typically intramurally (see Fig. 27-1). The trajectory is short. In a series of 20 children, the fistula was at C5-6 in 2, C6-7 in 3, C7–T1 in 8, T1-2 in 3, and T2-3 in 1.[19] Rarely, there is a second fistula.[200]

Clinical Presentation

Respiratory symptoms, especially choking, usually occur immediately after birth during drinking. Sometimes, there are unexplained cyanotic spells. Symptoms subside when the child is fed by a nasogastric tube. Often the abdomen is distended with air, and flatulence may be present. This is caused by air going down through the fistula during crying. Older children present with recurrent pneumonia, especially of the right upper lobe. Often symptoms can be traced back to the neonatal period. Sometimes symptoms present later in life.[201-203]

Diagnosis

There has been considerable debate on the optimal method for diagnosis. Obviously, awareness is of key importance. A contrast swallow using a water-soluble, low osmolar contrast medium seems to be the best initial investigation and demonstrates the fistula in 80% of the cases (Fig. 27-17).[19] In the remaining 20%, contrast material during swallowing is seen in the trachea. Tracheoscopy is another imaging modality to be considered, but even then the fistula can be missed.[204] CT esophagography is another option but has the disadvantage of radiation exposure.[203]

Therapy

A cervical approach can be used in most (80%) cases.[205] With the use of a feeding tube placed through the fistula by tracheoscopy and pulled out of the esophagus, even these lower H-type fistulas can be pulled up and approached through the neck as well.[206,207] The classic approach is that from the right through a small low cervical incision (Fig. 27-18). The sternal head of the sternocleidomastoid muscle may need transection. The esophagus is easily identified and separated from the trachea, taking care not to injure the recurrent laryngeal nerve. The left recurrent laryngeal nerve is vulnerable as well. The proximal esophagus, as well as the fistula, are encircled with separate vessel loops and so is the distal esophagus. Traction sutures are placed at the upper and lower ends of the fistula, which is transected close to the esophagus. The trachea is closed longitudinally and the esophagus transversally with interrupted absorbable sutures. Because fistula recurrence is rare, there is no need for interposition of tissue.

It is obvious that less trauma is inflicted when a thoracotomy can be avoided. The availability of thoracoscopy indeed obviates the need for a thoracotomy, thus making a cervical approach for the extremely low H-fistulas less imperative. Several case reports of thoracoscopically closed fistulas have been published.[208,209] Alternatively, a thoracoscopically assisted approach

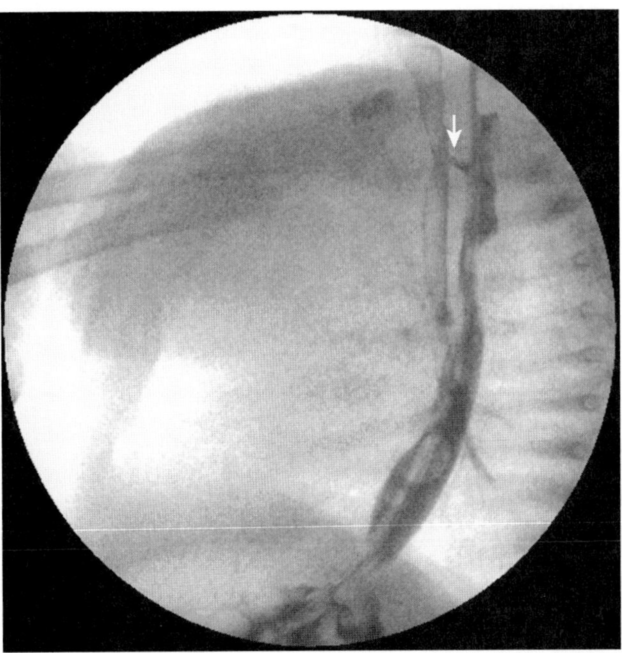

Figure 27-17. Imaging for an H-type TEF. A contrast swallow is performed using a low osmolar, water-soluble medium. The fistula (*arrow*) is clearly seen on the lateral chest film. The fistula is at the level of the thoracic inlet. Contrast material entered the trachea and bronchial tree.

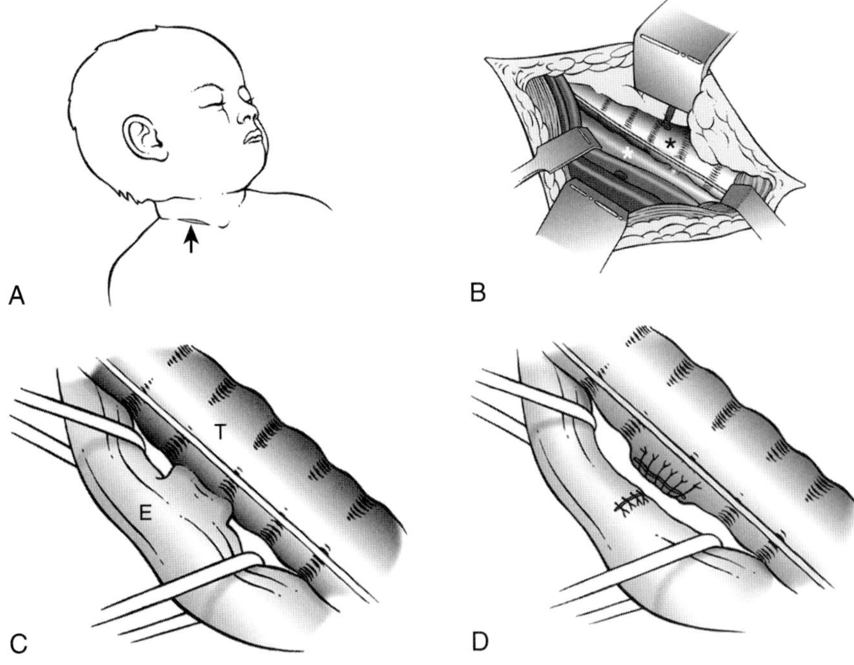

Figure 27-18. Cervical approach used to repair an H-fistula. **A,** Low right transverse cervical incision (*arrow*). **B,** The esophagus (*white asterisk*) is approached medial to the carotid artery and jugular vein. Care is taken not to injure the recurrent laryngeal nerve on either side. The trachea is marked with a *black asterisk.* **C,** The esophagus (E) is encircled both above and below the fistula. The fistula will be transected close to the trachea (T). **D,** The tracheal opening is closed vertically, and the esophageal defect is closed transversely.

can be used in which the fistula is dissected from below but repaired from above through the neck. As a matter of interest, EA repair through the neck has been reported as well.[210,211] Whether a fistula should be primarily approached from the neck or the chest depends on the location of the fistula based on preoperative imaging.

COMMUNICATING BRONCHOPULMONARY FOREGUT MALFORMATIONS

Communicating bronchopulmonary foregut malformations (CBPFMs) are rare congenital malformations characterized by a fistula between an isolated portion of the respiratory tissue and the esophagus, stomach, or even pancreas.[212,213] CBPFMs belong to the broader group of bronchopulmonary foregut malformations, which also includes intralobar and extralobar pulmonary sequestrations and bronchogenic cysts. The classification system for these anomalies is seen in Table 27-4.[212]

Patients with CBPFMs commonly have other associated malformations that contribute significantly to an increased morbidity and mortality.[212,214] Tracheal stenosis may be part of the anomaly.[214,215] Awareness of the possible existence of a CBPFM is essential for making an early diagnosis and treatment plan.

LARYNGEAL AND LARYNGOTRACHEOESOPHAGEAL CLEFT

Laryngeal and laryngotracheoesophageal clefts are rare congenital anomalies with an incidence of approximately 1 in 10,000 to 20,000 live births.[216] The cleft consists of a midline communication of the larynx, trachea, and even bronchus with the pharynx and upper esophagus. Its embryology is poorly understood. Originally, it was thought to be the consequence of a failure of the tracheoesophageal septum to fuse in the caudocranial direction. However, this theory of tracheoesophageal separation by fusion of a tracheoesophageal septum has been challenged.[21-24]

Table 27-4 Classification System for Congenital Bronchopulmonary Foregut Malformations (CBPFMs)

I. CBPFMs are associated with esophageal atresia
   A. The entire lung is involved
   B. Only part of the lung is involved

II. One lung originates from the lower esophagus

III. An isolated lobe or segment of the lung communicates with the esophagus or stomach.
   The arterial supply comes from either the pulmonary artery or an independent branch from the aorta, or both. The venous drainage is to the pulmonary vein, portal vein or azygos system.

IV. A portion of the normal bronchial system communicates with the esophagus.
   The communicating bronchus has a systemic blood supply.

From Srikanth MS, Ford EG, Stanley P, et al: Communicating bronchopulmonary foregut malformations: Classification and embryogenesis. J Pediatr Surg 27:732-736, 1992.

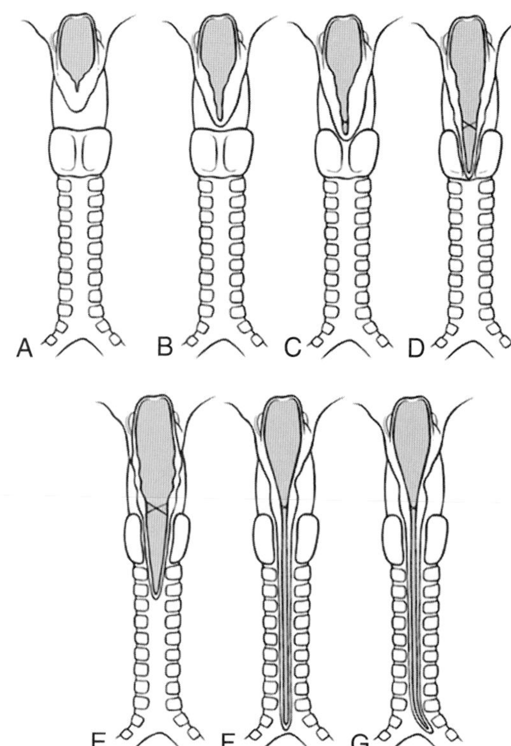

Figure 27-19. This schematic depicts the classification of laryngotracheoesophageal clefts described by Myer and colleagues.[222] The laryngoesophageal clefts are seen in the top drawing **(B-D)**, and the laryngotracheoesophageal clefts are seen on the bottom **(E-G)**. **A,** Normal anatomy. **B,** Interarytenoid cleft (LI). **C,** Partial cricoid cleft (LII). **D,** Complete cricoid cleft (LIII). **E,** Cleft extends into trachea (LTEI). **F,** Cleft extends into the carina (LTEII). **G,** Cleft extends into the bronchus (LTEIII, proposed).

Many congenital malformations can coexist, including congenital heart disease, gastrointestinal and genitourinary tract abnormalities, and midline defects.[217] Familial occurrence has been described.[218] Clefts may be part of the Opitz-Frias syndrome and the Pallister-Hall syndrome.[219] TEFs have been described in 20% to 37% of the patients.[217] Several classifications have been described (Fig. 27-19) and can be seen in Table 27-5.[220-222]

Symptoms vary according to the extension of the cleft. Patients may be symptomatic immediately from birth as a result of drowning in their saliva (Fig. 27-20). Secretions are increased, and there may be choking and cyanosis. A typical symptom is hoarseness. Drinking aggravates the symptoms, and recurrent aspiration pneumonia can occur. The clinical picture may be blurred by associated anomalies, such as EA with distal fistula.

Contrast radiographs may be diagnostic, although it can be difficult to differentiate between overflow or aspiration and the direct entrance of contrast as a result of the cleft. Tracheobronchoscopy is diagnostic. The diagnosis may well be missed, especially in less

Table 27-5 Three Classification Systems for Laryngotracheoesophageal Clefts

Pettersson[220]	Ryan et al.[221]	Myer et al.[222]
I: Cleft limited to the cricoid II: Cleft extending beyond the cricoid into the trachea III: Cleft involving the whole cricoid and trachea	As described by Pettersson but with the addition of: IV: Cleft extending the whole way down into one of the main bronchi	Laryngeal clefts Interarytenoid: LI Partial cricoid: LII Complete cricoid: LIII Laryngotracheoesophageal Into trachea: LTEI To carina: LTEII

Comment: The classification of Myer and colleagues seems best suited because it is more specific regarding the anatomic region involved. Extension into the bronchus, however, is not part of this classification. It could be added as LTEIII.

severe cases. A high degree of suspicion is required for making the diagnosis in these patients. Pressure of the scope on the arytenoids will open the cleft.

Management varies according to the type of cleft and the associated anomalies. Aspiration should be avoided by nasogastric feeding, antireflux medication, or gastrostomy in combination with antireflux surgery.

Using the Myer classification system,[222] LI may need no treatment other than antireflux therapy. If still symptomatic, these patients may need an open or endoscopic repair. LII, LIII, and LTEI are best managed through anterior laryngotomy. LTEII and LTEIII are best treated by a combined cervical and thoracic approach.[223] A lateral cervical approach provides suboptimal access.[224] An anterior approach under cardiopulmonary bypass has also been used.[224,225] Repair under extracorporeal membrane oxygenation may be the best option.[224,226]

This is a rare anomaly, and reported series are small. Tracheal instability, tracheomalacia, and GER with recurrent aspiration have been noted. The anastomotic leak rate is high, and hospitalization is often prolonged.

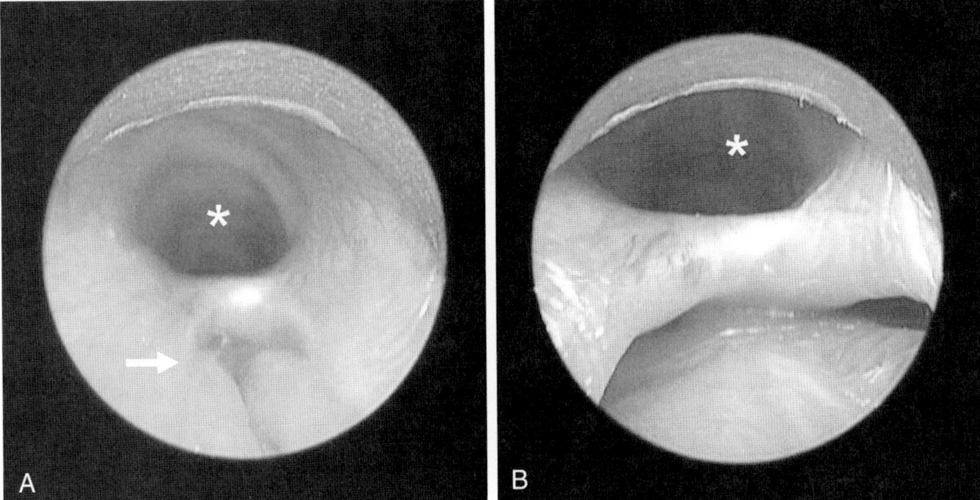

Figure 27-20. This newborn began to have respiratory distress shortly after birth. Clinically, it was felt that the baby might have a tracheoesophageal fistula without esophageal atresia as a small nasogastric tube was able to be passed into the stomach. The bronchoscopic examination is shown. In both figures, the trachea is identified with the asterisk. On the left **(A)**, the laryngotracheoesophageal cleft is visualized. The esophagus is marked with the arrow. On the right **(B)**, the distal end of the laryngotracheoesophageal cleft is easily seen with the trachea anteriorly (asterisk) and the esophagus posteriorly. According to the classification of laryngotracheoesophageal clefts described by Meyer, this would be an LTE-1 (see Fig. 27-19E).

chapter 28

THORACOSCOPY IN INFANTS AND CHILDREN

Steven S. Rothenberg, MD

Thoracoscopy is a technique that has been in use since the early 1900s but has undergone an exponential increase in popularity and growth over the past 2 decades. The first experience in humans was reported by Jacobeus in 1910 and consisted of inserting a cystoscope through a rigid cannula into the pleural space to lyse adhesions and cause complete collapse of a lung as treatment for patients with tuberculosis. He later reported the first significant experience with a series of over 100 patients.[1] During the next 70 years, thoracoscopy gained some favor, primarily in Europe, for the biopsy of pleural-based tumors and limited thoracic explorations in adults. However, widespread acceptance was minimal.[2,3]

In the 1970s and 1980s, the first significant experience in children was reported.[4,5] Equipment modified for pediatric patients was used to perform biopsies, evaluate various intrathoracic lesions, and perform limited pleural debridement in patients with empyema.[6] However, even though there was an increasing recognition of the morbidity associated with a standard thoracotomy, especially in small infants and children, there was little acceptance or adoption of these techniques.[7] It was not until the early 1990s, with the dramatic revolution in technology associated with laparoscopic surgery in adults, that more advanced diagnostic and therapeutic procedures were performed in children.[8] The development of a high-resolution microchip, and now digital and high-definition cameras, smaller instrumentation, and better optics, has enabled pediatric surgeons to perform even the most complicated intrathoracic procedure thoracoscopically.[9]

INDICATIONS

Today there are a wide variety of indications for thoracoscopic procedures in children (Table 28-1), and the number continues to expand with advances and refinements in technology and technique. Currently, thoracoscopy is being used extensively for lung biopsy and wedge resection in patients with interstitial lung disease and metastatic lesions.[10,11] More extensive pulmonary resections, including segmentectomy and lobectomy, are now being routinely performed for infectious diseases, cavitary lesions, bullous disease, lobar emphysema, congenital pulmonary airway malformations (CPAM), and neoplasms.[12-17] Thoracoscopy is also extremely useful in the evaluation and treatment of mediastinal masses.[18] It provides excellent access and visualization for biopsy and resection of mediastinal structures, such as lymph nodes, thymic and thyroid lesions, cystic hygromas, foregut duplications, ganglioneuromas, and neuroblastomas.[19-21] Other advanced intrathoracic procedures such as decortication for empyema, patent ductus arteriosus closure, division of vascular rings, repair of hiatal hernia and congenital diaphragmatic defects, esophageal myotomy for achalasia, thoracic sympathectomy for hyperhidrosis, anterior spinal fusion for severe scoliosis, and, most recently, primary repair of esophageal atresia have been described in children.[22-31]

Table 28-1 Indications for Thoracoscopy in Infants and Children

Lung biopsy	Ligation of patent ductus arteriosus
Lobectomy	Thoracic duct ligation
Sequestration resection	Esophageal atresia repair
Cyst excision	Tracheoesophageal fistula
Decortication	Aortopexy
Foregut duplication resection	Mediastinal mass excision
Esophageal myotomy	Thymectomy
Anterior spine fusion	Sympathectomy
Diaphragmatic hernia/ plication	Pericardial window

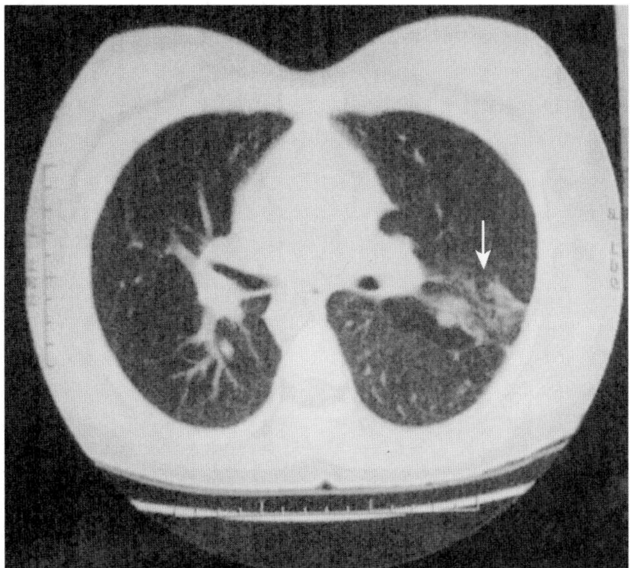

Figure 28-1. CT scan of a patient with interstitial lung disease. The areas of greatest involvement *(arrow)* can be identified for biopsy.

PREOPERATIVE WORKUP

The preoperative workup varies significantly depending on the procedure to be performed. Most intrathoracic lesions require routine radiography as well as computed tomography (CT) or magnetic resonance imaging (MRI). A thin-cut high-resolution CT scan is especially helpful in evaluating patients with interstitial lung disease because it can identify the most affected areas and help determine the site of biopsy (Fig. 28-1), since the external appearance of the lung is usually not helpful. CT-guided needle localization can also be used to direct biopsies for focal lesions that may be deep in the parenchyma and therefore not visible on the surface of the lung during thoracoscopy. This is usually performed just before the thoracoscopy, with the radiologist marking the pleura overlying the lesion with a small blood patch or dye (Fig. 28-2). On occasion, a wire may be placed, as in breast biopsies, but it may become dislodged during collapse of the lung with the pneumothorax. As intraoperative ultrasound imaging improves, this may provide a more sensitive way for the surgeon to detect lesions deep to the surface of the lung and compensate for the lack of tactile sensation. Unfortunately, in its current state, this technology is still unreliable.[32] MRI may be more useful in evaluating vascular lesions or masses, which may arise from or encroach on the spinal canal, or in infants with vascular rings. These studies can be extremely important in determining positioning of the patient and initial port placement.

Another major consideration for the successful completion of most thoracoscopic procedures is whether or not the patient will tolerate single-lung ventilation, thus allowing for collapse of the ipsilateral lung to ensure adequate visualization and room for manipulation. Unfortunately, there is no specific preoperative test that will yield this answer. However, most patients, even those who are ventilator dependent, can tolerate short periods of single-lung ventilation. This should allow adequate time to perform most diagnostic procedures such as lung biopsy. In cases in which single-lung ventilation cannot be tolerated, other techniques can be used (see later).

PREOPERATIVE PREPARATION

Anesthetic Considerations

Whereas single-lung ventilation is achieved relatively easily in adult patients using a double-lumen endotracheal tube, the process is more difficult in the infant or small child. The smallest available double-lumen tube is a 28 Fr, which can generally not be used in a patient weighing less than 30 kg. Another option is a bronchial blocker. This device contains an occluding balloon attached to a stylet on the side of the endotracheal tube. After intubation, the stylet and tube are advanced into the bronchus to be occluded and the balloon is inflated. Unfortunately, size is again a limiting factor because the smallest blocker currently available is a 6.0-mm tube. In smaller patients, a Fogarty balloon catheter can be placed adjacent to a standard endotracheal tube or through the lumen of the tube to achieve occlusion of the desired bronchus. For the majority of cases in infants and small children, selective main-stem intubation of the contralateral bronchus with a standard uncuffed endotracheal tube is

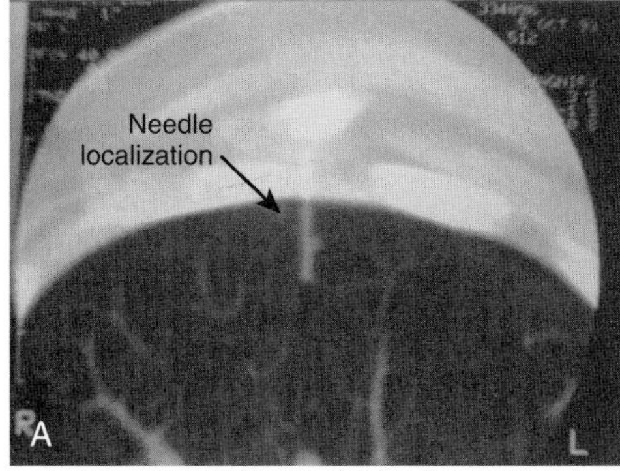

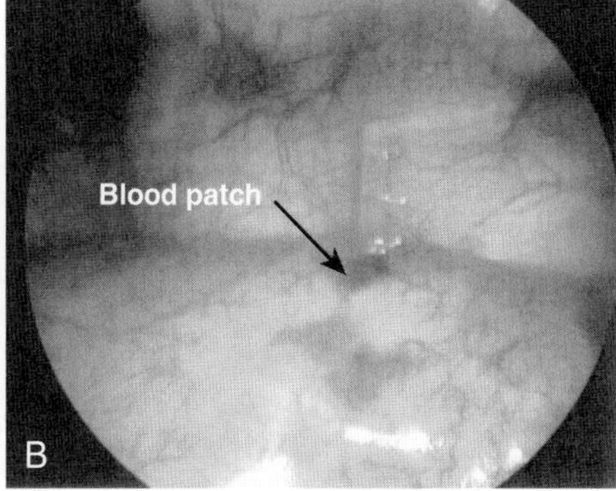

Figure 28-2. A, Needle localization of a presumed metastatic lesion under CT guidance. **B,** Small blood patch visible on the pleural surface marking the underlying nodule.

effective. This can usually be done blindly without the aid of a bronchoscope simply by manipulating the head and neck. It is also important to use an endotracheal tube one-half to one size smaller than the anesthesiologist would pick for a standard intubation or the tube may not pass into the main-stem bronchus, especially on the left side.

At times, this technique will not lead to total collapse of the lung because there may be some overflow ventilation because the endotracheal tube is not totally occlusive. This problem is overcome by the routine use of a low flow (1 L/min), low pressure (4 mm/Hg) CO_2 infusion during the procedure to help keep the lung compressed. If adequate visualization is still not achieved, then the pressure and flow can be gradually increased until adequate lung collapse is achieved. Pressures of 10 to 12 mm Hg can be tolerated without significant respiratory or hemodynamic consequences in most cases. This requires the use of a valved cannula rather than nonvalved port. This technique can also be used on patients who cannot tolerate single-lung ventilation. By using small tidal volumes, lower peak pressures, and a higher respiratory rate, enough lung collapse can be achieved to allow for adequate exploration and biopsy. In neonates with esophageal atresia with or without fistula, or with other congenital malformations, CO_2 insufflation alone can be used to deflate the lung. Once the lung is collapsed, it will remain compressed until the anesthesiologist makes a conscious effort to re-expand it. The surface tension of the collapsed alveoli in the newborn keeps the lung collapsed without excessive pressures being used. Another option is to place the neonate on a high-frequency ventilator, which minimizes airway pressures used and may be tolerated better by some neonates than single-lung ventilation.[33] This may be a better solution, especially in institutions in which the anesthesiologists are not as experienced or comfortable with single-lung ventilation or isolation.

CO_2 insufflation is also useful if bilateral procedures are being performed, such as in the case of sympathectomy.[34] A slight tension pneumothorax gives adequate exposure to visualize the sympathetic chain without the need for changing the double-lumen tube or bronchial blocker. Whatever method is chosen, it is imperative that the anesthesiologist and surgeon have a clear plan and good communication to prevent problems with hypoxia and excessive hypercapnia and to ensure the best chance for a successful procedure.[35]

Patient Positioning

Patient positioning depends on the site of the lesion and the type of procedure. Most open thoracotomies are performed with the patient in the lateral decubitus position. Thoracoscopic procedures should be performed with the patient in a position that allows for the greatest access to the area of interest and uses gravity to aid in keeping the uninvolved lung or other tissues out of the field of view.

For routine lung biopsies or lung resections, the patient can be positioned in a standard lateral decubitus position (Fig. 28-3). This position provides for excellent visualization and access to all surfaces of the lung. This position is also optimal for decortication, pleurodesis, and other procedures when the surgeon may need access to the entire pleural or lung surface.

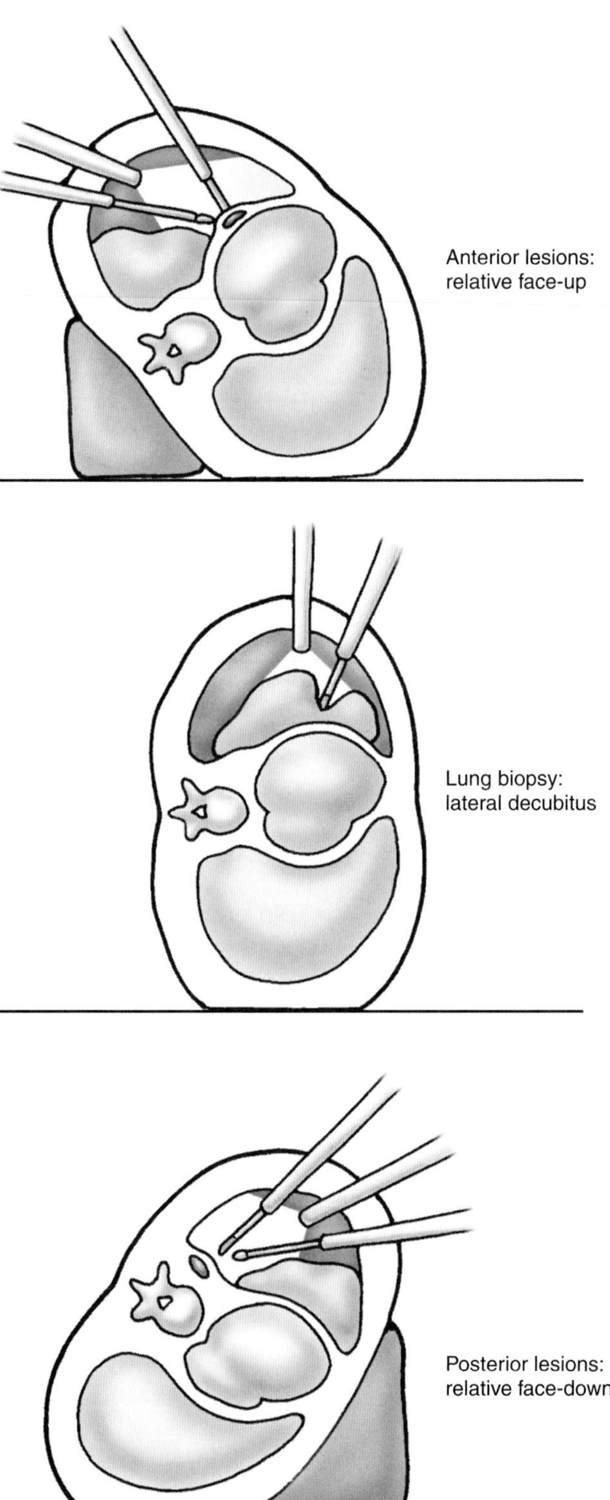

Figure 28-3. Patient positioning for the thoracoscopic approach to mediastinal and pulmonary lesions in children is important. The relative positions of the three cannulas also are illustrated for these lesions.

For anterior mediastinal masses, the patient should be placed supine with the affected side elevated 20 to 30 degrees (see Fig. 28-3). This allows for excellent visualization of the entire anterior mediastinum while allowing gravity to retract the lung posteriorly without the need for extra retractors. The surgical ports may then be placed between the anterior and midaxillary lines, giving clear access to the anterior mediastinum. This position should be used for thymectomy, aortopexy, or biopsy or resection of anterior tumors or lymph nodes. For posterior mediastinal masses, foregut duplications, esophageal atresia, and work on the esophageal hiatus, the patient should be placed in a modified prone position (see Fig. 28-3). This maneuver again allows for excellent exposure without the need for additional retractors. The patient can then be placed in the Trendelenburg or reverse Trendelenburg position as needed to help keep the lung out of the field of view.

Once the patient is appropriately positioned and draped, the monitors can be situated. For most thoracoscopic procedures, it is advantageous to use two monitors, one on either side of the table. The monitors should be situated between the patient's shoulders and hips, depending on the site of the lesion. As with any endoscopic procedure, the goal is to keep the surgeon in line with the camera, in line with the pathologic process, and in line with the monitor. This allows the surgeon to work in the most efficient and ergonomic way. In some cases, such as decortication, the field of interest may constantly change. In this case, the monitors should be placed at shoulder level and moved as necessary.

The majority of operations can be performed with the surgeon and one assistant. The surgeon should stand on the side of the table opposite the area to be addressed so that he or she can work in line with the camera. In most lung cases such as biopsies, it is preferential to have the assistant on the same side of the table as the surgeon so that the surgeon is not working in a paradox (against the camera). This concept is even more important when the field of dissection is localized. Cases such as resection of mediastinal masses, esophageal atresia repair, or more complicated lung resections require greater surgical skill. It is imperative that both the surgeon and the assistant are working in line with the field of view to prevent clumsy or awkward movements. In cases such as decortication, where the field of view and dissection are constantly changing and the majority of movements are relatively gross, having the surgeon and assistant on opposite sides of the table is appropriate and may actually expedite the procedure.

Port Placement

Positioning of the cannulas varies widely with the procedure being performed and the site of the lesion. Thoughtful positioning of the ports is more important than with laparoscopic surgery because the chest wall is rigid. Therefore, the mobility of the instruments will be somewhat restricted as compared with procedures on the abdomen. In general, the camera port should be placed slightly above and between the working ports to allow the surgeon to look down on the field of view, much as in open surgery. This will also minimize instrument "dueling," which can be a significant problem in smaller infants. For example, for lung biopsies, the cannulas should usually be placed between the fourth and eighth intercostal spaces. The camera port is usually in the midaxillary line at the fifth or sixth interspace. If an endoscopic stapler is being used, it requires a 12-mm cannula. Therefore, it should be situated in the lowest interspace possible, especially in smaller children, because these are the widest interspaces and better able to accommodate the larger port. If the lesion is anterior, it should be positioned closer to the posterior axillary line and vice versa. This is to allow the greatest amount of space between the chest wall insertion and the lesion because the working head of the stapler requires at least 45 to 50 mm of space. The third or grasping port is placed closer to the lesion and provides traction on the lesion during biopsy. This arrangement allows the surgeon, camera, and primary working port to be in line with the area to be sampled.

The midaxillary port should be placed first to allow for modification of the other two ports once an initial survey of the chest cavity has been completed. A triangular arrangement of the cannulas has also been recommended because it allows for rotation of the telescope and instruments between the three ports, giving excellent access to all areas. However, the surgeon can then be working against the camera, a situation that can make the simplest procedure very difficult. Also, especially in children, the number of large ports should be limited. Therefore, thoughtful planning regarding port placement is important. Generally, the cannula placement can be tentatively planned based on preoperative imaging studies and then modified once the initial port is inserted.

Instrumentation

The equipment used for thoracoscopy is basically the same as that for laparoscopy. In general, 5-mm and 3-mm instruments are adequate in size. In most cases, valved cannulas are used for the reasons previously discussed. Basic equipment should include 5-mm 0-degree and 30-degree telescopes. If procedures are being performed in smaller children and infants, it is also helpful to have smaller telescopes such as a short (16 to 18 cm) 3- or 4-mm wide-angle 30-degree telescope and specifically designed shorter instruments. These tools enable the surgeon to perform much finer movements and dissection, allowing advanced procedures to be performed in infants as small as 1 kg. A high-resolution digital camera and light source are also extremely important to allow for adequate visualization, especially when using smaller telescopes that transmit less light. Basic instrumentation should include curved dissecting scissors, curved dissectors (Maryland), atraumatic clamps (i.e., 3- and 5-mm atraumatic bowel clamp), a fan retractor, a suction/irrigator, and needle holders. Disposable

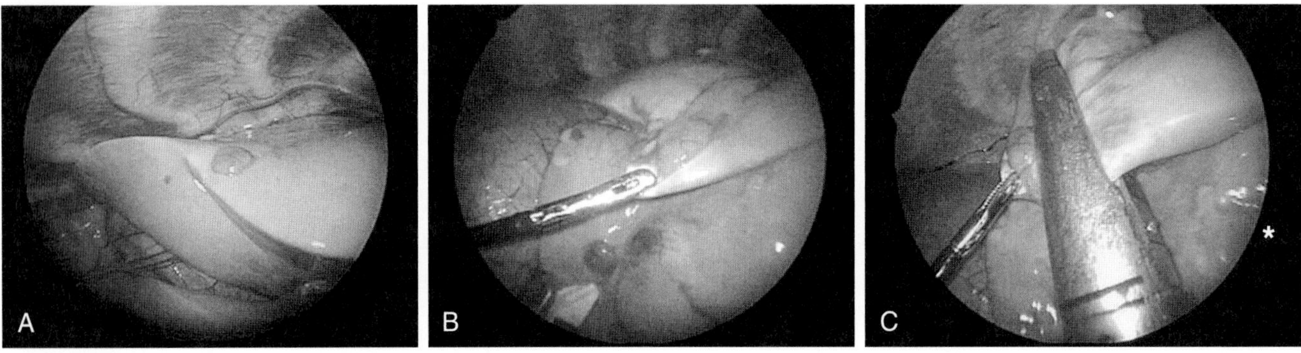

Figure 28-4. A 5-year-old with Wilms' tumor developed suspected metastatic lesions in the left upper lobe. **A,** The lesion is visualized on the inferior border of the left upper lobe. **B,** The edge of the left upper lobe is grasped to place the desired specimen on stretch. **C,** The stapler is then situated across the base of the lung containing the desired specimen and fired. As in this case, more than one firing often is required to remove the desired lesion. (From La Quaglia MP, Rothenberg SS: Thoracoscopic lung biopsy. In Holcomb GW III, Georgeson KE, Rothenberg SS [eds]: Atlas of Pediatric Laparoscopy and Thoracoscopy. Philadelphia, Elsevier, 2008, pp 247-251.)

instrumentation that should be available includes 5-mm hemostatic clips, endoloops (pre-tied ligatures), and an endoscopic linear stapler. It lays down six to eight rows of staples and divides the tissue between them, providing an air- and water-tight seal (Fig. 28-4). This is an excellent tool for performing wedge resections of the lung. Unfortunately, its current size requires placement of a 12-mm port, precluding its use in patients much under 10 kg because of the limited size of the thoracic cavity. There are also a number of energy sources available that provide hemostasis and divide tissue. These include monopolar and bipolar cautery, the ultrasonic coagulating shears, and the Ligasure (Valleylab, Boulder, CO), all of which can be helpful in difficult dissections. It is also helpful to have one of the various tissue glues available for sealing lung and pleural surfaces.

EMPYEMA

Empyema is a relatively common intrathoracic problem encountered by pediatric surgeons. Traditionally, it has been treated by antibiotics and varying degrees of chest drainage, including pleurocentesis, tube thoracostomy, mini-thoracotomy, and formal thoracotomy. Recent evidence has shown that fibrinolytic therapy is effective in 85% of patients.[36,37] When needed, thoracoscopic debridement offers an opportunity to diminish the morbidity and recovery period associated with an empyema while limiting the surgical trauma and recovery.[38,39] The patient's condition should be optimized with fluid resuscitation, aggressive pulmonary care, and antibiotics. In many cases, it is helpful to have a preoperative ultrasound evaluation or CT scan (Fig. 28-5). This will help make the decision to proceed with thoracoscopy by determining the amount of loculated fluid and inflammatory peel and to look for evidence of septations.

Although it is unusual to have significant blood loss during the procedure, the patient should undergo blood typing and crossmatching for a unit of blood as a precaution. Many of these patients are anemic, and preoperative transfusion may be necessary to help with preoperative stabilization.

The procedure is performed using general anesthesia. Single-lung isolation with either a double-lumen endotracheal tube or main-stem intubation of the

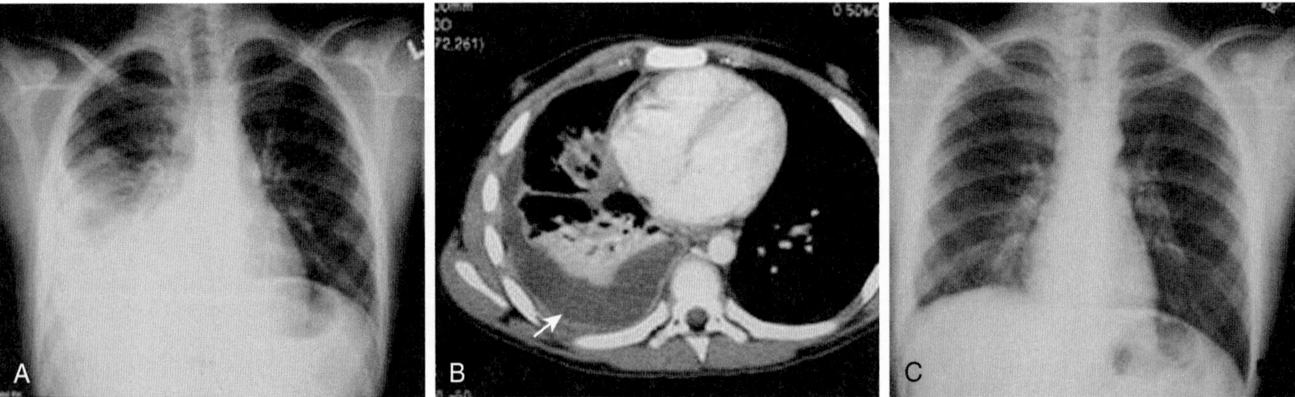

Figure 28-5. **A,** This 10-year-old was found to have a right parapneumonic effusion on the chest radiograph. **B,** CT revealed fluid (*arrow*) loculated in the right base. However, septations were also identified and the patient required thoracoscopic debridement and decortication. **C,** Six weeks after the operation, the chest radiograph is completely clear. (From Arca MJ, Holcomb GW III: Thoracoscopic decortication and debridement for empyema. In Holcomb GW III, Georgeson KE, Rothenberg SS [eds]: Atlas of Pediatric Laparoscopy and Thoracoscopy. Philadelphia, Elsevier, 2008, pp 266-269.)

contralateral side is preferable but not mandatory. Single-lung isolation may help in preventing cross contamination of the airways during manipulation of the affected side. It also aids in maintaining an adequate working space by preventing inflation of the trapped lung as the peel is removed. However, CO_2 insufflation usually is adequate to maintain lung collapse until attempts are made to actively re-expand the lung with positive pressure. The patient's respiratory status should not be compromised further, and excessive time should not be wasted in trying to get single-lung isolation.

The procedure is best performed with the patient in a lateral decubitus position. This allows the greatest access to the entire pleural cavity. The patient is supported on a bean bag or with rolls. As with all procedures performed in a lateral decubitus position, it is important to place an axillary roll and sufficient padding at all pressure points. Tape or a strap can be used to enhance this support. Patients with severe pulmonary disease may not tolerate having their good lung compromised by being in a dependent position. In these cases, a modified supine position can be used with the affected side elevated 25 to 30 degrees.

In this operation, the surgeon and assistant are positioned opposite each other. This facilitates the procedure as the entire pleural cavity needs to be explored. The scrub nurse may be positioned toward the patient's feet on whichever side is convenient. As previously mentioned, monitors should be placed on both sides, at approximately the level of the shoulders. Port placement can be somewhat variable depending on the size of the patient and the area of the chest cavity most involved. In general, the operation can be performed with just two ports. These are placed in the anterior and posterior axillary lines at the fifth or sixth interspace. If necessary, a third cannula can be inserted as needed to reach an area not readily accessible by the other two or if lung retraction is necessary. If the child is large enough, one of the ports should be 10 mm to facilitate removal of the infected peel. However, it is important to remember that the larger the port size, the more limited may be the range of motion of the instrument at that site because of the thoracic cage. The primary goal of the operation is to remove as much of the infected fluid and fibrous peel as possible, break down any septa, allow for re-expansion of the lung, and provide adequate drainage. All of this should be accomplished in an efficient manner without taking excessive time.

Mobilization of the fibrous peel can begin in a systematic manner under direct vision. A blunt grasper or ring forceps is used to grasp some of the peel, and a sweeping motion is used to strip as much as possible off the lung surface or chest wall (Fig. 28-6). The more fibrous the peel, the easier it is to remove it. This inflammatory tissue can almost be removed in strips. If the peel is less fibrous, much of it may be able to be broken up and removed with the suction device alone.

The surgeon should proceed in a clockwise fashion to ensure that all areas are addressed. When an area becomes difficult to visualize, the telescope and grasper can be exchanged, usually giving a better view and exposure to the area. If the surgeon is working through the smaller port and the peel cannot be easily exteriorized through the port, it can simply be mobilized, left in the pleural cavity, and then removed through the larger port when convenient.

The monitors may also need to be repositioned to try and keep the surgeon in line with the camera and the area of focus. Once the majority of the peel is removed and all loculations broken down, the chest cavity is irrigated with copious amounts of saline with or without antibiotics.

The goal of the operation is to remove the majority of infected fluid and tissue, lyse all loculations, free and re-expand the trapped lung, and establish adequate drainage. It is not necessary to remove every piece of the peel. The operative time should be kept to a minimum to avoid a prolonged anesthetic. If adequate drainage and lung re-expansion is achieved, then the residual infected peel will be re-absorbed as long as the patient's clinical picture improves. This procedure

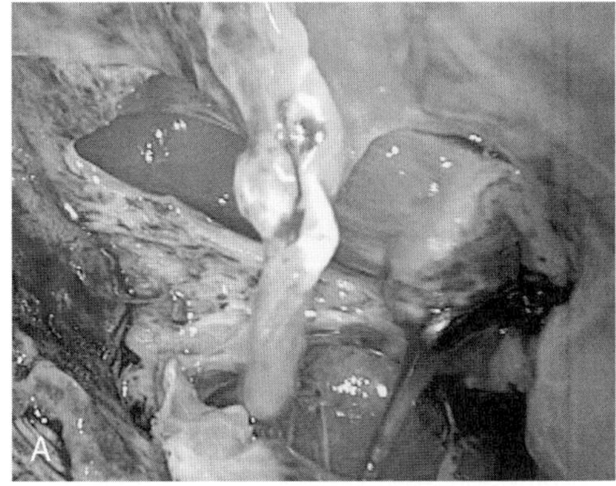

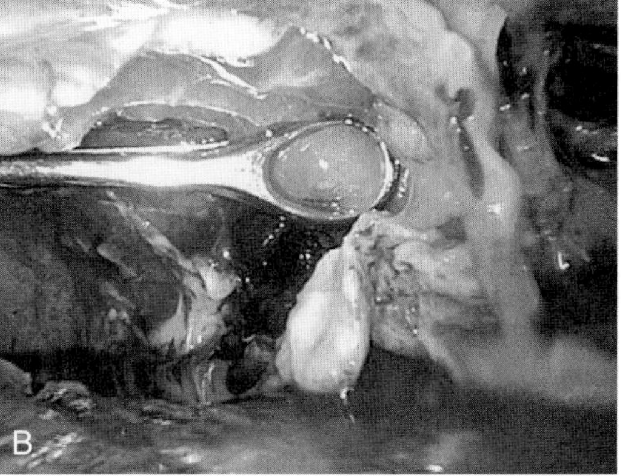

Figure 28-6. The typical appearance of the inflammatory peel in a patient with empyema is seen. **A,** Note the thick fibrinous exudate hanging from the parietal pleura. **B,** Ring forceps have been introduced through a 10-mm incision to allow grasping of the purulent exudate. Note the collapsed lung at the bottom of the photograph. (From Arca MJ, Holcomb GW III: Thoracoscopic decortication and debridement for empyema. In Holcomb GW III, Georgeson KE, Rothenberg SS [eds]: Atlas of Pediatric Laparoscopy and Thoracoscopy. Philadelphia, Elsevier, 2008, pp 266-269.)

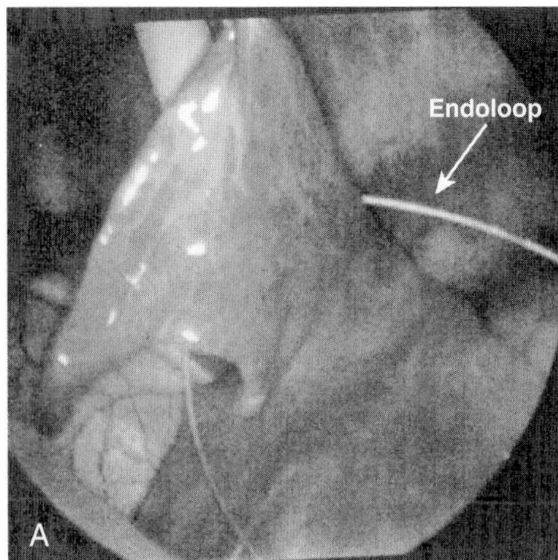

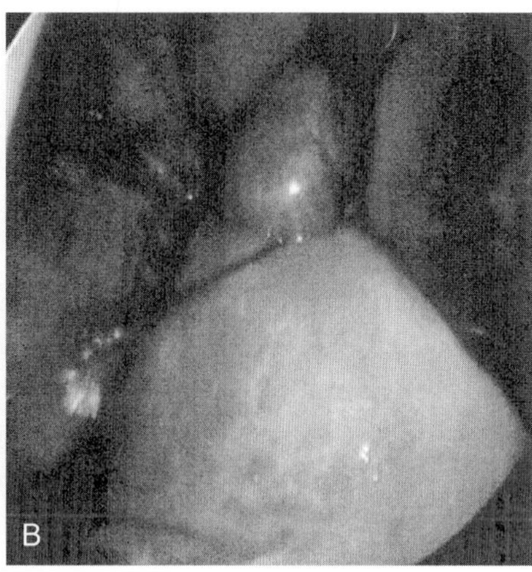

Figure 28-7. **A,** An endoloop is being applied to a tongue of lung tissue for lung biopsy in a small child. **B,** A second endoloop is being snared down to provide an air- and water-tight seal.

should not take more than 60 minutes and, in most cases, requires less time.

After irrigation, the ports are removed. A single chest tube is placed through the posterior port site and positioned posteriorly so it lies in a dependent position. Two drainage tubes are rarely needed. The small incisions are closed in layers with absorbable suture. If the patient is stable, it is best to extubate at the end of the procedure. The limited surgical trauma allows aggressive postoperative physiotherapy.

LUNG BIOPSY

Lung biopsy is one of the most common thoracoscopic procedures, and it will be described here to illustrate basic techniques. The side for the biopsy is chosen based on the chest radiograph and CT findings. With the patient under general anesthesia, single-lung ventilation is obtained as previously described. The patient is then placed in a lateral decubitus position and prepped and draped. Low flow (1 L/min), low pressure (4 mm Hg) CO_2 insufflation is used to collapse the lung, allowing for better visualization. In general, three cannulas are sufficient and the ports are placed as previously described. The first port is inserted in the midaxillary line in the fifth or sixth intercostal space. This site is chosen because it allows good access to the entire pleural cavity for the initial survey and because this insertion site is unlikely to cause injury to the lung, diaphragm, or other structures. After the initial survey, the other two ports are introduced. In small children, 3- or 5-mm ports can be used. In children 10 kg or larger, a single 12-mm cannula is introduced so that the stapler may be used. If a biopsy specimen is being taken from the ventral surface of the lung, the telescope should be placed through the midaxillary cannula, the grasper in the anterior port, and the stapler in the inferior and posterior port. For biopsies on the posterior surface of the lung, the positions of the scope and grasper are reversed. In smaller patients whose chest cavity cannot accommodate the stapler, endoloops are used to snare and ligate a small area of lung. Two consecutive loops are placed at the base of the specimen and the tissue is sharply excised distal to the ligatures (Fig. 28-7). This provides a hemostatic and air-tight seal equivalent to that obtained with the stapler.[40] Specimens of 2 to 3 cm can be obtained in this manner and are more than adequate for diagnosis. Biopsy samples can easily be obtained from all five lobes using this technique.

For metastatic lesions, port placement is altered depending on the site of the lesion. Although the majority of nodules are peripheral, lesions less than 1 cm in diameter or deep in the lung parenchyma may not be readily visible on the pleural surface. In these cases, preoperative CT-guided localization as previously described should be performed (see Fig. 28-2). At the time of surgery with the lung collapsed, the marked area can easily be identified. If the lesion itself is not visible, then the area underlying the blood patch can be wedged out. A frozen section should be performed to ensure the lesion is included with the specimen. Ongoing improvements in endoscopic ultrasound probes should eventually become the preferred technique for localization.

Resection of bullae or infectious cavitary lesions can be accomplished using a similar technique (Fig. 28-8). The minimal morbidity associated with thoracoscopy has shifted the algorithm for treatment, and earlier surgical intervention is often indicated (Fig. 28-9). In the case of bullous disease presenting as a spontaneous pneumothorax, it is usually advisable to combine excision with a limited pleurodesis or pleurectomy. This can easily be accomplished by abrading the parietal pleura (usually the apex) with an endoscopic peanut or a small sponge placed through one of the port sites. In recurrent or severe cases, a formal pleurectomy may be needed. Some surgeons prefer the use of a chemical or talc pleurodesis, and these agents can be used as well. However, only in the case of malignant effusions is chemical pleurodesis usually needed.

Any potentially malignant or infectious lesion that will not fit through the inner channel of the port should be placed in an endoscopic specimen bag to prevent possible seeding.[41] Once the intrathoracic

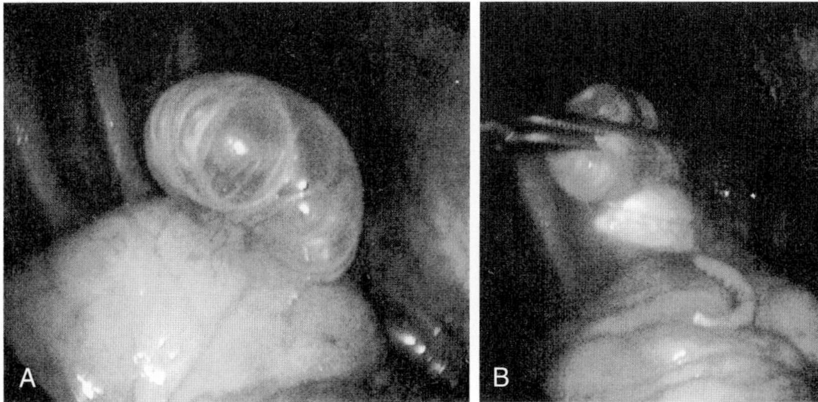

Figure 28-8. **A,** An apical bleb is seen in a patient with a spontaneous pneumothorax. **B,** The stapler has been used to resect the bleb.

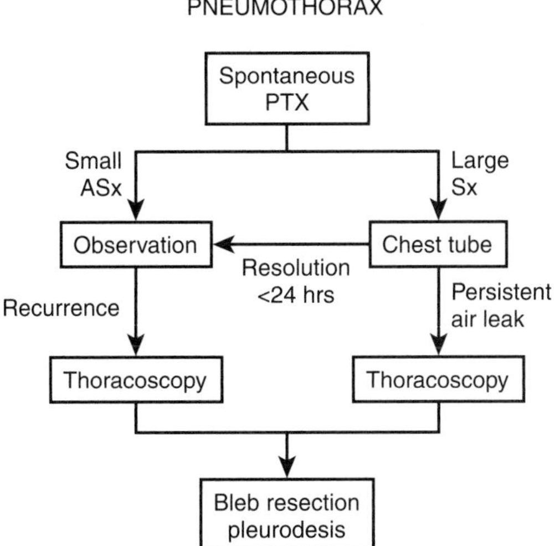

Figure 28-9. Algorithm for the treatment of spontaneous pneumothorax (PTX) in children. Sx, symptomatic; ASx, asymptomatic.

procedure has been completed, a small chest tube is introduced through one of the port sites and the collapsed lung is ventilated. In most cases, when there is no concern over adequate hemostasis or malignant effusion, the chest tube can be removed before extubation in the operating room if there is no evidence of an air leak.[42] This avoids the considerable discomfort associated with the chest tube in the postoperative period. A chest radiograph is obtained in the recovery room. If the lung is fully expanded, no further follow-up films are needed.

THORACOSCOPIC LOBECTOMY

Initial experience with minimally invasive lobectomy required a video-assisted approach. This utilized two to three cannulas and standard laparoscopic instruments with a mini-thoracotomy through which standard thoracic instruments and staplers could be more easily passed.[14] These operations were technically demanding and often arduous but did spare the patient the morbidity of a formal thoracotomy. The mini-thoracotomy was placed in the midaxillary line and used a muscle-sparing technique. With improvement in endoscopic staplers as well as energy sources that can seal both pulmonary vessels and lung parenchyma, the need to employ a mini-thoracotomy has been eliminated. These procedures can now be done completely thoracoscopically through 3-, 5-, 10-, and 12-mm ports in a safe and efficacious manner.[15-17]

Sealing devices such as the Ligasure allow the surgeon to seal the main pulmonary vessels in smaller patients without the need for suture ligation, clips, or staples. It also seals lung tissue, preventing both bleeding and air leak. In larger patients, the articulating stapler can be used to complete the fissure as well as ligate and divide the main pulmonary vessels and bronchi. These technical advances have enabled the surgeon to accomplish a lobectomy completely in an endoscopic manner. However, the surgeon's view is limited to a two-dimensional plane. Moreover, it is difficult to manipulate the lobe to look at both the anterior and posterior aspects in an attempt to gain a three-dimensional perspective. Therefore, it is critical that the surgeon have a good understanding of the anatomic spatial relationships between the vessels, lung tissue, and bronchus because these structures may not be visible and cannot be palpated (Figs. 28-10 and 28-11). The operation is performed with the patient in a lateral decubitus position, and the surgeon works from anterior to posterior. In general, the pulmonary artery branches are taken before the vein to minimize lung congestion, which can make the lobe even more difficult to manipulate (Fig. 28-12). Lower lobectomies are generally easier than upper resections because dissection can proceed along the major fissure. Any vessel or bronchus crossing it is considered an end vessel and can be ligated and divided. Upper lobectomies are much more difficult because dissection must proceed along the main pulmonary artery, sacrificing each segmental branch to the upper lobe as it comes off and taking care not to injure the main trunk. Once the lobectomy is completed, the lower port site is widened slightly and the lung is removed in a piecemeal fashion, if necessary. A chest tube is left overnight but can usually be removed on the first postoperative day.

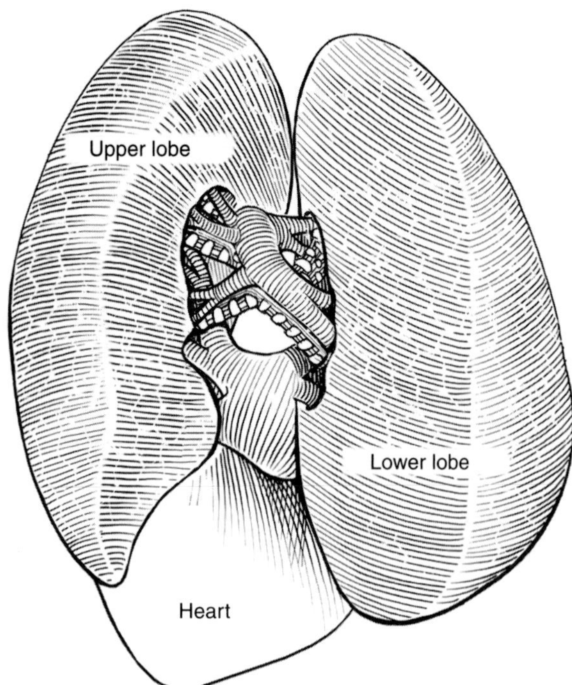

Figure 28-10. The anatomy seen by the surgeon when the contents of the fissure between the left upper and lower lobes are exposed. The arteries are visualized first within the fissure, and the bronchial structures are behind the arteries. The pulmonary veins exit from the inferior portion of these lobes and drain into the heart. (From Rothenberg SS: Thoracoscopic lobectomy. In Holcomb GW III, Georgeson KE, Rothenberg SS [eds]: Atlas of Pediatric Laparoscopy and Thoracoscopy. Philadelphia, Elsevier, 2008, pp. 253-260.)

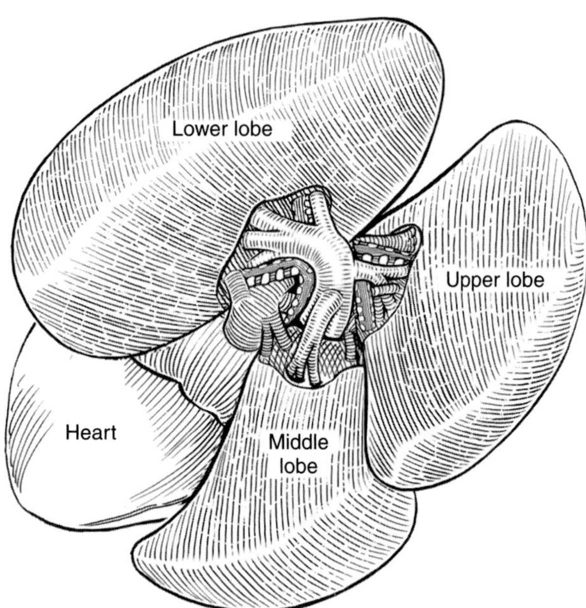

Figure 28-11. The anatomy as seen by the surgeon when dissecting in the major and minor fissures of the right lung. The arteries are the first structures seen in the fissure, and the bronchial structures are behind the arteries. The pulmonary veins are inferior to the arteries and bronchial structures and drain into the heart. (From Rothenberg SS: Thoracoscopic lobectomy. In Holcomb GW III, Georgeson KE, Rothenberg SS [eds]: Atlas of Pediatric Laparoscopy and Thoracoscopy. Philadelphia, Elsevier, 2008, pp. 253-260.)

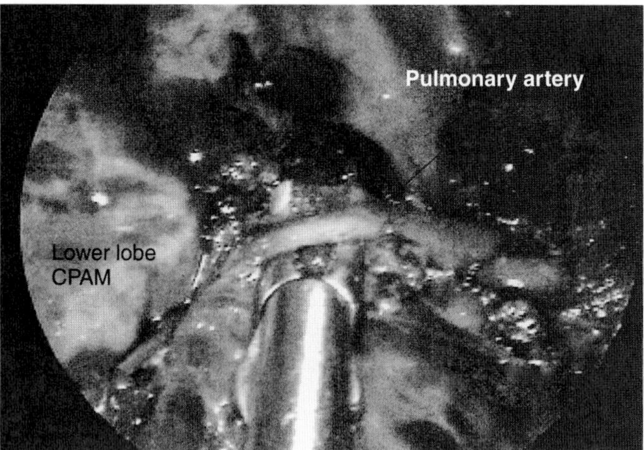

Figure 28-12. Isolation of the pulmonary artery as it transverses the major fissure during excision of a right lower lobe congenital pulmonary airway malformation is seen.

POSTERIOR MEDIASTINAL AND ESOPHAGAL LESIONS

In dealing with extrapulmonary lesions such as mediastinal masses or esophageal pathologic processes, the patient should be positioned to allow gravity to retract the lung. This usually is accomplished by placing the patient in a modified supine or prone position as already described. In thinking about port placement, the surgeon should put the telescope in a position that allows the best visualization of the area to be addressed. The working ports are then positioned so that the surgeon is working in line with the camera. The cannulas should not be placed too close together because the instruments and telescope will end up "dueling," making the dissection much more difficult. If possible, the telescope should be situated superior to the working ports to avoid this problem. A 30- to 45-degree scope allows the surgeon to look down on the instruments, much as in open surgery, and is extremely helpful when the working space is limited.

When working in the posterior mediastinum or on the esophagus, it is useful to have a flexible gastroscope, bougie, or nasogastric tube in the esophagus during the dissection. This helps to identify the esophagus by illumination or by palpation of the intraesophageal stent with the instruments. It may also be useful in identifying any iatrogenic injuries to the esophagus. This is especially true in performing a myotomy for achalasia. Having the esophagoscope in place during the myotomy not only aids in identifying the esophagus and checking for mucosal perforations but also with internal visualization, which can help to determine whether the myotomy has been extended far enough distally. This is evident by the relaxation of the lower esophageal sphincter as seen intraluminally. The myotomy can be performed using a number of different instruments, but most surgeons find a hook cautery or sharp dissection work extremely well. Care must be taken not to cause thermal injury to the mucosal lining when using the hook or other energy

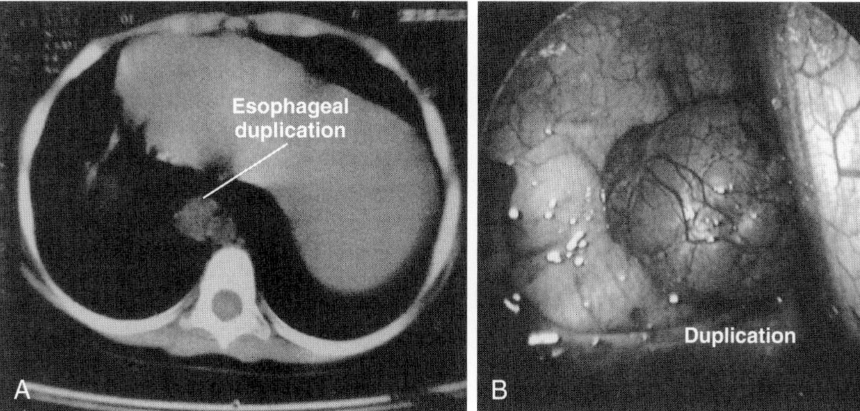

Figure 28-13. A foregut duplication cyst is seen on a CT scan (**A**) and at thoracoscopy (**B**).

devices. The main question surrounding thoracoscopic esophagomyotomy is whether it is appropriate to perform the myotomy without the addition of a partial fundoplication to prevent postoperative gastroesophageal reflux. Most authors now believe that there is a significant risk of severe gastroesophageal reflux after myotomy and therefore recommend performing a partial wrap with the myotomy. This is best achieved using a laparoscopic approach.

The same exposure can be used to approach the esophageal hiatus in cases of hiatal or paraesophageal hernias. This is especially useful in patients who have undergone a previous abdominal fundoplication and whose wrap is intact but has herniated into the mediastinum. This technique allows the surgeon to approach the hiatus without having to go through a previously operated field and avoids the need of taking down the wrap to get adequate exposure. Both the right and left crus can be exposed from the left chest, and an excellent hiatal repair can be achieved.

Other esophageal procedures that have been successfully completed and reported include resection of duplications, diverticula, and esophageal wall tumors. Foregut duplications are relatively common entities that are easily approached thoracoscopically (Fig. 28-13). Once identified, the lesion is circumferentially freed from the overlying parietal pleura. This can be done either with sharp dissection because the plane is generally avascular or with the use of various energy sources. There is generally a well-defined stalk at the base of the cyst, although most do not have a luminal connection and can simply be dissected off the muscular wall of the esophagus without breeching the mucosal lining. If there is a connection, this can be sutured. In larger patients, an endoscopic stapler can be used to divide and seal the tract. Even if there is not a mucosal connection, there will be a defect in the muscular wall of the esophagus because of the common wall. This should be closed primarily to prevent later development of a diverticulum.

Bronchogenic cysts are approached in much the same fashion with dissection of the cyst down to its common wall with either the membranous trachea or bronchus. However, in these cases, the common wall often cannot be separated without causing injury or perforation of the membranous portion of the trachea. Therefore, it is usually better to leave the small common portion on the back wall of the cyst intact and either excise or ablate the retained mucosal lining.

In the last few years, successful thoracoscopic repair of esophageal atresia and tracheoesophageal fistula has become commonplace.[43-45] A multi-institutional review of 106 patients suggested that the procedure is equivalent, if not better, than the standard open technique.[31] These procedures are performed with the infant in a modified prone position with the right side slightly elevated. A three-port technique with the telescope and camera in the posterior axillary line and the working ports in the midaxillary line allows excellent exposure. In general, CO_2 insufflation alone is adequate to cause collapse of the right lung and time should not be wasted trying to obtain single-lung isolation. The operative technique follows the same course as in open surgery with a few minor differences. The first is cauterization and division of the azygos vein, which provides a good landmark for the location of the fistula. The lower esophageal segment is isolated and dissected proximally to its insertion into the membranous trachea (Fig. 28-14). This is actually seen much better thorascopically than via a thoracotomy because the telescope is at right angles to the fistula and the view is magnified. A 5-mm surgical clip or suture can be used to ligate the fistula at its insertion into the trachea. The upper esophageal pouch is then identified by having the anesthesiologist provide downward pressure on the oroesophageal tube. The upper pouch is mobilized well up into the thoracic inlet. The distal tip of the upper pouch is resected, and an end-to-end anastomosis is performed. The posterior wall is approximated first with a series of interrupted simple sutures with the knots lying intraluminal. This is done with 4-0 or 5-0 PDS (Ethicon, Inc., Somerville, NJ) suture. Once the back row is secure, a small nasogastric tube is passed into the lower segment (Fig. 28-15). Then, the anterior wall anastomosis is completed. A chest drain is inserted through the lowest cannula site to a point adjacent to the anastomosis. A contrast study is obtained on day 4 to rule out a leak, and oral feedings are then started.

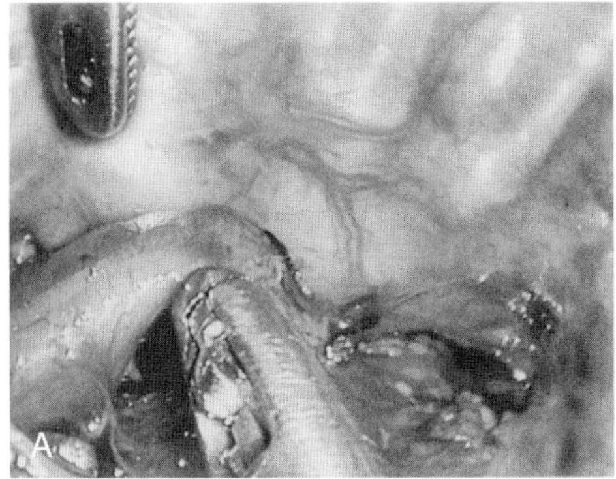

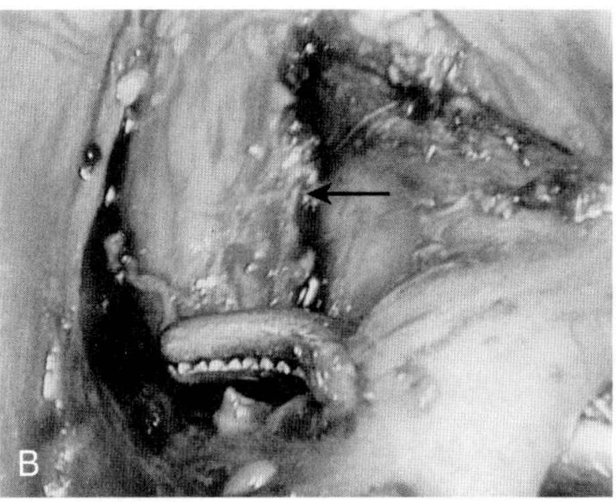

Figure 28-14. A, The distal esophagus is being mobilized near its insertion into the membranous fistula. **B,** The angled telescope is rotated to visualize the back side of the tracheoesophageal fistula. The distended proximal esophagus also is seen (*arrow*).

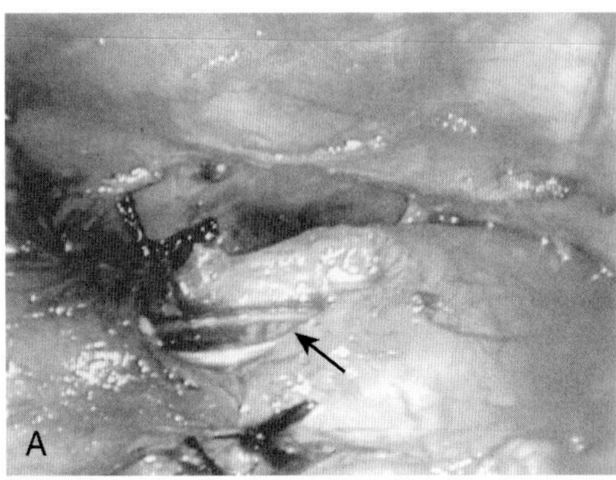

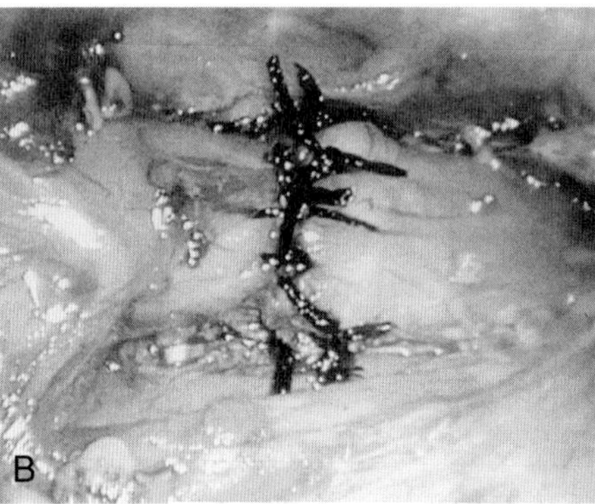

Figure 28-15. A, The posterior row of the esophageal anastomosis has been accomplished, and a small feeding catheter (*arrow*) is advanced through the anastomosis into the stomach. **B,** The completed anastomosis is seen on the right.

ANTERIOR MEDIASTINAL PROCEDURES

The entire anterior mediastinum can be well visualized thoracoscopically and provides excellent access to anterior mediastinal, paratracheal, and hilar adenopathy. This is an excellent approach for node biopsy and can avoid a more invasive anterior mini-thoracotomy, Chamberlain procedure, or a more limited and dangerous mediastinoscopy, which provides far less visualization and access. These biopsy samples can usually be performed with three 3- or 5-mm ports. The patient is placed in a modified supine position, and the ports are situated between the third and fifth interspaces and between the anterior and midaxillary lines. The mass can usually be easily visualized, and a resection or biopsy can be obtained without difficulty (Fig. 28-16). Care should be taken in all anterior mediastinal procedures to avoid injury to the phrenic nerve, which can be easily seen. Teratomas and mediastinal thyroid tumors have also been excised using this approach with excellent results. Occasionally, a mini-thoracotomy is necessary to remove the specimen.

Thymectomy for myasthenia gravis is perfectly suited to a thoracoscopic approach.[20] This can be approached from either the right or left chest depending on surgeon preference. The ports are placed in a similar position as for other anterior mediastinal masses. The ipsilateral inferior horn is dissected first, taking care to avoid the phrenic nerve. Dissection is carried up to the isthmus, and then the upper pole is mobilized. There is usually a posterior thymic vessel draining into the innominate vein. Once this is sealed and divided, the contralateral horns are easily retracted to the surgeon's side and can be fully mobilized under direct vision. The contralateral pleura should not be breached. The specimens can be removed by slightly enlarging one of the cannula sites, usually in the midaxillary line, which results in a very cosmetic incision.

PATENT DUCTUS ARTERIOSUS CLOSURE

Closure of a persistent patent ductus arteriosus has been routinely performed through a standard posterolateral thoracotomy incision with either suture or clip ligation. Over the past decade, an increasing experience with intravascular occlusive devices such as coils and plugs developed, but this technique is often limited by the size of the patient and the diameter of the ductus.[46] Thoracoscopic closure offers an alternative approach and affords many of the same benefits as seen in other thoracoscopic procedures.

The procedure is performed with the patient in a modified prone position with the left side elevated approximately 30 degrees. Two 3-mm ports and one 5-mm port are used to perform the operation. A right main-stem intubation is obtained, and the collapsed left lung is retracted anteriorly by gravity, exposing the ductus. Starting in the middle of the aorta, the pleura overlying the ductus is dissected and retracted

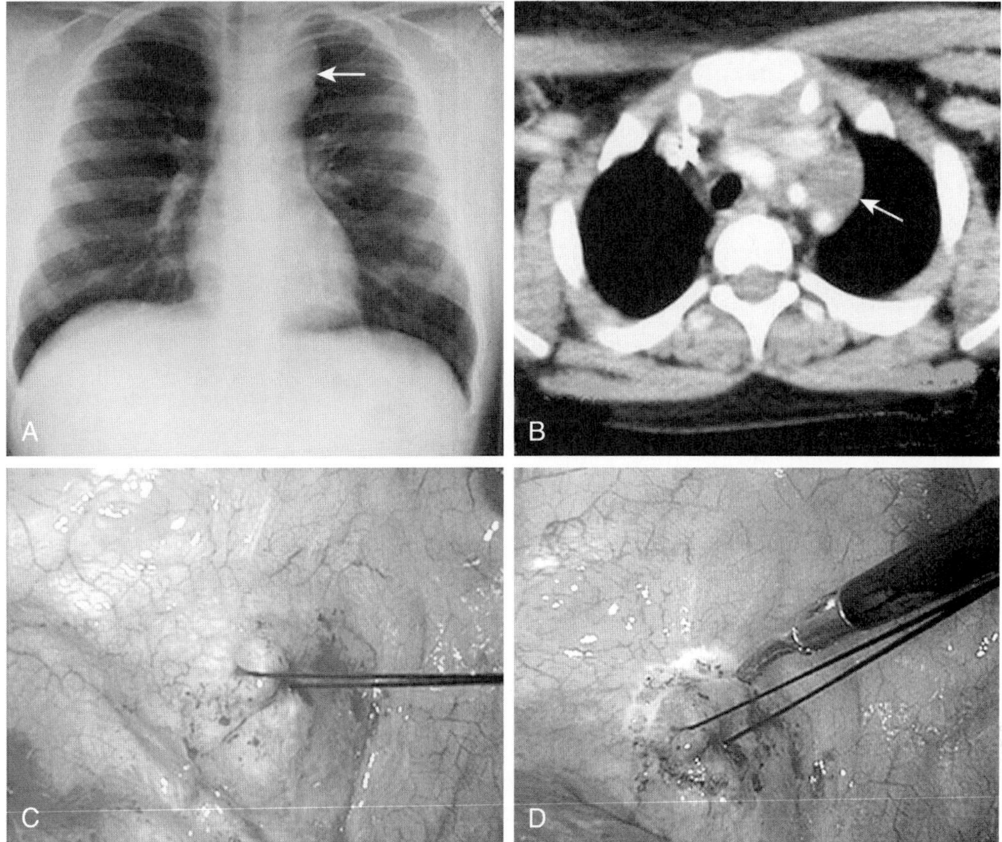

Figure 28-16. **A,** In this patient the chest radiograph reveals a left mediastinal mass (*arrow*). **B,** On the chest CT scan, the vascular structures are seen to be medial and inferior to the mass (*arrow*). **C,** A silk suture has been placed in a figure-of-eight fashion through the mass to help manipulate the specimen without traumatizing it. **D,** The biopsy site is being outlined with a Maryland dissecting instrument connected to cautery. Scissors were used to excise a piece of the mass for the biopsy. (From Little DC, Holcomb GW III: Thoracoscopic biopsy of a mediastinal mass. In Holcomb GW III, Georgeson KE, Rothenberg SS [eds]: Atlas of Pediatric Laparoscopy and Thoracoscopy. Philadelphia, Elsevier, 2008, pp 275-278.)

medially. This exposes the ductus and pulls the vagus nerve out of the field of dissection. The endoscope allows excellent visualization of the ductus and the recurrent laryngeal nerve, which should help prevent injury to this structure. A 5-mm endoscopic clip can then be safely applied to the ductus, thereby occluding flow (Fig. 28-17). In some cases, it is necessary to use a larger clip or perform suture ligation. In these cases, the 5-mm port is removed and a standard hemoclip can be placed through an enlarged port incision. To date, excellent results have been obtained with this technique with minimal morbidity and a significant decrease in recovery and hospitalization.

SYMPATHECTOMY

Thoracic sympathectomy for hyperhidrosis is an accepted technique in patients who have debilitating sweating in their upper extremities. The ability to perform the procedure thoracoscopically has removed the majority of the morbidity associated with the

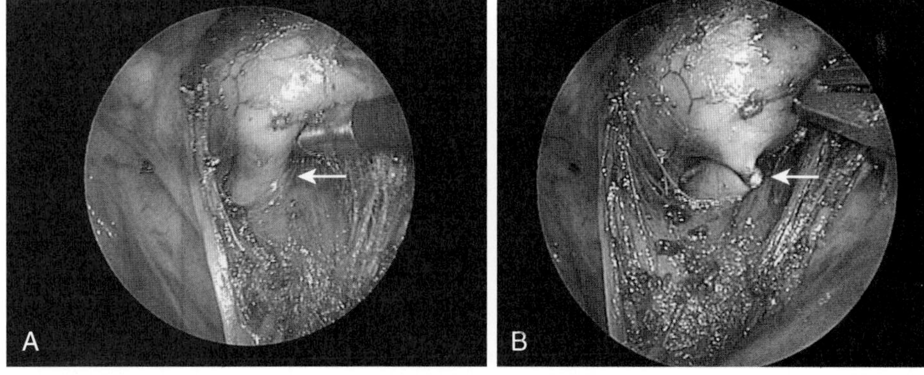

Figure 28-17. **A,** A patent ductus arteriosus (PDA) (*arrow*) is being isolated. **B,** The PDA has been occluded with two 5-mm endoscopic clips (*arrow*).

procedure.[47] Generally, bilateral sympathectomies are performed at the same operative session. These can be done either with the patient in a lateral decubitus position with ports placed in the axilla or with the patient supine and in relatively steep reverse Trendelenburg position.

The first option gives slightly better exposure but requires repositioning the patient to move to the other side. The supine position allows both sides to be accomplished without moving the patient.

CO_2 insufflation is usually sufficient to create lung collapse to expose the upper thoracic sympathetic chain. The procedure consists of interruption of the upper sympathetic chain, below the stellate ganglion, usually from T2 to T4. This can be accomplished by exposing the sympathetic chain and resecting a small segment or simply cauterizing the second and third thoracic ganglion. This can be performed using either two or three ports. A single-port technique utilizing a hook cautery has also been used. Care must be taken to prevent injury to the stellate ganglion to avoid Horner syndrome.

ANTERIOR SPINAL PROCEDURES

The treatment for severe scoliosis and kyphosis in children has involved extensive dissection with significant associated pain and morbidity. These procedures are usually a joint endeavor between the pediatric surgeon and the pediatric orthopedist and consist of an anterior discectomy and release, followed by posterior correction and fixation with rods. Many of these children already have severe pulmonary compromise and these procedures can be associated with significant morbidity and even death. Over the past 10 years, the anterior part of the operation has been performed thoracoscopically.[48] The patient has thus avoided a painful thoracotomy.

The patient is placed in a modified lateral decubitus position tilted slightly prone to aid in keeping the lung out of the visual field. The anterior release can usually be performed through four or five small incisions ranging from 5 to 10 mm (Fig. 28-18). The position of the incisions depends on the number and level of the discs to be removed. In general, the initial port is placed near the apex of the spinal deformity in the midaxillary line. The disc spaces can then be counted and the other ports positioned appropriately. Often, two discs can be extracted using one incision. All ports are kept in the midaxillary line so that the scope and instruments can be interchanged as the spine surgeon moves up and down along the spine.

The first step is exposure of the disc spaces by incising and then clearing the overlying pleura at each level. The segmental vessels can either be preserved or ligated and divided depending on the preference of the spine surgeon. The spine surgeon then performs the discectomy using modified spine instrumentation and packs the disc space with tricortical allograft or other bone graft to enhance fusion. The disc spaces from T2 to T12 can be extracted thoracoscopically. The diaphragm can be mobilized to give access to the first and second lumbar vertebrae, if needed.

A single chest tube is inserted through one of the lower port sites, and the other sites are closed. The operative time for this approach is now shorter than the open operation. The postoperative recovery has markedly improved, and the time needed for chest tube drainage has significantly diminished. Some centers have even started placing anterior instrumentation using a thoracoscopic-assisted approach, but the experience is very limited. Other spinal procedures, including vertebral body biopsies and hemi-vertebrectomy can also be accomplished.

POSTOPERATIVE CARE

The postoperative care in the majority of patients is straightforward. After biopsy or limited resection, most patients can be admitted directly to the surgical floor with limited monitoring (i.e., a pulse oximeter for 6 to 12 hours). These patients are generally 23-hour observation candidates, and a number are actually ready for discharge the same evening. If a chest tube is left, it can usually be removed on the first postoperative day. Pain management has not been a significant problem. Local anesthetic is injected at each port site before insertion of the port and then one or two doses of intravenous narcotic are given in the immediate postoperative period. By that evening or the following morning, most patients are comfortable on oral analgesics. It is very important, especially in the patients with compromised lung function, to start early and aggressive pulmonary toilet. The significant decrease in postoperative pain associated with the thoracoscopic approach results in much less splinting

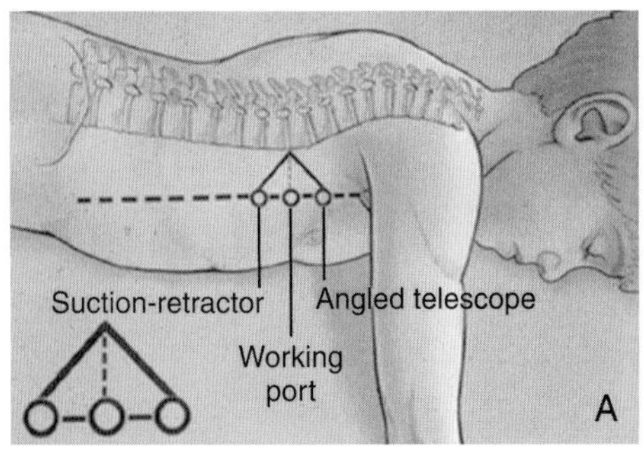

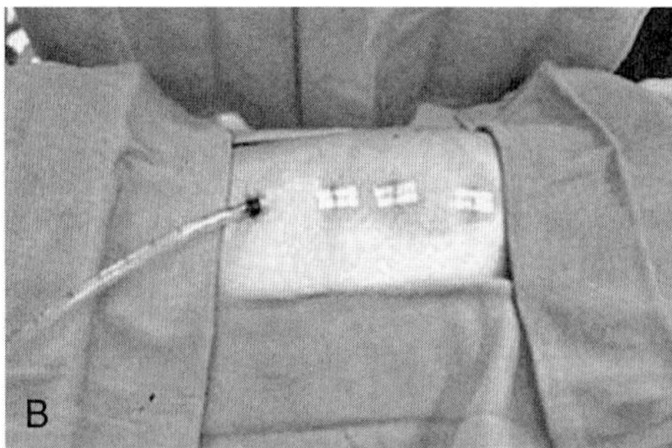

Figure 28-18. The incisions for a thoracoscopic anterior release, discectomy, and fusion are seen. In general, four incisions are needed for release, discectomy, and fusion at five disc levels. **A,** The instruments are rotated among the ports so that the working port is at a 90-degree angle to the disc space. **B,** Operative photograph shows the incisions. The chest tube has been exteriorized through the most caudal incision.

and allows for more effective deep breathing. This has resulted in a decrease in postoperative pneumonias and other pulmonary complications.

Although a thoracoscopic approach may not always result in a significant decrease in hospitalization, it usually results in a significant decrease in the overall morbidity for the patient. The thoracoscopic approach has clearly shown significant benefits over standard open thoracotomy in many cases. With continued improvement and miniaturization of the equipment, the procedures we can perform and the advantages to the patient should continue to grow.

section 4

ABDOMEN

chapter 29

GASTROESOPHAGEAL REFLUX

Daniel J. Ostlie, MD • George W. Holcomb III, MD, MBA

Gastroesophageal reflux (GER) is a disease that is commonly encountered in infants and children. In general, the episodes of GER that are seen in infants and children are not clinically significant and will have no identifiable etiology. In addition, 60% to 65% of children with GER will undergo spontaneous symptom resolution by 2 years of life, regardless of any medical treatment.[1] However, some children will have pathologic gastroesophageal reflux disease (GERD) that will result in either failure to grow appropriately, respiratory complications, or apparent life-threatening events (ALTE). This is the population that will require medical and/or surgical intervention.

HISTORY

The effects of GERD in pediatric patients have been reported for over a century.[2-6] Before the introduction of proton pump inhibitors (PPIs) in the 1990s, the medical management of GER in children and adults was relatively ineffective and based on antacids and histamine antagonists. Because of this limited spectrum of medical management in the 1950s and 1960s, several surgeons developed operative approaches for GER management. Lortat-Jacob, Hill, Belsey, Nissen Rosetti, and Thal all contributed greatly to the surgical management of GERD.[7-13]

These antireflux procedures were initially developed in adults and were effective in controlling GER. Subsequently, they were applied to infants and children with good success.[7,14,15] The overall management of GERD has progressed significantly over the past 2 decades with more effective PPIs and refinement in the surgical technique. Clearly, the most important surgical advance occurred in 1991 when Dallemagne reported his experience with laparoscopic fundoplication.[16] An expected evolutionary cascade led to the use of laparoscopy in children by Georgeson and Lobe.[17,18] Because of these pioneers, and the many researchers that followed, we now know that laparoscopic fundoplication is safe and effective in treating GERD with few complications and excellent control of symptoms in infants and children.

PATHOPHYSIOLOGY

GERD is defined as the pathologic effects of involuntary passage of gastric contents into the esophagus. Ultimately, the pathophysiologic alteration that is responsible for the development of GERD is incompetence of the antireflux barriers that exist between the lower esophagus and the stomach. The result of this incompetence is the presence of gastric refluxate (acid and pepsin) in direct contact with the esophageal mucosa. The pathologic events that occur because of GERD are due to one or multiple failures of the normal physiologic barriers that exist to prevent gastric contents from entering the esophagus, or to limit injury to the esophagus as a result of gastric refluxate, or to clear the refluxate that enters the esophagus (Table 29-1).

In adults, the consequence of this refluxate in the esophagus is primarily limited to erosive esophagitis, esophageal stricture, and Barrett's esophagitis. In children, its detrimental effects are much broader. Also, associated physiologic, anatomic, and developmental abnormalities co-exist in children that make GERD and its consequences much more complex. Many children with GERD have significant neurologic impairment. These children can have increased

Table 29-1 Mechanisms That Either Prevent Gastroesophageal Reflux, Limit the Esophageal Injury, or Clear the Refluxate

Prevent Gastric Reflux	Limit Esophageal Injury	Clear Esophageal Refluxate
Lower esophageal sphincter	Saliva	Esophageal peristalsis
Angle of His	Amount of gastric acid	Saliva
Length of intra-abdominal esophagus	Pepsin	Gravity
Elevated intra-abdominal pressure	Trypsin	
	Bile acids	

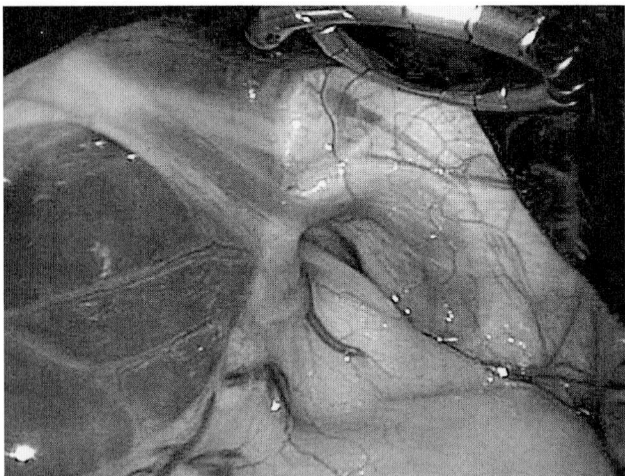

Figure 29-1. This intraoperative photograph depicts a de-novo hiatal hernia in a 13-month-old infant. Note the enlarged hiatus. A portion of the upper stomach has herniated into the chest.

spasticity with retching and related increased abdominal pressures. Poor swallowing mechanisms lead to gagging and choking, which add to this intermittent increased abdominal pressure. Sometimes, a hiatal hernia develops (Fig. 29-1), further predisposing to GERD. Congenital anomalies such as esophageal atresia with or without tracheoesophageal fistula (EA/TEF), duodenal and proximal small bowel atresias, congenital diaphragmatic hernia (CDH), and gastroschisis/omphalocele all predispose to the development of GERD. The consequences of GERD in children lead to the same complications seen in adults (erosive esophagitis, stricture, and Barrett's esophagitis) but also include pulmonary effects (reactive airway disease and pneumonia), potential malnutrition secondary to the inability to maintain adequate caloric intake, and apneic episodes leading to ALTE spells.

Barriers against GERD

The most important factor for preventing reflux of gastric contents into the esophagus is the lower esophageal sphincter (LES). Embryologically, the LES arises from the inner circular muscle layer of the esophagus, which is asymmetrically thickened in the distal esophagus. This thickened muscle layer creates a high pressure zone that can be measured manometrically. In addition, this muscular thickening extends onto the stomach more prominently on the greater than lesser curvature.[19] The phrenoesophageal membrane, arising from the septum transversum of the diaphragm and the collar of Helvetius, holds the LES in position. The result is an LES that lies partially in the chest and partially in the abdomen. This positioning is important for the normal barrier function against GER. Esophageal manometry can identify this transition (which is known as the respiratory inversion point) from the thoracic to the abdominal esophagus.

The LES is an imperfect valve that creates a pressure gradient in the distal esophagus. The ability to prevent GER is directly proportional to the LES pressure and its length, provided that LES relaxation is normal. In an adult study, LES pressures greater than 30 mm Hg prevented GER, as documented by 24-hour pH study, whereas pressures between 0 and 5 mm Hg correlated with abnormal pH studies in more than 80% of patients.[20] Also, GER is statistically significantly more likely to develop in adults if the LES pressure falls below 6 mm Hg at the respiratory inversion point or if the overall LES length is 2 cm or less.[21] As noted previously, the LES is relatively fixed across the esophageal hiatus by its surrounding attachments. Malposition of the LES, which can occur with a hiatal hernia or abnormal development, results in loss of the protective function of the LES, resulting in GER. Finally, LES relaxation occurs with esophageal peristalsis initiated by the swallowing mechanism. This relaxation is normal and must occur. Inappropriate LES relaxations, referred to as transient LES relaxations, have been shown to occur sporadically, unassociated with the swallowing mechanism. Interestingly, when children with symptoms of GER were studied with pH and manometry simultaneously, reflux episodes rarely correlated with decreased LES pressures. Rather, the majority of reflux episodes occurred during transient LES relaxations, and no reflux episodes were identified during LES relaxation after swallowing with normal peristaltic sequence.[22,23] There continues to be growing support that these transient LES relaxations are the primary mechanism for GER.

In summary, although the barrier function of the LES is imperfect, it can be highly effective. Short LES length, abnormal smooth muscle function, increased frequency of transient LES relaxations, and LES location within the chest can contribute individually (or in combination) to LES failure and GER.

Another barrier to the development of symptomatic GER is the intra-abdominal length of the esophagus.[24] Although no absolute effective intra-abdominal esophageal length has been identified that prevents GER, correlation between several lengths and GER have been identified. In one report, an intra-abdominal length of 3 to 4.5 cm in adults with normal abdominal pressure provided LES competency 100% of the time.[20] A length of 3 cm was sufficient in preventing reflux in 64% of individuals, whereas less than 1 cm of intra-abdominal esophagus resulted in reflux in 81% of patients. It is believed that failure to mobilize adequate esophageal length for intra-abdominal positioning can lead to less than successful results or recurrent GER in adults. However, whether these data are applicable in infants and children is unclear.

A third barrier to reflux is the angle of His, which is the angle at which the esophagus enters the stomach. The usual orientation is that of an acute angle, which creates a flap valve at the gastroesophageal junction. Although the actual functional component of the angle of His is not well known, it has been shown to provide resistance to GER. Experimentally, when this angle is more obtuse, GER is more prone to develop. Conversely, accentuation of the angle inhibits GER.[25]

The ability of the angle of His to prevent GER may be diminished as a result of abnormal development or may be iatrogenic, as occurs after gastrostomy placement. When a normal angle of His is present, there is a convoluted fold of mucosa present at the gastroesophageal junction. This mucosa creates a rosette-like configuration that collapses on itself with increases in intragastric pressure or negative pressure in the thoracic esophagus, thus acting as an additional weak antireflux valve.[26,27]

Patients with increased abdominal pressure as a result of neurologically related retching, physiologic effects (ascites, peritoneal dialysis), or anatomic abnormalities (gastroschisis, omphalocele, CDH) are at increased risk for developing GERD owing to the effects of chronic pressure from the abdomen into the thorax.[28-35] Finally, certain congenital defects such as congenital short esophagus, congenital hiatal hernia, and EA/TEF predispose to GERD. In patients with EA/TEF, the esophagus has abnormal peristalsis and the LES is incompetent. It has been reported that up to 30% of these patients will require antireflux surgery after repair of their EA/TEF.[36-38] Regarding CDH, anatomic abnormalities of the esophageal hiatus and the esophagus predispose to GERD, with 15% to 20% of surviving patients undergoing an antireflux operation for GERD.[33-35]

Once the barrier to GER has been overcome (or failed), mechanisms for esophageal clearance become important in preventing damage associated with exposure of the esophageal mucosa to the gastric refluxate. The primary mechanism for esophageal clearance remains esophageal motility. However, gravity and saliva contribute to the ability of the esophagus to clear the refluxate.[39,40] There are three types of esophageal contractions: primary, secondary, and tertiary. Primary contraction waves are initiated with swallowing and are responsible for the clearance of refluxed contents in 80% to 90% of reflux episodes. Secondary waves occur when material is refluxed into the esophagus and clearance is required, especially when the reflux occurs during sleep.[41,42] Tertiary waves have nothing to do with esophageal clearance and are sporadic, nonpropagating contractions. When impaired esophageal motility is present as a result of either abnormal smooth muscle function, impaired vagal stimulation, or obstruction, refluxed gastric contents are not moved caudad into the stomach in a timely manner. This prolonged exposure can lead to esophageal mucosal injury and can potentiate the motility disturbance due to vagal and/or smooth muscle inflammation or injury. Saliva neutralizes refluxed material, and patients with GERD have been found to have decreased salivary function. It has also been shown that positional effects of GERD treatment may be related to gravity assisting in the clearance of esophageal refluxate.[43-46]

The final element for prevention of esophageal injury related to GERD is the ability to limit injury once refluxed contents have reached the esophagus. In addition to functioning as a neutralizing agent, saliva also aids in lubricating the esophageal contents, thus making it easier to clear any retained refluxate. Acid exposure has been postulated to cause the most significant injury. When combined with pepsin, esophageal mucosal injury occurs.[47,48] The injury related to gastric acid is not strictly due to the low pH but also to the volume of acid that is refluxed. Some pediatric patients with documented GERD have been shown to have increased acid secretion.[49,50] To this end, the role of PPIs in controlling GERD in this population is very important because they have the dual effect of decreasing pH while simultaneously decreasing the acid volume.[51-53] Regarding substances that increase esophageal mucosal injury, bile salts, pepsin, and trypsin are the most important components in the refluxate that need to be neutralized. When combined with acid, bile salts are injurious to the esophageal mucosa. In addition, they increase the permeability of the esophageal mucosa to existing acid, thus further potentiating injury.[54,55] Pepsin and trypsin are both proteolytic enzymes that can injure the esophageal mucosa. Both of these enzymes are more toxic at lower pH levels and, hence, are more injurious in the presence of acid.[56,57]

Table 29-2 Frequency of Symptoms in Patients with Gastroesophageal Reflux

Symptom	Frequency
Regurgitation/vomiting	81%
Pulmonary symptoms	41%
Dysphagia/pain	30%
Hemorrhage	7%

Adapted from Tovar JA, Olivares P, Diaz M, et al: Functional results of laparoscopic fundoplication in children. J Pediatr Gastroenterol Nutr 26:429-431, 1998.

CLINICAL MANIFESTATIONS

The presentation of GERD in infants and children is variable and depends on the patient's age and overall medical condition. The surgeon must consider both this variability and the patient characteristics when evaluating a child with symptoms for possible GERD. Although the symptoms of GERD are variable for each patient, the actual frequency of symptoms seen in infants who have required surgical intervention for GERD has been reported (Table 29-2).[58]

When considering the symptoms associated with GERD, persistent regurgitation is the most common complaint reported by parents of children with GERD.[59] However, in infants, vomiting is often physiologic and can be "normal." This type of vomiting is termed *chalasia of infancy* and is seen early in life, usually during burping, after feeding, or when placed in the recumbent position.[60] Chalasia does not interfere with normal growth or development and rarely leads to other complications. It is a self-limited process with most infants transitioning to being asymptomatic by 2 years of age or near the time of initiating solid foods.[1] No treatment is necessary in patients who have chalasia, and no diagnostic evaluation should be pursued. However, when persistent regurgitation is the result of

GER, it can lead to complications, including significant malnutrition and growth failure due to insufficient caloric intake.

In infants, another presenting symptom is irritability due to pain. Painful esophagitis can be the result of the acid refluxate. Discomfort leads to crying despite consoling measures.[61,62] Occasionally, small volumes of feeds briefly assist in alleviating pain. However, this is generally not a lasting effect.[24,25] In contrast to infants, children with pathologic GER more often present with complaints of pain. As in adults, the pain is retrosternal in nature, often described as "heartburn." Long-standing GER with esophagitis can lead to chronic inflammation or even ulcer formation with eventual scarring and stricture. Dysphagia develops as a result of a narrowed esophageal lumen, as well as possible esophageal dysmotility secondary to long-standing mucosal inflammation. Obstructive symptoms and pain are the two most common associated complaints when an esophageal stricture is present.[63,64]

Barrett's esophagitis is a premalignant condition that is associated with prolonged GERD. It occurs when metaplasia develops in the esophageal squamous epithelium that is replaced with columnar epithelium. In adults, it is thought to be the result of chronic esophageal injury by gastric acid reflux.[65-67] Although uncommon in infants and children, when it does develop, serious complications often result. In addition to the increased risk for adenocarcinoma, approximately 50% of these patients will develop stricture and many patients will develop ulcers.[68,69] Aggressive GER management, along with vigilant long-term surveillance via yearly esophagogastroscopy, must be pursued to minimize these often difficult and possibly fatal complications.

Respiratory symptoms are commonly seen in infants and children. Delineating the role of GER as an etiologic agent for ongoing respiratory complaints can be difficult because of the similiarity of the symptoms that are seen with other pulmonary diseases. Chronic cough, wheezing, choking, apnea, or near sudden infant death syndrome (SIDS) can all be symptoms attributable to GER. Recurrent bronchitis or pneumonia can occur from aspiration of the refluxate.[70] Esophageal stimulation via acidification of the esophageal mucosa causes vagally mediated laryngospasm and bronchospasm, which clinically presents as apnea or choking or mistakenly as asthma.[71,72] Esophageal inflammation, as seen with esophagitis, likely enhances this mechanism.[73,74] The effects of GER on premature infants with respiratory problems have been studied.[75] Most of these infants were intubated for varying periods owing to respiratory distress syndrome or bronchopulmonary dysplasia. In the former group, GER was responsible for deteriorating pulmonary status requiring intubation. In the latter, deterioration of pulmonary status plus failure to thrive and anorexia led to the diagnosis of GER. All improved with correction of the GER.[76]

Although uncommon, hemorrhage can be a presenting symptom of GER. Esophagitis, gastritis, and ulcer formation can lead to hematochezia or melena in a small percentage of infants or children.[58]

DIAGNOSTIC EVALUATION

As noted in the previous section, the clinical history is an invaluable asset when evaluating for the presence of GERD and determining the need for antireflux therapy. Once the concern for GER as the etiologic cause of the patient's complaints has been raised, diagnostic evaluation should be initiated. Upper gastrointestinal radiography is the most frequent initial study employed. Evidence for reflux is sometimes seen on the examination. However, the absence of reflux is an extremely poor indicator of GER as a cause of the patient's symptoms. The contrast study is most useful for delineating the anatomy of the esophagus and esophagogastric junction. It also evaluates esophageal clearance and assesses esophageal and gastric motility. The contrast study can identify the presence of esophageal strictures, webs, or distal obstructions, such as duodenal obstruction, antral web, or malrotation, as the cause of the reflux symptoms.

Twenty-four-hour pH monitoring is the gold standard for establishing the diagnosis of GER, especially in infants and children whose history is unclear. It provides the diagnosis of GER in cases in which the clinical history cannot be obtained or is confusing, such as a patient presenting with respiratory symptoms only. The study is performed by placing an electrode 2 to 3 cm proximal to the gastroesophageal junction and measuring the pH in the distal esophagus. Although initially developed in adults, its use in children is now accepted and invaluable.[77,78]

The accuracy of the pH examination is dependent on the cessation of all antireflux medication. PPIs should be withheld for 7 days, and histamine receptor blockers are stopped 48 hours before the study. A reflux episode is considered to have occurred if the esophageal pH is recorded as less than 4. Ideally, the examination should occur over an uninterrupted 24-hour period. The pH is continuously monitored via the esophageal electrode while the patient's position (upright and supine) and activities (awake, asleep, eating) are simultaneously recorded. The final score is calculated based on the percent of total time that the pH was less than 4, the total number of reflux episodes, the number of episodes lasting longer than 5 minutes, and the longest reflux episode.[79,80] A normal range of values has been established that is easily reproducible and reliable.[81]

The 24-hour pH monitoring study is indicated in the following specific circumstances:

1. Infants who have respiratory symptoms (apnea, ALTE spells)
2. Infants who are irritable, intractably crying, and anorexic
3. Children who have reactive airway disease (asthma) or unexplained or recurrent pneumonia
4. Children who are unresponsive to medical measures and in whom the role of GER in their symptoms is uncertain

The study also should be done in those children who again become symptomatic after fundoplication. Conversely, the study generally is not useful or necessary for infants with uncomplicated regurgitation, children with esophagitis already found by endoscopy and biopsy, and children with dysphagia or heartburn thought to be caused by GER.

Three patterns of reflux have been described in symptomatic infants, as determined by extended esophageal pH monitoring: continuous, discontinuous, and mixed.[82] Those infants with the discontinuous type rarely required a surgical antireflux operation, whereas approximately half of those with the other two types did. One should keep in mind that medical treatment at the time of this study was much less effective than in the late 1990s. Nonetheless, this study indicates that pH monitoring can be useful in sorting out infants with GER who may or may not require an antireflux procedure.[81,83] Incidentally, all of the infants in this study, including the "normal controls," experienced reflux frequently in the first 2 hours after being given apple juice.

It has been assumed that the retrograde flow of acid/pepsin material from the stomach into the esophagus is the basic pathologic event of reflux disease. It is becoming clear that the situation is not this straightforward. Attempts to correlate symptoms (other than spitting up and vomiting) to pH-probe–detected reflux episodes have been particularly problematic. For example, in infants with spells of choking or colic, a close association between pH-probe–detected acid reflux and these symptoms cannot be routinely demonstrated. Some spells coincide with reflux episodes, but many do not. Similar questions can be raised when looking at pH-probe data on the relation between acid reflux episodes and apnea/bradycardia spells of premature infants or between wheezing, coughing, dental erosion, sleep disturbance, and all the other myriad symptoms attributed to reflux.

By using one "old" diagnostic technique and one "new" one, some of the disparities between pH-probe observations and "events" may be better understood. This is based on the recent observation that some reflux of acid into the lower esophagus occurs while the intraesophageal pH is still less than 4 due to a traditional acid-reflux episode. This is called "acid re-reflux" (ARR) and will be missed by using only pH-monitoring techniques.[84] ARR is most likely to occur in patients with severe esophagitis, postprandially, and in the recumbent posture. It is now thought to be a common cause of prolonged acid contact. Detecting ARR provides a better estimation of the incompetence of the antireflux barrier than does traditional pH-probe evaluations.

Two methods may be used to evaluate ARR. The first is scintigraphy, which directly measures radiolabeled liquid gastric contents flowing into the esophagus, independent of the pH of the refluxate or the esophageal lumen. The second is multichannel intraluminal impedance (MII), a method that recognizes the flow of gastric contents into the esophagus by detecting decreases in impedance from high (the esophagus) to low (the stomach) values across electrode pairs placed throughout the esophagus and in the stomach. MII also can distinguish liquid from gas refluxate.[85-87]

Recent studies using MII suggest that measuring acid reflux (pH study) may not be the best method of evaluating GERD.[88-91] These studies indicate that the pH probe does not simultaneously detect the majority of reflux events as defined by impedance monitoring, presumably because the re-reflux boluses are not acidic. When MII and pH monitoring are used simultaneously, there are significant reflux episodes that are not identified with pH monitoring alone because the episodes are actually non-acid reflux episodes with a pH greater than 4.[89] These non-acid reflux episodes are less common in untreated GERD patients than in normal patients. MII has shown that GERD patients more commonly have liquid-type reflux events, whereas non-GERD patients generally have more gas-type reflux events.[90] Additionally, MII data suggest that treatment with PPIs does not decrease the amount of reflux but rather converts the reflux to non-acid or weakly acidic in nature.[91]

Although essential in adults, esophageal manometry is infrequently utilized in the pediatric population. When employed, the study measures the motility of the esophagus and the pressure at the LES via a multiple-port pressure transducer placed in the esophagus and traversing the LES. The clinical data accumulated in adult patients have revealed several important points that are likely applicable to infants and children with GERD. First, it has been shown that pharyngeal swallowing and primary peristaltic contractions are responsible for the majority of the esophageal clearance of refluxed gastric contents, rather than by secondary and tertiary peristalsis as previously believed.[92] Additionally, through the use of a concomitant 24-hour pH study and esophageal manometry, it has been shown that there is a direct relationship between worsening esophagitis secondary to GERD and deterioration of esophageal motility. Manometric evaluation has been particularly useful in documenting abnormal distal esophageal motility in infants after repair of EA/TEF.[93] It is hoped that, as technology continues to provide more appropriately sized instruments for sophisticated manometric studies in infants and children, the usefulness and feasibility of such studies will increase our knowledge of the physiology and abnormalities associated with GERD in this population.

Endoscopic evaluation of the esophagus and stomach is occasionally needed in the diagnosis of GERD in infants and children. Hematemesis, dysphagia, or irritability in infants, or dysphagia with or without heartburn in children, should prompt esophagogastroscopy to determine if esophagitis is present. Other complications, such as ulcer formation, esophageal stricture, and Barrett's esophagus, can also be diagnosed during the endoscopic examination. Mucosal biopsy should be performed to stage the severity of esophagitis or to histologically exclude dysplasia or malignancy in Barrett's esophagus.[94,95]

The relationship between delayed gastric emptying (DGE) and GERD in infants and children has been extensively studied and continues to be one of the more controversial aspects of antireflux surgery. The evaluation for DGE is undertaken using radionuclide scanning via a technetium-99-labeled meal. When documented preoperatively, DGE has not been shown to significantly improve when an emptying procedure is performed at the time of an antireflux procedure.[96] In fact, one study evaluating patients with DGE undergoing fundoplication showed significantly improved gastric emptying for both solids and liquids after fundoplication alone.[97] Neurologically impaired children with GERD have been shown to have DGE more often than neurologically normal children. Conflicting data regarding the benefit and complication rates for these patients undergoing emptying procedures at the time of their fundoplication have been reported as well.[98] Based on these data, it is not recommended that an empting procedure be performed for a patient with DGE and GERD unless a second operative intervention would place the patient at significant morbidity or mortality.

At our institution, the evaluation for GERD includes an upper gastrointestinal contrast study and 24-hour pH monitoring for most patients suspected of having GERD. The main exceptions are the neurologically impaired patient in the intensive care unit who needs a gastrostomy for feeding and for whom the intensivists request a fundoplication to protect the airway from aspiration. Esophagogastroscopy and esophageal manometry are employed only when circumstances suggest that the information they will provide will dictate changes in the operative management. An example of this situation is the patient with symptoms of GER but a normal pH study. When esophagitis or other complications of GERD are found after esophagogastroscopy or manometry, surgical intervention is usually recommended. Preoperative gastric emptying studies are not performed on a routine basis, primarily owing to the improvement that has been seen and reported in gastric emptying after fundoplication.[96,97] If symptoms of DGE persist after antireflux surgery, gastric emptying studies can be performed with a subsequent emptying procedure, if necessary. However, all patients requiring a second fundoplication undergo an emptying study to be sure their recurrent symptoms are not exacerbated by DGE.

TREATMENT

Once GERD has been diagnosed, the question becomes: should medical or surgical treatment be applied?[15] This decision needs to be individualized based on the patient's age, anatomic information, disease severity, and social environment (which will affect compliance with a treatment regimen). In the majority of cases, nonoperative treatment is the initial therapy of choice.

Medical Management

Position and Feeding

Nonoperative therapy for GERD in infants and children has been based on postural changes and dietary modification for many years. It is important to know the caloric needs of the patient so that a reduction in feeding volume in an attempt to limit reflux does not result in caloric deprivation. Postural and dietary modifications alone will result in clinical improvement in the vast majority of infants with GERD.[99,100] In older children, dietary alterations should include a diet low in fat and the elimination of chocolate, coffee, tea, carbonated drinks, and spicy foods.

The seated semi-upright position (approximately 45 degrees) for an infant with reflux has been recommended since the 1950s. In the 1960s, Carré showed that 60% of children with GERD treated in this way improved by approximately 2 years of age and an additional 30% improved by age 4 years.[1,101]

Failure of postural therapy may be related to social problems, chronic infections, or impaired gastric clearance. In older patients, postural treatment is impractical because of the virtual impossibility of maintaining the desired semi-sitting posture for sleep. Close attention to the details of postural therapy by the family members is most important to its success.[102]

Pharmacologic Therapy

If symptoms persist despite a well-monitored program of postural therapy and dietary modifications, pharmacologic measures should be added. Medical therapy includes the administration of one or more drugs that increase esophageal peristalsis, increase LES pressure, increase gastric emptying, or lessen gastric acid production.

Prokinetic Agents

Historically, prokinetic agents have been utilized in an attempt to increase LES pressure, enhance esophageal peristalsis, and accelerate gastric emptying. The use of cisapride and, more recently, metoclopramide, has been questioned with regard to their safety.[103-105] Both randomized controlled trials and meta-analyses have shown no clinically relevant improvement in children receiving cisapride or metoclopramide.[103,104,106,107] Therefore, the current recommendation regarding prokinetic agents in the management of GERD is that there is no beneficial effect and their use is not advantageous.

Acid Alteration

Measures to reduce gastric acidity should be given to patients with complicated reflux, especially with esophagitis.[108] Alterations in gastric acid may be accomplished by neutralization with antacids, by competition with histamine-2 (H_2)-receptor antagonists, or by PPIs. Because of the superiority of PPIs in controlling acid production, H_2-receptor antagonists or antacids are being utilized less frequently.

PPIs inhibit the final step of gastric acid secretion by blocking proton production by bonding and deactivating H^+,K^+-ATPase (or proton pump) by traversing the parietal cell membrane and accumulating in the secretory canaliculi.[109] The PPI omeprazole has been demonstrated to reduce gastric acid production to zero.[110-112] It is a very powerful medicine that affects gastric acid production for 72 hours after cessation of administration. A prospective study determined that, within the therapeutic dose range (0.7 to 3.5 mg/kg/day), omeprazole was both efficacious and safe for children.[111] In this study, omeprazole was found to be highly effective in severe (grade IV) esophagitis and patients refractory to other medical therapy. A dosage of 0.7 mg/kg/day healed 45% of patients, and 1.4 mg/kg/day healed another 30%. On a body weight basis, the dosages required in children are generally higher than those in adults.[112] For children unable to swallow the whole capsule, it is suggested to open the capsule and give the granular contents in a weakly acidic vehicle such as orange juice, yogurt, or cranberry juice. The granules are stable in acid but are degraded in a neutral or alkaline pH. Newer PPIs (lansoprazole, rabeprazole, pantoprazole, esomeprazole) hold promise as better medical therapeutic possibilities.[113-116]

Operative Management

Operative management usually follows failed medical management for growth failure (failure to thrive or gain weight appropriately), most respiratory symptoms, and other symptoms such as pain and esophagitis. However, in selected circumstances, it may be best to proceed with fundoplication without a trial of medical therapy. These selective situations include the previously mentioned patient in an intensive care unit who requires gastrostomy and the neurologically impaired patient with a similar need for gastrostomy and concern for aspiration. This latter scenario is commonly seen in infants and children, and the decision for or against fundoplication at the time of gastrostomy should be individualized. For example, in a 2- or 3-year-old (or older) neurologically impaired patient who begins to have difficulty with oral intake and requires tube feedings but has no reflux symptoms and a normal pH study, gastrostomy alone without fundoplication is very reasonable. On the other hand, a neurologically impaired infant who cannot swallow and requires tube feedings in the intensive care unit probably should have a fundoplication in addition to a gastrostomy.

Another scenario is the infant who presents with an ALTE spell and GER is documented but no other etiology is identified. This patient may be best served with a fundoplication as the initial therapy. In a review from our institution involving 81 infants presenting with ALTE, their symptoms resolved with fundoplication in 78.[117] The median follow-up in this study was 1738 days. Two required a second fundoplication when their symptoms recurred, and one needed a pyloromyotomy. Interestingly, 96.3% of these patients had been treated with antireflux mediation and 87.7% were taking antireflux medications at the time of their ALTE. Therefore, medical management may not be effective in this population.

Barrett's esophagitis and esophageal stricture are the two other conditions in which initial operative therapy is recommended. The changes of Barrett's esophagus will usually resolve in adolescents after fundoplication, although lifelong postoperative endoscopic surveillance will be needed. Regarding a stricture, dilation can be performed at the time of fundoplication. Subsequent dilations may be needed in severe cases. Finally, children with a known hiatal hernia and symptomatic GER are not likely to respond to medical management. Initial fundoplication is a reasonable choice in these patients.

Laparoscopic Nissen Fundoplication

The patient is placed at the end of the operating table so that the surgeon can stand at the foot of the bed and the assistant to his or her right. The scrub nurse stands to the surgeon's left (Fig. 29-2). For infants, the legs should be placed in a frog-leg position. For

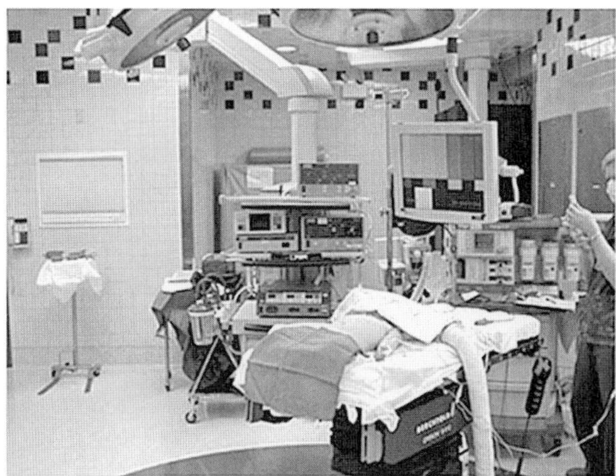

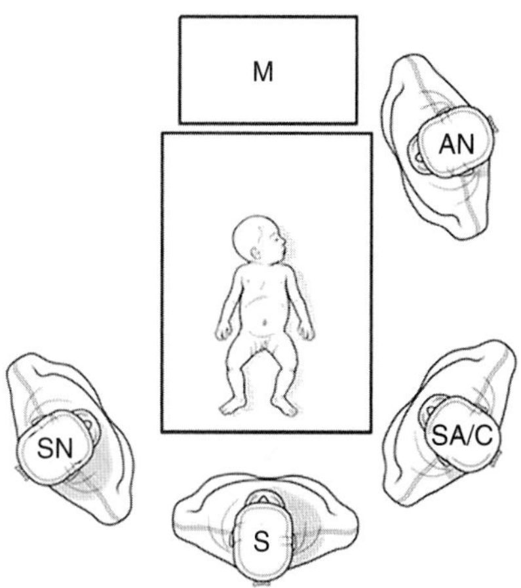

Figure 29-2. For laparoscopic fundoplication, the patient is placed supine on the operating table. Infants and young children are positioned at the foot of the bed in a frog-leg position and the foot of the bed is dropped. The surgeon (S) and surgical assistant/camera holder (SA/C) stand next to the patient at the end of the bed. The scrub nurse (SN) is to the surgeon's left. A single monitor (M) is placed over the patient's head. AN, anesthesiologist. (From Holcomb GW III: Laparoscopic Nissen fundoplication. In Holcomb GW, Georgeson KE, Rothenberg SS [eds]: Atlas of Pediatric Laparoscopy and Thoracoscopy. Philadelphia, Elsevier, 2008, pp 15-20.)

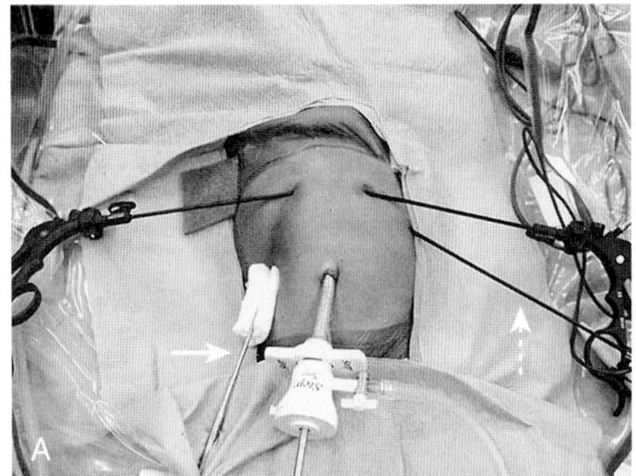

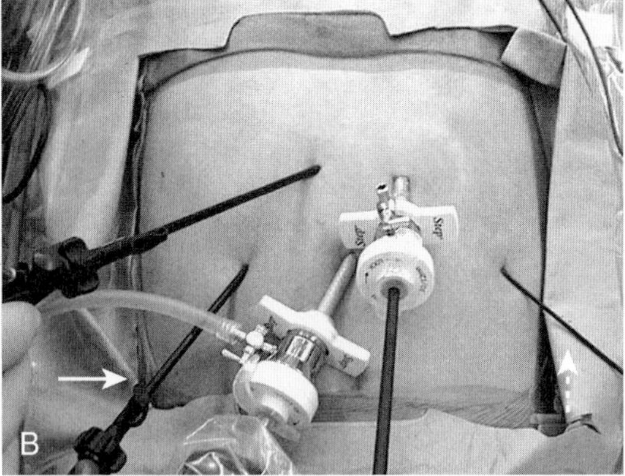

Figure 29-3. There are a number of ways to orient the instruments when performing a laparoscopic fundoplication. With our technique, a 45-degree angled, 5-mm telescope is introduced after insertion of the 5-mm umbilical cannula. The liver retractor is introduced in the patient's right subcostal region (*solid arrow*). The two main working ports are in the left and right epigastrium. The main working port for the surgeon is the one in the patient's left epigastric region. It is through this incision that dissecting instruments, needle holder, and suture are introduced. The instrument utilized by the surgical assistant is in the patient's left subcostal region (*dotted arrow*). The stab incision technique can be utilized for both infants (**A**) and adolescents (**B**). (From Holcomb GW III: Laparoscopic Nissen fundoplication. In Holcomb GW, Georgeson KE, Rothenberg SS [eds]: Atlas of Pediatric Laparoscopy and Thoracoscopy. Philadelphia, Elsevier, 2008, pp 15-20.)

older children, the legs can be positioned in stirrups. Although a single monitor placed over the patient's head is usually sufficient, two monitors, placed to the right and the left of the patient's head, can be used as well. An orogastric tube is introduced by the anesthesiologist to decompress the stomach. The bladder is usually emptied using a Credé maneuver.

After prepping and draping, a 5-mm vertical incision is made in the center of the umbilicus and carried down through the umbilical fascia. A Step sheath (Covidien, Mansfield, MA) is gently introduced into the abdominal cavity, followed by introduction of a cannula with a blunt-tipped trocar through the sheath. By using this open technique, injury to the underlying viscera should be extremely rare. The sheath can be secured to the umbilical skin for stabilization should the surgeon desire. A pneumoperitoneum is created to a pressure of 12 to 15 mm Hg, and diagnostic laparoscopy is performed with a 5-mm, 45-degree angled telescope. Four stab incisions are then placed in infants, and three stab incisions and a 5-mm port for the ultrasonic scalpel are utilized in children older than 5 years of age. The arrangement of these cannulas is seen in Figure 29-3. A liver retractor is introduced through the lateral right port. The two main working sites are the instruments positioned on either side of the midline. The assistant's instrument is in the patient's left lateral abdomen.

We have standardized our technique and have utilized it for the past 8 years.[118-123] Initially, the superior short gastric vessels are ligated and divided. Cautery connected to a Maryland dissecting instrument is used in the younger patients. As previously mentioned, the ultrasonic scalpel is used in older children. The retroesophageal window is initially made from the patient's left side because it is quite easy

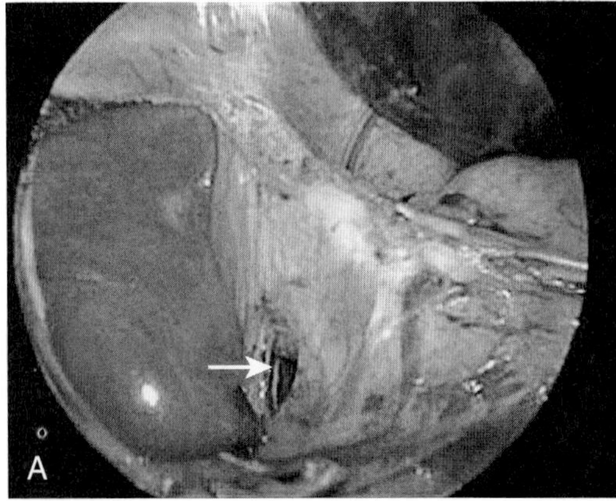

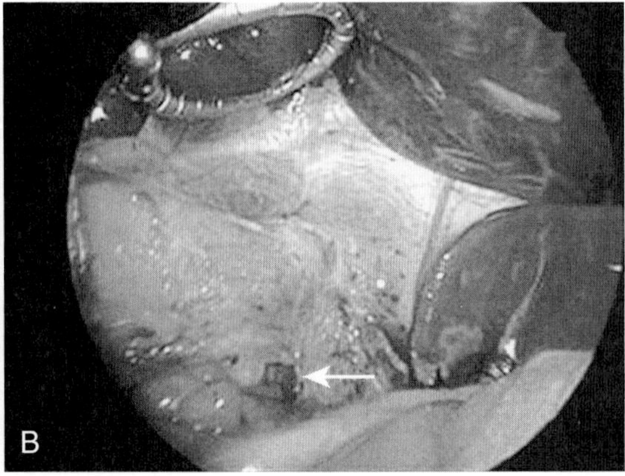

Figure 29-4. If an adequate length of intra-abdominal esophagus is present, then as little dissection as possible is performed to help prevent migration of the fundoplication wrap through an enlarged esophageal hiatus. The phrenoesophageal ligament is kept intact on both the patient's right side of the esophagus (**A**) and the patient's left side of the esophagus (**B**). Note creation of the retroesophageal window has been initiated (*arrows*). (From Holcomb GW III: Laparoscopic Nissen fundoplication. In Holcomb GW, Georgeson KE, Rothenberg SS [eds]: Atlas of Pediatric Laparoscopy and Thoracoscopy. Philadelphia, Elsevier, 2008, pp 15-20.)

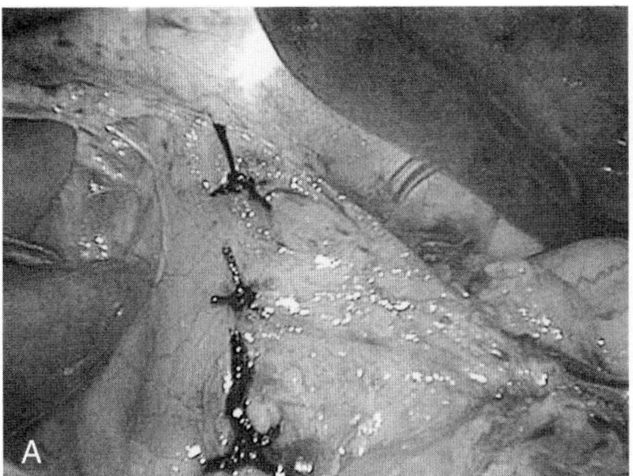

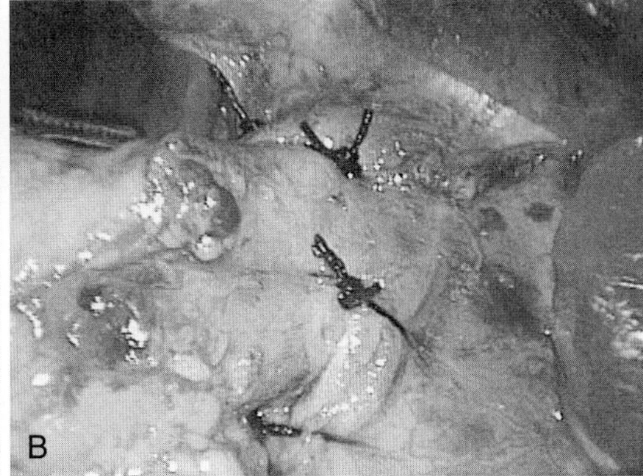

Figure 29-5. Following closure of the esophageal hiatus with a 2-0 silk suture placed posterior to the esophagus, esophagocrural sutures are placed at the 7-, 11-, 1-, and 5-o'clock positions around the esophagus. These photographs show the right (**A**) and left (**B**) sides of the patient's esophagus. The purpose of these sutures is to secure the esophagus in the intra-abdominal position to reduce the incidence of postoperative reflux and also to obliterate the space between the esophagus and crura in an effort to prevent transmigration of the fundoplication wrap.

to accomplish after mobilization and ligation of the superior short gastric vessels. We do not mobilize the esophagus very much to help reduce postoperative transmigration of the fundoplication wrap. (This will be discussed later.) Once the left side of the patient's gastroesophageal junction has been identified, the stomach is flipped to the patient's left and attention is turned toward the right aspect of the esophagus and upper stomach. The gastrohepatic ligament is incised to expose the esophagus and stomach on the right side. Great care must be taken to always know the location of the left gastric artery. It is imperative that the fundoplication wrap is positioned above the left gastric artery rather than inferior to it. The opening in the retroesophageal window is then completed from the right side so that the fundus can be brought through it for the Nissen fundoplication. Again, as little esophageal mobilization as possible is performed at the gastroesophageal junction (Fig. 29-4). Essentially, this means that the phrenoesophageal membrane is incised minimally, if at all.

At this point, usually a single suture is placed posterior to the esophagus to close a small hiatal hernia that may have either been present initially or created during the dissection. This is usually accomplished with a 2-0 silk suture. After placement of this suture and tying it, a small bite of the esophagus at the 7-o'clock position is then taken with the same needle and tied to help obliterate the space between the posterior esophagus and the posterior crural closure. Next, esophagocrural sutures are then created with 3-0 silk at the 8-, 11-, 1-, and 5-o'clock positions to further obliterate the space between the esophagus and the crura to prevent transmigration of the fundoplication wrap (Fig. 29-5).[121] After placement of these crural sutures, the bougie is then introduced. A table describing the appropriate bougie size for neonates weighing less than 15 kg has been developed (Table 29-3).[118] The fundoplication is then performed using a standard Nissen technique. Usually, three 2-0 sutures are utilized to perform the fundoplication. The most superior suture also incorporates a small portion of the anterior esophagus. The length of the fundoplication is measured. Usually a length of approximately 2 cm is desired.[118] For older children, 2.5 to 3.0 cm may be appropriate.

Bupivacaine is instilled in the incisions, and the umbilical fascia and skin are closed. Steri-strips are usually utilized for closure of the stab incisions.

Gastrostomy

If a gastrostomy is also needed, the stab incision or cannula site in the patient's left midepigastric area is the one utilized for exteriorization of the gastrostomy button. If a fundoplication has not been performed, then the same site is used for locating the button. In either event, this site is marked before insufflation so as not to distort its location when the abdomen is distended with CO_2.

A red rubber catheter is introduced by the anesthesiologist into the stomach and the stomach is insufflated with 30 to 60 mL of air to prevent incorporating the back wall of the stomach with the suture utilized to secure the stomach to the anterior abdominal wall. The anterior wall of the stomach is grasped with a locking grasper and brought toward the anterior abdominal wall. The technique for laparoscopic gastrostomy is

Table 29-3 Recommended Bougie Size for Esophageal Calibration in Patients Weighing Less Than 15 kg

Weight (kg)	Bougie Size
2.5-4.0	20-24
4.0-5.5	24-28
5.5-7.0	28-32
7.0-8.5	32-34
8.5-10.0	34-36
10.0-15.0	36-40

From Ostlie DJ, Miller KA, Holcomb GW III: Effective Nissen fundoplication length and bougie diameter size in young children undergoing laparoscopic Nissen fundoplication. J Pediatr Surg 37:1664-1666, 2002.

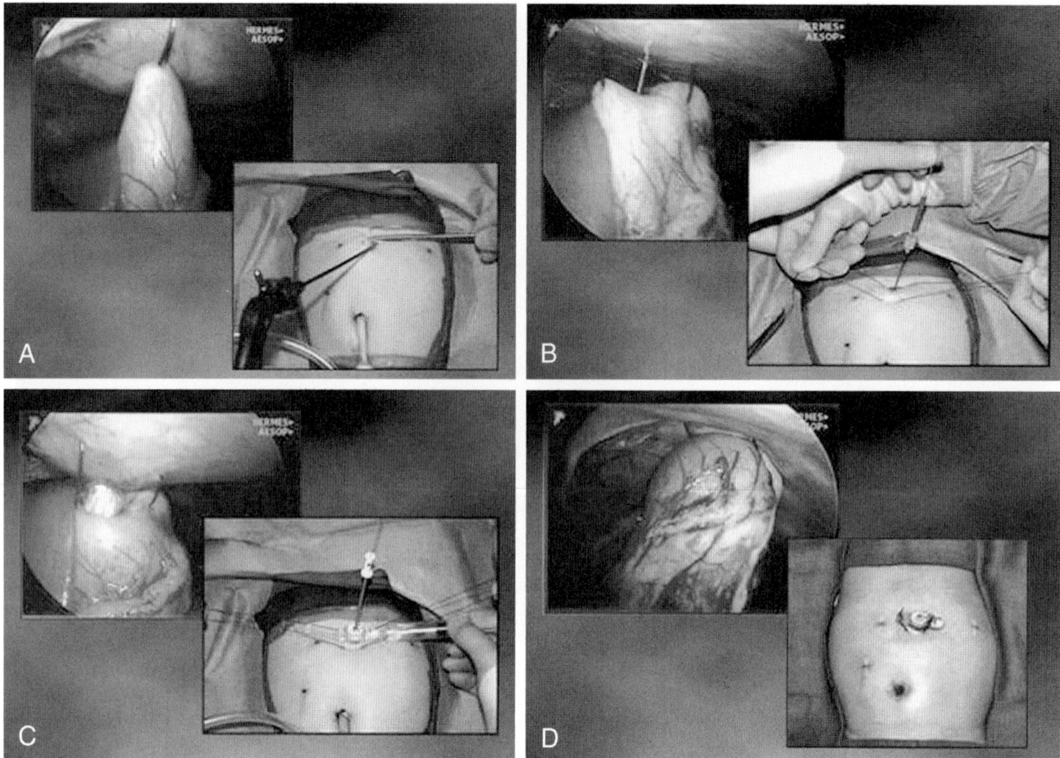

Figure 29-6. **A,** After approximation of the stomach to the anterior abdominal wall, two sutures of 2-0 or 0 PDS (depending on the patient's age) are placed extracorporeally through the abdominal wall, through the stomach, and out through the abdominal wall inferior to the gastrostomy. **B,** After placing the extracorporeal sutures, an 18-gauge needle is introduced through the left epigastric incision and into the stomach under direct visualization. Following a rush of air through the needle, a guide wire is inserted through the needle and the needle is removed. With the guide wire in place, the tract is serially dilated using the Cook Vascular Dilator Set (Cook, Inc., Bloomington IN). These dilators come in 8-Fr, 12-Fr, 16-Fr, and 20-Fr sizes. **C,** After dilating the tract and gastrostomy with the 20-Fr dilator, the 8-Fr dilator is placed through the Mic-Key gastrostomy button and is introduced over the guide wire and into the stomach. **D,** After placement of the button within the stomach, the balloon on the button is inflated, the guide wire and dilator are removed, and the extracorporeal sutures are tied over the button to secure it to the anterior abdominal wall. (From Holcomb GW III: Gastroesophageal reflux in infants and children. In Fischer JE [ed]: Mastery of Surgery, 5th ed. Philadelphia, Lippincott Williams & Wilkins, 2007, pp 650-651.)

seen in Figure 29-6. Two 2-0 PDS sutures (Ethicon, Inc., Somerville, NJ) are placed through the anterior abdominal wall cephalad to the grasper, through the stomach, and out through the anterior abdominal wall inferior to the instrument that has been used to grasp the stomach. Next, a needle followed by a guide wire is introduced through the abdominal wall and stomach in the center of the square formed by the two PDS sutures. Dilators from a Cook Vascular Dilator Set (Cook, Inc., Bloomington, IN) are used to serially dilate the anterior abdominal wall and gastrotomy. In infants, a 16-Fr dilator is usually the largest needed. In older children, the 20-Fr dilator may be required. The gastrostomy button is then placed over the guide wire and into the stomach. Under visualization, the balloon on the Mic-Key (Ballard Medical Products, Draper, UT) gastrostomy button is inflated. Attention must be paid to be sure that the button is, in fact, in the stomach and not external to the stomach. This can also be confirmed with the angled telescope by looking around each side of the stomach with the button in place. The PDS sutures are then secured over the button to prevent its dislodgement. Our protocol is to cut these sutures in 5 days. Others may cut them sooner. This technique was initially described by Georgeson and Owings, and details about complications have been published.[124,125]

Postoperative Care

Postoperatively, if a gastrostomy button was placed with the fundoplication (or if a button was placed primarily), feedings are usually started several hours later and advanced over the evening and the next morning. Most (90%) patients are ready for discharge the day after the operation. The parents will have been instructed on the use of the gastrostomy during the patient's 24-hour hospitalization and can advance the feedings as needed. The patient can also be seen in the clinic should further questions or issues arise.

If the patient did not need a gastrostomy, then liquids are allowed several hours after the procedure. It is very important to mention to the family that there is initial edema around the fundoplication. Therefore, for the first 3 weeks, the diet should be a mechanical soft diet that has the consistency of pudding, apple sauce, mashed potatoes, and so on. Essentially, meats and pizza should not be allowed because these food substances can become lodged above the fundoplication wrap. After 3 weeks, the edema usually resolves

Table 29-4 Operative Results after Open Operations for Management of GERD

Study	No. Patients	% Reoperation	Herniation	Wrap Dehiscence	Other
Wheatley et al. (Michigan) 1974-1989	242	12% (29)	3	14	3
Caniano et al. (Ohio State) 1976-1988	358	6% (21)	16	2	3
Dedinsky et al. (Indiana) 1975-1985	429	6.7% (29)	29	0	0
Fonkalsrud et al. (UCLA) 1976-1996	7467	7.1%	Not mentioned	Not mentioned	Not mentioned

and small portions of meats and pizza can be added to the diet.

Patients are seen 2 weeks, 3 months, 6 months, and 1 year after the operation. An upper gastrointestinal contrast study is performed at 1 year to evaluate for transmigration of the wrap or any other abnormalities.

Outcomes

Our group has been interested in the efficacy of laparoscopic fundoplication for the past 10 years. A number of articles have been published from our institution detailing our thoughts about indications, complications, the operative technique, and ways to improve the results.[117-123,126-130] A number of other authors have been interested as well and have published their experience with laparoscopic fundoplication.[131-136]

In early 2002, in looking at our outcomes from January, 2000, through March, 2002, we believed that the need for repeat fundoplication was higher than desired.[121] In 130 patients undergoing laparoscopic Nissen fundoplication during that time, the incidence of repeat fundoplication was 12%. All patients who required a repeat operation had transmigration of the fundoplication wrap. During that time period, the esophagus was being extensively mobilized to try to create at least a 2-cm length of intra-abdominal esophagus. Moreover, there was no attempt to obliterate the space between the esophagus and the crura. These principles derived from prior training as well as literature reports in adults.[20,21] Although the operations proceeded nicely and no conversions were needed, this 12% incidence of re-do procedures seemed high. However, historical reports for the open operation have also documented a relatively high incidence of repeat fundoplications from 6% to 12% (Table 29-4).[59,137-139]

In an attempt to reduce the incidence of postoperative transmigration of the wrap, two modifications were made in the operative technique beginning in April, 2002. First, there was minimal mobilization of the esophagus. It was believed that the main reason for wrap transmigration was that the esophagus was being mobilized and a space was being created between the esophagus and crura to allow for the transmigration to occur. Therefore, the phrenoesophageal membrane was kept as intact as possible to try to obliterate this space. Second, to further obliterate this space, sutures were placed between the esophagus and crura. Initially, only two sutures were used, but eventually four sutures have come to be placed for the purpose of further obliterating this space (see Fig. 29-5). No other modifications in the operative technique were made. In looking at the results from April, 2002, through December, 2004, the incidence of transmigration was reduced to 5%.[121] This was actually reduced even further when looking at the patients in whom four esophageal crural sutures were utilized rather than two or three.

In 2005, in conversations with Georgeson and colleagues at the University of Alabama-Birmingham, it was evident that similar observations had been made by the Alabama group. Therefore, it was decided to join together and perform a prospective, randomized trial looking at the operative technique.[140] Initially, it was believed that the efficacy of esophageal mobilization should be evaluated. The primary endpoint was transmigration of the wrap. A power analysis based on the difference between the 12% and 5% repeat fundoplication rate previously mentioned was made and the study was powered at 360 patients. The patients were randomized on the day of the surgery. One group was randomized to receive minimal esophageal mobilization with placement of four esophagocrural sutures. The other group was randomized to extensive esophageal mobilization to create a 2-cm length of intra-abdominal esophagus along with the four esophagocrural sutures. In addition, all patients would receive an upper gastrointestinal series at 1-year postoperatively to evaluate for transmigration of the fundoplication wrap. Other variables were also captured.

The two surgical groups have met twice yearly since 2005. At the midpoint of the study, 172 patients had been entered. The data were overwhelmingly in favor of minimal esophageal mobilization and placement of the four esophagocrural sutures. At the time of the interim analysis, almost all of the re-do operations had occurred in patients undergoing extensive esophageal mobilization and placement of the four esophagocrural sutures. Therefore, it was believed that ethically the study could not continue and was closed. The upper gastrointestinal studies for all the enrolled patients should be completed late in 2009. A final report will be available in 2010.

Repeat Fundoplication

As mentioned previously, the goal of the initial fundoplication is to control symptomatic GER but also to prevent the need for a second operation.[141] In 2006,

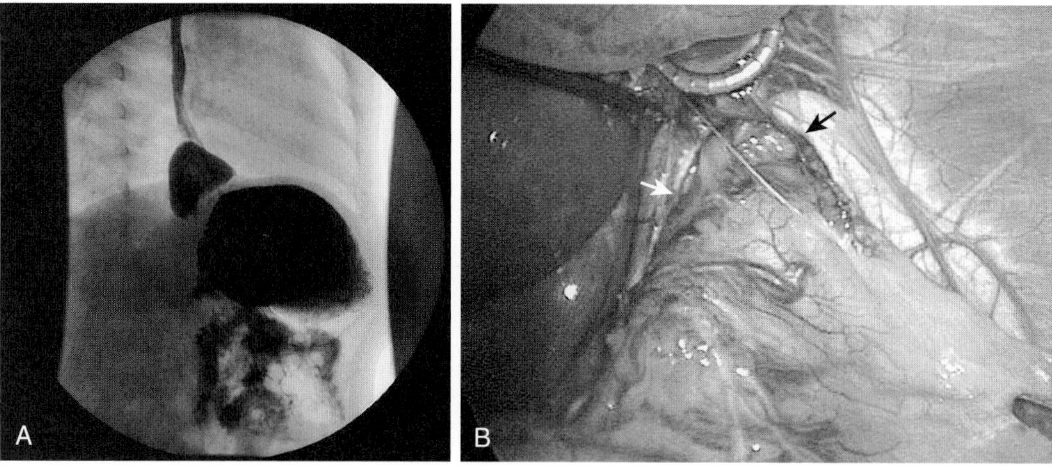

Figure 29-7. In 5% to 10% of patients undergoing laparoscopic fundoplication, reoperation becomes necessary. **A,** In our experience, almost all reoperations are due to transmigration of the fundoplication wrap, which is seen on this upper gastrointestinal study. **B,** The intraoperative photograph shows a large esophageal hiatus (*arrows*) with transmigration of the fundoplication wrap and upper stomach into the lower mediastinum. Note the significant lack of adhesions after the initial laparoscopic fundoplication. (From Ostlie DJ, Holcomb GW III: Reiterative surgery for gastroesophageal reflux. Semin Pediatr Surg 16:252-258, 2007.)

our group looked at our experience with re-do fundoplications.[142] Of 273 patients who underwent laparoscopic fundoplication by the senior surgeon (GWH) between January, 2000, and April, 2006, 21 required a re-do fundoplication (Fig. 29-7).[142] The repeat operative technique generally fell into two groups. In one group, it was performed laparoscopically without the use of mesh to reinforce the large hiatal closure that had developed after transmigration of the wrap. In the other group, Surgisis (Cook, Inc, Bloomington, IN) was used to reinforce the hiatal closure because it was believed that a great deal of tension was needed to close the large muscular defect (Fig. 29-8). Initially 4-ply Surgisis was used, but 8-ply Surgisis was employed when it became available. In the patients undergoing the second operation without Surgisis, three required a second re-do or third overall fundoplication. To date, no patient has required another repeat operation in which Surgisis was placed at the time of the initial repeat procedure.[142]

At the same time as our concept developed about reinforcing the hiatal closure with Surgisis, a multi-institution, prospective randomized trial was being performed in adult patients.[143] The investigators were looking at the efficacy of placing 4-ply Surgisis at the time of initial repair of a large paraesophageal hernia defect to help prevent recurrence. This trial also closed early because of the marked disparity in results favoring the use of Surgisis to help close the large diaphragmatic defect. The study included 71 patients in each arm. The primary outcome variable was recurrence of the paraesophageal hernia. The study closed at 108 total patients because, at the time of interim review, 12 patients (24%) had developed a recurrence in the arm in which Surgisis was not used and only 4 patients (9%) had a recurrent paraesophageal hernia in the Surgisis arm.

Laparoscopic fundoplication has evolved into the preferred technique for surgical management of GERD. Although the Nissen operation is generally performed, similar good results have been noted with the Thal operation.[144-147] It is only through critical evaluation of one's experience that advances are made in improving the results. There is no doubt that patients have less discomfort and earlier discharge from the hospital after the laparoscopic operation.[130] Moreover, there is a faster return to regular activities as well. However, the operative technique continues to need ongoing evaluation with proper data collection and critical analysis to improve these results.

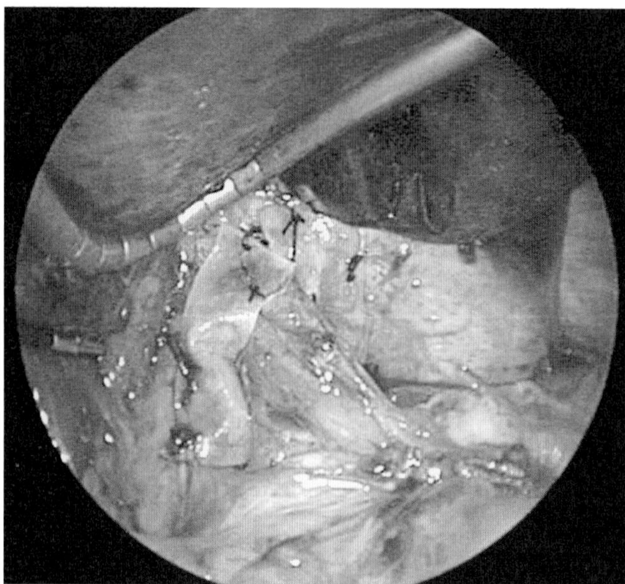

Figure 29-8. This intraoperative photograph shows the 8-ply Surgisis that has been wrapped around the esophagus and is overlapped anterior to the esophagus. The 8-ply Surgisis is secured to the esophagus medially and the diaphragm laterally with interrupted 3-0 silk sutures. It is employed to help reinforce the closure of the crura at the time of repeat fundoplication.

chapter 30

LESIONS OF THE STOMACH

Curt S. Koontz, MD • Mark Wulkan, MD

The stomach forms from the foregut and is recognizable by the fifth week of gestation. It then elongates, descends, and dilates to form its familiar structure by the seventh week of gestation. The vascular supply to the stomach is very robust, and ischemia of the stomach is rare. The stomach is supplied by the right and left gastric arteries along the lesser curvature, the right and left gastroepiploic arteries along the greater curvature, and the short gastric vessels from the spleen. There is also contribution from the posterior gastric artery, which is a branch of the splenic artery, as well as the phrenic arteries.

In this chapter, we discuss common and unusual conditions of the stomach that are treated surgically. Some topics relevant to the stomach, such as gastroesophageal reflux and obesity, are covered elsewhere.

HYPERTROPHIC PYLORIC STENOSIS

Hypertrophic pyloric stenosis (HPS) is one of the most common surgical conditions of the newborn.[1-9] It occurs at a rate of 1 to 4 per 1000 live births in white infants but is seen less in non-white children.[1-4] Males are affected more often with a 4:1 male-to-female ratio. Risk factors for HPS include family history, gender, younger maternal age, being a first-born infant, and maternal feeding patterns.[4,9,10] Premature infants are diagnosed with HPS later than term or post-term infants.[4]

Etiology

The cause of HPS is unknown, but genetic and environmental factors appear to play a large role in the pathophysiology. Circumstantial evidence for a genetic predisposition includes race discrepancies, the increased frequency in males, and the birth order (first-born infants with a positive family history). Environmental factors associated with HPS include the method of feeding (breast vs. formula), seasonal variability, exposure to erythromycin, and transpyloric feeding in premature infants.[5-7] Additionally, there has been interest in several gastrointestinal peptides or growth factors that may facilitate pyloric hypertrophy. Some of these include excessive substance P, decreased neurotrophins, deficient nitric oxide synthase, and gastrin hypersecretion.[8,9] Thus, the etiology of HPS is likely multifactorial with environmental influences.

Diagnosis

The classic presentation of HPS is nonbilious, projectile vomiting in a full-term neonate who is between 2 and 8 weeks old. Initially, the emesis is infrequent and may appear to be reflux. However, over a short period of time, the emesis occurs with every feeding and becomes forceful (i.e., projectile). The contents of the emesis are usually the recent feedings, but signs of gastritis are not uncommon ("coffee-ground" emesis). On physical examination, the neonate usually appears well if the diagnosis is made early. However, depending on the duration of symptoms and degree of dehydration, the neonate may be gaunt and somnolent. Visible peristaltic waves may be present in the mid to left upper abdomen. To palpate the pyloric mass (i.e., "olive"), the neonate must be relaxed. Techniques for relaxing the patient include bending the neonate's knees and flexing the hips and using a pacifier with sugar water. These techniques should be attempted after the stomach has been decompressed with a 10-Fr to 12-Fr orogastric tube. After palpating the liver edge, the examiner's fingertips should slide underneath the liver in the midline. Slowly, the fingers are pulled back down, trying to trap the "olive." Palpating the pylorus requires patience and an optimal examination setting. The definitive diagnosis can be made in a considerable number of patients with this examination. However, if the diagnosis is unclear after a thorough physical examination, radiologic evaluation is warranted.

Ultrasonography has become the standard technique for diagnosing HPS and has supplanted the physical examination at most institutions. The diagnostic criteria for pyloric stenosis is a muscle thickness of greater than or equal to 4 mm and a length of greater than or equal to 16 mm (Fig. 30-1).[10] A thickness of more than 3 mm is considered positive if the neonate is younger than 30 days of age.[11] The study is dependent on the expertise of the ultrasound technician and radiologist.

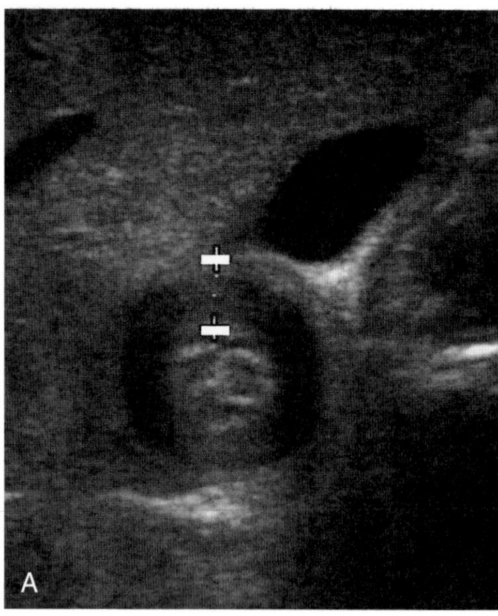

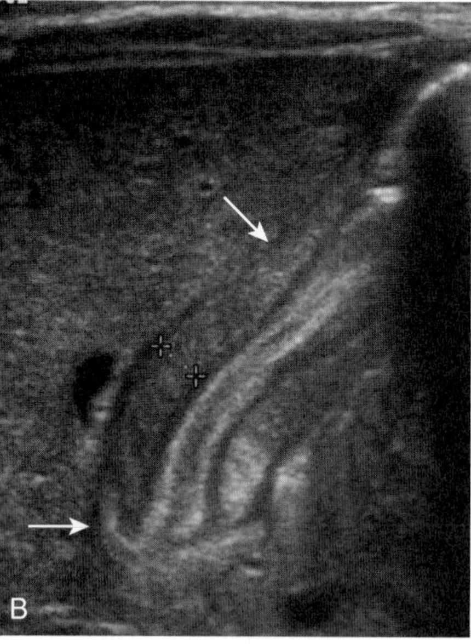

Figure 30-1. Ultrasonography has become the standard imaging study for diagnosing pyloric stenosis and has supplanted physical examination at most institutions. The transverse (**A**) and longitudinal (**B**) views of hypertrophic pyloric stenosis are seen here. Muscle thickness greater than or equal to 4 mm on the transverse view or a length greater than or equal to 16 mm on the longitudinal view is diagnostic of pyloric stenosis. On this study, the pyloric wall thickness was 5 mm and the length (*arrows*) was 20 mm.

Availability of skilled personnel can also be a problem at night. There are reports of non-radiologists performing ultrasonography for diagnosing HPS, which would obviously reduce the need for the ultrasound technician.[12,13] If the ultrasound findings are equivocal, then an upper gastrointestinal series can be helpful in confirming the diagnosis (Fig. 30-2). It is, however, important to evacuate the contrast agent after the study to reduce the risk of aspiration and deleterious pulmonary complications.

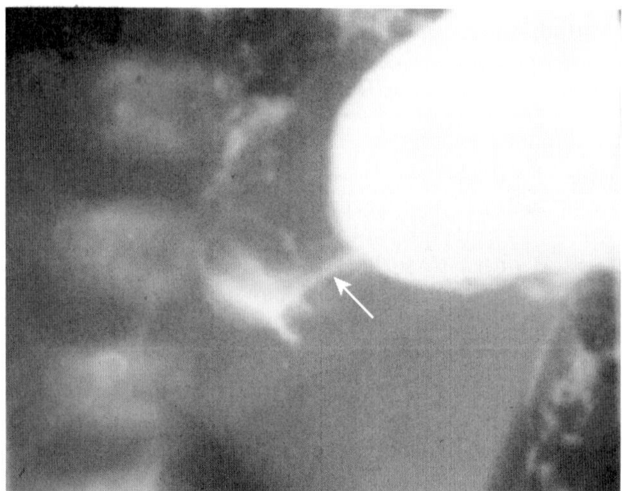

Figure 30-2. At some hospitals outside of urban centers, ultrasound technicians and radiologists proficient in performing an ultrasound study for pyloric stenosis are not available. Also, in some instances, an ultrasound study can be equivocal. An upper gastrointestinal series can be helpful in making the diagnosis of pyloric stenosis or confirming an equivocal ultrasound study. In this upper gastrointestinal study, note the "string sign" indicating a markedly diminished pyloric channel (*arrow*) and subsequent gastric outlet obstruction. It is important to evacuate the contrast material after this study to reduce the risk of aspiration and pulmonary complications.

In the past, the diagnosis was often delayed and profound dehydration with metabolic derangements was common. Today, however, primary care physicians are more aware of the problem and the availability of ultrasonography facilitates an earlier diagnosis and treatment of HPS. The differential diagnosis for nonbilious vomiting, however, should be considered. This includes medical causes such as gastroesophageal reflux, gastroenteritis, increased intracranial pressure, and metabolic disorders. Anatomic causes would include an antral web, foregut duplication cyst, gastric tumors, or a tumor causing extrinsic gastric compression.

Treatment

The mainstay of therapy is typically resuscitation followed by pyloromyotomy. There are reports of medical treatment with atropine and pyloric dilation, but these treatments require long periods of time and are often not effective.[14-18]

Once the diagnosis of HPS is made, feedings should be withheld. Gastric decompression is usually not necessary but occasionally may be required for extreme cases. If a barium study was performed, it is important to remove all of the contrast material from the stomach to prevent aspiration.

The hallmark metabolic derangement of hypochloremic, hypokalemic metabolic alkalosis is usually seen to some degree in most patients. Profound dehydration is rarely seen today, and correction is usually achieved in less than 24 hours after presentation. A basic metabolic panel should be ordered and the resuscitation should be directed toward correcting the abnormalities. Most surgeons use the serum carbon dioxide (<30 mmol/L), chloride (>100 mmol/L), and potassium (4.5-6.5 mmol/L) levels as markers of resuscitation. Initially, a 10- to 20-mL/kg bolus of normal saline should be given if the electrolyte values are abnormal. Then D5/½NS with 20 to 30 mEq/L of potassium chloride is started at a rate of 1.25 to 2 times the maintenance rate. Electrolytes should be checked every 6 hours until they normalize and the alkalosis has resolved. Then the patient can safely undergo anesthesia and operation. It is important to appreciate that HPS is not a surgical emergency and resuscitation is of the utmost priority.

After general anesthesia has been induced, an abdominal examination should be performed to physically check for an "olive" if one was not detectable preoperatively. The pyloromyotomy may be performed by the standard open technique or by the minimally invasive approach. The anesthesiologist should pass and leave a suction catheter in the stomach for decompression and for instilling air after the pyloromyotomy to check for a leak.

The Open Approach

Several incisions have been described for the open approach. The typical right upper quadrant transverse incision seems to be used most commonly (Fig. 30-3). An alternate, more cosmetically pleasing incision involves an omega-shaped incision around the superior portion of the umbilicus followed by incising the linea alba cephalad. With either incision, the pylorus is exteriorized through the incision. A longitudinal serosal incision is made in the pylorus approximately 2 mm proximal to the junction of the duodenum and is carried onto the anterior gastric wall for approximately 5 mm. Blunt dissection is used to divide the firm pyloric fibers. This can be performed using the handle of a scalpel. Once a good edge of fibers has been developed, a pyloric spreader or hemostat can be used to spread the fibers until the pyloric submucosal layer is seen. The pyloromyotomy is then completed by ensuring that all fibers are divided throughout the entire length of the incision. This is confirmed by visualizing the circular muscle of the stomach proximally as well as a slight protrusion of the mucosa. The most common point of mucosal disruption is at the distal part of the incision at the duodenal-pyloric junction. Therefore, care must be exercised when dividing the fibers in this region. The pyloromyotomy can be checked for completeness by rocking the superior and inferior edges of the myotomy back and forth to ensure independent movement. The mucosal integrity can be checked by instilling air through the previously placed suction catheter. If there are no leaks, the air should be suctioned. Minor bleeding is common and should be ignored because it will cease after the venous congestion is reduced when the pylorus is returned to the abdominal cavity. The abdominal incision is then closed in layers.

The Laparoscopic Operation

Neonatal laparoscopy has grown in popularity with the refinement in technique and smaller instruments. The first reported laparoscopic pyloromyotomy in the English language was in 1991 (the authors had reported the first case in the French literature in 1990).[19] Since then, this procedure has been accepted by most pediatric surgeons. Critics of the procedure argue that laparoscopic pyloromyotomy exposes the patient to undue risks compared with the open technique. However, recent randomized prospective trials have not shown any difference in complication rates.[20,21] Operative times can vary depending on the laparoscopic experience of the surgeon. The minimally invasive approach is similar to laparoscopic appendectomy in terms of acceptance and has become the standard technique for pyloromyotomy in many centers.

The technique involves entering the abdomen through an umbilical incision. A Veress needle is placed at the base of the umbilicus between the umbilical arteries. It is paramount to ensure proper placement of the Veress needle before insufflation. This can be done by several simple methods, including the "blind man's cane" sweep and the water drop test. Alternatively, an open approach can be used to introduce the umbilical cannula. The abdomen is then insufflated to a pressure of 10 mm Hg and a 3- or 5-mm port is introduced for the telescope and camera. Two stab incisions are made. One incision is in the right paramedian side of the abdomen at the level of the umbilicus, and the other is in the left paramedian side of the abdomen just superior to the umbilicus.

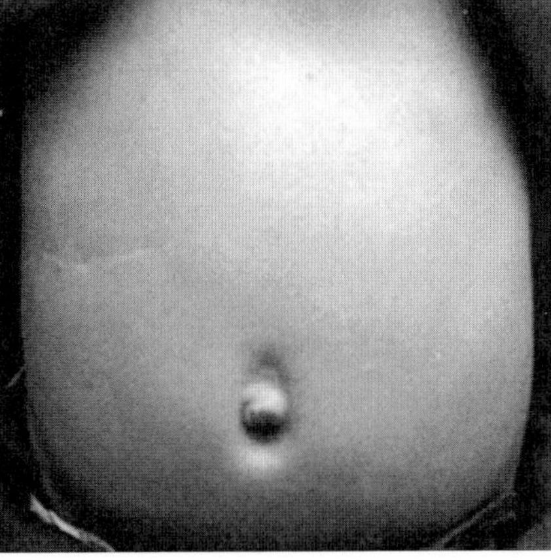
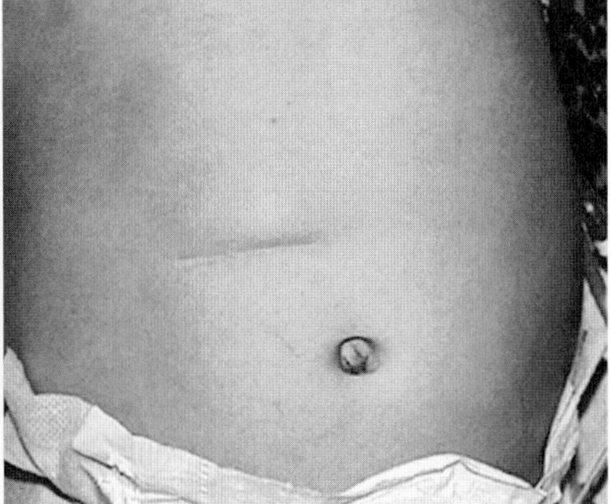

Figure 30-3. These two children underwent open pyloromyotomy through a right upper quadrant transverse incision. Over time, the cosmetic appearance of their incision is not as attractive as that seen after the laparoscopic operation.

Local anesthesia is used at all incisions. An atraumatic bowel grasper is placed through the left incision, and an arthrotomy knife is introduced through the right incision (Fig. 30-4). The duodenum is grasped firmly just distal to the pylorus, and the pylorus is maneuvered into view. Occasionally, a transabdominal stay suture wrapping around the falciform ligament is helpful to elevate the liver away from the pylorus. A pyloromyotomy is then made with the knife in a similar manner as the open technique (Fig. 30-5). The closed arthrotomy knife can be used to separate the muscle fibers similar to the scalpel handle. A laparoscopic pyloric spreader or a box-type grasper can be used to complete the myotomy. Completeness of the myotomy and mucosal integrity is checked in a similar manner as the open technique. Omentum can be placed over the myotomy to help with hemostasis. The pneumoperitoneum is evacuated after the instruments are removed. The umbilicus is closed with absorbable suture, and the stab incisions are closed with skin adhesive.

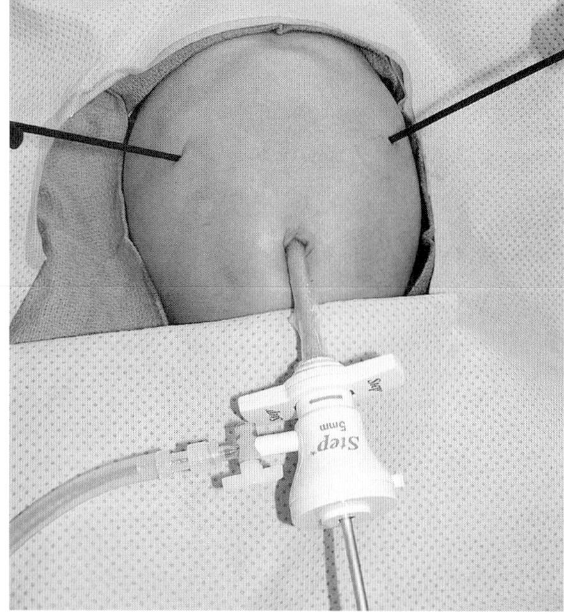

Figure 30-4. For laparoscopic pyloromyotomy, a 3- or 5-mm cannula is introduced through the umbilicus and insufflation achieved to a pressure of 10 mm Hg. Through a stab incision in the right upper abdomen, an atraumatic bowel grasper is introduced for grasping and stabilizing the duodenum. The arthrotomy knife and pyloric spreader are introduced through the stab incision in the patient's left upper abdomen.

Postoperative Care

Postoperative care is similar for both surgical techniques, assuming the mucosal integrity is intact. Complicated feeding regimens have been advocated in the past. However, recent studies support the use of ad libitum feeds in the early postoperative period. This results in a faster time to full feeds and quicker discharge.[22,23] If postoperative emesis is encountered, it is suggested to "feed through it." At our institution, we limit the feedings to a maximum of 3 oz every 3 hours. There are data to suggest that the degree and duration of metabolic derangement affects postoperative feeding. Patients who required more complicated resuscitation tend to take longer to reach full feeds and discharge.[24]

Pain is usually controlled with acetaminophen. Intravenous fluids are discontinued when the patient tolerates a 2-oz feeding twice. The infant can be

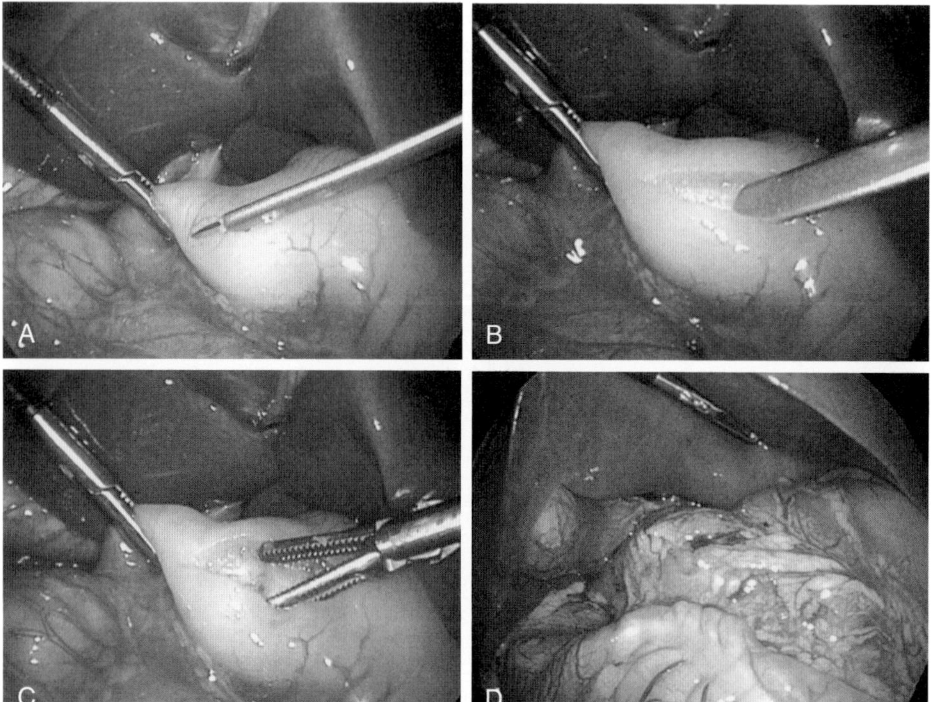

Figure 30-5. Technique of laparoscopic pyloromyotomy. **A,** With the duodenum stabilized, a seromuscular incision is made in the hypertrophied pylorus with the arthrotomy knife. **B,** Next, the knife is returned to its sheath and the sheath is used to further bluntly divide the hypertrophied fibers. **C,** Then a pyloric spreader can be introduced to completely divide the hypertrophied muscle. **D,** After pyloromyotomy, omentum can be placed over the myotomy to help with hemostasis.

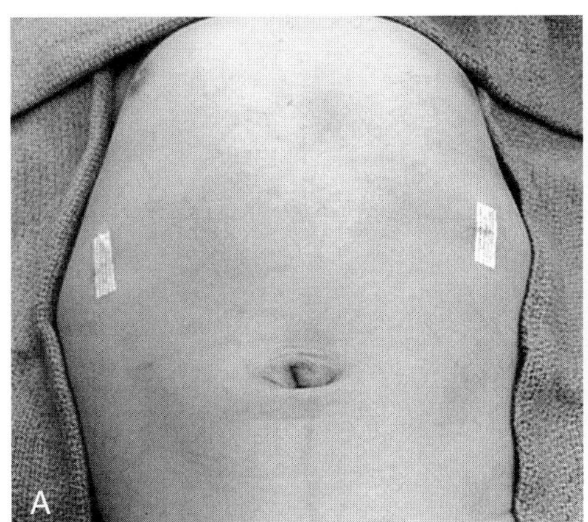

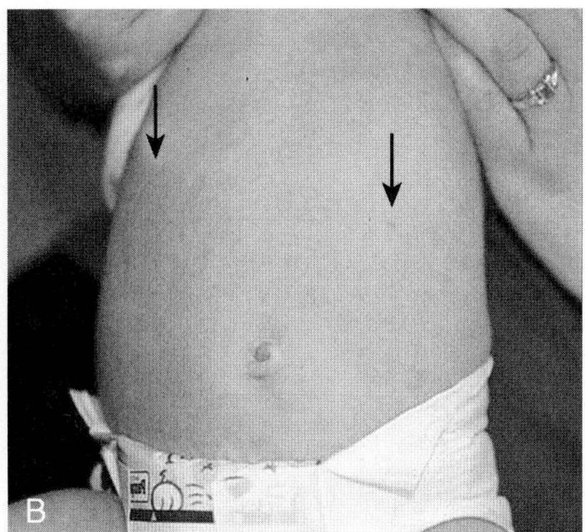

Figure 30-6. The cosmetic advantage of the laparoscopic approach cannot be overemphasized. **A,** Incisions after a laparoscopic pyloromyotomy. **B,** Incisions (*arrows*) 3 weeks after the operation. Often after 6 months the incisions cannot be easily seen.

discharged when tolerating full feeds, which is usually on the first postoperative day.

Complications

The major complications of pyloromyotomy include mucosal perforation, wound infection, incisional hernia, prolonged postoperative emesis, incomplete myotomy, and duodenal injury. There have been retrospective studies that do not show any difference in complication rates between the laparoscopic and open techniques.

Mucosal perforation occurs in 1% to 2% of cases.[20,21] If the disruption occurs at the duodenopyloric junction, a simple interrupted absorbable suture can be placed to close the defect and a patch of omentum can be used to bolster the repair. This can be accomplished laparoscopically depending on the experience of the surgeon. Otherwise, the laparoscopic case should be converted to open. If the perforation is large or in the middle of the myotomy, then the myotomy should be closed with absorbable suture. A new myotomy can then be made 90 to 180 degrees from the original incision. Repairing this injury would be difficult to perform laparoscopically. Feedings should be held for 24 hours and then restarted. A water-soluble contrast study can be performed if desired.

Duodenal injuries also can occur with either the laparoscopic or open approach. In a 25-year retrospective review of 901 open pyloromyotomies performed between 1969 and 1994, there were 39 duodenal perforations that were recognized intraoperatively and repaired. There were no unrecognized duodenal perforations that developed after the operation.[25]

Wound infections also occur in 1% to 2% of cases.[20,21] There are no data to support the use of prophylactic perioperative antibiotics because a pyloromyotomy is considered a clean procedure. Local wound care is usually sufficient to treat these infections.

Incisional hernias and wound dehiscence occurs in approximately 1% of cases.[20] Most hernia defects require repair at some point. Laparoscopically, port site hernias usually involve omentum protruding through the incision. This can sometimes be managed at the bedside by cleansing the area with povidone-iodine (Betadine), ligating and trimming the extracorporeal omentum, elevating the abdominal wall to get the omentum back into the peritoneal cavity, and using fine absorbable suture to close the skin.

Postoperative emesis is common, occurring in up to 80% of patients at some point. Prolonged emesis is less common and ranges in incidence from 2% to 26%. Most commonly, this is due to gastroesophageal reflux (24%-31%) but can be secondary to incomplete myotomy (0-6%). It has been suggested that the laparoscopic approach may be a risk factor for inadequate myotomy, but this is likely related to surgical experience with this technique.[21]

Outcome

In the past, the mortality from pyloric stenosis was considerable and approached 50%. Today, however, mortality is nearly zero with improvement in neonatal resuscitation and anesthesia as well as surgical techniques. Morbidity is also significantly lower than in the past, with an overall complication rate between 1% and 2%. Additionally, with more pyloromyotomies being performed laparoscopically, the cosmetic advantage of the minimally invasive techniques cannot be overemphasized (Fig. 30-6).

PYLORIC ATRESIA

Pyloric atresia is a rare disease (1:100,000 live births) and presents as symptoms of gastric outlet obstruction. The disease is difficult to characterize because it is so rare. However, several generalizations can be made from looking at larger series. Pyloric atresia may be associated with epidermolysis bullosa and other gastrointestinal anomalies, such as duplications.[26-33] Pyloric atresia is diagnosed with a "single bubble" on the abdominal radiograph (Fig. 30-7). The diagnosis may be confirmed with a contrast study. Pyloric atresia may occur as a web, a cord, or

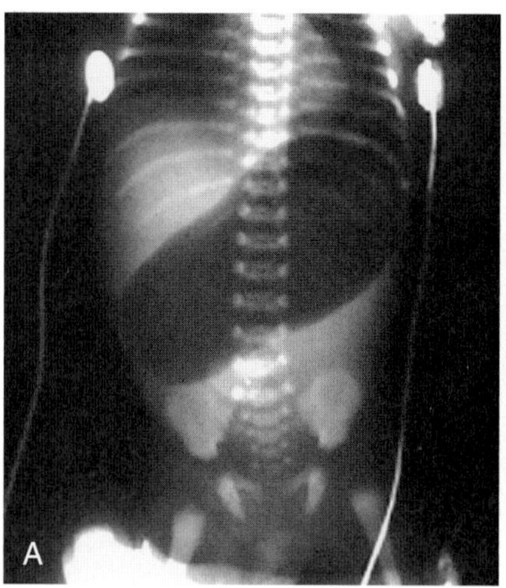

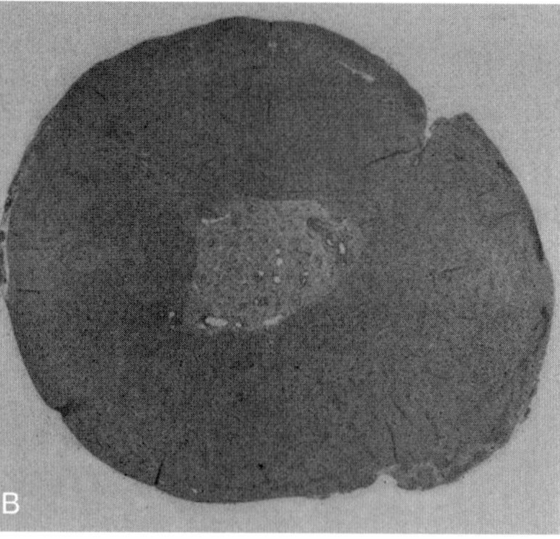

Figure 30-7. **A,** In contrast to duodenal atresia in which a "double bubble" sign is the pathognomonic finding on the abdominal radiograph, pyloric atresia is diagnosed with a "single bubble" on the abdominal film. **B,** A cross-sectional histologic view of an infant with pyloric atresia. Note the obliterated lumen and the enlarged muscular layer.

a gap between the antrum of the stomach and the first portion of the duodenum. Repair is performed after resuscitation. These infants may have similar electrolyte abnormalities to infants with hypertrophic pyloric stenosis. Repair is usually with a Billroth type I (gastroduodenostomy) anastomosis. Morbidity and mortality are usually related to the associated anomalies.

GASTRIC PERFORATION

The causes of gastric perforation are spontaneous perforation of the newborn, iatrogenic perforation from instrumentation, peptic ulcer disease, and trauma. Gastric perforation usually presents as abdominal distention and signs of sepsis or shock related to the perforation. The diagnosis is suspected when a large amount of extraluminal gas is seen on an abdominal radiograph.

Neonatal gastric perforations most commonly occur in premature infants. About half of neonatal perforations are spontaneous, and the other half are iatrogenic from instrumentation.[34] Prematurity is associated with an increased mortality.[35] The perforations are usually managed with laparotomy or laparoscopy. The perforation can usually be closed primarily with or without an omental patch.

Gastric perforation due to peptic ulcer disease in infants and children is very rare. Typically, perforation occurs at the site of a prepyloric ulcer. Again, this may be repaired primarily via laparotomy or laparoscopy with or without an omental patch.[36]

PEPTIC ULCER DISEASE

Peptic ulcer disease and its complications are rarely seen in children. However, there have been reports of neonatal and pediatric perforated ulcers as well as gastric outlet obstruction in children due to peptic ulcer disease.[36-38] Peptic ulcer disease appears to be associated with *Helicobacter pylori* in the majority of pediatric cases. Treatment is primarily directed at acid reduction and eradication of *H. pylori.* Triple therapy with a proton pump inhibitor, amoxicillin, and clarithromycin is typically used initially. For strains that are resistant to clarithromycin, metronidazole is substituted.[39] Operative treatment is usually reserved for complications of peptic ulcer disease, such as perforation or gastric outlet obstruction (Fig. 30-8).

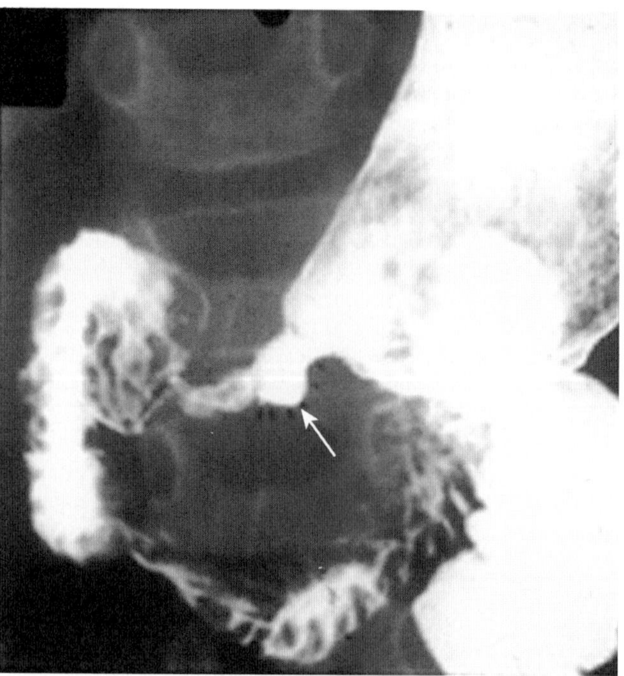

Figure 30-8. A 10-year-old presented with abdominal pain and vomiting. She was found to have a prepyloric ulcer (*arrow*) on the upper gastrointestinal study. In addition, there was evidence of gastric outlet obstruction. She underwent antrectomy and Billroth I reconstruction.

If ulcer perforation is suspected, it is reasonable to start with exploratory laparoscopy because there are reports of successful laparoscopic treatment in children.[37] A gastric resection operation is not usually needed since the development of effective proton pump inhibitors.

GASTRIC DUPLICATIONS

Gastric duplications are rare anomalies that generally occur along the greater curvature (Fig. 30-9). If the lesion is near the pylorus, the presentation may be very similar to hypertrophic pyloric stenosis. The diagnosis can be differentiated from pyloric stenosis by ultrasonography. The lesion rarely communicates with the lumen. If it does, the patient may present with hematemesis or melena. Gastric duplications represent approximately 4% of all gastrointestinal duplications. Ectopic gastric mucosa is common in other duplications throughout the gastrointestinal tract. These are not considered gastric duplications. Approximately half are discovered in the neonatal period and are seen when the neonate presents with vomiting, poor feeding, and an epigastric mass.[40]

Treatment of gastric duplications is complete resection of the cyst. There have been gastric duplications associated with pancreatic ductal abnormalities.[41] In this case, care must be taken during the dissection not to injure normal pancreas, although it may be necessary to resect an accessory pancreas.

MICROGASTRIA

Congenital microgastria is a rare disorder that usually occurs in conjunction with other congenital anomalies or, more rarely, alone (Fig. 30-10). Associated anomalies include the VACTERL association (Vertebral anomalies, Anorectal atresia, Cardiac anomalies, TracheoEsophageal fistula and esophageal atresia, Renal and Limb anomalies), tracheoesophageal cleft, malrotation, and asplenia. There are currently only three reported cases of isolated microgastria.[42,43] Microgastria is usually temporized with jejunal feedings. Operative intervention consists of jejunal feeding tubes and Hunt-Lawrence gastric augmentation. There are a few patients who have been reported with successful follow-up after a Hunt-Lawrence pouch.[42,44,45]

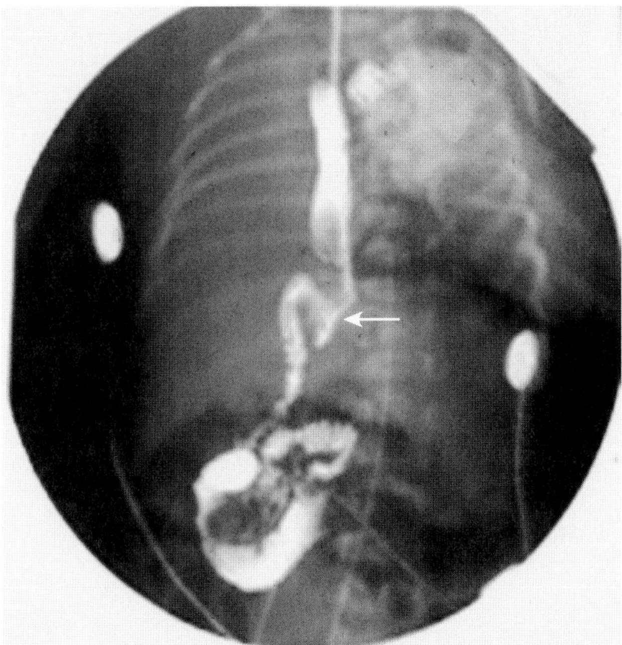

Figure 30-10. This neonate was born with congenital microgastria. Note the dilated esophagus and the extremely small stomach (*arrow*). There is also malrotation. The patient underwent creation of a Hunt-Lawrence pouch and was doing well at 1-year follow-up.

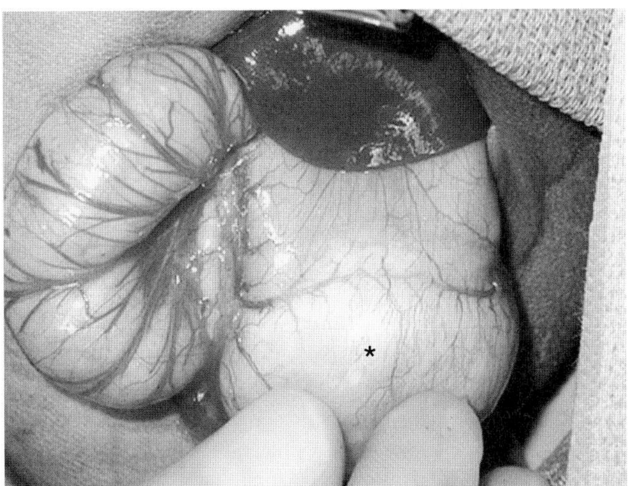

Figure 30-9. This intraoperative view shows a gastric duplication (*asterisk*) emanating from the greater curvature of the stomach. This lesion was able to be removed without compromising the native stomach.

ANTRAL WEB

The first modern description of an antral web was in 1969.[46] Early case reports in children described incomplete gastric outlet obstruction due to an antral web.[47-50] The etiology is unknown and is generally thought to be congenital or the result of an inflammatory process. In adults there has been a case report that strongly suggested peptic ulcer disease can lead to antral web.[51] The patient presents with a typical gastric outlet obstruction. In the infant, antral web may be confused with hypertrophic pyloric stenosis. The patient with antral web may have a normal abdominal sonogram. However, an upper gastrointestinal series will show the lesion. The abdominal examination may be normal.

Treatment of an antral web consists of resuscitation (see earlier section on pyloric stenosis) and operative correction (Fig. 30-11). The procedure can be completed with laparotomy or laparoscopically. This is a diagnosis that may be amenable to endoluminal treatment.

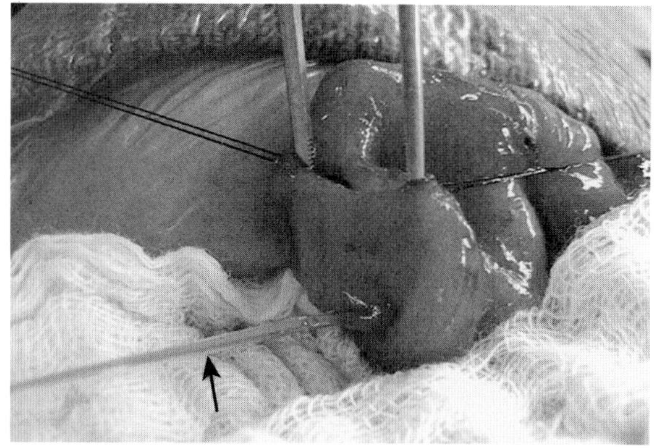

Figure 30-11. This neonate developed nonbilious emesis shortly after birth and was thought to have an antral web. At laparotomy, the antral web is visualized. The forceps are proximal to the web and the feeding tube (*arrow*) has been placed through the web. After resection of the web, the patient recovered uneventfully and has not developed any further problems.

GASTRIC VOLVULUS

Gastric volvulus can occur from primary or secondary causes. Primary gastric volvulus is thought to be due to laxity of the gastric ligaments. Secondary disease may occur due to a paraesophageal hernia or other diaphragmatic hernia. The presenting symptoms can be intermittent or complete gastric obstruction, ischemia, pain, and/or bleeding. The most common signs and symptoms of gastric volvulus in children include acute abdominal pain, intractable retching, and the inability to pass a nasogastric tube into the stomach lumen.[52,53]

The average age at presentation is 2.5 years. Equal numbers of males and females are affected.[52] Gastric volvulus is classified into categories based on the axis of gastric rotation. Mesenteroaxial gastric volvulus is rotation about the gastric short axis, transecting the greater and lesser curvatures. Organoaxial gastric volvulus is rotation around the long axis of the stomach (Figs. 30-12 and 30-13).

Treatment consists of patient resuscitation, nasogastric decompression, and surgical correction. The volvulus is reduced. Any diaphragmatic defects are repaired in secondary gastric volvulus. A gastropexy is then performed. This has traditionally been accomplished with a gastrostomy tube or button. However, there have been several recent reports of successful laparoscopic gastropexy in which the anterior stomach, along the greater curvature, is sutured to the abdominal wall.[54]

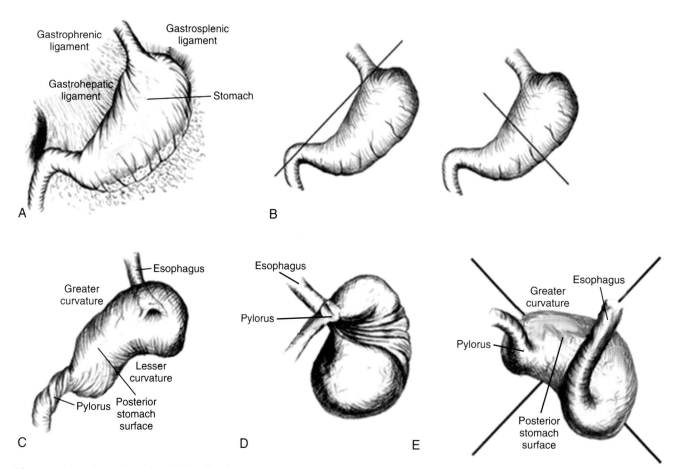

Figure 30-12. These drawings depict the development of a gastric volvulus. **A,** Normal anatomy. **B,** The axis of rotation for an organoaxial volvulus is seen on the left and a mesoaxial volvulus is on the right. **C,** Demonstration of an organoaxial volvulus. **D,** Demonstration of a mesoaxial volvulus. **E,** Combined mesoaxial and organoaxial volvulus. (Reprinted with permission from Cribbs RK, Gow KW, Wulkan ML: Gastric volvulus in infants and children. Pediatrics 122:e752-e762, 2008.)

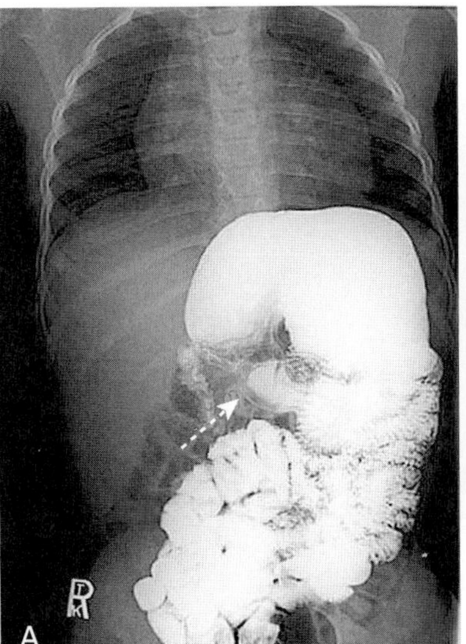

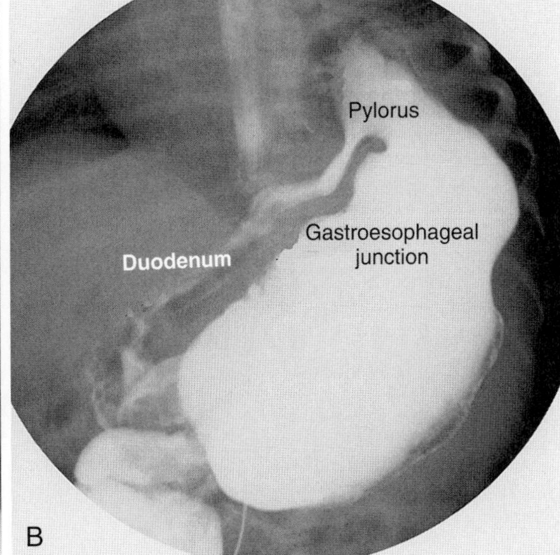

Figure 30-13. These two contrast studies depict a gastric volvulus. **A,** This contrast study depicts an organoaxial volvulus in which the stomach has rotated on its long axis. Note the relatively normal position of the pylorus (*arrow*). **B,** This contrast study shows a mesoaxial volvulus. In this study, the pylorus is in the left upper abdomen due to rotation around the short axis of the stomach. In both studies, the gastroesophageal junction is in a relatively normal position.

FOREIGN BODIES AND BEZOAR

Foreign bodies in the stomach can be generally ignored. If the foreign body passed through the esophagus, it will likely pass out the rectum. Even razor blades and other sharp objects usually safely pass. The exception would be button batteries, which have a high incidence of leakage and should be removed if they have not passed through the pylorus. Otherwise, watchful waiting is a reasonable strategy. Occasionally larger coins, such as quarters, can remain in the stomach and cause intermittent gastric outlet obstruction. It is also reasonable to remove the object in this circumstance. Most gastric foreign bodies are removed endoscopically with a snare, grasper, or bag. The surgeon should consider using an overtube to extract large sharp objects that may injure the esophagus upon retrieval.

Gastric bezoars are relatively uncommon causes of gastric outlet obstruction and chronic abdominal pain in children. Phytobezoars are made up of vegetable matter. Trichobezoars are made up of hair that is swallowed. This is referred to as the Rapunzel syndrome.[55] The hair usually fills the stomach and extends into the duodenum. However, it can extend to the ileum. Attempts at gastroscopic removal are usually futile, except in cases of small bezoars. The bezoar has been typically removed through a gastrotomy at laparotomy. However, there are recent reports of laparoscopic removal.[56,57] At our institution, we recently removed a large gastric trichobezoar laparoscopically with the aid of an endoscopic bag (Fig. 30-14).

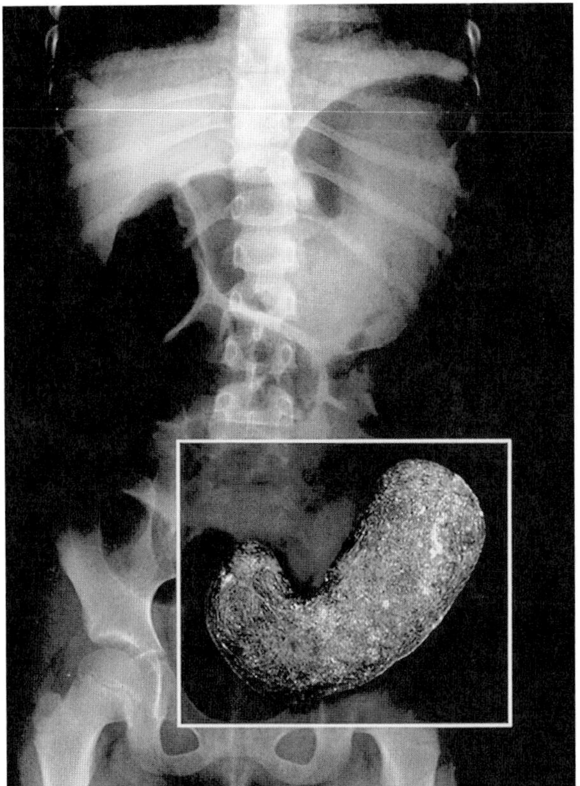

Figure 30-14. A young girl presented with gastric outlet obstruction and was found to have a trichobezoar. The preoperative radiograph shows the outline of the bezoar in the stomach. **Inset,** The bezoar after removal.

chapter 31

DUODENAL AND INTESTINAL ATRESIA AND STENOSIS

Pablo Aguayo, MD • Daniel J. Ostlie, MD

Congenital intestinal obstruction occurs in approximately 1:2000 live births and is one of the most common causes of admission to a neonatal surgical unit, accounting for up to one third of all admissions.[1] Morphologically, congenital defects related to continuity of the intestine can be divided into either stenosis or atresia. Together, they constitute one of the most common causes of neonatal intestinal obstruction.[2-4]

PYLORIC ATRESIA

Pyloric atresia is a rare congenital anomaly that occurs in approximately 1:100,000 live births and constitutes less than 1% of all gastrointestinal atresias.[5,6] Although usually occurring as an isolated lesion, an associated congenital anomaly rate of 30% to 44% has been reported. Epidermolysis bullosa is the most common associated lesion, but associations with aplasia cutis congenita and multiple intestinal atresias have also been found.[7-12] Familial occurrence has also been reported, with a suggestion of autosomal recessive transmission.[11]

Three anatomic variants of pyloric atresia have been described. In type I, there is a mucosal membrane or web. In type II, the pyloric channel is a solid cord (Fig. 31-1). In type III, there is a gap between the stomach and the duodenum.[6] Clinically, neonates with pyloric atresia present with nonbilious vomiting. There is a single stomach bubble in 98%, polyhydramnios in 63%, and epigastric distention in 68%.[13] The diagnosis is made with the appearance on plain abdominal radiographs of a solitary gas-filled bubble representing the distended stomach with no distal air in the gastrointestinal tract (see Fig. 31-1). A long, stretched-out beak at the pylorus is regarded as a pathognomonic sign of complete pyloric obstruction.[14] The differential diagnosis includes proximal duodenal atresia, malrotation with midgut volvulus, gastric volvulus, pyloric duplication, retrograde duodenogastric intussusception, and aberrant pancreatic tissue plugging the pylorus.[15-17]

The operative management of pyloric atresia depends on the anatomic type. The recommended treatment for a pyloric web (type I) is excision with Heinecke-Mikulicz pyloroplasty. For solid pyloric atresia (types II or III), a Finney or Heinecke-Mikulicz pyloroplasty is performed if the atresia is short. A Billroth I gastroduodenostomy may be needed if the solid core or gap is long.[13,18] Reports of successful treatment of solid segment atresias with gastroduodenal mucosal advancement have also been described.[19] Gastrojejunostomy should be avoided because there is a 60% failure rate and a reported mortality rate of 55%.[20]

Long-term outcomes in cases of isolated pyloric atresia are excellent. However, cases of pyloric atresia associated with epidermolysis bullosa are usually fatal, with death occurring from septicemia, electrolyte imbalances, protein loss, and failure to thrive secondary to the exudative skin lesions. Reported cases of long-term survival of neonates with epidermolysis bullosa and surgically treated pyloric atresia exist.[21] Therefore, aggressive surgical intervention for these patients should not be withheld.

DUODENAL ATRESIA AND STENOSIS

Congenital duodenal atresia and stenosis is a frequent cause of intestinal obstruction, occurring in 1 per 5000 to 10,000 live births and affecting boys more commonly than girls.[22] More than 50% of affected patients have associated congenital anomalies, with trisomy 21 occurring in approximately 30% of patients.[23,24] At present, either laparoscopic or open duodenoduodenostomy, with or without tapering duodenoplasty, has become standard with early postoperative survival rates of greater than 90%.[24-31]

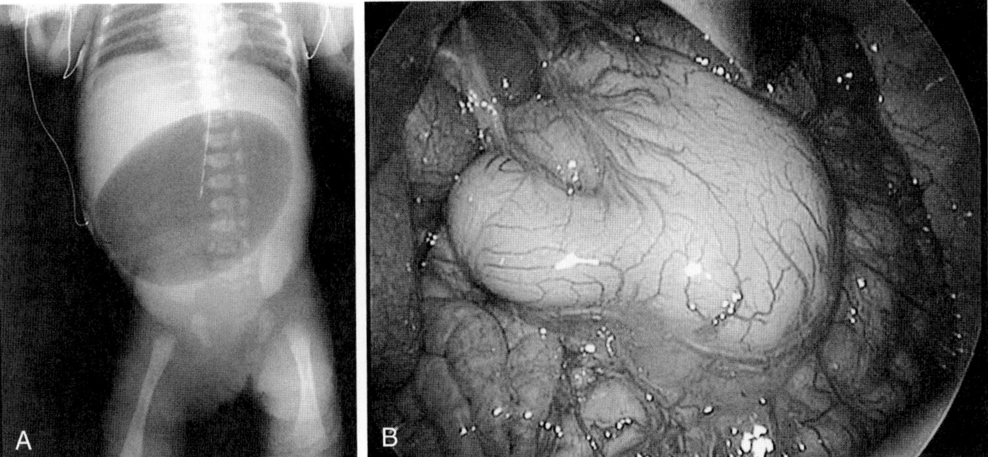

Figure 31-1. **A,** Abdominal radiograph of a newborn with pyloric atresia. The diagnosis is made by the large single gastric bubble with no distal intestinal air. **B,** Laparoscopic view of the stomach in this infant with pyloric atresia. The entire length of the pylorus was a solid core and required resection with a Billroth I reconstruction. The infant has recovered uneventfully.

Etiology

Congenital duodenal obstruction can present due to an intrinsic or extrinsic gastrointestinal lesion.[32] The most common cause of duodenal obstruction is atresia.[24] This intrinsic lesion is most commonly believed to be caused by a failure of recanalization of the fetal duodenum, resulting in complete obstruction. Early in the 4th week of gestation, the duodenum begins to develop from the distal foregut and the proximal midgut. During the 5th and 6th weeks of gestation, the duodenal lumen temporarily obliterates owing to proliferation of its epithelial cells. Vacuolation due to degeneration of the epithelial cells during the 11th week of gestation then leads to recanalization of the duodenum.[33] An embryologic insult during this period can lead to an intrinsic web, atresia, or stenosis. The extrinsic form of duodenal obstruction is due to defects in the development of neighboring structures such as the pancreas, a preduodenal portal vein, or secondary to malrotation and Ladd's bands.[34,35]

Although annular pancreas is an uncommon etiology for duodenal obstruction, it warrants special mention because this form of obstruction is likely due to failure of duodenal development rather than a true constricting lesion. Thus, the presence of an annular pancreas is simply a visible indicator for an underlying stenosis or atresia.[27,36] Between the fourth and eighth weeks of gestation, the pancreatic buds merge. In annular pancreas, the tip of the ventral pancreas becomes fixed to the duodenal wall forming a nondistensible, ring-like or annular portion of pancreatic tissue surrounding the descending part of the duodenum.[33] In annular pancreas associated with duodenal obstruction, the distal biliary tree is often abnormal and may open proximal or distal to the atresia or stenosis.[37,38] Other reported biliary abnormalities associated with duodenal obstruction include biliary atresia, gallbladder agenesis, stenosis of the common bile duct, and choledochal cyst.[39-44]

Classification

Anatomically, duodenal obstructions are classified as either atresias or stenoses. An incomplete obstruction due to a fenestrated web or diaphragm is considered a stenosis. Most stenoses involve the third and/or fourth part of the duodenum. Atresias, or complete obstruction, are further classified into three morphologic types (Fig. 31-2). Type I atresias account for more than 90% of all duodenal obstructions and contain a

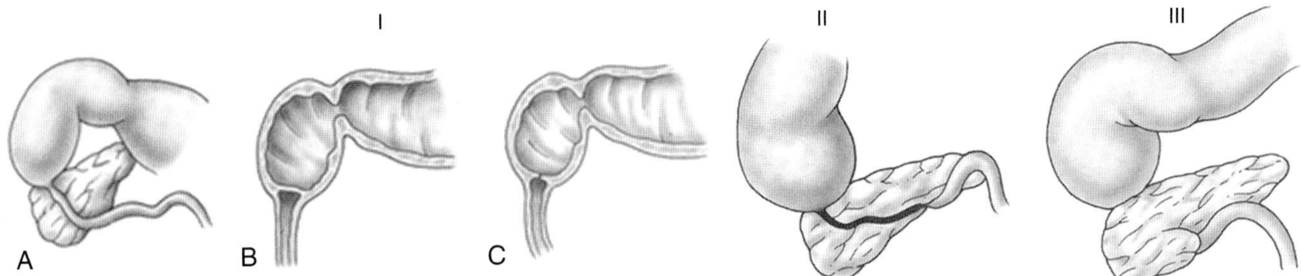

Figure 31-2. Duodenal atresia (and stenosis) is depicted. In type I, either a membrane (B) or web (C) causes the intrinsic duodenal obstruction. There is no fibrous cord and the duodenum remains in continuity. Type II is characterized by complete obliteration of a segment of the duodenum with the proximal and distal portions attached via a fibrous cord. Type III is associated with complete separation of the dilated proximal duodenum from the collapsed distal duodenum.

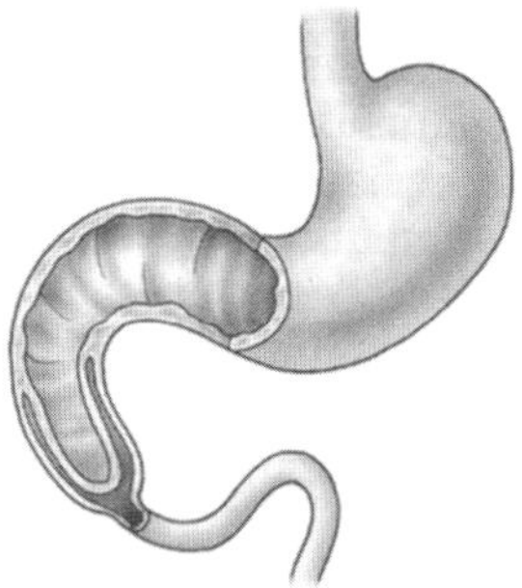

Figure 31-3. Illustration of the "windsock" deformity, a variant of type I duodenal atresia. Note the actual position of the origin of the web in relation to the extent of proximal duodenal dilation and the distal collapsed duodenum.

luminal diaphragm that includes mucosal and submucosal layers. A diaphragm that has ballooned distally ("windsock") is a type I atresia.[45,46] The "windsock" deformity is of particular concern because a portion of the dilated duodenum may actually be distal to the actual obstruction (Fig. 31-3). Type II atresias are characterized by a dilated proximal and collapsed distal segment connected by a fibrous cord. Type III atresias have an obvious gap separating the proximal and distal duodenal segments.[47]

More than 50% of affected patients with duodenal atresia have associated congenital anomalies.[48] Approximately 30% are associated with trisomy 21, 30% with isolated cardiac defects, and 25% with other gastrointestinal anomalies.[49,50] Approximately 45% of patients are premature, and about one third exhibit growth retardation.[23,24]

Pathology

The obstruction can be classified as either preampullary or postampullary with approximately 85% of obstructions located distal to the ampulla of Vater.[51] With complete or almost complete obstruction, the stomach and proximal duodenum become significantly dilated. The pylorus is usually both distended and hypertrophic. As expected, the bowel distal to the obstruction is collapsed. The exception is a "windsock" deformity, where the distal bowel is dilated to a variable length depending on the length of the "windsock" (see Fig. 31-3). In most cases of duodenal obstruction, the gastrointestinal tract can be decompressed proximally, with perforation rarely occurring.[52] With complete obstruction of the duodenum, the incidence of polyhydramnios ranges from 32% to 81%.[1,52-55] Growth retardation is also common, presumably from nutritional deprivation from the swallowed amniotic fluid.

Diagnosis

There are multiple benefits to the antenatal diagnosis of duodenal obstruction including parent counseling and further investigations to exclude associated congenital abnormalities. The diagnosis can often be suggested by prenatal ultrasonography. Sonographic evaluation in fetuses of mothers with a history of polyhydramnios can detect two fluid-filled structures consistent with a double bubble in up to 44% of cases.[56-58] Although most cases of duodenal atresia are detected at between 7 and 8 months of gestation, one report described duodenal obstruction before the 20th week of gestation.[59] Despite duodenal obstruction usually occurring by week 12, the reason for failure of early prenatal detection is not entirely clear. The prevailing thought is that immature gastric emptying may contribute to low gastric pressures failing to dilate the proximal duodenum until later in gestation. Both circular and longitudinal muscle layers are present in the stomach by week 8 of gestation, but pressure amplitudes at 25 weeks are only 60% of term gastric pressures.[60,61]

Clinically, the presentation of the neonate with duodenal obstruction varies depending on whether the obstruction is complete or incomplete, and on the location of the ampulla of Vater in relation to the obstruction. The classic presentation is that of bilious emesis within the first hours of life in an otherwise stable neonate. In about 10% of cases, however, the atresia is preampullary and the emesis is nonbilious.[35] Abdominal distention may or may not be present. In neonates with duodenal atresia, the abdomen is scaphoid. Aspiration via a nasogastric tube of more than 20 mL of gastric contents in a newborn suggests intestinal obstruction as normal aspirate is less than 5 mL.[62] For patients with stenosis, the diagnosis is often delayed until the neonate has started on enteral feeds and feeding intolerance develops with emesis and gastric distention. A delay in diagnosis can result in dehydration and acid-base disorders.

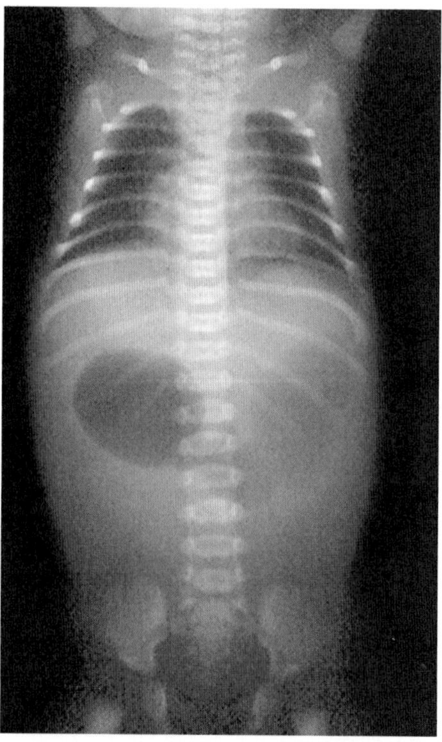

Figure 31-4. Classic "double bubble" sign. This abdominal radiograph in a newborn shows a markedly distended stomach and duodenal bulb without evidence of distal intestinal air.

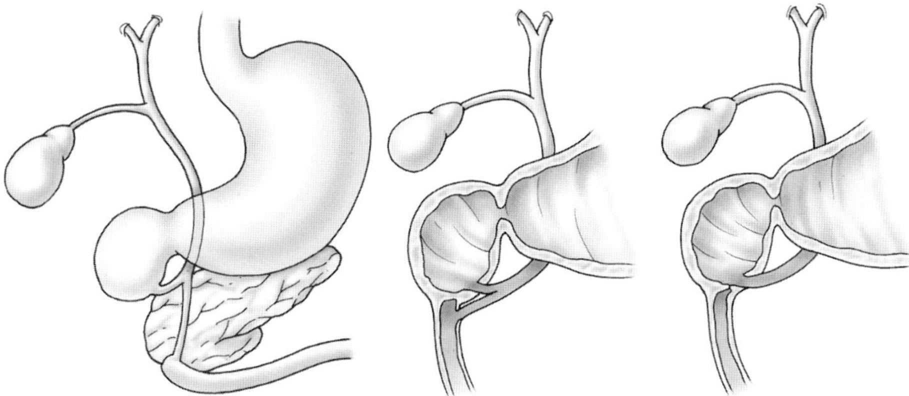

Figure 31-5. Variations in biliary ductal anatomy seen in infants with duodenal atresia.

In antenatally suspected cases of duodenal obstruction, as well as in neonates with a clinical presentation consistent with a proximal bowel obstruction, an upright abdominal radiograph is usually sufficient to confirm the diagnosis of duodenal atresia. The diagnostic radiographic presentation of duodenal atresia is that of a "double bubble" sign with no distal bowel gas (Fig. 31-4). The proximal left-sided bubble represents the air- and fluid-filled stomach, whereas the dilated proximal duodenum represents the second bubble to the right of midline.[63] In almost all cases of duodenal atresia, the distal bowel is gasless. The presence of distal gas, however, does not necessarily exclude the diagnosis of atresia because there are reports of bifid common bile ducts with an insertion both proximal and distal to the atretic segment allowing the air to bypass the atresia.[64] In neonates whose stomach has been decompressed by either nasogastric aspiration or vomiting, 40 to 60 mL of instilled air into the stomach will reproduce the "double bubble."[47] Rarely, the biliary tree is air filled, and a variety of pancreatic and biliary anomalies have been demonstrated (Fig. 31-5).[64] At our institution, neonates who present with bilious emesis and a decompressed stomach on plain abdominal films receive a limited upper gastrointestinal contrast study to exclude malrotation and volvulus. With duodenal stenosis, a "double bubble" sign is usually not present and the diagnosis is usually made with a contrast study (Fig. 31-6).

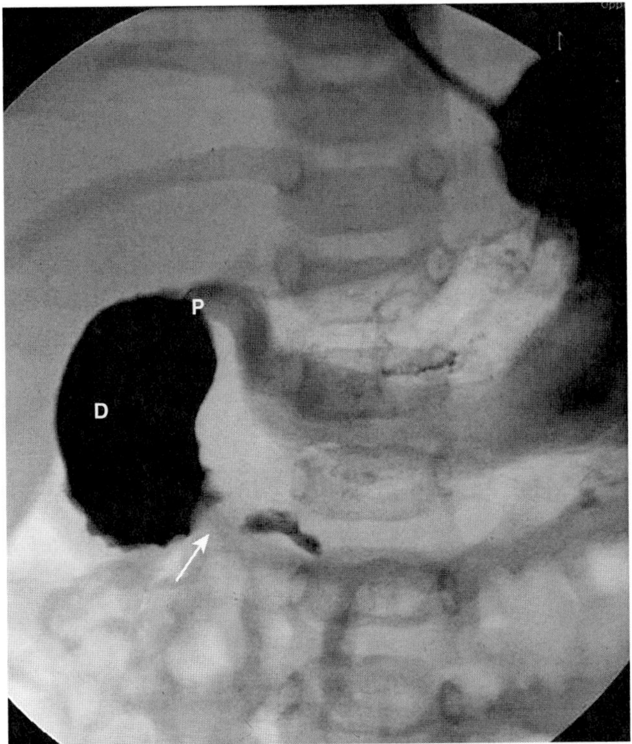

Figure 31-6. An upper gastrointestinal contrast study is shown illustrating a duodenal web. Contrast medium outlines the markedly dilated proximal duodenum (D) with a collapsed distal segment. Note the absence of contrast agent at the location of the tiny web (*arrow*). P, pylorus.

Management

After the diagnosis is made, appropriate resuscitation is required with correction of fluid balance and electrolyte abnormalities in addition to gastric decompression. At our institution, all neonates diagnosed with duodenal obstruction receive a complete metabolic profile, complete blood cell count, coagulation studies, an abdominal and spinal ultrasound evaluation, and two-dimensional echocardiography before any surgical intervention. Emergent surgery is only performed in cases in which malrotation with concurrent volvulus cannot be excluded.

Prior to the mid 1970s, duodenojejunostomy was the preferred technique for correcting duodenal atresia or stenosis.[24,65,66] The various techniques utilized since then include side-to-side duodenoduodenostomy, diamond-shaped duodenoduodenostomy, partial web resection with Heineke-Mikulicz–type duodenoplasty, and tapering duodenoplasty.[65-67] The long side-to-side duodenoduodenostomy, although effective, is associated with a high incidence of anastomotic dysfunction and prolonged obstruction.[50] Blind-loop syndrome appears to be more common in patients treated with duodenojejunostomy.[68] Gastrojejunostomy should not be performed because it is associated with a high incidence of marginal ulceration and bleeding.[47]

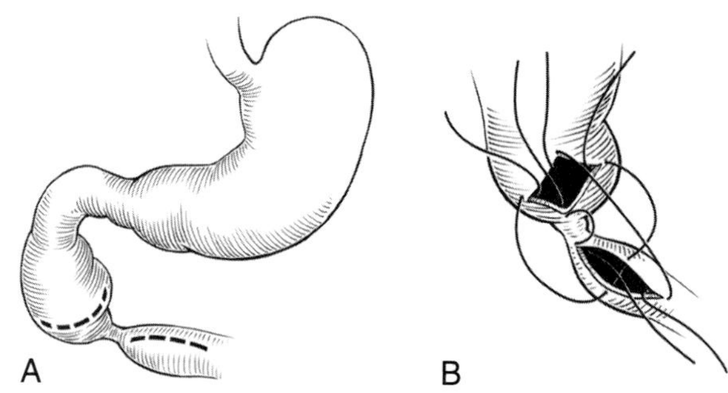

Figure 31-7. **A** and **B**, The technique of duodenoduodenostomy. A diamond-shaped anastomosis is created via the proximal transversely oriented and distal vertically oriented duodenotomies.

Today, the procedure of choice is either laparoscopic or open duodenoduodenostomy.[29-31,50] Originally, a side-to-side anastomosis was performed. Currently, a proximal transverse to distal longitudinal, or diamond-shaped, anastomosis is preferred.[24,65,66,69,70] For the open approach, a right upper quadrant supraumbilical transverse incision is made. After mobilizing the ascending and transverse colons to the left, the duodenal obstruction is readily exposed. Malrotation should be evaluated at this point because it can occur in association with congenital duodenal obstruction in up to 30% of patients.[1] A sufficient length of duodenum distal to the atresia is mobilized to allow for a tension-free anastomosis. A transverse duodenotomy is made in the anterior wall of the distal portion of the dilated proximal duodenum, and a duodenotomy of similar length is made in a vertical orientation on the antimesenteric border of the distal duodenum. The anastomosis is then fashioned by approximating the end of each incision to the appropriate midportion of the other incision (Fig. 31-7).[71] Tapering duodenoplasty is usually not necessary as the proximal duodenal dilation frequently resolves after relief of the obstruction. Muscular continuity of the duodenal wall suggests a "windsock" deformity or diaphragm and calls for extra vigilance in the operative correction, because dilated and collapsed bowel, both distal to the "windsock," have been anastomosed in error.[45,72]

The laparoscopic approach was first described by Rothenberg.[29] The standard laparoscopic approach begins with the patient supine, and the abdomen is insufflated through the umbilicus. Two other instruments are inserted: one in the infant's right lower quadrant and one in the right midepigastric region. A liver retractor can be placed in the right or left upper quadrant if necessary. Alternatively, the liver can be elevated by placing a transabdominal wall suture around the falciform ligament and tying it outside the abdomen (Fig. 31-8). The duodenum is mobilized, and the location of obstruction is identified. By using the same principles that have been described for the open approach, a standard diamond-shaped anastomosis is created. Although some surgeons will perform the laparoscopic anastomosis with interrupted sutures, this can be technically demanding because of the significant number of sutures required. We recently reported our results using Nitinol U-clips (Medtronic, Minneapolis, MN) to create the duodenoduodenostomy with no leaks and more rapid initiation of feeds when compared with the traditional open approach (Fig. 31-9).[30,31] The main advantage of using U-clips is a reduction in the time to complete the anastomosis.

Early postoperative mortality for duodenal atresia repair has been reported to be as low as 3% to 5%, with the majority of deaths occurring secondary to complications related to associated congenital abnormalities.[73] Long-term survival approaches 90%.[24,74-76] Long-term complications have been noted after repair and include delayed gastric emptying, severe gastroesophageal reflux, bleeding peptic ulcer, megaduodenum, duodenogastric reflux, gastritis, blind-loop syndrome, and intestinal obstruction related to adhesions.[50]

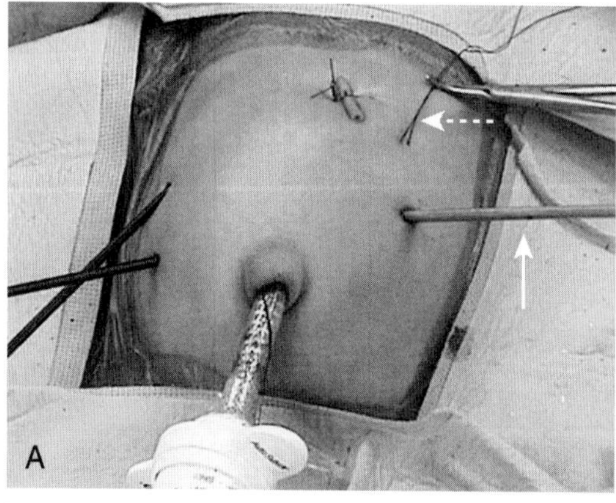

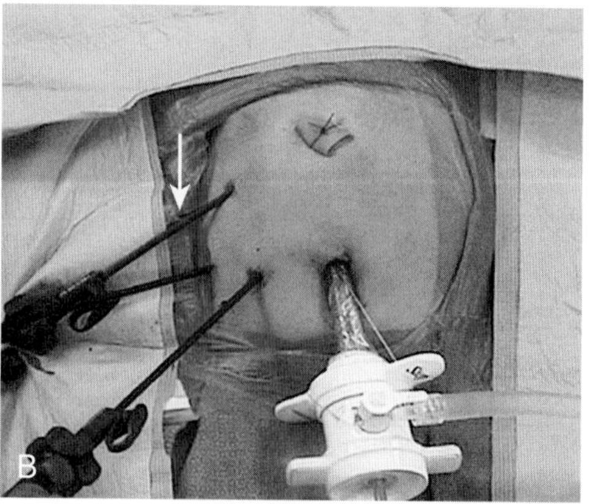

Figure 31-8. Two approaches to placement of the instruments for a laparoscopic duodenal atresia repair. **A**, The two right-sided instruments are the primary working sites for the surgeon. The liver retractor (*arrow*) has been placed in the left midepigastric region. The falciform ligament has been elevated by a suture placed under it and tied over the red rubber catheter, which is used as a bolster. The suture (*dotted arrow*) exteriorized in the infant's left upper abdomen was placed in the dilated proximal duodenum so that it could be easily manipulated. **B**, This is a similar configuration except the instrument elevating the liver (*arrow*) is placed in the infant's right upper abdomen rather than the left upper abdomen. The suture that was placed through the proximal dilated duodenum in **A** was not needed in this particular case.

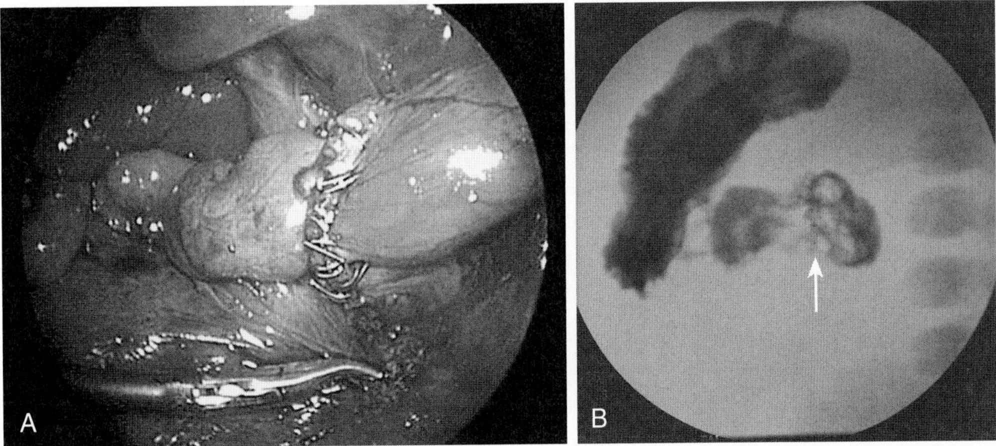

Figure 31-9. **A,** Laparoscopic view of a completed duodenoduodenostomy using the Nitinol U-clips. **B,** A postoperative contrast study at 5 days showed no evidence of obstruction or leak at the anastomosis. The U-clips (*arrow*) can be seen marking the anastomosis.

JEJUNOILEAL ATRESIA AND STENOSIS

Etiology

Jejunoileal atresia occurs in approximately 1 in 5000 live births. It occurs equally in males and females, and about one in three infants is premature.[73] Although the majority of cases are thought to occur sporadically, familial cases of intestinal atresias have been reported.[77] It is generally accepted that jejunoileal atresia occurs as a result of an intrauterine ischemic insult to the midgut affecting single or multiple segments of the already developed intestine.[33,73,78-84] Intrauterine vascular disruption can lead to ischemic necrosis of the bowel with subsequent resorption of the affected segment or segments (Fig. 31-10).

The hypothesis that most cases of jejunoileal atresia occur secondary to vascular disruption during fetal life has been derived from experimental as well as clinical evidence. Isolated mesenteric vascular insults and interference with the segmental blood supply to the small intestine were created in fetal dogs and resulted in different degrees and patterns of intraluminal obstruction, reproducing the spectrum of stenosis and atresia found in humans.[81-83,85-88] Moreover, the presence of bile, lanugo hair, and squamous epithelial cells from swallowed amniotic fluid distal to an atresia, as well as evidence of intrauterine fetal intussusception, midgut volvulus, thromboembolic occlusions, transmesenteric internal hernias, and incarceration or snaring of bowel in an omphalocele or gastroschisis have contributed to wide acceptance of this hypothesis.[79,88-93]

The presence of associated extra-abdominal organ abnormalities in jejunoileal atresia is low (<10%), owing to its occurrence later in fetal life and the localized nature of the vascular compromise.[94,95] In rare instances, jejunoileal atresia has been found to be associated with Hirschsprung's disease, cystic fibrosis, malrotation, Down syndrome, anorectal and vertebral anomalies, neural tube defects, congenital heart disease, and other gastrointestinal atresias.[73,94-96] Methylene blue, previously used for amniocentesis in twin pregnancies, has been implicated in causing small bowel atresia.[97]

Although jejunoileal atresias are usually not hereditary, there is a well-documented autosomal recessive

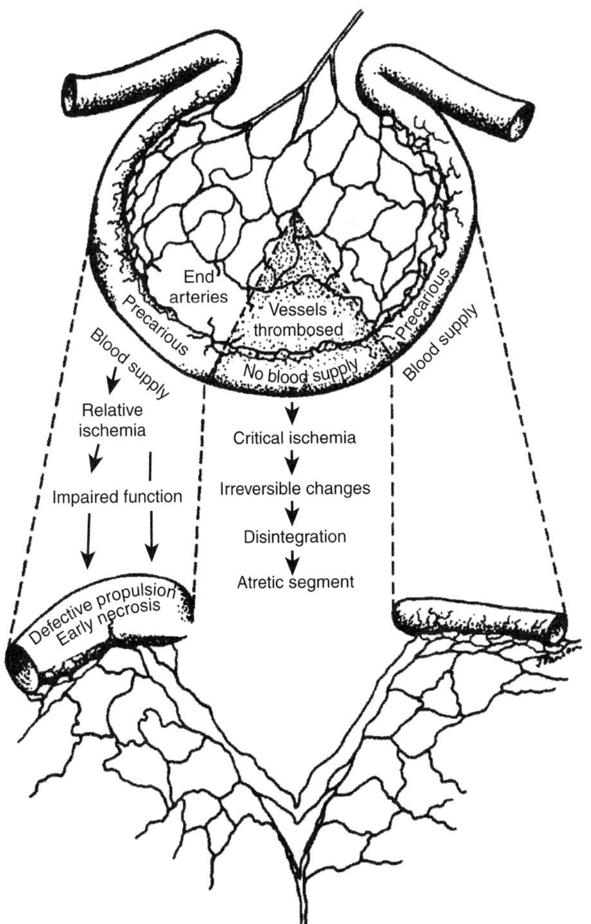

Figure 31-10. Proposed mechanism of vascular compromise and subsequent development of jejunoileal atresia.

pattern of inheritance of multiple atresias first documented in Montreal and later identified elsewhere.[98] In these cases of inherited jejunoileal atresia, rotation was normal, mesenteric defects were never observed, and lanugo hairs and squamous cells were not identified distal to the most proximal atresia, suggesting an early intrauterine event. This disorder is uniformly lethal even with successful bowel resection. No correlations have been found between jejunoileal atresia and parental or maternal disease. However, the use of maternal vasoconstrictive medications as well as maternal cigarette smoking in the first trimester of pregnancy has been shown to increase the risk of small bowel atresia.[99] Chromosomal abnormalities are seen in less than 1% of the patients.[100]

Pathology

Following the Grosfeld classification, the defects of jejunoileal atresia are separated into four groups based on the type of atresia, with an additional consideration for type III(b) ("apple peel" or "Christmas tree" appearance) (Fig. 31-11E).[4] This classification has significant prognostic and therapeutic value because it emphasizes the importance of associated loss of intestinal length, abnormal collateral intestinal blood supply, and concomitant atresia or stenosis.[101] Regarding classification, the most proximal atresia determines whether the atresia is classified as jejunal or ileal atresia. Multiple atresias are found in up to 30% of patients.[73,102]

Stenosis

Stenosis is defined as a localized narrowing of the intestinal lumen without disruption in the intestinal wall or a defect in the mesentery (see Fig. 31-11A). At the stenotic site, a short, narrow, somewhat rigid segment of intestine with a small lumen is found. Often the muscularis is irregular and the submucosa is thickened. Stenosis may also take the form of a type I atresia with a fenestrated web. Patients with jejunoileal stenosis usually have a normal length of small intestine.

Type I Atresia

In type I atresia, the intestinal obstruction occurs secondary to a membrane or web formed by both mucosa and submucosa while the muscularis and

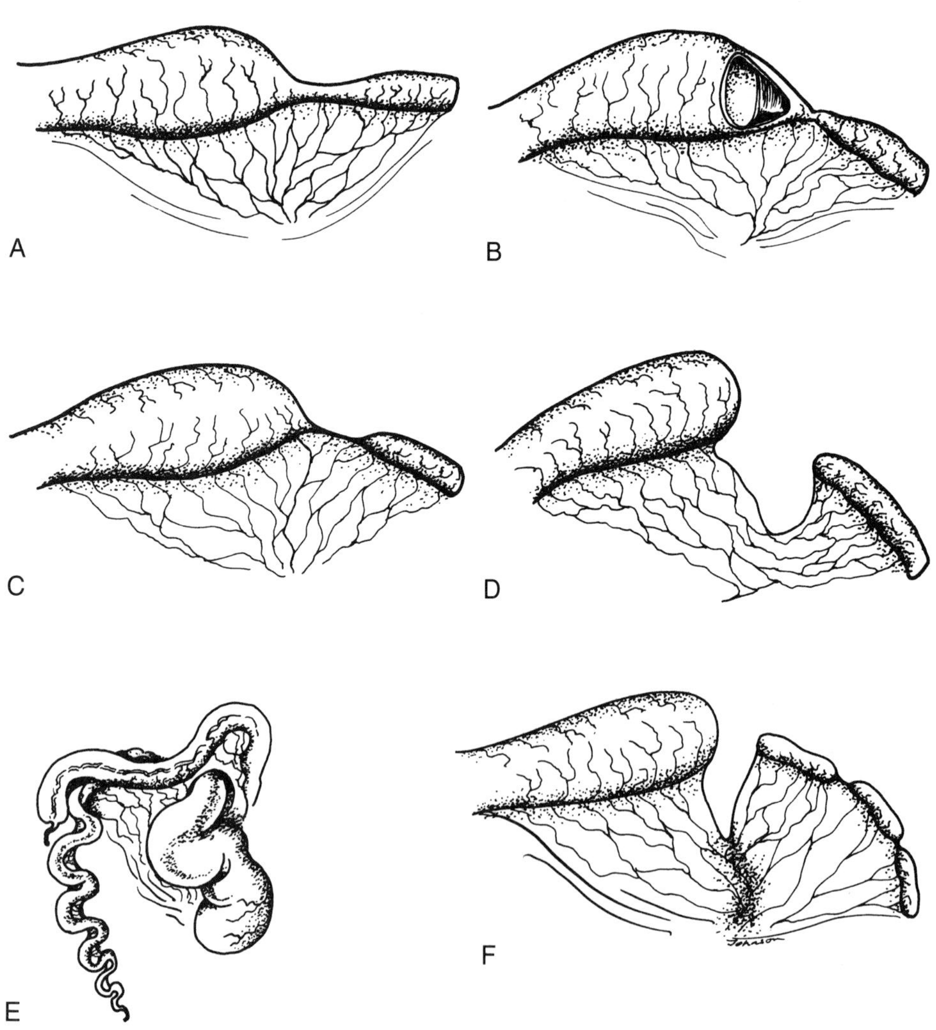

Figure 31-11. The classification for jejunoileal atresia and stenosis. **A,** Stenosis. **B,** Type I. **C,** Type II. **D,** Type III(a). **E,** Type III(b). **F,** Type IV.

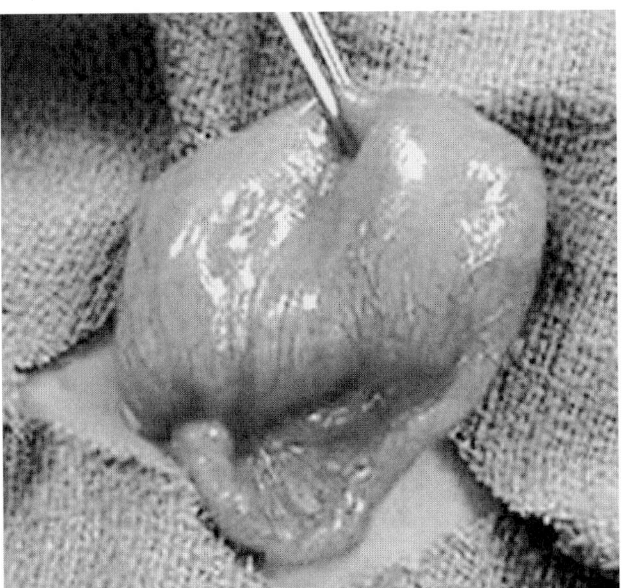

Figure 31-12. In this infant with abdominal distention and evidence of a congenital bowel obstruction, a type I jejunal atresia was found. Note the mesentery is intact and the small, distal jejunum is connected to the very dilated, proximal jejunum.

serosa remain intact (see Figs. 31-11B and 31-12). On gross inspection, the bowel and its mesentery appear to be in continuity. However, the proximal bowel is dilated while the distal bowel is collapsed. With the increased intraluminal pressure in the proximal bowel, bulging of the web into the distal intestine can create a windsock effect. As with stenosis, there is no foreshortening of the bowel in type I atresias.

Type II Atresia

The clinical findings of a type II atresia are a largely dilated, blind-ending proximal bowel loop connected by a fibrous cord to the collapsed distal bowel with an intact mesentery (see Fig. 31-11C). Increased intraluminal pressure in the dilated and hypertrophied proximal bowel may lead to focal proximal small bowel ischemia. The distal collapsed bowel commences as a blind end, which sometimes assumes a bulbous appearance owing to the remains of an intussusception. Again, the total small bowel length is usually normal.

Type III(a) Atresia

In type III(a) atresia, the atresia ends blindly with no fibrous connecting cord to the distal intestine. A V-shaped mesenteric defect of varying size is present between the two ends of intestine (see Figs. 31-11D and 31-13). The dilated, blind-ending proximal bowel is often aperistaltic and frequently undergoes torsion or becomes overdistended, with subsequent necrosis and perforation occurring as a secondary event.[103] In this scenario, the total length of the small bowel is variable (but usually less than normal), owing to intrauterine resorption of the affected bowel.

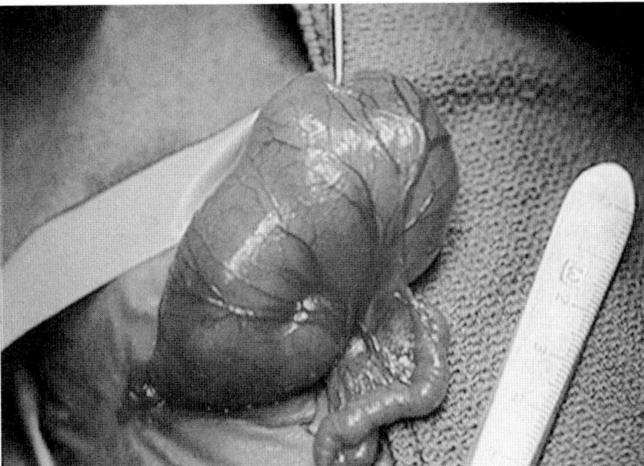

Figure 31-13. In this infant with congenital small bowel obstruction, a type III(a) jejunal atresia was found. Note the atresia ends blindly without a connection to the distal intestine. Moreover, there is a V-shaped mesenteric defect between the two segments of intestine.

Type III(b) Atresia

Type III(b) atresia ("apple peel," "Christmas tree," or "maypole" deformity) consists of a proximal jejunal atresia, absence of the superior mesenteric artery beyond the origin of the middle colic branch, agenesis of the dorsal mesentery, a significant loss of intestinal length, and a large mesenteric defect (see Fig. 31-11E). The decompressed distal small bowel lies free in the abdomen and assumes a helical configuration around a single perfusing vessel arising from the ileocolic or right colic arcades (Fig. 31-14). Occasionally, additional type I or type II atresias are found distally. Also,

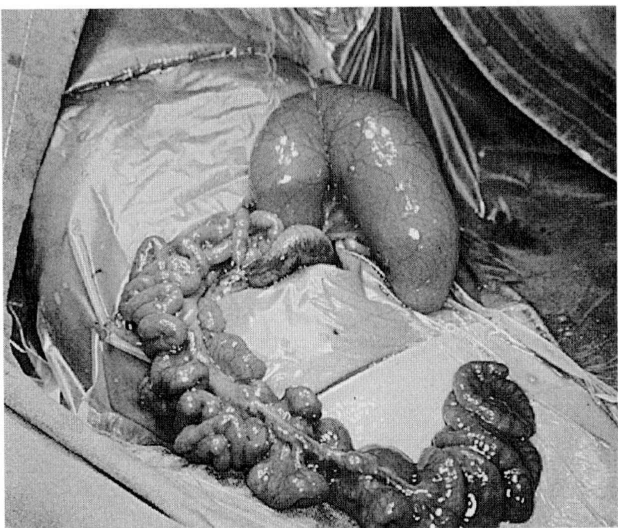

Figure 31-14. The operative findings in a neonate with type III(b) intestinal atresia are seen. Note the classic "apple core" or "Christmas tree" deformity associated with a type III(b) atresia and the wide mesenteric gap between the proximal dilated bowel and distal decompressed ileum. Also, the colon and distal small bowel are perfused through a single artery running through the coils of the bowel.

the vascularity of the distal bowel is often impaired. This type of atresia has been found in families with a pattern suggestive of an autosomal recessive mode of inheritance. It also has been encountered in siblings with identical lesions and in twins.[84,103-107]

The occurrence of intestinal atresia in other siblings, the association of multiple atresias (15%), and the discordance in a set of apparently monozygotic twins may point to more complex genetic transmission with an overall recurrence rate of 18%.[104,108-110] Infants with this anomaly are often premature. Up to 50% may have malrotation. Short bowel syndrome is present in nearly 75% of cases. Accordingly, there is increased morbidity (63%) and mortality (54%) in this population.[104,111] Type III(b) atresias are most likely the consequence of a proximal superior mesenteric arterial occlusion with extensive infarction of the proximal segment of the midgut. Also, it can develop from a midgut volvulus.[79,104,105,112] Primary failure of development of the distal superior mesenteric artery has also been suggested as an etiologic factor. However, this is unlikely because meconium is usually found in the bowel distal to the atresia. This finding indicates that the atresia develops after bile secretion begins, which occurs around week 12 of intrauterine life. The superior mesenteric artery develops much earlier than 12 weeks.[113]

Type IV Atresia

Multiple-segment atresias or a combination of types I to III are classified as type IV (see Fig. 31-11F). Twenty to 35 percent of infants affected with jejunoileal atresia present with multiple atresias.[73,102] A familial form of multiple intestinal atresia involving the stomach, duodenum, and both the small and large bowel has been described.[98,114] It is associated with prematurity and shortened bowel length. To date, it has been uniformly fatal. It is associated with type I and II atresias, with type II predominating. An autosomal recessive mode of transmission has been suggested for this familial form of hereditary multiple intestinal atresia because it is unlikely that an isolated prenatal vascular accident would be responsible for such extensive involvement of the gastrointestinal tract. In addition, infants affected with this familial form are found to have long segments of completely occluded small or large intestine without a recognizable lumen.[114-116] Another pathognomonic feature seen in familial multiple intestinal atresia is the sieve-like appearance of the intestine on histologic examination in which multiple lumens are surrounded by epithelial cells and muscularis mucosa.[102]

The majority of cases of multiple-segment atresias are sporadic with no other family history of gastrointestinal defects. They are likely a result of multiple vascular insults to the mesentery, intrauterine inflammatory processes, or a malformation of the gastrointestinal tract occurring during embryonic development.[102,117] Embolic material from a nonviable fetus to a living monochorionic twin through placental vascular connections could also account for single or multiple intestinal atresias.[118] Associated defects, particularly abnormalities of the central nervous system, have been noted in approximately 25% of patients without familial multiple intestinal atresia.[102] Multiple atresias have also been seen in association with severe immunodeficiency.[119]

Pathophysiology

The vascular and subsequent ischemic insult not only causes morphologic abnormalities but also adversely influences the structure and subsequent function of the remaining proximal and distal bowel.[78-81,84,120] The blind-ended proximal bowel is dilated and hypertrophied with histologically normal villi, but without effective peristaltic activity. A deficiency of mucosal enzymes and muscular adenosine triphosphatase has also been found. At the level of the atresia, the ganglia of the enteric nervous system are atrophic with minimal acetylcholinesterase activity. These changes are most likely secondary to local ischemia.[84,121] Obstruction alone can elicit similar, but less severe, morphologic and functional abnormalities.[122]

Immunohistochemical stains of human intestinal tissue have revealed discrepancies of neural components both proximal and distal to the atretic intestinal segment. Quantification of the density of the myenteric plexus during the antenatal period has shown a decreased density proximal to the atresia despite an increase in the number of glial cells when compared with gestational age-matched controls.[88] Thus, these results cannot be ascribed solely to distention and obstruction proximal to the atresia. Similarly, staining for neurons and ganglion cells in the myenteric plexus was significantly decreased in the proximal and distal segments, suggesting a perturbation in the maturation of different components of the enteric nervous system.[88]

Experimental studies showing that the intestinal atresia results from ischemic necrosis of the intestine also imply that there is a precarious blood supply to the proximally dilated bowel. This has been confirmed with postmortem injection of barium sulfate into the mesenteric vessels.[79,81,113] However, it has also been postulated that the intestine is not ischemic at birth but rather becomes so only with swallowing air. Distention and increased intraluminal pressure or torsion can then occur. The good results obtained with tapering procedures without resection of the bulbous portion would support the contention that the blood and nerve supply to the bowel adjacent to the atresia is normal.[79] However, this ischemic insult may interfere with mucosal and neural function. Defective peristalsis is commonly noticed in the atretic area, thus supporting resection of the dilated bulbous proximal end for better function. Because the proximal end of the distal atretic bowel has been subjected to a similar insult, a small portion of it should be resected at the time of surgical correction as well.

Insufficient bowel length, excessive removal of residual bowel, or ischemic insult to the remaining bowel can lead to short gut syndrome with long-term sequelae for growth and development. Postoperative complications or the inappropriate use of hyperosmolar feeding or medication can predispose to these complications as well.

Clinical Manifestations

Prompt recognition of intestinal obstruction in the neonate is paramount due to the possibility of midgut volvulus or an internal hernia with subsequent ischemia. Although ultrasonography is more reliable at detecting duodenal atresia, in recent years it has become useful in diagnosing jejunoileal atresia as well. The ultrasonographic findings include dilated loops of bowel and polyhydramnios. Polyhydramnios may not be present early in gestation or with very distal obstructions. Although these findings may be suggestive of atresia, they are not pathognomonic and other diagnoses must be entertained. However, abnormal findings should elicit a search for familial gastrointestinal abnormalities as well as referral for prenatal evaluation. The vast majority of patients with jejunoileal atresia will not be diagnosed prenatally.

Type III(b) and multiple intestinal atresias also have a familial tendency. A 3.4% incidence of anomalies in siblings has been reported in a large survey of children with jejunoileal atresias as well as an 18% recurrence rate in siblings of patients with multiple intestinal atresias.[104,111]

In neonates with atresia or stenosis, the presenting symptoms are consistent with bowel obstruction, including bilious emesis and abdominal distention. Although the meconium may appear normal, it is more common to see gray plugs of mucus passed via the rectum.[123] Occasionally, if the distal bowel in type III(b) atresia is ischemic, blood may be passed through the rectum.

Intestinal stenosis is more likely to create diagnostic difficulty when compared with intestinal atresia. Intermittent partial obstruction or malabsorption may improve without treatment.[89,124,125] Clinical investigations may initially be normal. However, these infants usually develop failure to thrive and ultimately progress to complete intestinal obstruction and require exploration.

Diagnosis

The diagnosis of jejunoileal atresia can usually be made by radiographic examination of the abdomen with only swallowed air as contrast.[124,125] Swallowed air reaches the proximal bowel by 1 hour and the distal small bowel by 3 hours in a normal vigorous infant in whom its passage is blocked, but this pattern may be delayed in premature or sick infants with poor sucking.[126,127] Jejunal atresia patients have a few gas-filled and fluid-filled loops of small bowel, but the remainder of the abdomen is gasless (Fig. 31-15). When the atresia is associated with cystic fibrosis, fewer air-fluid levels are evident, and the typical ground-glass appearance of inspissated meconium is present. A limited-contrast meal may be useful if intestinal stenosis is suspected.

Because haustral markings are rarely seen in neonates, distal ileal atresia may be difficult to differentiate from colonic atresia (Fig. 31-16). A contrast enema reveals an unused appearance to the colon. Reliance on intraoperative injection of saline into the large bowel to confirm distal bowel patency may fail to identify an associated colonic or rectal atresia.[128,129] If the small bowel atresia occurred late in gestation, the bowel distal to the atresia may have a more normal caliber. Occasionally, air and meconium can accumulate proximal to an atresia, mimicking the radiologic appearance

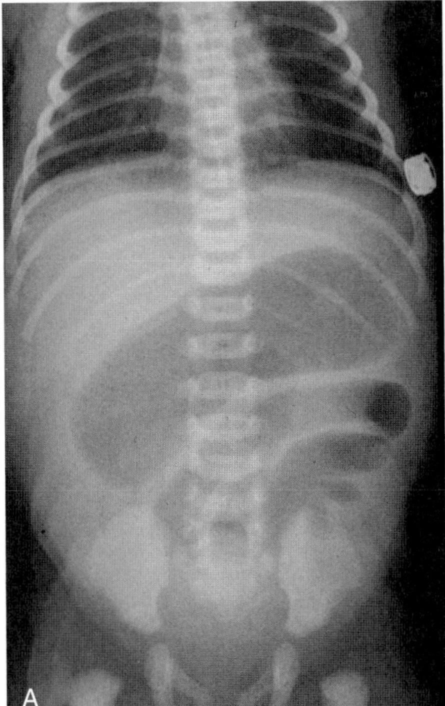

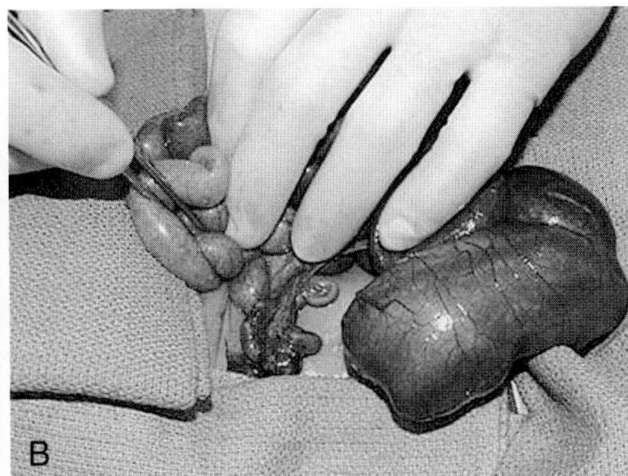

Figure 31-15. **A,** The abdominal radiograph in this neonate shows several proximally dilated intestinal loops consistent with jejunal atresia. **B,** A type III(a) distal atresia was found at operation.

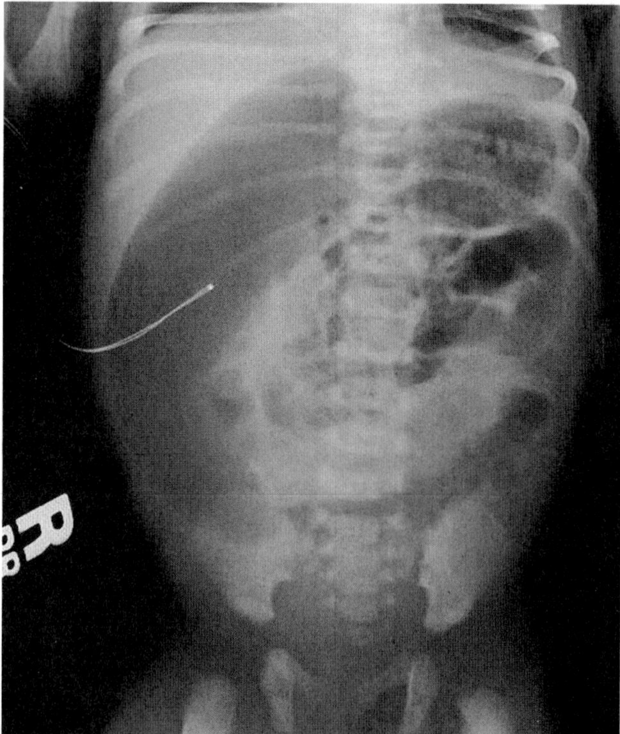

Figure 31-16. The diagnosis of colonic atresia can be difficult on the plain abdominal radiograph. This radiograph shows multiple dilated intestinal loops and appears similar to the findings shown in Figure 31-15. At operation, the infant was found to have atresia of the transverse colon (see Fig. 31-19).

of meconium ileus. Additionally, total colonic aganglionosis may be difficult to differentiate from atresia.

Ten percent of infants with jejunoileal atresia present with meconium peritonitis.[4,125] The intestinal perforation usually occurs proximal to the obstruction at the bulbous blind end. The radiologic appearance of a meconium pseudocyst containing a large air-fluid level is related to the late intrauterine perforation of bowel. Intraluminal calcification of meconium or intramural dystrophic calcification in the form of diffuse punctate or rounded aggregations has been reported with intestinal stenosis or atresia.[130] Meconium calcification in patients with hereditary familial multiple intestinal atresia produces a "string of pearls," which is pathognomonic of this condition.[98,116]

The clinical and radiologic picture of jejunoileal stenosis is determined by the level and degree of stenosis. The diagnosis may be delayed for years.[111,124] Morphologic and functional changes in the proximal obstructed intestine vary depending on the degree of obstruction.

Differential Diagnosis

Diseases that mimic jejunoileal atresia include colonic atresia, midgut volvulus, meconium ileus, duplication cysts, internal hernias, ileus due to sepsis, birth trauma, maternal medications, prematurity, and hypothyroidism.[4,85,124,131,132] Special investigations, including an upper gastrointestinal contrast study, contrast enema, rectal biopsy, and a ΔF508 gene deletion assay or sweat test to exclude associated cystic fibrosis, may be needed.[131,133]

Management

Delay in diagnosis may lead to impairment of intestinal viability (50%), frank necrosis and perforation (10% to 20%), fluid and electrolyte abnormalities, and sepsis.[103,123,124] Preoperative management involves insertion of a nasogastric or orogastric tube to decompress the stomach and fluid resuscitation to correct electrolyte abnormalities and hypovolemia. Antibiotics should be initiated if there is any concern for perforation or infection.

Surgical Considerations

The surgical management of intestinal atresias is based on the location of the lesion, anatomic findings, associated conditions noted at operation, and the length of the remaining intestine.[73] Resection of the dilated and hypertrophied proximal bowel, with primary end-to-end anastomosis with or without tapering of the proximal bowel, is the most common surgical technique.[4,79-81,85,103]

As recently as the 1950s, the surgical mortality for neonates with intestinal atresia was 80% to 90%.[85,124] The poor prognosis early in the 20th century was mostly related to late presentation and dysmotility of the proximal dilated portion of the bowel, which led to complications related to chronic obstruction and inanition. The current survival rate is greater than 90%.[73] Understanding that the proximal bowel is dysfunctional, improvements in the anastomotic technique and suture material, and the development of total parenteral nutrition are the primary reasons for this significantly improved survival in recent years. Only infants with severe associated congenital abnormalities or short bowel syndrome should not have a good prognosis.

Operative Considerations

The repair of small intestinal atresia can be undertaken via several approaches. One option is to evaluate using a laparoscopic approach, with subsequent resection and anastomosis performed in an extracorporeal fashion. Although this approach seems attractive, it can be difficult to identify the atresia due to the markedly dilated small intestine and the small working space of the neonate's abdominal cavity. Because of these limitations, we have begun to explore the abdomen through the umbilicus. With this approach, the umbilical skin is incised and the fascia is opened vertically in the midline to the extent allowed by the umbilical skin incision. A Lonestar (CooperSurgical, Inc., Trumbull, CT) retractor can be inserted to obtain exposure and allow for evisceration of the bowel (Fig. 31-17). The traditional transverse supraumbilical or infraumbilical incision is also appropriate. Regardless of the approach, access to the entire intestine and peritoneal cavity is necessary. If perforation has

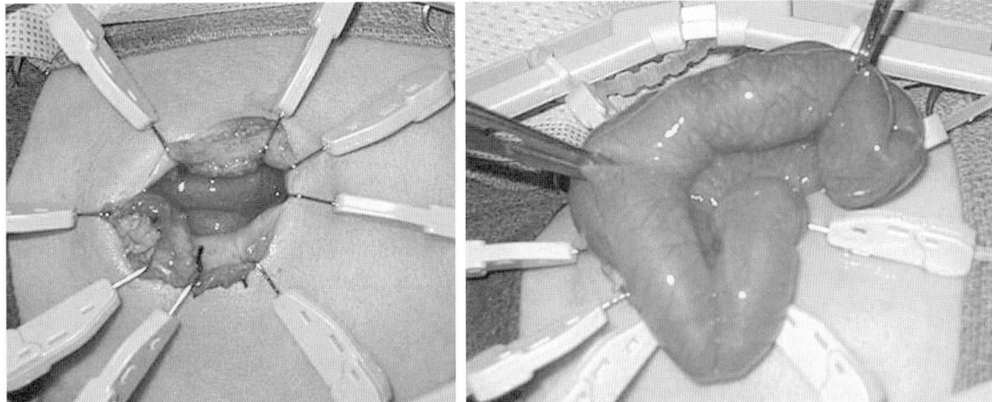

Figure 31-17. The operative approach through the umbilical ring allows for complete evaluation of the intestine and repair of an atresia. Shown here is the technique using the Lonestar retractor to maintain exposure during repair of a type IIIa jejunal atresia.

occurred, it should be controlled and the abdomen irrigated with normal saline. Careful inspection of the entire bowel is performed and the site and type of obstruction should be noted as well as any other abnormalities. In addition, the length of bowel should be assessed. The most distal limb of the atretic bowel should then be cannulated with a red rubber catheter and irrigated with warm saline to evaluate for distal obstruction. Continuity of the colon can be established preoperatively by a contrast enema or with a prepositioned transrectal catheter placed before prepping.[134] Failure to adequately evaluate for distal obstruction or stenosis can lead to postoperative complications such as an anastomotic leak. If present, malrotation should be corrected with a Ladd procedure. Because the length of functional bowel has important prognostic significance and determines the most appropriate method of repair, this length of functional bowel should be carefully measured along the antimesenteric border.

Delayed intestinal function in the blind proximal atretic segment as well as functional obstruction after performance of a side-to-side anastomosis without resection of the dilated proximal atretic bowel has been discussed.[84,132] In addition, it has been reported that the inciting ischemic event that led to the atresia may lead to a deficiency in mucosal enzymes for a distance of 10 to 20 cm proximal to the atresia.[135] Therefore, if the length of functional bowel is adequate, the bulbous hypertrophied proximal bowel should be resected to approximately normal-caliber bowel.[79,103] Ultimately, the goal is to restore bowel continuity while maintaining both intestinal function and length.[84] In high jejunal atresias, this proximal bowel resection may extend into the second portion of the duodenum, requiring de-rotation of the duodenum and mobilization of the right colon to the left. Intestinal imbrication has also been shown to be an effective method to reduce the caliber of the distended bowel while maintaining mucosal absorptive surface.[136] Distally, a short segment (4 to 5 cm) of the bowel is removed obliquely, leaving the mesenteric side longer than the antimesenteric aspect. An incision along the antimesenteric border to create a "fish mouth" may be needed to create an adequate distal enterotomy for the anastomosis (Fig. 31-18).[80,84,134]

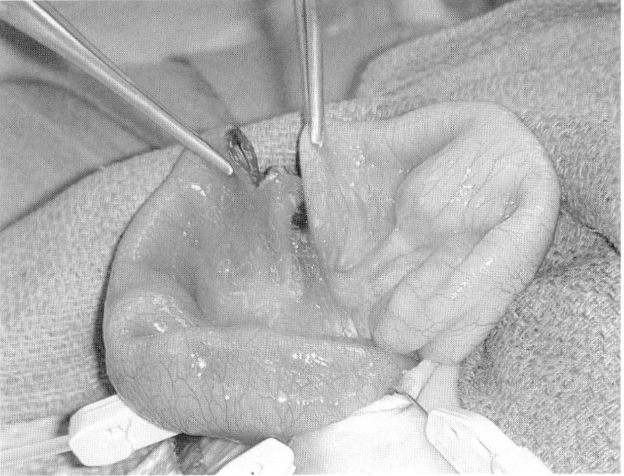

Figure 31-18. The intestinal anastomosis in the infant seen in Figure 31-17 is shown. At the time of repair, there can be a significant size discrepancy between the proximal and distal bowel. The proximal bowel has been resected to a point that will allow for a more appropriately sized intestinal anastomosis.

Although there are multiple techniques for the anastomosis, a one-layer modification of the end-to-back technique using 5-0 or 6-0 monofilament absorbable sutures has been shown to be safe and effective.[100,103] Once the anastomosis is completed, the suture line is tested for leaks and reinforcing sutures are placed as needed. The mesenteric defect is repaired with careful attention to avoid rotation or kinking of the anastomosis or injury to the blood supply. A temporary enterostomy should be performed in cases of perforation with significant contamination or meconium peritonitis or if there is a question of bowel viability.[73] However, neither decompressive gastrostomy nor transanastomotic stents are usually needed.[137,138]

Similar techniques are used for stenosis and jejunoileal membranes. Procedures such as transverse enteroplasty, excision of the membrane, and bypassing techniques are not recommended, primarily because they fail to remove the abnormal segments of bowel and may produce blind-loop syndromes.

Prognostic Factors

The normal small bowel length in term neonates is approximately 250 cm. In preterm infants, it ranges from 160 to 240 cm. With the development of total parenteral nutrition, special enteral diets, and pharmacologic management of short gut syndrome, previous estimates that a small bowel length of 100 cm or more is necessary to sustain oral intake and survival may no longer be applicable.[81] Regardless, preservation of bowel length at the expense of a poorly functioning anastomosis should be avoided.

If proximal resection will lead to significant, or unacceptable, bowel loss, tapering or plication of the dilated bowel is a useful technique.[72,135-140] Tapering enteroplasty as proximal as the second portion of the duodenum can be accomplished by resecting an antimesenteric strip of the dilated proximal bowel.[141] During tapering duodenojejunoplasty, particularly with type III atresias, the duodenum is de-rotated and the cecum moved to the left to avoid kinking of the anastomosis.[142] The tapering can be safely performed up to 35 cm.[140] The tapered bowel may be anastomosed to the distal bowel or exteriorized as a stoma.

Plication or infolding along the antimesenteric border is preferred by some surgeons because it conserves mucosal surface area and may facilitate the return of bowel function.[140] Plication also reduces the risk of leak from the antimesenteric suture line that can occur with a tapering enteroplasty. More than 50% of the bowel circumference can be imbricated into the intestinal lumen over an extended length without causing obstruction. However, breakdown of the suture line results in a functional obstruction.[73] The plication may be less likely to disrupt if a longitudinal antimesenteric seromuscular strip is resected before the plication.[143,144]

A primary anastomosis may be contraindicated in cases of peritonitis, volvulus with vascular compromise, meconium ileus, and type III(b) atresia.[145,146] Under these circumstances, exteriorization of both ends of the atresia may be needed.

Atresia encountered in gastroschisis may be single or multiple and may be located in either the small or large bowel.[91] In a series from our institution, 12.6% of 199 patients with gastroschisis had an associated atresia.[147] The most common location for the atresia was jejunoileal, and most were type III(a). Our current management algorithm for patients with gastroschisis and atresia is to first assess the extent of reactive change of the intestine (peel). If there is minimal intestinal peel, a primary anastomosis may be considered. This is rare and should be considered only in the most optimal situations. In most instances, the atresia should be left undisturbed at the initial operation. After fascial closure is accomplished, management should include nasogastric decompression and total parenteral nutritional support with subsequent repair of the atresia 4 to 6 weeks later.[147]

Although isolated type I atresias are usually managed by primary resection and anastomosis, multiple diaphragms have been successfully perforated and dilated by passing a bougie along the entire length of the small intestine.[80,111]

With type III(b) atresia, restricting bands along the free edge of the distal coiled and narrow mesentery should be divided to optimize the blood supply. The bowel should be returned to the abdomen with careful inspection of the mesentery to prevent torsion of the single marginal artery and vein.[148] In cases of questionable intestinal viability, improved long-term results have been achieved with resection and tapering of the dilated proximal bowel with limited resection of the distal bowel.[149,150]

Bowel length conservation methods, such as multiple anastomoses for multiple atresias, may result in increased morbidity.[81,123] An absorbable silicone (Silastic) catheter stent can be used with multiple primary anastomoses and serves as a conduit for radiologic evidence of anastomotic integrity, luminal patency, and enteral feeding.[151] If multiple atresias are grouped closely together and there is adequate bowel length, a single resection and anastomosis can be performed.[134]

There is no place for bowel lengthening procedures at the initial operation. However, such procedures may ultimately obviate the need for prolonged total parenteral nutrition in patients with short gut syndrome associated with intestinal atresias.

Postoperative Care

Parenteral nutrition is mandatory and should begin as soon as possible. It should continue until the infant is tolerating full enteral feeding.

The return of bowel function varies. Generally, a more proximally located anastomosis takes longer to function. Enteral feedings can be initiated when the gastric aspirate is clear, output is minimal, and the infant is producing stools. At our institution, enteral feeding is usually started through the nasogastric feeding tube at a rate of 20 mL/kg/day of breast milk or formula in a continuous fashion. The feeds are increased by 20 to 30 mL/kg/day. Oral intake is started when the infant is alert, able to suck, and tolerating at least 8 mL of tube feeds per hour.

Any clinical findings suggestive of an anastomotic leak require immediate re-exploration. At operation, it is important to once again confirm patency of the distal bowel.

Transient gastrointestinal dysfunction is frequently observed in infants with jejunal and ileal atresia, and its etiology is multifactorial.[4,89,103,152] Lactose intolerance, malabsorption (owing to stasis with bacterial overgrowth), and diarrhea may be significant in infants who have undergone repair of type III(b) atresia or in those with short bowel syndrome after surgery for multiple atresias. Regular monitoring for clinical signs of intestinal overload or intolerance is required. Water-loss stools, increasing frequency of stooling, hematochezia, fecal-reducing substances, or a decreased stool pH warrant biochemical evaluation of the stool for disaccharide or monosaccharide intolerance.[153] Unintentional injury to the mucosa can be caused by sugars, high-osmolarity feeds, oral medications, and bacterial or viral infections. Pharmacologic control of altered gastrointestinal function may hasten adaptation. Loperamide decreases intestinal peristaltic activity, and cholestyramine is effective in binding bile salts.[152,154] Cholestyramine should not be used unless water-loss stools are evident. Vitamin B_{12} and folic acid should be given regularly to the patient without a terminal ileum to prevent megaloblastic anemia.

Functional outcome ultimately depends on the following factors: (1) the location of the atresia (the ileum adapts to a greater degree than the jejunum), (2) the maturity of the intestine (the small intestine in a premature infant still has time for maturation and growth), and (3) the length of the small intestine, which can be difficult to determine accurately after birth.[155] The ileocecal valve is critically important because it allows for more rapid intestinal adaptation when the residual small bowel length is short.

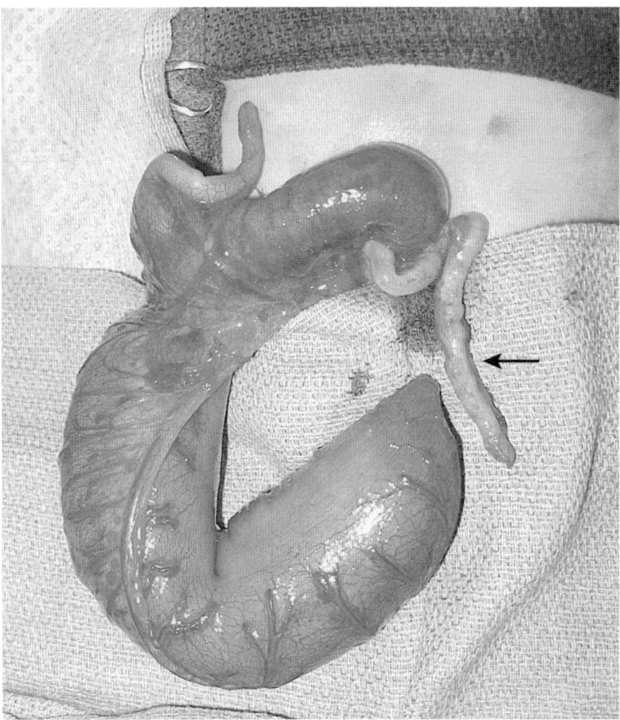

Figure 31-19. A type III colonic atresia was found at operation in this infant with intestinal obstruction. Note the cecum and appendix and the very dilated right colon. Also, note the extremely small distal colon (*arrow*). A colostomy was performed as the initial procedure in this infant.

COLONIC ATRESIA

Colonic atresia is a rare cause of intestinal obstruction and comprises 1.8% to 15% of all gastrointestinal atresias.[156,157] The reported incidence of colonic atresia varies greatly from 1:5000 to 1:60,000 live births.[158-161] The accepted incidence is approximately 1 in 20,000 live births. Although it is most commonly reported as an isolated anomaly, approximately one third of infants have associated congenital lesions.[158,159,162] There are various classifications of colonic atresia, but the one most commonly used divides colonic atresia into three types. Type I consists of mucosal atresia with an intact bowel wall and mesentery. In type II the atretic ends are separated by a fibrous cord. In type III the atretic ends are separated by a V-shaped mesenteric gap (Fig. 31-19).[4,101,131] In the ascending and transverse colon, type III colonic atresias predominate. Types I and II are seen more commonly distal to the splenic flexure.[158,163] Type III lesions are the most commonly occurring lesions overall.

The rate of associated anomalies with colonic atresias is much smaller when compared with other atresias. Colonic atresias have been found in approximately 2.5% of neonates with gastroschisis.[147] There are fewer than 25 published cases of colonic atresia and Hirschsprung's disease.[147,162,164] Complex urologic abnormalities, multiple small intestinal atresias, an unfixed mesentery, and skeletal anomalies have also been reported to occur with colonic atresia.[158,163,165,166] Similar to small bowel atresias, a vascular insult to the fetal intestine continues to be the accepted cause for all types of colonic atresia.[167,168]

Prenatal diagnosis is of great importance in the management of colonic atresia. On prenatal ultrasonography, the colon has a relatively characteristic appearance. The presence of an obstruction can usually be determined when the diameter of the colon is larger than expected for gestational age.[169]

The characteristic clinical features of colonic atresia are abdominal distention, bilious emesis, and failure to pass meconium. On plain radiographs, air-fluid levels are usually appreciated as well as dilated intestinal loops of large bowel often associated with a "ground-glass" appearance of meconium mixed with air.[122] Occasionally, the dilation can be so massive that it mimics pneumoperitoneum (Fig. 31-20). The diagnosis is made with a contrast enema showing a small-diameter distal colon that comes to an abrupt halt at the level of the obstruction (Fig. 31-21).

The diagnosis of colonic atresia is an indication for urgent surgical management because the risk for perforation is higher than is seen in small intestinal atresias. The operative approach depends on the clinical status of the patient, the level of the atresia, any associated small intestinal atresias, and the patency of the bowel distal to the atresia. It is important to exclude other intestinal atresias and stenoses at the time of operation because they occur with some frequency.[49,61,62,170] A diagnosis of associated Hirschsprung's disease, although rare, must be made by frozen section analysis of rectal biopsy specimens during the initial surgery because unrecognized Hirschsprung's disease can lead to anastomotic leak or functional obstruction.

A staged surgical approach consisting of colostomy with mucous fistula is generally preferred. Because

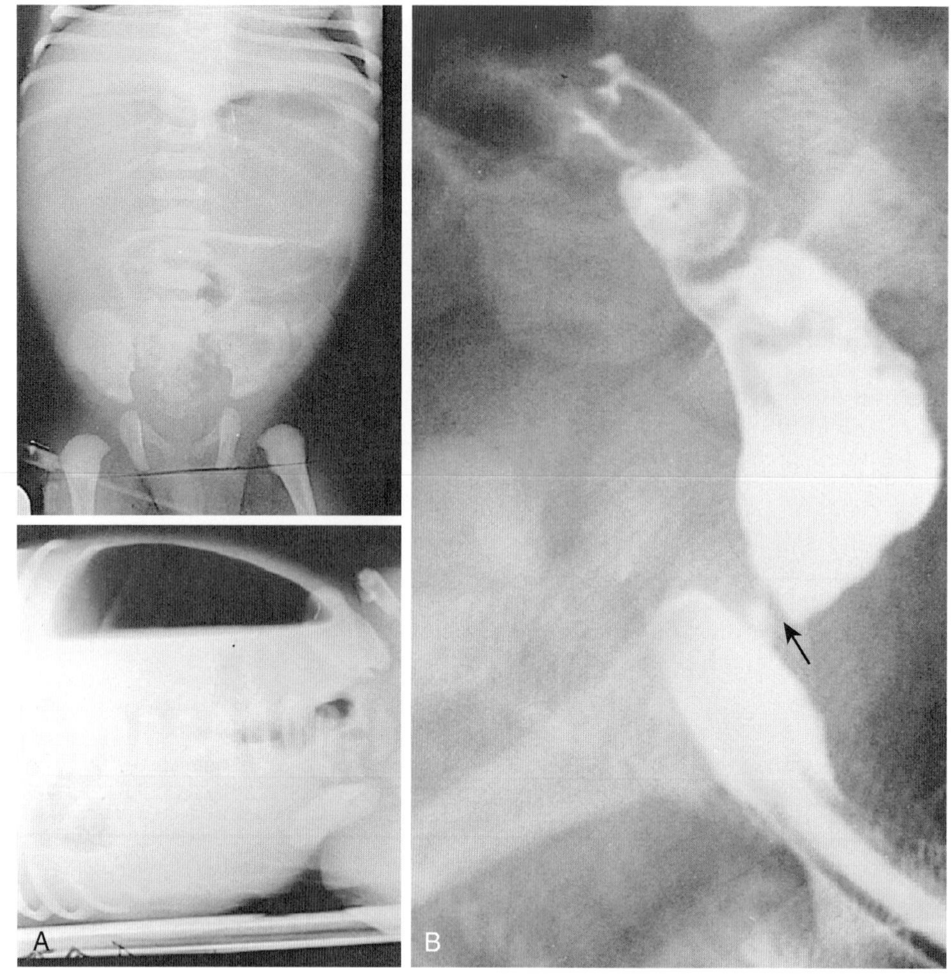

Figure 31-20. **A,** Abdominal radiograph of colonic atresia showing huge air-filled proximal colon mimicking a pneumoperitoneum. **B,** Right colonic atresia with rectal stenosis (*arrow*) is seen on this retrograde contrast study.

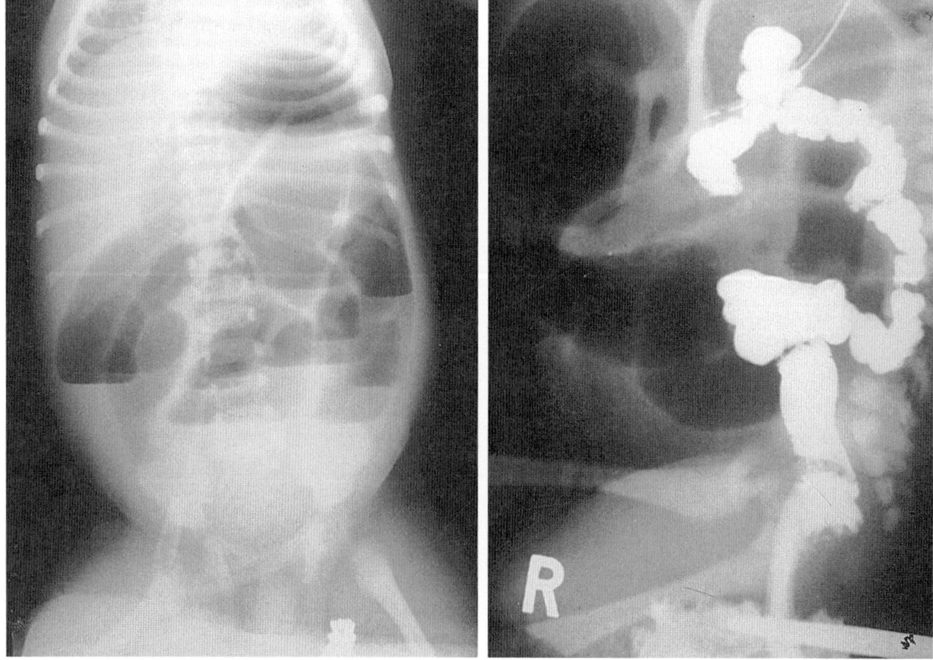

Figure 31-21. The contrast enema (*right*) in a patient with a distal intestinal obstruction (*left*) shows a small colon and failure of the contrast agent to move proximally past the mid-transverse colon.

the proximal and distal ends adjacent to the atresia are abnormal in both innervation and vascularity, resection of the bulbous proximal colon as well as a portion of the distal microcolon is suggested.[171-175] Primary resection with anastomosis has a higher incidence of complications, usually due to undiagnosed distal pathology.[160,175]

In the absence of other serious co-morbidities, the prognosis in colonic atresia is excellent. If diagnosed early, the overall mortality is less than 10%.[162] A delay in diagnosis beyond 72 hours, however, may result in a mortality of greater than 60%.[164,166] This high mortality is due, in part, to the formation of a closed loop obstruction between an intact ileocecal valve and the atresia, leading to massive colonic distention and perforation.

chapter 32

MALROTATION

Danny C. Little, MD • Samuel D. Smith, MD

Normal rotation of the human intestine requires transformation from a simple, straight alimentary tube into the mature fixed and folded configuration present at birth. Through precise embryologic events, the duodenojejunal junction becomes fixed in the left upper abdomen while the cecum is anchored in the right lower quadrant. The midgut, defined as the portion of the intestine supplied by the superior mesenteric artery, is thus suspended from a wide mesenteric base. In children with malrotation, the bowel is not fixed adequately and is thus held by a precariously narrow-based mesentery. Rotational anomalies create a spectrum of anatomic conditions with critical importance to the pediatric surgeon. Clinical disorders may arise when intestinal rotation either fails to occur or is incomplete. Rotational anomalies may be isolated or occur as an intrinsic component of gastroschisis, omphalocele, or congenital diaphragmatic hernia. Additionally, malrotation may present as an incidental, subtle finding discovered during the radiographic evaluation of another diagnosis or with septic shock from a catastrophic midgut volvulus.

The earliest descriptions of intestinal development were from Mall in 1898 and later expanded upon by Frazer and Robbins in 1915.[1,2] Eight years later, Dott translated these preliminary embryologic observations into problems encountered clinically.[3] In his 1932 landmark surgical paper, Ladd described the evaluation and surgical treatment of malrotation.[4] He described a relatively simple solution to a complicated problem. In his 1941 textbook entitled *Abdominal Surgery of Infancy and Childhood*, Ladd warned that unfamiliarity with this lesion would quickly lead to surgical confusion.[5] Over 200 postmortem studies had been reported previous to Ladd's paper, yet he was the first to emphasize the importance of placing the duodenum along the right abdominal wall, widening the mesenteric base, and moving the cecum to the left upper abdomen. With the exception of the laparoscopic approach, the original Ladd procedure has remained relatively unchanged.

EMBRYOLOGY

The development of the midgut begins with the differentiation of the primitive intestinal tract into the foregut, midgut, and hindgut at the fourth week of gestation.[6] The mature alimentary tract and all associated digestive organs are formed from this primitive tube. The most accepted model of midgut maturation involves four distinct stages: (1) herniation, (2) rotation, (3) retraction, and (4) fixation. Normal fixation of the duodenum and colon is illustrated in Figure 32-1. The intestinal loop can be divided into the cephalic (duodenojejunal) limb and the caudal (cecocolic) limb, which rotate separately but in parallel. The superior mesenteric artery serves as the fulcrum with the omphalomesenteric duct at the apex. Because of disproportional growth and elongation of the midgut during the fourth gestational week, the intestinal loop herniates into the extraembryonic coelom. Next, the bowel enters a critical period of rotation when the prearterial and postarterial limbs make three separate 90-degree turns, all in the counterclockwise direction around the superior mesenteric artery. The first 90-degree rotation occurs outside the abdomen. The second 90-degree rotation commences during the return of the intestine into the abdominal cavity during the 10th gestational week. The duodenojejunal junction now passes posterior to the superior mesenteric artery. The last rotation occurs in the abdomen. The primitive intestine has thus completed a 270-degree counterclockwise rotation, allowing the duodenojejunal limb to be positioned to the left of the superior mesenteric artery while the cecocolic limb is on the right. Fixation of the ascending and descending colon now occurs. Disruption of any of these vital steps leads to the spectrum of malrotation encountered clinically.

Alternatively, Kluth has proposed another model of intestinal rotation based on rat embryo studies.[6] In this model, the rapid growth and subsequent duodenal lengthening forces the tip of the duodenojejunal loop to grow under the mesenteric root. Simultaneously,

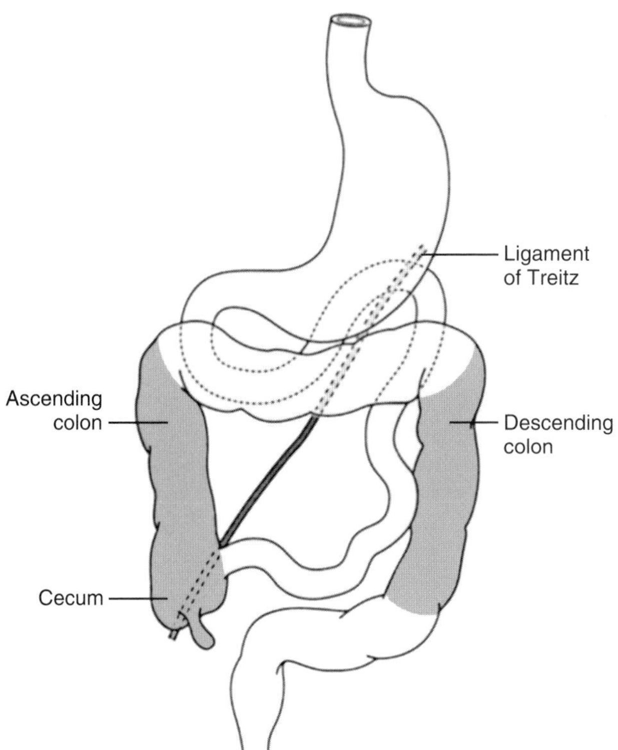

Figure 32-1. Normal intestinal anatomy results in fixation of the duodenojejunal junction in the left upper quadrant and the cecum in the right lower quadrant. This allows a wide breadth to the mesentery of the small bowel.

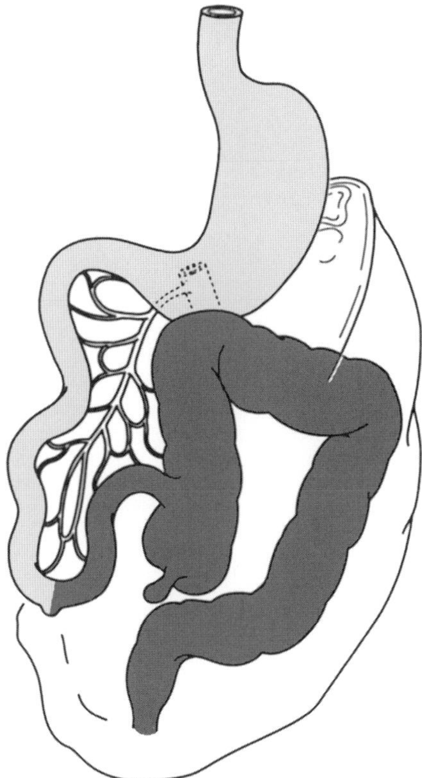

Figure 32-2. Illustration of nonrotation. The prearterial midgut (*lightly shaded*) is found on the right side of the abdomen, while the postarterial midgut (*darkly shaded*) remains on the left. Neither segment has undergone appropriate rotation. Volvulus is a risk.

the distal midgut is also growing, forcing the cecum from a caudal to cranial position. In this hypothesis, cecal and colonic positioning is a passive process with final location of the midgut being based on a process of differential growth rather than active rotation.

The most common forms of rotational disorders include nonrotation (Fig. 32-2), incomplete rotation (Fig. 32-3), and reversed rotation. Right and left mesocolic hernias can also occur. In nonrotation, there is failure of the normal intestinal 270-degree counterclockwise rotation around the superior mesenteric artery. Thus, the duodenojejunal limb lies in the right hemi-abdomen with the cecocolic limb in the left hemi-abdomen. Midgut volvulus due to a narrow mesenteric pedicle and extrinsic duodenal obstruction secondary to abnormally positioned cecal attachments are significant risks. In cases of incomplete rotation, normal rotation has been arrested at or near 180 degrees. The cecum will usually reside in the right upper abdomen. Obstructing peritoneal bands are present. With reversed rotation, an errant 90-degree clockwise rotation occurs, which leaves a tortuous transverse colon to the right of the superior mesenteric artery, passing through a retroduodenal tunnel dorsal to the artery and in the small bowel mesentery.[7,8] The duodenum will assume an anterior position. Reverse rotation with volvulus may occur with obstruction of the transverse colon. Paraduodenal hernias are rare and result from failure of the right or left mesocolon to fuse to the posterior body wall. A potential space is created. Subsequently, the small intestine may become sequestered and potentially obstructed. A significant delay in diagnosis is often encountered.

PRESENTATION

The incidence of malrotation has been estimated at 1 in 6000 live births. An increased incidence of 0.2% has been found in barium swallow studies,[9] whereas autopsy studies estimate that the true incidence may be as high as 1% of the total population.[10] Associated anomalies are common (Table 32-1).[11] Rotational disorders are also known to coexist with heterotaxia but rarely with situs inversus.[12] Intestinal malrotation occurs along a wide spectrum of anatomic variants and clinical presentations, including midgut volvulus and chronic duodenal obstruction. In-utero volvulus may lead to intestinal atresia.

Classic malrotation with midgut volvulus is often discovered in a previously healthy term neonate. Up to 75% of patients present during the first month of life. Another 15% will present within the first year.[13-15] Volvulus, intestinal gangrene, and mortality have been noted regardless of the patient's age or chronicity of symptoms.[16] Bilious vomiting remains the cardinal sign of neonatal intestinal obstruction, and malrotation must be the presumed diagnosis until

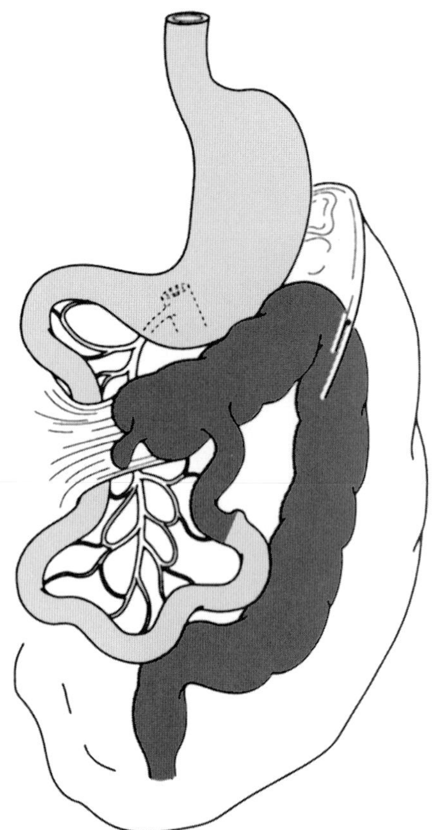

Figure 32-3. Illustration of incomplete rotation. Both the prearterial (*lightly shaded*) and postarterial (*darkly shaded*) segments have undergone partial, yet not complete, rotation. Ladd's bands are seen attaching the cecum to the right posterior abdominal wall. The duodenum becomes compressed and possibly obstructed. Volvulus is a risk.

proven otherwise. Delays in diagnosis can be devastating. Other signs in the neonate include abdominal pain and distention. The inconsolable infant may rapidly deteriorate as metabolic acidosis quickly advances to hypovolemic shock. Late signs include abdominal wall erythema and hematemesis or melena from progressive mucosal ischemia. Laboratory investigation may reveal leukocytosis or leukopenia, hyperkalemia, and thrombocytopenia. Mesenteric vascular compromise rapidly leads to peritonitis, sepsis, shock, and death.

Many other cases will present less dramatically. Failure to thrive, gastroesophageal reflux, early satiety,

Table 32-1	Incidence of Associated Anomalies (by percent) with Malrotation
Intestinal atresia	5-26%
Imperforate anus	0-9%
Cardiac anomalies	7-13%
Duodenal web	1-2%
Meckel's diverticulum	1-4%
Hernia	0-7%
Trisomy 21	3-10%

Rare: esophageal atresia, biliary atresia, mesenteric cyst, craniocynostosis, Hirschsprung's disease, intestinal duplication.

and mild abdominal discomfort are routinely reported. Partial volvulus leads to mesenteric venous and lymphatic obstruction and subsequently impairs nutrient absorption. The diagnosis becomes more challenging with the older child or teenager because the symptoms are often very vague and seemingly unrelated to the abdomen.[17]

The discordant incidence of malrotation between clinical cases and autopsy studies suggests that many patients are asymptomatic but "anatomically at risk" for midgut volvulus. Although most cases will present in the neonatal period or infancy, presentation in children or adults is not uncommon.[18] Anomalies of intestinal rotation may be discovered incidentally in the teenager or adult during investigation for upper abdominal complaints. Yet, it is important to remember that these patients possess a narrow small bowel mesentery and thus remain susceptible to midgut volvulus.

DIAGNOSIS

Radiologic studies play a critical role in establishing a diagnosis of intestinal malrotation. Initial evaluation will usually begin with a plain anteroposterior abdominal flat plate combined with a lateral decubitus or upright view (Fig. 32-4). Variable, nonspecific findings are common. However, gastric and/or duodenal distention ("double bubble" sign) may be observed. Additionally, bowel wall thickening and edema may be present secondary to vascular compromise. A gasless

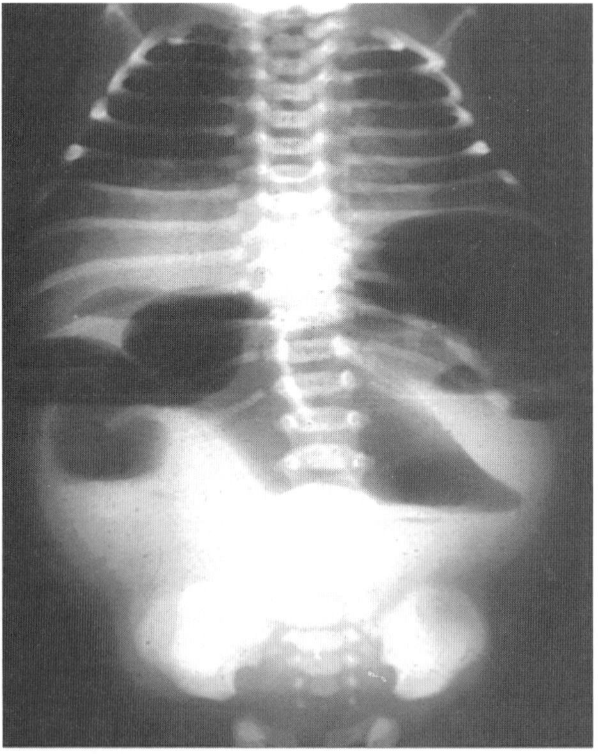

Figure 32-4. Upright abdominal film in an infant demonstrating proximal small bowel dilatation. This infant had a midgut volvulus.

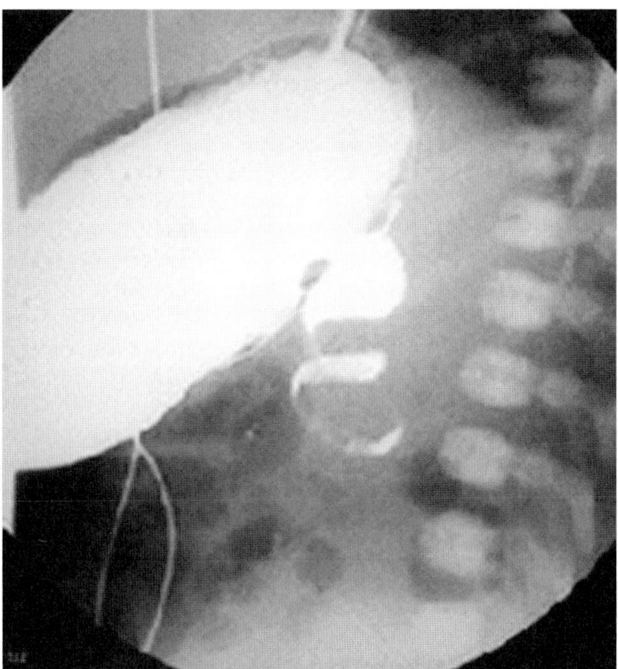

Figure 32-5. Lateral image on upper gastrointestinal series in an infant with malrotation and midgut volvulus showing the "corkscrew" appearance of the obstructed duodenum.

abdomen is particularly worrisome because the compromised bowel may be filled with fluid alone. Of particular importance is the presence of rectal gas in the newborn, which essentially excludes duodenal atresia (but not duodenal stenosis or web). If the diagnosis remains in doubt, an emergent upper gastrointestinal contrast study is needed to document the position of the ligament of Treitz. Delineation of the duodenojejunal junction remains the most important diagnostic tool with high sensitivity and is preferred over barium enema.[19] The duodenum should be seen traveling across the spine to the left. Additionally, the lateral film will show the duodenum obtaining a retroperitoneal, posterior position. Abnormal findings include positioning of the duodenojejunal flexure to the right of the spine, obstruction of the duodenum, and the "coil spring," "corkscrew," or "beak" appearance of the obstructed proximal jejunum (Figs. 32-5 and 32-6). In some settings, color Doppler ultrasound imaging is favored and may reveal a dilated duodenum with inversion of the superior mesenteric artery and vein (the whirlpool sign) in cases of acute volvulus.[20,21-23] Moreover, with ultrasonography, it is now possible to diagnose intestinal volvulus in utero.

The patient with suspected or confirmed midgut volvulus should be aggressively resuscitated, given intravenous broad-spectrum antibiotics, and taken to the operating room for immediate exploration. Delaying surgery for confirmatory testing should be discouraged when the diagnosis is likely based on clinical grounds. Prompt diagnosis and exploration is paramount to limit the complications and mortality of massive bowel resection. Clinicians should counsel the family preoperatively, but an intraoperative discussion is also advisable in certain cases.

MANAGEMENT

Management of children with radiographically proven symptomatic malrotation is relatively straightforward. A discussion of the open and laparoscopic techniques is presented later. Malrotation is an integral part of abdominal wall defects and congenital diaphragmatic hernia. Operative correction of these defects creates intra-abdominal adhesions. These patients are considered to be protected from volvulus. Therefore, Ladd's procedure is not generally required.

The dilemma arises when an abnormality is discovered on imaging, and the child is labeled as a "malrotation variant." To exclude malrotation, the duodenojejunal flexure must be located to the left of the spine at the level of the duodenal bulb. Defined as the ligament of Treitz, this flexure may be in an equivocal position. Symptoms are generally mild and could easily be attributed to several diagnoses. Volvulus or internal hernia is usually not seen with malrotation variants. These children are usually referred, leaving the surgeon with the dilemma to decide whether the symptoms are truly related to the radiographic findings. Given the higher rate of persistence of symptoms after operation and an overall increase in postoperative complications in general, close observation or repeated contrast study has been suggested in these equivocal cases.[24,25]

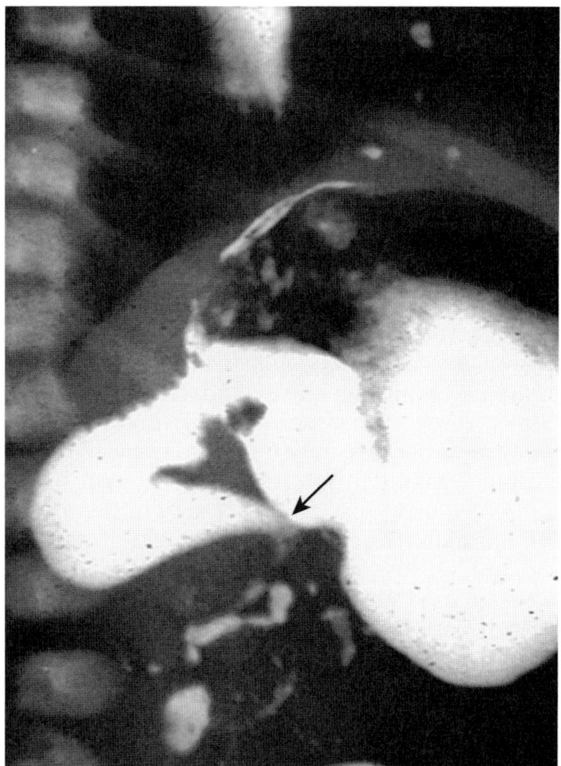

Figure 32-6. Lateral image on upper gastrointestinal series in infant with malrotation and midgut volvulus showing the "beak" (*arrow*) appearance of the obstructed duodenum. Note that a small amount of contrast agent has progressed through the volvulus.

Table 32-2	Six Key Elements in Operative Correction of Malrotation

1. Entry into abdominal cavity and evisceration (open)
2. Counterclockwise detorsion of the bowel (acute cases)
3. Division of Ladd's cecal bands
4. Broadening of the small intestine mesentery
5. Incidental appendectomy
6. Placement of small bowel along the right lateral gutter and colon along the left lateral gutter

Open Surgical Technique

There has been little change from Ladd's original description of the operative technique for correction of malrotation with or without acute volvulus. Preoperative discussion with the family is crucial. The six essential/critical steps are summarized in Table 32-2. Prolonged resuscitation efforts are not warranted. Preincision broad-spectrum antibiotics should be administered in cases of suspected volvulus. The surgeon's primary goal is to prevent the catastrophic loss of portions of the entire midgut. Entry into the abdomen through a right upper quadrant transverse approach is preferred, although a midline incision is also reasonable. In suspected cases of acute volvulus, time to detorsion is critical. Chylous ascites secondary to lymphatic obstruction and rupture of mesenteric lacteals is often encountered. When turbid fluid is seen, contamination should be suspected and peritoneal cultures taken. The bowel and mesentery should be eviscerated. One will commonly encounter two or three complete clockwise revolutions. The bowel will be often discolored and congested, although frankly gangrenous or perforated bowel is not uncommon. The bowel wall is fragile, and manipulation should be delicate. Care with counterclockwise detorsion is needed to prevent serosal or full-thickness injury (Fig. 32-7). The bowel may remain dusky. After detorsion, release of inflammatory mediators and lactic acid is common and may require aggressive fluid resuscitation and the temporary use of vascoactives. Once detorsion has been accomplished, warm soaked lap pads are placed on the bowel, and the surgeon should patiently observe for reperfusion. Twenty or 30 minutes of intraoperative rewarming may be required. If perfusion remains in question, the surgeon has several options, including (1) assessment of the antimesenteric vascular integrity with the use of a Doppler probe and (2) intravenous administration of fluorescein with Wood's lamp evaluation.

After a period of observation, a limited segment of intestine may remain gangrenous and resection should proceed. However, when longer segments are of questionable viability, the principles of intestinal salvage and preservation should be remembered. Resection of clearly necrotic bowel should be performed while leaving bowel of uncertain perfusion in the abdomen (clip and drop) to be re-evaluated at a second-look operation 24 to 48 hours later. At the second exploration, recovery of questionable bowel or demarcation of necrotic bowel requiring resection is usually obvious. Unfortunately, an occasional patient will have complete infarction of the midgut. Closure of the abdomen, without bowel resection and comfort care, may be considered after intraoperative family discussion. The development of intestinal and multiple-viscera transplantation makes this approach less clear.

Assuming bowel viability has been confirmed, the breadth of the mesentery must be widened. This is accomplished through a series of maneuvers, including excision of cecal peritoneal bands traversing the duodenum (Ladd's bands) and kocherization of the duodenum. The dissection then continues to the base of the superior mesenteric artery and vein by incising the anterior mesenteric leaflet. When properly opened, the mesentery is maximally broadened and the possibility of postoperative volvulus is reduced, although not completely eliminated.

Most surgeons will complete the procedure with an appendectomy. Owing to the subsequent malposition of the cecum in the left upper quadrant, failure to remove the appendix could lead to diagnostic uncertainty and delay if appendicitis developed. Standard or inversion appendectomy is equally acceptable. Finally, as the surgeon prepares for closure, the duodenum and small intestine are positioned toward the right abdomen with the colon in the left abdomen. A final check to rule out mesenteric torsion is advisable. Suture fixation of the bowel to the lateral abdominal wall is not recommended.[26,27]

In patients without evidence of volvulus or obstruction, a nasogastric tube is not required. Bowel function generally returns in 1 to 5 days. However, older patients with chronic obstruction are likely to have a prolonged ileus, and thus nasogastric drainage and parenteral support should be considered. Antibiotics are not required. Feedings can be advanced per the surgeon's discretion. Patients with extended or subtotal small bowel resection pose a special problem. Total parenteral nutrition is essential to sustain these patients until adaptation and compensatory growth of the residual bowel can occur.[28] Small bowel or multiple-viscera transplantation should be considered. Postoperative intussusception has been noted in 3.1% of all patients who underwent a Ladd procedure, compared with 0.05% following other laparotomies.[29] The incidence of recurrent volvulus is low. Finally, up to 10% of patients may develop an adhesive small bowel obstruction requiring laparotomy after the procedure.[26,27,30]

Laparoscopic Approach

The laparoscopic treatment for intestinal rotation anomalies in neonates, infants, and children with or without midgut volvulus has been proposed by several authors since van der Zee's original report in 1995.[31] The previously published reports have been single-institution case reports or small case series. Clinical outcomes for the laparoscopic technique have been favorable.

The patient is placed supine in the reversed Trendelenburg position, on a shortened operating room

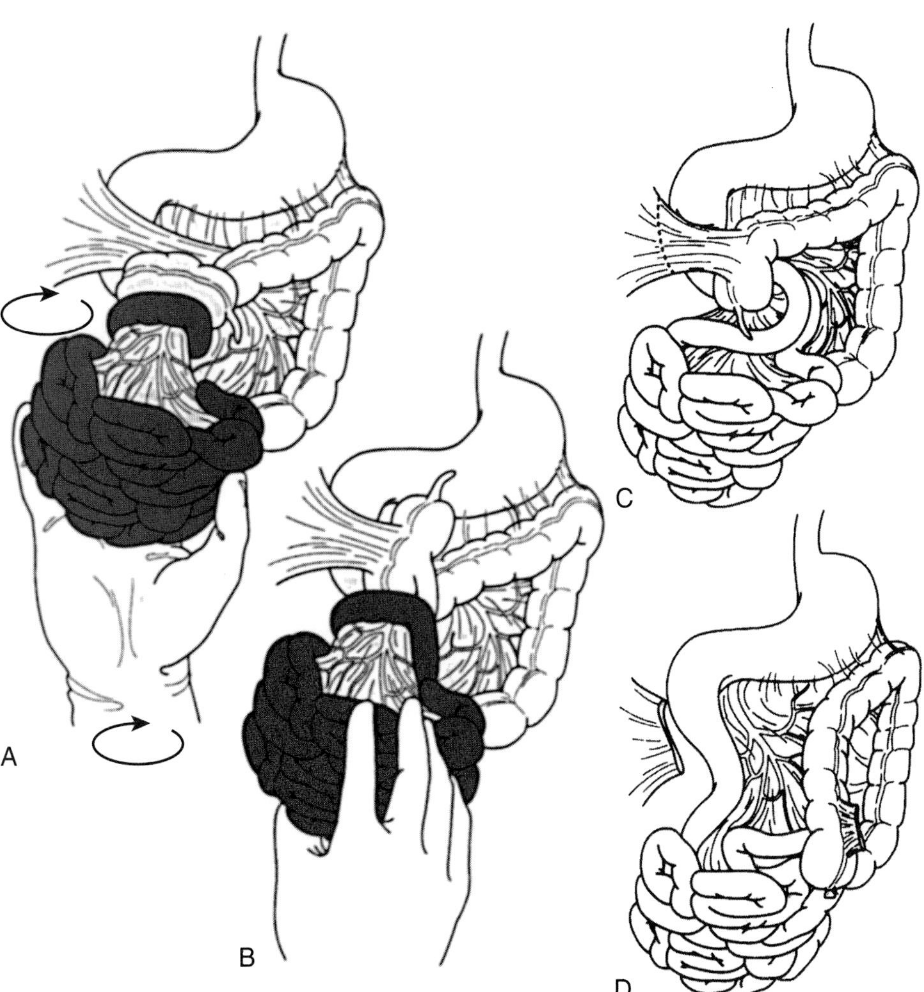

Figure 32-7. Open correction of malrotation. **A** and **B,** Initial appearance of the malrotated bowel during exploration. The surgeon first will perform counterclockwise detorsion of the midgut. **C,** Next, Ladd's bands from the cecum to the right abdominal wall are divided. **D,** Last is the critical step of broadening the small bowel mesentery. An appendectomy is also performed.

table, if available. The surgeon will stand at the child's feet with the assistant positioned to the surgeon's left. Alternatively, the surgeon may stand at the patient's right with the assistant and camera holder to the left. The stomach and bladder are decompressed. The child's arms are tucked. A four-port technique provides adequate visualization with cannulas placed at the umbilicus, right and left mid abdomen, and subxiphoid region (for the liver retractor, if required). Gentle insufflation with carbon dioxide to a pressure of 8 to 12 mm Hg with flow at 2 to 5 L/min is generally well tolerated.[31-33] Muscle relaxation will allow an optimal working space. Full abdominal exploration may reveal internal hernias, which are associated with malrotation. The surgeon's first goal is to determine if malrotation is actually present and thus confirm preoperative imaging (Figs. 32-8 and 32-9). Tilting the table 30 degrees may help identify the ligament of Treitz and the ileocecal junction. Findings are variable but may include a high and medial cecal position and an elongated, tortuous duodenum. Although there are no specific guidelines established to predict whether a future volvulus will occur, a mesenteric base extending more than half the diameter of the abdomen is generally sufficient to prevent volvulus.[34]

Owing to the necessity of rapid detorsion, the laparoscopic approach for acute volvulus is controversial. In these acute cases, a clockwise volvulus is easily recognized. The expeditious dissection may progress by identifying the second portion of the duodenum and excising restricting peritoneal bands. Next the surgeon may proceed with reduction of the volvulus (if present), mobilization of the duodenum and jejunum, and incision of the anterior mesenteric leaflet. The friable, ischemic bowel may be injured by the laparoscopic instruments. In older children with long-standing duodenal obstruction, the proximal bowel may be molded into a cocoon-like deformity (Fig. 32-10).[33] Lastly, the appendix is brought out through the umbilicus for an extracorporeal appendectomy (Fig. 32-11). Alternatively, an intracorporeal appendectomy may be performed through the 5-mm ports using bipolar cautery and endoloops, or the surgeon may proceed with a standard stapled intracorporeal appendectomy if a 12-mm umbilical cannula has been placed. The ports are removed under direct visualization, and the

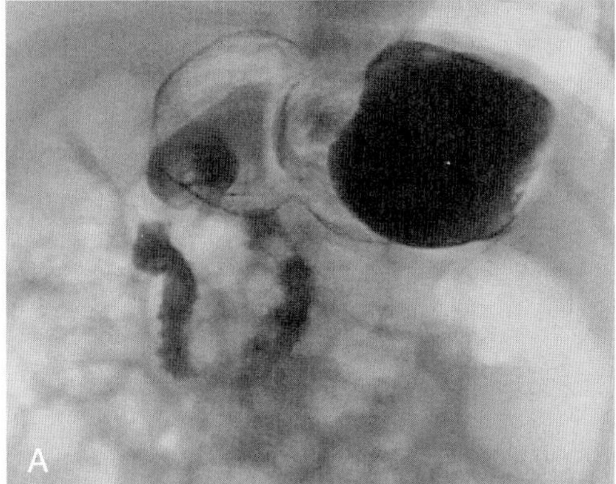

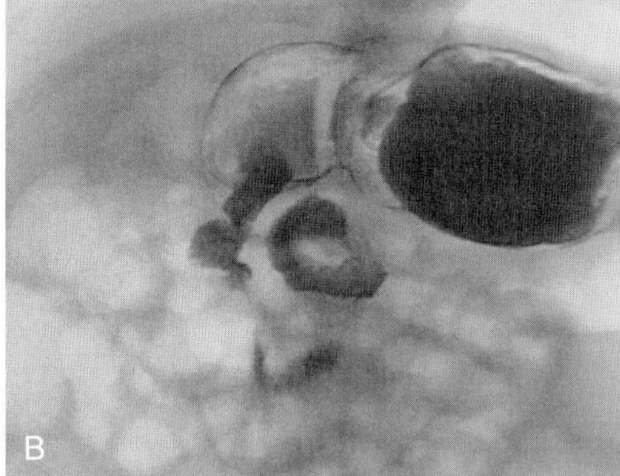

Figure 32-8. An upper gastrointestinal study was performed in this infant who presented with vomiting. **A** and **B,** The radiologic interpretation was that the duodenum was entirely on the patient's right side and the ligament of Treitz was at the level of pylorus. Also, the ligament of Treitz did not cross the midline. There was no evidence of obstruction. This patient underwent diagnostic laparoscopy and was found to have normal anatomy with correct positioning of the ligament of Treitz and the cecum (see Fig. 32-9).

incisions are closed in layers with absorbable suture. Postoperative management is similar to that for the open approach. Most children may begin clear liquids on the day of surgery. Discharge on day 1 or 2 is expected.[33]

Although each procedure will present its own challenges, several recommendations may expedite the procedure, decrease the conversion rate, and reduce surgeon frustration. For elective cases, decreasing stool burden with a gentle bowel preparation will improve visualization. Furthermore, it is important to position the working sites as far away as possible from the congenital bands, which increases the intra-abdominal working space. Direct handling of the bowel increases the risk of serosal tears so gentle manipulation is important. The majority of the dissection may be accomplished by grasping the congenital bands or appendix.

Since van der Zee's initial report, other authors have described variations in technique and have published their positive results.[35-38] Successful laparoscopic management of a 15-day-old with acute midgut volvulus has been described.[39] The authors carefully reduced the acute volvulus, divided the Ladd's bands, incised the anterior mesentery, and performed an appendectomy. However, the majority of patients undergoing laparoscopic repair of intestinal malrotation have been elective cases without volvulus.[36,37,40] Operative times have been reported to average 111 to 120 minutes.[36,40] In one report, the time to a regular diet was 2 days (median) and resolution of symptoms was found in 5 of 7 patients at 15 months.[36]

In another series, 12 neonates and infants, weighing 3 to 7 kg, underwent a three-port laparoscopic Ladd's procedure.[35] Presentation included intermittent upper intestinal obstruction, and the diagnosis was eventually confirmed by contrast study. Three 3.5-mm ports were placed in the infraumbilical ring and in the right and left abdomen. Operative time was equivalent to published open results, ranging from 35 to 120 minutes (mean, 58 minutes). Feedings were started on postoperative day 1 or 2, and the patients were discharged at a mean of 2 days. All symptoms had resolved on postoperative evaluation.

In a review of 21 adults undergoing both an open and laparoscopic Ladd procedure, comparative results were favorable for the laparoscopic group for resumption of oral intake (1.8 days vs. 2.7 days), shorter

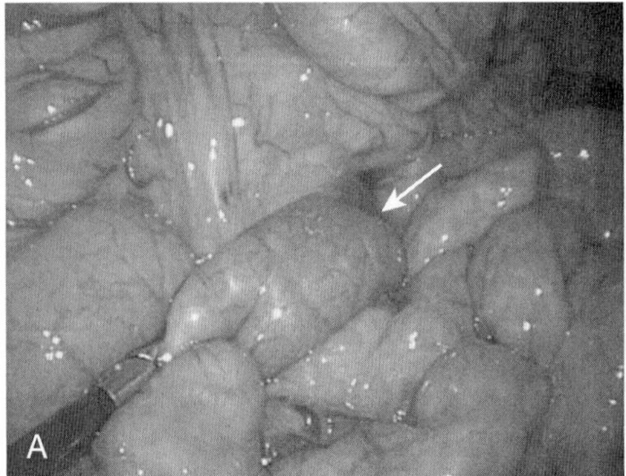

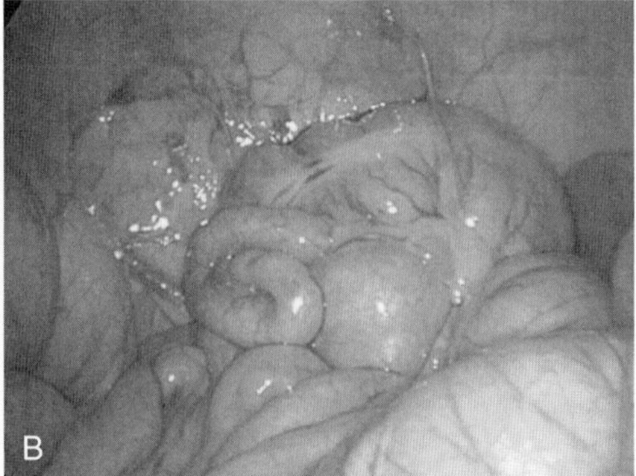

Figure 32-9. At times, the upper gastrointestinal study can be equivocal for possible malrotation (see Fig. 32-8). In such patients, diagnostic laparoscopy is a useful technique to ascertain whether the patient actually has malrotation. **A,** In such patients, the position of the ligament of Treitz (*arrow*) to the patient's left of midline is important. **B,** In addition, the location of the cecum in the right lower quadrant also helps verify that the patient does not have malrotation.

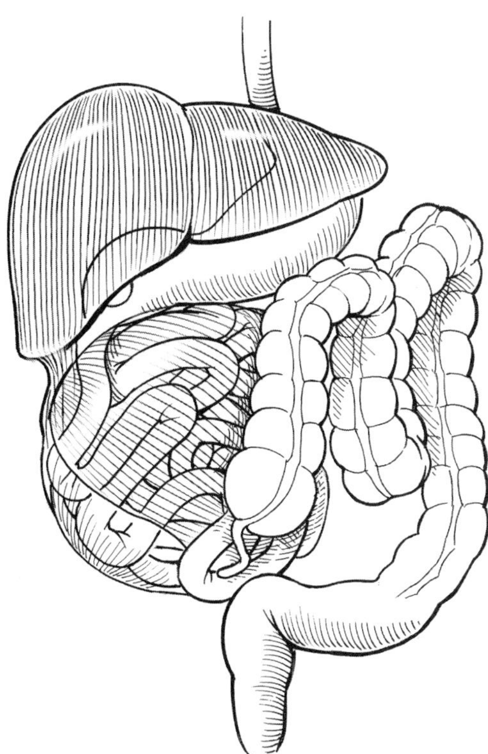

Figure 32-10. In older children with long-standing partial obstruction or internal herniation, the Ladd bands may cause the bowel to form into a cocoon-like deformity. (From Moir CR: Laparoscopic Ladd procedure. In Holcomb GW III, Georgeson KE, Rothenberg SS [eds]: Atlas of Pediatric Laparoscopy and Thoracoscopy. Philadelphia, Elsevier, 2008, pp 55-60.)

hospitalization (4 days vs. 6.1 days), and decreased requirements for intravenous narcotics on postoperative day 1 (4.9 mg vs. 48.5 mg).[41] Operative times, however, averaged 51 minutes longer for the laparoscopic patients (194 minutes vs. 143 minutes). Conversion to an open operation occurred in 25% of the patients undergoing a laparoscopic procedure. No patients required a second operation.

One additional value of laparoscopy is found in cases of malrotation variants when the ligament of Treitz is in an equivocal position on preoperative imaging (see Fig. 32-8). Radiographic terms such as "wandering duodenum," "low ligament of Treitz," and "abnormal rotation" are frequently encountered in the radiologist's vernacular. Such "soft" radiologic findings place the responsibility of excluding malrotation directly on the surgeon. In equivocal cases, laparoscopy may be used to determine the position and fixation of the cecum and the overall breadth of the mesenteric pedicle (see Fig. 32-9). Additionally, when performing open exploration based on these preoperative descriptives, a surgeon may find relatively normal rotation that is not suggestive of malrotation or prone to volvulus. The laparoscopic approach allows excellent visualization of the width and fixation of the mesentery and the presence of Ladd's bands. Questionable cases are thus stratified regarding whether operative correction is required.[42] If the mesentery is noted to be narrow, the patient will be prone to volvulus and requires operative correction. The procedure may continue with laparoscopic correction, or the surgeon may wish to convert to an open procedure at this point.

The formation of intra-abdominal adhesions has generally been viewed as necessary to prevent postoperative volvulus. Through open exploration and direct manipulation of the bowel, adhesions are created. Concerns have been raised that adhesion formation may be limited with laparoscopy, as is seen in other laparoscopic procedures. Initial reports have not validated these concerns.

Laparoscopic correction of malrotation is an accepted procedure but still remains a technical challenge. In patients with acute volvulus, the working space will be limited owing to bowel edema and chylous ascites. Although many cases can be accomplished with these minimally invasive techniques, conversion to an open procedure should be considered if significant progress has not been made after 60 minutes. As a collection, the available literature supports consideration of laparoscopy. Further prospective studies with large sample sizes, possible randomization, and long-term follow-up should be conducted to confirm the advantages and disadvantages of the laparoscopic approach.

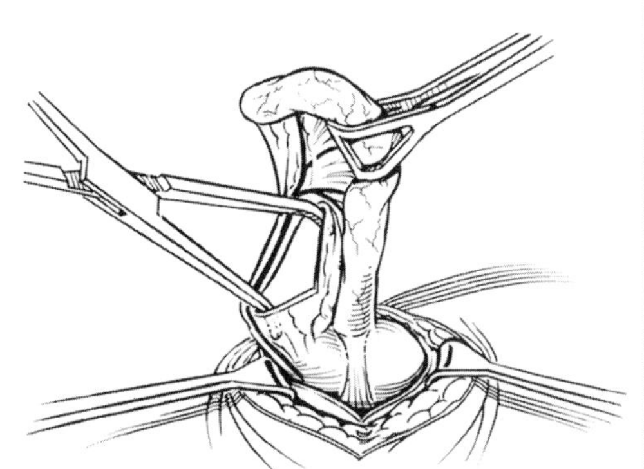

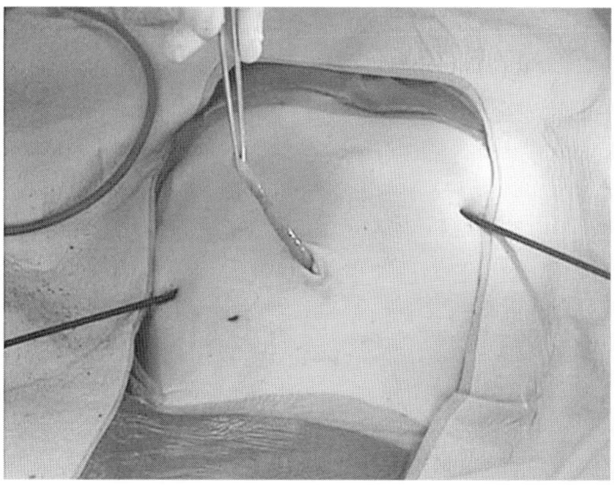

Figure 32-11. When performing a laparoscopic Ladd procedure, an extracorporeal appendectomy eliminates the need for a large port for the endoscopic stapler. The appendix is grasped with one of the intracorporeal instruments and brought into view through the umbilicofascial defect, where it is grasped and exteriorized. (From Moir CR: Laparoscopic Ladd procedure. In Holcomb GW III, Georgeson KE, Rothenberg SS [eds]: Atlas of Pediatric Laparoscopy and Thoracoscopy. Philadelphia, Elsevier, 2008, pp 55-60.)

THE OLDER PATIENT

Malrotation is occasionally diagnosed in the teenager or adult, yet the symptoms are often vague, including vomiting, diarrhea, early satiety, bloating, dyspepsia, and ulcer disease.[43-46] After a lengthy period of medical evaluation, some of these patients are labeled with functional or psychiatric disorders.[10,44,45] The diagnosis may require multiple imaging modalities, including barium studies, computed tomography, magnetic resonance imaging, and angiography. Furthermore, preoperative imaging may also delineate vascular and/or hepatobiliary anatomic irregularities that are associated with rotational disorders.[47] In the acute symptomatic patient, only emergent laparotomy can provide the correct diagnosis in a timely fashion. Given that adult surgeons may have little experience with this disorder, it is common for pediatric surgeons to be asked for intraoperative consultations.

Outcomes in patients younger than 16 years old have been compared with those of patients older than 16.[48] When compared with younger patients, the older patients experienced longer delays in diagnosis, endured a higher percentage of postoperative complications, and required a higher percentage of reoperation. No patients in the adult group were diagnosed correctly at the time of initial presentation.

The question arises whether an incidental discovery of malrotation in the older child or adult should be repaired at all. A candid discussion on the risk-benefit ratio with these older patients is important. The principle of "watchful waiting" has been suggested.[49] Currently, there are no diagnostic modalities that can assess an individual's future risk for midgut volvulus. Up to 20% of adult patients undergoing operative repair of malrotation will have an acute volvulus or bowel ischemia, both potentially life-threatening presentations.[50] Furthermore, even in patients who are believed to be asymptomatic, preoperative symptoms attributable to malrotation have retrospectively been noted, and postoperative improvement has been seen.[37,48,51]

As noted by Ladd in 1932, malrotation is a "condition rare enough that it is likely to escape the mind, and it is common enough to be important."[4] This advice is especially true in older patients. The subtle presentation may lead to unnecessary or ineffective treatment. A high index of suspicion is required to prevent a delay in diagnosis, counsel patients effectively, and improve outcomes. Operative correction in the symptomatic and asymptomatic older patient is currently recommended.[45,48,52,53]

chapter 33

MECONIUM DISEASE

Michael G. Caty, MD • Mauricio A. Escobar, MD

Intestinal obstruction in the neonate is one of the most common diagnoses requiring admission to the neonatal intensive care unit, accounting for as many as one third of all admissions.[1] Failure to pass meconium within the first 24 to 48 hours of life, feeding intolerance, abdominal distention, and bilious emesis are hallmarks of intestinal obstruction in the newborn period and evoke a differential diagnosis of obstruction based on anatomic, metabolic, and functional considerations. Strictly speaking, the term *meconium disease* refers to meconium ileus and meconium plug syndrome. These conditions are considered here separately from functional or anatomic causes of neonatal intestinal obstruction such as Hirschsprung's disease, intestinal atresia, and anorectal malformations.

MECONIUM ILEUS

Meconium ileus is one of the most common causes of intestinal obstruction in the newborn, accounting for 9% to 33% of neonatal intestinal obstructions.[2] It is characterized by extremely viscid, protein-rich, inspissated meconium causing an intraluminal obturator-type obstruction of the distal ileum. It is the earliest clinical manifestation of cystic fibrosis (CF), occurring in approximately 16% of patients with that disease.[3] Although meconium ileus may occur with rare conditions such as pancreatic aplasia and total colonic aganglionosis, it is considered pathognomonic for CF[4,5] and may be an early indication of a more severe phenotype of CF. This has been suggested due to significantly lower pulmonary function found in children with a history of meconium ileus compared with age- and sex-matched children with CF who did not have meconium ileus.[6]

Due to abnormalities of exocrine mucus secretion and pancreatic enzyme deficiency, the meconium in meconium ileus differs from normal meconium in that it has less water content (meconium ileus, 65%; normal, 75%), lower sucrase and lactase levels, increased albumin, and decreased pancreatic enzymes.[7-9] Additionally, concentrations of sodium, potassium, magnesium, and heavy metals in meconium are reduced in CF patients. Concentrations of protein nitrogen are increased and composed of abnormal mucoproteins, and concentrations of carbohydrate are reduced.[10-12] Thus, more viscous intestinal mucus in the absence of degrading enzymes results in thick, dehydrated meconium that obstructs the intestine.[13] An understanding of CF guides the clinical management of patients with meconium ileus.

Cystic Fibrosis

The association of inspissated meconium in a newborn with pathologic changes of the pancreas was first described in 1905.[14] In 1936, the term *cystic fibrosis* was first used to describe the combination of pancreatic insufficiency and chronic pulmonary disease in childhood.[15] Two years later, the coexistence of meconium ileus and CF was described and the histologic lesions in the pancreas were noted to be identical in both conditions.[16] Inspissation of meconium, caused by abnormal intestinal mucus, was first suggested in 1946.[17] Chemical analysis of inspissated meconium from infants with meconium ileus was carried out as early as 1952.[18] In 1953, the abnormally viscid nature of meconium in meconium ileus was attributed to abnormal mucus secreted by the intestine of patients with CF.[19]

Incidence

CF is the most common potentially lethal genetic defect affecting whites, with approximately 1200 infants with CF born each year. Approximately 30,000 children and young adults live with CF in the United States.[4] It is an inherited autosomal recessive disease with a 4% to 5% carrier rate and occurs in 1:3000 to 1:2000 live births yearly. The incidences of CF in non-white populations are 1 in 15,000 African-American births (much lower in native Africans), 1 in 31,000 in Asian-American births, 1 in 10,500 Native American Aleut (Eskimo) births, and 1:13,500 in Hispanic-white births.

Genetics

In 1989, the CF locus was localized through linkage analysis to human chromosome 7q31.[20,21] Mutations in the cystic fibrosis transmembrane (conductance) regulator gene (*CFTR*) result in CF.[22,23] The cell membrane protein coded by *CFTR* is a 3′,5′-cyclic adenosine monophosphate (cAMP)-induced chloride channel, which also regulates the flow of other ions across the apical surface of epithelial cells. The alteration in *CFTR* results in an abnormal electrolyte content in the environment external to the apical surface of epithelial membranes. This leads to desiccation and reduced clearance of secretions from tubular structures lined by affected epithelia.

The most common mutation of the *CFTR* gene, the ΔF508 mutation, is a 3–base pair deletion that results in the removal of a phenylalanine residue at amino acid position 508 of the *CFTR*. Over 1000 *CFTR* mutations have been reported to the CF Genetic Consortium. The ΔF508 mutation is responsible for approximately 70% of abnormal CF genes.[20,21,23] Genetically, families with meconium ileus have a significantly higher occurrence rate than the expected 25% for an autosomal recessive genetic disorder.[15,24] In one series, for the few CF patients for whom genetic analysis was available, 79% with the ΔF508 mutation presented with abdominal complaints including meconium ileus rather than pulmonary complaints.[4] However, there is no evidence of distinct allelic frequencies or haplotypic variants in CF patients with meconium ileus compared with those without[25] or in those CF patients with significant liver disease.[26,27]

Gastrointestinal Pathophysiology

Cystic fibrosis is characterized by mucoviscidosis of exocrine secretions throughout the body resulting from abnormal transport of chloride ions across the apical membranes of epithelial cells.[28-30] The clinical result is chronic obstruction and infection of the respiratory tract, insufficiency of the exocrine pancreas, and elevated sweat chloride levels.[31] Other variants can have minimal other manifestations, such as patients with chronic sinusitis or men with congenital bilateral absence of the vas deferens (CBAVD) (Fig. 33-1).[32-34] In patients with CBAVD, the *CFTR* genotype usually includes at least one mild mutation not typical of CF patients. The mild-mutation allele is frequently associated with a severe mutation on the other allele, such as the ΔF508 mutation.[6,35] CBAVD has been described in a patient with ΔF508 and G551D mutations,[36] both of which are categorized as severe. The allele G551D is the third most common CF-associated mutation.[7,37]

Development of both the pancreas and intestinal tract in fetuses with CF is abnormal. In patients with CF, abnormal pancreatic secretions obstruct the ductal system leading to autodigestion of the acinar cells, fatty replacement of pancreatic parenchyma, and fibrosis. Although the process begins in utero, it occurs variably over time. Pancreatic insufficiency is prevalent in young infants with CF and has a significant impact on growth and nutrition.[26]

Investigations have also suggested that pancreatic insufficiency plays a central role in the pathogenesis of meconium ileus. Congenital stenosis of the pancreatic ducts is associated with meconium-induced bowel obstruction. This is further supported by the fact that two thirds of infants found to have CF by neonatal screening are pancreatic insufficient at birth. However, approximately 10% of patients with CF are pancreatic sufficient and will tend to have a milder course. Pancreatic lesions are also variable at birth and are more severe in children with CF older than 1 year of age. This suggests that pancreatic insufficiency is not the leading cause of abnormal meconium in meconium ileus. In fact, histologic data have shown that a prevalence of intestinal glandular abnormalities contributed more significantly to the production of the abnormal meconium. In CF, intestinal disease is characterized by a glandular abnormality in which hyperviscous mucus is produced. The lack of concordance between meconium ileus and the severity of pancreatic disease and preponderance of intestinal glandular lesions implies that intraluminal intestinal factors contribute more to the development of meconium ileus than absence of pancreatic secretions.[17-19,38-42]

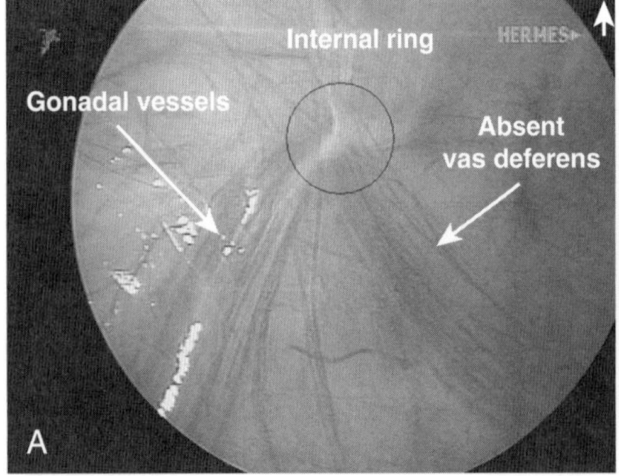

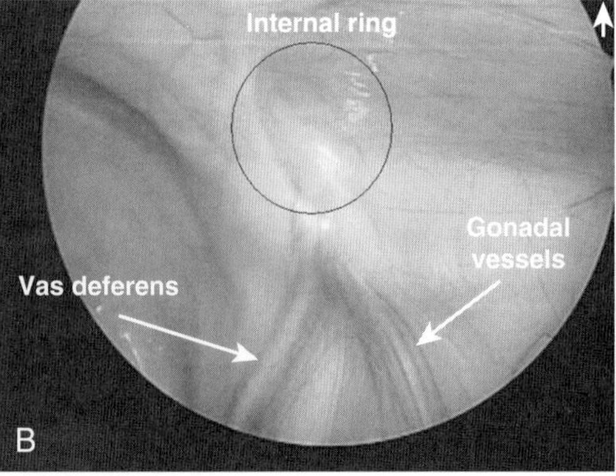

Figure 33-1. Congenital bilateral absence of the vas deferens (CBAVD). **A,** Laparoscopic view of a patient's left internal ring. **B,** Compare with a laparoscopic view of a similar-aged patient's right internal ring with a normal vas deferens. (From Escobar MA, Lau ST, Glick PL: Congenital bilateral absence of the vas deferens. J Pediatr Surg 43:1222-1223, 2008.)

Abnormal intestinal motility may also contribute to the development of meconium ileus. Some patients with CF have prolonged small intestinal transit times.[43,44] Non-CF diseases associated with abnormal gut motility, such as Hirschsprung's disease and chronic intestinal pseudo-obstruction, have been associated with meconium ileus-like disease, signifying that decreased peristalsis may allow for increased reabsorption of water and the development of abnormal meconium.[45-47] Moreover, the *CFTR* ion channel defect results in an exocrine secretion abnormally rich in sodium and chloride, leading to further dehydration of intraluminal contents and their impaired clearance.[9]

Prenatal Diagnosis and Screening

The antenatal diagnosis of meconium ileus can be made in two different groups, a high-risk group and a low-risk group. In the low-risk group the diagnosis is suspected when the sonographic appearances of meconium ileus are found on routine prenatal ultrasonography when there is no previous family history of CF. All pregnancies subsequent to the birth of a CF-affected child are considered high risk, and parents of a child with CF are considered to be obligate carriers of a CF mutation.

Pediatric surgeons are often asked to provide prenatal consultations to parents of fetuses suspected of bowel obstruction. Meconium ileus must be considered in the differential diagnosis, particularly in the high-risk fetus. An algorithm has been established that may be useful in counseling and management of the fetus suspected of having meconium ileus (Fig. 33-2).[48-50] The obvious advantage of establishing a prenatal diagnosis is that it allows clinicians to prepare for the medical and psychological needs of the parents, fetus, and newborn before, during, and after delivery. In a pregnancy in which CF is suspected, sonographic examinations should be performed on a monthly basis until delivery. This evaluation allows the early detection of potential complications as they occur and prepares the physicians for special or urgent medical or surgical needs upon delivery.

Ultrasound Evaluation

Sonographic characteristics associated with meconium ileus include a hyperechoic, intra-abdominal mass (inspissated meconium) (Fig. 33-3), dilated bowel, and nonvisualization of the gallbladder. Normal fetal meconium, when visualized in the second and third trimesters, is usually hypoechoic or isoechoic to adjacent abdominal structures.[51-56] The sensitivity of intra-abdominal echogenic masses in the detection of meconium ileus is reported to be between 30% and 70%. As a sonographic marker of meconium ileus, this finding is plagued by difficulties, including the subjective assessment of echogenicity and the lengthy associated differential diagnosis. In addition to meconium ileus,[51-54,57,58] hyperechoic bowel has been reported with Down syndrome,[59,60] intrauterine growth retardation,[51,53,54,59-61] prematurity,[62] in-utero cytomegalovirus infection,[63] intestinal atresia, abruptio placentae, and fetal demise.[61] The importance of hyperechoic fetal bowel is related to gestational age at detection, ascites, calcification, volume of amniotic fluid, and the presence of other fetal anomalies.[56] Furthermore, the prenatal diagnosis of meconium ileus using the sonographic feature of hyperechoic bowel must take into account the a priori risk of the parents. The positive predictive value of hyperechoic masses in a high-risk fetus is estimated to be 52%, whereas it is only 6.4% in the low-risk fetus.[51]

Reviews of pregnancies with a 1 in 4 risk of CF show a 25% to 60% association between hyperechoic

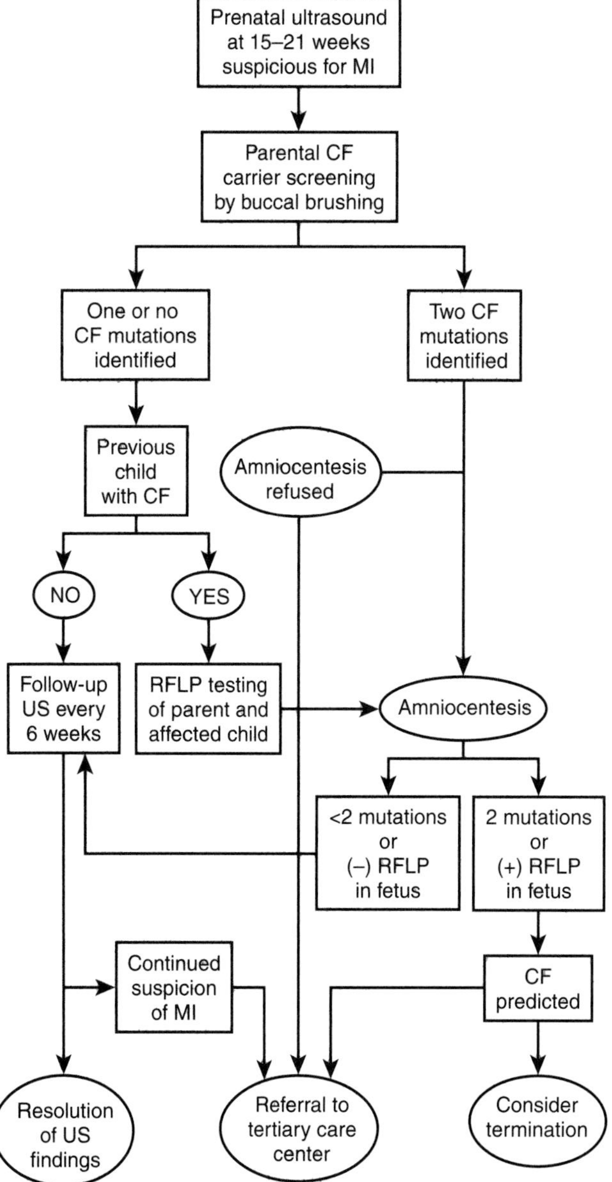

Figure 33-2. Suggested algorithm for antenatal management of suspected meconium ileus (MI) and cystic fibrosis (CF). US, ultrasonography; RFLP, restriction fragment length polymorphism. (From Irish MS, Ragi JM, Karamanoukian H, et al: Prenatal diagnosis of the fetus with cystic fibrosis and meconium ileus. Pediatr Surg Int 12:434-436, 1997.)

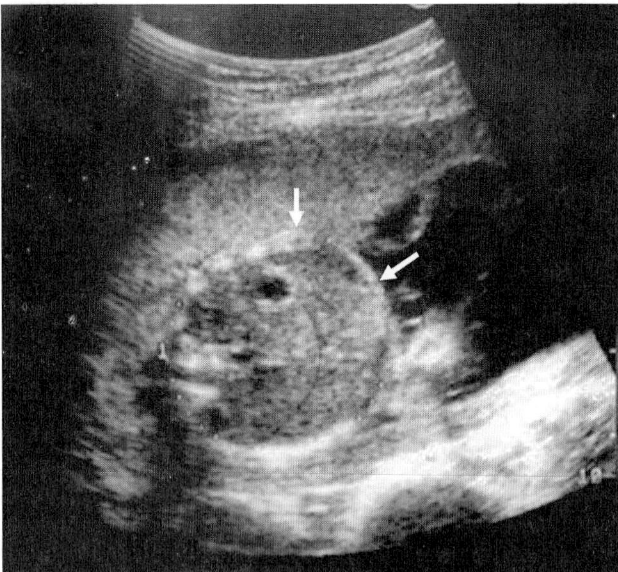

Figure 33-3. Ultrasound image of a 22-week gestation demonstrating a 2 × 3-cm intraluminal (distal ileum) mass (*arrows*) consistent with meconium inspissation (meconium ileus). (From Irish MS, Ragi JM, Karamanoukian H, et al: Prenatal diagnosis of the fetus with cystic fibrosis and meconium ileus. Pediatr Surg Int 12:434-436, 1997.)

bowel and CF.[58,62] However, this association is less prevalent in the general population. In a review of 12,776 fetal ultrasound examinations performed after 14 weeks' gestation, hyperechoic bowel was noted in only 30 fetuses (0.2%)[51] and CF was found in 13.3%. Whereas an echogenic bowel wall noted in the third trimester is often thought to be diagnostic, it is crucial to note that hyperechoic bowel has been found to be a normal variant in both the second and third trimesters.[55,56,64]

The finding of dilated bowel on prenatal ultrasonography, in association with CF, has been reported less frequently than that of hyperechoic bowel. In meconium ileus, bowel dilation is caused by obstruction from meconium but mimics findings in midgut volvulus, congenital bands, intestinal atresia, intestinal duplication, internal hernia, meconium plug syndrome, and Hirschsprung's disease.[65] The correlation of dilated fetal bowel and meconium ileus suggests that dilated fetal bowel warrants parental testing for CF and continued sonographic surveillance of the fetus.

Inability to visualize the gallbladder on fetal ultrasonography has also been associated with CF.[66] Combined with other sonographic features, nonvisualization of the gallbladder can be useful in the prenatal detection of the disease. However, caution should be exercised in the interpretation of an absent gallbladder because the differential diagnosis also includes biliary atresia, omphalocele, and diaphragmatic hernia.

Sonographic characteristics of fetal bowel obstruction are neither sensitive nor specific for meconium ileus, but the interpretation of these findings must include consideration of the risk of the fetus having CF. Certainly findings suggesting meconium ileus in the high-risk fetus indicate a high probability of CF.[66] In the low-risk fetus, suspicious ultrasound findings warrant consideration of prenatal screening by DNA testing or, at the very least, serial follow-up examinations.

The utility of prenatal screening for CF in fetuses with intestinal obstruction was recently examined by prospectively reviewing patients with meconium ileus, meconium plug syndrome, meconium peritonitis, jejunoileal atresia, and volvulus. Prenatal sonographic signs were correlated with postnatal findings of CF and the type of bowel obstruction. Immunoreactive trypsin measurement, genetic studies, and sweat tests were performed to evaluate for CF. Of the 80 patients reviewed, 30 (37.5%) had a prenatal diagnosis of an intestinal anomaly. The overall incidence of CF with a prenatal diagnosis of an intestinal anomaly was 13%, or 333 times the estimated risk of CF in the general population. A hyperechoic pattern with dilated bowel was associated with higher specificity for CF (100%), followed by hyperechoic bowel with ascites (75%). These authors suggest that prenatal screening for CF is indicated in all pregnancies with ultrasound patterns of specific intestinal disorders, and all neonates with any type of neonatal intestinal obstruction should be screened for CF.[67] Neonatal screening has also been noted to lead to better preservation of lung function in the long term, prevents severe malnutrition, and improves long-term growth in CF patients.[68]

Clinical Presentation

Meconium ileus is categorized as either simple or complicated. Thickened meconium begins to form in utero. As it obstructs the mid-ileum, proximal small bowel dilatation and bowel wall thickening occur. Approximately one half of these neonates present with a simple uncomplicated obstruction.[4] The remaining patients present with complications of meconium ileus, including volvulus, gangrene, atresia, and perforation, which may result in meconium peritonitis and giant cystic meconium peritonitis.[18,40,69-76]

Simple Meconium Ileus

In simple meconium ileus, the terminal ileum is filled with firm concretions, is small in diameter, and molds around the inspissated lumps of meconium. Proximally, the ileum becomes dilated and filled with thick sticky meconium with gas and fluid found within the small bowel proximal to this area.[4] Newborns with uncomplicated meconium ileus can appear healthy immediately after birth. However, within 1 to 2 days, they develop abdominal distention and bilious vomiting. Normal meconium will not be passed. Dilated loops of bowel become visible on examination and have a "doughy" character that indents on palpation.[77] The rectum and anus are often narrow, a finding that may be misinterpreted as anal stenosis.[78] The presentation of the patient with meconium ileus is similar to that of many types of neonatal small bowel obstructions. Therefore, the clinician should simultaneously consider and evaluate for malrotation, small intestinal atresia, colonic atresia, and meconium plug syndrome.

The history, physical examination, and contrast enema help make the distinction between these conditions.

Complicated Meconium Ileus

Complicated meconium ileus may present dramatically and immediately after birth. In others, symptoms will develop within 24 hours of birth. Signs of peritonitis (abdominal distention, tenderness, abdominal wall erythema), as well as clinical evidence of sepsis, may be present on the initial neonatal examination as a result of in-utero perforation or bowel compromise. Abdominal distention can be so severe as to cause immediate respiratory distress. A palpable mass suggests pseudocyst formation, which results from in-utero bowel perforation.[77,78] Often the neonate is in extremis and needs urgent resuscitation and surgical exploration.

Historically, segmental volvulus was reported to be the most common complication of meconium ileus.[71,72] Prenatal volvulus of the meconium-distended segment of ileum may lead to occlusion of the mesenteric blood flow and subsequent ischemic necrosis, intestinal atresia with an associated mesenteric defect, or perforation. When prenatal perforation occurs, most of the sterile meconium is reabsorbed, with trace amounts becoming calcified. Atretic segments are common in meconium ileus, and the affected bowel may appear viable with no evidence of perforation or gangrene. Twelve to 17 percent of neonates born with jejunoileal atresia have CF.[4,79,80] These observations indicate that all neonates with jejunoileal atresia and abnormal meconium presentation (e.g., meconium ileus, meconium plug syndrome, giant cystic meconium peritonitis) should undergo a sweat chloride test.[4]

The incidence of CF in neonates with meconium peritonitis is reported to be 15% to 40%. Four types of meconium peritonitis have been recognized, including adhesive meconium peritonitis, giant cystic meconium peritonitis or pseudocyst, meconium ascites, and infected meconium peritonitis.[81] Each form of meconium peritonitis shares a common etiology, namely, bowel perforation. The differences in clinical presentation are secondary to the timing of perforation and whether the perforation seals spontaneously. The site of perforation is usually closed by birth. However, mortality is increased in cases in which the perforation remains patent.[82] Initially, meconium peritonitis is a nonbacterial, chemical and foreign body peritonitis occurring during intrauterine or early neonatal life.[83] As meconium escapes from the obstructed bowel, a sterile chemical peritonitis ensues. After delivery, however, bacterial superinfection may occur with colonization of the gastrointestinal tract. It is important to note that meconium peritonitis may also occur without meconium ileus and is not pathognomonic for CF.[4,76]

Radiographic Features

Uncomplicated meconium ileus is characterized by a pattern of unevenly dilated loops of bowel with the variable presence of air-fluid levels on abdominal radiography.[73,84,85] The absence of air-fluid levels is due to the increased viscosity of the meconium not allowing an air interface with the fluid. As swallowed air mixes with the tenacious meconium, bubbles of gas develop. This ground-glass appearance (Fig. 33-4) depends on the viscosity of the meconium and is not a constant feature.[73,84] Although each of these features alone is not diagnostic of meconium ileus, collectively with a family history of CF, they strongly suggest the diagnosis.[86]

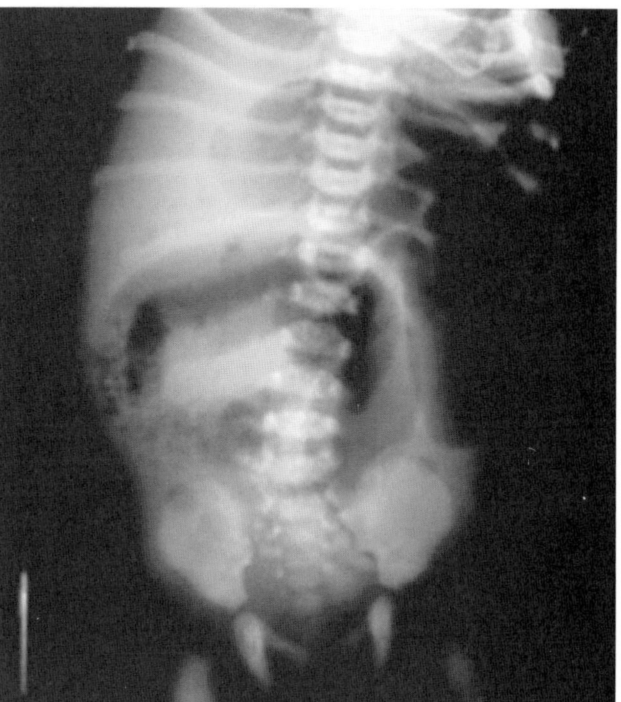

Figure 33-4. This abdominal radiograph in a neonate with meconium ileus shows the typical ground-glass appearance in the right lower abdomen. Also note the different-sized loops of distended small bowel.

Radiographic findings in complicated meconium ileus vary with the complication. Prenatal ultrasound findings include ascites, intra-abdominal cystic masses, dilated bowel, and calcifications.[87] Neonatal radiographic findings may include peritoneal calcifications, free air, and/or air-fluid levels (related to atresia).[4] Air-fluid levels may be few or absent, misleading the clinician to make an incorrect diagnosis of uncomplicated meconium ileus. Speckled calcification on abdominal plain films is highly suggestive of intrauterine intestinal perforation and meconium peritonitis. A large dense mass with a rim of calcification implies a pseudocyst (Fig. 33-5). When present, these calcium deposits are linear, coursing from the parietal peritoneum to the serosal surface of the visceral organs.[88] Interestingly, one third of cases of complicated meconium ileus have no radiologic findings suggesting a complication of meconium ileus.[89]

A contrast enema should be performed when there is evidence of a low intestinal obstruction in the newborn. We advocate a hyperosmolar, water-soluble contrast enema for both diagnosis and treatment. In

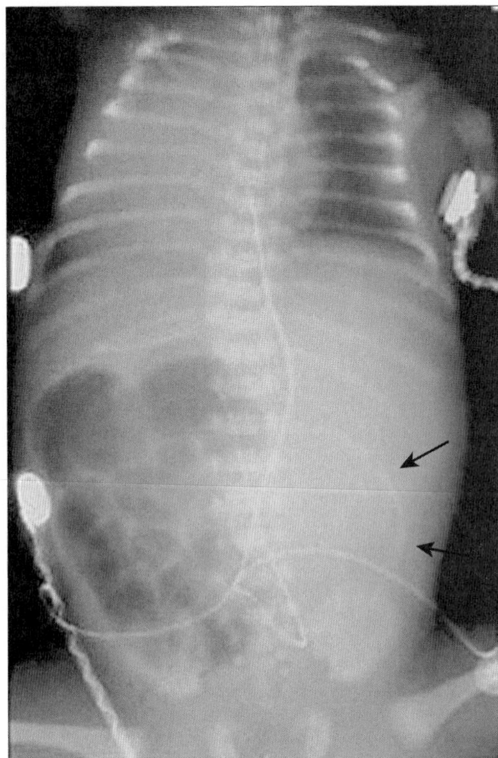

Figure 33-5. This neonate presented with evidence of meconium peritonitis. A mass effect in the left abdomen with a rim of calcification (*arrows*) implies in-utero perforation and a pseudocyst.

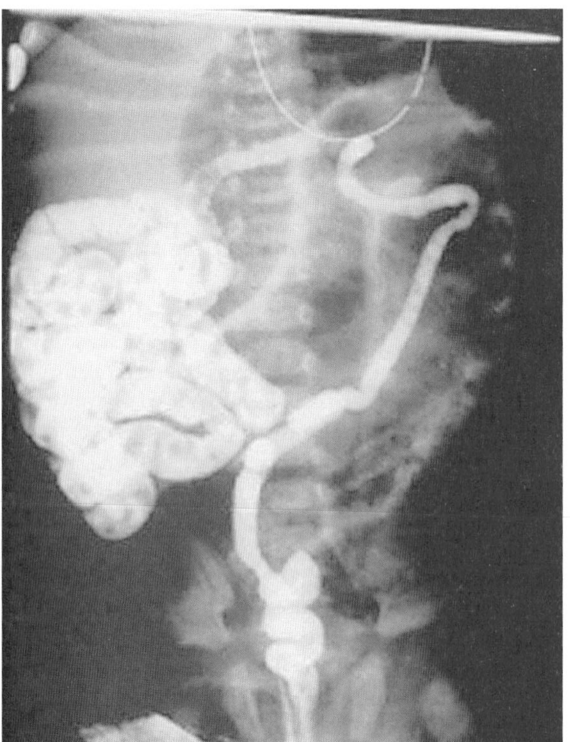

Figure 33-6. Classic radiographic findings of meconium ileus are seen on this retrograde contrast study. First, a "microcolon of disuse" is seen. The colon is extremely small and unused. Second, inspissated pellets (filling defects) of meconium are seen in the more proximal small bowel. Third, note there is a small bowel obstruction as the contrast material has not reached the markedly dilated loops of small bowel.

meconium ileus, the contrast enema reveals a small-caliber colon, a "microcolon of disuse," which often contains small, inspissated "rabbit pellets" of meconium (Fig. 33-6). If contrast medium cannot be refluxed into the dilated small bowel, operative exploration is required for diagnosis and therapy.

Diagnostic Testing

The diagnosis of CF is established with a sweat test at several weeks of life. A concentration of 60 mmol/L in 100 mg of sweat is diagnostic of CF with 40 to 60 mmol/L being intermediate (but more likely to be diagnostic in infants) and less than 40 mmol/L being normal. To ensure an adequate sweat sample, the test is typically performed at several weeks of life.[90] Neonatal CF screening programs using the Guthrie blood spot test for raised concentrations of immunoreactive trypsinogen are available in many countries but must be confirmed in a two-stage approach incorporating *CFTR* mutation analysis.[91,92] Genetic testing for *CFTR* mutations is available, but commercial assays test for a limited number of mutations. Most regional laboratories will provide the results for the four or five most common mutations for the relevant ethnic group or geographic region in their area using the amplification refractory mutation system (ARMS) technique.[91] Stool analyses for albumin, trypsin, and chymotrypsin are available, and abnormal values coupled with operative findings indicate CF.[18]

Neonates with meconium ileus who fail to respond to nonoperative measures may be treated by appendectomy and irrigation with a hyperosmolar contrast medium into the small bowel via the appendiceal stump or small bowel.[93] The appendix (or intestinal biopsy) may be sent for histologic examination. Pathognomonic findings for CF include goblet cell hyperplasia and accumulated secretions within the crypts or lumen.[94]

Treatment

Nonoperative Management of Simple Meconium Ileus

Treatment of meconium ileus has evolved over the past 55 years. Neonates should initially be managed as having a newborn intestinal obstruction. Volume resuscitation, gastric decompression, and mechanical respiratory support should be provided as necessary. Correction of any coagulation disorders and empirical broad-spectrum antibiotic coverage complete this initial management. When meconium ileus is suspected or diagnosed, a diagnostic enema or hyperosmolar enema is performed initially to exclude other causes of neonatal intestinal obstruction. Many newborns with meconium ileus can be managed nonoperatively with hyperosmolar enema washouts (Table 33-1).

Table 33-1 Commonly Used Contrast Materials for Meconium Ileus Patients

	Gastrografin (Bracco)	Conray 43 (Mallinckrodt)	Omnipaque 240 (GE Healthcare)	Omnipaque 300 (GE Healthcare)
Chemical Structure	Ionic	Ionic	Iohexol	Iohexol
Anion	Diatrizoate	Iothalamate	Nonionic	Nonionic
Cation	Meglumine sodium	Meglumine	None	None
% Salt Concentration	6610	43	24	30
% Iodine Concentration	37	20.2	24	30
Iodine + (mg I/mL)	370	20.2	240	300
Viscosity + 25° C (cps)		≈3	5.8	11.8
Viscosity + 25° C (cps)	8.4	≈2	3.4	6.3
Osmolality (mOsm/kg H_2O)	1940	≈100	520	672

On instillation, fluid is drawn into the intestinal lumen, hydrating and softening the meconium mass. Both transient osmotic diarrhea and diuresis follow. Thus, adequate resuscitation and hydration anticipating these fluid losses is important. Additionally, they should receive appropriate electrolyte repletion and maintenance of normothermia. These enemas are contraindicated in patients with complicated meconium ileus. The hypertonic enema must be performed under fluoroscopic control. Close surgical supervision, from the initial evaluation and throughout the hospital course, is mandatory, and the patient should be prepared for immediate operation should complications develop.[89]

Under fluoroscopic control, a 25% to 50% dilution of the hyperosmolar enema is slowly infused at low hydrostatic pressure through a catheter inserted into the rectum. Balloon inflation should be avoided to minimize the risk of rectal perforation. Usually there is rapid passage of meconium "pellets" followed by semiliquid meconium, which continues in the ensuing 24 to 48 hours. On completion of the enema, the catheter is withdrawn and an abdominal radiograph is obtained to evaluate for perforation. The infant is then returned to the neonatal care unit for intensive monitoring and fluid resuscitation. Warm saline enemas containing 1% *N*-acetylcysteine (Mucomyst; Apothecon, Princeton, NJ) may be given to help complete the meconium evacuation.[77] Radiographs should be taken in 8 to 12 hours, or as clinically indicated, to confirm evacuation of the obstruction and to exclude late perforation. If evacuation is incomplete, or if the first attempt at hyperosmolar enema evacuation does not reflux contrast medium into dilated bowel, a second enema may be necessary. However, if progressive distention, signs of peritonitis, or clinical deterioration occurs, surgical exploration is indicated. After two failed attempts at nonoperative hyperosmolar washout, operative intervention is needed.

After successful evacuation and resuscitation, 5 mL of a 10% *N*-acetylcysteine solution may be administered every 6 hours through a nasogastric tube to liquefy upper gastrointestinal secretions. Feedings, with supplemental pancreatic enzymes for those infants confirmed with CF, may be initiated when signs of obstruction have subsided.[95] The success rate of babies with uncomplicated meconium ileus treated with hyperosmolar enemas ranges between 63% and 83%.[96]

Several potential complications exist with the use of hyperosmolar enemas in treating meconium ileus. The risk of rectal perforation can be avoided by careful placement of the catheter under fluoroscopic guidance and not inflating the balloon-tipped catheter. A 23% perforation rate has been demonstrated in patients when inflated balloon catheters were used.[97] Early perforation, occurring during the administration of the enema, is usually apparent under fluoroscopy. The risk of perforation increases with repeated enemas.[98] Late perforation, occurring between 12 and 48 hours after the enema, can occur. Potential causes for late perforation include severe bowel distention by fluid osmotically drawn into the intestine or by direct injury to the bowel mucosa by the contrast medium.[98] The former appears to be the etiology in experimental models.[99,100] Delayed perforation associated with extensive bowel necrosis has been reported.[101,102] The pathogenesis of intestinal perforation associated with necrotizing enterocolitis is believed to be the ischemia produced by intestinal distention.[101] Hypovolemic shock is also a risk when delivering hypertonic enemas. Ischemia caused by overdistention is worsened by hypoperfusion caused by hypovolemia due to inadequate fluid resuscitation. Adequate fluid resuscitation (150 mL/kg/day, minimum) with anticipation of fluid losses due to osmotic diarrhea and diuresis is mandatory and should be initiated at the time of the enema.[101]

Operative Management

Simple Meconium Ileus

The indications for operative management of simple meconium ileus are inadequate meconium evacuation or a complication of the contrast enema (e.g., perforation). Failure of nonoperative treatment with hyperosmolar enemas may result from the technical inability to advance the enema column for a sufficient distance into the ileum or from an unsuspected, associated intestinal atresia. If the enema fails to promote passage of meconium within 24 to 48 hours, or two attempts at washout are unsuccessful, an operative approach is indicated.

Before the widespread acceptance of enemas and an initial nonoperative approach, several operative strategies predominated as initial therapy.[50] Many of these techniques involved the use of proximal and distal stomas. This approach provided for decompression of the dilated proximal intestine and provided access for intestinal irrigation.

In 1948, the first successful operative management of five infants with meconium ileus by intraoperative meconium disimpaction with saline via a tube enterostomy coupled with a limited small bowel resection was reported.[103] Enterotomy and intraoperative saline irrigation for mechanical separation of the pellets from the bowel wall and evacuation of the meconium continues to be the mainstay of operative therapy for simple meconium ileus.

With either operative approach, manual evacuation of the inspissated meconium can be aided by intraoperative instillation of 2% or 4% *N*-acetylcysteine or 50% hyperosmolar solutions. A purse-string suture is placed in the antimesenteric wall of the small bowel proximal to the obstruction, and a red rubber catheter is inserted through a small incision within the purse-string. This is followed by gentle instillation of the solution into the terminal ileum. Often the thick tenacious meconium must be removed directly through the enterotomy (Fig. 33-7), while the dissolved meconium and the pellets can be either removed directly or milked into the colon. A similar technique was reported in 1989 in which an appendectomy was performed and a cecostomy catheter was placed through the appendiceal stump to irrigate and evacuate impacted meconium.[93] With either technique, the surgeon must take care to avoid exposure of the meconium to the peritoneal cavity. Once the meconium is cleared, the enterotomy or appendiceal stump can be closed. In some situations, an indwelling intestinal catheter or a T-tube may be left in the enterotomy for the purpose of postoperative bowel irrigation, decompression, pancreatic enzyme instillation, and/or feeding.[104] The T-tube or enterostomy tube should be left at the junction of the proximal dilated bowel and collapsed distal ileum. The irrigations are begun in the early postoperative period. After successful clearance of meconium, the tubes are removed and the enterocutaneous fistula is allowed to close spontaneously.[69,74,77,93,105-108]

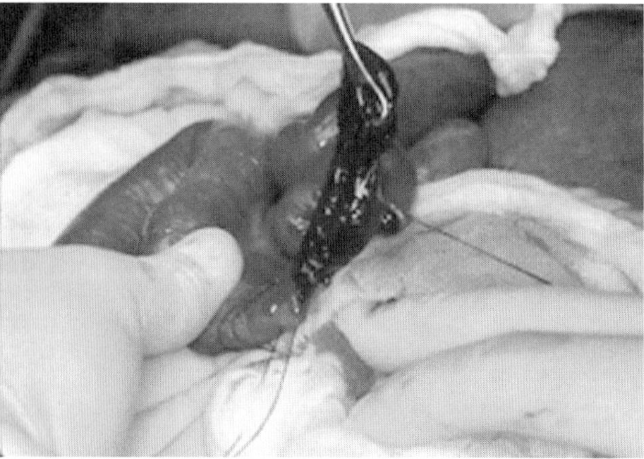

Figure 33-7. At operation, the meconium in a neonate with cystic fibrosis is very thick and tenacious.

Resection with primary anastomosis was first described in 1962.[108] Anastomotic leakage complicated early attempts with this approach. Since then improved results have been reported.[109,110] An alternative to this approach was small bowel resection with creation of a stoma and eventual closure of the stoma with an end-to-end anastomosis. Successful outcome after resection with primary anastomosis depends on adequate resection of compromised bowel, complete proximal and distal evacuation of meconium, and preservation of adequate blood supply to the anastomosis.

Alternative surgical techniques involve resection, anastomosis, and temporary enterostomy through which postoperative irrigations may be delivered (Fig. 33-8). The Mikulicz double-barreled enterostomy has three distinct advantages. First, operative and anesthesia times are reduced because complete evacuation of inspissated meconium is not necessary. Second, an intra-abdominal anastomosis is averted, avoiding the risk of anastomotic leakage. Third, the bowel is opened after complete closure of the abdominal wound, thereby reducing the risk of intraperitoneal contamination. Solubilizing agents are administered postoperatively through both the proximal and distal limbs of the stoma as well as per rectum or via a nasogastric tube.[86,106] As classically described, a spur-crushing Mikulicz clamp may be applied to the two limbs to create continuity for distal flow of intestinal fluids. The clamp-induced anastomosis may spontaneously close after relief of the distal obstruction (inspissated meconium). Disadvantages of this and other procedures employing resection and stoma(s) are potential postoperative fluid losses through high volume stomas, bowel shortening by resection, and the need for a second procedure to re-establish intestinal continuity.

A distal chimney enterostomy (the Bishop-Koop procedure) involves resection with anastomosis between the end of the proximal segment and the side of the distal segment of bowel approximately 4 cm from the opening of the distal segment. The distal end is brought out as the ileostomy.[105] This technique allows for normal gastrointestinal transit while providing a means for management of the distal obstruction through the ileostomy should it occur. The reverse of the distal chimney enterostomy is the Santulli and Blanc proximal enterostomy. After resection, the end of the distal limb is anastomosed to the side of the proximal limb. The end of the proximal limb is brought out as the enterostomy.[74,111] With this arrangement, proximal irrigation and decompression are enhanced and it is not necessary to evacuate the proximal small bowel at the time of surgery. Like the distal chimney enterostomy, catheter access to the distal limb is achieved through the stoma, thus providing a means of irrigating the distal bowel. The apparent disadvantage of this technique is the presence of a high-output stoma and the inherent risk of dehydration and electrolyte derangement.

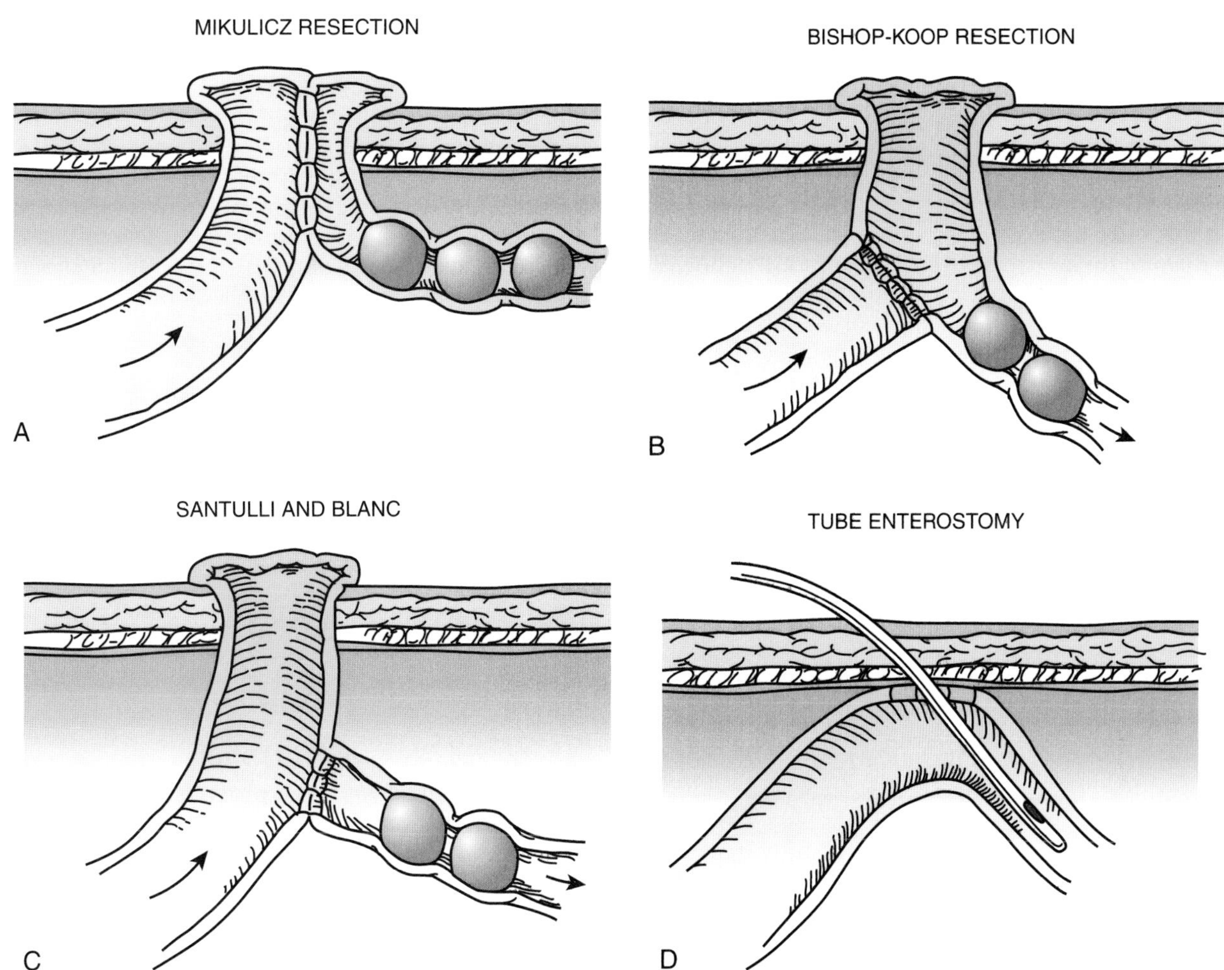

Figure 33-8. There are a number of options for surgical management of a neonate with meconium ileus. Options for creation of an ileostomy include the double-barrel ileostomy (Mikulicz enterostomy) (**A**), the Bishop-Koop ileostomy (**B**), and the Santulli ileostomy (**C**). Both the Bishop-Koop and Santulli ileostomies require an intra-abdominal anastomosis. Another option is to place a red rubber catheter into the uninvolved proximal small bowel for postoperative irrigations (**D**).

Care must be taken to replenish fluids, electrolytes, and nutrients in accordance with the stoma output. Re-instillation of stoma output from the proximal to the distal limb is often performed via the indwelling catheter.[74,86]

Complicated Meconium Ileus

An operation is almost always indicated in cases of complicated meconium ileus. One exception is a rare in-utero spontaneously sealed perforation with intact intestinal continuity and extraluminal intraperitoneal calcified meconium.[73] Additional findings seen later in life include calcified meconium identified in a patent processus vaginalis during herniorrhaphy or incidentally on an abdominal radiograph. Indications for operation include peritonitis, persistent intestinal obstruction, an enlarging abdominal mass, and ongoing sepsis. Surgical management includes early diagnosis, debridement of necrotic material, pseudocyst resection, diverting stoma(s), antibiotics, and meticulous postoperative care.[76] Creation of an ostomy is the fastest and safest course, alleviating concern over bowel discrepancy, anastomotic breakdown, and return of bowel activity. Decortication of the cyst wall is recommended, if possible.

Whereas meconium peritonitis is best managed in this fashion, both segmental volvulus and intestinal atresia in stable patients without peritoneal contamination may be managed with resection, irrigation of the bowel to remove inspissated contents, and an end-to-end or end-to-oblique anastomosis depending on the size of the intestine. The goal of operative management is the relief of intestinal obstruction and the preservation of maximal intestinal length.

Postoperative Management

The initial postoperative management involves ongoing resuscitation. Maintenance fluids and replacement of insensible fluid losses, as well as gastrointestinal losses (nasogastric suction and ileostomy) must be carefully monitored. Instillation of 2% or 4% *N*-acetylcysteine via a nasogastric tube or ileostomy will help solubilize residual meconium. In the patient with fetal or neonatal bowel obstruction, CF must be suspected, and diagnostic tests should be performed as soon as possible. Stomas placed in the course of surgical management should be closed as soon as possible (4 to 6 weeks) to help avoid prolonged problems with fluid, electrolyte, nutritional losses, and cholestatic jaundice.

Nutritional Management

With relief of the obstruction and resumption of bowel function, infants with uncomplicated meconium ileus and CF may be given breast milk or infant formula, along with supplemental pancreatic enzymes and vitamins.[112,113] Caution must be used when prescribing enteric enzyme medication to patients with meconium ileus and CF. Treatment failures and complications, such as fibrosing colonopathy from excessive enzyme doses[112] and meconium ileus equivalent, or distal intestinal obstruction syndrome (DIOS),[47] from inadequate enzyme therapy or generic substitutions for proprietary medications have been reported.[114-116] Those with a complicated surgical course will require either continuous enteral feeds or total parenteral nutrition (TPN). Dilation of the small bowel by the obstructing meconium may lead to mucosal damage that could contribute to poor peristalsis or malabsorption. In patients with complicated meconium ileus or in those with significant loss of intestinal length, we recommend beginning feeding with predigested, diluted formula at low continuous volumes. If this is well tolerated, the strength may be increased followed by the volume, while observing for signs of feeding intolerance (i.e., abdominal distention, heme-positive stools, and/or emesis). Once enteral feedings are begun, pancreatic enzymes must be given (even with predigested formula) starting at 2000 to 4000 lipase units per 120 mL of full-strength formula. Capsules containing enteric-coated microspheres can be opened and the contents mixed with formula or applesauce in older infants. The microcapsules should not be crushed because this will expose the enzymes to the acid of the stomach where they will be destroyed. Uncrushed pancreatic enzymes should be given, even with medium-chain triglyceride/oil-containing formulas.[117]

Infants with meconium ileus are at increased risk for cholestasis, particularly if they have had, or are receiving TPN. Alkaline phosphatase, alanine aminotransferase, aspartate aminotransferase, and bilirubin should be monitored weekly. The fluid and nutritional status of infants who have had significant bowel resection (greater than one third) may be difficult to manage. In addition, the presence of an ileostomy may lead to excessive losses of fluid and sodium. Again, stomas should be closed as soon as possible. In the interim, if access to the distal, defunctionalized bowel is feasible, drip feeds of glutamine-enriched formula or instillation of the effluent from the proximal stoma may be tried at low volumes to enhance bowel growth and help prevent bacterial translocation.

Gastric acid hypersecretion is seen in patients who have short bowel syndrome.[118] An acidic intestinal environment inactivates pancreatic enzymes and prevents dissolution of enteric-coated microcapsules. Histamine-2 (H_2)-receptor antagonists or proton pump inhibitors may be used as an adjunct to pancreatic enzyme therapy in patients who have had significant bowel resections. Patients with excessive sweat and intestinal sodium losses may develop a total body sodium deficit. Urine sodium should be measured in infants with ileostomies, especially when there is failure to grow, even if serum sodium levels are normal. Those with urine sodium less than 10 mEq/L will need sodium (and possibly bicarbonate) supplementation.[119]

Pulmonary Management

Although clinical lung disease does not usually develop early, mucus plugging and atelectasis can be seen. Prophylactic pulmonary care with chest physiotherapy is initiated immediately postoperatively. The head-down position should not be used because this increases the risk of gastroesophageal reflux and aspiration. Infants should receive nebulized albuterol (2.5 mg) twice a day followed by chest physiotherapy. Prophylactic antibiotics are not necessary, and antibiotic therapy is directed by respiratory tract cultures if needed.

Prognosis

Prior to the mid 1900s, the prognosis for infants with meconium ileus was uniformly poor despite surgical treatment. Early reports showed mortality rates of 50% to 67%.[70,71,105,106] Improved survival in infants with meconium ileus can be attributed to many factors. Because of advances in prenatal diagnosis, pulmonary and neonatal intensive care, nutrition, antibiotics, anesthesia, operative management, and an improved understanding of the pathophysiology and treatment of the complications of CF, the prognosis for infants with both complicated and simple meconium ileus has improved dramatically.[25,120] Survival rates of 85% to 100% have been reported in uncomplicated meconium ileus[4,86] and up to 93% in complicated cases.[4,70]

Some argue that long-term follow-up of patients with meconium ileus shows pulmonary function at age 13 years to be no different between those born with meconium ileus and those without meconium ileus.[25] However, a recent prospective study found CF children with meconium ileus have worse lung function and more obstructive lung disease than those without meconium ileus.[121] Furthermore, comparison of the nutritional status of a similar population of patients with CF suggests that those who presented with meconium ileus suffer long-term nutritional complications as well as other problems.[122]

MECONIUM PLUG SYNDROME

Meconium plug syndrome, a cause of newborn colonic obstruction, was first described in 1956.[123] It was hypothesized that either colonic motility or the character of the meconium was altered, thereby preventing normal passage and decompression of the colon in the newborn period. Under normal conditions, the terminal 2 cm of neonatal meconium is firm in texture, forming a whitish cap. Most newborns pass this cap of meconium before, during, or shortly after delivery. One in 500 newborns will have a longer, more tenacious obstructive plug. Failure to pass this plug results in meconium plug syndrome and the term *plugged-up babies* was coined.[123]

The presentation of meconium plug syndrome is similar to that of meconium ileus. Signs include failure to pass meconium, bilious vomiting, and abdominal distention with an obstructive pattern on plain abdominal radiographs. Often, the meconium plug may become dislodged after digital stimulation of the anus and rectum. Fortunately, colon function is generally preserved and returns to normal after passage of the plug. Ultimately, most of these infants are found to be healthy.

Pathologic causes of meconium plug syndrome include CF, small left colon syndrome, and Hirschsprung's disease.[118,124,125] Less common causes include congenital hypothyroidism, maternal narcotic addiction, and neuronal intestinal dysplasia. Affected newborns should undergo contrast enemas, which may be therapeutic as well as diagnostic. After resolution, a sweat test should be performed to evaluate for CF and a thyroid-stimulating hormone level should be checked. All patients with slow passage of meconium require close observation of their stool pattern. Historically, a rectal biopsy has been recommended to rule out Hirschsprung's disease.[77,118] A recent report documents a 13% incidence of Hirschsprung's disease in a neonate with meconium plug syndrome. Therefore, a suction biopsy could be reserved for those neonates with an abnormal stooling pattern.[126]

COMPLICATIONS OF MECONIUM ILEUS AND CYSTIC FIBROSIS

Gastroesophageal Reflux Disease

Gastroesophageal reflux disease (GERD) occurs with increased prevalence in patients with CF. Moreover, aspiration in children with CF may aggravate failure to thrive, may adversely affect pulmonary function, and may account for the predilection of CF lung disease for the right upper lobe.[127,128] Pathologic reflux with endoscopic and histologic esophagitis is present in over 50% of CF patients, and the incidence of GERD in patients with CF is approximately 81% in patients younger than 60 months.[129] Many children with CF lung disease are managed with theophylline, which causes a decrease in lower esophageal sphincter pressure and may contribute to the development of GERD.[127] It is clear that early diagnosis and treatment of this condition is of prime importance if the complications of pathologic reflux are to be curtailed and respiratory function maximized because reflux may also worsen the respiratory status of the CF patient.

Antireflux medications, modification of chest physiotherapy, and eliminating the 30-degree head-down tilt may all decrease the incidence of GERD in this population.[130] Children unresponsive to medical management may benefit from a surgical evaluation for an antireflux procedure.[129,130] Our antireflux procedure of choice is a laparoscopic Nissen fundoplication. Recent data suggest that a fundoplication may improve respiratory function (improved FEV_1 slope) in CF children with mild versus moderate disease.[131] Patients with symptomatic reflux requiring an antireflux procedure may benefit from concurrent placement of a gastrostomy tube if inadequate caloric intake is a problem. Barrett's esophagus, a rare finding in children, has been reported in older children with CF.[4,132] Although an antireflux procedure may halt the advancement of metaplasia, if dysplasia is present the malignant potential remains.[128] Frequent endoscopic monitoring is the same for patients with CF as those without.[133] In adults, if high-grade dysplasia is confirmed by two pathologists and aggressive medical therapy fails to eliminate the dysplasia, esophagectomy is recommended. With so little data available in children with CF, it is reasonable to suggest that those patients with CF who have dysplastic esophageal changes should be evaluated for an antireflux procedure.[128]

Biliary Tract Disease

Multiple macroscopic cysts may replace the pancreas in CF.[30] Although it was classically thought that hepatic and pancreatic dysfunction occurred together, hepatic dysfunction may occur in patients with maintained pancreatic function.[128] The most common hepatic complications of CF are steatosis, fibrosis, biliary cirrhosis, atretic gallbladder, cholelithiasis, sclerosing cholangitis, and biliary dyskinesia. Obstruction of intrahepatic biliary ductules by abnormal mucoid secretions or inspissated bile, resulting from absence of functional CFTR in bile duct epithelial cells, leads to cirrhosis in patients with CF.[134] The classic liver histology in CF is focal biliary fibrosis with progression to multilobular, biliary cirrhosis.[134] Prolonged cholestatic liver disease in CF patients may lead to cirrhosis, portal hypertension, and, ultimately, liver failure and death without liver transplantation.

Although more common in older patients with CF, intrahepatic cholestasis can be seen in the neonate. In extreme neonatal forms with early profound intrahepatic cholestasis, this process can be associated with a marked decrease in ductal diameter, varying from hypoplasia to atresia. Additionally, these neonates are at increased risk for cholestatic jaundice when they are not being fed enterally. This condition is suggested by prolonged jaundice unresponsive to choleretics, nondilated bile ducts and gallbladder on ultrasonography, absent biliary excretion on nuclear scan, and characteristic liver biopsy.[135-137]

End-stage liver disease (ESLD) is manifest by loss of synthetic function, growth failure, or portal hypertension presenting as variceal hemorrhage.[128] Although abnormal results of liver function tests have been noted in 12.9% of CF patients, only 4.2% manifest overt liver disease.[138] However, the prevalence is reported as high as 37% depending on the definition of liver disease.[139] Surgical portosystemic shunts, transjugular intrahepatic portosystemic shunts (TIPS), partial splenectomy, and endoscopic injection sclerotherapy have been advocated in treating CF patients with portal hypertension.[140] Other surgical options for these patients are direct ligation of the varices, esophageal transection, or the Sugiura procedure (gastric devascularization).[141,142] These procedures are all palliative. The only curative treatment for portal hypertension and ESLD is orthotopic liver transplantation.

Liver transplantation has been successfully carried out in CF patients with ESLD who did not have respiratory failure.[128,140] Successful reports exist of combined liver and intestinal transplantation, combined liver and pancreas transplant, kidney transplant after combined heart and lung transplants, and triple-organ transplant (pancreas, liver, and kidney) in patients with exocrine pancreatic insufficiency and insulin-dependent diabetes related to CF.[4,143,144] Liver, pancreas, kidney, intestine, and multiple-viscera transplantation are valid options for children with CF.

Gallbladder disease is prevalent in the CF population and includes cholelithiasis in up to 24%[139,145]; microgallbladder, atretic cystic duct,[139] abnormal cholecystograms in 46%[146]; and hyperviscous mucus.[147] Many CF patients with gallstones are asymptomatic,[128] with symptomatic gallbladder disease encountered in only approximately 4% of patients.[148] Ultrasonography (not computed tomography) is recommended in patients with CF[139,149] because the stones are radiolucent.[148] Bile in patients with CF is not cholesterol supersaturated, and the stones are composed of protein and calcium bilirubinate.[145]

Patients with symptomatic gallbladder disease (symptomatic cholelithiasis and acute cholecystitis) should undergo prompt cholecystectomy.[149,150] Experience with laparoscopic cholecystectomy is positive, and it is the recommended approach.[4,151] The incidence of common bile duct stones in CF is very low,[149-151] and routine intraoperative cholangiograms or preoperative endoscopic retrograde cholangiopancreatography is not usually needed.[128] In fact, the biliary tract abnormalities often encountered in patients with CF make penetration of radiocontrast dye into the biliary tract during endoscopic retrograde cholangiopancreatography difficult.[139] Intraoperative cholangiography is recommended if jaundice, pancreatitis, cholangitis, dilated common bile duct, or palpable stones in the common bile duct are present.[128]

Distal Intestinal Obstruction Syndrome

Distal intestinal obstruction syndrome (DIOS, formerly called meconium ileus equivalent) is a recurrent, partial or complete intestinal obstruction unique to teenage and young adult patients with CF that occurs secondary to abnormally viscid mucofeculent material in the distal ileum and right colon.[152-156] The etiology of DIOS is unclear, but these patients are more likely to have a history of steatorrhea from pancreatic exocrine insufficiency, despite adequate enzyme therapy. A number of aspects particular to gastrointestinal function of the CF patient may help to explain this syndrome. In addition to inherently slow intestinal motility, other contributing factors may include thickening of chyme secondary to the presence of undigested protein and fat,[157] precipitation of undigested protein and bile acids in duodenal fluid with reduced pH,[157-159] lower water content of pancreatic and duodenal secretions, hyperviscosity of mucus resulting from abnormal ion and water transport,[158,159] abnormal regulation of mucin secretion,[160] and altered biochemical properties of mucus glycoprotein.[157-160] Precipitating factors include sudden withdrawal of, or noncompliance with, adequate enzyme supplementation, immobilization, dehydration, respiratory tract infections, and recovery from surgery. However, in the majority of cases, no identifiable cause will be found.[4]

DIOS occurs in 15% to 37% of patients with CF, particularly those with associated pancreatic insufficiency with malabsorption and severe pulmonary limitation.[124,161-168] One study noted a 12% incidence in children with CF, but the majority (63%) had meconium ileus as an infant.[4] Children with normal fat absorption are rarely affected.

Patients with DIOS present with crampy abdominal pain often localized to the right lower quadrant and a decreased frequency of defecation. They may complain of an insidious, debilitating abdominal pain. Physical examination in uncomplicated DIOS usually reveals abdominal distention and a tender mass in the right lower quadrant with no evidence of peritonitis. Typically, there is no fecal impaction on rectal examination and the stool is Hemoccult negative. Different degrees of obstruction will be present, from partial, which is most common, to complete, with vomiting, abdominal distention, and obstipation.

A supine and erect abdominal radiograph is the most helpful initial investigation when DIOS is suspected (Fig. 33-9). This will show distended small bowel with scattered air-fluid levels and a granular, bubbly pattern of intestinal gas representing the mixing of air and inspissated meconium in the right lower quadrant similar to infants with meconium ileus.

Inspissated material in the right colon and distal ileum can be demonstrated with a water-soluble contrast enema. In doing so, ileocolic intussusception, which is also seen in CF patients, can be excluded and the investigation itself may prove therapeutic in some cases.

The diagnosis of DIOS must take into consideration other potential causes of abdominal pain and intestinal obstruction in CF patients. This constellation of signs and symptoms has historically been a diagnostic dilemma in patients with CF. Intussusception, mechanical small bowel obstruction due to adhesions, appendicitis, Crohn's disease, and biliary tract disease may present similarly.

In the absence of mechanical small bowel obstruction due to adhesions, intussusception, or appendiceal disease, a trial of medical management aimed at relieving the inspissated distal bowel obstruction is recommended. After adequate volume resuscitation

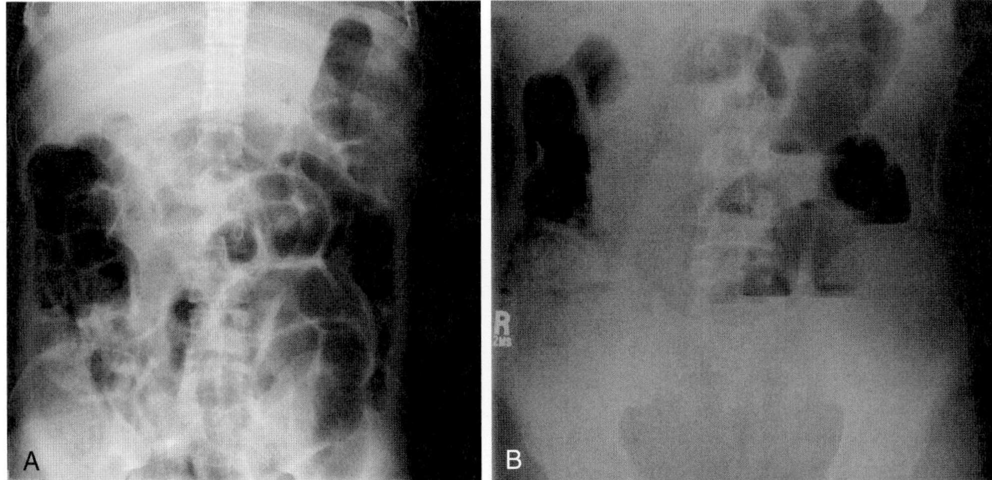

Figure 33-9. This 18-year-old with cystic fibrosis presented with crampy abdominal pain that was localized to the right lower abdomen. In addition, he also had a decreased frequency of defecation. **A,** The ground-glass appearance in the loops of bowel on the right side are typical findings in a patient with distal intestinal obstruction syndrome. **B,** The upright abdominal film shows air-fluid levels. This patient responded nicely to a contrast enema with relief of his symptoms.

and colonic enema washout, a balanced polyethylene glycol-electrolyte solution can be given orally or by nasogastric tube. The dose is 20 to 40 mL/kg/hr with a maximum of 1200 mL/hr. Alternatively, ingestion of a nonabsorbable intestinal lavage solution such as a hyperosmolar solution may produce the most striking results.[169] A single oral dose is successful in the majority of patients. Careful attention to the fluid status is vital. Oral administration of the hyperosmolar solution should be withheld in patients with preexisting dehydration, obstruction, or peritoneal signs. Younger patients will usually require nasogastric tube placement, whereas older children are able to ingest sufficient volumes of lavage solution to relieve the impacted material.

The passage of stool, resolution of symptoms, and the disappearance of a previously palpable right iliac fossa mass implies successful treatment. Sequential abdominal radiographs will help to document the resolution of DIOS, but if symptoms persist then the differential diagnoses already outlined must be considered. Some authors have recommended prophylaxis with the use of scheduled laxatives and high dietary roughage.[124,161]

When there is complete obstruction or evidence of peritonitis, surgical intervention is necessary and all oral or rectal therapies are contraindicated. A nasogastric tube should be placed to help with decompression and adequate resuscitative measures initiated. At laparotomy, the bowel wall will feel thickened and filled with tenacious material. It can be decompressed and irrigated with hyperosmolar solution through a small catheter placed through the appendiceal stump, as previously described for uncomplicated meconium ileus. It is also possible to leave an irrigating tube in situ to irrigate the bowel postoperatively. Some children may require lysis of adhesions and/or bowel resections with either a primary anastomosis or creation of an ostomy.[4]

Appendicitis

Abdominal pain is a common complaint of patients with CF. Because they are often already being treated with antibiotics and corticosteroids, the classic clinical signs and symptoms of appendicitis are often masked and the diagnosis missed. This results in a high incidence of perforation and substantial morbidity in this patient group. Despite the blunting of clinical signs, there may still be evidence of fever and leukocytosis. Depending on the location of the appendix, a contrast enema may show deformity of the cecum with an associated mass effect and not the typical inspissated material features of DIOS. Abdominal ultrasonography or computed tomography will show free fluid or an abscess collection in the region of the cecum. In such cases of perforated appendicitis, treatment should then proceed with percutaneous drainage of the abscess and interval appendectomy. Appendectomy is required in acute nonperforated appendicitis. If the diagnosis is still in doubt, diagnostic laparoscopy may be indicated. Many surgeons perform incidental appendectomy during other abdominal operations.

Intussusception

Intussusception occurs in approximately 1% of children with CF with the average age at onset being 9.5 years.[170] In contrast, the average age at onset in children with idiopathic intussusception in the general pediatric population is 6 to 18 months.[126] Toddlers and older children presenting with intussusception and a history of recurrent pulmonary infections should be tested for CF.[127] The most common site for intussusception is ileocolic, but it may be ileoileal, cecocolic, or colocolic.[128] The abnormally thick stools adhering to the bowel wall or the appendix may act as a lead point.[170,171] Controversy exists over conservative management of intussusception in CF patients, with some reporting high rates of successful hydrostatic reduction[172] in the majority of patients. However, others report poor results.[170] If the intussusception is unable to be reduced operatively, bowel resection with anastomosis is necessary. Regardless, the appendix should be removed at operation in cases of intussusception.[170]

Fibrosing Colonopathy

Fibrosing colonopathy is a result of colonic strictures, and these children present with the signs and symptoms of DIOS.[112,113,153,173-175] Findings include colonic strictures with histopathologic changes of post–ischemic ulcer repair, an erythematous cobblestone appearance to the mucosa, mucosal and submucosal fibrosis, and destruction of the muscularis mucosa. In some patients, a change from conventional enteric-coated pancreatic enzymes to high-strength products 12 to 15 months earlier has been described. In the largest case-control study reported, the absolute dose of pancreatic enzymes, rather than the type of enzyme, was the strongest predictor of fibrosing colonopathy.[176]

The diagnosis of fibrosing colonopathy should be considered in CF patients who have been exposed to high doses of pancreatic enzymes and present with symptoms of abdominal pain, distention, chylous ascites, change in bowel habit, or failure to thrive. Continued diarrhea may also be a prominent feature, which unfortunately may prompt the family to increase supplemental enzymes further. On occasion, the diarrhea may be bloody. A barium enema may reveal mucosal irregularity, loss of haustral markings with a foreshortened colon, and varying degrees of stricture formation. In some cases the whole colon is involved. Colonoscopy may show an erythematous mucosa and areas of narrowing, from which it is advisable to take multiple biopsy samples.[173]

Initial management should include reduction of the enzyme dosage to the recommended levels of 500 to 2500 lipase units/kg per meal. This should be accompanied with adequate nutritional supplementation, which may be enteral elemental feeding or even TPN for a time. Those patients who show signs of unrelenting failure to thrive, obstruction, uncontrollable diarrhea, or chylous ascites will need surgical intervention.

When surgery is planned electively for patients with intractable symptoms, a gentle bowel preparation can be given preoperatively. The aim of surgical intervention is to resect the affected bowel and perform a primary anastomosis. Unfortunately, this is not possible in the event of total colonic or rectal involvement. As a result the patient may require an ileostomy or colostomy. It is also not clear if this condition completely resolves with a reduction in enzyme dosage and surgical resection. Therefore, the operated group also requires regular follow-up for any signs of deterioration or recurrence.

CONCLUSION

The operative mortality in patients with CF has decreased considerably in the past 3 decades. The average mortality rate for meconium ileus and peritonitis was 55% in the 1960s and 1970s.[177] During this time there was a significant decrease in survival in the first year of life compared with those patients with CF who did not have meconium ileus.[178] After the first year, survival among infants with meconium ileus approached that of other infants with CF. Over the past few years, these statistics have improved dramatically. There are now reports stating a 100% early survival and 86% late survival in 42 patients with meconium ileus[127] and a 91.6% survival for uncomplicated meconium ileus and 85% for complicated cases at 1 year.[70] Most recently, survival for patients with simple meconium ileus was reported at 93% (early 100%, late 93%) and that for those with complicated meconium ileus at 89% (early 96%, late 93%).[4]

Discussing the long-term needs of the patient with meconium ileus means discussing the long-term needs of a patient with CF. A multidisciplinary approach to the management of the surgical patient with CF, including respiratory care, nutrition support, and pancreatic enzyme therapy, allows for a low operative morbidity and mortality. Children with meconium ileus need long-term follow-up because they are prone to develop DIOS and fibrosing colonopathy. Furthermore, patients may be more prone to develop mechanical bowel obstructions later in life if operated on as an infant for meconium ileus.[4] Other late complications of meconium ileus, including gallstones, cirrhosis of the liver, and male sterility, may also be viewed as late complications of CF in general.[4] Many patients with CF are now surviving into the third and even fourth decades of life, and many of the surgical complications of CF occur later in life.

chapter 34

NECROTIZING ENTEROCOLITIS

Marion C. W. Henry, MD, MPH • R. Lawrence Moss, MD

The earliest reports of necrotizing enterocolitis (NEC) in the United States originated in the early 1960s.[1,2] Santulli and his colleagues published the first significant surgical experience with NEC when they described a disease of low birth weight infants with high mortality rates that required early, aggressive surgical management.[1] In the half-century since these early reports, many investigators have devoted careers to helping better define this challenging disease and improve our strategies of treatment and prevention. Despite these efforts, NEC remains a difficult and elusive disease. We continue to struggle to best delineate which premature infants are most at risk, to maximize our prevention strategies, to determine the optimal treatment strategies, and to understand and treat the long-term sequelae faced by survivors of this disease.

EPIDEMIOLOGY

Several large population-based studies have found incidence rates of 0.7 to 1.1 cases of NEC per 1000 live births and occurrence rates of 3% to 7% in selected populations (Table 34-1). An 8-year population-based study in the state of New York found an average annual incidence of 0.72 case per 1000 live births. The highest incidence was in those infants weighing 750 to 1000 g, and this incidence decreased with increasing birth weight.[3] A database query of 98 neonatal intensive care units (NICUs) in 24 states across the United States found an NEC rate of 3% among infants of 23 to 34 weeks' gestational age. In this group, low birth weight was the most significant risk factor for NEC.[4] The Vermont Oxford network reported rates of 6% to 7% between 1991 and 1999.[5] A study of 17 tertiary NICUs in Canada found an incidence of 6.6% stage 2 NEC among very low birth weight (VLBW) infants, defined as weight less than 1500 g, and 0.7% among those weighing more than 1500 g. NEC was associated with lower gestational age and birth weight, with the highest incidence in the group weighing less than 1000 g.[6]

Rates have remained stable for VLBW infants cared for at centers of the National Institute of Child Health and Human Development (NICHD) Neonatal Research Network. Between 1999 and 2001, 7% of VLBW infants developed proven NEC. Half of these infants required surgery.[7] A database of neonatal hospitalizations in 2000 found a rate of 1.1 cases of NEC per 1000 live births.[8] These studies all showed that the incidence of NEC and its fatality rates increase with decreasing birth weight and gestational age.[3,6-9]

Mortality from NEC remains high, with rates ranging from 15% to 30%.[3,4,7-10] Higher fatality rates are associated with lower birth weight and younger gestational age.[9,10] In a study summarizing trends for mortality and NEC in the United States between 1979 and 1992, there were 6692 deaths from NEC or an average of 474 deaths per year.[10] This equaled a death rate of 12.4 deaths per 100,000 live births. The highest mortality was in VLBW infants who were black and male.[3,8,10]

Although the majority of cases of NEC are managed medically, 20% to 40% will require surgical intervention.[4,6,9,11] The mortality rate markedly increases when surgical intervention is necessary and has been reported to be as high as 50%. The highest fatality rates in this subgroup are also in the lowest birth weight and youngest gestational age infants.[12]

NEC is primarily a disease of prematurity, with over 90% of cases occurring in preterm infants. However, there are occasional reports of NEC in full-term infants. Although the clinical and pathologic findings are similar in preterm and term infants, the initiating factors are likely different. Term infants who develop NEC are more likely to have predisposing risk factors such as congenital heart disease, respiratory disease, or reported hypoxic events.[13-16] A study from a multi-hospital health care system between 2001 and 2006 found that 0.5% of term infants developed stage II or greater NEC.[14]

PATHOPHYSIOLOGY

Despite recent insights into the multifactorial pathogenesis of NEC, a complete understanding of its pathophysiology remains elusive. The classic histologic findings of inflammation and coagulation necrosis are present

TABLE 34-1 Population-Based Epidemiologic Studies on Necrotizing Enterocolitis (NEC)

Author	Year	Population	No. Studied	No. NEC	%	Rate per 1000 Live Births	Fatality Rate
Llanos	2002	New York State	117,892	85		0.72	19%
Guthrie	2003	Pediatrix Medical group	15,072 (23-34 wks gestation)	390	3%		12%
Sankaran	2004	Canadian Neonatal network	18,234 (3628 VLBW)	336	7% VLBW	1.8	
Luig and Lui	2005	New South Wales NICU Study	4649 (24-31 wks gestation)	178	4%		30%
Guillet	2006	NIHCD Neonatal research network	11,936 VLBW	787	7% VLBW		24%
Holman	2006	Hospital discharges in USA: 2000—children inpatient database	Sample of all neonatal hospitalizations (4,058,814 live births)	4464		1.1	15%

VLBW, very low birth weight.

in over 90% of surgical specimens.[17] As patients progress along the clinical spectrum of suspected NEC to advanced stage III disease, radiologic and clinical findings also give hints as to the pathologic processes that are unfolding. The development of pneumatosis intestinalis (air within the intestinal wall) is thought to be due to gas produced by overgrowth of enteric bacteria.[18] The progression to portal venous or lymphatic gas suggests extension of the process along vessels draining the affected intestine. Pneumoperitoneum indicates necrosis with complete disruption of the intestinal wall.

As greater understanding into the pathophysiology of NEC evolves, a unifying concept is emerging that allows for a working model to understand the many factors that play a role in the pathogenesis of this complex disease. This unifying concept is based on the concept that NEC represents an overexuberant or inappropriate inflammatory response to some type of insult. The nature of this insult is not defined. It may be a global ischemic insult from congenital heart disease, an infectious insult from abnormal bacterial colonization, an insult related to formula feeding or the absence of any enteral feeding, or simply the response of translocation of normal bacterial flora in a genetically predisposed host.

This insult leads to a disruption of the intestinal epithelial barrier, with translocation of bacteria, which subsequently results in an exaggerated or inappropriate response, likely owing to the immature nature of the intestine. Stress pathways become activated, and perhaps even overactivated, whereas pathways that normally suppress the immune system are inhibited. The end result is the activation of the host immune system and the release of circulating cytokines, leading to a global and detrimental inflammatory response.

The Intestinal Barrier

The pathologic features of NEC suggest that failure of the intestinal barrier is crucial in its development. Therefore, an understanding of the critical components of the normal intestinal barrier, and how these components differ in the immature intestine, may lead to a better understanding of the pathogenesis of NEC. The normal intestinal barrier is composed of both mechanical and nonmechanical factors that contribute to its impermeable nature. The mechanical factors include intestinal peristalsis, the mucous coat, and tight junctions between epithelial cells.

Intestinal Motility and Digestion

Intestinal motility normally develops during the third trimester of pregnancy but may not be fully mature until the eighth month of gestation.[19-22] The mechanical action of intestinal motility not only aids in digestion but also serves as the first step in epithelial barrier integrity by limiting the amount of time any substance is in contact with the surface of the enterocytes. In premature infants, the immature intestinal motility leads to an increased exposure of the epithelium to potentially noxious substances with poor clearance of bacteria and subsequent bacterial overgrowth. Additionally, the immature intestine has decreased nutrient digestion and absorption, which may lead to direct epithelial injury through a lowered pH level.[23-25]

Other studies suggest that increased ileal bile acid levels may play a role in the pathogenesis of NEC. The accumulation of bile acids in the intestinal lumen and in enterocytes may be due to immature levels of the ileal bile acid–binding protein, which is crucial for transporting bile acids through the enterocyte and into the portal circulation,[26] as well as suppression of these bile acid transporters by proinflammatory cytokines such as tumor necrosis factor-α (TNF-α).[27-29] Two other risk factors for NEC also may contribute to abnormal bile acid levels. Formula feeding elicits more toxic bile acids than breast feeding,[30] and the formation of secondary bile acids, which have been found in animals with NEC, requires bacterial-induced deconjugation.[31]

The Mucous Coat

The mucous coat overlying the intestinal epithelium plays a key role in the barrier function of the epithelium. The mucous layer is composed of water, mucin, lipids, and peptides, such as trefoil factor.[32] The glycoprotein mucin, as well as the peptide trefoil factor, is secreted by goblet cells interspersed within the epithelial layer.[33-35] Mucin aids in lubrication, mechanical protection, protection against the acidity of gastric and duodenal secretions,[36] and fixation of pathogenic bacteria, viruses, and parasites.[37] The effectiveness of mucin as a protectant is related to the maturity of the mucin,[36] because mature mucins have a higher viscosity, better pH buffering, and resistance to breakdown by bacteria.[36-38] The amount of mucin production, as well as its composition, also changes with gestational age, bacterial challenges, and colonization by commensal organisms.[39] Immaturity of goblet cells may also lead to a deficiency in the production of mucus.[40,41] Deficits in the production or composition of mucin may contribute to the ability of bacteria to invade the intestinal epithelium and thus contribute to the pathogenesis of NEC.[32,42-44]

Tight Junctions

Tight junctions create fusion points between epithelial cells, thus forming an intact barrier that maintains the semipermeable properties of these cells. Mature tight junctions are composed of the transmembrane proteins occludin, claudin, and junctional adhesion protein.[45] Immaturity in the composition of tight junctions likely plays a role in some of the increased permeability of the epithelium in the newborn intestine.[46]

Additionally, cytokines that are produced in response to bacteria and their products, such as lipopolysaccharide, may also interfere with tight junctions, promoting the translocation of bacteria.[47] Inflammatory mediators such as TNF, interferon (IFN)-γ, and interleukin (IL)-1β further cause epithelial dysfunction by upregulating inducible nitric oxide synthase (iNOS), overproducing nitric oxide (NO), and generating the reactive nitrogen intermediate peroxynitrite (ONOO−), which has been associated with increased epithelial cell apoptosis and death.[48] NO has been shown to play a role in mediating the decrease in the localization and expression of tight junction proteins as well as occludin.[49] Disruption of tight junctions by these inflammatory mediators may lead to increased intestinal permeability that gives way to bacterial translocation and the activation of the immune system.

Immunologic Defenses of the Gastrointestinal Tract

The gastrointestinal tract contains the greatest amount of lymphoid tissue in the body and coordinates the immunologic defense mechanisms of both the adaptive and innate immune systems.[50] The gut-associated lymphoid tissue (GALT) consists of lymphocytes, macrophages, dendritic cells, M cells overlying Peyer's patches, and Paneth cells in the crypts. Macrophages and dendritic cells act as the antigen-presenting cells while M cells and epithelial cells may also play a role in presenting antigens to resident lymphocytes.[51]

In neonates, the processing and presenting of antigens is less efficient, thus reducing the ability of the immune system to respond to pathogenic organisms. Peyer's patches are also fewer and smaller and lack germinal centers in preterm infants, thus impairing the systemic and intestinal immune system.[32] Paneth cell activation by bacteria or components of bacterial cell walls leads to secretion of a variety of antibacterial substances, primarily α-defensins, which play an important role in selecting and limiting the growth of both pathologic and commensal bacteria.[52,53] Thus the decreased production of these peptides in premature infants may predispose infants to bacterial overgrowth, allowing NEC to develop.

IgA is normally synthesized by plasma cells of the lamina propria and secreted into the mucin layer where it binds bacteria and viruses so that they cannot attach to the epithelium. Neonates can also obtain IgA through passive transfer from breast milk. The newborn lamina propria is largely devoid of the IgA-secreting plasma cells, which may contribute to the susceptibility of the newborn to mucosal infections.[54,55]

Regenerating the Intestinal Barrier

The pathologic findings of NEC arise not only from alterations in the integrity of the intestinal barrier but also from an impaired ability to regenerate properly.[56] Premature infants have a reduced capacity for intestinal repair, and this may contribute to the pathogenesis of NEC.

Lipopolysaccharide

Lipopolysaccharide (LPS) is the endotoxin portion of the gram-negative bacterial cell wall. It is one of the most abundant proinflammatory stimuli in the gastrointestinal tract and has been seen in high levels in clinical NEC.[18] LPS impairs intestinal barrier function by causing inhibition of intestinal restitution and by promoting the release of signaling molecules such as NO and IFN-γ from enterocytes.[57] LPS increases the activity of signaling molecule RhoA, which leads to an inhibition in cell movement.[56] LPS also causes an increase in the expression and function of integrins on the cell surface, resulting in an increase in cell adhesion to the basement membrane.[58] LPS stimulates the release of proinflammatory cytokines, including NO, IFN-γ, and cyclooxygenase-2 (COX-2), which promote intestinal injury through direct cytopathic effects on the enterocytes.[59,60] LPS also compounds the effects of platelet-activating factor (PAF).[61,62]

Nitric Oxide

NO is a key mediator of numerous physiologic and pathologic systems. Low levels of NO may be important for maintaining vasodilation, but excessive levels of NO can lead to the production of toxic nitrogen intermediates. Thus, NO has competing and dose-dependent roles in intestinal physiology.

NO is a highly reactive free radical formed by the conversion of arginine to citrulline by NO synthase (NOS), of which three isoforms exist.[63] These three isoforms include the constitutive neuronal isoform, nNOS, the inducible isoform, iNOS, and the constitutive endothelial isoform, eNOS. The presence of the constitutive forms of NOS in the gastrointestinal tract suggests that NO has a normal physiologic role in gut function. The constitutive calcium-dependent eNOS isoform maintains intestinal homeostasis by enhancing mucosal blood flow and maintaining microvascular tone and will be discussed later.[64]

Whereas low levels of NO may play a homeostatic role in the gastrointestinal tract, when it is produced by iNOS under inflammatory conditions in high concentrations, NO may lead to cellular damage and failure of the intestinal barrier. Excess NO reacts with superoxide anion (O_2^-) to produce the highly toxic ONOO−, which causes much of the cytopathic damage that is attributed to NO.[65,66] The activities of NO may be compounded in the presence of high levels of LPS, which leads to increased iNOS expression and function within the intestine.[66,67]

Studies have linked NO with the pathogenesis of NEC. The expression of iNOS has been shown to be upregulated in critically ill patients and in patients with NEC.[48,68] NO may also inhibit intestinal restitution by blocking enterocyte migration.[57,69]

Platelet-Activating Factor

PAF is an endogenous phospholipid mediator of inflammation that is produced by inflammatory, endothelial, and lamina propria cells.[70] PAF has a short half-life and is regulated by the PAF-degrading enzyme acetyl hydrolase (PAF-AH). The cytotoxic effects of PAF are likely due to reactive oxygen radical formation. PAF-induced bowel injury is associated with the production of oxygen-derived free radicals and with neutrophil migration, activation, and capillary leakage.[71]

Various studies have shown the importance of PAF in the pathogenesis of NEC. Higher concentrations of PAF have been found circulating in NEC patients compared with age- and disease-matched controls.[72,73] PAF-AH activity has been shown to be deficient in sick infants with NEC, and the administration of PAF-AH in animal models of NEC reduces the degree of intestinal injury.[72,74]

Maintaining Intestinal Barrier Homeostasis

Epidermal Growth Factor

Epidermal growth factor (EGF) plays an important role in the development, maturation, and maintenance of gut homeostasis.[75-80] Additionally, EGF is important in the prevention and treatment of inflammatory conditions. EGF enemas given to patients with left-sided colitis have been shown to be effective treatment, resulting in significant improvement in the scoring of disease activity and histologic grading of injury compared with controls treated with a placebo.[81]

Other studies have shown that EGF has a role in adaptive bowel regeneration after intestinal loss. After 50% small bowel resection in mice, salivary EGF levels were increased with increased enterocyte receptor (EGFR) activity, which is the receptor on which EGF acts.[82] Sialoadenectomy before bowel resection resulted in an inhibition of this response, but exogenous EGF administration resulted in rescue.[83] Mice with a dysfunctional EGFR have an impaired adaptation response, whereas those with overexpression of EGFR or stimulation of EGFR have improved adaptation.[84-88]

EGF is believed to play an important role in the pathogenesis of NEC. Decreased levels of EGF have been demonstrated in the saliva and serum of premature infants with NEC.[89] Furthermore, additional studies have shown that salivary levels of EGF in the first 2 weeks of preterm life may have a predictive value for the occurrence of NEC.[90] Mice that are unable to express EGFR either die in utero or shortly after birth from hemorrhagic enteritis that closely resembles NEC in humans.[91] A potentially therapeutic role for EGF was reported on an infant suffering from intestinal necrosis resembling NEC who received a continuous infusion of EGF that resulted in the complete recovery of the damaged intestine.[92] These investigators subsequently treated a small group of neonates with stage II and III NEC in a randomized, double-blind, prospective trial with recombinant EGF and found that repair of the intestinal epithelium was seen at 4, 7, and 14 days, as inferred from rectal biopsy specimens.[93] One limitation of this study, however, is the extrapolation of changes in the distal colon to the upper intestine.

EGF may also have a role as a potential preventive strategy for NEC. In a mouse model of NEC, supplementation with EGF has been shown to decrease the incidence of NEC, downregulate the production of inflammatory cytokines, and decrease apoptosis at the site of injury.[94-96] The enteral administration of EGF appears to decrease the overproduction of the proinflammatory mediator IL-18 and increase production of the anti-inflammatory cytokine IL-10 in the ileum.[48] Therefore, EGF may have a protective effect by altering the balance of these pro- and anti-inflammatory cytokines in the pathogenesis of NEC. EGF may also play a role in decreasing bacterial translocation from the intestine, another key factor in the pathogenesis of NEC.

Neonatal Vasculature and the Pathogenesis of NEC

The newborn intestinal circulation is characterized by a low resting vascular resistance, particularly in comparison with older subjects.[97,98] This results in a relative increase in blood flow and oxygen delivery. The control of this vascular resistance involves both intrinsic and extrinsic control mechanisms.[99] The extrinsic mechanisms are mediated by the autonomic nervous system. The intrinsic regulation is mediated by two vascular effector mechanisms produced and released within the intestine–one vasoconstrictive and one vasodilatory.[100,101] Endothelin (ET)-1 is the primary vasoconstrictor stimulus in the newborn intestine and is produced by the endothelium.[102,103] Although constitutively produced, it can also be stimulated by decreased flow, hypoxia, and various inflammatory cytokines.[104-106] The production of ET-1 is age specific, being greater in younger subjects.[102]

NO is the primary vasodilator stimulus in the newborn intestinal circulation.[97,98] eNOS is also continuously produced, but like ET-1 the rate of production can be increased in response to a variety of stimuli.[100] In the neonate, the balance of these two products favors vasodilation due to an increased production of NO, thus generating the characteristic low vascular resistance. In pathologic states, however, endothelial dysfunction leads to ET-1– mediated vasoconstriction, which can cause compromised blood flow, intestinal ischemia, and injury (Fig. 34-1). The vasoconstrictor ET-1 has been linked to intestinal tissue injury in several studies.[102,107] Increased expression of ET-1 has been found in intestine removed from infants with NEC, and the amount of ET-1 increased proportionally to the degree of intestinal injury.[101]

In summary, the intestinal circulation of the newborn is unique, with a dynamic balance between constrictor (ET-1) and dilator (NO) stimuli maintaining basal vascular resistance. Disruption of the intestinal endothelial function can alter the delicate balance, favoring ET-1–dependent vasoconstriction over the normal state of vasodilation, leading to significant intestinal ischemia and tissue injury.

Bacterial Colonization

NEC most commonly is diagnosed during the second week of life, after intestinal colonization has been established. Therefore, bacteria likely play a role in the pathogenesis of NEC. Not attributable to a single infectious agent, NEC more likely arises from an unfavorable balance between commensal and pathogenic bacteria.

Abnormal colonization may alter the balance of pathogenic and beneficial bacteria, favoring an increase in pathogenic bacteria and resulting in a loss of the beneficial role of commensal bacteria. This could lead to an increase in the inflammatory response due to a loss of the inhibition that commensal bacteria provide. Furthermore, the immature immune system of premature infants may not be able to respond appropriately to normal colonization of bacteria, much less abnormal flora.[108]

CLINICAL DIAGNOSIS

The diagnosis of NEC is based on clinical findings as well as characteristic radiographic findings. The clinical course can vary from a slow, indolent process to

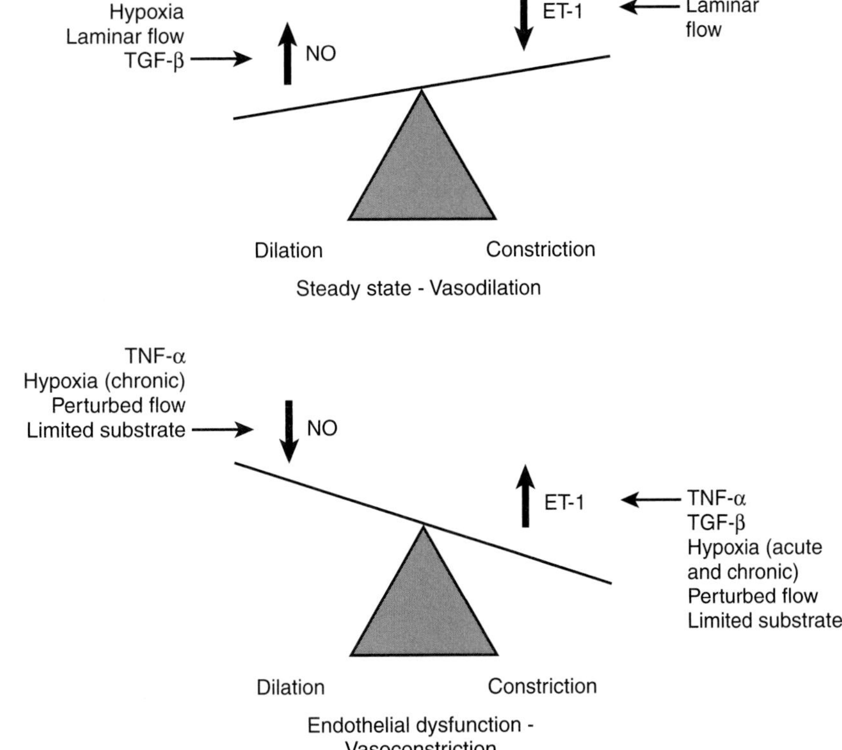

Figure 34-1. Characterization of the dynamic balance between nitric oxide (NO) and endothelin-1 (ET-1) in determining intestinal vascular resistance in the newborn. Many exogenous stimuli play a role in the regulation of NO and ET-1. Under steady-state conditions, the balance heavily favors vasodilation secondary to the copious production of endothelium-derived NO. However, endothelial dysfunction would alter the balance, thus favoring ET-1–mediated vasoconstriction leading to ischemia and tissue injury.

one that progresses rapidly to death in a few hours. Early signs are nonspecific, including apnea, bradycardia, lethargy, and temperature instability. Feeding intolerance, demonstrated by high gastric residuals, and occasionally bilious vomiting, is the most common gastrointestinal symptom of NEC. The most common presenting sign is abdominal distention. Gross or occult blood in the stool may be found.

The gastrointestinal signs progress from initial abdominal distention to tenderness suggestive of peritoneal irritation. Palpable loops of intestine may become evident as the ileus worsens. Localized disease may progress to generalized peritonitis or may worsen in a focal area with evidence of severe disease, including discoloration or ecchymotic changes of the skin and the presence of an abdominal mass (Fig. 34-2). When they are present, the findings of a fixed abdominal mass and erythema of the abdominal wall are strongly predictive of NEC. However, these findings are present in only 10% of patients with NEC.[109] Ascites may also become evident on physical examination as the disease progresses. A sudden need for increased ventilatory support that cannot otherwise be explained may also serve as a harbinger of NEC.[110] This is due to increased metabolic requirements in combination with increased intra-abdominal pressure.

Confirmation of the diagnosis of NEC combines the signs and symptoms described earlier with radiologic findings that are described later. All of the findings have been combined into the clinical staging system proposed by Bell that aids in describing the severity of disease (Table 34-2).[111,112]

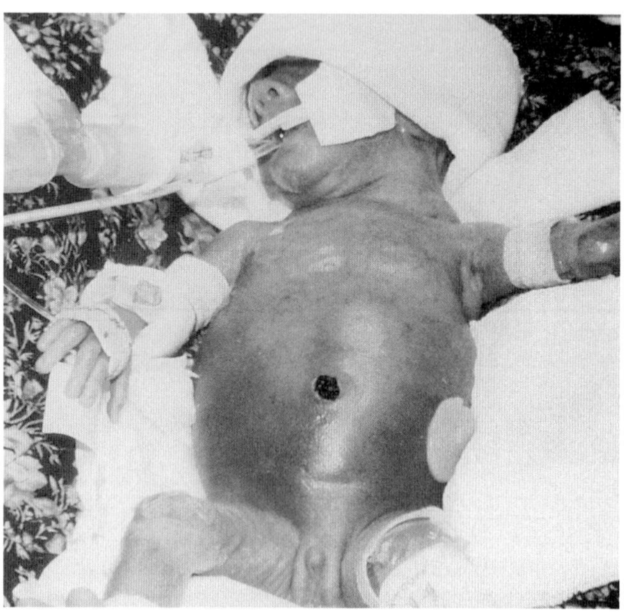

Figure 34-2. An infant with NEC. Note the abdominal wall ecchymosis extending from the suprapubic region to above the umbilicus and laterally to the flanks.

Laboratory Studies

Laboratory studies reveal nonspecific indicators of an inflammatory or infectious process such as leukocytosis with bandemia. Thrombocytopenia and metabolic acidosis are also common. A rapid fall in platelet count is a poor prognostic factor.[113]

Several studies have tried to identify an accurate biochemical marker that might identify neonates who are at risk for NEC, thus avoiding prolonged periods without enteral nutrition as well as the use of unnecessary tests and antibiotics.[114] Serum acute phase proteins and cytokines have been investigated for an association with high levels and the severity of a course of NEC. Increased levels of IL-6, IL-10, and C-reactive protein (CRP) have been documented in premature infants with NEC, with the highest levels of IL-10 in those patients who did not survive.[115] CRP has also been associated with NEC when the levels rose quickly after the diagnosis was suspected. A failure of the levels to return to normal was also associated with complications, including abscesses, strictures, and sepsis.[116] In a prospective study, CRP levels were elevated in infants with stage II and III NEC and might

Table 34-2 Modified Bell's Staging for NEC

Stage	Clinical Findings	Radiographic Findings	Gastrointestinal Findings
I—Suspected	Apnea, bradycardia, temperature instability	Gas pattern of mild ileus	Increased gastric residuals, occult blood in stool, mild abdominal distention
IIa—Definite	Apnea, bradycardia, temperature instability	Ileus gas pattern with one or more dilated loops, focal pneumatosis	Grossly bloody stools, prominent abdominal distention, absent bowel sounds
IIb	Thrombocytopenia, mild metabolic acidosis	Widespread pneumatosis, ascites, portal venous gas	Abdominal wall edema with palpable loops and tenderness
IIIa—Advanced	Mixed acidosis, oliguria, hypotension, coagulopathy	Prominent bowel loops, worsening ascites, no free air	Worsening wall edema, erythema and induration
IIIb	Shock, deterioration in laboratory values and vital signs	Pneumoperitoneum	Perforated bowel

be useful in discriminating between stage II NEC and other gastrointestinal disorders.[117]

Activation of the Thomson-Friedenreich cryptantigen (TCA), a naturally occurring antigen on red blood cells, occurs when *N*-acetyl neuraminic acid is cleaved from a bacterially produced neuraminidase. Such activation, in the setting of NEC, is diagnostic of the involvement of neuraminidase-producing anaerobic organisms and correlates with the severity of disease.[113]

Multiple other potential markers have been studied–gastrointestinal tonometry, urinary D-lactate levels, exhaled breath hydrogen, endotoxin elevations in stool, plasma intestinal fatty acid binding proteins–but none of these has yielded the sensitivity or specificity required for a diagnostic tool.[58,118-120] Currently, no biochemical markers have been adequately predictive of the patient's clinical course or outcome to be clinically useful.

Radiographic Findings

Radiography

The cornerstone of the radiographic diagnosis of NEC relies on standard anteroposterior and cross-table lateral or left lateral decubitus radiographs. The most specific radiographic finding is pneumatosis intestinalis, either cystic or linear, as seen in Figure 34-3. Other radiographic findings that are often found include air-fluid levels, gas-filled loops of bowel, persistently dilated loops of bowel, thickened bowel walls, portal venous gas, and pneumoperitoneum. Although most commonly seen in NEC, pneumatosis intestinalis has also been reported in cases of Hirschsprung's enterocolitis, severe diarrhea, and carbohydrate intolerance. Portal venous gas (Fig. 34-4) is a less common radiographic finding but is generally considered a poor prognostic sign. Several studies have noted a high incidence of diffuse or "pan" necrosis associated with portal venous gas and a high associated mortality rate. Nevertheless, many patients with portal venous gas recover fully with medical management.

Other Imaging Modalities

Although plain radiography is the current standard for diagnosing and evaluating NEC, recent studies have examined ultrasonography as an adjunctive measure for the diagnosis and management of infants with NEC. Abdominal ultrasound evaluation emerged as a potential modality in the treatment of NEC after a report in 2005 that assessed bowel viability using color Doppler imaging in neonates with NEC.[121,122] This publication established critical data for bowel wall thickness, echogenicity, peristalsis, and perfusion in both normal neonates and those with NEC. Additional studies corroborated the usefulness of ultrasonography as a means of diagnosing NEC.[122,123] Ultrasonography offers some potential advantages over radiography in that it can depict bowel wall thickness and echogenicity, free and focal fluid collections, peristalsis, and the presence or absence of bowel wall perfusion by using Doppler imaging.[124-126]

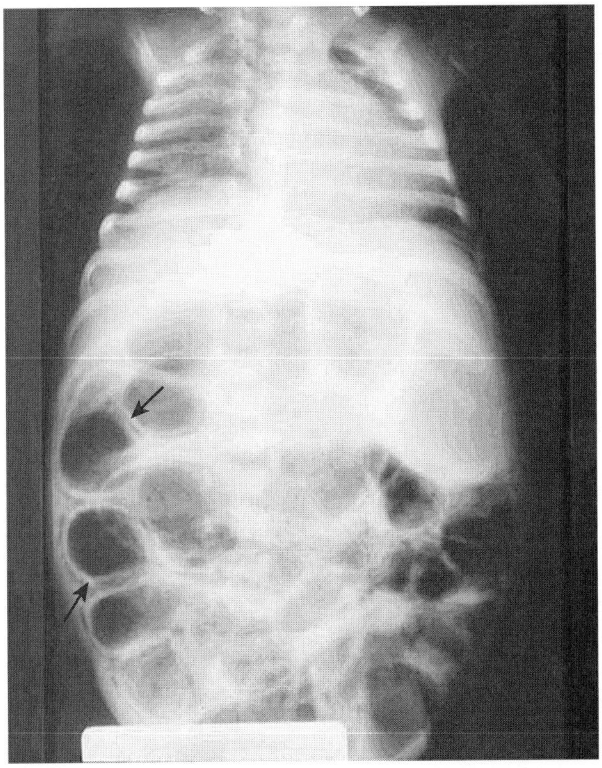

Figure 34-3. Pneumatosis intestinalis (*arrows*) is seen on this abdominal radiograph.

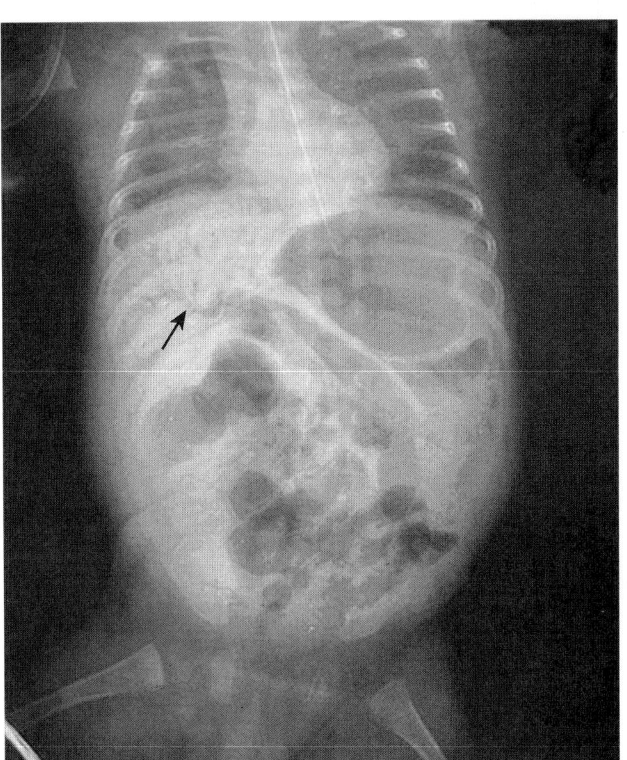

Figure 34-4. Portal venous gas (*arrow*) is seen on this radiograph.

The presence of pneumatosis on plain abdominal radiographs helps clinch the diagnosis in cases of suspected NEC. However, in the setting of nonspecific, possibly mild findings and radiographs without intramural gas, the diagnosis may be more difficult. Abdominal ultrasonography may be a useful adjunct in this population because it may be able to detect small amounts of intramural gas not visible on plain films or changes in bowel wall thickness, peristalsis, or perfusion that could confirm or exclude the diagnosis of NEC.[127] The time frame for when to perform ultrasonography initially or when to use it during follow-up has not been established.

In addition to assisting with the diagnosis in difficult cases as just described, ultrasound evaluation has been suggested as an adjunct modality in two other groups of patients: those in whom the evolution of changes in the radiographs does not match the clinical course and those whose condition is deteriorating without evidence of pneumatosis on plain films.[127] Finally, some have suggested that ultrasonography may be useful in helping to decide the appropriate time to re-initiate and advance feeding.[122] At this time, ultrasonography does not yet have a well-defined or established role in the management of NEC.

Contrast examinations of the gastrointestinal tract in the acute setting, computed tomography, and magnetic resonance imaging have not been found to be clinically useful modalities in clinical practice in treating infants with NEC.[128-132]

DIFFERENTIAL DIAGNOSIS

The most clinically relevant differential diagnosis in a premature infant with abdominal distention is distinguishing between NEC and sepsis with ileus. In the absence of clinical signs of peritonitis or radiographic signs of NEC, the two conditions may well be clinically indistinguishable and only differentiated after observing the course of the disease. The differential diagnosis also includes other conditions that may cause abdominal distention, including Hirschsprung's disease, ileal atresia, volvulus, meconium ileus, and intussusception.

A subset of premature infants presents with bowel perforation while not exhibiting any other symptomatology of NEC nor pneumatosis on radiographs. Some investigators have defined this as spontaneous, isolated, or focal intestinal perforation (FIP). FIP tends to occur in extremely low birth weight infants, very early in life (usually the first 7-10 days), and sometimes in association with indomethacin treatment.[133-139] Whether these infants have a "limited" form of NEC or a distinct entity is controversial. Some reports contend that FIP is a different disease than NEC, but definitive evidence is lacking.[138-141] As expected, neonates with a bowel perforation have better outcomes in the absence of extensive disease.[137,142,143] Increasing recognition of the differences between these entities may warrant an improved classification of neonatal intestinal diseases and new criteria for their description.[144]

MEDICAL MANAGEMENT

Medical management of NEC begins with the suspicion of disease. Infants are initially treated with bowel rest, gastric decompression, intravenous fluid resuscitation, and broad-spectrum antibiotic therapy, including anaerobic coverage. Blood, urine, and sputum cultures should be obtained before the initiation of antibiotic therapy. Adjunctive therapy such as cardiovascular support with pressors, pulmonary support with oxygen and ventilation, and hematologic support with the transfusion of blood products may all be necessary. A critical component of medical management is ongoing close observation with serial abdominal examinations and serial radiographs. As long as the clinical situation is stable or improving, expectant management can continue. Clinical deterioration or worsening radiographic features may indicate the need to consider surgical intervention.

Experimental Medical Treatments—Heparin-Binding EGF

Heparin-binding EGF-like growth factor (HB-EGF) is a member of the EGF family. Endogenous HB-EGF is increased in response to hypoxia, stress, and during wound healing.[145-150] HB-EGF mRNA is induced after intestinal ischemia/reperfusion injury in vivo[151] and is involved in epithelial cell repair, proliferation, and regeneration in the early stages after injury.[152] Based on these findings that endogenous HB-EGF is involved in the promotion of healing, it has been theorized that exogenous HB-EGF may also play a role protecting the intestinal mucosa from injury.

Multiple studies have demonstrated that exogenous administration of HB-EGF can protect cells and organs from injury both in vitro and in vivo. HB-EGF can protect enterocytes from proinflammatory cytokine-induced apoptosis[153] and renal tubule cells from acute oxidant-induced apoptosis.[154] Intestinal epithelial cells pretreated with HB-EGF before hypoxia showed less necrosis with maintenance of the cytoskeletal structure and improved recovery ability.[155] HB-EGF also downregulates the production of NO[156,157] and blocks (NF-κB) activation in intestinal epithelial cells after cytokine stimulation.[157] In a neonatal rat model of NEC, the administration of HB-EGF reduced the severity and incidence of NEC with preservation of gut barrier integrity.[158] These findings were consistent with studies showing EGF reducing the severity and incidence of NEC, decreasing the overproduction of IL-18 and increasing the production of anti-inflammatory IL-10.[159] HB-EGF is the only compound with imminent plans for investigation in humans. A host of other therapeutic agents have shown promise but not yet reached the stage of clinical testing.

Surgical Management

Although many infants can be managed medically, 20% to 40% will require surgical intervention. In some cases, indication for operation develops during observation, while in others it is found at presentation. The only absolute indication for surgical intervention is evidence of intestinal perforation either on abdominal radiograph or via paracentesis that is positive for stool or bile.[160] Relative indications for surgical intervention include deterioration of the infant's clinical condition despite maximal medical management. Findings can include oliguria, hypotension, worsening metabolic acidosis, worsening thrombocytopenia, leukopenia or leukocytosis, and ventilatory failure. Radiographic relative indicators for surgical intervention include portal venous gas or persistently abnormal "fixed" loops of bowel on serial radiographs.

Ideally, surgical intervention would occur when intestinal gangrene is imminent but before actual perforation or necrosis occurs. However, this theoretical ideal time for intervention has been difficult to identify; thus, perforation has consistently been considered the only absolute indication for surgery. One study has tried to evaluate the sensitivity and specificity of 12 different findings in an attempt to identify earlier indicators for surgery.[109] Three findings had specificity and a positive predictive value (PPV) close to 100% with prevalence greater than 10%. These were deemed "best" indications and included pneumoperitoneum, portal venous gas, and positive paracentesis (Table 34-3). Three indicators had specificity and PPV close to 100% but prevalence less than 10%. These indicators were, therefore, considered "good" and included a fixed loop on abdominal radiograph, erythema of the abdominal wall, and a palpable abdominal mass. One indicator, severe pneumatosis, was deemed "fair" because it had a specificity and PPV above 90% and 20% prevalence. The five remaining indicators were considered "poor" because the specificities were less than 90% and the PPVs less than 80%. This probability analysis can be used to assist in the complex decision-making process of when surgical intervention is warranted.

NEC can affect any segment of the gastrointestinal tract. Most commonly, both large and small bowel are involved.[17] Isolated small intestinal lesions occur with the next greatest frequency. It is as common to have a single affected area as to have multiple-segment disease.[17,161,162] A small subgroup of NEC patients may have massive necrosis of the entire intestine, known as "NEC totalis."[161]

Traditional surgical management has consisted either of laparotomy with limited resection of the affected bowel and the creation of stomas or of peritoneal drainage. Much of the attention of surgical investigators of NEC has focused on the relative benefits of these procedures.

Peritoneal drainage was first reported in 1977 as a salvage treatment for perforation in VLBW infants who were believed to be too unstable for laparotomy (Fig. 34-5).[163] Initially, this strategy was intended as a temporizing procedure in the sickest and smallest patients. However, it rapidly evolved into a widely utilized option for primary treatment of perforated NEC. After many years of conflicting results comparing outcomes of the two approaches, a meta-analysis was attempted to synthesize these disparate data into a treatment recommendation. This study found such significant bias in the assignment of patients to one treatment or another that the techniques could not be adequately or effectively compared.[164] A need existed for a prospective randomized controlled trial.

Three prospective studies have recently evaluated laparotomy and peritoneal drainage to determine which surgical procedure is associated with better outcomes. The NICHD Neonatal Research Network conducted a prospective observational cohort study at 16 centers.[165] In this study, 156 infants with either NEC or FIP underwent either laparotomy or drainage. Overall 50% (n = 78) of the patients died and 72% (n = 112) either died or had some element of neurologic impairment at 18 to 22 months. The patients in this study were not randomized to their treatment groups. The treating surgeons and neonatologists chose which therapy to use for each infant. However, unlike other nonrandomized studies, extensive prospective data were collected, allowing for risk-adjusted

Table 34-3 Probability Analysis of Various Indications for Operation in NEC (%)

Indication	Sensitivity	Specificity	PPV	NPV	Prevalence
Pneumoperitoneum	48	100	100	52	31
Portal venous gas	24	100	100	43	16
Fixed loop (on radiograph)	12.5	100	100	46	7
Fixed abdominal mass	12.5	100	100	46	7
Erythema of abdomen	8	100	100	45	5
Positive paracentesis*	87	100	97	60	72
Severe pneumatosis	31	94	91	43	20
Clinical deterioration	39	89	78	59	25
Platelet count < 10^5	38	83	73	54	28
Severe gastrointestinal hemorrhage	12	83	50	42	14
Abdominal tenderness	29	72	58	43	29
Gasless abdomen/ascites	0	94	0	41	2

PPV, positive predictive value; NPV, negative predictive value.
*Positive paracentesis was defined as brown fluid and/or bacteria noted on Gram stain.
From Kosloske AM: Indications for operation in necrotizing enterocolitis revisited. J Pediatr Surg 29:663-666, 1994.

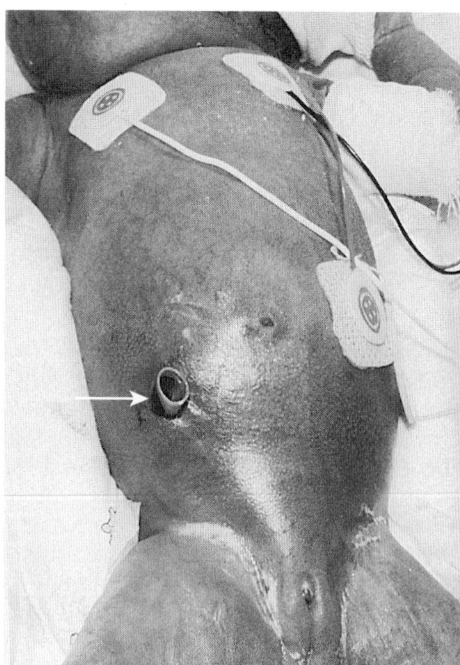
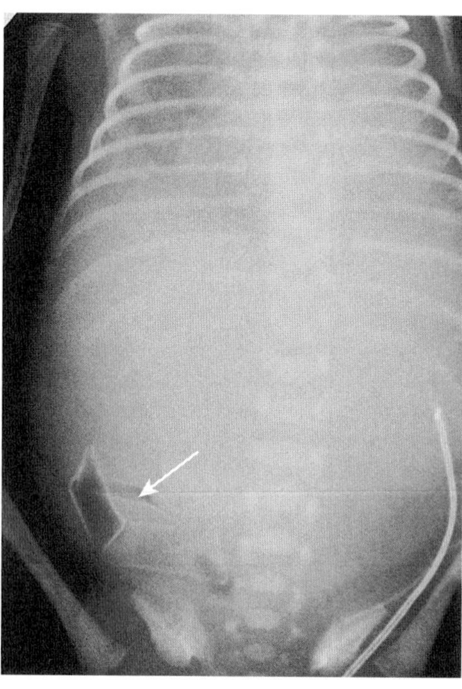

Figure 34-5. A micropremature infant with NEC and perforation is shown with her corresponding abdominal radiograph. A percutaneous drain (*arrows*) has been placed in the right lower quadrant for drainage of the intestinal perforation. Note that the drain is placed at a position below the level of the umbilicus to avoid injury to the lower edge of the right lobe of the liver.

multivariable regression analyses to be performed. This strategy enabled the investigators to account for the differences between the treatment groups. The odds ratio for death after adjusting for differences in the two treatment groups was 0.97 for laparotomy compared with peritoneal drainage (95% confidence interval [CI]: 0.43-2.20). The odds ratio for the combined outcome of death or neurodevelopmental impairment at 18 to 22 months was 0.44 for laparotomy compared with drainage (95% CI: 0.16-1.2). Although not statistically significant, there is some suggestion in this study that overall outcomes at 18 to 22 months of age may be improved by laparotomy rather than drainage.

The first randomized trial evaluating laparotomy versus peritoneal drainage was the NECSTEPS trial.[166] In this trial, 117 VLBW infants at 15 North American tertiary care centers were randomized to either treatment group. The primary outcome variable was mortality at 90 days. There was no difference in mortality at 90 days between the two treatment groups (34.5% vs. 35.5%) (Fig. 34-6). Secondary outcomes were the need for parenteral nutrition at 90 days and the length of hospitalization and were also similar between the two groups. This study only focused on short-term outcomes. However, within those limits, the results suggest that the method of surgical intervention does not impact the outcome.

A second randomized trial comparing laparotomy and peritoneal drainage in infants with perforated NEC has also been completed.[167] The NET trial was a multinational trial conducted at 31 centers in 13 countries. The primary outcome variable was mortality at 1 and 6 months. Sixty-nine patients weighing less than 1000 g were enrolled and randomized. There was a trend toward better survival in the laparotomy group (65% survival) compared with the drainage group (51%), with a relative risk of mortality of 0.5 (95% CI: 0.2-1.5). These findings were not statistically significant, with a P value of 0.2, but the sample size does limit their power to detect a difference. The authors concluded that there was no evidence from the trial to support the benefit of primary peritoneal drainage in extremely LBW infants with intestinal perforation.

Overall, both of these randomized trials suggest that the method of surgical management does not affect the ultimate outcome of infants with perforated NEC. The impact of choice of operation on the outcome of infants who underwent operation for an indication other than perforation is not known. Most commonly, these infants are treated with laparotomy.

When laparotomy is performed, stomas are usually created. Because of concerns about the high morbidity associated with enterostomies, a few centers have advocated primary anastomosis at the time of initial laparotomy. The data, however, to support such management are nonrandomized and retrospective. In actuality, the majority of stomal complications are easily managed and early closure is well tolerated.[168] One study found that survival was 72% with intestinal diversion but only 48% in those undergoing primary anastomosis.[169]

Diffuse intestinal involvement poses the most difficult situation for the surgeon. Those infants who survive may develop short bowel syndrome and have some level of dependency on total parenteral nutrition given the extensive amount of affected bowel. Surgical strategies focus on trying to preserve as much intestine as possible while still resecting enough bowel to stabilize the patient. Second-look laparotomies have been proposed as a way to minimize the amount of bowel resected.[170] The "clip and drop back" technique is another option with a similar strategy.[171] All nonviable

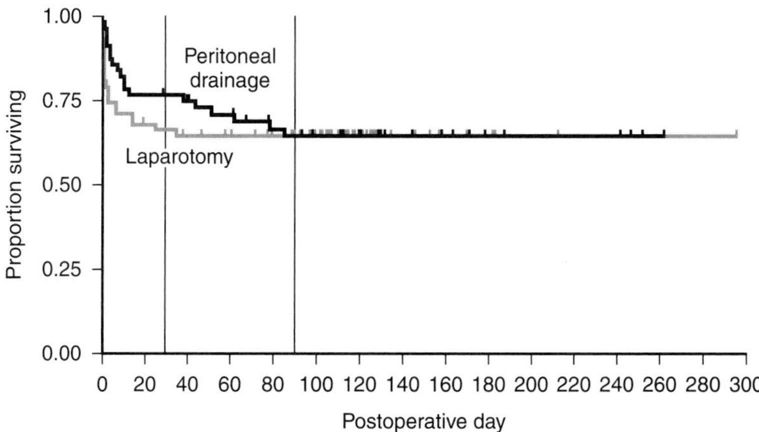

Figure 34-6. Survival outcomes of patients treated by laparotomy and peritoneal drainage in the NECSTEPS trial. There was no difference in mortality at 90 days between the two treatment groups.

intestine is resected initially but no ostomies or anastomoses are created. Blind-ending segments are left in the abdomen, and continuity is restored or ostomies are created on re-exploration in 48 to 72 hours. Proximal diversion alone has also been used to treat "pan" necrosis without reported worsened survival and with recovery of much of the bowel by the time of ostomy closure.[172] However, none of these approaches has been prospectively evaluated. Thus, no single technique can be strongly advocated.

OUTCOMES

Recurrence

Recurrence can occur after NEC, although the incidence is low, only occurring about 5% of the time.[173,174] There is no apparent correlation between the site of disease and the site of recurrence. Usually recurrent disease can be managed nonoperatively.[160,174-179]

Length of Hospitalization

Hospital stays are longer for infants who suffer from NEC when compared with other infants of the same gestational age. Furthermore, those who require surgical intervention tend to have even longer and more expensive hospitalization. Multiple studies have shown hospital stays averaging 2 to 3 months for medically treated NEC and 4 to 5 months for surgically treated NEC.[180-182] There was no difference in length of hospitalization between the two treatment groups in the NECSTEPS trial.[166]

Mortality

Estimates of mortality from NEC have remained steady over the past 2 decades at 15% to 30% despite the fact that the postsurfactant era has led to a rise in the incidence of disease.[3,4,7-10,180,181,183,184] Surgical mortality has seen improvement though, with a decline from 70% mortality in the 1960s[185] to more recent rates of 20% to 50%.[4,8,10,180,183,186,187] The main predictor of mortality in NEC is gestational age. As mentioned previously, the highest mortality occurs in the youngest, smallest infants and black male VLBW infants are at greatest risk. Additionally, infants with a greater extent of bowel affected by the disease tend to also have a higher mortality rate.[188,189] Patients who were discharged from their primary hospitalization had more than an 80% chance of long-term survival.[180]

Gastrointestinal Outcomes

Short Bowel Syndrome

NEC is the leading disease responsible for short bowel syndrome in children, accounting for half of all pediatric cases. Furthermore, short bowel syndrome develops in a fourth of all patients who suffer from NEC.[190] This condition develops when an infant is left with inadequate intestine to absorb enteral nutrients that are required for growth. Inadequate intestine can result from the extent of the resection at the time of operation or from poor function of the remaining intestine. Traditional teaching based on early reports has suggested that a minimum of 40 cm of small intestine is required for a patient to have a chance of weaning from total parenteral nutrition.[191] Despite these observations, experience has shown that the functional outcome is much more important to this disease rather than the specific length of intestine.

The portion of intestine resected is also important for subsequent gastrointestinal functioning. Patients with ileal or jejunal disease have a higher mortality rate than those with colonic disease.[187,188,192,193] Patients with extensive jejunal resection fare better than those with extensive ileal resection. These outcomes are due to the differing abilities of the intestinal regions to undergo adaptation. The ileum has the greatest capacity to undergo adaptive changes and increase its absorptive capacity. Therefore, infants who undergo jejunal resection but retain their ileum are much better off compared with those who have an ileal resection.

Preservation of the ileocecal valve has been considered important for minimizing the risk of short bowel syndrome.[194] Some studies have suggested that dependence on parenteral nutrition is lessened when

Table 34-4 Options for Enterostomy Formation

Type of Stoma
End stoma, single opening
Double-barrel (Mikulicz) stoma
End stoma with anastomosis below abdominal wall
Loop stoma over a small catheter or skin bridge
Exit of Stoma and Mucous Fistula
Through celiotomy incision
Through separate opening
Proximal and distal limbs together
Proximal and distal limbs separated
Multiple stomas

Table 34-5 Enterostomal Complications

Enterostomal Complications
Prolapse
Stricture
Retraction
Wound separation or dehiscence
Wound infection
Parastomal hernia
Intestinal obstruction
Intestinal torsion
Fistula formation
Skin excoriation, candidiasis, dermatitis
Electrolyte imbalance
Dehydration

the ileocecal valve was preserved,[195-198] but others have found no difference.[180,199-202] Recent data suggest that the actual length and functional capacity of the remaining ileum is far more important than the presence of the valve itself.

Stoma Complications

Creation of a properly constructed stoma can be lifesaving in the management of NEC. Stomas are used for both decompression and diversion. However, enterostomies can also be fraught with early and late complications. Thus, a number of strategies have been proposed for optimal stoma creation, including what type of stoma to create as well as how to exteriorize the stoma (Table 34-4). End stomas, double-barrel (Mikulicz) stomas, and a loop enterostomy have all been advocated. However, small studies comparing complication rates between these various strategies have not found differences in complications, including retraction, prolapse, hernias, or wound infections.[203-205] Many surgeons bring the stoma and mucous fistula out through the surgical incision, some at one end, others at opposite ends of the incision. Others advocate a separate incision, citing concerns about increased incidences of wound infection. Another consideration for a separate incision is whether the stoma needs to remain for a prolonged period of time.[203] Most surgeons do not recommend maturing a stoma owing to potential interference with an already tenuous blood supply.[203]

Stomal complications of both the small and large intestine can lead to significant morbidity (Table 34-5). Studies have shown complication rates exceeding 50%.[187,206-209] The most serious complications include prolapse, stricture, and retraction, all of which may require surgical intervention. Proximal jejunostomies can cause significant electrolyte and fluid losses that can lead to problems with fluid balance and weight gain.[194,210] Furthermore, fluid losses from jejunostomies can cause peristomal skin complications. However, with an aggressive approach to fluid and electrolyte replacement and meticulous skin care, proximal jejunostomies can be a viable option for the management of NEC.[194,211]

The timing of enterostomy closure remains controversial. Recommendations vary from as early as 1 month to as late as 4 months after surgery.[212-215] Most suggest waiting 1 to 2 months after the initial operation, and until a weight of 2000 g is reached, as long as adequate feeding and growth is being maintained.[194,210,213] Earlier closure may be necessary with very proximal stomas due to fluid and electrolyte losses and inability to gain weight. Coexisting medical problems must also be considered in determining the optimal time to closure.

Intestinal Strictures

Intestinal strictures are a common occurrence after both medically and surgically managed NEC. The incidence of stricture formation has been reported from 12% to 35%.[130,207,216-221] This incidence does not differ between patients treated by primary anastomosis or enterostomies.[160,186,187,199,206,207,212,215-227] In one series of patients treated for severe NEC by proximal diverting enterostomy, the incidence was 55%.[217] Most post-NEC strictures occur in the colon, specifically the left colon (Fig. 34-7).[161,212,219,226,228]

Resection of strictures is standard management, although not all lesions are symptomatic and spontaneous resolution has been reported.[130,224,229,230] Therefore, other approaches have been proposed, including close radiographic follow-up of asymptomatic patients.[130] Balloon catheter dilatation has also been tried for focal, nonobstructing lesions, although this technique has not been studied in a large number of patients.[230]

Patients who have been treated by laparotomy and stoma creation for NEC should undergo routine imaging of the distal intestine before enterostomy closure to evaluate for a possible stricture. However, patients managed medically, by peritoneal drainage, or with primary anastomosis may also develop strictures. Some patients remain asymptomatic and others present acutely in distress due to perforation.[219] Cautionary tales of these acute incidences presenting after completion of medical treatment have led some surgeons to advocate routine contrast studies in these NEC patients.[130,218,219,221] However, the potential for

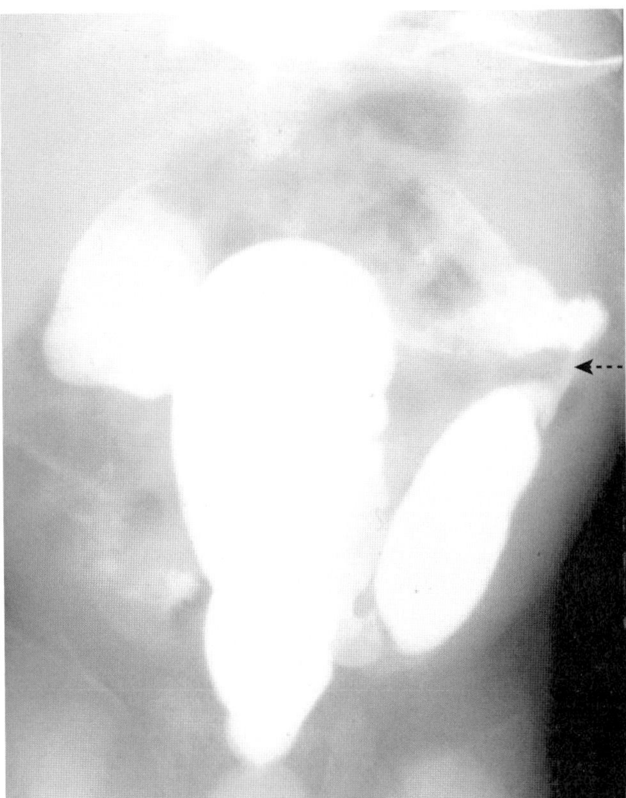

Figure 34-7. This contrast enema demonstrates a stricture in the left colon (*arrow*) after medical treatment for NEC.

false-negative results and the invasiveness of the procedure prevent this practice from being common.

Despite a relatively high incidence of stricture formation after NEC, little evidence exists regarding the impact of this complication on long-term outcomes. For those infants requiring ostomy closure, strictures can usually be addressed at that time. For those managed without ostomies initially, stricture resection requires a new operation with subsequent prolongation of recovery and time to full enteral feeding. Resection of additional bowel may also ultimately impact gastrointestinal functional outcomes.

Growth

Impaired growth rates may be a long-term problem after NEC. Several small observational studies have shown that children treated for NEC fall below the 50th percentile for height and weight even into their grade-school years.[231-233] Although not all studies have had the same findings,[234,235] this growth retardation seems particularly to affect those who suffered from stage III NEC. Additionally, the problem is much more severe in those children who develop short bowel syndrome as a result of NEC. Long-term evaluations of growth are required to evaluate the impact that birth weight, NEC severity, operative strategy, and subsequent outcomes may play in ultimate growth outcomes for these children.

Neurodevelopmental Outcomes

In infants surviving NEC, adverse neurodevelopmental outcomes remain an important challenge. Concerns were first raised in a groundbreaking study in 1980 that reported that less than half of children surviving NEC were neurodevelopmentally normal at 3-year follow up.[236] Subsequently, multiple observational studies have cited "intellectual delays,"[237] "moderate-to-severe developmental delay with speech and motor impairment,"[183] "developmental delay requiring special educational classes,"[231] and delays in "locomotor," "hearing and speech," "intellectual performance" and "personal and social" skills.[234]

A large multicenter cohort study from the NICHD Neonatal Research Network evaluated neurodevelopmental outcomes in 1100 extremely low birth weight survivors.[238] This study confirmed that NEC is associated with increased odds of having a delayed score on psychomotor developmental assessment as well as increased odds of cerebral palsy. This study found that almost all of these abnormalities occurred in patients with surgically treated NEC.[239]

Two systematic reviews have confirmed these findings of an increased risk of neurodevelopmental impairment in VLBW infants who develop NEC.[240,241] Additionally, they found that the risk for those treated surgically is almost twice the risk for those treated medically (Fig. 34-8). Most infants with NEC who are treated medically develop like age-matched premature infants without NEC, whereas those with more severe disease requiring surgical intervention have a significantly increased risk of poor neurodevelopmental outcomes.

PREVENTION

Prevention of NEC has become a major focus of research because management strategies have had little impact on mortality. Prevention has focused on two main aspects of care: feeding strategies and infectious characteristics of the gastrointestinal tract.

Human Milk

Human milk has a variety of antimicrobial, anti-inflammatory, and immunomodulating properties that may be protective for the gastrointestinal mucosa. Additionally, it furnishes mucosal antibody via secretory IgA as well as macrophages, lactoferrin, and EGF. Because of these properties, it has been postulated that breast milk is protective against developing NEC. However, there are major challenges in evaluating the efficacy of human milk in preventing this disease. One issue lies in a lack of standardization of what is considered human milk: maternal preterm milk, donor preterm milk, donor term milk, and unfortified or fortified human milk. Another lies in the fact that many infants receive supplementation with formula or donor milk when there is insufficient maternal milk. Thus, determining how much human milk is fed and what

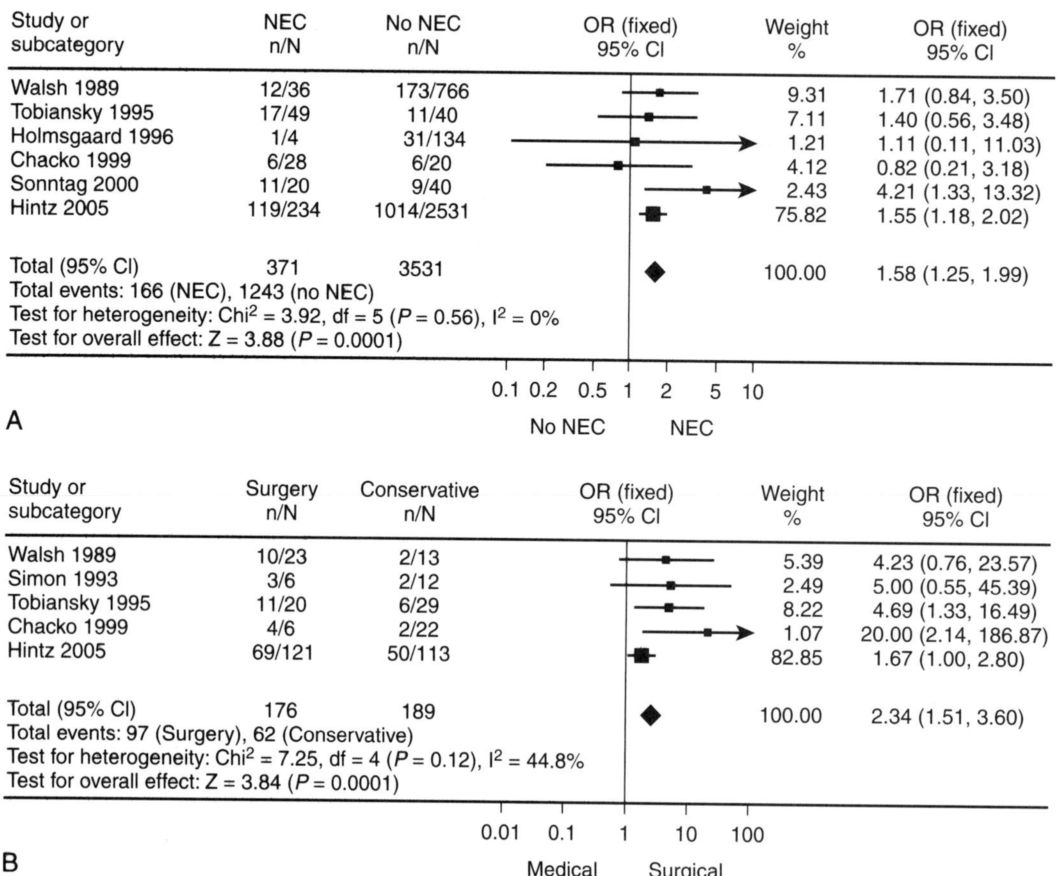

Figure 34-8. Summary data from systematic reviews examining the relationship between NEC and neurodevelopmental outcome. **A,** Data comparing infants with NEC with those without NEC. **B,** Data comparing infants with NEC requiring surgical treatment with those with NEC who were treated medically.

constitutes human milk feeding versus formula feeding has not been standardized. Finally, recent practices in the NICU often involve fortifying human milk to increase the caloric and nutritional content.

Four small (n = 36 to 81) randomized or quasi-randomized studies in the 1980s evaluated the incidence of NEC in infants fed either human milk or formula.[242-245] None of these studies showed a significant difference in NEC between the two groups.

An additional randomized study was done as part of a larger prospective observational study in the United Kingdom.[246] The randomized portion of this study included 159 infants who were fed exclusively either donor breast milk or preterm formula. The incidence of all cases and confirmed cases of NEC was slightly lower in the breast milk group, but the odds ratio did not reach significance. These investigators subsequently looked at all 926 patients who were part of the prospective observational study being conducted. They divided the patients into three groups based on what they had been fed: formula only, formula plus mother's milk, and human milk only. The formula group had a 10% incidence of NEC versus 4% in the human milk only group. When only considering confirmed cases, the formula group had 7% versus 1% in the human milk group. The overall study design entailing two separate studies, with one conducted at two centers and one at five centers, may have confounded the findings. However, adjustments for the effects of different centers did not affect the overall outcomes.

Two systematic reviews and meta-analyses have subsequently been published, combining the results of the four initial studies as well as the results from 159 randomized patients from the later study.[247,248] Both of these meta-analyses found that combining the evidence from these studies suggests that human milk reduces the risk of NEC with findings of a relative risk of 0.21 (95% CI: 0.06-0.76) in one and 0.25 (95% CI: 0.06-0.98) in the other. However, these findings must be evaluated with some caution. One of the meta-analyses is based on 13 cases of NEC in 268 infants and the other one had 13 cases of NEC in 343 infants. The studies included in the meta-analyses also had significant variation in the incidence of NEC (0-20%), the type of human milk (donor, maternal, term, or preterm) and the timing of feeding. Furthermore, one of the included studies was not truly randomized but used an alternate assignment allocation and none of the studies was blinded to allocation or outcome. The diagnosis of NEC was also not uniform among the studies.

Fortification of human milk is commonly practiced to improve caloric and nutrient content of the human milk received. Fortification has been shown to result in increases in weight, length, and head circumference.[249] A Cochrane review did not show an increase in NEC in the group fed fortified milk.[249] Additionally, a nonrandomized study evaluated 108 infants fed either fortified human milk or preterm formula. In this study, there was a significantly lower incidence of NEC in those fed human milk compared with those fed formula.[250] Given the apparent association of human milk in decreasing rates of NEC, and the lack of clear data reflective of contemporary neonatal practices, large randomized controlled trials examining the rates of NEC in premature infants fed fortified human milk seem warranted.

Feeding Strategies

Early initiation of enteral feedings in preterm infants helps to promote growth and decreases the need for parenteral nutrition. However, there have been concerns that early feeding may be associated with an increased risk of NEC. A systematic review found only two small, randomized studies with a total of 82 infants.[251] In these studies, early feeding had no effect on the incidence of NEC. Given the small sample size, important effects of either strategy may have been missed. In one large prospective study, early feeding of human milk appeared protective against NEC while early feeding of formula was linked to an increased incidence.[246] These investigators found that for each day earlier formula feeds were started, the risk of developing NEC increased 20%. Among those infants who received breast milk there was no association between the day of life that feeds were begun and the risk of NEC.

After starting feeds, the rate at which to advance feeds is another concern with regard to NEC. For infants to quickly regain their birth weight and achieve full feeds, rapid advancement is advocated.[252] However, concerns have been raised about the safety of this strategy with regard to increasing the incidence of NEC. In one randomized trial, the study was terminated early due to a higher incidence of NEC in the group that had their feeds rapidly advanced.[253] The results from this study were confounded by a questionable randomization model, an unusually high incidence of NEC, and the early termination of the study itself. Additionally, 4 patients were excluded from the study who died or developed intestinal perforation, which may have introduced bias into the patient population. A systematic review of rapid versus slow advancement of feeds examined 372 patients in three separate trials and did not find any difference in the relative risk of developing NEC.[252]

Amino Acid Supplementation

Arginine is the sole substrate for nitric oxide synthase. As described earlier, NO plays an important role in the proper functioning of the gastrointestinal tract. Therefore, supplementation with arginine has been considered as a potential preventive measure for avoiding NEC. One randomized controlled trial of 152 preterm infants found a significant reduction in NEC in those infants receiving supplementation.[254] However, because this was a small study that was unable to evaluate stage II and III NEC independently, further research on this possible preventive measure needs to be performed to confirm these results.[255]

A deficiency of serum glutamine has also been correlated with NEC.[256] Glutamine is a key fuel for enterocytes and promotes the growth and integrity of the intestinal epithelium. Therefore, glutamine has also been postulated as having protective effects against NEC. However, two large multicenter randomized trials did not show a benefit for those who received glutamine.[257,258] A Cochrane systematic review of five trials also did not show any benefit to the group receiving glutamine.[259]

Oral Antibiotics

Given the role of bacteria in the pathogenesis of NEC, enteral antibiotics have been considered as possible NEC prophylaxis. The use of antibiotics, of course, also increases the potential for the development of resistant bacteria. Five randomized trials have examined the effects of prophylactic therapy with enteral antibiotics. The primary outcome variable in each study was the occurrence of NEC. Although no individual study found a significant reduction in NEC, when the five were combined together in a meta-analysis there was a significant reduction in the incidence of NEC in those who received the antibiotics.[260] Unfortunately, these studies did not report on the potential harmful effects of such widespread use of enteral antibiotics. Without sufficient evidence regarding the safety of using enteral antibiotics as prophylaxis, an endorsement of this prophylactic measure cannot be made.

Probiotics

Probiotics have been proposed as a potential means of promoting the healthy colonization of the premature gut and, therefore, possibly protecting the immature intestine against NEC. Defined as "live microorganisms which when administered in adequate amounts confer a health benefit on the host,"[261] these supplements contain potentially beneficial bacteria or yeasts, most commonly *Lactobacillus, Bifidobacterium,* and *Streptococcus* strains.[262] They can enhance the mucosal barrier by reducing permeability, increasing the production of mucus, inhibiting bacterial translocation, and strengthening tight junctions, all problems in the immature intestine.[39,263-268] Furthermore, colonization with these organisms can reduce the ability of pathogenic bacteria to adhere to the intestinal mucosa.[269,270] Probiotics have also been shown to increase the production of mucosal IgA and short-chain fatty acids that help the immature immune system.[271-273] Additionally, they decrease intestinal inflammation through the reduction of proinflammatory cytokines, the increase of anti-inflammatory cytokines, and the increase of cytokine production by T cells.[274-277]

Studies have examined the ability of probiotics to normalize intestinal flora and to prevent NEC. One randomized controlled trial showed that administration of *Bifidobacterium breve* within the first 24 hours and continued for 28 days can change the intestinal colonization rates, with increased levels of *Lactobacillus* and decreased counts of *Enterobacter*.[278] Another study showed that administering *Bifidobacterium* probiotics to preterm infants lowered the levels of pathogenic species such as *Enterobacter* and *Clostridium* in their intestines compared with controls who did not receive the probiotics.[279] In a study that differentiated between infants under 1500 g and those of 1500 to 1999 g, the infants with the lower birth weight had lower stool colonization rates than the higher birth weight group, despite being given *Lactobacillus casei* subspecies for 2 weeks longer.[280] These studies all suggest that the use of probiotic supplementation can influence intestinal colonization, although the success may vary with birth weight and gestational age.

Once it was shown that such changes in intestinal flora could be manipulated, the next step lay in determining what clinical effect this might have on these preterm infants. One large prospective cohort study using historical controls evaluated whether newborns given *Lactobacillus acidophilus* and *Bifidobacterium infantis* would have reduced rates of NEC.[281] They studied 1237 infants over 1 year with a mean gestational age of 35 weeks and mean birth weight of 2040 g. These infants were treated with each probiotic daily until discharge. The results were compared with those in the 1282 infants hospitalized the year before. During the treatment year, they had an incidence of NEC of 3% compared with 6.6% the year before ($P < .0002$). Furthermore, no side effects were noted.

Subsequently, there have been three randomized prospective trials specifically looking at rates of NEC in infants treated with probiotics. In the first study, 585 preterm infants were randomized to receive *Lactobacillus GG* or no probiotics.[282] The three main outcomes for this study were NEC, sepsis, and urinary tract infection. There were no differences between the two groups in any of these three outcomes. However, the study may not have had adequate power to detect any difference in NEC because the observed baseline incidence was very low (2.8% in the controls).

Another study of 367 infants weighing less than 1500 g randomized those infants who survived beyond 1 week of life and were receiving enteral feeds to either *Lactobacillus acidophilus* and *Bifidobacterium infantis* or no supplementation until discharge.[283] The incidence of NEC in the study group was 1.1% compared with 5.3% in the control group ($P = .04$). Additionally, the study infants had less severe NEC and there were no deaths due to NEC in the study group.

The third randomized study examined the effectiveness of a combination of *Bifidobacterium infantis, Streptococcus thermophilus,* and *Bifidobacterium bifidus* in 145 infants weighing less than 1500 g.[284] These infants were entered into the study at the time they started enteral feedings, and the two groups had no difference in the time it took to reach full feedings. The study group received probiotic supplementation until they reached 36 weeks' gestational age. The study group showed a lower incidence of NEC (4% vs. 16.4%, $P = .03$), less severe NEC, and no NEC-related deaths.

These three randomized trials specifically evaluating the incidence of NEC were combined with four other trials that evaluated NEC as a secondary outcome in a systematic review and meta-analysis (Table 34-6).[285] In the combined analysis, there were 690 infants who received no treatment and 703 who received probiotics. After combining the individual study results using meta-analysis, the relative risk for NEC in the group that received probiotics was 0.36 (95% CI: 0.20-0.65). However, these results must be considered with caution because this meta-analysis combined studies that had many significant differences. This heterogeneity normally would preclude the method of meta-analysis.[286] There was considerable variability among the studies in the demographics of the patients, the age at commencement of treatment, and the type, dose, and duration of probiotic treatment. Additionally, although this meta-analysis found no increased risk of sepsis in the treatment group, the issue of side effects of probiotics was not adequately addressed owing to the lack of power to detect serious infections.

Table 34-6 Clinical Trials Evaluating Probiotics and the Incidence of NEC*

Study (1st Author)	Population	No.	Probiotic	Incidence of NEC		P value	Comment
				Study Group	*Control*		
Dani[290]	<33 wks or <1500 g	585	LBG	4/295 (1.4%)	8/290 (2.8%)		
Lin [291]	<1500 g	367	LBA, BI	2/180 (1.1%)	10/187 (5.3%)	0.04	
Bin-Nun [292]	≤ 1500 g	145	BI, BBB, ST	3/72 (4%)	12/73 (16.4%)	0.031	
Kitajima [293]	<1500 g	91	BB	0/45	0/46	1	NEC a secondary outcome measure
Costalos [294]	28-32 wks	87	SB	5/51 (9.8%)	6/36 (16%)	0.5	NEC a secondary outcome measure
Manzoni[295]	< 1500 g	80	LBC	1/39	3/41	0.51	NEC a secondary outcome measure
Mohan [296]	< 37 wks	38	BBL	2/21	1/17		NEC a secondary outcome measure

BB, *Bifidobacterium breve;* LBG, *Lactobacillus* GG; SB, *Saccharomyces boulardii;* BI, *Bifidobacterium infantis;* BBB, *Bifidobacterium bifidus;* LBA, *Lactobacillus acidophilus;* LBC, *Lactobacillus casei;* BBL, *Bifidobacterium lactis;* ST, *Streptococcus thermophilus.*
*See references for further information.

Given the high-risk population in which these probiotics might be used, the issue of safety is crucial.

The results of this meta-analysis suggest that probiotic supplements might reduce the risk of NEC. These results are promising and call for additional large well-designed randomized trials to confirm these results before implementing this strategy in the prevention of NEC. However, additional trials must evaluate both short-term and long-term safety considerations.

Epidermal Growth Factor

As discussed earlier, EGF plays an important role in the pathogenesis of NEC. Furthermore, premature infants in general, and infants with NEC, specifically, have been shown to have decreased salivary concentrations of EGF.[89] Because EGF is known to support the maintenance of the intestinal barrier and down-regulate proinflammatory cytokines,[121] it could help to prevent NEC. A preliminary study of neonates already diagnosed with NEC has shown that administration of EGF will promote the repair of the intestinal epithelium. In animal models, supplementation with EGF has decreased the incidence of NEC.[287] Heparin-binding epidermal growth factor (HB-EGF) has been shown to have similar effects. Trials to test both EGF and HB-EGF as preventive strategies are planned.[288]

CONCLUSION

Despite many advances in the care of premature infants, NEC remains a challenging disease with a relatively constant incidence rate over the past 4 decades. The only clearly established risk factor is prematurity. Much insight has been gained into the pathophysiology of this disease, with a unifying hypothesis emerging: an excessive and uncontrolled inflammatory response by the neonatal intestine after exposure to some inciting event. Future research efforts will focus on further elucidating the underlying causes and the molecular mechanisms that occur early in this pathogenic process. Because clinical parameters alone have not helped identify which children are at risk for developing the disease and progressing to serious disease,[289] advanced approaches using proteomic and genomic techniques should be considered to compare those who develop NEC with those who do not, as well as those who progress to severe disease with those who have a mild course. Novel treatment strategies such as growth factors should be evaluated. Any trial of treatment should include evaluation of both long- and short-term outcomes. Finally, because no treatment for NEC will be uniformly effective once the disease is established, research efforts should focus on approaches to prevent this disease.

chapter 35

HIRSCHSPRUNG'S DISEASE

Keith E. Georgeson, MD

Harold Hirschsprung, a Danish pediatrician, is credited with the first definitive description of the disease that bears his name.[1] Many earlier scattered reports can be found in the literature that describe children who had symptoms and findings consistent with Hirschsprung's disease (HD), but these descriptions are not definitive enough to be certain of the diagnosis. Some historians give credit to Fredericus Ruysche, a Dutch anatomist, who, in 1691, described a 5-year-old girl with abdominal pain and constipation who eventually died and was noted at autopsy to have megacolon.[2] An understanding of the cause of the constipation and megacolon in HD did not develop until the 1920s when Valla and his associates described the absence of ganglion cells in the myenteric plexus of the distal colon in two brothers with megacolon.[3] Over the next 30 years, poorly understood procedures that were intended to reduce sympathetic hyperactivity of the colon were reported to be, at least temporarily, successful in treating HD. Drs. Swenson, Neuhauser, and Pickett recognized the spastic rectum and distal rectosigmoid colon that defined the site of obstruction in patients with congenital megacolon using fluoroscopy and a barium enema.[4] They established the barium enema as a useful diagnostic tool in HD. Swenson performed a proximal colostomy in six patients with severe constipation and a barium enema demonstrating a classic transition zone. The colostomy was therapeutic in these patients. Later, closure of the colostomy in three of these patients resulted in recurrence of their obstructive symptoms. Based on the findings of the spastic distal colon and the careful clinical observation that the obstructive symptoms recurred with closure of a colostomy proximal to this spastic segment, Swenson conceptualized and performed the first pull-through procedure in a patient with HD.[5] Duhamel, Soave, and others have described operations that differed from Swenson's but clearly integrated concepts that he defined for successful management of HD. Despite the relative success of all of these procedures, the precise etiology and many of the complexities of this disorder remain unknown. Important contributions regarding the etiology, genetics, pathophysiology, epidemiology, and management of patients with HD have been made in the past 50 years. The diagnosis and treatment of HD are discussed in this chapter. A description is also provided of some aspects of HD that remain poorly understood and are confusing to both researchers and clinicians.

ETIOLOGY

Cellular and molecular abnormalities in the development of the enteric nervous system, along with incomplete migration of the neural crest cells, are a major part of the cause of HD.[6-8] Neural crest-derived neuroblasts appear in the developing esophagus at about 5 weeks' gestation in the human fetus. These cells then migrate in both a cranial and caudal direction into the rest of the developing gut between 5 and 12 weeks' gestation.[6,9] The Hirschsprung phenotype is variable owing to a wide range of possible abnormalities during the development of the enteric nervous system and the different times at which arrest occurs in the migration of the neural crest-derived cells. The earlier the arrest in neural crest migration, the longer the segment of aganglionosis.[8-10] Many other factors, such as an altered extracellular matrix, abnormalities in neurotrophic factors, and neural cell adhesion molecules have also been suggested as contributing to the development of HD.[9,11]

GENETIC FACTORS

HD often occurs as an isolated phenotype. However, there are strong associations that support a genetic etiology for the disease. Siblings of children with HD have an increased risk of being born with HD.[12-14] There is an unbalanced gender ratio of approximately 4:1 favoring males over females. HD is also associated with known chromosomal anomalies.[12-16] Genetic studies have documented at least 10 mutations in different genes associated with its development. The more common genetic mutations that have been identified

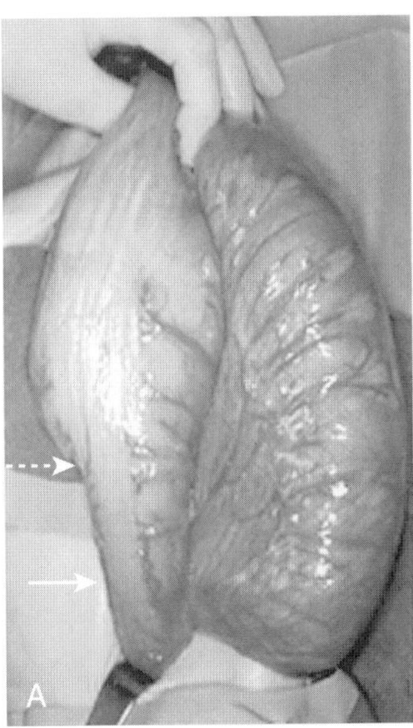

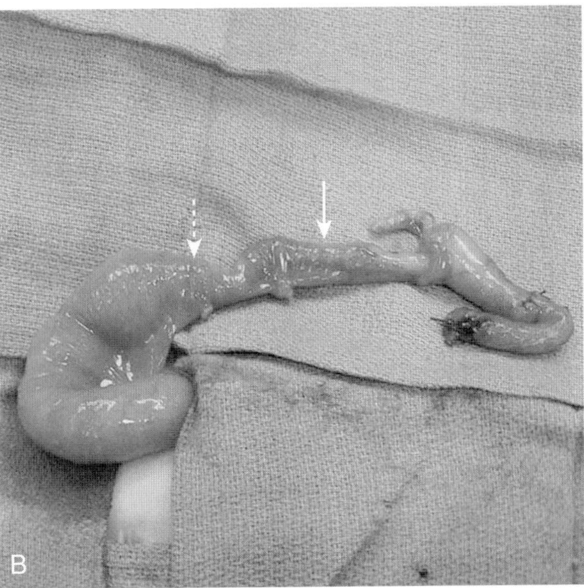

Figure 35-1. **A,** Classic case of rectosigmoid Hirschsprung's disease in a 2-year-old child. Note the contracted rectum (*solid arrow*) and the dilated proximal rectum and sigmoid colon. The transition zone is marked with the *dotted arrow.* **B,** A very small, contracted right colon, cecum, and terminal ileum (*solid arrow*) in a neonate with total colon aganglionosis. The normal, dilated ileum is noted proximal to the transition zone (*dotted arrow*).

include the *RET* gene (7%-35% of sporadic cases), the *EDNRB* gene (7%), and the *END3* gene (<5%). More than 20 mutations have been described in the *RET* proto-oncogene. Some polymorphisms in this gene are associated with particular HD phenotypes. HD has been associated with other genetic abnormalities, such as trisomy 21, cardiac septal defects, congenital central hypoventilation syndrome, multiple endocrine neoplasia type 2, neurofibromatosis, Waardenburg's syndrome, and anorectal malformations. Trisomy 21 is reported in approximately 7% of children with HD. HD has a complex inheritance with penetrance being highly variable. Studies have reported the risk of HD in the siblings of the proband to be 4%.[14,17]

PATHOPHYSIOLOGY

The primary clinical feature of HD is obstruction caused by a lack of propagation of the peristaltic wave. This lack of propagation is associated with the absence of ganglion cells in the myenteric and submucosal plexus.[18] The cause of the spasm in the aganglionic bowel is unclear. Cholinergic hyperenervation, inadequate distribution of nitric oxide synthetase, and abnormalities of the interstitial cells of Cajal have all been reported to be associated with HD.[19-21] A comprehensive understanding of how these factors work to cause the disease has not been achieved. The majority (75%) of patients with HD have ganglion cells down to the level of the rectosigmoid colon (Fig. 35-1A). Long-segment HD, which describes aganglionosis of the descending colon, splenic flexure, or transverse colon, occurs in approximately 15% of patients.[12,22-24] Also, even longer segment cases have been described, including total colon aganglionosis, which occurs in 5% to 7% of patients (see Fig. 35-1B). A small number of infants with no ganglion cells at all in the entire gastrointestinal tract have been noted.

The incidence of HD is approximately 1 in 5000 live births. Asian children seem to have the highest incidence at almost 3 per 5000 live births. However, HD is seen in almost all racial groups.[25] It is possible that differences in the recognition of HD occur because of differences in diagnostic capabilities and reporting mechanisms. Although the male-to-female ratio of HD is approximately 4:1, it is 2:1 in longer-segment disease.[16] In medically sophisticated cultures, the diagnosis of HD is often made in the first few weeks or months of life. Delayed passage of meconium in the newborn, constipation with intermittent diarrhea, a distended abdomen with bilious vomiting, and feeding intolerance with poor weight gain or even weight loss are frequent clinical signs of HD.

Most neonates pass a meconium stool in the first 48 hours of life.[26] However, the majority of children with HD fail to pass meconium in the first 48 hours of life.[27-29] The onset of explosive, foul-smelling stools associated with fever and abdominal distention heralds the onset of HD enterocolitis.[30-32] If unrecognized, HD-associated enterocolitis is a potentially fatal complication. In patients with a rectosigmoid colon transition zone, prompt saline irrigation of the sigmoid colon along with fluid resuscitation and antibiotic therapy are important measures to decrease the risk of death in these patients. Infants and children with longer segment disease and a more proximal transition zone are not as effectively treated by rectal irrigation. Some of these patients will require immediate exploration with a colostomy proximal to the aganglionic bowel. A delayed diagnosis of HD may lead to an increased risk of serious and occasionally fatal enterocolitis.[27,33]

DIAGNOSIS

Infants and children who failed to pass meconium in the first 24 to 48 hours of life, who suffer from severe constipation with bouts of intermittent diarrhea, who

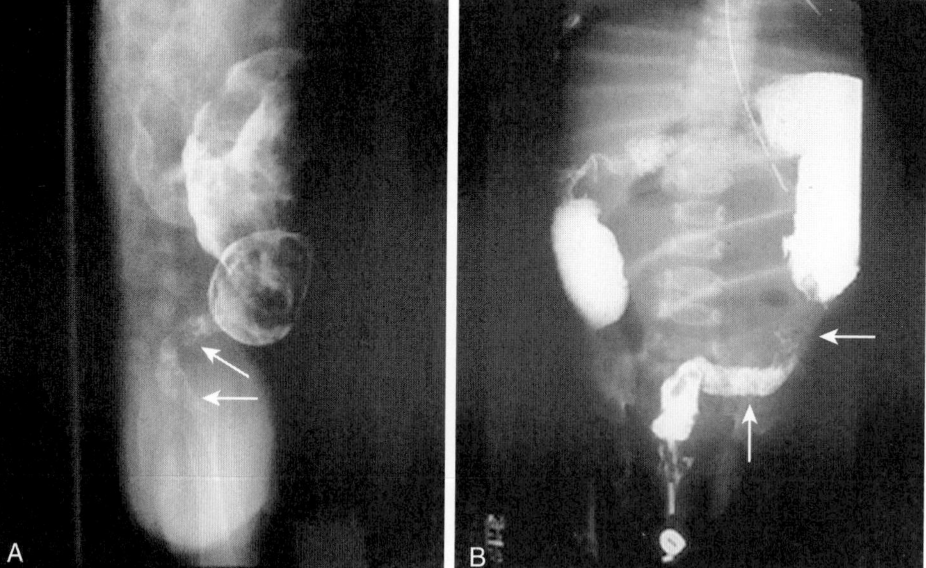

Figure 35-2. **A** and **B,** These two barium enema examinations in different infants demonstrate Hirschsprung's disease. The aganglionic rectum (*arrows*) in both studies is small and contracted. The proximal ganglionic colon is dilated. A transition zone between the aganglionic and ganglionic colon is nicely seen in the both studies.

have abdominal distention, or who present with bilious vomiting are likely candidates for the diagnosis of HD. Diagnostic tests include full-thickness rectal biopsy (gold standard), contrast enema (sensitivity [SN] 65%-80%, specificity [SP] 65%-100%), anorectal manometry (SN 75%-100%, SP 85%-95%) and rectal suction biopsy (SN > 90%, SP > 95%).[34-42] Typically, patients with HD show gaseous distention of the colon and small bowel. In patients with a classic rectosigmoid transition zone, the sigmoid colon is often noted to be redundant and dilated. A contrast enema often shows the presence of a transition zone and irregular colonic contractions in the distal, aganglionic segment (Fig. 35-2). Often, irregular mucosal ulcerations are seen on the contrast enema due to enterocolitis. Some authors have reported an even lower sensitivity for detecting HD with a contrast enema in neonates and believe that a contrast enema in the neonatal period should be cautiously interpreted.[43-45]

Although anorectal manometry is rarely used in neonates to establish the diagnosis,[46,47] it is a useful technique in older children.[48] The classic finding is the absence of the rectoanal inhibitory reflex when the rectum is distended. In normal children, distention of the rectum results in a transient increase in rectal pressure with a reduction in the anal internal sphincter pressure. Children with HD lack this inhibitory reflex and relaxation of the internal sphincter (Fig. 35-3).[48]

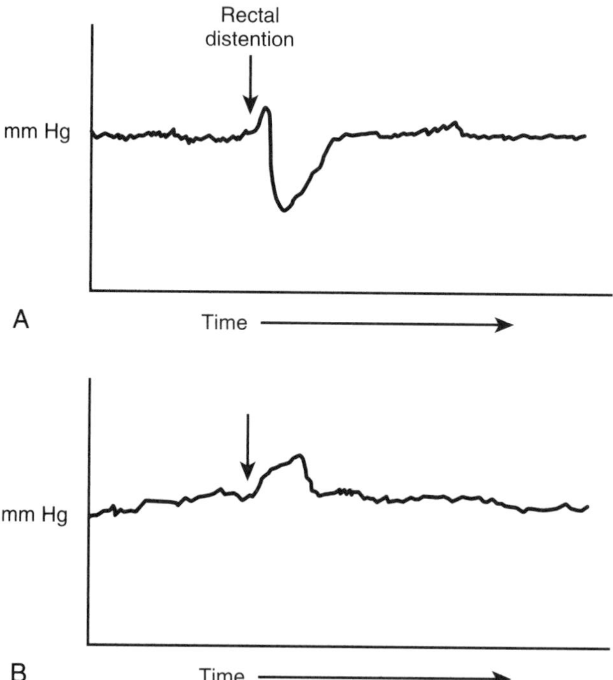

Figure 35-3. **A,** In the child undergoing anorectal manometry without Hirschsprung's disease, the rectoanal inhibitory reflex is normal. Note the drop in the internal sphincter pressure with rectal distention. **B,** A child with Hirschsprung's disease is seen to have abnormally increased contraction of the anal canal and no relaxation of the internal sphincter with rectal distention. (The *arrow* points to the initiation of rectal distention in both **A** and **B.**)

The standard diagnostic tool for documenting HD is an open or suction rectal biopsy. Normal colon has demonstrable myenteric and submucosal ganglion cells (Fig. 35-4A). The absence of ganglion cells in both the myenteric and submucosal plexus and the finding of hypertrophic nerve fibers are diagnostic of HD (see Fig. 35-4B). Additionally, the presence of increased acetylcholinesterase staining in the submucosa and mucosa is confirmatory of HD (see Fig. 35-4C). In some pediatric centers, the presence of increased staining of acetylcholinesterase in the mucosa and submucosa is adequate to confirm the diagnosis in a patient with typical symptoms and a contrast enema that demonstrates a transition zone. A suction rectal biopsy, at least 2 cm or more above the dentate line, is the commonly used method for confirming HD in most centers. The presence of

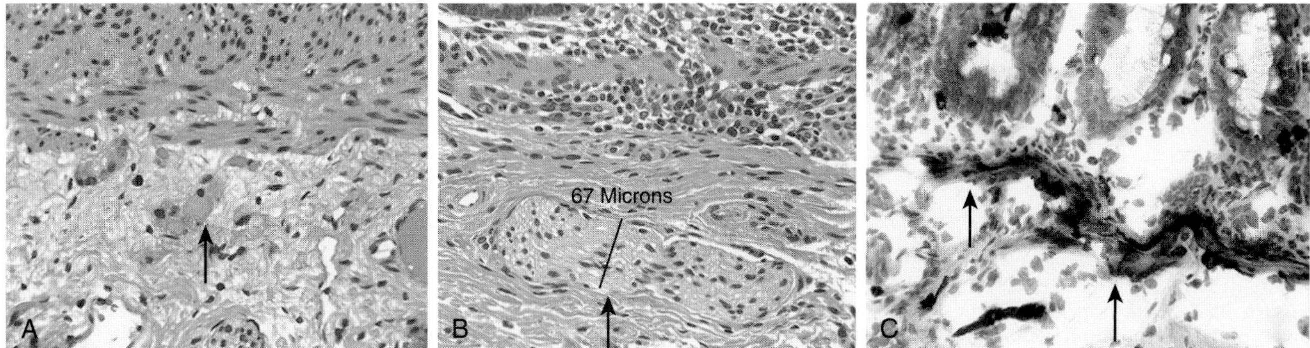

Figure 35-4. **A,** This biopsy specimen of normal ganglionated bowel has been stained with hematoxylin and eosin. A ganglion cell (*arrow*) is seen in the submucosa. **B,** This rectal biopsy specimen in a neonate with Hirschsprung's disease has been stained with hematoxylin and eosin. Ganglion cells cannot be found in the wall of the rectum. Also, the submucosal nerve trunks (*arrow*) are noted to be greater than 40 μm in diameter, which strongly correlates with aganglionosis. **C,** This rectal biopsy specimen in a neonate with Hirschsprung's disease has been stained with acetylcholinesterase. The increased staining in the mucosa and submucosa (*arrows*) is diagnostic of Hirschsprung's disease. (Courtesy of Dr. D. Kelly, Children's Hospital of Alabama, Birmingham, AL.)

ganglion cells within 2 cm of the dentate line is variable. Both the absence of ganglion cells and an increase in acetylcholinesterase staining can be determined on these specimens.[49] However, it is more difficult in older children to acquire adequate material on suction biopsy and these children usually require an open biopsy to obtain adequate tissue for diagnosis. Other enzyme-staining techniques have also been used to diagnose HD, such as lactate dehydrogenase, succinic dehydrogenase, and NADPH-diaphorase enzyme histochemistry.[50]

There also have been reports describing the use of rapid frozen section analysis for determining enzymatic activity of the ganglion cells in the transition zone because anatomically normal-appearing ganglion cells may lack normal enzymatic activity.[42] With this approach, the transition zone is defined as the point where the ganglion cells have normal enzymatic activity. The proximal point of this enzymatically determined transition zone is then used as the neorectum for the coloanal anastomosis. Using the enzymatic activity of the ganglion cells to determine the proximal part of the transition zone has been reported to result in a lower incidence of complications and enterocolitis after pull-through for HD. Nakao and coworkers reported a 91% sensitivity using acetylcholinesterase staining for the diagnosis of HD and a false-negative rate of 8%.[42] Rectal suction biopsy is clearly more sensitive than both anorectal manometry and contrast enema for the diagnosis of HD. However, the biopsy should be deep enough to show the absence of ganglion cells and the presence of hypertrophic nerve fibers. Interestingly, children with total colon HD can have elevated acetylcholinesterase activity in the rectum and left colon but may show near-normal levels of acetylcholinesterase activity proximal to the splenic flexure.

Histologic grading of enterocolitis has been proposed by Teitelbaum and coworkers.[51] However, this grading system has not been widely used. Some authors have suggested that an initial histologic enterocolitis index of grade 2 or greater predicts a higher risk of subsequent clinical enterocolitis.[52] However, other reports have not confirmed this finding.[53]

TREATMENT

Surgical approaches to HD should only be considered after the diagnosis has been firmly established by either suction or open rectal biopsy. Historically, a two- or three-stage repair was performed with the first stage consisting of a diverting colostomy usually leveled at the point where the transition zone was identified by seromuscular biopsy. The second stage, performed 3 to 12 months later, consisted of resection of the aganglionic bowel with a coloanal anastomosis. The colostomy was closed either during the pull-through operation or subsequently as a third-stage procedure.

Surgical Techniques

Multiple operative approaches have been described for managing HD. All these operations conform to the original concepts for correcting HD espoused by Swenson. These principles for effective surgical treatment include resection of the aganglionic portion of bowel and identification of normally ganglionated proximal bowel with a leveled coloanal or enteroanal anastomosis. Additionally, the operation should preserve both fecal and urinary continence and normal sexual function. The most commonly used operations for HD have been developed by Swenson, Duhamel, and Soave.[4,54,55]

The Swenson technique utilizes a near-total proctectomy with the dissection plane close to the outside of the muscular wall of the rectum (Fig. 35-5). Swenson believed a diagonal resection of the distal rectum resulted in fewer strictures at the anastomotic line.[4]

The Duhamel technique employs dissection behind the rectum and leaves the aganglionic rectum in place. The aganglionic proximal rectum and colon are then resected. The ganglionated bowel is brought down behind the rectum, creating two parallel cylinders

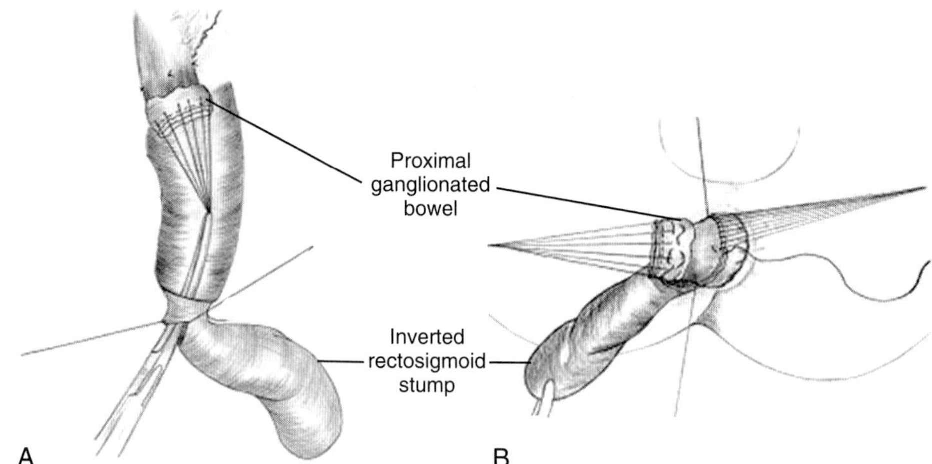

Figure 35-5. The principles of the Swenson pull-through procedure are seen in these drawings. **A,** The proximal ganglionated bowel is grasped through an incision in the prolapsed rectosigmoid stump. **B,** The ganglionated bowel is then sewn to the anus.

(Fig. 35-6). The lumen of the neorectum is sutured end to side to the lumen of the native rectum, approximately 2 cm above the dentate line. The septum between the two cylinders of bowel is then ablated. Initially, this ablation was performed using large clamps placed in parallel with the handles of the clamps protruding out of the anus for up to 2 weeks. This technique has been modified several times. Currently, the stapler is used to incise the septum between the neorectum and native rectum. Additionally, the native rectal stump can be cut short, minimizing the redundancy above the common channel to avoid a fecal impaction in the backwater portion of the aganglionic rectum.[54]

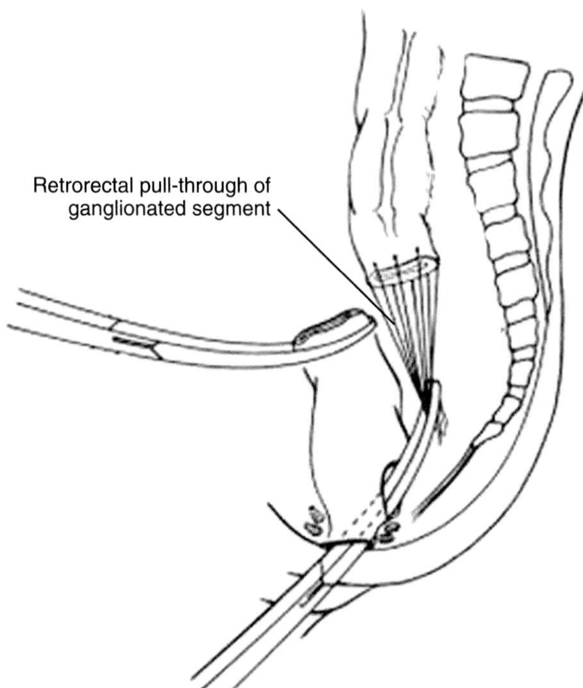

Figure 35-6. With the Duhamel technique, the ganglionated bowel is delivered through an incision in the posterior aspect of the native aganglionated rectum and sewn to the anus. The septum between the ganglionated pull-through colon and the aganglionated native rectum is then divided using a stapler.

The Soave technique utilizes a mucosectomy of the rectum, leaving a muscular cuff (Fig. 35-7). Soave originally described exteriorizing the neorectum out the anus and leaving it as a protuberant stump. The stump was trimmed 2 to 3 weeks later.[55] Boley described a similar approach with a primary anastomosis.[56] All of these procedures have a laparoscopic or transanal counterpart.

In 1980, So and co-workers introduced the concept of primary pull-through for HD.[57] A single-stage procedure avoids the complications associated with a colostomy and the need for another operation to close the colostomy. A primary single-stage pull-through is appropriate for most infants and children diagnosed with HD.

When indicated, I perform an end colostomy just proximal to the biopsy-documented transition zone. The Brooke technique is utilized to mature the colostomy. The colon should be carefully secured to the inner abdominal wall for a distance of at least 4 cm to avoid prolapse of the colostomy because the proximal colon often shrinks in size after colostomy formation. The distal colon is left as a Hartman pouch unless the transition zone is at or above the splenic flexure.

The single-stage pull-through for HD became more popular with the introduction of the laparoscopic-assisted transanal endorectal pull-through (LATEP).[58] The LATEP allowed the pull-through to be performed without a large abdominal incision. Subsequently, de la Torre described a transanal pull-through (TAP) without abdominal exploration or biopsy.[59] The LATEP and the TAP have become the two most popular methods for primary repair of HD in infants and children. At the Children's Hospital of Alabama, the LATEP is preferred in neonates and children undergoing a primary operation for two reasons. First, laparoscopic biopsies allow confirmation of the extent of the aganglionosis before any division of the colonic mesentery or rectal ablation occurs. This is especially advantageous in the neonate in whom the contrast enema can be somewhat unreliable in predicting the level of the transition zone.[43-45] If a long segment of aganglionosis is identified, delaying the definitive operation until the histopathologic

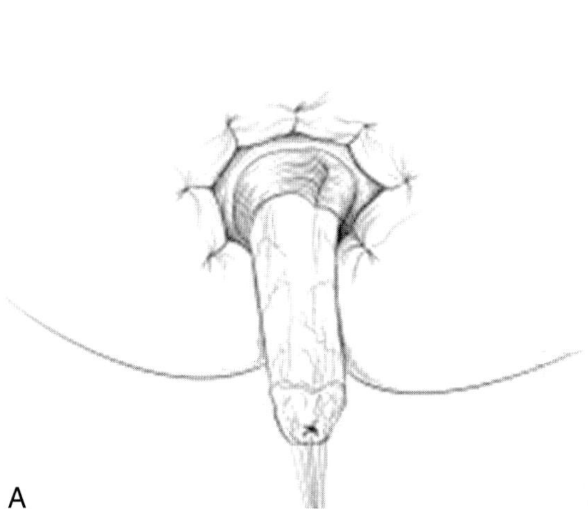

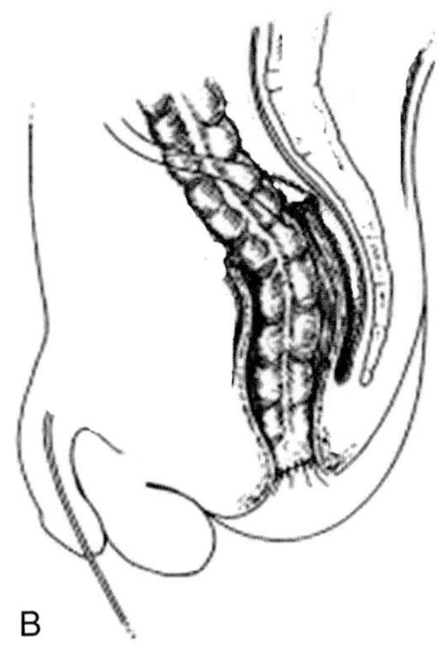

Figure 35-7. **A,** For the Soave operation, there is extramucosal dissection of the rectum after circumferential incision of the rectal mucosa. **B,** The ganglionated colon is pulled through the aganglionic rectal cuff, and a coloanal anastomosis is performed.

results are available from the permanent sections may prevent unnecessary resection of long segments of colon due to errors in frozen section analysis. Second, the use of laparoscopy helps in performing a tension-free coloanal anastomosis by releasing the restraining ligaments to the descending colon and ensuring that there is no twisting of the pull-through colon during the anastomosis. At the Children's Hospital of Alabama, neonates with total colon aganglionosis are managed with an initial leveling small bowel enterostomy, followed 6 to 12 months later by a laparoscopic-assisted Duhamel procedure. The Duhamel technique offers the advantage of creating a larger rectal reservoir in patients with near-total or total colonic HD. Performing an initial ileostomy and delaying the procedure for 6 to 12 months also reduces the incidence of the severe postoperative diaper rash associated with a pull-through of the small intestine in the newborn.

In a neonate, unless contraindications are present, LATEP is performed as soon as the diagnosis is confirmed by suction rectal biopsy.[60] Contraindications to a neonatal primary pull-through include the following:

- Severe enterocolitis
- Massive proximal dilatation
- Inability to determine the transition zone
- Life-threatening comorbidities

Preoperative decompression of the bowel is performed by a combination of finger dilation of the rectum and irrigation of the colon with saline through a rectal tube with the tip of the tube positioned above the transition zone. The neonates are hydrated intravenously. Two doses of an oral antibiotic regimen consisting of erythromycin and neomycin are given 8 and 4 hours before the scheduled operation. Intravenous administration of a broad-spectrum antibiotic is given immediately before the patient is taken into the operating room.

Laparoscopic Pull-Through

Infants are positioned transversely near the end of the operating table to allow for access to both the abdomen and the perineum. Positioning works best if the patient's head is turned to the right side and toward the anesthetist. With this arrangement, the laparoscopic surgeon has better access to the patient's sigmoid and left colon. The laparoscopic portion of the procedure is performed after a thorough body prepping below the nipples. The legs and feet are draped in the operating field after prepping. The pneumoperitoneum is obtained using an open cut-down technique through the umbilicus. Pressures of 10 to 12 mm Hg are well tolerated in all age groups. Modest hyperventilation is useful to prevent hypercarbia in these patients. A 4-mm, 30-degree telescope is used in infants, and a 5-mm, 30-degree scope is helpful in larger patients. Port placement is illustrated in Figure 35-8. As mentioned, the initial cannula (5 mm) is inserted through the umbilicus. A second (4 or 5 mm) cannula is introduced in the right upper abdominal quadrant just below the liver margin. The telescope is then moved to this site. The third port is placed in the right lower abdomen just anterior to the anterior axillary line. The transition zone between ganglionated and aganglionic bowel is identified visually when possible. Seromuscular biopsy specimens for histologic analysis can be obtained using laparoscopic Metzenbaum scissors or by exteriorizing the colon through the umbilicus (Fig. 35-9). For an intracorporeal biopsy, it is best for the surgeon to use a sharply pointed instrument in the left hand to elevate the seromuscular wall. Broader-tipped instruments can lead to a full-thickness biopsy. Once the biopsy is obtained, it is best to delay further dissection until the transition zone is determined. Visual identification of the transition zone can be inaccurate, especially in infants.

Assuming a rectosigmoid transition zone is found, a window is created through the rectosigmoid mesocolon. This window can be made either with a hook cautery or using an ultrasonic scalpel placed through the 5-mm port in the umbilicus. The mesenteric window should be extended to the peritoneal reflection of the pelvis. In older children, the dissection can be extended below the peritoneal reflection, which makes the transanal dissection easier. However, in infants younger than 1 year of age, the transanal dissection

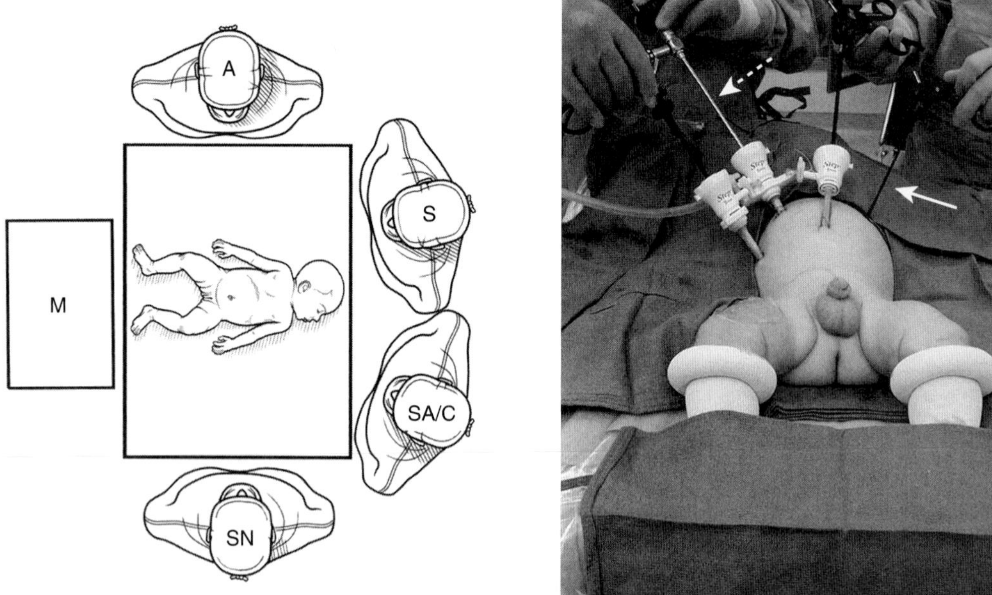

Figure 35-8. The surgeon (S) and surgical assistant/camera holder (SA/C) stand above the patient's head with the monitor (M) positioned beyond the infant's feet. The scrub nurse (SN) can be positioned according to the surgeon's preference, although being positioned at the foot of the operating table appears to be ideal. A, anesthesiologist. The photograph shows port placement for this operation. Usually three or four ports are required. The umbilical port is inserted using an open technique, and the other ports are introduced under direct visualization. The telescope (*dotted arrow*) is placed through the 5-mm port in the right upper abdomen. The surgeon's two primary working ports are the umbilical port for the left hand and the right lower abdominal port for the right hand. A retracting instrument (*solid arrow*) is often helpful and can be inserted through a stab incision in the infant's left upper abdomen. A urinary catheter has been introduced to help decompress the bladder. (From Morowitz MJ, Georgeson KE: Laparoscopic assisted pull-through for Hirschsprung's disease. In Holcomb GW, Georgeson KE, Rothenberg SS [eds]: Atlas of Pediatric Laparoscopy and Thoracoscopy, Philadelphia, Elsevier, 2008, pp 101-108. Reprinted with permission.)

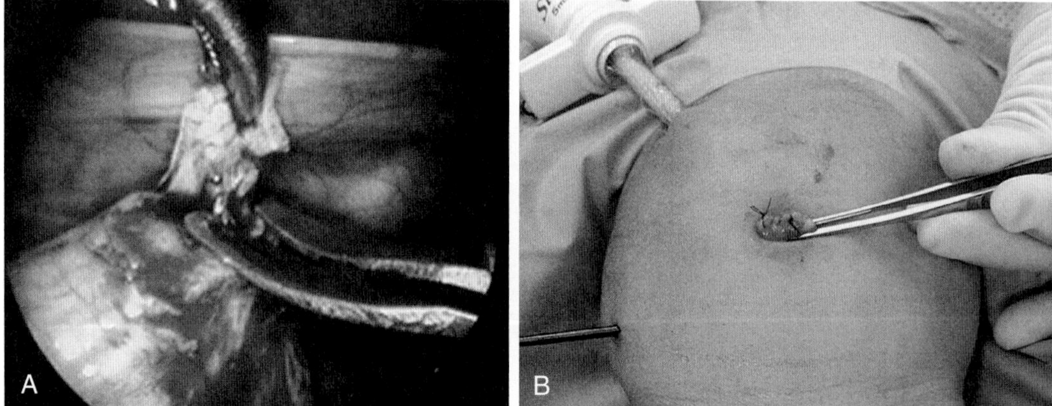

Figure 35-9. A, An intracorporeal biopsy is being performed on the sigmoid colon. A fine-tipped grasping forceps has been used to grasp the biopsy site, and Metzenbaum scissors are used to obtain the biopsy specimen. **B,** This biopsy was performed through the umbilical incision. One port and another instrument have been introduced through the infant's abdominal wall. A site on the colon for the biopsy was visualized and delivered just under the umbilical cannula. The umbilical cannula was removed, and this portion of the colon was grasped and exteriorized. An extracorporeal biopsy was obtained and the biopsy site was closed. This is an alternative means for obtaining the biopsy. (From Morowitz MJ, Georgeson KE: Laparoscopic assisted pull-through for Hirschsprung's disease. In Holcomb GW, Georgeson KE, Rothenberg SS [eds]: Atlas of Pediatric Laparoscopy and Thoracoscopy, Philadelphia, Elsevier, 2008, pp 101-108. Reprinted with permission.)

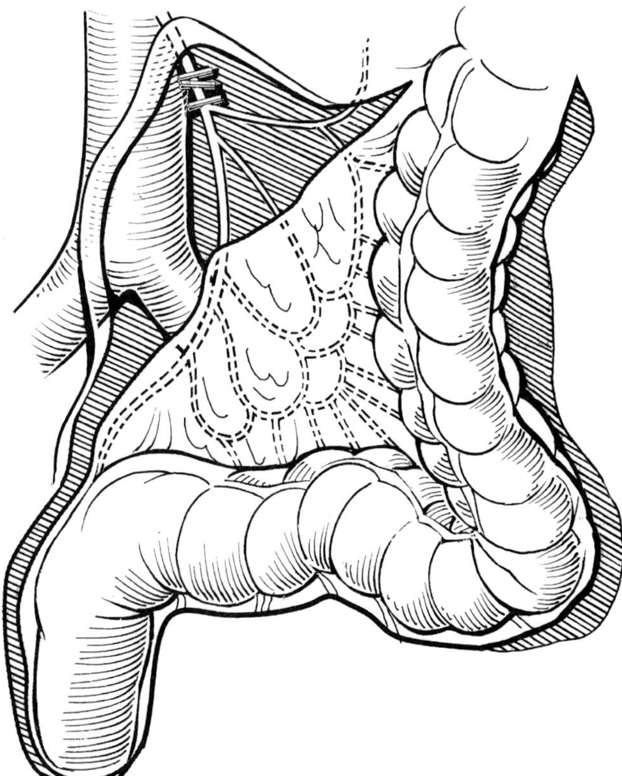

Figure 35-10. When the transition zone is proximal to the mid-sigmoid colon, a pedicled colon flap must be developed for the endorectal pull-through. In this situation, the pull-through colon will derive its vascular supply from the marginal artery. Therefore, to mobilize the descending colon and splenic flexure, it is necessary to ligate and divide either the inferior mesenteric artery just distal to its origin from the aorta (as seen in this drawing) or the left colic artery just after it arises from the inferior mesenteric artery. By ligating these vessels at these sites, the arterial supply through the marginal artery is not compromised. (From Morowitz MJ, Georgeson KE: Laparoscopic assisted pull-through for Hirschsprung's disease. In Holcomb GW, Georgeson KE, Rothenberg SS [eds]: Atlas of Pediatric Laparoscopy and Thoracoscopy, Philadelphia, Elsevier, 2008, pp 101-108. Reprinted with permission.)

is not difficult. The distal branches of the inferior mesenteric artery and vein should be preserved to prevent potential ischemic scarring of the seromuscular cuff after the mucosal sleeve resection.

Infants and children with a longer transition zone (above the proximal sigmoid colon) require pedicle formation for the pull-through of the ganglionated colon. The vascular pedicle is formed by preserving the marginal artery (Fig. 35-10). The lateral fusion fascia and other restraining ligaments should also be divided so that there is no tension on the colon or its vascular pedicle when it is pulled down for the coloanal anastomosis. The appropriate length for the pedicle can be determined by pulling the intended site of anastomosis down into the pelvis and allowing a few extra centimeters for a tension-free coloanal anastomosis.

I usually extend the resection of the aganglionic segment for a distance of 5 to 10 cm proximal to the histologically identified transition zone. This extension allows for removal of dilated, dysfunctional bowel that may be present proximal to the transition zone. If available, rapid frozen evaluation of the enzymatic activity of the ganglion cells is used to accurately level the pull-through colon pedicle. Once the endoscopic dissection has been completed, attention is turned to the transanal dissection. Six to eight perianal retraction sutures are used to evert the anus and expose the rectum (Fig. 35-11A). It is important to avoid overstretching the internal sphincter while placing these sutures. Overstretching of the internal sphincter will lead to long-term fecal soiling and diminish the quality of life for patients with HD. The dissection is always performed outside the anus using downward traction to keep the dissection plane outside the anus. This will avoid the tendency to stretch the internal sphincter by using retractors in the anorectal canal. Moreover, retractors are usually not necessary when the dissection is performed properly. Mucosal traction sutures are usually placed in a vertical orientation before incising the mucosa. These traction sutures should be tied snugly before the transanal dissection to co-apt

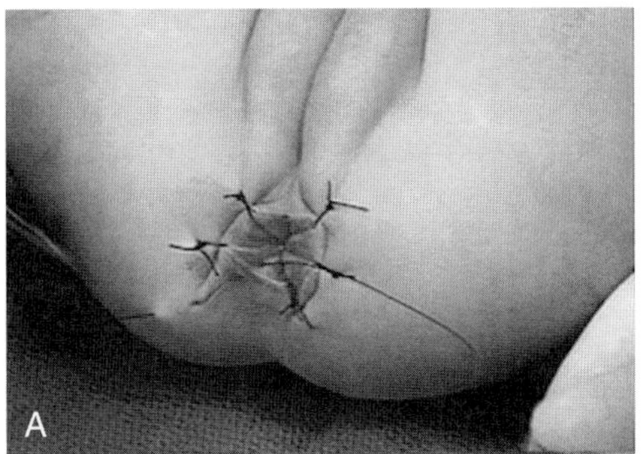

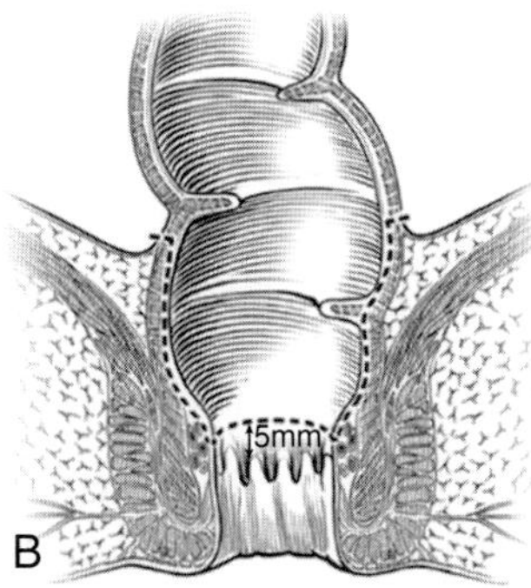

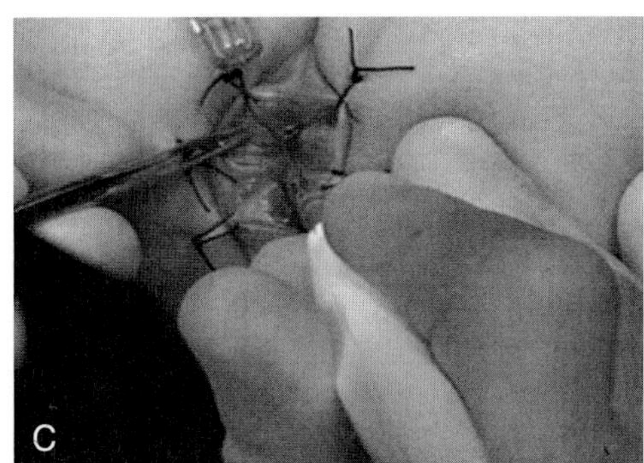

Figure 35-11. A, The perineal dissection begins with the placement of circumferential 2-0 silk traction sutures from the dentate line to the perineum 2 to 3 cm outward from the anus. **B** and **C,** A needle-tipped electrocautery is used to circumferentially incise the rectal mucosa approximately 5 mm proximal to the anal columns. Fine silk traction sutures are then placed in the rectal mucosa to help retract the mucosa during circumferential dissection. (From Morowitz MJ, Georgeson KE: Laparoscopic assisted pull-through for Hirschsprung's disease. In Holcomb GW, Georgeson KE, Rothenberg SS [eds]: Atlas of Pediatric Laparoscopy and Thoracoscopy, Philadelphia, Elsevier, 2008, pp 101-108. Reprinted with permission.)

the anus and prevent soiling during the dissection. Also, this allows more robust traction for defining the submucosal plane. A circular incision is made at the anorectal line near the top of the rectal columns (see Fig. 35-11B, C). This submucosal plane is then developed using both blunt and sharp dissection. Generous use of the electrocautery for hemostasis is helpful. It seems best to dissect the two side planes initially and then to connect them with the anterior and posterior planes. The dissection is continued circumferentially proximally until bleeding ceases because of the previous separation of the mesentery from the colon during the laparoscopic mobilization. Another sign of adequate transanal dissection is the increasing ease of withdrawing the colon out through the anus.

After the colorectum has been exteriorized through the anus, the peritoneal cavity is entered posteriorly. This dissection is continued circumferentially by dividing the seromuscular wall using cautery. The posterior wall of the cuff is split down to the intended point of anastomosis. This division of the cuff allows for the creation of a larger neorectal reservoir. The colon is pulled down to a point where the biopsies have indicated an appropriate transition zone. As previously mentioned, an additional 5- to 10-cm margin of ganglionated bowel is resected when possible. The colon is transected and the coloanal anastomosis is performed (Fig. 35-12). In some cases of longer segment HD, a mini-reservoir can be developed by using the Heineke-Mikulicz technique (Fig. 35-13). A vertical incision is made in the pull-through colon, beginning 1.5 cm above the point of intended anastomosis and extended 3 cm proximally. The incision is then closed transversely like a Heineke-Mikulicz pyloroplasty. A watertight anastomosis is then performed between the anus and the neorectum at the anorectal line. It is important that the neorectum is relatively lax so that a new anorectal angle forms. If the neorectum is pulled down under tension, the anorectal angle is lost and the patient may have a more difficult time developing continence later in life. This is more problematic with the transanal approach when compared with the laparoscopic assisted technique. Also, this lack of tension at the anastomosis helps to avoid ischemia of the distal colon pedicle and/or retraction of the colon pull-through.

Once the anastomosis is completed, the pneumoperitoneum is re-established and the abdominal cavity is inspected laparoscopically. The rectal cuff should also be inspected to make certain it is straight and not folded down into the anorectal canal. If there is a potential internal hernia space under the pedicle of the neorectum, it should be closed with interrupted sutures. The pedicle should also be observed for twisting. If the pedicle is twisted, the anastomosis should be taken down and performed again. In most instances, an oral diet is started 1 to 2 days after the pull-through.

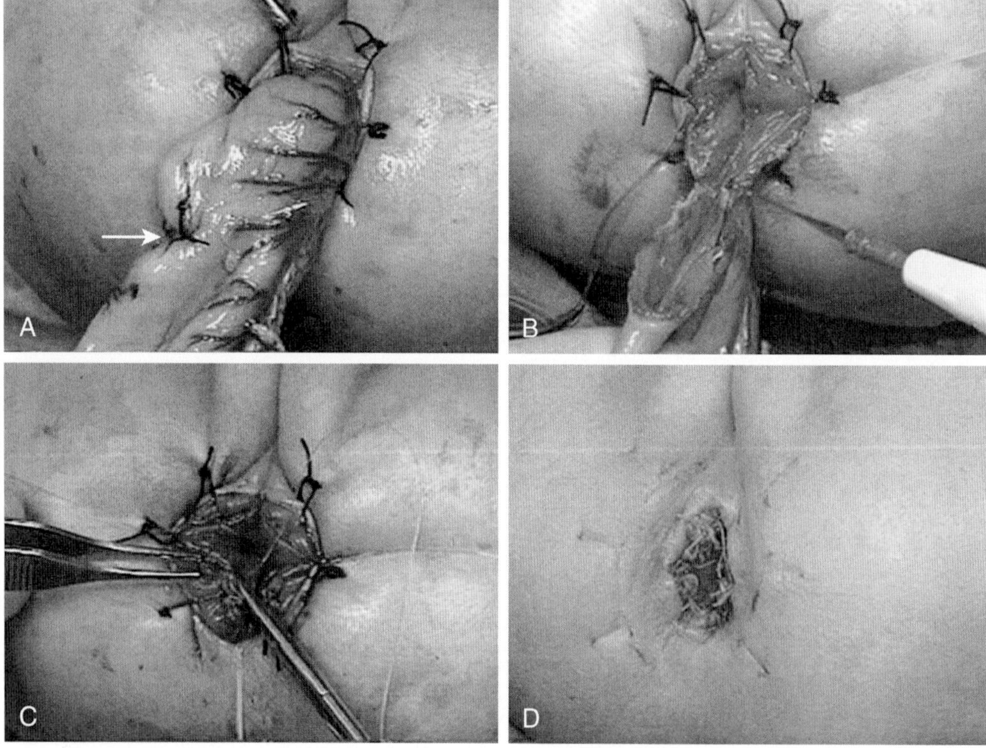

Figure 35-12. **A,** The muscular cuff of the rectum has been divided and the ganglionic colon has been exteriorized through the anal canal. Note that the anastomosis will be performed proximal to the biopsy site (*arrow*). **B,** The pull-through colon is being completely transected above the biopsy site and made ready for the coloanal anastomosis. **C,** The anastomosis is being performed with interrupted 4-0 absorbable sutures. **D,** The everting stay sutures have been cut, allowing the anastomosis to retract cephalad. (From Morowitz MJ, Georgeson KE: Laparoscopic assisted pull-through for Hirschsprung's disease. In Holcomb GW, Georgeson KE, Rothenberg SS [eds]: Atlas of Pediatric Laparoscopy and Thoracoscopy, Philadelphia, Elsevier, 2008, pp 101-108. Reprinted with permission.)

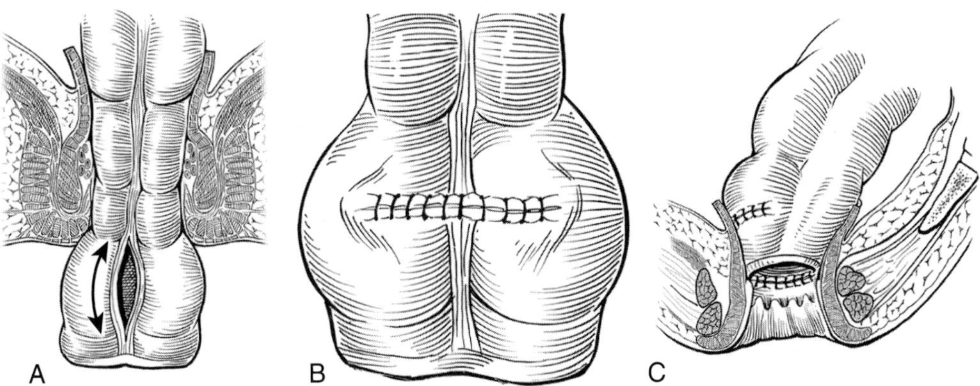

Figure 35-13. **A,** To create the mini-reservoir, a full-thickness linear incision is made through the anterior wall of the ganglionic colon beginning 1.5 cm above the transected bowel and continuing for 3 cm proximally. **B,** The linear incision is then closed transversely in a Heineke-Mikulicz fashion. **C,** The coloanal anastomosis and the reservoir closure are seen. (From Morowitz MJ, Georgeson KE: Laparoscopic assisted pull-through for Hirschsprung's disease. In Holcomb GW, Georgeson KE, Rothenberg SS [eds]: Atlas of Pediatric Laparoscopy and Thoracoscopy, Philadelphia, Elsevier, 2008, pp 101-108. Reprinted with permission.)

The length of postoperative hospitalization is about 4 days unless the patient has other medical problems.[60] A clinic visit is scheduled 2 weeks after the operation. During this visit, an interval history and physical examination, including a digital rectal examination, is performed. Postoperative anorectal dilatations are sometimes needed at home.

TAP (without laparoscopic assist) is almost identical to the previously described transanal dissection of the LATEP. Some pediatric surgeons prefer the prone jackknife position similar to the position for a posterior sagittal anorectoplasty for the TAP.[61] Other surgeons prefer the supine position and advocate initial leveling biopsies by way of a transumbilical celiotomy.[62] A randomized, long-term study comparing the LATEP and the TAP has not been reported.

POSTOPERATIVE ISSUES

Complications after pull-through can be classified as either early (weeks to months) or late (months to years). Early postoperative complications include anastomotic leak and cuff abscess, bowel obstruction, perineal excoriation, stoma complications, and wound infection. Late complications include bowel obstruction, constipation, enterocolitis, incontinence, and stricture. There is some overlap between the early and late complications. An anastomotic leak has been reported in 5% to 10% of cases, and a cuff abscess is seen in about 5% of cases. Factors that increase the risk of these complications include tension on the anastomosis or ischemia of the pull-through segment. Anastomotic leaks are usually treated by surgical exploration and diverting colostomy.[63-66]

Bowel obstruction is seen in both the early and late postoperative periods. It occurs in 5% to 10% of children after pull-through.[66,67] It is sometimes responsive to bowel decompression without the necessity of operative release, but may require urgent operative exploration in some circumstances. Factors increasing the risk of adhesions include prior operations, use of the open pull-through technique, and an anastomotic leak. Some authors have suggested that the laparoscopic or transanal approaches decrease the incidence of adhesive bowel obstruction.[66] I have not yet seen an adhesive obstruction as the cause of a postoperative bowel obstruction after a LATEP for HD.

Perineal excoriation due to an increase in stool frequency is common after the definitive repair of HD. It is frequently seen after a Swenson or Soave pull-through and may be less common after the Duhamel operation. Protective creams and antifungal agents (topical and oral) help to prevent or treat the excoriated skin. Neoanal prolapse, retraction, and peristomal skin breakdown are infrequent postoperative complications. Usually, mild strictures of the anal anastomosis can be easily corrected by daily postoperative dilatation by the parent beginning 3 weeks after the primary pull-through and continuing for 1 to 2 months.

Enterocolitis is a major cause of morbidity after surgery for HD. However, its pathogenesis is not completely understood.[68,69] Obstruction at the level of the anus certainly plays a role, particularly if it causes intestinal stasis and leads to proliferation of luminal pathogens. However, the very high incidence of Hirschsprung enterocolitis cannot be explained by partial obstruction alone. The reported incidence of Hirschsprung enterocolitis varies widely, but seems to be in the 30% to 40% range in carefully conducted studies.[31,68,70] In one recent retrospective study, it was reported that an initial admission for Hirschsprung enterocolitis was unusual beyond 2 years after the pull-through.[53] Risk factors for Hirschsprung enterocolitis are reported to be diagnosis at a young age, anastomotic stricture, and malnutrition.[31,53] Some researchers have suggested that a short rectal muscular cuff may also decrease the incidence of enterocolitis by reducing the obstruction caused by the spastic cuff.[70] It seems that keeping the cuff as short as possible and splitting the remaining cuff posteriorly during the primary pull-through operation may help reduce postoperative enterocolitis.

Yamataka has described resection of the posterior half of the muscle cuff to avoid infolding and stricture of the cuff in an attempt to reduce the secondary constipation and enterocolitis.[71] Intestinal stasis combined with immature mucosal immunity seems to contribute to the development of enterocolitis.[72]

An anastomotic stricture after the definitive pull-through procedure is another important postoperative complication. The incidence of anastomotic stricture varies widely depending on the method of reporting. The risk factors include anastomotic ischemia, cuff ischemia, anastomotic leak, and a small circular anastomosis.[73,74] As previously noted, Swenson believed that performing an oblique coloanal anastomosis may help to prevent stricture formation.[4] Stricture formation has been consistently associated with a higher risk of postoperative enterocolitis.[53] Most strictures can be managed by daily home dilatation. A few strictures require more aggressive measures such as the injection of mitomycin after aggressive dilatation. Occasionally, surgical ablation of the stricture or a re-do pull-through are needed to ameliorate the problem.

Stool frequency is high (10 or more per day) during the immediate postoperative period after pull-through. This frequency generally improves with time. By 6 months to 1 year after surgery, the stool frequency has usually declined to two to four times per day.[74] An algorithm for evaluation of post–pull-through soiling or constipation at my institution is shown in Figure 35-14. Constipation is sometimes seen a few months after pull-through and may depend on the type of operation. A higher incidence of constipation has been noted after the Duhamel or Rehbein technique.[66,73] Post–pull-through constipation has been reported in as low as 8% to 10% of children, but this incidence is probably underestimated. In one published study, it was reported that 37% of children had difficulty in evacuating stool after an operation for HD.[75] This functional form of constipation may be managed with nonoperative measures such as a high-fiber diet, laxatives, and enemas, but may require more aggressive management such as placement of a cecostomy or sigmoidostomy button, or even a re-do pull-through in the most severe cases.[74,76,77]

Fecal continence is best assessed after 4 years of age. In a series of carefully evaluated patients, the incidence of soiling was much higher than previous reports have indicated.[76] Most surgeons likely underestimate the presence of fecal soiling and incontinence in their patients. Catto-Smith and coworkers assessed continence after operation for HD in a cohort of 84 children with a mean age of 12 years.[75] They noted that fecal urgency was common (58%), and many patients were unable to hold back their stool or discriminate stool consistency (32%). Loose (liquid or pasty) stools were more common in children with long segment disease. Also, nearly 20% of the children were using continence aids or kept extra underwear available beyond the toilet training years.

Specific food intolerance is common after operation, with 44% of children using modified diets to avoid loose stools or constipation.[75,77] Anorectal manometry

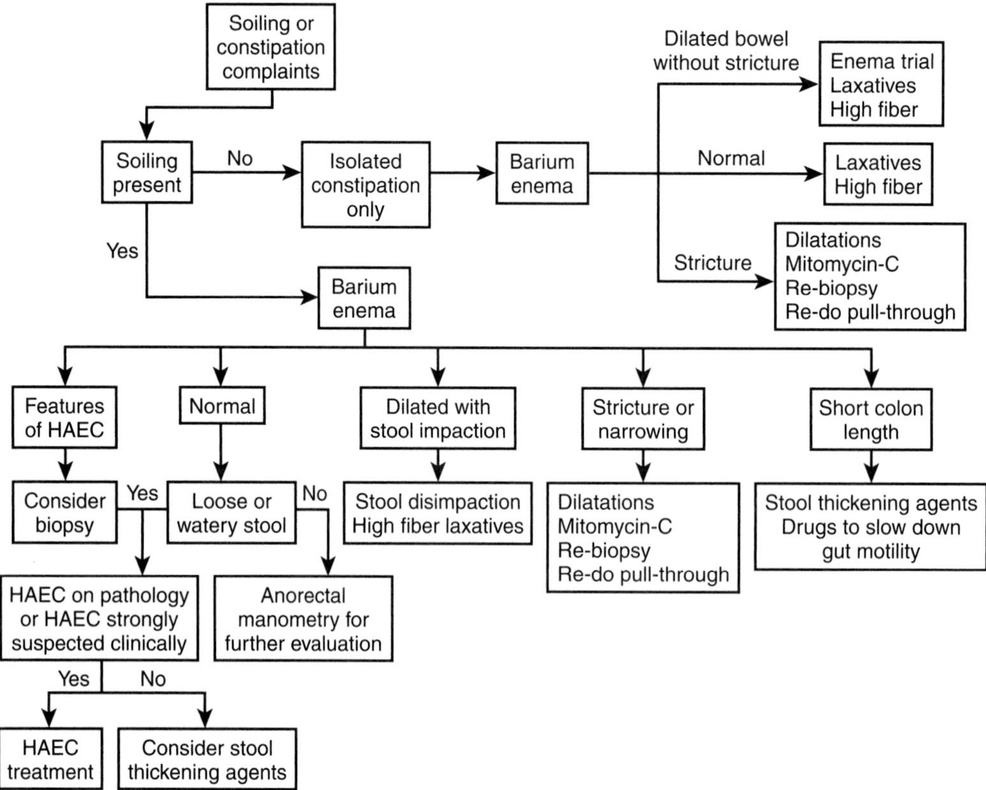

Figure 35-14. This algorithm is useful for evaluation of post pull-through soiling and constipation. HAEC, Hirschsprung-associated enterocolitis.

results showed higher baseline sphincter pressures and marked blunting of the sensation of rectal distention in children with significant soiling.[73,75] These authors, however, noted that continence and stool consistency improved with age. Enuresis has been reported in 5% to 26% of children and has been attributed to pelvic nerve injuries or neuropathy.[73,75]

Late mortality has been reported to be between 1% and 5% of the children undergoing operation for HD.[63,78] Although the exact cause of death is not consistently reported, a large percentage of the deaths are associated with enterocolitis (Fig. 35-15). With improvement in the recognition and treatment, mortality due to enterocolitis should decrease.

Stooling issues including constipation, incontinence, and enuresis may have the most impact on the postoperative quality of life of the child with HD and their parents. A trend toward improvement in stooling problems as the child gets older has been noted in several studies.[75,78] Improvement in continence as the child ages is probably due to the increased sophistication of the child as he or she grows, and to a better understanding of bowel management by pediatric surgeons and gastroenterologists. The presence of long-segment disease has been associated with a worse quality of life.[75,79] Children seem to cope with their disease in later years by developing stronger psychosocial skills.[80] The goal of the surgeon, however, should be to minimize these problems by providing meticulous operative, postoperative, and long-term care. HD is a lifelong disorder and should be thoughtfully explained to the family before any surgical procedures. Mechanisms for adequate long-term follow-up care should be in place at the time of postoperative discharge.

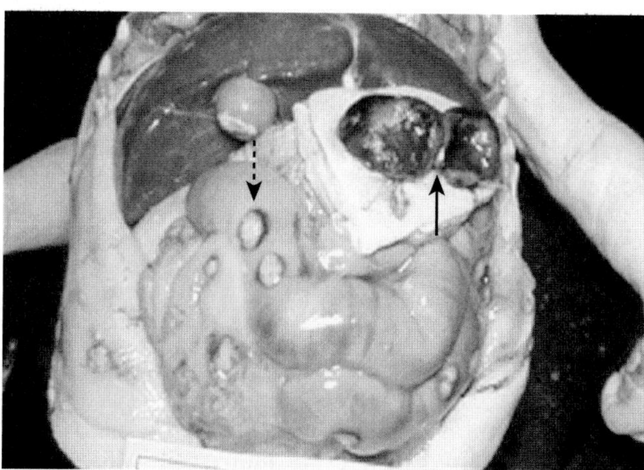

Figure 35-15. Enterocolitis can be a major cause of morbidity and mortality, both before any operative procedure for Hirschsprung's disease and in the postoperative period. Most of the deaths in the postoperative period are related to enterocolitis. In this autopsy specimen, note the several areas of perforation (*dotted arrow*) along the colon due to significant enterocolitis. Also note that the patient had undergone a diverting colostomy and had a mucous fistula (*solid arrow*).

chapter 36

IMPERFORATE ANUS AND CLOACAL MALFORMATIONS

Marc A. Levitt, MD • Alberto Peña, MD

"Imperforate anus" has been a well-known condition since antiquity.[1-3] For many centuries, physicians, as well as individuals who practiced medicine, tried to help these children by creating an orifice in the perineum. Many patients survived, most likely because they suffered from a type of defect that is now recognized as "low." Those with a "high" defect did not survive treatment. In 1835, Amussat was the first to suture the rectal wall to the skin edges, which could be considered the first actual anoplasty.[2] During the first 60 years of the 20th century, most surgeons performed a perineal anoplasty without a colostomy for the so-called low malformations. A colostomy performed during the newborn period was followed by an abdominal perineal pull-through for the treatment of high malformations. The decision to create the colostomy was based mainly on the radiologic information obtained by an invertogram.[4] During the era of the abdominoperineal pull-through operation, the specific recommendation was to pull the bowel as close to the sacrum as possible to avoid trauma to the genitourinary tract. Stephens made a significant contribution by performing the first objective anatomic studies in human specimens. In 1953, he proposed an initial sacral approach followed by an abdominoperineal operation, if necessary.[5] The purpose of the sacral stage of the procedure was to preserve the puborectalis sling, considered a key factor in maintaining fecal incontinence. Since then, different surgical techniques have been proposed.[6-9] Their common denominator is the protection and use of the puborectalis sling.

The posterior sagittal approach for the treatment of imperforate anus was performed first in 1980, and its description was published in 1982.[10,11] This new approach allowed direct exposure of this important anatomic area. Also, the unique opportunity arose to correlate the external appearance of the perineum with the operative findings and, subsequently, with the clinical results. Since its original description, significant innovations in terminology and classification have emerged.

INCIDENCE, TYPES OF DEFECTS, AND TERMINOLOGY

Anorectal atresia occurs in one of every 4000 to 5000 newborns and is slightly more common in males.[12-14] The estimated risk for a couple having a second child with an anorectal malformation is approximately 1%.[15-18] The most frequent defect in male patients is anorectal atresia with a rectourethral fistula,[19] and is anorectal atresia with a rectovestibular fistula in females.[19] Imperforate anus without a fistula is a rather unusual defect. It occurs in about 5% of the entire group of malformations, and is associated with Down syndrome.[19,20] Historically, persistent cloaca was considered an unusual defect, whereas a high incidence of rectovaginal fistula was reported in the literature.[21] In retrospect, it seems that the presence of a cloaca is a much more common defect in females.[22] A cloaca is the third most common defect in female patients after vestibular and perineal fistulas, whereas a rectovaginal fistula actually is a rare defect, present in fewer than 1% of all cases.[22,23] It is likely that most patients suffering from a persistent cloaca were erroneously thought to have a rectovaginal fistula. Many of these patients underwent surgery with repair of the rectal component but were left with a persistent urogenital sinus.[22,24] Additionally, most rectovestibular fistulas were erroneously called "rectovaginal fistula."[22] A recto-bladder neck fistula in male patients is the only true supralevator malformation and occurs in about 10% of male patients.[19] Because it is the only malformation in males in which the rectum is unreachable through a posterior sagittal incision, it requires an abdominal approach (either laparotomy or laparoscopy) in addition to a perineal approach.

Anorectal malformations represent a wide spectrum of defects. The terms "low," "intermediate," and "high" are arbitrary and not useful in therapeutic or prognostic terms. Within the group of anorectal malformations traditionally referred to as "high," there are defects included with different therapeutic and

Table 36-1	Classification
Males	
Cutaneous (perineal fistula)	
Rectourethral fistula	
Bulbar	
Prostatic	
Recto–bladder neck fistula	
Imperforate anus without fistula	
Rectal atresia	
Females	
Cutaneous (perineal fistula)	
Vestibular fistula	
Imperforate anus without fistula	
Rectal atresia	
Cloaca	
Complex malformations	

prognostic implications.[25] For instance, retroprostatic fistula and recto-bladder neck fistula were both considered high, yet the first can be repaired with a posterior sagittal approach alone and the second requires an additional abdominal approach. Furthermore, the prognosis for each type is completely different. Therefore, a more therapeutic and prognostically oriented classification is depicted in Table 36-1.

MALE ANORECTAL DEFECTS

Rectoperineal Fistulas

Rectoperineal fistula is what traditionally was known as a "low defect." The rectum is located within most of the sphincter mechanism. Only the lowest part of the rectum is anteriorly mislocated (Fig. 36-1). Sometimes, the fistula does not open into the perineum but rather follows a subepithelial midline tract, opening somewhere along the midline perineal raphe, scrotum, or even at the base of the penis. This diagnosis is established by perineal inspection. No further investigations are required. Usually, the anal fistula opening is narrow (stenotic). The terms *covered anus, anal membrane, anteriorly mislocated anus,* and *bucket-handle malformations* all refer to perineal fistulas.

Rectourethral Fistulas

Imperforate anus with a rectourethral fistula is the most frequent defect in male patients.[19] The fistula may be located at the lower (bulbar) (Fig. 36-2A) or the higher (prostatic) part of the urethra (see Fig. 36-2B).

Immediately above the fistula, the rectum and urethra share a common wall. The lower the fistula, the longer is the common wall. This is an important anatomic fact with significant technical and surgical implications. The rectum is usually distended and surrounded laterally and posteriorly by the levator muscle. Between the rectum and the perineal skin, a portion of striated voluntary muscle called the muscle complex is present. The contraction of these muscle fibers elevates the skin of the anal dimple. At the level of the skin, a group of voluntary muscle fibers, called parasagittal fibers, are located on both sides of the midline. Lower urethral fistulas are usually associated with good-quality muscles, a well-developed sacrum, a prominent midline groove, and a prominent anal dimple. Higher urethral fistulas are more frequently associated with poor-quality muscles, an abnormally developed sacrum, a flat perineum, a poor midline groove, and a barely visible anal dimple. Of course, exceptions to these rules exist. Occasionally, the infant passes meconium through the urethra, which is an unequivocal sign of a rectourinary fistula.

Recto-Bladder Neck Fistulas

In this defect, the rectum opens into the bladder neck (Fig. 36-3). The patient usually has a poor prognosis for bowel control because the levator muscles, the striated muscle complex, and the external sphincter frequently are poorly developed. The sacrum is often deformed and short. In fact, the entire pelvis seems to be underdeveloped. The perineum is often flat, which is evidence of poor muscle development. About 10% of males with anorectal atresia fall into this category.[19]

Imperforate Anus without Fistula

Interestingly, most patients with this unusual defect have a well-developed sacrum and good muscles, and have a good prognosis in terms of bowel function.[19] The rectum usually terminates approximately 2 cm from the perineal skin. Although the rectum and urethra do not communicate, these two structures are separated only by a thin, common wall. About half of

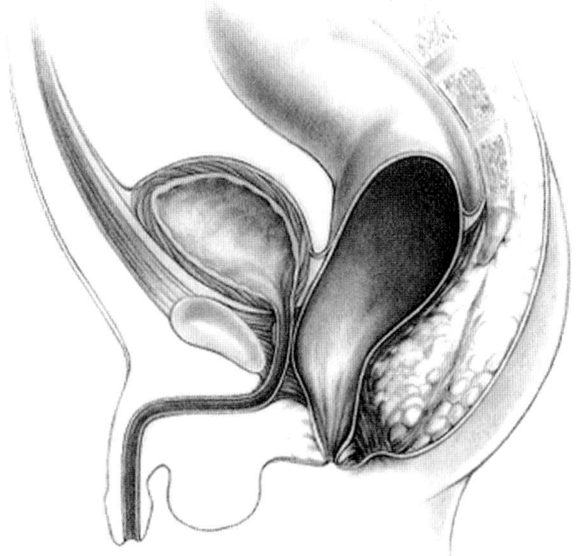

Figure 36-1. This drawing shows the course of a perineal fistula in a male. The rectum is located within most of the muscle complex. Only the most distal aspect of the rectum is misplaced.

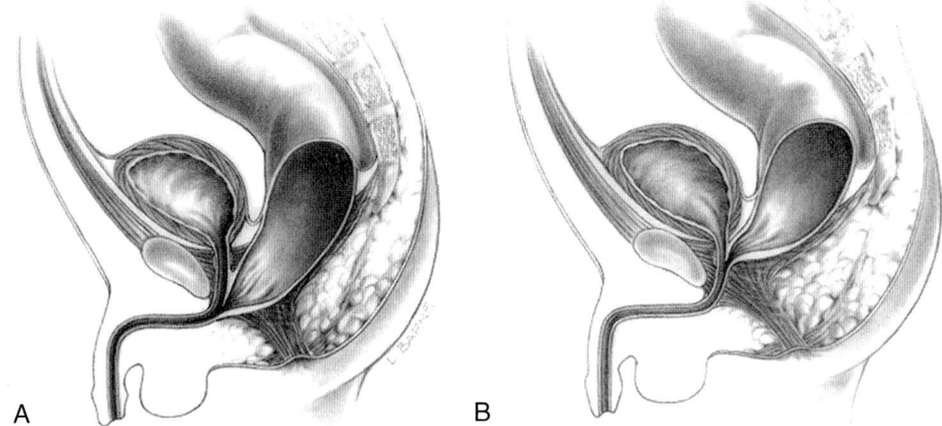

Figure 36-2. These drawings depict anorectal atresia with rectourethral fistulas. **A,** Rectourethrobulbar fistula **B,** Rectourethroprostatic fistula.

the patients with no fistula also have Down syndrome, and more than 90% of patients with Down syndrome and imperforate anus have this specific defect, suggesting a chromosomal link.[18,20] The fact that these patients have Down syndrome does not seem to interfere with their good prognosis for bowel control.[20]

Rectal Atresia

In this extremely unusual defect in male patients (~1% of the entire group of malformations), the lumen of the rectum is totally (atresia) or partially (stenosis) interrupted.[19] The upper pouch is represented by a dilated rectum, whereas the lower portion is represented by a small anal canal that is in the normal location and is 1 to 2 cm deep (Fig. 36-4). These two structures may be separated by a thin membrane or by dense fibrous tissue. The repair involves a primary anastomosis between the upper pouch and anal canal (see Fig. 36-4B) and is ideally approached posterior sagittally. Patients with this defect have all the necessary elements to be continent and have an excellent functional prognosis. Because they have a well-developed anal canal, they have normal sensation in the anorectum and have almost normal voluntary sphincters. Patients with rectal atresia must be screened for a presacral mass.[26]

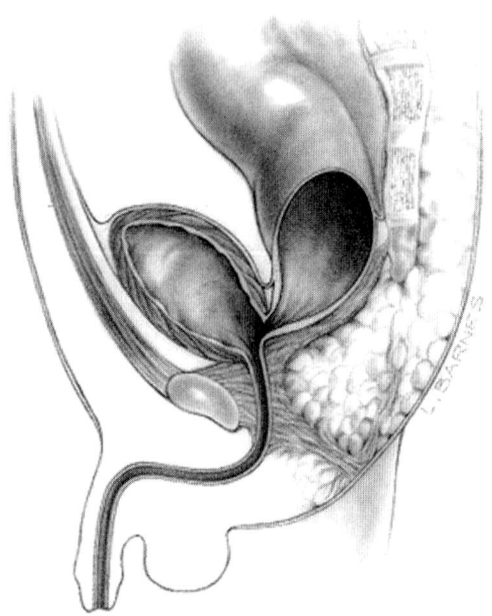

Figure 36-3. Schematic representation of a recto-bladder neck fistula. Note that the fistula enters into the bladder neck near the junction between the urethra and the bladder.

FEMALE ANORECTAL DEFECTS

Rectoperineal Fistulas

From the therapeutic and prognostic viewpoint, this common defect is equivalent to the perineal fistula described in the male patient.[19] The rectum is well positioned within the sphincter mechanism, except for its lower portion, which is anteriorly located. The rectum and vagina are well separated (Fig. 36-5). The key anatomic issues are the anal opening in relation to the sphincter mechanism, and the length of the perineal body.

Rectovestibular Fistulas

Rectovestibular fistula is the most common defect in girls and has an excellent functional prognosis. The diagnosis is based on clinical examination. A meticulous inspection of the neonatal genitalia allows the clinician to observe a normal urethral meatus and a normal vagina, with a third hole in the vestibule, which is the rectovestibular fistula (Fig. 36-6). About 5% of these patients will have two hemivaginas with a vaginal septum.

A number of pediatric surgeons repair this defect without a protective colostomy. This is a well-recognized trend in the management of anorectal malformations.[27-30] The advantage of this approach is

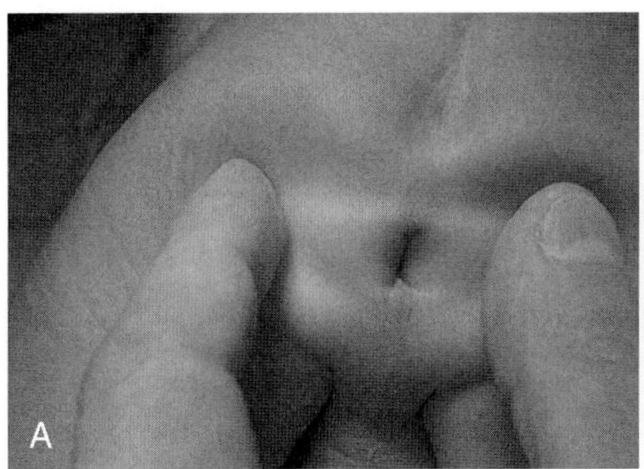

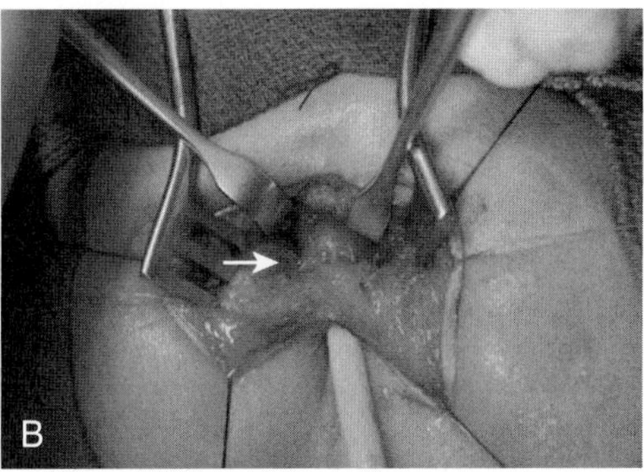

Figure 36-4. This newborn was found to have rectal atresia. **A,** Note the normal anal position and short depth of the anal canal. **B,** Operative repair. A dilator has been inserted into the anus and the anastomosis (*arrow*) is identified just proximal to the distal anal canal.

that it avoids the potential morbidity of a colostomy and reduces the number of operations to one from as many as three (colostomy, main repair, and colostomy closure). Many patients do very well with a primary neonatal operation without a protective colostomy. However, a perineal infection followed by dehiscence of the anal anastomosis or perineal body, or recurrence of the fistula provokes severe fibrosis that may interfere with the sphincter function. If these complications occur, the patient may have lost the best opportunity for an optimal functional result because secondary operations do not render the same prognosis as a successful primary operation.[31] Thus, a protective colostomy is still the best way to avoid these complications. The decision to perform a colostomy or primary repair in these cases must be made individually by the surgeon, taking into consideration his or her experience and the clinical condition of the patient. At our institution, neonates born with this anomaly, without significant associated defects, undergo operation without a colostomy.

The term *vaginal fistula* is frequently erroneously used in patients who actually have a vestibular fistula or a cloaca. A true vaginal fistula occurs in less than 1% of all cases[22] and is not considered part of the proposed classification.

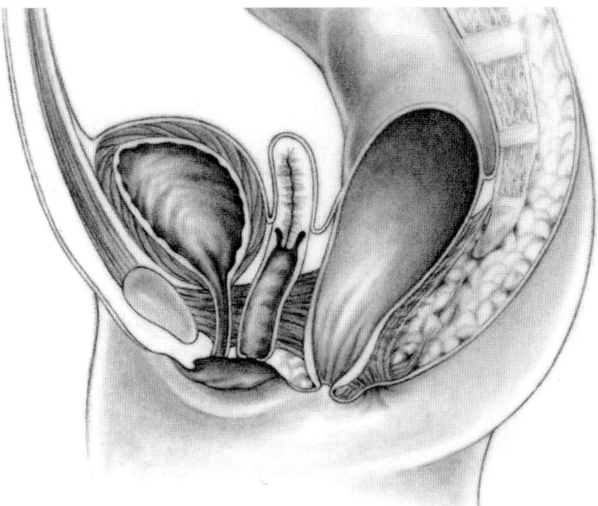

Figure 36-5. Schematic drawing of a perineal fistula in a female. Most of the rectum is in the muscle complex. Only the most distal aspect of the rectum is anteriorly positioned.

Imperforate Anus without Fistula

This defect in female patients carries the same therapeutic and prognostic implications as described for male patients.

Persistent Cloaca

This group of defects represents the extreme in the spectrum of complexity of female malformations. A cloaca is defined as a defect in which the rectum, vagina, and urinary tract meet and fuse, creating a single common channel.

The diagnosis of persistent cloaca is a clinical one. This defect should be suspected in a female born with imperforate anus and small-looking genitalia. Careful separation of the labia discloses a single perineal orifice. The length of the common channel varies from 1 to 7 cm. This distance has technical and prognostic implications. Common channels longer than 3 cm usually are associated with complex defects (Fig. 36-7A). Mobilization of the vagina is difficult in such cases. Therefore, in patients with a long common channel, some form of vaginal replacement is often needed during the definitive repair. A common channel of less than 3 cm usually means that the defect can be repaired with a posterior sagittal operation without opening the abdomen (see Fig. 36-7B). When the rectum opens high into the dome of the vagina (Fig. 36-8), an abdominal approach must be utilized to mobilize the bowel. Frequently, the vagina is abnormally distended and full of secretions (hydrocolpos) (Fig. 36-9A). The distended vagina compresses the trigone and interferes with drainage of the ureters and is frequently associated with megaureters. This condition may be diagnosed prenatally.[32,33] The dilated vagina can also become infected (pyocolpos) and may lead to perforation and peritonitis. However, such a large vagina may represent a technical advantage for the repair, providing more vaginal tissue to facilitate the reconstruction. A frequent finding in cloacal malformations is the presence of different degrees of vaginal and uterine septation or duplication (see Fig. 36-9B). The rectum usually enters between the two hemivaginas. Rarely, patients may have cervical atresia. During puberty, they are unable to drain menstrual blood through the vagina. These patients accumulate menstrual blood in the peritoneal cavity and often require

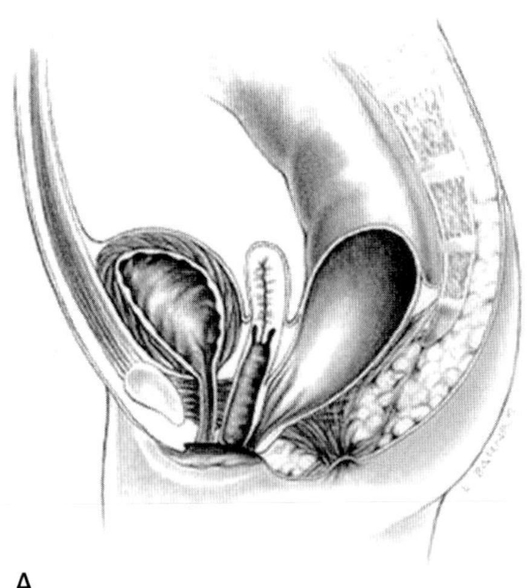

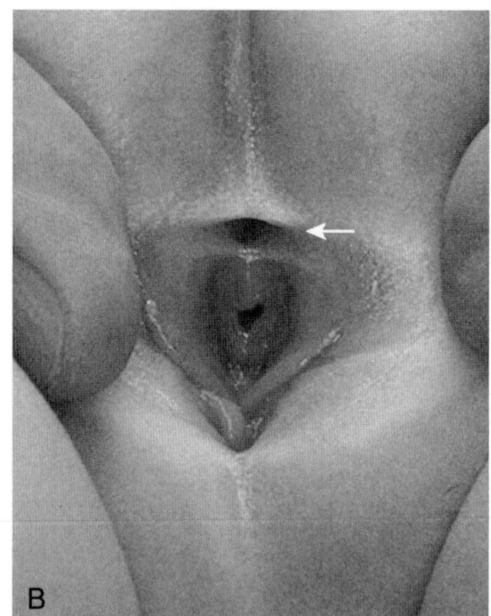

Figure 36-6. **A,** Schematic drawing of a rectovestibular fistula. **B,** A female neonate with a rectovestibular fistula. Note the patient is in the prone position and the rectal fistula (*arrow*) is located in the posterior aspect of the vestibule.

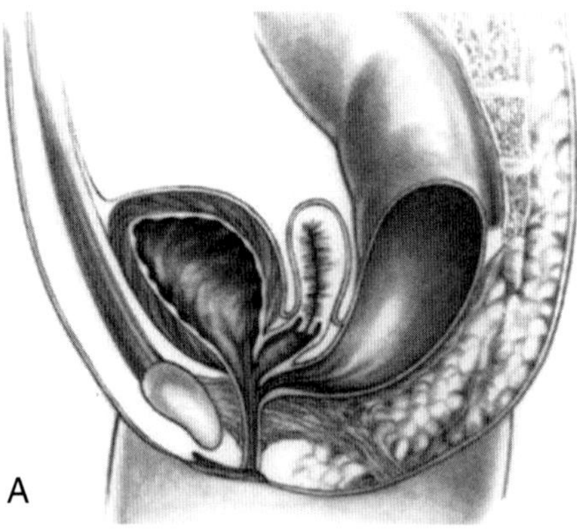

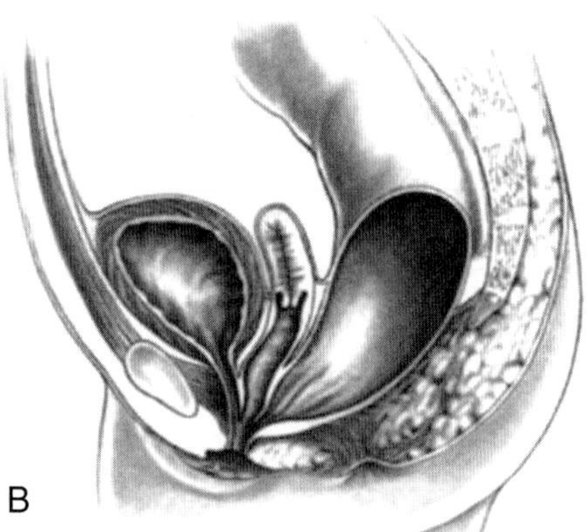

Figure 36-7. **A,** Schematic diagram of a long common channel in a female with a cloacal anomaly. **B,** The more commonly encountered short common channel cloaca is depicted.

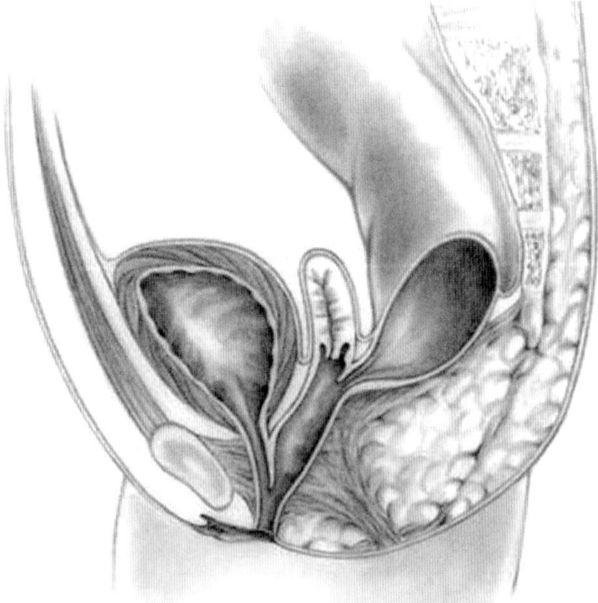

Figure 36-8. A schematic diagram of the rectum inserting high into the posterior vagina with a short common urethral and vaginal channel is shown.

emergency operations.[34] An evaluation of a patient's müllerian anatomy, either at the time of the definitive repair or at the colostomy closure, is vital and can prevent future problems. Low cloacal malformations (<3 cm) are usually associated with a well-developed sacrum, a normal-appearing perineum, and adequate muscles and nerves. Therefore, a good functional prognosis should be expected.

Complex Malformations

Unusual and bizarre anatomic arrangements can be seen. Each case represents a unique challenge to the surgeon, with different prognoses and therapeutic implications. No general guidelines can be drawn for the management of these patients. Each case must be individualized.

ASSOCIATED DEFECTS

Sacrum and Spine

Sacral deformities appear to be the most frequently associated defect.[35] One or several sacral vertebrae may be missing. A single missing vertebrae does not

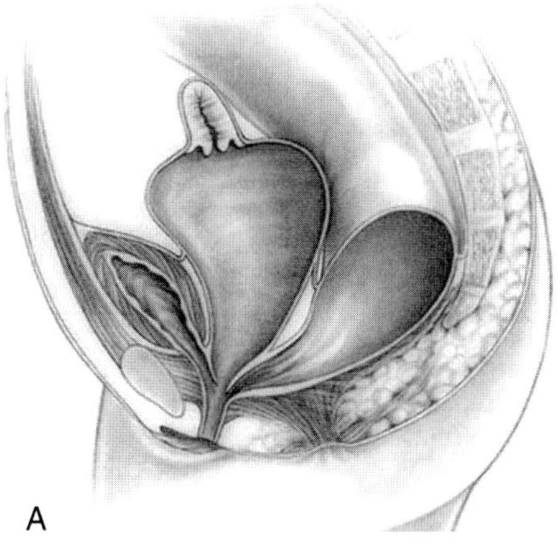

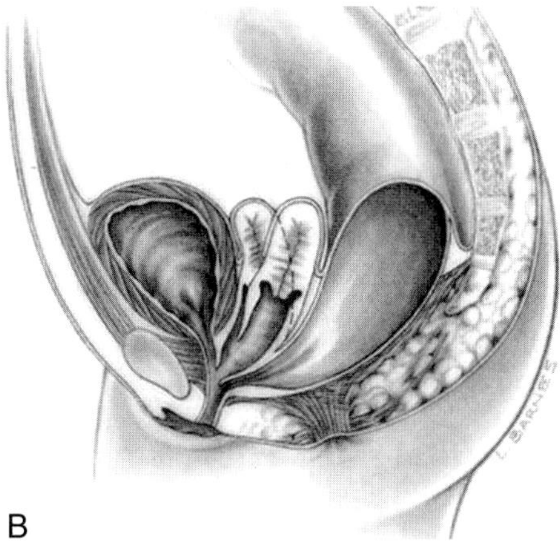

Figure 36-9. **A,** Schematic depiction of a cloacal anomaly with insertion of the rectum into the common channel and subsequent vaginal obstruction with hydrocolpos. **B,** Schematic depiction of a cloacal anomaly and uterine duplication. The rectum is shown entering between the two hemivaginas.

seem to have any important prognostic implications.[19] However, more than two absent sacral vertebrae represent a poor prognostic sign in terms of bowel continence and, sometimes, urinary control. A hemisacrum is usually associated with a presacral mass and poor bowel control.[26] Other sacral abnormalities, such as spinal hemivertebra, have a negative implication for a patient's bowel control.

A sacral ratio allows for a more objective evaluation of the sacrum (Fig. 36-10). The normal sacral ratio in children is 0.77. Children with anorectal malformations suffer from different degrees of sacral hypodevelopment, and the sacral ratio can vary from 0.0 to 1.0. We have never seen a patient develop good bowel control with a sacral ratio of less than 0.3.

Emphasis has been placed on the diagnosis and treatment of a tethered cord, which is a defect frequently associated with anorectal malformations.[36-44] It has been assumed that the presence of a tethered cord is associated with poor functional prognosis in these children. A review of our own series showed that 25% of patients with an anorectal malformation suffer from tethered cord.[45] Although it is true that most of these children have a poor prognosis, the presence of a tethered cord by itself coincides with a very high defect, very abnormal sacrum, or spina bifida. Therefore, it is difficult to know whether the tethered cord itself is responsible for the poor prognosis. Also, we have not found evidence that the operation to release the tethered cord changes the functional bowel prognosis of the patient.[42-45]

Genitourinary Defects

The frequency of associated genitourinary defects varies from 20% to 54%.[46-58] The accuracy and thoroughness of the urologic evaluation may account for the reported variation.

In our experience, 48% of patients (55% girls and 44% boys) had associated genitourinary anomalies.[52] These figures may not reflect the real incidence of genitourinary defects because our hospital is a referral

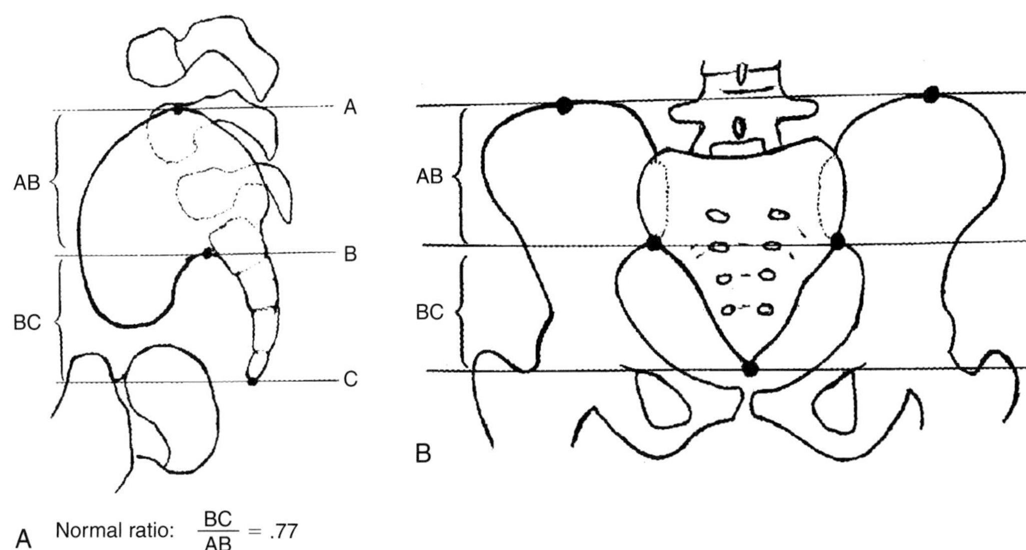

Figure 36-10. Drawings with landmarks necessary for the calculation of the sacral ratio. **A,** Lateral view. **B,** Anteroposterior view. The normal ratio is 0.77.

center where we see a high proportion of complex malformations that are not necessarily representative of the entire spectrum of defects.

The higher the malformation, the more frequent are the associated urologic abnormalities. Patients with persistent cloacas or recto-bladder neck fistulas have a 90% chance of having an associated genitourinary abnormality.[52] Conversely, children with low defects (perineal fistulas) have less than a 10% chance of having an associated urologic defect. Hydronephrosis, urosepsis, and metabolic acidosis from poor renal function represent the main sources of morbidity in infants with anorectal malformations. Thus, a thorough urologic investigation is mandatory in cases of high defects, but is not as urgent in cases of rectovestibular and rectourethral fistulas. The evaluation in every child with imperforate anus must include an ultrasonographic study of the kidneys and abdomen to evaluate for the presence of hydronephrosis or any other urologic obstructive process. In patients with a cloaca, this study is especially important to exclude the presence of hydrocolpos. If this study is abnormal, further urologic evaluation is necessary.

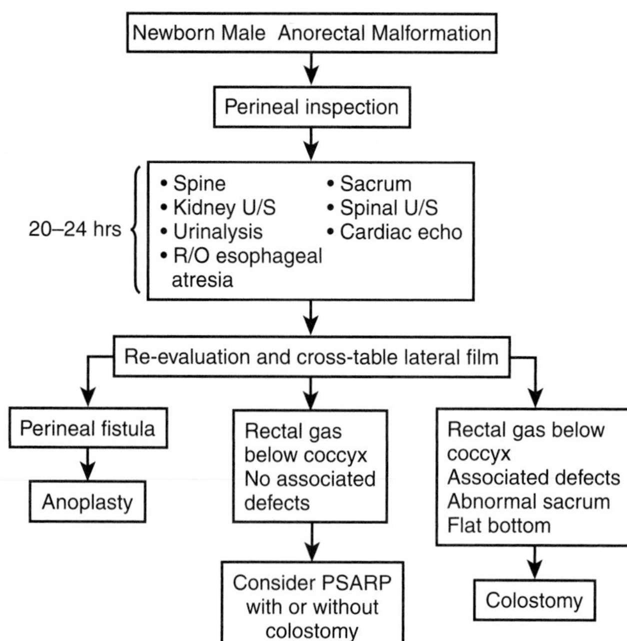

Figure 36-11. Algorithm for the management of male newborns with anorectal malformations based on the physical examination and radiographs. PSARP, posterior sagittal anorectoplasty; U/S, ultrasonography; R/O, rule out.

NEWBORN MANAGEMENT

A decision-making algorithm for the initial management in male patients is seen in Figure 36-11. During the past few years, the tendency by the pediatric surgical community has been to operate on patients with anorectal malformations primarily without a protective colostomy.[27-30,59,60] We promote this trend, but also alert all surgeons to the potential negative consequences of performing these operations without the necessary preoperative evaluation and experience.

When asked to evaluate a male newborn with an anorectal malformation, a thorough perineal inspection must be performed. This usually gives the key clues to the type of malformation. It is important not to make a decision about a colostomy or a primary operation before 24 hours of life. The reason is that significant intraluminal pressure is required for the meconium to be forced through a fistulous orifice. Passage of meconium through a fistula will be the most valuable sign for the location of that fistula. If meconium is seen on the perineum, a perineal fistula is present. If there is meconium in the urine, a rectourinary fistula exists. Radiologic evaluations may not show the correct anatomy before 24 hours because the rectum is collapsed. It takes a significant amount of intraluminal pressure to overcome the muscle tone of the sphincters that surround the lower part of the rectum. Therefore, radiologic evaluations done too early (before 24 hours) most likely will show a "very high rectum" and may lead to an incorrect diagnosis.

During the first 24 hours, the neonate should receive intravenous fluids and antibiotics and be evaluated for associated defects that may represent a threat to life. These include cardiac malformations, esophageal atresia, and urinary defects.[35,61] A radiograph of the lumbar spine and the sacrum should be obtained as well as a spinal ultrasonogram to evaluate for a tethered cord. Ultrasonography of the abdomen will evaluate for hydronephrosis.

If the neonate has signs of a perineal fistula, we recommend that an anoplasty, without a protective colostomy, be performed during the first 48 hours of life. After 24 hours, if there is no meconium on the perineum, we recommend obtaining a cross-table lateral radiograph with the patient in the prone position. If air in the rectum is located below the coccyx, (Fig. 36-12) and the patient is in good condition with no significant associated defects, one may consider performing a posterior sagittal operation without a protective colostomy. A more conservative alternative would be to perform the posterior sagittal repair and a protective colostomy at the same stage.

Conversely, if the rectal gas does not extend beyond the coccyx, or the patient has meconium in the urine, an abnormal sacrum, or a flat bottom, we strongly recommend a colostomy. This allows for a future distal colostogram, which will precisely delineate the anatomy. We would then perform a posterior sagittal anorectoplasty 1 to 2 months later, provided the neonate is gaining weight appropriately.

Performing the definitive repair at age 1 to 3 months has important advantages, including less time with an abdominal stoma, less size discrepancy between the proximal and distal bowel at the time of colostomy closure, and easier anal dilation (because the infant is smaller). In addition, at least theoretically, placing the rectum in the right location early in life may represent an advantage in terms of the potential for acquired local sensation.[62]

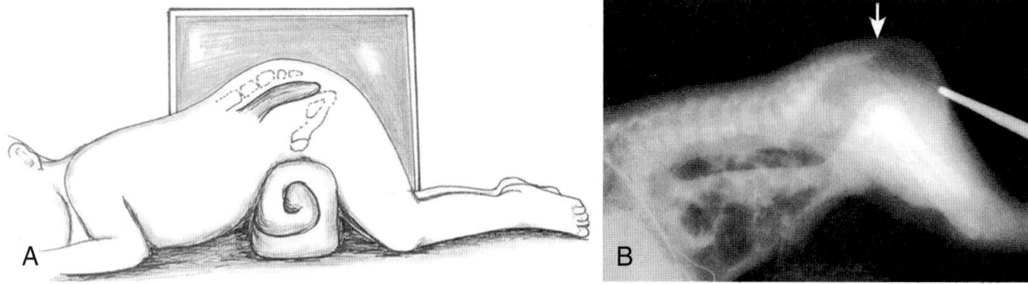

Figure 36-12. Technique for a cross-table lateral radiograph. **A,** A roll has been placed beneath the hips of the infant to elevate the buttocks and allow air to migrate superiorly to the end of the rectum. **B,** Actual cross-table lateral radiograph. Air is visualized distal to the coccyx (*arrow*).

All of these potential advantages of an early operation must be weighed against the possible disadvantages of an inexperienced surgeon who is not familiar with the minute anatomic structures of an infant's pelvis.

A temptation to repair these defects without a protective colostomy always exists.[27,28,59,60] Repair without a colostomy limits the anatomic information (provided by a distal colostogram) that may be very helpful to the surgeon. The worst complications involve patients operated on without a colostomy or a properly performed distal colostogram.[63] Proceeding with the posterior sagittal approach looking blindly for the rectum has resulted in a spectrum of serious complications, including damage to the urethra, complete division of the urethra, pull-through of the urethra, pull-through of the bladder neck, injury to the ureters, and division of the vas deferens or seminal vesicles.[63]

A decision-making algorithm for the initial management of newborn females is seen in Figure 36-13. Again, the perineal inspection is the most important step to guide diagnosis and decision making. The first 24 hours should also be used to evaluate for serious associated defects, as previously described. The perineal inspection may disclose the presence of a single perineal orifice. This single finding establishes the diagnosis of a cloaca, which carries a high risk of an associated urologic defect. The patient needs a complete urologic evaluation, including abdominal and pelvic ultrasonography, to look for hydronephrosis and hydrocolpos.

Patients with a cloaca require a colostomy. It is important to perform the divided sigmoid colostomy in such a manner as to leave enough redundant, distal rectosigmoid colon to allow for the subsequent pull-through (Fig. 36-14). When performing the colostomy, it is mandatory to drain the hydrocolpos when present. This can be achieved with a red rubber catheter. Because a significant number of these patients have two hemivaginas, the surgeon must be certain that both

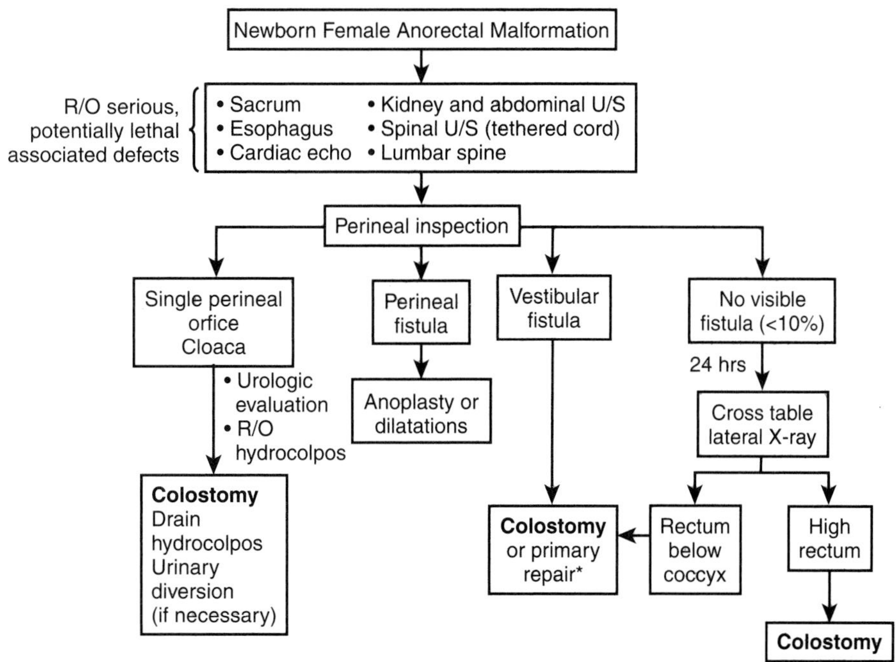

Figure 36-13. Decision-making algorithm for female newborns with anorectal malformations. U/S, ultrasonography; R/O, rule out.

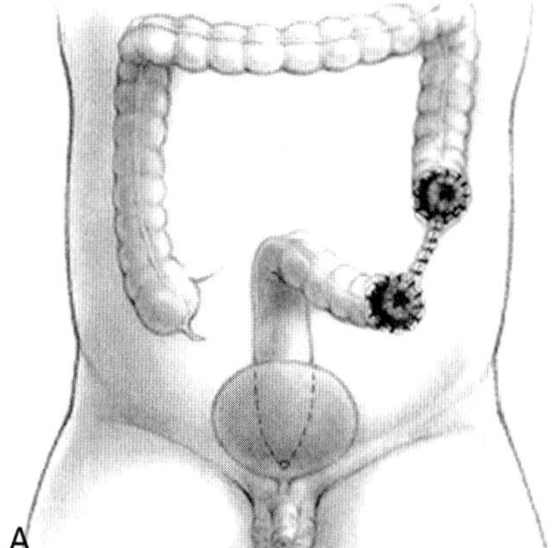

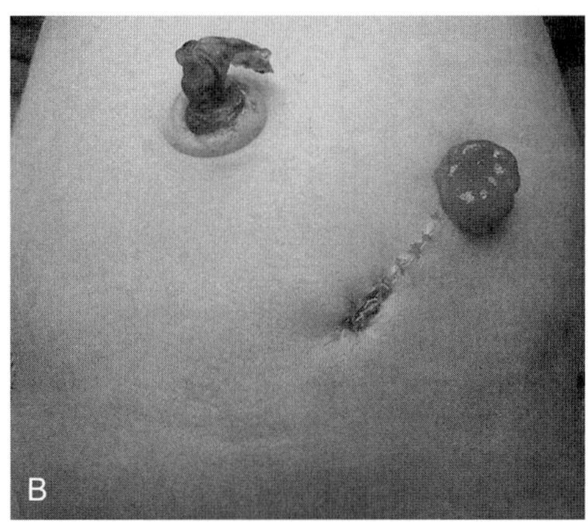

Figure 36-14. An ideal colostomy for infants with high anorectal malformations is seen in the drawing (**A**) and infant (**B**). Note the colostomy and mucous fistula are separated and that adequate distal colonic length remains for the subsequent rectal pull-through.

hemivaginas are drained. Occasionally, a vaginovaginostomy in the vaginal septum will have to be created to drain both hemivaginas with one catheter. At times, the hydrocolpos is so large that it may produce respiratory distress. It is the hydrocolpos that compresses the trigone and causes bilateral hydronephrosis, and drainage of the hydrocolpos allows for decompression of the urologic system. Rarely, if the common channel is very narrow and does not allow the bladder to drain, the neonate may require a vesicostomy or suprapubic cystostomy to decompress the bladder. However, in the vast majority of cases, drainage of the hydrocolpos is all that is required. Endoscopic examination of the cloaca is recommended to delineate the anatomy. This is best done later (in several months) during a separate anesthetic because the neonatal perineum is swollen and endoscopy is difficult.

The presence of a vestibular fistula represents the most common finding in female patients (see Fig. 36-6). When newborns with a vestibular fistula undergo primary repair at our institution, we keep the patient 5 to 7 days, do not allow any oral intake, and use parenteral nutrition. Conversely, when the patient undergoes a primary repair of a vestibular fistula or perineal fistula without colostomy later in life, we are very strict about preoperative bowel irrigation 24 hours preoperatively to ensure that the intestine is completely clean. We then keep the patient on parenteral nutrition 7 to 10 days with nothing by mouth, all in an attempt to avoid a perineal infection.

The perineal inspection may show the presence of a perineal fistula. When present, we recommend performing a primary anoplasty without a colostomy. In fewer than 5% of girls, there is no visible fistula and there is no evidence of meconium after 24 hours of observation. This small group of patients requires a cross-table lateral prone radiograph (see Fig. 36-12). If the radiograph shows gas in the rectum very close to the skin, it means that the patient very likely has a very narrow perineal fistula. Conversely, if the distal extent of the rectal gas is located 1 to 2 cm above the skin, the patient most likely has an imperforate anus with no fistula. If the patient is in stable condition, one can perform a primary operation without a colostomy, depending on the surgeon's experience. Most of these patients with no fistula also have Down syndrome.[20] In the event that associated conditions make the rectal repair unfeasible in the newborn period, a colostomy should be performed, with definitive repair later.

Occasionally, if the infant with a rectoperineal or rectovestibular fistula has severe associated defects or is ill, the surgeon may elect to dilate the fistula to facilitate emptying of the colon while these other issues are addressed. Definitive repair can be performed in a few months.

A divided descending colostomy is ideal for the management of anorectal malformations (see Fig. 36-14). The completely diverting colostomy provides bowel decompression as well as protection for the final reconstruction of the malformation. In addition, the colostomy is used for the distal colostogram, which is the most accurate diagnostic study to determine the detailed anatomy of these defects.[64]

The descending or upper sigmoid colostomy has definitive advantages over a right or transverse colostomy.[65] It is important to have a relatively short segment of defunctionalized distal colon, but not too short as to interfere with the subsequent pull-through. The ideal location is just at the point where the proximal sigmoid comes off the left retroperitoneum. In some patients, atrophy of the bowel can occur distal to a more proximal colostomy. Mechanical cleansing of the distal colon at the time of colostomy creation is much less difficult when the colostomy is located in the descending portion of the colon. In the case of a large rectourethral fistula, the patient frequently passes urine into the colon. A more distal colostomy allows urine to escape through the distal stoma without significant absorption. With a more proximal colostomy, the urine remains in the colon and is absorbed, leading to metabolic acidosis. A loop colostomy permits the passage of stool from the proximal stoma into the distal bowel. This can lead to urinary tract infections, distal rectal pouch dilation, and fecal impaction (Fig. 36-15). Prolonged distention of the rectal pouch may produce an irreversible hypomotility disorder, leading to severe constipation later in life. Also, the problem of colostomy prolapse is more frequent in loop colostomies.[66] The most common error we have seen is a colostomy established in the lower rectosigmoid that

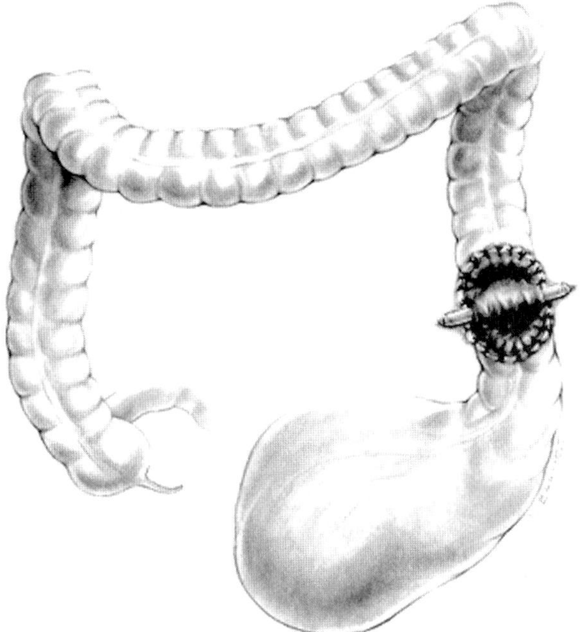

Figure 36-15. A markedly dilated distal rectal pouch secondary to fecal impaction.

interferes with the mobilization of the rectum during the pull-through (Fig. 36-16).

Historically, there have been many surgical techniques to repair anorectal malformations. These include endorectal dissection,[6,8,9] anterior perineal approaches,[67] and many different types of anoplasties.[68] Most pediatric surgeons now use the posterior sagittal approach with or without laparotomy or laparoscopy to repair these malformations. The debate recently has been centered more on the possibility of performing these operations primarily without a colostomy, or for which cases a laparoscopic approach is best suited.

The patient is placed in the prone position with the pelvis elevated. An electrical stimulator is used to elicit muscle contraction during the operation. The demonstrated contraction serves as a guide to keep the incision in the midline, leaving an equal amount of muscle on both sides. The length of the incision varies with the type of defect and can be extended to achieve the necessary exposure needed to have a satisfactory repair. Thus, a perineal fistula requires a minimal posterior sagittal incision (2 cm), whereas higher defects may require a full posterior sagittal incision that runs from the lower portion of the sacrum toward the base of the scrotum in the male or to the single perineal orifice in females with a cloaca. The incision includes the skin and subcutaneous tissue and splits the parasagittal fibers, muscle complex, and levator muscles in the midline. In simple defects (perineal and vestibular), the incision divides only the parasagittal fibers and the muscle complex in the midline. It is not usually necessary to open the levator muscle. Once the sphincter mechanism has been divided, the next most important step of the operation is the separation of the rectum from the urogenital structures, which represents the most delicate part of the procedure. Any kind of blind maneuver at this point in the operation exposes the patient to the possibility of serious injury.[63]

About 90% of defects in boys can be repaired via a posterior sagittal approach without opening the abdomen and without laparoscopy. Each case has individual anatomic variants that mandate technical modifications. An example is the size discrepancy frequently seen between an ectatic rectum and the space available for the pull-through. If the discrepancy is significant, the surgeon must tailor the rectum to fit. As repairs are being performed earlier in life and patients undergo

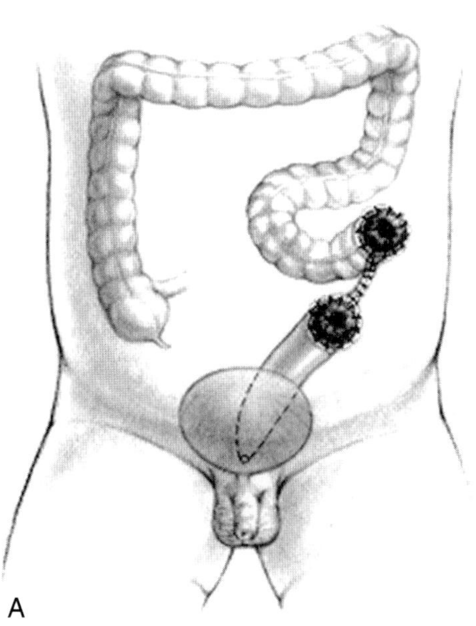

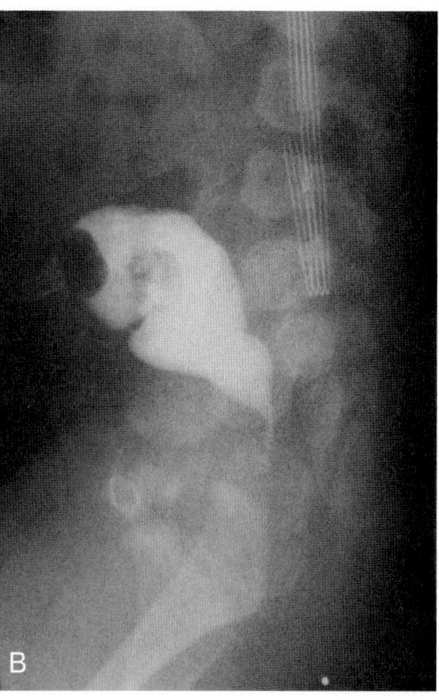

Figure 36-16. **A,** It is important not to create the colostomy too distal because there will not be sufficient rectal length to allow for pull-through. **B,** This problem is seen on the lateral view of the barium enema, where there is insufficient distal rectal length for the pull-through. This is because of an inappropriately placed colostomy and mucous fistula.

adequate colostomies, rectal dilatation is less commonly seen. Therefore, tapering is less frequently required.

If a colostomy has been done, the posterior sagittal approach should never be attempted without a technically adequate high-pressure distal colostogram to determine the exact position of the rectum and the fistula.[64] Attempting the repair without this important information significantly increases the potential damage to the seminal vesicles, prostate, urethra, and bladder innervation.[63]

REPAIR OF SPECIFIC DEFECTS IN MALE INFANTS

Perineal Fistula

The operation in these infants is performed in the prone position with the pelvis elevated. Multiple 6-0 silk stitches are placed in the fistula orifice. An incision is created dividing the sphincter mechanism located just posterior to the fistula. The incision usually measures about 2 cm in length. The sphincter is divided, and the posterior rectal wall is identified by its characteristic whitish appearance. This plane is easy to find. Dissection of the rectum continues laterally following this specific plane. The last part of the dissection consists of separating the anterior rectal wall from its intimate relation to the urethra. The most common and serious complication in these relatively simple operations involves injury to the urethra.[63] The patient must have a urinary catheter inserted preoperatively. The best way to avoid urethral injury is to continuously be aware of the fact that the common wall has no plane of dissection and that the surgeon must create two walls out of one.

Rectourethral Fistulas

A urinary catheter is inserted. In about 20% of cases, this catheter goes into the rectum rather than into the bladder. Under these circumstances, the surgeon may attempt the bladder catheterization again using a Coudé catheter or catheter guide, or can relocate the catheter into the bladder under direct visualization during the operation.

The incision is performed as previously described (Fig. 36-17). The parasagittal fibers, muscle complex, and levator muscle fibers are completely divided in the midline. Sometimes, the coccyx can be split in the midline with cautery, particularly in those cases of a rectoprostatic fistula when the surgeon requires more exposure in the upper part of the incision. The higher the malformation, the deeper the levator muscle. When the entire sphincter mechanism has been divided, the surgeon should identify the rectum. It is at this point in the operation that the importance of a good high-pressure distal colostogram cannot be overstated. If the radiologic image showed the presence of a bulbourethral fistula (Fig. 36-18), the rectum is going to be found just below the levators, with little risk of inadvertent injury to the urinary tract. In this

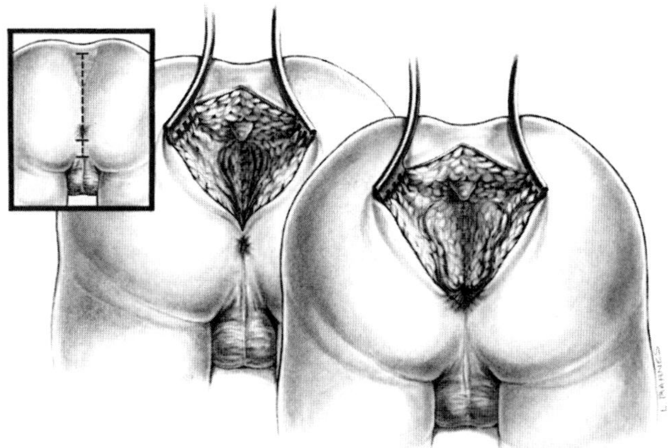

Figure 36-17. This drawing shows a posterior sagittal incision in a male patient with a rectourethral fistula. Separation of the parasagittal fibers and exposure of the muscle complex are shown.

situation, the rectum actually bulges through the incision when the sphincter mechanism is divided (Fig. 36-19). Mobilization of the rectum is rather minimal because only a short gap exists between the rectum and perineum.

Conversely, if the preoperative distal colostogram shows a rectoprostatic fistula, the surgeon must be particularly careful because the rectum joins the urinary tract much higher (Fig. 36-20). The initial search for the rectum should be near the coccyx. Looking for the rectum lower than the coccyx risks injury to the bulbar urethra. If the colostogram shows a recto-bladder neck fistula, the posterior sagittal approach is not appropriate as a means of identifying the distal bowel.

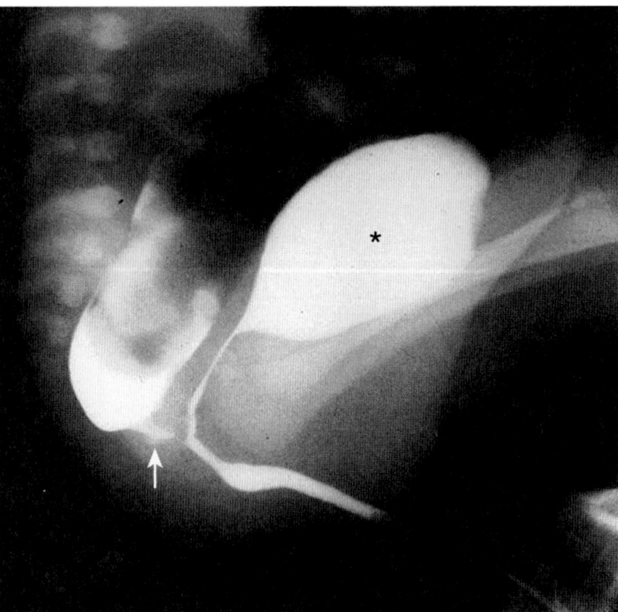

Figure 36-18. A lateral view of a high pressure, distal colostogram shows a rectobulbar urethral fistula (*arrow*). The bladder (*asterisk*) also filled during the study.

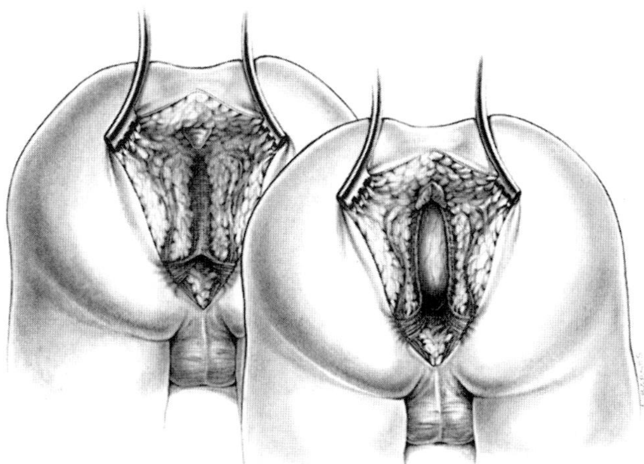

Figure 36-19. Schematic drawing of the posterior sagittal approach. The muscle complex and the levator muscles have been divided, and the rectum is visualized below the levator muscle complex.

The rectum must be identified and separated from the urinary bladder through an abdominal approach.

In all cases in which the rectal fistula is at the bulbar level or higher, silk traction sutures are placed in the posterior rectal wall on both sides and the rectum is opened in the midline. The incision is extended distally, exactly in the midline, down to the fistula. Additional silk traction sutures are situated around the edges of the opened posterior rectal wall. When the fistula opening is visualized, silk sutures are placed around the orifice of the fistula as well.

The anterior rectal wall above the fistula is part of a common wall, with no natural plane of separation between the urinary tract and the rectum. The plane of separation must be created in the common wall. For this, multiple 6-0 silk traction stitches are placed in the rectal mucosa immediately above the fistula orifice. The rectal mucosa is then separated from the urethra for 5 to 10 mm above the fistula (Fig. 36-21). This is a submucosal dissection. It is this dissection that is the source of the most serious complications during this repair. We recommend creating a lateral plane of dissection on either side of the rectum to help delineate the rectal wall from the urethra and prostate. The rectum is covered by a thin fascia that contains fat, vessels, and nerves that must be preserved on the back side of the bladder. This tissue should be completely stripped from the rectum to be sure that one is working as close as possible to the rectal wall. This is the only way to prevent denervation of the bladder or injury to the vas deferens. Once the rectum is fully separated from the deep structures of the urinary tract, a circumferential perirectal dissection is performed to gain enough rectal length to reach the perineum.

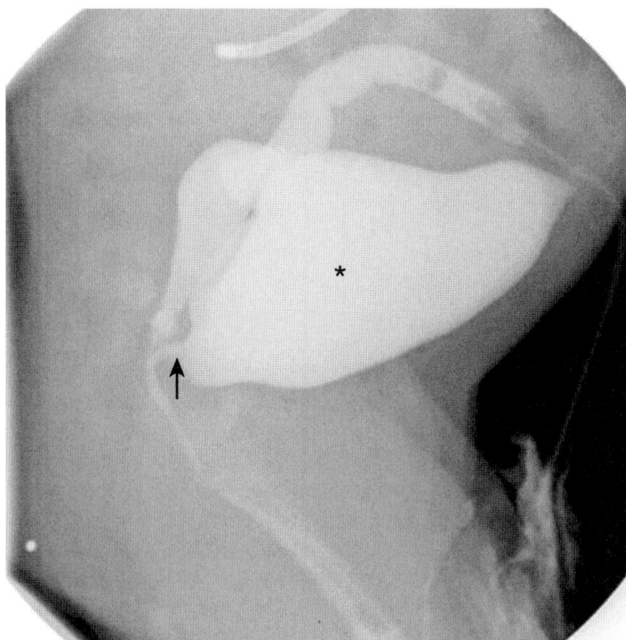

Figure 36-20. This distal colostogram shows the rectum entering the prostatic urethra (rectoprostatic urethral fistula) (*arrow*). Note filling of the bladder (*asterisk*) as well.

In cases of a rectoprostatic fistula, the perirectal dissection is considerably more difficult. During this dissection, uniform traction is applied on the multiple silk traction sutures that were originally placed on the rectal edges and also on the mucosa above the fistula. Uniform traction shows the rectal wall and allows identification of fibrous bands and vessels that hold the rectum in the pelvis. These bands must be carefully separated from the rectal wall using cautery because they contain vessels that tend to retract into the pelvis once divided. The rectum should be dissected as close as possible to the rectal wall without injuring the rectal wall itself. Perhaps in these cases, a surgeon with advanced laparoscopic skills would feel more comfortable with this dissection performed laparoscopically.[60,69-71]

At the completion of the dissection in prostatic fistula cases, many of the extrinsic vessels that supply the rectum have been sacrificed. The rectum should be viable, however, provided the intramural blood supply was preserved by not injuring the rectal wall. One might think that this denervation would provoke a motility disorder, leading to severe constipation, but this has not been our experience. Patients with lower defects (who undergo less dissection) are bothered by more severe postoperative constipation than are patients with higher defects.[19] We do not have an explanation for this, unless there is an inherent motility disorder that is more prevalent in lower defects.

The circumferential dissection of the rectum must continue until the surgeon feels that enough length has been gained to allow for a rectoperineal anastomosis without tension. At this point, the size of the rectum can be evaluated and compared with the available space. If necessary, the rectum can be tapered, removing part of the posterior wall. In such cases, the rectal wall is reconstructed with two layers of interrupted long-lasting absorbable stitches. The anterior rectal wall is frequently thinned to some degree as a consequence of the mucosal separation between the rectum and urethra. To reinforce this wall, both smooth muscle layers

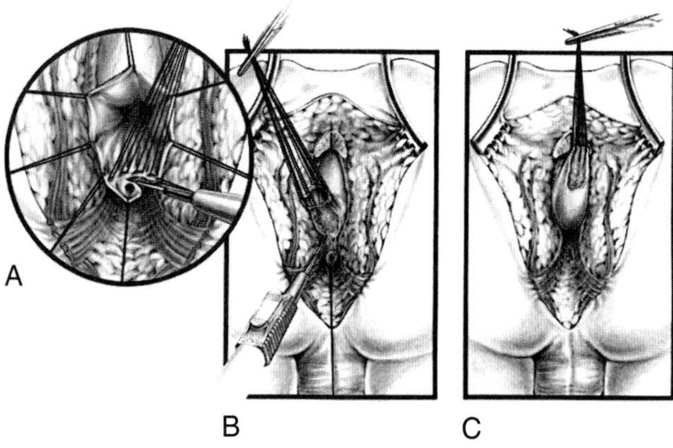

Figure 36-21. A schematic representation of the separation of the rectal fistula from the urethra is shown. **A,** Separation of the rectum from the urethra using silk traction stitches in the rectum. **B,** Proximal dissection of the rectum from the urethra. **C,** Depiction of the rectum completely separated from the underlying urethra.

can be approximated with interrupted 5-0 long-lasting absorbable stitches. The urethral fistula is closed with the same suture material. The rectal tapering should never be performed anteriorly because this would leave a rectal suture line adjacent to the urethral fistula repair and may lead to a recurrent fistula.

The limits of the sphincter mechanism are electrically determined and marked with temporary silk stitches at the skin level. Sometimes, in patients with a good sphincter mechanism, these limits are easily visible, even without electrical stimulation. The limits of the sphincter are represented by the crossing of the muscle complex with the parasagittal fibers. These are the voluntary muscles that run from the levator all the way down to the skin parallel with the direction of the rectum. This muscle structure crosses the parasagittal fibers that run perpendicular and lateral to the muscle complex and parallel to the posterior sagittal incision. The perineal body is reconstructed, bringing together the anterior limits of the sphincter previously marked with the temporary silk stitches. The rectum must then be placed in front of the levator and within the limits of the muscle complex (Fig. 36-22). Long-lasting 5-0 absorbable stitches are placed on the posterior edge of the levator muscle.

The posterior limit of the muscle complex must also be reapproximated behind the rectum. These stitches should incorporate part of the rectal wall to anchor it to avoid rectal prolapse (see Fig 36-22B).[72] An anoplasty is performed with 16 interrupted long-lasting absorbable stitches. The ischiorectal fossa and the subcutaneous tissue are reapproximated, and the wound is closed with subcuticular 5-0 absorbable monofilament suture material (Fig. 36-23).

All these patients have a urinary catheter inserted before the beginning of the operation that remains in place for 7 to 10 days. The patient receives broad-spectrum antibiotics for 24 hours. These patients can be fed after recovery from anesthesia because they have a diverting colostomy.

Recto-Bladder Neck Fistulas

In these patients, the rectum connects to the bladder neck approximately 2 cm below the peritoneal reflection. A very important anatomic feature that must be remembered is that the higher the malformation, the shorter the common wall between the rectum and the urinary tract. This means that in these cases the rectum joins with the urinary tract at nearly a right angle, with little common wall. Thus, separation of the rectum from the bladder is much easier. The laparoscopic approach provides an excellent view of the peritoneal reflection, the ureters, and the vas deferens, which must be kept under direct vision to prevent injury to them.

For this repair, a total body preparation is performed. The entire lower part of the patient's body is included in the sterile field, and the operation is begun laparoscopically.

We recommend dividing the peritoneum around the distal rectum to create a plane of dissection to be followed distally. The dissection should stay right on the rectal wall. The rectum rapidly narrows as it reaches its communication with the bladder neck, at which point it is divided and the bladder side of the fistula is sutured or ligated with an endoloop. The vessels that supply the distal rectum are divided with electrocautery or between ligatures until there is enough length to pull the rectum comfortably down to the perineum. These vessels should be divided close to the rectal wall, preserving the inferior mesenteric artery trunk because the arcade may have been disrupted by the initial colostomy. This dissection preserves perfusion to the rectum because the rectum has an excellent intramural blood supply. In these cases, the distal rectum can be very ectatic and may require tapering. If the colostomy was created too distal in the sigmoid, it

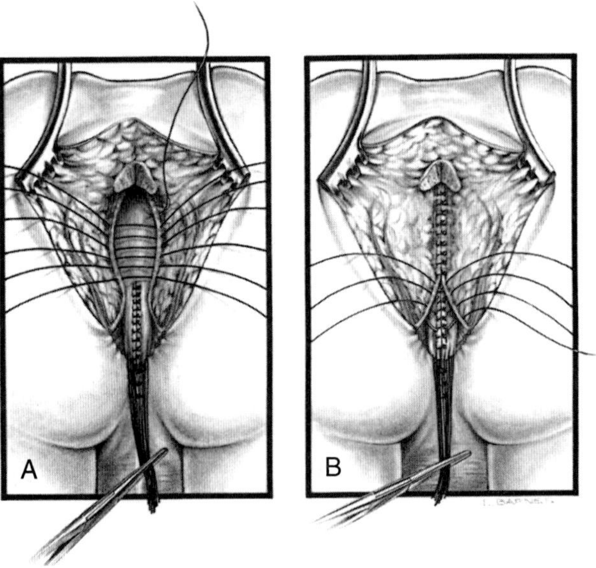

Figure 36-22. Position of the rectum after separation from the urethra is shown. **A,** Technique of passing the rectum in front of the levator muscle complex. **B,** Technique of anchoring the rectal wall to the levator complex to avoid rectal prolapse.

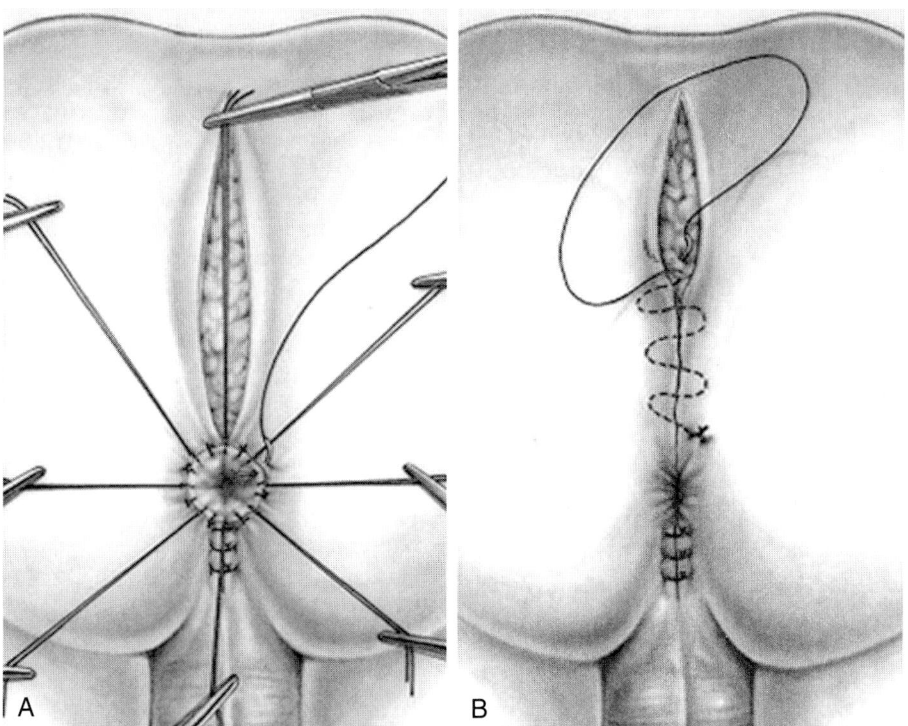

Figure 36-23. **A,** Technique of anoplasty. Four quadrant stay sutures are placed followed by three sutures between each quadrant. **B,** Subcuticular skin closure.

may interfere with this mobilization. Once the rectum is mobile, a cannula with blunt trocar or mosquito clamp is passed through the perineum, just anterior to the coccyx. Great care must be taken to avoid passing the cannula and trocar too anteriorly because injury to the bladder neck or ectopic ureters could occur. The distal rectum is grasped and pulled through to be situated in the center of the sphincter mechanism. Often, in these patients, the center of the sphincter is quite anterior, near the base of the scrotum. Traction on the rectum from below can help demonstrate further lines of tension that must be divided to allow the rectum to reach the perineum. We prefer a small posterior sagittal incision so that the posterior edges of the muscle complex can be visualized and tacked to the posterior rectal wall.[72]

Imperforate Anus without Fistula

In these cases, the blind end of the rectum is usually located at the level of the bulbar urethra and easily reachable from the posterior sagittal approach. The rectum must be carefully separated from the urethra because both structures have a common wall, even though no fistula is present. The rest of the repair is performed as described for the rectourethral fistula defect.

Rectal Atresia and Stenosis

The approach to these malformations is also posterior sagittal. The upper rectal pouch is opened as is the small distal anal canal. An end-to-end anastomosis is performed under direct visualization (see Fig. 36-4), followed by a meticulous reconstruction of the sphincter mechanism posterior to the rectum. If a presacral mass is identified, it is removed with presacral dissection at the time of this operation.

REPAIR OF SPECIFIC DEFECTS IN FEMALE INFANTS

Rectoperineal Fistulas

This defect is repaired in the same way as described for male patients. The rectum is not usually attached to the vagina. Therefore, the chance of a vaginal injury is low.

Vestibular Fistulas

The complexity of this defect is frequently underestimated. Multiple 5-0 silk stitches are placed at the mucocutaneous junction of the fistula. The incision is shorter than the one used to repair the male recto-urethral fistula. The incision continues down to and around the fistula into the vestibule. Once the entire sphincter mechanism is divided, the surgeon identifies the posterior rectal wall by its characteristic whitish appearance. The fascia that surrounds the rectum must be removed to be sure that the dissection is as close as possible to the rectal wall. The dissection is aided by working along each side of the rectum, as well as from below, while applying tension on multiple silk traction sutures. A long common wall exists between the vagina and the rectum, and two walls must be created out of one by using a meticulous, delicate technique. The dissection continues cephalad until the rectal and vaginal walls are fully separated and an areolar plane

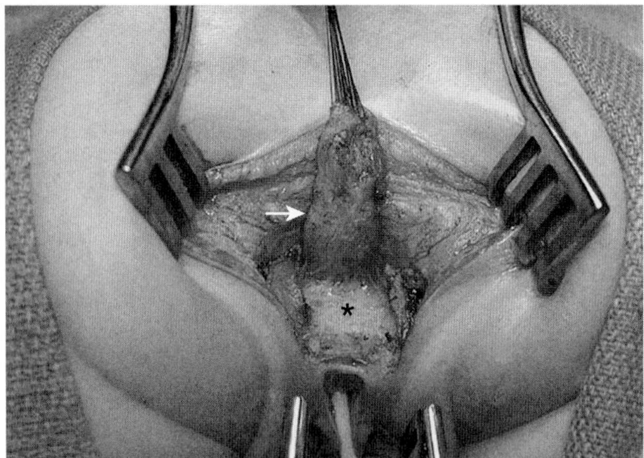

Figure 36-24. In this operative photograph of a female patient undergoing repair of a rectovestibular fistula, note the complete separation of the rectum (*arrow*) from the anteriorly positioned vagina (*asterisk*). A catheter has been inserted into the vagina.

between the two is encountered (Fig. 36-24). If the rectum and the vagina are not completely separated, a tense anal anastomosis predisposes the patient to dehiscence, retraction, and stricture.[31]

Once the dissection is complete, the perineal body is repaired (Fig. 36-25A). The anterior edge of the muscle complex is reapproximated as previously described. The sutures include the posterior edge of the muscle complex and the posterior rectal wall to avoid rectal prolapse.[72] The anoplasty is performed as previously described (see Fig. 36-25B,C).

Cloaca Repair

Before undertaking repair of a cloaca, the surgeon should perform an endoscopic study, with the specific purpose of determining the length of the common channel. A review of over 400 patients identified two well-characterized groups of patients with cloaca.[73] These two groups have different technical challenges and must be recognized preoperatively. The first is represented by patients who are born with a common channel shorter than 3 cm. Fortunately, these patients comprise the majority and they can usually undergo repair with a posterior sagittal approach alone, avoiding a laparotomy. The operation to repair this particular variant is reproducible and can be accomplished by most general pediatric surgeons. The second group is represented by patients with a long common channel (>3 cm). These patients usually need a laparotomy for correction. In this group of patients, intraoperative decision-making requires a large experience and special training in urology. Therefore, referral to a specialized center is in the best interest of the patient.

Cloacas with a Common Channel Shorter Than 3 cm

The incision extends from the middle portion of the sacrum down to the single perineal orifice (Fig. 36-26A). The sphincter mechanism is divided in the midline. The first structure that the surgeon finds after division of the sphincter mechanism is the rectum (see Fig. 36-26B). However, because of the complexity of these malformations, bizarre anatomic arrangements of the rectum and vagina are sometimes encountered. The rectum is opened in the midline (see Fig. 36-26C), and silk sutures are placed along the edges of the posterior rectal wall. The incision is extended distally through the posterior wall of the common channel. Placing a mosquito clamp into the single perineal orifice facilitates this midline split. The entire common channel is exposed, which allows for measurement and confirmation of its length under direct vision. The separation of the rectum from the vagina, which share

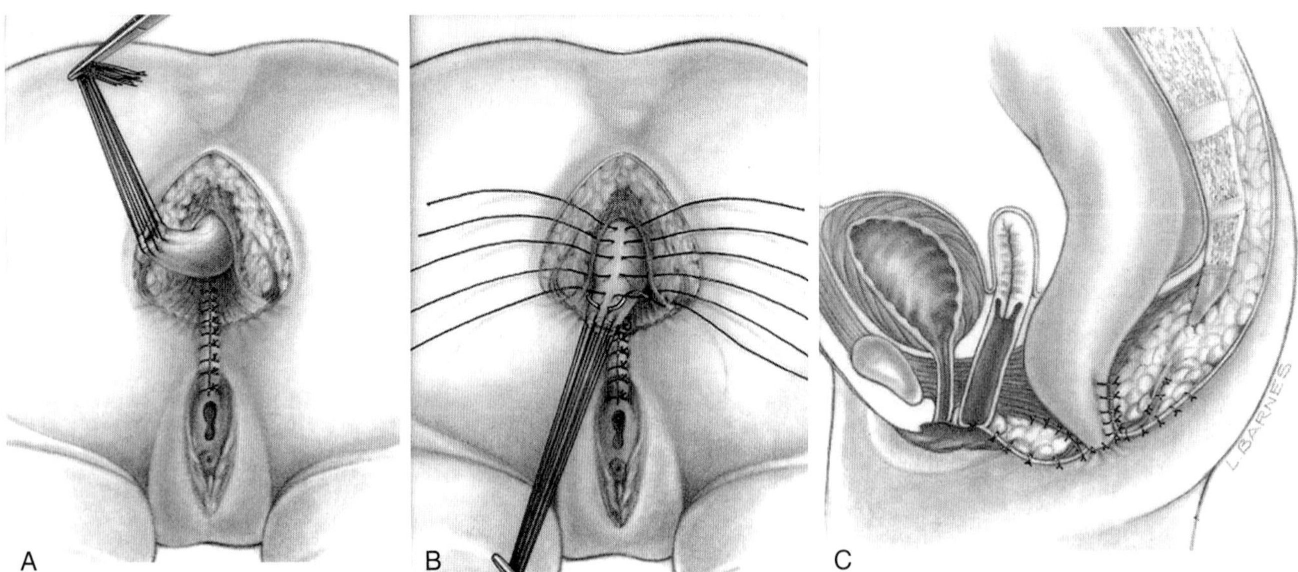

Figure 36-25. Schematic drawings of the final stages of the repair of a rectovestibular fistula in a female. **A,** Reconstruction of the perineal body. **B,** Positioning the rectum in front of the levator muscle complex. **C,** Sagittal view of the completed operation.

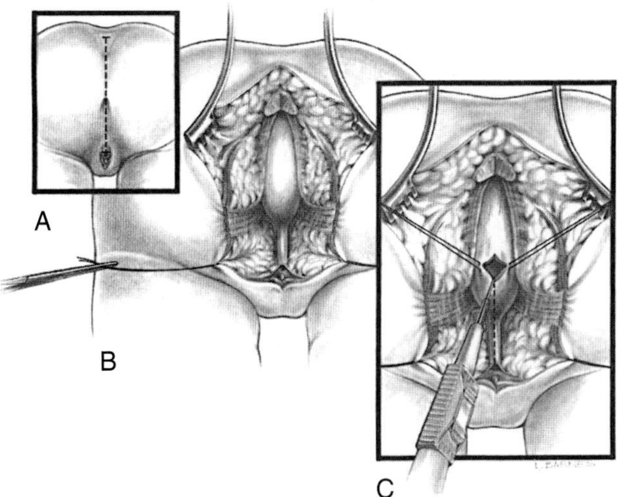

Figure 36-26. Drawings of the initial steps of the posterior sagittal approach for cloacal repair. **A,** The incision extends from the sacral prominence to the common orifice. **B,** The exposure of the rectum and common channel above the levator complex. **C,** The technique of opening the rectum and placement of traction sutures in the rectal opening.

a common wall (Fig. 36-27), is performed as described for the repair of a rectovestibular fistula.

Once the rectum has been completely separated from the vagina, the total urogenital mobilization begins.[74] Before developing this approach, we tried to separate the vagina from the urinary tract, which was technically challenging and had significant morbidity, with most concern being for a urethrovaginal fistula. The total urogenital mobilization consists of bringing both vagina and urethra to the perineum as a single unit.

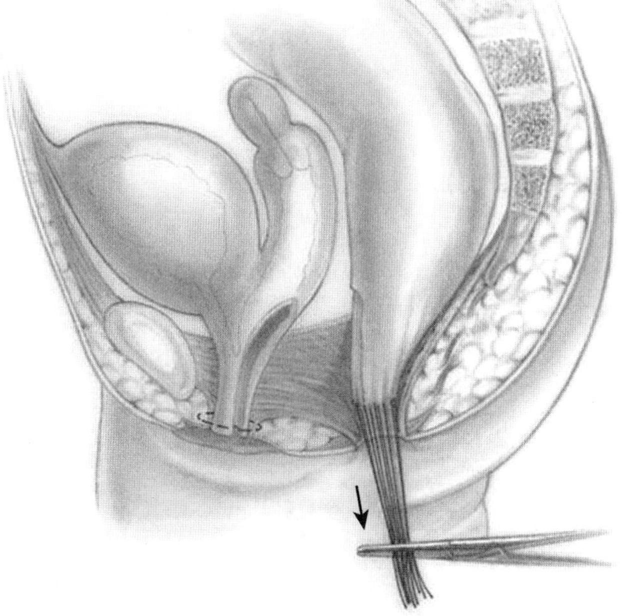

Figure 36-27. A schematic representation of total urogenital sinus mobilization with separation of the rectum from the vagina. (From Peña A: Total urogenital mobilization: An easier way to repair cloacas. J Pediatr Surg 32:263-268, 1997.)

After the rectum has been dissected away from the urogenital complex, multiple silk traction sutures are placed at the edge of the vagina and the common channel in order to apply uniform traction on the urogenital sinus as it is mobilized. Another series of fine traction sutures is placed transversely approximately 5 mm proximal to the clitoris (Fig. 36-28). The urogenital sinus is transected between the last row of silk stitches and the clitoris. The anterior aspect is dissected full thickness from the pubic symphysis, taking advantage of the fact that a natural plane exists between it and the pubis. This dissection is usually easy and relatively bloodless. At the upper edge of the pubis, there are fibrous, avascular suspensory ligaments that give support to the vagina and bladder. While applying traction to the multiple urogenital sinus sutures, the suspensory ligaments are divided, providing 2 to 3 cm of additional mobilization. Lateral and posterior dissection of the urogenital sinus will provide an additional 0.5 to 1.0 cm in length, allowing for complete urogenital mobilization (Fig. 36-29). Both the urethral meatus and the vaginal introitus can then be anastomosed to the perineum in the appropriate positions. Approximately 60% of all cloacas can be satisfactorily repaired with this technique. This technique has the additional advantage of preserving an excellent blood supply to both the urethra and vagina while placing the urethral opening and the smooth-walled urethra in a visible location to facilitate intermittent catheterization when necessary (Fig. 36-30). What used to be the common channel is divided in the midline, creating two lateral flaps that are sutured to the skin, creating the new labia. The vaginal edges are mobilized to reach the skin to create a surprisingly natural-looking introitus. The limits of the rectal sphincter are electrically determined, and the perineal body is reconstructed, bringing together the anterior limits of the sphincter. The rectum is placed within the margins of the sphincter (Fig. 36-31). Because they have a colostomy, these neonates can eat the same day, and their pain is usually easily controlled. They are discharged 48 hours after surgery with their urinary catheter in place.

Cloacas with a Common Channel Longer than 3 cm

When endoscopy shows that the patient has a long common channel, the surgeon must be prepared to face a significant technical challenge. In the presence of a long common channel, the patient should be prepped so that the entire lower body is accessible because it is likely that the patient will require a laparotomy after initial exploration by the posterior sagittal approach. As before, the rectum is separated from the vagina and urethra and the length of the common channel of the urogenital sinus is determined.

A midline laparotomy is recommended. The bladder is opened in the midline, and feeding tubes are placed into the ureters to protect them. The ureters run through the common wall between the vagina and bladder, and the stents allow for their identification

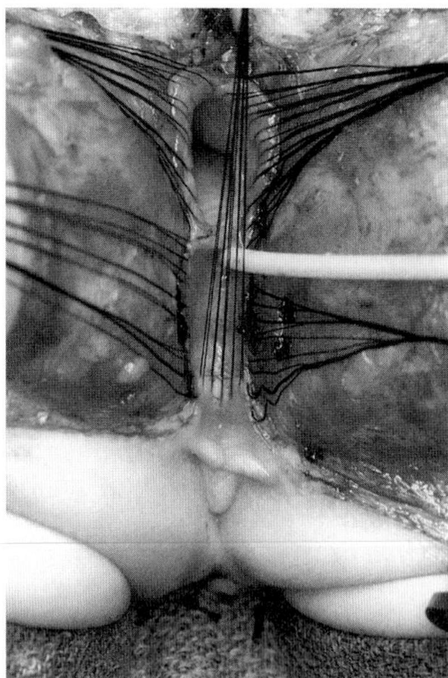

Figure 36-28. Total urogenital mobilization. The patient is in the prone position. Silk sutures have been placed around the vagina (*top*) and transversely across the dissection plane near the clitoris (*bottom*). A catheter has been inserted in the urethra.

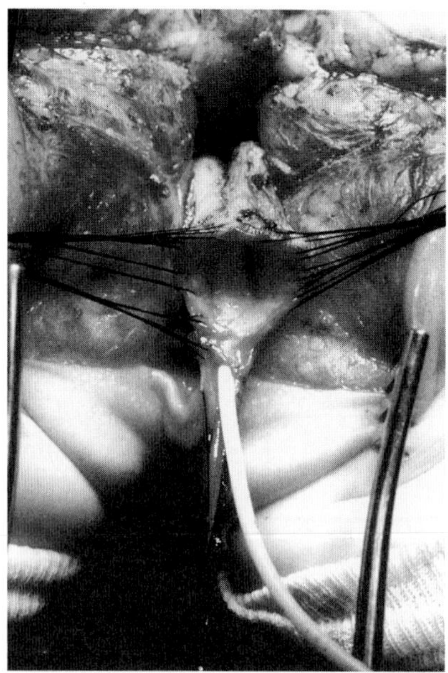

Figure 36-29. In this female infant with a cloaca who is in the prone position, the urogenital sinus has been fully mobilized and freed from all of its lateral, anterior, and posterior attachments. The catheter is in the urethra.

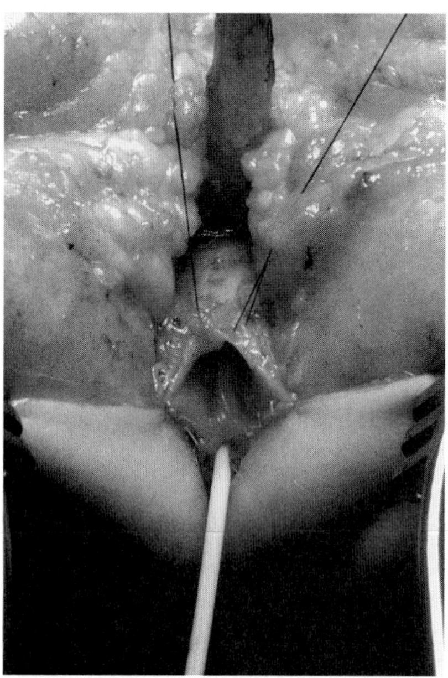

Figure 36-30. A nearly completed cloacal repair. The urethral meatus (with catheter) and vaginal introitus have been anastomosed to the perineum in their appropriate positions. The patient is in the prone position.

during the difficult dissection of vaginas from the bladder neck.

We also confirm the patency of the müllerian structures by injecting saline through a 3-Fr feeding tube through the fimbriae of the fallopian tubes. If one of the tubes is not patent, we recommend excising it, along with its hemiuterus if the system is bifid. The ovary and its blood supply are preserved.[34]

When both müllerian structures are atretic, we recommend leaving both in place and informing the parents. Once the patient develops breast buds, menstruation usually occurs 1 to 2 years thereafter and ultrasonography is used to follow the size of these structures. At that point, laparoscopic inspection or intervention for nondraining structures may be reasonable.

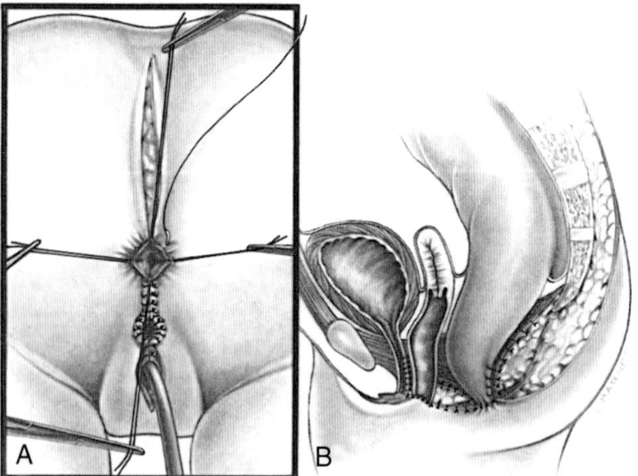

Figure 36-31. Drawings showing the final stages of cloacal repair. **A,** The repaired urethra and vagina and the anoplasty are being completed. **B,** Sagittal depiction of the finished cloacal repair. (From Peña A: Atlas of Surgical Management of Anorectal Malformations. New York, Springer-Verlag, 1990, p 69.)

With the abdomen open, surgical decisions must be based on the anatomic findings. In the presence of a single vagina of normal size, the surgeon must separate the vagina from the urinary tract, being sure to preserve its blood supply that comes from the uterine vessels. It is brought to the perineum, and the introitus is constructed. When the vagina is found to be too short, the patient requires some form of vaginal replacement that can be performed using the rectum, colon, or small bowel.

The presence of a common channel longer than 5 cm means that total urogenital mobilization from below will not be enough to repair this malformation. In this scenario, it is advisable to leave the common channel intact for use as the urethra, which will eventually be used for intermittent catheterization. The two small hemivaginas are separated from the urinary tract, and the posterior wall of the previous common channel is closed with interrupted absorbable sutures. This is a very delicate, meticulous, and tedious maneuver. With this dissection, one can gain separation of the vagina from the urinary tract for approximately 2 cm. In other cases, when the vaginas are larger, the entire urogenital mobilization can be delivered into the abdomen. If further dissection does not allow it to reach, then the vaginas can be separated from the urinary tract and the urethra can be tubularized.

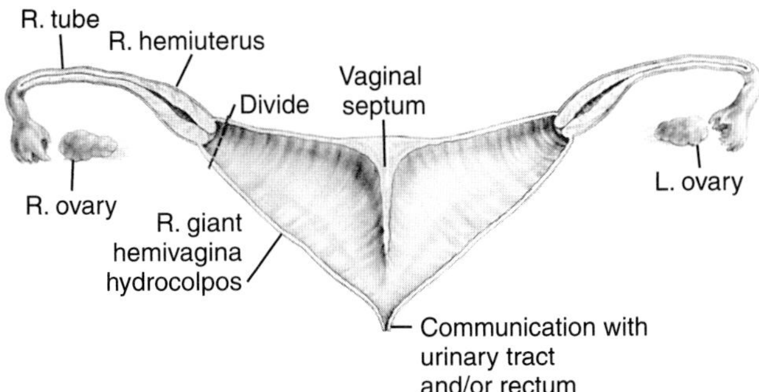

Figure 36-32. Diagram shows the constellation of persistent cloaca with hydrocolpos in the presence of hemivaginas and hemiuterus. Bilateral hydrocolpos is present with a very high vagina. This circumstance is the ideal anatomy for a subsequent repair via a vaginal switch maneuver. (From Kiely EM, Peña A: Anorectal malformations. In O'Neil JA, Rowe MI, Grosfeld JL, et al [eds]: Pediatric Surgery. St. Louis, Mosby–Year Book, 1998, p 1442.)

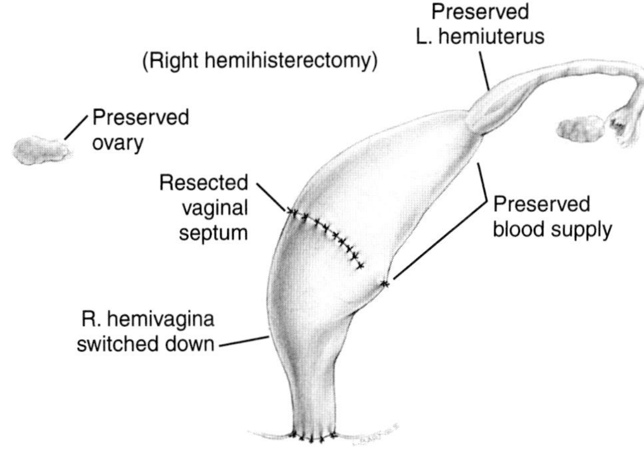

Figure 36-33. Technique of vaginal reconstruction using a vaginal switch maneuver. (From Kiely EM, Peña A: Anorectal malformations. In O'Neil JA, Rowe MI, Grosfeld JL, et al [eds]: Pediatric Surgery. St. Louis, Mosby–Year Book, 1998, p 1442.)

Vaginal Switch Maneuver

There is a specific group of patients who are born with hydrocolpos and two hemivaginas. The hemivaginas are very large, and the two hemiuteri are separated. The distance between one hemiuterus and the other is longer than the vertical length of both the hemivaginas. In these cases, it is ideal to perform a maneuver called a "vaginal switch" (Figs. 36-32 and 36-33). To perform the "vaginal switch," one of the uteri and its fallopian tube are resected (see Fig. 36-32), preserving the ovary and its blood supply. The blood supply of the ipsilateral hemivagina must be sacrificed, but collateral vessels from the opposite vagina should support both. The vaginal septum is resected, creating a single long vagina. The cut end of the ipsilateral vagina is turned down to the perineum (see Fig. 36-33). This is an excellent technique for constructing a viable and functional vagina.

Vaginal Augmentation and/or Replacement

A short vagina can be augmented or a totally absent vagina constructed from a bowel segment. The intestinal choices are rectum, colon, or small bowel.

1. *Vaginal reconstruction with rectum.* The vagina can be constructed with the rectum when the patient has a megarectum that can be divided longitudinally, preserving the mesenteric blood supply (Fig. 36-34). Occasionally, when there is adequate length, the rectum can be divided transversely, maintaining vascular pedicles for both rectum and vagina. The blood supply of the rectum will be provided transmurally from branches of the inferior mesenteric vessels.
2. *Vaginal replacement with colon.* The colon is an ideal substitute for the vagina. When available,

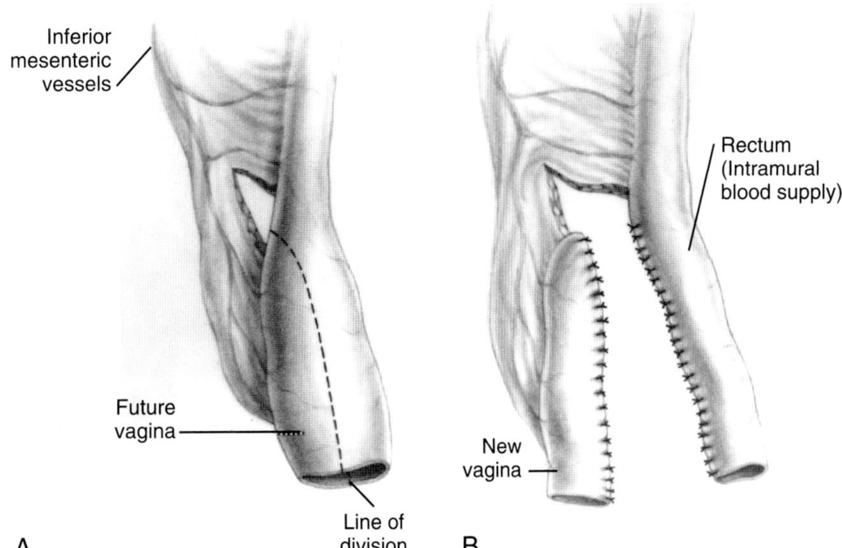

Figure 36-34. The technique of vaginal replacement using the rectum is depicted. The presence of a megarectum is necessary for successful vaginal reconstruction. **A,** The portion of the existing rectum that will become the vagina. **B,** Division of the rectum and creation of the vagina and remaining rectum.

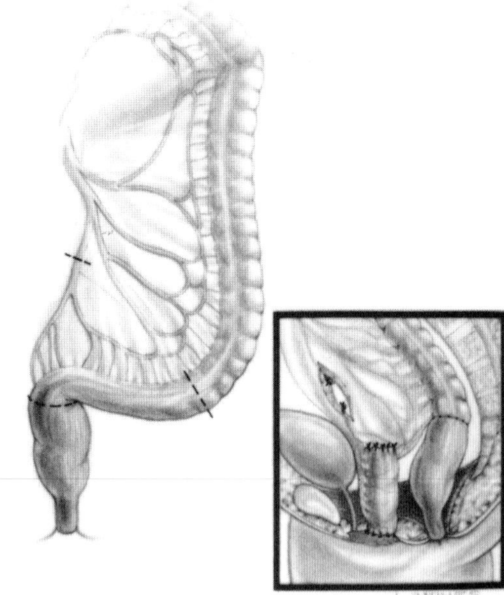

Figure 36-35. Schematic representation of a vaginal replacement using sigmoid colon.

the sigmoid colon is preferable. At times, the location of the colostomy interferes with this type of reconstruction. The most mobile portion of the colon usually has a long mesentery. When the patient has internal genitalia or a little cuff of vagina or cervix, the upper part of the bowel used for replacement must be sutured to the vaginal cuff. When the patient has no vagina and no uterus, the neovagina is closed at its upper end and is used only for sexual purposes (Fig. 36-35).

3. *Vaginal reconstruction with small bowel.* If a colon segment is not available, the most mobile portion of the small bowel is utilized for vaginal reconstruction. Generally, the ileum located approximately 15 cm proximal to the ileocecal valve (Fig. 36-36A) is isolated and pulled down, preserving its blood supply (see Fig. 36-36B, C).

We do not use skin flaps or vaginal flaps for vaginal replacement because we have found that these other maneuvers give better results.

The most difficult type of cloacal malformation is one in which two little hemivaginas are attached to the bladder neck or even to the trigone of the bladder. In these cases, the rectum also opens in the trigone (Fig. 36-37). Separation of these structures is performed in the abdomen, and the patient is frequently left with a nonfunctional bladder neck. The surgical decision now lies between an attempt to reconstruct the bladder neck or to close it permanently. In the first situation, most of the patients will need intermittent catheterization to empty the bladder. If permanent closure of the bladder neck is elected, a vesicostomy is created, delaying a continent diversion until the patient is 3 to 4 years old. With this type of malformation, vaginal replacement should be performed using one of the substitutes described previously.

POSTOPERATIVE MANAGEMENT AND COLOSTOMY CLOSURE

Postoperatively, the patients generally have a smooth course. Pain is rarely a complaint except for those who have undergone a laparotomy. After cloaca repair, the urinary catheter remains for 2 to 3 weeks until the perineum is no longer swollen, and the patient can be recatheterized, if necessary. In very complex malformations, as with a bladder neck reconstruction, we prefer to leave a suprapubic tube. In patients in whom the bladder neck was closed, we establish a vesicostomy. Male patients with repaired rectourethral fistulas should have urinary catheter drainage for 7 days. If the catheter becomes dislodged, the patients often can void without difficulty and do not require replacement of the catheter.

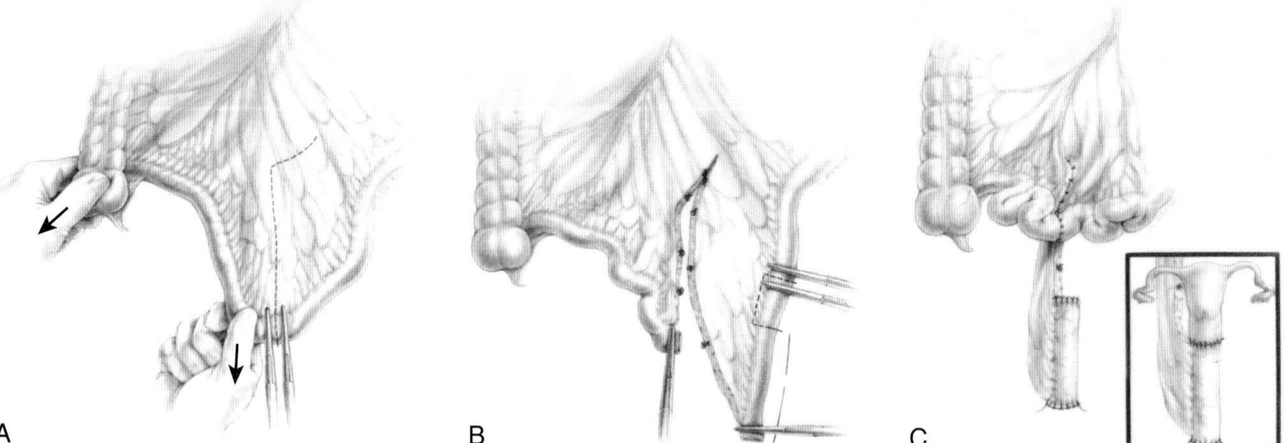

Figure 36-36. Technique of vaginal replacement using small bowel. **A,** A segment of small bowel is chosen that has adequate mesenteric length for transposition to the pelvis. **B,** The mesentery has been divided, the segment of small bowel chosen for vaginal reconstruction is identified, and the blood supply is evaluated to ensure adequate perfusion. **C,** The completed anastomosis.

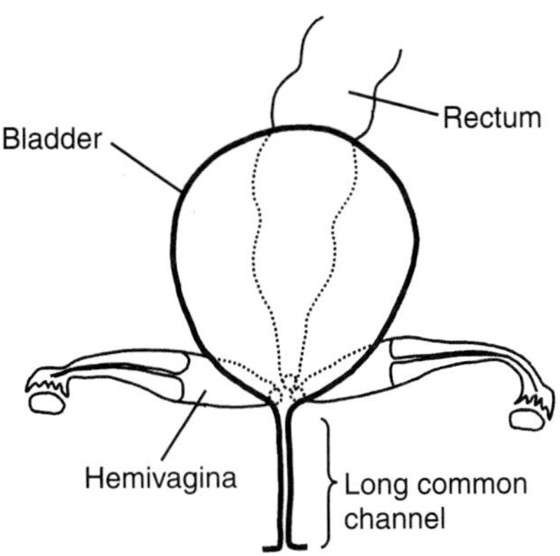

Figure 36-37. This diagram shows the association between a cloaca with an extremely long channel with hemivaginas and the rectum entering the bladder neck (Drawing by George Rodriguez).

Intravenous antibiotics are administered for 48 hours and antibiotic ointment is applied to the perineal suture line for 7 days. Most patients are discharged 2 days after posterior sagittal repair and 3 to 4 days after a laparotomy.

Anal dilatations are started 2 weeks after the repair with a dilator that fits gently into the anus. Dilation is performed twice daily by the parents, and the size of the dilator is increased weekly until the rectum reaches the desired size, which depends on the patient's age (Table 36-2). Once this desired size is reached, the colostomy can be closed. The frequency of dilatation can be reduced once there is no resistance using the final dilator size. After that, the parents follow a tapering dilatation schedule that is once a day for 1 month, every third day for 1 month, twice a week for 1 month, once a week for 1 month, and once a month for 3 months.

Anal strictures occur in cases in which the blood supply of the distal rectum is insufficient, or when the anoplasty is performed under tension.[31]

At the time of colostomy closure in patients who have undergone cloacal repair, we perform an endoscopy to evaluate the repair. After the colostomy is closed, the patient may have multiple bowel movements and may develop perineal excoriation. A constipating diet may be helpful in the treatment of this problem. After several weeks, the number of bowel movements decreases and most patients will develop constipation. After 1 to 3 months, the patient develops a more regular bowel movement pattern. A good prognosis can usually be predicted in a patient who has one to three bowel movements per day, remains clean between bowel movements, and shows evidence of feeling or pushing during bowel movements. This type of patient can be toilet-trained. A patient with multiple bowel movements or one who passes stool constantly without showing any signs of sensation or pushing usually has a poor functional prognosis.

In our series, about 20% of the patients with a cloacal malformation and a common channel shorter than 3 cm require intermittent catheterization to empty their bladder. Patients with common channels longer than 3 cm require intermittent catheterization 70% to 80% of the time. Therefore, we leave the urinary catheter until the perineal incisions are healed sufficiently to allow catheterization. Once we are able to see the urethral orifice, we remove the urinary catheter and observe the patient to see if she is capable of spontaneous bladder emptying. A kidney and bladder ultrasonogram can assess this emptying and should be done 2 to 3 weeks after the catheter is removed. If she cannot pass urine, or does not empty her bladder well, we teach the parents how to perform intermittent catheterization. In cases of very long common channels, we prefer to utilize a suprapubic tube. One month after surgery, we perform a suprapubic cystogram and begin clamping the tube. We measure the residual urine, which is an indicator of bladder function. The suprapubic tube remains until we have evidence of good bladder function or the parents learn to catheterize the bladder when needed.

Most patients with persistent cloaca have a flaccid, smooth, large bladder that does not empty completely.[77] Fortunately, most patients with cloacas have a competent bladder neck. The combination of a competent bladder neck with a flaccid bladder makes these patients ideal candidates for intermittent catheterization, which keeps them completely dry. Two exceptions to this rule exist. One is represented by patients who have a very long common channel, with the hemivaginas attached to the bladder neck, leading to a bladder neck that is damaged during the reconstruction. The second group is represented by a small number of patients who are born with separated pubic bones, a condition that can be described as a "covered exstrophy."[78,79] These patients have congenital absence of the bladder neck and will eventually require a continent urinary diversion.

Table 36-2 Size of Dilator According to Age

Age	Hegar Dilator (No.)
1-4 mo	12
4-12 mo	13
8-12 mo	14
1-3 yr	15
3-12 yr	16
>12 yr	17

FUNCTIONAL DISORDERS AFTER REPAIR OF ANORECTAL MALFORMATIONS

Most patients who undergo repair of an anorectal malformation suffer from some degree of a functional defecating disorder.[75,76]

Fecal continence depends on three main factors:

1. *Voluntary muscle structures.* These structures are represented by the levator muscle, the striated muscle complex, and the external sphincter. Normally, they are used only for brief periods when the rectal fecal mass, pushed by the involuntary peristaltic contraction of the rectosigmoid,

reaches the anorectal area. This contraction occurs only in the minutes prior to defecation. The voluntary muscle structures that close around the anus are used only occasionally during the rest of the day and night. Patients with anorectal malformations have abnormal voluntary striated muscles with different degrees of underdevelopment. Voluntary muscles can be used only when the patient feels that it is necessary to use them. For that sensation, the patient needs information that can only be derived from an intact sensory mechanism, a mechanism that many patients with anorectal malformations lack.

2. *Sensation.* Exquisite sensation in normal individuals resides in the anal canal. Except for patients with rectal atresia, most patients with anorectal malformations are born without an anal canal. Therefore, sensation does not exist or is rudimentary. Distention of the rectum, however, can be felt in many of these patients, provided the rectum has been located accurately within the muscle structures. This sensation (proprioception) seems to be a consequence of stretching of the voluntary muscle. The most important clinical implication of this is that liquid stool or soft fecal material may not be felt by the patient with anorectal malformations as the rectum is not distended. Thus, to achieve some degree of sensation and bowel control, the patient must be able to (or helped to) form solid stool.
3. *Bowel motility.* Perhaps the most important factor in fecal continence is bowel motility. However, the impact of motility has been largely underestimated. In a normal individual, the rectosigmoid remains quiet for variable periods of time (one to several days), depending on an individual's defecation habits. During that time, anorectal sensation and voluntary muscle structures are almost unnecessary because the stool remains in the rectosigmoid if it is solid.

The patient normally feels the rectosigmoid's peristaltic contraction. Voluntarily, the normal individual can relax the striated muscles, which allows the rectal contents to migrate down into the highly sensitive area of the anal canal. There, accurate information is provided concerning the consistency and quality of the stool. The voluntary muscles are used to push the rectal contents back up into the rectosigmoid and hold them if desired, until the appropriate time for evacuation. At the time of defecation, the voluntary muscle structures relax, allowing the fecal mass to pass into and through the anorectum.

The main factor that initiates emptying of the rectosigmoid is a massive involuntary peristaltic contraction that is helped sometimes by a Valsalva maneuver. Most patients with an anorectal malformation have a disturbance of this sophisticated bowel motility mechanism. Patients who have undergone a posterior sagittal anorectoplasty or any other type of sacroperineal approach, in which the most distal part of the bowel was preserved, often show evidence of an overefficient bowel reservoir (megarectum) (Fig. 36-38).

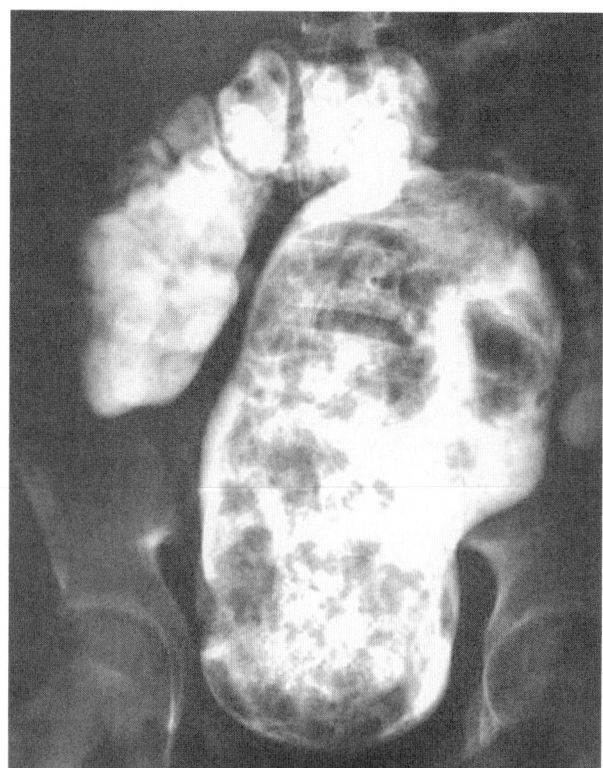

Figure 36-38. A barium enema is shown in a patient with a megarectum. Note the markedly dilated rectum in relation to the more proximal normal-sized colon.

The main clinical manifestation of this is constipation, which seems to be more severe in patients with lower defects. Females with a vestibular fistula, in particular, are more prone to this problem. A loop colostomy can cause this problem by allowing for a fecal impaction in the blind rectal pouch. The enormously dilated rectosigmoid has normal ganglion cells, but behaves like it has a myopathic type of hypomotility disorder. The overflow fecal incontinence based on rectosigmoid constipation in patients with potential for bowel control can be managed with the appropriate dose of laxatives. Those with a poor sacrum, poor muscles, and thus with no potential for bowel control are treated with a daily enema.

Those patients treated with techniques in which the most distal part of the bowel was resected (endorectal dissection)[6,9] behave clinically as individuals without a rectal reservoir (Fig. 36-39). This is a situation equivalent to a perineal colostomy. Depending on the amount of colon resected, the patient may have loose stools. In these cases, medical management consisting of a daily enema and a constipating diet, with medications to slow down the colonic motility, is indicated.

EVALUATION OF RESULTS

Each defect described in this chapter has a different prognosis. The patients with lower defects usually have excellent results, except when technical errors

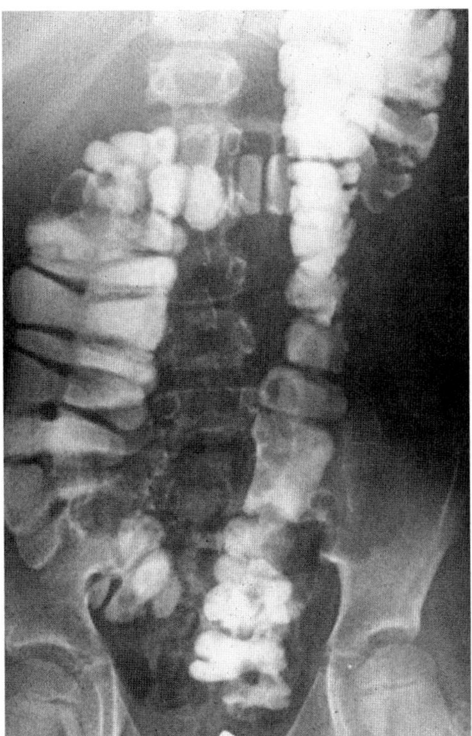

Figure 36-39. This barium enema was performed in a patient who has had the rectosigmoid colon resected. Note the straight position of the colon to the anus with no evidence of a rectal reservoir.

have been made, or if they have associated sacral or spinal problems.

Tables 36-3 and 36-4 shows the results obtained in our series. The patients with a sacral ratio of less than 0.3 and flat perineums have fecal incontinence regardless of the type of malformation or quality of the repair.

Because persistent cloacas represent another spectrum of defects, they must be subclassified on the basis of potential for bowel and urinary control. The length of the common channel seems to be the most important prognostic factor.

Table 36-4 Urinary Incontinence

	No. Patients	%
Rectal atresia or stenosis	0/8	0
Perineal fistula	0/38	0
Bulbourethral fistula	2/85	2.4
Imperforate anus without fistula	1/37	2.7
Prostatic fistula	7/85	8.2
Bladder neck fistula	7/38	18.4
Cloaca: short common channel	5/18	27.8
Vaginal fistula	1/5	20
Cloaca: long common channel	37/48	77.1

Complications

There are several complications related to operative intervention and repairs of anorectal malformations in general. Wound infection in the immediate postoperative period can occur and, fortunately, usually affects only the skin and subcutaneous tissue. All heal secondarily without functional sequelae. Anal strictures may be the consequence of failure to follow the protocol of dilatations. When trying to prevent discomfort for the patient, some surgeons dilate the anus once a week, frequently under anesthesia. This protocol can eventually create a severe, intractable fibrous stricture. Strictures can also occur with devascularization of the rectum during the rectal mobilization.[31] Constipation is the most common functional disorder observed in patients who undergo a posterior sagittal anorectoplasty (see Table 36-3). Patients with the best prognosis have the highest incidence of constipation. Patients who underwent tapering do not have more constipation than those without a tapering procedure. Patients with a very poor prognosis, such as with bladder neck fistula, have a low incidence of constipation

Table 36-3 Global Functional Results

	Voluntary Bowel Movement		Soiling		Totally Continent		Constipated	
	No. Patients	*%*	*No. Patients*	*%*	*No. Patients*	*%*	*No. Patients*	*%*
Perineal fistula	39/39	100	3/43	20.9	35/39	89.7	30/53	56.6
Rectal atresia or stenosis	8/8	100	2/8	25	6/8	75	4/8	50
Vestibular fistula	89/97	92	36/100	36	63/89	70.8	61/100	61
Imperforate anus without fistula	30/35	86	18/37	48.6	18/30	60	22/40	55
Bulbourethral fistula	68/83	82	48/89	53.9	34/68	50	52/81	64.2
Prostatic fistula	52/71	73	67/87	77.1	16/52	30.8	42/93	45.2
Cloaca: short common channel	50/70	71	50/79	63.3	25/50	50	34/85	40
Cloaca: long common channel	18/41	44	34/39	87.2	5/18	27.8	17/45	34.8
Vaginal fistula	3/4	75	4/5	80	1/3	33.3	1/5	20
Bladder neck fistula	8/29	28	39/43	90.7	1/8	12.5	7/45	15.6

and a high rate of incontinence. Colostomies that do not allow cleaning and irrigation of the distal colon can lead to megarectum. Patients require proactive aggressive treatment of constipation after colostomy closure to avoid significant problems. Rectal prolapse occurs on occasion and is more prevalent in higher malformations with poor sphincters and is impacted by postoperative constipation.[72] Finally, transient femoral nerve palsy can occur as a consequence of excessive pressure on the groin during the operation. This problem can be avoided by adequate cushioning.

Specific to cloacal repairs, urethrovaginal fistulas had been the most common and feared complication prior to the introduction of the total urogenital mobilization technique.[74] In cases in which vaginal mobilization and separation from the neourethra result in opposing suture lines, 90-degree rotation of the vagina can decrease the incidence of a postoperative fistula. Fibrosis of the vagina can develop secondary to an excessive dissection during the mobilization of a high vagina.

Regarding male patients, a review of over 500 patients showed significant urologic injuries.[63] Failure to obtain a good distal colostogram to delineate the anatomy precisely was the most important reason for these complications. Neurogenic bladder in male patients, as a result of the anorectal malformation or the repair itself, must be extremely unusual because it only happens in patients with a very abnormal sacrum (see Table 36-4).[77] In the presence of a relatively normal sacrum, it may reflect a poor surgical technique with denervation of the bladder and bladder neck during the repair.[63]

Finally, fecal incontinence is a very common sequelae of any anorectal malformation repair and is discussed in Chapter 37.

chapter 37

FECAL INCONTINENCE AND CONSTIPATION

Marc A. Levitt, MD • Alberto Peña, MD

Fecal incontinence represents a devastating problem for all who suffer from it. It often prevents a person from becoming socially accepted, which, in turn, provokes serious psychological sequelae. It is a problem that impacts more children than previously thought, affecting those born with anorectal malformations and Hirschsprung's disease as well as children with spinal cord problems or spinal injuries.

True fecal incontinence must be distinguished from overflow pseudoincontinence. Pediatric patients with true fecal incontinence include some surgical patients with anorectal malformations, those with Hirschsprung's disease, and those with spinal problems, either congenital or acquired. In patients with pseudoincontinence, who have the potential for bowel control but who soil, most often their problem results from severe constipation (encopresis) and sometimes from hypermotility.

Most patients who undergo an anorectal malformation repair suffer from some degree of a functional defecation disorder, and all suffer from an abnormality in their fecal continence mechanism. Approximately 25% of patients are deficient enough in these mechanisms that they are fecally incontinent and cannot have a voluntary bowel movement. The others are capable of having voluntary bowel movements but may require treatment of an underlying dysmotility disorder, which most often manifests as constipation.[1] A small, yet significant, number of patients with Hirschsprung's disease (<5%) suffer from fecal incontinence possibly because of a lost anal canal or damaged sphincters that occurred during surgical repair.[2] Patients with spinal problems or injuries can lack the capacity for voluntary bowel movements or may have this ability to varying degrees.

Patients with true fecal incontinence require an artificial way to be kept clean and in normal underwear. This regimen is termed *bowel management* and involves a daily enema. Patients with pseudoincontinence require proper medical treatment of either constipation or loose stools. This involves getting the stool to the right consistency so that they can have a bowel movement that they voluntarily control. Understanding this major differentiation is the key to deciding the correct management.

MECHANISM OF CONTINENCE

Fecal continence depends on three factors: voluntary sphincter muscles, anal canal sensation, and colonic motility.[1]

Voluntary Muscle Structures

In the normal patient, the voluntary muscle structures are represented by the levators, the muscle complex, and the parasagittal fibers. Normally, they are used only for brief periods of time when the rectal fecal mass, pushed by the involuntary peristaltic contraction of the rectosigmoid colon, followed by relaxation, reaches the anorectal area. This voluntary contraction occurs only at the time of defecation. These muscles are used only occasionally during the rest of the day and night.

Patients with anorectal malformations have abnormal voluntary striated muscles with different degrees of hypodevelopment. Patients with Hirschsprung's disease may have suffered damage to this sphincter mechanism, and patients with spinal problems may have deficient innervation of these muscles.

Anal Canal Sensation

Voluntary muscles are used only when the patient has the sensation that it is necessary to use them. To appreciate that sensation, the patient needs information that can only be derived from an intact anal sensory mechanism.

Exquisite sensation in normal individuals resides in the anal canal. Except for patients with rectal atresia, most patients with anorectal malformations are born without an anal canal. Therefore, sensation does not exist or is rudimentary. Patients with spinal problems may lack this anal canal sensation as well. Patients with Hirschsprung's disease are born with a normal anal canal, but this can be injured if not meticulously

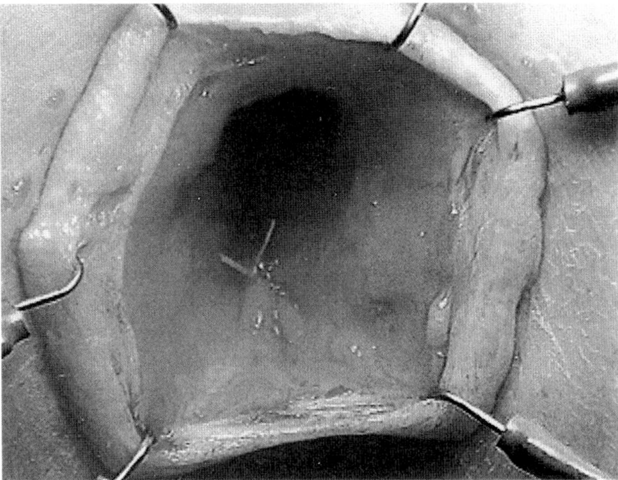

Figure 37-1. Loss of the anal canal (with no visible dentate line) is seen after a Soave pull-through operation. In this patient, the anal dissection was begun too distally.

preserved at the time of their colonic pull-through procedure (Fig. 37-1). Patients with perineal trauma may have an injured or destroyed anal canal.

It seems that patients can perceive distention of the rectum, if the rectum has been properly located within the muscle structures. This surgical point is quite important for patients undergoing pull-through procedures for imperforate anus. This sensation seems to be a consequence of stretching of these voluntary muscles (proprioception). The most important clinical implication is that patients might not feel liquid stool or soft fecal material because such stool consistency does not distend the rectum. Thus, to achieve some degree of sensation and bowel control, the patient must have the capacity to form solid stool. This point is quite relevant in children with ulcerative colitis who have undergone an ileoanal pull-through procedure. They may suffer from varying degrees of incontinence due to the incapacity to form solid stool. Their normal sphincter muscles and anal canal allow them to overcome this problem. Also, some need the help of medications that bulk up the stool.

Bowel Motility

Perhaps the most important factor in fecal continence is bowel motility. However, the impact of motility has been largely underestimated. In a normal individual, the rectosigmoid remains quiet for variable periods of time (1 to several days), depending on specific defecation habits. During that time, sensation and voluntary muscle structures are almost not necessary because the stool, if it is solid, remains inside the colon. The patient feels the peristaltic contraction of the rectosigmoid that occurs before defecation. Voluntarily, the normal individual can relax the striated rectal muscles, which allows the rectal contents to migrate down into the highly sensitive area of the anal canal. There, the anal canal provides accurate information concerning stool consistency. The voluntary muscles are used to push the rectal contents back up into the rectosigmoid and to hold them until the appropriate time for evacuation. At the time of defecation, the voluntary muscle structures relax.

The main impetus for rectosigmoid emptying is a massive involuntary peristaltic contraction sometimes helped by a Valsalva maneuver. Most patients with an anorectal malformation suffer from a disturbance of this sophisticated bowel motility mechanism. Patients who have undergone a posterior sagittal anorectoplasty (or any other type of sacroperineal approach in which the most distal part of the bowel was preserved) can show evidence of an overefficient bowel reservoir (megarectum) (Fig. 37-2). The main clinical manifestation of a megarectum is constipation, which seems to be more severe in patients with lower defects.[3] Constipation that is not aggressively treated, combined with an ectatic distended colon, eventually leads to severe constipation. A vicious cycle ensues, with worsening constipation leading to more rectosigmoid dilation, leading to more severe constipation. The enormously dilated rectosigmoid, which has normal ganglion cells, behaves like a myopathic type of hypomotile colon.[1]

Patients with an anorectal malformation, treated with techniques in which the most distal part of the bowel was resected (Fig. 37-3), behave clinically as individuals without a rectal reservoir. This is a situation equivalent to a perineal colostomy. Depending on the amount of colon removed, the patient may have loose stools. In these cases, medical management consisting of enemas, a constipating diet, and medications to slow down the colonic motility is indicated.

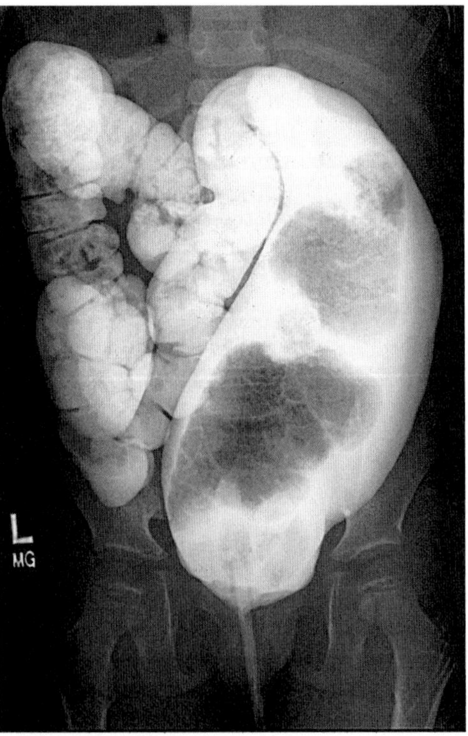

Figure 37-2. This contrast enema shows a megarectosigmoid colon. (From Peña A, Levitt M: Colonic inertia disorders in pediatrics. Curr Prob Surg 39:681, 2002).

Patients with Hirschsprung's disease undergo operative resection of the distal aganglionic colon and rectum. However, their normal anal canal and sphincter mechanism allows the vast majority of them to be continent despite the lack of a rectal reservoir. Some patients with Hirschsprung's disease have bowel hypermotility and need medications to slow the colon. Amazingly, some patients with an injured anal canal and sphincters (perineal trauma) can be continent if their motility is normal, because the regular contraction of the rectosigmoid can translate into a successful voluntary bowel movement.

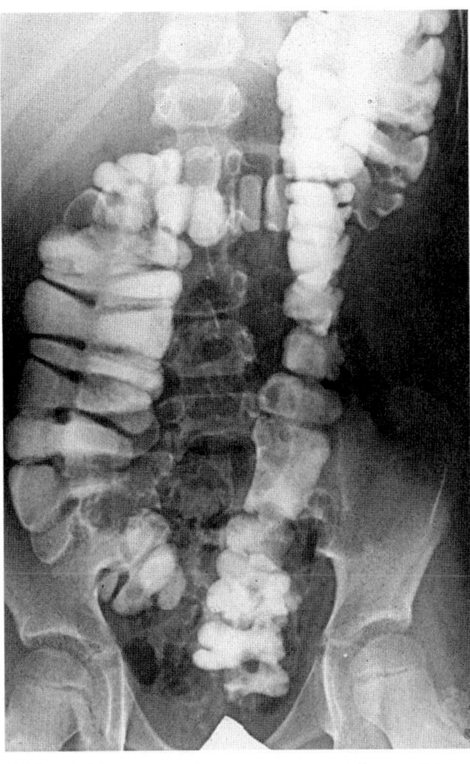

Figure 37-3. This contrast enema was performed in a patient who had resection of the rectosigmoid colon. Often these patients act like they do not have a rectal reservoir. (From Levitt MA, Peña A: Treatment of chronic constipation and resection of the inert rectosigmoid. In: Anorectal Malformations in Children. Heidelberg, Springer, 2006, p 417).

TRUE FECAL INCONTINENCE

For patients with true fecal incontinence, the ideal approach is a bowel management program consisting of teaching the patient and the parents how to clean the colon once daily with an enema so as to stay completely clean for 24 hours until the next cleanout. This is achieved by keeping the colon quiet between enemas. These patients cannot have voluntary bowel movements and require an artificial mechanism (a daily enema) to empty their colon. The program, although simplistic, is ideally implemented by trial and error over a period of 1 week. The patient is seen each day and an abdominal radiograph is taken so that they can be monitored for the amount and location of any stool left in the colon. The presence or absence of stool in the underwear is also noted. The decision as to whether the type and/or quality of the enemas should be modified, as well as changes in their diet and/or medication, can thus be made daily (Fig. 37-4).[4]

Which Pediatric Patients Have True Fecal Incontinence?

In children with anorectal malformations, 75% who have undergone a correct and successful operation have voluntary bowel movements after the age of 3 years.[3] About half of these patients occasionally soil their underwear. These episodes of soiling are usually related to constipation. When the constipation is treated properly, the soiling frequently disappears.

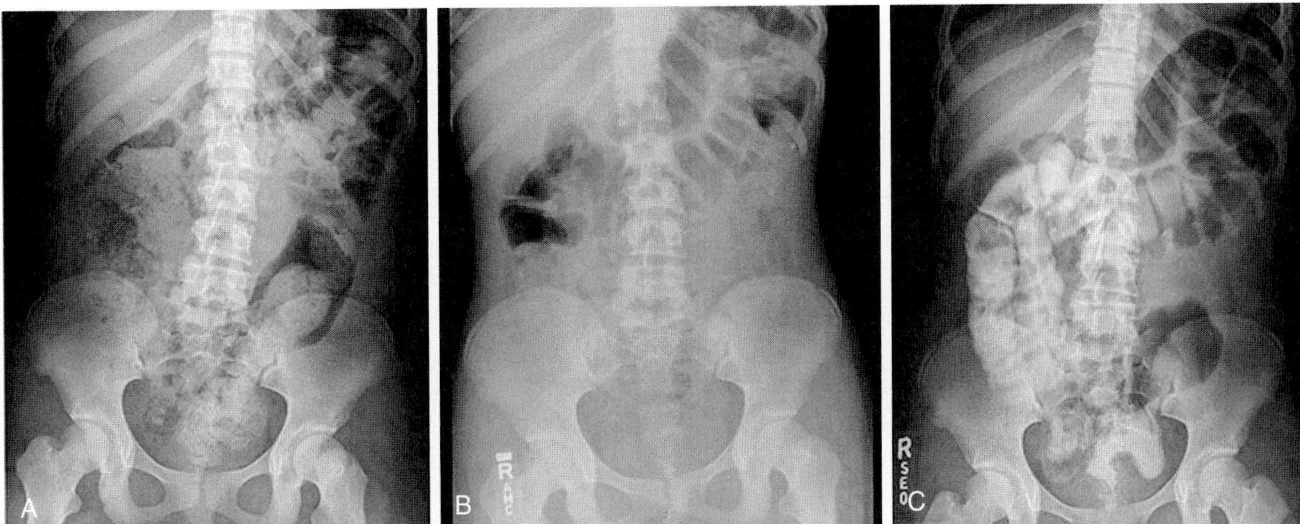

Figure 37-4. A to C, This series of abdominal radiographs was obtained during inpatient bowel management showing progression toward a completely clean colon with daily adjustment of the enema. After 5 days, a post-contrast abdominal film (C) shows minimal evidence of retained fecal material.

Table 37-1 Prognostic Signs in Patients with Anorectal Malformations

Good Prognosis Signs	Poor Prognosis Signs
Good bowel movement patterns: 1-2 bowel movements per day—no soiling in between	Constant soiling and passing of stool
Evidence of sensation with passing stool (pushing, making faces)	No sensation (no pushing)
Urinary control	Urinary incontinence, dribbling of urine

Thus, approximately 40% overall have voluntary bowel movements and no soiling. In other words, they behave like normal children. Children with good bowel control still may suffer from temporary episodes of fecal incontinence, especially when they experience diarrhea.

Some 25% of all patients with anorectal malformations suffer from true fecal incontinence, and are the patients who need bowel management to be kept clean. As noted, certain patients with Hirschsprung's disease and those with spinal problems can suffer from true fecal incontinence as well. For these patients, similar principles of bowel management learned from treatment of patients with anorectal malformations can be applied.[4]

For children with anorectal malformations, the surgeon should be able to predict in advance which patients may have a good functional prognosis and which children may have poor prognosis. Table 37-1 shows the most common indicators of good and poor prognosis. After primary repair and colostomy closure, it is possible to establish the functional prognosis (Table 37-2). Parents should be given the information regarding their child's realistic chances for bowel control to avoid needless frustration at the age of toilet training. To avoid creating false expectations for the parents, it is imperative to establish the functional prognosis for each child as early as possible, which is sometimes possible even in the newborn period.

Table 37-2 Predictors of Prognosis in Patients with Anorectal Malformations

Good Prognostic Signs	Poor Prognostic Signs
Normal sacrum	Abnormal sacrum
Prominent midline groove (good muscles)	Flat perineum (poor muscles)
Some types of anorectal malformations:	Some types of anorectal malformations:
Rectal atresia	Rectal/bladder neck fistula
Vestibular fistula	Cloacas with a common channel > 3 cm
Imperforate anus without a fistula	Complex malformations
Cloacas with a common channel < 3 cm	
Less complex malformations: perineal fistula	

Once the diagnosis of the specific anorectal defect is established, the functional prognosis can be predicted. If the child's defect is associated with a good prognosis (e.g., a vestibular fistula, perineal fistula, rectal atresia, rectourethral bulbar fistula, or imperforate anus with no fistula), one should expect that the child will have voluntary bowel movements by the age of 3 years (provided the sacrum and spine are normal). These children will need careful supervision to avoid fecal impaction, constipation, and soiling.

If the child's defect is associated with a poor prognosis (e.g., a very high cloaca with a common channel longer than 3 cm, a recto-bladder neck fistula, or a very hypodeveloped sacrum), the parents must understand that their child will most likely need a bowel management program to remain clean. This should be implemented when the child is 3 to 4 years of age and before starting school. Children with rectoprostatic fistulas have an almost 50-50 chance of having voluntary bowel movements or of being incontinent. In these children, an attempt should be made to achieve toilet training by the age of 3 years. If this proves to be unsuccessful, bowel management should be implemented. Each summer, after school is finished, further attempts can be made to assess the child's ability to toilet train.

In patients who have undergone repair of imperforate anus and who have fecal incontinence, a reoperation to relocate a misplaced rectum with the hope of obtaining good bowel control should be considered if the child was born with a good sacrum, a good sphincter mechanism, and a malformation with good functional prognosis. A repeat posterior sagittal anorectoplasty can be performed and the rectum relocated within the limits of the sphincter mechanism. Approximately 50% of the children who undergo reoperation under these very specific circumstances have a significant improvement in bowel control.[5]

Patients with true fecal incontinence and a tendency toward constipation cannot be treated with laxatives but instead need bowel management for fecal incontinence. In fact, laxatives in such patients make their soiling worse. This population usually consists of those patients born with a bad prognosis type of defect and with associated defects of the sacrum, a poor muscle complex, or an abnormal spine.

Children operated on for imperforate anus who suffer from true fecal incontinence can be divided into two well-defined groups that require individualized treatment plans. The first and larger group is those with fecal incontinence and a tendency toward constipation. The second group is fecally incontinent with a tendency toward loose stools. Patients with fecal incontinence after operations for Hirschsprung's disease and those with spinal disorders usually fall into the first group and have a tendency toward constipation. A small group of Hirschsprung's patients fall into the hypermotile group. These patients have multiple daily stools and a nondilated colon seen on a constrast enema.

Table 37-3 Food Products and Stool Consistency

Foods that produce loose stools	Foods that promote constipation
Milk or milk products	Apple sauce
Fats	Apple without skin
Fried foods	Rice
Fruits	White bread
Vegetables	Bagels
Spices	Soft drinks
Fruit juices	Banana
French fries	Pasta
Chocolate	Pretzels
	Tea
	Potato
	Jelly (not jam)
	Boiled, broiled, baked meat, chicken or fish

Children with True Fecal Incontinence and Constipation (Colonic Hypomotility)

In these children, the motility of the colon is slow. The basis of the bowel management program in these patients is to clean the child's colon once a day with an enema. No special diet or medications are necessary. The fact that they suffer from constipation (hypomotility) is helpful, because it helps them to remain clean between enemas. The real challenge is to find the appropriate enema capable of evacuating the colon completely. Definitive evidence that the colon is empty after an enema requires a plain abdominal radiograph (see Fig. 37-4). Soiling episodes or "accidents" occur when there is incomplete cleaning of the bowel with feces that progressively accumulates.

Children with True Fecal Incontinence and Loose Stools (Colonic Hypermotility)

The great majority of children with anorectal malformations who suffer from this problem were repaired before the introduction of the posterior sagittal technique. The older procedures frequently included a rectosigmoid resection.[6,7] Therefore, this group of children has an overactive colon because they lack a rectal reservoir (see Fig. 37-3). Rapid transit of stool results in frequent episodes of diarrhea. This means that even when an enema cleans their colon rather easily, stool keeps passing fairly quickly from the cecum to the descending colon and into the anus. For treatments, a constipating diet and/or medications to slow down the colon are necessary. Also, eliminating foods that further loosen bowel movements will help the colon slow down (Table 37-3). A small subset of patients with Hirschsprung's disease behaves like they have hypermotility and can be managed similarly.

The keys to success of the bowel management program are dedication and sensitivity from the medical team. The basis of the program is to clean the colon and keep it quiet, thus keeping the patient clean for the 24 hours after the enema. This program is an ongoing process that is responsive to the individual patient and differs for each child. It is usually successful within a week, during which time the family, patient, physician, and nurse undergo a process of trial and error, tailoring the regimen to the specific patient. More than 95% of the children who follow this program are artificially clean and dry for the whole day and can have a completely normal life.[4]

One should embrace the philosophy that it is unacceptable to send a child with fecal incontinence to school in diapers when his or her classmates are already toilet trained. Proper treatment to prevent this is perhaps more important than any surgical procedure.

BOWEL MANAGEMENT: KEY STEPS

The first step is to perform a contrast enema with hydrosoluble material. The study should never be done with barium. It is very important to obtain a postevacuation film. This contrast study shows the type of colon that is present: dilated-constipated (see Fig. 37-2) or nondilated-tendency toward loose stool (Figs. 37-3 and 37-5). The enema volume and type can be estimated from this study.

The bowel management program is then implemented according to the patient's type of colon, and

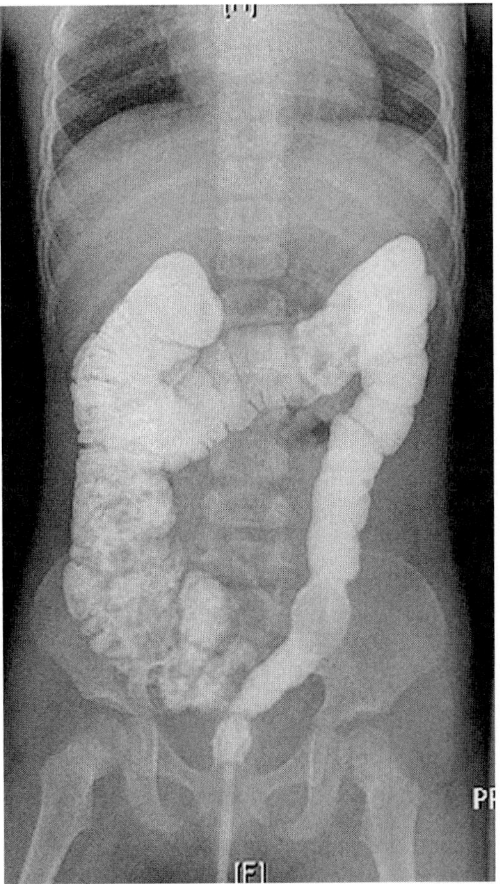

Figure 37-5. This contrast study shows a nondilated colon.

the results are evaluated daily. Changes in the volume and content of the enema are made until the colon is successfully cleaned. For this, an abdominal radiograph that is obtained every day is invaluable in determining whether the colon is empty (see Fig. 37-4).

There are different types of solutions to use for enemas: some are ready made and can be bought in a drugstore. Some can be prepared at home based on water and salt (0.9% saline can be made by adding 1.5 teaspoons of salt to 960 mL of water). The use of phosphate enemas is most convenient because they are available in prepared containers. However, saline enemas are often just as effective, and some families find them easier and less expensive. Occasionally, children will complain of cramping with the phosphate enema but often have no complaints with saline enemas. Children should never receive more than one phosphate enema a day because of the risk of phosphate intoxication. Others with impaired renal function should avoid them entirely. The saline enema can be mixed with glycerin and/or soap to make it more effective.

The daily enema should result in a bowel movement within 30 to 45 minutes, followed by a period of 24 hours of complete cleanliness. If a single enema is not sufficient to clean the colon (as demonstrated by a radiograph) or if the child keeps soiling, then the child requires more aggressive treatment. Administering the enema with a balloon catheter helps prevent enema leakage (Fig. 37-6). The "right" enema is the one that can empty the child's colon and allow him or her to stay clean for the following 24 hours. This can be achieved only by trial and error and learning from previous attempts.

Children with loose stools have an overactive colon. Most of the time they do not have a rectal reservoir. This means that even when an enema cleans their colon rather easily, new stool passes quickly from the cecum to the descending colon and the anus. To prevent this, a constipating diet, bulking agents (e.g., pectin), and/or medications (e.g., loperamide) to slow down the colon are used. Eliminating foods that loosen bowel movements will help the colon to move more slowly (see Table 37-3).

Parents should be provided with a list of constipating foods to utilize and a list of laxative foods to avoid. The constipating diet is rigid: banana, apple, baked bread, white pasta with no sauce, boiled meat, and so on. Fried foods and dairy products must be avoided (see Table 37-3). Most parents learn which meals provoke loose stools and which constipate their child. To determine the right combination, treatment is initiated with enemas, a very strict diet, loperamide, and pectin. Most children respond to this aggressive management within 1 to 2 weeks. The child should remain on a strict diet until clean for 24 hours for 2 to 3 days in a row. They can then choose one new food every 2 to 3 days and the effect of this new food on the child's colonic activity is observed. If the child soils after eating a newly introduced food, that food must be eliminated from the diet. Over several months, the most liberal diet possible should be sought. If the child remains clean with a liberal diet, the dose of the medication can gradually be reduced to the lowest effective dose to keep the child clean for 24 hours.

In children in whom a successful bowel management program has been implemented, the parents frequently ask if this program will be needed for life. The answer is "yes" for those patients born with no potential for bowel control. However, because there is a spectrum of defects, there are patients with some degree of bowel control. These patients are subjected to the bowel management program to avoid embarrassing accidents of uncontrolled bowel movements. As time goes by, the child becomes more cooperative and more interested in his or her problem. It is conceivable that later in life, a child may be able to stop using enemas and remain clean by following a specific regimen of a disciplined diet with regular meals (three meals per day and no snacks) to provoke bowel movements at a predictable time. Every summer, children with some potential for bowel control can try to find out how well they can control their bowel movements without the help of enemas. This is attempted during vacations to avoid accidents at school or during a time that they can stay home and try some of the toilet training strategies.

For patients with a colostomy and no potential for bowel control, a key question is whether to perform a pull-through operation or leave the permanent

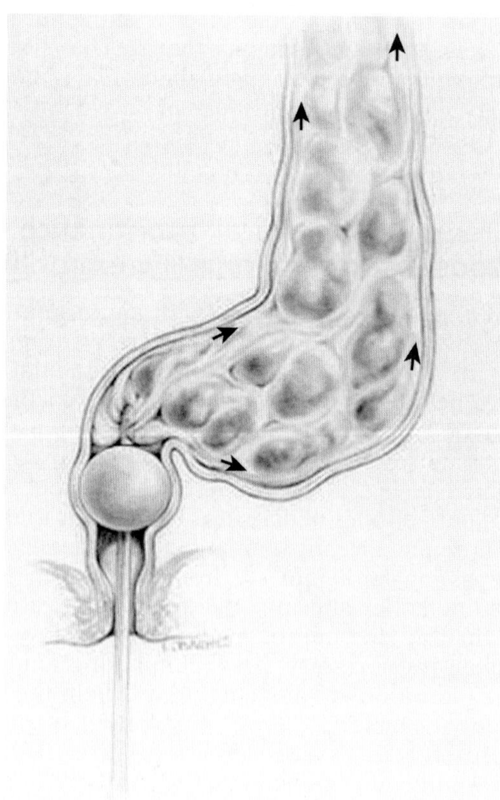

Figure 37-6. Note that inflation of the balloon on the catheter helps prevent enema leakage in this retrograde contrast study.

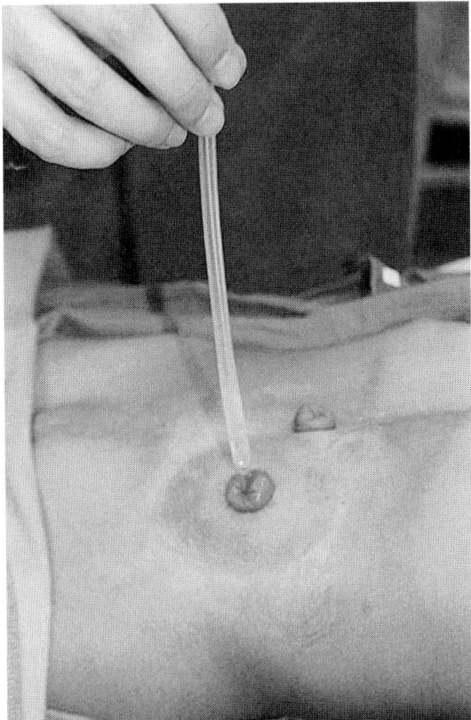

Figure 37-7. Some patients have the capacity to have good bowel control with a daily enema administered through their colostomy.

stoma. We believe that if the patient has the capacity to form solid stool, a pull-through procedure can be performed and a daily enema given thereafter helps to keep them clean. For these patients, we believe that successful bowel management provides a better quality of life compared with a permanent stoma. Thus, for this group of patients, bowel management is initiated with a daily enema via the stoma (Fig. 37-7). If the stoma remains quiet for 24 hours between enemas, then that stoma could be pulled through and a daily enema using the Malone technique utilized (Fig. 37-8).[8]

Most preschool- and school-age children enjoy a good quality of life while undergoing the bowel management program. However, when they reach puberty, many express dissatisfaction. They believe that their parents are intruding on their privacy by giving them enemas. It is feasible, but rather difficult, for them to administer the enema themselves. For this specific group of children, a continent appendicostomy or Malone procedure has been developed (see Fig. 37-8).[8] Using the appendix, a valve mechanism is created and connected to the umbilicus. The appendicostomy can be catheterized to administer the enema fluid but will avoid leakage of stool through it. If the child has had the appendix removed, it is possible to create a new one from a colonic flap (a continent neoappendicostomy).

The Malone procedure is just another way to administer an enema. Therefore, before performing it, the child has to be perfectly clean with a bowel management regimen.

PSEUDOINCONTINENCE

Pseudoincontinence occurs when a patient behaves like he or she is fecally incontinent but really has severe constipation and overflow soiling. Once the disimpaction is treated and the patient receives enough laxatives to avoid constipation, he or she starts having voluntary bowel movements.

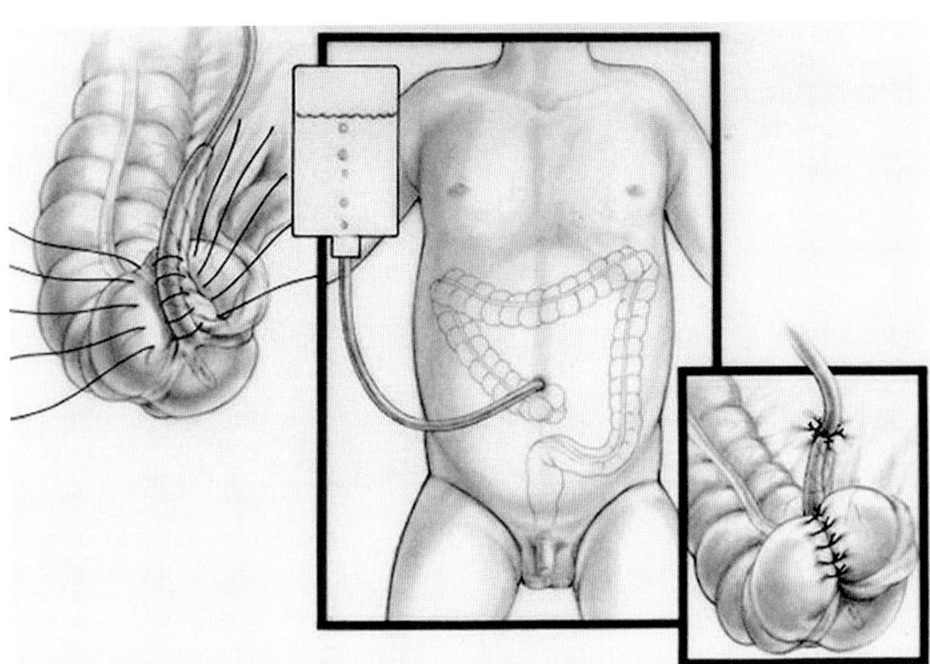

Figure 37-8. Some patients are able to have bowel continence with a daily prograde enema administered through an appendicostomy. (From Levitt MA, Soffer SZ, Peña A: Continent appendicostomy in the bowel management of fecal incontinent children. J Pediatr Surg 32:1631, 1997.)

The colon absorbs water from the stool and serves a reservoir function. These processes depend on colonic motility, which is an area of physiology that is not well understood and for which treatments of problems are limited. In normal individuals, the rectosigmoid stores the stool. Every 24 to 48 hours, it develops active peristaltic waves, indicating that it is time to empty. A normal individual feels this sensation and decides when to relax the voluntary sphincter mechanism.

If a child is fecally continent, then management involves treatment of constipation, using laxatives, which helps to provoke peristalsis and to overcome the dysmotility. Patients who have undergone successful surgery for Hirschsprung's disease or for anorectal malformations (good prognosis type) with a normal spine should be fecally continent.

Constipation in children with anorectal malformations is extremely common, particularly in the more benign types.[3,9] It is also common in patients after successful surgery for Hirschsprung's disease and occurs in a large group of patients considered to have idiopathic constipation.[1] When left untreated, constipation can be extremely incapacitating. Although diet impacts colonic motility, its therapeutic value is negligible in the most serious forms of constipation. While it is true that many patients with severe constipation suffer from psychological disorders, a psychological origin for the constipation cannot explain the severe forms, because it is not easy to voluntarily retain stool when an autonomous rectosigmoid undergoes peristalsis. Passage of large, hard pieces of stool may provoke pain and make the patient behave like a stool retainer. This may complicate the problem of constipation, but it is not the original cause.

Constipation is a self-perpetuating disease. A patient who suffers from a certain degree of constipation and is not treated adequately will only partially empty the colon, leaving larger and larger amounts of stool inside the rectosigmoid. This results in greater degrees of distal colonic enlargement. It is clear that dilation of a hollow viscus produces poor peristalsis. This explains why constipation leads to fecal retention, leading to megacolon, which exacerbates the constipation. In addition, the passage of large, hard pieces of stool may produce anal fissures, leading to painful stooling and a reluctance by the patient to have bowel movements.

The clinician must decide which type of patient is being treated. Patients with anorectal malformations and Hirschsprung's disease with good prognosis for bowel control are those more likely to have constipation. In these patients, an aggressive, proactive treatment of their constipation is the best approach. Additionally, the child must be deemed capable of being fecally continent and having the capacity for voluntary bowel movements before initiating treatment for constipation because laxatives will make an incontinent constipated child worse.

When children with anorectal malformations and Hirschsprung's disease are managed early with aggressive treatment of constipation, children with good prognosis should toilet train without difficulty. When constipation is not managed properly, they behave much like children with idiopathic constipation and may have overflow pseudoincontinence. Because of a hypomotility disorder that interferes with complete emptying of the rectosigmoid, most of these patients suffer from different degrees of dilation of the rectum and sigmoid, a condition known as megarectosigmoid (see Fig. 37-2).[1] These can be children who were born with a good prognosis type of anorectal defect and who underwent a technically correct operation, but did not receive appropriate treatment for constipation. Subsequently they developed fecal impaction and overflow pseudoincontinence. These may also be children with severe idiopathic constipation who have a very dilated rectosigmoid.

First, the impaction needs to be removed with enemas and colonic irrigations to clean the megarectosigmoid. Subsequently, once the colon is clean, the constipation is treated with the administration of large doses of laxatives. The dosage of the laxative is increased daily until the right amount of laxative is reached to completely empty the colon every day.

If medical treatment proves to be extremely difficult because the child has a severe megasigmoid and requires an enormous amount of laxatives to empty, the surgeon can offer a segmental resection of the colon. After the resection, the amount of laxatives required to treat these children can be significantly reduced or even eliminated. Before performing this operation, it is mandatory to confirm that the child is definitely suffering from overflow pseudoincontinence rather than true fecal incontinence with constipation. Failure to make this distinction may lead to an operation in which a fecally incontinent constipated child is changed to one with a tendency to have loose stool, which will make the patient's condition much more difficult to manage.

The dysmotility of the colon in patients with Hirschsprung's disease, even after successful surgery to remove the aganglionic bowel, is not understood. These patients can also benefit from proactive medical treatment of their constipation. The clinician must understand that the dysmotility observed is essentially incurable. It is, however, manageable, but requires careful follow-up for life. Treatments cannot be given on a temporary basis. If they are tapered or interrupted, the constipation will recur.

Some clinicians treat these patients with colostomies or colonic washouts via a catheterized stoma or button device, and monitor the improvement of colonic dilatation with contrast studies.[10] Once the distal colon regains a normal caliber, the physician assumes that the patient is cured and discontinues the washouts or closes the colostomy. Unfortunately, these patients' symptoms quickly recur. Washouts are often ineffective in such patients because they simply retain the fluid. We believe that washouts are really only for patients with true fecal incontinence who are incapable of having voluntary bowel movements and thus require a daily irrigation to empty their colon. On the other hand, the patient with pseudoincontinence is capable of emptying the colon with the help of adequate doses of laxatives and thus does not need washouts.

Determining which patient the clinician is managing can be a challenge. If the patient is incontinent, washouts with a bowel management regimen are appropriate. If the patient is continent, then aggressive management of the constipation after ensuring disimpaction is the treatment choice.

Fecal impaction is a stressful event resulting from retained stool for several days or weeks, crampy abdominal pain, and sometimes tenesmus. When laxatives are prescribed to such a patient, the result is exacerbation of the crampy abdominal pain and sometimes vomiting. This is a consequence of increased colonic peristalsis (produced by the laxative) acting against a fecally impacted colon. Therefore, disimpaction, proven by radiograph, must precede initiation of laxative therapy.

Soiling of underwear is an ominous sign of severe constipation. A patient who is old enough to have bowel control, but soils the underwear day and night and does not have spontaneous bowel movements, may have overflow pseudoincontinence. These patients behave similarly to fecally incontinent individuals. When the constipation is treated adequately, the great majority of these pseudoincontinent children regain bowel control. Of course, this clinical presentation may also occur in a patient with true fecal incontinence. When uncertain, the clinician can start the 3- to 4-year-old who is having trouble with toilet training on a daily enema. Once clean with this regimen, and if the child has the potential for bowel control, then an attempt at a laxative program can be tried.

A contrast enema with hydrosoluble material (never barium) is an extremely valuable study. In the constipated patient, it usually shows a megarectosigmoid with dilation of the colon all the way down to the level of the levator mechanism (see Fig. 37-2). There is usually a dramatic size discrepancy between a normal transverse and descending colon and the dilated megarectosigmoid. The size of the colon guides the dosing of the laxatives. It seems that the more localized the dilatation of the rectosigmoid, the better the results of a colonic resection in reducing or eliminating the laxative requirement.

Rectal and colonic manometry is sometimes used in the evaluation of these patients. Manometry is performed by placing balloons at different levels in the colon and recording the waves of contraction or the electrical activity.[11,12] Scintigraphy, a nuclear medicine study, is also being used to assess colonic motility.[13] These are sophisticated studies that do not yet help guide therapeutic decisions. The key information the surgeon needs to know is if and where a colonic resection would prove beneficial to the patient who requires enormous doses of laxative to empty the bowel.

Histologic studies of the colon in these patients mainly show hypertrophic smooth muscle in the area of the dilated colon and normal ganglion cells. In the near future, it is hoped more sophisticated histopathologic research will enhance our knowledge about colonic dysmotility.

TREATMENT

Patients with anorectal malformations, severe constipation, and the potential for bowel control, as well as those with severe idiopathic constipation in whom dietary measures or gentle laxatives do not work, require a more aggressive regimen. Drugs that are designed to increase the colon's motility (containing senna) are best when compared with medications that are only stool softeners. Softening of the stool without improving the colonic motility will likely make the patient worse. With soft stool they no longer have control, whereas they do reasonably well with solid stool that allows them to feel rectal distention. This is a common misconception. Often the switch from stool softener to laxative makes an enormous difference.

In many cases, the laxative regimen we employ uses the same medications that have been tried previously but were unsuccessful. This is because the protocol is different in that the laxatives are only started with a radiographically clean colon and the dosage is adapted to the patient's response. The response is monitored daily with an abdominal radiograph with the laxative dose adjusted, if necessary. Almost always, the patient previously had received a lower dose than what was really needed.

Disimpaction

The disimpaction process is a vital and often neglected step. This includes the administration of enemas three times a day until the patient is disimpacted, which is confirmed radiologically. The contrast enema using water-soluble material not only shows the anatomy, but also is a helpful tool for cleaning the colon. If the patient remains impacted after 3 days, then he or she is given a balanced electrolyte solution via nasogastric tube in the hospital and the enema regimen is continued. If this is unsuccessful, a manual disimpaction under anesthesia may be necessary. It is important to remember not to prescribe laxatives to a patient who is fecally impacted. To do so may provoke vomiting and crampy abdominal pain. In addition, the patient will become reluctant to take laxatives because of the fear of these symptoms.

Determining the Laxative Requirement

Once the patient has been disimpacted, an arbitrary amount of laxative, usually a senna derivative, is started. The initial amount is based on the information that the parents give about the previous response to laxatives and the subjective evaluation of the megasigmoid on the contrast enema. An empirical dose is given, and the patient is observed for the next 24 hours. If the patient does not have a bowel movement in the 24 hours after giving the laxative, it means the laxative dose was not strong enough and must be increased. An enema is also required to remove the stool produced during the previous 24 hours. Stool

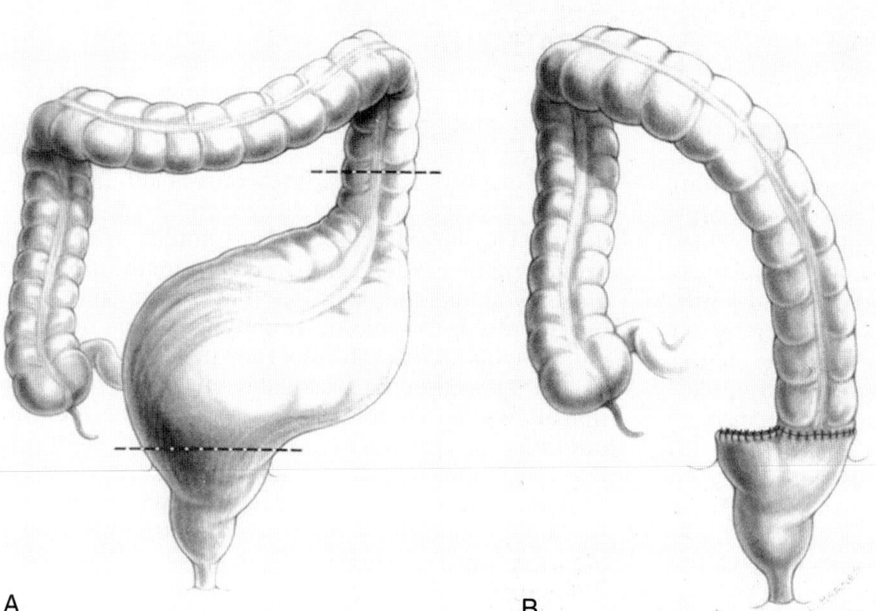

Figure 37-9. **A** and **B,** These drawings show resection of a dilated sigmoid colon, which can be very effective in select patients with an anorectal malformation and severe constipation.

in these extremely constipated patients should never remain in the rectosigmoid for more than 24 hours.

The routine of increasing the amount of laxatives and giving an enema, if needed, is continued every night until the child has a voluntary bowel movement and empties the colon completely. Ideally, this routine is checked with a daily radiograph. Each day that the patient has a bowel movement (which is usually with diarrhea), a radiograph should confirm that the bowel movement was effective, meaning that the patient completely emptied the rectosigmoid. If the patient passed stool but did not empty completely, the dose of laxative should be increased. If the patient passed stool and successfully emptied the colon, then that laxative dose should be continued on a daily basis. If the patient passed multiple stools and the abdominal film is clear, then the laxative dose can be reduced slightly.

It is important to remember that this condition covers a wide spectrum and patients may have laxative requirements much larger than the manufacturer's recommendation. Occasionally, in the process of increasing the amount of laxatives, patients throw up or feel nauseated and cramping with the medication before reaching any positive effect. In these patients, a different medication can be tried. Some patients vomit all kinds of laxatives and are unable to reach the amount of laxative that produces a bowel movement that empties the colon. Such a patient is considered to have an intractable condition and is a candidate for surgical intervention. Usually, however, the dosage that the patient needs to empty the colon completely (as demonstrated radiologically) can be achieved. At that dose, the patient should stop soiling because he or she is successfully emptying the colon each day. Because the colon is empty, the patient remains clean until the next voluntary bowel movement.

At this point, the patient and the parents have the opportunity to evaluate the quality of life that they have with this kind of treatment, understanding that this treatment will most likely be lifelong. For many of these patients, a sigmoid or rectosigmoid resection can provide symptomatic improvement leading to significant reduction or complete elimination of laxatives.

Rectosigmoid Resection

For the past 15 years, we have been performing a sigmoid resection for the treatment of select patients with severe constipation and voluntary bowel movements.[14] The megarectosigmoid is resected and the descending colon is anastomosed to the rectum (Fig. 37-9). In a recent review of our patients with anorectal malformations, 315 who suffered from severe constipation were fecally continent but required significant laxative doses to empty the colon.[15] Of these, 53 underwent a sigmoid resection with preservation of the rectum. Of those undergoing sigmoid resection, 10% of patients no longer required laxatives, had daily bowel movements, and did not soil. Thirty percent of patients decreased their laxative requirement by 80% and the remaining 60% of patients decreased their laxative requirement by 40%. These patients must be followed closely because the condition is not cured by the operation. The remaining rectum is most likely abnormal. Without careful observation and treatment of constipation, the colon can re-dilate.

In patients with anorectal malformations, keeping the rectum intact is vital because they need it for continence. It is their reservoir in which they feel the distention of the stool. In contrast, patients with idiopathic constipation who have not undergone any rectal surgery and have a normal anal canal and sphincters, the rectum and sigmoid can be resected with preservation of fecal continence. The resection of the

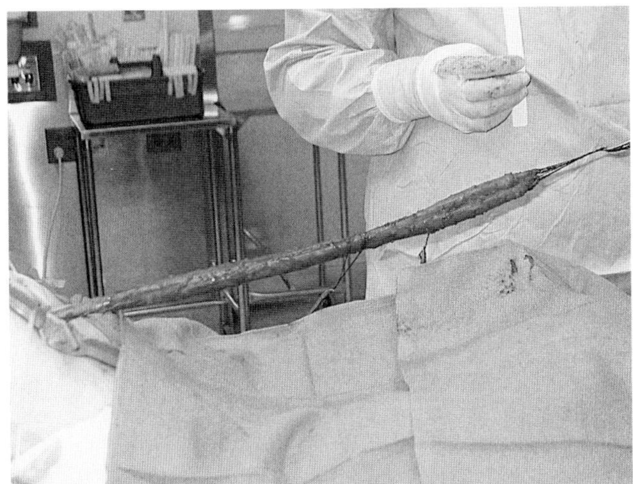

Figure 37-10. In patients with idiopathic constipation who have not undergone previous operations and have a normal anal canal and sphincter, an extensive resection of the rectosigmoid colon can be performed transanally.

rectosigmoid down to the pectinate line can be done in a similar manner used for patients with Hirschsprung's disease, with anastomosis of the nondilated colon (that is assumed to have normal motility) to the rectum above the pectinate line (Fig. 37-10). An extensive rectosigmoid resection can be done completely transanally.[16] We have performed this operation in 25 patients and have seen dramatic improvement in their ability to empty their colon.

The most dilated part of the colon is resected because it seems to be the most seriously affected and the nondilated part of the colon is assumed to have a more normal motility. Unfortunately, we lack a more scientific way to assess the dysmotile anatomy. Perhaps emerging colonic motility studies will help with surgical planning. It seems that the patients who improve the most are those who have a more localized form of megarectosigmoid. Patients with more generalized dilation of the colon do not respond as well and may require a more extensive resection.

chapter 38

ACQUIRED ANORECTAL DISORDERS

Casey M. Calkins, MD • Keith T. Oldham, MD

PERIANAL AND PERIRECTAL ABSCESS

Perianal or perirectal abscesses are often encountered during infancy. The majority of patients in a pediatric surgical practice are seen prior to 12 months of age. The abscess typically presents as a fluctuant, tender mass in the perianal region (Fig. 38-1). Patients are usually otherwise well. A history of stool abnormalities is typically not elicited, either before development of the abscess or during its maturation. Perianal abscesses are much more common in male infants and are infrequent in toddlers and older children.[1] Crohn's disease, immunodeficiency, glucose intolerance, and perianal trauma can be causative stimuli. It is unusual to find complex ischiorectal abscesses in children unless associated with chronic inflammatory bowel diseases. During infancy, abnormal crypt architecture may predispose the patient to the development of an infection within the crypts of Morgagni.[1] However, some have disputed the role of abnormal crypt architecture in the development of perianal abscess and subsequent fistula-in-ano.[2]

Sitz baths (or their equivalent for the infant) are prescribed if the abscess does not appear to be fluctuant and in need of immediate drainage. Approximately one third of abscesses thus treated resolve without recurrence.[3] Approximately two thirds require incision and drainage. This continues to be the mainstay of surgical therapy, albeit recent reports have surfaced that describe favorable outcomes for patients treated with needle aspiration and oral antibiotic therapy.[4] Although surgical drainage can be accomplished in the infant without anesthesia or with a topical anesthetic ointment, we prefer a brief anesthetic to allow for adequate drainage and optimal patient comfort. Considerable debate exists with regard to making an effort to delineate a fistula at the time of abscess drainage.[5,6] We prefer simple abscess drainage as the initial step in an infant with a perianal abscess. A small wick of gauze is typically left within the cavity. Removal of the packing along with sitz baths is undertaken on the first postoperative day.

FISTULA-IN-ANO

As many as 40% to 50% of perianal abscesses progress to a fistula-in-ano.[7] Fistula-in-ano also appears predominantly in male infants.[8] The child is usually seen after two or more flareups of a perianal abscess that either continues to drain or forms a small pustule that ruptures, only to form again (Fig. 38-2).[9] The fistula is commonly located lateral to the anus rather than in the midline. Occasionally, two fistulas may occur simultaneously in one child. In a few patients, fistulas have occurred in a serial fashion. An intriguing theory has been suggested that fistula-in-ano results from infection in abnormally deep crypts that are under the influence of androgens.[1] The fact that fistula-in-ano almost never follows a perianal abscess in female children lends credence to this theory.[10]

The preferred surgical procedure for fistula-in-ano is fistulotomy. With the patient under general anesthesia, the anus is gently serially dilated with Hegar dilators and a small nasal speculum suffices as an anoscope. A fine malleable probe is inserted through the fistula and gently advanced until it is visualized to exit the base of the involved crypt (Fig. 38-3A), remembering that the tract is direct and does not follow Goodsall's rule for fistulas seen in adult patients. An incision is made along the probe and is deepened through the superficial portion of the external sphincter (see Fig. 38-3B). The base of the exposed fistula is denuded of granulation tissue with a curet. The wound is left open, which provides some distress on the part of the parents but little discomfort on the part of the child (see Fig. 38-3C). Although suture closure has been reported to result in satisfactory healing without infection, we prefer to leave the tract open.[1] We instruct the parents to provide a sitz bath after each bowel movement, at least twice daily, and to separate the skin edges of the fistulotomy site during bathing to promote healing by secondary intention. We reserve cryptectomy and tract excision for patients with recurrence, which is rare after an adequate fistulotomy.

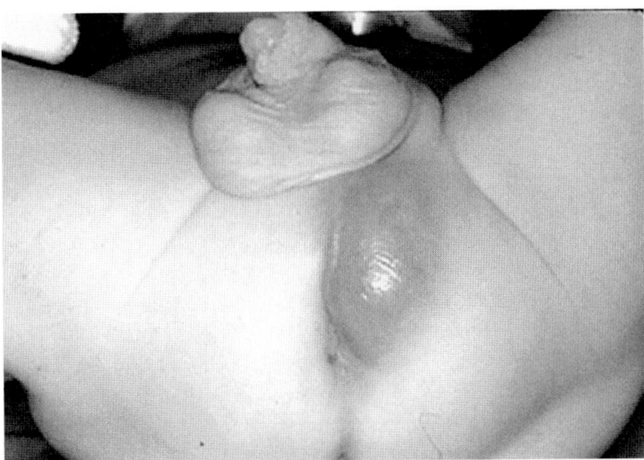

Figure 38-1. Perianal abscesses are often seen in male infants. The abscess typically presents as a fluctuant, tender mass in the perianal region. Incision and drainage is the initial management of these abscesses.

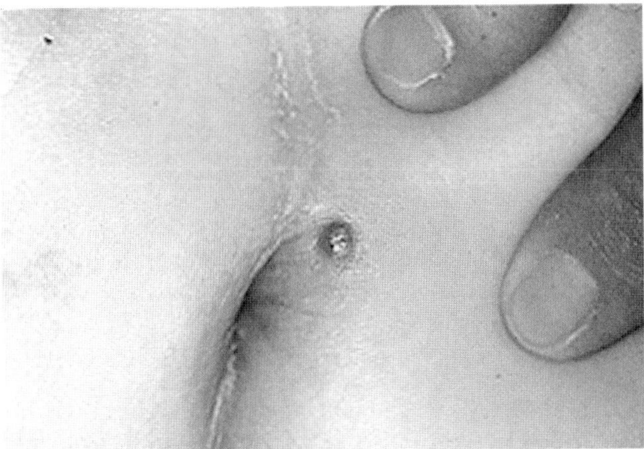

Figure 38-2. As many as one half of the perianal abscesses progress to a fistula-in-ano. In this photograph, the fistula is seen at 1 o'clock when the infant is in the lithotomy position.

ANAL FISSURE

An anal fissure commonly develops in a toddler whose diet changes from liquid to solid and whose stool consistency changes from soft to firm. A period of constipation often precedes a hard, bulky stool that results in a posterior midline tear in the anoderm below the mucocutaneous junction. The discomfort in having a bowel movement associated with the fissure often leads to further constipation, which, in turn, aggravates the fissure with each stool and prevents healing. Anal fissure in the pediatric population is typically seen in the toddler who is capable of repressing the urge to defecate because of this anticipated pain. The diagnosis is made through the history of blood streaking on the stool, the child's crying during bowel movements, and the recognition of a split in the anoderm. Operative interventions such as lateral internal sphincterotomy[11] or fissurectomy[12] are rarely necessary. We prefer to manage these patients with sitz baths and an osmotic stool softener such as polyethylene glycol, although any form of stool softener is sufficient. Sitz baths promote good anal hygiene and relax the anal sphincter. Although 0.2% nitroglycerin ointment has become a popular treatment for anal fissure in adults, its use in children is still limited, although some studies have shown promising efficacy.[13-15] Nevertheless, we believe its use should be entertained for the older child without evidence of inflammatory bowel disease. The same is true for chemical sphincterotomy by botulinum toxin, which has gained popularity in adults. However, it has not been demonstrated to be superior to topical nitroglycerin and has not been well studied in children.[14]

An anal fissure in an older child or a teenager is often associated with chronic inflammatory bowel disease, usually Crohn's.[16] Demonstration of an anal fissure often precedes the diagnosis of Crohn's disease. Medical treatment of Crohn's disease typically results

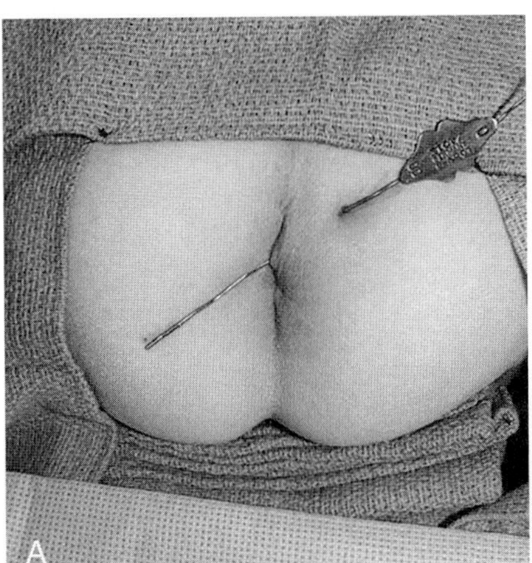

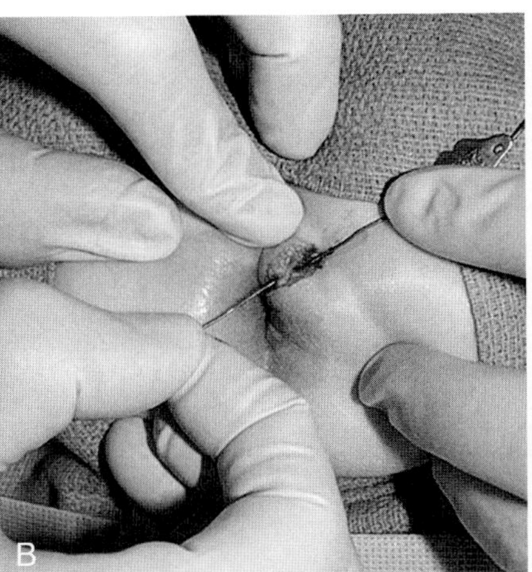

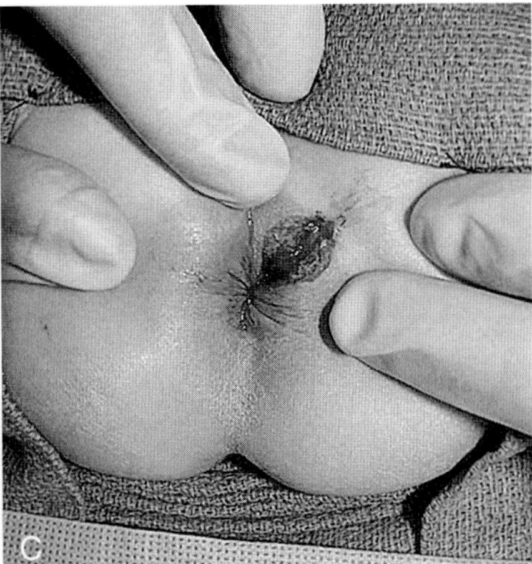

Figure 38-3. **A,** At the time of operation, a small, fine, malleable probe is inserted through the fistula and can usually be gently advanced until it is visualized to exit the base of the involved crypt. **B,** An incision is then made along the probe and is deepened through the superficial portion of the external sphincter. **C,** After complete unroofing of the tract, the incision is usually left open, which may provide some distress on the part of the parents but usually does not cause much discomfort for the child.

in healing of the fissure.[17,18] Also, topical application of tacrolimus ointment is a promising new therapy.[19] Internal sphincterotomy appears to be a relatively safe undertaking in this patient population when local measures and immunomodulator therapy fail.[16,20]

ANAL SKIN TAGS AND HEMORRHOIDS

A perianal skin tag is rarely an indication of other disease, although it may result from a healed fissure. Although it is generally of no consequence, when large enough it can be bothersome and can affect adequate perianal hygiene. In these cases, local excision is reasonable.

Hemorrhoids are uncommon in the pediatric population, and rarely is surgical therapy a necessary aspect of treatment. External hemorrhoids are located in the distal one third of the anal canal and covered by anoderm. Symptoms from external hemorrhoids are generally due to thrombosis, and examination reveals a tender, bluish mass at the mucocutaneous junction (Fig. 38-4). Treatment consists of incision of the hemorrhoid and extrusion of the clot with subsequent sitz baths, dietary modification (fiber supplementation), and stool softeners. Internal hemorrhoids are extremely rare in children unless associated with portal hypertension. The treatment of bleeding from internal hemorrhoids due to portal hypertension should be aimed at decreasing portal pressure, either pharmacologically or surgically. In patients without portal hypertension, initial treatment of internal hemorrhoids should be focused on conservative measures such as provision of stool bulking agents and topical treatment (sitz baths and topical pharmaceutical preparations). Rubber band ligation or operative hemorrhoidectomy is performed when conservative measures fail.

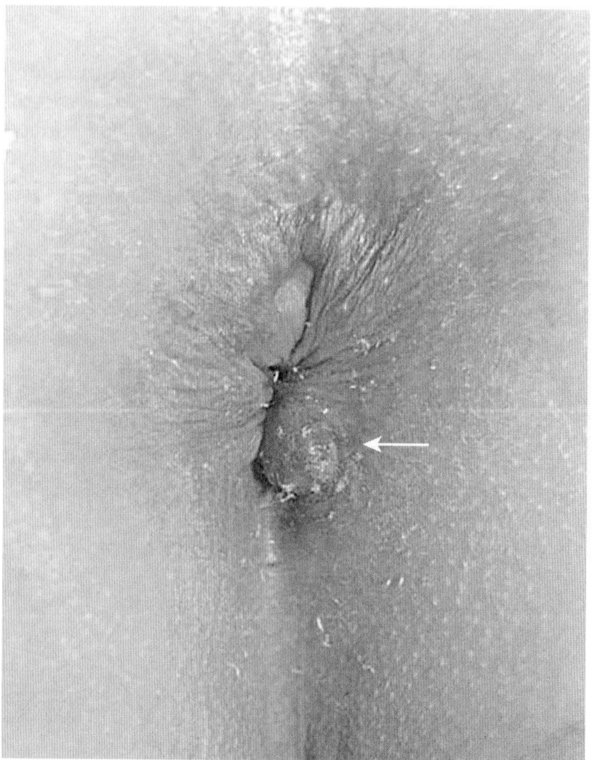

Figure 38-4. This adolescent presented with pain secondary to thrombosis of an external hemorrhoid (*arrow*). The hemorrhoid was incised and the clot extruded.

RECTAL PROLAPSE

Rectal prolapse is a relatively common problem in young children and causes great distress to the child and the parents. Prolapse can range from an intermittent mucosal prolapse that occurs during defecation and reduces spontaneously to full-thickness prolapse of the rectum, which requires manual reduction. Worse is if the prolapse cannot be reduced, which may result in vascular compromise. Rectal prolapse in children is likely precipitated by weakness of the pelvic supporting musculature (levator mechanism) and loosely attached rectal submucosa to the underlying muscularis. The latter may improve with time (especially in cases where the weakness is due to malnutrition or dehydration),[21] whereas a weak and dilated pelvic floor may not. Straining during stooling and long periods of sitting on the toilet, because of protracted diarrhea or constipation (which may occur in cystic fibrosis), allows stretching of the pelvic diaphragm and other less well-defined suspensory structures of the rectum, resulting in prolapse.[22] Up to 20% of cases of rectal prolapse initially seen between 6 months and 3 years of age will later be diagnosed with cystic fibrosis.[23] A chloride sweat test should be undertaken to substantiate the diagnosis when there is no apparent underlying cause.[24]

The diagnosis is usually made by the parent, who notices a rosette of mucosa when the child complains of discomfort at the anus while defecating. Bleeding is occasionally noted as the primary symptom. Rarely is rectal prolapse in children the source of significant disability. The prolapse either reduces spontaneously as the child gets off the toilet or the parent pushes it back in. Many 3-year-old children very quickly learn to reduce their own prolapse. It generally does not recur until the next stool. It is uncommon for the child to be able to produce the prolapse in the examining room. Occasionally, the prolapse can be demonstrated during a brief session on the commode. The typical prolapse is a rosette of mucosa, sometimes slightly longer posteriorly than anteriorly (Fig. 38-5). One should be able to slip a finger alongside the prolapse and feel the sulcus 1 to 2 cm up inside the anus. Sometimes what appears to be rectal prolapse is an intussusception of the sigmoid colon.[25] In these cases, an intact rectal suspension system exists but a dilated levator mechanism produced by straining at stool, coupled with a redundant sigmoid colon, allows for its intussusception. A deeper sulcus suggests sigmoid intussusception rather than rectal prolapse. It is often difficult to differentiate the two clinically, even in the face of rectal examination at the time of prolapse or radiologic defecography and/or barium enema obtained to clarify the situation.

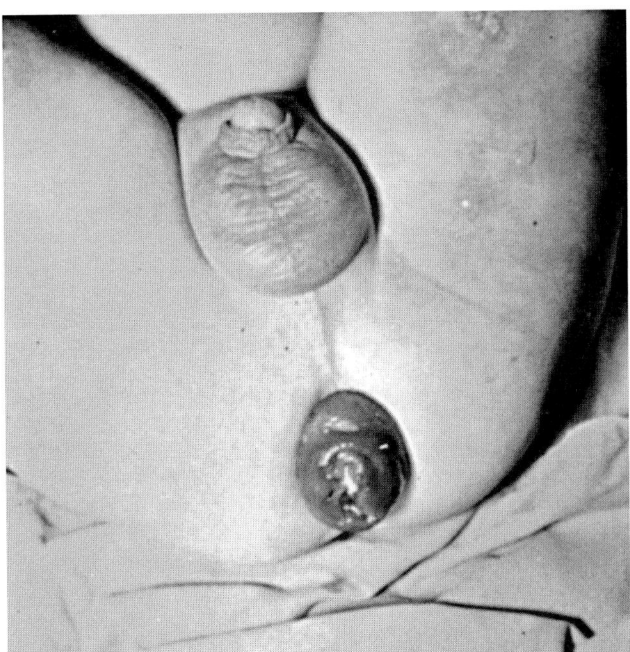

Figure 38-5. Rectal prolapse occurring in a child who had severe burns on his legs. Despite its being reduced repeatedly for several weeks, this prolapse continued to occur several times daily and required surgical correction.

The pelvic diaphragm is a muscular structure. If the prolapse is prevented from recurring, the muscle fibers shorten and the situation may be self-limiting. However, if the child continues straining during stooling once the pelvic diaphragm and rectal sphincters have been stretched, there is little chance that the prolapse will correct itself.

The nonoperative treatment of rectal prolapse consists of attempts to alter the disorder that led to the prolapse. A change in defecation habits and provision of stool softeners that eliminates the persistent urge to defecate may allow the pelvic musculature to resume its normal tone. One of the early reports advised against allowing the child to use the commode until the problem was resolved, suggesting that the child defecate in a squatting position on a newspaper.[26] We advocate that patients with rectal prolapse be restricted from spending prolonged periods of time on the commode. In addition, a child-specific commode or a step stool in front of an adult commode will assist the child in toilet training and may eliminate straining-like behaviors. In patients who are identified with cystic fibrosis, enzymatic supplementation and addressing malnutrition may be all that is required to eliminate episodes of prolapse.[27]

Surgical therapy has taken a number of forms. Perianal cerclage tightens the anal outlet and prevents prolapse from recurring while the musculature of the pelvic floor re-establishes its normal anatomic relationship.[24] The fact that the cerclage procedure is commonly used bespeaks its effectiveness, although one must be cautious to avoid placing the cerclage too tightly to avoid erosion of the anus. This is typically avoided by tying the cerclage over an appropriately sized Hegar dilator.[28] Sclerotherapy with any number of compounds (30% saline, Deflux, 25% glucose, 5% sodium morrhuate) injected into the retrorectal space produces an inflammatory response and scar that theoretically prevents the rectum from sliding downward. Whatever the injection material, it sometimes must be repeated.[29-33] We have found sclerotherapy to be especially effective in children with mucosal prolapse when combined with stool softeners and behavior modification. An open sclerosing procedure, in which the retrorectal space is developed and packed with gauze, is not performed routinely today.[34,35] It was performed through an incision posterior to the anus but anterior to the coccyx. The gauze packing is removed gradually over a 10-day period. The packing produces enough inflammatory response that the rectum remains suspended.

Various methods of cauterization therapy have been tried for rectal prolapse.[22,36,37] Endorectal cauterization or mucosal stripping as an alternative to suspension and plication procedures may be effective by allowing restoration of the suspensory apparatus. However, there is little evidence that rectal prolapse is due to mucosal overabundance, and we do not recommend this approach as a primary form of surgical therapy.

In patients with full-thickness prolapse, or for those who have failed other surgical forms of therapy, operative fixation techniques are generally needed. Transanal suture fixation of the rectum (initially described in 1909) has recently been used in a group of children with good success.[38,39] Its benefit probably derives from prevention of recurrent prolapse, while inflammation produced by the mattress suture, which extends from the rectal lumen to the skin, produces adhesions. An extensive plication or reefing of the posterior rectal wall via a coccygectomy incision has recently been reported to have good results, but the morbid potential for fistula formation makes this a technique that we do not routinely employ.[40] Laparoscopic rectopexy is an alternative to standard open rectopexy and is performed with two operating ports and a port for laparoscopic visualization.[41,42] The rectum is mobilized and sutured to the periosteum of the sacral promontory in multiple locations with nonabsorbable suture. The operation has been successfully completed in children as young as 10 months of age, and early results are encouraging.

Open posterior rectopexy has been advocated as the primary therapeutic modality for rectal prolapse not responsive to more conservative measures.[43] Through a natal cleft incision, the coccyx is removed, the muscular hiatus is narrowed, and the rectum is suspended from the cut edge of the sacrum so that it cannot slide downward (Fig. 38-6). This maneuver immediately re-establishes the levator ani suspensory mechanism and narrows the anorectal hiatus, which is the ultimate therapeutic intention of all the methods of treatment. Ashcraft and colleagues reported this technique in 46 patients over a 17-year period.[44] Of these patients, 42 had satisfactory resolution of their rectal prolapse. The operation can be performed

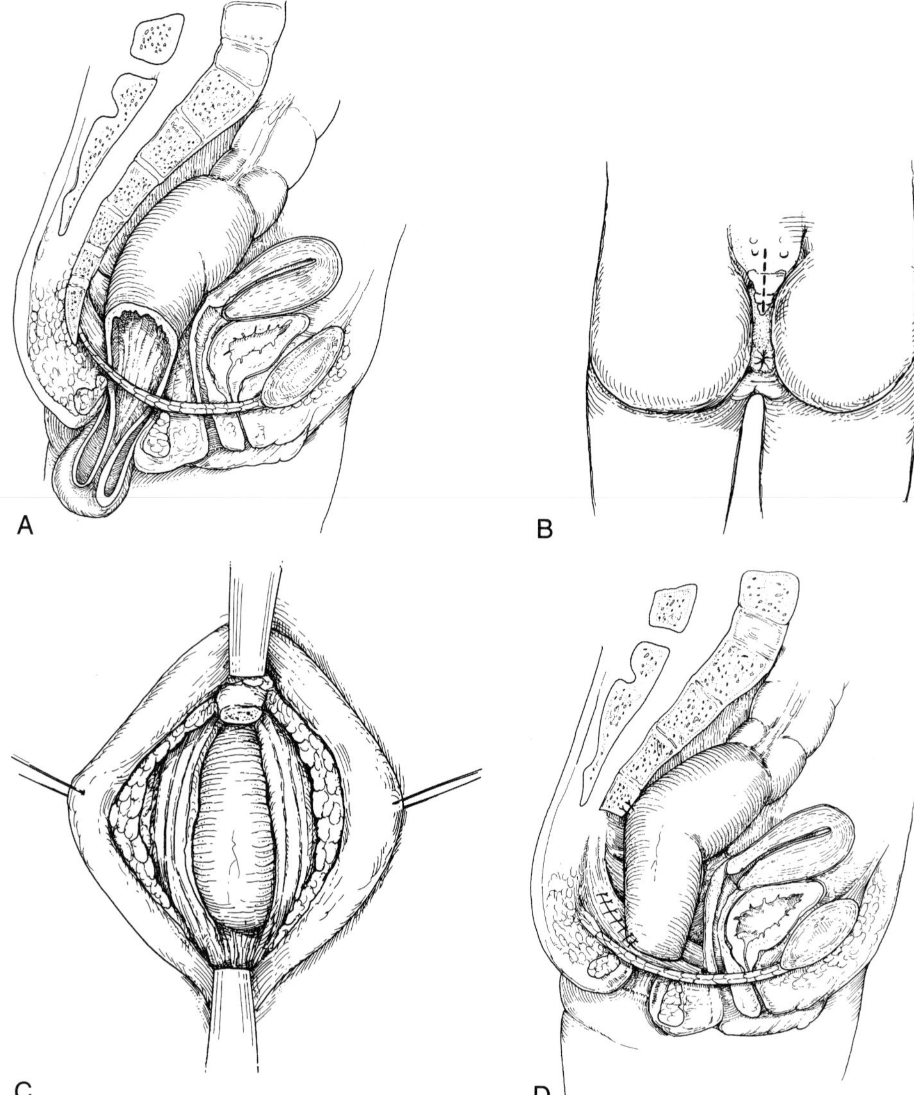

Figure 38-6. **A,** A cut-away sagittal view illustrates the failure of the rectal suspensory mechanism to hold the rectum within the pelvis. **B,** The posterior sagittal incision is depicted. **C,** The coccyx has been removed and the posterior rectal wall exposed. **D,** The pelvic diaphragm is closed posterior to the reduced rectum. The rectum is sutured laterally to the pelvic diaphragm. The rectum is further suspended from the cut edge of the sacrum. (**A** and **D** redrawn from Ashcraft KW, Amoury RA, Holder TM: Levator repair and posterior suspension for rectal prolapse. J Pediatr Surg 12:241-245, 1977; **B** and **C** from Ashcraft KW: Atlas of Pediatric Surgery. Philadelphia, WB Saunders, 1994, p 217.)

satisfactorily as an outpatient procedure. Modification of this approach by tapering a redundant and patulous rectum has considerable merit when the size of the rectum limits the ability to adequately narrow the anorectal hiatus.[45]

RECTAL TRAUMA

Rectal trauma in pediatric patients generally occurs by one of two mechanisms. The first is by way of penetrating trauma after an accidental impalement injury or, occasionally, a gunshot (Fig. 38-7). The second, and more common, occurs as the result of sexual abuse. Digital or penile penetration of the anorectum or other instrumentation may cause bleeding or bruising. The most common clinical presentation is that of a chronic stellate laceration of the anus with edema (Fig. 38-8).

Perianal condylomata are a common sequelae in cases of sexual abuse. Careful questioning may reveal that a male member of the immediate family has penile condylomata. However, as many as 25% of males who carry human papillomavirus in the urethra have no external evidence of the virus.[46]

The patient with an accidental injury to the anus usually is seen immediately after the incident occurs. An accurate and consistent history of the mechanism of injury is critical. Sexual abuse is suspected when an inconsistent history of the mechanism of injury is elucidated. As with other forms of sexual abuse involving genital penetration in female patients or manipulation in male patients, difficulty is often encountered in obtaining an adequate history from the victim owing to fear, threats of retaliation, or guilt. Unexplained injuries to the rectum must be considered a manifestation of sexual abuse until proven otherwise and must be investigated through the appropriate social service authorities.[47-49]

The child who has an acute traumatic rectal injury is often difficult to examine adequately, owing to the associated discomfort. Penetration of a foreign object by impalement typically requires rectal examination and sigmoidoscopy under general anesthesia. A retrograde urethrogram and/or voiding cystourethography

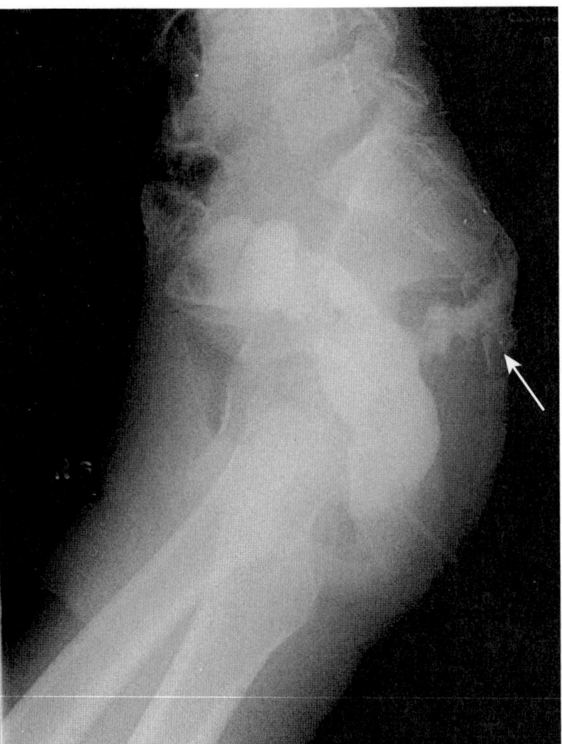

Figure 38-7. This teenager sustained a gunshot wound to the buttocks with a suspected injury to the rectum. He underwent sigmoidoscopy followed by a diverting colostomy. Several days postoperatively, this contrast study was performed and revealed extravasation (*arrow*) from the rectal injury.

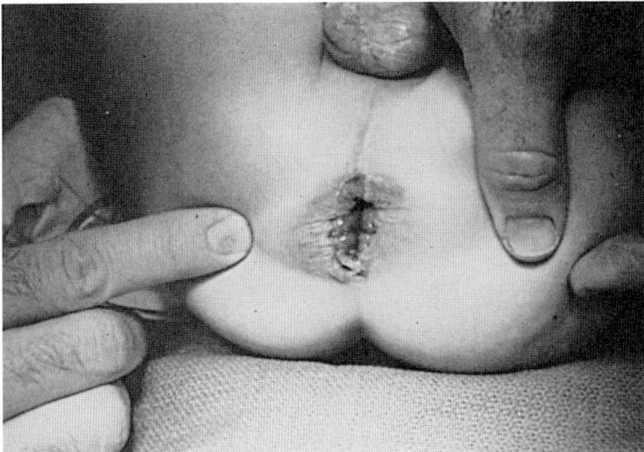

Figure 38-8. This male child was the victim of chronic sexual abuse and shows the typical stellate lacerations of the anal mucosa and skin.

should be obtained when there is suspicion of urethral and/or bladder injury. Although a child who is sexually abused and who has either condylomata or lacerations of a more chronic nature can be examined while awake, we prefer to examine the child using general anesthesia to make a complete assessment of the nature and extent of the injury and to proceed with surgical treatment, when necessary. Photographs are taken to document the extent of the findings for medicolegal purposes.

Treatment of penetrating rectal injuries often requires a diverting colostomy.[50] However, primary repair without fecal diversion can be performed safely in select cases.[51,52] When in doubt, one should always divert the fecal stream to avoid the consequences of perineal sepsis after repair of an anorectal injury. In general, isolated intraperitoneal rectal injuries can be treated with primary repair. Injuries to the proximal two thirds and accessible distal one third of the extraperitoneal rectum can be managed with repair and selective fecal diversion. Inaccessible or severe distal extraperitoneal rectal injuries should be treated by fecal diversion and presacral drainage.[53] Accessible injuries of the distal rectum and anal canal can be repaired with the intent of reapproximating the underlying sphincter muscle mechanism and the overlying mucosa. When the injury is full thickness in nature, fecal diversion should be undertaken. When fecal diversion is necessary, closure of the colostomy is performed once satisfactory healing is demonstrated.

Treatment of sexual abuse lesions involves interruption of the abuse pattern, which may require removal of the child from the home environment. Immediate consultation with child protective services or the local equivalent is mandatory. In the sexual abuse victim who is found to have an acute laceration extending up the rectal wall, it is rarely necessary to perform a diverting colostomy, because these lacerations are not usually full thickness. However, patients with a full-thickness injury should be managed by repair and diverting colostomy. When present, treatment of condylomata depends on the extent of disease. Although small lesions may be responsive to repeated applications of topical agents such as podophyllin or imiquimod, more extensive lesions require surgical removal. Intralesional interferon may be a useful adjunct to surgical methods to decrease recurrence.[54]

chapter 39

INTUSSUSCEPTION

Romeo C. Ignacio, Jr., MD • Mary E. Fallat, MD

Intussusception is one of the most frequent causes of bowel obstruction in infants and toddlers. Nevertheless, an individual pediatrician may encounter this condition only rarely. It was first described in 1674 by Paul Barbette of Amsterdam and was defined by Treves in 1899 as the prolapse of one part of the intestine into the lumen of the immediately adjoining part.[1] John Hutchinson reported the first successful operation for intussusception in 1873.[2] In 1876, Harold Hirschsprung described hydrostatic reduction, which led to a 23% reduction in mortality.[3] Ravitch popularized the use of contrast enema reduction for intussusception, which gradually became the accepted initial treatment for pediatric intussusception in stable patients.[4]

PATHOPHYSIOLOGY

Intussusception is the acquired invagination of one portion of the intestine into the adjacent bowel. It is described by the proximal, inner segment of intestine (intussusceptum) first and the outer distal, receiving portion of intestine (intussuscipiens) last. Eighty to 95 percent of pediatric intussusceptions are ileocolic. The ileoileal, cecocolic, colocolic, and jejunojejunal varieties occur with increasing rarity.[5] Occasionally, an intussusception may have an identifiable lesion that serves as a lead point, drawing the intussusceptum into the distal bowel by peristaltic activity. As the mesentery of the proximal bowel is drawn into the distal bowel, it is compressed, resulting in venous obstruction and edema of the bowel wall. If reduction of the intussusception does not occur, arterial insufficiency will ultimately lead to ischemia and bowel wall necrosis. Although spontaneous reduction undoubtedly occurs, the natural history of an intussusception is to progress to a fatal outcome as a result of sepsis unless the condition is recognized and treated appropriately. For many reasons, the morbidity and mortality rates have decreased dramatically at children's hospitals in North America since the mid 1940s.[6]

Idiopathic (or Primary) Intussusception

The vast majority of cases of intussusception do not have a pathologic lead point and are classified as primary or idiopathic intussusceptions. In idiopathic intussusception, the lead point is generally attributed to hypertrophied Peyer's patches within the ileal wall.[5] Intussusception occurs frequently in the wake of an upper respiratory tract infection or an episode of gastroenteritis, providing an etiology for the enlargement of the lymphoid tissue. Adenoviruses, and to a much lesser extent rotaviruses, have been implicated in up to 50% of cases.[7,8] Most cases of primary intussusception occur in children between the ages of 6 to 36 months of age when there is a high susceptibility to these viruses. Other contributing evidence that viruses might play a role in idiopathic intussusception includes the rise in cases during seasonal respiratory viral illnesses and the documented increase in the incidence of intussusception associated with previous rotaviral immunization.[9] The most recent immunization, Rotashield, has not been associated with a similar increase in intussusception.[10-12]

Secondary Intussusception

An intussusception may have an identifiable lesion that serves as a lead point, drawing the proximal bowel into the distal bowel by peristaltic activity. These anatomic lead points tend to increase in proportion to age, especially after 2 years of age.[5,13,14] The incidence of a definite anatomic lead point ranges from 1.5% to 12%.[6,12,13] The most common pathologic lead point is a Meckel's diverticulum followed by polyps and duplications (see Fig. 41-6). Other benign lead points are the appendix, hemangiomas, carcinoid tumors, foreign bodies, ectopic pancreas or gastric mucosa, hamartomas from Peutz-Jeghers syndrome (Fig. 39-1), and lipomas. Malignant causes, which are very rare, include lymphomas, lymphosarcomas, small bowel tumors, and melanomas.[15] The occurrence of malignant lesions increases with age. Small bowel

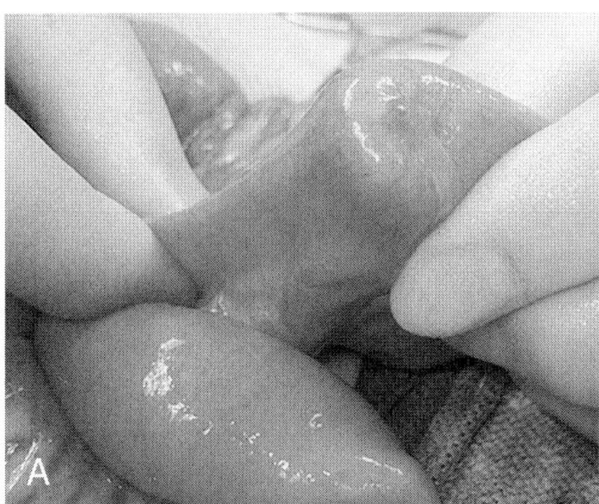

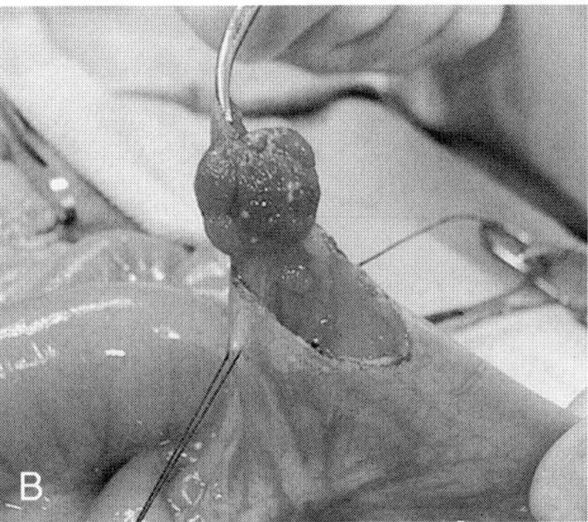

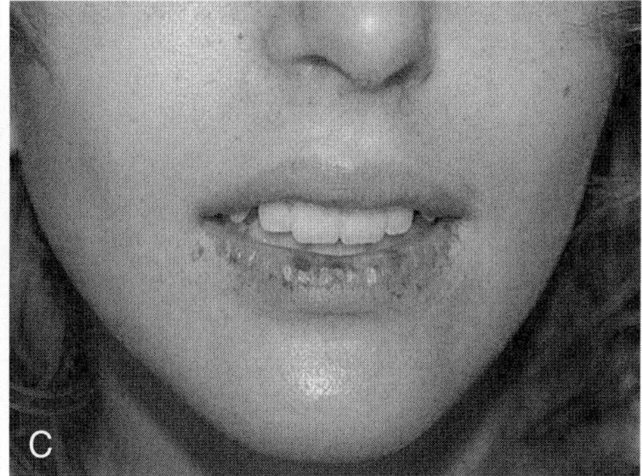

Figure 39-1. **A,** Operative view of the outside of the jejunum shows a palpable mass as the lead point of a reduced intussusception. **B,** A hamartomatous polyp is characteristic of Peutz-Jeghers syndrome. **C,** Mucocutaneous macular lesions are seen in this patient with Peutz-Jeghers syndrome. Note extension of the pigmentation beyond the vermilion border.

intussusceptions related to gastrojejunostomy tubes also have been described.[16]

Various systemic diseases, such as Henoch-Schönlein purpura and cystic fibrosis, may also be complicated by intussusception. The majority of abdominal complaints in Henoch-Schönlein purpura are due to vasculitis in the gastrointestinal tract. However, submucosal hemorrhages within the bowel wall can function as lead points in Henoch-Schönlein purpura and cause similar abdominal complaints. Patients with cystic fibrosis are prone to intussusception due to the inspissated secretions and thick fecal matter in the intestinal lumen. This thick, tenacious stool acts as a lead point to produce repeated intussusceptions, more typically seen in children aged 9 to 12 years.[5] Other rare diseases associated with intussusception are celiac disease and *Clostridium difficile* colitis.[17]

INCIDENCE

Idiopathic intussusception can occur at any age. However, the greatest incidence occurs in infants between ages 5 and 10 months.[18] The incidence of intussusception is highest in the first and second years of life and is uncommon below 3 months of age and after 3 years of life. The condition has been described in premature infants and has been postulated as the cause of small bowel atresia in some cases.[19] Most patients are well-nourished, healthy infants. Approximately two thirds are male.[5]

CLINICAL PRESENTATION

The classic presentation of intussusception is a young child with intermittent, crampy abdominal pain associated with "currant jelly" stools and a palpable mass on physical examination, although this triad is seen in less than a fourth of children.[20] The abdominal pain is sudden in onset in a child who was previously comfortable. The child may stiffen and pull the legs up to the abdomen. Hyperextension, writhing, and breath holding may be followed by vomiting. The attack often ceases as suddenly as it started. Between attacks, the child may appear comfortable or may fall asleep. After some time, the child becomes lethargic between episodes of pain. The symptoms are associated with anorexia and dehydration. Small or normal bowel movements may result initially from the straining as the colon evacuates distal to the obstruction. As the obstruction worsens, the child will have bilious emesis and worsening abdominal distention. Later in the course, the stools may be tinged with blood. The progression of bowel ischemia, sloughing of mucosa, and compression of the mucous glands within the intussusceptum leads to the evacuation of dark, red mucoid clots or "currant jelly" stools. The latter is often a late sign. A diagnostic pitfall is to wait for this sign to occur.

PHYSICAL EXAMINATION

The child's vital signs are usually normal early in the course of the disease. During painless intervals, the child might look comfortable and the physical examination will be unremarkable. Based on the benign clinical appearance, this may lead to an erroneous diagnosis of constipation or gastroenteritis. However, the cramping episodes usually occur every 15 to 30 minutes. When the pain occurs, the child may be difficult to examine. There may be audible peristaltic rushes, and a mass might be palpable anywhere in the abdomen or even visualized if the child is relatively thin (Fig. 39-2). The right lower abdominal quadrant may appear flat or empty (Dance's sign) as the intussuscepted mass is pulled up. The mass is often curved because it is tethered by the blood vessels and mesentery on one side. On rectal examination, blood-stained mucus or blood may be encountered. The longer the duration of symptoms, the more likely the probability of identifying gross or occult blood. Palpation of the intussuscepted mass on bimanual examination is possible but rare.

Prolapse of the intussusceptum through the anus is a grave sign, particularly when the intussusceptum is ischemic. An ileocolic or colocolic intussusception can progress to the rectosigmoid and through the anus. Such a patient would undoubtedly exhibit signs

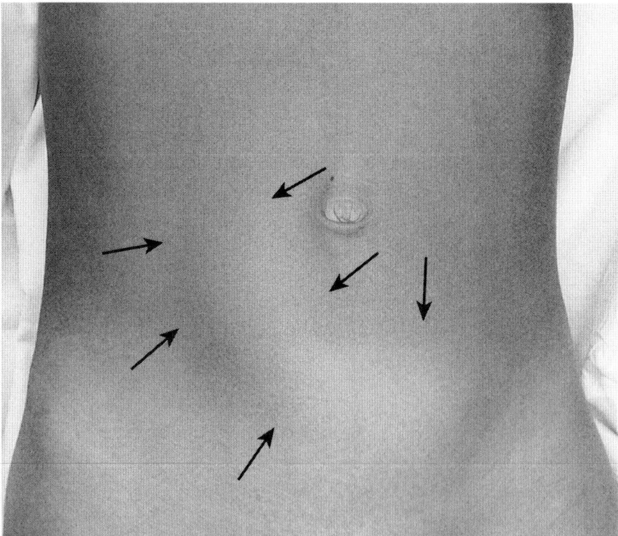

Figure 39-2. This 10-year-old boy has a palpable sausage-shaped mass (*arrows*) due to an intussusception.

of systemic illness. The greatest danger in a case of prolapse of the intussusceptum is that the examiner will misdiagnose the condition and attempt to reduce what is thought to be a rectal prolapse. Careful physical examination of the intussusceptum through the anus is mandatory to avoid this potentially life-threatening error in diagnosis. This is done by inserting a lubricated tongue blade along the side of the protruding mass before reduction is attempted. If the blade can be inserted more than 1 or 2 cm into the anus alongside of the mass, the diagnosis of intussusception should be considered. Rectal prolapse, while producing discomfort, is not generally accompanied by vomiting or signs of sepsis.

If the obstructive process worsens and bowel ischemia has occurred, dehydration, fever, tachycardia, and hypotension can develop in quick succession as a result of bacteremia and bowel perforation. In the absence of a rapid diagnosis, fluid resuscitation, and operation, a fatal outcome is likely.

DIAGNOSIS

Laboratory Studies

Although there are no specific laboratory studies that aid with the specific diagnosis of intussusception, as the process progresses there may be associated electrolyte abnormalities due to dehydration, anemia, and/or leukocytosis.

Abdominal Radiography

In about half of cases, the diagnosis of intussusception can be suspected on plain flat and upright abdominal radiographs (Fig. 39-3). Suggestive radiographic abnormalities include an abdominal mass, abnormal distribution of gas and fecal contents, sparse large

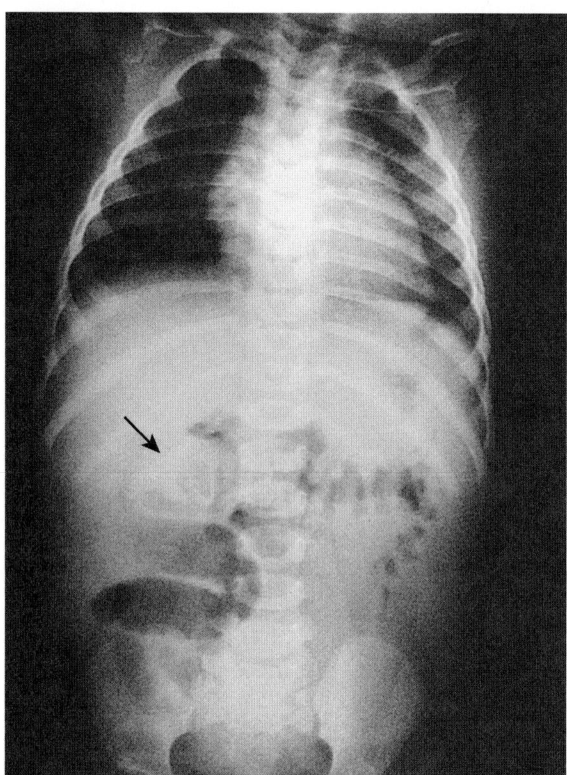

Figure 39-3. Abdominal radiograph showing dilated loops of small bowel in the right lower quadrant and a soft tissue mass density in the vicinity of the transverse colon near the hepatic flexure (*arrow*).

bowel gas, and air-fluid levels in the presence of bowel obstruction.[21] The "target" sign or "coiled spring" sign denotes a cross-sectional appearance of the invaginated mesentery and bowel into the intussuscipiens, appearing as concentric lucencies on plain film. The "meniscus" sign is a crescent-shaped lucency in the colon outlining the distal end of the intussusception. However, plain films have limited value in confirming the diagnosis and cannot be used as the sole diagnostic test.[22]

Ultrasonography

The use of abdominal ultrasound for the evaluation of intussusception was first described in 1977.[23] Since then, many institutions have adopted its use as a screening tool because of the lack of radiation exposure and decreased cost.[24] The intussusception is usually discovered in the right side of the abdomen. A transverse sonographic image of the bowel consists of alternating rings of low and high echogenicity representing the bowel wall and mesenteric fat within the intussusceptum. This characteristic finding has been referred to as a "target" or "doughnut" lesion (Fig. 39-4). The "pseudokidney" sign is seen on a longitudinal section and appears as superimposed hypoechoic and hyperechoic layers (Fig. 39-5). This pattern is similar to a sandwich and represents the edematous walls of the intussusceptum within the intussuscipiens. Ultrasonography can also guide the therapeutic

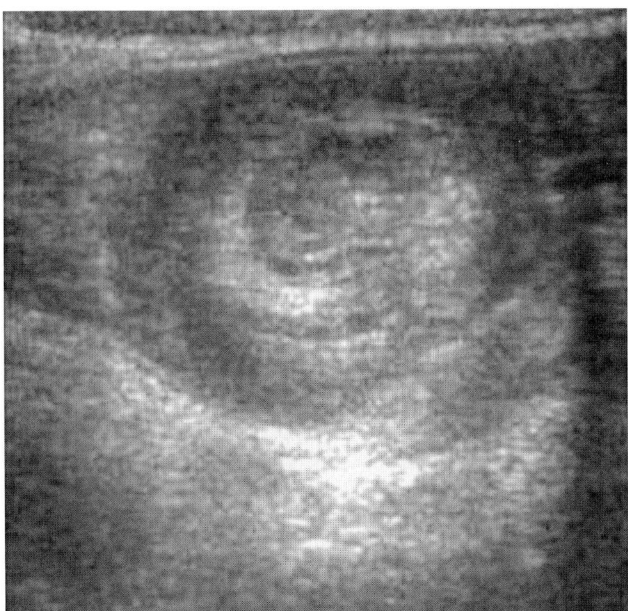

Figure 39-4. This transverse sonographic image shows the alternating rings of low and high echogenicity due to an intussusception. This finding has been called a "target" sign.

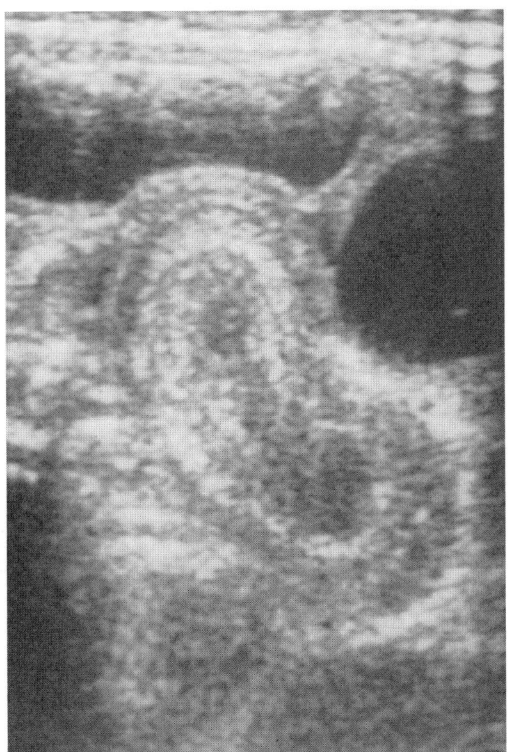

Figure 39-5. Sonogram showing the "pseudokidney" sign seen with intussusception on longitudinal section.

reduction of an intussusception by using a 10% meglumine iothalamate enema in a balanced salt solution or using sonographically guided pneumatic pressure.[24,25] Successful reduction results in a smaller "donut," with an echogenic rim representing the edema of the terminal ileum and ileocecal valve. Equivocal findings using this modality should mandate a conventional contrast or air enema.[26]

Computed Tomography and Magnetic Resonance Imaging

Neither computed tomography (CT) nor magnetic resonance imaging (MRI) are routinely used in the evaluation of a patient with intussusception, although either may reveal possible pathologic causes for intussusception, such as a malignancy (i.e., lymphoma). The characteristic finding is a target or doughnut sign (invaginated bowel within the contiguous bowel loop) (Fig. 39-6). Transient small bowel intussusceptions that are discovered on CT or MRI are usually not clinically significant.[27] These "incidental" intussusceptions involve a small segment of bowel with no pathologic lead point. Repeat imaging usually demonstrates resolution of the intussusception. Radiographic or surgical treatment should be based on clinical findings in symptomatic patients.[28] Laparoscopy is an excellent means to evaluate these patients if surgical intervention is needed.

NONOPERATIVE MANAGEMENT

If the diagnosis of intussusception is suspected, a nasogastric tube may be needed to decompress the stomach. Bowel rest and intravenous fluid resuscitation should be initiated. A complete blood cell count and serum electrolytes are obtained. An air or contrast enema is the study of choice for diagnosis and potential first-line treatment. The complications with hydrostatic or pneumatic reduction are minimal as long as certain guidelines are followed. Absolute contraindications to nonoperative reduction are intestinal perforation (free intra-abdominal air), peritonitis, or persistent hypotension. Findings of peritonitis or bowel perforation warrant surgical exploration.

Hydrostatic Reduction

The methodology for hydrostatic reduction has not changed significantly since its first description in 1876.[3] Although hydrostatic reduction with barium under fluoroscopic guidance has been the historic method since the mid 1980s,[22] most pediatric centers use water-soluble isotonic contrast because of the potential hazard of barium peritonitis in patients with intestinal perforation.

A large, lubricated catheter is inserted into the rectum, and a seal is attempted by firmly taping the buttocks together. Balloon catheters are avoided by most radiologists owing to the risk of perforation and potential for a closed-loop obstruction. The "rule of threes" is commonly described, consisting of (1) hydrostatic reduction kept at a height of 3 feet above the patient and (2) no more than three attempts, with (3) each attempt no more than 3 minutes each. Under fluoroscopic evaluation, the contrast agent is observed until a concave filling defect is seen (Fig. 39-7). Occasionally, a curvilinear spiral pattern can be seen as the contrast

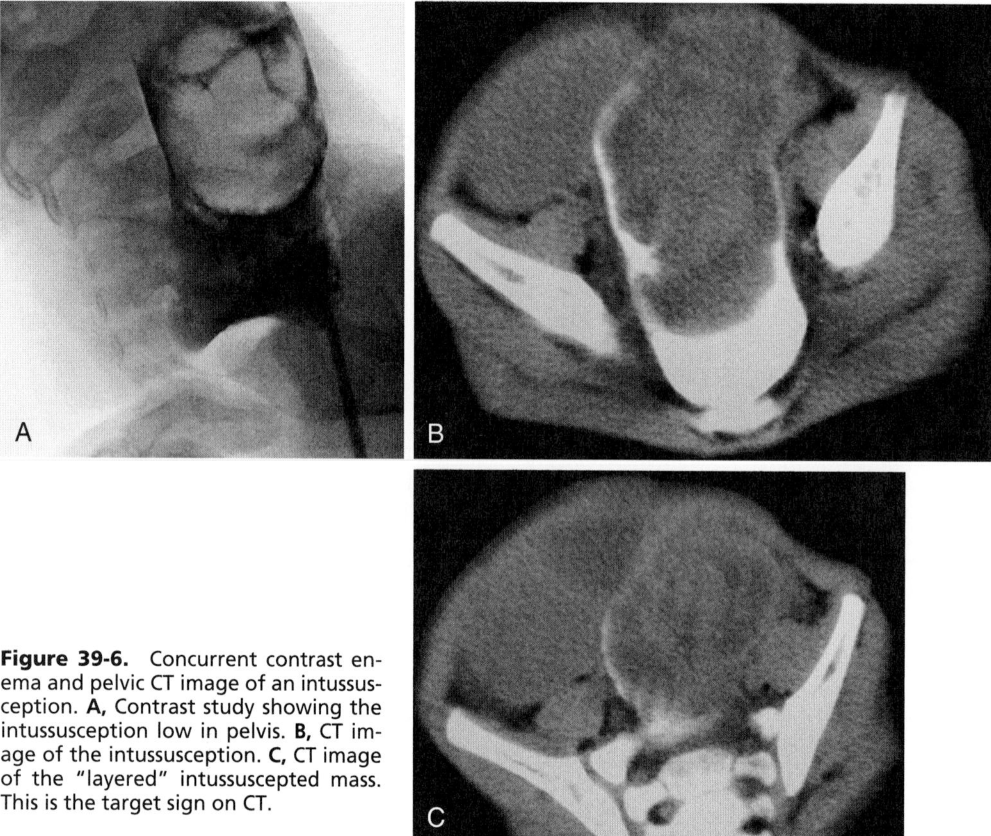

Figure 39-6. Concurrent contrast enema and pelvic CT image of an intussusception. **A,** Contrast study showing the intussusception low in pelvis. **B,** CT image of the intussusception. **C,** CT image of the "layered" intussuscepted mass. This is the target sign on CT.

medium surrounds the intussusceptum. Constant hydrostatic pressure is continued as long as reduction is occurring. Additional attempts can be repeated a second or third time.

Hydrostatic reduction is complete when the contrast medium freely flows through the ileocecal valve into the terminal ileum. Successful reduction in uncomplicated patients is seen in about 85% of cases and ranges from 42% to 95%.[29] There is less success with long-segment intussusceptions,[30] patients with symptoms for more than 24 hours, and those with pathologic lesions. The advantages of nonoperative over operative reduction are decreased morbidity, cost, and length of hospitalization.

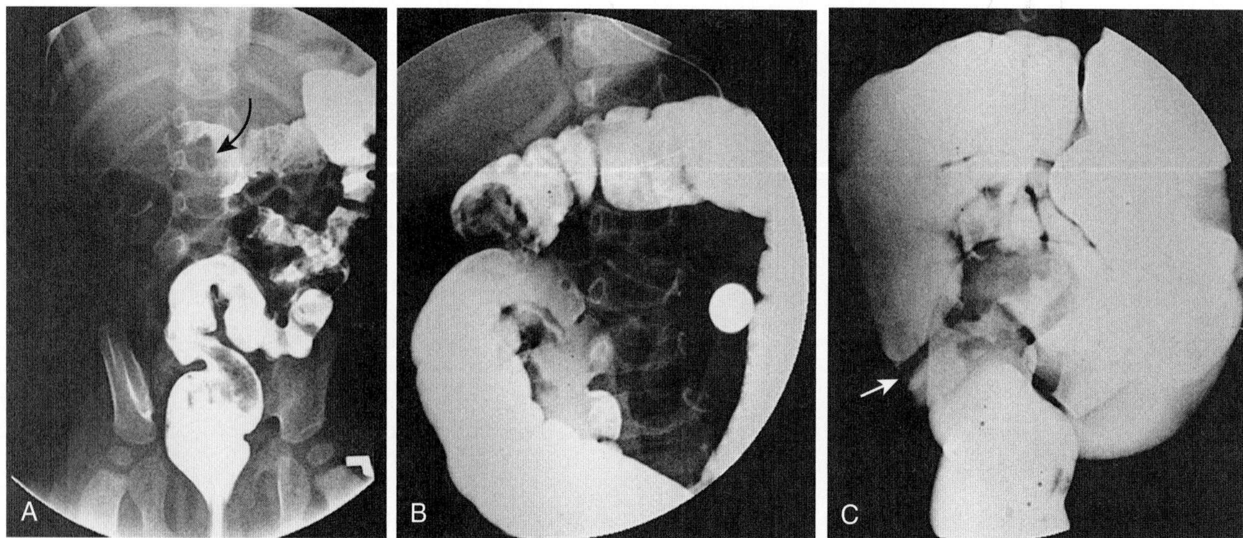

Figure 39-7. Fluoroscopic examination using isotonic contrast for hydrostatic reduction of intussusception. **A,** Intussusception (*arrow*) seen in midtransverse colon. **B,** Reduction has occurred to the hepatic flexure. **C,** Complete reduction with reflux of contrast medium into the terminal ileum. Note the edematous ileocecal valve (*arrow*).

Pneumatic Reduction

Air reduction of intussusception was first described in 1897.[31] Pneumatic reduction gained popularity in the late 1980s, owing to the higher rates of successful reduction reported in large international series.[32] Success rates of reduction reported between 1980 and 1991 using hydrostatic techniques were 50% to 78% compared with 75% to 94% between 1986 and 1991 using pneumatic reduction.[5] Advocates of the air enema believe that the method is quicker and safer, is less messy, and decreases the exposure time to radiation.[32] The procedure is fluoroscopically monitored as air is insufflated into the rectum (Fig. 39-8). The maximum safe air pressure is 80 mm Hg for younger infants and 110 to 120 mm Hg for older infants. Carbon dioxide can be used instead of air because of the advantages of rapid reabsorption and less abdominal discomfort. Accurate pressure measurements are possible, and reduction rates are higher than with hydrostatic techniques.[33] Potential drawbacks of pneumatic reduction include the possibility of development of a tension pneumoperitoneum, poor visualization of lead points, and relatively poor visualization of the intussusception and reduction process, resulting in false-positive reductions.[33-35] Rates of perforation range from 0.4% to 2.5%.[36]

Several studies have shown improved reduction rates by a second attempt after waiting between 30 minutes to 24 hours after the initial attempt.[37-39] However, the risks of the increasing radiation burden must be weighed against the risks of emergency surgery and anesthesia.[40] If nonoperative reduction is successful either by hydrostatic or pneumatic technique, the patient should be admitted for observation and should receive a short period of bowel rest and intravenous fluids. Any clinical signs of abdominal pain after reduction could be a sign of ischemic bowel or recurrent intussusception (see later).

OPERATIVE TREATMENT

Open Approach

Surgery is indicated when nonoperative reduction is unsuccessful or incomplete (Fig. 39-9), for signs of

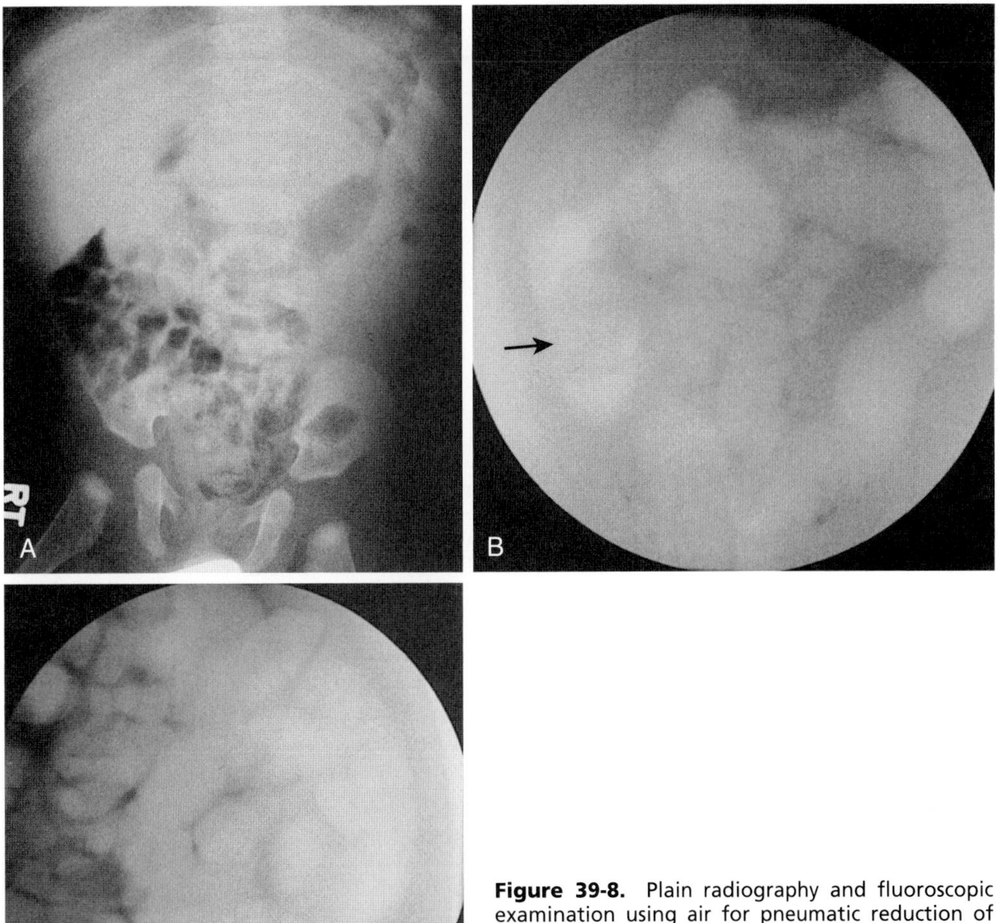

Figure 39-8. Plain radiography and fluoroscopic examination using air for pneumatic reduction of an intussusception. **A,** Plain radiograph showing a mass effect in the right upper quadrant. **B,** Pneumatic reduction to the vicinity of the cecum with the intussusception still present (*arrow*). **C,** Complete reduction with reflux of air into multiple loops of small intestine. (Courtesy of Charles Maxfield, MD.)

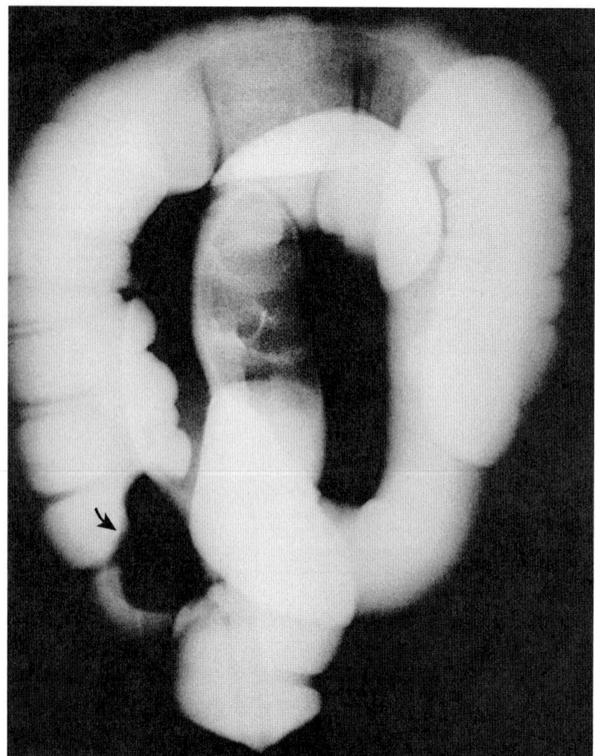

Figure 39-9. Contrast enema view after hydrostatic reduction of an intussusception to the ileocecal junction. A persistent filling defect (*arrow*) is present without free reflux into the terminal ileum.

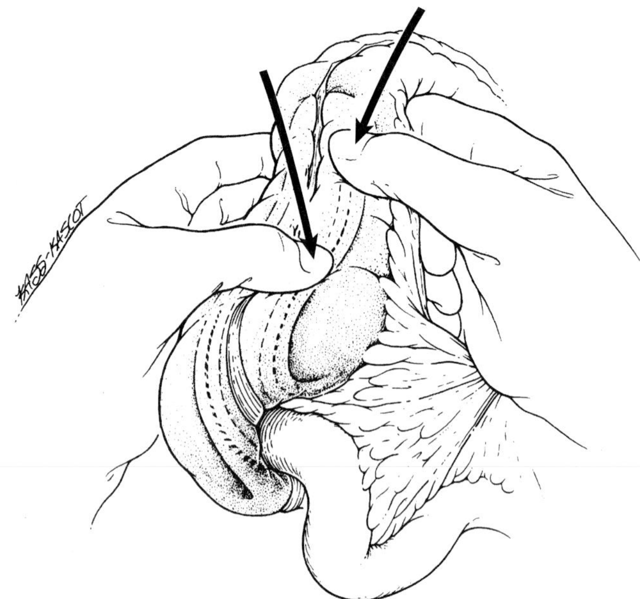

Figure 39-10. A right lower quadrant muscle-splitting incision allows delivery of the intussusception through the incision. Gentle and continuous massage from distal to proximal usually results in reduction of the intussusception.

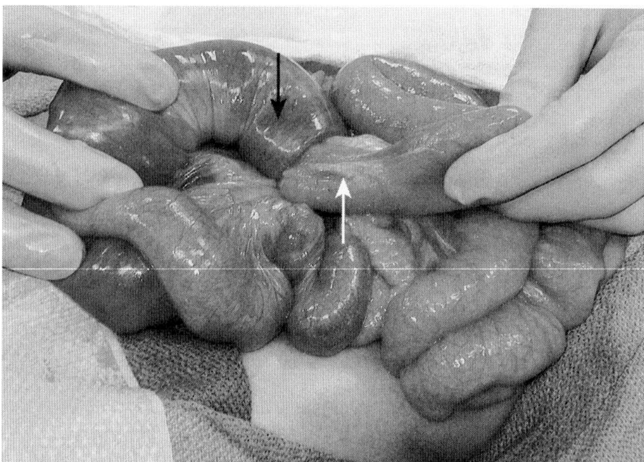

Figure 39-11. This operative view shows an incompletely reduced intussusception with the intussusceptum (*white arrow*) telescoping into the intussuscipiens (*black arrow*). A pathologic lead point due to Hodgkin's lymphoma was found.

peritonitis, for the presence of a pathologic lead point, or for radiographic evidence of pneumoperitoneum. Preoperative preparation includes administration of broad-spectrum antibiotics, intravenous fluid resuscitation, and placement of a nasogastric tube for decompression.

Open exploration of the abdomen and intestines has been traditionally performed through a right lower quadrant incision. Moderate serous ascites may be encountered owing to the obstructive lesion. Usually, the intussusception involves the cecum and terminal ileum, which can be delivered through the incision. Care must be taken to evaluate the extent of the intussusceptum before delivering it, because it can extend into the rectosigmoid region in severe cases. Extension of the incision is often required in such cases.

Once the leading edge of the intussusceptum is identified, it is gently manipulated back toward its normal position in the terminal ileum (Fig. 39-10). Excessive force or pulling is avoided to prevent injury or perforation of the bowel and subsequent contamination. Inability to manually reduce the intussusception, the finding of ischemic bowel, or identification of a pathologic lesion requires surgical resection and bowel anastomosis or diversion, depending on the condition of the bowel and child (see Figs. 39-1 and 39-11).

If surgical reduction is possible, the bowel is then evaluated for viability, perforation, or a pathologic lead point (especially in children older than 2 years of age). Questionable ischemic bowel can be warmed with saline-soaked laparotomy pads and reevaluated by the coloration of the bowel, peristalsis, presence of Doppler signals, or Wood's lamp evaluation using fluorescein. After complete reduction of the intussusception, an incidental appendectomy is usually performed because the location of the abdominal scar is similar to an open appendectomy incision.

Laparoscopic Approach

Initially, the use of laparoscopy in intussusception was strictly diagnostic and used in cases with equivocal radiographic studies or those with suspected

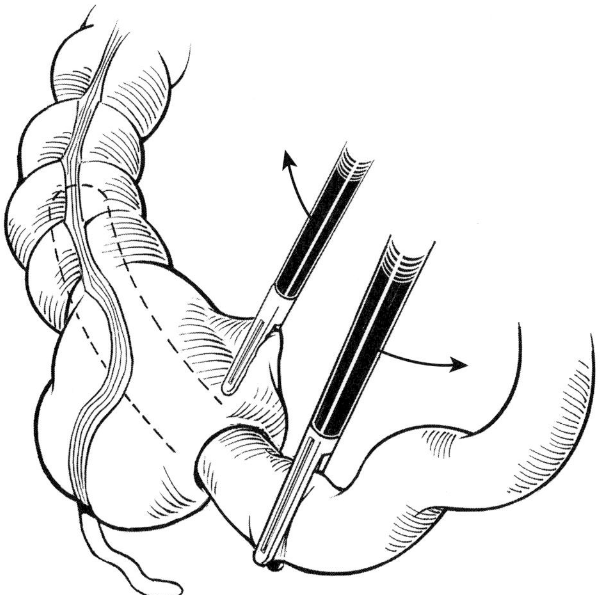

Figure 39-12. For laparoscopic reduction of an ileocolic intussusception, the small bowel (intussusceptum) is grasped with an atraumatic bowel clamp. It is best to completely grasp across the entire intussusceptum so that the bowel is not torn when attempting to distract it from the colon. A larger clamp (5 vs. 3 mm) is therefore often helpful. The cecum is then pushed away from the small bowel with an intestinal grasping forceps. (From Georgeson KE: Laparoscopic management of ileocolic intussusception. In Holcomb GW, Georgeson KE, Rothenberg SS [eds]: Atlas of Pediatric Laparoscopy and Thoracoscopy. Philadelphia, Elsevier Saunders, 2008, pp 71-73.)

pathologic lesions. Once the diagnosis was confirmed, the operation was converted to a laparotomy. Recent small studies have demonstrated laparoscopic reduction of intussusception with variable degrees of success.[41-46]

Various techniques have been reported, but a majority of minimally invasive approaches describe the use of three abdominal ports: one in the infraumbilical region with two other ports along the left side of the abdomen. Laparoscopic reduction is accomplished by applying gentle pressure distal to the intussusceptum using atraumatic graspers. Although counterintuitive to the conventional open method, traction is usually required proximal to the intussuscipiens to complete the reduction (Figs. 39-12 and 39-13). Careful inspection is then performed to evaluate for any signs of ischemia, necrosis, or perforation. If a resection is required, this can sometimes be accomplished by exteriorizing the bowel through the periumbilical incision. If this cannot be accomplished safely, the operation should be converted to an open laparotomy.

RECURRENT INTUSSUSCEPTION

Recurrent intussusception has been described in 2% to 20% of cases (average about 5%), with about one third occurring within 24 hours and the majority within 6 months of the initial episode.[7,47-49] Recurrences usually have no defined lead point, and they are less likely to occur after surgical reduction or resection. Multiple recurrences can occur in the same patient. Success rates with enema reduction after one recurrence are comparable to those with the first episode and are better if the child did not previously require operative reduction. Patients tend to be seen earlier with recurrent intussusception, and they have fewer symptoms. Irritability and discomfort may be the only clues during the early stage of a recurrence.

An overriding concern in recurrent intussusception is occult malignancy, although multiple recurrences are not a contraindication to attempted radiologic reduction.[48] Unfortunately, the clinical findings or pattern of recurrence do not predict the presence of a pathologic lead point. A careful imaging search is mandatory, and ultrasonography has been recommended as the imaging study of choice.[50] Indications for operation include (1) irreducible recurrence, (2) clinical evidence to suggest a pathologic lead point, (3) documentation of a pathologic lead point by an imaging procedure, or

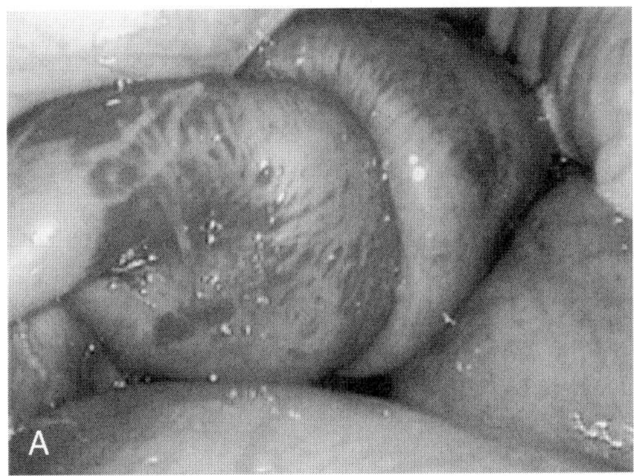

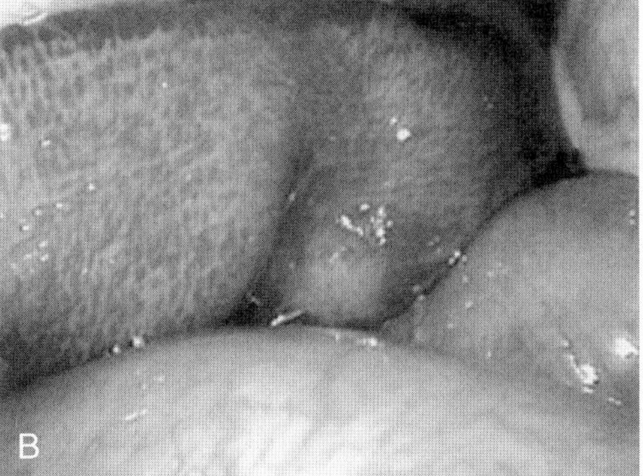

Figure 39-13. **A,** Ileoileal intussusception remaining after reduction of the ileum from the colon. **B,** The ileoileal intussusception has been completely reduced. Note the edema and induration in the wall of the small bowel in both photographs. (From Georgeson KE: Laparoscopic management of ileocolic intussusception. In Holcomb GW, Georgeson KE, Rothenberg SS [eds]: Atlas of Pediatric Laparoscopy and Thoracoscopy. Philadelphia, Elsevier Saunders, 2008, pp 71-73.)

(4) persistence of clinical symptoms after the completion of the enema.[47]

POSTOPERATIVE INTUSSUSCEPTION

Intussusception accounts for 3% to 10% of cases of postoperative bowel obstruction during childhood and may occur after operations performed for a variety of conditions.[51] Thoracic and abdominal operations have been followed by latent intussusception. Because ileus and adhesive obstruction more frequently come to mind as a cause for postoperative intestinal obstruction, these intussusceptions may not be diagnosed preoperatively, although ultrasonography has proved to be a successful diagnostic modality.[51] Most postoperative intussusceptions occur within a month of the initial procedure. An interval of about 10 days between initial operation and development of symptoms is average.[52] Most postoperative intussusceptions are ileoileal and respond to operative reduction without resection.[51,52]

chapter 40

ALIMENTARY TRACT DUPLICATIONS

Scott J. Keckler, MD • George W. Holcomb III, MD, MBA

Alimentary tract duplications are relatively rare congenital anomalies that may be found anywhere along the gastrointestinal tract from the mouth to the anus. If they are symptomatic, intestinal obstruction or bleeding can occur. Asymptomatic duplications can be discovered incidentally. Most duplications are benign conditions, but ectopic gastric mucosa and rare malignant degeneration remain secondary concerns. The majority of duplications are diagnosed by 2 years of age, but more are being diagnosed in utero with prenatal ultrasonography.

The surgical goal is to remove the duplication and prevent its recurrence. Duplications share a common vascular supply with the native alimentary tract, and simple resection is usually adequate. The management of thoracoabdominal or long tubular abdominal duplications can be challenging. Radical resections are rarely indicated and often not in the patient's best interest. After surgical resection, the prognosis is generally favorable, but the severity of the presenting illness and morbidity and mortality of any associated malformations will factor into the overall outcome.

HISTORY

The first published report of alimentary tract duplication was by Calder in 1773, who described a duodenal duplication.[1] The first to use the term *duplication* was Reginald Fitz, who applied it to an omphalomesenteric duct remnant.[2] In the ensuing years, multiple terms such as *ileum duplex* and *enterogenous cyst* to describe these anomalies appeared in the literature. William Ladd applied the term *duplication of the alimentary tract* to a series of 10 patients that he described in 1937.[3] In this series, three common findings were noted regardless of location: a well-developed coat of smooth muscle, an epithelial lining, and attachment to the alimentary tract. This nomenclature was supported by the first large series to appear in the literature by Gross and associates in 1952.[4]

EMBRYOLOGY

Alimentary tract duplications may be seen at any age but most commonly appear before age 2. Two types are seen: cystic or tubular. The incidence has been reported to be 1 in 4500 births.[5] Duplications are considered congenital malformations because they are thought to arise from disturbances in embryonic development.

Multiple theories have been proposed regarding the etiology of duplications. A persistent embryonic diverticulum from the developing alimentary tract was the first postulated theory.[6] Decades later, it was postulated that duplications resulted from aberrant recanalization of the alimentary tract lumen.[7] Also, the coincidence of colonic and genitourinary tract duplications and similar findings in conjoined twins led to the partial twinning theory.[8,9] The role of hypoxia in the development of fetal defects[10] was also applied to the development of alimentary tract duplications.[11,12] The association of enteric duplications and spinal anomalies led to the "split notochord" theory,[13] and the notochord has been recently shown to be involved in both foregut and hindgut malformations.[14,15]

Alimentary tract duplications are found in association with vertebral, spinal cord, and genitourinary anomalies in 30% to 50% of patients.[4,16] They have also been found in patients with malrotation and intestinal atresias.[17] All these findings suggest a multifactorial process for development and possibly different mechanisms depending on location. To date, no single unifying theory for their development has been described.

CLINICAL PRESENTATION AND DIAGNOSIS

Alimentary tract duplications do not have a classic presentation but can manifest a variety of symptoms, including abdominal distention and/or pain, vomiting, bleeding, chronic respiratory complaints, or a painless abdominal mass. In general, symptoms are related to

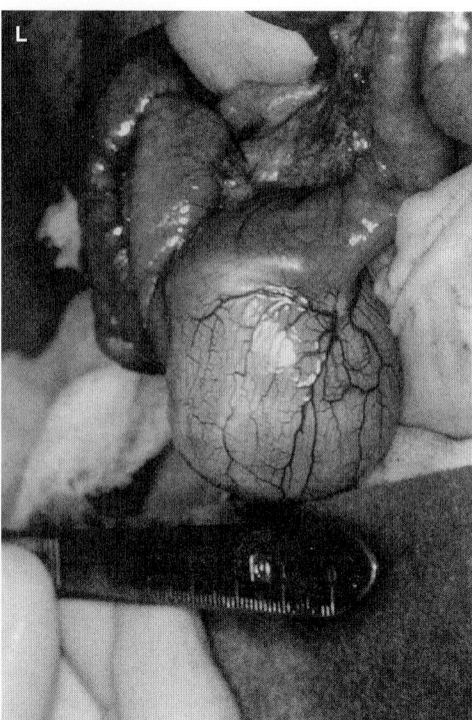

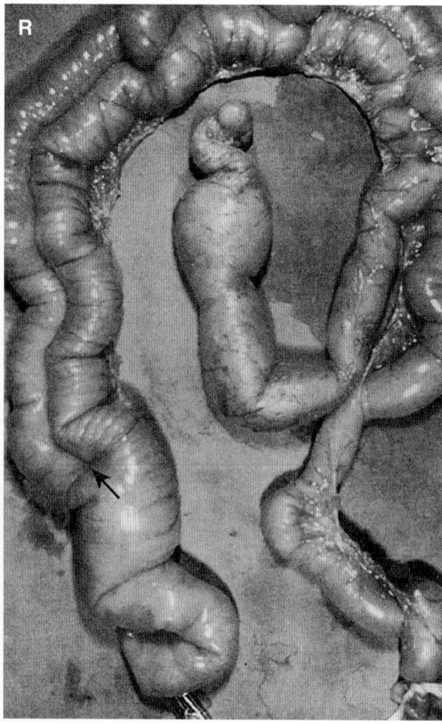

Figure 40-1. Left, Most alimentary tract duplications are cystic. **Right,** A tubular duplication is seen. Note that the native bowel is bifurcated (*arrow*) into the tubular duplication and native intestine.

location, size, shape, and type of mucosa. The majority of patients (80%) present prior to 2 years of age, with over half (60%) seen before 6 months of age.[17,18] However, duplications may be found at any age from the fetus to the geriatric patient.[19,20] Of the two types, the vast majority are cystic, whereas a small minority are tubular (Fig. 40-1). The most common location is the jejunum/ileum, followed by the esophagus (Table 40-1). Histologically, most duplications are lined by the mucosa native to the lesion, but ectopic tissue is present in 25% to 30% of specimens.[4,17] The most common type of ectopic tissue is gastric followed by both exocrine and endocrine pancreatic tissue (Table 40-2).[21] However, any type of epithelial mucosa can be found. Peptic ulceration causing perforation or hemorrhage may occur in duplications with ectopic gastric mucosa (Fig. 40-2). In children, duplications are considered benign lesions, but malignancy has been detected in adults.[22]

DIAGNOSIS OF SUSPECTED DUPLICATIONS

A variety of imaging studies are useful to make the diagnosis. Plain radiographs may demonstrate a posterior mediastinal mass, suggesting an esophageal duplication. Contrast studies may reveal a mass effect from the adjacent duplication or communication with the alimentary tract. In cases in which a combined thoracoabdominal duplication is suspected, computed tomography (CT) is beneficial. An enhancing rim of tissue surrounding a fluid-filled cyst is diagnostic of alimentary tract duplications. Ultrasonography is a noninvasive, radiation-free modality for diagnosis of suspected duplications and is currently the most common imaging study for diagnosing small bowel duplications.[23] The typical sonographic appearance of duplications is an inner hyperechoic rim of mucosal-submucosal tissue and an outer hypoechoic muscular layer (Fig. 40-3).[24] Duplication cysts are being discovered in utero owing to the use of routine prenatal ultrasonography.[25] The presence of ectopic gastric mucosa may be discovered by technetium-99m (^{99m}Tc) scintigraphy if there is a history of bleeding or anemia.[26,27] Suspected esophageal duplications with vertebral anomalies should be further investigated. CT myelography may be beneficial but is invasive. Magnetic resonance imaging (MRI) is less invasive but may require sedation or general anesthesia in young children.[28]

CLASSIFICATION AND TREATMENT BY LOCATION

To better understand the variety of presentations and surgical management of alimentary tract duplications, they will be discussed according to their anatomic location. A compilation of the major case series from 16 institutions in the past 60 years is seen in Table 40-1.[4,12,16-18,29-39] Multiple duplications were found in approximately 8% of patients.

Oropharyngeal Duplications

Oropharyngeal duplications are rare and account for 1% of all duplications. Most are asymptomatic, but they may present as feeding difficulties.[36] The most

Table 40-1 Alimentary Tract Duplications by Location as Described In Literature Reports

1st Author	Institution	No. D (No. Pts)	Oral	Esophagus	Thoraco-abdominal	Stomach	Duodenum	Jejunum/ Ileum	Colon	Rectum	Other
Gross, 1952	Children's, Boston	68 (67)	1	13	3	2	4	32	10	3	0
Basu, 1960	A. H. Children's, Liverpool	33 (28)	0	7	0	1	3	16	4	2	0
Grosfeld, 1970	Children's, Columbus	23 (23)	0	4	2	1	0	9	7	0	0
Favara, 1971	Children's, Denver	39 (37)	1	6	0	3	4	20	4	0	1
Bower, 1977	Children's, Pittsburgh	78 (64)	0	15	1	6	6	34	12	2	2
Hocking, 1981	RHSC, Glasgow	60 (53)		8	2	8	1	32	4	5	0
Ildstad, 1988	Children's, Cincinnati	20 (17)	0	6	0	1	0	5	8	0	0
Bissler, 1988	Children's, Akron	11 (11)	0	1	0	1	2	4	2	1	0
Holcomb, 1989	Children's, Philadelphia	101 (96)	0	21	3	8	2	47	15	5	0
Pinter, 1992	Hungary	30 (28)		6	2	4	3	9	3	3	0
Bajpai, 1994	IIMS, New Delhi, India	15 (14)	0	8	1	0	1	1	3	1	0
Stringer, 1995	Hospital for Sick Children, London	77 (72)	2	15	6	10	3	21	10	6	4
Iyer, 1995	Children's, Los Angeles	29 (27)	2	0	0	3	1	9	8	6	0
Yang, 1996	NTUH, Taipei, China	20 (17)	0	2	0	1	0	14	3	0	0
Karnak, 2000	Ankara, Turkey	42 (38)	1	7	2	1	3	17	9	2	0
Puligandla, 2003	Montreal Children's	73 (73)			0	6	7	51	5	4	0
TOTALS		719 (665)	7 (1%)	119 (17%)	22 (3%)	56 (8%)	40 (6%)	321 (45%)	107 (15%)	34 (6%)	7 (1%)

No. D, number of duplications;
No. Pts, number of patients.

Table 40-2 Ectopic Gastric Mucosa by Location

1st Author	Esophageal	Small Bowel	Colorectal
Gross, 1952	7/16	8/36	0/10
Favara, 1971	3/6	6/24	0/4
Bower, 1977	7/16	5/40	0/14
Hocking, 1981	5/10	21/33	2/9
Ildstad, 1988	2/6	5/13	0/8
Holcomb, 1989	8/24	12/49	1/20
Bajpai, 1994	9/9	2/2	1/4
Stringer, 1995	9/21	7/24	0/16
Puligandla, 2003		30/58	3/9
TOTALS	50/108 (46%)	96/279 (34%)	7/94 (7%)

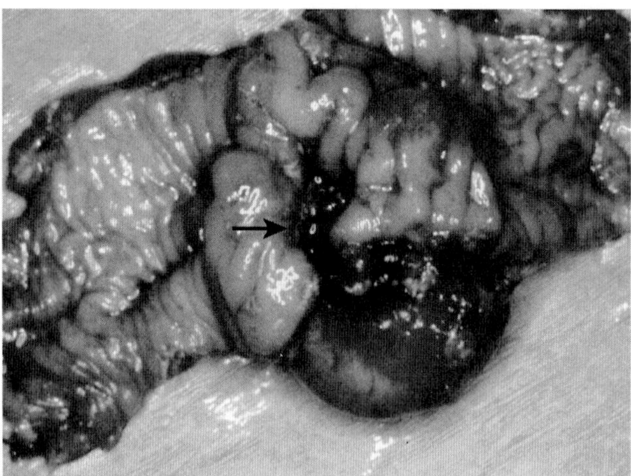

Figure 40-2. Most intestinal bleeding from duplications is caused by tubular duplications with communication to the intestine. However, in this case, the bleeding was due to mucosal ulceration (*solid arrow*) secondary to an adjacent cystic duplication. (From Holcomb GW III, Gheissari A, O'Neill JA, et al: Surgical management of alimentary tract duplications. Ann Surg 209:167-174, 1989.)

common site is the floor of the mouth, and these duplications frequently contain gastric or colonic mucosa. Treatment involves an oral approach with resection of the cyst and reapproximation of the oral mucosa.[40]

Esophageal Duplications

Approximately 20% of all duplications are esophageal. They may occur anywhere along the esophagus. Although duplications of the cervical esophagus are reported, the majority occur on the right side of the thoracic esophagus. Most esophageal duplications are cystic and do not share a muscular wall or communicate with the esophageal lumen. Extrinsic compression of the trachea may cause respiratory distress or pneumonia, or an incidental mass may be found on a chest radiograph. In older patients, dysphagia may occur. Esophageal duplication cysts should be in the differential diagnosis of any mediastinal mass. Because approximately half of esophageal duplications contain gastric mucosa, hematemesis or occult anemia may develop. Communication with the spinal column has been described in 20% of these patients.[16] Once suspected on chest radiography or esophagography, further imaging to clarify the anatomic details is usually warranted either with CT or MRI (Fig. 40-4). Because some esophageal duplications extend through the diaphragm, abdominal imaging may be necessary as well. Also, abdominal ultrasonography is a useful screening tool for intestinal duplications because 25% of patients with an esophageal duplication also had an intestinal duplication in the largest study published.[17] Historically, esophageal duplications limited to the thorax were excised through a right thoracotomy. However, owing to the benign nature of duplications, thoracoscopic excision leads to less morbidity and can usually be accomplished without significant complications.[41-43] Some authors have recommended against thoracoscopy if mediastinal

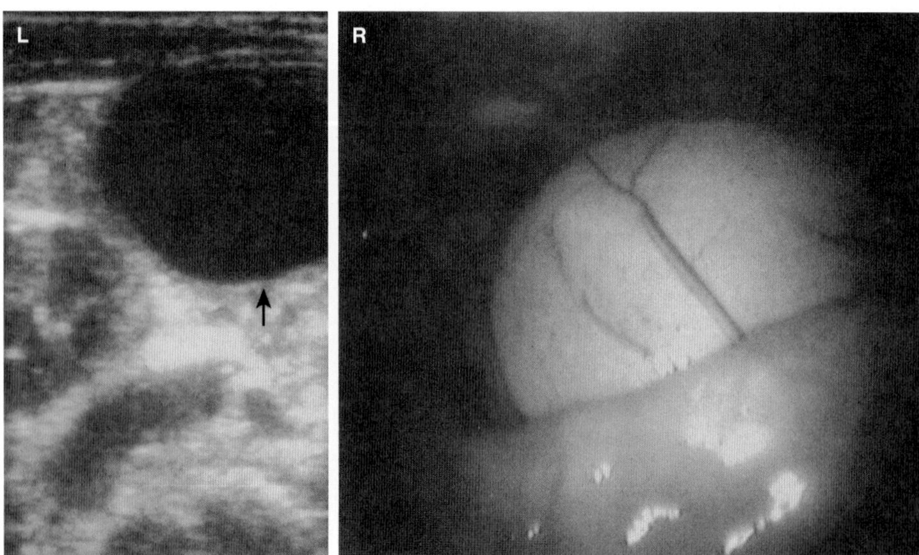

Figure 40-3. Ultrasonography is a frequent imaging modality for diagnosing abdominal duplications. **Left,** This ultrasound image shows a cystic mass (*arrow*) in an infant with symptoms of intestinal obstruction. **Right,** The laparoscopic view in this same patient shows a cystic duplication of the ileum.

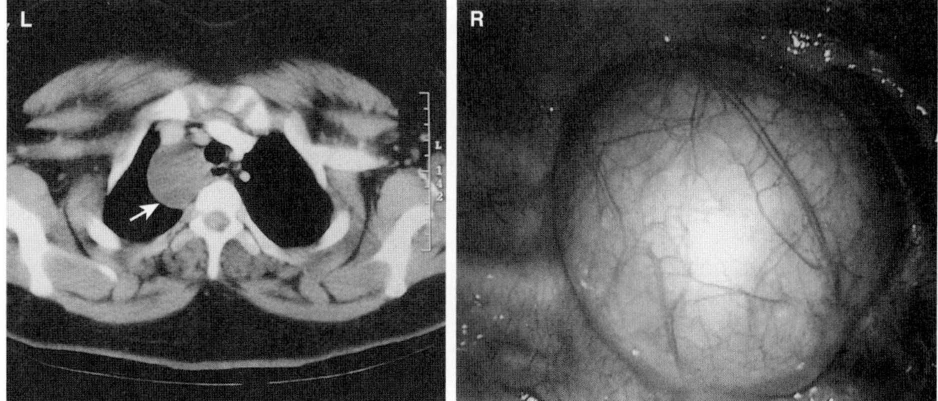

Figure 40-4. This 16-year-old was found to have a posterior mediastinal mass on a chest radiograph. **Left,** CT scan shows the duplication (*arrow*) to be adjacent to the trachea and the esophagus. **Right,** View of the duplication as seen at thoracoscopy.

shift or lung compression is present,[41] but others have found that thoracoscopy can be performed safely after cyst decompression.[43]

Thoracoabdominal Duplications

Extension of an esophageal duplication through the diaphragmatic hiatus into the abdomen is known as a thoracoabdominal duplication. These are uncommon and represent 3% of all duplications. The duplication has a variable length of intra-abdominal extension with connections to the stomach, duodenum, pancreas, and jejunum all being reported. Jejunal connections are the most common.[16,17] These duplications are all tubular, and a high percentage have ectopic gastric mucosa. As with isolated esophageal duplications, they may be asymptomatic. Likewise, symptomatic duplications will most often present as dyspnea or dysphagia. Hemorrhage and death from ectopic gastric mucosa has been described.[29] The two largest series of thoracoabdominal duplications in the literature report an 88% incidence of vertebral anomalies in these patients.[16,17] This high association warrants further workup through either MRI or CT to exclude neuroenteric communication (Fig. 40-5). The current treatment is a one-stage combined thoracoabdominal approach for resection.

Gastric Duplications

Gastric duplications account for about 8% of all duplications and usually become symptomatic in early childhood.[17] Unlike other duplications, a female predilection is seen.[8,44] Pain, hematemesis, melena, or anemia are the most frequent presenting symptoms. Gastric duplications are most often cystic and located along the greater curvature (Figs. 40-6 and 40-7), although there are reports of duplications along the

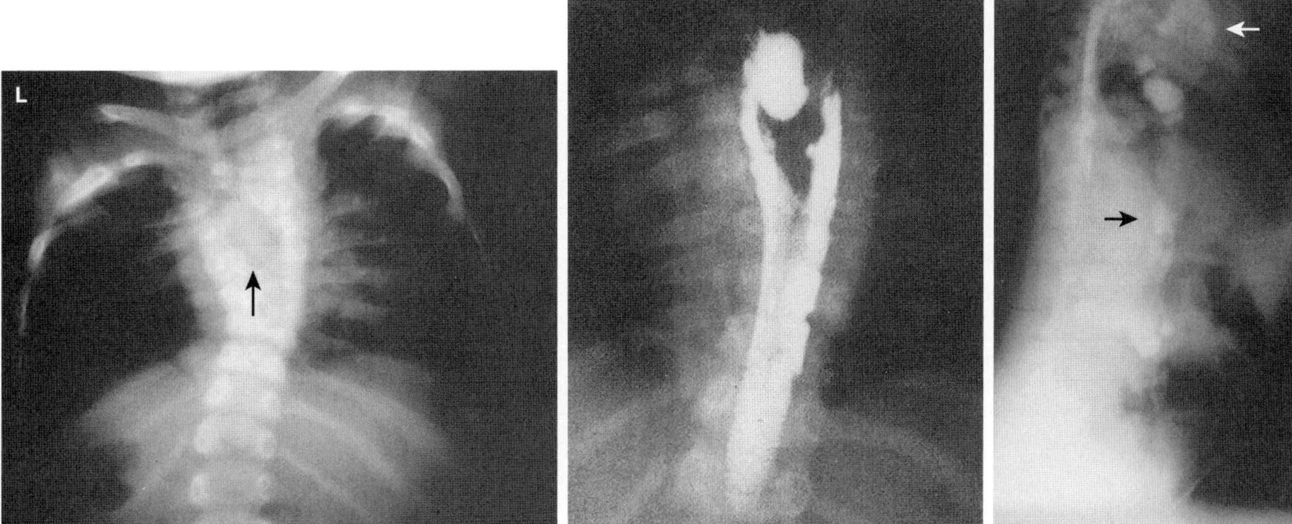

Figure 40-5. A 3-year-old was found to have a right paravertebral mass. **Left,** A large anterior defect in the vertebral bodies of the upper thoracic spine (*arrow*) is seen. **Middle,** This myelogram shows the filling defect caused by a neuroenteric cyst. **Right,** The contrast agent from the myelogram is seen in the neuroenteric cyst (*upper arrow*) with extension subdiaphragmatically (*lower arrow*) into the distal small intestine. (From Holcomb GW III, Gheissari A, O'Neill JA, et al: Surgical management of alimentary tract duplications. Ann Surg 209:167-174, 1989.)

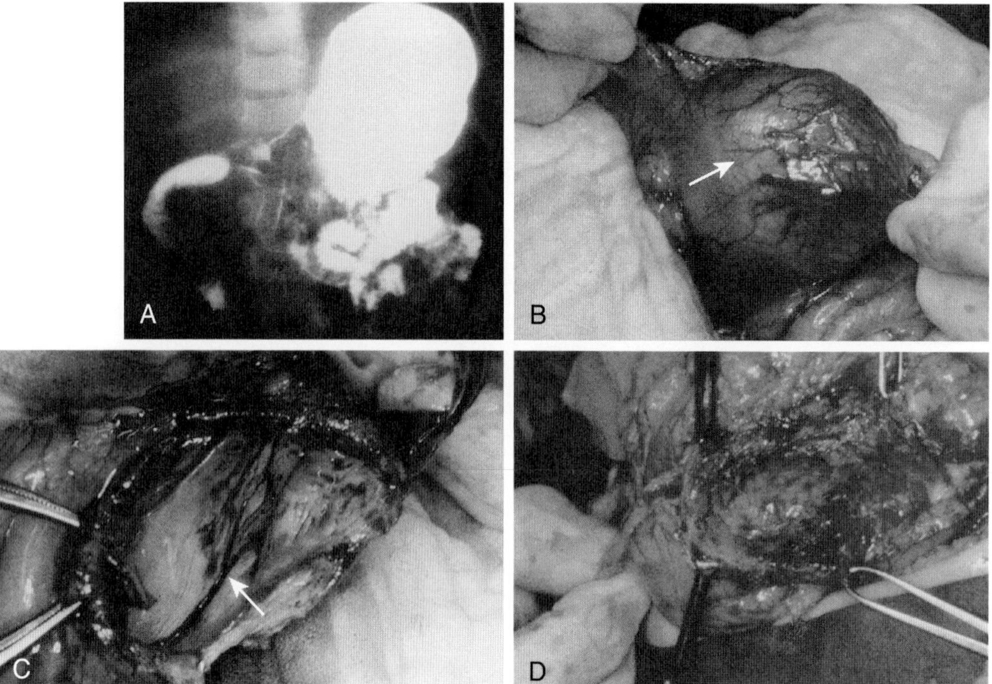

Figure 40-6. **A,** This patient had nonbilious emesis and was found to have a mass effect on the antrum with extrinsic compression of the second portion of the duodenum on this contrast study. **B,** A gastric duplication (*arrow*) was found emanating from the inferior aspect of the greater curvature of the gastric antrum at operation. It was thought best to marsupialize the duplication, because a significant partial gastrectomy would be required to remove this lesion completely. **C,** The duplication has been marsupialized, and the mucosa (*arrow*) of the duplication lying on the common wall with the stomach is seen. **D,** The mucosa has been stripped, leaving intact the common wall between the duplication and the gastric antrum. (From Holcomb GW III, Gheissari A, O'Neill JA, et al: Surgical management of alimentary tract duplications. Ann Surg 209:167-174, 1989.)

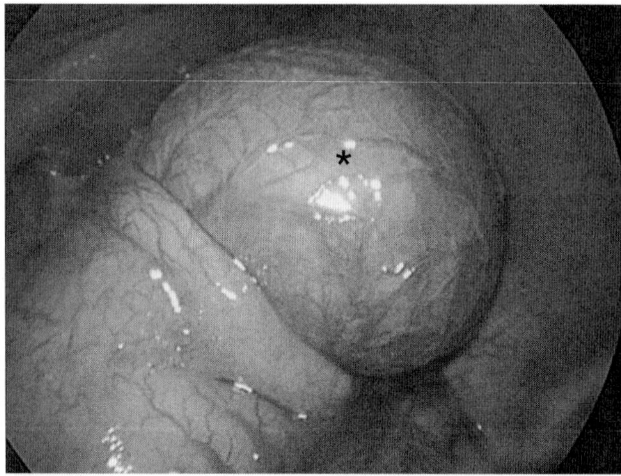

Figure 40-7. A neonate was found to have pyloric atresia and underwent laparoscopic correction. At laparoscopy, a large gastric duplication (*asterisk*) was seen emanating from the greater curvature of the stomach. The duplication was excised and the greater curvature closed. The patient recovered uneventfully and did not develop any postoperative problems.

lesser curvature and the pylorus. Although the majority do not communicate with the lumen, if intraluminal communication is present, peptic ulceration with hemorrhage or perforation can occur.

Diagnostic evaluation is directed toward symptoms, with abdominal ultrasonography as the initial study. Typically, the ultrasound image shows a duplication and differentiates it from pyloric stenosis.[24] Pancreatic pseudocysts or a choledochal cyst may be confused with a gastric duplication. Abdominal CT scan or an upper gastrointestinal series may be needed to further delineate the anatomy. All gastric duplications regardless of symptoms should be excised to prevent future gastrointestinal bleeding. Excision without violating the lumen is the preferred approach, but large or complex duplications may require partial gastrectomy. If this type of resection is considered too radical, then mucosal stripping of the common wall will prevent subsequent ulceration (see Fig. 40-6).[17] Adenocarcinoma has been reported in an adult with a gastric duplication.[22]

Duodenal Duplications

Like gastric duplications, duodenal duplications are uncommon and account for about 6% of reported duplications.[17] Partial intestinal obstruction with emesis or gastrointestinal bleeding can be seen, but these lesions may also be asymptomatic. The presence of ectopic gastric mucosa has been reported at 13%.[45] Most duplications on the mesenteric side are found in the first or second portion of the duodenum. The majority are cystic, but tubular variants are occasionally seen.[46] The anatomic location of these duplications may obstruct the biliopancreatic ducts, causing jaundice or pancreatitis.

Abdominal ultrasonography or CT is the preferred imaging modality for these lesions. The location of duodenal duplications and their tenuous blood supply dictate the operative plan. Simple excision is preferred as long as the blood supply to the duodenum can be maintained. The intimate relationship to the biliopancreatic ducts may necessitate a Roux-en Y cystojejunostomy to preserve the blood supply.[47] If the duplication is large and contains gastric mucosa on frozen section, duodenal resection may be necessary to decrease the risk of future gastrointestinal hemorrhage.

Pancreatic Duplications

The rarest form of alimentary tract duplications are pancreatic, with only 43 reported in the literature.[48] The most common presentation is abdominal pain (67%), followed by nausea/vomiting and a palpable abdominal mass. The radiologic workup is similar to gastric and duodenal duplications, with pancreatic duplications often mistaken for a pancreatic pseudocyst. Anatomically, the pancreatic head is the most common location (51%), with the remainder equally distributed in the body and tail. At operation, the presence of a smooth muscle lining on frozen section will distinguish pancreatic duplications from pseudocysts. Treatment ranges from cystectomy to more complex procedures, including cystojejunostomy, pancreaticoduodenectomy, or partial pancreatectomy, depending on the location.[48]

Small Bowel Duplications

Small bowel duplications account for almost half of all reported duplications. They may be cystic or tubular, with the majority being cystic (Fig. 40-8).

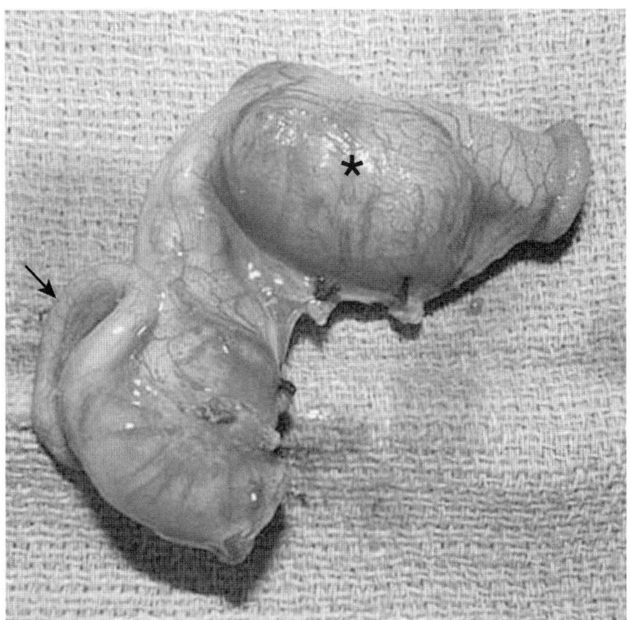

Figure 40-8. This small bowel duplication (*asterisk*) was located in the terminal ileum and required removal of the terminal ileum as well as the cecum. Note the appendix (*arrow*) attached to the cecum. A primary anastomosis was performed.

Tubular duplications vary in size from a few centimeters to the entire length of the bowel (Fig. 40-9). Small bowel duplications may be separate from the native bowel or share a common wall. They arise from the mesenteric side of the bowel and share a common blood supply. The most common location is the ileum (34%).[16-18]

Small bowel duplications are frequently seen in early childhood secondary to emesis, hematochezia, melena, anemia, or a palpable abdominal mass. The duplication may lead to volvulus, which is sometimes seen in neonates. In older children, intussusception is more common, with the duplication acting as the lead point.[17] Abdominal ultrasonography is usually the initial imaging study to evaluate these lesions. The presence of ectopic gastric mucosa is seen in 80% of tubular and 20% of cystic duplications.[39] This ectopic gastric mucosa may lead to ulceration and gastrointestinal bleeding or perforation. Also, such duplications can be mistaken for a Meckel's diverticulum on technetium scanning. Small bowel follow-through or CT scans are probably less helpful and lead to unnecessary radiation exposure. Recently, laparoscopy has been advocated for both diagnosis in uncertain cases as well as treatment, thereby eliminating open exploration and decreasing the length of postoperative hospitalization (see Fig. 40-3).[39,49]

Surgical management of small bowel duplications will vary because of the heterogeneity of these malformations. Small bowel resection with primary anastomosis is the usual approach. Infrequently, small cystic duplications can be treated with enucleation without sacrificing the native blood supply. Long tubular duplications may be more difficult to manage because of the intimate blood supply to the native bowel. Resections of large lengths of bowel will increase complications and can pose the risk of short gut syndrome. In this situation, mucosal stripping, sometimes through multiple enterotomies, will preserve bowel length and decrease the chance of ulceration and hemorrhage from the ectopic gastric mucosa.[50] Another approach is to anastomose the tubular duplication containing gastric mucosa to the stomach, allowing the gastric acid to drain and preserving bowel length.[51]

Colonic Duplications

Colonic duplications account for approximately 15% of all duplications. Most occur in the cecum and are cystic. However, tubular duplications can also be found and will vary in length and complexity (see Fig. 40-9). Sometimes multiple tubular duplications are seen. Colonic duplications are found along the mesenteric border of the bowel. Large bowel obstruction secondary to compression, intussusception, and volvulus are the usual presenting symptoms. Because colonic duplications usually do not contain ectopic gastric mucosa, gastrointestinal bleeding is rare. However, a higher number of associated anomalies are present in patients with tubular colonic duplications. With total colonic tubular duplications, other duplicate structures such as bladder, vagina, and external genitalia are described,

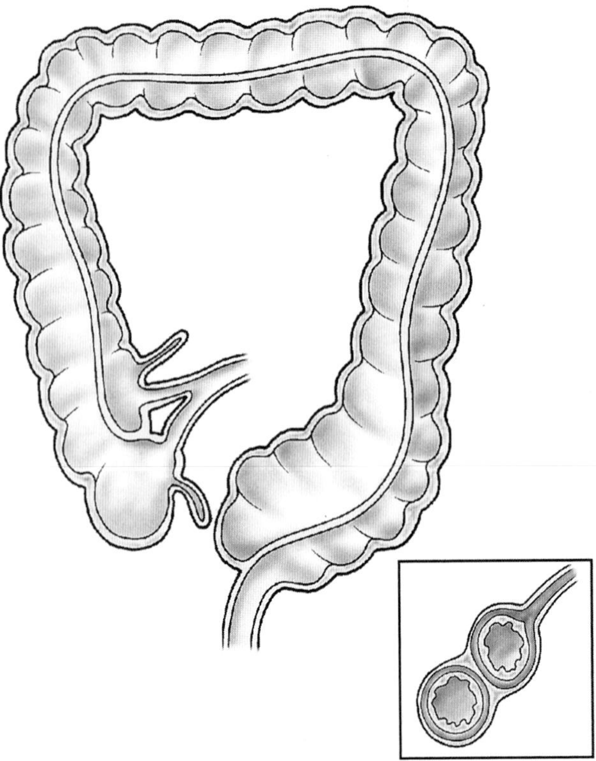

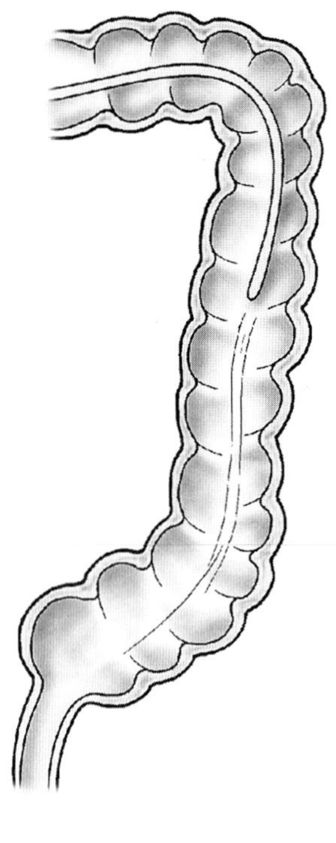

Figure 40-9. Ileal and colonic tubular duplications vary in length and complexity. **Left,** The terminal ileum is seen to bifurcate into native colon and duplicated colon, which is medial to the native colon. In this scenario the duplicated colon ends blindly in the upper rectum. **Right,** In this drawing, the duplicated colon communicates with the native colon and forms a common descending colon.

supporting the partial twinning theory of embryogenesis.[52,53] The wide variety of tubular colonic duplications and associated anomalies has led some to state that no two are alike.[54] To better categorize tubular colonic duplications, a classification system has been described. Type I colonic duplications are limited to the alimentary tract, whereas type II duplications are associated with genital or urinary tract duplications.[55]

With colonic duplications, plain radiographs are usually nonspecific. Other studies including ultrasonography, CT, or contrast enema are usually ordered based on symptoms. A contrast enema may demonstrate a duplication and communication with the native colonic lumen, if present. Sometimes, colonic duplications are discovered at exploration for other reasons.

The treatment of colonic duplications will vary depending on the type and extent. Cystic duplications are managed with resection and anastomosis. Small cystic duplications can sometimes be enucleated. Tubular duplications are usually more challenging. For symptomatic tubular duplications, resection is preferred, if possible. If resection is considered too aggressive, a distal communication between the duplication and native colon can be created to relieve the obstruction. For large tubular duplications that are asymptomatic and with a distal communication, conservative management with stool softeners is appropriate. Although rare, carcinoma has been reported in adults with both cystic and tubular colonic duplications, but this has not been reported in duplications with a distal colonic communication.[22,56,57] Because colonic duplications rarely contain ectopic gastric tissue, mucosal excision is usually not needed. Resection of a fistula tract to the bladder or uterus should be performed.

Rectal Duplications

Rectal duplications account for approximately 6% of all duplications and are commonly found in the presacral space, posterior to the rectum (Fig. 40-10). A perirectal abscess may develop if a perineal fistula is present. Chronic constipation is commonly found in patients with rectal duplications because of the posterior mass effect. Digital rectal examination may be used to identify this presacral mass. Treatment will vary from marsupialization through a transanal approach, division of the septum between the duplication and rectum, or excision using a posterior sagittal approach. An initial colostomy may be needed in some patients.

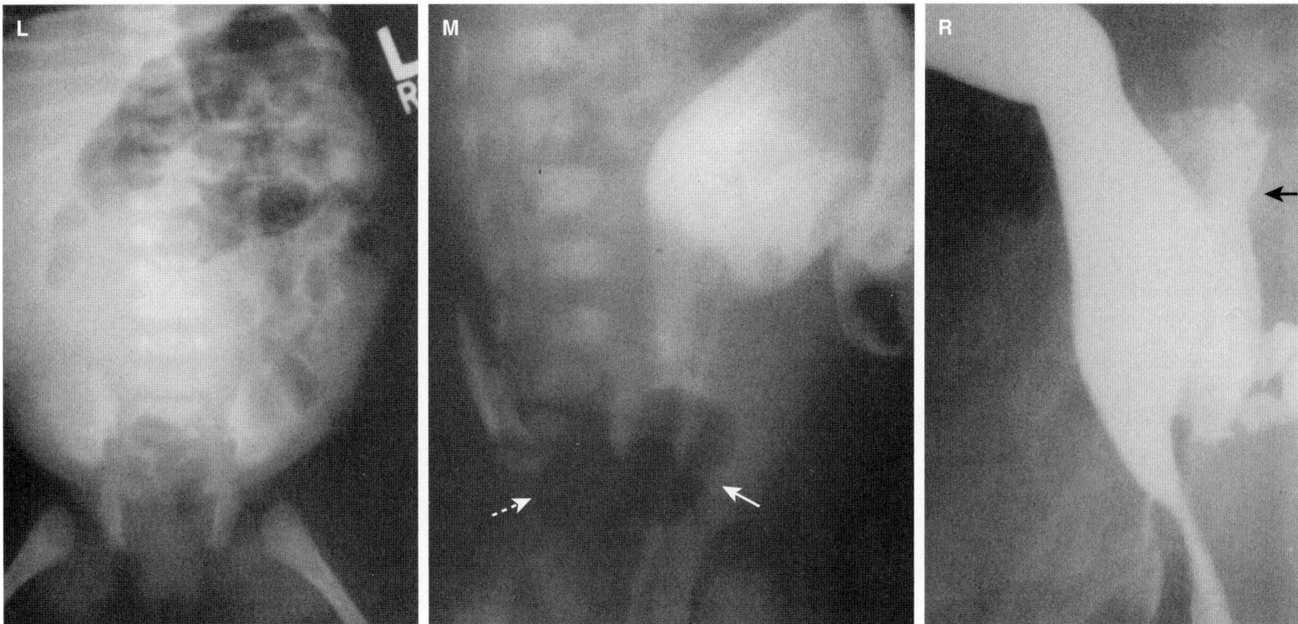

Figure 40-10. **Left,** Radiograph of a neonate with abdominal distention and evidence of a pelvic mass. On rectal examination, a mass was palpable posterior to the rectum. **Middle,** A contrast study in which an 8-Fr Foley catheter was introduced into the rectum, and the balloon was inflated with air (*solid arrow*). Posterior to the rectum and compressing it is a rectal duplication with air (*dotted arrow*), indicating communication to the gastrointestinal tract. A colostomy was initially performed because of the rectal obstruction. **Right,** A barium enema was performed at age 6 months in this patient. On this lateral radiograph, filling of the posterior rectal mass is seen (*arrow*). (From Holcomb GW III, Gheissari A, O'Neill JA, et al: Surgical management of alimentary tract duplications. Ann Surg 209:167-174, 1989.)

chapter 41

MECKEL'S DIVERTICULUM

Kurt P. Schropp, MD • Carissa L. Garey, MD

Meckel's diverticulum was first described by its namesake, the German anatomist Johann Meckel, in 1809. It is the most common congenital anomaly of the gastrointestinal tract and is a remnant of the vitelline (omphalomesenteric) duct. In utero, the vitelline duct connects the fetal gut to the yolk sac. The duct usually involutes during the fifth to sixth weeks of gestation. When the portion of the vitelline duct that is on the antimesenteric border of the ileum fails to regress, it forms a true diverticulum (Fig. 41-1). Its persistence may be present in a number of anatomic variations. These anomalies may be asymptomatic or the cause of a number of complications.

Although this malformation has been known for many years, controversies still persist, such as the best method for diagnosing a bleeding diverticulum and the proper treatment of an incidentally discovered malformation.

INCIDENCE

Because the majority of patients who have a Meckel's diverticulum are asymptomatic, its true incidence is unknown. Most studies report the incidence to be around 2% of the general population, with an increased incidence in patients with certain congenital anomalies of the umbilicus (patent vitelline duct, omphalocele), alimentary tract, central nervous system, and cardiovascular system.[1] Overall, about 4% of patients with a Meckel's diverticulum become symptomatic, meaning that about 8 in 10,000 people will manifest complications.[2] The male-to-female complication rate ratio is about 3:1, and 50% to 60% of all cases of a symptomatic Meckel's diverticulum are discovered in the first 2 years of life.[3] Only about 15% of children initially seen with a symptomatic Meckel's diverticulum are older than 4 years of age.[4]

Heterotopic tissue is the cause of most of the complications, consisting mostly of gastric mucosa but less commonly of pancreatic, jejunal, or colonic tissue.[3] Symptomatic Meckel's diverticula have a 10-fold increased incidence of heterotopic tissue, but it is estimated that only 50% to 60% of patients with ectopic tissue become symptomatic.[5]

PATHOPHYSIOLOGY

A wide spectrum of omphalomesenteric abnormalities may be present, depending on the degree of involution of the vitelline duct (Fig. 41-2).[6] Anatomically, the classic description is that the Meckel's diverticulum is found on the antimesenteric border of the ileum 2 feet proximal to the ileocecal valve, 2 cm in diameter, 2 inches in length, and not attached to the abdominal wall. Bleeding secondary to heterotopic tissue is the most common complication. Occasionally, heterotopic tissue can act as a lead point for an intussusception, resulting in a bowel obstruction. Also, intestinal obstruction may be caused by a Meckel's diverticulum that is attached to the umbilicus by a mesodiverticular band. This may lead to a volvulus around the band and may be difficult to diagnose because the patient usually will not have undergone any previous abdominal

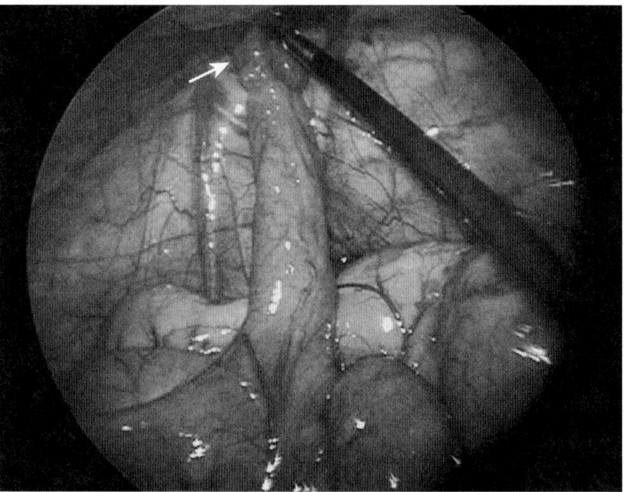

Figure 41-1. This laparoscopic view shows a long Meckel's diverticulum emanating from the antimesenteric border of the ileum. This is a true diverticulum and contains ectopic mucosa at the tip of the diverticulum (*arrow*).

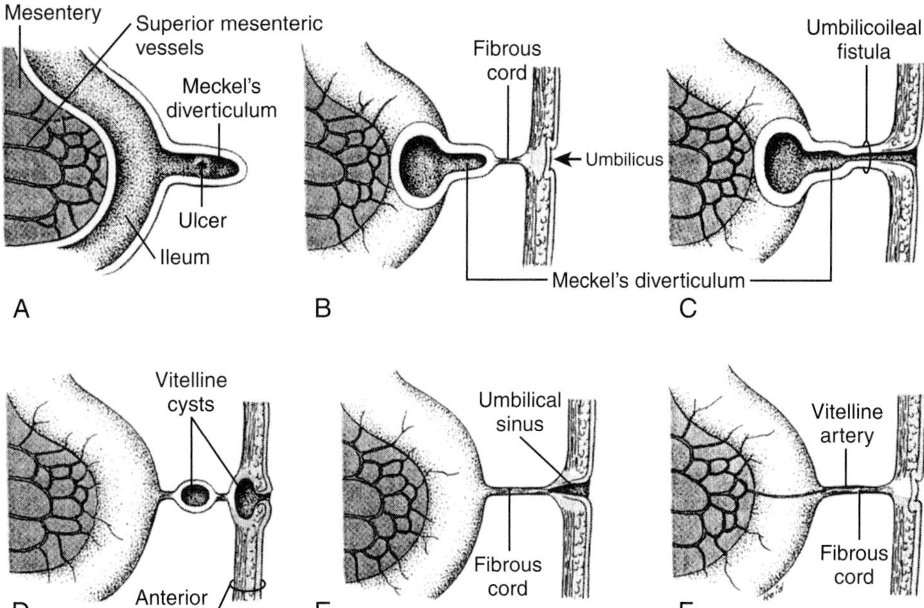

Figure 41-2. A to F, Drawings illustrating Meckel's diverticulium and other remnants of the yolk sac. (From Moore KL: The Developing Human. Philadelphia, WB Saunders, 1988.)

operations and adhesive bowel obstruction is not high on the differential diagnosis. Similarly, a persistent vitelline artery, which is an end artery from the superior mesenteric artery, may cause obstruction and/or volvulus. Often this will cause a fibrous band from the base of the mesentery across the ileum and onto the diverticulum.

Because of the association of *Helicobacter pylori* and gastroduodenal ulceration, it had been suggested that the gastritis and ulceration/bleeding of Meckel's diverticula may be due to colonization with *H. pylori*. Eradicating the *H. pylori* potentially would decrease the bleeding associated with ectopic gastric tissue. Recently, however, studies have shown a very low colonization rate with *H. pylori* in children with Meckel's diverticulum.[7,8] These studies also concluded that the majority of symptomatic Meckel's diverticula do not have colonization. Therefore, *H. pylori* may incidentally colonize a Meckel's diverticulum and most likely has a minor role in pathophysiology.[9]

In a recent report about an asymptomatic Meckel's diverticulum in a patient with Beckwith-Wiedemann syndrome, nesidioblastosis was found in ectopic pancreatic tissue.[10] Moreover, being composed mostly of small bowel mucosa, the Meckel's diverticulum also may contain a wide variety of tumors, such as carcinoid, leiomyoma, gastrointestinal stromal tumor, angioma, and neurofibroma, which are often found incidentally but may be the cause of serious complications.

CLINICAL PRESENTATION

The clinical presentation in symptomatic patients with a Meckel's diverticulum is quite varied and dependent on the configuration of the Meckel's diverticulum and whether it has ectopic tissue. The three main forms of presentation are hemorrhage (40%-60%), obstruction (25%), and diverticulitis (10%-20%).[3] The classic presentation of a child with a bleeding Meckel's diverticulum is a preschool patient with painless rectal bleeding. This may consist of dark, tarry stools or red, gross blood if bleeding is heavy. The hemorrhage is episodic and usually ceases without treatment. Rarely will a child need immediate operation to control the bleeding. Sometimes the hemorrhage is insidious and not appreciated by the family. A young child with hemoglobin-positive stools and a chronic iron deficiency anemia must be investigated for a bleeding Meckel's diverticulum. The hemorrhage is often at the junction of the gastric and ileal mucosa. Hemorrhage can also originate on the mesenteric border of the ileum, especially with a short, wide-based diverticulum.

Patients seen with obstruction secondary to an intussusception usually have classic signs and symptoms of an idiopathic intussusception, including crampy abdominal pain, progressing to bilious vomiting and obstipation. They will often have currant-jelly stools. Patients with artery/band obstruction also demonstrate bilious vomiting and abdominal distention but may be in extremis if volvulus and ischemia develop. As mentioned earlier, the intussusception or obstruction is often diagnosed preoperatively but a Meckel's diverticulum is usually not the cause.

Patients with diverticulitis often have symptoms that resemble appendicitis. Periumbilical pain is usually the first presenting symptom. They usually do not have the same amount and intensity of nausea and vomiting as do children with appendicitis. Moreover, their point of maximal tenderness may migrate across the abdomen as the child moves. Many of these children have been previously hospitalized with similar symptoms but did not undergo exploration because the diagnosis of a Meckel's diverticulum was not entertained.

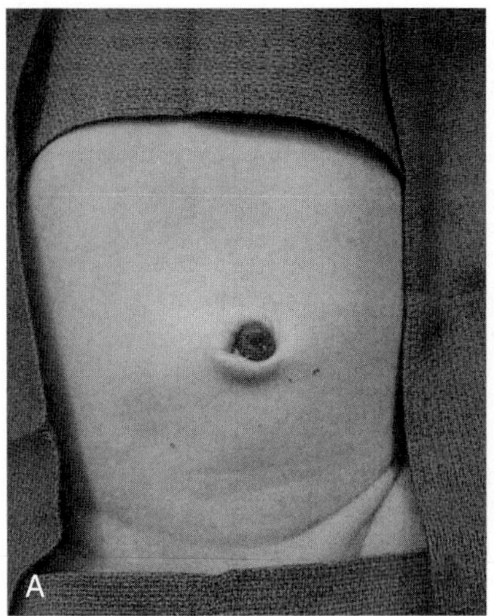

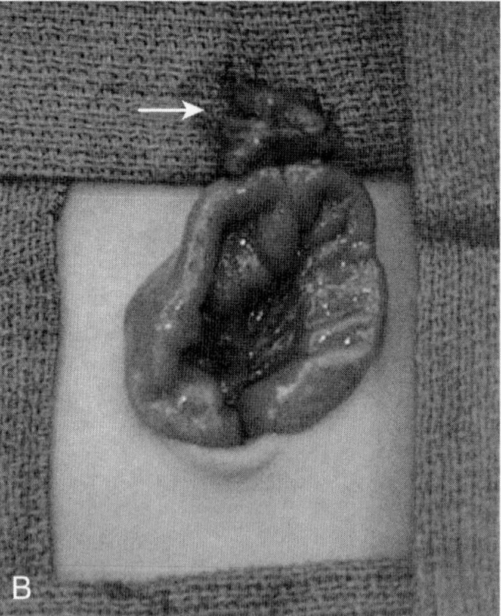

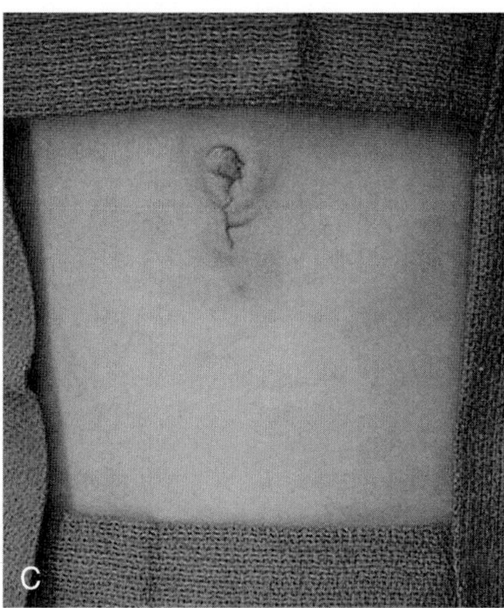

Figure 41-3. This neonate was born with an obvious patent omphalomesenteric duct. **A,** Meconium was seen to emanate from the stoma. **B,** A circumumbilical incision was made, and the duct (*arrow*) was dissected to its connection with the ileum. **C,** The duct was amputated from the ileum and the umbilical incision closed. The patient recovered uneventfully and has not developed any further problems.

Finally, a Meckel's diverticulum may be found in a number of less common, unusual presentations. A neonate can be found with an obvious patent vitelline duct (Fig. 41-3). Littre's hernia is an inguinal hernia with an incarcerated Meckel's diverticulum. It also can be incarcerated in a spigelian hernia,[11] be a cause of intra-abdominal hemorrhage,[12] or be a cystic mass.[13] Finally, it has been diagnosed in a neonate only 4 hours old.[14]

DIAGNOSIS

The diagnosis of a symptomatic Meckel's diverticulum is dependent on the anatomic configuration of the diverticulum and its presentation, signs, and symptoms. Routine history and physical examination are probably the most important diagnostic methods. For example, patients with lower gastrointestinal bleeding need a complete description of the quality and frequency of the bloody stools. A nasogastric tube should be placed to help exclude gastric bleeding as the cause. Rectal examination, and occasionally lower endoscopy, is useful in identifying other causes of lower gastrointestinal bleeding, such as polyps and rectal tears. Radiologic examination may be helpful in diagnosing the complications of a Meckel's diverticulum, such as obstruction caused by the Meckel's diverticulum that has formed an intussusception or intestinal inflammation caused by Meckel's diverticulitis. However, of the three most common presentations, a bleeding diverticulum is probably most often diagnosed preoperatively by radiographic procedures.

Technetium-99m (^{99m}Tc) pertechnetate scintigraphy of the abdomen is commonly used to help detect ectopic gastric tissue in a Meckel's diverticulum. Unfortunately, ectopic gastric mucosa also may be found in intestinal duplications and in the small bowel separate from a Meckel's diverticulum. The ^{99m}Tc pertechnetate is secreted by the tubular gland cells of gastric mucosa. Therefore, any Meckel's diverticulum with ectopic gastric mucosa potentially may be diagnosed with scintigraphy. Unlike many other invasive and noninvasive tests for bleeding, an active hemorrhage is not a prerequisite for a positive diagnosis.

The scintigraphic study is fairly easily performed. If possible, the child should fast for 3 to 4 hours before the scan. Optimally, no barium studies should have been performed in the preceding 24 hours, nor should enemas or laxatives have been utilized. After the injection of the ^{99m}Tc pertechnetate, the only focal accumulation of tracer should be in the urinary tract or the stomach. A positive study is characterized by a focal tracer uptake that appears simultaneous with the stomach and increases in intensity over time (Fig. 41-4).[15] A number of causes of false-positive results may be found, including intussusception, inflammation of the bowel, intestinal duplication, an abnormal urinary collecting system, a hemangioma, or an arteriovenous malformation. False-negative scans are probably even more problematic. They may result from having only a small amount of gastric mucosa, residual barium from a previous study, or a Meckel's diverticulum that is low in the pelvis and obscured by the bladder.

Controversy exists as to the utility of pharmacologic enhancement of the isotope uptake to increase the accuracy of scintigraphy. The most commonly used medications for this purpose are pentagastrin and histamine-2 (H_2) blockers. Pentagastrin enhancement works by stimulating acid production by parietal cells. H_2-blocker enhancement works by decreasing the washout of pertechnetate from the gastric glands, thus enhancing the visualization of the scan. Because no conclusive evidence exists that pharmacologic enhancement clearly increases accuracy, many use these agents only when a study is inconclusive (not clearly positive or negative).

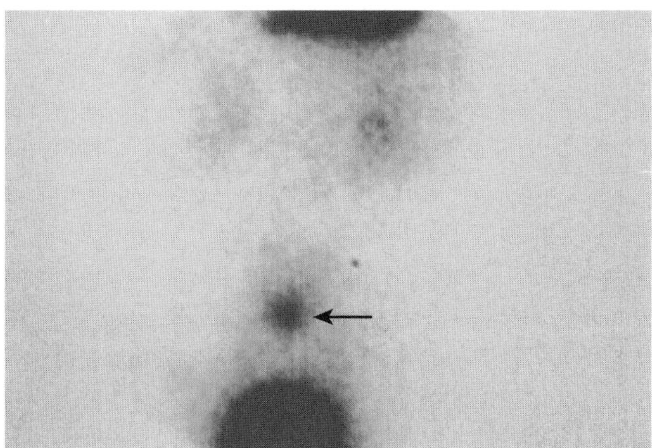

Figure 41-4. Technetium-99m pertechnetate scan of a patient with a Meckel's diverticulum. Note the blush (*arrow*) above the bladder. (Courtesy of Kyo Lee, MD.)

Even though the presence of ectopic gastric mucosa in a patient with a bleeding Meckel's diverticulum approaches 100%, the accuracy of ^{99m}Tc scanning does not. The specificity of scintigraphy is probably about 95% or higher, but the sensitivity is significantly worse at around 60%. Therefore, a negative scan result does not necessarily exclude a bleeding Meckel's diverticulum. A number of authors advocate laparotomy, or more recently, laparoscopy, to exclude Meckel's diverticulum as the cause of bleeding in a patient with a negative scintigram but a high clinical suspicion of a bleeding Meckel's diverticulum.[16]

Some authors have touted the utility of angiography for a bleeding Meckel's diverticulum if high suspicion exists in the presence of a negative scintigram.[17] One difficulty with angiography, besides being very invasive, is that the ulcer must be actively bleeding for the study to be accurate.

A new, noninvasive diagnostic technique that may aid in the diagnosis of a bleeding Meckel's diverticulum is wireless capsule endoscopy.[18] With this study, the patient swallows a capsule and numerous pictures of the intestine are taken. Obscure gastrointestinal bleeding is the usual indication for this study. Data in the pediatric population are limited, but one study found relevant lesions in 60% of children with obscure bleeding that were not detectable with previous studies.[19] One limitation of this diagnostic tool is that it requires a child to swallow an 11 × 26-mm capsule. There is the option of delivering the capsule by endoscopy, but this makes the study more invasive. Complications such as delayed passage can also occur. A short course of corticosteroids and bowel preparation has been used to aid success in passage. Obstruction is another complication. In one study, 20% had delayed passage of the capsule and two patients had acute small bowel obstruction requiring surgical bowel resection for removal of the capsule.[19] There has been advancement with the recent invention of a capsule that will disintegrate within 40 hours. In conclusion, the current pediatric gastrointestinal community has recommended a role for capsule endoscopy in older children with obscure gastrointestinal bleeding.

The patient with a nonhemorrhaging Meckel's diverticulum will have a low incidence of heterotopic gastric mucosa. In this setting, scintigraphy will not be useful. Patients with obstruction secondary to an intussuscepted Meckel's diverticulum can often be diagnosed with an air enema. On occasion, the air enema will reduce the ileocolic portion of the intussusception and an unrecognized ileoileal component will remain. This component often will not be reducible with the enema. If it does reduce, it will often recur. Ultrasonography remains fairly reliable in skilled hands to diagnose the intussusception. It also may demonstrate an inflamed Meckel's diverticulum. Sometimes a combination of ultrasonography, computed tomography, and contrast enema may aid in the diagnosis of complicated, scintigraphy-negative Meckel's diverticulum.[20]

TREATMENT

The treatment of a symptomatic Meckel's diverticulum begins with adequate resuscitation. If the patient presents initially with bleeding, adequate resuscitation to an appropriate hemoglobin level should be accomplished before operation.

Resection can be accomplished by either a simple diverticulectomy or by a partial ileal resection. This decision is based on the key principle of resecting all the ectopic tissue. Most authors believe that it is important to resect the ulcer, if present, caused by the gastric secretions. Because most narrow-based lesions have the gastric tissue at the tip, the ulcer is usually in the Meckel's diverticulum itself. A simple diverticulectomy by resecting transversely across the base would be appropriate in this setting. Conversely, some believe that resection of the ulcer is not necessary as long as all the gastric mucosa has been removed. If the diverticulum is wide based, then an increased chance exists the ectopic mucosa could be anywhere in the diverticulum. Therefore, an ileal resection should probably be performed.

For the past decade, most surgeons have advocated laparoscopy as the optimal approach for elective diverticulectomy for a bleeding Meckel's diverticulum. Multiple techniques have been described. The two primary techniques are laparoscopic intracorporeal and laparoscopic-assisted extracorporeal diverticulectomy.[21] The intracorporeal method utilizes an umbilical cannula large enough to allow a stapler (12 mm) and two additional 5-mm cannulas. These smaller cannulas are usually placed in the left upper and left lower abdominal quadrants, similar to port placement for laparoscopic appendectomy. Once the cecum is located, the ileocecal valve is identified and the small bowel can then be inspected in a retrograde fashion until the diverticulum is located. The decision can then be made whether a simple diverticulectomy or ileal resection is warranted. For diverticulectomy, a stapler is used to transect the Meckel's diverticulum at the base. Partial ileal resection can be accomplished intracorporeally by stapling across the ileum on

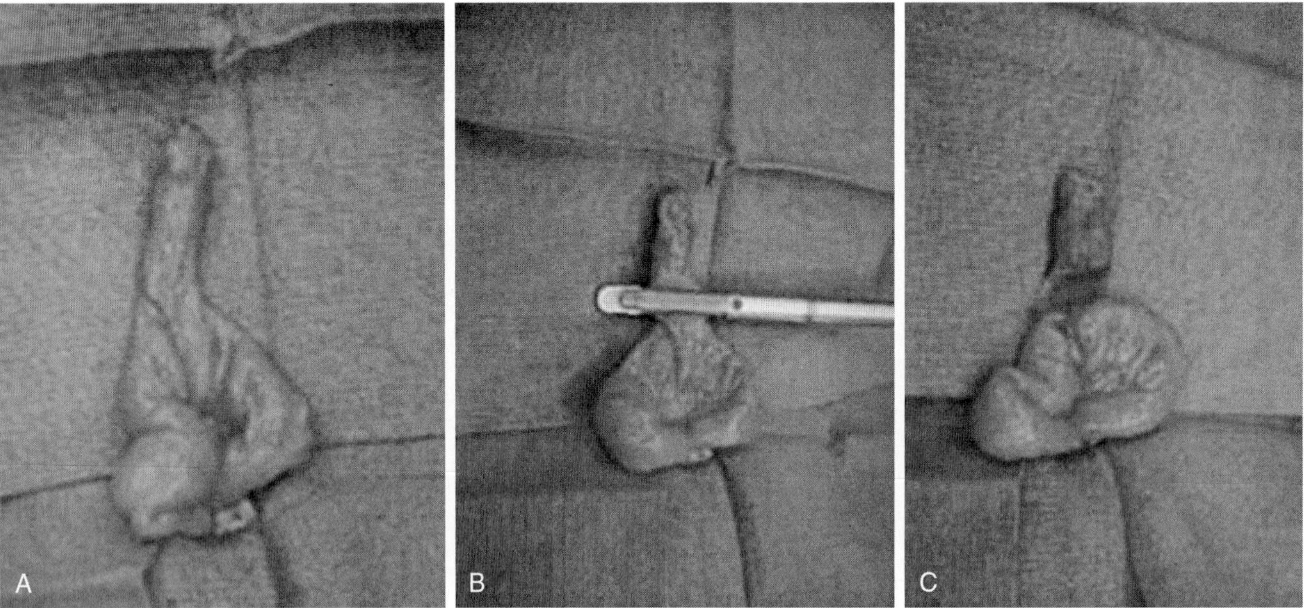

Figure 41-5. **A,** When diagnosed, Meckel's diverticulum can be managed either totally intracorporeally or exteriorized through the umbilical incision. **B** and **C,** The diverticulum and a small segment of the ileum just proximal and distal to the diverticulum were exteriorized through the umbilicus and the diverticulum was excised using the endoscopic stapler. The excision was done in an oblique direction to avoid narrowing the ileum at the site of the diverticulectomy.

either side of the diverticulum and then performing a stapled intracorporeal anastomosis. After removal from the abdomen in an endoscopic bag, the diverticulum should be opened to ensure that the ulcer is resected.

Because this procedure is often needed in infants and small children, adequate working space for endoscopic stapling is limited, and laparoscopic-assisted extracorporeal diverticulectomy is preferred by many surgeons.[22] This method also has the benefit of palpating the Meckel's diverticulum to determine ectopic tissue location, which assists in the decision for an ileal resection.[23] With the extracorporeal approach, a 10- to 12-mm cannula is inserted through an umbilical incision (Fig. 41-5). One additional smaller cannula is then inserted in the left lower quadrant. The Meckel's diverticulum is identified and exteriorized through the umbilical incision. Diverticulectomy or ileal resection is then performed extracorporeally, and the bowel is then returned to the abdominal cavity.

Because the other presentations of Meckel's diverticulum often are found unexpectedly at operation, the feasibility of resection is determined on a case-by-case basis. For example, if an intussuscepted Meckel's diverticulum can be reduced, it may or may not be wise to staple across the base of the diverticulum, depending on the thickness of the base, the appearance of the intussusceptum itself, its ease of removal, and any damage that occurred because of the intussusception (Fig. 41-6).

Postoperatively, if the procedure is performed laparoscopically with simple diverticulectomy, the child may be fed almost immediately. If an ileal resection is needed, it is best to wait until bowel function returns before feeding is resumed.

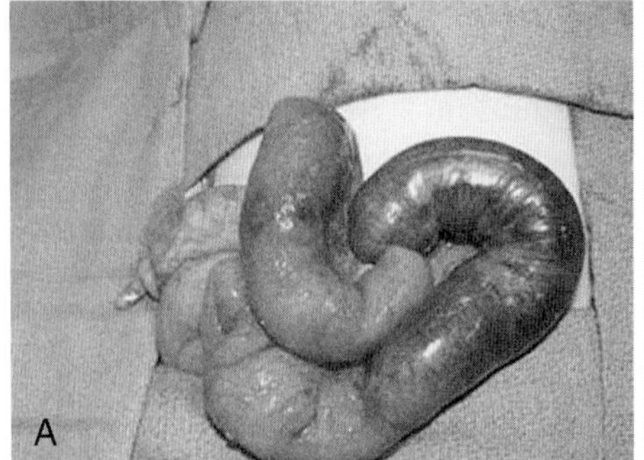

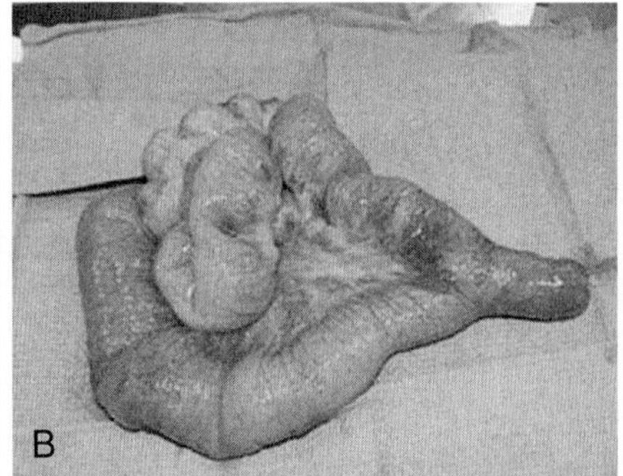

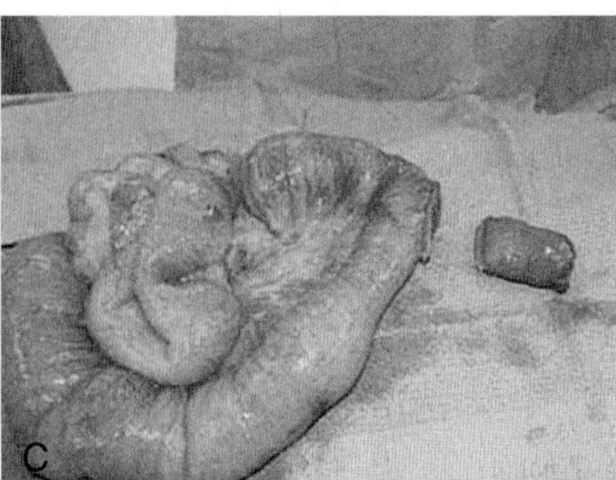

Figure 41-6. A 4-year-old presented with an irreducible intussusception and required an operative reduction. **A,** Note the small bowel intussuscepted into the large bowel. **B,** After reduction of the ileum, a Meckel's diverticulum was found to be the lead point for the intussusception. **C,** The diverticulum was excised with an endoscopic stapler.

CONTROVERSIES

The major controversy is whether to resect an incidentally discovered Meckel's diverticulum at operation for another indication. In adults, some evidence exists that more morbidity occurs with resection than does the risk that a complication will be found in the future from the diverticulum.[24] Others argue that, because it is difficult to predict who will become symptomatic and because of the low incidence of surgical morbidity, no contraindication to removal exists.[25] If palpable gastric mucosa is noted in the tip and simple excision is feasible, it seems reasonable that the Meckel's diverticulum should be removed. In young children, because of a life-long potential for complications and the low morbidity with resection, an incidentally encountered Meckel's diverticulum probably should be resected.

chapter 42

INFLAMMATORY BOWEL DISEASE AND INTESTINAL CANCER

Christopher R. Moir, MD

Children with inflammatory bowel disease (IBD) present with distinct clinical patterns that have important implications for surgical care. The overall incidence of IBD is four to six cases per 100,000 population.[1,2] Pediatric surgeons are becoming more involved because up to one third of patients who develop IBD experience their first symptom in childhood and surgical intervention occurs, on average, 2 years later.[1,3,4] Furthermore, operative treatment is more likely in Crohn's disease (CD), which is now twice as prevalent in children.[5,6]

Surgeons should be aware that up to 65% of children with IBD younger than age 8 present with pancolitis regardless of their eventual diagnosis.[1,4,6] Ulcerative colitis or indeterminate colitis is the most typical diagnosis in children between 3 and 5 years of age whereas CD becomes increasingly more prevalent after age 6, rising to a childhood peak at 15 years.[1,7,8] The diagnostic dilemma of pancolitis in the young child may not be sorted out until the mid-teens when the adult distribution pattern of CD is established.[7,9] To further cloud the situation, boys are now at higher risk than girls for CD by a ratio of 2:1, a reversal of the adult trend.[4,6] The surgeon evaluating a child with colitis must be aware that the disease location may change with age, which ultimately changes the choice of operation.[10]

The classic association of abdominal pain with CD is a less helpful differentiating factor in pediatric IBD. Many children with chronic ulcerative colitis (CUC) present with abdominal pain as the main complaint rather than rectal bleeding. Increased stool frequency and urgency are commonly seen as well.[1,3,11] Growth failure is often associated with CD but also occurs in CUC.[3,12]

A genetic predisposition is found in 12% to 44% of children depending on their age at presentation. The younger the child, the higher is the familial incidence of IBD.[3,11,13] Genetic polymorphism associated with colitis and familial disease is more frequent in pediatric-onset CD. This polymorphism in the NFκβ binding site of the tumor necrosis factor-alpha (TNF-α) promoter is more strongly associated with colonic disease than ileal or small bowel involvement.[14] The latter is classically associated with *NOD2/CARD15* mutations.[15] These genetic findings may help explain the relatively high prevalence of colonic involvement in young children who have yet to be exposed to major environmental influences. The *NOD2/CARD15* mutations confer a more likely need for operation secondary to stricturing disease in older children and adults with longer exposure to environmental pathogens.[15,16]

CROHN'S DISEASE

Whereas earlier versions of this textbook chapter started the discussion with CUC, it seems appropriate in this edition to begin with CD because it is the most prevalent form of childhood IBD owing to a marked increase in its incidence. CD affects children in both urban and rural settings and occurs in all minority groups and ethnicities. A child diagnosed with CD has a 78% probability of the need for operation within 20 years.[17] This risk is higher for ileocolic disease (92%). Approximately two thirds of patients with small bowel involvement and slightly less than 60% of patients with colonic disease will require operation. Pediatric surgeons planning the first operation should realize that 50% of their patients will return for another procedure.[17,18]

Medical Therapy

Even though the incidence of CD is increasing and the probability of operation is a near certainty over time, the need for an early initial operation is decreasing. Improved responses to medical therapy and a general reluctance to proceed with operation in smaller children may explain this change.[9,19] Pediatric patients at higher risk for early surgical intervention include those with anti-*Saccharomyces cerevisiae* antibody (ASCA)-positive disease, hypoalbuminemia, poor growth velocity, female gender, and stricture disease.[20,21] Interestingly, children with predominantly colonic CD and those on long-term therapy with aminosalicylates are less likely to undergo early operation.[20] In adults, smoking increases the risk for operation,[22] particularly in genetically susceptible individuals. On the other hand, prior appendectomy has been found to have a curiously protective effect.[23]

Enteral nutrition and corticosteroids are the mainstays of medical therapy for children with CD.[24] Nutritional therapy in children may avoid the growth delay and osteoporotic effects of corticosteroids while maintaining a more normal lifestyle and school attendance. With more palatable formulas and good compliance, enteral nutrition is associated with a reduction in inflammatory mediators and healing of CD lesions.[25] The best results have been obtained in the United Kingdom and in some European and Canadian centers. In the United States, enteral nutrition is used less frequently. Patient and physician noncompliance, variable insurer coverage, and frequent relapse are common reasons for a lack of widespread acceptance in the United States.[26]

The success of exclusive enteral nutrition therapy in children differs with the site of disease. Improvement is seen in 80% to 90% of children with primarily ileal or ileocolonic disease versus 50% of children with colitis. These findings may be related to a different genetic phenotype in patients with isolated Crohn's colitis and the interaction with colonic bacteria.[27]

Corticosteroid treatment remains an important induction therapy for children despite the well-known side effects. Milder cases may respond to mesalamine and antibiotics. Budesonide, a topically active corticosteroid with fewer systemic side effects, has also shown efficacy in children with ileocolonic disease. Unfortunately, these alternative therapies are effective for select subgroups only. Available data suggest a limited efficacy of mesalamine and related products in children with active disease and a limited ability to prevent postoperative recurrence.[28] Metronidazole and ciprofloxacin work best for patients presenting with perianal disease and can be useful for maintaining remission after operation as well.[29] Budesonide has been effective in adults who were previously corticosteroid dependent.[30]

Despite high initial response rates to systemic corticosteroids, a recent population-based study reported 58% of children remained corticosteroid dependent or required operation by 1 year. The response rates were similar for colonic and ileocolic disease, whereas small bowel disease was twice as likely to improve.[31] These recent data demonstrate the need for early implementation of second-line treatment strategies for children with CD. For example, early addition of azathioprine or mercaptopurine reduced the need for surgery and produced a 50% prolonged response in one study.[31] Oral tacrolimus also showed promise but did not produce long-term remission in another study.[32] A Danish population-based study of infliximab in children identified 71% with treatment benefit. This therapy was associated with a 29% long-term response, whereas 42% were infliximab dependent. Twenty-five percent of children had no response. Forty-two percent of the children in this study had Crohn's colitis.[33]

Indications for Operation

Refractory illness and complications of disease are the most common indications for operation in children with CD.[34] Strictures and local perforation/penetration are most commonly identified in children who present with small bowel and ileocolic disease.[15] Children with colonic CD do not often contract the common complications of abscess, perforation, or obstruction. In these patients, symptomatic disease and growth failure predominate.[20] Colonic strictures are the next most common indication and raise the possible spectre of colorectal carcinoma in patients with long-standing disease.[35]

Nearly 50% of children require their first operation to relieve refractory illness. The decision to operate represents a balance of medical and surgical factors designed to relieve symptoms and reduce treatment toxicity. Operative considerations include the site of disease, ease of resection, and the possibility of needing a stoma. The medical therapy of CD has evolved so rapidly that a treatment algorithm is proposed (Fig. 42-1).[26]

Choice of Operation

The ability of the surgeon to select an appropriate operation and reduce recurrence risk in children with CD depends on specific patterns of disease. Isolated small bowel and localized ileocecal disease with clear proximal and distal margins present the least difficult surgical decision. Colonic disease is more complex. Children with significant ileal involvement will experience higher reoperation rates after right colectomy due to small bowel and anastomotic recurrence. Similarly, the presence of rectal ulceration portends recurrence and eventual proctocolectomy in patients undergoing an initial left colon or subtotal resection with reanastomosis. Anoperineal disease with rectal involvement is a particularly poor prognostic finding in children with colonic disease and is associated with the highest risk of permanent ileostomy.[36-38] Because most patients will have evidence of some forms of these conditions, operative judgment is very important.

A complete history and physical examination to detect perianal disease and the extent of small bowel and colon involvement is important. Before operation, a contrast study of the small intestine is needed to evaluate for proximal disease (Fig. 42-2). All patients should undergo upper gastrointestinal endoscopy and colonoscopy with ileal intubation and biopsy to determine the extent of ileal involvement. CT enterography and capsule endoscopy have shown promise in selected patients. However, a blinded four-way comparison of these techniques did not identify significant benefits of capsule endoscopy over CT enterography, small bowel follow-through studies, or endoscopy.[39]

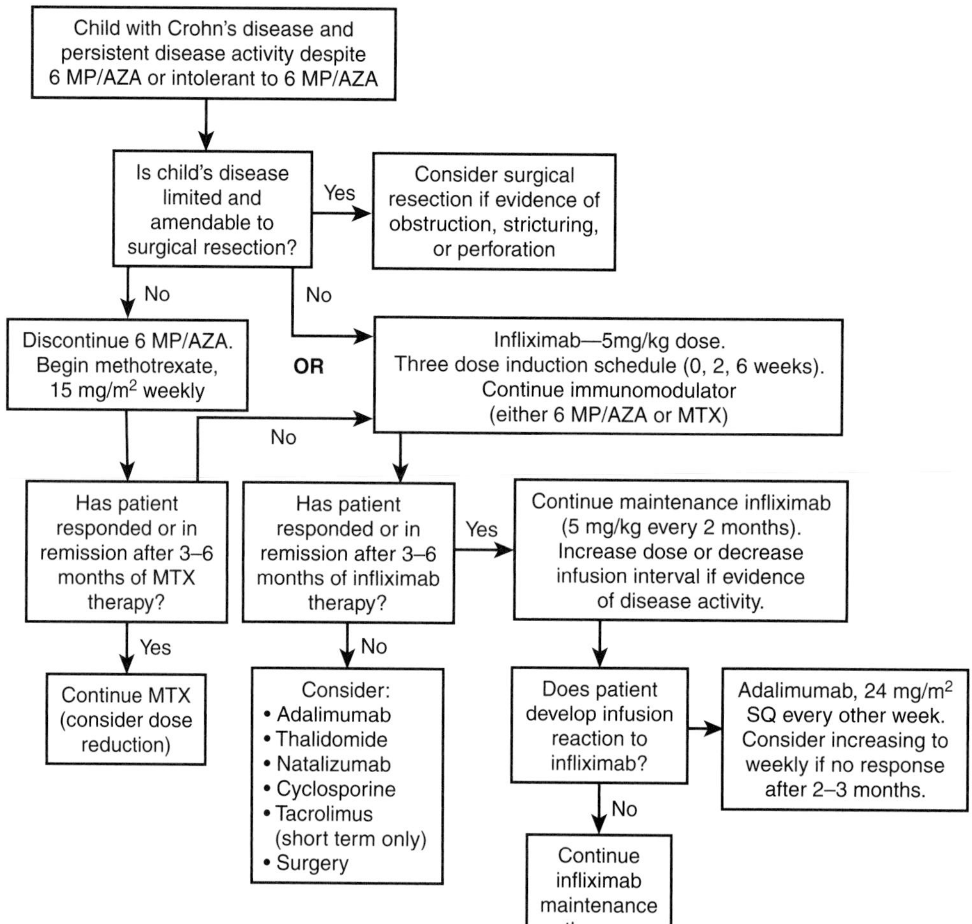

Figure 42-1. This treatment algorithm for medical therapy for Crohn's disease is utilized at the Mayo Clinic in the child with persistent disease who is either intolerant to mercaptopurine/azathioprine (6MP/AZA) or has persistent disease with these medications. MTX, methotrexate.

The need for operative resection depends on the site of disease and age of the patient. In a population-based study of 1,936 patients in Sweden with 99% follow-up after 14.9 years, children were found to have the lowest incidence of operative therapy when compared with other age groups. Colorectal presentation had the lowest need for operation with a relative risk of 1.0. Small bowel or ileocecal CD had the highest relative risk of 3.2 whereas high intestinal and discontinuous ileal and colonic disease had intermediate surgical risks of 1.7 and 1.8, respectively.[9] The overall incidence of surgical recurrence was 33% at 5 years and 44% at 10 years. Again, small bowel and ileocolonic recurrences were more likely to need operation when compared with isolated colonic disease (1.5 and 1.8 vs. 1.0). Female gender and perianal disease also significantly increased the risk of recurrence in patients with colonic disease. Interestingly, diagnosis and an initial operation at a young age did not increase the risk of recurrence, nor was there a decrease in recurrence in the more recent years of the study.[9]

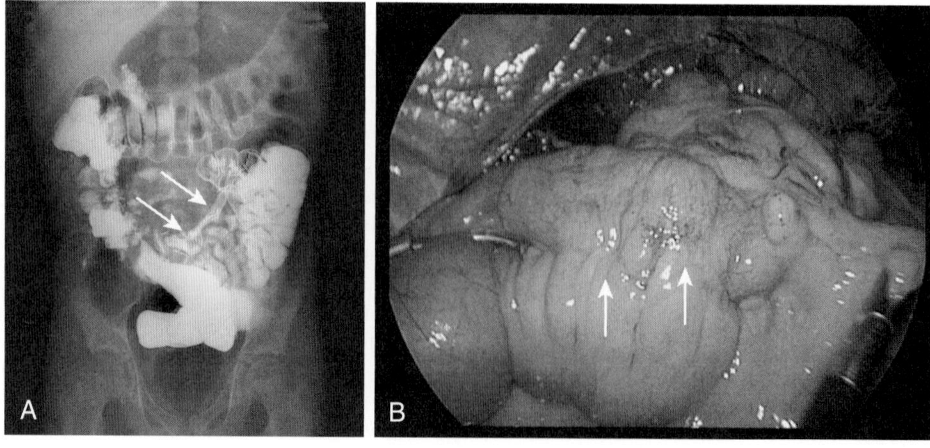

Figure 42-2. A, This upper gastrointestinal and small bowel follow-through contrast study shows a significant stricture (*arrows*) of the terminal ileum in a patient with persistent and symptomatic Crohn's disease despite medical therapy. **B,** The laparoscopic view shows active inflammation with creeping fat (*arrows*) along the terminal ileum in this patient.

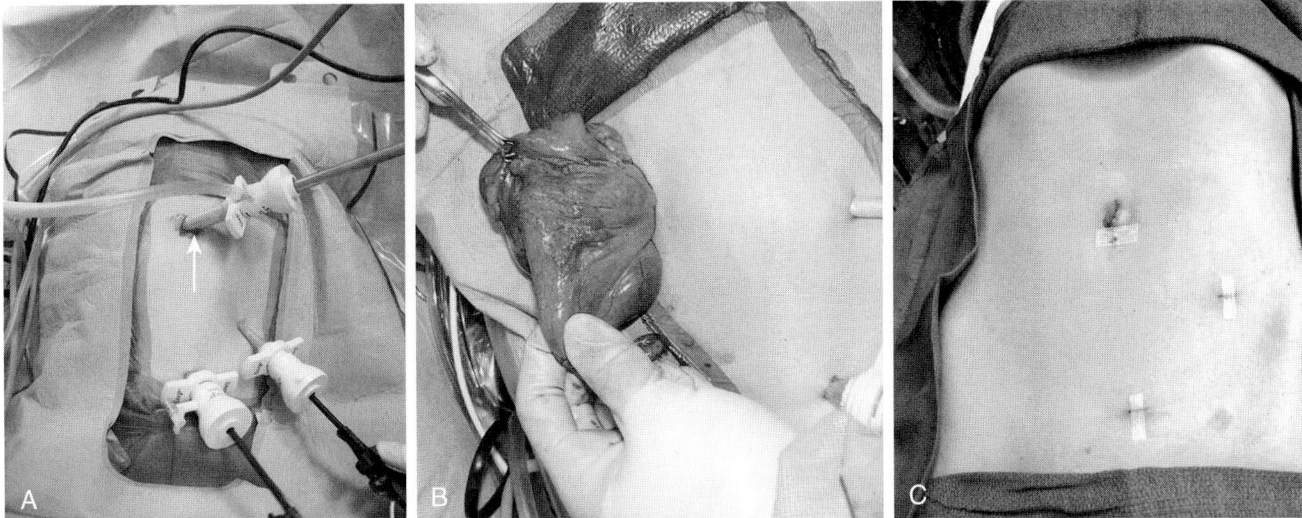

Figure 42-3. **A,** The port placement for a patient undergoing a laparoscopic ileocolectomy is seen. A 12-mm port is placed in the umbilicus (*arrow*), and two 5-mm ports are introduced in the left lower abdomen and suprapubic area. **B,** The diseased small bowel has been exteriorized through the umbilicus for an extracorporeal resection and anastomosis. Note the inflamed bowel and creeping fat in the exteriorized portion of the small bowel. **C,** The appearance of the incisions after the laparoscopic ileocolectomy. The intestinal resection and anastomosis was performed extracorporeally through the umbilical incision.

Ileocecal Resection

Pediatric surgeons most often perform ileocecal resections when operating for CD. This disease pattern is most likely to be associated with clear margins and an excellent disease-free interval. The need for a stoma is not likely, and postoperative complications are less likely than with colonic, pelvic, or long segment disease.

Laparoscopic-assisted surgery obviates the issue of where to make the incision.[40] Repeat laparoscopy is also feasible. The degree of obstruction, the presence of intraperitoneal adhesions, or a retroperitoneal, penetrating mass, along with the persistence of the surgeon, will determine the success of the laparoscopic approach. Intestinal reconstruction is accomplished using either an intracorporeal anastomosis or a laparoscopic-assisted technique with extraction of the bowel through one of the incisions for anastomosis or stricturoplasty (Fig. 42-3). In one small series, the laparoscopic approach resulted in longer recurrence-free intervals.[41] However, given consistent recurrence rates over time, it is possible that concomitant advances in medical management may have decreased recurrence in the short term.

An important principle of CD surgery is to create a widely patent anastomosis. Patients with ileocolic resections are natural candidates for a stapled side-to-side anastomosis that can be twice as large as the end-to-end technique (Fig. 42-4). Studies of stapled versus hand-sewn anastomoses have shown improved recurrence-free intervals using the stapler.[42,43] A similar technique is now recommended for other small bowel anastomoses. Although such widely patent anastomoses may be expected to reflux colonic contents into the small bowel, whether this colonic reflux has a detrimental effect on growing children is unknown. Caution should be exercised in younger children in whom issues of growth and development are paramount.

Small Intestine Surgery

Open or laparoscopic segmental resection is the standard approach to limited small intestine disease. The principles are identical to ileocecal resection. However,

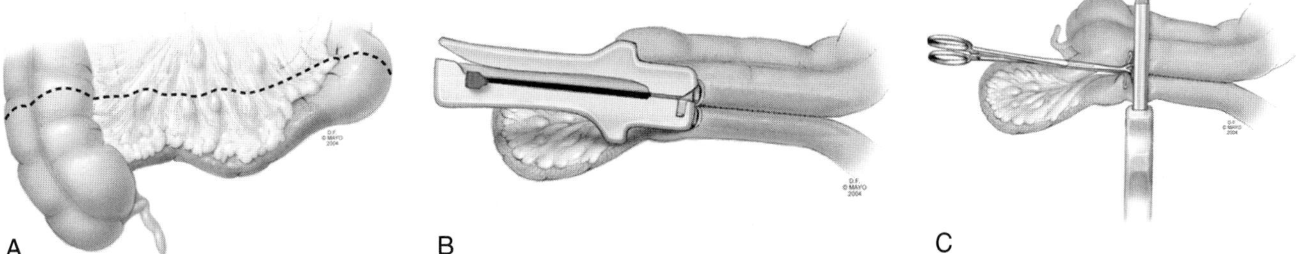

Figure 42-4. Patients undergoing an ileocolic resection are ideal candidates for a stapled side-to-side anastomosis that can be twice as large as an end-to-end anastomosis. **A,** The mesentery is divided to visually normal bowel. **B,** The normal-appearing proximal ileum is then anastomosed to the normal-appearing ascending colon using a long linear stapler. **C,** The diseased ileocecal region is then resected. A second application of the stapler is utilized, if needed.

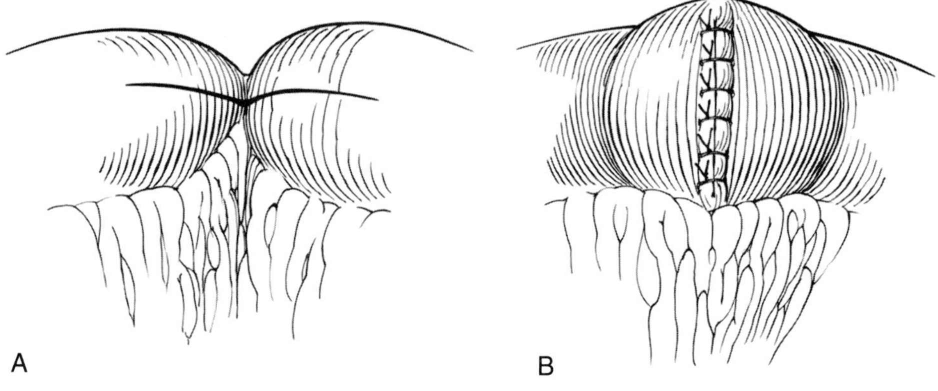

Figure 42-5. This schematic depicts a Heineke-Mikulicz strictureplasty for a very short segment of active disease or for fibrotic strictures in a patient with multicentric Crohn's disease. The incision that transverses the stricture (**A**) is then closed in a vertical direction (**B**) to enlarge the intestinal lumen.

the opportunity for such procedures is less due to a decreased incidence of this disease pattern and the tendency for small intestinal disease to be multifocal.

Strictureplasty for active disease, as well as for fibrotic strictures, remains an excellent option for patients with multicentric activity. The length of the stricture and the noninflammatory nature of the obstruction are the two strongest factors determining success.[44] Such length-sparing procedures are particularly attractive for children with extensive disease and skip areas.[45] There are no data yet to support the relative contraindication of leaving persistent disease behind in developing children. Adverse effects on growth and the risk of malignancy have not been quantified.[46,47]

The strictureplasty technique resembles a Heineke-Mikulicz pyloroplasty (Fig. 42-5). The procedure is best suited for short fibrotic strictures less than 10 cm in length without surrounding inflammation and adjacent normal bowel.[48] The reoperative rate for strictureplasty approaches 25% and 30% at 5 and 10 years, respectively.[49] A meta-analysis suggests the Finney technique may have a lower recurrence rate.[50]

Most pediatric studies demonstrate improved growth velocity after resection of all disease.[37,38,51] The increased morbidity and recurrence rates of stricturoplasty suggest that selective use for isolated short segments is the best approach.[44]

Colonic Resection

Because refractory disease is the main operative indication for Crohn's colitis, the decision to operate represents a balance between the effects of ongoing therapy and the consequences of resection. Crohn's colitis represents the highest risk for a permanent ileostomy. The 20-year risk of needing a stoma ranges from 14% to 44%.[19,38] This risk increases in children with significant rectal and perianal inflammation,[37] high pediatric CD activity index scores, and female gender.[36,38,52] On the other hand, a history of long-standing disease before operation may reduce this risk.[20,38] Data from large studies (that include adult patients) indicate that patients with colonic CD without major ileal or rectal involvement may experience similar success with bowel-sparing procedures as patients with isolated small bowel disease.[36,53] Furthermore, there is insufficient evidence that infliximab or other immunotherapies have reduced the need for permanent stomas. However, these therapies do offer hope for temporary bowel-sparing procedures that may improve the quality of life.

Segmental Resections

Segmental resections of the colon involve modifications of right and left hemicolectomies with primary reanastomosis. These procedures are ideal for laparoscopic-assisted mobilization, resection, and reanastomosis, depending on the degree of scarring and mesenteric mobility.[54] The affected portion of the colon is mobilized and resected to grossly normal margins. A primary ileocolonic or colocolonic anastomosis is then performed. However, long-term follow-up of children undergoing segmental colonic procedures report high recurrence rates, and a permanent ileostomy rate of 36% to 50%.[55,56] Despite nearly universal recurrence, 60% of pediatric surgeons surveyed in the United Kingdom favored segmental resection over total colectomy.[57] This optimism may be based on recent studies that indicate a trend toward decreased postoperative recurrence and increased salvage rates after colonic resections. Long-lasting remissions are most likely in patients with minimal or no anorectal disease.[36,53,54]

These results are similar to a large study of 84 patients undergoing segmental colonic resection.[33] In that study, with a follow-up of 9 years, 16% had a permanent ileostomy. The risk of colonic recurrence after segmental resection was 20% at 5 years and 35% at 10 years, substantially lower than a similar study from the Mayo Clinic (55%).[58] Of the 26 patients undergoing segmental resections, repeat resections were possible in 17 whereas colectomy with ileorectal anastomosis occurred in 5. The segmental colonic resections included 55% right-sided procedures and 40% left-sided operations and a combination of the two in 5%. The anastomotic leak rate was 7%, which is similar to other reports. Whether the resection margin is positive for disease has no effect on the leak rate or recurrence.[36]

Strictureplasty is not recommended for colonic involvement because of the cancer risk. Stricture disease is difficult to survey, and biopsy specimens may not be representative.

Total Colectomy with Ileorectal Anastomosis

For children with pancolonic disease, an ileorectal anastomosis is performed primarily or as a staged procedure depending on the indication for operation.[34,51] Emergent colectomy for life-threatening complications such as hemorrhage, sepsis, or perforation precludes immediate reconstruction. When an ileostomy is created, it is wise to leave a generous rectal stump. The bowel is usually divided with a stapler, preserving a portion of the sigmoid colon and rectum when possible. The proximal stapled end of rectum or sigmoid is attached to the anterior fascia for ease of identification 3 to 6 months later. Without significant attachment to the anterior abdominal wall, most stumps will retract well into the pelvis and require additional time for mobilization at the second operation.

When an ileorectal anastomosis is possible, less than 20% of patients with mild to moderate rectal disease progress to completion proctocolectomy.[59] Again, the significance of preexisting rectal or perianal disease is the highest predictor for failure.

There does not appear to be a linear relationship between the severity of disease and failure of the rectum, unless there is a significant lack of distensibility of the rectal wall.[60] Similarly, perianal involvement, if responsive to treatment, does not necessarily predict a poor outcome.[37] Significant ileal disease predicts a higher rate of recurrence, but the rectal failure is more related to the colonic disease rather than the small bowel involvement. Patients are able to undergo re-resection of the small bowel with repeat ileorectal anastomoses to preserve the intestinal tract.[58]

Ileal Pouch Anal Anastomosis

Most patients with chronic CD undergoing an ileal pouch/anal anastomosis (IPAA) were initially misdiagnosed as having CUC or came to operation with the diagnosis of indeterminate colitis. There is a much higher rate of serious complications after this procedure. Families may expect repeat visits for anal dilation or control of perianal disease. Short-term success may not predict long-term outcome. Patients with indeterminate colitis may expect good functional outcome in 73% to 85% of cases compared with 89% for CUC.[61] Known CD patients have a failure rate of at least 45%.[62]

Proctocolectomy with End Ileostomy

Complete removal of the colon and rectum with establishment of an end ileostomy carries the lowest rate of surgical recurrence in patients with Crohn's colitis.[19] Complications requiring surgery still occur at the stoma, but this option remains the best choice for patients with extensive colonic disease that involves the rectum and the anus. Perianal disease portends a poor outcome for more limited colon resections.[37] Although families understand the prognosis, they may prefer a staged approach without a permanent ileostomy for as long as possible. In centers advocating bowel-sparing procedures, proctocolectomy with end ileostomy is performed as an initial procedure in approximately 20% of patients.[36,53]

Removal of the residual rectal stump via an abdominoperineal approach is reserved for patients with the most resistant disease.[63] Management of the perineal wound can be particularly problematic. A standard intersphincteric proctectomy is performed with a secure water-tight closure of the pelvic floor and placement of vascularized tissue, such as omentum. It is important to separate the remaining small bowel from the pelvic floor to reduce the possibility of perineal fistulas. The perineal wound is closed over a catheter irrigation system placed into the pelvis from the perineum. The catheter is passed through the ischiorectal fossa and levator musculature to irrigate and drain the pelvis. The technical challenge of such procedures is surpassed only by the difficulty of caring for a nonhealing perineal wound. Multiple return visits for debridement, packing, and curettage may be necessary. Definitive closure with myocutaneous flaps can still have high recurrence rates.

Anorectal Disease

Almost two thirds of patients with CD will develop perianal complications.[64] Most develop within 10 years of intestinal symptom onset, and 25% occur as the first sign of disease.[65] Symptoms are most pronounced in children whose colonic disease is anorectal. These children form a distinct genetic subtype identified on chromosome 5.[66]

The most common conditions are fistula-in-ano, anal fissures, and hypertrophy of the perianal skin.[67] These conditions combine to produce painful lesions that drain, bleed, and develop recurrent abscesses. Anal sphincter spasm complicates their presentation. Ongoing surveillance of symptoms is necessary for the early identification of surgical conditions. Perianal sepsis may progress to severe regional infection, including gangrene. Fortunately, complications are rare, because most interventions are performed in a timely fashion.[68,69]

Should there be a question of more extensive fistulization, magnetic resonance imaging is the investigation of choice. It is a highly sensitive (97%) and specific (100%) tool for detection of fistulas and quantification of surgical success.[70] Magnetic resonance fistulography is superior to endoanal ultrasonography but is more expensive and lacks the advantage of portability. The ultrasound probe can be utilized in the examination room, but the procedure can be quite painful.[71]

Examination and treatment is best performed under anesthesia. This allows for confirmation of the findings, endoscopy of the distal rectum, and identification of the internal fistulous openings. Drainage of abscesses and surgical debridement of chronic cavities are also important. In teenage girls with CD, a Bartholin cyst should be diagnosed cautiously. Most vaginal or vulvar masses are the result of perianal fistulization rather than a separate disease process.

After the treatment has been established, local wound care remains an important part of symptom relief. Perianal hygiene with daily wound therapy, including debridement and application of barrier creams and ointments, is effective. Patients may purchase or create specialized cushions for sitting. Bowel management is also helpful for constipation or diarrhea.

A draining seton suture is effective for prevention of abscess and recurrent pain.[67] The goal is to produce a well-established draining tract without obstruction or sepsis. The seton is placed in a noncutting fashion using a soft silicon vessel loop or monofilament suture (Fig. 42-6). With the addition of immune and biologic therapy, the seton suture technique provides excellent control of disease and will lead to healing in most circumstances.[72]

Injection of "fibrin glue" into the remaining fistula tract has also been moderately successful.[73] The internal fistula opening may be sutured closed at the time of "fibrin glue" injection. There should be minimal to no granulation tissue left within the tract. Should a cavity persist, the seton suture technique affords the best chance for healing.

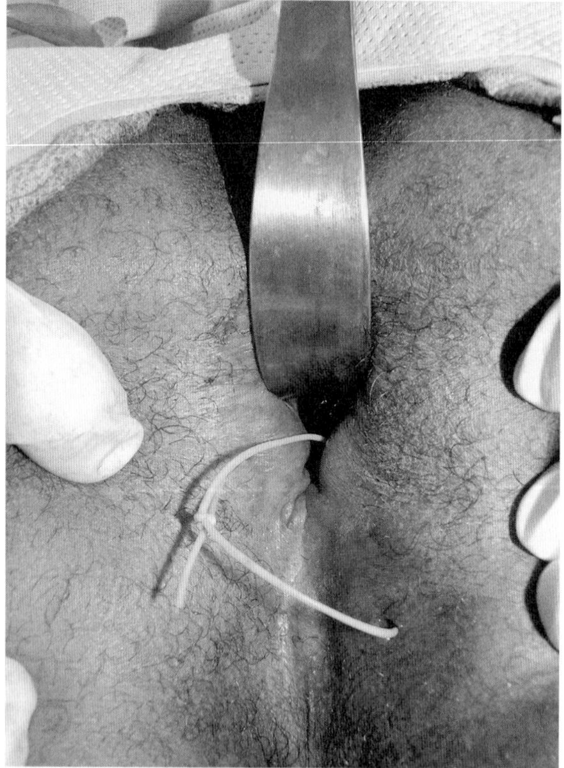

Figure 42-6. This teenager with refractory Crohn's disease developed a perianal abscess that was quite painful. Examination under anesthesia confirmed the fistula and underlying abscess that was drained. A soft, noncutting silicon vessel loop (seton) was then placed. This technique allows excellent control of the perianal disease and leads to healing in most circumstances.

Fistulotomy is the definitive procedure for a persistent anal fistula. Healing occurs in 73% to 81% of patients with low fistulas laid open in the traditional fashion.[68] The risk of incontinence and poor wound healing is high in children with a transsphincteric or complex fistula. If there has been a good response to medical therapy, advancement flaps may be a reasonable consideration. Rectal mucosal flaps preserve continence and provide healing in 64% to 71% of patients with transsphincteric abscesses. In this setting, ileostomy is often required for healing.[67,74]

Rectovaginal fistulas may also be cured with advancement flaps. In one study, healing was successful in 54% of patients.[75] After reoperation, the success rate increased to 60% during follow-up of 5 years. A transvaginal approach is recommended for those with persistent rectal disease. Success rates of 90% may be achieved with this approach in patients with controlled disease.[67] Rectal dissection is also successful when the disease has improved after fecal diversion. Cutaneous advancement flaps for persistent mucosal disease have also been advocated. Under the best of circumstances, a 70% healing rate may be possible.[76]

Recurrent Crohn's Disease

Recurrence at the anastomosis is a feature of the disease process rather than the presence of microscopic residual disease at the margins. Grossly negative resection margins are all that is necessary for an initial success.[51,77] Symptomatic recurrence is usually preceded by a long interval of subclinical disease at the resection margin. Symptom onset can be expected to occur earlier for patients with diffuse intestinal disease, perianal CD, and those who had postoperative surgical complications.[78] At least 85% of surgical patients have histologic evidence of recurrence by 3 years after surgery. The high prevalence of microscopic disease does not mean all postoperative patients will develop endoscopically obvious lesions, nor does endoscopic recurrence necessarily mean reoperation is imminent. Most studies report 10-year reoperative rates of approximately 50% for ileocolic disease and 45% each for isolated colonic or small bowel CD.[17,37]

Initial perforation developing from CD represents a group that is at high risk for perforation again. The absolute risk of recurrence is similar to obstructing CD.[79] Older adolescents who smoke represent another high-risk group.

Indications for reoperation are based on the intensity of symptoms, treatment toxicity, and interference with quality of life.

Subfertility

Subfertility was thought to be a complication of the underlying disease. Recent studies have shown a stronger correlation to operative sequelae rather than the disease process itself.[80] Perianal disease, dyspareunia, and the risk of incontinence may reduce the desire for intercourse. Tubal factors are also extremely important. There is evidence that fertility may be reduced by as much as 80% to 90% after ileoanal procedures. The most important factors are the location of the dissection and the development of pelvic sepsis. Patients with polyposis or those undergoing appendectomy for uncomplicated appendicitis do not share the same tubal infertility risks as patients undergoing deep pelvic procedures for CD or CUC. Although colon resection and ileorectal anastomosis for CD remain an excellent operation, care should be taken to reperitonealize the pelvis and protect the fallopian tubes from damage.[81-83]

CHRONIC ULCERATIVE COLITIS

The surgical options for children with CUC are well studied, and the expectation for disease eradication is high. Complete surgical resection leaves little chance of recurrence unless some disease has been left behind. Segmental resection of the most involved portion of the colon is not recommended. In general, more limited forms of CUC respond well to medication whereas those with refractory pancolitis require proctocolectomy.

Optimal surgical management of pediatric patients includes restoration of bowel function after removal of the colon and rectum.[84-86] Significant postoperative complications and pouch failures still occur in patients treated in high volume centers. Nevertheless, children do well despite the high morbidity.[87]

The timing of operation is a balance between the risk of ongoing disease and the risk of complications associated with proctocolectomy. Laparoscopic procedures have the potential to improve outcome by reducing perioperative morbidity and improving social adaptation important to developing teenagers.[88] Questions concerning the patient's quality of life are paramount. Because the long-term results of pouch function and the effects of the operation on the patient's life are uncertain, families and their physicians may be hesitant to risk the possibility of the need for a permanent ileostomy.

Medical Therapy

In contrast to CD, the incidence and presentation of CUC in childhood is stable. Population studies identify 1 child per 100,000 with disease, compared with CD, which is 2 to 4/100,000.[5,6,89] As noted previously, a higher proportion of children with CD now present with pancolitis. The colonic predilection for CD means a child with pancolitis undergoing an ileoanal procedure could have CD.[4,10] These issues and the differentiating factors have been discussed previously.

The need for surgery for CUC is much less than with CD. Less than half of affected patients will require colectomy during their lifetime. The increased incidence of pancolitis in childhood produces relatively more treatment resistance, but durable remissions and good medical control is still possible. The introduction of TNF-α inhibitors is the latest alternative to surgery. Despite these advances, early involvement of the surgical team to discuss the surgical options and outcomes is important for an informed decision by the parents.

CUC is a cyclic disease characterized by flares and remission. Aminosalicylates and corticosteroids are the foundation of therapy. Immune modulation with azathioprine, mercaptopurine, and cyclosporine form a second line of therapy that is augmented by the TNF inhibitors infliximab and adalimumab.[90] Surgical therapy is needed in patients whose disease is resistant to these medications.

Further investigation into genetic and environmental factors may produce innovative new therapies. The high rate of familial disease with IBD in children makes this population ideal for future study of gene-targeted therapy. Environmental factors also play a role, especially the bacterial environment and the unusually protective association of appendectomy. The reproducible correlation of tobacco use and IBD is not only of great interest to parents, but may figure prominently in amelioration of pouchitis.[91-93]

Indications for Operation

Refractory disease, defined as treatment resistance or the inability to wean from corticosteroids, is the most common indication for operation. Children are particularly sensitive to long-term corticosteroid therapy. Not only are there implications for growth and development, but bone mineralization and the risk of fracture are important considerations for the active child.[3] Middle and high school adolescents are acutely aware of their social limitations and look to surgery to restore a more normal life. Preoperative discussions center on the expected quality of life and psychosocial issues associated with bowel functional outcome.

In contrast to adults, acute-onset, unremitting, fulminant colitis is a presentation more common in children.[4,6] Most of these desperately ill children require urgent colectomy and ileostomy. Pouch reconstruction is deferred for several months. The consistent occurrence of this pattern suggests a genetic or immune etiology. Other indications for operation include medication toxicity, growth retardation, and carcinoma prophylaxis. Quality of life instruments may help guide surgical decision-making.

Before operation, children are evaluated for the presence of toxic colitis, anemia, hypoalbuminemia, elevated C-reactive protein levels, and coagulopathic states.[94-96] Correction of mild abnormalities should not preclude complete reconstruction, but seriously ill children should have a staged procedure. Recent data from adult studies suggest a deleterious effect of infliximab on pouch healing.[97] A delay in constructing the pouch is suggested when infliximab has been administered within 2 months of operation.

Mechanical bowel preparation is beneficial when possible. Perioperative intravenous antibiotics are administered within 1 hour of surgery and continued postoperatively at the surgeon's discretion. Preoperative oral (luminal) antibiotics are no longer necessary.

Patients who are corticosteroid dependent require a "steroid prep" that includes a high initial bolus of intravenous corticosteroids followed by a postoperative taper over several weeks or months. When truncal obesity precludes safe pouch construction, weight reduction is discussed as a postoperative bridge to successful restoration of function. Laparoscopy is size independent and recommended in such patients.[94] Currently, many centers utilize a laparoscopic-assisted approach.[98] Preoperative evaluation of the child's abdomen helps determine whether a Pfannenstiel or periumbilical incision is most appropriate for specimen removal and pouch construction.

Choice of Operation

The colectomy may be accomplished laparoscopically, be laparoscopically-assisted, or via an open approach. The reconstruction can occur in one, two, or three stages, and with or without a variety of pouches that are stapled or hand sewn to the anus. These choices reflect the need to tailor the operative approach to the individual needs of the patient.

For children with severe refractory disease, laparoscopic colectomy and end ileostomy is a good option. The colon is removed through the ileostomy or umbilical cannula site. Newer intracorporeal ligating devices have reduced the amount of mesenteric manipulation, limiting the risk of bleeding or perforation in critically ill children. Postoperative recovery is still prolonged owing to the patient's condition, but the procedure is effective and safe. The ensuing months allow for recovery, tapering of corticosteroid therapy, and differentiation from Crohn's disease. Later, ileal pouch construction may be performed without an ileostomy provided there are no technical concerns, such as bleeding or tension on the anastomosis. Three-stage procedures have become less common but remain an option for some patients undergoing emergent colectomy.[99]

Colectomy and immediate reconstruction is possible for most children with stable, but corticosteroid-dependent disease. A diverting loop ileostomy is usually performed, followed by ileostomy closure 6 to 8 weeks later as the final procedure. Despite the relatively short time with a stoma, teens may be concerned about returning to school and may want to prolong the decision for the initial colectomy. Ironically, any delay in operation may actually increase the need for a stoma because the corticosteroid doses may need to be increased concomitantly.

An informed family may present for operation at an earlier stage of disease to avoid the need for ileostomy. Although such an approach is possible in highly selected patients with low corticosteroid exposure and normal nutritional parameters, single-stage procedures should be unusual. An anastomotic leak and pelvic sepsis are too high a risk in most children.[88,98,100]

Although the double-stapled ileoanal anastomosis is the standard technique for adults and older adolescents undergoing reconstruction,[99-101] there is a short segment of involved mucosa that requires surveillance. Small children may require a hand-sewn

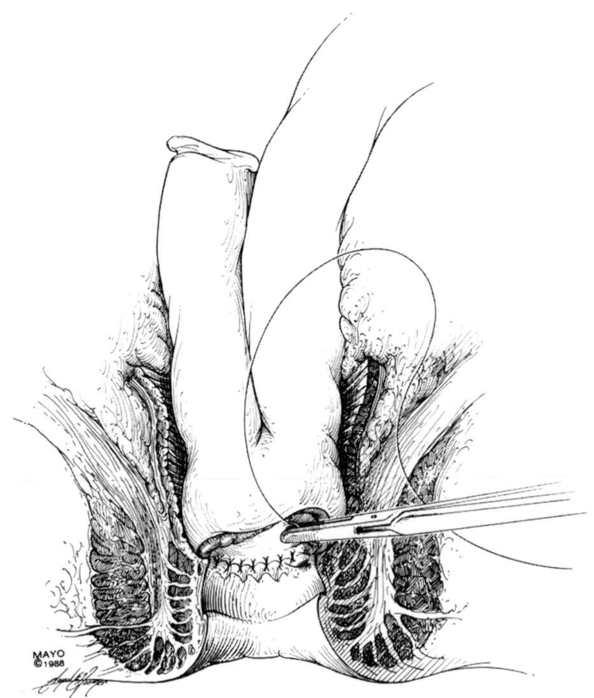

Figure 42-7. In small patients, the double-stapled ileoanal anastomosis using the endoscopic circular stapler may not be possible. Also, some surgeons prefer the hand-sewn ileoanal anastomosis. The rectal mucosectomy begins approximately 5 mm above the dentate line and continues proximally to the completed pelvic dissection. The J-pouch is then pulled through the muscle cuff and anastomosed to the anal mucosa, just above the dentate line with interrupted sutures. (Copyrighted and used with permission of Mayo Foundation for Medical Education and Research, all rights reserved.)

anastomosis with similar concerns for retained islands of mucosa and the later development of cuff adenocarcinoma (Fig. 42-7).[102] Pediatric surgeons caring for children with Hirschsprung's disease have extensive experience with mucosectomy and hand-sewn coloanal anastomosis. It is expected that this experience will help reduce this risk in children.

Not all children require an ileal pouch. The success of straight ileoanal procedures is a testimony to the tremendous long-term adaptability of children.[94,103] Relatively equivalent stool frequencies are achieved with fewer reports of pouchitis. The postoperative time necessary to achieve a reasonable stool frequency is significantly longer than in those children with pouch construction. Therefore, ileal J-pouches have become the standard technique for reconstruction in children. Other methods, such as the S-, W-, and lateral pouches, have also been utilized in leading pediatric centers.[96] Whereas each has its advocates and may be necessary in certain situations, the J-pouch is the easiest to construct and can be performed laparoscopically.[91,98,99,104]

Laparoscopic Technique

The laparoscopic approach utilizes a standard laparoscopic total abdominal colectomy followed by a laparoscopic proctectomy. The patient is positioned in a low lithotomy position and prepared for synchronous

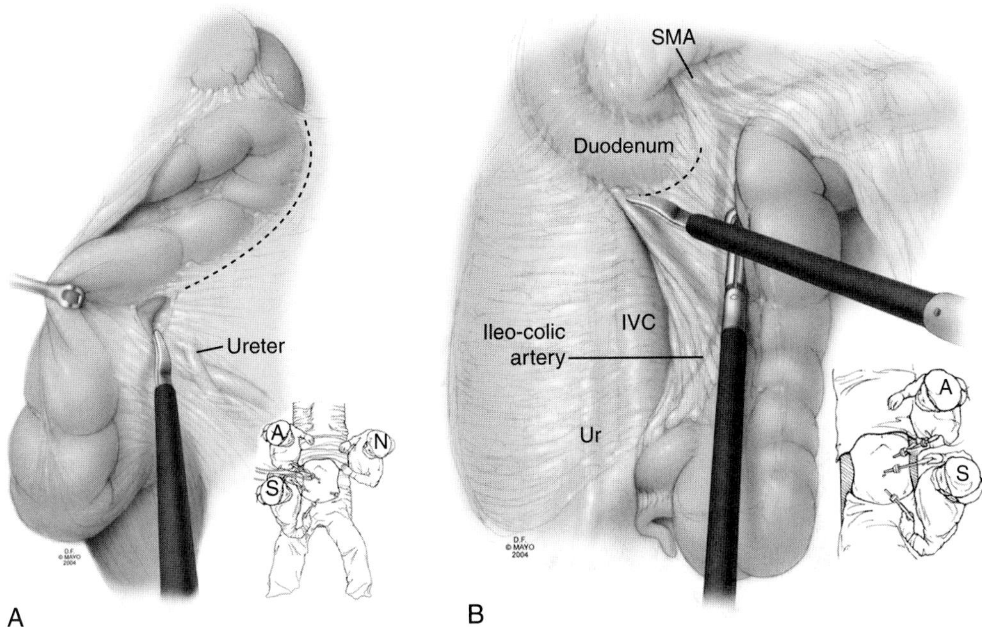

Figure 42-8. In a child undergoing a laparoscopic colectomy and ileoanal anastomosis at the same setting, the patient is placed in a low lithotomy position and prepared for synchronous abdominal and perineal procedures. **A,** For mobilization of the upper rectum and left colon, the surgeon (S) can stand along the patient's right lower abdomen (see *inset*) or between the patient's legs. The left lateral peritoneal attachments are then divided sharply, taking care not to injure the left ureter. **B,** For mobilization of the right colon, a similar technique is employed. The *inset* show the surgeon (S) and assistant (A) positioned along the patient's left side. Again, the location of the right ureter is important. N, scrub nurse. (Copyrighted and used with permission of Mayo Foundation for Medical Education and Research, all rights reserved.)

abdominal and perineal procedures. The initial cannula is placed in the umbilicus. After diagnostic laparoscopy, three additional ports are inserted under direct vision. If desired by the surgeon, the cannula sites can be situated such that they are incorporated within a future Pfannenstiel incision, depending on the body habitus of the patient. The stoma site should be marked preoperatively by the enterostomal therapist. The left and right lateral peritoneal attachments of the colon are mobilized, and mesenteric windows are created (Fig. 42-8). The omentum is preserved by entering the lesser sac and freeing the anterior attachments from the transverse colon. The mesocolon is then divided intracorporeally (Fig. 42-9). In older children, the proctectomy can be completely performed laparoscopically, with division of the rectum just above the level of the levator complex using a roticulating laparoscopic stapler. In younger or smaller children, when the pelvis is too narrow or too small to allow for the insertion of a roticulating stapler down to the level of the levators, the rectum can be divided at a location that will allow for a stapled transection. In a three-stage procedure, the specimen is removed through the ileostomy site and an end stoma is created. For a two-stage operation, the remainder of the laparoscopic dissection is completed distal to the level of the levator complex and the rectum is everted out through the anus. After everting the rectum out the anus, the rectum is divided externally using a standard stapler. The small anal cuff is then inverted back into the pelvis. The colon and rectum are removed either transanally or through an enlarged umbilical incision, or at the site of the

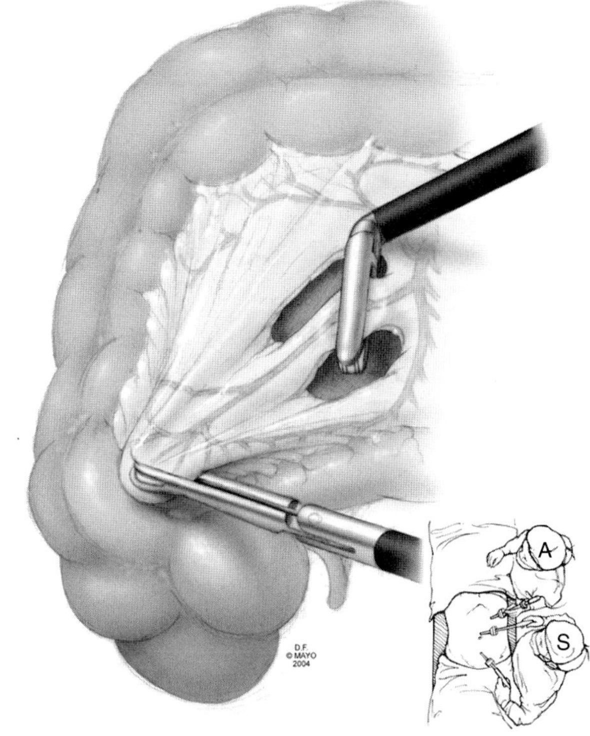

Figure 42-9. Once the right and left peritoneal attachments are incised, mesenteric windows are created for application of the stapler, as seen in this schematic. Other devices such as the ultrasonic scalpel and Ligasure can also be used, especially in patients with a thin mesentery. Again, it is often advantageous for the surgeon (S) to stand between the patient's legs or along the patient's left side as shown in the *inset*. A, assistant. (Copyrighted and used with permission of Mayo Foundation for Medical Education and Research, all rights reserved.)

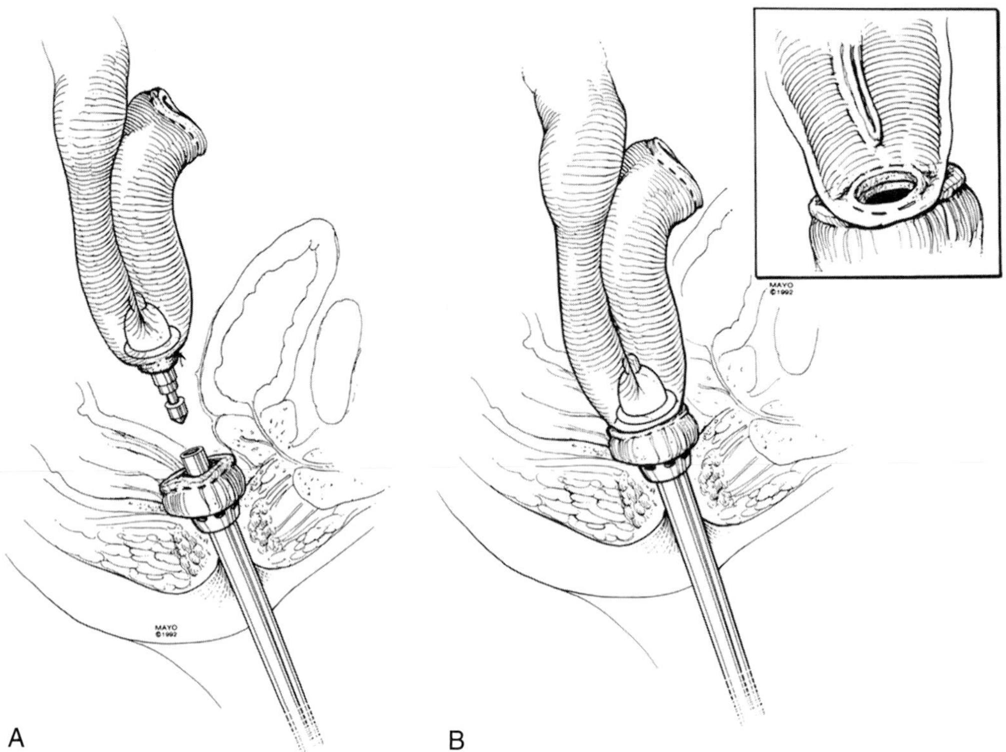

Figure 42-10. The double-stapled technique for the pouch/anal anastomosis has shown similar results as the hand-sewn technique. **A,** The anvil has been placed into the pouch and is being brought close to the circular stapler, which has been introduced through the anus. **B,** The anus and pouch have been approximated and the circled, stapled anastomosis performed (*inset*). There is usually about a 5-mm to 1-cm cuff of native rectal mucosa remaining that requires lifetime surveillance. (Copyrighted and used with permission of Mayo Foundation for Medical Education and Research, all rights reserved.)

protecting ileostomy. The J-pouch is created using a stapled technique through an enlarged umbilical incision, the ileostomy site, or a low suprapubic incision. The J-pouch can be stapled to the anal cuff using an appropriately sized circular endoscopic stapler or hand sewn, depending on surgeon preference (Fig. 42-10). A diverting loop ileostomy is created and exteriorized at one of the port sites in the right lower quadrant.

The laparoscopic approach using a circular endoscopic stapler for creation of the pouch/anal anastomosis has shown similar results as the hand-sewn technique. However, in one report, the double-staple technique resulted in less night-time soiling and produced better postproctectomy anal resting pressures.[105]

On occasion, some children have insufficient mesenteric length to safely perform an ileoanal anastomosis. Sufficient length can be measured by stretching the folded terminal ileum over the pubis. An adequate length is reliably predicted if the terminal ileum extends beyond the inferior margin of the symphysis. Body habitus and the influence of corticosteroids can predispose patients to mesenteric infiltration and edema. Also, uncontrolled disease activity may temporarily shorten the mesentery by reducing elasticity and increasing fragility. In these circumstances, it is usually best not to perform the ileoanal anastomosis at the time of the colectomy.

Several options are available for patients without adequate mesenteric length for primary pull-through. A straight ileoanal anastomosis has acceptable long-term functional results in children. Storage capacity is limited but improves over the ensuing years to provide a good quality of life.[94] Creation of an S-pouch is an alternative to the use of a J-pouch in selected patients. However, prior experience with S-pouch creation and an understanding of the optimal length of the efferent limb is essential for good results.[106]

Some patients will have already undergone a rectal mucosectomy before discovering the ileum will not reach the anus. An ileostomy is then created at the first stage. At the second stage, reoperation is more difficult owing to scarring in the muscle cuff. The pelvic dissection can be aided by inserting a dilator through the anus to identify the top of the muscle cuff. The cuff is then opened farther and expanded to allow passage of the pouch. It is usually necessary to split the muscle cuff posteriorly. It is important to preserve the deep pelvic nerves by staying within the cuff. If the scarring is too intense, partial cuff resection can be performed transabdominally beginning at the distal extent of the prior dissection.

After the operation, total parenteral nutrition is continued, especially for children who had fulminant colitis preoperatively. Once a diet is tolerated, antibiotics are discontinued and the corticosteroid dosage is tapered. Ileostomy dysfunction is common. Problems include prolapse, stenosis, and bleeding. Preoperative counseling is suggested for children concerned about returning to school with a stoma. Most children are capable of engaging in school activities and sports within 3 to 4 weeks of the operation, but are reluctant to do so. Contact with peers who have undergone operations for CUC is helpful.

Postoperative Course

There is a persistently high (30%-66%) incidence of perioperative complications.[107] Infection, obstruction, and ileoanal anastomotic strictures predominate along with the temporary, but sometimes acute, complications associated with the ileostomy. The practice of at-home anal dilation is difficult in children with chronic disease. Many opt for outpatient procedures under sedation.

Long-term complications center on the high rate of pouchitis and chronic problems with the ileoanal anastomosis.

Pouchitis

Pouchitis is a nonspecific mucosal inflammation that develops in 26% to 47% of children postoperatively. The incidence increases with longer follow-up.[86,107] Each episode is characterized by increased stool frequency, night-time incontinence, pain, urgency, and bleeding. Extraintestinal symptoms include arthralgias and erythema nodosum. Pouchitis is not life threatening nor is it usually life limiting. However, the symptoms represent the perception of return of disease. Patients feel ill, and their quality of life is affected.[108-110]

Treatment is directed at identifying causative factors and symptom relief. Patients with persistent disease should be investigated for anal stricture, retained rectal mucosa, small volume pouch, medication-induced irritability, and CD.[70] These conditions require a different therapeutic approach than idiopathic pouchitis.[104,111] Children without risk factors usually respond to oral antibiotics, and symptomatic improvement is generally seen within 12 to 24 hours of therapy with oral metronidazole or ciprofloxacin. A gradual reduction in the dose is possible within days of treatment.

Chronic pouchitis is controlled with low-dose antibiotics that may be alternated on a weekly or monthly schedule. Amoxicillin and vancomycin have also been successful. Probiotics and other measures have been tried for pouchitis, but their effectiveness remains in question.[112] Investigation of lifestyle and over-the-counter medication usage is important when treating pouchitis. Smoking, caffeine use, stress, and nonsteroidal anti-inflammatory drugs contribute to pouch irritability.

Approximately 10% of ileoanal procedures fail secondary to severe pouchitis that is resistant to medical therapy,[113] and pouch excision may be necessary. Chronic antibiotic use has been tried in an attempt to avoid a permanent stoma. The long-term effects of years of low-dose antimicrobial agents in children have not been established. Dysplasia in chronically inflamed pouches has also been raised as a concern for children who have a long life expectancy. A relatively short-term follow-up study did not identify problems.[114]

Functional Outcome

Pediatric studies have identified lower incontinence rates and less frequent stooling than is seen in most adult studies.[85] Also, children score well when evaluated for functional outcomes, including night-time continence, completeness of defecation, and the lack of dietary restrictions. Importantly, the presence of postoperative surgical complications has not been shown to have a negative effect on functional outcome.[5,108] The two most common negative outcomes identified were chronic pouchitis and night-time incontinence.

Randomized trials investigating the laparoscopic approach in adults have demonstrated similar efficacy and safety compared with the open operation. These techniques have also been applied to children. Laparoscopic and laparoscopic-assisted proctocolectomy with ileal pouch/anal anastomosis (IPAA) began in the late 1990s. Preliminary data suggest functional outcomes are similar to those with the open approach.[85]

Quality of Life

A patient's quality of life after a major surgical procedure can be measured and correlates with bowel functional outcomes. A study of children undergoing IPAA procedures at our institution revealed normal assessment scores despite major surgery and change in bowel function.[86] Pouchitis and night-time stooling correlated with lower quality of life scores. Parental anxiety regarding their child's ongoing health remained higher than U.S. norms, reflecting a higher level of parental concern for the child's well-being. This anxiety did not dissipate over time.

Effect of Aging

Families often wonder if the good functional outcomes found in children will decline with age. A recent 15-year follow-up study has shown durable pouch function without a decline in continence or quality of life.[115] Follow-up studies in children will continue to be important for evaluating the real incidence of pouch failure and long-term quality of life.

Reoperation

The risk of pouch-related failure increases with time to approximately 10% at 10 years.[113] Technical complications with pouch construction and the ileoanal anastomosis are the most common reason for a poor outcome.[116] Early pelvic or anastomotic sepsis increases the failure rate by a factor of 5.[108] A pouch/anal anastomotic stricture can result in urgency, frequent bowel movements, inability to fully evacuate, night-time incontinence, and poor sleep. These secondary symptoms directly correlate with a poor quality of life.[86,100]

The risk of sepsis after ileoanal procedures decreases with increased surgeon experience. Identification of the complication before ileostomy closure allows for antibiotic management and percutaneous drainage of an abscess. Occasionally, multiple local procedures are necessary before stoma closure. Once eradicated, long-term pouch success rates are similar to those in patients who did not develop pelvic sepsis (92%).[108] Patients with severe infection requiring abdominal reoperation for infection control have a guarded outlook. More than 50% will lose their pouch, and fewer than one third have good long-term function. Similarly, 30% of patients with extensive anastomotic dehiscence have long-term failure, despite reoperation.[116] Fortunately, most of the anastomotic disruptions are localized, and minor revisions allow good long-term results.

Patients have reverted to ileostomy to avoid the ongoing symptoms of stool frequency, bleeding, mucus discharge, urgency, night-time incontinence, and extra-intestinal manifestations such as arthralgias and erythema nodosum. Prompt treatment will usually ameliorate these symptoms. Treatment resistance usually leads to a diagnostic workup for CD.

Intra-abdominal conditions above the level of the pouch are a rare cause of failure. Patients may have kinking at the small bowel/pouch interface or present with intermittent small bowel obstruction secondary to adhesions. Both of these conditions produce abdominal distention, cramping, and poor pouch evacuation. The difference in these symptoms from the usual pouch-associated symptoms of urgency and incontinence helps the surgeon differentiate these diagnoses.

When complications from the IPAA procedure become chronic, the quality of life for the patient is poor. Frequent defecation and loss of night-time control seriously impair the abilities of the adolescent or young adult to attend school or embark on a professional career.[86] These problems eventually outweigh the stigmata of an ileostomy. When surveyed, patients with permanent ileostomies still prefer a restorative pull-through, but have quality of life indicators similar to those without an ileostomy. It is helpful to set goals for therapy and establish a time line for re-evaluation. Although not ideal, an ileostomy remains an excellent long-term solution for patients with chronic problems after colectomy.[108,113]

Subfertility and Pregnancy

Studies have demonstrated decreased fertility in patients after proctocolectomy and IPAA.[82,83] Reperitonealization of the pelvis at the time of pouch construction is recommended to prevent entrapment of the fallopian tubes and ovaries. Pregnancy and vaginal delivery are possible and recommended for women after pouch procedures without serious pouch- or anastomosis-related complications. One review showed no difference in birth weight, pregnancy, or delivery complications before or after IPAA procedures.[117] However, there was a higher rate of planned cesarean sections and day-time stool frequency.

Indeterminate Colitis

Indeterminate colitis is a distinct clinical and pathologic entity diagnosed in 5% to 15% of patients requiring surgery for IBD. With long follow-up, these patients gradually differentiate into ulcerative colitis or Crohn's categories.[118] Also, there is greater morbidity after an IPAA procedure in patients with the diagnosis of indeterminate colitis. Adults with indeterminate colitis have a higher rate of serious postoperative complications (20%)[119] than those with CUC (3.5%-10%), but still less than patients with CD (35%).[108] The long-term success of IPAA for indeterminate colitis is 73% to 85% compared with 89% for CUC. These results make a fairly good case for IPAA in the setting of indeterminate colitis.[61] However, indeterminate colitis patients with features favoring CD may benefit from delayed IPAA 6 to 12 months after colectomy. Operative decisions are based on the age of the child, severity of disease, and the urgency of the operation. Surgeons who see a child younger than age 8 years with indeterminate colitis should proceed cautiously before full reconstruction.

INTESTINAL CANCER

Secondary Intestinal Cancer

Hematologic malignancy is the most common childhood cancer and is the most common cancer of the gastrointestinal tract as well. Small bowel lymphomas and colonic tumors, such as Burkitt's lymphoma of the ileocecal region, comprise 75% to 80% of intestinal malignancies in children. Two reports describing 82 pediatric gastrointestinal malignancies identified lymphoma as the only small bowel tumor and Burkitt's lymphoma as the major colonic tumor.[120,121] In these reviews, the remaining tumors were colorectal carcinoma and gastric sarcomas. Although appendiceal carcinoid was more common than lymphoma, carcinoma, or sarcoma, it was alternatively classified as benign or malignant and excluded in these reviews. Surgical therapy for lymphoma, when necessary, involves tissue diagnosis and treatment of complications such as perforation, obstruction, or stricture. With Burkitt's lymphoma, resection of all gross disease in the abdomen (intestine and mesentery) results in a limited chemotherapy regimen (6 weeks compared with 6 months) in the current Children's Oncology Group protocol.

Primary Intestinal Cancer

Adenocarcinoma

Colon cancer is the third most common cause of cancer-related deaths in adults. In children, the disease remains rare. Primary adenocarcinoma of the colon does occur in young adults, but most have a familial link or other special features. Pediatric surgeons are most concerned with prevention of this fatal condition. Surgery for children with familial polyposis syndromes is the most visible example of this approach. Other conditions that may require prophylactic resection include chronically active IBD (CUC and CD) and inherited colorectal cancer (hereditary nonpolyposis colorectal cancer [HNPCC] or Lynch syndrome). The genetics of these disorders are known, and some cases overlap. Mutations are found in the adenomatous polyposis coli (*APC*) tumor suppressor gene in the autosomal dominant form of polyposis and in the *MYH* repair gene for the recessive version. The *MYH* defect promotes somatic mutations in the tumor *APC* gene. Nonpolyposis cancer patients have mutations in the DNA mismatch repair genes, especially *MSH2, MLH1,* and *PMS2*.[122-124] Screening of children with a family history of early-onset colorectal cancer could uncover defects that lead to prophylactic colon resection. Because the entire colon mucosa is at risk, the best available procedure is total proctocolectomy with IPAA.

Children who progress from dysplasia to colorectal cancer tend to present with a late stage of disease and with the more aggressive subtypes (mucinous or poorly differentiated adenocarcinoma). In a recent small review of seven children from Italy, the overall survival at 5 years was 23%, despite the fact that it was possible to achieve total gross resection in 5 of 7 patients.[125] Only one patient is currently disease free.

Because there are not enough pediatric cases for separate clinical studies, treatment of pediatric colorectal cancer is based on adult clinical trials. The surgical principles of complete resection with clear margins and a wide regional node dissection apply. Most children receive postoperative chemotherapy. Neoadjuvant chemotherapy may salvage some unresectable tumors. Major chemotherapeutic agents include 5-fluorouracil, oxaliplatin, and irinotecan. Targeted therapies with bevacizumab and cetuximab are under investigation.[126] If possible, early screening of children from families with known colorectal malignancies may improve current results. Unfortunately, the poor prognosis in children continues to be based on an advanced stage of disease and the inability to achieve a complete resection.

Small bowel adenocarcinoma is so rare in children that only a few case reports exist.[127] Celiac disease in childhood has been reported to result in small intestine cancer or non-Hodgkin's lymphoma later in life.[128]

Inflammatory Bowel Disease

The risk of colorectal cancer with CUC is an indication for colectomy when the disease has been active for more than 10 years. The commonly quoted figure is an annual increase in cancer risk of 0.5% to 1% per year after 8 to 10 years of pancolitis.[129] A meta-analysis in children who developed CUC reported higher overall probabilities of cancer, which has been estimated at 5.5% at 10 years, 11% at 20 years, and 16% at 30 years.[130] Population-based estimates identify colon cancers arising two to three times more frequently in CUC patients.[131,132] These data influence surgical decision-making for families considering colectomy and IPAA during the teenage years. If colectomy is deferred, colonoscopic surveillance is mandatory. Patients at higher risk for developing colorectal cancer include those diagnosed at an early age and those with a family history of colon cancer, with findings of inflammatory pseudopolyps or strictures, or with the presence of sclerosing cholangitis.[130] In addition, removal of the colon does not completely remove the risk of disease. A stapled anastomosis preserves transitional mucosa that may later become dysplastic.[133] A hand-sewn anastomosis reduces this concern, but there are case reports of cancer developing in the retained rectal mucosa on the muscle cuff.[103]

The risk of adenocarcinoma developing in CD patients is less than in those with CUC or indeterminate colitis. In 1251 patients with CD followed in Stockholm County, Sweden, the cancer risk was 1.15 times higher than the general population.[134] This increase was mainly in small intestine cancer with a standardized morbidity ratio over 15. Patients with CD are also at higher risk for developing other intestinal malignancies, particularly lymphoma. Persistent perianal disease could predispose to squamous cell carcinoma as well.[135,136]

Familial Polyposis Syndromes

A summary of the childhood polyposis syndromes is found in Tables 42-1 and 42-2. Adenomatous polyps are by definition dysplastic and have a distinct propensity for malignant degeneration. The sheer number of polyps (sometimes in the thousands) combined with a long duration of illness leads to inevitable malignancy. Large polyps are more prone to malignant degeneration than smaller ones. Most children have tubular adenomatous polyps smaller than 1 cm, with a reassuring low cancer risk of less than 5%. Once the polyps advance beyond 2 cm, the risk of cancer increases to 35%. Villous architecture is even more concerning, with a malignant risk of over 50% in 2-cm polyps.[137]

Most children with polyps are asymptomatic. The average age at discovery of nonfamilial polyposis coli is 29 years, but earlier identification occurs when children develop mucus in their stools, blood per rectum, frequency, and change in bowel habit. Generally, when the family history is known, children present to the surgeon for colectomy at an early age. Although treatment is suggested by symptoms, the symptoms themselves are rarely severe enough to warrant colectomy. Rather, it is the cancer risk that is of most concern. The average age at cancer development is 39 years, but this varies by family, depending on the specific *APC* gene mutation within affected family members. Children who have more than 1000 colon polyps can be expected to have a higher risk of early cancer. There are case reports of children as young as 5 and 9 years old developing adenocarcinoma.[138,139] A recent worldwide survey of selected polyposis registries identified 14 patients with cancer younger than 20 years, leading to a calculated risk of 1/471 pediatric cases.[124]

Table 42-1 Features of Gastrointestinal Polyps in Children

Syndrome	Gene Defect	Population Frequency	Gastrointestinal Cancer Risk	Defining Features
Common juvenile polyps	Unknown	1:50-1:100 (1%-2% of children)	None known	Hamartoma
Juvenile polyposis	*SMAD4* (18q21.1) *PTEN* Autosomal dominant	1:100,000	Up to 50%	50-200 hamartomas; 5- to 50-mm diameter
Peutz-Jeghers syndrome	*LKB1* (19p13.3) Autosomal dominant	1:120,000	20%-40%	Muscle polyp core, mucocutaneous pigment
Familial adenomatous polyposis	*APC* (5q21) Autosomal dominant or spontaneous mutation	1:5,000-1:17,000	100%	Adenomatous polyps in colon and small bowel

The timing of operation is based on symptoms, the risk of cancer, and the expected outcome. The prophylactic nature of the operation has prompted some families and physicians to consider waiting until the child is old enough to participate in the decision. Such an approach may be possible in patients with late-onset disease and a low polyp burden, but may not be advisable in younger children with larger numbers of polyps of significant size.

Essential investigations before operation include genetic or biologic confirmation of the diagnosis, obtained by gene testing and colonoscopic biopsy. The presence of desmoid tumors in the family should prompt a search in the child as well. The most common locations for desmoid tumors are the truncal muscle or the mesentery. When desmoid tumors are found preoperatively, the risk of postoperative recurrence is high and must be weighed against the preventative nature of an operation. A more cautious approach is suggested for these patients, especially when the polyp load is small and the risk of cancer is low. Treatment of desmoids remains difficult, although newer chemotherapeutic agents offer optimism.

Surgical management in children with familial adenomatous polyposis (FAP) is aimed at removal of all polyp-bearing tissue combined with preservation of continent gastrointestinal function. This is accomplished by a standard proctocolectomy and IPAA, as discussed previously. Long-term complications, such as pouchitis, are much less common in patients with FAP. Functional outcome data demonstrate excellent pouch function with the stool frequency averaging three to four per day. There is usually no night-time stooling or incontinence. Children rate their quality of life as equal to that of their peers.

Subtotal colectomy with ileorectostomy is an alternative to total proctocolectomy. Candidates for this procedure recognize the need for life-time surveillance of the remaining rectal mucosa. Endoscopy and polypectomy may be reasonable alternatives for patients with attenuated forms of the syndrome (AFAP) and a low polyp burden that typically spares the rectum. Preservation of the rectum is useful in children with nonadenomatous polyps and those with a contraindication to the proctocolectomy and IPAA such as children with pelvic abnormalities that preclude surgery or perineal disorders of continence that affect outcome.

Other Intestinal Malignancies

Carcinoid Tumor

A carcinoid tumor is most often diagnosed at or following an appendectomy. The estimated incidence of such an event is 2 to 5/1000 operations.[140] Carcinoid tumors are the next most common intestinal tumor after lymphoma.[120] The indolent behavior of these small tumors suggests they should be classified as benign in most circumstances. Appendiceal carcinoids are usually found at the distal tip of the appendix but can occur anywhere along its course (Fig. 42-11).

Table 42-2 Features of the Variants of Familial Adenomatous Polyposis

Syndrome	Germline Mutation	Cancer Risk	Clinical Features
Familial adenomatous polyposis (FAP)	*APC*	100% by age 40 yr	CHRPE, desmoid tumors, thyroid and liver cancer risk
Gardner's syndrome	*APC*	Same as FAP	Osteomas, lipomas, sebaceous cysts, dental lesions, desmoids
FAP-related Turcot's syndrome	*APC*	Same as FAP	Medulloblastomas
Attenuated FAP	*APC*	70% by age 65 yr	<100 right-sided colon and fundic polyps, exclude *MYH* mutation

CHRPE, congenital hypertrophy of retinal pigment epithelium.

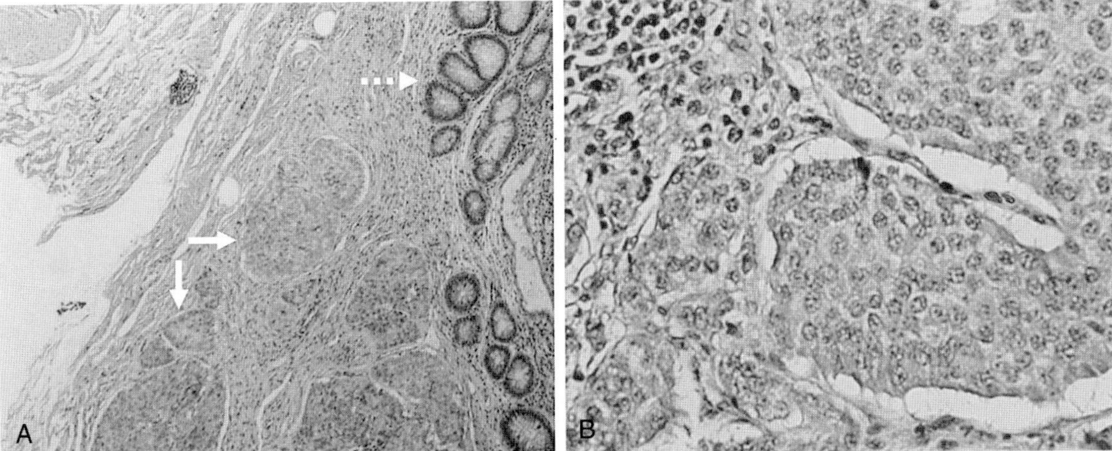

Figure 42-11. This 14 year old girl presented with acute appendicitis and underwent laparoscopic appendectomy. Histologic examination of the appendix revealed a carcinoid tumor in the mid-portion of the appendix. The tumor was less than 2 cm in size. **A,** A low power view shows the nests of tumor cells (solid arrows) invading the muscularis mucosa. The normal appendiceal glands are noted by the dotted arrow. **B,** A higher power view shows the solid islands of uniformed oval to polygonal tumor cells with minimal pleomorphism. Mitotic figures are not seen.

The usual location does not account for the relatively high incidence of appendicitis. The tumor can infiltrate the appendiceal wall and mesenteric fat, creating significant concern for regional nodal and distant metastasis. The carcinoid syndrome is not seen until hepatic implantation has occurred and has not been reported in childhood. Malignant carcinoid tumors are slow-growing, slow-spreading lesions without meaningful cure rates until decades have passed.

Longitudinal follow-up of appendiceal carcinoid tumors found in children has shown that appendectomy is curative for all tumors less than 2 cm in diameter. Very little data are available for larger tumors. Traditional teaching suggests patients with larger tumors should undergo right hemicolectomy and regional mesenteric node excision. A combined review of 124 children identified only 7 patients with 2-cm tumors.[140] Of the 4 undergoing hemicolectomy, one tumor recurred. The three who had appendectomy alone have remained free of disease. In our experience, we have found that lesions larger than 2 cm may be safely resected by appendectomy alone.[141] However, it is difficult to draw conclusions from such limited data on a tumor known to take decades to reappear.

Tumor invasion into the periappendiceal fat or vessels has also been considered an indication for hemicolectomy. In adults, metastatic disease is observed more frequently when these characteristics are found.[142] However, the pediatric data do not necessarily support this conclusion because no recurrence was noted in 16 patients with tumor margins outside the wall.[141] An exception should probably be made for lesions near the base of the appendix where wide local excision is not possible.

Laboratory and radiologic studies are usually unremarkable and are not helpful in the decision for hemicolectomy. Unless hepatic metastases are already established, serum and urine markers for serotonin metabolites will be negative. Similarly, chromogranin A levels will be normal. Octreotide scans may be more sensitive for metastatic disease and can be confirmed by magnetic resonance imaging of the liver for larger lesions.[143] Carcinoid tumors may occur elsewhere in the gastrointestinal tract in children, most commonly in the terminal ileum. These tumors tend to have a higher malignant potential and should be excised with a wide margin of mesentery, including the lymph nodes. Carcinoids of the colon and rectum have not been described in children.[141]

Gastrointestinal Stromal Tumor

Gastrointestinal stromal tumors (GISTs) have emerged from obscurity as a rare, but leading cause of pediatric intestinal malignancies. Once thought to be leiomyomas or sarcomas, electron microscopy and immunohistochemistry have identified an overlap of muscle and neural elements inconsistent with a smooth muscle tumor. CD34 was found to be positive. Later, KIT tyrosine kinase became the phenotypic marker for this tumor. Recent studies have also identified a less common but causative role for platelet-derived growth factor receptor A (PDGFRA) mutation.[144] These features suggest a common stem cell origin with the interstitial cells of Cajal (ICC).

Pediatric GISTs tend to express fewer KIT and PDGFRA mutations than adults, have a higher female predominance, and may be associated with pulmonary chordomas and paragangliomas. The majority of pediatric GISTs are found in the stomach. Small bowel and colorectal locations are rare. Tumors in these locations have a worse prognosis than those in the stomach.

GIST behavior varies by size, location, and mitotic index. The risk of complications, such as local recurrence and regional spread, is stratified by these indicators into low, medium, and high risk. Surgical resection remains the best form of therapy. Even low-risk tumors may recur at the margins, mandating a cancer operation for every GIST tumor regardless of risk assignment. The typical pattern begins with local recurrence, followed by serosal spread and hematogenous liver metastasis. Distant disease is late, and lymphatic spread is not characteristic.

Low-risk tumors have excellent survival, but late recurrences are still possible. High-risk GISTs recur early and spread indiscriminately throughout the abdomen. Chemotherapy has been disappointing, but therapy targeting KIT activation and the downstream effects may yet hold promise. Early results are promising despite the lower expression of KIT in children.[145]

chapter 43

APPENDICITIS

Shawn D. St. Peter, MD

Over 70,000 cases of appendicitis are seen in children in the United States each year, making it the most common acute surgical condition.[1,2] A lifetime risk of appendicitis has been estimated at 8.7% for boys and 6.7% for girls.[3] The age-specific incidence progresses from extremely low in the neonatal period to a peak incidence between ages 12 and 18 years. Although the disease is common enough to make familial predisposition difficult to identify, there are data to suggest a higher family risk in children who suffer appendicitis before 6 years of age.[4]

NATURAL HISTORY

Appendicitis is simply a version of diverticulitis in which the appendix represents a long, true diverticulum with a narrow lumen. Inflammation of the appendix is initiated as the result of an obstructive process within the lumen. This was initially demonstrated in an experimental model 70 years ago.[5] The offending mechanism obstructing the lumen can be lymphoid hyperplasia, inspissated fecal matter, a foreign body, or parasites. There is a temporal relationship aligning the incidence of appendicitis with the development of submucosal lymphoid follicles at and near the base of the appendix. These collections of reactive immune cells are sparse at birth but increase with age to a peak in adolescents followed by a sharp decline after age 30.[6] An epidemiologic association between fecaliths and appendicitis is seen in developed countries with a high consumption of low-fiber diets where both are more common than in developing nations with high-fiber diets.[7]

After appendiceal obstruction, intraluminal pressure increases from the accumulation of undrained mucus and contained bacterial proliferation. This pressure progresses until lymphatic and venous drainage are impaired, directly resulting in local edema. If untreated, this congestion will limit arterial inflow and thereby limit cellular substrate exchange. This results in impaired tissue integrity to the end point of necrosis with subsequent perforation. However, luminal obstruction is not always found on histologic examination, in which case the obstruction may be physiologic or static and not mechanical. Alternatively, the tissue may be locally inflamed as the result of a noxious inciting agent. *Yersinia, Salmonella,* and *Shigella* and viruses such as mumps virus, coxsackievirus B, and adenovirus have been implicated in appendicitis.[8,9] In children with cystic fibrosis, painful distention of the appendix may develop from abnormal production of mucus without inflammation.[10] Appendicitis in neonates is rare and warrants evaluation for cystic fibrosis as well as Hirschsprung's disease.[11] Neonatal appendicitis also can be indistinguishable from focal necrotizing enterocolitis confined to the appendix.[12]

Although the natural history of untreated appendicitis is usually perforation and abscess development, this course is not assured because resolution without treatment can occur.[13] Early inflammation that does not progress to perforation appears to be the mechanism behind the clinical phenomena of relapsing or chronic appendicitis.[14] When the disease does progress to perforation, the patient will present with peritoneal irritation. If the presentation is further delayed, the patient may present with an abscess. Young children have less ability to understand or articulate their developing symptomatology compared with adolescents. Therefore, they more commonly present with perforation. Perforation rates have been reported to be as high as 82% in children younger than 5 years and nearly 100% of 1-year olds.[15] However, all perforation rates reported in the literature must be viewed with caution because these rates are reported without a consistent definition of perforation. This accounts for the wide range of 20% to 76% perforation rates reported from 30 pediatric hospitals in the United States.[16]

Delays in presentation or diagnosis causing elevated perforation rates have been documented to occur for reasons other than age. Children with perforation are much more likely to have been initially referred to a pediatrician rather than a surgeon.[17] It would logically follow that patients who do not have good access to medical care would be more likely to present with perforation. In adults, lack of insurance or financial coverage status has been shown to be related to an increase in perforation.[18] In children, a review of a national database reports perforation disproportionately affects minority children with a 24% to 38% higher rate of rupture than white children, adjusting for age and gender.[19] A separate database review also found the rate of rupture in school-aged children was associated with race and lack of health insurance.[20] Encouragingly, a more recent single institution study found no relation to race or financial status.[21]

CLINICAL PRESENTATION

The clinical course of appendicitis in its simplest and classic presentation begins with anorexia and vague periumbilical pain. This pain is of visceral origin and is referred to the common dermatome of the 8th to 10th thoracic dorsal ganglia, which results in the periumbilical pain. It is important to remember that inflammation of any midgut derivative will cause similar symptoms. The description of periumbilical pain migrating to the right lower quadrant is not a true migration of the pain nor is it migration of the inflammatory source. Localization occurs when the inflammation of the appendix progresses to irritate the peritoneum, which has potent somatic sensation. More typically, nausea leading to vomiting follows the onset of pain, but this is not a reliable finding in children. Diarrhea is more commonly seen with perforated appendicitis but is also more common in infants and toddlers, which may direct the diagnosis toward gastroenteritis.[22] In general, gastroenteritis is more likely with a history of repeated episodes of vomiting and diarrhea starting at a similar time or preceding the onset of pain, particularly when the abdominal pain is the minor symptom, is not localized, and is without focal tenderness on examination.

The most discrete physical finding is tenderness, exhibited by the objective demonstration of pain such as wincing, moving, or flexing on gentle pressure applied in the right lower quadrant near McBurney's point. This point was originally described as "one and a half to two inches from the anterior superior iliac process along a line drawn from the process to the umbilicus."[23] If the patient is under the influence of narcotic analgesia at the time of examination, tenderness in the right lower quadrant is considerably of more concern for appendicitis. Narcotic analgesics improve the level of comfort but do not change the inflammatory focus, which may still be tender on palpation. However, a negative examination done on a patient on analgesics does not exclude appendicitis.

The search for rebound tenderness, by deep palpation with abrupt removal of pressure, is inherently uncomfortable for the patient and is a poor indicator of peritonitis and should be avoided. Gentle pressure applied to the left side of the abdomen or placing a hand in the center of the abdomen with mild shaking of the abdomen will elicit tenderness in the setting of peritonitis. If these maneuvers precipitate sharp pain in the right lower quadrant, acute appendicitis is extremely likely. A palpable mass in the right lower abdomen is difficult or impossible to identify in the patient with guarding or rigidity. (This mass often becomes evident on the operating table after anesthesia has been induced.) It is important to remember that localized symptoms depend on peritoneal irritation that is detectable by examination. Therefore, obesity, a retrocecal appendix, or a medial appendix walled off by omentum, mesentery, or small intestine may never localize and the patient may maintain vague symptoms. One or more of these factors are often present in patients who present with perforation or abscess.

Examination of a crying, resistant child can be difficult. This requires patience, deflection of the child's attention, and/or a reassuring parent. However, sedation may be necessary. Despite previous dogma, a rectal examination is a traumatizing and nonspecific adjunct that is unlikely to contribute to the evaluation.[24] Even in the setting of a suspected pelvic abscess or ovarian pathologic process, these diagnoses cannot be affirmed without imaging. Bowel sounds are also quite nonspecific but may be absent with perforation compared with being hyperactive with gastroenteritis.

Fever is common and is usually low grade in acute appendicitis. However, a lack of documented fever does little to exclude the disease. High fever is more common after appendiceal rupture due to the inflammatory response of peritoneal contamination. A patient with high fever and no peritoneal signs is less likely to have appendicitis and should alert the physician toward a viral infection or urinary tract condition.

Serum studies are generally not very sensitive nor specific for appendicitis. A mild elevation of the leukocyte count (11,000 to 16,000/mm^3) is the most common finding. A markedly elevated leukocyte count suggests perforation or another diagnosis. A case-control series has shown that patients with perforated appendicitis have, on average, a significantly higher leukocyte count than those with acute appendicitis.[25] This series also found that the leukocyte differential count showing neutrophilia and lymphopenia were both fairly predictive of appendicitis. However, a normal leukocyte count does not exclude appendicitis.

The urine is usually free of bacteria, whereas a few or moderate number of red or white blood cells are common because the inflammation may affect the ureter or bladder. Because patients are often dehydrated, a concentrated urine is expected with ketones from decreased oral intake and the release of insulin-antagonizing inflammatory mediators. Serum electrolytes, liver enzymes, and liver function studies are usually normal. C-reactive protein is usually increased and becomes markedly elevated with perforation.[26,27] However, this finding is less reliable in children compared with adults, and no studies have yet demonstrated C-reactive protein to be superior to the leukocyte count. As with a leukocyte count, a normal C-reactive protein does not exclude appendicitis, even when combined with a normal leukocyte count.[28] Therefore, C-reactive protein is not routinely measured.[27,29]

Whereas the aforementioned clinical picture represents the most common manifestation of appendicitis, it must be recognized that children often present with wide deviations from the classic picture, which makes a confident diagnosis often unlikely without imaging. Moreover, the location of the appendix is not consistent, owing to the variation in the position of the cecum. The appendix can be in the right upper abdomen if the patient has an incomplete rotation. Likewise, if the patient has untreated nonrotation, the appendix could lie anywhere in the abdomen. Because there are commonly one or more components of the presentation not consistent with appendicitis, several groups have attempted to apply clinical scoring systems utilizing elements of the history, physical examination, and laboratory studies to quantitate the sum of the clinical features that are consistent with the diagnosis. One series found scoring to be rather accurate,[30] whereas others have found their overall sensitivity and specificity to be only modest with little advantage over experienced clinical judgment.[31,32] Recently, a scoring system was used to stratify which patients should have surgical consultation (high score), proceed to imaging (moderate score), or be discharged (low score).[32] This is the most applicable use of a scoring system because imaging has become an important adjunct in patients with unclear symptoms.

RADIOLOGIC IMAGING

Misdiagnosis can lead to an extremely prolonged delay in treatment due to family reassurance from the first caregiver interaction, which may delay them from seeking further care. This results in an increase in morbidity from advanced disease. Epidemiologic data have shown the risk of a missed diagnosis in children to be higher in hospitals with a volume of less than one pediatric appendectomy per week.[33] Parents should be encouraged to take their children to pediatric hospitals for abdominal pain when possible. Historically, negative appendectomy rates of 10% to 20% were not only considered appropriate but advisable to minimize the number of patients with a missed diagnosis. More recently, some authors have questioned this philosophy, citing the risk and expense of an avoidable operation.[34] Diagnostic imaging is necessary if physicians are going to balance minimizing the risk of negative appendectomy and the risk of a missed diagnosis. Currently, data from children's hospitals demonstrate extremely low negative appendectomy rates with the use of diagnostic imaging.[16,35]

Plain films may demonstrate a fecalith in 5% to 15% of patients.[36-38] However, these studies are extremely nonspecific and almost never serve as the determinant for operation. Therefore, they fruitlessly consume time and resources and are not recommended unless bowel obstruction, or free peritoneal air is suspected.[39]

Ultrasonography offers the advantages of being an efficient bedside technique that is noninvasive, requires no contrast, and emits no radiation. Graded compression ultrasonography is performed by placing pressure on the transducer to displace bowel loops and identify the appendix. The pressure is adequate if the psoas muscle and the iliac vessels are identified, which assure the range of view is posterior to the appendix. The common signs of appendicitis include a fluid-filled, noncompressible appendix, a diameter greater than 6 mm, appendicolith, periappendiceal or pericecal fluid, and increased periappendiceal echogenicity caused by inflammation.[40,41] Results from multiple pediatric series totaling more than 5000 patients have documented that the sensitivity of ultrasonography ranges from 78% to 94% and the specificity ranges from 89% to 98%.[42-50] However, ultrasonography is operator dependent. Thus, the published results must be interpreted relative to local experience and expertise with this imaging modality. The effectiveness of ultrasonography is hindered by abdominal wall thickness and fat, which accounts for the generally inferior results reported in the adult literature.[51-56] Causes of false-positive results include a normal large appendix, the psoas muscle being mistaken for the appendix, and inspissated stool. A false-negative study can result from a retrocecal appendix, perforated appendix, gas-filled appendix, involvement of only the tip, and, most importantly, the inability to visualize the appendix.[37,40] Whereas a normal appendix must be visualized to exclude appendicitis, ultrasonography is not typically efficacious in identifying the normal appendix, because early reports showed only 10% to 50% of normal appendices could be identified in children.[37,40] However, as with other modalities, appendicitis is effectively excluded by the inability to identify the appendix in combination with the identification of a pathologic process that explains the symptoms.[57] Furthermore, recent data from a large series employing upward graded compression, posterior manual compression, left oblique lateral decubitus position, and a low frequency convex transducer, demonstrated that nearly all appendices could be identified with over 98% accuracy for diagnosing appendicitis.[58] Another recent report in 50 patients using contrast-enhanced power Doppler ultrasound imaging demonstrated similar accuracy.[59]

Computed tomography (CT) provides a complete three-dimensional image of the entire abdomen and pelvis, is not operator dependent, and is extremely accurate. Although there is some overlap in the ranges of sensitivity and specificity reported for CT with the ranges reported for ultrasonography, most series report both sensitivity and specificity around 95% or greater for CT.[33,43,53,60-66] These data are difficult to interpret because of the range in sample sizes, quality of patient selection for imaging, and institutional variation in technology and expertise. Therefore, more insight is gained by examining intrainstitutional comparative series between US and CT, which have almost universally found CT to be significantly more accurate than ultrasonography.[33,43,53,60,62,67] There are, however, several concerns with CT. Some protocols require a delay in the emergency department for contrast agent administration, and the smaller children may require sedation. Radiation has become a growing concern with the wide application of CT. It has been estimated that a complete abdominal CT is equivalent to 25.7 months of natural background radiation exposure.[68]

The risk of radiation-induced malignancy from a CT scan decreases with age.[69] The lifetime risk of a fatal radiation-induced malignancy is estimated at 0.18% for a 1-year-old child. Stated another way, one malignancy would result from a CT scan done on 555 one-year-old patients, whereas about twice as many 15-year-olds would need to be scanned to equal that risk. Although this risk may appear miniscule, it is important information when evaluating a patient with the classic symptoms of appendicitis.

Magnetic resonance imaging (MRI) is an intriguing nonradiation alternative to CT and is extremely accurate in diagnosing appendicitis.[70] The current version of this technology makes it impractical for widespread application, but future generations of scanners could allow this technology to be the initial imaging study.

Radionuclide-labeled white blood cell scans have been employed, but the reported diagnostic capacity appears to offer little advantage over the aforementioned modalities and they have the disadvantage of being more cumbersome to obtain.[71]

Imaging is invaluable in the evaluation of children with abdominal pain, allowing for an accurate diagnosis, avoiding unnecessary operations, and decreasing the risk of a repeat presentation with perforation. Perhaps the most important contribution of imaging is the ability to pinpoint an alternative diagnosis that entirely redirects therapy.[19,37,40,72]

DIFFERENTIAL DIAGNOSIS

In the patients with lower abdominal pain, the workup toward a diagnosis of appendicitis must also consider the alternative possible causes. Causes of acute right lower quadrant pain that is indistinguishable from appendicitis without laboratory or imaging studies include a tubo-ovarian pathologic process, Crohn's disease, mesenteric adenitis, cecal diverticulitis, Meckel's diverticulitis, constipation, viral gastroenteritis, and regional bacterial enteritis (*Yersinia* and *Campylobacter,* particularly). Lower abdominal pain or vague nonfocal pain can result from a urinary tract infection, kidney stone, ureteropelvic junction obstruction, uterine pathologic process, right lower lobe pneumonia, sigmoid diverticulitis, cholecystitis, pancreatitis, gastroenteritis, vasculitis, bowel obstruction, and malignancy (lymphoma). The most common diagnosis made in the presence of missed appendicitis has been reported to be gastroenteritis.[17] Although many of these conditions may seem easily distinguished from appendicitis, they all possess a spectrum of presentation that overlaps the possible symptoms of appendicitis.

TREATMENT

Medical Management

The treatment of appendicitis begins with intravenous fluids and antibiotics. The antibiotic regimen must provide broad-spectrum coverage of enteric organisms. In simple, acute appendicitis, a single dose of antibiotics is adequate preoperative coverage. After appendectomy, patients with acute appendicitis are usually discharged within 24 hours. Current evidence suggests that an additional dose of antibiotics after appendectomy is not necessary or recommended.[73,74]

The patients with perforated appendicitis will require antibiotic therapy postoperatively until clinical resolution has occurred. The antibiotic regimen employed in this situation has traditionally been triple-antibiotic therapy (ampicillin, gentamicin, and clindamycin), which is still practiced in many pediatric surgery centers despite several reports of simpler antibiotic regimens.[75-77] Monotherapy with piperacillin/tazobactam for intra-abdominal infections has recently been shown to be equally efficacious as traditional triple-antibiotic therapy.[75,76] Similarly, cefotaxime, a third-generation cephalosporin, has been shown to be equal to the monotherapy schedule of piperacillin/tazobactam in children with complicated perforated appendicitis when combined with metronidazole.[77] Monotherapy has the disadvantage of being costly and requires three to four doses per day.

The financial charges to the patient are inseparably linked to the dosing schedule. This impact of decreased dosing on antibiotic expenses has been emphasized by several authors.[78-82] In several studies, a decrease in expense has been shown with once-daily dosing of ceftriaxone compared with broad-spectrum monotherapeutic agents in the penicillin and cephalosporin families.[80-87] A retrospective comparative study found once-daily dosing with ceftriaxone and metronidazole was as effective as traditional triple-antibiotic therapy with cost benefits.[88] This was confirmed in a prospective, randomized trial.[89] Therefore, current best evidence suggests once-a-day dosing with ceftriaxone at 50 mg/kg/day and with metronidazole at 30 mg/kg/day provides the simplest and least expensive regimen.

The length of time required for antibiotic treatment or the mode of delivery for perforated appendicitis has yet to be delineated. A multicenter case-control study suggests that the patient who is clinically well by postoperative day 3 is unlikely to develop an abscess.[90] A retrospective comparative series found early transition to oral antibiotics as effective as a prolonged course of intravenous antibiotics.[91] However, prospective trials will be required to clarify this issue.

Surgical Management

A discussion of the surgical management of appendicitis must be separated into the three distinct categories of disease at presentation. These categories are those with appendicitis with no evidence of perforation, those with perforated appendicitis, and those with a well-defined abscess.

Acute Appendicitis

Acute, nonperforated appendicitis is cured with prompt appendectomy, which is the rationale for why an early operation has always been the standard of care. We now understand that, as a version of diverticulitis, acute appendicitis can be treated effectively to the point of disease resolution and hospital discharge with antibiotics alone.[92-94] This fact has been proven by large prospective, randomized trials in adults comparing antibiotics alone to appendectomy for appendicitis.[94,95] Therefore, once antibiotics have been initiated, the operation is not an emergency or even necessary in the immediate setting. Appendectomy in the middle of the night is no longer justified.[92-94,96-98] Not only is the operation elective once antibiotic therapy has been initiated, this information may be useful in easing family anxiety during the time they await surgical intervention.

Perforated Appendicitis

Appendectomy for perforated appendicitis is currently a topic of debate. There are three general strategies possible for this situation: antibiotics only, antibiotics followed by interval appendectomy, and appendectomy on presentation.

The logic of treating initially with antibiotics is to avoid a difficult operation in the presence of severe inflammation that obliterates the normal anatomy and creates dense adherence of the surrounding structures. Once the infection is controlled with antibiotics, allowing an operation to be more simple and safe, the decision becomes whether to perform the appendectomy. Those who do not perform appendectomy believe there is a low risk of recurrent appendicitis, which short-term data suggest are 8% to 14%.[99,100] However, not only is there short-term follow-up in these studies, these are retrospective reviews of patients already treated, meaning they were specifically selected for this management. It would be expected that a prospective application of antibiotics alone to all patients with evidence of perforation on CT would yield a much higher failure rate. Furthermore, all pediatric follow-up data, even to age 18, is relatively short term considering the current life expectancy is nearly 80 years. Therefore, it is impossible to estimate the lifetime risk of leaving the appendix in situ as these patients mature through adulthood because we do not know what the recurrence curves would look like decade by decade. However, assuming a stable rate, and assuming the current series are accurate in estimating the short-term risk of recurrence at 1% to 3% per year, this is an unfavorable prognosis when the typical pediatric patient has 60 to 80 years of expected life remaining.

Some authors have noted a high rate of pathologic findings in interval appendectomy specimens.[101,102] These cases augment the concern over the lifetime risk of not performing the appendectomy. In addition, most pediatric surgeons perform the interval appendectomy in patients who were initially managed medically. A survey of the American Pediatric Surgical Association (APSA) found that 86% of the responders perform interval appendectomy routinely after nonoperative management of perforated appendicitis.[103]

Regarding nonoperative management of perforated appendicitis, one group found a high failure rate in patients with more than 15% band forms in the differential white cell count on presentation.[104] Another group found failure was more common when an appendicolith was present on imaging.[105] Others have found that evidence of disease or contamination beyond the right lower quadrant on imaging is a predictor of failure.[106] Finally, when choosing among treatment options, the surgeon should remember that some cases are difficult to categorize accurately as perforated or nonperforated preoperatively.

Although the logic of antibiotic therapy first is to avoid a difficult and potentially dangerous operation, most experienced surgeons can perform this operation safely through a minimally invasive approach. Laparoscopic appendectomy has been shown to be reliably feasible and safe in both children and adults who present with a phlegmonous mass in the right lower quadrant.[107,108]

In the discussion about whether to perform an operation, the most important factor is deciding if the patient has a perforation. The presence or absence of perforation cannot be accurately predicted by preoperative imaging, but not all patients will have preoperative imaging performed. In these cases, perforation is diagnosed intraoperatively. This is another source of controversy. Surgeons polled with photographs have extreme incongruence on which patients would be considered to have a perforation.[109] Furthermore, a survey of APSA members demonstrated the majority of members reported that they based their practice approaches on their individual preferences.[110] Because surgeons do not agree on what constitutes perforation, and because each surgeon holds his or her own opinion, this means almost all of the data published on the topic of perforated appendicitis must be viewed with caution because we do not know the composition of the study populations. In reality, a definition of perforation is not as important as the ability to identify which patients possess a high risk of developing a postoperative abscess. Emerging prospective evidence suggests defining perforation as an identifiable hole in the appendix or as a fecalith in the abdomen clearly separates high-risk from low-risk patients.[111] Moreover, this distinction prevents overtreating patients with purulent disease who actually have a good prognosis from the outset.

Abscess on Presentation

Patients presenting with a well-defined abscess that is identified on imaging are clinically challenging. Historically, the operations were difficult and required large incisions with high morbidity. Treatment of the abscess with percutaneous drainage with or without drain placement (Fig. 43-1), followed by interval appendectomy when the inflammation has resolved, allows for a less morbid operation. This approach was initially described over 25 years ago and has become an important part of contemporary practice.[103,112-116] However, the advancement of laparoscopic skills has also allowed the operation to be performed with minimal morbidity. There are no concurrent comparative

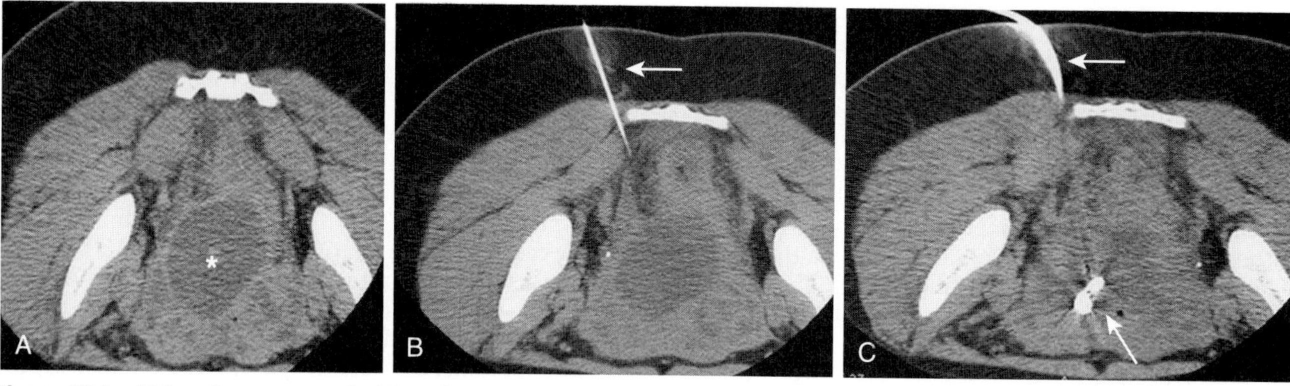

Figure 43-1. This patient presented with perforated appendicitis and a well-defined abscess. She underwent initial nonoperative management (abscess drainage, antibiotics) followed by a laparoscopic interval appendectomy 10 weeks later. These CT scans show the large pelvic abscess (*asterisk,* **A**) followed by needle placement (*arrow,* **B**), and drainage with a percutaneous drain (*arrow,* **C**). The drainage resulted in resolution of the abscess.

data available describing how the patients with percutaneous drainage fare in comparison to a cohort undergoing early operation. The practice of percutaneous drainage with interval appendectomy also carries the risk of complications and employs considerable medical resources.[117] Furthermore, there are no data available on the stress of the medical burden placed on the families treated with a long medical course involving antibiotics, drainage, and a long wait for the interval operation. This topic is an important one to address with a prospective trial, which is currently underway.[118]

Regardless of whether the abscess is drained under radiologic guidance or is opened at operation, culture of the fluid has not been shown to be helpful.[119,120] One study demonstrated that children whose treatment followed the cultures did somewhat worse than those whose fluid was not cultured.[120] In addition, peritoneal lavage with saline or antibiotic solution has never been shown to reduce the incidence of postoperative abscess.[121] Similarly, the use of drains has not proved useful except in cases of walled-off abscess cavities.[122,123] Injection of bupivacaine into the wound has been shown to reduce postoperative pain significantly in a randomized controlled trial in children.[124]

The Laparoscopic Approach

The traditional method of appendectomy was a muscle-splitting, right lower quadrant incision. Laparoscopic appendectomy typically involves a camera site at the umbilicus with two additional working ports (Fig. 43-2). During the initial experience with laparoscopy for perforated appendicitis, some authors found a higher postoperative abscess rate than had been seen with the open operation.[125-127] However, this literature also suffers from the lack of a substantative definition of perforation. Alternatively, this finding may have been the result of the early experience with laparoscopy.

Since the last edition of this book, there has been a plethora of evidence from around the world documenting no difference in intra-abdominal abscess risk between the open and laparoscopic approaches.[128-146] This evidence includes a multitude of level 1, 2, and 3 studies, including multiple prospective trials,

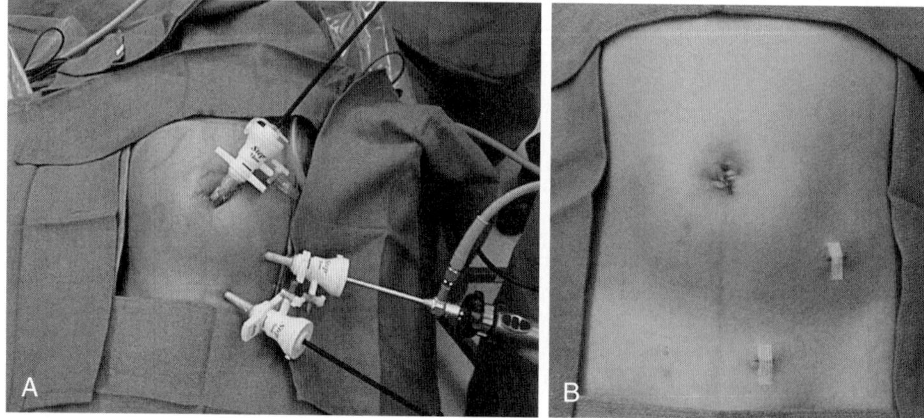

Figure 43-2. **A,** Port positions for a laparoscopic appendectomy. Typically three cannulas are used, with the endoscopic stapler introduced through the 12-mm umbilical port. The appendix is removed through this site as well. **B,** Postoperative appearance.

meta-analyses, and large multi-institutional comparative series from several countries. This is important because the risk of postoperative abscess was the potential justification for the open approach.

Laparoscopy possesses several advantages. This approach effectively removes the concern for wound infections, which has been a formidable problem in some patients with the open operation. The wound infection rate is substantially lower with laparoscopy owing to the small incisions and protection of the tissues by the cannulas.[128-132,135,136,142-144,146,147] When a wound infection occurs with laparoscopy, the morbidity is quite minimal owing to the size of the incision.[89] This effect is amplified in obese patients in whom the laparoscopic incision size remains the same but the open operation requires a much larger incision that results in the contamination of an abundance of poorly vascularized subcutaneous tissues.[148,149] Also, the length of hospitalization has been repeatedly shown to be shorter with laparoscopy.[129,130,132-137,140-145,147] Laparoscopy has been shown to allow for an earlier return to full activity in several studies, including an earlier return to sports and work.[141,142,144,145,147]

One prospective, randomized trial documented a superior quality of life at 2 weeks after laparoscopic appendectomy compared with the open operation.[137] A large database study involving 43,757 patients found a lower rate of gastrointestinal complications and overall complications with laparoscopy.[143] Similarly, the laparoscopic operation has also been shown to reduce the rate of postoperative adhesive small bowel obstruction.[150] Multiple authors have expressed the point that laparoscopy offers the substantial advantage of allowing excellent visualization of the entire abdominal cavity, removing therapeutic concerns of an alternative diagnosis.[132-134,141,144,147,151] The most recent Cochrane review concluded that laparoscopy should be the primary approach for suspected appendicitis, if available.[147]

The concern about laparoscopy requiring longer operative time is becoming dated. As with the early experience of all laparoscopic operations, it is likely that a longer operating time was the result of surgeons comparing an approach they were beginning to apply against one they had practiced for decades. Several recent comparative studies, including two prospective, randomized trials, have failed to show laparoscopy as taking longer.[130,136,138,139,141] The most recent meta-analysis found no difference in operative time.[136] One prospective trial in patients with acute appendicitis and another large comparative series in patients with perforated appendicitis found the laparoscopic approach to have a shorter operating time.[130,138] Most of the early studies documenting longer operating times for laparoscopy were reporting operating times of over 1 hour. The recent studies report times of less than 50 minutes. In the most recent prospective, randomized trial in children with perforated appendicitis, who all underwent laparoscopic appendectomy, the mean operating time was 44 minutes, with many cases requiring 30 minutes or less.[89] If these times are found in the setting of perforation, a straightforward appendectomy can easily be done in 20 minutes with good laparoscopic experience.

In spite of the fact that appendicitis is the most common acute surgical condition in children, there are many unresolved management issues that will require prospective studies to delineate.

Technique

The patient is placed supine on the operating table, and the abdomen is prepped widely. A 12-mm cannula is introduced through an umbilical incision, and pneumoperitoneum is established. Diagnostic laparoscopy is then performed. Two 5-mm ports are then placed, one in the left midabdomen and one in the left suprapubic area (see Fig. 43-2). A 5-mm 45-degree telescope is introduced through the umbilical port, and the two 5-mm ports are the working ports until introduction of the stapler. Once the appendix is identified, a window is made in the mesoappendix. At this point, the telescope is rotated from the umbilical port to the left midabdominal port and an endoscopic stapler is inserted through the 12-mm umbilical cannula. Usually, the appendix is ligated and divided first (Fig. 43-3), followed by ligation and division of the mesoappendix. On occasion, however, it may be more expedient to ligate the mesoappendix first.

If the appendix can be delivered through the cannula, an endoscopic bag is not used. However, so as not to drag the appendix through the umbilical incision, an endoscopic bag is utilized if the appendix is too large for the cannula.

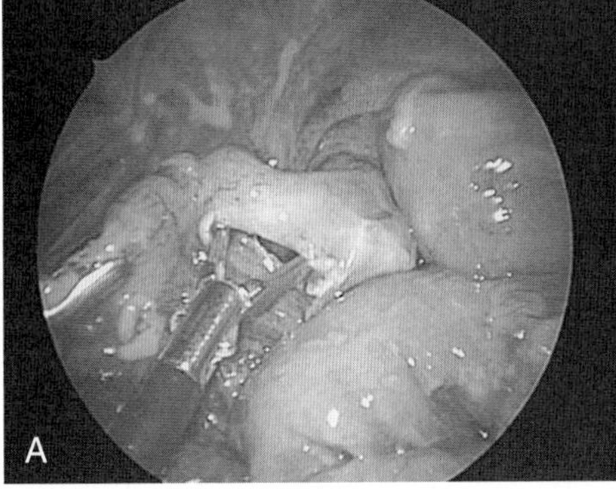

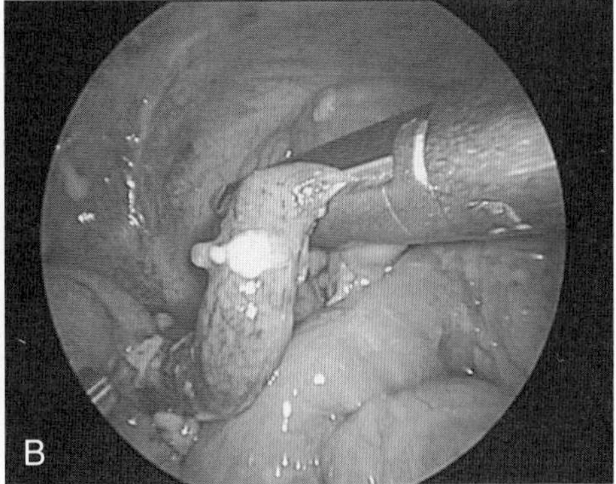

Figure 43-3. **A,** Initially, a window is made in the mesoappendix. **B,** Usually, the appendix is ligated and divided with the stapler first, followed by ligation/division of the mesoappendix.

chapter 44

BILIARY TRACT DISORDERS AND PORTAL HYPERTENSION

Atsuyuki Yamataka, MD, PhD • Yoshifumi Kato, MD, PhD • Takeshi Miyano, MD, PhD

BILIARY ATRESIA

Biliary atresia is a relatively rare obstructive condition of the bile ducts causing neonatal jaundice. The etiology is unknown but is the result of a progressive obliterative process of variable extent. Reliable incidence figures are available from Europe (1 in 18,000 live births), France (1 in 19,500 live births), the United Kingdom and Ireland (1 in 16,700 live births), Sweden (1 in 14,000 live births), and Japan (1 in 9640 live births),[1-6] but the highest recorded incidence is in French Polynesia (1 in 3124 live births).[7] No significant seasonal variation or clustering appears. In most large series, a slight female preponderance is found.

In the late 1950s, Morio Kasai reported the presence of patent microscopic biliary channels at the porta hepatis in young infants with biliary atresia. He postulated that by exposing these channels through radical excision of the atretic extrahepatic biliary remnants, then effective drainage of bile could be possible in some cases, especially if such surgery was performed within 8 weeks of birth. Although the Kasai portoenterostomy has become accepted as the standard initial operation for biliary atresia, this disease remains the foremost indication for liver transplantation in infants and children.

History

Biliary atresia appeared as a distinct disease entity in the *Edinburgh Medical Journal* in 1891.[8] In 1916, the concepts of "correctable" and "noncorrectable" types of disease were introduced after a comprehensive review of all reported cases.[9] Successful surgical treatment for the correctable type was reported for the first time in 1928.[10] However, over the next 3 decades there were only a few long-term survivors, all of whom had the favorable correctable type.[11,12]

For the majority with "noncorrectable" type disease, a number of procedures designed to relieve biliary obstruction, including impalement of the liver with metal tubes, incisions into the hilum with a cardiac valvulotome, partial hepatectomy to create biliary fistulas, and lymphatic drainage through the thoracic duct were developed.[13-17] Despite occasional hopeful reports, all techniques failed to provide adequate biliary decompression. Timing of surgical intervention was controversial, with some surgeons recommending that all infants with obstructive jaundice undergo early diagnostic laparotomy and cholangiography to identify those with correctable variants, whereas others concluded that early age was a contraindication for surgical treatment.[18,19] This latter group emphasized that neonatal hepatitis could be worsened by surgical intervention and recommended that surgical procedures should be postponed until at least 4 months of age. The argument for early surgical correction also was weakened by reports describing "spontaneous" cure.[20,21] Finally, second-look surgical exploration became recommended because of a rather mystical belief that a totally fibrotic extrahepatic ductal system might subsequently become patent.[22]

In 1959, the now common Kasai hepatic portoenterostomy procedure was reported for the first time and ended a long, hopeless era for patients with the noncorrectable-type disease.[23] Kasai's original report was in Japanese and received little attention until it was published in English in 1968.[24] Although effective bile drainage could be achieved after portoenterostomy in about 50% of patients, early surgical repair was crucial and needed to be performed before the age of 2 months. Conversely, effective bile drainage was observed in only 7% if correction was performed after the age of 4 months.[25] The portoenterostomy procedure gradually gained popularity in the United States during the 1970s. In the 1990 report of the Biliary Atresia Registry, more than 90% of infants with biliary atresia had undergone the procedure.[26]

Etiology and Pathogenesis

Despite intensive interest and investigation, the cause of biliary atresia remains unknown. Two different forms are described.[27] In syndromic biliary atresia (also known as the embryonic type), associated congenital anomalies are found, such as an interrupted inferior vena cava, preduodenal portal vein, intestinal malrotation, situs inversus, cardiac defects, and polysplenia. In this variety, which accounts for 10% to 20% of all cases, biliary atresia is likely to be due to a developmental insult occurring during differentiation of the hepatic diverticulum from the foregut of the embryo. A possible relation between syndromic biliary atresia and maternal diabetes has been reported.[28] Nonsyndromic biliary atresia (also known as the perinatal type) may have its origins later in gestation and may have a different clinical course, with biliary obstruction being progressive.

No ideal animal model exists for biliary atresia, a fact that has slowed the understanding of its pathogenesis. Various etiologic mechanisms have been postulated, including intrauterine or perinatal viral infection, genetic mutation, abnormal ductal plate remodeling, vascular or metabolic insult to the developing biliary tree, pancreaticobiliary ductal malunion, and immunologically mediated inflammation. Recent observations would suggest that biliary atresia is not a single disease entity. Some infants even have pigmented stools at birth.

Reovirus type 3 infection, rotavirus, cytomegalovirus (CMV), papillomavirus, and Epstein-Barr virus have all been proposed as possible etiologic agents, but conclusive evidence is lacking. CMV infection has been found in 4 of 10 patients with biliary atresia, and reovirus infection has been found in the livers of up to 55% of biliary atresia patients versus 10% to 20% in a control group.[29,30] Reovirus type 3 can cause an inflammatory cholangiopathy in recently weaned mice, but the condition is not progressive and the animals recover. The identification of viruses in children with biliary atresia is inconsistent in the literature, and several viruses have been used to create animal models that may be valuable for assessing the pathogenesis and treatment of biliary atresia.

Generally, biliary atresia is not considered an inherited disorder. However, genetic mutations that result in defective morphogenesis may be important in syndromic biliary atresia. Transgenic mice with a recessive deletion of the inversin gene have situs inversus and an interrupted extrahepatic biliary tree.[27,31] Mutations of the *CFC1* gene, which is involved in left-right axis determination in humans, have recently been identified in a few patients with syndromic biliary atresia.[32] The importance of the macrophage migration inhibitory factor (MIF) gene, which is a pleiotropic lymphocyte and macrophage cytokine in biliary atresia pathogenesis, has also been reported.[33] Other studies have identified abnormalities in laterality genes in a small number of subjects with biliary atresia, including the transcription factor ZIC3.[34] A high incidence of polymorphic variants in the jagged-1, keratin-8, and keratin-18 genes have been reported in a series of 18 children with biliary atresia.[35,36] Taken together, the increased incidence of nonhepatic anomalies in children with biliary atresia and genetic mutations reported in subsets of patients with laterality defects suggest that multiple genes are involved, each affecting a small number of patients.

Intrahepatic bile ducts are derived from primitive hepatocytes that form a sleeve (the ductal plate) around intrahepatic portal vein branches and associated mesenchyme in early gestation. Remodeling of the ductal plate in fetal life results in the formation of the intrahepatic biliary system. This is supported by similarities in cytokeratin immunostaining between biliary ductules in biliary atresia and normal first-trimester fetal bile ducts.[37] These findings suggest that nonsyndromic biliary atresia might be caused by a failure of bile duct remodeling at the hepatic hilum, with persistence of fetal bile ducts poorly supported by mesenchyme.

Several studies have investigated whether bile duct epithelial cells are susceptible to an immune/inflammatory attack because of abnormal expression of human leukocyte antigen (HLA) antigens or intracellular adhesion molecules on their surfaces.[38,39] A greater than threefold increase in HLA-B12 antigen is found in patients with biliary atresia compared with controls, particularly in those with no associated malformations and increased incidence of haplotypes A9-B5 and A28-B35.[40] Aberrant expression of class II HLA-DR antigens on biliary epithelial cells and damaged hepatocytes in patients with biliary atresia may render these tissues more susceptible to immune-mediated damage by cytotoxic T cells or locally released cytokines.[41] Increased expression of intercellular adhesion molecule-1 (ICAM-1) is noted on bile duct epithelium in patients with biliary atresia, a finding that may play a role in immune-mediated damage.[39] Strong expression of ICAM-1 also has been found on proliferating bile ductules, endothelial cells, and hepatocytes in biliary atresia.[42] A direct relationship exists between the degree of ductular expression of ICAM-1 and disease severity, suggesting that ICAM-1 might be important in the development of cirrhosis.

More recently, interest has focused on co-stimulatory molecules. Two processes are involved in the activation of T lymphocytes by antigen-presenting cells (APCs). One relates to the expression of major histocompatibility complex class II molecules, which interact directly with T-cell receptors. The other depends on the expression of B7 antigens on APCs and provides the second (co-stimulatory) signal to T lymphocytes through CD28.[43] In postoperative biliary atresia patients with good liver function, co-stimulatory antigens (B7-1, B7-2, and CD40) are expressed only on bile duct epithelial cells, whereas in patients with failing livers these markers are found on the surfaces of Kupffer cells, dendritic cells, and sinusoidal endothelial cells and in the cytoplasm of hepatocytes.[44] This suggests that the biliary epithelium and hepatocytes in biliary atresia are susceptible to immune recognition and destruction. Agents that block or prevent co-stimulatory pathways might offer a new therapeutic approach to controlling liver damage. Two studies performed comprehensive molecular and cellular surveys of liver biopsies and found a proinflammatory gene expression signature, with increased activation of interferon-γ, osteopontin, tumor necrosis factor-α, and other inflammatory mediators.[45,46] These studies may prove to be instrumental in dissecting the molecular networks responsible for the proinflammatory response and autoimmunity thought to be involved in the pathogenesis of biliary atresia. However, none of these mechanisms appears to be mutually exclusive. Moreover, it is not clear which signs and symptoms are primary and which are secondary. One current hypothesis is that the etiology of nonsyndromic biliary atresia is due to a viral or other toxic insult to the bile duct epithelium that induces the expression of new antigens on the surfaces of biliary epithelial cells.[47] Coupled with a genetically predetermined susceptibility that is mediated via histocompatibility antigens, these neoantigens are recognized by circulating T lymphocytes, resulting in a cell-mediated, immune, fibrosclerosing bile duct injury.

Classification and Histopathology

Although the term *biliary atresia* implies a static process with complete obstruction or absence of bile ducts, it is more a dynamic process of progressive bile duct obliteration and sclerosis. The areas that are affected and the degrees of fibrosis are variable and presumably reflect different sites of primary involvement by an as yet unknown cause.

The disease can be classified by using macroscopic appearance and cholangiography findings according to three main categories: (1) main type, (2) subtypes according to the pattern of distal bile ducts, and (3) subgroups according to the pattern of hilar hepatic radicles. Types I, II, and III are defined as atresia at the site of the common bile duct (CBD), at the site of the hepatic duct, and up to the porta hepatis, respectively. Most patients have type III. Cystic dilatation at the distal end of a patent duct is seen in some cases of type I biliary atresia (Fig. 44-1). Of the subtypes, patent distal ducts through the gallbladder to the duodenum are seen in 20% and atretic distal ducts are seen in 62% of cases. In these subgroups, a patent duct that can be anastomosed to the intestine at the porta hepatis is present in 5% of cases (i.e., "correctable" type). In more than 90% of cases, however, no normal ductal structures are seen at the porta hepatis (i.e., "noncorrectable" type).[48]

Early in the course of biliary atresia, the liver is enlarged, firm, and green. The gallbladder may be small and filled with white mucus, or it may be completely atretic (Fig. 44-2). Microscopically, the biliary tracts contain inflammatory and fibrous cells surrounding miniscule ducts that are probably remnants of the original embryonic duct system. The liver parenchyma is fibrotic and shows signs of cholestasis. Proliferation of biliary neoductules is seen (Fig. 44-3). This process develops into end-stage cirrhosis if good drainage cannot be achieved. These early changes are often nonspecific and may be confused with neonatal hepatitis and metabolic disease.

It is generally accepted that the pathologic changes seen in biliary atresia are panductal, affecting the intrahepatic biliary tree as well as the extrahepatic bile duct system. Moreover, the intrahepatic bile ducts can be narrowed, distorted in configuration, or irregular in shape.[49-51] However, some authors believe that secondary damage occurs only to the extrahepatic biliary system as a result of obliteration of extrahepatic bile ducts during development of the liver.[52] This

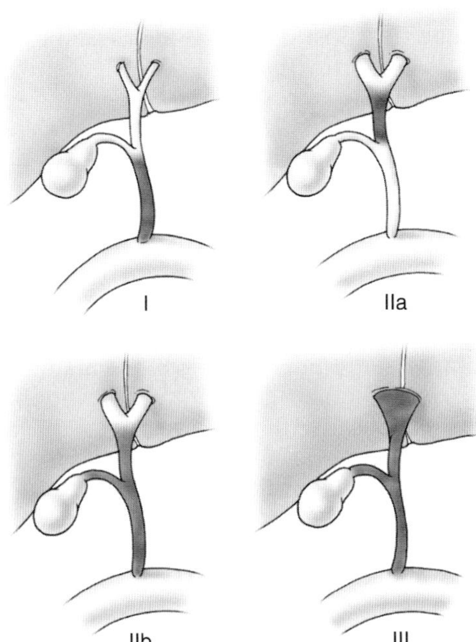

Figure 44-1. Morphologic classification of biliary atresia based on macroscopic and cholangiographic findings. Type I, occlusion of common bile duct; type IIa, obliteration of common hepatic duct; type IIb, obliteration of common bile duct, hepatic and cystic ducts, with cystic dilatation of ducts at the porta hepatis, and no gallbladder involvement; type III, obliteration of common, hepatic, and cystic ducts without anastomosable ducts at porta hepatis. (From Lefkowitch JH, et al: Biliary atresia. Mayo Clin Proc 73:99, 1998.)

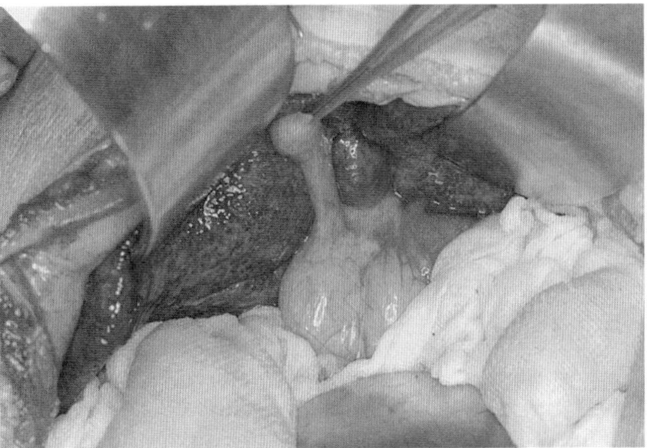

Figure 44-2. Type III biliary atresia with an enlarged, firm, green liver and hypoplastic small gallbladder was found in this infant.

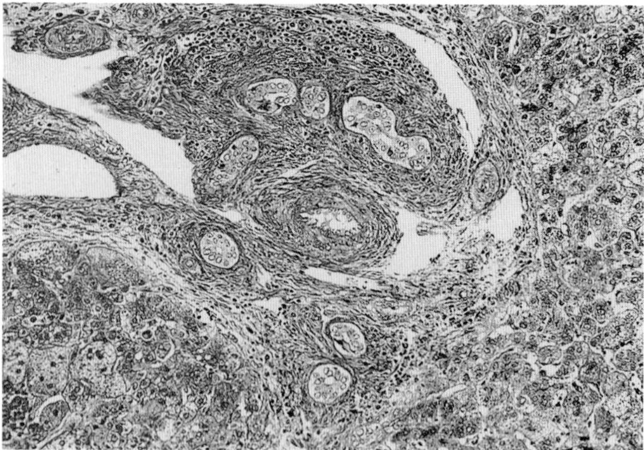

Figure 44-3. Photomicrograph of the portal tract of the liver in a 60-day-old infant with biliary atresia. Ductal plate malformation can be seen in the center of the portal space with portal fibrosis. Note ductal metaplasia of hepatocytes (Azan stain, ×100).

theory is strongly supported by the fact that outcome is better if corrective surgery is performed early. In any case, the intrahepatic biliary tree is important not only pathologically but also clinically. The degree of damage that is present in the intrahepatic biliary system is actually responsible for much of the morbidity after hepatic portoenterostomy. Ductal proliferation includes ductal plate malformations, such as a disturbance of adequate remodeling of the ductal plate as well as ductular metaplasia of hepatocytes.[53] Paucity or absence of intralobular bile ducts along with architectural disturbances, even in jaundice-free infants after successful hepatic portoenterostomy, has been observed by some investigators.[54] The nature and fate of the intrahepatic biliary involvement is still a subject of great controversy.

Diagnosis

The cardinal signs and symptoms of biliary atresia are jaundice, clay-colored stools, and hepatomegaly. However, meconium staining is normal in most patients. In the neonatal period, feces are yellowish or light yellowish in more than half of patients.[55] The newborn's urine becomes dark brown. Although the neonates are active, and their growth is usually normal for the first few months, anemia, malnutrition, and growth retardation develop gradually because of malabsorption of fat-soluble vitamins. In this period, jaundice that persists beyond 2 weeks should no longer be considered physiologic, particularly if the elevation in bilirubin is mainly in the direct fraction. Neonatal hepatitis and interlobular biliary hypoplasia are most likely to be confused with biliary atresia. Conventional liver function tests alone are useless for establishing a definitive diagnosis of biliary atresia.

A number of diagnostic protocols have been published, but the emphasis must always be on early diagnosis (Table 44-1).[56,57] For definitive diagnosis of biliary atresia, further investigations, including special biochemical studies, tests to confirm the patency of

Table 44-1 Clinical Findings and Examination for Diagnosis of Biliary Atresia

Routine Examinations
Color of stool
Consistency of the liver
Conventional liver function tests, including test for γ-glutamyl transpeptidase
Coagulation times (PT, aPTT)
Special Examinations
Special biochemical studies
Hepatitis A, B, C serologic studies
TORCH titers
α_1-Antitrypsin level
Serum lipoprotein-X
Serum bile acid
Confirmation of patency of extrahepatic bile ducts
Duodenal fluid aspiration
Ultrasonography
Hepatobiliary scintigraphy
Endoscopic retrograde cholangiopancreatography
Near-infrared reflectance spectroscopy
Needle biopsy of the liver for histopathologic studies
Laparoscopy
Surgical cholangiography

PT, prothrombin time; aPTT, activated partial thromboplastin time; TORCH, toxoplasmosis, other viruses, rubella, cytomegalovirus, and herpes simplex virus.

the extrahepatic bile ducts, and needle biopsy of the liver are often required. Several authors consider liver biopsy to be the most reliable test for establishing the diagnosis.[58,59] Serum lipoprotein-X is positive in all patients with biliary atresia, although it also is positive in 20% to 40% of patients with neonatal hepatitis. Serum bile acid levels increase in infants with cholestatic disease, but both the total bile acid level and the ratio of chenodeoxycholic acid to cholic acid have no value for differentiating biliary atresia from other cholestatic diseases.[60] Hyaluronic acid, which has been considered as a serum marker for liver function, has been reported to be a biochemical marker for evaluating infants with biliary atresia.[61] Duodenal fluid aspiration is recommended as an easy, noninvasive, and rapid test because biliary atresia can be excluded if typical yellow bilirubin-stained fluid is aspirated.[62] Hepatobiliary scintigraphy with technetium-labeled agents is widely used for differentiating biliary atresia from other cholestatic diseases. In biliary atresia, nucleotide uptake by hepatocytes is rapid but excretion into the bowel is absent, even on delayed images. In hepatocellular jaundice, isotope uptake is delayed owing to parenchymal disease and excretion into the intestine may or may not be demonstrated.

Ultrasonography, a safe and noninvasive test, should be performed in all jaundiced infants. Hepatobiliary ultrasonography will exclude other surgical causes of jaundice such as choledochal cyst and inspissated bile. In biliary atresia, the intrahepatic ducts are not dilated on ultrasonography because they are affected by the

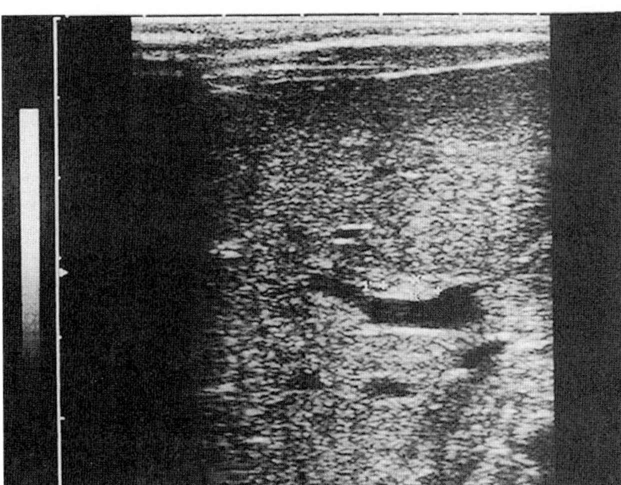

Figure 44-4. Ultrasonography shows a well-defined triangular area of high echogenicity at the porta hepatis, corresponding to fibrotic ductal remnants (the "triangular cord" sign).

inflammatory process. Various sonographic features have been targeted in an attempt to distinguish biliary atresia from other causes of conjugated hyperbilirubinemia in infants.[63-67] In biliary atresia, the gallbladder is small, shrunken, and noncontractile and there is increased echogenicity of the liver. The presence of other associated anomalies of the polysplenia syndrome is pathognomonic of biliary atresia.[68] Differentiation from choledochal cyst and type I biliary atresia also is rapid and simple with ultrasonography.[69] Irrespective of interobserver variation, failure to visualize the CBD is not diagnostic of biliary atresia, because a patent distal CBD can be found in up to 20% of biliary atresia cases. However, an absent gallbladder or one with an irregular outline is suggestive of biliary atresia.[67] In some cases, a well-defined triangular area of high reflectivity is seen at the porta hepatis, corresponding to fibrotic ductal remnants (the "triangular cord" sign) (Fig. 44-4).[64,65]

Nonvisualization of the fetal gallbladder may indicate abnormalities ranging from gallbladder agenesis to biliary atresia.[70] Amniotic fluid digestive enzymes, which are synthesized by the biliary epithelium, gradually decrease until 24 weeks of gestation. Because it is no longer possible to differentiate between abnormally low and physiologically low levels of the enzymes after 24 weeks of gestation, the prenatal diagnosis of biliary atresia is very difficult.[71]

Most patients with biliary atresia can be correctly diagnosed by using an appropriate combination of the investigations just listed. However, to differentiate accurately among biliary atresia, biliary hypoplasia, and severe neonatal hepatitis, cholangiography is usually required.

Recently, laparoscopy-assisted cholangiography has been used to accurately display the anatomic structure of the biliary tree with minimal surgical intervention.[72] Percutaneous cholecystocholangiography has also been considered as a useful option to prevent unnecessary laparotomy in infants whose cholestasis is caused by diseases other than biliary atresia.[73]

Treatment

Preoperative Management

Daily doses of vitamin K are usually given for several days before operation. The bowel should be prepared with oral kanamycin. Oral feeding is discontinued 24 to 48 hours before surgical intervention, and glycerin enemas are given. Preoperative broad-spectrum antibiotics are administered preoperatively.

Surgical Technique

Hepatic Portoenterostomy

The patient is placed supine on an operating table with facilities for intraoperative cholangiography. An extended right subcostal incision, dividing the muscle layers, is used to expose the inferior margin of the liver. After division of the falciform and triangular ligaments, the liver is delivered from the abdominal cavity. This procedure provides an excellent operative field for dissection of the porta hepatis. Cholangiography is needed to determine if biliary atresia is present and the correct anatomy (Fig. 44-5). The fundus of the gallbladder is mobilized from the liver bed, and a 4- to 6-Fr feeding tube is passed into the gallbladder through a small incision. If bile is detected on aspiration of the gallbladder, a small amount of contrast material is injected.

Unless normal anatomy of the intrahepatic biliary system is seen, a hepatic portoenterostomy should be performed.[24,74] At some point, a liver biopsy is performed on the right lobe to obtain histopathologic data for prognostic purposes.[75-77] To begin the portoenterostomy, the cystic artery is ligated and divided and the gallbladder is dissected from the liver bed. The mobilized gallbladder is used as a guide for locating the fibrous remnant of the CBD. After the caudal end of the CBD is ligated and divided at the upper border of the duodenum, the cephalad portion of the CBD with the gallbladder attached is dissected

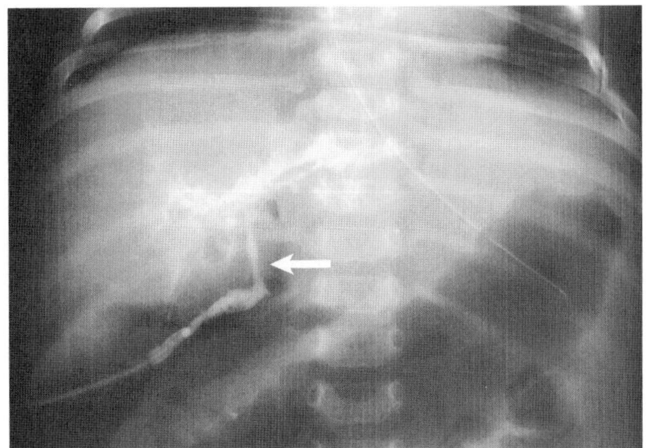

Figure 44-5. Intraoperative cholangiogram, type III biliary atresia. Note the almost atretic common bile duct (arrow).

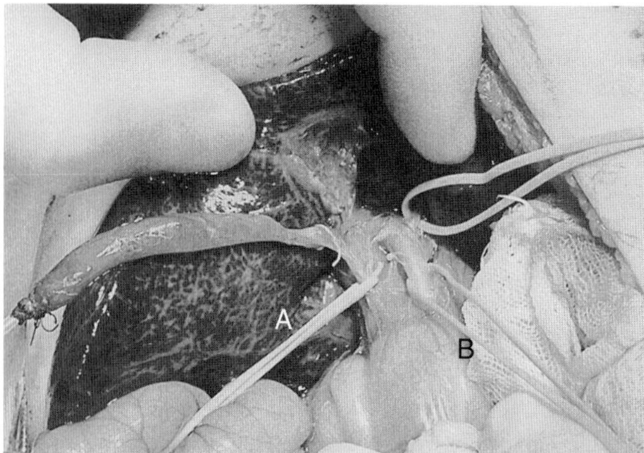

Figure 44-6. Type III biliary atresia. The vessel loops are around the atretic common bile duct (A) and hepatic artery (B).

cephalad above the bifurcation of the portal vein. The portal vein and the hepatic arteries are exposed along their entire course. For better portal dissection, the right and left hepatic arteries and the right and left portal branches are individually encircled by vessel loops (Fig. 44-6). The fine veins extending between the portal vein and the base of the portal fibrous mass are carefully ligated and divided. After dissecting up to the right and left portal vein branches, the portal fibrous mass is transected at its border with the liver. Transection can be performed very accurately by using scissors or a scalpel. The liver parenchyma should be avoided to prevent obstruction of the remnant bile duct by scar tissue. For use during the portoenterostomy anastomosis, 5-0 absorbable sutures are usually placed in the liver surface of the posterior side of the remnant fibrous mass before transection. It is important to have enough distance between these sutures and the remnant fibrous mass. Bleeding points are controlled by packing with gauze. Diathermy electrocautery is not used because it can cause damage to the remnant bile ducts (Fig. 44-7). Intraoperative histopathology of the transected portal fibrous plate is important. If openings of microscopic bile duct structures are present at the transected surface, additional transection of the portal fibrous mass should be performed. A 30- to 40-cm Roux loop is prepared by transecting the jejunum 15 to 25 cm downstream from the ligament of Treitz (Fig. 44-8). The distal end may be oversewn or left open and is passed in a retrocolic position to the hepatic hilum. Small bowel continuity is established with an end-to-side enteroenterostomy. The hepatic portoenterostomy is performed in an end-to-side or end-to-end fashion using interrupted 5-0 sutures. Using the previously placed 5-0 sutures, the posterior anastomosis is performed first. The anterior margin of the jejunum is then sutured to the surface of the liver. There should be adequate separation between the anterior margin and the remnant fibrous mass. A small drain is positioned in the foramen of Winslow through a separate stab incision in the right abdominal wall and the incision is closed.

Hepaticoenterostomy

In "correctable" biliary atresia, a Roux-en-Y hepaticojejunostomy is usually performed. Although a wide and deep portal dissection is not required, excision of the patent CBD to the liver hilum is needed. Any cyst-like structure should be excised and must not be used for anastomosis to the intestine. Failure to remove all abnormal duct tissue results in an anastomotic stricture and cholangitis.[78]

Repeated Hepatic Portoenterostomy

Pediatric surgeons have reached a consensus about repeated hepatic portoenterostomies.[79] Bile drainage after reoperation is significant only in patients with good bile excretion after the initial surgery.[80] Because liver transplantation is a treatment option, repeated hepatic portoenterostomy should be considered only in patients in whom good bile flow suddenly ceases.

Minimally Invasive Surgery

The first laparoscopic Kasai procedure was described in 2002, and there have been few other reports.[81] One reason for the lack of information on minimally invasive surgery for this condition may be related to the difficult nature of the procedure, the apparent increased incidence of postoperative complications, and the worse early clinical outcome.[82] At the 2007 International Pediatric Endosurgery Group meeting in Buenos Aires, a consensus panel of experts in biliary atresia surgery and minimally invasive surgery concluded that minimally invasive surgery should not be utilized for this operation at this time because the results are not as good.

Postoperative Management

Patients are given oxygen and intravenous fluids, and nasogastric tube drainage is used. Broad-spectrum antibiotics are continued postoperatively to prevent cholangitis. Corticosteroids are also given intravenously or orally. Some studies have reported improved outcomes with high-dose corticosteroid therapy after a Kasai procedure and the effectiveness of standardized protocols that include corticosteroids.[83] Both antibiotic and corticosteroid use are largely empirical but corticosteroids are used both for their choleretic effect and to decrease scarring at the anastomosis site.[84,85] Ursodeoxycholic acid may be useful in augmenting bile flow, but only in the presence of patent bile ductules. Fat-soluble vitamins (A, D, E, and K) and formula feeds enriched with medium-chain triglycerides are also used.

Complications

Cholangitis

Cholangitis is the most frequent complication occurring after portoenterostomy and occurs most commonly during the first 2 years. Approximately 40% of infants are affected. All conduits become colonized within a month of surgery. Cholestasis is the main risk

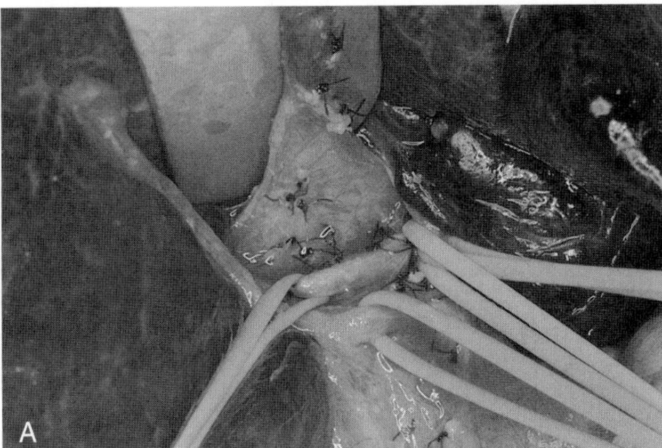

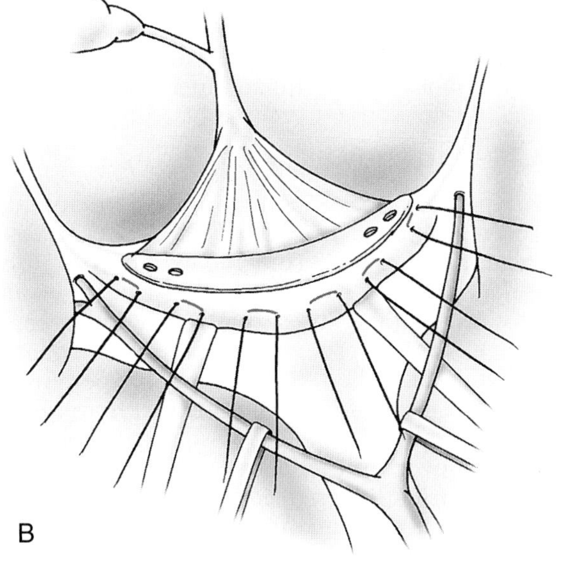

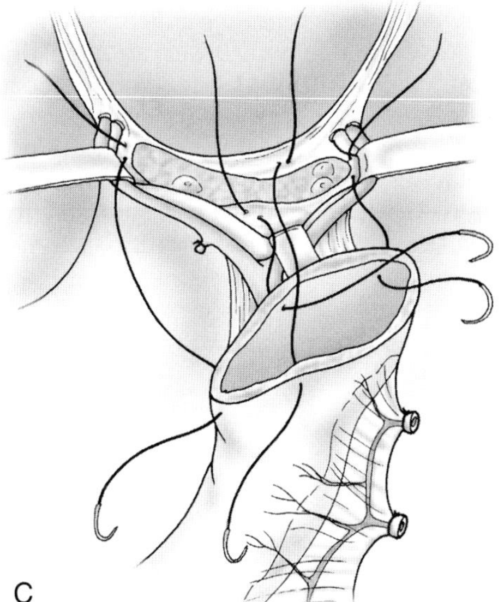

Figure 44-7. The portoenterostomy operation. **A,** Photograph of the initial mobilization of the gallbladder and atretic bile ducts and dissection/exposure of the porta hepatis. After the common bile duct remnants are severed from the duodenal side, the proximal end is pulled up and the portal bile duct remnants are freed from underlying structures. The portal vein and hepatic artery are encircled with vessel loops. Several small vessel branches between the portal vein to the fibrous remnants can be identified and should be divided between ligatures. **B,** The portal bile duct remnants must be dissected 5 or 6 mm proximal to the anterior branch of the right hepatic artery on the right side and to the umbilical point of the left portal vein on the left side. After completion of the portal dissection, the portal bile duct remnants should be transected at the site of the line that has been drawn. **C,** The end of the Roux-en-Y limb is anastomosed around the transected end of the portal bile duct remnants. Sutures should not be placed into the transected surface of the bile duct remnant because minute bile ducts may be present. (B and C from O'Neill JA, Rowe MI, Grosfeld JL, et al: Pediatric Surgery, 5th ed. St. Louis, Mosby–Year Book, 1998, vol 2, p 1471.)

factor for cholangitis, and all patients with biliary atresia have very small ducts.

Cholangitis presents initially as fever, decreased quantity and quality of bile, elevations in serum bilirubin, and a variety of signs associated with any infection. Nonetheless, prompt treatment is necessary because recurring attacks cause progressive liver damage. After initial blood cultures, broad-spectrum antibiotics with good gram-negative coverage are started and a favorable response is usually prompt. If stools become acholic, a pulse of corticosteroids is useful. To decrease the risk for cholangitis, Roux-en-Y biliary reconstruction has been modified by various maneuvers, including lengthening the Roux-en-Y limb from 50 to 70 cm, total diversion of the biliary conduit, intestinal valve formation, and the use of a physiologic intestinal valve.[86-90] An intussusception-type intestinal valve may be associated with a lower incidence of cholangitis. Stomas complicate liver transplantation, which may be required later. At this time, the antireflux intussusception valve may be the modification of choice. A gallbladder conduit is not recommended when the lumen of the patent duct is narrow or when pancreaticobiliary anomalies are demonstrated on cholangiography.

Cessation of Bile Flow

Loss of fecal bile pigment in a patient with a well-functioning portoenterostomy is an ominous sign. Prompt re-establishment of bile flow is imperative to avoid liver damage. Parents should be encouraged to report changes in stool color or signs of cholangitis. If cessation of bile flow occurs, a pulse of corticosteroids is tried because corticosteroids both augment bile flow and reduce inflammation.[84,85] If bile flow is re-established, then the corticosteroid dosage is reduced.

If bile flow is not re-established, corticosteroids are stopped. If bile flow was initially good, it is reasonable to consider reoperation. However, multiple attempts at reoperation are not useful and increase the technical difficulties for subsequent transplantation.

Portal Hypertension

Portal hypertension is common after portoenterostomy, even in infants with good bile flow. The basic inflammatory process affecting the extrahepatic ducts also damages the intrahepatic branches, albeit at variable rates. Continuing fibrosis has been demonstrated in some children despite successful portoenterostomy.[91] Clinical manifestations of portal hypertension include esophageal variceal hemorrhage, hypersplenism, and ascites (Fig. 44-9). Of special note is the finding that, over time, the susceptibility to complications of portal hypertension seems to decrease, resulting in reduced frequency and severity of variceal bleeding. This observation is difficult to explain and may be related to improvement in hepatic histology or the development of spontaneous portosystemic shunts. In any case, this general observation justifies a nonsurgical approach to the management of portal hypertension, as long as hepatic function is preserved (i.e., the patient remains anicteric with no coagulopathy and normal serum albumin level). In the presence of poor hepatic function, however, complications of portal hypertension are an indication for liver transplantation.

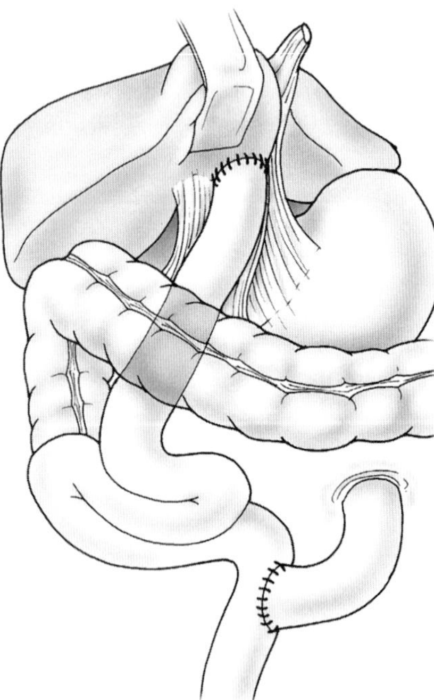

Figure 44-8. A 40-cm Roux-en-Y loop is prepared by transecting the jejunum 20 to 30 cm downstream from the ligament of Treitz. The distal end is oversewn and passed in a retrocolic position to the hepatic hilum. (From Tagge DU, Tagge EP, Drongowski RA, et al: A long-term experience with biliary atresia. Ann Surg 214:591, 1991.)

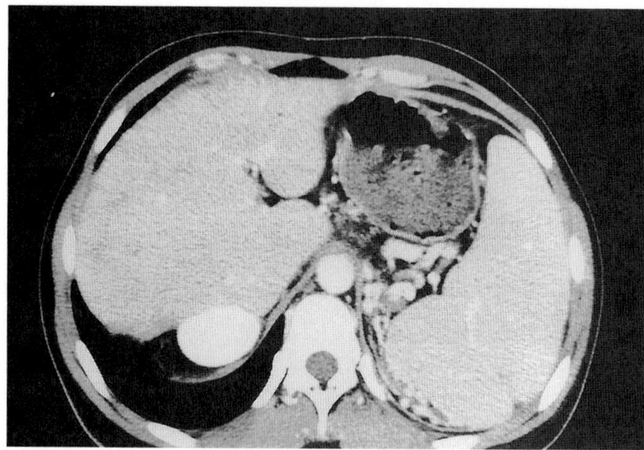

Figure 44-9. CT scan of a 20-year-old woman in whom severe portal hypertension developed. Note marked atrophy of the left lobe of the liver, severe splenomegaly, and varices around the stomach.

Intrahepatic Cysts

Biliary cysts or "lakes" may develop within the livers of long-term survivors and cause recurring attacks of cholangitis (Fig. 44-10).[92] Prolonged antibiotic treatment and ursodeoxycholic acid may be helpful in preventing cholangitis, but unremitting infection is an indication for liver transplantation.

Hepatopulmonary Syndrome

Diffuse intrapulmonary shunting may occur as a complication of chronic liver disease in children with biliary atresia, probably as a result of vasoactive compounds from the mesenteric circulation bypassing sinusoidal inactivation. The syndrome is characterized by cyanosis, dyspnea on exertion, hypoxia, and finger clubbing. It is more prevalent in children with syndromic biliary atresia. The diagnosis is confirmed by using a combination of arterial blood gas estimations with and without inspired oxygen, radionuclide lung scans with

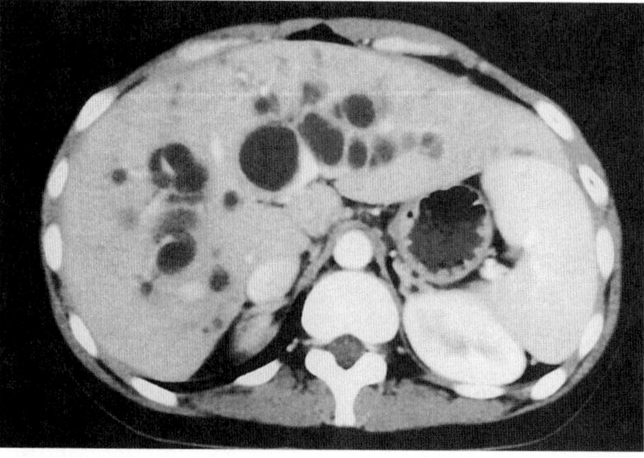

Figure 44-10. CT scan of a 17-year-old with biliary atresia. Multiple biliary cysts or "lakes" have developed within the liver of this long-term survivor and caused recurrent attacks of cholangitis.

macroaggregated albumin to quantify the degree of shunting, and contrast bubble echocardiography. This complication is progressive and can usually be reversed by liver transplantation. Pulmonary hypertension is a rarer complication but also may develop in long-term survivors after portoenterostomy.

Hepatic Malignancy

Rarely, malignant change (hepatocellular carcinoma or cholangiocarcinoma) may complicate long-standing biliary cirrhosis after portoenterostomy. A case of hepatocellular carcinoma has been reported in a 19-year-old young man after Kasai instrumentation for biliary atresia,[93] indicating the need for a high index of suspicion for the development of carcinoma, even in young patients.

Other Complications

Because of the presence of residual hepatic disease, metabolic problems associated with malabsorption of fat, protein, vitamins, and trace minerals can occur postoperatively because of impairment of bile flow to the gut.[94,95] Weight gain after surgical correction may be retarded if hepatic dysfunction persists. Essential fatty acid deficiencies and rickets are common problems related to metabolic derangements.[96] Long-term monitoring of clinical symptoms and adequate nutritional supplementation are required. Ectopic intestinal variceal bleeding and pulmonary arteriovenous fistulas are sometimes seen in long-term survivors with incomplete relief of impaired liver function.[37,46]

As more postoperative biliary atresia patients are reaching adulthood, the issue of pregnancy in females is becoming more common. In untransplanted postoperative biliary atresia patients, preterm cesarean delivery at around the 34th week appears to be reasonable because the pregnancy is high risk in a patient with poor hepatic reserve. Conversely, abdominal delivery at full term may be possible for selected patients with favorable liver function.[97]

Results and Prognosis

Without question, the Kasai hepatic portoenterostomy has greatly improved the prognosis of infants with biliary atresia and the results of surgical treatment have improved steadily over the past 30 years. However, a wide discrepancy exists in reported long-term postoperative results. One study from Japan found postoperative outcome to be excellent, with a 10-year survival rate of more than 70% if corrective surgery was performed before 60 days of age.[98] However, a nationwide survey of the Surgical Section of the American Academy of Pediatrics found that long-term survival was only 25%.[26] Other reported survival rates include 40% to 50% from the United Kingdom and 68% for a French national study on 10-year overall survival.[1,99] Results are considerably worse if the infant is older than 100 days at the time of portoenterostomy because obliterative cholangiopathy and hepatic fibrosis are more advanced.[99,100] The major determinants of satisfactory outcome after portoenterostomy are (1) age at initial operation, (2) successful achievement of postoperative bile flow, (3) presence of microscopic ductal structures at the hilum, (4) the degree of parenchymal disease at diagnosis, and (5) technical factors of the anastomosis. The age at which the surgical drainage is performed is the single most widely quoted prognostic variable. A favorable outcome is expected if the procedure is performed before 60 days of age because cirrhosis can develop by 3 to 4 months of age.[85] Infants who show a significant decrease in serum bilirubin and have fecal signs of good bile excretion also have improved results. The serum bilirubin value at 3 months after surgical correction can be used to predict long-term survival.[101]

The presence of microscopic ducts at the hilum is somewhat controversial. Some authors have suggested that duct size is important. However, not all agree.[102,103] Types I and II biliary atresia generally have good prognosis if treated early. In the more typical type III biliary atresia, the presence of larger bile ductules at the porta hepatis (>150 mm in diameter) is associated with a better prognosis. The subgroup of infants with syndromic biliary atresia have worse outcomes in terms of both clearance of jaundice and overall mortality.[1,28] The latter is related to associated malformations, particularly congenital heart disease, a predisposition to developing hepatopulmonary syndrome, and possibly immune compromise from functional hyposplenism. Anecdotal evidence suggests that infants with concomitant CMV infection fare less well after a portoenterostomy.

The importance of surgical technical experience was demonstrated by a British survey in which patients who underwent treatment at centers treating one case per year had significantly worse outcome than patients who underwent surgical treatment at centers performing more than five cases per year.[104] Thus, the level of surgical skill and the experience with postoperative management are critical factors for optimizing outcome.

Certain substances may act as prognostic factors in biliary atresia. Serum levels of interleukin (IL)-6, IL-1ra, insulin-like growth factor-1 (IGF-1), vascular cell adhesion molecule-1 (VCAM-1), and ICAM-1 correlate with liver dysfunction in postoperative biliary atresia patients.[42,105,106] Immunohistochemically, a reduction in the expression of CD68 and ICAM-1 at the time of portoenterostomy is associated with a better postoperative prognosis.[107] The presence of ductal plate malformation in the liver predicts poor bile flow after hepatoportoenterostomy in infants with biliary atresia.[108] Growth failure and poor mean weight z-scores 3 months after hepatoportoenterostomy were associated with a poor clinical outcome.[109]

Liver Transplantation

Biliary atresia is the most common indication for liver transplantation in children, and the majority of affected children will eventually come to transplant. Infants whose jaundice is not cleared after portoenterostomy, or those with complications associated with end-stage chronic liver disease that develops despite initially successful portoenterostomy, require liver transplantation. Most of these cases require transplantation within the first few years of life. The indications for liver transplantation in postoperative biliary atresia patients are (1) no bile drainage at all, because major clinical deterioration will be inevitable; (2) the presence of signs of developmental retardation or their sequelae if they become uncontrollable; and (3) complications/side effects being socially unacceptable.

A high hepatic artery resistance index measured on Doppler ultrasonography is an indication for relatively urgent transplantation. Deterioration in hepatic status may be precipitated by adolescence or pregnancy.[110] However, as many as 20% of patients undergoing portoenterostomy will remain well and reach maturity with good native liver function.

The dramatic improvement in survival with the use of cyclosporin and tacrolimus immunosuppression after liver transplantation raises the question of transplantation becoming a more conventional form of surgical treatment for biliary atresia. The donor supply is always a problem, alleviated to some extent by reduced-size liver transplantation. Favorable experience with living-related liver transplantation at Kyoto University in Japan has been widely reported.[111]

Five-year survival after liver transplantation for biliary atresia is currently 80% to 90%, and techniques such as split-liver grafting and living-related liver transplantation have decreased waiting times. The combination of Kasai portoenterostomy and liver transplantation has transformed a disease that was almost invariably fatal in the 1960s into one with an overall 5-year survival of about 90%. Furthermore, long-term studies of postoperative biliary atresia patients have shown that survivors have an acceptable to good quality of life.[112,113] A more recent study summarized the largest series (n = 464) of post–Kasai portoenterostomy biliary atresia patients who had undergone living-related liver transplantation. The outcome of living-related liver transplantation in adult biliary atresia patients was significantly worse than in the pediatric patients. The overall 5- and 10- year survival rates were 70% and 56% in adults versus 87% and 81% in pediatric patients, respectively.[114] On the other hand, there is another report concluding that living-related liver transplantation for post-Kasai portoenterostomy can be performed safely in adults with a long-term survival rate equivalent to that for pediatric patients.[115] Longer immunosuppression might ultimately lead to increased co-morbidity, including higher rates of cancer, infection, and metabolic diseases later in life. In addition, in living-related liver transplantation, the risk to the donor is also a matter of concern.[116] The optimal timing of transplantation for successful long-term outcome in post-Kasai portoenterostomy biliary atresia patients has yet to be established.

Despite the debate over whether hepatic portoenterostomy or primary liver transplantation should be performed as the initial surgical procedure for biliary atresia, the consensus among pediatric surgeons all over the world is that hepatic portoenterostomy is still the most reasonable first choice. However, liver transplantation plays an important role in the long-term management of biliary atresia.

CHOLEDOCHAL CYST

Choledochal cyst was first reported by Douglas in 1852.[117] This condition is relatively rare, with an estimated incidence in Western populations of 1 in 13,000 to 15,000 live births.[118] However, it is far more common in the East, with rates as high as 1 per 1000 live births having been described in Japan. Although the etiology remains unknown, choledochal cyst is likely to be congenital. Pathologic features frequently include an anomalous junction of the pancreatic duct and CBD (pancreaticobiliary malunion [PBMU]), intrahepatic bile duct dilatation with or without downstream stenosis, and varying degrees of hepatic fibrosis.

Choledochal cyst is usually classified into three groups, based on anatomy.[119] However, other forms and subgroups have been described, based on cholangiographic findings of intrahepatic ducts or the presence of a long common duct shared by the liver and the pancreas (PBMU).[120,121] Based on our experience, we prefer to classify choledochal cyst into groups according to the presence or absence of PBMU (Fig. 44-11). The vast majority of cases of choledochal cyst are associated with PBMU. Thus, the following comments are related primarily to cystic (saccular), fusiform, and forme fruste choledochal cysts (FFCC).

Pathogenesis

A number of theories have been proposed for the etiology of choledochal cyst. Congenital weakness of the bile duct wall, a primary abnormality of proliferation during embryologic ductal development, and congenital obstruction have been postulated.[122-124] An early obstructive factor has gained popularity after an experimental study in which cystic dilatation of the CBD was produced by ligation of the distal end of the CBD in neonatal lambs, but not at later stages of development.[125]

In 1969, the "long common channel theory" was proposed.[126] It was postulated that PBMU allows reflux of pancreatic enzymes into the CBD, which leads to disruption of the duct walls. This theory is supported by the high amylase content of fluid that is usually aspirated from choledochal cyst. In theory, the CBD could become obstructed distally because of edema or fibrosis caused by refluxed pancreatic fluid.

We support the "long common channel theory" anatomically because almost all cases of choledochal cyst have PBMU, but we cannot agree with the hypothesis that weakness of the choledochal wall is due to reflux of pancreatic fluid. Our experimental data in puppies showed that the chemical reaction initiated by refluxed pancreatic fluid in the CBD is extremely mild.[127] In addition, there are a number of patients with PBMU and high gallbladder amylase levels with

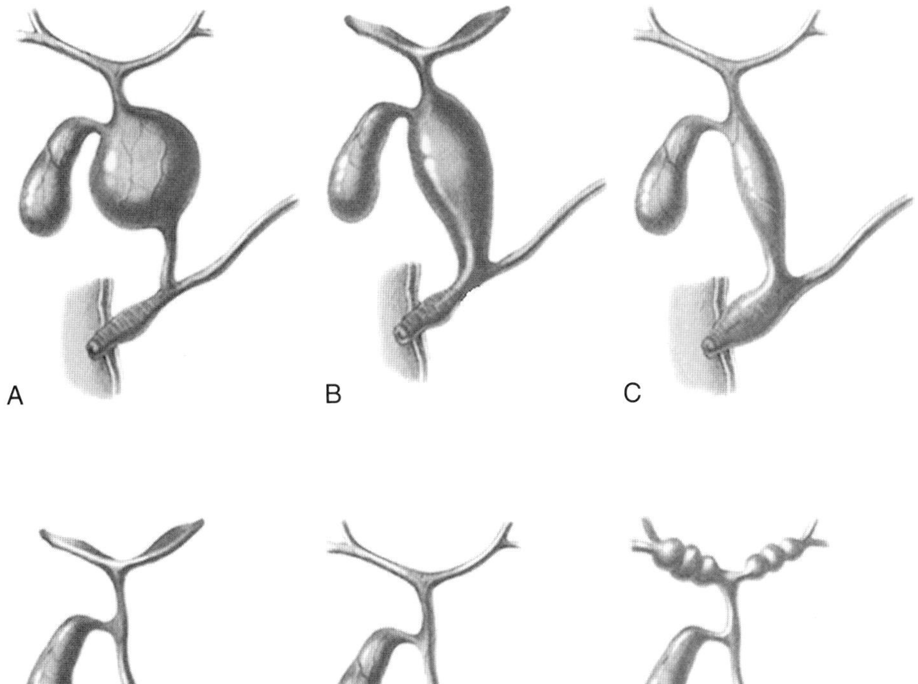

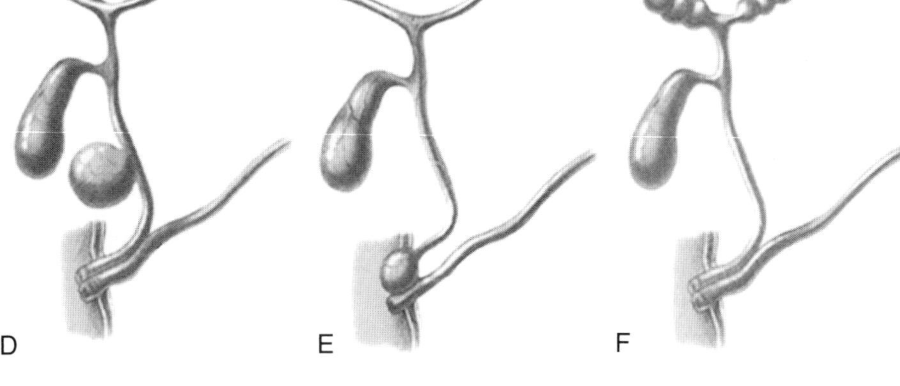

Figure 44-11. Classification of choledochal cysts with pancreaticobiliary malunion (PBMU). **A,** Cystic dilatation of the extrahepatic bile duct. **B,** Fusiform dilatation of the extrahepatic bile duct. **C,** Forme fruste choledochal cyst without PBMU. **D,** Cystic diverticulum of the common bile duct. **E,** Choledochocele (diverticulum of the distal common bile duct). **F,** Intrahepatic bile duct dilatation alone (Caroli's disease).

no dilation of the CBD. Also, choledochal cyst can be diagnosed as early as the fifth month of gestation. At this time in gestation, the fetal pancreas does not produce functional enzymes. Thus, the exact role of the pancreatic fluid is unclear.

From research on human fetuses, the pancreaticobiliary ductal junction has been demonstrated to be outside the duodenal wall before the eighth week of gestation and then migrates normally toward the duodenal lumen. Thus, PBMU may persist as a result of arrest in this migration.[128]

Based on these studies, we believe that PBMU and congenital stenosis are the basic causative factors of choledochal cyst rather than destruction caused by reflux of pancreatic fluid.

Clinical Presentation

Choledochal cyst can present at any age, but more than half of patients are initially seen within the first decade of life. Clinical manifestations differ according to the age at onset. Young infants may have obstructive jaundice, acholic stools, and hepatomegaly, resembling biliary atresia, and may even have advanced liver fibrosis. At cholangiography, there is a patent communication with the duodenum and a well-developed intrahepatic bile duct (IHBD) tree. Young infants may also present with a large upper abdominal mass without jaundice. In young children, presenting symptoms can be divided roughly into two groups: a right upper quadrant mass with intermittent jaundice due to biliary obstruction, seen in patients with saccular choledochal cyst, and abdominal pain due to pancreatitis, which is characteristic of fusiform choledochal cyst or FFCC. In adolescence and adulthood, choledochal cyst has often been misdiagnosed for many years as cholelithiasis, cirrhosis, portal hypertension, hepatic abscess, and biliary carcinoma. Surgical treatment in this group is much more difficult than in children. The incidence of postoperative complications is quite high, even after primary cyst excision.[129]

Pathology

In choledochal cyst, bile duct mucosa shows erosion, epithelial desquamation, and papillary hyperplasia with regenerative atypia.[130] Bile duct mucosal dysplasia without carcinoma can also be found frequently.[131] Additionally, metaplastic changes, such as mucous cells, goblet cells, and Paneth cells can be seen. Hyperplasia and metaplasia increase with age and can progress to carcinoma in adults. These changes are seen in all types of choledochal cyst.[132]

The gallbladder mucosa in patients with PBMU shows cholecystitis, cholesterolosis, adenomyosis or adenomyomatosis, polyp including adenoma, and epithelial hyperplasia. The gallbladder mucosa in FFCC is characterized by diffuse epithelial hyperplasia, with or without metaplasia of the pyloric glands, goblet cells, and Paneth cells.

Diagnosis

For the diagnosis of choledochal cyst, it is important to detect not only dilatation of the extrahepatic bile duct but also PBMU.

Currently, abdominal ultrasonography is probably the best screening method in patients who are suspected of having choledochal cyst. In recent years, the number of patients who are diagnosed by antenatal ultrasonography is increasing. Ultrasonography also clearly demonstrates IHBD dilatation and the state of the liver parenchyma.

Preoperatively, endoscopic retrograde cholangiopancreatography (ERCP) can accurately visualize the configuration of the pancreaticobiliary ductal system in fine detail. However, it is invasive and therefore unsuitable for repeated use and is contraindicated during acute pancreatitis.

Magnetic resonance cholangiopancreatography (MRCP) can provide excellent visualization of the pancreaticobiliary ducts, allowing detection of narrowing, dilatation, and filling defects with medium to high degrees of accuracy (Fig. 44-12).[133,134] MRCP is noninvasive and can be useful for delineating the pancreatic and biliary ducts proximal to an obstruction. However, in children younger than 3 years, MRCP may not visualize the pancreaticobiliary ductal system because of the small caliber. Percutaneous transhepatic cholangiography is also available, especially for patients with IHBD dilatation and severe jaundice. Also, intraductal ultrasonography has been applied successfully to delineate the distal parts of the CBD and pancreatic duct, which is useful for diagnosing choledochal cyst.[135]

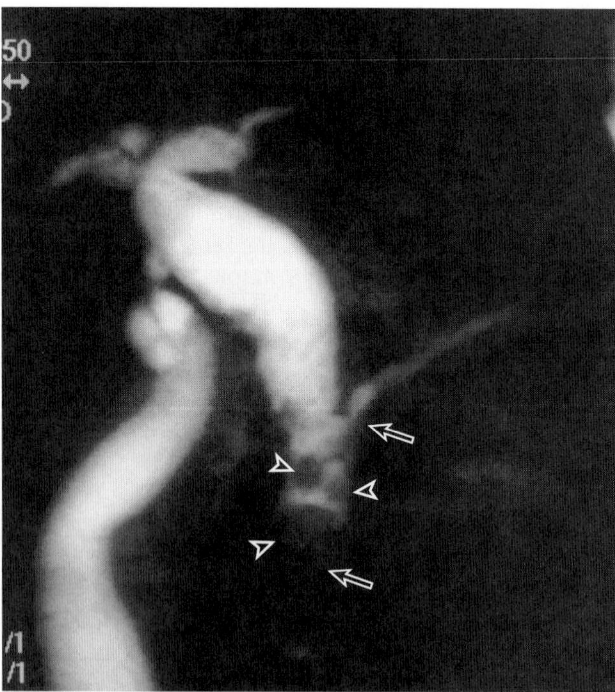

Figure 44-12. Magnetic resonance cholangiopancreatography in a patient with a choledochal cyst, showing fusiform dilatation of the extrahepatic bile duct, long common channel (between *arrows*), protein plugs (*arrowheads*), and pancreatic duct. (From Miyano T, Yamataka A: Choledochal cysts. Curr Opin Pediatr 9:285, 1997.)

Intraoperative cholangiography is unnecessary if the entire biliary system has been delineated before cyst excision, but it should be used if the pancreaticobiliary ductal system has not been completely visualized.

Treatment

Cyst excision is the definitive treatment of choice for choledochal cyst because of the high morbidity and high risk for carcinoma after internal drainage, a commonly used treatment in the past. Recently, more attention has been paid to the treatment of intrahepatic and intrapancreatic ductal diseases such as IHBD dilatation, focal stenosis, debris in the IHBD, and protein plugs or stones in the common channel.[136,137] The transection level of the common hepatic duct and excisional level of the intrapancreatic bile duct also are highly controversial.[136,138]

The Common Bile Duct

Usually more adhesions are found between a saccular choledochal cyst, the portal vein, and hepatic artery than with a fusiform choledochal cyst, especially in older children. In adolescents and adults, adhesions are often very dense and great care is required during cyst excision.

Before excision, we always open the anterior wall transversely (Fig. 44-13). After opening the anterior wall, the posterior wall is visible from the inside, facilitating the dissection of the portal triad. If the cyst is extremely inflamed and the adhesions are very dense, mucosectomy of the cyst (Figs. 44-14 and 44-15) should be performed rather than attempting full-thickness dissection to minimize the risk for injuring the portal vein and hepatic artery.

The Distal Common Bile Duct

To prevent postoperative pancreatitis or stone formation, or both, in a remnant cyst, the caudal CBD should be resected as close as possible to the pancreaticobiliary ductal junction. In saccular choledochal cyst, the caudal CBD is sometimes so narrow that it cannot be identified and it is quite unlikely that a residual cyst will develop within the pancreas. In contrast, in fusiform choledochal cyst, delineation of the diseased duct is more difficult, because the caudal CBD is still wide at the pancreaticobiliary ductal junction and the likelihood of leaving some remnant of the CBD is high. If the caudal CBD is resected along line 1 shown in

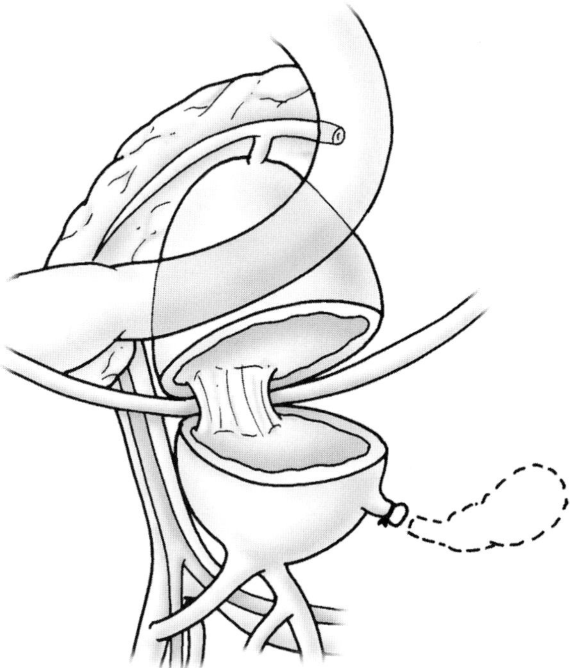

Figure 44-13. Schema showing transection of a choledochal cyst. (From Miyano T: Congenital biliary dilatation. In Puri P [ed]: Newborn Surgery. Oxford, UK, Butterworth-Heinemann, 1996, p 436.)

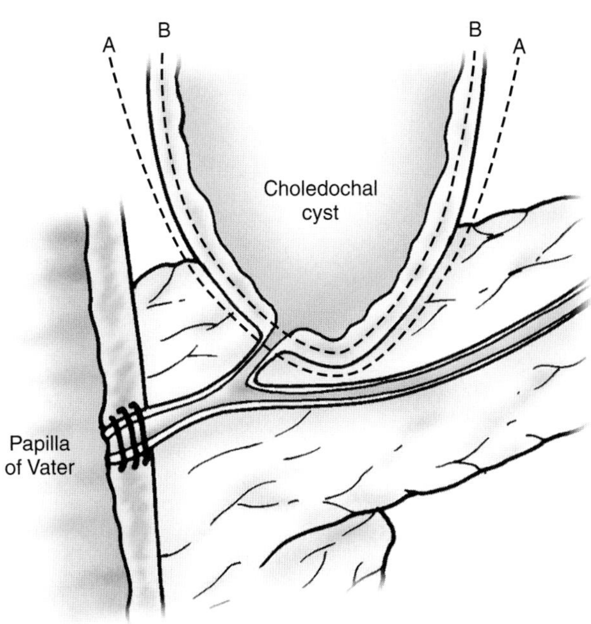

Figure 44-15. Operative technique for excision of the distal portion of choledochal cyst. A, full-thickness layer; B, mucosectomy layer. (From Miyano T: Congenital biliary dilatation. In Puri P [ed]: Newborn Surgery. Oxford, UK, Butterworth-Heinemann, 1996, p 437.)

Figure 44-16, over time a cyst will re-form around the distal CBD left within the pancreas, leading to recurrent pancreatitis, stone formation, or malignancy in the residual cyst (Fig. 44-17). In contrast, if the distal duct is resected along line 2 in Figure 44-16, just above the pancreaticobiliary ductal junction, cyst re-formation due to residual duct within the pancreas is unlikely.[120]

Before the introduction of intraoperative endoscopy, it was difficult to excise the pancreatic portion of a fusiform choledochal cyst completely and safely because of the risk for injury to the pancreatic duct. Endoscopy now allows safe excision of most of the wall of a fusiform choledochal cyst in the pancreas without damaging the pancreatic duct. We believe this reduces the risk for postoperative complications.

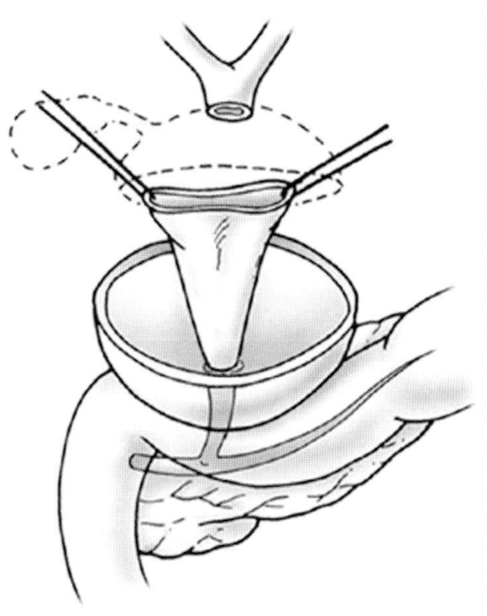

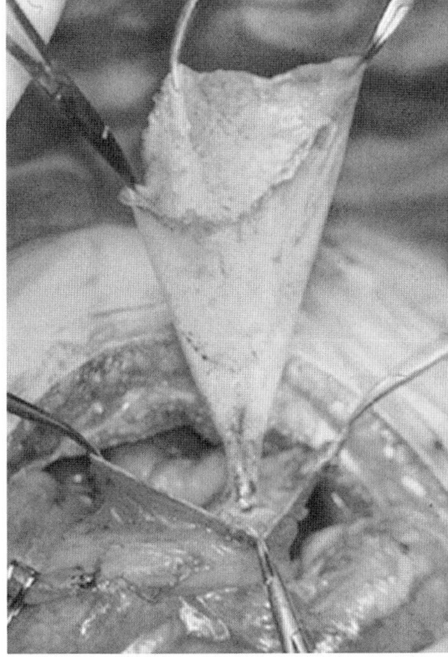

Figure 44-14. If there is significant inflammation surrounding the choledochal cyst that precludes mobilization of the cyst from the hepatic artery and portal vein posteriorly, mucosectomy of the distal portion of the cyst is an alternate operative technique.

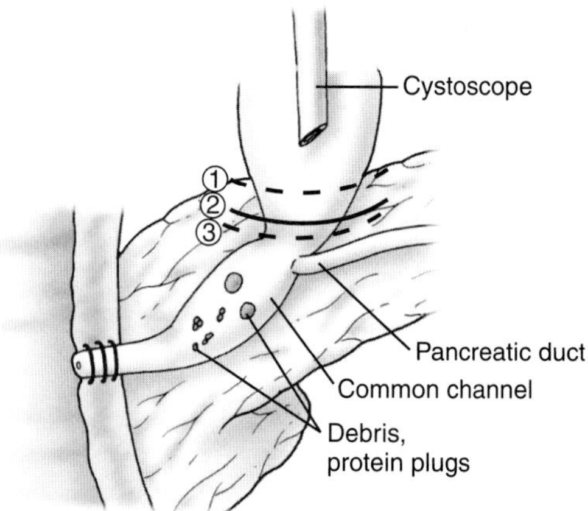

Figure 44-16. Diagram of intraoperative endoscopy of the bile duct distal to a cyst with debris and protein plug. After identification of the orifice of the pancreatic duct, the cyst is excised. Level 1, High likelihood of leaving some residual cyst. Level 2, Adequate excision level of the cyst. Level 3, High likelihood of injuring the pancreatic duct. (From Miyano T, Yamataka A, Long Li: Congenital biliary dilatation. J Pediatr Surg 9:190, 2000.)

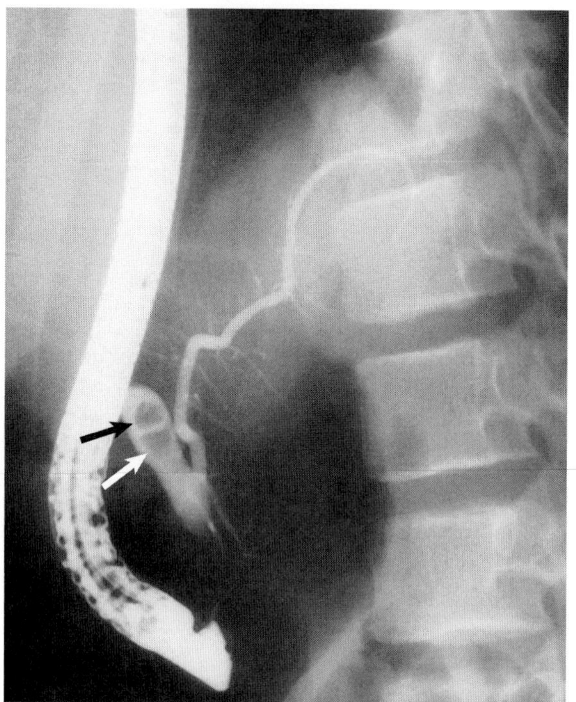

Figure 44-17. Endoscopic retrograde cholangiopancreatography showing stones (*arrows*) in the residual intrapancreatic terminal choledochus after excision of fusiform-type choledochal cyst. (From Yamataka A, Ohshiro K, Okada Y, et al: Complications after cyst excision with hepaticoenterostomy for choledochal cyst and their surgical management in children versus adults. J Pediatr Surg 32:1099, 1997.)

The Proximal Common Bile Duct

The common hepatic duct is transected at the level of distinct caliber change. Because any remaining proximal cyst mucosa is prone to malignant changes, care must be taken to excise it completely, especially when a large anastomosis is performed (Fig. 44-18).

Dilatation of the peripheral IHBD in patients with choledochal cyst may be associated with late complications such as recurrent cholangitis, stone formation, and anastomotic stricture. Severe dilatation of the IHBD can be managed by segmentectomy of the liver, intrahepatic cystoenterostomy, or balloon dilatation of a stenotic lesion at the time of cyst excision.[139-142] However, the incidence of late complications appears to be low, especially in younger children, so such excessive surgical intervention may be unnecessary, except in specific cases. If IHBD dilatation persists after definitive surgery, careful follow-up is mandatory.

Intraoperative endoscopy is also useful for examining for the presence of debris in the dilated IHBD (Fig. 44-19). Recently, we found a high incidence of IHBD debris that was not detected by preoperative radiologic investigations, and some debris that had been shown in preoperative studies that had been overlooked.[143] These facts indicate that intraoperative endoscopy is extremely useful at the time of cyst excision. Another striking finding was that this debris could be present even in the absence of IHBD dilatation, although this was uncommon. We believe endoscopic inspection of the IHBD to be so valuable that it should be a routine part of the operative treatment of choledochal cyst.

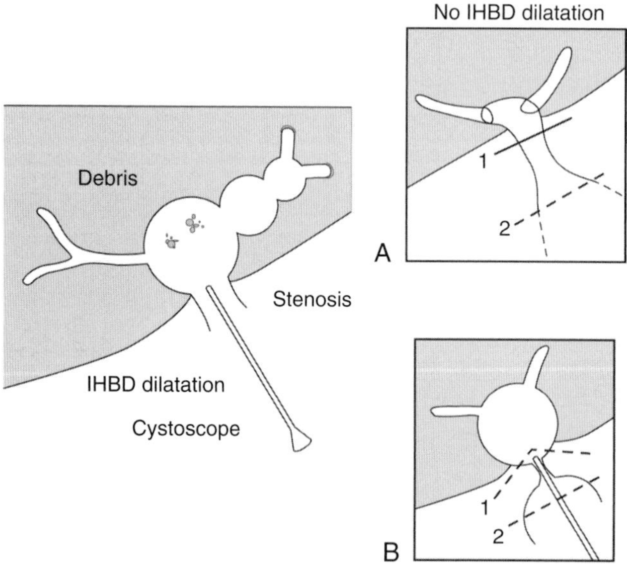

Figure 44-18. Diagrams of intraoperative endoscopy of the bile duct proximal to a cyst. **A,** Ideal level of resection of the common hepatic duct is safely determined without injuring the orifices of the intrahepatic duct and without leaving any redundant common hepatic duct. **B,** Stenosis of the common hepatic duct near the hepatic hilum is safely excised, and a wide anastomosis is made. Level 1, Adequate level of resection of the common hepatic duct. Level 2, Inadequate level of resection. (From Miyano T, Yamataka A, Long Li: Dilatation of the intrahepatic duct. Semin Pediatr Surg 9:187-195, 2000.)

The Anastomosis

An end-to-end anastomosis of the jejunum to the cephalad remnant of the CBD is recommended if the ratio between the diameters of the CBD and the proximal Roux-en-Y jejunum is less than or equal to 1 (common hepatic duct) to 2.5 (jejunum) (Fig. 44-20). If the

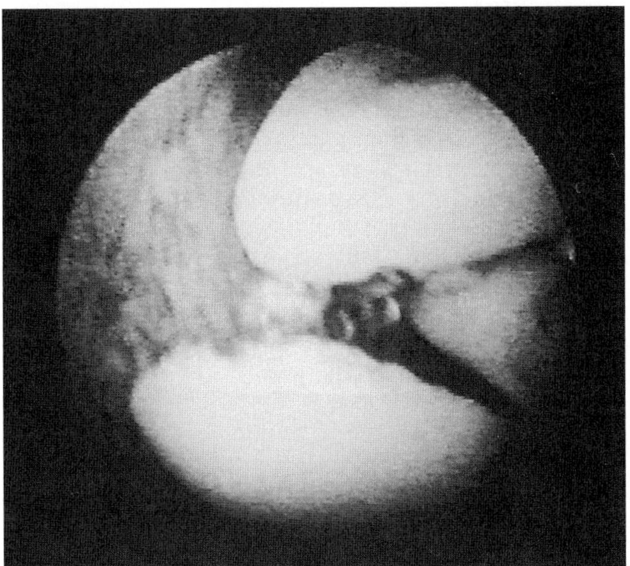

Figure 44-19. Massive debris in the intrahepatic bile duct observed through the pediatric cystoscope. (From Shima H, Yamataka A, Yanai T, et al: Intracorporeal electrohydraulic lithotripsy for intrahepatic bile duct stone formation after choledochal cyst excision. Pediatr Surg Int 20:70-72, 2004.)

biliary duct is too small, then an end-to-side anastomosis is preferred. The anastomosis should be as close as possible to the closed end of the jejunal limb (see Fig. 44-20, inset). An end-to-side anastomosis that is performed away from the closed end of the proximal jejunum will allow a blind pouch to form as the child grows (Fig. 44-21). Bile stasis in the blind pouch can lead to intrahepatic stone formation, especially if the intrahepatic ducts are dilated. We believe that using an end-to-end hepaticojejunostomy and our end-to-side jejunojejunostomy technique will help prevent both stone formation and ascending cholangitis.

Some surgeons predetermine the length of the Roux-en-Y jejunal limb without considering the size of the child. This causes the Roux-en-Y jejunal limb to be unnecessarily long, especially in infants and younger children. Redundancy of the Roux limb is likely as the patient grows. This leads to bile stasis in the limb itself which, in turn, leads to cholangitis or stone formation. Construction of the Roux-en-Y as shown (see Fig. 44-20) should prevent redundancy of the Roux limb. We recommend securing the jejunal limb from the ligament of Treitz to the Roux limb in a side-to-side fashion for about 8 cm proximal to the end-to-side anastomosis to ensure smooth flow of bile and bowel contents distally. Without using this technique, the jejunojejunostomy will tend to be T shaped, promoting reflux of jejunal contents into the Roux limb, a situation we recently encountered in a patient who had surgery elsewhere (see Fig. 44-21).[144]

Laparoscopic Surgery

In 1995, the first laparoscopic choledochal cyst excision in a child was reported.[145] Since then, the number of reports has increased. Intraoperative bile duct endoscopy can also be performed laparoscopically.[146] Recently, robot-assisted laparoscopic resections of choledochal cyst have been reported by several centers.[147,148]

Results

Satisfactory surgical outcome with low morbidity in the short to mid-term is expected in patients after cyst excision. However, in the long term, many complications have been reported and careful long-term follow-up is mandatory.

In an American survey in 1981, 14 of 198 patients with choledochal cyst were reported to have died of biliary atresia, cholangitis with sepsis, hepatic failure, or carcinoma.[149] Other late and serious complications were cholangitis, obstructive jaundice, pancreatitis, stone formation, and portal hypertension. Thirty-six patients had been lost to follow-up, and only 115 patients were alive without liver disease.

In 1997, we reported 200 children who were 15 years old or younger at the time of cyst excision.[129] The onset of symptoms was 5 years or earlier in 175 children and between 6 and 15 years in the remaining 25 children. The mean age when initial symptoms began was 3 years. The mean age at cyst excision was 4.2 years. Primary cyst excision was performed in 176 children, 5 had cyst excision converted from internal drainage,

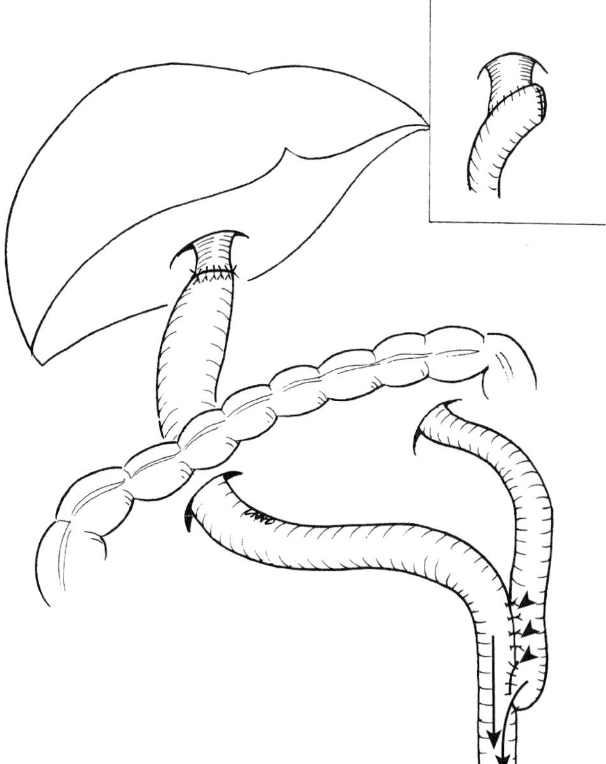

Figure 44-20. Adequate Roux-en-Y hepaticojejunostomy at the time of cyst excision. *Arrowheads,* Approximated native jejunum and distal Roux-en-Y limb. *Arrows,* Smooth flow without reflux of small bowel contents. (From Yamataka A, Kobayashi H, Shimotakahara A, et al: Recommendations for preventing complications related to Roux-en-Y hepaticojejunostomy performed during excision of choledochal cyst in children. J Pediatr Surg 38:1830-1832, 2003.)

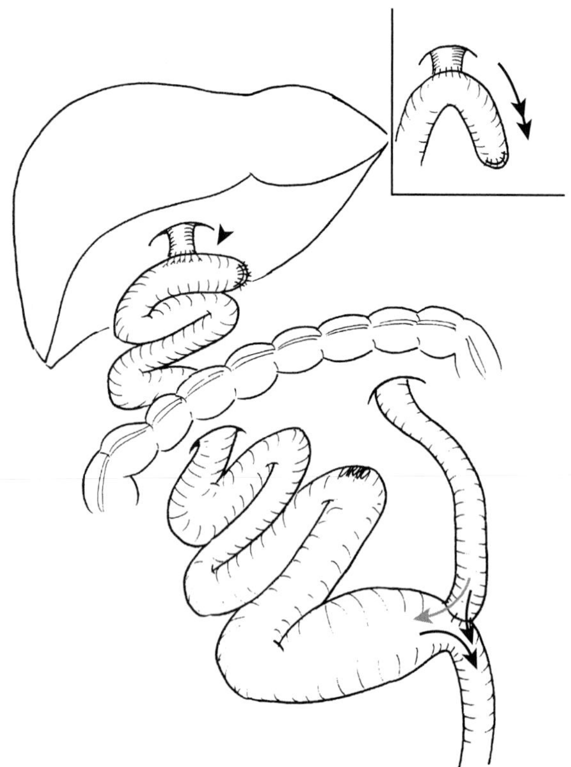

Figure 44-21. Inadequate Roux-en-Y hepaticojejunostomy at the time of cyst excision. Note hepaticojejunostomy far from the closed end of the blind pouch (*arrowhead*). *Double arrows in the inset,* Elongation of the blind pouch. *Shaded arrow,* Reflux of jejunal contents into the Roux-en-Y limb through a T-shaped Roux-en-Y jejunojejunostomy. (From Yamataka A, Kobayashi H, Shimotakahara A, et al: Recommendations for preventing complications related to Roux-en-Y hepaticojejunostomy performed during excision of choledochal cyst in children. J Pediatr Surg 38:1830-1832, 2003.)

and 19 had cyst excision converted from other biliary surgery such as percutaneous transhepatic cholangiodrainage, T-tube drainage, and cholecystectomy. Intraoperative endoscopy was performed in 70 children. The mean follow-up period was 10.9 years. Roux-en-Y hepaticojejunostomy was performed in 188 patients, 11 had standard hepaticoduodenostomy, and 1 had a jejunal interposition hepaticoduodenostomy. There was no operative mortality. Eighteen (9%) children had 25 complications after cyst excision, including ascending cholangitis, intrapancreatic terminal CBD calculi, pancreatitis, and bowel obstruction (Table 44-2). Fifteen of the 18 children required further surgical intervention such as revision of the hepaticoenterostomy, percutaneous transhepatic cholangioscopic lithotomy, excision of the residual intrapancreatic terminal CBD, endoscopic sphincterotomy, pancreaticojejunostomy, or laparotomy for bowel obstruction. Neither stone formation, anastomotic stricture, nor cholangitis was seen in the 70 children who had intraoperative endoscopy. No malignancy was found.

In patients who underwent cyst excision when aged 5 years or younger, no major complications such as intrahepatic stones, intrapancreatic terminal CBD calculi, or stricture of the hepaticoenterostomy were seen. Thus, early diagnosis followed by cyst excision and intraoperative endoscopy is extremely important to prevent postoperative complications.

Even after primary cyst excision, malignancy can arise from the intrapancreatic terminal CBD,[150] the hepaticojejunostomy anastomosis site,[151] and the IHBD.[152] Of the 40 adult patients in our series who had cyst excision at age 16 years or older, 2 died of cholangiocarcinoma. One of these patients had had primary cyst excision at 25 years of age.

Table 44-2 Complications after Cyst Excision in Children versus Adults

Incidence in 200 Children	Complication	Incidence in 40 Adults
3	Ascending cholangitis	9
3	Intrahepatic bile duct stones	5
3*	Intrapancreatic terminal choledochus calculi	1
1	Pancreatic duct calculus	1
1*	Stones in the blind pouch of the end-to-side Roux-en-Y hepaticojejunostomy	0
9†	Bowel obstruction	3‡
0	Cholangiocarcinoma	2
0	Liver dysfunction	1
5	Pancreatitis	5
25 (18)	TOTAL	27 (17)

Note: The numbers in parentheses indicate the patients who had complications after cyst excision (18 children and 17 adults had 25 and 27 complications after cyst excision, respectively).
*One patient with intrapancreatic terminal choledochus calculi also had a stone in the blind pouch of the end-to-side hepaticojejunostomy.
†Adhesions in 6 patients and intussusception in 3 patients.
‡Adhesions in all 3 patients.
From Yamataka A, Ohshiro K, Okada Y, et al: Complications after cyst excision with hepaticoenterostomy for choledochal cysts and their surgical management in children versus adults. J Pediatr Surg 32:1098, 1997, with permission.

In the past 18 years, we have performed a total of 92 Roux-en-Y hepaticojejunostomies (70 end-to-end and 22 end-to-side) by using our cyst excision technique with intraoperative endoscopy and the Roux-en-Y hepaticojejunostomy technique mentioned previously. We reviewed these patients after a mean follow-up period of 8.0 years (range: 9 months to 16 years), and there were no major complications.[144]

OTHER BILIARY TRACT DISORDERS

Biliary Hypoplasia

Biliary hypoplasia is a lesion characterized by an exceptionally small but grossly visible and radiographically patent extrahepatic biliary duct system. The diagnosis is made at the time of surgical exploration for the investigation of jaundice in infancy. Biliary hypoplasia is not a specific disease entity but a manifestation of a variety of hepatobiliary disorders: neonatal hepatitis, α_1-antitrypsin deficiency, intrahepatic biliary atresia, Alagille syndrome, and nonsyndromic paucity of IHBDs. Biliary hypoplasia cannot be improved by surgical maneuvers. The prognosis is highly variable and depends on the primary disease. Some patients die in infancy and others live to adolescence, often with jaundice, pruritus, and stunted growth. Still, others recover fully.

Alagille syndrome is a genetic defect that results in a typical constellation of features: peculiar facies with a high, prominent forehead and deep-set eyes, chronic cholestasis, posterior embryotoxon, butterfly-like vertebral arch defects, and heart disease (usually peripheral pulmonary stenosis) (Fig. 44-22). These patients often respond to supportive measures such as treatment with ursodeoxycholic acid and phenobarbital.[153] They often have hypercholesterolemia and may eventually require liver transplantation because of ongoing hepatic scarring and the development of hepatocellular carcinoma.

Nonsyndromic paucity of bile ducts may be associated with liver changes similar to those seen in Alagille syndrome but without the associated findings. Treatment is similar for both conditions.

Idiopathic Perforation of Bile Ducts: Bile Ascites

Bile ascites typically is first seen with gradually worsening abdominal distention and jaundice in a neonate. The disease may be associated with an episode of sepsis or ABO blood group incompatibility. More typically, it is an isolated finding, probably related to duct malformation. Although the almost universal site of perforation is at the junction of the cystic duct with the CBD, spontaneous rupture of the intrahepatic duct has been also reported, especially at the left IHBD.[154] The diagnosis is made by hepatobiliary scan, demonstrating radioactivity in the free peritoneal cavity. There is a report that radiologic demonstration of the degree of leakage by ERCP is useful and that internal stenting can be performed laparoscopically.[155]

At operation, sterile bile ascites and bile staining are found. An operative cholangiogram should be performed throughout the gallbladder. The lesion is usually self-limiting, and the perforation seals with drainage. Aggressive surgical intervention is not indicated because the small, delicate, presumably

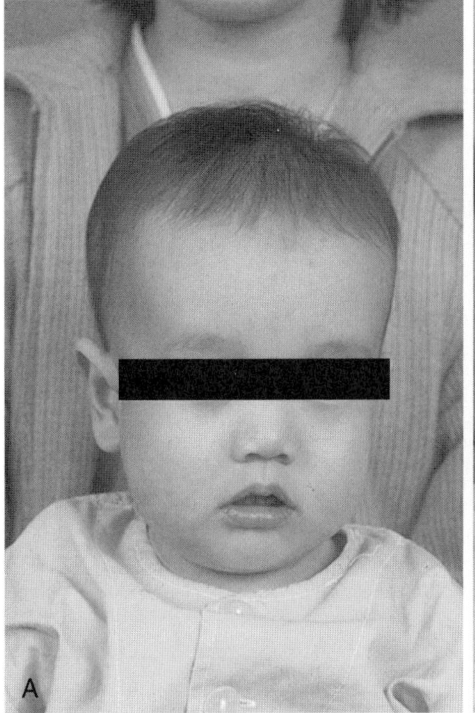

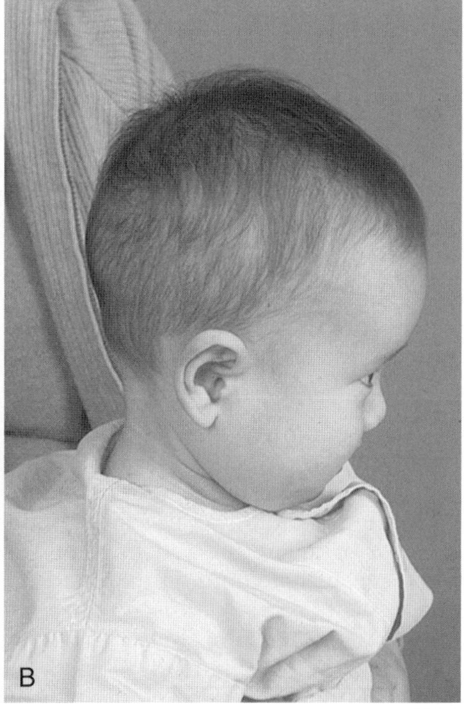

Figure 44-22. This photograph shows an infant with Alagille syndrome. Note the high prominent forehead and deep-set eyes.

congenitally weakened bile duct may be further damaged during attempts at anastomosis.[156]

Gallbladder Disease

Gallbladder disease in children is being diagnosed with increasing frequency. This is related both to increased detection associated with more widespread use of routine ultrasonography and to an increased incidence secondary to dietary changes that have developed. Biliary dyskinesia is being diagnosed more frequently in the pediatric population, and these patients do well with laparoscopic cholecystectomy.[157,158] Gallbladder disease also may develop in infants supported with total parenteral nutrition.

Hydrops of the Gallbladder

Acute distention with edema in the wall of the gallbladder has been reported in association with a number of septic or shock-like states, including Kawasaki disease, severe diarrhea with dehydration, hepatitis, scarlet fever, familial Mediterranean fever, leptospirosis, and mesenteric adenitis. Hydrops is suspected if a palpable mass of the gallbladder is confirmed by ultrasonography. In most cases, hydrops resolves spontaneously. If symptoms intensify, cholecystectomy may be necessary.[159]

Acalculous Cholecystitis

Hydrops and acalculous cholecystitis are probably manifestations of the same disease entity and usually arise after a patient has been resuscitated from a state of primary sepsis or shock. Presumably, asymptomatic hydrops of the gallbladder then develops and becomes secondarily infected. Patients are often intubated in an intensive care unit setting, so early manifestations of the disease are not evident. The most common presentation is one of deterioration and signs of sepsis in a previously stable patient. If suspected, the diagnosis can be confirmed by ultrasonography, which demonstrates gallbladder distention and intraluminal echogenic debris. Hepatobiliary scans show nonfunction of the gallbladder. Treatment in mild cases can be conservative with antibiotics. However, if the patient's condition deteriorates, cholecystectomy is indicated. In patients who are very ill, percutaneous or open cholecystostomy may be a useful temporary measure.

Hemolytic Cholelithiasis

Historically, the usual cause of gallstones in children has been hemolytic disease. Hereditary spherocytosis, sickle cell anemia, and thalassemia are the most common hemolytic disorders resulting in the development of gallstones. Jaundice also may occur intermittently because of hemolysis and therefore does not necessarily mean that common duct calculi are present. In patients with spherocytosis, ultrasonography is recommended before splenectomy. Demonstration of stones dictates that simultaneous cholecystectomy should be performed. In sickle cell disease, the incidence of stones progresses from 10% to 55% as the child grows older. Unless symptomatic, cholecystectomy is currently not recommended for children with sickle cell disease, unless symptomatic. Also, cholecystectomy should be performed electively rather than as an emergency procedure during a hemolytic crisis.[160] In the past, partial exchange transfusion was performed before operation to reduce the hemoglobin S level to less than 40%. Alternatively, preoperative transfusion to a hemoglobin of 10 mg/dL is currently being utilized in many centers. In patients with thalassemia major, the incidence of gallstones has now dropped to 2% to 3% because of hypertransfusion regimens.

Cholesterol Cholelithiasis

Cholesterol gallstones appear to occur in children and adolescents because of the same pathophysiologic disturbances that cause such stones in adults. In most North American institutions, the incidence is increasing and has come to surpass hemolytic disease as the leading cause of cholelithiasis in pediatric patients. The typical patient is a markedly obese young girl. The clinical symptoms are usually vague abdominal pain and minimal physical findings. The classic history of fatty food intolerance is often not present. The diagnosis is usually made at ultrasonography, and the treatment is typically laparoscopic cholecystectomy. Cholesterol stones can occur in infants on prolonged total parenteral nutrition or after ileal resection. Cholecystectomy is still the treatment of choice, although these patients typically have had multiple previous operations and laparoscopy may be more difficult.

Congenital Deformities

A variety of abnormal configurations and locations of the gallbladder such as gallbladder agenesis, duplication, bi-lobation, floating gallbladder, diverticula, and ectopia have been reported. They are usually of no real clinical relevance unless they impair gallbladder emptying. In such cases, calculi are frequent and treatment is almost always cholecystectomy.

PORTAL HYPERTENSION

Portal hypertension in children produces some of the most uniquely challenging problems encountered in clinical pediatric practice. Although the predictable consequences of increased pressure in the portal system (bleeding esophageal varices, hypersplenism, and ascites) are the same in adults and children, their etiology, outcome, and appropriate management are very different. For example, the onset of bleeding esophageal varices in an adult is often a preterminal event or, at best, a grave prognostic indicator of impending clinical deterioration. In children, at least half of all esophageal variceal bleeding occurs as an isolated, albeit life-threatening, problem in a setting of normal liver metabolism in which portal hypertension has resulted from portal vein thrombosis. Even when portal hypertension has resulted from cirrhosis, the overall outcome in children is much better than in adults. For these reasons, palliation per se is almost never the treatment goal in children. Rather, the aim is for growth, development, and improvement in quality and length of life. Modern therapeutic management of isolated manifestations of portal hypertension should not limit any chance a child has for liver transplantation. As a result, treatment has moved increasingly away from shunting toward nonshunt management, such as esophageal variceal endosclerosis, splenic embolization, vigorous nutritional support, and diuretics.

Pathophysiology

Portal hypertension results from an increase in resistance to venous flow through the liver. The site of obstruction is categorized anatomically as being prehepatic, intrahepatic, or suprahepatic. Prehepatic causes of portal hypertension are relatively unique to the pediatric age group, and hepatic parenchymal function is well maintained. Moreover, coagulopathy plays no role in the bleeding episodes. Intrahepatic and suprahepatic causes typically have associated liver dysfunction, which increases the risk for bleeding resulting from coagulopathy, increases the formation of ascites, and affects all aspects of a patient's care.

The hemodynamic effects of portal venous obstruction are complex. In experimental animals, it has been shown that, in addition to portal venous obstruction, an increase in mesenteric arterial flow is required to cause an increase in portal venous pressure.[161] The interplay of these hemodynamic changes, coupled with the development of collateral vessels in the growing child, makes any prediction of long-term outcome after therapy difficult and emphasizes the importance of long-term follow-up.

Prehepatic Obstruction

In the past, portal vein thrombosis was the most common cause of portal hypertension in children.[162] Now, with extended survival achieved through operative bile drainage in children with choledochal cyst, intrahepatic obstruction (hepatic fibrosis) nearly equals portal vein thrombosis as a cause for portal hypertension in children.[163] Portal vein thrombosis may result from perinatal omphalitis, cannulation of the umbilical vein in the newborn period, intra-abdominal sepsis, or dehydration. However, in more than half the cases, no causal event is known. In contrast to those with cirrhosis, patients with portal vein thrombosis usually have normal liver synthetic function (bilirubin, prothrombin time, albumin), but manifestations of portal hypertension (variceal hemorrhage and hypersplenism) are pronounced.

Intrahepatic Obstruction

Biliary atresia is the single most common cause of intrahepatic obstruction leading to portal hypertension in children. Even when bile drainage is achieved, histopathologic studies show that the liver is affected by hepatic fibrosis of varying degrees, even in the newborn period. Approximately one third of patients with choledochal cyst with successful bile drainage do well, have normal liver function, and continue normal growth and development. The remaining two thirds have clinical evidence of liver disease, with half requiring liver transplantation to survive, and the other half growing, but with clinical or laboratory manifestations of liver dysfunction. In the last group, postsinusoidal obstruction is the result of hepatic venous compression by regenerating nodules.

Congenital hepatic fibrosis may occur as an isolated disease of the liver characterized by hepatosplenomegaly that becomes manifest at age 1 to 2 years or in association with multiple forms of kidney disease, the most common of which is infantile polycystic disease. The disease is defined histopathologically by the presence of linear fibrous bands within the liver that result in pre-sinusoidal obstruction. Although hepatomegaly is present, no stigmata of chronic liver disease are seen. In the liver, the parenchyma is spared (pre-sinusoidal obstruction), hepatocellular function is preserved, and serum bilirubin, transaminase, and alkaline phosphatase levels, and prothrombin time are usually normal. Portal hypertension is the most frequent complication of congenital hepatic fibrosis.[164] Often, children are first seen with hepatosplenomegaly and frequently have bleeding esophageal varices.

Other causes of intrahepatic portal hypertension in children include focal biliary cirrhosis, α_1-antitrypsin deficiency, chronic active hepatitis, and complications secondary to irradiation or chemotherapy. The incidence of focal biliary cirrhosis with portal hypertension occurring in patients with cystic fibrosis ranges from 0.5% to 8% in children and from 5% to 20% in adolescents and young adults.[165]

Suprahepatic Obstruction

Obstruction of the hepatic veins (Budd-Chiari syndrome) is a rare cause of portal hypertension in children. This syndrome may be seen in association with coagulation disorders, use of oral contraceptives, malignant disease, autoimmune disorders, and hepatic vein webs. The course is typically insidious, with a long interval between the onset of hepatomegaly, abdominal pain, and ascites and the recognition of the syndrome. If symptoms develop urgently, they can be associated with sudden severe liver enlargement and liver damage with central lobular congestion and necrosis.

Clinical Presentations

Variceal hemorrhage occurs most commonly from the distal esophagus. Increased portal pressure leads to dilation of the portosystemic collateral veins, the most important of which link the coronary vein to the short gastric vein and the submucosal plexus of the lower esophagus. As blood flow through the system increases, esophageal varices develop and can be frighteningly large. The typical presentation is one of vomiting bright red blood, but melena also may occur. Retroperitoneal, periumbilical, and hemorrhoidal collaterals also develop. Although these can be large, they do not tend to cause significant bleeding.

After control of an acute hemorrhage, the cause for the bleeding (i.e., portal hypertension) is sought. In a patient without stigmata of liver disease, portal vein thrombosis is by far the most likely diagnosis. Physical examination typically shows an enlarged spleen and a normal-sized liver. Doppler ultrasound imaging is nearly 100% diagnostic. In contrast, patients with concurrent liver disease usually have signs of liver failure, and the liver is almost always firm and enlarged, with associated malnutrition, splenomegaly, ascites, and jaundice.

Occasionally, splenomegaly and hypersplenism are the first signs of portal hypertension in children. Splenic size does not correlate with the degree of venous pressure elevation, but the hematologic effects of hypersplenism do correlate with the size of the spleen. All formed blood elements may be affected. Long-standing portal hypertension can cause splenic fibrosis, which then reduces the hematologic consequences. This also makes the effects of subsequent shunting less efficacious.

Diagnosis and Treatment

The initial management of upper gastrointestinal hemorrhage is the same regardless of etiology and involves fluid-volume resuscitation, nasogastric tube placement for gastric lavage, and stabilization. Accurate monitoring of cardiovascular parameters and urine output and frequent laboratory determination of blood counts necessitate an intensive care setting. Balloon tamponade with a Sengstaken-Blakemore tube may be necessary initially to control the hemorrhage, and children often require tracheal intubation, sedation, and ventilation. Once the patient's condition has stabilized, endoscopic and Doppler ultrasonography are used to delineate the status of the portal vein. Ultrasonography can accurately document portal venous thrombosis as well as cirrhosis with hepatofugal flow and can quantify arterial inflow. Liver function tests document hepatic functional status. Esophagoscopy can be performed electively to document clinical status and for therapeutic purposes.

Endoscopic varix sclerosis in children requires deep sedation and tracheal intubation. Short-term results are typically excellent in experienced hands.[166] Patients with acute hemorrhage are re-injected every 2 to 3 days until bleeding ceases. Patients who are not actively bleeding should have repeated endoscopy at 6-week intervals until all varices are obliterated. Nearly complete control of bleeding can be achieved using this regimen. Minor complications include superficial esophageal ulceration, pleural effusion, and atelectasis. Occasionally, very serious complications of varix injection can occur. These include esophageal stricture, perforation, spinal cord paralysis, systemic venous thrombosis, and respiratory distress syndrome related to the use of excessive volumes of sclerosant.[167,168]

An alternative to sclerosants is band ligation of esophageal varices. It is just as effective for controlling bleeding and has fewer systemic complications (Fig. 44-23).[169] Therapeutic endoscopic variceal clipping is now widely used to control hemorrhage secondary to portal hypertension in elective or emergency conditions, even in the case of rupture.[170]

Other therapy after acute esophageal bleeding is dependent on the underlying pathophysiology. Portal hypertension resulting from intraparenchymal liver disease most likely will require liver transplantation. Evaluation for transplantation has usually already started, and variceal bleeding usually expedites assessment of these patients. Conversely, if patients are found to have good liver function with either suprahepatic or portal venous obstruction, other surgical interventions may be more appropriate. For patients who have a prehepatic cause for portal hypertension, shunt therapy should be considered after the first hemorrhage and is specifically indicated if repeated bleeding occurs despite sclerotherapy.[171,172] Because these patients typically have good liver function, the incidence of post-shunt encephalopathy is low.[173,174] Selective

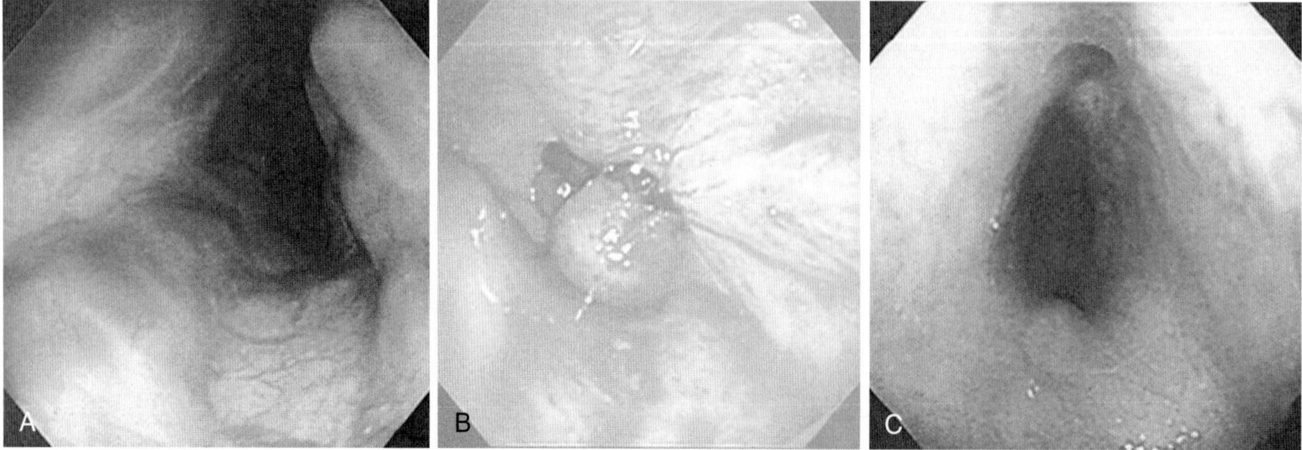

Figure 44-23. Endoscopic variceal ligation. **A,** Preoperative photograph. **B,** Ligation with rubber band. **C,** Postoperative photograph.

splenorenal shunting also is a satisfactory option.[175] However, the increased complexity of this procedure, coupled with the observations that most children at the time of shunt surgery already have hepatofugal flow in the portal vein, and the fact there is loss of selectivity of the distal splenorenal shunt over time usually work against its use in pediatric patients.[176]

Of special consideration are those patients who bleed from varices in the stomach, small bowel, or colon. These vessels are not amenable to sclerotherapy. Thus, these patients may require earlier intervention with shunt therapy. In 1998, a new operative technique using direct bypass of an extrahepatic portal venous obstruction (a cavernoma) was discribed.[177] In this procedure, the obstructive lesion was bypassed by interposing a venous jugular autograft between the superior mesenteric vein and the distal portion of the left portal vein (Rex shunt). Although this procedure is restricted to those patients in whom the intrahepatic left portal branch can be confirmed to be patent by Doppler ultrasonography, it is certainly an option and may be utilized more frequently in the future.

Long-standing splenomegaly is occasionally accompanied by clinically significant hypersplenism. Because of the recognized hazard of postsplenectomy sepsis in children, embolization methods aimed at eliminating hypersplenism while conserving splenic immune function have been developed. Maddison was the first to perform embolization for hypersplenism in 1973.[178] Since then, improvements in materials and methods have made splenic embolization the treatment of choice for hypersplenism in children. The technique usually involves injection of surgical gel particles until 60% to 80% splenic infarction has been achieved. The immediate postembolization morbidity rate is high, with fever and pain being present in all children. Ileus, pleural effusion, and atelectasis also are common. However, major complications such as splenic rupture and splenic abscess are rare, and postsplenectomy sepsis has not developed with long-term follow-up.[179]

ASCITES

Children can have severe ascites, typically associated with end-stage liver disease, and portal hypertension. Ascites may contribute to respiratory embarrassment because of elevation of the diaphragm and to malnutrition because of protein loss. Occasionally, chylous ascites may develop as a result of portal hypertension and liver disease. Long-term total parenteral nutrition and the use of somatostatin analogs reduce the volume of fluid produced.[180] Conservative management consists of dietary sodium and water restriction, spironolactone, furosemide, and periodic paracentesis. In the absence of infection in the ascitic fluid, coagulopathy, and primary cardiac failure, peritoneovenous shunt procedures can return the ascitic fluid to the circulating blood volume, but this is rarely performed in the pediatric age group. Most patients with refractory ascites require liver transplantation, and therapy should be directed at preparing the patient for that procedure.

chapter 45

SOLID ORGAN AND INTESTINAL TRANSPLANTATION

Frederick C. Ryckman, MD • Maria H. Alonso, MD • Jaimie D. Nathan, MD • Greg Tiao, MD

The ability to undertake successful solid organ transplantation in children has led to a remarkable improvement in survival and quality of life. Although the vast majority of solid organ transplant recipients are adults, the innovative techniques that have been developed to meet the challenges of pediatric transplantation and the unique demands of immunosuppression in infancy continue to be a forum for the advancement of transplant care. In this chapter we examine each of the solid organ transplant procedures with their indications, operative procedures, and postoperative complications that are relevant to the practicing pediatric surgeon.

LIVER TRANSPLANTATION

Few subspecialties have undergone the dramatic improvements in survival that have occurred in pediatric liver transplantation. In the early 1980s, survival rates of 30% limited the enthusiasm for this costly and work-intense operation. The introduction of more effective immunosuppression along with refinements in the operative and postoperative management of infants and children improved survival rates to greater than 90%. When compared with the universally fatal outcome these patients would experience without transplantation, it is not surprising that liver transplantation has been embraced as the preferred therapy for several conditions.

Along with this improved survival rate has come an increasing need for donor organs suitable for pediatric recipients of all ages and sizes. This wide spectrum of needs, coupled with the national shortage of transplant donor organs, has stimulated the pioneering development of surgical procedures such as reduced-size liver transplantation, "split-liver" transplantation, and living donor (LD) liver transplantation. However, the excellent survival and organ availability offered by the complementary use of these transplant options cannot overshadow the need for comprehensive evaluation and selective application of liver transplantation.

Indications

The primary aim of the evaluation process is to define which patients require or would benefit from orthotopic liver transplantation (OLT) and when such therapy should be undertaken. Evaluation is directed toward the identification of (1) progressive deterioration of hepatocellular function, (2) portal hypertension and gastrointestinal bleeding, and (3) nutritional and growth failure. Referral for transplantation should occur when progressive deterioration is noted and before the development of life-threatening complications.

The most common clinical presentations prompting transplant evaluation in children can be classified as follows: (1) primary liver disease with the expected outcome of hepatic failure, (2) stable liver disease with significant morbidity or known mortality, (3) hepatic-based metabolic disease, (4) fulminant hepatic failure, and (5) hepatic malignancy, particularly hepatoblastoma, when the lesion is not resectable by conventional means. In addition, children with diffuse and extensive arteriovenous anomalies or benign vascular tumors leading to irreversible heart failure should also be considered for hepatectomy and transplantation.

Table 45-1 reviews the primary diagnoses leading to pediatric liver transplantation. These disease entities define a bimodal age distribution of pediatric transplant recipients. Infants and children with biliary atresia and, occasionally, rapidly progressive hepatic failure secondary to metabolic abnormalities, such as neonatal tyrosinemia and hemochromatosis, or neonatal hepatic vascular tumors are the patients who may require transplantation early in life. Patients with metabolic disturbances, fulminant hepatic failure, and cirrhosis present as older children and adolescents requiring OLT.

Table 45-1 Indications for Liver Transplantation at Cincinnati Children's Hospital Medical Center, 1986-2007

Primary Diagnosis	No. Patients	% Total
Biliary atresia	173	42.5
Fulminant liver failure	62	15.2
α_1-Antitrypsin deficiency	38	9.3
Hepatoblastoma/tumor	16	3.9
Cryptogenic cirrhosis	16	3.9
Alagille syndrome	11	2.7
Tyrosinemia	11	2.7
Autoimmune hepatitis	11	2.7
Urea cycle defects	10	2.5
Primary sclerosing cholangitis	10	2.5
Glycogen storage disease	5	1.2
Neonatal hepatitis	5	1.2
TPN cholestasis/short gut	5	1.2
Primary hyperoxaluria	4	1.0
Cystic fibrosis	3	0.7
Wilson's disease	3	0.7
Gastroschisis	2	0.5
Hemangioendothelioma	2	0.5
Neonatal hemochromatosis	2	0.5
Other	18	4.4
Total Primary Transplants	407	
Retransplantation	50	
Second allograft	42	
Third allograft	5	
Primary transplant elsewhere	3 (1 each, 2nd, 3rd, 4th allograft)	
Total Transplants	457	

Biliary Atresia

Children with extrahepatic biliary atresia constitute about 50% of the pediatric liver transplant population. Successful biliary drainage achieving an anicteric state after the Kasai portoenterostomy is the most important factor affecting preservation of liver function and long-term survival. Primary transplantation without portoenterostomy is not recommended in patients with biliary atresia unless the initial presentation is at more than 120 days of age and the liver biopsy shows advanced cirrhosis.[1,2] We believe that the Kasai portoenterostomy should be the primary surgical intervention for all other infants with extrahepatic biliary atresia. Patients with progressive disease after a Kasai procedure should be offered early OLT. The sequential use of these two procedures optimizes overall survival and organ use.[2]

Patients with extrahepatic biliary atresia who are seen for transplantation form several cohorts. Infants with a failed Kasai procedure have recurrent bacterial cholangitis, ascites, rapidly progressive portal hypertension, malnutrition, and progressive hepatic synthetic failure. Most require OLT within the first 2 years of life. Children with the successful establishment of biliary drainage have an improved prognosis, but this alone does not preclude the development of progressive cirrhosis, with eventual portal hypertension, hypersplenism, variceal hemorrhage, and ascites formation. These patients are seen in later childhood for OLT. Individual patients with mild hepatocellular enzyme and bilirubin elevation and mild portal hypertension can be safely observed with ongoing medical therapy. Approximately 20% of all patients with biliary atresia do not require OLT.[3,4]

Alagille Syndrome

Alagille syndrome (angiohepatic dysplasia) is an autosomal dominant genetic disorder manifest as bile duct paucity leading to progressive cholestasis and pruritus, xanthomas, malnutrition, and growth failure. Liver failure occurs late, if at all. Occasionally, severe growth retardation, hypercholesterolemia, and pruritus can compromise the patient's overall well-being to the point that transplantation is valuable. Specific criteria for OLT are difficult to quantitate. Evaluation must include assessment for congenital cardiac disease and renal insufficiency, both of which are associated with this syndrome. Hepatocellular carcinoma has also been seen in occasional patients.[5,6]

Experience using external biliary diversion or internal ileal bypass accompanied by ursodeoxycholic acid therapy has demonstrated a significant decrease in both pruritus and complications of hypercholesterolemia.[7] Both of these procedures may ameliorate or decrease the rate of ongoing parenchymal destruction and cirrhosis, obviating the need for liver transplantation. The vast improvement in growth and nutrition and the resolution of pruritus, hypercholesterolemia, and xanthoma allow these quality of life issues to be criteria for consideration for OLT.[8-10]

Metabolic Disease

The leading indication for hepatic transplantation in older children is hepatic-based metabolic disease. In these patients, OLT not only is lifesaving but also accomplishes phenotypic and functional cure. A review of these diseases and their mode of presentation can be seen in Tables 45-2 and 45-3.

Hepatic replacement to correct the metabolic defect should be considered before other organ systems are affected and before complications develop that would preclude transplantation, such as in patients with tyrosinemia, in whom there is a high risk of hepatocellular carcinoma.[11] Although results of transplantation are excellent in the metabolic disease subgroup, replacement of the entire liver to correct single enzyme deficiencies is an inefficient but presently necessary procedure. Current research efforts may demonstrate that orthotopic partial hepatic replacement, hepatocyte transplantation, and gene therapy may better serve this patient population in the future.[12-16] Patients with primarily extrahepatic manifestations of their disease, such as cystic fibrosis, are occasionally helped by liver transplantation, although their prognosis is most often determined by their primary illness.[17]

Table 45-2	Indications for Transplantation for Metabolic Disease in Children
Wilson's disease	
α_1-Antitrypsin deficiency	
Crigler-Najjar syndrome (type I)	
Tyrosinemia	
Cystic fibrosis	
Glycogen storage disease type IV	
Branched-chain amino acid catabolism disorders	
Hemophilia A	
Protoporphyria	
Homozygous hypercholesterolemia	
Urea cycle enzyme deficiencies	
Primary hyperoxaluria	
Iron storage disease	

Reprinted from Balistreri WF, Ohi R, Todani T, et al: Hepatobiliary, Pancreatic and Splenic Disease in Children: Medical and Surgical Management. Amsterdam: Elsevier Science, 1997, pp 395-399.

Fulminant Hepatic Failure

Patients with fulminant hepatic failure without recognized antecedent liver disease present diagnostic and prognostic difficulties. Rapid clinical deterioration frequently makes establishment of a definitive diagnosis impossible before there is an urgent need for transplantation. Acute viral hepatitis of undefined type makes up the largest group, followed by drug toxicity and toxin exposure. Previously unrecognized metabolic disease must also be considered. Recently, an immune-based defect has been recognized as a cause of fulminant liver failure. This population needs to be identified because these children may require a combination of bone marrow and liver transplantation to achieve long-term survival. When acceptable clinical and metabolic stability make liver biopsy safe, diagnostic information allowing directed treatment of the primary liver disease is helpful. The presence of ongoing coagulopathy often dictates the need for an open approach to biopsy.

The prognosis of patients with fulminant liver failure is difficult to predict, and neurologic outcome is potentially suboptimal.[15,18,19] Use of intracranial pressure monitoring in patients with progressive encephalopathy has allowed early recognition and directed treatment of increased intracranial pressure. Monitoring should be instituted for patients with advancing grade III encephalopathy and in all patients with grade IV encephalopathy. Intracranial monitoring is continued intraoperatively and for 24 to 48 hours after OLT because significant increases in intracranial pressure have been identified throughout the entire clinical course. Failure to maintain a cerebral perfusion pressure of more than 50 mm Hg and an intracranial pressure less than 20 mm Hg has been associated with very poor neurologic outcome.[19] Survival after transplantation is significantly decreased in patients who reach grade IV encephalopathy. Efforts to identify and perform transplantation in children before this deterioration are obviously important. When candidates are identified before they develop irreversible neurologic abnormalities, the results of transplantation can be dramatic. Hepatocyte transplantation can provide neurologic protection during organ acquisition or while awaiting spontaneous recovery.[16,18,20]

Liver Tumors

Transplantation for hepatoblastoma is recommended for individuals who, after the administration of several cycles of chemotherapy, have a neoplasm confined to the liver that is unresectable by conventional means. Children who had prior isolated metastasis that disappeared while undergoing preoperative chemotherapy can be considered in selected instances. Factors associated with a favorable prognosis include (1) absence of prior surgical resection attempts, (2) unifocal rather than multifocal involvement, (3) absence of vascular invasion, and (4) fetal histology compared with anaplastic or embryonal histology. In addition to these staging factors, a favorable response to pretransplant chemotherapy suggests a more favorable long-term

Table 45-3 Mode of Presentation*

Cirrhosis	Liver Tumor	Life-Threatening Progressive Liver Disease	Failure of Secondary Organ, Normal Liver
α_1-Antitrypsin deficiency	Tyrosinemia	Urea cycle defect	Type 1 hyperoxalosis
Wilson's disease	GSD type I	Protein C deficiency	Hypercholesterolemia
Hemochromatosis	Galactosemia	Crigler-Najjar syndrome type 1	
Byler's disease	FHD	Niemann-Pick disease	
Cystic fibrosis	Hemochromatosis	Hemochromatosis	
Tyrosinemia	α_1-Antitrypsin deficiency	Tyrosinemia	
GSD type IV		BCAA	
FHD			
EPP			

*Classification of inherited metabolic disorders according to clinical modes of presentation.
BCAA, branched-chain amino acid catabolism disorders; EPP, erythropoietic protoporphyria; FHD, fumaryl hydrolase deficiency; GSD, glycogen storage disease.
Reprinted from Balistreri WF, Ohi R, Todani T, et al: Hepatobiliary, Pancreatic and Splenic Disease in Children: Medical and Surgical Management. Amsterdam, Elsevier Science, 1997, pp 395-399.

prognosis. Historically, recurrent disease has accounted for 50% of postoperative mortality.[21] However, in our experience, transplantation for unresectable hepatoblastoma followed by postoperative chemotherapy has led to an overall survival of 88%.[22] The role of transplantation has evolved such that in an upcoming Children's Oncology Group treatment study in the management of children who have hepatoblastoma, early referral for transplant evaluation is recommended for those children who present with large lesions that appear unresectable by conventional surgery.

Transplantation for hepatocellular carcinoma is complicated by less successful chemotherapy options and frequent extrahepatic involvement. The reported 2-year survival rates of 20% to 30% compare unfavorably to the recent experience with hepatoblastoma. Most deaths are due to recurrent carcinoma within the allograft or to extrahepatic tumor involvement. When primary hepatocellular carcinoma is discovered incidentally within the cirrhotic native liver at the time of hepatectomy, the overall prognosis is unaffected by the tumor.[23]

Vascular tumors represent a group of patients with diffuse pathology who can benefit from transplantation. Children with progressive, intractable congestive heart failure, even when caused by non-neoplastic arteriovenous malformations or hemangioendothelioma, offer a unique opportunity for complete removal of the vascular malformation and correction of congestive heart failure. In our experience, transplantation in these patients offers significantly better long-term survival compared with embolization or hepatic artery occlusion that can precipitate sudden and widespread hepatic necrosis. Pretransplant biopsy is essential in large or complex lesions to exclude angiosarcoma.

Contraindications

Contraindications to transplantation include (1) extrahepatic unresectable malignancy, (2) malignancy metastatic to the liver, (3) progressive terminal nonhepatic disease, (4) uncontrolled systemic sepsis, and (5) irreversible neurologic injury.

Relative contraindications to transplantation that need to be individually evaluated include (1) advanced or partially treated systemic infection, (2) advanced hepatic encephalopathy (grade IV), (3) severe psychosocial difficulties, (4) portal venous thrombosis extending throughout the mesenteric venous system, and (5) serology positive for human immunodeficiency virus.

Donor Considerations

Donor Options

The single factor limiting the availability of OLT is the supply of donor organs. The number of patients awaiting liver transplantation has increased by 11-fold since 1991. Available donor resources have not kept pace. Because of this donor shortage, the time to transplant (waiting time) for all pediatric age groups has increased significantly. Infants and young children have been most affected (Figs. 45-1 and 45-2). This severely limited supply of available donor organs has driven the advancement of many innovative liver transplant surgical procedures. The development of reduced-size liver transplantation allowed significant expansion of the donor pool for infants and small children. This has not only improved the availability of donor organs but has also allowed access to donors with improved stability and organ function. Evolution of these operative techniques has allowed the development of both split liver transplantation and LD transplantation.

In the hands of experienced transplant teams, these procedures all have equivalent success to whole-organ transplantation. Furthermore, access to these many donor options has reduced the waiting list mortality rate to less than 5%. Infants and children requiring transplantation benefit greatly from having access to

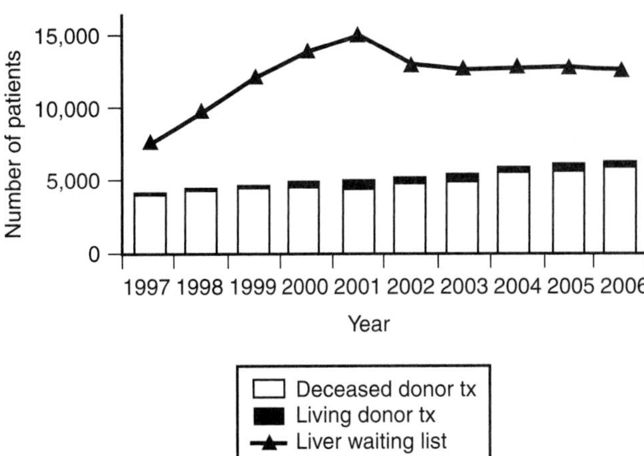

Figure 45-1. Number of patients on the United Network of Organ Sharing (UNOS) waiting list for liver transplantation compared with the number of cadaver donors and cadaver liver recipients, 1988 to 2006. (From Organ Procurement Transplant Network—2007 Annual Report.)

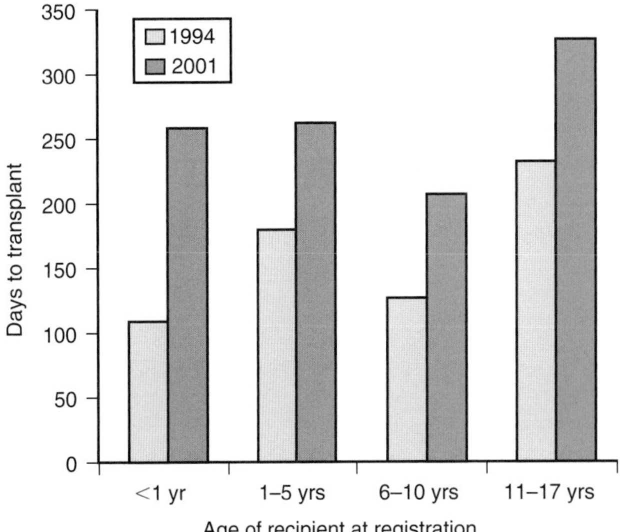

Figure 45-2. Time to transplant (waiting time) for pediatric liver transplant recipients subdivided by age at the time of registration. Comparison of 1994 and 2001 waiting times.

all of these transplant options to minimize waiting time and optimize organ use.

Organ Allocation

In 1998, the "Final Rule" established by the Health Resources and Service Administration (HRSA) mandated the formation of a system for candidate stratification based on a continuous severity score reflecting 90-day waiting list mortality (i.e., outcome).[24] The system that was developed for pediatrics, the Pediatric End-Stage Liver Disease (PELD) score, was created using analysis of the prospective registry of children listed for transplantation by the Studies of Pediatric Liver Transplantation (SPLIT). The parameters selected included total bilirubin, international normalized ratio (INR), albumin, age younger than 1 year, and evidence of failure to thrive (Table 45-4). The assumption was that this score would allow equitable stratification of children by severity of disease and mortality risk and allow integration with the adult Model for End-Stage Liver Disease (MELD) system. The primary function of PELD is the stratification of candidates for transplantation by risk of 90-day waiting list mortality, allowing optimal use of donor organs. When death rates for all children listed were analyzed, PELD was an accurate predictor of mortality risk and demonstrated progressive risk until high scores were reached (>35) (Fig. 45-3).[25]

Donor Selection

Assessment of donor organ suitability is undertaken by evaluating clinical information, static biochemical tests, and dynamic tests of hepatocellular function. The clinical factors reviewed identify donors who are at the limits of age, have had prolonged intensive-care hospitalization with potential sepsis, and have vasomotor instability requiring excessive vasoconstricting inotropic agents. Static biochemical tests identify preexisting functional abnormalities or organ trauma but do not serve as good benchmarks to differentiate among acceptable and poor donor allografts. Donor liver biopsy is helpful in questionable cases to identify preexisting liver disease or donor liver steatosis. The shortage of donor organs has led to expanded efforts to use individuals of advanced age and marginal stability, termed *extended-criteria donors.*

Anatomic replacement of the native liver in the orthotopic position requires selection or surgical preparation of the donor liver to fill but not to exceed available space in the recipient. When using full-sized allografts, a donor weight range 15% to 20% above or below that of the recipient is usually appropriate, taking into consideration body habitus and factors that would increase recipient abdominal size such as ascites and hepatosplenomegaly.

Table 45-4 Pediatric End-Stage Liver Disease (PELD) Score

PELD score = 0.436 × (age) − 0.687 $\log_e$ (albumin [g/dL])
+ 0.480 $\log_e$ (total bilirubin [mg/dL]) + 1.857 $\log_e$ (INR) + 0.667 (growth failure)

INR, International normalized ratio.
Age: Age < 1, score = 1; age > 1, score = 0.
Growth failure: Growth > 2 standard deviations below mean, score = 1; growth < 2 standard deviations below mean, score = 0.
Equation based on age, growth, and serum total bilirubin, INR, and albumin.

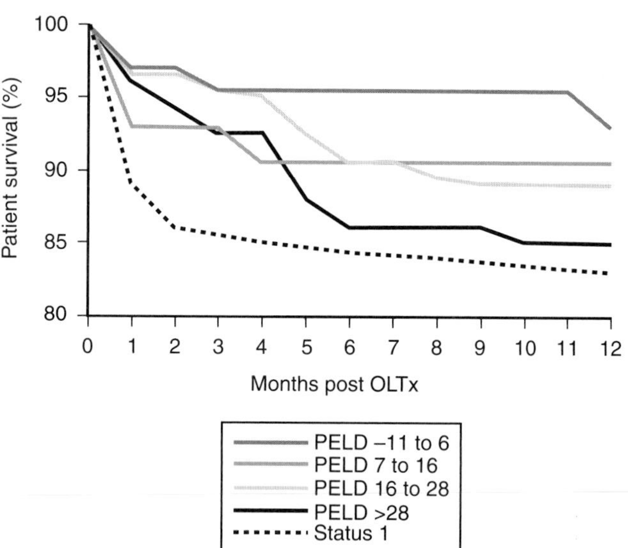

Figure 45-3. PELD score predictive of survival after transplantation. (Redrawn from Barshes NR, Lee TC, Udell IW, et al: The PELD model as a predictor of survival benefit and of post transplant survival in pediatric liver transplant recipients. Liver Transpl 12:475-480, 2006.)

Surgical preparation of reduced-size liver allografts is based on the anatomy of the hepatic vasculature and bile ducts. Prolonged cold ischemic preservation allows for the safe application of the extensive hypothermic bench surgery necessary for reduction techniques. The need for this preparation also limits the acceptability of extended-criteria donors for these procedures. The three primary reduced-size allografts used are the right lobe, the left lobe, and the left lateral segment, all prepared by ex vivo hepatic resection.

The right lobe graft, using segments V to VIII, can be accommodated when the weight difference is no greater than 2:1 between donor and recipient. The thickness of the right lobe makes this allograft of limited usefulness in small recipients. Similar anatomic grafts from LDs have become widely used in adults. The left lobe, using segments I to IV, is applicable with a donor-to-recipient (D:R) disparity from 4:1 to 5:1. A left lateral segment graft (segments II and III) can be used up to a 10:1 D:R weight difference. For a left or right lobe graft, the parenchymal resection follows the anatomic lobar plane through the gallbladder fossa to the inferior vena cava (IVC).[26,27] A crush and tie technique is preferred to achieve good closure of vascular and biliary structures. The middle hepatic vein is retained with the graft in all left lobe and many right lobe preparations. The bile duct, portal vein, and hepatic artery are divided and ligated at the right or left confluence. The vena cava is left incorporated with the allograft in both right and left lobe preparation. Vena caval reduction by posterior caval wall resection and closure is only occasionally necessary. Resection of the inferior protruding portion of the caudate lobe is necessary during left lobe preparation to reduce the likelihood of arterial angulation, which can result in arterial thrombosis. This also facilitates shortening of the IVC to fit in a small recipient.[28]

When using left lateral segment (LLS) allografts, the parenchymal dissection follows the right margin of the falciform ligament with preservation of the left hilar structures. Direct implantation of the left hepatic vein into the combined orifice of the right and middle/left hepatic veins in the recipient IVC is preferred. The donor vena cava is not retained with this segmental allograft. Further reduction of the LLS graft to a monosegmental graft may be necessary in very small recipients. Resection of the distal LLS is technically easier than an anatomic segment II/III division.

Biliary reconstruction in all allograft types is achieved through an end-to-side choledochojejunostomy. Primary bile duct reconstruction is not used with reduced-size allografts owing to the risk of ischemia in the common bile duct. The bile ducts are perfused by a dense arterial plexus, which travels within the common connective tissue "vasobiliary sheath."[29] Dissection should be limited to that necessary to identify the bile duct for anastomosis.

The use of LDs has increased as the safety and success of this procedure has been demonstrated (Fig. 45-4).[30-32] One of the critical elements of LD transplantation is the proper selection of a donor, usually a parent or relative. This procedure is performed on the assumption that donor safety can be assured and that the donor's liver function is normal. Donors should be 21 to 55 years of age, have an ABO compatible blood type, and have no acute or chronic medical condition. Careful attention must be paid to proper living donor consent. Parental concerns to help their ill child make true informed consent a challenge. A dedicated "donor advocate" not directly associated with the transplant team should assist with this process. Independent medical assessment of the donor is essential. The United

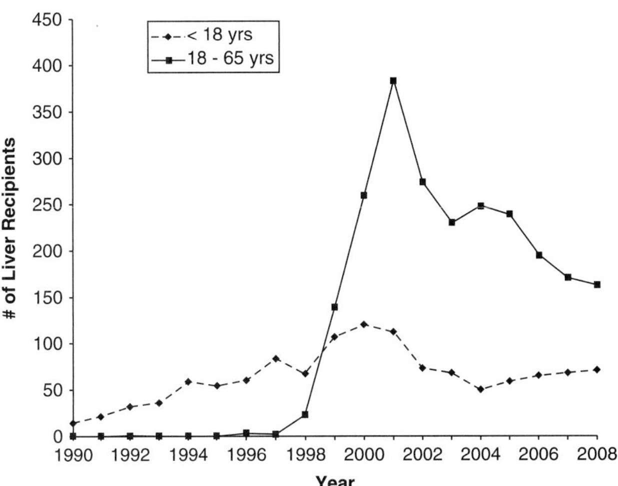

Figure 45-4. Number of living donor transplants per year subdivided by the age of the transplant recipient, 1991-2008 (From Organ Procurement Transplant Network data).

Table 45-5 Estimation of Allograft Size for Living Donor Transplant

Urata Formula
ELV (mL) = 706.2 × BSA (m^2) + 2.4 ELV (mL) = 2.223 × BW (kg)$^{0.425}$ × BH (cm)$^{0.682}$
Revised Urata Formula
ELV (mL) = 1072.8 × BSA (m^2) – 345.7 (white population)

Graft estimate to weigh ≥ 1% body weight of recipient.
Best to weigh 2%-3% of recipient body weight.
BW, body weight; ELV, estimated liver volume; BSA, body surface area.

Network for Organ Sharing (UNOS) has recently established clear criteria for this process. After a satisfactory medical and psychological examination by a physician not directly involved with the transplant program, computed tomography (CT) is used to measure the volume of the potential donor segment to ensure that it will meet the metabolic needs but not exceed the space available in the recipient (Table 45-5). If acceptable, CT angiography or arteriography is undertaken to assess the hepatic arterial anatomy, thereby excluding potential donors with multiple arteries to segments II and III and facilitating minimal hilar vascular dissection at the time of OLT. When donors were deemed unacceptable, experience has shown that 90% of patients were excluded on the basis of history, examination, laboratory screening, and ABO type. Donor safety has been excellent in all pediatric LD series.[33-35]

In most pediatric patients, the LLS donated from an adult is used as the graft. At the time of harvest, the left hepatic vein is divided from the IVC and the left branch of the portal vein and proper hepatic artery are removed with the allograft.[33] Vascular continuity of the hepatic arterial branches to segment IV is maintained if possible. Recently, increased experience has been gained using the right lobe as an LD allograft for larger recipients such as adolescents and adults.[30,36,37] This more extensive operation has proven to be a challenge to the donor and recipient alike, with a complication and mortality rate significantly exceeding that of left lateral segmentectomy. Although the number of right lobe LD recipients now greatly exceeds the number of children receiving LD grafts, several publicized donor deaths and increased interest in "split-liver" cadaveric procurement have slowed the enthusiasm for right lobe donation.

Split-liver grafting involves the preparation of two allografts from a single donor. Two techniques have been used to accomplish hepatic division in the donor with similar overall success. The ex situ split procedure divides the right lobe allograft (segments V to VIII) from the LLS allograft (segments II and III) after the whole donor organ has been procured. Because this division is undertaken under vascular hypothermic conditions without hepatic perfusion, the vascular integrity of segment IV is difficult to assess and it is frequently discarded. Conventional techniques for implanting the respective allografts are then used.[29] The successful experience with in situ division of the LD left lateral segment is the basis for the in situ split procedure. Here the LLS is prepared identically to that of a living related donor. The viability of segment IV can be examined at the time of the division, and it is usually incorporated with the right lobe graft to increase the cellular mass of the allograft. Because this procedure adds considerably to the donor procurement time, and the necessary skill of the donor team, it is more demanding and occasionally difficult to successfully orchestrate. However, despite these considerations, this is the preferred method for split-liver donor preparation.[30,32,38,39]

The benefits of split-liver transplantation are best achieved when ideal donors are selected. Strict restrictions on age, vasopressor administration, predonation hepatic function, and limited donor hospitalization have been used to select optimal candidates for this donor procedure. When these donors are selected, the results from both in situ and ex situ techniques are similar, with both techniques now having patient survival for both allografts of 90% to 93% and graft survival rates of 86% to 89%.[40]

The selection of a donor segment with an appropriate parenchymal mass for adequate function is critical to success. However, the minimal mass necessary for recovery is not yet established. Any calculation must take into account loss of function after preservation damage, acute rejection, and technical problems. When the D:R weight range falls within the normal 8:1 to 10:1 ratio, risk is minimal. Estimates of donor graft to recipient body weight ratio (GRWR) may prove to be a more accurate predictor of adequate graft volume. When the GRWR is less than 0.7%, overall allograft and patient survival suffered. In extreme cases in which small-for-size grafts are used, excessive portal flow can lead to hemorrhagic necrosis of the graft. Large-for-size allografts (GRWR > 5.0%) have a less deleterious effect.[41] A review of these donor anatomic options is shown in Figure 45-5.

Creative use of the techniques refined for reduced-size liver transplantation has allowed additional donor options in individual cases. Resection of the left lobe of the native liver followed by auxiliary partial orthotopic transplantation of a reduced-size LLS allograft has been successfully undertaken for patients with metabolic disease (ornithine transcarbamylase deficiency, Crigler-Najjar syndrome) and fulminant hepatic failure.[42,43]

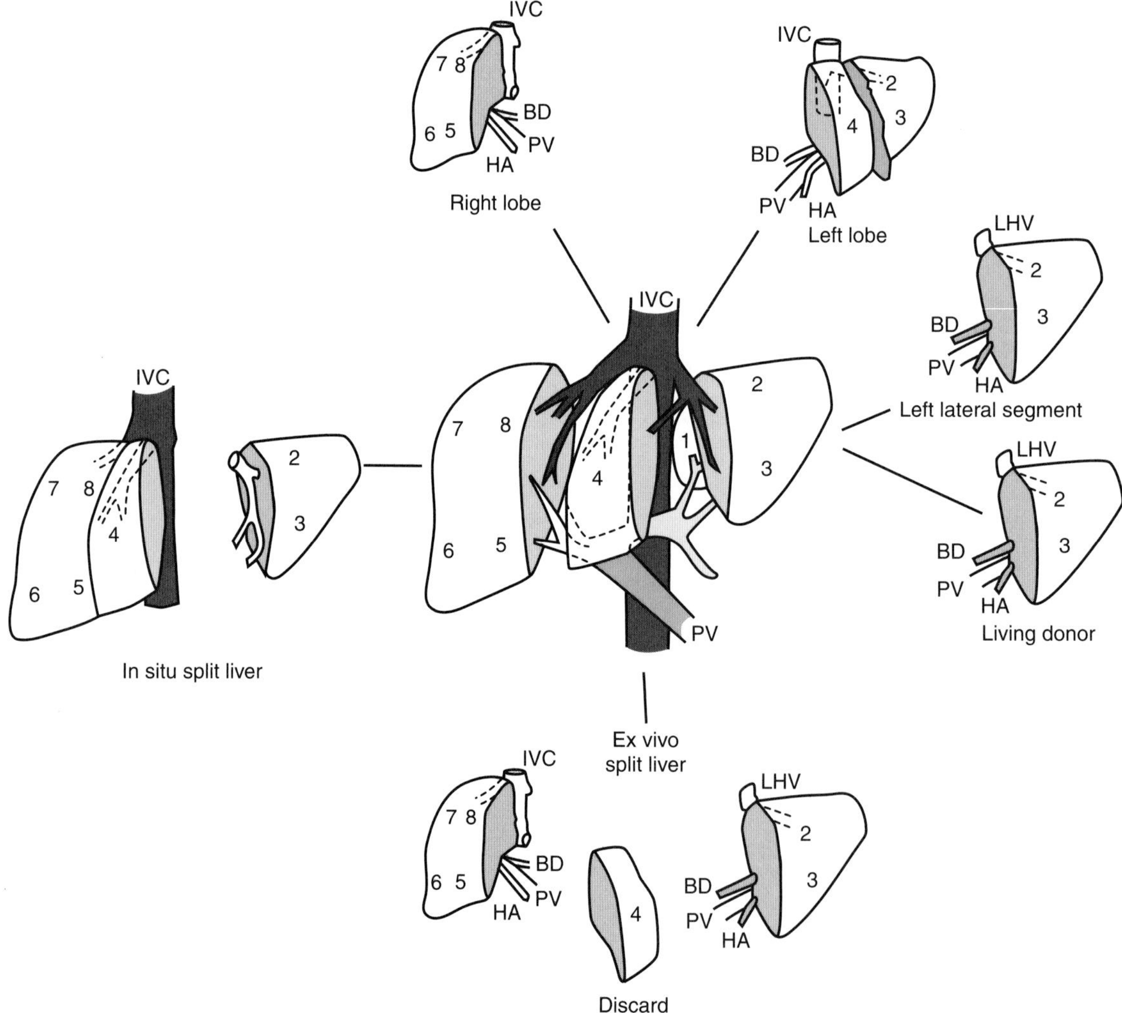

Figure 45-5. Anatomic donor options available through surgical reduction. The numbers correlate to the segmental hepatic anatomy as defined by Couinaud. IVC, inferior vena cava; BD, bile duct; PV, portal vein; HA, hepatic artery; LHV, left hepatic vein.

This provides for normal hepatic synthesis and function while leaving the right lobe of the donor liver in situ. The auxiliary partial OLT technique has also been undertaken using an LD for similar indications.[44] Auxiliary placement of a reduced-size allograft has also been successfully performed for fulminant hepatic failure in patients deemed too unstable for OLT. In these cases, recovery of the recipient native liver function can ultimately allow discontinuation of immunosuppression and atrophy of the donor allograft if it is no longer required to supplement organ function.[45,46]

Preoperative Preparation

Efforts to correct abnormalities noted during candidate evaluation decrease both the operative risk and postoperative complications. Complications of portal hypertension and malnutrition are vigorously treated. Assessment of prior viral exposure and meticulous attention to the delivery of all normal childhood immunizations, particularly the live-virus vaccines, are imperative, if time allows, before OLT. Additionally, patients receive a one-time inoculation with pneumococcal vaccine and appropriate administration of hepatitis B vaccine. Preoperative assessment of specific cardiopulmonary reserve and hepatic vascular anatomy is also necessary.

The Transplant Procedure

The transplant procedure is carried out through a bilateral subcostal incision with midline extension. Meticulous ligation of portosystemic collaterals and vascularized adhesions is necessary to avoid slow but relentless hemorrhage. Dissection of the hepatic hilum, with division of the hepatic artery and portal vein above their bifurcation, allows maximal recipient vessel length to be achieved. The bile duct, when present, is divided high in the hilum to preserve the length and vasculature of the distal duct in case it is needed for primary reconstruction in older recipients. Preservation of the Roux-en-Y limb in biliary atresia patients who have undergone Kasai portoenterostomy simplifies later biliary reconstruction. Complete mobilization of the liver, with dissection of the suprahepatic vena cava to the diaphragm and the infrahepatic vena cava to the renal veins, completes the hepatectomy.

In children with serious vascular instability who cannot tolerate caval occlusion, and in LD transplantation, "piggy-back" implantation is necessary. In this procedure, the recipient vena cava is left intact and partial caval occlusion allows end-to-side implantation of a combined donor hepatic vein patch. Access to the infrarenal aorta to implant the celiac axis of the donor liver or iliac artery vascular conduits, provided by mobilizing the right colon and duodenum, is our preference for arterial reconstruction in complex allograft recipients.

Control of hemorrhage is essential during the recipient hepatectomy and requires meticulous surgical technique. Coagulation factor assays (V, VII, VIII, fibrinogen, platelets, prothrombin time, partial thromboplastin time) allow specific blood product supplementation to improve clotting function. The use of venovenous bypass is reserved for recipients weighing more than 40 kg who demonstrate hemodynamic instability at the time of venous interruption. Early institution of venovenous bypass combined with high-dose vasopressin (0.2 to 0.6 units/min) is occasionally used in patients with marked friable retroperitoneal variceal hypertension before completing hepatic mobilization.

Removal of the diseased liver is completed after vascular isolation is achieved. Retroperitoneal hemostasis is achieved before implanting the donor liver. In standard OLT, the suprahepatic vena cava is prepared by suture ligating any large phrenic orifices and creating one caval lumen from the confluence of the IVC and hepatic vein orifices. The donor liver is implanted using conventional vascular techniques and monofilament suture for the vascular anastomosis. In small recipients, interrupted suture techniques, monofilament dissolving suture material, and a "growth factor" knot have all been used to allow for vessel growth. When LLS reduced-size grafts are used, the left hepatic vein orifice is anastomosed directly to the anterolateral surface of the infradiaphragmatic IVC using the combined right-middle hepatic vein orifices. The LLS allograft is later fixed, when necessary, to the undersurface of the diaphragm to prevent torsion and venous obstruction of this anastomosis. Similar fixation is not necessary with right or left lobe allografts or with whole-organ transplants.

Before completing the vena caval anastomosis, the hyperkalemic preservation solution is flushed from the graft using 500 to 1000 mL of hypothermic normokalemic intravenous solutions. When using full-sized grafts in older patients, we prefer to complete all venous anastomoses before reconstructing the hepatic artery. In reduced-size allografts and in small recipients in whom we prefer to use direct aortic vascular inflow reconstruction, the hepatic arterial anastomosis is completed before reconstructing the portal vein to improve visibility of the infrarenal aorta without placing traction on the portal vein anastomosis. We prefer to complete all anastomoses during vascular isolation before organ reperfusion, although some transplant teams reperfuse after venous reconstruction is complete.

Before re-establishing circulation to the allograft, anesthetic adjustments must be made to address the large volume of blood needed to refill the liver and the presence of hypothermic solutions released at reperfusion. Inotropic support using dopamine (5 to 10 μg/kg/min) is begun. Calcium and sodium bicarbonate are administered to combat the effects of hyperkalemia from any remaining preservation solution and systemic acidosis after aortic and vena caval occlusion. Sufficient blood volume expansion, administered as packed red blood cells to raise the central venous pressure to 15 to 20 cm H_2O and the hematocrit to 40%, minimizes the development of hypotension with unclamping and prevents dilutional anemia. Cooperative communication between the surgical and

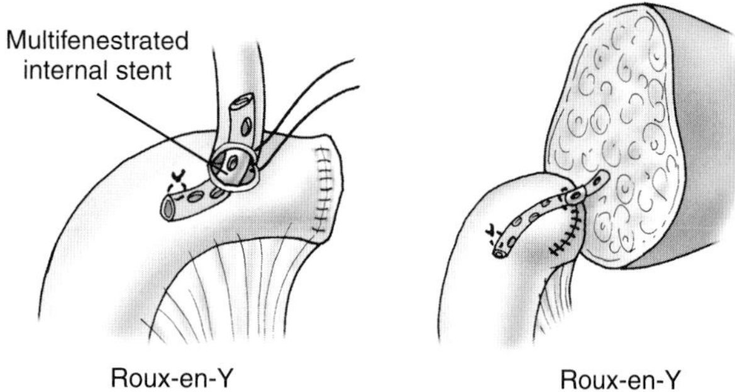

Figure 45-6. Bile duct reconstruction is shown using the common hepatic duct in whole organ transplants (left) and segmental hepatic ducts into a Roux-en-Y intestinal limb for reduced-sized liver transplants (right). An internal multi-fenestrated stent is used in both situations. (From Ryckman F: Liver transplantation. In Ziegler MM, Azizkhan RG, Weber T [eds]: Operative Pediatric Surgery. New York, McGraw-Hill, 2003, p 1275.)

anesthesia teams facilitates a smooth sequential reestablishment of vena caval, portal venous, and then arterial recirculation to the allograft.

Biliary reconstruction in patients with biliary atresia or in those weighing less than 25 kg is achieved through an end-to-side choledochojejunostomy using interrupted dissolving monofilament sutures. A multifenestrated Silastic internal biliary stent is placed before completing the anastomosis (Fig. 45-6). In most cases, the previous Roux-en-Y jejunal limb can be used, with a 30- to 35-cm length being preferred. Primary bile duct reconstruction without stenting is used in older patients with whole-organ allografts.

When closing the abdomen, increased intra-abdominal pressure should be avoided. In many cases, avoidance of fascial closure and the use of mobilized skin flaps and running monofilament skin closure are advisable. Musculofascial abdominal closure can be completed before patient discharge.

Immunosuppressive Management

Most centers use an immunosuppressive protocol based on the administration of multiple complementary medications. All use corticosteroids and cyclosporine or tacrolimus. Additional antimetabolites (azathioprine, mycophenolate) are used when more treatment is needed. Prior protocols using polyclonal or monoclonal induction therapy have been abandoned in most cases owing to the extent of the immunosuppressive potency. The recent introduction of humanized monoclonal antibodies to interleukin-2 (basiliximab, daclizumab) has stimulated interest in induction immunosuppression protocols because these agents appear to have a low risk of associated opportunistic infections. The role that they will play in the future is not clear at present. A sample protocol is given in Table 45-6.

Postoperative Complications

Most postoperative complications present as cholestasis, increasing hepatocellular enzyme levels, and, on occasion, fever, lethargy, and anorexia. This nonspecific symptom complex requires specific diagnostic evaluation before instituting treatment. Therapy directed at the specific causes of allograft dysfunction is essential. Empirical therapy for presumed complications is fraught with misdiagnoses, morbidity, and mortality. A flow diagram outlining this evaluation is shown in Figure 45-7.

Primary Nonfunction

Primary nonfunction of the hepatic allograft implies the absence of metabolic and synthetic activity after transplantation. Complete nonfunction requires immediate retransplantation before irreversible coagulopathy and cerebral edema occur. Lesser degrees of allograft dysfunction occur more frequently and can be associated with several donor, recipient, and operative factors (Table 45-7).

The status of the donor liver contributes significantly to the potential for primary nonfunction. Ischemic injury secondary to anemia, hypotension, hypoxia, or direct tissue injury is often difficult to ascertain in the history of multiple trauma victims. Donor liver steatosis has also been recognized as a factor contributing to severe dysfunction or nonfunction in the donor liver. Macrovesicular steatosis on donor liver biopsy is somewhat more common in adult than pediatric donors and, when severe, is recognized grossly by the enlarged yellow, greasy consistency of the donor liver. The risk of primary nonfunction increases as the degree of fatty infiltration increases. Microscopic findings are classified as mild if less than 30% of the hepatocytes have fatty infiltration, moderate if 30% to 60% are involved, and severe if more than 60% of the hepatocytes have fatty infiltration. Livers with severe fatty

Table 45-6 Immunosuppression Protocol Utilized for Liver Transplantation

Day/ Week	Methylprednisolone (mg/kg/day)	Tacrolimus (mg/kg/ day)	Tacrolimus Target Level
Intra-Op	15	0	
1	10	0.3	
2	8	0.3	
3	6	0.3	
4	4	0.3	12-18
5	3	0.3	
6	2	0.3	
7	1	0.3	
Week 2	0.9	Adjust as needed	12-18
Week 3	0.8		
Week 4	0.7		
Week 5	0.6		8-14
Week 6	0.5		
Week 7	0.4		
Week 8	0.3		
Week 9	0.2		
Week 10	0.1		
Week 11	0.1		
Week 12	D/C		6-12
>1 year			3-7

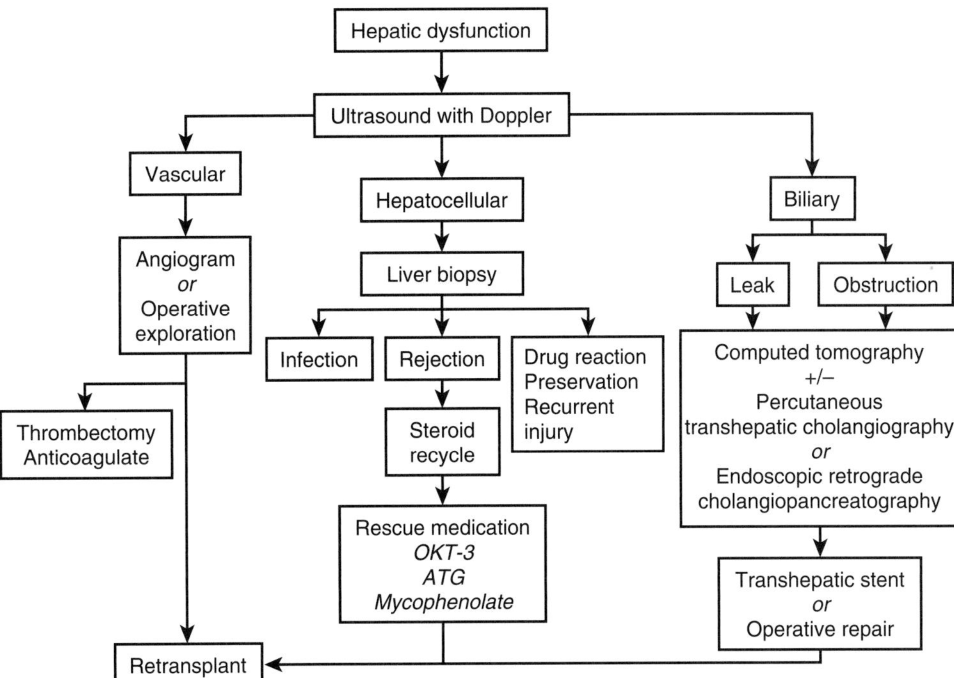

Figure 45-7. Schematic flow diagram for management of postoperative liver allograft dysfunction. ATG, antithymocyte globulin; OKT-3, monoclonal antibody.

infiltration should be discarded. Donors with moderate involvement are used with some concern, with the degree of steatosis and the condition of the recipient determining use of the allograft. Microvesicular steatosis is not related to primary nonfunction.[47-53]

Immediate post-transplant immunologic events, such as humoral antibody-mediated hyperacute rejection, can occur but are uncommon after OLT. Initial reports suggested that a positive cytotoxic antibody crossmatch between the donor and recipient did not affect the viability or function of the allograft.[54] However, more recent experience with crossmatch positive donors has demonstrated significantly decreased allograft and patient survival.[55,56]

Table 45-7	Factors Related to Primary Nonfunction
Donor Factors	
Preexisting disease or injury to donor, anemia, hypoxia, hypotension before organ harvest	
Donor organ steatosis (>60% macrovesicular fat)	
Transplant Factors	
Prolonged cold ischemic storage (>8-12 hr)	
Prolonged warm ischemic time at implantation	
Complex vascular anastomosis requiring surgical revision	
Significant size discrepancy between donor and recipient	
Recipient Factors	
Post-reperfusion hypotension	
Vascular thrombosis	
Immunologic factors	
ABO incompatible, positive crossmatch	

The use of ABO-incompatible donors has been controversial. Allograft and patient survival rates in adult recipients have not been comparable to those achieved using ABO-identical or ABO-compatible donors.[57,58] However, pediatric recipients of ABO-incompatible allografts have achieved survival rates equivalent to those using ABO-compatible and ABO-identical donors, using either cadaver donors (CDs) or LDs.[59-61]

Documentation of functional hepatic recovery is best undertaken by evaluating the ongoing hepatic output of clotting factors (V, VII) with improvement in coagulation parameters (prothrombin time, partial thromboplastin time) and the synthesis of bile. Hepatic biopsies assist in the documentation of histologic and immunologic events, but they cannot accurately predict the likelihood of recovery.

Vascular Thrombosis

Hepatic artery thrombosis occurs in children three to four times more frequently than in adult transplant series, occurring most often within the first 30 days after transplantation. Factors influencing the development of hepatic artery thrombosis are listed in Table 45-8.

Hepatic artery thrombosis presents as a variable clinical picture that may include (1) fulminant allograft failure, (2) biliary disruption or obstruction, or (3) systemic sepsis. Doppler ultrasound imaging has been accurate in identifying arterial thrombosis. It is used as the primary screening modality to assess blood flow after transplantation or whenever complications arise. Acute hepatic artery thrombosis with allograft failure most often requires immediate retransplantation. Successful thrombectomy and allograft salvage is possible if undertaken before allograft necrosis.[62] Biliary

Table 45-8 Factors Affecting Vascular Thrombosis

Donor/Recipient Age/Weight Allograft Type
Whole organ > reduced size Living donor ≥ reduced size
Anastomotic Anatomy
Primary hepatic artery > direct aortic
Allograft Edema—Increased Vascular Resistance
Ischemic injury secondary to prolonged preservation; prolonged implantation Rejection Fluid overload
Recipient Hypotension and/or Hypercoagulability
Administration of coagulation factors, fresh-frozen plasma Procoagulant factor deficiencies

complications are particularly common after hepatic artery thrombosis. Ischemic biliary disruption with intraparenchymal biloma formation or anastomotic disruption presents as cholestasis associated with systemic sepsis. The development of systemic septicemia or multifocal abscesses in sites of ischemic necrosis secondary to gram-negative enteric bacteria, *Enterococcus*, anaerobic bacteria, or fungi can also be seen. Antibiotic therapy directed toward these organisms, along with surgical drainage, is indicated when specific abscess sites are identified. Percutaneous drainage and biliary stenting may control bile leakage and infection until retransplantation is possible.

Late postoperative thrombosis can be asymptomatic or present as slowly progressive bile duct stenosis. Rarely, allograft necrosis occurs. Arterial collaterals from the Roux-en-Y limb can provide a source of revascularization of the thrombosed allograft through hilar collaterals. These collateral channels develop during the first postoperative months, often making late thrombosis a clinically silent event. Conversely, disruption of this collateral supply during operative reconstruction of the central bile ducts in patients with hepatic artery thrombosis can precipitate hepatic ischemia and parenchymal necrosis. When hepatic artery thrombosis is asymptomatic, careful follow-up alone is indicated.

Prevention of hepatic artery thrombosis requires meticulous microsurgical arterial reconstruction at the time of transplantation. Anatomic reconstruction is preferred in whole-organ allografts. Direct implantation of the celiac axis into the infrarenal aorta is recommended for all reduced-size liver allografts. All complex vascular reconstructions of the donor hepatic artery should be undertaken ex vivo whenever possible using microsurgical techniques before transplantation. When vascular grafts are required, they should also be directly implanted into the infrarenal aorta.[63] We do not routinely use systemic anticoagulation, but aspirin (20 to 40 mg/day) is administered to all children for 100 days. Complex protocols administering both procoagulants and anticoagulants have also been very successful.[49]

Portal vein thrombosis is uncommon in whole-organ allografts unless prior portosystemic shunting has altered the flow within the splanchnic vascular bed or unless severe portal vein stenosis in the recipient has impaired flow to the allograft. Preexisting portal vein thrombosis in the recipient can be overcome by thrombectomy, portal vein replacement, or extra-anatomic venous bypass. In biliary atresia recipients, preexisting portal vein hypoplasia is best corrected by anastomosis to the confluence of the splenic and superior mesenteric veins in the recipient. When inadequate portal vein length is present on the donor organ, iliac vein interposition grafts are used. Early thrombosis after transplantation requires immediate anastomotic revision and thrombectomy. Discrepancies in venous size imposed by reduced-size allografts can be modified to allow anastomotic construction.[64,65] Deficiencies of anticoagulant proteins, such as protein C and S, and antithrombin III deficiency in the recipient must also be excluded as a contributing cause for vascular thrombosis.[66] Failure to recognize portal vein thrombosis can lead to either allograft demise or, on a more chronic basis, to significant portal hypertension with hemorrhagic sequelae or intractable ascites.

Biliary Complications

Complications related to biliary reconstruction occur in approximately 10% of pediatric liver transplant recipients. Their spectrum and treatment is determined by the status of the hepatic artery and the type of allograft used. Although whole and reduced-size allografts have an equivalent risk of biliary complications, the spectrum of complications differs.[67,68]

Primary bile duct reconstruction is the preferred biliary reconstruction in adults, but it is less commonly used in children. It has the advantages of preserving the sphincter of Oddi, decreasing the incidence of enteric reflux and subsequent cholangitis, and not requiring an intestinal anastomosis. Early experience using primary choledochocholedochostomy without a T-tube has been favorable.[69] Late complications after any type of primary ductal reconstruction include anastomotic stricture, biliary sludge formation, and recurrent cholangitis. Endoscopic dilation and internal stenting of anastomotic strictures has been successful in early postoperative cases. Roux-en-Y choledochojejunostomy is the preferred treatment for recurrent stenosis or postoperative leak.

Roux-en-Y choledochojejunostomy is the reconstruction of choice in small children and is required in all patients with biliary atresia. Recurrent cholangitis, a theoretical risk, suggests anastomotic or intrahepatic biliary stricture formation or small bowel obstruction within the Roux limb or distal to the Roux-en-Y anastomosis. In the absence of these complications, cholangitis is uncommon.

Reconstruction of the bile ducts in patients with reduced-size allografts is more complex. Division of the bile duct in close proximity to the cut-surface margin of the allograft, with careful preservation of the biliary duct collateral circulation, decreases but does not eliminate ductal stricture formation secondary to ductal ischemia. In our early experience, in 14% of patients with left lobe reduced-size allografts, a short segmental stricture developed requiring biliary anastomotic revision (Fig. 45-8). Operative revision of the biliary anastomosis and reimplantation of the bile ducts into the Roux-en-Y limb are necessary. Percutaneous transhepatic cholangiography is essential to define the intrahepatic ductal anatomy before operative revision, and temporary catheter decompression of the obstructed bile ducts allows treatment of cholangitis and elective reconstruction. Operative reconstruction is accompanied by transhepatic passage of exteriorized multifenestrated biliary ductal stents, which remain until reconstructive success is documented. Late stenosis is unlikely. Dissection away from the vasobiliary sheath in the donor has significantly decreased the incidence of this complication.

Biliary complications have been seen with an increased frequency after living donation in pediatric recipients. The left lateral segment II and III bile ducts are frequently separate at the plane of parenchymal division. The need for individual drainage of these small biliary ducts makes the development of late anastomotic stenosis more frequent. Individual segmental strictures may not lead to jaundice in the recipient but rather are identified by elevated γ-glutamyltransferase enzymes or through ultrasound surveillance. Reoperation after ductal dilatation allows for easier reconstruction owing to the increased caliber of the segmental bile duct.

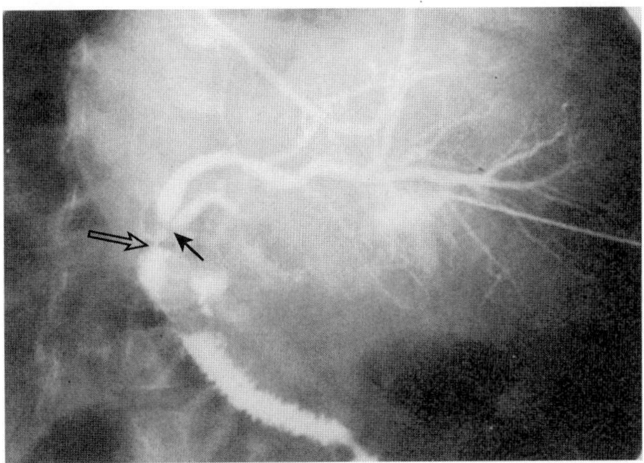

Figure 45-8. Segmental bile duct stricture at the junction of the left lateral and left medial segmental bile ducts in a left lobe reduced-size allograft. *Solid arrow*, bile duct stricture; *open arrow*, Roux-en-Y loop and bile duct anastomosis. (From Ryckman FC: Liver transplantation in children. In Suchy FJ [ed]: Liver Disease in Children. St. Louis, CV Mosby, 1994, p 941.)

Acute Cellular Rejection

Allograft rejection is characterized by the histologic triad of endothelialitis, portal triad lymphocyte infiltration with bile duct injury, and hepatic parenchymal cell damage.[70] Allograft biopsy is essential to establish the diagnosis before treatment. The rapidity of the rejection process and its response to therapy dictates the intensity and duration of antirejection treatment.

Acute rejection occurs in approximately two thirds of patients after OLT.[71] The primary treatment of rejection is a short course of high-dose corticosteroids. Administration of bolus doses over several days with a rapid taper to baseline therapy is successful in 75% to 80% of cases.[72] When refractory or recurrent rejection occurs, antilymphocyte therapy using the monoclonal antibody OKT-3 (Ortho Biotech Products, Bridgewater, NJ) or Thymoglobulin (Genzyme Transplant, Cambridge, MA) is successful in 90% of cases.[28]

Chronic Rejection

Uniform diagnosis and management of chronic rejection are complicated by the lack of a consistent definition or clinical course. Chronic rejection occurs in 5% to 10% of transplanted patients. Its incidence appears to be decreasing in all transplant groups, perhaps related to better overall immunosuppressive strategies. There is some suggestion that the use of primary tacrolimus-based immunosuppression is a key element in this apparent decrease.[73,74] Risk factors for its development are many, and no factor predicts the outcome of treatment. The chronic rejection rate was significantly lower in recipients of living-related grafts than in recipients of cadaver grafts. African-American recipients had a significantly higher rate of chronic rejection than did white recipients. In addition, the number of acute rejection episodes, transplantation for autoimmune disease, occurrence of post-transplant lymphoproliferative disease (PTLD), and cytomegalovirus (CMV) infection were also significant risk factors for chronic rejection.[75] The primary clinical manifestation is a progressive increase in biliary ductal enzymes (alkaline phosphatase, γ-glutamyltransferase) and progressive cholestasis. This course can be initially asymptomatic or often will follow an unsuccessful treatment course for acute rejection. The syndrome can occur within weeks of transplantation or later in the clinical course.

Chronic rejection can follow one of two clinical forms.[76] In the first, the injury is primarily to the biliary epithelium and the clinical course is typically slowly progressive with preservation of synthetic function. Histologic evidence shows interlobular bile duct destruction in the absence of ischemic injury or the presence of hepatocellular necrosis. In full expression, this lesion is characterized as acute vanishing bile duct syndrome, defined by severe ductopenia in at least 20 portal tracts.[77,78] The eventual spontaneous resolution in up to one-half of affected patients with tacrolimus therapy has led to the development of enhanced immunosuppression protocols for this patient subgroup.[76] Retransplantation is occasionally necessary but rarely emergent.

The second subtype is characterized by the early development of progressive ischemic injury to both bile ducts and hepatocytes, leading to ductopenia and ischemic necrosis with fibrosis. The clinical picture of cholestasis is accompanied by significant synthetic dysfunction with superimposed vascular thrombosis or biliary stricture formation. The vascular endothelial injury responsible for the progressive ischemic changes is characterized by the development of subintimal foam cells or fibrointimal hypertrophy. The clinical course is relentlessly progressive and nearly always requires retransplantation. Unfortunately, recurrence of chronic rejection in the retransplanted allograft is common.[77]

The immunologic nature of this process is emphasized by the primary target role played by the biliary and vascular endothelium. These are the only tissues in the liver that express class II antigen. Other interdependent cofactors such as CMV infection, HLA mismatching, positive B-cell crossmatching, and differing racial demographics of the donor to recipient combination have all failed to show consistent correlation with the development of chronic rejection.[76,77]

Renal Insufficiency

The long-term success of liver transplantation has been related to effective immunosuppression with calcineurin inhibitors (CNI), such as cyclosporine and tacrolimus. However, nephrotoxicity associated with their long-term use has become a major problem and affects up to 70% of all nonrenal recipients. Renal insufficiency can present in many ways after CNI administration and liver transplantation. When this occurs during the initial post-transplant weeks, it is most often related to transient excessive blood levels and is reversible with appropriate dose correction. Impaired glomerular filtration rate (GFR) seen in pediatric recipients with stable graft function represents a more serious problem. Up to 20% may have a drop in their GFR to below 50 mL/min/1.73 m^2, and 5% may progress to end-stage renal disease (ESRD). Adult studies have shown a progressive increase in chronic renal failure from 0.9% at year 1 to 8.6% at year 13 after OLT.[79] Similarly, ESRD rose from 1.6% at year 1 to 9.5% at year 13 post OLT, yielding a total incidence of renal dysfunction of 18%. The presence of an elevated serum creatinine value before OLT and at 1-year post transplant and the presence of hepatorenal syndrome before transplant were all identified risk factors.[79,80] Cyclosporine and tacrolimus both appear to have a similar risk.

In a recent review from our program, in children who were more than 3 years post liver transplant, we found that 32% had a GFR less than 70 mL/min/1.73 m^2.[22] The primary factors related to lower GFR were the presence of an elevated creatinine at 1-year post transplant and the length of time after transplantation. Our data supported the concept of a continued decline in renal function after liver transplantation. Considering the long survival for children undergoing liver transplantation, the possibility of progressive asymptomatic renal insufficiency leading to severe kidney disease poses a critical challenge.

Efforts to reverse ongoing renal insufficiency using protocols that include instituting non-nephrotoxic agents, such as mycophenolate mofetil, while decreasing the CNI dose, have shown some limited success in improving GFR while protecting against acute rejection at the time of immunosuppressive drug conversion.[81] Efforts have also been undertaken to use the new class of monoclonal anti-CD25 antibodies for induction therapy coupled with mycophenolate mofetil and corticosteroids in an effort to avoid administration of CNI during the first post-transplant week. These agents appear to afford sufficient protection against rejection to successfully allow the late administration of CNI. Whether these efforts will prevent the later development of renal insufficiency is unknown.[82]

Efforts to completely eliminate CNI administration have been complicated by acute or ductopenic rejection. Present efforts suggest that earlier staged reduction of calcineurin inhibitors before the development of severe GFR reduction will decrease but not eliminate this complication. Once established, chronic renal failure does not appear to resolve with calcineurin inhibitor dose adjustment. Although calcineurin inhibitor toxicity is now appreciated, the association of both hepatic and renal disease in many metabolic diseases of childhood may also contribute to the identified GFR abnormalities seen in post-transplant patients.

Infection

Infectious complications have become the most common source of morbidity and mortality after transplantation. Multiple organism infection is common as are concurrent infections by different infectious agents.

Bacterial infections occur in the immediate post-transplant period and are most often caused by gram-negative enteric organisms, *Enterococcus*, or *Staphylococcus* species. Intra-abdominal abscesses or infected collections of serum along the cut surface of the reduced-size allograft are best addressed with extraperitoneal or laparotomy drainage. Percutaneous drainage is less successful in our experience. Intrahepatic abscesses suggest hepatic artery stenosis or thrombosis, and treatment is directed by the vascular status of the allograft and associated bile duct abnormalities. Sepsis originating at sites of invasive monitoring lines can be minimized by replacing or removing all intraoperative lines soon after transplantation. Antibacterial prophylactic antibiotics are discontinued as soon as possible to prevent the development of resistant organisms.

Fungal sepsis represents a significant potential problem in the early post-transplant period. Aggressive protocols for pretransplant prophylaxis are based on the concept that fungal infections originate from organisms colonizing the gastrointestinal tract of the recipient. Selective bowel decontamination was successful in eliminating pathogenic gram-negative bacteria from the gastrointestinal tract in 87% of adult patients.[83,84] Moreover, *Candida* was eliminated in all patients. However, these protocols have not been practical in pediatric patients because there is a long waiting time for pediatric organs and the taste of the oral antibiotics is poorly accepted. These regimens are, however, commonly used in the preoperative preparation for combined liver/small intestinal transplantation. Fungal infection most often occurs in patients requiring multiple operative procedures and those who have had multiple courses of antibiotics. Development of fungemia or urosepsis requires renal and cardiac investigation and a search for renal fungal involvement. Antifungal therapy should be promptly undertaken because severe fungal infection has a mortality greater than 80%. All patients undergoing OLT should receive antifungal prophylaxis with fluconazole.

The majority of early and severe viral infections are caused by viruses of the Herpesvirus family, including Epstein-Barr virus (EBV), CMV, and herpes simplex virus (HSV). CMV transmission dynamics are well studied and serve as a prototype for herpesvirus transmission in the transplant population. The likelihood that CMV infection will develop is influenced by the preoperative CMV status of the transplant donor and recipient.[85,86] Seronegative recipients receiving seropositive donor organs are at greatest risk, with seropositive donor to recipient combinations at the next greatest risk. Use of various immune-based prophylactic protocols including intravenous IgG or hyperimmune anti-CMV IgG, coupled with acyclovir or ganciclovir/valganciclovir, have all achieved success in decreasing the incidence of symptomatic CMV infection. However, seroconversion in recipients of seropositive donor organs inevitably occurs.

The clinical diagnosis of CMV infection is suggested by the development of fever, leukopenia, maculopapular rash, hepatocellular abnormalities, respiratory insufficiency, or gastrointestinal hemorrhage. Hepatic biopsy or endoscopic biopsy of colonic or gastroduodenal sites allows early diagnosis with immunohistochemical recognition. Rapid blood and urine assays for CMV can also expedite diagnosis. In suspected cases, treatment should be instituted while awaiting culture or biopsy results, owing to the potential rapidity and severity of this infection in a previously uninfected child. The treatment of CMV has been greatly improved by the development of ganciclovir. Early treatment with intravenous IgG and ganciclovir is successful in most cases.

HSV syndromes, similar to those seen in nontransplant patients, require treatment with acyclovir when diagnosed. Other viral infections leading to significant post-transplant infectious complications include adenovirus infection, hepatitis, varicella, and enterovirus-induced gastroenteritis. Recurrent viral hepatitis is an uncommon problem in pediatric transplantation, but it is commonly seen in adult patients. *Pneumocystis* infection has been nearly eliminated by the prophylactic administration of sulfamethoxazole-trimethoprim or aerosolized pentamidine.

EBV infection occurring in the perioperative period represents a significant risk to the pediatric transplant recipient.[87] It has a varying presentation, including a mononucleosis-like syndrome, hepatitis-simulating rejection, extranodal lymphoproliferative infiltration with bowel perforation, peritonsillar or lymph node enlargement, or encephalopathy. In small children, its primary portal of entry is often the tonsils, making asymptomatic tonsillar hypertrophy a common initial presentation.[88] EBV infection can occur as a primary infection or after reactivation of a past primary infection. When serologic evidence of active infection exists, an acute reduction in immunosuppression is indicated. It has become clear that continuous surveillance is necessary because the presentation is often nonspecific and the prognosis is related to early diagnosis. Screening by determination of EBV blood viral load by quantitative PCR appears to be the best current predictor of risk. However, viral loads have been identified in asymptomatic patients and patients recovering from PTLD, limiting the specificity of this test. The balance between viral load, measured by quantitative polymerase chain reaction (PCR) and specific cellular immune response, perhaps mediated by CD8 T-cells specific to EBV, may explain this lack of specificity to viral load alone.[89-91]

Many pediatric transplant centers now use serially measured quantitative EBV-DNA PCR as an indication for primary immunosuppression modulation. We recommend monthly EBV-DNA PCR counts to monitor increased genomic expression. Increasing viral load levels warrant more frequent monitoring on an every 2-week or 1-week basis. In the EBV seronegative pretransplant patients, more than 40 genomes/10^5 peripheral blood leukocytes and more than 200 genomes/10^5 peripheral blood leukocytes identify patients for reduction in primary immunosuppression by 25% to 100%. Institution of antiviral therapy with ganciclovir and CMV-IgG is also used in most cases, although only nonrandomized observational studies support their use. Both agents are active in vitro against linear replicating forms of the EBV but have no activity against the circular episome in immortalized B cells. Treatment should be continued until symptoms of lymphadenopathy have resolved and viral EBV-DNA PCR has returned to baseline.[87,92] However, it should be cautioned that PTLD can develop and progress without increases in EBV-PCR viral load.[93]

PTLD, a potentially fatal abnormal proliferation of B lymphocytes, can occur in any situation in which immunosuppression is undertaken. The importance of PTLD in pediatric liver transplantation is a result of the intensity of the immunosuppression required, its lifetime duration, and the absence of prior exposure to EBV infection in 60% to 80% of pediatric recipients. PTLD is the most common tumor in children after transplantation and represents 52% of all tumors, compared with 15% in adults. About 80% of cases occur within the first 2 years after transplantation.[90]

Multiple studies analyzing immunosuppressive therapy and the development of PTLD have shown a progressive increase in the incidence of PTLD with (1) the increase in total immunosuppressive load, (2) EBV-negative recipients, and (3) intensity of active viral load.[94] No single immunosuppressive agent has been directly related to PTLD, although high-dose cyclosporine, tacrolimus, polyclonal antilymphocyte sera (MALG, ALG), and monoclonal antibodies (OKT-3) have all been implicated. Immunosuppressive strategies using these agents as sequential therapy in low doses have not produced an increase in PTLD when successful induction prevents recurrent high-dose or long-duration immunotherapy for rejection. However, prolonged treatment with anti–T-cell agents and the increased duration, intensity, and total immunosuppressive load are the origin of the defective immunity that creates the background for neoplasia.

The second pathogenic feature influencing PTLD appears to be EBV infection. Primary or reactivation infections usually precede the recognition of PTLD. Active EBV infection, whether primary or reactivation, involves B-cell proliferation. A simultaneous increase in cytotoxic T-cell activity is the normal primary host mechanism preventing EBV dissemination. Loss of this natural protection, as a result of the administration of T-cell inhibitory immunotherapy, allows polyclonal B-cell proliferation to progress. Polyclonal proliferation of B lymphocytes occurs after EBV viral replication and release. These EBV proliferating cells express specific viral antigens that represent possible targets for the immune system, thereby explaining the well-described regression of PTLD after immunosuppressive tapering. With time, transformation of a small population of cells results in a malignant monoclonal aggressive B-cell lymphoma.[89,95-97]

Most tumors seen in children are large cell lymphomas, 86% being of B-cell origin. Extranodal involvement, uncommon in primary lymphomas, is seen in 70% of PTLD cases. Extranodal sites include central nervous system (27%), liver (23%), lung (22%), kidney (21%), intestine (20%), and spleen (13%). Allograft involvement is common and can mimic rejection. T-cell and B-cell immunohistochemical markers of the infiltrating lymphocyte population define the B-cell infiltrate and assist in establishing an early diagnosis.

Treatment of PTLD is stratified according to the immunologic cell typing and clinical presentation.[98] Documented PTLD requires an immediate decrease or discontinuation of immunosuppression and institution of anti-EBV therapy. We prefer to use intravenous ganciclovir for initial antiviral therapy, owing to the high incidence of concurrent CMV infection. Acyclovir is used for long-term treatment. The development of newer antiviral alternatives such as valganciclovir may offer better long-term treatment options in the future.[99] Patients with polyclonal B-cell proliferation frequently show regression with this treatment.[87,92] If tumor cells express B-cell marker CD20 at histology, the anti-CD20 monoclonal antibody rituximab can be administered as weekly infusions of 375 mg/m^2. Although associated in many cases with significant reduction in tumor mass, patients have frequently experienced reversible neutropenia requiring granulocyte colony-stimulating factor and hypogammaglobulinemia requiring supplementation.[100] Acute liver rejection has frequently been reported during rituximab treatment. Patients with aggressive monoclonal malignancies have poor survival even with immunosuppressive reduction, acyclovir, and conventional chemotherapy or radiation therapy. These additional treatment modalities often precipitate the development of fatal systemic infection. Efforts to reconstitute the EBV-specific cellular immunity using partially HLA-matched EBV-specific cytotoxic T-cells may offer improved treatment outcomes for advanced cases, and future development of an anti-EBV vaccine may decrease the current significant risks of this unique complication of pediatric transplantation.[101,102] When treatment is successful, careful follow-up to identify recurrent disease or delayed central nervous system involvement is essential.

Retransplantation

The vast majority of retransplantation procedures in pediatric patients are done as a result of acute allograft demise caused by hepatic artery thrombosis or primary nonfunction. Acute rejection, chronic rejection, and biliary complications are more uncommon causes. Many of these complications are associated with concurrent sepsis, which further complicates reoperation and compromises success. Survival after transplantation is directly related to prompt identification of appropriate patients and acquisition of a suitable organ. When retransplantation is promptly undertaken for early graft failure, in our experience the patient survival rate is 73%. However, when retransplantation is undertaken for chronic allograft failure, often complicated by multiple organ system failure (MOSF), the survival rate is only 45%.[22]

Similar findings were reported by UNOS Region I in their combined experience. Patients undergoing retransplantation for acute organ failure had twice the overall survival rate as those undergoing retransplantation for chronic disease.[103] In addition, acute retransplantation survival was significantly influenced by the time to acquire a retransplant organ, with a more than 3-day wait decreasing the survival rate from 52% to 20%. The overall incidence of retransplantation is 15% in our series and compares with others' experience of 8% to 29%. This incidence is similar when primary whole-organ allografts are compared with primary reduced-size allografts. Reduced-size allografts are frequently used when retransplantation is required in view of their greater availability and their decreased incidence of allograft-threatening complications.[28,104,105] These findings emphasize the need for early identification of children requiring retransplantation and expeditious reoperation before the development of MOSF or sepsis.

Outcome

Although the potential complications after liver transplantation are frequent and severe, the overall results are rewarding. Improvements in organ preservation, operative management, immunosuppression, and treatment of postoperative complications have all contributed to the excellent survival rate that currently exists. Factors influencing the survival of children undergoing transplantation are detailed in

Table 45-9 Factors Affecting Transplant Survival
Medical status at orthotopic liver transplantation
Primary diagnosis
Age and size
Comorbid conditions
Encephalopathy
Infection
Multiple organ dysfunction

Table 45-9. Most successful transplant programs have reached overall 1-year survival rates of 90%, with greatly decreased risk thereafter.[106,107] Similar, if not better results, have resulted from living donor transplantation, especially for small recipients.[108-110] Infants younger than 1 year of age or weighing less than 10 kg have historically had reported survival rates of 65% to 88% overall, an improvement over initial reported rates of 50% to 60% during the early era of OLT development.[104,111,112] Survival rates in infants now equal those seen in older children.[113] Improved survival in these small recipients is consistent throughout all levels of diseases and results from a decrease in life-threatening and graft-threatening complications, such as hepatic artery thrombosis and primary nonfunction, in the reduced-size donor organ.

Patients with fulminant hepatic failure have an overall survival rate that is significantly lower than other diagnostic groups, with patients having metabolic disease having the highest survival rate. Prior surgical procedures, especially in patients who have undergone multiple reoperations, and the presence of multiple episodes of subacute bacterial peritonitis prior to OLT influence the incidence of complications, especially bowel perforation, but do not adversely affect overall survival in most cases. However, the most important factor determining survival is the severity of the patient's illness at the time of transplantation.[28,114] When stratified for illness by PELD scores, Pediatric Risk of Mortality (PRISM) score, and the previous UNOS score, the PRISM score was the most accurate in predicting both survival and morbidity during the perioperative period.[115] Present efforts to use surgically altered allografts, such as reduced-size orthotopic liver transplant (RSOLT), LD-OLT, and split-liver OLT, have shown similar survival rates as those for whole-organ recipients (Fig. 45-9).[104,116]

The increased donor availability for small recipients achieved with the use of surgically reduced, split-liver, or LD organs has also brought about a significant decrease in waiting list mortality. In our center, the mortality rate for patients awaiting transplantation has decreased from 29% to 2%, and similar results have been reported by other pediatric centers.[104,105,117] Efforts to enhance donor availability are essential before major improvements in postoperative survival rates will occur.

The significant success now achieved after liver transplantation cannot overshadow the need for improved management of post-transplant consequences of immunosuppression and pre-OLT chronic disease. In our program, the most significant factors contributing to long-term failure of the allograft or patient death are consequences of immunosuppressive medications, such as late infection, PTLD, and chronic rejection of the allograft.[107,118-120] Our ability to successfully address these challenges will determine the lifelong success of transplantation for our youngest recipients.

Follow-up

The overriding objective of liver transplantation in children is complete rehabilitation with an improved quality of life. Factors contributing to the attainment of this goal include improved nutritional status with appropriate growth and development as well as enhanced motor and cognitive skills, allowing social reintegration.

Nutrition and Growth

Optimal postoperative nutrition significantly facilitates recovery and rehabilitation. This initially requires 100 to 130 calories/kg/day in recipients weighing less than 10 kg. Hepatic synthetic function, gut absorption, and appetite all improve after successful pediatric liver transplantation.

Despite these improvements, growth disturbances do not immediately resolve.[121-123] In the first year after transplantation, very little catch-up growth occurs. During the second and third year after transplantation patients usually show significant catch-up growth, with the potential for catch-up growth being directly correlated with the degree of preoperative growth retardation. Decreased corticosteroid administration accelerates this recovery. This growth is further improved by the use of alternate-day corticosteroids or complete corticosteroid withdrawal in patients with stable allograft function 2 years after OLT.[124] The "steroid-sparing" effects of new immunosuppressive agents, such as tacrolimus, could diminish this unwanted consequence of immune modulation.

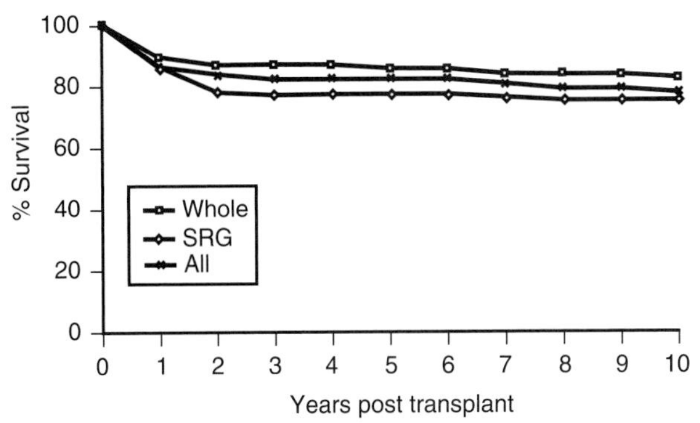

Figure 45-9. 10-Year patient and allograft survival subdivided by whole and surgically reduced grafts (SRG). (Data from Cincinnati Children's Hospital Medical Center, Liver Care Center.)

Neuropsychological Outcome

Although most pediatric transplant recipients are returning to normal age-appropriate activities (e.g., accomplishing normal developmental milestones, restarting school), recent studies indicate that they may be experiencing subtle functional difficulties.[125-127] Neuropsychological function studies of children after transplantation demonstrate multiple deficits involving learning and memory, abstraction, concept formation, visuospatial function, and motor function. The well-documented neurologic and cerebral abnormalities associated with chronic cirrhosis precede transplantation but certainly influence these results.[126,128-130]

The long-term impact that transplantation has on the psychosocial and financial health of the entire family unit is also the subject of much concern. Long-term pediatric liver transplant survivors need in-depth, multicenter longitudinal studies to clarify these issues.

Health Related Quality of Life (HRQOL) surveys of post-transplant families and patients demonstrate improved health and physical perception compared with their pretransplant status. However, as can be imagined, the overall impact on the family is significant. In one study, HRQOL in pediatric liver transplant recipients was lower than that reported for healthy children but similar to that for children with other chronic illness.[131] Age at transplantation, the time elapsed since transplantation, hospitalizations within the previous year, maternal education, and race were significant predictors of physical health. Age at transplantation and maternal education also predicted psychosocial function.

Both younger children and adolescents continue to have self-confidence and body image concerns, and their participation in out-of-family activities and sports is often limited. Caregivers and mothers, in particular, are heavily impacted by the need for care of their chronically ill children before and after transplant. Many have experienced job losses, career changes, and significant family stress.

MULTIVISCERAL/ISOLATED INTESTINAL TRANSPLANTATION

Intestinal failure is a significant problem in the pediatric population. Total parenteral nutrition (TPN) remains the first line of therapy of children who have a loss of gastrointestinal function and is a proven, effective means of treatment. However, complications of long-term parenteral alimentation such as TPN-induced cholestatic liver disease, a paucity of access due to venous thrombosis, and recurrent catheter sepsis may preclude its continued use. When complications of long-term TPN become life threatening, the only alternative is intestinal transplantation. Although the exact incidence of intestinal failure in children is unclear, more than two thirds of the patients who are currently on the national intestinal transplantation waiting list are in the pediatric age group.[132]

Recent developments in the use of immunosuppression and the technical aspects of surgery have improved the outcome of patients who have undergone intestinal transplantation.[133,134] With the improved outcome, the role of intestinal transplantation has evolved from a heroic last effort to salvage patients with no remaining treatment options to a standard part of the armamentarium in the management of patients with intestinal failure. As a result, in October 2000, the Centers for Medicare and Medicaid Services issued a memorandum approving federal reimbursement for intestinal transplantation for selected indications.[135] In this section, we review the role of intestinal transplantation in pediatric patients with intestinal failure.

Indications

Intestinal failure is the inability of the native gastrointestinal tract to provide nutritional autonomy. Patients who suffer from intestinal failure require TPN to maintain a normal state of nutrition, fluid and electrolyte balance, as well as growth and development. The cause of intestinal failure can be divided into three categories: short bowel syndrome, intestinal dysmotility syndromes, and congenital epithelial mucosal disorders. Short bowel syndrome, usually caused by the loss of intestinal length due to surgical resection for an intra-abdominal catastrophe, is the most common cause of intestinal failure. Disease processes necessitating surgical intervention that may result in short bowel syndrome range from necrotizing enterocolitis and gastroschisis in the newborn to Crohn's disease and traumatic injury to the main intestinal blood supply in the older population. Midgut volvulus, another frequent cause of short bowel syndrome, may occur at any age, although the majority of cases occur in infants.

The intestinal dysmotility syndromes include total intestinal aganglionosis (Hirschsprung's disease) and the constellation of disorders known as chronic idiopathic intestinal pseudo-obstruction. Congenital epithelial mucosal diseases, which through impaired enterocyte absorption lead to intractable diarrhea, include microvillus inclusion disease, epithelial dysplasia, and autoimmune enteritis. Although these disorders are rare, affected children face life-long difficulty with gastrointestinal function and require TPN for survival.

TPN is the standard treatment for patients who experience acute intestinal failure. Bowel rehabilitation should be tried because intestinal adaptation may result in eventual enteral autonomy. Bowel rehabilitation programs utilizing a combination of TPN, gradual re-introduction of enteral feeds, and intestinal antimotility agents are successful in achieving enteral autonomy in some patients.[136,137] Bowel lengthening procedures may be beneficial in selected patients.[138] Survival and complete return of gastrointestinal function may be predicted when the postresection length of intestine exceeds 5% of normal for gestational age, when the ileocecal valve remains or is greater than 10% of normal if the ileocecal valve has been lost.[139]

Unfortunately, a subset of patients will fail bowel rehabilitation and require life-long TPN for survival.

Although TPN is lifesaving, complications of long-term TPN may eventually preclude its use. The current Medicare-approved indications for intestinal transplantation are shown in Table 45-10.[135]

Impending liver failure from TPN-induced cholestasis is associated with a significant mortality. Unless the TPN can be stopped, it is a strong indication for combined liver/intestinal transplantation. Studies have shown that the presence of hyperbilirubinemia of more than 3 mg/dL or bridging fibrosis and cirrhosis found on liver biopsy in an infant dependent on TPN is associated with a 1-year survival of less than 30%.[140] All of the remaining indications reflect patients with chronic problems from continued TPN use and are relative indicators for intestinal transplantation.

Currently, with improved outcomes after intestinal transplantation, some centers advocate early intestinal transplantation before the onset of TPN-induced complications.[133,134] These groups believe that graft and patient survival after intestinal transplantation may improve if recipients undergo transplantation before the onset of secondary organ damage, especially liver disease. Furthermore, the quality of life in patients who have undergone successful intestinal transplantation may be better than that of patients who require long-term TPN. This issue is controversial and requires further study because TPN is a well-established and effective means of treatment for intestinal failure. A better understanding of the natural history of long-term TPN use and the progression at which TPN induces complications is necessary.

Contraindications

The contraindications to intestinal transplantation are similar to those for any other solid organ transplantation. The presence of an active nonresectable malignancy, severe neurologic disabilities, or life-threatening extraintestinal illness precludes intestinal transplantation.

Operative Considerations

Currently, there are three types of intestinal grafts: multivisceral, liver/small bowel composite, and small bowel alone. The type of intestinal transplant utilized is dictated by the needs of the individual patient. The biggest limitation to intestinal transplantation is the need for size-matched grafts. Patients with intestinal failure generally have limited abdominal domain (due in part to a lack of intestine volume), which necessitates near-identical-size donors. Recent developments using reduced-size liver grafts have increased the flexibility of recipient to donor size match.[141] However, between 40% and 50% of patients on the intestinal transplant waiting list die before undergoing transplantation owing to the lack of appropriate donors.[132,142] In the past, it was believed that recipients who were CMV negative should not receive intestinal grafts from CMV-positive donors because they experienced severe, potentially life-threatening CMV infection after transplantation.[143] However, with current antiviral therapy, it appears this barrier has been overcome.

Table 45-10 Medicare-Approved Indications for Intestinal Transplantation

1. Impending or overt liver failure due to TPN-induced liver injury. Liver failure defined as increased serum bilirubin or liver enzyme levels or both, splenomegaly, thrombocytopenia, gastroesophageal varices, coagulopathy, stomal bleeding, hepatic fibrosis, or cirrhosis
2. Thrombosis of two or more central veins (subclavian, jugular, or femoral)
3. The development of two or more episodes of systemic sepsis secondary to line infection that requires hospitalization or a single episode of line-related fungemia, or septic shock or acute respiratory distress syndrome or both
4. Frequent episodes of severe dehydration despite intravenous fluid supplementation in addition to TPN

TPN, total parenteral nutrition.

An ileostomy is created in all recipients so that surveillance endoscopy and biopsy of the small bowel mucosa can be performed to monitor the allograft for rejection. If absent, a Stamm gastrostomy, placed for gastric decompression, can be used for access to the gastrointestinal tract.

Multivisceral Graft

Multivisceral transplantation entails transplantation of the stomach, duodenum, pancreas, small intestine, and if necessary, the liver. In the pediatric population, the primary indications for multivisceral transplantation are the intestinal dysmotility syndromes. On occasion, a giant desmoid tumor of the mesentery that extensively infiltrates the mesentery may require this form of transplantation. Exenteration of the native intra-abdominal viscera is followed by transplantation of the multivisceral graft using arterial inflow through the donor celiac and superior mesenteric artery. Venous outflow occurs via the transplanted liver placed in the standard orthotopic position.

Liver/Small Bowel Composite Graft

A liver/small bowel composite graft is a modification of the multivisceral graft in which the stomach is removed during procurement. This form of transplantation is indicated in patients with intestinal failure and impending or overt TPN-induced liver failure and is the most common type of intestinal transplant currently utilized (Fig. 45-10). The recipient's liver and residual small intestine are removed while the native stomach, duodenum, pancreas, and spleen are left intact. A portacaval shunt from the native portal vein to the inferior vena cava is necessary to provide venous outflow from the recipient's foregut organs (Fig. 45-11). The donor celiac and superior mesenteric artery remain the source of arterial inflow to the transplanted organs. The donor portal vein and biliary tree are intact, having not undergone dissection during procurement. As a result, no portal vein or bile duct reconstruction is necessary. The pancreas is left intact to protect the peribiliary ductal vessels and to prevent the possibility of pancreatic leak from a divided surface. Venous outflow from the transplanted organs is once again provided by the donor liver placed in a standard orthotopic position. If the liver is too large, an ex vivo hepatic lobectomy can be performed usually removing the right lobe of the liver (Fig. 45-12). Luminal continuity from the patient's stomach and duodenum to the newly transplanted bowel is achieved by anastomosis of the recipient's duodenum to the donor jejunum. If the recipient has any colon, a donor ileum to recipient colonic anastomosis is created distal to the ileostomy.

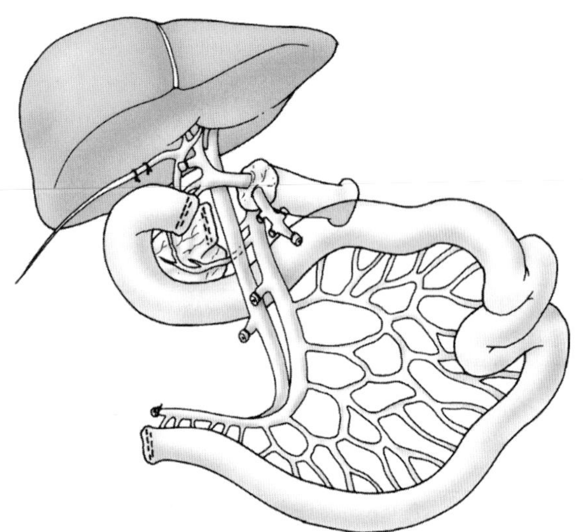

Figure 45-10. Schematic diagram of liver/intestine composite allograft. (From Abu-Elmagd K, Reyes J, Todo S, et al: Clinical intestinal transplantation: New perspectives and immunologic considerations. J Am Coll Surg 186:512-527, 1998.)

Small Intestine Graft

Transplantation of the small intestine alone entails procurement of only the jejunum and ileum. During procurement, the superior mesenteric artery and vein are divided just below the third portion of the duodenum at the root of the mesentery, generating a graft of jejunum and ileum (Fig. 45-13). This type of transplant is indicated in patients with intestinal failure without other organ dysfunction. Depending on space requirements, the recipient's residual small bowel is removed. Arterial inflow is provided by anastomosis of the superior mesenteric artery to the recipient's aorta. Venous drainage of the transplanted intestines is either directly into the inferior vena cava or the native superior mesenteric vein. Initially it was believed that venous drainage into the native portal circulation was beneficial to the liver, but recent studies suggest minimal benefit.[144] Therefore, currently the most common form of venous reconstruction is an end-to-side anastomosis of the donor superior mesenteric vein to the native vena cava. Luminal continuity is restored by

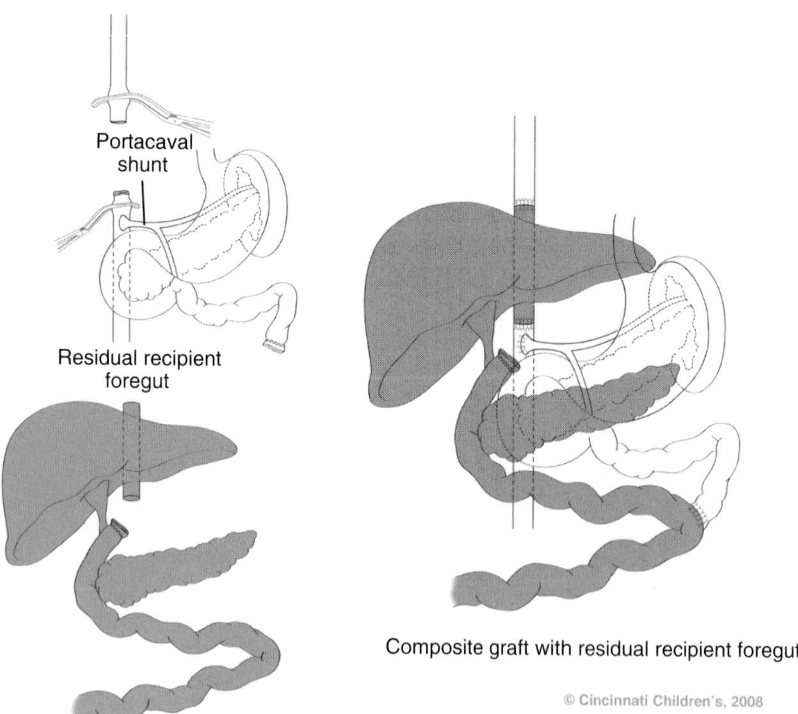

Figure 45-11. Schematic diagram of liver/intestine composite allograft with native portacaval shunt. (© Cincinnati Children's, 2008.)

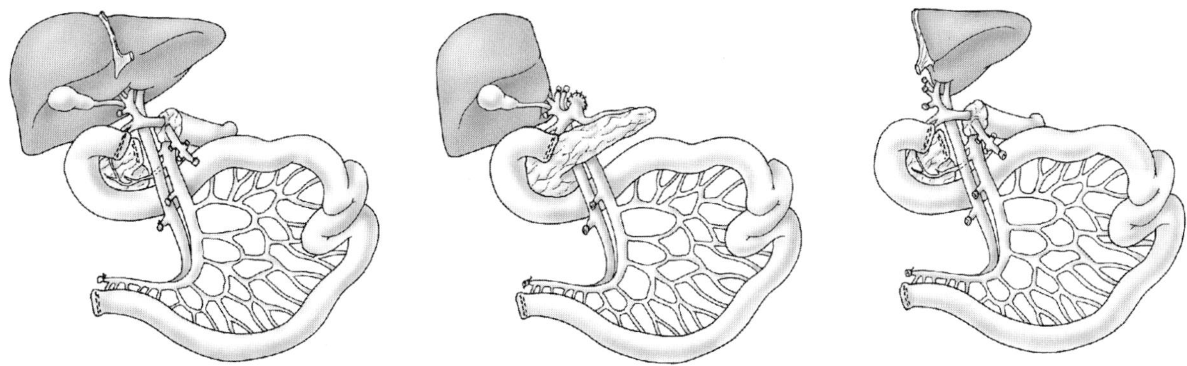

Figure 45-12. Schematic diagram of reduced-size liver/intestine composite allograft. (From Reyes J, Mazariegos GV, Bond GMD, et al: Pediatric intestinal transplantation: Historical notes, principles and controversies. Pediatr Transplant 2002:6:193-207.)

anastomosis of the recipient's proximal bowel to the transplanted jejunum. Once again, if residual colon is present, a donor ileum to colonic anastomosis is created downstream from the ileostomy.

Postoperative Complications

Although the success rate after intestinal transplantation continues to improve, postoperative complications are common. A breakdown of intestinal integrity either at sites of anastomosis or in areas of mucosal injury from ischemia and reperfusion will necessitate re-exploration. Bowel perforation may also occur during surveillance endoscopy. Patients with a significant amount of peritoneal contamination after bowel perforation may require serial operative exploration to clear foci of intra-abdominal infection. Postoperative bleeding is frequent, especially in patients who undergo liver/small intestine composite grafts, because preexisting portal hypertension results in varices throughout the abdomen. Chylous leaks are also frequent because lymphatic drainage may be disrupted during both the procurement and the recipient operative procedure. Most chylous leaks can be managed conservatively. Almost all patients who undergo intestinal transplantation will require re-exploration at some point in the postoperative period.

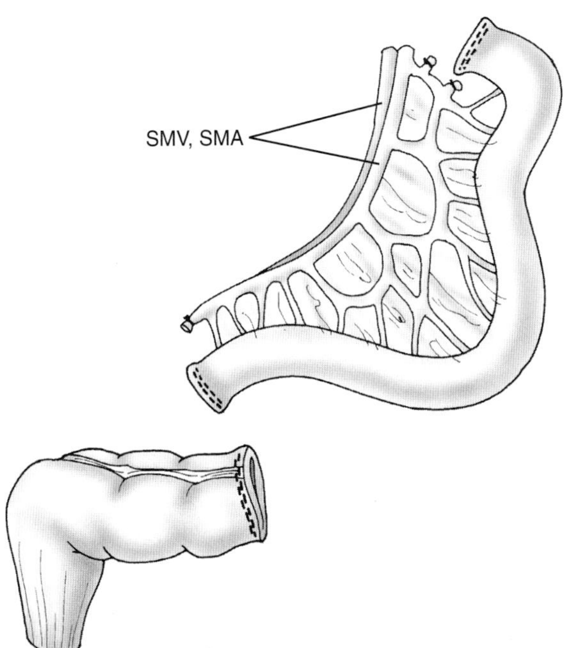

Figure 45-13. Schematic diagram of isolated small intestinal transplant. SMV, superior mesenteric vein; SMA, superior mesenteric artery. (Adapted from Abu-Elmagd K, Fung J, Bueno J, et al: Logistics and technique for procurement of intestinal, pancreatic, and hepatic grafts from the same donor. Ann Surg 232:680-687, 2000.)

Immunosuppression/Rejection

The most significant advances in the management of an intestinal transplant recipient have occurred in the use of immunosuppression. Rejection remains the most common complication after intestinal transplantation with virtually every patient experiencing an episode of rejection in the first 6 months after transplantation. Overwhelming rejection was one of the most frequent causes of graft loss during the initial experience with intestinal transplantation due, in part, to the limited number of immunosuppressive agents available. Before tacrolimus was developed, high-dose immunosuppression was necessary to prevent rejection. Infections and PTLD, side effects of high-dose immunosuppression, became frequent causes of a poor outcome. The goal of current immunosuppressive regimens is to use just enough immunosuppression to prevent rejection but not so much that infections and PTLD become common. The management of immunosuppression in patients who undergo intestinal transplantation remains the most challenging aspect of patient care.

Surveillance endoscopy and biopsy is initiated 5 days after transplantation to evaluate for rejection and is performed at least two to three times per week for the first month. Significant progress in the definition of the histologic characteristics of small bowel rejection has been achieved. If rejection is diagnosed, a short course of high-dose corticosteroids is administered. If rejection persists, anti–lymphocyte antibody immunosuppression using agents such as OKT-3 or thymoglobulin is required. In an effort to achieve tolerance, some centers are using a combination of thymoglobulin, graft irradiation, and bone marrow transplantation.[145]

Infections

Owing in large part to the high level of immunosuppression needed after intestinal transplantation, bacterial and fungal infections are common in the postoperative period. Patients with intestinal failure are frequently colonized with antibiotic-resistant bacteria due to recurrent infections while on TPN. As mentioned previously, because intestinal perforation is common, peritonitis is a frequent complication often requiring repeat intra-abdominal explorations to completely clear the peritoneum.

CMV, EBV, and adenovirus are the most frequent viral pathogens found in the postoperative period. PTLD, an EBV-driven process, remains a significant problem because most infants are EBV negative at the time of transplantation. Surveillance for CMV and EBV using PCR, followed by aggressive treatment when detected, has diminished the impact of these dangerous pathogens on patient outcome. All patients are maintained on prophylactic antiviral agents in the perioperative period.

Outcome

The initial experience of patients who underwent intestinal transplantation was dismal with few long-term survivors.[146] Thus, because TPN was so successful at treating patients with intestinal failure, the interest in intestinal transplantation was limited. As long-term use of TPN increased, the complications of TPN became increasingly apparent. As a result, renewed interest in intestinal transplantation occurred. With the development of tacrolimus, intestinal transplantation became a viable alternative. Currently, over 70% of patients survive 1 year and 50% survive 5 years after transplantation.[146-148] Recent data from the University of Pittsburgh have shown that in children using a combination of thymoglobulin induction followed by tacrolimus monotherapy, graft and patient survival of 100% at 1 year can be achieved.[149] Such results support the conclusion that the role of intestinal transplantation in the management of children with intestinal failure has moved from experimental to an integral part of the treatment for intestinal failure.[150]

RENAL TRANSPLANTATION

Indications

Acute renal failure in infants is most often the consequence of hemodynamic instability, with poor perfusion or hypoxia resulting in acute tubular necrosis (ATN). Most of these patients either recover sufficient renal function for normal long-term survival or die of multisystem failure.

Chronic renal failure is uncommon in infants, with the estimate of infants with ESRD placed at 0.2 per million total population for infants younger than 1 year of age.[151,152] Congenital lesions, such as renal dysplasia, obstructive malformations, or complex urogenital malformation, and congenital nephrosis are the most common causes of ESRD in children younger than 5 years of age. These diseases account for about half the cases. Glomerulonephritis, including focal segmental glomerulosclerosis, membranoproliferative glomerulonephritis, and lupus nephritis, as well as recurrent pyelonephritis, are common causes of ESRD in older children (Table 45-11).[153] Hereditary causes of renal failure should be identified to plan an appropriate overall treatment strategy, including evaluating other family members and providing

Table 45-11 Primary Diagnoses in Children Requiring Renal Transplantation (NAPRTCS, 2008)

Primary Diagnosis	No. Patients	Percentage
Aplasia/hypoplasia/dysplasia of kidney	1564	15.9
Obstructive uropathy	1538	15.6
Focal segmental glomerulosclerosis	1154	11.7
Reflux nephropathy	515	5.2
Chronic glomerulonephritis	328	3.3
Polycystic disease	287	2.9
Medullary cystic disease	271	2.8
Hemolytic uremic syndrome	260	2.6
Prune belly syndrome	254	2.6
Congenital nephrotic syndrome	254	2.6
Familial nephritis	225	2.3
Cystinosis	201	2.0
Pyelo/interstitial nephritis	173	1.8
Membranoproliferative glomerulonephritis type I	171	1.7
Idiopathic crescentic glomerulonephritis	171	1.7
Systemic lupus erythematosus nephritis	150	1.5
Renal infarct	136	1.4
Berger's (IgA) nephritis	127	1.3
Henoch-Schönlein nephritis	110	1.1
Membranoproliferative glomerulonephritis type II	81	0.8
Wegener's granulomatosis	55	0.6
Wilms' tumor	52	0.5
Drash syndrome	52	0.5
Oxalosis	52	0.5
Membranous nephropathy	44	0.4
Other systemic immunologic disease	32	0.3
Sickle cell nephropathy	16	0.2
Diabetic glomerulonephritis	11	0.1
Other	962	9.8
Unknown	608	6.2
TOTAL	9854	100.0

genetic counseling when needed. Recently, because the number of patients who have undergone renal transplantation in childhood has increased, chronic rejection after renal transplantation has become a frequent cause of ESRD.

Knowledge of the etiology of the ESRD is important to allow assessment of the potential for recurrence within a transplant allograft and consideration of LD transplantation. Patients with a "structural/congenital" etiology without an immunologic component also enjoy better graft survival rates than those patients with glomerulonephritis.[154]

Pretransplant Management

Pretransplant management is critical in infants and children with ESRD. Children with ESRD beginning in infancy or early childhood experience significant complications from growth retardation, renal osteodystrophy, and neuropsychiatric developmental delay. Recent advances in dialysis regimens, nutritional supplementation, and recombinant human erythropoietin and growth hormone have significantly improved the pretransplant management of these patients.

Dialysis

Dialysis is indicated when complications of ESRD occur despite optimal medical management, specifically hyperkalemia, volume overload, acidosis, intractable hypertension, and uremic symptoms such as vomiting. In older children, lethargy and poor school performance can signal the need for more aggressive treatment. In addition, dialysis may be necessary to facilitate the administration of adequate protein as part of an extensive nutritional resuscitation plan.

When dialysis is needed, the use of peritoneal dialysis is preferred for the following reasons: (1) it avoids the multiple blood transfusions associated with hemodialysis; (2) it allows a gradual correction of electrolyte abnormalities, preventing cerebral disequilibrium syndrome in small infants; (3) it allows for easier control of osteodystrophy; (4) it optimizes nutrition; and (5) it is easy to administer.

Hemodialysis is used when there is an unsuitable peritoneal cavity secondary to prior surgery or multiple peritoneal infections. However, the construction and maintenance of adequate long-term vascular access sites in small infants and children is difficult. Use of central venous catheters, rather than arteriovenous fistulas, is our preferred mode for temporary hemodialysis access in infants and small children, although infection and vascular thromboses complicate this therapy. Access via the internal jugular veins is preferred over subclavian routes to avoid venous occlusion from the upper extremity, which compromises future arteriovenous fistula sites. Although dialysis and its complications, such as infection, have a great influence on the complexity of care, they do not affect the ultimate results of renal transplantation.[155]

Nutritional Support

The need for vigorous nutritional support of the infant with uremia has been well documented by the growth retardation seen in infants and children with ESRD. The etiology of this growth disturbance is multifactorial, including anorexia that leads to protein and calorie insufficiency, renal osteodystrophy, aluminum toxicity, uremic acidosis, impaired somatomedin activity, and growth hormone and insulin resistance.[156] Because the most intense period of growth occurs during the first 2 years of life, careful nutritional support during that time is essential.

With extensive nutritional efforts, the mean weight at the time of transplantation for all patients has improved from 2.2 standard deviation (SD) to 1.6 SD below the appropriate age-adjusted and gender-adjusted mean for normal children in the recent North American Pediatric Renal Transplant Cooperative Study (NAPRTCS).[157] Similar height deficits occurred. This growth deficit was greater (2.8 SD) in children younger than 5 years of age. Transplantation afforded a +0.8 SD increase in growth over the first post-transplant year. However, this accelerated growth then reaches a stable plateau. After 2 to 3 years, the mean weight values were comparable to those in normal children.[153] Children 6 years of age and older show no improvement in their height deficit 5 years after transplantation.[158,159] These limitations to "catch-up" growth emphasize the need for early transplantation in young ESRD patients. If epiphyseal closure has occurred (bone age >12 years), additional bone growth is often not achieved.[152,160,161] Normalization of growth rarely occurs with the introduction of either hemodialysis or peritoneal dialysis.

The importance of normalizing nutritional parameters is emphasized by the adverse impact of uremia on the developing nervous system in the infant. The significance of this problem was emphasized in a study in which progressive encephalopathy, developmental delay, microcephaly, hypotonia, seizures, and dyskinesia developed in 20 of 23 children with ESRD before 1 year of age.[162] All of these patients had significant growth impairment. Monitoring of the head circumference has been suggested to identify the infant at risk, with the intent to initiate dialysis, nutritional support, or transplantation if this parameter deviates from the normal curve.[152]

Transplant Management

Preoperative Evaluation

In preparation for transplantation, an extensive evaluation of the patient's urinary tract and immunologic status is necessary. The increased frequency of urinary tract abnormalities as the primary cause of ESRD in infants and children necessitates the investigation of the urinary tract for sites of obstruction, presence of ureteral reflux, and functional state and capacity of the urinary bladder.[163] This investigation is best accomplished by ultrasonography or intravenous pyelography of the upper urinary tract and a voiding cystourethrogram to assess bladder and reflux parameters. Any questions related to bladder function or structure require urodynamics and cystoscopy.

In patients with long-standing oliguric ESRD, the bladder capacity may appear very small. In the absence of abnormal obstructive or neuromuscular bladder pathology, adequate enlargement of the bladder in the presence of normal urinary production is to be expected. Any surgical correction of urethral obstruction or bladder augmentation should be undertaken far in advance of the kidney transplant. Preoperative sterilization of the urinary tract and development of unobstructed urinary outflow should be the ultimate goals of evaluation and reconstruction. Although complex anomalies of the urogenital tract often require many extensive operative procedures to augment, reconstruct, or create an acceptable lower urinary tract, virtually all such children can undergo successful reconstruction with continent urinary reservoirs without the use of intestinal conduits.[164]

Immunologic assessment includes tissue typing and panel reactive antibody analysis. Patients should be monitored periodically for the development of a positive crossmatch to their potential LD or a positive cytotoxic antibody to a panel of random donors to assess immunologic reactivity. In addition, reactivity to CMV, EBV, HSV, and hepatitis should be investigated. Childhood immunizations should be current, and immunization against hepatitis B virus should be instituted. Any immunizations with live virus vaccines should be given well in advance of transplantation because their use is contraindicated in the early post-transplant period.

Selection of the appropriate donor for transplantation is a decision for the transplant team and family to consider together. A related immediate family member (LD) has the advantage of a low incidence of postoperative acute tubular necrosis, an improved histologic matching (leading to fewer rejection episodes and the need for less immunosuppression), and the possibility of extended organ function. In addition, any operative procedures required for recipient preparation, as well as the transplant procedure, can be scheduled around the needs of the patient, simplifying preoperative care and potentially avoiding the complications of dialysis. Parents form the majority of donors. Siblings younger than 18 years of age are rarely considered unless they are identical twins. At present, 60% of children receive a related LD kidney.[158] Complete evaluation of the potential donor to exclude intrinsic renal anomalies, vascular anomalies, and systemic illness is necessary.

Cadaver donor (CD) kidneys are used for 40% of renal transplants. The unpredictability of donor organ availability and the need to establish a negative antibody crossmatch for CD transplantation make surgical planning impossible. The size of a potential allograft, whether CD or LD, is also important. Kidneys from small adult donors can be transplanted into infants as small as 5 kg with good technical success.[165] CD organs from pediatric donors 5 years of age or older also yield an excellent survival rate. However, a progressive decrease in 1-year graft survival has been noted when kidneys from donors younger than 3 to 4 years of age have been used.[166,167] This decrease in graft and patient survival rate is related to the donor organ source. Children 2 to 5 years of age have a similar survival rate as the overall pediatric population when living related donors are used. Recognition of this potential risk has led to reluctance by most centers to use donors younger than 5 years of age. An effect of donor age on graft survival has been attributed to an increased rate of both graft thrombosis and acute rejection.[153]

The decision to use a CD is often strengthened by the possibility of disease recurrence within the transplanted kidney. The incidence of disease recurrence after transplantation and the risk of graft loss are listed in Table 45-12.[168] The decision to proceed with LD transplantation in small children is influenced by the recent improvements in outcomes that show similar 1-year graft survival for all age groups.

Preemptive Transplantation

The desire to begin preemptive transplantation before undertaking dialysis is often fueled by the patient's or parents' desire to avoid the surgical procedures, potential infections or cardiovascular complications, and psychological impairment inherent with dialysis.

Table 45-12 Recurrence Rates and Graft Loss from Recurrent Disease in Children

Disease	Recurrence Rate (%)	Clinical Severity	% of Those with Recurrence Whose Graft Failed
FSGS	25-30	High	40-50
MPGN type I	70	Mild	12-30
MPGN type II	100	Low	10-20
SLE	5-40	Low	5
HSP	55-85	Low/mild	5-20
HUS			
Classic	12-20	Moderate	0-10
Atypical	±25	High	40-50

FSGS, focal segmental glomerulosclerosis; HSP, Henoch-Schönlein purpura; HUS, hemolytic uremic syndrome; MPGN, membranoproliferative glomerulonephritis; SLE, systemic lupus erythematosus.

From Fine RN, Ettenger R. In Morris PJ (ed): Kidney Transplantation: Principles and Practice, 4th ed. Philadelphia, WB Saunders, 1994, p 418.

A recent NAPRTCS review found 26% of primary transplantations were performed without prior dialysis.[168] Most cases used LDs rather than CDs. There was no difference in patient or graft survival in this group when compared with patients who undergo dialysis before transplantation. Preemptive transplantation is not possible when uncontrolled hypertension, massive proteinuria, or recurrent infection require prior native kidney removal or when oliguric renal failure requires immediate dialysis.

Operative Procedure

Preparation for transplantation should include placing adequate large-bore intravenous lines and using the largest urinary catheter possible. Central venous lines are used in all infants and children to ensure vascular access, hemodynamic monitoring, and a route for postoperative immunosuppressive delivery. Perioperative prophylactic antibiotics are administered. Arterial pressure monitoring lines are only necessary in small infants and patients with hemodynamic compromise, allowing preservation of future hemodialysis access sites.

Transplantation in infants and small children can be undertaken through a generous retroperitoneal approach or transabdominal placement of the allograft within the peritoneal cavity posterior to the right or left colon. An extraperitoneal approach to the retroperitoneum allows the maintenance of postoperative peritoneal dialysis and should be strongly considered when size permits. The arterial anastomosis is constructed end-to-side into the distal aorta or common iliac artery, and venous outflow of the allograft should be into the IVC or common iliac vein (Fig. 45-14) Ureteral implantation using the Lich extravesical ureteroneocystostomy avoids the presence of a cystotomy and minimizes postoperative blood clots within the bladder, which may obstruct the urinary catheter. When larger donor kidneys are used in small recipients, the vessels must be shortened to avoid redundancy when the kidney is positioned in the retroperitoneum. The internal iliac artery is not used in pediatric transplants so that pelvic blood flow is preserved. Ureteral "double-J" stents are used when small ureter size may lead to obstruction.

Anesthetic management of the infant and small child during kidney transplantation is complicated by preexisting electrolyte abnormalities and the large fluid fluxes that occur in the operating room. Intravascular blood volume must be augmented during allograft implantation to allow maintenance of normal systemic blood flow when allograft blood flow is re-established. Perfusion of the allograft with hypothermic lactated Ringer's solution before implantation to remove any remaining hyperkalemic graft preservation solution is necessary in infants and small children to avoid massive potassium infusion with establishment of allograft perfusion. Blood volume loading to a central venous pressure of 13 to 15 cm H_2O and administration of bicarbonate, calcium, and low-dose vasopressors (dopamine, 5 μg/kg/min) should be started before graft reperfusion.

Postoperative Management

Post-transplant management requires careful screening for technical complications, rejection, recurrence of the primary renal disease, and prevention of immunosuppression-related complications.

Frequent fluid and electrolyte monitoring is necessary immediately after transplantation because larger kidneys can excrete the equivalent of the infant's blood volume within a single hour. Careful attention to serum concentrations of calcium, phosphorus, magnesium, and electrolytes is necessary. Urine output is initially replaced isovolumetrically and is then tapered as the high-output state subsides. Glucose-free urine replacement fluids minimize hyperglycemia and attendant osmotic diuresis in the recipient. Selection of appropriate electrolyte concentrations is guided by urinary electrolyte excretion, which is regularly monitored. Central venous filling pressures

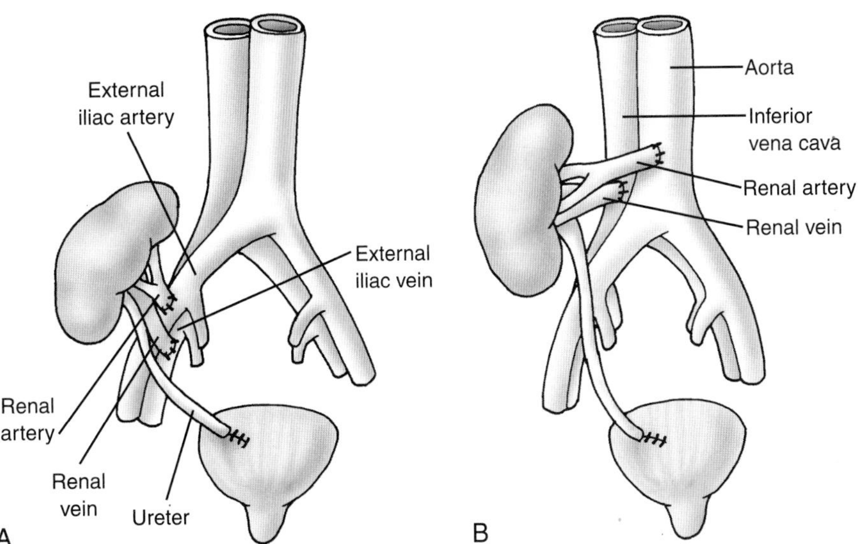

Figure 45-14. Schematic diagram showing the transplant arterial and venous anastomosis to the illiac vessels (**A**) or the aorta and vena cava (**B**). Ureteral implantation using the Lich extravesical ureteroneocystostomy is preferred.

should be maintained at 7 to 10 cm H_2O to ensure adequate intravascular volume. In patients with high-output renal failure, urine losses from both the native and transplant kidneys need to be replaced to avoid hypoperfusion and thrombosis. Maintenance of catheter patency is essential. Any episode of decreased urinary output should be rapidly investigated to exclude urinary catheter occlusion and bladder distention. An algorithm for the evaluation of early postoperative oliguria is shown in Figure 45-15.

Technical Complications

Vascular thrombosis still accounts for graft loss in up to 13% of initial transplants and 19% of repeat transplants in children. Graft thrombosis is significantly more frequent in children younger than 2 years of age and is directly related to the age of both the donor and the recipient. In addition, prolonged cold ischemic preservation time (>24 hours) and the related presence of ATN with delayed graft function also increase this risk. Prior transplantation and more than five pretransplant blood transfusions have also been shown to be independent risk factors. Immediate post-transplant Doppler ultrasound vascular imaging is helpful in confirming suitable allograft blood flow after abdominal closure, especially when large allografts are implanted into small recipients. Adequate hydration is important to maintain suitable perfusion. Anticoagulation has not been used in most series.

Urinary leak, most often at the neocystostomy site, presents as oliguria and persisting uremia. Ultrasound or nuclear imaging can be used to identify an extravesical fluid collection. Direct operative repair is necessary to prevent urinoma formation and its potential infectious complications. Urinary collections must be differentiated from lymphoceles at the transplant site. Unresolving lymphoceles are best opened into the peritoneal cavity using laparoscopy.

Hypertension

Hypertension after renal transplantation is common. One month after transplantation, 72% of patients require treatment, although this percentage decreases to 53% at 30 months. Careful attention to the pretransplant control of hypertension and dietary management improves post-transplant control. Hypertension presents a significant risk to possible renal function when using small allografts. Hypertension in the early postoperative period is most often due to fluid overload or acute rejection, but it can also originate from the native kidneys.

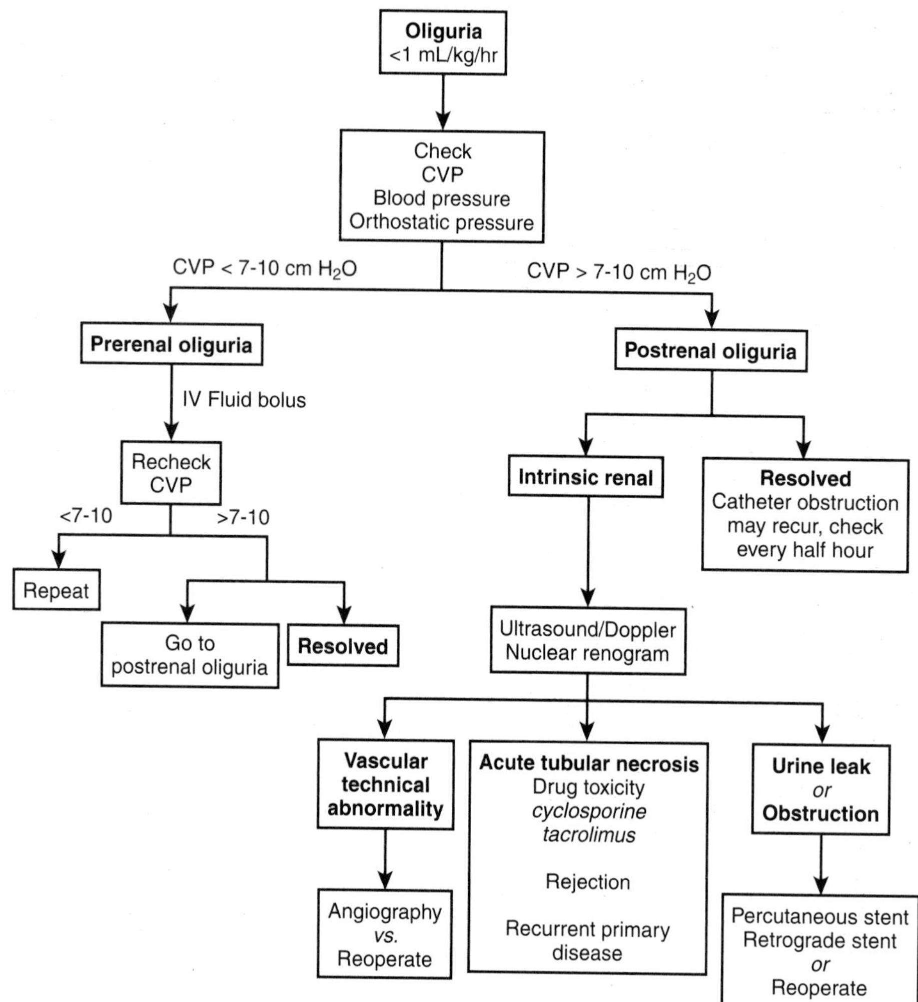

Figure 45-15. Algorithm for the evaluation of early postoperative oliguria after pediatric renal transplant. CVP, central venous pressure.

Preexisting hypertension is augmented by the immunosuppressive drugs cyclosporine, tacrolimus, and prednisone. The development of hypertension more than 3 months after transplantation suggests possible renal artery stenosis and warrants Doppler ultrasound flow studies for initial evaluation. Arteriography is needed in questionable cases. Transluminal angioplasty has been successful in managing the majority of these cases when recognized. Surgical correction is reserved for angioplasty failures and vessels with a complex arterial anastomosis.

Infection

Most long-term complications are related to infection and occur within the first 6 post-transplant months. During this time, immunosuppression is intense and susceptibility to life-threatening infection is increased. The frequent use of organs from donors who have had prior exposure to CMV and EBV in infants and children who are seronegative enhances the risk of these specific infections. Expanded use of antiviral prophylaxis using ganciclovir and acyclovir has decreased the intensity of these infections and their associated morbidity or mortality. Trimethoprim-sulfamethoxazole is used for *Pneumocystis jiroveci* pneumonia prophylaxis as well.

Immunosuppression

Many immunosuppressive regimens are available, and all share similar strategy. Most regimens include corticosteroids, cyclosporine or tacrolimus, and azathioprine or mycophenolate. Polyclonal or monoclonal antilymphocyte antibodies are used when ATN is anticipated or for retransplantation in highly presensitized patients. Significant efforts to decrease or discontinue corticosteroids have been attempted to enhance growth and development. At 4 years after transplantation, 31% of LD and 23% of CD recipients were receiving alternate-day prednisone.[153]

Overall, there has been a decrease in the frequency of acute rejection, with 12-month probabilities in LD recipients of 32% and CD recipients of 36%. The risk of rejection is similar for LD and CD recipients in the first few post-transplant weeks. Factors that increase the likelihood of rejection or long-term graft loss include receiving a graft from a CD rather than a related LD, receiving a graft from a donor younger than 5 years of age, having the graft in cold storage for more than 24 hours, being an African-American recipient, and delayed graft function from ATN.[153] The ability to treat rejection has also improved with complete reversal of acute rejection in 65% of episodes. The rate of success in treating rejection declines with each successive rejection episode, increased recipient age, and late rejection episodes.[153] Most rejection episodes can be treated with corticosteroid administration alone (78%). Monoclonal anti–T-cell agents such as OKT-3 are needed in 32%. In patients who remain rejection free for the first post-transplant year, the risk of rejection in the following year is 20%.[155]

Results

The overall results of renal transplantation in children are steadily improving. Overall 1-year transplant graft survival rates of 88% to 100% have been reported for LD allografts, with results for CD allografts being 50% to 72%.[152,165-168] In the 2008 NAPRTCS report, 1-, 3-, and 5-year graft survival rates were as follows: CD, 93%, 84%, and 77%; LD, 95%, 91%, and 85%, respectively (Fig. 45-16).

Chronic rejection has become the most common cause of graft failure, accounting for 27% of all graft losses. With improved immunosuppressive treatments, acute rejection accounts for only 15% of failures. Recurrence of the original disease caused graft failure in 6%, and vascular thrombosis accounted for 12% of graft failures. Long-term graft survival after pediatric renal transplantation continues to deteriorate after 10 years despite low patient mortality rates. Death of the recipient with a functioning graft is an uncommon problem. When this occurs, death results primarily from infection (40%) or cardiovascular causes (21%). Young recipients (birth to 1 year of age) and patients with early graft failure are at the highest

GRAFT SURVIVAL BY ALLOGRAFT SOURCE AND TRANSPLANT YEAR

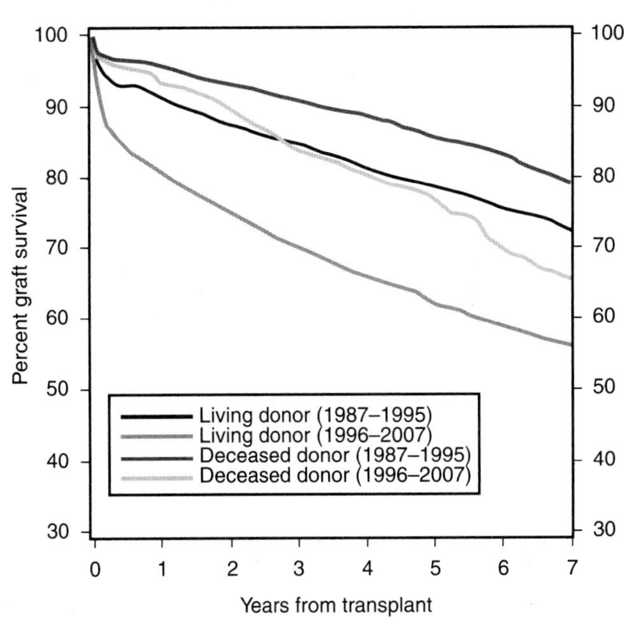

	Years post transplant							
	Year 1		Year 3		Year 5		Year 7	
	%	SE	%	SE	%	SE	%	SE
Living donor (1987–1995)	91.2	0.59	84.6	0.76	78.9	0.89	72.2	1.05
Living donor (1996–2007)	95.3	0.41	90.9	0.62	85.4	0.91	78.9	1.40
Deceased donor (1987–1995)	80.7	0.81	70.5	0.96	62.4	1.06	56.2	1.16
Deceased donor (1996–2007)	93.4	0.57	83.8	0.99	77.3	1.31	65.3	2.05

Figure 45-16. Renal allograft survival over 5 years from a living donor compared with a cadaveric donor. (From 2008 North American Pediatric Renal Transplant Cooperative Study Report.)

risk. Progressive loss of renal function may be secondary to complications of hypertension, hyperfiltration, hypercholesterolemias, chronic indolent immunologic damage leading to chronic rejection, and progressive primary renal disease. All of these contribute to long-term graft loss.[154,168] Methods to circumvent this progressive graft loss will greatly improve the long-term prognosis.

The overall half-life of pediatric renal transplants is about 25 years for LD grafts and 16 years for CD grafts. Many recipients require second transplants in their lifetime. Overall graft survival for second transplants using LDs was equivalent to primary CD allografts. The factor exerting negative influence on survival in CD grafts was donor age younger than 6 years. Better donor-recipient matching has improved graft survival. The rapidity of first allograft loss, immunologic protocol at retransplant, and race of recipient are not significant factors. Thus, use of cadaveric kidneys from young donors for these procedures is not recommended.

PANCREAS TRANSPLANTATION

Children have rarely been candidates for pancreas transplantation. In the past, the results after pancreas transplantation have not justified the risks associated with immunosuppression and operation. However, recent improvements in the operative procedure and follow-up have occurred. Overall 1-year patient survival rate exceeds 90%, and graft survival with complete insulin independence exceeds 70% in patients in whom combined kidney and pancreas transplantation is undertaken. The survival rate is approximately 50% in isolated pancreas transplantation.[169,170]

The addition of pancreas transplantation with kidney replacement for diabetic nephropathy does not subject the patient to additional immunosuppressive risks, and it is better accepted. The use of isolated pancreas transplantation is reserved for patients who have extremely labile glucose control or experience hypoglycemic unawareness syndrome.[169] As the results of this procedure improve in the future, the role of this operation in children will need to be reviewed.

Pancreatic islet transplantation has also become possible in children. However, its role in the treatment of juvenile diabetes in childhood is still limited. This procedure has been undertaken in children after pancreatic resection when the cellular autotransplant does not require immunosuppressive treatment. Results have been excellent. Further expansion of this treatment option awaits firm documentation that hypoglycemic correction retards the systemic complications of diabetes.

chapter 46

LESIONS OF THE PANCREAS

Marcus M. Malek, MD • George K. Gittes, MD

ANATOMY AND EMBRYOLOGY

The pancreas originates in week 4 of gestation as paired evaginations of the foregut.[1] The dorsal pancreatic bud gives rise to the body and tail of the pancreas, the minor duct (Santorini) and minor papilla, and the continuation of the main duct (Wirsung) into the body and tail. The dorsal pancreas arises as a diverticulum from the dorsal aspect of the duodenal anlage. The ventral pancreatic bud arises from the biliary diverticulum and swings around the dorsal aspect of the duodenal anlage during gut rotation to give rise to the head of the pancreas, as well as the proximal portion of the main pancreatic duct (Fig. 46-1).

The two pancreatic buds fuse to form one pancreas at approximately 7 weeks' gestation, although it appears that complete fusion of the two ducts to form the main pancreatic duct is delayed until the perinatal period.[2] The endocrine component of the pancreas, the islets of Langerhans, starts to differentiate before evagination of the pancreatic buds from the wall of the foregut.[3] The islets make up 10% of the pancreas during early embryonic and fetal life, but that figure decreases to less than 1% in the adult. Fetal pancreatic islets appear to play an important role in fetal homeostasis. Pancreatic acini begin to form at 12 weeks and begin to accumulate organelles and zymogen granules characteristic of acinar cells. These cells do not secrete appreciable amounts of enzyme until the time of birth.[1]

The pancreas is retroperitoneal and is light pink in children. The acini can be seen with low-power loupe magnification, as can the septa dividing the lobulations. The head of the pancreas lies in the C-loop of the duodenum while the uncinate process, emanating from the posteromedial portion of the head, projects under the superior mesenteric artery and vein. The neck of the pancreas is defined as that portion of the pancreas anterior to these vessels.[4] The body and

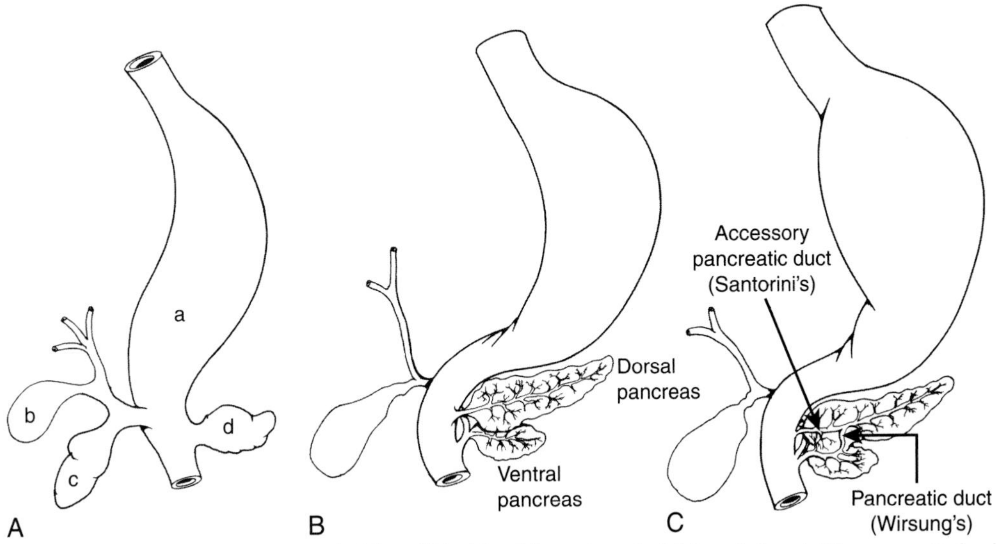

Figure 46-1. Pancreatic embryology. **A,** Stomach (a), gallbladder (b), and ventral (c) and dorsal (d) pancreatic buds develop separately at embryologic week 4. The pancreas develops as an evagination of the developing foregut. The dorsal bud evaginates directly off of the duodenal anlage. **B,** The ventral bud evaginates from the biliary bud and then swings around to the left, with gut rotation occurring simultaneously. **C,** The main pancreatic duct of Wirsung and the minor accessory duct of Santorini are shown.

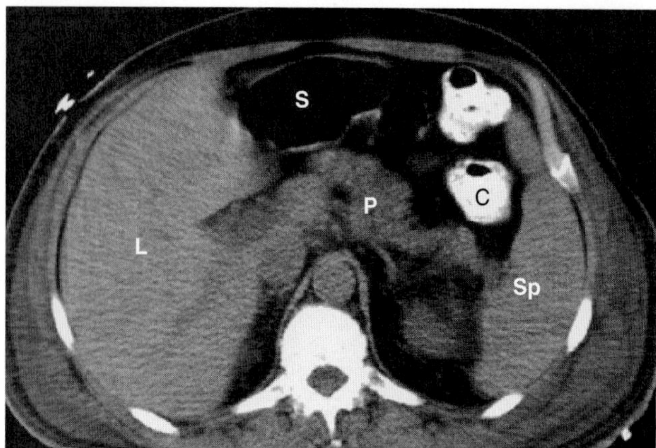

Figure 46-2. CT scan showing the cross-sectional anatomy of the pancreas. The pancreas (P) lies convexly across the lumbar spine with the tail of the pancreas next to the spleen (Sp) and the hilum of the left kidney. The head of the pancreas lies to the right of the spine near the hilum of the right kidney. L, Liver; S, stomach; C, colon. (From Maher MM, Hahn PF, Gervais DA, et al: Portable abdominal CT: Analysis of quality and clinical impact in more than 100 consecutive cases. AJR Am J Roentgenol 183:663-670, 2004.)

tail, to the left of these vessels, angle sharply upward toward the hilum of the spleen. The main pancreatic duct runs along the posterior aspect of the gland and curves downward in the head to run alongside the common bile duct, which runs in a groove posterior to the pancreas or within the substance of the posterior gland. The main pancreatic duct and common bile duct may fuse to form a "common channel" before entry into the duodenum.

The pancreas is quite convex, with its midportion being reflected over the anterior surface of the upper lumbar vertebrae and aorta and the lateral portions falling posteriorly toward each kidney (Fig. 46-2). The arterial supply of the pancreas is from the celiac and superior mesenteric arteries, which form the pancreaticoduodenal arcade. The pancreas also has anastomoses from the splenic artery.

CONGENITAL ANOMALIES

Ectopic pancreatic rests are frequently encountered along foregut derivatives, such as the stomach and the duodenum, as well as along the jejunum, ileum, and colon.[5] These lesions are found in approximately 2% of autopsy series and represent the most common anomaly of the gastric antrum. Moreover, they may cause gastric outlet obstruction.[6] Their origin is unknown, but one possible explanation is aberrant epithelial-mesenchymal interactions, leading to the transdifferentiation of heterotopic embryonic epithelium into pancreatic epithelium. Some recent studies have implicated defects in "hedgehog" signaling, which may antagonize normal pancreatic development, as the cause of the formation of ectopic pancreatic tissue.[7,8] Ectopic rests are typically asymptomatic and are encountered incidentally at laparotomy. They can be identified as pancreatic tissue because the surface has the same granular acinar appearance as the normal pancreas. These ectopic pancreatic rests usually do not become inflamed, possibly because they contain numerous small drainage ducts rather than a large single duct, which might become obstructed more easily. Occasionally, an ectopic pancreatic rest produces obstruction or bleeding. When encountered at laparotomy, ectopic rests should probably be excised unless the excision would entail significant risk of morbidity.

Annular pancreas is thought to result from faulty rotation of the ventral pancreatic bud in its course around the posterior aspect of the duodenal anlage. The duodenum is encircled and often obstructed by normal pancreatic tissue containing normal-functioning acini, ducts, and islets of Langerhans.[9,10] The prevailing theory of pathogenesis is that half of the ventral bud migrates anteriorly and half migrates posteriorly. Abnormal endodermal expression patterns of Sonic hedgehog (Shh) and Indian hedgehog, potent intercellular signaling proteins that demarcate a molecular boundary between the pancreas and the adjacent gastrointestinal tract, may be responsible for the formation of annular pancreas.[7,8] The ductal drainage of this system is variable and complex. Duodenal atresia and stenosis, intestinal malrotation, and trisomy 21 can often be found in combination with annular pancreas.[11] The clinical significance relates primarily to duodenal obstruction, typically with bilious vomiting. Radiographic studies may reveal the classic finding of a "double-bubble" sign.[12] Management consists of surgical bypass of the obstructing lesion with a duodenoduodenostomy. If such a bypass is not technically feasible, a duodenojejunostomy can be performed. Resection or division of the annular pancreas should not be done.

Cystic fibrosis is an autosomal recessive condition, seen primarily in the white population, and is found in about 1 in 2500 live births.[13] It is caused by mutations in the cystic fibrosis transmembrane conductance regulator (*CFTR*) gene that encodes a protein expressed in the apical membrane of exocrine epithelial cells. Cystic fibrosis leads to significant pancreatic insufficiency. The pancreatic secretions generally have a reduced amount of bicarbonate, a lower pH, and a lower overall exocrine fluid volume. The inspissated secretions lead to blockage of the ducts, with subsequent duct dilatation and obstruction of pancreatic exocrine flow. The acinar cells degenerate, leading to pancreatic fibrosis. The result is impaired digestion of fats and proteins.[14]

PANCREATITIS

Acute Pancreatitis

Acute pancreatitis is an acute inflammation of the pancreas, varying in severity from mild abdominal pain that may go undiagnosed to fulminant necrotizing pancreatitis and death. Episodes of acute inflammation may completely resolve and then recur. In such cases the term *acute relapsing pancreatitis* is applied to the clinical course. It is thought that complete interval resolution of morphology and function occurs as opposed to the occurrence of irreversible changes in the pancreas in cases of chronic pancreatitis.

The causes of acute pancreatitis include trauma, biliary tract stone disease, choledochal cyst, ductal developmental anomalies, drugs, metabolic derangements, and infections. Most commonly the cause is not apparent and it is termed *idiopathic.*

Because the pancreas is fixed against the lumbar spine, trauma to the upper abdomen (classically a bicycle handlebar) fractures the pancreas or injures the major duct at that point (Fig. 46-3). Biliary stone disease, as in adults, may lead to pancreatitis from transient pancreatic duct obstruction, with or without bile reflux. Choledochal cysts produce pancreatitis by pancreatic duct compression or bile reflux resulting from a long common biliary-pancreatic duct within the head of the pancreas.

Pancreas divisum is an anomaly present in 10% of the population and is thought to result from failure of the dorsal duct to fuse with the ventral duct. In pancreas divisum, the majority of the exocrine secretions of the pancreas, including those from the entire body and tail, must drain through the small minor duct of Santorini into the duodenum. The resulting relative obstruction may cause recurring episodes of pancreatitis.[15] These symptomatic patients should undergo a sphincteroplasty of the minor papilla. Endoscopic stenting with or without sphincterotomy has been described but requires particular skill with the endoscope cannulating the small ducts encountered in children.[16] Other rare ductal anomalies may result in obstruction and recurring bouts of pancreatitis. Biliary tract stones are not as common in children, but when present they may lead to pancreatitis. Data extrapolated from the adult literature indicate that removal of impacted stones in gallstone pancreatitis in children should be performed endoscopically.[17,18] Choledochal cysts may produce pancreatitis from transient pancreatic duct compression or from bile reflux. Drugs that are thought to induce pancreatitis include asparaginase and valproic acid.[19,20] Systemic illnesses and metabolic conditions, such as cystic fibrosis with inspissation of pancreatic secretions in the ducts, Reye syndrome, Kawasaki disease, hyperlipidemias, and hypercalcemia, may cause pancreatitis. Infections with viruses (e.g., coxsackievirus and rotavirus) and generalized bacterial sepsis also can cause pancreatitis.[21]

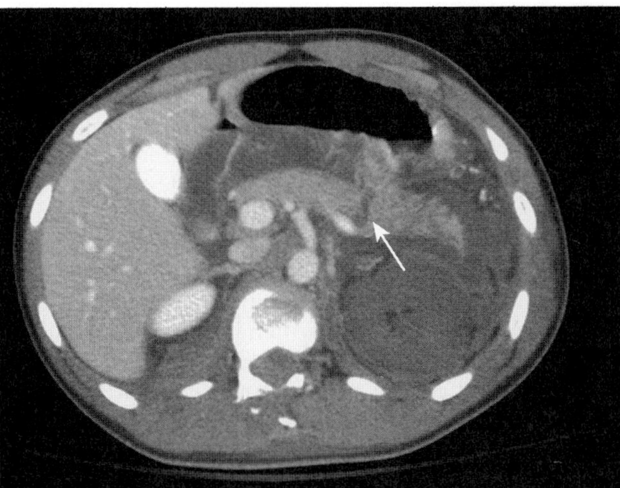

Figure 46-3. A teenager sustained blunt trauma to his epigastrium and was found to have complete transection of his pancreas (*arrow*). He underwent distal pancreatectomy and has recovered uneventfully.

Clearly, the pathogenesis of acute pancreatitis entails the inappropriate activation of proenzymes, leading to autodigestion of the pancreas. The cellular mechanisms leading to acute pancreatitis are not known, but they are the subject of intense scientific investigation. Pancreatic enzymes can cause destruction at distant sites either by vascular dissemination or by release from the pancreas of cytokines such as tumor necrosis factor-α, free radicals such as superoxide, and vasoactive substances such as histamine and kallikrein.

The mechanism by which inappropriate activation of pancreatic enzymes occurs is not known. Possibilities include (1) reflux of duodenal enterokinase into the pancreas to activate trypsin, which then inappropriately activates other proenzymes in the pancreas; (2) ductal obstruction with extravasation of enzyme-rich ductal fluid into the parenchyma of the pancreas; or (3) fusion of lysosomes with zymogen granules inside acinar cells to allow lysosomal enzyme activation of the proenzymes. Once activated, elastase, phospholipase, and superoxide free radicals are thought to be the principal mediators of tissue damage.

Acute pancreatitis usually is initially seen with the sudden onset of midepigastric pain associated with back pain, severe vomiting, and low-grade fever.[22,23] The abdomen is diffusely tender with signs of peritonitis, and distention occurs with a paucity of bowel sounds. In severe cases of necrotizing or hemorrhagic pancreatitis, hemorrhage may dissect from the pancreas along tissue planes, appearing as ecchymosis either in the flanks (Grey Turner's sign) or at the umbilicus (Cullen's sign) (Fig. 46-4). These ecchymoses typically take 1 to 2 days to develop.

Elevated amylase levels are helpful in the diagnosis, although normal serum amylase levels do not exclude pancreatitis from the differential diagnostic possibilities. The degree of serum amylase elevation does not correlate with severity of the disease. Amylase is excreted in the urine, but, as is true with glucose, tubular reabsorption results in amylase levels in the urine only after significant hyperamylasemia occurs.[24] In addition, the half-life of amylase is approximately 10 hours. Thus, moderately elevated levels of serum amylase may not be detectable in the urine.

Hyperamylasemia or hyperamylasuria may be caused by conditions other than pancreatitis, most notably salivary inflammation or trauma; intestinal disease including perforation, ischemia, necrosis, or inflammation; renal failure; and macroamylasemia. Alterations in renal excretion are accounted for by

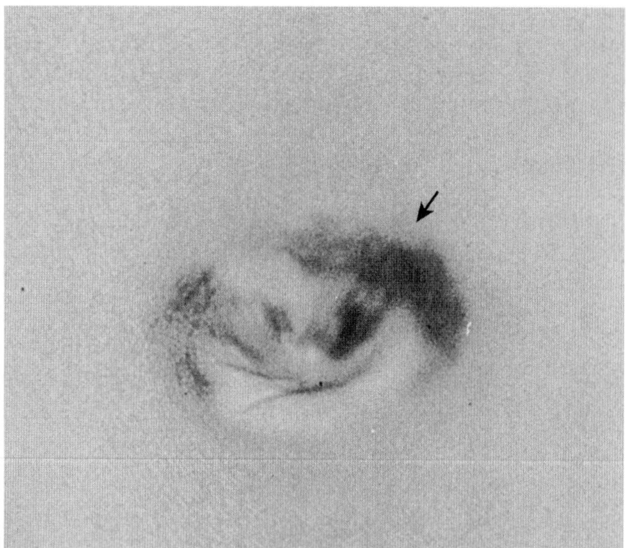

Figure 46-4. Positive Cullen's sign, with periumbilical ecchymosis (*arrow*), in a patient with hemorrhagic pancreatitis.

measuring the ratio of the clearance of amylase to that of creatinine. The ratio requires measurement of simultaneous spot levels of serum amylase and creatinine and urine amylase and creatinine:

$$(U_{amy}/Serum_{amy})(Serum_{Cr}/Urine_{Cr}).$$

Ratios greater than 0.03 are significant. Lipase levels have been proposed as a more specific test of pancreatic tissue damage, although intestinal perforation does cause an elevation of lipase through reabsorption via the peritoneum. Lipase is produced only in the pancreas, and its measurement is particularly helpful for distinguishing pancreatic trauma from salivary trauma.[25]

Imaging the abdomen is important as part of the evaluation of the patient with abdominal pain. In the patient with pancreatitis, plain abdominal radiographs may reveal an isolated loop of intestine in the vicinity of the inflamed pancreas, the so-called sentinel loop. Other findings suggesting pancreatitis include local spasm of the transverse colon with proximal dilation, known as the colon cut-off sign. Pancreatic calcifications suggest chronic pancreatitis. Plain chest radiographs should be performed in all patients with acute pancreatitis to look for evidence of pleural effusion and pulmonary edema.

Abdominal ultrasonography may show a decrease in echogenicity of the pancreas due to pancreatic edema, but such a finding is not reliable in determining the diagnosis or severity.[26] The main utility of ultrasonography is to demonstrate gallstones as a possible cause of pancreatitis and to look for improvement in edema or peripancreatic fluid collections. Abdominal computed tomography (CT) offers much better resolution than ultrasonography in determining the size of the pancreas, the degree of edema, and the presence of fluid collections.[27] The size of the pancreatic duct can often be estimated much more accurately with CT than with ultrasonography, and the presence of complications such as pancreatic abscess or pseudocyst may be delineated. The use of dynamic CT pancreatography has been advocated because of its ability to differentiate perfused from nonperfused (necrotic) pancreas. By using a bolus of contrast with rapid scanning in fine cuts through the pancreas, a precise assessment of the percentage of the pancreas that is either underperfused or nonperfused can be made. If necessary, CT can also be used for interventional procedures for diagnosis or drainage of fluid collections. Endoscopic retrograde cholangiopancreatography (ERCP) may also be used in children with acute pancreatitis. The literature would suggest that the complication rates in children are higher than those in the adult patient population.[28] However, it may be potentially helpful in children with severe refractory biliary pancreatitis who may have a stone impacted in the ampulla, as well as in trauma patients in whom a ductal injury is suspected or a pancreatic pseudocyst has formed. Magnetic resonance cholangiopancreatography (MRCP) is a relatively new, noninvasive technique for evaluating the biliary tree and the pancreatic duct. This technique is particularly attractive because the procedure is noninvasive and spares the patient the potential complications of ERCP. In addition, the study is less expensive and does not require radiation or contrast administration, which are routinely needed with ERCP. One disadvantage of MRCP is that it does not allow therapeutic interventions. However, it may help direct the type of therapeutic intervention best suited to the patient's pathologic process.[29] Another problem is that MRCP tends to overestimate the stenosis of the main pancreatic duct in patients with pancreatitis. Regardless, MRCP is now the initial imaging study of choice in the evaluation of pancreatic ductal anatomy in children with unexplained or recurrent pancreatitis.[16]

Key features in treating patients with acute pancreatitis are aggressive fluid replacement to maintain a good urine output (2 mL/kg/hr), usually measured with the aid of an indwelling urinary catheter, and a very low threshold for transferring the patient to an intensive care unit.[30,31]

Acute pancreatitis causes diffuse tissue damage throughout the body as a result of the release of active mediators, including phospholipase A_2, elastase, histamines, kinins, kallikreins, and prostaglandins. Extracellular fluid losses can be enormous. Constant monitoring is necessary to avoid the development of severe hypovolemia. Patients with acute pancreatitis should be kept at bowel rest with nasogastric suction. Most patients receive histamine-2 (H_2) receptor antagonists to prevent exposure of the duodenal secretin-producing cells to gastric acid, which is a potent stimulator of pancreatic secretion. These antagonists also may help prevent the stress ulceration seen in patients with pancreatitis. This therapeutic regimen is logical but empirical, because no studies have shown improvement in outcome with these interventions. Clinical trials have, however, shown an improved outcome in acute pancreatitis by using long-acting somatostatin analogs. It is probably reasonable to use these analogs in moderate-to-severe cases of pancreatitis.[32]

Adequate analgesia is critical to minimize the additional stress from pain. Meperidine (Demerol) is thought to be a better analgesic in pancreatitis because morphine causes spasm of the sphincter of Oddi. In turn, this sphincter spasm increases pancreatic duct pressure and potentially worsens the pancreatitis. To date, the superiority of meperidine over morphine in acute pancreatitis has not been proved in an outcome-based comparison. In fact, morphine may actually provide a longer period of analgesia with a lower seizure risk.[33] An important caveat is that the diagnosis of pancreatitis must be certain before giving the patient significant doses of narcotics because the ability to diagnose serious nonpancreatic problems, such as intestinal ischemia or perforated ulcer, may be lost.

As cases of severe pancreatitis progress, patients need to be monitored closely for signs of the development of multisystem organ failure. Pleural effusions and pulmonary edema can progress to severe adult respiratory distress syndrome with hypoxia, requiring endotracheal intubation. The tense abdominal distention associated with pancreatitis frequently contributes to the hypoventilation. Hypocalcemia, hypomagnesemia, anemia from hemorrhage, hyperglycemia, renal failure, and late sepsis can be seen in these patients and require close monitoring. Disagreement exists concerning the use of prophylactic antibiotics. In general, mild or moderate cases probably do not benefit from antibiotics. More severe cases of pancreatitis, however, may benefit because of the high rate of sepsis, although confirmatory data in such patients are lacking. Some advantage has been demonstrated with the use of imipenem, with reduction in the incidence of pancreatic sepsis in patients with necrotizing pancreatitis.[17]

Nutrition is critically important in patients with pancreatitis. An early positive nitrogen balance has been shown to improve survival rates. This need for aggressive nutrition should come in the form of early parenteral hyperalimentation. The hyperalimentation should include lipid formulations, despite the known association of hyperlipidemia and pancreatitis, although a close monitoring of the serum lipid levels should be maintained to avoid triglyceride levels greater than 500 mg/dL. In general, the resumption of enteral nutrition should be cautious, usually after complete resolution of the abdominal pain and preferably after normalization of the serum enzyme levels.

Surgical intervention in acute pancreatitis is usually not necessary. Other than surgery for pancreatic pseudocyst or papillotomy in the case of pancreas divisum, surgical intervention for acute pancreatitis is restricted to patients with severe necrotizing pancreatitis needing debridement or to patients with a pancreatic abscess.[34,35] In some instances, pancreatitis is discovered when laparotomy or laparoscopy is performed for a preoperative diagnosis of appendicitis (Fig. 46-5). In this circumstance, the best course is to palpate the gallbladder for stones. If the pancreatitis is mild and gallstones are present, cholecystectomy is reasonable. If the pancreatitis is severe, the safer course may be to perform a cholecystostomy, which allows later access to the biliary stones. If no gallstones are present, but the patient has severe necrotizing pancreatitis, limited debridement is acceptable. Also, simply leaving large sump drains in place may be adequate. Early pancreatic lavage, pancreatic drainage, and pancreatic resection have not been shown to improve survival rates in cases of severe pancreatitis.

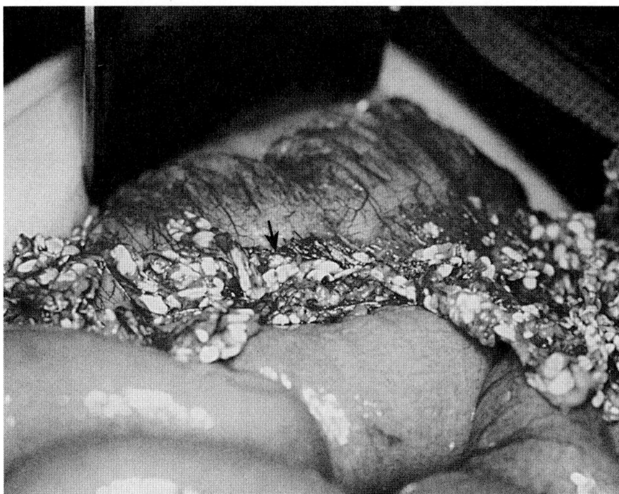

Figure 46-5. Severe peritoneal and omental fat saponification, seen as white fatty deposits (*arrow*) in a patient with acute pancreatitis. The preoperative diagnosis was acute appendicitis.

A pancreatic abscess may result from infection of the necrotic pancreatic tissue or infection of a peripancreatic fluid collection. Pancreatic abscess increases the mortality from pancreatitis threefold and is an absolute indication for surgical therapy.[36,37] Differentiating a pancreatic abscess from an uninfected pancreatic fluid collection is important because pancreatitis itself can make the patient appear "septic." The diagnosis of pancreatic abscess is established by Gram stain and culture of the suspected abscess by CT-guided needle aspiration. The indication for aspiration is fever and leukocytosis persisting more than 7 to 10 days after onset of the pancreatitis. Patients shown to have pancreatic necrosis by dynamic CT pancreatography are candidates for aspiration because pancreatic necrosis usually precedes the development of a pancreatic abscess. The surgical therapy for a pancreatic abscess is debridement of clearly necrotic tissue and placement of large sump suction drains. Some mechanism must be in place for ongoing removal of the infected material postoperatively, either by reoperation or by the sump drains. In some cases it is impossible to differentiate an infected pancreatic pseudocyst from an abscess. In this case, a laparotomy or laparoscopy should be performed with sump drainage of the fluid collection.

Pancreatic pseudocyst is a complication of trauma or pancreatitis that entailed damage to the pancreatic ductal system. The extravasated pancreatic enzymes and digested tissue are contained by the formation of a cavity composed of fibroblastic reaction and inflammation, but without an epithelial lining. Pseudocysts may be acute or chronic. The acute pseudocyst has an irregular wall on CT scan, is tender, and usually develops shortly after an episode of acute

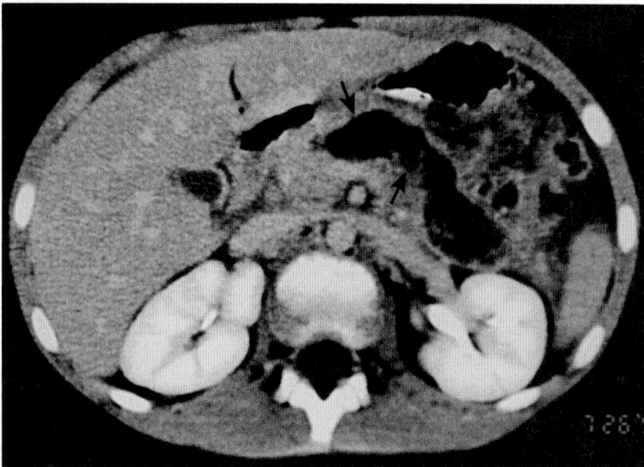

Figure 46-6. CT scan of an acute pseudocyst in a patient after a severe motor vehicle accident. The wall (*arrows*) is irregular with nonloculated fluid inside.

pancreatitis or trauma (Fig. 46-6). Chronic pseudocysts are usually spherical with a thick wall and are commonly seen in patients with chronic pancreatitis. The distinction between these two types of pseudocysts is important because 50% of acute pseudocysts resolve without therapy, whereas chronic pseudocysts rarely spontaneously resolve. An acute pseudocyst develops a thick fibrous wall in 4 to 6 weeks. Pseudocysts smaller than 5 cm in diameter usually disappear without intervention. When compared with those in adults, pseudocysts in children tend to resolve more frequently with medical therapy alone.[38] Some evidence exists that somatostatin may help resolve pancreatic pseudocysts in children.[39]

Pancreatic pseudocysts that persist require either internal drainage (preferred), excision (distal pseudocysts only), or external drainage (infected or immature cysts). A minimally invasive approach to cystogastrostomy has been described in which intragastric laparoscopic ports were used.[40] Other minimally invasive strategies for pancreatic pseudocysts include transesophageal endoscopic cystogastrostomy and percutaneous drainage.[41] These endoscopic procedures should be performed at institutions with significant experience with these techniques.[42,43] Percutaneous drainage is the treatment of choice for infected pseudocysts because these cysts typically have thin, weak walls that are not amenable to internal drainage.

The three major complications of pancreatic pseudocysts are hemorrhage, rupture, and infection. Hemorrhage is the most serious complication and usually results from pressure and erosion of the cyst into a nearby visceral vessel (e.g., splenic, gastroduodenal). These patients require emergency angiography with embolization. Rupture or infection of a pseudocyst is uncommon. In both cases, external drainage is indicated.

Pancreatic ascites in children usually follows trauma or pancreatic surgery.[44] These patients may be seen with ascites or with pancreatic pleural effusions. Free fluid results from the uncontained leakage of a major pancreatic duct. Treatment initially consists of bowel rest with hyperalimentation and use of long-acting somatostatin analogs. In many cases, ascites resolves spontaneously with this treatment. If not, ERCP or MRCP should be performed to determine the site of the ductal injury.[45] For distal duct injuries, simple distal resection is adequate, but proximal duct injury requires Roux-en-Y jejunal onlay anastomosis to preserve an adequate amount of pancreatic tissue.

Pancreatic fistula is a postoperative complication. Most low-output fistulas close spontaneously but may drain for several months. Long-acting somatostatin analogs decrease the fistula output and accelerate the rate of closure, but they do not appear to induce closure of fistulas that would not have otherwise closed. Managing a pancreatic fistula centers around (1) maintaining adequate nutrition, with hyperalimentation if enteral feeding results in high-volume output, and (2) making sure the fistula tract does not become obstructed. In fistulas that do not close, surgical intervention with a Roux-en-Y jejunostomy to the leak point is recommended.[46]

Chronic Pancreatitis

Chronic pancreatitis is distinguished from acute pancreatitis by the irreversibility of the changes associated with the inflammation.[47] Chronic pancreatitis is either calcifying or obstructive. The calcifying form, most commonly caused by hereditary pancreatitis, is more common than the obstructive form in children and is associated with intraductal pancreatic stones, pseudocysts, and a more aggressive scar formation with more significant damage (Fig. 46-7). The obstructive type of chronic pancreatitis, which is associated with anatomic obstructions (most commonly pancreas divisum), is generally less severe with less scar formation than calcifying pancreatitis. The pancreatic architecture in the obstructive type may be partially reversible with correction of the obstruction.[48]

Chronic pancreatitis is distinctly uncommon in children. The most common cause in North America is hereditary or familial pancreatitis.[49] The inheritance is autosomal dominant with incomplete penetrance. The genetic mutations responsible for hereditary pancreatitis have been isolated to chromosome 7q35. The majority of these patients express one of two mutations in the cationic trypsinogen (*PRSS1*) gene. It has been suggested that these mutations lead to an alteration in the trypsin recognition site that prevents deactivation of trypsin within the pancreas. Autodigestion occurs, resulting in pancreatitis. In certain cases of idiopathic pancreatitis, it may be worthwhile to perform genetic screening for the cationic trypsinogen gene mutation.[50,51] The clinical presentation is typically one of recurrent attacks resembling acute pancreatitis. Familial pancreatitis has no distinguishing characteristics other than pancreatic calcification and its occurrence in other family members. These patients typically begin to have symptoms at about age 10 years, and pancreatic insufficiency, both exocrine and endocrine, slowly develops. Other complications include diabetes mellitus, ascites with pleural effusion, portal

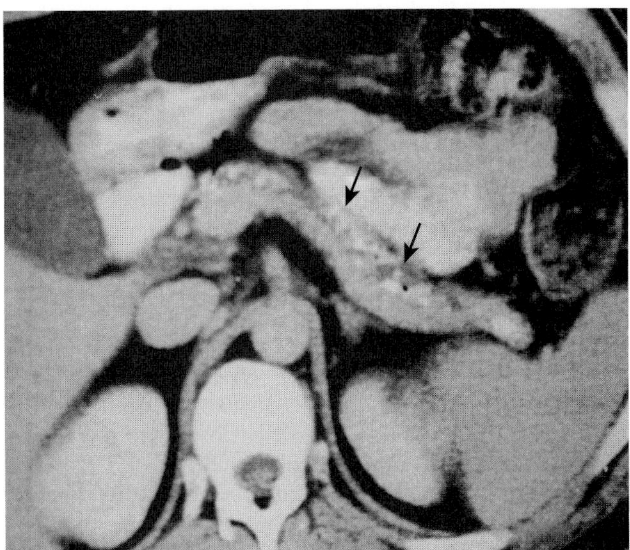

Figure 46-7. CT scan of a pancreas with chronic calcifying pancreatitis. A dilated duct can be seen within the pancreas, further supporting the diagnosis of chronic pancreatitis. Calcified stones (*arrows*) can be seen in the dilated duct.

hypertension, dilatation of the pancreatic ducts, and thrombosis of the portal and splenic vein.[17] Pseudocysts tend to occur more often in patients with hereditary pancreatitis. Such patients have a 40% lifetime risk of developing adenocarcinoma of the pancreas.[51]

In some patients with familial pancreatitis who have severe, intractable pain, ERCP or MRCP may help locate surgically correctable lesions, such as large stones or a stricture with distal ductal dilation. Surgical options in this form of pancreatitis include excision of the localized pancreatitis, subtotal pancreatectomy, lateral pancreaticojejunostomy (modified Puestow procedure), and sphincteroplasty. Although the results of surgical therapy in these patients are generally disappointing, evidence exists that complicated cases of hereditary pancreatitis treated with a modified Puestow procedure may experience an improved quality of life, with subsequent improvement in pancreatic function and nutritional status (Fig. 46-8). Unlike adults with hereditary pancreatitis, some reversal of the steatorrhea may be seen in children.[52]

Obstructive pancreatitis due to pancreas divisum or choledochal cyst is best treated by relieving the obstruction. The association between pancreas divisum and chronic pancreatitis remains controversial. Some patients with ductal dilation clearly improve with sphincterotomy or sphincteroplasty. Other cases may be difficult to diagnose, and functional tests of duct pressure after secretin stimulation have been suggested. Surgical results in patients with functional obstruction are often not satisfying.

The diagnosis of chronic pancreatitis does not depend on amylase or lipase determination. Even though mild serum enzyme elevations are commonly seen during an exacerbation, they are inconsistent and frequently are normal. The diagnosis of chronic pancreatitis relies on a characteristic pain, diminished pancreatic function, and changes in radiographic appearance. Increased stool fat, diabetes mellitus, and steatorrhea are signs of pancreatic insufficiency. Frequently on CT scan the pancreas has microcalcifications throughout the parenchyma and calcified stones in the duct (see Fig. 46-7). Additionally, pancreatic pseudocysts or inflammation may be seen on CT scan. ERCP offers the best view of ductal anatomy and can confirm the diagnosis of pancreas divisum as a probable cause of chronic pancreatitis. MRCP provides a less invasive alternative to better define the pancreatic ductal anatomy.[29] Papillotomy may be accomplished endoscopically as well.

Therapy for chronic pancreatitis is directed toward palliation of symptoms. Initial therapy for acute exacerbation is pain control and hydration. Steatorrhea indicates the need for pancreatic enzyme replacement. In general, these patients do better with small, frequent meals. The diabetes mellitus that results from chronic pancreatitis seems to be unusually brittle, with a propensity for severe hypoglycemic episodes after even low doses of insulin. This hypersensitivity to insulin may be due to loss of entire islets. Unlike autoimmune diabetes mellitus, in which specific destruction of the insulin-producing beta cells of the islets of Langerhans occurs, entire islets, including the glucagon-producing alpha cells, are destroyed in chronic pancreatitis. Thus, the important insulin-opposing effects of glucagon are lost in these patients.

Surgical or endoscopic therapy is indicated for bile or pancreatic duct obstruction or for pancreatic pseudocyst complications (Fig. 46-9).[53] Patients with intractable pain who do not have an identifiable anatomic problem will likely not benefit from surgical intervention. Relief of obstruction may be achieved by endoscopic sphincterotomy, ductal stenting, or open surgical drainage with Roux-en-Y lateral pancreaticojejunostomy (a modified Puestow procedure) (see Fig. 46-8). Pancreatic resection, starting with distal resection only, but extending to subtotal or even total pancreatectomy,

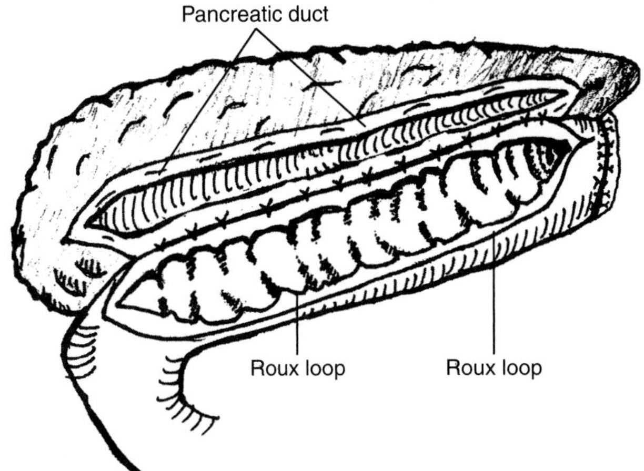

Figure 46-8. Modified Puestow procedure. The pancreatic duct is opened longitudinally and a side-to-side anastomosis to a Roux loop of jejunum is performed. (Adapted from Mayo-Smith WW, Iannitti DA, Dupuy DE: Intraoperative sonographically guided wire cannulation of the pancreatic duct for patients undergoing a Puestow procedure. AJR Am J Roentgenol 175:1639-1640, 2000.)

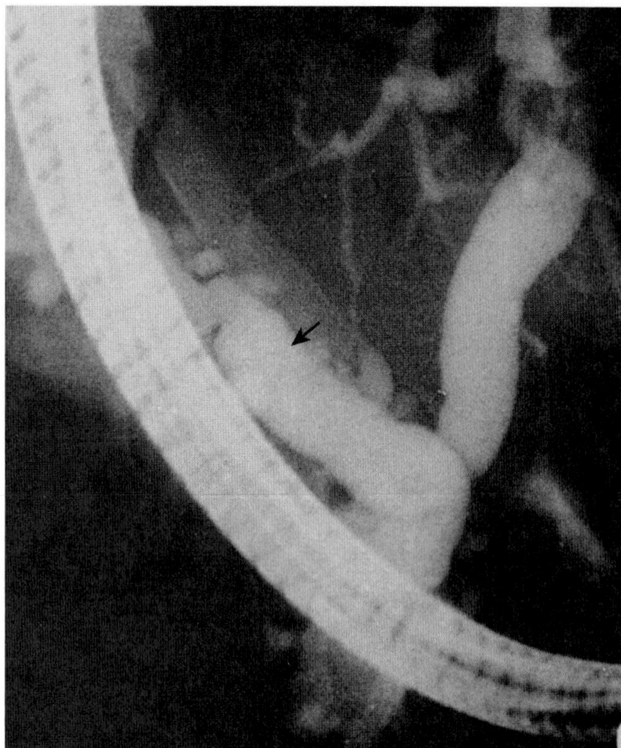

Figure 46-9. Endoscopic retrograde cholangiopancreatography in a patient with chronic pancreatitis with dilation of the biliary and pancreatic ducts (*arrow*).

has been advocated for intractable pain. These patients trade the sequelae of further, and perhaps complete, pancreatic insufficiency for anticipated pain relief.

FUNCTIONAL PANCREATIC DISORDERS

The causes of persistent hypoglycemia in children vary greatly with age. In newborns and young infants, the major causes are:

1. Persistent hyperinsulinemic hypoglycemia of infancy (PHHI), previously called nesidioblastosis
2. Lack of substrate for gluconeogenesis (e.g., glycogen storage disease)
3. Inadequate gluconeogenic hormones (e.g., hypothyroidism or growth hormone deficiency)

In children with the onset of hypoglycemia after 1 year of age, the causes are different, with insulinoma being the most common.

Persistent Hyperinsulinemic Hypoglycemia of Infancy

Nesidioblastosis comes from the Greek *nesidio*, meaning "island," and *blast*, meaning "new formation." Nesidioblasts are thought to be progenitor cells in the wall of the pancreatic ducts, normally giving rise to islets in physiologic states requiring more islets, such as during pregnancy or after pancreatic resection. It has been postulated that these nesidioblasts overproliferate in patients with PHHI.[54] This postulate was based on what had been thought to be atypical pathology of nesidioblastosis. However, it has been shown that the proliferation of nesidioblasts in the periductular regions of the pancreas is actually a normal variant in neonates.[55]

The defect in patients with PHHI appears to be related to four genes that are responsible for the ability of the beta cell to regulate insulin secretion through the adenosine triphosphate (ATP)-sensitive potassium channels, which normally consist of heteromultimers of the sulfonylurea receptors (SURs).[56-58] More specifically, the four genes are the sulfonylurea receptor (*ABCC8*), the potassium channel (*KCNJ11*), glutamate dehydrogenase (*GULDI*), and glucokinase (*ADPGK*) located on chromosome 11p15.1.[59] Some PHHI patients have been found to have a truncation mutation of the second nucleotide-binding fold on the *ABCC8* of the ATP-sensitive potassium channel. Mutations in this receptor channel prevent the normal feedback regulation of insulin production by serum glucose. Oral hypoglycemic agents act by binding the sulfonylurea receptor and activating insulin release.

The two forms of PHHI are a focal and a diffuse type. Because both forms have the same clinical presentation, the difference between the two types can be seen only after histologic analysis. The focal type is associated with the loss of a maternal allele from chromosome 11p15, with inheritance of a paternal mutation of *ABCC8*. It is characterized by a localized tumor-like aggregation of islets and also is referred to as focal adenomatous islet-cell hyperplasia. The accumulation of the large islet clusters are separated by thin rims of acinar cells or strands of connective tissue.[60] It represents about one third of the cases of PHHI. The diffuse type of PHHI represents a recessively inherited mutation of the ABCC8/KCNJ11 protein that presents as a diffuse pancreatic beta cell functional abnormality. The distinction between the two forms of PHHI is important because patients with focal PHHI may be spared the extensive pancreatic resection required in patients with diffuse PHHI.[61,62]

PHHI patients typically have hypoglycemia shortly after birth, although adult cases have been reported (probably not of the same origin).[63] Symptoms are those of hypoglycemia, with behavioral changes such as jitteriness and seizures. It is critical to measure serum insulin and glucose levels simultaneously because the absolute insulin level may be normal but the ratio of insulin to blood glucose is not normal. These patients differ from insulinoma patients in that adenoma patients usually have high absolute insulin levels. In addition, the hyperinsulinemia of PHHI is more easily suppressed with somatostatin and somatostatin analogs.

Initial treatment of PHHI should be frequent feeding, or even a drip-feeding regimen, with the addition of intravenous glucose as needed. Central venous access is advised because adequate venous access is lifesaving, and high concentrations of glucose infusion may be necessary. When the glucose infusion rate necessary to prevent hypoglycemia is more than 15 mg/kg/hr, PHHI is likely. When onset occurs after the newborn period, the patients may have only intermittent hypoglycemia and the diagnosis may be more difficult. Owing to the much higher incidence of insulin-producing adenoma, patients older than 1 year at the onset of hypoglycemia should undergo evaluation, which may include exploratory laparotomy or laparoscopy.

Initial medical treatment of PHHI should include a long-acting somatostatin analog such as octreotide or an antisecretory drug such as diazoxide. Diazoxide acts primarily by activating the potassium ATP channel through ABCC8 to inhibit insulin secretion. Octreotide activates beta cell potassium channels to inhibit insulin secretion. The main drawback of octreotide is that it requires subcutaneous injection. Other medical therapy includes glucocorticoids to promote insulin resistance and streptozotocin (beta cell–specific toxin) to decrease the number of insulin-secreting cells. In addition, glucagon can be used as a temporizing agent to control hypoglycemia.[64] These drugs seem to be most effective for treating milder cases or older children with PHHI. Medical failure to control hypoglycemia necessitates surgical resection.

In patients with diffuse-type PHHI, adequate surgical treatment consists of a 90% to 95% pancreatectomy, which entails leaving a residual remnant of pancreas on the common bile duct along the C-loop of the duodenum (Fig. 46-10).[65] It is important, especially in patients out of the newborn period, to inspect the pancreas closely for evidence of an insulin-producing adenoma, because finding an adenoma would allow significant preservation of pancreatic tissue and obviate potential endocrine and exocrine insufficiency. Postoperatively, these patients are often transiently hyperglycemic. All patients after resection of a large part of the pancreas are at significant risk for developing diabetes mellitus in later years. A 95% pancreatectomy has approximately a 75% rate of eventual diabetes mellitus.[66] For this reason, some strategies have been suggested to minimize the effects of a near-total pancreatectomy. These strategies include a nonsurgical approach using long-term hyperalimentation, continuous gastric tube feeding, and octreotide administration; a 75% pancreatectomy with a plan for a near-total pancreatectomy in the future if symptoms persist; and a near-total pancreatectomy in all patients, with isolation of the islets from the excised pancreas and cryopreservation for later autotransplantation to control diabetes.

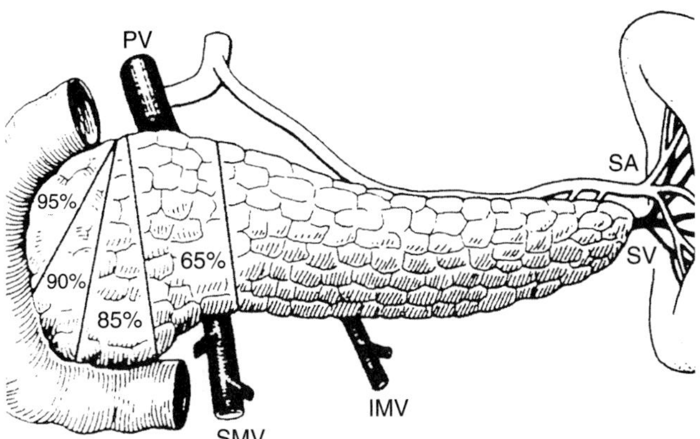

Figure 46-10. Various degrees of pancreatectomy may be indicated for persistent hyperinsulinemic hypoglycemia of infancy. Typically, a 95% pancreatectomy, as shown here, leaves behind a cuff of pancreas along the C-loop of the duodenum. IMV, inferior mesenteric vein; PV, portal vein; SA, splenic artery; SMV, superior mesenteric vein; SV, splenic vein.

In contrast, patients with focal-type PHHI may be treated with a more topographically guided pancreatic resection. The difficulty lies in distinguishing between focal and diffuse types. Recent series have shown that arterial calcium stimulation with venous sampling and transhepatic portal venous sampling can help distinguish between focal and diffuse PHHI. After a more localized exploration during laparotomy or laparoscopy and with the addition of frozen-section analysis, the pancreatic resection may be limited to the region of involvement.[61,62] In this manner, the complications of extensive pancreatic resection can be avoided in patients with focal-type PHHI.

The long-term outlook for these patients depends primarily on the age at onset, which relates to severity of disease, and on an expeditious diagnosis, because a late diagnosis results in a higher incidence of neurologic deficits.[67] Most patients seem to "grow out of the disease" after several years, implying diminished activity of the beta cells. This natural history may explain the development of diabetes mellitus in some of these patients during their school-age years.

Glycogen Storage Disease

Glucose-6-phosphatase deficiency (glycogen storage disease type I) classically appears as severe hypoglycemia in neonates and infants and is caused by the inability to dephosphorylate glycogen subunits into glucose.[68] The hypoglycemia becomes apparent when the time between feedings increases, requiring the liver to generate glucose from glycogen stores. Diagnosed clinically by the low insulin levels and hepatomegaly, ketosis and cutaneous xanthomas develop as a result of compensatory high lipid levels. Such patients often have fasting glucose levels less than 20 mg/dL. Central venous access is needed to allow continuous infusion of highly concentrated glucose. An increased incidence of hepatic adenoma is found in patients who survive to adulthood, with a 10% risk of malignant transformation.[69] Liver transplantation has become the treatment of choice for these patients.

PANCREATIC TUMORS AND CYSTS

Pancreatic Endocrine Tumors

The endocrine cells of the mature human pancreas are confined to the islets of Langerhans (Fig. 46-11), although pancreatic neurons are known to secrete locally active peptide hormones such as vasoactive intestinal peptide (VIP). Four main hormones are produced by the islets: insulin from the centrally located beta cells, which make up more than 90% of the islet; glucagon from the peripheral mantle of alpha cells;

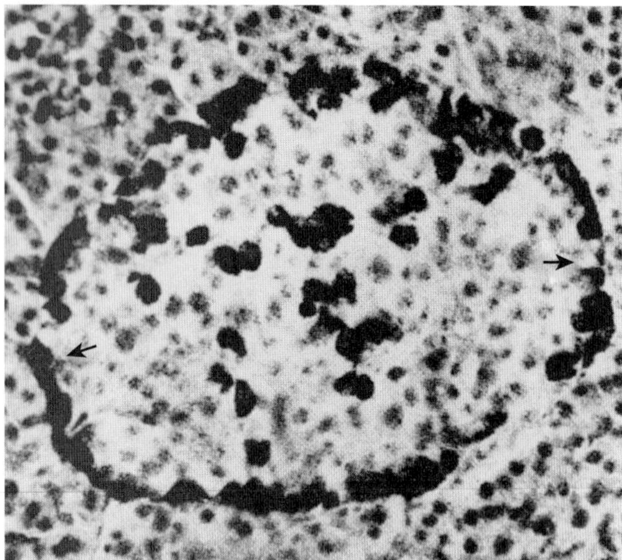

Figure 46-11. Mature islet in the pancreas. Immunohistochemical stain shows the peripheral location of the glucagon cells (alpha cells, *arrows*). The insulin-producing cells (beta cells) are located in the central portion of the islet. (From Fawcett DW [ed]: Textbook of Histology. New York, Chapman & Hall, 1994, p 699.)

and somatostatin and pancreatic polypeptide from the delta cells and pancreatic polypeptide (PP) cells scattered throughout. A small population of endocrine cells accounts for the production of ghrelin, gastrin, and other peptide hormones. Currently, it is believed that pancreatic endocrine tumors arise from cells located in the islets, although some evidence indicates that precursor cells in the pancreatic ducts or acini may give rise to these tumors as well.[70] Only insulinoma, gastrinoma, and VIPoma are known to occur in children.

Insulinoma is the most common pancreatic endocrine tumor in children, although it is still quite rare, with an estimated incidence of one case per 250,000 patient-years. Only 10% of insulinomas are malignant, and these metastasize to surrounding tissues.[71,72] This tumor causes symptoms of hypoglycemia, including dizziness, headaches, sweating, and seizures. The classic Whipple's triad was described in patients with insulinoma and consists of the following: symptoms of hypoglycemia with fasting, glucose level less than half of normal when fasting, and relief of symptoms with glucose administration.

Patients are typically older than 4 years, although neonates have been described with insulinoma. The lesions are usually solitary, except in multiple endocrine neoplasia type 1 (MEN 1) in which multiple insulinomas may be found.

Insulinoma is diagnosed by demonstrating an insulin-to-glucose ratio of more than 1.0 (microunits of insulin per milliliter/milligrams of glucose per deciliter). Normal should be less than 0.3. Levels of insulin C-peptide should always be measured because its absence indicates exogenous administration of insulin. The distinction between benign and malignant lesions is difficult and is based on tumor size (<2 cm tend to be benign) and the presence of metastases.

Tumor localization preoperatively can be difficult.[73] Extrapancreatic insulinomas are rare, and thin-slice CT of the pancreas will identify more than half of the tumors. Small hypervascular tumors may be visualized by angiographic blush, but angiography is probably not warranted with the advent of newer imaging techniques. Magnetic resonance imaging (MRI) and endoscopic ultrasonography allow visualization of very small tumors. Selective portal venous sampling may help localize the tumor for blind pancreatic resections. All patients should undergo surgical resection. The tumors are pink and firm, appear encapsulated, and are usually amenable to simple enucleation. At operation, occult tumors may be localized by intraoperative ultrasonography.[74] Failure to localize the tumor by any of the aforementioned techniques is unlikely, but because insulinomas tend to be located in the tail of the pancreas, distal pancreatectomy is the best "blind" procedure. Patients with MEN 1 and multiple adenomas require a 95% pancreatectomy. Malignant insulinomas require chemotherapy, usually with the beta cell–toxic drug streptozotocin. When malignant tumors have metastasized to the liver, chemoembolization is widely used and should be combined with somatostatin analogs. The overall prognosis for these latter patients is very poor.

Fetal gastrin-producing cells in the pancreas are believed to give rise to pancreatic gastrinoma. The pancreas is the primary source of gastrin in the fetus. After birth, the gastric antrum becomes the principal gastrin source. The Zollinger-Ellison syndrome consists of gastric hypersecretion with severe peptic ulcer disease and a gastrin-producing tumor, which classically is located in the pancreas. The pancreas is the most common site for gastrinomas, which are malignant in 65% of cases and usually produce the 17-amino-acid form of gastrin. Unlike adults, children with gastrinoma have not been reported to have MEN 1.[75,76]

The diagnosis of a gastrinoma is based on hypergastrinemia and gastric hypersecretion. Gastrin levels are usually greater than 500 pg/mL, but equivocal cases can be diagnosed by using 2 U/kg of IV secretin as a stimulation test. A gastrinoma responds with a 200 pg/mL or more increase in serum gastrin. Localization of gastrinomas can be difficult because these tumors may be outside the pancreas. CT, MRI, endoscopic ultrasonography, and selective portal venous sampling have all been used to help localize the tumors. Occult tumors have been shown most often to be located in the duodenum and may require a duodenotomy.

The medical treatment for gastrinoma is omeprazole, the inhibitor of acid secretion that selectively blocks the ATP-dependent hydrogen-potassium proton pump necessary for acid secretion. All patients with potentially resectable disease should undergo exploration, although most pancreatic tumors are not resectable. Only patients who undergo complete resection are cured.

Non-neoplastic Cysts

Although most cystic lesions of the pancreas are pseudocysts and are acquired, congenital cysts may be first seen at an early age as a symptomatic mass with compression of surrounding structures.[77] Alternatively, these congenital cysts may be noted incidentally on physical examination or radiographic studies. Congenital cysts contain cloudy straw-colored fluid with normal pancreatic enzyme levels. The cysts are most often found in the distal pancreas and are amenable to local resection with a rim of normal pancreas. Lesions in the head of the pancreas should be internally drained with a Roux-en-Y cystojejunostomy. Congenital duplications of the intestine also may be sequestered in the pancreas. They have a gastric mucosal lining but maintain pancreatic ductal communication. The gastric acid may cause episodes of pancreatitis. The mass is usually small and identified only on CT. Surgical resection is necessary, either in the form of enucleation, distal pancreatectomy, or even pancreaticoduodenectomy.

Acquired non-neoplastic cysts of the pancreas are called retention cysts and seem to represent ectasia of the pancreatic ducts (Fig. 46-12). The cysts contain fluid rich in pancreatic enzymes. The preoperative distinction of a retention cyst from other types of cysts or pseudocysts may be difficult. ERCP or MRCP may demonstrate a communication with the ductal system and may help in determining the surgical approach (resection versus Roux-en-Y cystojejunostomy).

Pancreatic Exocrine Tumors

The pancreatic exocrine system consists of the pancreatic ducts, centroacinar cells, and acini. Tumors arising from this system include pseudopapillary tumors, ductal adenocarcinomas, acinar cell carcinomas, or pancreatoblastomas. Cystic tumors of the pancreas, which include serous cystadenoma, mucinous cystadenoma, and cystadenocarcinoma, are well characterized in the adult population. In children, however, rare cases have been described in the literature, but overall they are poorly characterized.[77] A recent review of the literature suggests that no documented case of cystadenocarcinoma has been described in children. Moreover, with one exception, the few cases of cystadenoma are dissimilar to the adult lesions. These cases of cystadenomas may represent a developmental malformation and not neoplasms.[78]

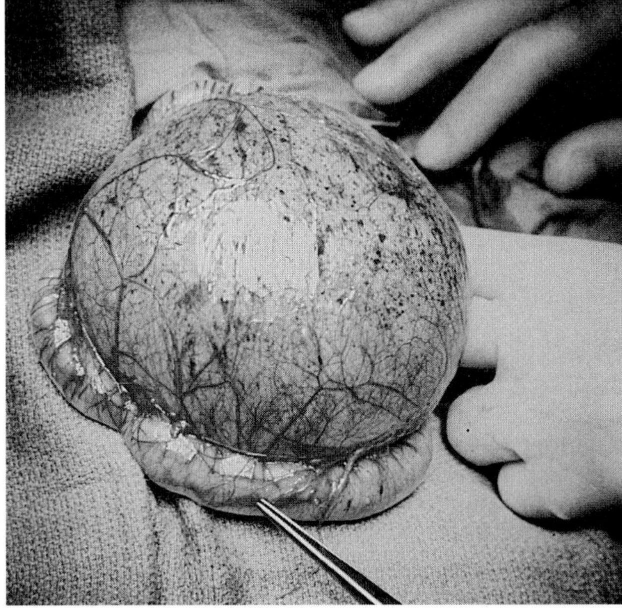

Figure 46-12. Large pancreatic cyst (retention cyst) emanating from the pancreatic parenchyma. The cyst was filled with clear fluid. (Courtesy of Howard B. Ginsburg, MD.)

Adenocarcinoma/Pancreatoblastoma

In general, pancreatic cancers are rare in children. Children with malignant pancreatic exocrine tumors generally have a much better overall prognosis after surgical resection than malignant pancreatic exocrine tumors in adults. Ductal adenocarcinoma is the most common adult form of pancreatic cancer. It has been described in children, but most of the reported cases are in the older literature. As the pancreatic tumors of childhood have become better characterized, these previous diagnoses of ductal adenocarcinoma have been questioned. Because these lesions have become rare in recent years, it appears that many of these tumors may have been previously misdiagnosed.[78] Acinar cell adenocarcinoma is more often seen in children and tends to have a less aggressive behavior with a better prognosis. Treatment is complete surgical resection for both ductal adenocarcinoma and acinar cell carcinoma.

Another variant of adenocarcinoma seen in infants and younger children has been termed *pancreatoblastoma* and represents the most common exocrine tumor of the pancreas in childhood. It is seen more often in boys than in girls and is thought to be of embryonic origin, similar to Wilms' tumor and hepatoblastoma. An allelic loss occurs on chromosome 11p, suggesting a common genetic relationship among pancreatoblastoma, Beckwith-Wiedemann syndrome, and related embryonal malignancies.[79] Pancreatoblastomas are of low malignancy and often arise in the head of the pancreas (two thirds). They may represent a tumor of immature duct cells.[80,81] Even large tumors have a relatively benign course. Metastases are reported in one third of the patients, with the liver and lung being the most common sites. α-Fetoprotein levels may be elevated in pancreatoblastoma and may be used to monitor patients for recurrence.[82] The prognosis is relatively good with complete resection of the tumor. Recurrence is common, so close follow-up is mandatory.

A Frantz tumor is a papillary-cystic tumor, also referred to as solid pseudopapillary tumor, seen in girls and young women. It is derived from exocrine cells. Histologically, no acinar or ductal structures appear to be present. Degenerative changes result in the formation of pseudopapillae, and a fibrous capsule is usually seen.[83] Solid pseudopapillary tumor is less malignant than pancreatoblastoma, and metastases are rarely present. The prognosis is good even with just local resection. Although solid pseudopapillary tumor is a relatively indolent tumor, at the present time aggressive resection is advocated, given that the tumor is curable.[84]

chapter 47

SPLENIC CONDITIONS

Frederick J. Rescorla, MD

The role of the spleen as an important functional organ in health and disease has been well documented. An early observation was the recognition by King and Schumacher in 1952 of the susceptibility of splenectomized infants to infection.[1] The essential role of the spleen led pediatric surgeons to introduce nonoperative management of splenic injuries in children, which evolved into the preferred method for treating not only children but also adults.[2] Currently, the primary role of surgery for the spleen involves the management of hematologic disorders. Perhaps the most significant change has been the introduction of laparoscopic splenectomy in adults by Delaitre and Maignon and subsequently in children by Tulman and Holcomb.[3,4] The laparoscopic approach has quickly emerged as the preferred technique for the management of splenic disorders.

EMBRYOLOGY, ANATOMY, AND PHYSIOLOGY

The splenic primordium develops as a mesenchymal bulge in the dorsal mesogastrium between the stomach and the pancreas, initially observed at the 8- to 10-mm embryo stage. A true epithelium is noted at the 10- to 12-mm stage as sinusoids communicate with capillaries. The spleen produces white and red cells by the fourth month of fetal life, although this function ceases later in gestation. The anatomic arrangement of the spleen is consistent with the various functions of the spleen. The splenic artery branches into segmental vessels, which further branch into trabecular arteries. After further bifurcations, small arteries enter the white pulp, which consists of lymphocytes and macrophages arranged as a germinal center around the central artery. The central artery delivers particulate material into the white pulp, an arrangement that may facilitate antibody formation in response to particulate antigens.[5-8] The red pulp consists of the endothelial cords of Billroth, which are functionally distal to the white pulp. The function of the spleen consists of red blood cell maintenance, immune function, and a reservoir.

The red pulp serves to destroy old and defective cells. The spleen also removes Howell-Jolly bodies (nuclear remnants), Heinz bodies (denatured hemoglobin), and Pappenheimer bodies (iron granules). These particles are noted on the peripheral smear after splenectomy. The immune response occurs in the white pulp as antigens come in contact with macrophages and helper T cells. T cells respond with cytokine synthesis, and activated T cells circulate to modulate the response. A humoral response occurs as macrophages and helper T cells come in contact with antigens.[9]

Splenic function also involves removal of particulate matter as well as production of nonspecific opsonins, which further activate the complement system. In addition, the spleen serves as a biologic filter. If little antibody is available for opsonization of bacteria, the spleen assumes a greater role. This may be a factor in the age-related differences in post-splenectomy infections in young children who can lack an adequate antibody response.[6] The spleen also serves as a reservoir for platelets and factor VIII.

ANATOMIC ABNORMALITIES

Asplenia and Polysplenia

Asplenia is often noted with complex congenital heart disease as well as bilateral "right-sidedness" such as bilateral three-lobed lungs and a right-sided stomach and central liver.[10] Intestinal malrotation has also been observed with asplenia.[11] These infants are at a risk for overwhelming infection and should receive antibiotics for prophylaxis.

Polysplenia usually consists of a cluster of very small splenic masses and is often associated with biliary atresia. Other associated conditions can include preduodenal portal vein, situs inversus, malrotation, and cardiac defects.[10] These children have adequate splenic immune function.

Wandering Spleen

This condition is characterized by a lack of ligamentous attachments to the diaphragm, colon, and retroperitoneum, resulting in a mobile spleen. This is

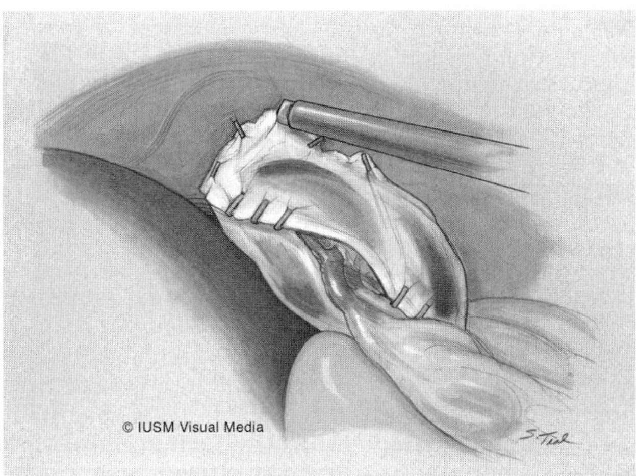

Figure 47-1. Drawing of a laparoscopic splenopexy with placement of the spleen between two sheets of absorbable mesh with fixation in the left upper quadrant. (© IUSM Visual Media.)

likely due to failure of development of the ligaments from the dorsal mesentery.[12] Children are occasionally noted with an abdominal mass and episodic pain but can also present with torsion and infarction.[13-17] Pancreatitis has also been noted as a presenting sign.[18] Splenopexy is the preferred method of treatment and can be performed with placement of the spleen into a mesh basket, suture splenopexy, colonic displacement with gastropexy, placement in an omental basket, or placement in an extraperitoneal pocket.[17,19-22] The laparoscopic approach is the preferred method, and the use of an absorbable or nonabsorbable mesh with fixation in the left upper quadrant is demonstrated in Figure 47-1.[23,24] Placement of the spleen in an extraperitoneal pocket is seen in Figure 47-2. Torsion with infarction requires splenectomy. Cases of chronic torsion have also been reported with massive splenomegaly,[25] which may necessitate splenectomy.

Accessory Spleens

Accessory spleens have been noted in 15% to 30% of children, with a recent series noting a 19% rate.[23] Accessory spleens likely originate from mesenchymal remnants that fail to fuse with the main splenic mass, with most (75%) located near the splenic hilum (Fig. 47-3). Other locations that must be evaluated during surgery include the lesser sac along the splenic vessels, omentum, and retroperitoneum. If an accessory spleen is noted, 86% are single, 11% have two, and 3% have three or more.[26,27] A missed accessory spleen at the time of planned total splenectomy can lead to recurrence of the primary disease process, which in cases of immune thrombocytopenic purpura is early and with hereditary spherocytosis is later.[28-30]

Splenic Gonadal Fusion

This condition in which the left gonad and the spleen are attached is a result of early fusion between the two structures before descent of the testis.[31] The remnant can be a continuous band or discontinuous with splenic tissue attached to the gonad. A remnant of spleen has also been noted totally separate in the left scrotum as an accessory splenic remnant type of abnormality.[32]

Splenic Cysts

Cysts of the spleen are most frequently primary splenic cysts containing an epithelial lining and are also referred to as epithelial or epidermoid cysts (Fig. 47-4). Post-traumatic pseudocysts are also occasionally seen. Inclusion of surface mesothelium into the splenic parenchyma is the most likely etiology of the epithelial cysts. They may present as symptoms related to their size with gastric compression or pain, an abdominal mass, rupture, or infection with abscess.[33-35] Simple cysts less than 5 cm may be observed, but cysts that are enlarging, symptomatic, or larger than 5 cm

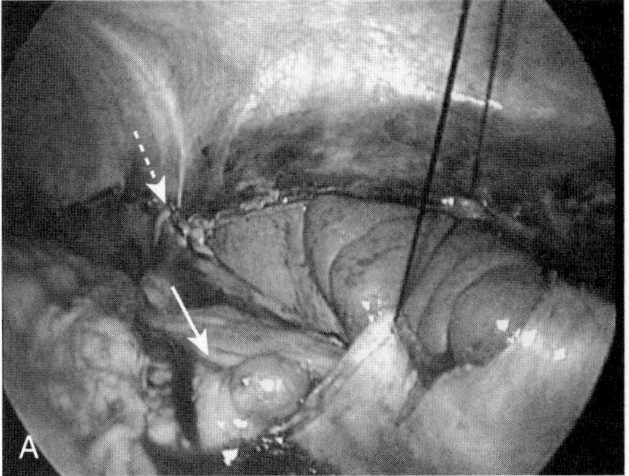

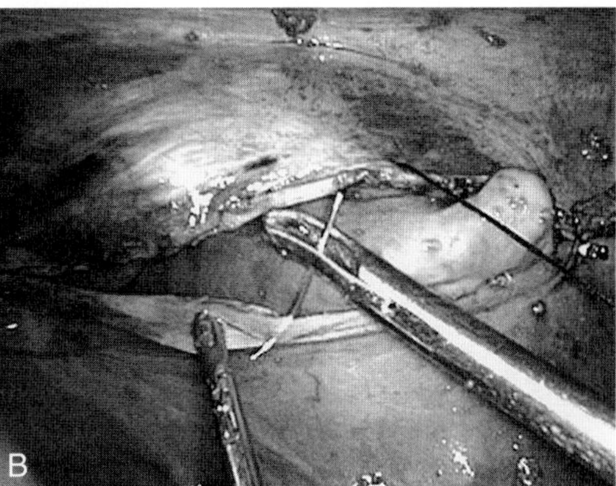

Figure 47-2. **A,** The upper pole of the spleen was placed in the retroperitoneal pouch, and the upper aspect of the pouch (*dotted arrow*) was closed with interrupted sutures. Note the splenic vessels (*solid arrow*) coursing into the spleen. A generous opening was left in the pouch for these vessels so that the vessels would not be compressed by closure of the pouch. **B,** One of the interrupted silk sutures is being placed to approximate the peritoneal flaps over the spleen. At this point, most of the spleen has been placed into the extraperitoneal pouch. (From Upadhyaya P, St. Peter SD, Holcomb GW III: Laparoscopic splenopexy and cystectomy for an enlarged wandering spleen and splenic cyst. J Pediatr Surg 42:E23-E27, 2007. Reprinted with permission.)

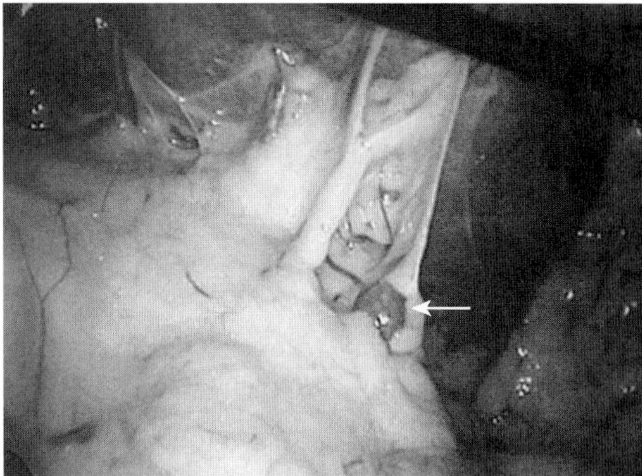

Figure 47-3. An accessory spleen (*arrow*) is seen in the lienocolic ligament in this patient.

require treatment. Most symptomatic cysts are larger than 8 cm.[33] Percutaneous aspiration and sclerosis utilizing alcohol or other agents have been reported with variable success.[36,37]

Marsupialization is commonly performed (Fig. 47-5) but has been associated with a high recurrence rate if an adequate segment of cyst is not removed.[38,39] In addition, a recent report noted a high recurrence rate with laparoscopic partial excision.[40] However, others have had good success with this technique, and many also recommend partial splenectomy associated with cyst resection.[41-45] Our group has reported good results with partial splenectomy, emphasizing a margin of normal spleen so that the cut surfaces of the cyst cannot be in opposition which might lead to recurrence.[23]

INDICATIONS FOR SPLENECTOMY

Hereditary Spherocytosis

Hereditary spherocytosis, an autosomal dominant condition, is the most common inherited red cell disorder among Northern European descendants, with approximately 25% of affected children representing new mutations. Defects in red cell proteins ankyrin or spectrin result in poorly deformable spherocytes. Most affected children have anemia, an elevated reticulocyte count, and a mild elevation in bilirubin concentration. The degree of hemolysis can vary, with some having only a mild anemia. Spherocytes on peripheral smear along with a positive osmotic fragility test confirms the diagnosis. Affected children may develop an aplastic crisis associated with parvovirus B19 infection with suppression of bone marrow red cell production and a very low hemoglobin concentration due to ongoing splenic red cell destruction.[46] Splenectomy is usually performed for moderate to severe anemia. If possible, splenectomy is delayed until 5 to 6 years of age to decrease the likelihood of post-splenectomy infection. Splenomegaly is common with this condition. Associated gallstones are also common, and an ultrasound evaluation of the gallbladder should be performed before splenectomy. A recent study noted the presence

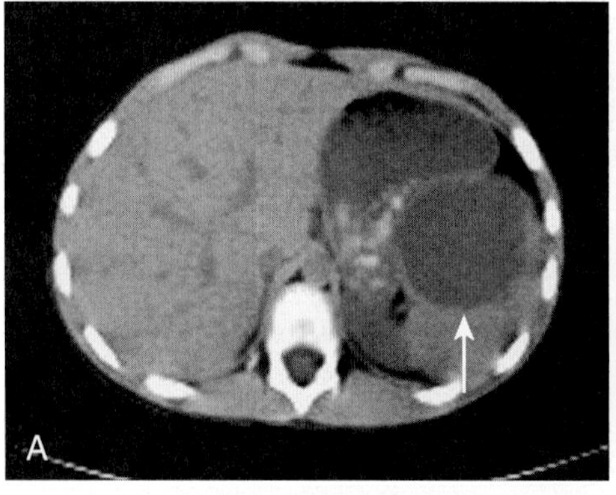

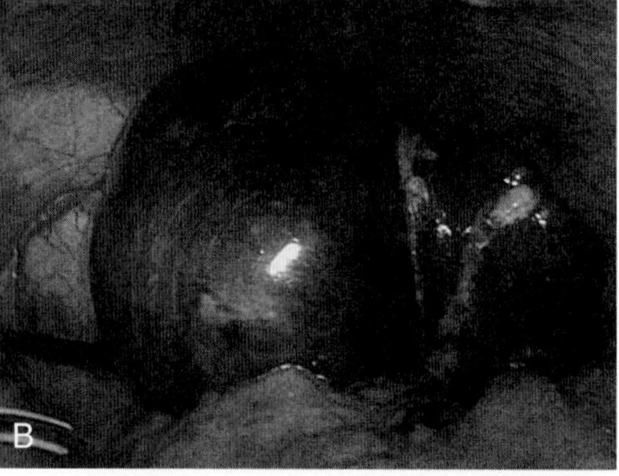

Figure 47-4. A, A large epithelial splenic cyst (*arrow*) is seen on the CT scan. **B,** At laparoscopy, the large cyst is seen to occupy most of the spleen.

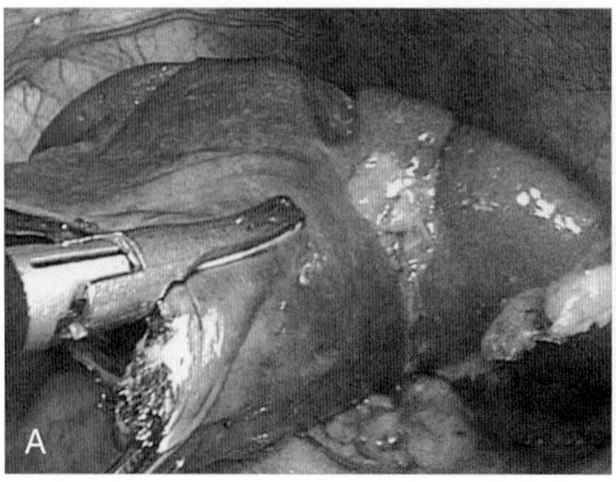

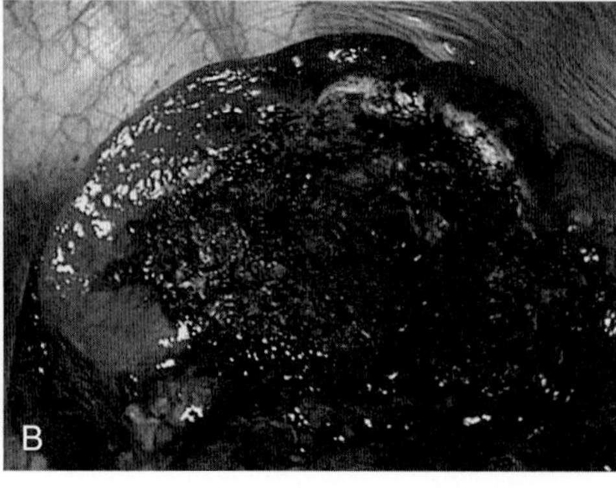

Figure 47-5. A, The wall of the large epithelial splenic cyst seen in Figure 47-4 is being excised. **B,** The cyst was marsupialized and the remnant lining of the cyst was ablated with the argon beam coagulator.

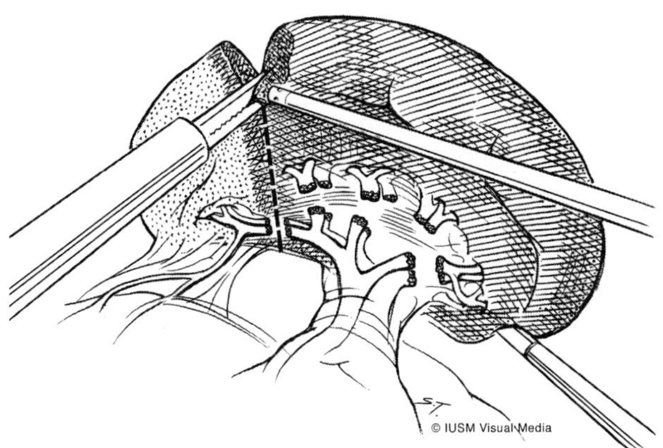

Figure 47-6. Laparoscopic partial splenectomy with preservation of blood flow to the spleen through the most superior short gastric vessel is depicted. Note division of the parenchyma about 1 cm to the right of the devascularized margin. (© IUSM Visual Media.)

of gallstones in children undergoing splenectomy to be 27% in those younger than age 10 years compared with 56% in those 10 years of age or older.[23] Partial splenectomy is an attractive alternative to a total splenectomy in an attempt to remove enough spleen to alleviate the anemia while preserving enough spleen to prevent overwhelming post-splenectomy infection (Fig. 47-6). This may be particularly useful in young children requiring splenectomy, but the long-term results are not known.

Immune Thrombocytopenic Purpura

Immune thrombocytopenic purpura (ITP) occurs due to antiplatelet autoantibodies binding with platelets and subsequently undergoing destruction in the spleen. In most children, it is primary (idiopathic), whereas in some it may be secondary to lupus, human immunodeficiency virus, malignancy, or hepatitis C infection. Most children (80%) have acute ITP that resolves with simple observation or medical management. Most treatment plans aim at decreasing platelet destruction. These include corticosteroids, which may have their effect by inhibiting the reticuloendothelial binding of platelet/antibody complexes; intravenous immunoglobulin (IVIG), which inhibits the Fc receptor binding of platelets by macrophages; or Rho(D) immunoglobulin in Rh-positive children, which bind red cells that then saturate the splenic receptors, allowing the platelets to avoid destruction. Response to corticosteroids, IVIG, or both, predicts excellent outcome with splenectomy.[47,48] Some children fail to respond to medical treatment or, more commonly, develop relapse when the treatment is stopped. In some cases, further therapy may include rituximab, a monoclonal antibody against CD20-positive B cells. This depletes the B cells and is somewhat of a "medical splenectomy." Other treatment modalities have included azathioprine, cyclophosphamide, danazol, and mycophenolate mofetil.[49] Platelet production may be decreased in ITP. Thus, the use of thrombopoietic agents has emerged[49] and successful therapy with agents such as AMG 531 (Amgen Inc., Thousand Oaks, CA) has been reported.[50]

Children with thrombocytopenia for longer than 6 months are considered to have chronic ITP and are candidates for splenectomy. The response to splenectomy is usually excellent in children who have responded to medical management. In adult patients, the response is not as high. Accessory spleens or residual splenic tissue has been identified in up to 50% of these patients with ITP, thus emphasizing both the importance of accessory spleen detection at exploration as well as the need to avoid parenchymal disruption.[28]

Sickle Cell Disease

Sickle cell disease results from an amino acid substitution in the β chain of normal hemoglobin A, which results in hemoglobin S. Children may be homozygous (sickle cell disease) or have less severe heterozygous types such as sickle-C or sickle-thalassemia. These cells become rigid as they pass through the hypoxic environment of the spleen, leading to splenic sequestration. Although in most children autoinfarction and atrophy lead to a functional asplenic state, some develop symptomatic sequestration. If the sequestration is severe, these children develop anemia and splenomegaly with associated thrombocytopenia known as acute splenic sequestration crisis. Because of the associated morbidity and mortality, severe or recurrent episodes merit consideration of splenectomy.

Thalassemia

The thalassemias are characterized by abnormal production of α or β chains of hemoglobin. Thalassemia major (β-thalassemia) is associated with the most severe clinical anemia among this group. Splenomegaly causes further red cell sequestration and the need for transfusion. Total or partial splenectomy has been used to decrease the need for transfusions in children with severe anemia.

Gaucher's Disease

Gaucher's disease is characterized by a deficiency of the enzyme β-glucocerebrosidase, resulting in excessive glucocerebroside in the macrophages of the spleen, liver, bone marrow, and lungs. Splenomegaly may be severe, and both partial and total splenectomy have been utilized to alleviate the symptomatic hypersplenism and decrease destruction of red cells, leukocytes, and platelets.[51] However, massive bleeding and death has been reported several months postoperatively in a child with Gaucher's disease who underwent partial splenectomy.[52]

SPLENECTOMY

Open Splenectomy

The open technique through a left upper quadrant incision is usually reserved for massive splenomegaly or partial splenectomy. The initial division of the splenorenal, splenocolic, and splenophrenic ligaments allows the spleen to be mobilized from the left upper quadrant and out of the abdominal cavity. The short gastric vessels are initially divided, followed by the hilar vessels. A careful search must be undertaken for accessory spleens. A lateral muscle-splitting approach has been reported with a 2.7-day length of stay, comparable to some early laparoscopic series but longer than more recent series.[23,53-56]

Laparoscopic Splenectomy

Laparoscopic splenectomy has evolved over the past 5 to 10 years to become the preferred technique for management of splenic disorders.[3,4] Less pain, shorter hospitalization, and smaller scars are the main advantages over open splenectomy. It is associated with longer operative time and can be difficult in cases of splenomegaly. The main technical advances have been the result of smaller instrumentation and advanced energy sources such as the Harmonic Scalpel (Ethicon Endosurgery Inc, Cincinnati, OH) and Ligasure (Valley Lab, Tyco Healthcare Group, Boulder, CO). At our institution, we primarily utilize the Ligasure because it allows division of vessels up to 7 mm.

Preoperative splenic artery embolization has been recommended in some adult series for spleens between 20 and 30 cm. However, complications such as pain, abscess, and retroperitoneal necrosis have been reported.[57,58] Although we have not found preoperative embolization necessary, on occasion we have been forced to divide the spleen in the abdomen to facilitate its removal. Hand-assisted procedures have been used in adults, but the large incision appears to eliminate the benefits of the laparoscopic approach in children.[59,60] Splenomegaly in children is usually associated with hereditary spherocytosis, but most cases are still amenable to the laparoscopic approach. A recent report confirmed the benefit of the laparoscopic technique in adults for spleens between 15 and 25 cm.[61]

The most significant initial concern of the laparoscopic approach related to accessory spleen detection. However, in adult studies, and comparison pediatric series, similar rates of accessory spleen detection at laparoscopic and open splenectomy have been noted.[28,29,54-56,62-64] For the laparoscopic operation, most surgeons utilize a lateral approach with slight elevation of the left flank. One technique to improve the ease of port placement is to have the patient's left side initially elevated approximately 45 degrees rather than the true lateral position. The operating table is tilted to the patient's left to achieve a flat position for the port placement and is then tilted to the patient's right to achieve a lateral position for the procedure (Fig. 47-7). The surgeon and assistant stand on the patient's right. In young children and with small spleens, the upper midline instruments can be inserted without cannulas because these instruments are not removed during the procedure (Fig. 47-8). The first assistant holds the two upper midline instruments and provides elevation of the spleen and traction on surrounding tissues. The surgeon holds the camera (5-mm, 30-degree telescope) in the left hand and the energy source in the right.

Initially, the splenocolic ligament is divided with the energy device, allowing the splenic flexure to fall away from the spleen. The inferior portion of the gastrosplenic ligament is divided, and the surgeon works in a cephalad direction dividing the short gastric vessels and opening the lesser sac (Fig. 47-9). The most superior short gastric vessels are often very short, and care must be taken to avoid injury to the stomach or diaphragm. The lesser sac should be inspected for the presence of accessory spleens. The splenophrenic ligament is divided to fully mobilize the upper pole. At this point, the hilum can be approached. It is often easiest at this time to divide the splenorenal ligament

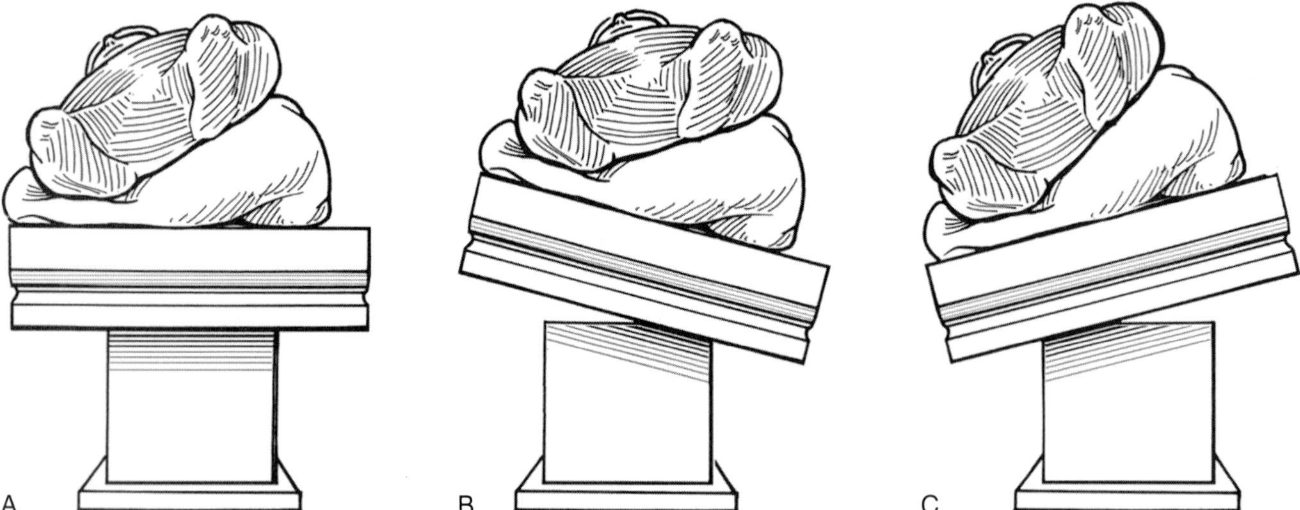

Figure 47-7. **A,** Initial positioning of the patient before any movement of the table. **B,** The table has been tilted to the patient's left to obtain a near supine position of the patient for port placement. **C,** The table is then rotated back to the patient's right to achieve a right lateral decubitus position for the operation. (From Rescorla FJ: Laparoscopic splenectomy. In Holcomb GW III, Georgeson KE, Rothenberg SS [eds]: Atlas of Pediatric Laparoscopy and Thoracoscopy. Philadelphia, Elsevier, 2008, pp 121-126. Reprinted with permission.)

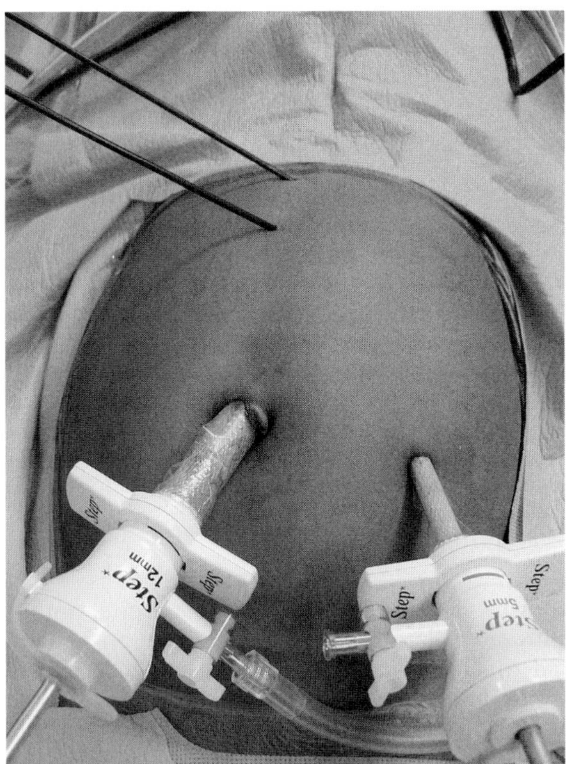

Figure 47-8. Placement in a child of 3-mm midline instruments without the use of cannulas. The umbilical port is 12 mm, and the left lower quadrant port is 5 mm.

because this allows the option to use the endovascular stapler on the hilum. The hilar vessels can be divided with clips, stapler, or the energy device (Fig. 47-10). One study comparing the endoscopic stapler to the Ligasure demonstrated safety and efficiency of both with a lower blood loss and conversion rate with the Ligasure.[65] At our hospital, we utilize the Ligasure to divide the individual segmental vessels, usually with one treatment applied toward the pancreas side without division and a second toward the spleen with division. Other reported adjuncts include use of a suction cup grasper to manipulate the spleen, a wall-lifting device, or umbilical tape around the hilum for splenic mobilization.[66-68]

The Endocatch II bag (Covidien, Norwalk, CT) is introduced through the 15-mm umbilical port with the telescope moved to the left lower quadrant site. This bag has a 13-cm diameter opening with a 23-cm depth and can accommodate most pediatric spleens. A smaller bag and umbilical cannula may be used for smaller spleens. The neck of the bag is delivered through the umbilical site, and either a finger or ring forceps is introduced to disrupt the capsule and remove the spleen piecemeal (Fig. 47-11). Use of an ultrasonic morcellator and liposuction has been reported but is usually unnecessary.[69] A coring device to remove portions of the spleen to decrease the size has also been described for children with sickle cell disease and splenomegaly.[70] This should not be utilized for hereditary spherocytosis because splenosis can lead to recurrent anemia.

These basic techniques are also utilized for the treatment of splenic cysts with excision and partial splenectomy as well as splenopexy for a wandering spleen. This approach is usually not applicable to traumatic splenic injuries because most of these children have unstable conditions and are in need of rapid control of the bleeding. However, a recent report described laparoscopic splenectomy after splenic artery embolization in a 15-year-old girl with a traumatic injury.[71]

Partial Splenectomy

Concerns of post-splenectomy infection have led to the concept of partial splenectomy. This is primarily utilized in children with hereditary spherocytosis but has also been utilized with Gaucher's disease, hypersplenism with cystic fibrosis, splenic hamartomas, and as previously noted for splenic cysts.[51,72,73] The principle of partial splenectomy in hereditary spherocytosis is to remove enough spleen to minimize hemolysis

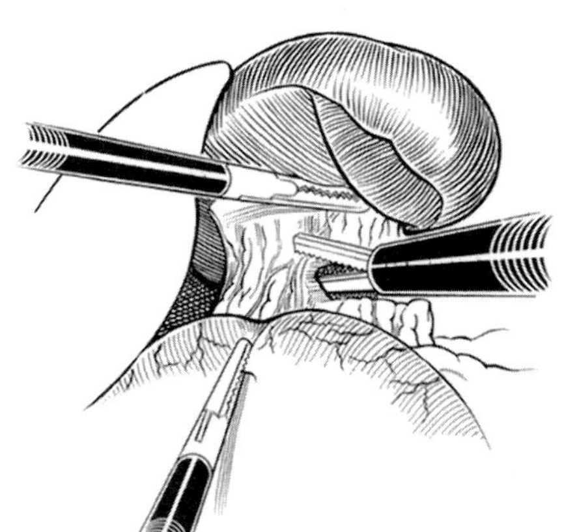

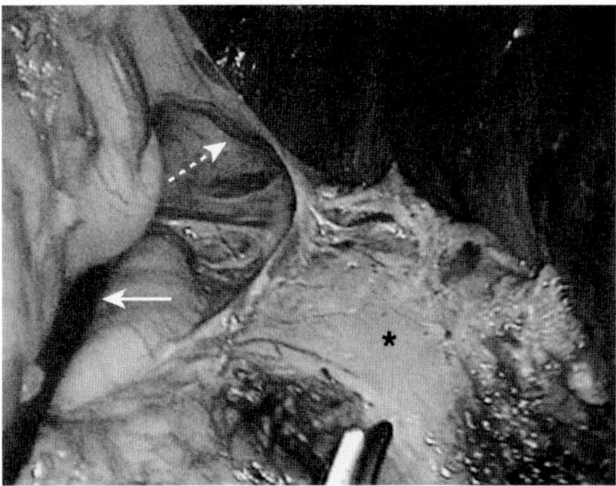

Figure 47-9. After division of the short gastric vessels using the ultrasonic scalpel, the lesser sac is entered. In the operative photograph, the stomach is being retracted by the assistant's instrument (*solid arrow*). The ultrasonic scalpel, at the bottom of the photograph, is approaching one of the intact short gastric vessels (*dotted arrow*). The pancreas is marked with an *asterisk*. (From Rescorla FJ: Laparoscopic splenectomy. In Holcomb GW III, Georgeson KE, Rothenberg SS [eds]: Atlas of Pediatric Laparoscopy and Thoracoscopy. Philadelphia, Elsevier, 2008, pp 121-126. Reprinted with permission.)

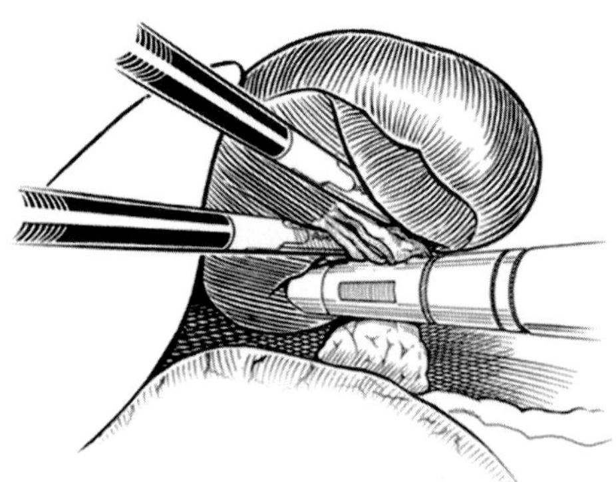

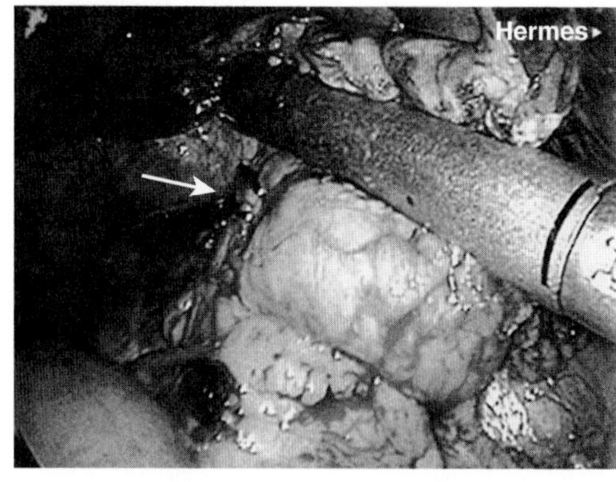

Figure 47-10. **Once the spleen has been mobilized and is attached only through the hilar vessels, the camera is rotated to the left lower quadrant port and the stapler is introduced through the umbilical port. It is then placed across the hilar vessels, taking care not to incorporate a portion of the pancreas in the tissue to be divided. In the operative photograph, note that the splenic artery has been ligated with clips (*arrow*) before hilar division because the spleen was extremely large.** (From Rescorla FJ: Laparoscopic splenectomy. In Holcomb GW III, Georgeson KE, Rothenberg SS [eds]: Atlas of Pediatric Laparoscopy and Thoracoscopy. Philadelphia, Elsevier, 2008, pp 121-126. Reprinted with permission.)

while preserving enough spleen to protect against overwhelming post-splenectomy infection. This generally involves removal of 85% to 95% of the spleen with preservation of approximately 25% of the normal splenic size. In this approach, the remnant spleen is supplied by one or two short gastric vessels with division of all of the hilar vessels (see Fig. 47-6). An alternative approach, depending on the anatomy of the segmental vessels, is to leave the uppermost segmental vessel as the only blood supply. Although most have been performed through an open technique, the laparoscopic approach is gaining popularity.[23,74,75]

The splenic parenchyma can be divided with a stapler, cautery, or energy device. Our institution recently reported 12 laparoscopic partial splenectomies.[23] In all cases, a combination of an energy device (Ligasure) and cautery were utilized, occasionally with a topical agent placed over the cut surface. After splenic vessel division, a clear line of demarcation is usually noted. We divide the spleen 1 cm onto the ischemic side to minimize bleeding. The upper splenorenal and splenophrenic ligaments are left in place in an attempt to avoid torsion. Another report of seven laparoscopic partial splenectomies utilized the harmonic scalpel for parenchymal division and also completely mobilized the spleen.[76] The authors utilized splenopexy to prevent torsion.

Most series have noted an increase in red cell half-life, higher hemoglobin levels, and lower reticulocyte and bilirubin levels after partial splenectomy for spherocytosis.[74,77] Lack of Howell-Jolly bodies on peripheral smear and a decreased number of pitted red cells is evidence of preservation of splenic phagocytic function. Normal levels of IgM- and IgG-specific antibody titers after *Streptococcus pneumoniae* have been observed. Splenic regeneration occurs in all patients although the degree of regrowth does not correlate with hemolysis.[75] The development of cholelithiasis varies from 7% to 22%, indicating ongoing hemolysis. Moreover, the need for total splenectomy has been reported.[74,78] Rice and

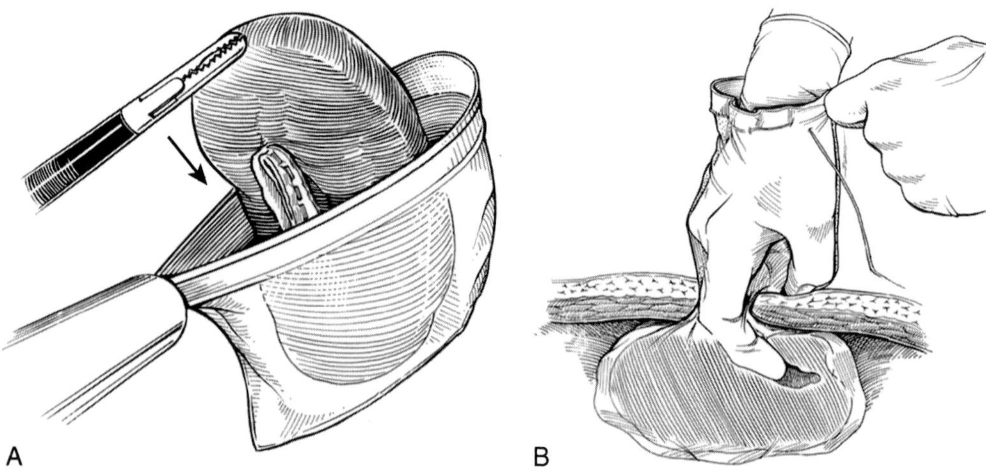

Figure 47-11. **A,** **After complete mobilization, the spleen is dropped into an endoscopic retrieval bag.** **B,** **The neck of the bag is then exteriorized through the umbilicus, and the surgeon's finger is used to fracture the splenic capsule. A combination of ring forceps and the surgeon's finger is then used to remove the splenic fragments.** (From Rescorla FJ: Laparoscopic splenectomy. In Holcomb GW III, Georgeson KE, Rothenberg SS [eds]: Atlas of Pediatric Laparoscopy and Thoracoscopy. Philadelphia, Elsevier, 2008, pp 121-126. Reprinted with permission.)

colleagues have popularized this procedure and recently summarized their experience in 29 children undergoing partial splenectomy.[75] They noted decreased transfusion requirements, elimination of splenic sequestration, as well as higher hematocrits and lower reticulocyte counts and bilirubin levels. An alternative technique has been described that leaves a 10-cm^3 remnant as a small cylinder supplied off one vessel.[79]

Complications and Controversies of Laparoscopic Splenectomy

Accessory Spleen Detection

The identification of residual splenic function in up to 50% of some selected adult patients after laparoscopic splenectomy has led to concern of the ability of laparoscopy to adequately detect accessory spleens.[28] Parenchymal disruption at the time of laparoscopic splenectomy has also been associated with a higher rate of residual splenic function.[28] Although preoperative computed tomography and splenic scintigraphy have been utilized, most surgeons have abandoned this approach.[80,81]

There are reports of equivalent detection rates of accessory spleens with laparoscopy.[28,82] A review of several comparative pediatric series demonstrated an accessory spleen rate of 20.3% with open splenectomy compared with 20.2% with laparoscopy.[54-56,62-64] A recent report of over 200 pediatric laparoscopic splenectomies noted an accessory spleen rate of 19%.[23] Laparoscopic removal of missed accessory spleens has been reported with good success.[83] Some have been identified years after splenectomy.[84]

Conversion to Open Splenectomy

Splenomegaly and bleeding are the main reasons for conversion from laparoscopy to an open operation and is reported in 1.3% to 2.8% of patients.[62,80,85-87] The largest pediatric series has a 1.7% rate.[23] Higher conversion rates have been noted with larger spleens, less surgeon experience, and obese patients.[57,87,88]

Operative Time

The laparoscopic approach has uniformly been associated with somewhat longer operative times than open splenectomy.[54-56,62-64] A recent report noted a decrease in time with experience from a mean of 110 ± 36 minutes in the early period to 86 ± 35 minutes in the later period.[23] This operative time is compared with 83 minutes for open splenectomy in a previous report from the same institution.[64]

Postoperative Hospitalization

Pediatric comparative studies have consistently demonstrated a lower duration of hospitalization with the laparoscopic compared with the open technique, ranging from 2.5 to 4.9 days for the open operation and 1.3 to 3.6 days for the laparoscopic approach.[54-56,62-64] Recent studies have noted a length of stay of 1.5 to 1.8 days.[23,62,63] Our recent series of over 200 cases noted the length of hospitalization to vary by diagnosis, with hereditary spherocytosis requiring 1.23 days, ITP, 1.20 days, and sickle cell disease, 2.37 days.[23] The increased length of hospitalization in sickle cell disease is secondary to the higher incidence of complications in these patients, such as acute chest syndrome. Splenomegaly itself, which is common in hereditary spherocytosis, does not appear to affect the length of stay. An unreported benefit of the shorter length of hospitalization is the effect on the parent's ability to return to work. One study noted children return to full activity faster with laparoscopy compared with open splenectomy.[56]

Complications

Most pediatric series have had relatively few complications with laparoscopic splenectomy. A meta-analysis of adult and pediatric studies reported between 1991 and 2002 noted a complication rate of 15.5% for laparoscopic and 26.6% for open splenectomy ($P < .0001$).[89] The laparoscopic group had fewer pulmonary, wound, and infectious complications but more hemorrhagic complications when conversions for bleeding were included. A large adult comparative study noted equivalent grade I and II complications (minor, potentially life threatening) but higher grade III and IV (residual or lasting disability, death) with the open technique compared with laparoscopy.[90] Our recent review of over 200 pediatric laparoscopic splenectomies reported an overall complication rate of 11% with no wound infections or deaths.[23] Postoperative ileus, acute chest syndrome, and bleeding requiring transfusion were the most common complications. The complication rate was 22% among the children with sickle cell disease and only 8.3% among those with other conditions ($P = .0083$). This report had one symptomatic portal vein thrombosis.

Splenic vein or portal vein thrombosis is a rare complication after splenectomy but may be more common than is clinically appreciated and is particularly common in cases of splenomegaly.[91,92] A recent small adult study identified a 50% incidence of portal or splenic vein thrombosis, with splenic weight being the strongest predictor of thrombosis.[93] Another prospective study in adults identified an incidence of 4.79% and noted spleen weight over 650 g and a platelet count over 650,000/mm^3 to be associated with portal system thrombosis.[94] A pediatric prospective series noted an incidence of 5.88% with the same risk factors.[95] Most authors recommend treatment with antithrombotic and antiplatelet therapy. Of the patients with total splenic vein thrombosis, over 50% were symptomatic with fever and abdominal pain, emphasizing the need to evaluate for this condition in symptomatic patients.

Post-splenectomy Sepsis

Overwhelming post-splenectomy infection (OPSI) was initially reported by King and Shumacher in a group of five infants undergoing splenectomy for hereditary spherocytosis.[1] The actual risk of OPSI is difficult to determine because most of the data was accumulated before routine vaccinations. Data from the 1990s note the rate of OPSI between 0.13% and 8.1% in children and adolescents younger than 15 years of age compared with 0.28% to 1.9% in adults.[96-98] Most authors quote the current rate between 3.5% and 4.4%.[75,97,98] Some have also noted a higher mortality in children younger than 4 years of age (8.1%) compared with a lower rate (3.3%) in older children. Most deaths occur within 4 years of splenectomy.[99,100] The causative organism is primarily *Streptococcus pneumoniae* which has been found in 50% to 90% of all infections.[101-104] Moreover, pneumococcus is responsible for 60% of all fatal infections followed by *Haemophilus influenzae,* meningococcus, and group A *Streptococcus.*[105] Vaccinations have been shown to decrease the risk of bacteremia.[105,106] Most studies and centers utilize post-splenectomy antibiotics, usually with penicillin.

A single institution study compared two time periods.[97] The first one was prior to immunizations and antibiotics. The second era (with a 70% immunization rate and 100% antibiotic prophylaxis rate) noted a decrease in OPSI (6% to 3.8%) and mortality (3.9% to 0.9%). This study noted an age difference with a rate of infection of 13.8% for those children younger than 6 years of age compared with 0.5% for older children. Although older studies noted mortality rates of 50% with OPSI, more recent studies have reported a rate of around 10%.[97,107-109] Routine immunization against *S. pneumoniae, H. influenzae,* and meningococcus as well as postoperative antibiotic prophylaxis are recommended by most authors. Although the optimal length of antibiotic prophylaxis is unclear, the highest rate of infection appears to occur within the first 2 years.[110]

chapter 48

CONGENITAL ABDOMINAL WALL DEFECTS

Cassandra Kelleher, MD • Jacob C. Langer, MD

Gastroschisis and omphalocele are the two most common congenital abdominal wall defects. These two conditions are often diagnosed on prenatal ultrasonography and are easily differentiated by the location of the defect and the presence or absence of a sac surrounding the eviscerated bowel. There is a differential rate of associated anomalies between infants with omphalocele and gastroschisis. The risk of an associated cardiac or genetic abnormality in an infant with omphalocele approaches 50% but is much lower in neonates with gastroschisis. The long-term outcome for neonates with omphalocele is often determined by these associated anomalies. Differences between gastroschisis and omphalocele are illustrated in Figure 48-1 and summarized in Table 48-1.

Gastroschisis occurs in 1 in 4000 live births.[1] The majority of pregnancies complicated by gastroschisis are diagnosed sonographically by 20 weeks' gestation.[2] Often an ultrasound evaluation is performed because of an abnormal maternal serum α-fetoprotein level, which is universally elevated in the presence of gastroschisis. Detection of bowel loops freely floating in the amniotic fluid and a defect in the abdominal wall to the right of a normal umbilical cord insertion are diagnostic of gastroschisis.[3] An increased incidence of gastroschisis in mothers younger than 21 years of age has been widely documented.[4] There has also been a significant increase in the overall incidence of gastroschisis in all age groups over the past 2 decades.[5,6] Preterm delivery is more frequent in infants with gastroschisis, with an incidence of 28% compared with 6% of normal deliveries.[7]

Concomitant bowel atresia is the most common associated anomaly in patients with gastroschisis, with rates ranging from 6.9% to 28% in recently reported series (Table 48-2).[8,9] Gastroschisis is also one of a constellation of disorders in the limb–body wall defect syndrome, also known as the amniotic band syndrome. In this rare syndrome, thoracic wall anomalies or gastroschisis are found associated with limb abnormalities, meningocele, abnormal genitalia, variable intestinal atresias, and umbilical cord abnormalities.[10,11]

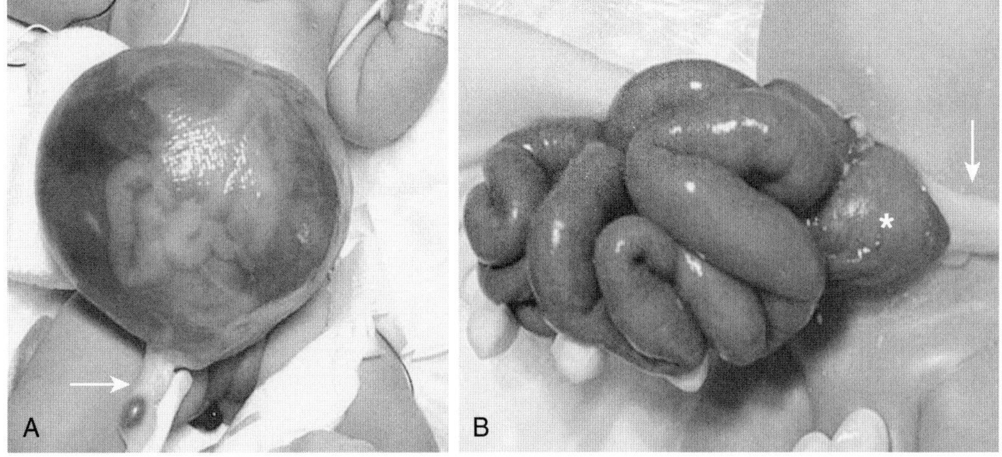

Figure 48-1. These two photographs nicely depict the differences between an omphalocele and gastroschisis. **A,** In an omphalocele both the liver and bowel can be herniated. A sac is always present and the umbilical cord (*arrow*) inserts onto the sac. Moreover, this is always a midline defect. **B,** With a gastroschisis, the liver is never herniated and a sac is absent. The location of the fascial defect is to the right of the umbilicus, and the umbilical cord (*arrow*) is attached to the umbilicus. In addition to the large and small intestine, the stomach (*asterisk*) can sometimes be herniated as well.

Table 48-1 Differentiating Characteristics between Gastroschisis and Omphalocele

Characteristic	Omphalocele	Gastroschisis
Herniated viscera	Bowel ± liver	Bowel only
Sac	Present	Absent
Associated anomalies	Common (50%)	Uncommon (<10%)
Location of defect	Umbilicus	Right of umbilicus
Mode of delivery	Vaginal/cesarean	Vaginal
Surgical management	Nonurgent	Urgent
Prognostic factors	Associated anomalies	Condition of bowel

Elevation of maternal serum α-fetoprotein is also present in many pregnancies complicated by fetal omphalocele, although not as commonly as with gastroschisis. The prenatal diagnosis of omphalocele can be made by 2D ultrasonography during the routine 18-week gestation ultrasound evaluation for dates.[2] Early first-trimester detection is possible if 3D ultrasonography is utilized. The incidence of omphalocele seen on ultrasonography at 14 to 18 weeks is as high as 1 in 1100.[12] Due to both spontaneous intrauterine fetal death and pregnancy termination, the incidence in live births is approximately 1 in 4000.[1]

Ultrasound evaluation is very useful for the detection of associated anomalies in infants with an omphalocele. An 18% to 24% incidence of cardiac anomalies is found and can be detected on fetal echocardiography.[1,12] Pulmonary hypoplasia is also commonly associated with omphalocele and may result in early respiratory distress requiring intubation and ventilatory support at the time of delivery. Recognized syndromes such as cloacal exstrophy and the pentalogy of Cantrell are diagnosed mainly on the basis of the physical examination. Chromosomal abnormalities occur in up to 48% of neonates with omphalocele.[13] Trisomy 13 and trisomy 18 are the most common. However, Down syndrome is also associated. The risk of a chromosomal abnormality is more common in infants with a central omphalocele and those containing only bowel, when compared with neonates with epigastric omphaloceles or those containing liver and bowel.[13] Infants with multiple anomalies are also more likely to have chromosomal abnormalities.

The delivery of an infant with a congenital abdominal wall defect requires prompt neonatal intervention. Immediate evaluation of respiratory and circulatory status, establishment of intravenous access, and resuscitation should be undertaken at birth. If pediatric surgical care is not available at the institution of delivery, urgent transfer should be arranged.

EMBRYOLOGY

The abdominal wall forms during the fourth week of gestation from differential growth of the embryo causing infolding in the craniocaudal and mediolateral directions. The lateral abdominal folds of the embryo meet in the anterior midline and surround the yolk sac, eventually constricting the yolk sac into a yolk stalk that becomes the site of the umbilical cord. During the sixth week of gestation, rapid growth of the intestine causes herniation of the midgut into the umbilical cord. Elongation and rotation of the midgut occurs over the ensuing 4 weeks. By week 10, the midgut has returned to the abdominal cavity and the first, second, and third portions of the duodenum and the ascending and descending colon assume their fixed, retroperitoneal positions.

An omphalocele occurs if the intestines fail to return to the abdominal cavity. Varying amounts of bowel may be contained within the omphalocele sac. Other intra-abdominal viscera including liver, bladder, stomach, ovary, and testis can also be found within the sac. The sac consists of the covering layers of the umbilical cord, which include amnion, Wharton's jelly, and peritoneum. The umbilical cord is attached to the sac itself.

The etiology of gastroschisis is less clear. One theory suggests that gastroschisis results from failure of the mesoderm to form in the anterior abdominal wall. A second theory posits that failure of the lateral folds to fuse in the midline leaves a defect to the right side of the umbilicus.[14] DeVries and associates and Hoyme and colleagues proposed that thrombosis of the right omphalomesenteric vein (umbilical vein) causes necrosis of the surrounding abdominal wall, leading to the right-sided defect.[15,16] This theory is supported by the observation that gastroschisis is sometimes associated with intestinal atresia, a condition that is also thought to be associated with an ischemic etiology.[17,18] Additionally, retrospective data have shown an increased

Table 48-2 Treatment Options in Patients with Gastroschisis and Intestinal Atresia

Study	No. Patients	Drop in	Anastomosis	Stoma
Amoury et al, 1977[93]	6		3	3
Pokorny et al, 1981[94]	5	1		4
Gornall, 1989[95]	5	1	3	1
Shah and Woolley, 1991[96]	4	3		1
Hoehner et al, 1998[97]	13		8	5
Fleet and de la Hunt, 2000[56]	10	6		4

risk of gastroschisis and intestinal atresia with maternal use of vasoconstrictive drugs such as ephedrine, pseudoephedrine, or cocaine, as well as with smoking.[19] In-utero rupture of an omphalocele has also been proposed as a mechanism of gastroschisis formation.[20,21] Most patients with congenital abdominal wall defects have some form of rotation abnormality, because the herniated bowel does not undergo the normal process of rotation and is not fixed in the appropriate retroperitoneal position during development.

GASTROSCHISIS

Perinatal Care

The optimal mode of delivery for fetuses with gastroschisis has been debated for many years. Proponents of routine cesarean delivery argue that the process of vaginal birth results in injury to the exposed bowel. However, the literature would suggest that both vaginal delivery and cesarean section are safe.[22] A recent meta-analysis by Segel and coworkers failed to demonstrate a difference in outcomes for infants delivered by cesarean section or vaginally.[23] Therefore, the delivery method of a neonate with gastroschisis should be at the discretion of the obstetrician and the mother, with cesarean section reserved for obstetric indications or fetal distress.

Early delivery of the fetus with gastroschisis has been advocated to limit exposure of the bowel to amniotic fluid in an attempt to reduce the inflammatory peel on the surface of the bowel. Poor motility of the bowel is thought to be related to exposure to the amniotic fluid and altered bowel wall cellular and extracellular matrix composition.[24,25] Interleukin-6, interleukin-8, and ferritin are elevated in the amniotic fluid in fetuses with gastroschisis when compared with controls.[26] Amniotic fluid cytokines and other proinflammatory mediators have been shown to damage the myenteric nerve plexus and interstitial cells of Cajal in animal models of gastroschisis.[27,28] Damage to the pacemaker cells and nerve plexuses may contribute to the profound dysmotility and malabsorption seen in patients with gastroschisis. Bowel edema and peel formation increase as pregnancy progresses, most significantly if the gastroschisis defect constricts venous outflow from the herniated bowel.[29] Early delivery may mitigate these effects, but the literature is mixed in terms of the benefit of preterm delivery. A recent randomized trial showed a shorter time to full enteral feeding or shorter hospital stay after induced early delivery.[30] Low birth weight does seem to impact outcome, with neonates weighing less than 2 kg having increased time to full enteral feeding, an increased number of ventilated days, and an increased length of parenteral nutrition compared with those weighing more than 2 kg.[31]

Some authors advocate selective preterm delivery based on the appearance of bowel distention and thickening on prenatal ultrasonography. The presence of dilated fetal bowel has been shown to correlate with poorer outcome, including fetal distress and demise in some series but not in others.[32-36] One confounding factor in the use of bowel dilatation to predict outcome is the lack of a common definition of "dilated," with values ranging from 7 to 25 mm being considered abnormal. The timing of fetal ultrasonography and bowel measurements also lack standardization. The presence of bowel atresia has also been correlated with worsening outcome by some authors but not by others.[37,38] Among those who advocate preterm delivery, there are some who suggest that delivery be done by routine cesarean section. Others attempt induction of labor at 36 to 37 weeks' gestation. We have found that labor can be successfully induced in gastroschisis pregnancies in a high percentage of cases, probably because of the inherent tendency toward preterm labor.[11] Most authors advocate delivery at a tertiary perinatal center so as to provide immediate access to neonatal and pediatric surgical expertise.

Neonatal Resuscitation and Management

Neonates with gastroschisis have significant evaporative water losses from the open abdominal cavity and exposed bowel. Appropriate intravenous access should be obtained and fluid resuscitation begun before transport to a tertiary referral center, if necessary. Nasogastric or orogastric decompression is important to prevent undue distention of the stomach and intestine. The herniated bowel should be wrapped in warm saline-soaked gauze and placed in a central position on the abdominal wall. The child should be positioned on the right side to prevent kinking of the mesentery and resultant bowel ischemia. The bowel should be wrapped with plastic wrap or the infant placed with the bowel and legs in a plastic bag to reduce evaporative losses and improve temperature homeostasis (Fig. 48-2). Although gastroschisis most often is an isolated anomaly, thorough examination of the neonate should be undertaken to exclude the coexistence of other

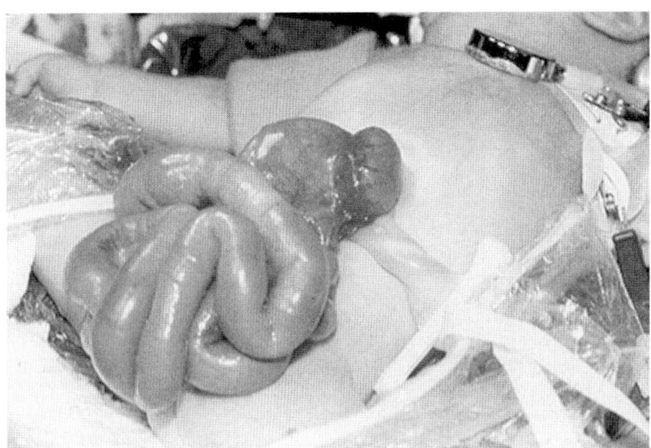

Figure 48-2. Photograph of a neonate with gastroschisis who has been transported wrapped with a bowel bag. The bag has been untied to allow inspection of the herniated bowel.

anomalies. In addition, the bowel must be carefully examined in a search for evidence of intestinal atresia, necrosis, or perforation.

Surgical Management

Surgical management of gastroschisis varies from center to center. The primary goal is to return the viscera to the abdominal cavity while minimizing the risk of damage to the viscera due to direct trauma or to increased intra-abdominal pressure. Options include silo placement, serial reductions, and delayed abdominal wall closure, primary reduction with operative closure, and primary or delayed reduction with umbilical cord closure. In addition, the timing and location of surgical intervention is controversial, ranging from immediate repair in the delivery room, to reduction and closure in the neonatal intensive care unit, to surgical closure in the operating room.[39,40] In all cases, inspection of the bowel for obstructing bands, perforation, or atresia should be undertaken. Bands crossing the bowel loops should be lysed before silo placement or primary abdominal closure to avoid subsequent bowel obstruction.

Because intestinal hypomotility is almost universally present in children with gastroschisis, central venous access should be established early. Options include a cuffed Broviac catheter or a peripherally inserted central catheter line.

Primary Closure

Historically, urgent primary closure of gastroschisis was advocated in all cases. This method of treatment is still commonly practiced for neonates in whom full reduction of the herniated viscera is thought to be possible. The procedure has traditionally been done in the operating room, but more recently some authors have advocated primary closure at the bedside without general anesthesia.[40] Multiple methods of closure have been described for children in whom primary fascial closure cannot be achieved. Many of these incorporate the umbilicus as an allograft.[41,42] Prosthetic options include nonabsorbable mesh or bioprosthetic materials such as dura or porcine small intestinal submucosa (Surgisis, Cook, Inc., Bloomington, IN). Once the fascial closure is completed, skin flaps can be mobilized to cover the abdominal wall closure. Breakdown of these flaps due to tension can occasionally occur. Thought can be given to leaving a skin defect and allowing healing by secondary intention.

Traditionally, most surgeons have excised the umbilicus during gastroschisis repair. However, many cases can be repaired with preservation of the umbilicus with an excellent cosmetic result (Fig. 48-3).[43] Another option in selected cases is to reduce the bowel and place a piece of Silastic sheeting under the abdominal wall to prevent evisceration (Fig. 48-4). This technique is useful in infants when the surgeon is concerned about worsening the pulmonary function with fascial and skin closure. The Silastic sheet is removed in 4 to 5 days, and the abdominal wall and skin are closed.

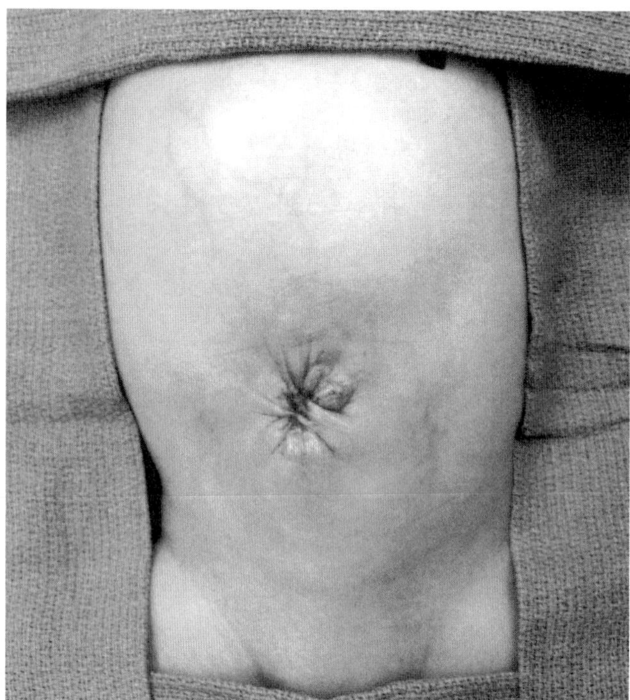

Figure 48-3. Nice cosmetic result after gastroschisis repair in which the umbilicus was preserved.

Intra-abdominal pressure, measured either as intravesical pressure using a bladder catheter or as intragastric pressure using the nasogastric tube, can sometimes be used to guide the surgeon during reduction. Pressures higher than 10 to 15 mm Hg indicate an elevated intra-abdominal pressure and are correlated with decreased perfusion to the kidneys and bowel.[44] Pressures higher than 20 mm Hg can lead to renal failure and bowel ischemia with ensuing infarction.[45] Similarly, an increase in central venous pressure greater than 4 mm Hg has been correlated with the need for silo placement or patch closure during attempted primary repair.[46] In the situation in which bladder pressure is higher than 20 mm Hg before or during visceral reduction, some authors advocate placing a silo or patch to maintain pressures less than 20 mm Hg.[47,48] Splanchnic perfusion pressure, defined as the difference between mean arterial pressure and intra-abdominal pressure, has also been used to guide surgeons during reduction, with a splanchnic perfusion pressure less than 44 mm Hg indicating decreased blood flow and the need for silo placement.[49]

Staged Closure

For many years, primary closure of gastroschisis was attempted in all cases. Multiple retrospective reviews of primary versus staged closure can be found in the literature, most of which documented better outcomes in those patients who underwent primary closure. However, this finding probably represents selection bias because those patients with the most intestinal damage were the most likely to require staged closure

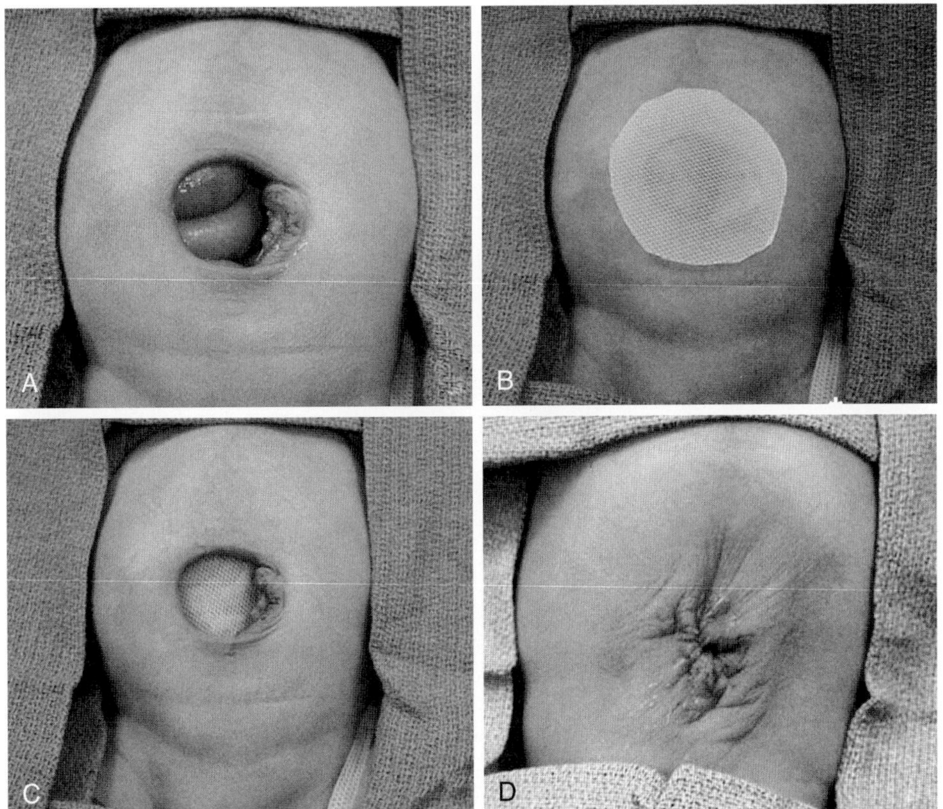

Figure 48-4. In selected cases, it may be possible to reduce the bowel back into the abdominal cavity (**A**), but the surgeon is concerned about worsening pulmonary function if the fascia and skin are closed. Therefore, one technique is to cut a circular piece of Silastic sheeting (**B**) and place it in the abdomen and on top of the reduced intestine (**C**). Four to 5 days later, after the neonate has become more stable and the pulmonary function has improved, the Silastic sheet is removed and the fascia and the skin are closed (**D**).

and were also the most likely to have a poor outcome. Recent data from the Canadian Pediatric Surgeons Network (CAPSNet) database confirm these thoughts, suggesting that infants who are able to undergo immediate primary reduction and closure have a shorter length of parenteral nutrition use and total length of stay when compared with those who required staged reduction and delayed repair.[37]

Originally, staged closure consisted of placing the bowel into a silo constructed of Silastic sheets sewn together and sutured to the abdominal wall. More recent introduction of a prefabricated silo with a circular spring that can be placed into the fascial opening, without the need for sutures or general anesthesia, has made it possible to insert the silo in the delivery room or at the bedside in the neonatal unit (Fig. 48-5). In either case, the bowel is reduced once to twice daily into the abdominal cavity as the silo is shortened by sequential ligation. When the eviscerated contents are entirely reduced, the definitive closure can be performed. This process usually takes between 1 and 14 days, depending on the condition of the bowel and the infant.

Over the past 2 decades, the routine use of a preformed silo with delayed closure of the abdominal wall defect has increasingly come into favor, with the theory being that avoidance of high intra-abdominal pressure will avoid ischemic injury to the viscera and permit earlier extubation. One study reported fewer days on mechanical ventilation for patients undergoing staged silo reduction when compared with primary closure.[50] However, there was no difference found in time to full feeds or days on parenteral nutrition. Another report showed a similar time to full enteral feedings but also showed that primary closure was associated with the need for higher mean airway pressures, oxygen requirement, vasopressor requirement, and decreased urine output in patients treated with primary closure.[51] In a prospective study using historical controls, our group demonstrated that the routine use of a spring-loaded silo was associated with a shorter time on the ventilator, lower postoperative airway pressures, shorter hospital stay, lower cost, and lower risk of complications.[52] In a recent randomized multicenter trial, the routine use of the spring-loaded silo was associated with a trend toward fewer days on the ventilator, with a similar incidence of other outcomes.[53] The main advantage of this approach would therefore appear to be repair of the defect in a more controlled and elective environment.

Definitive closure in the operating room consists of raising skin flaps around the fascial defect and primary fascial closure in the horizontal direction. Closure of the skin in a linear fashion creates a "keyhole" appearance with a horizontal scar to the right of the umbilicus. Some surgeons advocate a purse-string suture of the skin around the umbilicus to create a circular scar with improved cosmesis. Recently, the "plastic

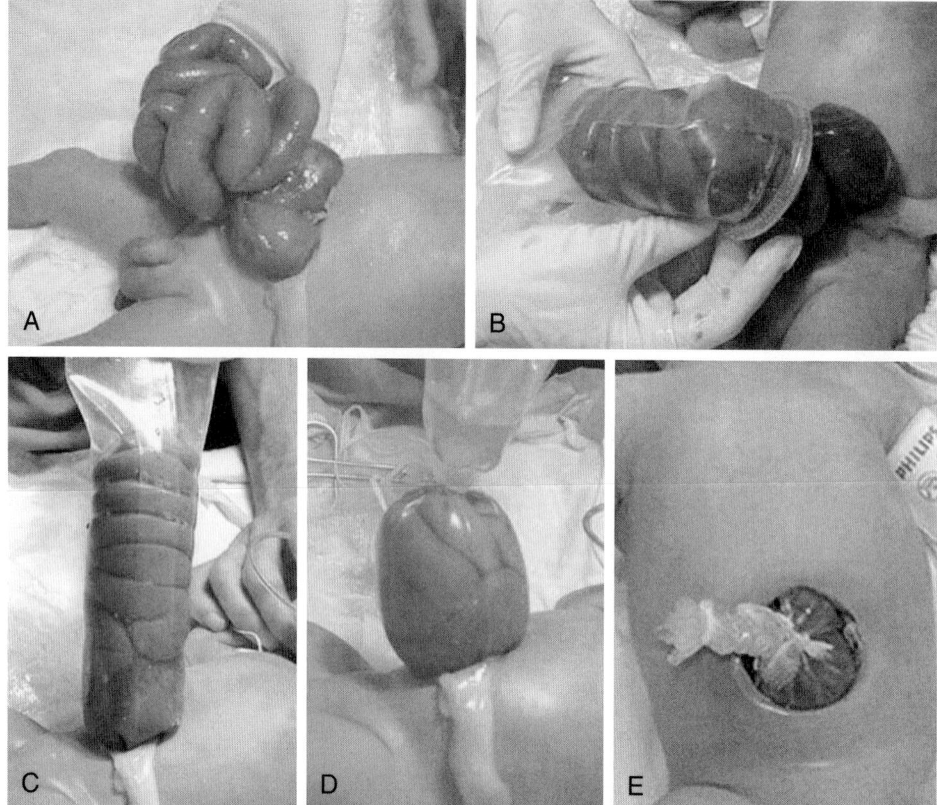

Figure 48-5. The use of a spring-loaded prefabricated silo is shown in these photographs. **A,** The gastroschisis defect is seen. **B,** An appropriate-sized spring-loaded silo is then placed over the eviscerated intestine. **C,** The ring of the silo has been positioned under the fascial defect and attached to an overhead support to keep the bowel from torquing, which may result in intestinal ischemia. **D,** Gradual reduction of the silo is performed. **E,** Finally, the bowel has been completely returned to the abdominal cavity and the neonate is ready for transport to the operating room for closure of the fascia and skin.

closure" method has been introduced in which the umbilical cord, if not too macerated or dried out, is tailored to fill the gastroschisis defect and is then covered with an adhesive dressing.[54] If the umbilical cord is not salvageable, the bowel can be directly covered with the dressing. In-growth of granulation tissue and epithelialization occurs over time. With this technique, an operation can be avoided entirely in many infants. Residual ventral hernia rates are reported to be 60% to 84%, the majority of which close spontaneously.[55]

Management of Associated Intestinal Atresia

Up to 10% of neonates with gastroschisis will have an associated atresia, most commonly jejunal or ileal. In a recent review of 4344 infants with gastroschisis, a 5% incidence of small bowel atresia and a 2% incidence of large bowel atresia was found.[8] These atresias can be treated at the time of abdominal wall closure with resection and primary anastomosis. If the condition of the bowel makes primary anastomosis inadvisable, the bowel can be reduced with the atresia intact and repair can be undertaken 4 to 6 weeks after the initial abdominal wall closure. Some surgeons have chosen to create a stoma in cases of atresia, particularly in the case of distal atresias.[56] If perforation is encountered, the perforated segment can be resected with primary anastomosis if the bowel inflammation is minimal. Alternatively, an ostomy can be created and primary closure undertaken with closure of the ostomy at a later date. In cases in which perforation has occurred and primary closure is impossible, a silo can be applied and the area of perforation exteriorized through a hole in the silo. Once the bowel has been reduced, a formal stoma can be created at the time of abdominal wall closure. There is no consensus in the literature about the optimal management of these complicated problems (see Table 48-2).

Intestinal atresia should be differentiated from "vanishing bowel" in infants with gastroschisis. This condition is usually associated with a very small abdominal wall defect and is characterized by necrosis and disappearance of some or all of the intestine (Fig. 48-6). Although this is a rare finding, it usually results in short bowel syndrome.

Postoperative Course

Gastroschisis is associated with abnormal intestinal motility and nutrient absorption, both of which gradually improve over time in most patients. Introduction of enteral feeding is often delayed for weeks while awaiting return of bowel function. During the period of dysmotility, nasogastric decompression and parenteral nutrition is required. When the nasogastric output is

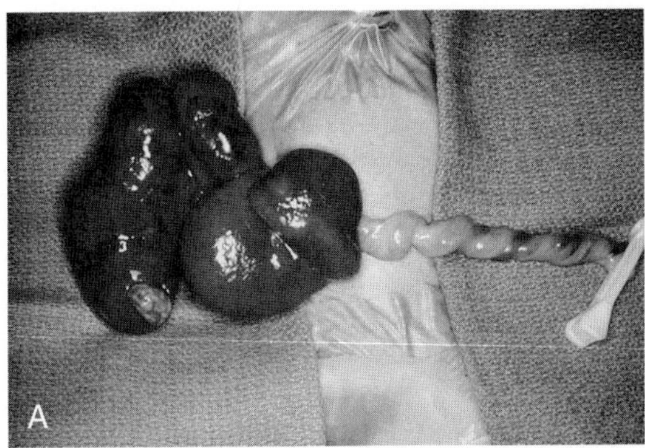
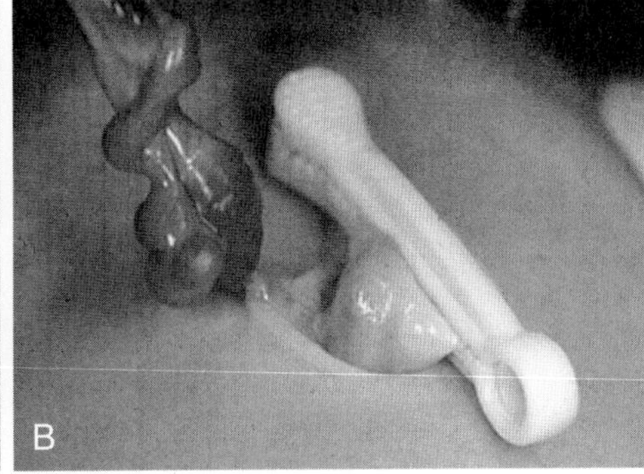

Figure 48-6. **A** and **B**, These two photographs show different neonates with the prenatal diagnosis of gastroschisis. In each instance, the herniated intestine has died. At exploration, each patient was found to have short bowel syndrome due to very little small intestine.

no longer bilious and bowel activity has begun, enteral feeds can be started and slowly advanced. Often there is initial intolerance with the need for slow progression of feeds. Holding feeds and restarting them a few days later due to feeding intolerance is often needed as well. Because progression to full enteral feeding can take weeks, secure central venous access is important. We also advocate early oral stimulation, because the sucking-swallowing reflex can be lost while awaiting bowel function.

The treatment of gastrointestinal dysmotility with prokinetics is often used to hasten initiation of feeding or time to full feeding. However, there is little documentation in the literature to support their use. Commonly utilized prokinetics include erythromycin, metoclopramide, domperidone, and cisapride. In a rabbit model of gastroschisis, only cisapride improved contractility of newborn intestine, whereas erythromycin improved motility in control adult tissue only.[57] A randomized controlled trial of erythromycin versus placebo similarly showed that enterally administered erythromycin did not improve time to achieve full enteral feedings over placebo.[58] However, a similar randomized trial examining the use of cisapride in postoperative neonates, most of whom had gastroschisis, did show a beneficial effect.[59] Cisapride is available on a compassionate use basis in North America. We have had success with its use in infants with severe dysmotility who had not responded to other agents.

A number of authors have recently attempted to stratify patients with gastroschisis according to risk, finding that intestinal damage predicts a more prolonged hospital course and increased morbidity and mortality. In one review of 103 infants with gastroschisis, the authors were able to document a significant increase in complications and mortality in those infants with a complex anomaly defined as the presence of atresia, volvulus, necrotic bowel segment or perforation. In the complex group, length of mechanical ventilation, time to the initiation and to full enteral feedings, infectious complications, and mortality (28% vs. 0%) were all increased when compared with the infants with simple conditions.[60] Using a classification of simple and complex conditions, one group showed similar increased morbidity and mortality in infants with complex gastroschisis in a review of 4344 patients.[8,61] Also, another study found a similar increased incidence of central venous catheter–related sepsis, a longer time to full enteral feeding, and a longer hospital stay in infants with gastroschisis complicated by atresia or necrotic bowel.[62] In a single institutional review, another group found that a significantly increased number of patients with complex gastroschisis required long-term enteral access for feeding difficulties.[63] In an additional analysis of 2003 inpatient data, the authors verified a risk stratification index that identifies patients with gastroschisis who are at the highest risk for death.[64] Infants with gastroschisis complicated by intestinal atresia, necrotizing enterocolitis, cardiac disease, or pulmonary hypoplasia/bronchopulmonary dysplasia are at a 2- to 14-fold increased risk of death, respectively. The ability to risk-stratify gastroschisis patients with respect to increased morbidity and mortality has utility in counseling families, predicting hospital utilization, and identifying a group of patients who would benefit from further strategies to improve outcomes.

Long-Term Outcomes

Long-term outcomes for patients born with gastroschisis are generally excellent. The presence of bowel atresia is the most important prognostic determinant for a poor outcome.[8,62,65] Patients with bowel atresia are significantly more likely to require prolonged parenteral nutrition with the associated risks of total parenteral nutrition–related cholestatic liver disease and central line–related sepsis. These complications lead to a 20-fold increased risk of death when compared with a patient without associated atresia.[62]

Necrotizing enterocolitis has been encountered in full-term infants with gastroschisis in higher than expected frequencies (up to 18.5%).[66,67] Significant bowel loss from necrotizing enterocolitis can predispose patients to short bowel syndrome and its associated hepatic and septic complications. On the other hand, another group found that in the patients with necrotizing enterocolitis after gastroschisis the clinical course was often uncomplicated.[66] There is a report suggesting that infants fed with breast milk have a lower incidence of necrotizing enterocolitis after gastroschisis repair than those infants fed with formula.[67]

Cryptorchidism is associated with gastroschisis with an incidence of 15% to 30%.[68,69] However, it is unclear from the literature if this is due to the testis being outside the abdomen through the abdominal wall defect, leading to testicular maldescent, or if the prematurity associated with gastroschisis is responsible.[68] Several retrospective analyses have shown that replacement of the herniated testis into the abdominal cavity will result in normal testicular descent into the scrotum in the majority of cases.[69,70] Our current practice is to allow a trial of spontaneous testicular descent after placement of the testis into the abdominal cavity. We then proceed with orchidopexy if the testis remains undescended by 1 year of age.

The majority of patients with gastroschisis will achieve normal growth and development after an initial catch-up period in early childhood.[9,71] If the umbilicus is sacrificed during the repair of the gastroschisis defect, up to 60% of children report psychosocial stress from the lack of an umbilicus.[71] Umbilical reconstruction can be undertaken when the child is healthy, if it is desired by the child or parents.

OMPHALOCELE

Perinatal Care

The delivery of patients with omphalocele, like those with gastroschisis, should be dictated by obstetric considerations, because neither vaginal delivery nor cesarean section has been shown to be superior.[72] However, despite the lack of data, most practitioners choose to deliver neonates with giant omphaloceles by cesarean section because of the fear of liver injury. In addition, most authors advocate delivery at a tertiary perinatal center to allow immediate access to neonatal and pediatric surgical expertise.

Neonatal Resuscitation and Management

After delivery, a thorough search for associated anomalies should be undertaken. The high risk of associated cardiac defects mandates a directed cardiac evaluation, including auscultation, four-limb blood pressures, and peripheral pulse examination. If there is suspicion of a cardiac defect, echocardiography should be obtained. Renal abnormalities can be detected on abdominal ultrasonography. Neonatal hypoglycemia should alert the practitioner of the possibility of Beckwith-Weidemann syndrome. Blood samples for genetic evaluation should be obtained, if indicated.

In preparing infants with omphalocele for transport, risks arising from associated anomalies should be specifically addressed. Adequate intravenous access should be obtained and fluid resuscitation begun. Infants with omphalocele do not have as significant fluid and temperature losses as those with gastroschisis but the losses are higher than those with an intact abdominal wall. The omphalocele itself can be dressed with saline-soaked gauze and an impervious dressing to minimize these losses. A nasogastric or orogastric tube should be inserted and placed to suction or gravity drainage. In some cases, the omphalocele sac may have ruptured either prenatally during delivery or postnatally (Fig. 48-7). In this situation, the surgical management should be the same as described for the infant with gastroschisis.

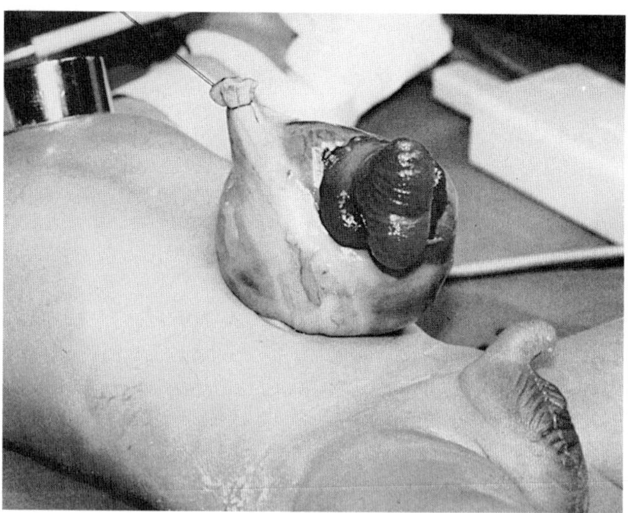

Figure 48-7. Neonate with an omphalocele sac that ruptured during delivery. Treatment was similar to that for gastroschisis, and a silo was constructed.

Surgical Management

Primary Closure

Treatment options in infants with omphalocele depend on the size of the defect, gestational age, and the presence of associated anomalies. In infants with small defects, the loss of abdominal domain may not be excessive and primary closure may be appropriate. This option is predicated on the ability of the patient to withstand an operation if associated cardiac disease is present. Primary closure consists of excision of the omphalocele sac and closure of the fascia and skin over the abdominal contents. It is not unusual for an omphalomesenteric duct remnant to be associated with a small omphalocele (Fig. 48-8). When dealing with a medium-sized omphalocele, care must be taken when excising the portion of the sac covering the liver, because the hepatic veins are located just under the epithelium/sac interface in the midline and can be inadvertently injured. Also, the sac is often adherent to the liver itself and significant hemorrhage can result from tears in Glissen's capsule. In this situation, it is best to leave part of the sac on the liver. The inferior portion of the sac covering the bladder can be quite thin, and excision of the sac in this area can lead to inadvertent bladder injury. As with gastroschisis, intra-abdominal pressure can be elevated during reduction, leading to abdominal compartment syndrome. Measurement of intra-abdominal pressure can be very useful to guide the surgeon. When reducing the contents, attention must be given to the position of the hepatic veins because kinking will result in acute obstruction.

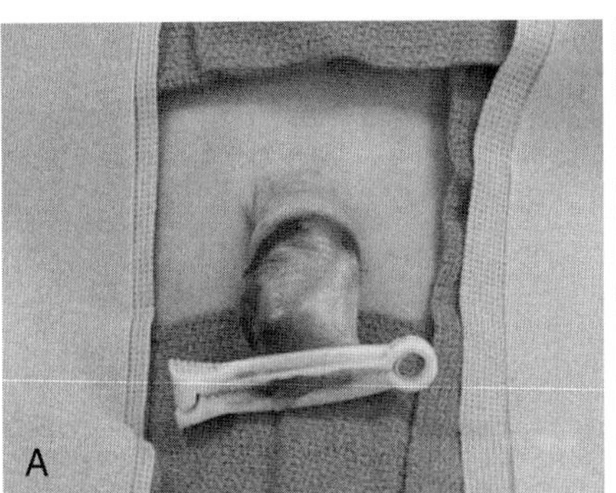

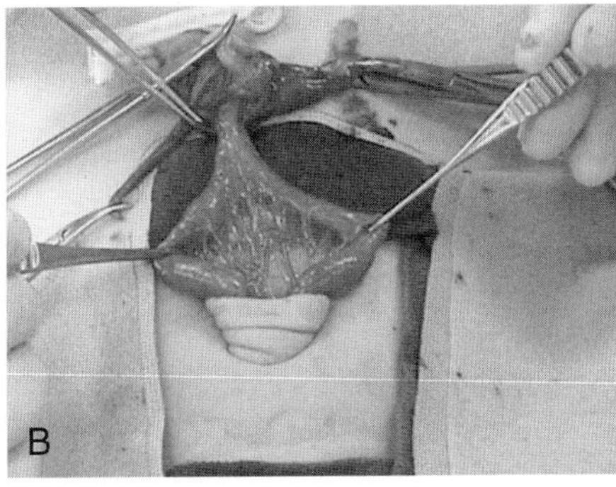

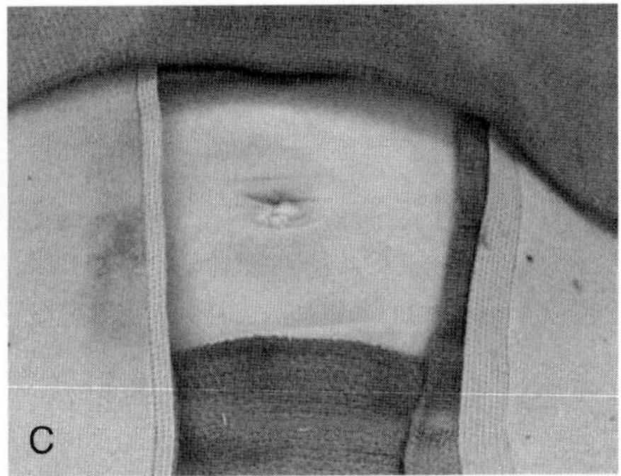

Figure 48-8. In patients with small omphaloceles (**A**), it is not unusual for an omphalomesenteric duct remnant to be found (**B**). **C**, The diverticulum was excised primarily and the fascia and skin closed. This neonate recovered uneventfully.

In many cases, the defect is large and the loss of domain in the peritoneal cavity prevents primary closure without an undue increase in intra-abdominal pressure (Fig. 48-9). Multiple methods have been proposed to obtain primary fascial closure of the abdominal wall in this setting. In the 1950s, Kearns and Clarke described a "cutis graft" composed of dermis and anterior rectus fascia.[73] Bilateral flaps that mobilize the muscle, fascia, and skin of the abdominal wall toward the midline and allow midline fascial closure have been used successfully.[74,75] Component separation at the level of the external oblique has also been described.[76] More recent approaches include the use of tissue expanders that are placed inside the abdominal cavity to reduce abdominovisceral disproportion.[77] Volume is added to the tissue expander over time until a primary fascial closure can be performed.

Some surgeons prefer to place a patch in the abdominal wall and close the skin over the patch. Experience with nonabsorbable materials such as Marlex, polypropylene mesh, and Gore-Tex have resulted in high rates of infection requiring removal of the mesh.[78] Recent introduction of bioabsorbable materials such as small intestine submucosa, dura, or human acellular dermis may represent promising alternatives.[79,80]

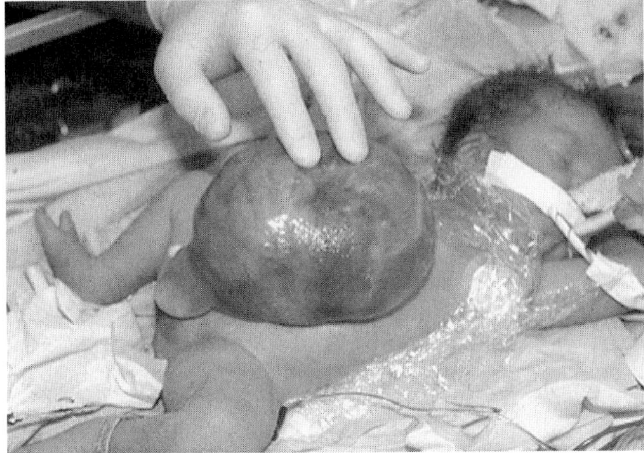

Figure 48-9. This neonate was born with a large omphalocele. As is evident, the abdominal cavity is quite small. Primary closure is not possible in such a patient.

Staged Closure

Historically, children with large omphaloceles were managed using skin flaps that were mobilized to cover the exposed viscera, leaving a large ventral hernia that would be closed in the future.[81,82] In 1967, Schuster first described the use of a silicone plastic "silo" to provide staged reduction for children with omphalocele.[83] With this approach, the infant is taken to the operating theater and the sac of the omphalocele is excised. Once the omphalocele sac has been removed, a Silastic silo can be sewn to the rectus fascia (Fig. 48-10A). In most instances, a short circumferential skin flap is raised so that the silo is sewn to the fascia only. Alternatively, the silo can be sewn to the full thickness of the abdominal wall. In our experience, the use of preformed spring-loaded silos in this setting is usually unsuccessful, owing to the relatively large size of the defect that prevents the silo from remaining in place. For moderate-sized omphaloceles with a relatively thick sac, sequential ligation of the sac itself can be used for gradual reduction of the viscera. Serial reductions, similar to that for gastroschisis, are performed on a once- to twice-daily schedule until definitive closure can be obtained. At this time, the infant is returned to the operating theater for definitive closure of the defect. If the fascial edges cannot be approximated at this time, prosthetic closure can be utilized (see Fig. 48-10B, C).

"Escharotic therapy," which results in gradual epithelialization of the omphalocele sac, is another form of staged closure that can be used for neonates who cannot tolerate operation due to prematurity, pulmonary hypoplasia, congenital heart disease, or other anomalies. Historically, mercurochrome was used as both a scarificant and a disinfectant (Fig. 48-11). Reports of deaths due to mercury poisoning led to abandonment of this treatment option.[84] Other options have included iodine, polymer membrane, silver sulfadiazine, and Nystatin powder. It usually takes many months for the sac to granulate and epithelialize (Fig. 48-12). Once that has occurred and the infant is stable enough to undergo anesthesia and surgery, the remaining ventral hernia can be repaired by one of the previously mentioned methods, usually requiring use of prosthetic mesh with skin flap coverage, especially

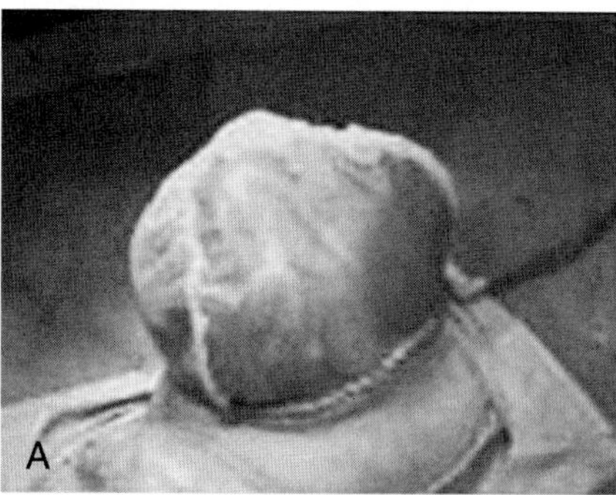

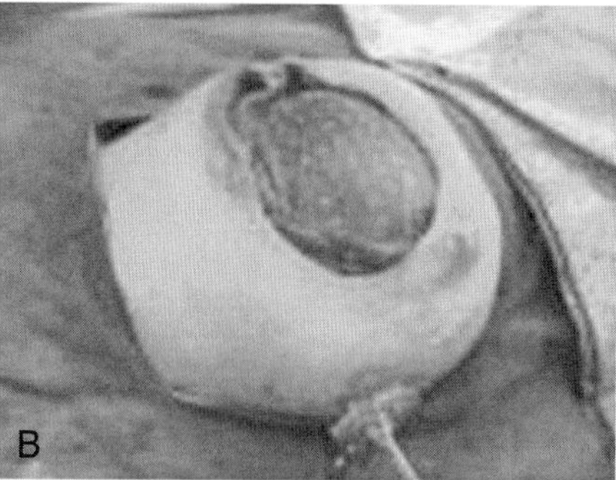

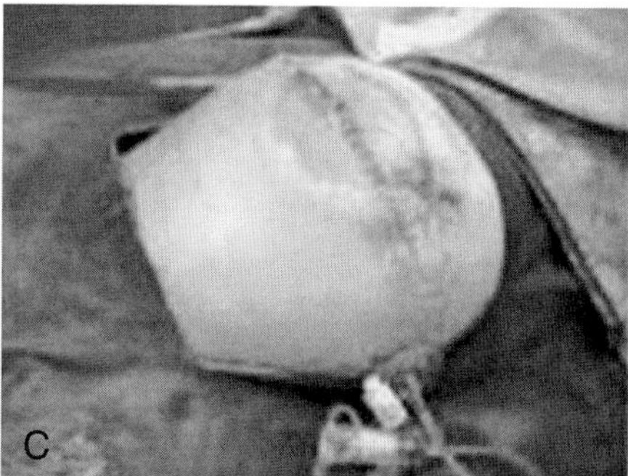

Figure 48-10. **A,** A Silastic silo has been sewn to the rectus fascia in this neonate with a large omphalocele. **B,** Serial reductions have been performed once or twice daily until the bowel has been reduced into the abdominal cavity. **C,** At that time, the silo is removed and fascia and skin are closed (if possible). If not, the skin is closed and the fascial defect is left open.

at the upper end of the defect. Again, tissue expanders have been used to create an abdominal cavity big enough to house the viscera (Fig. 48-13).[85]

Postoperative Course

If primary closure has been accomplished, the majority of patients will require mechanical ventilation for a number of days postoperatively. During this time, the abdominal wall and bowel wall edema will resolve and the intra-abdominal pressure will decrease. A nasogastric tube should be utilized for gastric decompression. Feeding can begin when the nasogastric tube output is no longer bilious, the volume is minimal, and bowel activity has occurred. Abdominal distention should have resolved by the time bowel function has returned. Antibiotics are administered postoperatively for 48 hours unless there are signs of wound infection, in which case they are continued. If a hernia develops, closure is usually possible after 1 year of age. A prosthetic mesh may be necessary in cases of large fascial defects.

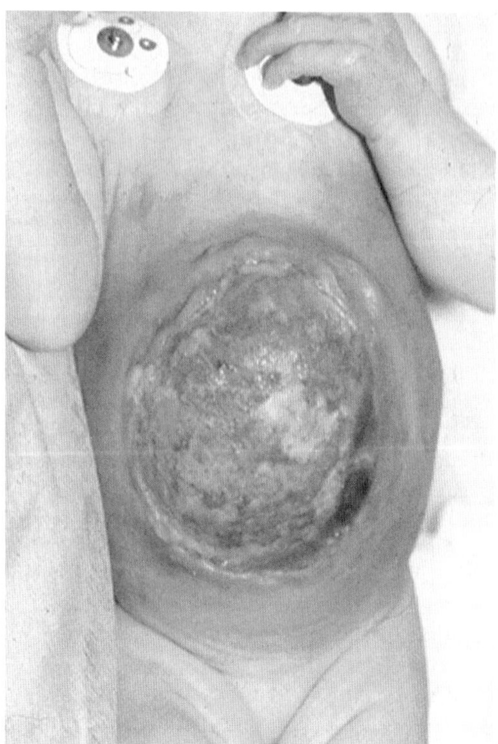

Figure 48-11. Photograph of an infant with a large omphalocele that was treated by scarification using mercurochrome. Note the intense inflammation on the abdominal wall surrounding the scarred sac. Reports of death due to mercury poisoning led to abandonment of this method.

The method of closure (primary, staged with delayed primary closure or prosthetic mesh) has not been shown to affect length of hospital stay. The time to resumption of enteral feeding, however, may be shorter with primary closure.[86] In a review of omphalocele treatment at one institution, the authors reported a 12% incidence of complications of increased intra-abdominal pressure after closure, including acute hepatic congestion requiring reoperation, renal failure requiring dialysis, and bowel infarction.[87] In this retrospective review, wound complications including skin and fascial dehiscence occurred in up to 25% of patients undergoing operative closure. It is likely that careful attention to avoiding excessive elevation in intra-abdominal pressure can minimize these types of complications.

Long-Term Outcomes

Most infants with a small omphalocele recover well and do not have any long-term issues. A number of long-term medical problems occur in patients with larger omphaloceles. These include gastroesophageal reflux, pulmonary insufficiency, recurrent lung infections or asthma, and feeding difficulty with failure to thrive.[88] In 23 patients with omphalocele, 43% were found to have gastroesophageal reflux disease by esophageal biopsy or pH monitoring. Patients younger than 2 years old had an increased rate of reflux compared with those older than 2 years of age. Patients with large defects also had an increased rate of reflux.[89] Only one of these children required a fundoplication, suggesting that reflux improves as the child ages. In children who are managed with escharotic therapy and who have persistent severe reflux, the fundoplication should be done at the time of definitive abdominal wall closure.

Feeding difficulties can occur in 60% of infants with a giant omphalocele.[88] Many of these children

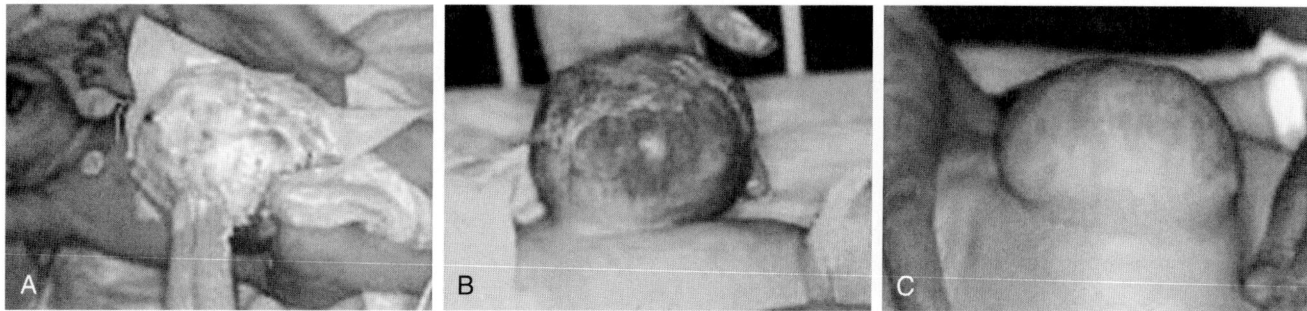

Figure 48-12. **A,** Options for scarification of the omphalocele sac include iodine, nystatin powder, polymer membrane, and sulfadiazine (shown above). **B,** Although it may take many months for the sac to granulate and epithelialize, eventually this does occur. **C,** The remaining ventral hernia can be repaired in multiple stages.

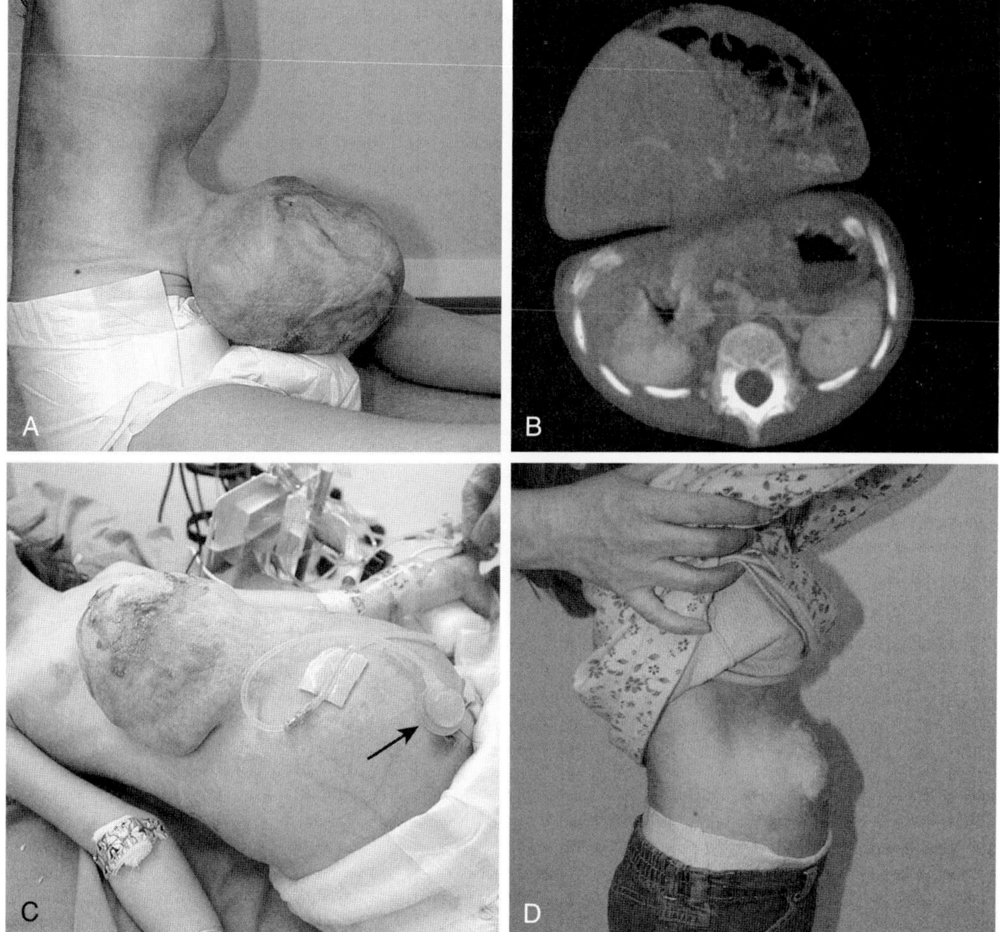

Figure 48-13. A 4-year-old girl was born with a number of anomalies including a diaphragmatic hernia, pulmonary hypoplasia and pulmonary hypertension, atrial septal defect, and a large omphalocele. She underwent repair of the diaphragmatic hernia shortly after birth, but no attempt was made to repair the large omphalocele because of its massive size and the disproportion between the extraperitoneal viscera and the peritoneal cavity. **A** and **B,** At 4 years of age, she was found to have loss of abdominal domain, a narrow neck to the omphalocele sac, and most of the viscera in the sac. **C,** She underwent placement of an intraperitoneal tissue expander in the pelvis. As an outpatient, the tissue expander was gradually filled to 900 mL of volume, through a catheter emanating from the expander (*arrow*). Over time, it was possible to expand the peritoneal cavity to the point that the abdominal muscles and fascia could be approximated. However, a biosynthetic patch was needed to complete the fascial closure. **D,** She has recovered uneventfully and has a very reasonable appearing abdomen. (A and B reprinted with permission from Foglia R, Kane A, Becker D, et al: Management of giant omphalocele with rapid creation of abdominal domain. J Pediatr Surg 41:704-709, 2006. Photos courtesy of Dr. Robert Foglia.)

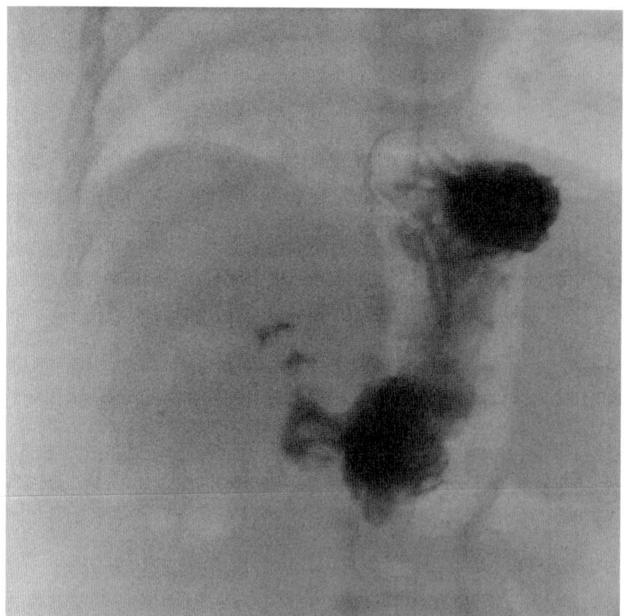

Figure 48-14. This upper gastrointestinal study in an infant born with a large omphalocele shows the stomach to be situated in the middle of the abdomen with a longitudinal rather than a horizontal orientation.

may require gastrostomy feeding. These difficulties seem to resolve by childhood, with height and weight measurements becoming similar to those of their peer group.[90] The respiratory insufficiency associated with giant omphaloceles may be secondary to abnormal thoracic development with a narrow thorax and small lung area leading to pulmonary hypoplasia.[91] Prolonged respiratory difficulties can occur in up to 20% of infants with giant omphaloceles, leading to increased time of mechanical ventilation and the need for supplemental oxygen during the neonatal period.[91] In a study looking at the long-term cardiopulmonary consequences of large abdominal wall defects, lung volumes and oxygen consumption were found to be normal.[92] Exercise tolerance, however, was reduced, possibly owing to a more sedentary lifestyle.

Many of the intra-abdominal organs in infants with omphalocele will be abnormally positioned. The liver sits in a medial position with the hepatic veins in variable locations. The stomach is also usually in the middle of the abdomen with a longitudinal rather than a horizontal orientation (Fig. 48-14). Rotation abnormalities of the bowel will also be present. When reoperation is necessary in patients with a previous omphalocele repair, the atypical organ position should be anticipated.

chapter 49

UMBILICAL AND OTHER ABDOMINAL WALL HERNIAS

Thomas R. Weber, MD

UMBILICAL HERNIA

Umbilical hernia is a common disorder in children that pediatric and general surgeons are frequently asked to evaluate and treat. Although the hernia defect is present at birth, unlike other hernias of childhood an umbilical hernia may resolve without the need for an operation. However, these hernias do not always resolve, and complications can develop that require an emergency operation. An understanding of the embryology, anatomy, incidence, natural history, and complications is important to any surgeon managing umbilical hernias in children.

Embryology

The 5-week embryo has a body stalk and yolk sac that enter the ventral aspect of the developing abdominal wall at the site of the umbilical cord. The omphalomesenteric duct forms from the yolk sac, whereas mesenchyme from the stalk forms the umbilical vessels. These structures enter the abdomen through the umbilical ring. The umbilical cord usually consists of two arteries, one vein, the omphalomesenteric duct and urachal remnants, and connective tissue.

After birth, closure of the umbilical ring is the result of complex interactions of lateral body wall folding in a medial direction, fusion of the rectus abdominis muscles into the linea alba, and umbilical orifice contraction aided by elastic fibers from the obliterated umbilical arteries. Fibrous proliferation of surrounding lateral connective tissue plates and mechanical stress from rectus muscle tension may also aid in closure.

Anatomy

Although "direct" and "indirect" umbilical hernias have been described, suggesting the existence of congenital and acquired lesions, virtually all pediatric umbilical hernias are congenital and form as a hernia through a persistent umbilical ring. The hernia sac is peritoneum, which is frequently adherent to the dermis of the umbilical skin. The actual fascial defect can range from several millimeters to 5 cm or more in diameter. The extent of the skin protrusion is not indicative of the size of the fascia defect. Frequently, small defects can result in alarmingly large "proboscis"-like protrusions (Fig. 49-1). Thus, it is important to palpate the actual fascia defect by reducing the hernia manually to assess whether operative or nonoperative treatment is appropriate.

Incidence

The incidence of umbilical hernia in the general population varies with age, race, gestational age, and coexisting disorders. In the United States, the incidence in African-American children from birth to 1 year old ranges from 25% to 58%, whereas white children in the same age group have an incidence of 2% to 18.5%.[1,2] Premature and low birth weight infants have a higher incidence than full-term infants, reported to be up to 75% in infants weighing 500 to 1500 g at birth.[3] Infants with certain other conditions, such as Beckwith-Wiedemann syndrome, Hurler's syndrome, various trisomy conditions (trisomy 13, 18, and 21), and congenital hypothyroidism, also have an increased incidence of umbilical hernia, as do children requiring peritoneal dialysis.[4,5]

Treatment

It has been known for many years that umbilical hernias will close spontaneously, and it seems very safe to simply observe the hernia until age 3 to 4 years to allow closure to occur. Pressure dressings and other devices to keep the hernia reduced do not speed the resolution and may result in skin irritation and breakdown and are therefore not advisable. Prospective studies in both white and African-American populations have shown spontaneous resolution rates of 83% to 95% by 6 years of age.[6-10] Another study has shown 50% of hernias still present at age 4 to 5 years will close by age 11 years.[9] One study suggests that hernias with fascial defects greater than 1.5 cm are unlikely to close by age 6 years,

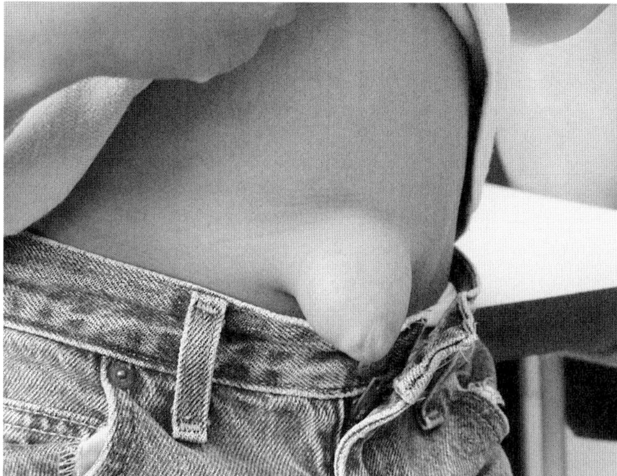

Figure 49-1. This 5-year-old child has a large proboscis-like umbilical hernia.

whereas other series suggest that even large defects will spontaneously resolve without operation.[8,11,12]

The primary danger associated with observation therapy is the possibility of incarceration or strangulation. Studies have shown these complications to be quite rare, with an incidence of less than 0.2%.[8,12,13] Patients with small fascial defects (0.5 to 1.5 cm in diameter) appear more prone to incarceration.[14] Strangulation with or without bowel infarction is even more rare. In general, informing the adult caregivers in the family regarding the signs and symptoms of incarceration, along with periodic follow-up, should ensure a safe observation period while waiting for spontaneous closure.

The operative closure of an umbilical hernia uses standard techniques, is generally straightforward, and can usually be completed as an outpatient procedure. Although a "minimally invasive" technique has been described using injection of a sclerosing agent,[15] most of these abnormalities are repaired using more traditional suture closure of the defect. Methods used commonly in the adult, such as prosthetic placement, are almost never needed in the child.

The most common method of repair is shown in Figures 49-2 and 49-3. A small transverse infraumbilical incision is made, usually placed in the redundant skin, which is inverted at the conclusion of the procedure, thereby burying the closed incision. The hernia sac is identified and dissected free from the dermis, underlying the umbilical cicatrix. Our technique includes excision of the sac to the fascial edges, although other authors have described a more limited excision or simple inversion of the sac through the fascial opening. Interrupted sutures of nonabsorbable or long-lasting absorbable sutures are placed and tied, closing the fascial defect in a transverse fashion. We leave the needle attached to the center fascia suture, which is then used to tack the underside of the umbilical cicatrix to the fascia. The skin incision is closed with an absorbable subcuticular suture, and a dressing is applied. Pressure dressings are generally unnecessary.[16]

Excision of the redundant skin is usually not performed because it tends to return to normal appearance after the

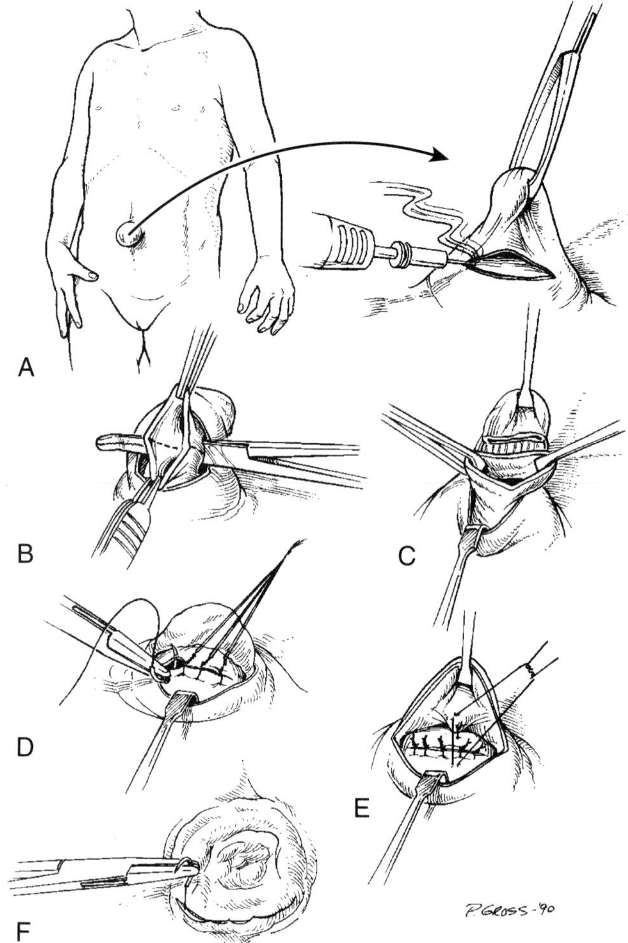

Figure 49-2. Diagram of technique for operative repair for umbilical hernia. **A,** An infraumbilical skin crease incision is made. **B,** The hernia sac is opened, leaving a portion of the sac attached to the umbilical skin for ease of subsequent umbilicoplasty. **C,** The umbilical sac has been completely divided and excised to strong fascia. D, The fascial defect is closed in a transverse fashion with interrupted, simple nonabsorbable sutures. E, The remaining umbilical sac, which is attached to the umbilical skin, is secured to the fascia with interrupted, absorbable sutures. **F,** The skin incision is closed with a subcuticular suture.

hernia is repaired. This can take up to 12 months to occur, and the family should be reassured appropriately. If the umbilicus fails to return to an acceptable appearance after 1 to 2 years, there are a number of techniques described to restore it to a more normal configuration.[17-19]

The complications of umbilical hernia repair are few and include seroma or hematoma formation, which are usually self-limited and resolve spontaneously. Wound infections can generally be treated with local care and antibiotics, whereas a recurrent hernia, occurring in less than 1%, is treated with reoperation.[14]

EPIGASTRIC HERNIA

Hernias of the abdominal wall through the midline linea alba, also termed *epigastric hernias,* are common in the pediatric age group. These hernias present as

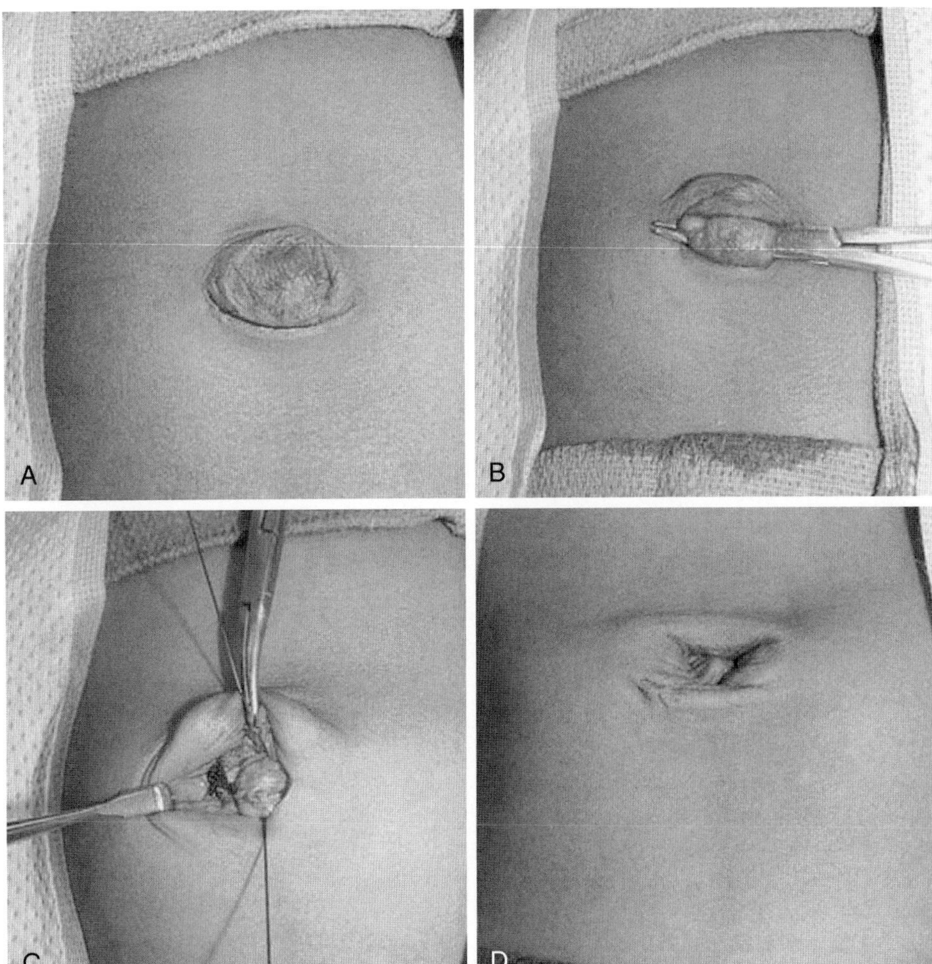

Figure 49-3. The steps depicted in the operative diagram in Figure 49-2 are shown. **A,** An infraumbilical incision is made. **B,** The umbilical hernia sac has been encircled with a hemostat. **C,** The umbilical hernia sac is excised, and transverse closure of the fascial defect is accomplished with interrupted long-lasting absorbable sutures. **D,** The umbilicus has been tacked to the fascial closure, and the skin is approximated with a subcuticular closure.

small masses, usually with incarcerated properitoneal fat, between the umbilicus and xiphoid process. An epigastric hernia should not be confused with diastasis recti, which is a generalized weakness in the linea alba from umbilicus to xiphoid and virtually always resolves by age 10 years. Incarcerated epigastric hernias can be painful. These hernias can also be multiple and associated with an umbilical hernia. Epigastric hernias do not resolve and should be repaired.

A small midline incision over the hernia is generally used, with suture repair of the defect after the contents (properitoneal fat) are reduced or excised. The site of the hernia should always be marked before anesthesia because the defect may be difficult to find with muscle relaxation. Recurrence is extremely rare.

SPIGELIAN HERNIA

Spigelian hernias are quite rare in children and can be difficult to detect and diagnose. The actual defect occurs at the intersection of the linea semicircularis, linea semilunaris, and the lateral border of the rectus abdominis muscle. It usually involves absence or attenuation of the transversus abdominis and internal oblique muscles. These hernias are more frequently found in girls and more commonly occur on the right side below the umbilicus.[20] They are also occasionally associated with skeletal abnormalities.[21] Pain in the area with a feeling of "fullness" or an actual mass are the most common symptoms. Ultrasonography may aid in the diagnosis. In extreme cases, computed tomography may be needed.

Repair consists of a transverse incision over the defect with excision of the sac and closure of the defect. Frequently, the sac is found below the external oblique muscle and may require prosthetic placement for secure repair if the defect is large. A tension-free closure is important to prevent recurrence in this area that has a high level of muscle tension.

LUMBAR HERNIA

Lumbar hernias are usually visible shortly after birth as a "bulge" in the area bordered by the 12th rib, sacrospinalis muscle, and internal oblique muscle. Occasionally, they extend inferiorly to the iliac crest. These hernias tend to develop at the site of penetration of the intercostal nerves and vessels or of the ilioinguinal, iliohypogastric, and lumbar nerves. The "bulge" is usually properitoneal fat. Therefore, the physical findings include a soft mass that is easily reducible. Although frequently asymptomatic, repair is advisable because the defect never resolves spontaneously and incarceration is possible.

Repair sometimes requires prosthetic reinforcement of the fascia or muscle closure because the tissue available for repair is usually thin and weak. We favor using absorbable mesh in the growing child that will not cause later scoliosis, which has been associated with the need for permanent prostheses. Recurrence is not uncommon because of the weak tissues involved. Repeat operations may be needed. Bilateral hernias can be repaired with either staged or simultaneous closures, depending on the surgeon's and family's preferences.

chapter 50

LAPAROSCOPY

George W. Holcomb III, MD, MBA

As opposed to 15 years ago, the benefits of the laparoscopic approach for infants and children are readily recognized today, and most training programs have, at the very least, one person who is adept with this technology. Also, laparoscopy is utilized commonly and almost exclusively for a number of common surgical conditions, such as appendectomy, cholecystectomy, fundoplication, pyloric stenosis, and splenectomy. Moreover, there are a number of reports describing this approach for relatively less common problems, such as excision of a choledochal cyst, cystogastrostomy for a pancreatic pseudocyst, colectomy for ulcerative colitis or polyposis syndromes, and gastric mobilization for a gastric pull-up operation. It has almost become the standard of care as part of the management for Hirschsprung's disease. Finally, many surgeons are utilizing this approach for high imperforate anus repair.

CONCERNS IN CHILDREN

Almost every abdominal operation performed by pediatric surgeons today has been accomplished using the laparoscopic approach. Regardless of the operation to be performed, a number of concerns are important for children. One major concern is the pliability and laxity of the abdominal wall, especially in young children. Because of this pliability, it is quite easy to introduce a cannula with a sharp trocar through the abdominal wall and into an underlying visceral or vascular structure, turning a routine operation into an emergency procedure. Therefore, it is imperative that the surgeon recognize this issue of the pliability of the abdominal wall and take great care not to injure the underlying structures when introducing a sharp trocar. One technique to avoid this problem is to direct the sharp stylet more in a transverse direction above the viscera once it has penetrated the peritoneum rather than continuing in an oblique or downward direction toward the viscera and major vessels. Injuries can occur with these sharp stylets whether or not a safety shield is attached to the trocar. Another technique used by many pediatric surgeons for safety reasons is the Step system (Covidien, Norwalk, CT). With this technique, after a small skin incision, a Veress needle with an expandable sheath is introduced through the abdominal wall into the peritoneal cavity. The Veress needle is then removed, and a cannula with a blunt-tipped trocar is introduced through the expandable sheath. It is unlikely that the blunt trocar will injure the underlying vasculature, and the expandable sheath stabilizes the cannula in the abdominal wall. This same Veress needle technique is used by some pediatric surgeons for the initial cannula entry, usually through the umbilicus. With this approach, an incision (3 mm, 5 mm, 10 mm, or 12 mm) is made in the umbilical skin and the Veress needle and sheath are introduced through the umbilical fascia and into the peritoneal cavity. Great care must be taken when introducing the Veress needle and cannula with this approach. Often it is helpful to grasp the abdominal wall manually and elevate it away from the underlying structures when introducing this Veress needle. A blind man's cane technique is then used by moving the Veress needle side to side, such as a blind man testing the surface in front of him before taking the next step. Once the surgeon is satisfied that the Veress needle is inside the abdominal cavity, insufflation is initiated, followed by removal of the Veress needle and introduction of a cannula with a blunt trocar through the expandable sheath. Other surgeons prefer a more direct cutdown approach by incising the umbilical skin and fascia, followed by introducing the cannula through the umbilical fascia into the peritoneal cavity. One modification of this approach is to insert only the expandable sheath (without the needle) through the umbilical fascial and peritoneal incision, followed by insertion of the cannula with the blunt-tipped trocar through the expandable sheath (Fig. 50-1). In experienced hands, all of these techniques for initial entry into the peritoneal cavity are safe, and few recent reports exist describing injuries to underlying viscera with careful introduction of cannulas in infants and children.

Once the initial cannula has been inserted and a pneumoperitoneum established, accessory instruments are introduced. Some surgeons prefer the use

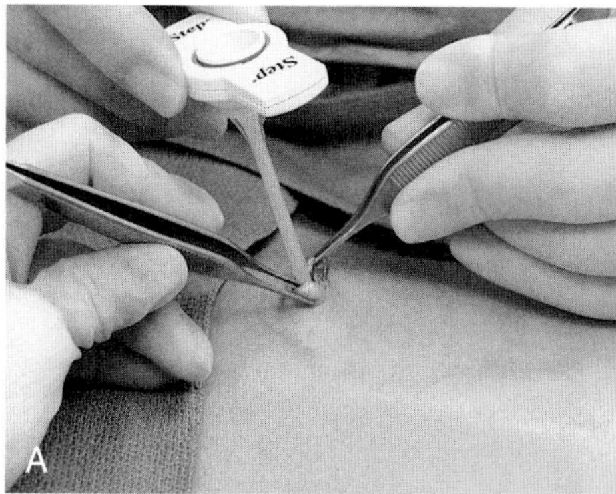
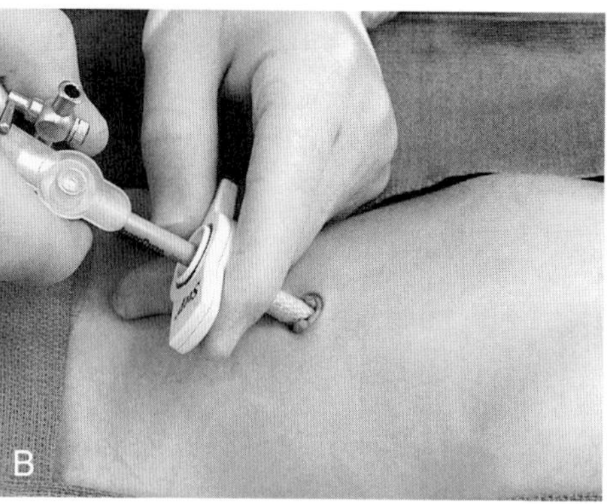

Figure 50-1. When introducing the initial umbilical cannula for laparoscopy, one approach is a direct umbilical cutdown technique, with insertion of the expandable Step sheath (**A**) followed by introduction of the cannula with a blunt trocar through the sheath (**B**). In this way, injuries from the use of the Veress needle technique are avoided.

of additional cannulas through which the instruments are inserted and removed from the peritoneal cavity. These accessory cannulas are either reusable, "reposable" (part reusable, part disposable), or completely disposable. The main disadvantage of the completely disposable cannula is the cost for one-time use. These ports vary in size from 2 to 15 mm, depending on the operation. For many procedures in children, 3-mm instruments are preferred, whereas for laparoscopic appendectomy in which the 12-mm stapler is used, a 12-mm port is necessary. Similarly, for laparoscopic splenectomy in which a 15-mm endoscopic retrieval bag is used, a 15-mm port is required. Whereas some surgeons prefer the use of cannulas for introduction of these accessory instruments, another technique is to introduce the instruments directly through the abdominal wall without the use of cannulas (Fig. 50-2).[1] With this technique, a stab incision is made with a No. 11 blade (Becton Dickinson, Franklin Lakes, NJ) through the skin and abdominal wall under telescopic visualization. The blade is removed, and the 3- or 5-mm instrument is inserted through the path created by the blade (Fig. 50-3). This technique is especially applicable for infants and young children when 3- and 5-mm instruments are used. It also is applicable for older children and adolescents with relatively thin abdominal walls for procedures in which instruments are not moved in and out of the abdominal wall during the operation. If instruments are exchanged frequently throughout the procedure, it is best to use a cannula at this site. Although a cosmetic advantage exists with this technique, the biggest advantage to the stab technique is the cost savings realized by not using either a reposable or disposable cannula system. In one study of 511 patients undergoing laparoscopic procedures using this stab incision technique, a total of $187,180 was saved in patient charges over a 3½-year period (Table 50-1).[1]

DIAGNOSTIC LAPAROSCOPY

Laparoscopy for diagnostic purposes in pediatric patients was reported in the early 1970s for several conditions, including evaluation of a contralateral patent processus vaginalis (CPPV).[2,3] Diagnostic laparoscopy also may be useful in boys with a nonpalpable testis. Moreover, it may be helpful in patients with cancer requiring a second-look procedure to determine the possibility of residual disease after chemotherapy (Fig. 50-4). In the cancer patient, laparoscopy is often used for determination of resectability as well as an adjunct for guided biopsy. Finally, diagnostic laparoscopy can be very useful in selected patients with penetrating trauma whose condition is stable and in whom a question exists of peritoneal penetration (Fig. 50-5). If no injury is found, the patient may be discharged within 24 hours, as opposed to the several days needed for recovery after laparotomy.

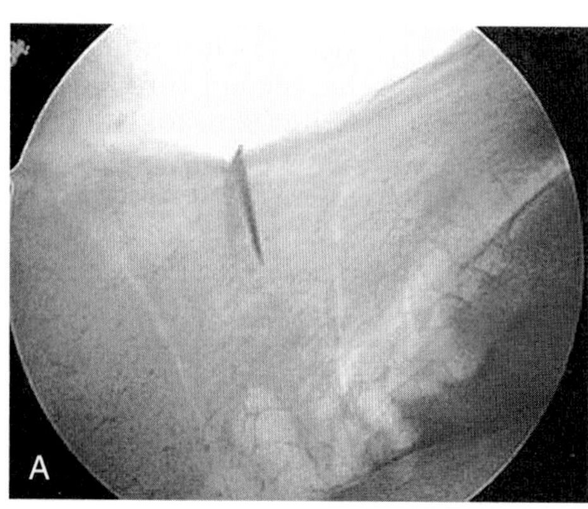
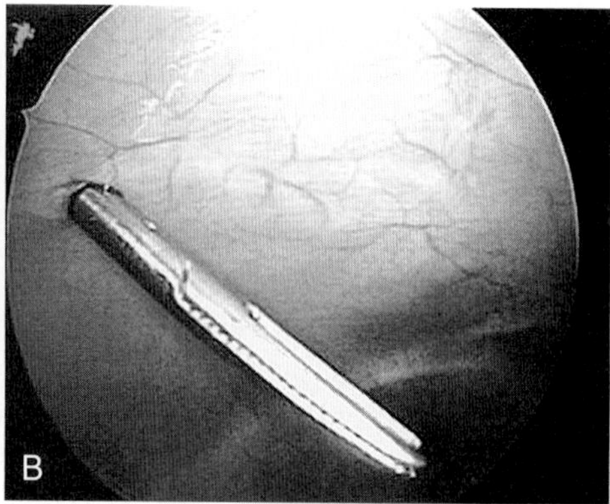

Figure 50-2. Technique for creating a transabdominal stab incision is shown. **A,** The No. 11 blade is seen to pass through the abdominal wall and into the peritoneal cavity. **B,** The No. 11 blade has been removed, and the instrument is directly introduced through the path created by the blade.

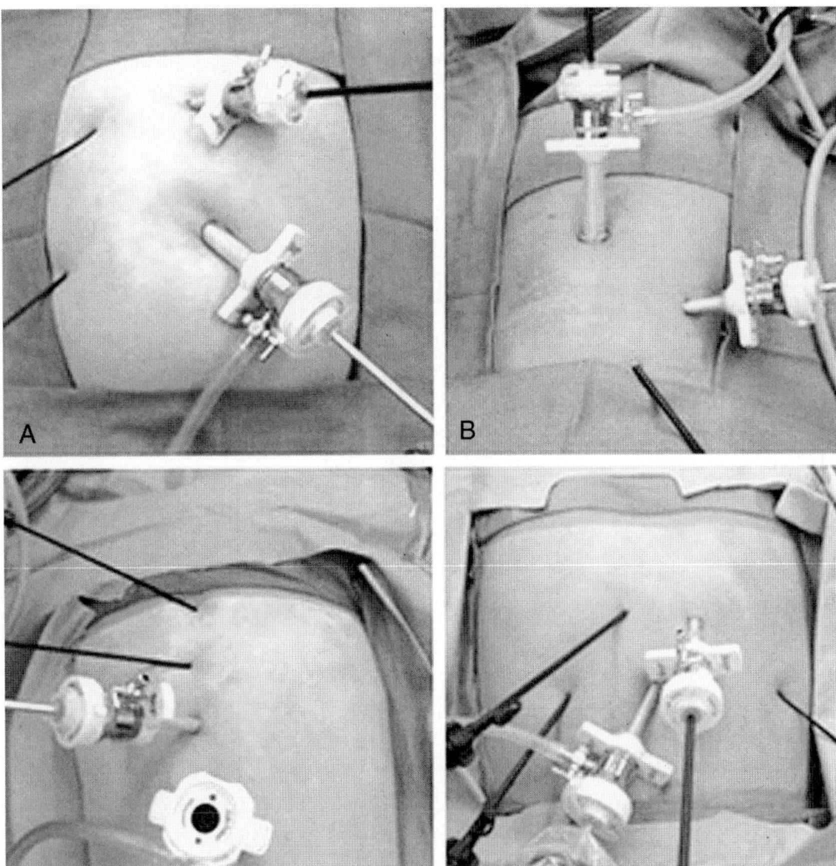

Figure 50-3. Depiction of the use of stab incisions with introduction of the instruments through the abdominal wall, without the use of accessory cannulas. In each photograph, an umbilical cannula appears through which the telescope is introduced and insufflation is achieved. **A,** A teenager is undergoing a laparoscopic cholecystectomy. Two 5-mm and two 3-mm instruments are placed directly through the abdominal wall. **B,** The patient is undergoing a laparoscopic appendectomy with a 5-mm instrument placed directly through the abdominal wall in the left suprapubic region. **C,** The patient is undergoing a laparoscopic splenectomy. A 12-mm cannula is placed in the umbilicus, and a 5-mm cannula is introduced in the midline epigastrium. Two 3-mm instruments are placed through stab incisions cephalad to the 5-mm cannula. **D,** An adolescent is undergoing a laparoscopic fundoplication. A second cannula has been placed in the patient's left upper abdomen through which the ultrasonic scalpel and needle holder are introduced.

Table 50-1 A Listing of Savings in Charges to the Patient and Cost to the Hospital Realized by Using the Stab Incision Technique with One or Two Step Cannulas

Procedure	Step Savings ($)		Ethicon Savings ($)	
	Patient	*Institution*	*Patient*	*Institution*
Nissen (209)	117,040	51,832	76,912	34,276
Nissen (14)	5,880	2,604	3,864	1,722
Appendectomy (102)	14,208	6,324	9,384	4,182
Pyloromyotomy (77)	21,560	9,548	14,168	6,314
Cholecystectomy (31)	8,680	3,844	5,704	2,542
Splenectomy (22)	5,880	2,604	3,864	1,722
Pull-through (20)	2,800	1,240	1,840	820
Ligation of testicular vessels (UDT) (15)	4,300	1,860	2,760	1,230
Esophagomyotomy (7)	2,940	1,302	1,932	861
Adrenalectomy (6)	1,680	744	1,104	492
Varicocele (5)	1,400	620	920	410
Ovarian (2)	560	248	368	164
Meckel's diverticulum (2)	280	124	184	82
TOTAL: 511 operations	$187,180	$82,894	$123,004	$54,817

Note: If Ethicon cannulas were used, the savings that would have occurred are seen as well (right column).
UDT, undescended testis.
From Ostlie DJ, Holcomb GW III: The use of stab incisions for instrument access in laparoscopic operations. J Pediatr Surg 38:1837-1840, 2003.

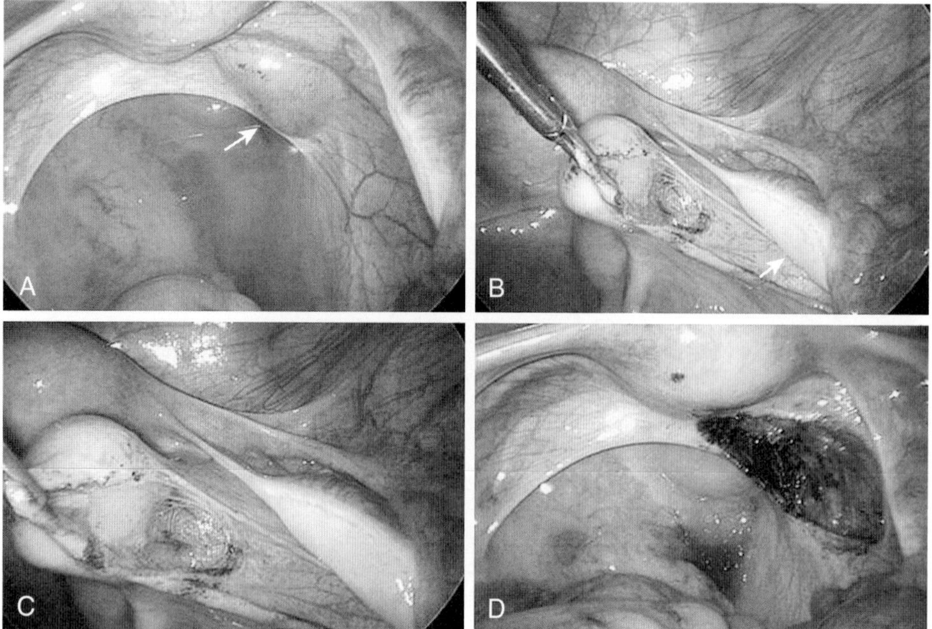

Figure 50-4. Second-look laparoscopy can be useful after adjuvant therapy in certain circumstances. In this teenage patient who previously had undergone laparotomy and resection of a large germ cell tumor, second-look laparoscopy was performed to determine whether evidence of residual disease existed. **A,** Residual disease is seen along the right pelvic side wall (*arrow*). **B,** This mass is being resected from the pelvic side wall. Note the normal right ovary (*arrow*). **C,** Further dissection of the mass is achieved. **D,** The mass has been completely excised, with hemostasis controlled by cautery.

Diagnostic Laparoscopy for Contralateral Patent Processus Vaginalis

In the early 1990s, two reports were published describing diagnostic laparoscopy through the umbilicus in children with a unilateral inguinal hernia to determine evidence of a CPPV.[4,5] Several years later, with the advent of 3-mm angled telescopes, it became apparent that this same information could be obtained through the ipsilateral hernia sac.[6] A number of reports have confirmed the efficacy of this technique to determine the presence of a CPPV, which may indicate the need for repair under the same anesthetic.[7-10]

The largest report describing laparoscopy for evaluating a CPPV described 1676 consecutive children presenting with a unilateral inguinal hernia who underwent diagnostic laparoscopy for evaluation for CPPV.[11] In 73 patients (4.49%), the sac was deemed too thin to perform laparoscopy. Therefore, 1603 patients underwent diagnostic laparoscopy. Within this group, 643 (40.1%) patients were found to have a patent processus vaginalis. Of those patients in whom a CPPV was not seen at laparoscopy, only 5 (0.70%) patients have returned with a symptomatic hernia. Of 446 patients thought to have a CPPV by examination under anesthesia, only 192 (43%) were found to have a CPPV at laparoscopy. On the other hand, 1157 patients were felt not to have CPPV by palpating a thickened cord on examination under anesthesia, but 451 (39%) actually did have a CPPV.

Although the accuracy of this technique approaches 99%, it is not possible to determine which patient with a CPPV will develop a symptomatic hernia. At the same time, it does subselect those patients who should undergo contralateral exploration based on a positive finding rather than subjecting all children with a unilateral inguinal hernia to contralateral exploration, as has been advocated in the past. A few surgeons have taken this approach one step further and are performing various types of laparoscopic hernia repairs in children. Laparoscopic hernia repair remains controversial because the recurrence rate has been cited to be 2% to 4% in several studies.[12-14]

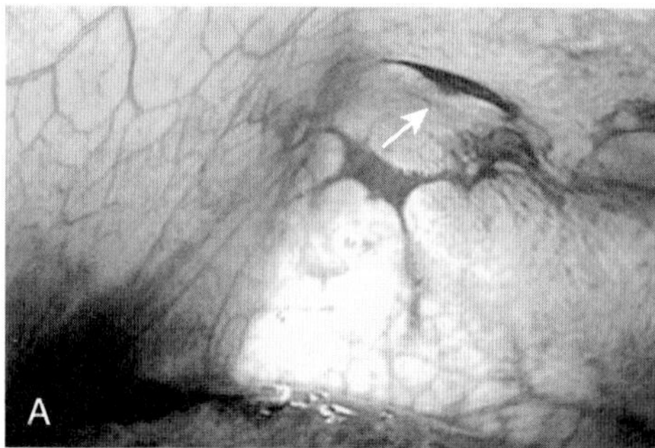

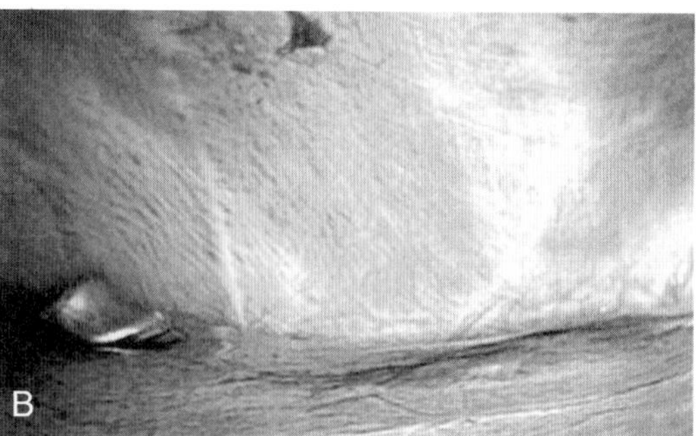

Figure 50-5. Laparoscopy can be useful in selected cases of penetrating trauma in which the patient appears to be uninjured, yet there is concern that the sharp object, or perhaps a bullet, has penetrated the abdominal cavity. **A,** An entrance wound from a bullet that entered the peritoneal cavity (*arrow*) is seen. **B,** The bullet is seen to lie on top of the left lobe of the liver just beneath the entry site. This patient did not have other injuries and was discharged the next day. A laparotomy was avoided in this patient.

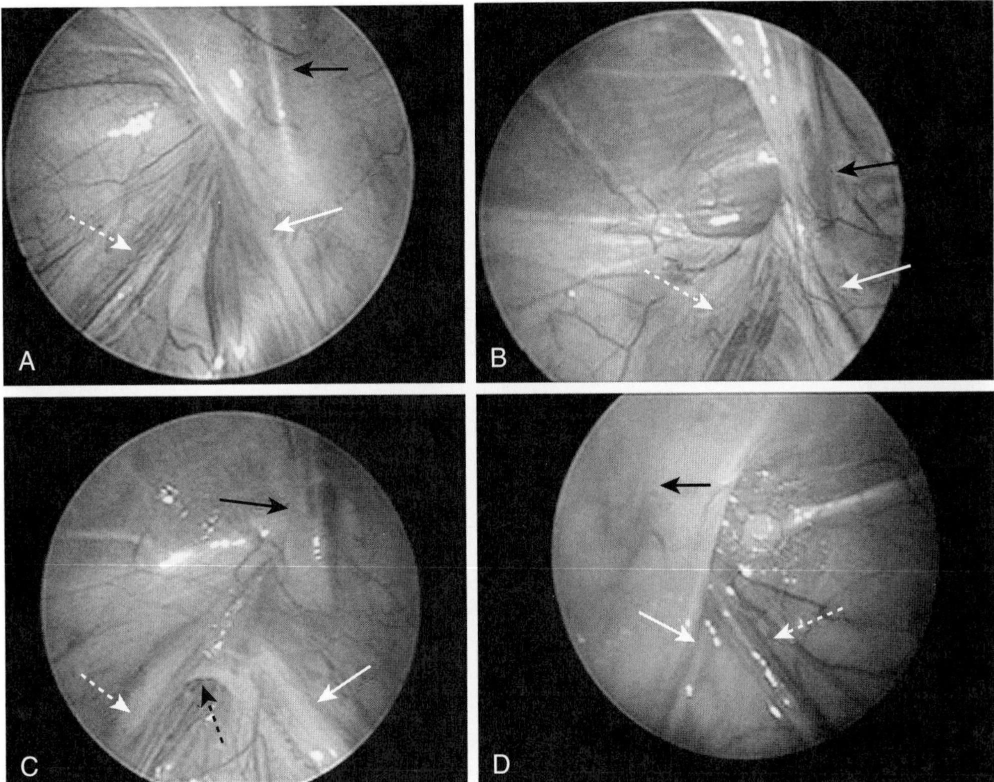

Figure 50-6. At laparoscopy for evaluation of a contralateral patent processus vaginalis, several findings are possible. In each of these photographs, the *dotted white arrow* depicts the testicular vessels and the *solid white arrow* depicts the vas deferens. An additional *black arrow* shows the inferior epigastric vessels. **A,** No evidence is seen for a left patent processus vaginalis. **B,** A large internal opening to a left patent processus vaginalis is found. **C,** A veil of peritoneum (*dotted black arrow*) covers the left testicular vessels and there appears to be a small opening to a patent processus vaginalis. In this setting, however, it is unclear how distal the small patent processus vaginalis extends. **D,** Air bubbles are seen emanating from the internal opening of right patent processus vaginalis when manual pressure is applied over the right inguinal canal.

The technique for evaluating the contralateral inguinal region involves creation of a pneumoperitoneum through the hernia sac, followed by diagnostic laparoscopy with an angled (usually 45- to 70-degree) telescope. Some surgeons insufflate the peritoneum by introducing a cannula into the abdomen through the hernia sac, whereas others use a catheter. Either technique appears to work well.

At laparoscopy, it is usually evident whether a CPPV is present (Fig. 50-6). However, on occasion, a veil of peritoneum may obscure the visualization of the contralateral inguinal ring. At times, the length of the CPPV may not be clear. A technique has been described in which a silver probe is percutaneously introduced on the contralateral side to retract the peritoneal veil to evaluate the length of the CPPV (Fig. 50-7).[15]

PROCEDURAL LAPAROSCOPY

Stomach and Solid Organs

Fundoplication

The laparoscopic operation for fundoplication has become the preferred approach for surgical management of gastroesophageal reflux for most pediatric surgeons. Any type of fundoplication, including a Nissen, Thal, Toupet, Boix-Ochoa, or other, can be performed by using the laparoscopic approach. It is my experience that the laparoscopic Nissen fundoplication is the easiest operation to perform laparoscopically and yields the best results, but this belief is not shared by all pediatric surgeons. Complications have been minimal, and results are very satisfactory. Transmigration (herniation) of the fundoplication wrap through the esophageal hiatus has been found to develop in 3% to 5% of patients undergoing laparoscopic fundoplication. It is possible that the lack of scarring near the esophageal hiatus after a laparoscopic fundoplication allows retraction of the esophagus and the fundoplication wrap through the esophageal hiatus. Because of this concern, I have taken additional steps in the technique I use to prevent this problem.

A 4- or 5-mm transumbilical cannula is placed in most patients. In adolescents, especially tall patients with a narrow costal margin, it may be more appropriate to place this initial cannula in the midepigastric region. After pneumoperitoneum, four additional instruments are introduced by using either cannulas or the stab incision technique. The short gastric vessels are divided beginning at a point midway along the greater curvature of the stomach and progressing to the esophageal hiatus (Fig. 50-8). The gastroesophageal junction is initially approached from the patient's

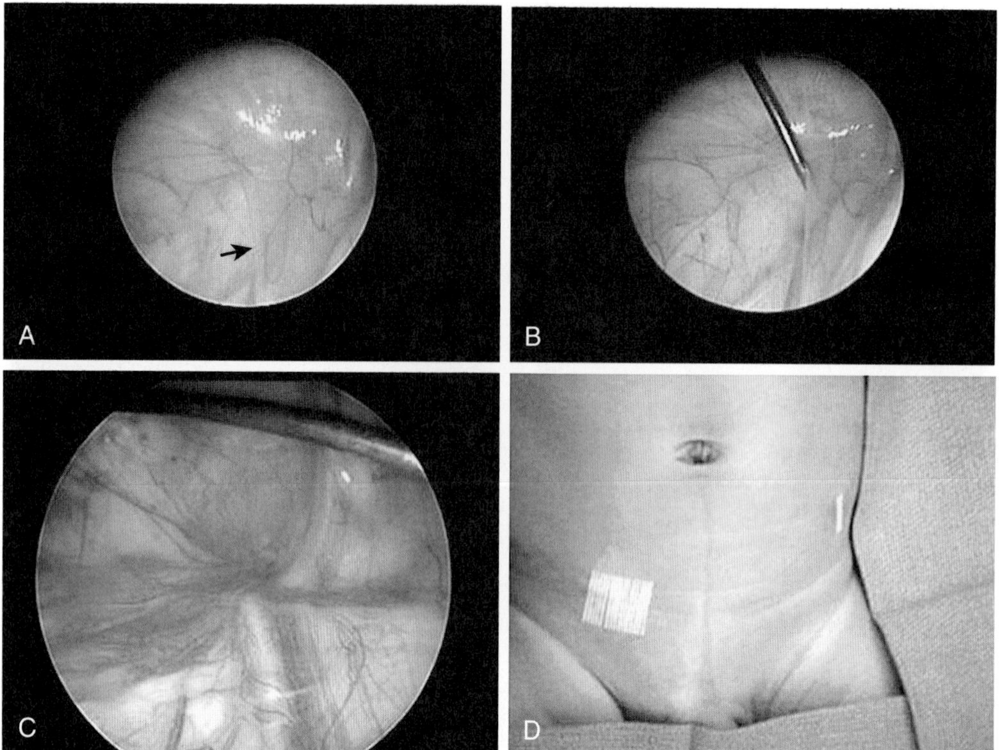

Figure 50-7. On occasion, it is not possible to determine accurately whether a significant contralateral patent processus vaginalis (CPPV) exists. **A,** A veil of peritoneum (*arrow*) covers the left internal ring structures, and even with a 70-degree telescope, it is not possible to determine whether a CPPV is present. **B,** A silver probe has been placed through a stab incision in the left lower abdomen. The tip of the silver probe is manipulated to retract the peritoneal veil, which, in **C,** shows a blind end to the internal ring. Thus, no evidence exists of a PPV on the left side. **D,** The Steri-strips are seen placed over the right inguinal crease incision. A single Steri-strip is used to approximate the skin where the silver probe was introduced through the left lower abdominal wall.

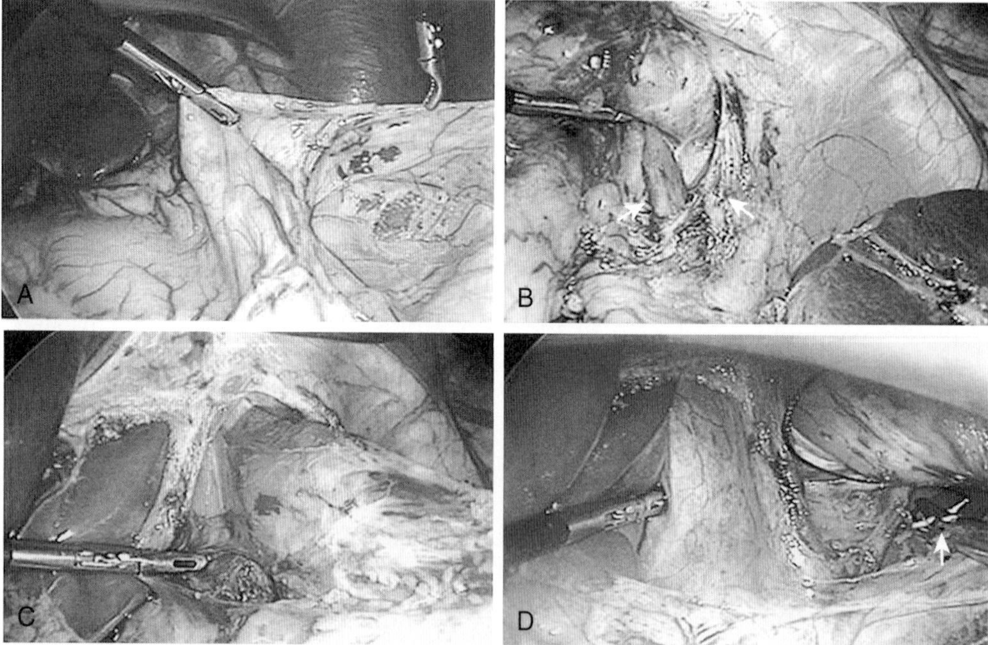

Figure 50-8. The initial steps for laparoscopic fundoplication are shown. **A,** The short gastric vessels are being ligated and divided by using the Maryland dissecting instrument, which is attached to cautery. **B,** The esophagus has been retracted anteriorly and to the patient's right, exposing the retroesophageal space. Note the right and left diaphragmatic crura (*arrows*). **C,** The patient's right diaphragmatic crus is being separated from the esophagus by using blunt dissection. **D,** A 2-0 silk suture attached to an RB-1 needle (*arrow*) is being placed through the patient's left diaphragmatic crus for approximation of the crura.

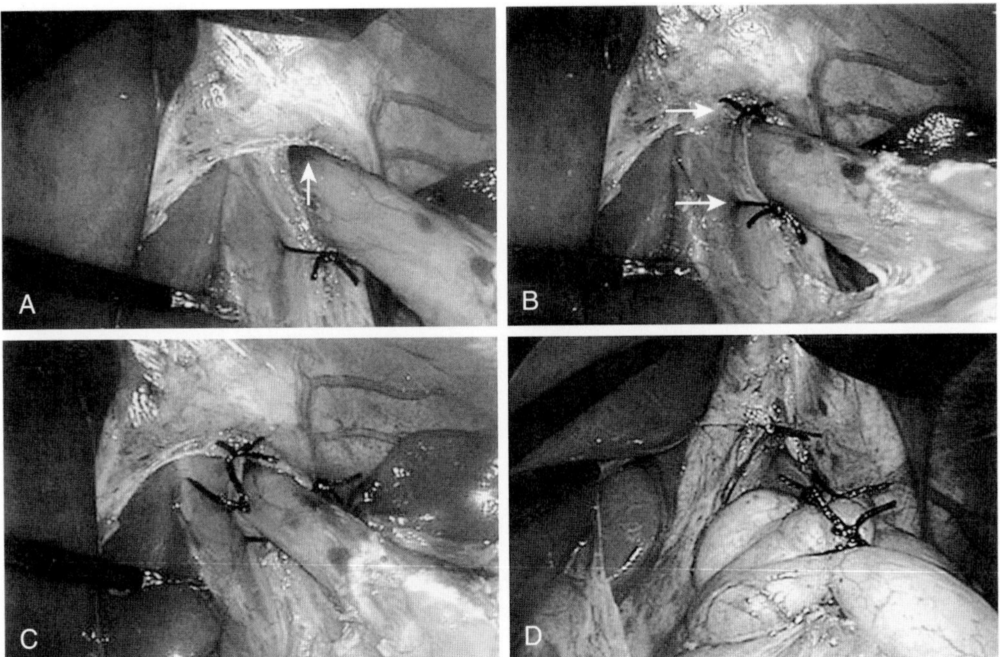

Figure 50-9. **A,** The diaphragmatic crura have been approximated posteriorly with a 2-0 silk suture. Note the small space anteriorly (*arrow*) that remains after posterior approximation of the crura. **B,** This space has been obliterated with an anteriorly placed 2-0 silk suture so that the diaphragmatic crura have been approximated both posteriorly and anteriorly (*arrows*). **C,** An esophagus-to-crura suture is seen at the 9-o'clock position. In addition, similar sutures are placed at the 3-o'clock position. **D,** The completed fundoplication.

left side, and the retroesophageal space is identified and opened. The esophagus is then freed from the diaphragmatic crura in all directions by using blunt and sharp dissection to create an adequate portion of intra-abdominal esophagus. After mobilizing the intra-abdominal esophagus, the diaphragmatic crura are usually approximated, at least with one suture, which is placed posterior to the esophagus (see Fig. 50-8). If the hiatus is greatly enlarged, a second suture may be needed anteriorly (Fig. 50-9). After crural repair, the esophagus is sutured to the narrowed hiatus at three or four sites several centimeters above the gastroesophageal junction (see Fig. 50-9). This suture fixation helps to prevent transmigration of the fundoplication wrap through the hiatus. After adding this modification to my technique, the incidence of transmigration of the wrap has markedly diminished. An appropriate-size transesophageal bougie is then introduced into the stomach. The fundus is wrapped around the intra-abdominal esophagus and sutured back to itself in a standard Nissen fundoplication fashion. In a recent study, a fundoplication length of approximately 2 cm was found to be effective in relieving symptoms.[16] Usually, three 2-0 silk sutures are used to create the fundoplication wrap. At this point, with hemostasis ensured, the operation is terminated and the cannulas/instruments are removed. Gastroesophageal reflux is discussed in detail in Chapter 29.

Gastrostomy

Laparoscopic gastrostomy may be performed either in conjunction with a laparoscopic fundoplication or as a separate procedure. When performed in conjunction with fundoplication, the site of placement of the gastrostomy button is the site of the main working port for the fundoplication in the left upper abdomen. This incision in the patient's left upper abdomen should be marked before creating the pneumoperitoneum. Otherwise, creation of the pneumoperitoneum will confuse the surgeon as to the appropriate location for the gastrostomy. For laparoscopic gastrostomy alone, the site can be marked as well. If laparoscopic gastrostomy is performed alone, a 4- or 5-mm cannula and telescope are introduced through the umbilicus. If it is performed after fundoplication, the telescope remains in place. A grasping forceps is introduced through the gastrostomy site incision in the left upper abdomen. It is often helpful to ask the anesthesiologist to insufflate the stomach. This maneuver reduces the likelihood that the posterior wall of the stomach will be caught by the fixation sutures, which are introduced next. After grasping a site for the gastrostomy on the anterior gastric wall near the greater curvature, the stomach is pulled anteriorly to approximate its serosa with the abdominal wall (Fig. 50-10). One 2-0 monofilament suture is placed on either side of the gastrostomy site. These sutures are placed in an extracorporeal manner through the skin and abdominal wall cephalad to the gastrostomy site, then through the anterior stomach wall, and then out through the abdominal wall and skin caudad to the gastrostomy. With the use of the Cook Vascular Dilator Set (Cook, Inc., Bloomington, IN), a needle is placed through the gastrostomy incision and into the stomach. A guide wire is inserted and, by using the Seldinger technique, the skin and gastrostomy are sequentially dilated using 8-, 12-, 16-, and 20-Fr dilators, which are introduced over the

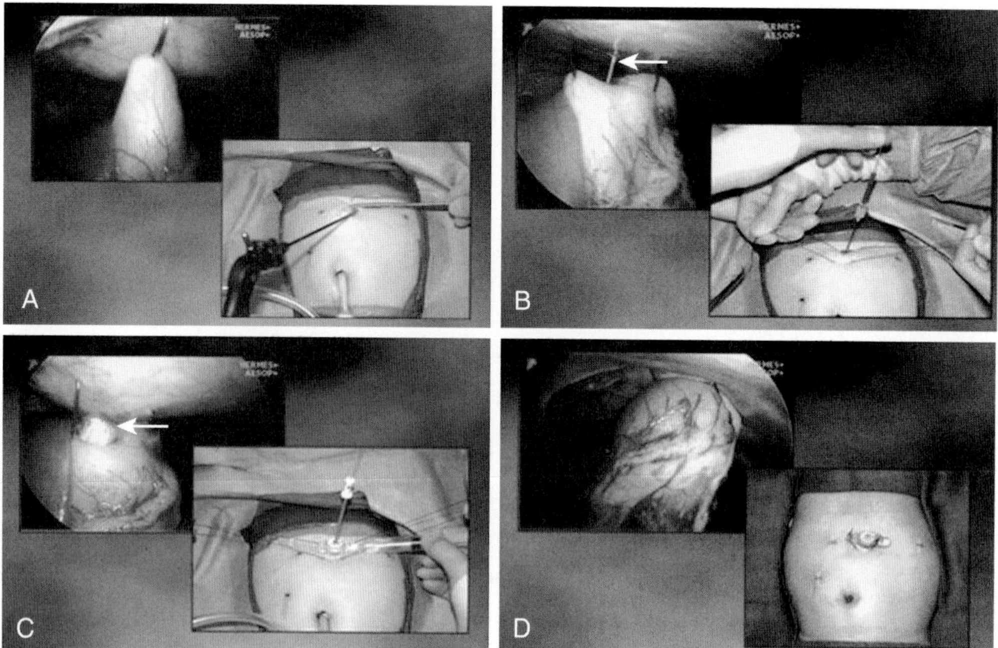

Figure 50-10. The technique for laparoscopic gastrostomy used by the author is shown. **A,** After fundoplication in this patient, a 3-mm instrument has been introduced through the left upper stab incision and the stomach has been grasped. Extracorporeal sutures are then placed on each side of this planned gastrostomy site. These sutures are introduced through the abdominal wall cephalad to the stomach, through the stomach, and exteriorized through the abdominal wall caudad to the gastrostomy site. **B,** With a suture on each side of the planned gastrostomy, a needle is introduced into the stomach (*arrow*) through the gastrostomy site, followed by advancement of a guide wire through the needle into the stomach. **C,** The tract is then serially dilated and a 14-Fr, 0.8-cm button (*arrow*) is introduced over the guide wire into the stomach. **D,** The balloon is inflated, and the extracorporeal sutures are tied over the button.

guide wire. The 8-Fr dilator is inserted through the gastrostomy button and used to introduce the button into the stomach. The balloon is inflated under telescopic visualization. The dilator is removed, and the sutures are tied over the button. It is important to ensure that the guide wire and the button are definitely inside the stomach. It is helpful to use an angled telescope to inspect the entire circumference of the gastrostomy to confirm that the button is not outside the stomach. The patient may be fed by using the gastrostomy several hours after its placement, if desired. The 2-0 monofilament sutures are removed 4 or 5 days later.

Esophagomyotomy

In preparation for a laparoscopic esophagomyotomy for achalasia, it is important to give the patient a liquid diet for several days. Usually the lower esophagus will empty itself of solid food during this time. After induction of anesthesia, it is important to suction the esophagus thoroughly to evacuate any retained food particles and to insert an esophageal bougie. In the event of entry into the esophageal lumen during the operation, gross spillage will not occur into the peritoneal cavity.

Placement of incisions for laparoscopic esophagomyotomy is almost identical to that for a laparoscopic fundoplication. In addition, because an anterior partial fundoplication, rather than a full fundoplication, is usually performed, only the most cephalad two or three short gastric vessels are ligated and divided. After ligation and division of these short gastric vessels, the wall of the anterior lower esophagus is grasped on each side. Through the primary working port in the left upper abdomen, either the ultrasonic scalpel or hook cautery is used to divide the distal esophageal muscle down to the submucosa (Fig. 50-11). Once the submucosa is visualized, the ultrasonic scalpel is used, with the "hot" blade turned anterior, to create the esophagomyotomy for a distance of 4 to 6 cm cephalad. The esophagomyotomy usually extends through the esophageal hiatus for 1 or 2 cm. By using the same technique, the myotomy is extended onto the stomach for 1 or 2 cm to ensure that the circular fibers of the lower esophageal sphincter are completely divided. If any question remains, esophagoscopy can be performed to verify this complete myotomy. Should entry into the lumen occur, it is often easy to see the bougie through the mucosal perforation. A perforation can usually be closed laparoscopically.

After the anterior esophagomyotomy, a partial fundoplication is usually performed. This can be either a partial posterior (Toupet) fundoplication or an anterior (Dor) fundoplication. The advantage of the Dor procedure is that it covers the just-completed esophagomyotomy. For this reason, I prefer this anterior fundoplication. With interrupted 2-0 silk, the cephalad portion of the greater curvature of the fundus is sutured initially to the left edge of the completed myotomy and the left diaphragmatic crus and then to the right edge of the completed myotomy and the

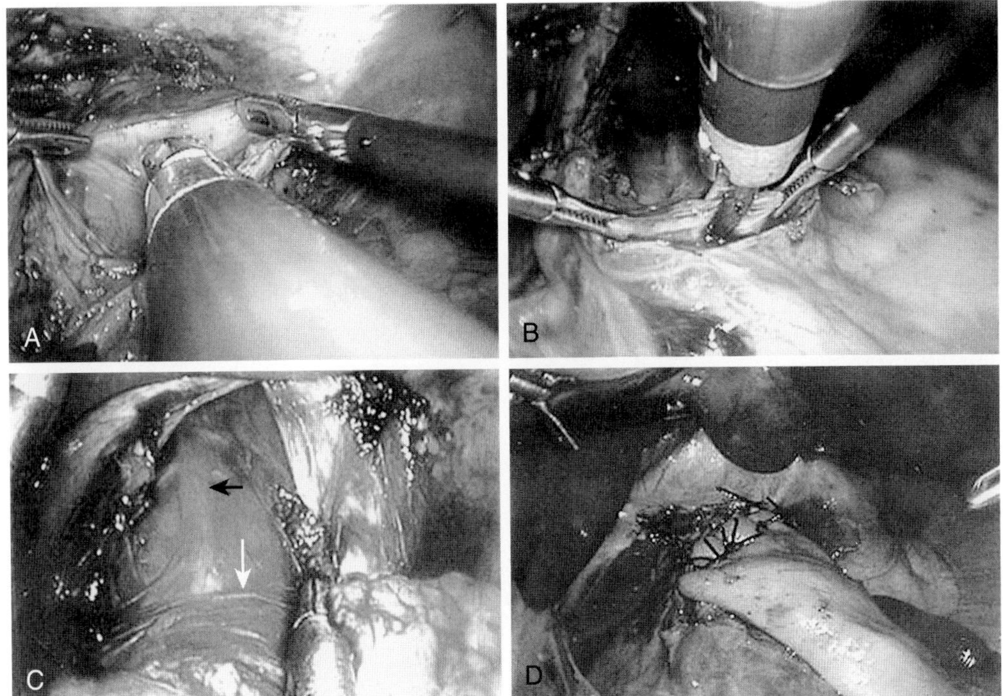

Figure 50-11. In a laparoscopic esophagomyotomy and anterior fundoplication, the placement of the ports and instruments is similar to that for a laparoscopic fundoplication. **A,** The muscle of the esophagus has been grasped on the lateral aspects of the esophagus, and a Maryland dissecting instrument is being used to develop a plane between the muscle down through the submucosa. **B,** This plane has been developed, and the ultrasonic scalpel is being used to ligate and divide the muscle. **C,** The longitudinal fibers of the esophageal muscle have been divided. Note the circular fibers (*white arrow*) of the lower esophageal sphincter in the lower aspect of the photograph. In addition, the anterior vagus nerve (*black arrow*) is seen to course vertically along the esophagus. **D,** An anterior (Dor) fundoplication has been performed to help prevent the development of gastroesophageal reflux in the postoperative period.

right crus. Approximately three sutures are taken on each edge of the myotomy along with the diaphragmatic crus. These sutures also help to separate each side of the myotomy to help prevent recurrence of symptoms.

Before initiating a clear liquid diet the next day, a water-soluble contrast study is performed to ensure that the esophageal mucosa is intact. Most patients are ready for discharge either the morning after the operation or on the second postoperative morning. Results with this operation in children have been favorable to date.[17-20] Achalasia is also covered in Chapter 26.

Pyloromyotomy

Laparoscopic pyloromyotomy is rapidly becoming the preferred approach for pyloromyotomy in infants. A prospective randomized trial comparing the laparoscopic and open approaches was recently completed in 200 infants.[21] The primary outcome variable was the operative time, which differed by 6 seconds. There was statistically significantly less pain medicine utilized in the laparoscopic group, and the length of postoperative hospitalization trended toward significance in the laparoscopic group as well. The authors believed there was a definite cosmetic advantage to the laparoscopic procedure.

A 4- or 5-mm cannula is positioned in the umbilicus, followed by insufflation and insertion of an angled telescope. With stab incisions in both the right and left upper abdominal quadrants, the duodenum is grasped with DeBakey endoscopic forceps placed through the patient's right upper abdominal stab incision. It is very important to grasp the duodenum securely because a few instances of injury to the duodenum with this technique have been reported.[22] Through the stab incision in the patient's left upper abdomen, an arthroscopy knife is introduced and the knife is extended to the second notch, which represents a 2-mm depth of penetration of the blade (Fig. 50-12). Because the ultrasonographic criterion for pyloromyotomy is 4 mm in depth, using a knife with a 2-mm blade should not allow entry into the mucosa. It is important to incise the serosa and muscle adequately on the initial pass to allow introduction of the pyloric spreader. The knife is then returned to its sheath and extracted, and a pyloric spreader is introduced through the same left upper abdominal stab incision. The pylorus is gently and carefully spread to disrupt the muscular fibers. The submucosa is visualized during this part of the operation to ensure that no evidence of mucosal injury is present. It is important that an adequate myotomy is performed. In one study, no evidence of incomplete pyloromyotomy was found in 171 patients in whom a mean pyloromyotomy incision length of 2.0 cm was achieved.[23] Conversely, in a few instances, an incomplete pyloromyotomy has been described, and it is postulated that inadequate extension onto the stomach was the reason.[22] After what appears to be a completed pyloromyotomy, it is often prudent to insufflate

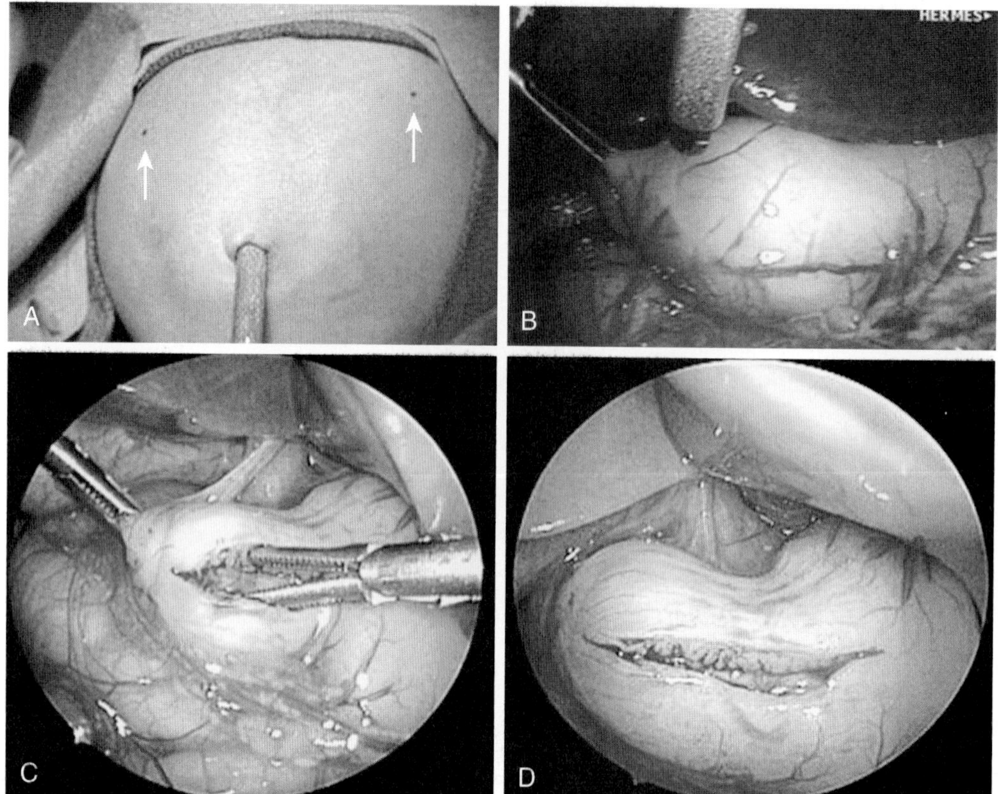

Figure 50-12. In an infant undergoing laparoscopic pyloromyotomy, a 5-mm cannula is inserted through an incision in the umbilical fascia. **A,** The sites of the stab incisions in the left and right upper quadrants are shown (*arrows*). **B,** With an arthroscopy knife, an incision will be made in the seromuscular portion of the hypertrophied pylorus. **C,** The knife is removed, a pyloric spreader is introduced through this same incision, and the hypertrophied muscle bluntly divided. **D,** The pyloromyotomy incision is usually approximately 2 cm long.

the stomach via a red rubber catheter to ensure that no evidence of unrecognized perforation exists. Placing omentum over the pyloromyotomy, as is commonly done in the open operation, may be advantageous. The instruments are then removed, and the umbilical fascia and skin are closed.

Splenectomy

The first report of a laparoscopic splenectomy in children was published in 1993.[24] A number of authors have described various techniques for elective removal of a spleen for hematologic diseases.[25-29] The largest report describes the outcomes in patients undergoing laparoscopy for splenic conditions.[30] These diseases are primarily idiopathic thrombocytopenic purpura, hereditary spherocytosis, and, occasionally, splenic sequestration from sickle cell disease. The patient is usually positioned with a roll under his or her left side so that he or she is in a 30- to 45-degree right decubitus position. Placement of the ports for this operation vary from surgeon to surgeon. A common denominator is the need for a 15-mm site through which the Endocatch II bag (Ethicon Endosurgery, Cincinnati, OH) can be inserted. In addition, a site for introduction of an angled telescope and two other accessory sites are necessary. One approach is to position the 15-mm cannula through a 15-mm incision in the umbilical skin and fascia and orient the accessory ports in the midline. The advantage of this positioning is that the largest incision is nicely hidden in the umbilicus, yet if conversion is required, the midline incisions can be incorporated in an upper midline incision (see Fig. 50-3). Stab incisions may be used for these accessory sites so that the only cannulas required are the 15-mm one in the umbilicus and a 5-mm port for introduction of the angled telescope. With the orientation described, the main working port is in the umbilicus, through which the ultrasonic scalpel is introduced. After insertion of all instruments, a thorough search is made for accessory spleens. The most common sites for these are in the splenic hilum or in the lienocolic region (Fig. 50-13). It is important to remove accessory spleens either separately or with the specimen. The lienocolic ligament is then incised with the electrocautery, taking great care to identify the transverse colon and splenic flexure. Once the left colon has been mobilized from the spleen, it can be gently pushed caudad, out of the way of future dissection. The dissection then proceeds along the greater curvature of the stomach, carefully ligating and dividing the short gastric vessels with the ultrasonic scalpel. During this part of the operation, it is often helpful to rotate the table to the patient's right, allowing the stomach to gravitate away from the spleen. Sometimes it is not possible to divide the most cephalad short gastric vessels completely until later in the operation. After exposing the splenic hilum, one approach is to dissect the main splenic artery and

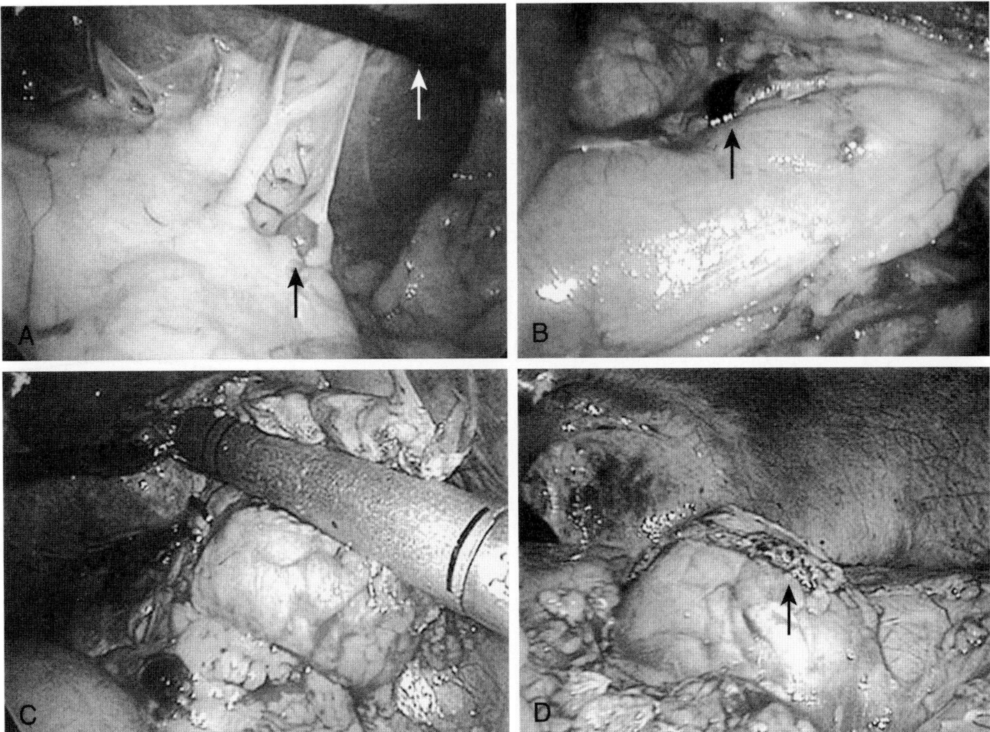

Figure 50-13. The technique for laparoscopic splenectomy is depicted. **A,** An accessory spleen is seen in a patient with idiopathic thrombocytopenic purpura (*black arrow*). In addition, one of the 3-mm instruments (*white arrow*) is being used to elevate the lower pole of the spleen for access to the lienocolic ligament. After ligation and division of the short gastric vessels, one technique is to isolate the artery and doubly clip it before dissection in the splenic hilum. **B,** Note the two clips (*black arrow*) on the splenic artery along the cephalad portion of the pancreas. **C,** Attachments of the spleen to the diaphragm and other structures have been divided, and an endoscopic vascular stapler is placed across the splenic hilum. The pancreas, noted below the stapler, has not been incorporated into the jaws of the stapler. **D,** The spleen has been removed. Note the intact staple line (*black arrow*) across the hilum of the spleen.

ligate it with an endoscopic clip before any further dissection. It is important to place this clip well away from the splenic hilum so that it does not later interfere with staple occlusion and division of the splenic veins. Occlusion of the arterial supply reduces the risk of dangerous hemorrhage and allows the splenic blood to "autotransfuse" the patient.

Attention is now turned to dissecting the pancreas from the splenic hilum by using the ultrasonic scalpel. Sometimes this is relatively straightforward, but it can be quite tedious. At this time, or perhaps earlier in the dissection, the attachments of the spleen to the lateral peritoneal wall are incised. The avascular cephalad peritoneal attachments to the diaphragm are divided by using scissors. It is important to be aware of the diaphragm, because it is possible to injure it while mobilizing the cephalad aspect of the spleen. Once the tail of the pancreas has been separated and the spleen has been detached from its peritoneal fixation, the spleen can be lifted on either side of the hilum with retracting instruments. A 15-mm articulating stapler is introduced through the 15-mm cannula and positioned across the hilum of the spleen (see Fig. 50-13). It is necessary to ensure that the pancreas is not incorporated in the stapler and to confirm that the stapler is completely across the splenic vessels. Once positioned, the stapler should be closed for 20 seconds, after which the stapler can be fired and then gently released. When releasing the stapler, be ready to grasp any vascular structures that may be bleeding. Once the spleen has been detached from its vascular and peritoneal attachments, the patient is placed into a deep Trendelenburg position and the Endocatch II bag is introduced. Then the patient is rotated into a reverse Trendelenburg position, allowing the spleen to fall into the open bag. The bag is closed after ensuring that no other structures have entered it, and the neck of the bag is exteriorized through the umbilical incision. The spleen is manually morcellated with sponge forceps and extracted in piecemeal fashion. During this part of the operation, it is very important to ensure that the bag is not perforated by overvigorous morcellation or extraction. It may take 10 to 20 minutes to accomplish splenic extraction. After removal of the bag and its contents, re-inspection of the area of dissection is performed to ensure that no evidence of complications is present. The incisions are then closed, and the patient is usually ready for discharge on the first or second postoperative day. Splenic diseases are also covered in Chapter 47.

Cholecystectomy

Laparoscopic cholecystectomy is becoming a common operation for pediatric surgeons.[31] Sometimes the development of cholelithiasis is due to hemolytic

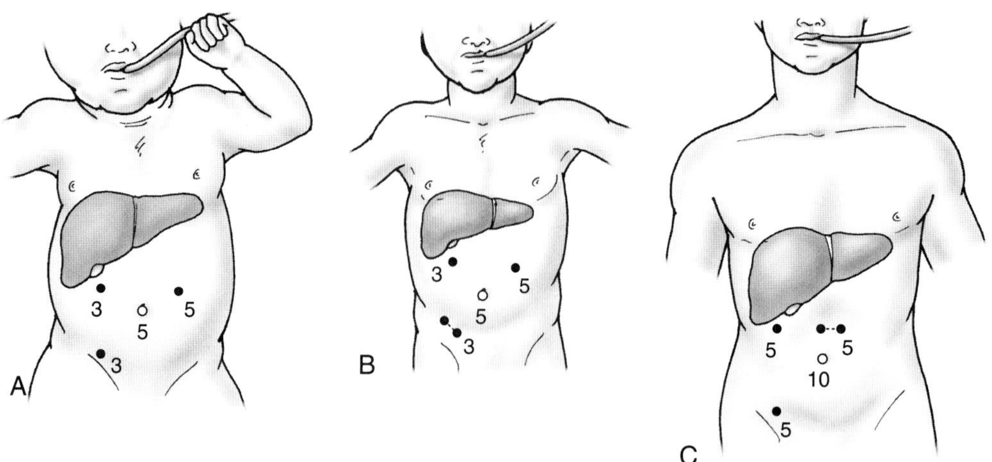

Figure 50-14. For laparoscopic cholecystectomy in infants and children, it is important to space the cannulas widely to create an adequate working space and not have the instruments inhibiting one another. **A,** A suggested diagram for location of the ports for an infant. **B,** The cannulas can be arranged as shown for a child between ages 3 and 10 years. **C,** Instruments can be positioned as they are for an adult.

disease, but often it is iatrogenic. Also, children presenting with biliary dyskinesia are being seen more frequently. Most pediatric patients undergoing laparoscopic cholecystectomy are in the adolescent age group. However, an occasional elementary school-age child will need this procedure, and, rarely, a preschool infant will be symptomatic from cholelithiasis.

When positioning the instruments and cannulas for the operation, it is important to space the cannulas widely for optimal working room (Fig. 50-14). This is especially true in the younger patient. The two right-sided instruments are usually for retracting purposes, with the most inferior instrument being used by the assistant and the most cephalad manipulated by the surgeon. These can often be inserted by using the stab incision technique (see Fig. 50-3). For the preschool patient a 5-mm umbilical port is placed, but for older patients a 10-mm port is usually necessary. The gallbladder will be extracted through this cannula or the umbilical fascial defect. For many pediatric patients, a 5-mm clip is used for ligation of the cystic duct and cystic artery, and therefore a 5-mm incision may be placed in the patient's epigastric region. For smaller patients, this incision should be positioned more in the patient's left epigastrium to ensure adequate working space. However, in the teenager, this incision is located just to the right of the patient's midline.

Regardless of the patient's age, the operative steps are similar. Any omental or peritoneal attachments to the gallbladder are bluntly divided, and the tip of the gallbladder is rotated ventrally over the liver, which exposes the infundibulum and cystic duct. It is very important to retract the infundibulum laterally, which orients the cystic duct at a right angle to the common bile duct (Fig. 50-15). If the infundibulum is retracted cephalad, the cystic duct approaches a more vertical orientation and the cystic duct and common duct can be misidentified. This may lead either to injury or to ligation of the common duct. With the infundibulum retracted laterally, the cystic duct is well visualized and then easily skeletonized. Cholangiography often is not necessary. However, if the surgeon desires cholangiography, several techniques are available. In older children, a lateral incision in the cystic duct can be

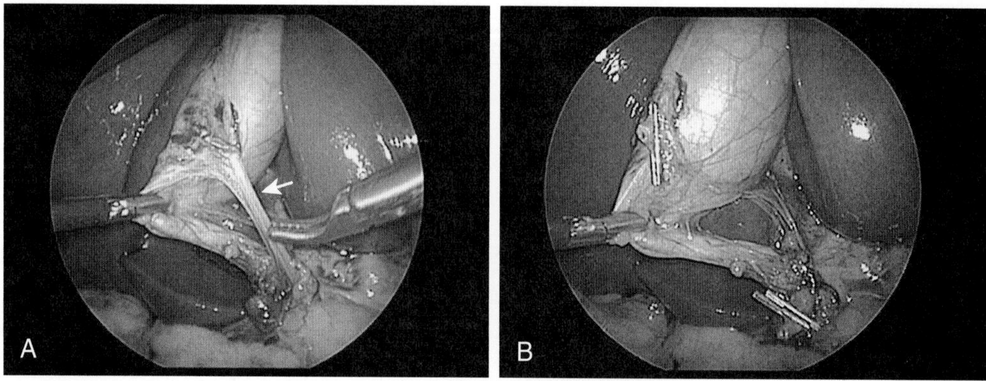

Figure 50-15. When dissecting in the triangle of Calot, it is important to retract the infundibulum laterally which orients the cystic duct at a right angle to the common duct. **A,** The cystic duct is being retracted laterally and the cystic artery (*arrow*) has not been divided. **B,** The cystic artery has been divided. If the infundibulum is retracted cephalad rather than laterally, the cystic duct approaches a more vertical orientation and the cystic duct and common duct can be misidentified.

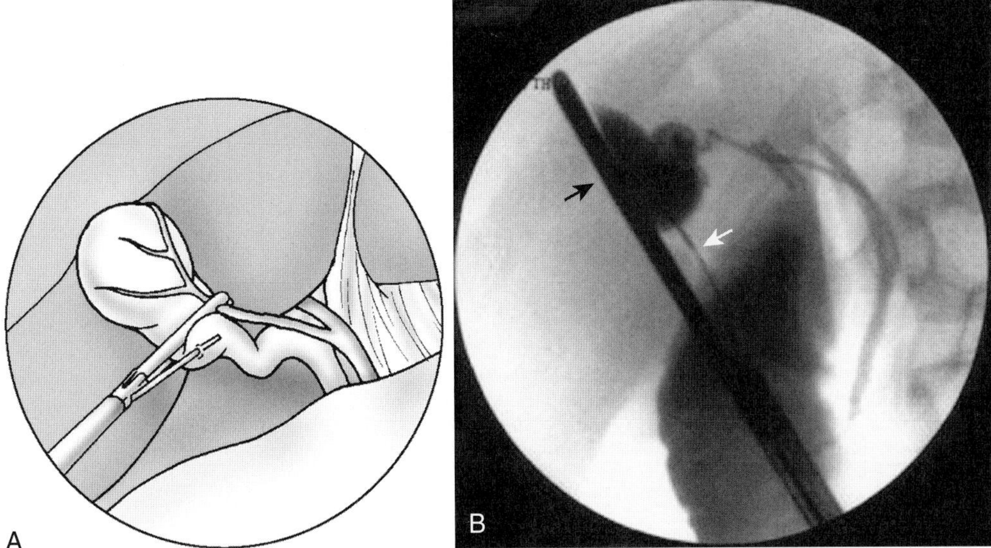

Figure 50-16. The cholangiography technique using the Kumar clamp is shown. **A,** An atraumatic clamp is placed across the gallbladder infundibulum. Through the side arm of the clamp, a sclerotherapy needle is introduced into the infundibulum and the dye is injected. **B,** The cholangiogram. Note the very small cystic duct entering a small common duct. The *black arrow* is oriented toward the atraumatic clamp, whereas the *white arrow* points to the sclerotherapy needle.

made, with insertion of a cholangiocatheter into the cystic duct, followed by cholangiography. In younger children, it is often easier to use the Kumar clamp technique, in which an atraumatic clamp is placed across the infundibulum and a sclerotherapy needle introduced through the side arm of the clamp into the infundibulum (Fig. 50-16).[32,33] After cholangiography, the sclerotherapy needle and cholangioclamp are removed. The advantage of this technique is that a lateral incision in a small cystic duct is technically very difficult, and this technique is much easier to accomplish in younger patients.

After cholangiography, if needed, the cystic duct is ligated and divided with endoscopic clips. Two clips are placed proximally near the junction of the cystic and common duct, and one clip is usually placed near the junction of the cystic duct and the infundibulum of the gallbladder. The cystic duct is then divided. In a similar fashion, the cystic artery is divided. The gallbladder is then dissected in a retrograde fashion from its attachments to the liver. A number of instruments can be used for this part of the operation, including the spatula cautery, the hook cautery, or the Maryland dissecting instrument attached to cautery. Regardless of the technique used, before complete detachment of the gallbladder, the area of dissection is carefully inspected again to ensure that hemostasis is adequate. Then the gallbladder is completely detached and extracted through the umbilical site. With a noninflamed gallbladder, it can sometimes be removed through the umbilical cannula. However, it is often necessary to remove the cannula and extract the gallbladder through the fascial defect. After extraction, the area of dissection is again inspected and hemostasis assured. The ports/instruments are removed, and the incisions are closed. Most patients are ready for discharge the following day. An occasional teenage patient may require an extra day of hospitalization. Gallbladder disease is also discussed in Chapter 44.

Adrenalectomy

Patients with adrenal diseases are being more frequently seen by pediatric surgeons. Usually these diseases are benign, although pheochromocytoma may be seen with very severe physiologic alterations.

The patient should be placed in a lateral decubitus position with the operative side up (Fig. 50-17). For this operation, a 10-mm incision is made in the flank and extended down through the subcutaneous tissue and muscles into the peritoneal cavity. A 10-mm cannula is directly introduced into the peritoneal cavity, and insufflation is achieved. With a 10-mm cannula for this initial site, the dissection is easier and the specimen can usually be extracted either through the cannula or through the incision. After insufflation, accessory ports are then placed. Usually the accessory ports are 5 mm in size, although one or two can be 3 mm. Sometimes it is necessary to divide the peritoneal attachments to the colon first to place the most posterior cannula, because the operative approach is usually from a more posterior direction toward the adrenal gland.

For a left adrenalectomy, the adrenal vein is usually ligated with endoscopic clips early in the operation (Fig. 50-18). Next, the gland is carefully dissected free from the kidney on its inferior and lateral aspect and the diaphragmatic attachments superiorly. Medially, it is dissected from the midline structures. The ultrasonic scalpel can be useful in making this dissection relatively bloodless.

For a right adrenalectomy, the adrenal vein is ligated as one of the last parts of the operation, because the right adrenal vein is very short and directly enters the vena cava. Therefore, it is usually necessary to divide the

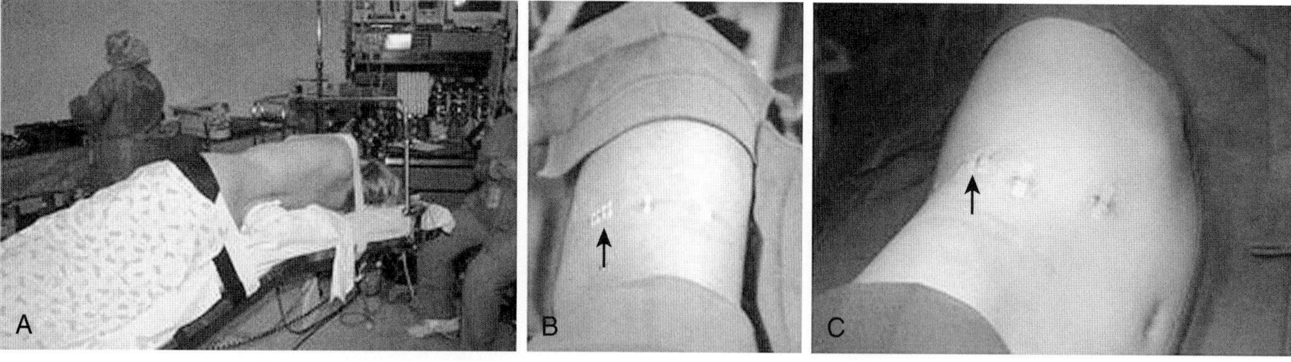

Figure 50-17. Patient positioning and sites of the incisions for laparoscopic adrenalectomy. **A,** The patient is usually positioned in a true lateral position. A roll is placed under the lumbar area, and the table is flexed. **B,** The incisions for a left laparoscopic adrenalectomy. The largest incision (*arrow*) is the site through which the intact specimen was removed in this patient. **C,** In a similar fashion, the incisions for a right laparoscopic adrenalectomy are visualized. Again, the intact specimen was removed through the largest incision (*arrow*), which was approximately 1.5 cm long.

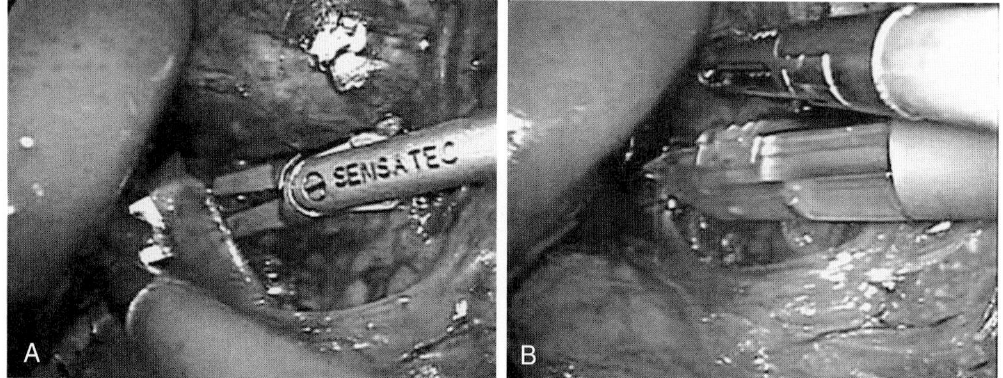

Figure 15-18. Although in a right adrenalectomy the vein is ligated as a final step, ligation of the adrenal vein is usually one of the early steps in a left adrenalectomy. **A,** The left adrenal vein entering the left renal vein is identified. **B,** It is doubly clipped on each side and will be divided between the middle clips. (From Holcomb GW III: Laparoscopic adrenalectomy. In Holcomb GW, Georgeson KE, Rothenberg SS [eds]: Atlas of Pediatric Laparoscopy and Thoracoscopy. Philadelphia, Elsevier, 2008, pp 135-141.)

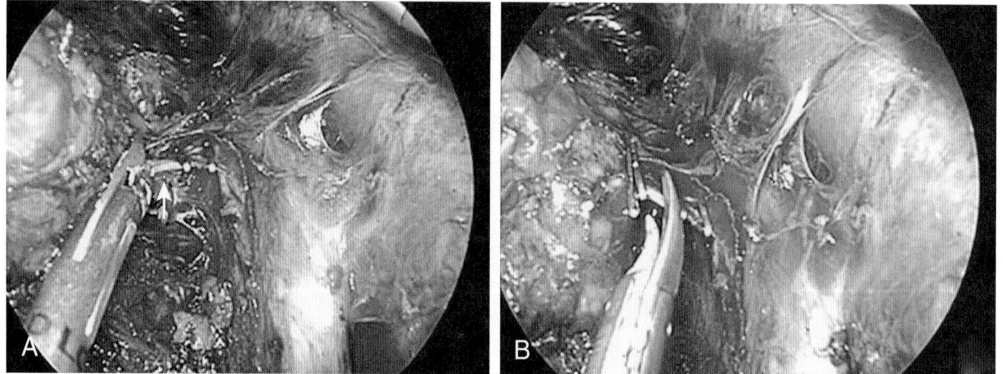

Figure 15-19. After identification and isolation of the right adrenal vein (*arrow*), it is doubly clipped on both the vena cava side and the adrenal gland side (**A**), and then divided between the middle two clips (**B**). The rest of the dissection can be completed easily with the ultrasonic scalpel. (From Holcomb GW III: Laparoscopic adrenalectomy. In Holcomb GW, Georgeson KE, Rothenberg SS [eds]: Atlas of Pediatric Laparoscopy and Thoracoscopy. Philadelphia, Elsevier, 2008, pp 135-141.)

right triangular ligament of the liver for access to the right adrenal gland. The right adrenal gland is circumscribed inferiorly, laterally, and superiorly by using the ultrasonic scalpel. With the right adrenal gland free on three sides, the right adrenal vein is carefully exposed medially. Endoscopic clips are placed on the adrenal vein as it enters the vena cava, the right adrenal vein is divided, and the specimen removed (Fig. 50-19).

Most patients are ready for discharge the day after the operation, although patients with pheochromocytoma often need to be monitored the first postoperative night in an intensive care setting. Usually these patients are ready for discharge on the second or third postoperative day.

Results of laparoscopic adrenalectomy in children have been favorable, with minimal morbidity and no mortality.[34-38]

Small Bowel

Duodenoduodenostomy

Laparoscopic repair of duodenal atresia and stenosis is becoming more frequently utilized.[38-41] In a recent report from my institution comparing 15 patients undergoing laparoscopic repair to 14 infants in a 3-year period having an open operation, the initiation of feedings and discharge was almost 7 days earlier for the laparoscopic group. There were no leaks in either group, but one patient in each group developed a symptomatic stenosis.[41]

Because the distal bowel is not distended, room exists within the infant's abdomen to perform the anastomosis. Familiarity with neonatal laparoscopic suturing is an important skill for surgeons performing this operation.

Four instruments are usually employed for repair of duodenal atresia/stenosis. A 5-mm port is introduced into the umbilicus and a 4- or 5-mm angled telescope is inserted for visualization. After the creation of a pneumoperitoneum, the two working ports for the surgeon are placed in the patient's right lower abdomen. An instrument utilized by the assistant is inserted in the patient's left abdomen. A suture can be placed around the falciform ligament to aid in retraction of the liver (Fig. 50-20). Usually, only one cannula is needed because the three instruments can be introduced through the stab incision technique in an infant with a very thin abdominal wall.

The operation is begun by identifying and mobilizing the dilated proximal duodenum. The distal duodenum is identified and mobilized on its antimesenteric side. If needed for better visualization of the proximal duodenum, a suture can be passed through the abdominal wall in the left upper quadrant, through the distal end of the proximal duodenal segment, and out

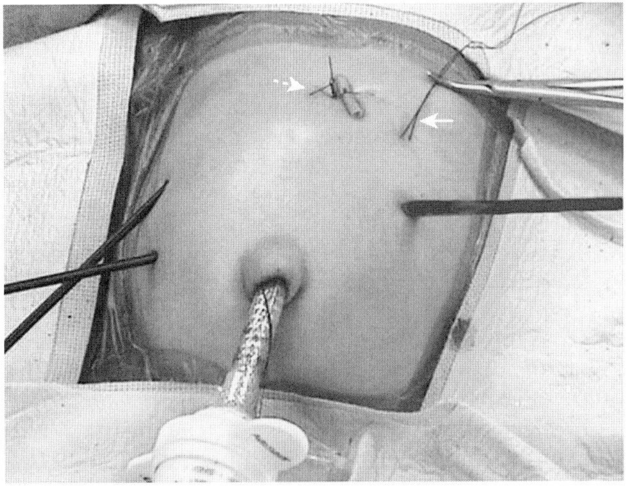

Figure 50-20. For a laparoscopic duodenal atresia/stenosis repair, a 5-mm port is placed in the umbilicus and secured with a suture to prevent its dislodgement. The two primary working ports for the surgeon are in the infant's right abdomen. The assistant's retracting port is in the left abdomen. In this photograph, a suture has been placed around the falciform ligament and tied over a bolster to help elevate the liver (*dotted arrow*). Also, a suture has been placed through the proximal duodenum to aid in its retraction for better visualization (*solid arrow*).

through the abdominal wall in the left upper quadrant (see Fig. 50-20). This suture is secured to a hemostat to allow mobilization of the proximal duodenal segment to aid in performing the anastomosis. A vertical incision is usually made with electrocautery or scissors in the distal duodenal segment, beginning at its blind end. An incision of similar length is made in the proximal duodenum at a right angle to the distal segment enterotomy. Tension on the traction suture on the proximal duodenal segment should be increased or decreased to line up the two duodenal enterotomies for the anastomosis. A diamond anastomosis is created in the traditional fashion. The anastomosis can be created using a continuous suture technique for both the anterior and posterior suture lines or an interrupted suture technique with silk, Vicryl, or U-clips (Fig. 50-21).[41] The anastomosis is begun in the

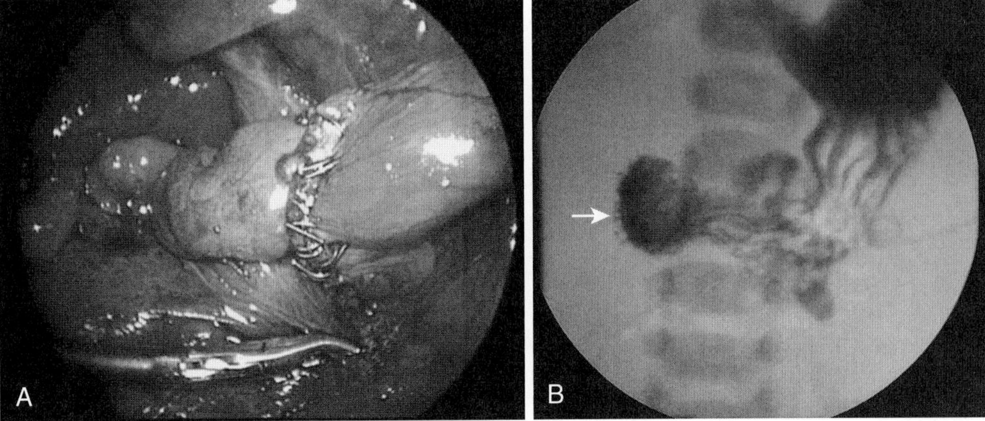

Figure 50-21. **A,** The duodenoduodenostomy can be performed using a continuous suture technique for both the anterior and posterior suture lines or an interrupted suture technique with silk, Vicryl, or U-clips. **B,** In the postoperative upper gastrointestinal study, the U-clips are well visualized (*arrow*). There was no evidence of a duodenal leak or stenosis on this study.

middle portion of the proximal duodenal enterotomy and the proximal end of the distal duodenal enterotomy. It is sometimes helpful to place stay sutures to hold the tissues of the proximal and distal duodenum in apposition for the anastomosis. If desired, the patency of the distal small bowel can be ascertained by using a saline injection technique. A 23-gauge needle is passed into the abdominal cavity attached to a 10-mL syringe. The distal bowel is grasped with a bowel grasper, and the needle is inserted through the abdominal wall and through the lumen of the distal bowel. Saline is injected and monitored visually. Two or three injections may be required more distally to follow the saline stream to the ileum.

The pneumoperitoneum is evacuated, and the instruments are removed. In neonates, even small fascial defects should be closed to prevent herniation of the omentum. The skin is approximated with sterile strips. Duodenal obstructions are discussed more fully in Chapter 31.

Malrotation

Malrotation anomalies offer an excellent opportunity for laparoscopic visualization and repair if the patient does not have volvulus.[42-45] Laparoscopic exploration is useful both in the neonate and in the teenage patient with malrotation diagnosed by an upper gastrointestinal contrast study but with uncertainty about the intestinal attachments to the posterior abdominal wall.[45]

The patient is usually placed in the reverse Trendelenburg position to allow the small bowel and colon to fall away. The laparoscopic operation is begun by the insertion of four instruments. Because I utilize the umbilicus for exteriorization of the appendix for an appendectomy (rather than introduction of a stapler for an intracorporeal appendectomy), I usually place a 5-mm cannula at the umbilicus through which the telescope is introduced. The main working ports for the surgeon are on the patient's right abdomen. A fourth instrument is placed in the patient's left abdomen for use by the camera holder/assistant. Although it is possible to accomplish the operation using three instruments, a fourth instrument utilized by the camera holder can be very helpful in manipulating the intestinal segments.

The presence of malrotation is confirmed by identifying the pylorus and advancing distally along the duodenum. The next step is to find the cecum and carefully separate it from the duodenum by dividing Ladd's bands. Both of these techniques are necessary to ascertain fully the presence of malrotation. If the patient has a volvulus, an attempt at rotating the bowel in a counterclockwise direction is reasonable. However, it is often necessary to convert to an open operation. If necrotic bowel is found, it is usually best to open the patient for further evaluation and surgical correction if possible.

After division of the bands connecting the cecum to the duodenum, the mesentery can be separated widely. Adhesions in the folded mesentery of the small bowel also should be released to allow a further broadening of the posterior mesenteric attachments. It is usually best to begin dividing the bands between the cecum and small bowel and then continue to divide these bands between the cecum, small bowel, and duodenum. The eventual goal of this dissection is to allow the cecum to fall freely into the left side of the peritoneal cavity and to release all subsequent adhesions in the small bowel mesentery. It is surprising that, even with very complex adhesions, an organized approach can unfold the adherent intestinal loops so that the proximal small bowel is retained in the right upper quadrant and the terminal ileum and colon naturally slide into the left side of the abdominal cavity.

An appendectomy is usually performed after the adhesions have been divided. The appendix is exteriorized through the umbilicus (Fig. 50-22) and an appendectomy performed per surgeon preference. Sometimes it is necessary to pull the cecum toward the right lower quadrant to return the appendiceal stump to the abdominal cavity.

The fascia of the incisions is then closed after the pneumoperitoneum has been evacuated. The patient is usually able to start feeding on the first or second postoperative day, unless a significant ischemic insult has occurred to the intestine.

Some pediatric surgeons have expressed concern that a laparoscopic Ladd procedure will not produce enough scarring of the colon and small bowel to prevent future volvulus. Volvulus following an open Ladd's procedure has been reported. I am unaware of midgut volvulus after a laparoscopic operation but this probably relates to the relatively small number of procedures performed. Malrotation is discussed in more detail in Chapter 32.

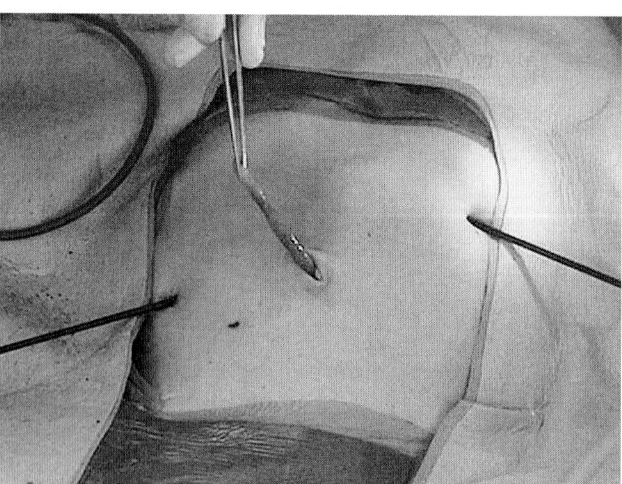

Figure 50-22. This young child is undergoing a laparoscopic Ladd procedure for malrotation. The appendix is being exteriorized through the umbilicus, and an extracorporeal appendectomy is performed. With this technique, 3-mm instruments can be utilized in small children and a large port is not needed for introduction of a stapler. Note two of the three instruments are seen inserted through the abdominal wall.

Reduction of Intussusception

Intussusception is usually diagnosed and treated with a contrast enema and hydrostatic reduction. In approximately 10-20% of patients, surgical reduction is needed. Laparoscopy is an excellent method for the surgical reduction of most intussusceptions that are not amenable to correction by contrast enema or pneumatic reduction.[46,47] Occasionally the intussusception has spontaneously reduced during the interval between failure of the contrast enema and induction of the anesthetic. These patients certainly benefit from visualization of the reduced intussusception, as opposed to an incision to discover the same information. However, in most cases, the intussusception must be reduced by laparoscopic manipulation.

Three incisions are used for laparoscopic reduction of an intussusception. The configuration of these incisions is similar to that used for a laparoscopic appendectomy (Fig. 50-23). The endoscope is passed initially through the umbilicus and then rotated to the port in the left lower abdomen equidistant from the anterior superior iliac spine and the umbilicus. The other site is located in the suprapubic region. The patient is secured to the operating table, and the table is tilted to the left side to allow the small bowel to fall toward the left, so the cecum is well visualized. After visualization of the intussusception, steady traction is used to squeeze the edema out of the intussusceptum so that it can be reduced (Fig. 50-24). Although the classic teaching has been that one should not pull the two segments apart, laparoscopic surgeons have discovered that this dogma is inaccurate. Steady traction on the ileum with countertraction on the cecum, sometimes taking as long as 10 to 15 minutes, results in decrease of the edema in the intussusceptum so that the small bowel can be reduced from the colon (see Fig. 50-24). The operating surgeon must be very careful not to tear or injure the small bowel or colon during this process. A Babcock clamp, which can be used to grasp around the bowel onto the mesentery, or a long, small bowel clamp is best for pulling on the small bowel and for countertraction on the colon. After 10 to 15 minutes, if no reduction of the intussusceptum has occurred, the operation should be converted to an open procedure. Additionally, if it is apparent that the intussusception cannot be reduced because the bowel is gangrenous, a laparoscopic ileocolectomy (described later) can be considered. In most cases, however, it is probably preferable to convert to an open procedure if reduction is not possible.

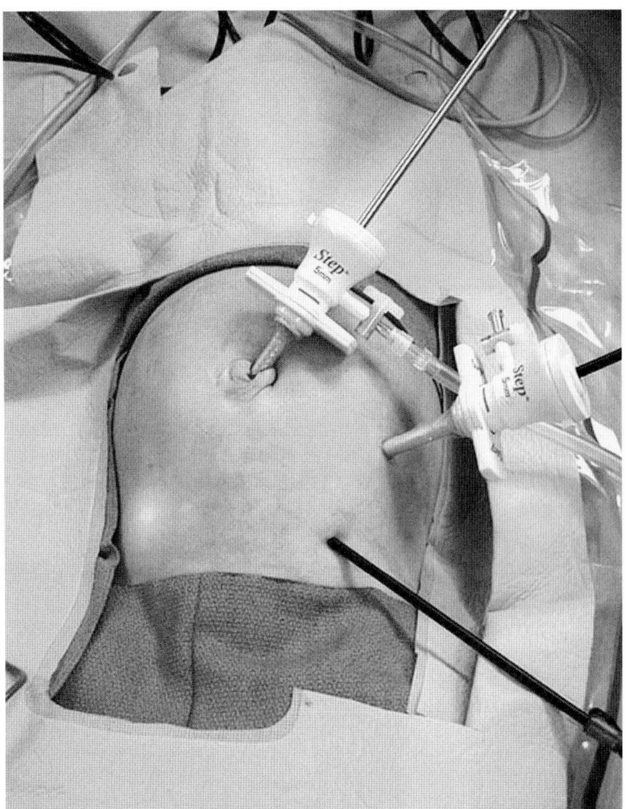

Figure 50-23. The incisions utilized for a laparoscopic reduction of an intussusception are similar to the configuration for a laparoscopic appendectomy. The 5-mm port in the umbilicus can be utilized for either a grasping forceps or the telescope and camera, depending on the surgeon's preference. The other two ports are the working ports through which the instruments are placed to help reduce the intussusception.

If the intussusception can be reduced laparoscopically, the pneumoperitoneum is evacuated. The fascia of the incisions should be closed to avoid herniation of the omentum.

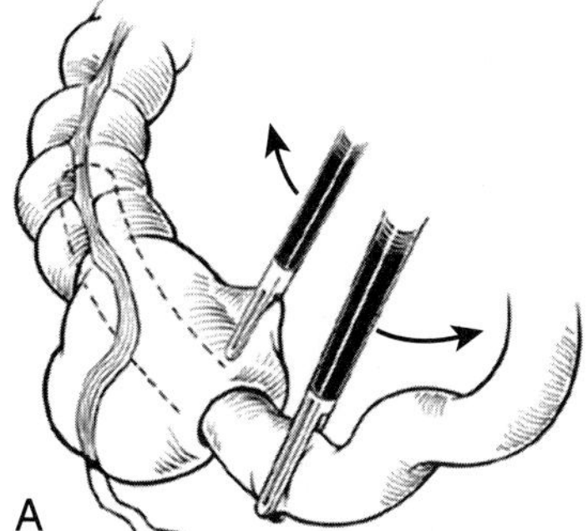

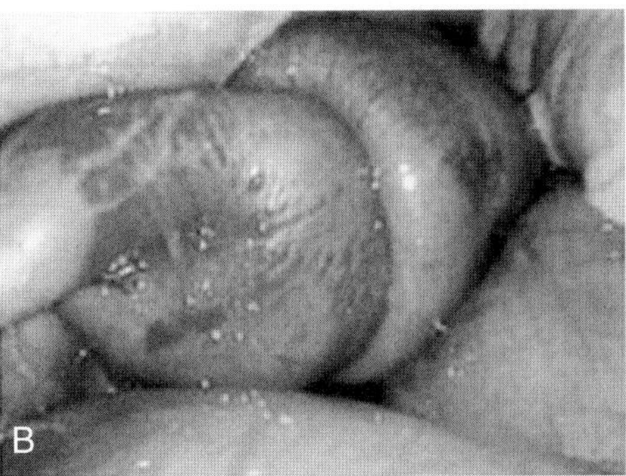

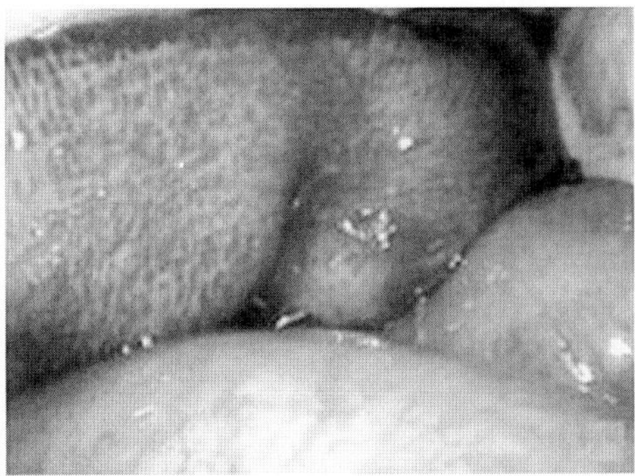

Figure 50-24. **A,** Laparoscopic reduction of an intussusception entails gently pulling the small bowel out of the colon. **B,** The resulting small bowel intussusception can usually be easily reduced. (From Georgeson KE: Laparoscopic management of ileocolic intussusception. In Holcomb GW III, Georgeson KE, Rothenberg SS [eds]: Atlas of Pediatric Laparoscopy and Thoracoscopy, Philadelphia, Elsevier, 2008, pp 71-73.)

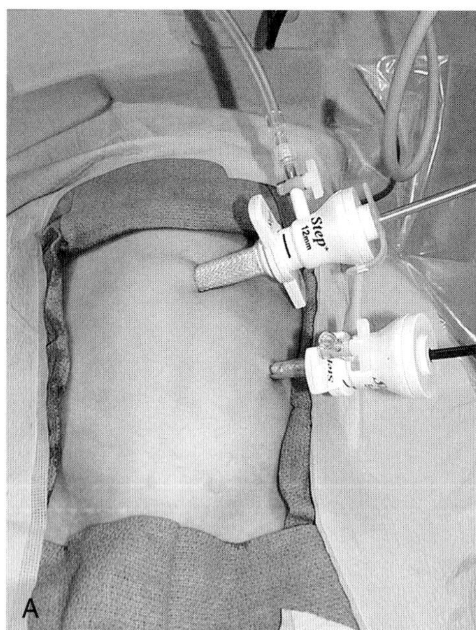
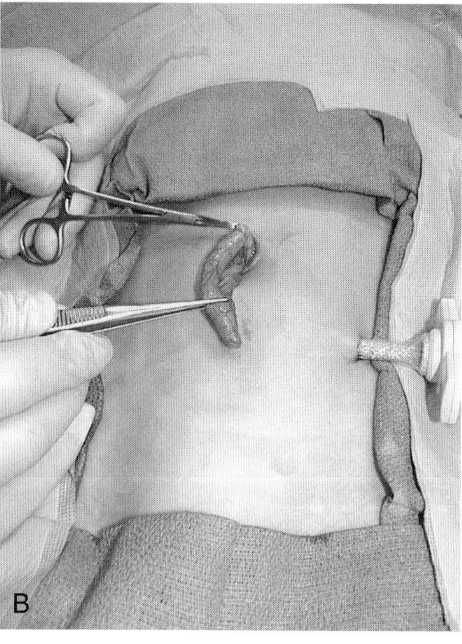

Figure 50-25. In this young patient, an extracorporeal appendectomy was performed. A, Only two incisions were needed because of the mobile appendix. B, The appendix was exteriorized through the umbilical port site, and the appendectomy was performed.

Oral feeding is usually initiated the day after operation. The reported incidence of recurrence is the same for laparoscopic or open surgical reduction. Appendectomy is not usually performed in these patients. Further information about intussusception can be found in Chapter 39.

Colon and Rectum

Appendectomy

Laparoscopic appendectomy is becoming the standard of care for both nonruptured and ruptured appendicitis. Two primary approaches are used for laparoscopic appendectomy. The "in" technique (intracorporeal) uses three ports and is described in this section. The "out" technique (extracorporeal) is commonly used in Europe. With the "out" procedure, the appendix is mobilized without dividing the mesoappendix. The appendix is exteriorized through the single umbilical port site, and the appendectomy is performed in a standard fashion externally through the umbilical incision (Fig. 50-25). The main problem with the "out" technique can be the bulbous size of the appendix, requiring enlargement of the umbilical port site. It also is sometimes difficult to mobilize the appendix and cecum adequately to pull the base of the appendix through the umbilicus. Some surgeons use a small right lower quadrant incision in these circumstances.

The technique most often used in the United States for laparoscopic appendectomy is performed within the peritoneal cavity by using three cannulas. The umbilical port is usually a 12-mm port. This large port is used anticipating that the bulbous, inflamed appendix will be removed through this cannula or the umbilical incision. Moreover, the stapler is inserted through this large port. The other two cannulas are positioned variably by laparoscopic surgeons. I prefer a left lower quadrant site for the endoscope and a suprapubic port site placement for the surgeon's left-hand grasping forceps (Fig. 50-26). With the appendix retracted caudad, a window is created in the

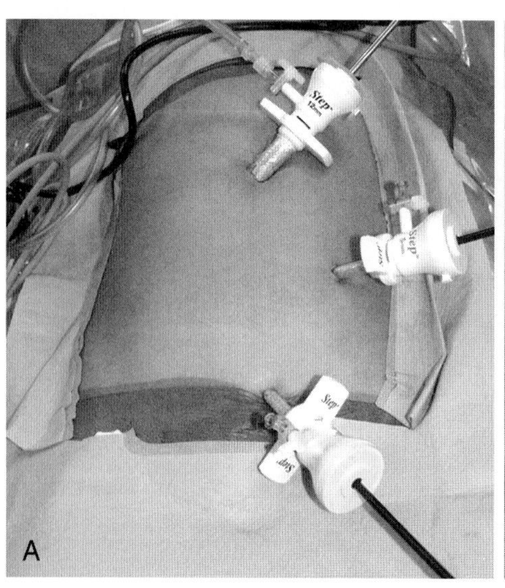
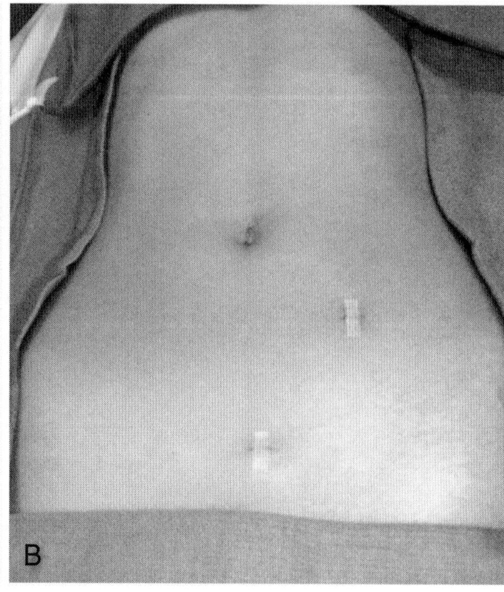

Figure 50-26. A, The typical cannula placement for a laparoscopic appendectomy. Initially the 5-mm telescope and camera are introduced through the larger umbilical port. When the stapler is ready to be introduced, the telescope and camera are rotated to the left midabdominal port and the stapler is introduced through the 12-mm umbilical port. B, Postoperative appearance.

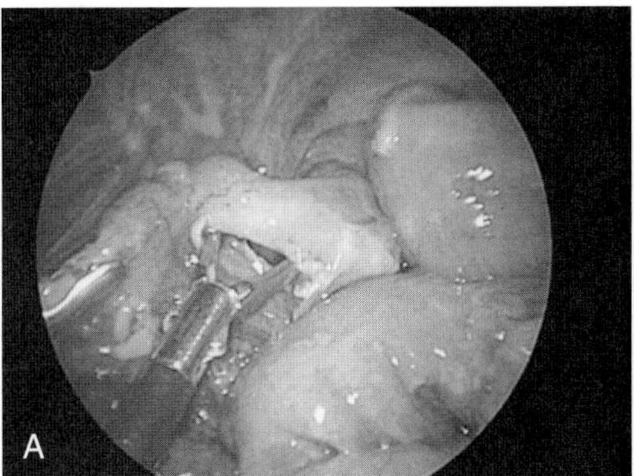

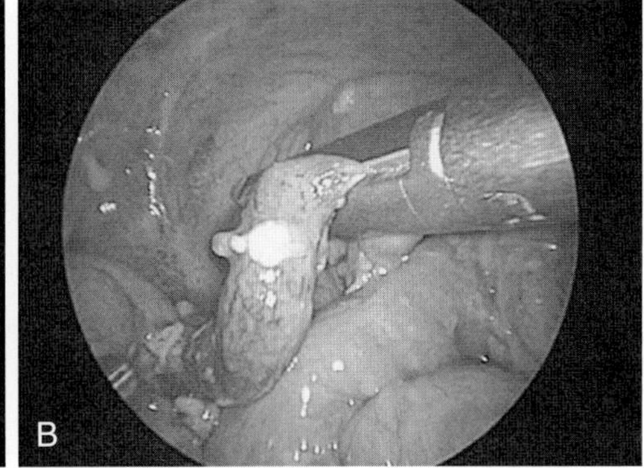

Figure 50-27. **A,** With the appendix retracted toward the pelvis, a window is created in the mesoappendix near the junction of the appendix and cecum. **B,** An endoscopic stapler is then inserted into the mesenteric window and the appendix is usually divided first, followed by ligation and division of the mesoappendix.

mesoappendix near the junction of the appendix and cecum (Fig. 50-27A). An endoscopic stapler is then inserted in this mesenteric window. I usually divide the appendix first followed by ligation and division of the mesoappendix (see Fig. 50-27B). The appendix is exteriorized through the 12-mm umbilical port. If it is too large, it is placed into a retrieval bag and exteriorized through the umbilical fascia and skin incision. Occasionally the fascia and skin of the umbilicus must be enlarged to allow removal of the appendix. This can be accomplished most easily by passing a grooved director both inferiorly and superiorly and by using electrocautery to increase the size of the opening in the umbilical skin and fascia. Once the appendix has been removed, the 12-mm cannula is replaced in the umbilical port site and then the abdomen and pelvis are thoroughly irrigated and aspirated. The ports are removed, and the pneumoperitoneum is evacuated. The umbilical fascia is closed, and the umbilical skin is approximated with absorbable suture.

A plethora of articles have addressed whether laparoscopic appendectomy is equivalent or superior to open appendectomy.[48-55] This controversy has been even more heated over the use of laparoscopic appendectomy for perforated appendicitis. Most of the early reports comparing laparoscopic with open appendectomy usually compared the learning curve for laparoscopic appendectomy with that for the open technique. However, as more large series have been reported, it is clear that the laparoscopic approach to appendectomy has some distinct advantages.[53-55] For my colleagues and I, the primary advantage for laparoscopic appendectomy for perforated and nonperforated appendicitis is a significantly lower wound infection rate. The incidence of intraperitoneal abscess formation seems to be about the same for both approaches. Cosmetic results appear to be better with the laparoscopic approach. For a more complete discussion on appendicitis, see Chapter 43.

Crohn's Disease

Although the medical management of patients with Crohn's disease has improved over the past few years, it is not uncommon for these patients to have irreversible obstruction of the terminal ileum, which can be an unremitting problem, even with appropriate medical management. Laparoscopic ileocolectomy can be performed using four port sites. These may be individualized per surgeon preference. I prefer a 12-mm cannula in the umbilicus and two 5-mm ports in the patient's left abdomen. Another 10- or 12-mm port is introduced in the right lower abdomen (Fig. 50-28). Bowel graspers are passed through the two left-side ports to help inspect the distal small bowel. A point is chosen to begin the resection. An endoscopic stapler with a vascular load is passed through the 12-mm umbilical cannula to divide the small bowel at the selected site. A second stapler is applied when needed. Either an ultrasonic scalpel or sequential vascular staple applications are used to divide the small bowel mesentery (Fig. 50-29). The appendix and cecum are mobilized by dividing the peritoneal attachments laterally. The entire cecum and part of the right colon are mobilized to make the subsequent ileocolic

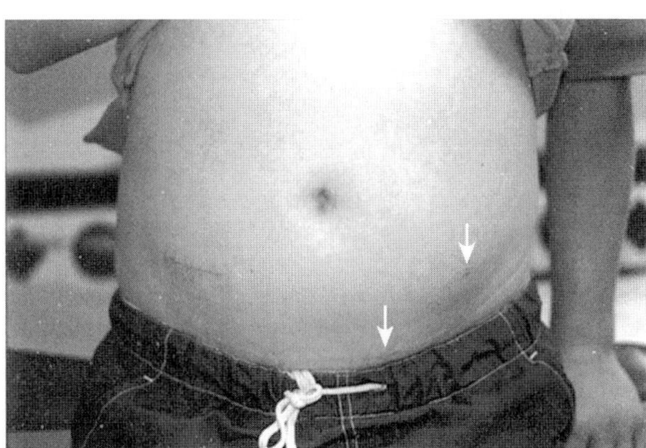

Figure 50-28. The port sites for performing a laparoscopic ileocolectomy for Crohn's disease can be individualized according to the surgeon's preference. It is my preference to place a 12-mm cannula in the umbilicus and two 5-mm ports (*arrows*) in the patient's left lower abdomen. Another 10- or 12-mm port is introduced in the right lower abdomen. This is the site that the specimen is exteriorized and an extracorporeal anastomosis performed. (From Rothenberg SS: Laparoscopic ileocolectomy for Crohn's disease. In Holcomb GW III, Georgeson KE, Rothenberg SS [eds]: Atlas of Pediatric Laparoscopy and Thoracoscopy. Philadelphia, Elsevier, 2008, pp 65-69.)

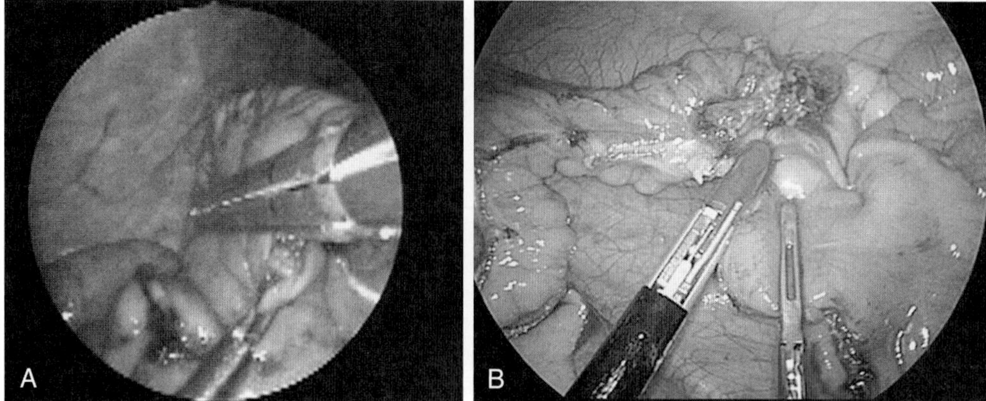

Figure 50-29. Ligation and division of the mesentery can be performed with a variety of instruments. Often, more than one instrument is used. **A,** The endoscopic stapler is used to ligate and divide the mesentery. **B,** The Ligasure is used for the same purpose in a different patient. (From Rothenberg SS: Laparoscopic ileocolectomy for Crohn's disease. In Holcomb GW III, Georgeson KE, Rothenberg SS [eds]: Atlas of Pediatric Laparoscopy and Thoracoscopy. Philadelphia, Elsevier, 2008, pp 65-69.)

anastomosis easier. Dissection of the intestinal mesentery is continued to the mid-cecum. The specimen is exteriorized through the 12-mm right lower port, and an extracorporeal anastomosis is performed. An intracorporeal anastomosis can be performed as well.

The incisions are closed in standard fashion. Nasogastric drainage is not routinely necessary. Oral feeding may begin as soon as evidence of gastrointestinal function is seen.

Although ileocecal resection for Crohn's disease has been performed in relatively small numbers of children and adolescents,[56-58] the adult experience has shown that this is a safe technique with significant cosmetic advantages. Otherwise, length of stay and complications are similar to those with the open technique. Further discussion about Crohn's disease can be found in Chapter 42.

Total Colectomy with J-Pouch Reconstruction

Approximately 20% of patients with ulcerative colitis have active symptoms before age 20 years (see Chapter 42). Some of these patients have unremitting symptoms that require urgent colectomy. Others have more chronic symptoms, such as persistent diarrhea, growth retardation, and delayed puberty. All of these patients are better managed with total colectomy with pouch reconstruction than with continued difficult medical management. Restorative proctocolectomy can be performed with a total laparoscopic technique or by laparoscopic colectomy with the proctectomy and J-pouch construction performed using a suprapubic incision. Moreover, because a proximal ileostomy is usually utilized to protect the pouch-anus anastomosis, the whole operative management can be in two or three stages.

The laparoscopic-assisted colectomy is begun with the surgeon standing to the patient's right. Four or five cannula sites are used (Fig. 50-30). The distal sigmoid colon is lifted anteriorly, and the sigmoid mesocolon is divided using an ultrasonic scalpel. The division of the mesocolon should be kept close to the colon to avoid bleeding. This dissection is carried cephalad to the descending colon. At this point, the lateral peritoneal attachments are divided up to the splenic flexure, followed by division of the descending mesocolon. The gastrocolic ligament is divided starting at the falciform ligament and extending toward the splenic flexure, followed by ligation and division of the lienocolic ligament. The transverse mesocolon is divided from the hepatic flexure toward the splenic flexure, where it joins the previous dissection of the descending mesocolon. At this point, the surgeon moves to a position between the patient's legs. The terminal ileum, appendix, cecum, and right colon are mobilized by dividing the lateral peritoneal attachments on the right side. The terminal ileum is divided with an endoscopic stapler. The mesocolon is divided close to the ascending colon, sparing the marginal artery, which is important for the future J-pouch. The surgeon divides the gastrocolic and hepatocolic ligaments on the right side of the abdomen, and the mesenteric division is completed. May be preferable to make a suprapubic incision for the proctectomy and pouch construction. After making the suprapubic incision, the rectosigmoid colon is divided with a gastrointestinal stapler, and the colon is removed. The remainder of the procedure is performed through an open approach.

Complication rates for total proctocolectomy and J-pouch pull-through are high (25%) for both the open and laparoscopic techniques. The most frequent complications are wound infection and small bowel obstruction.[59,60] The ileostomy is closed about 8 weeks after the initial operation.

Pull-through Procedure for Hirschsprung's Disease

One of the most dramatic changes in pediatric surgical procedures over the past several decades has been the ascendance of single-stage techniques in the treatment

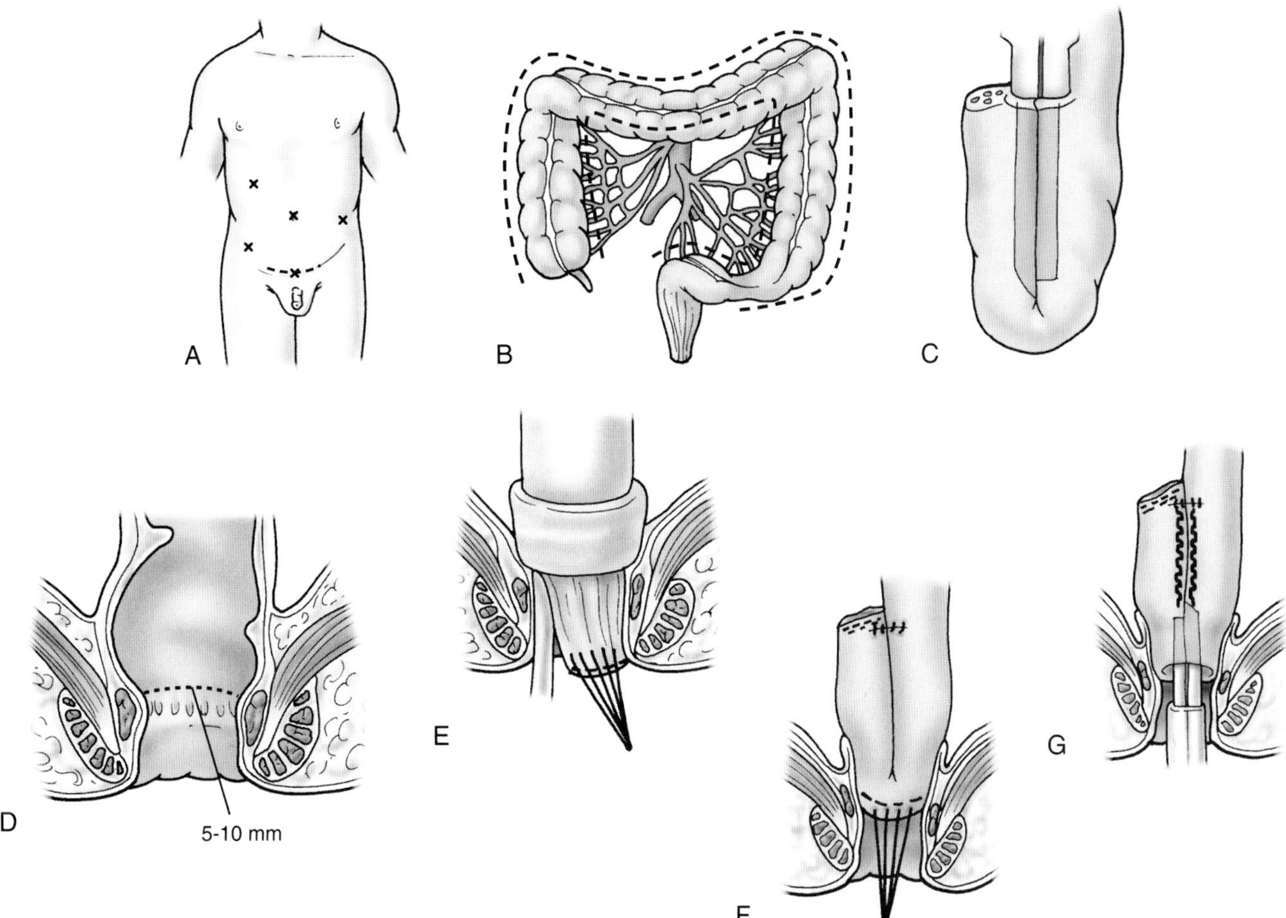

Figure 50-30. **A,** Four or five cannulas are placed as indicated for resection of the intra-abdominal colon. **B,** The intra-abdominal colon is separated from the lateral peritoneal attachments and its mesentery. **C,** An 8-cm J-pouch is formed with a stapler. **D,** The rectal mucosectomy is started near the top of the anorectal columns. **E,** Traction is applied to the mucosa, which is stripped away from the smooth muscle wall of the rectum. **F,** The J-pouch is passed through the muscular cuff without any twists. **G,** The lower portion of the J-pouch spur is divided at the time of closure of the ileostomy.

of Hirschsprung's disease. The primary pull-through procedure for Hirschsprung's disease was introduced in the early 1980s, but its popularity has increased since the late 1990s with the introduction of minimally invasive techniques.[61-65] The most popular technique now is the laparoscopic-assisted endorectal pull-through and its derivative, the transanal pull-through.[64] The laparoscopic technique offers several advantages over the pure transanal pull-through. Most significantly, the laparoscopic approach allows biopsy of the bowel above the apparent transition zone to confirm not only the presence of ganglion cells but also the absence of hypertrophic nerve fibers and the assessment of normally innervated smooth muscle above the transition zone. Because the mucosectomy is irreversible once completed, it is essential that confirmation of normal ganglion cells as well as the absence of hypertrophic nerve fibers be substantiated before initiating the rectal dissection.

A number of surgeons who have previously espoused the pure transanal pull-through now perform laparoscopy for biopsy. In one article, it was found that the transition zone defined by a barium enema was 90% accurate when the colorectal specimens were studied for histologic evidence for ganglion cells.[66] However, this also implies that in up to 10% of cases, the radiographic transition zone will not be correct. Therefore, biopsy of the colon seems best to avoid the unusual case of an infant with total colon Hirschsprung's disease undergoing a transanal pull-through. In this scenario, the surgeon must be ready to perform either a straight ileoanal anastomosis or create an ileal pouch. The biopsy can be performed either totally laparoscopically or through a laparoscopic-assisted technique in which the portion of the colon for biopsy is exteriorized through the umbilicus and the biopsy performed in an extracorporeal manner (Fig. 50-31). The advantage of this technique is secure closure of the biopsy site in case a full-thickness biopsy was performed.

Transanal pull-through is easiest in patients younger than age 6 months. With increasing patient size, the ease of transanal pull-through diminishes. By performing even minimal laparoscopic dissection to the peritoneal reflection, the transanal dissection is made much easier and requires significantly less anal retraction.[64]

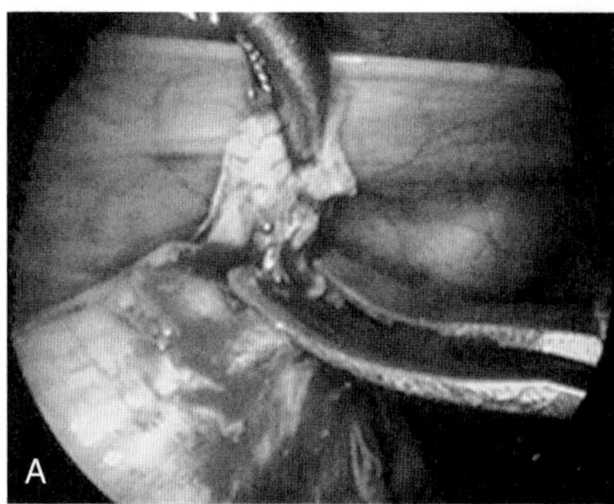

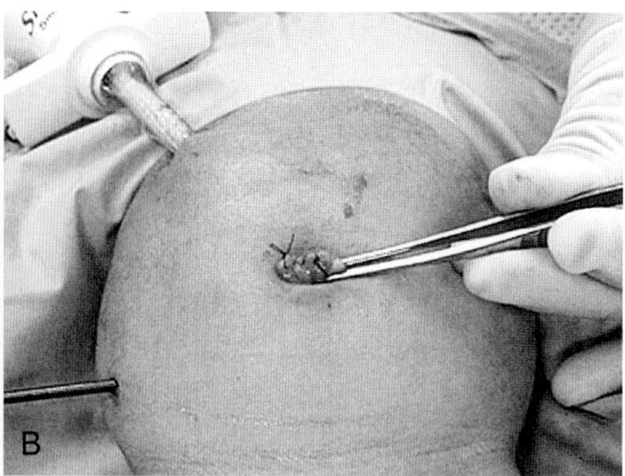

Figure 50-31. **A,** An intracorporeal biopsy is being performed on the sigmoid colon. A fine-tipped grasping forceps has been used to grasp the biopsy site, and Metzenbaum scissors are used to take the biopsy. **B,** An extracorporeal biopsy was performed through the umbilical incision in a different baby. One port and another instrument have been introduced through the infant's abdominal wall. A site on the colon for the biopsy was visualized and delivered just under the umbilical cannula. The umbilical cannula was removed, and this portion of the colon was grasped and exteriorized. An extracorporeal biopsy specimen was obtained and the biopsy site was closed. This is an alternative means for obtaining the biopsy specimen. (From Morowitz MJ, Georgeson KE: Laparoscopic-assisted pull-through for Hirschsprung's disease. In Holcomb GW III, Georgeson KE, Rothenberg SS [eds]: Atlas of Pediatric Laparoscopy and Thoracoscopy. Philadelphia, Elsevier, 2008, pp 102-108.)

Initially, a 5-mm umbilical port and a 5-mm right lower abdominal cannula are placed, followed by biopsy. If an appropriate transition zone is found, a right upper abdominal 5-mm port is inserted and the telescope rotated to this site. A 3-mm instrument is placed through a stab incision in the left upper abdomen for retraction by the assistant. The right lower abdomen site and the umbilical port become the primary working sites for the surgeon. A grasping instrument is inserted through the umbilical port and is manipulated by the surgeon's left hand. The endoscope is inserted through the right upper quadrant cannula, placed just below the liver in the anterior axillary line.

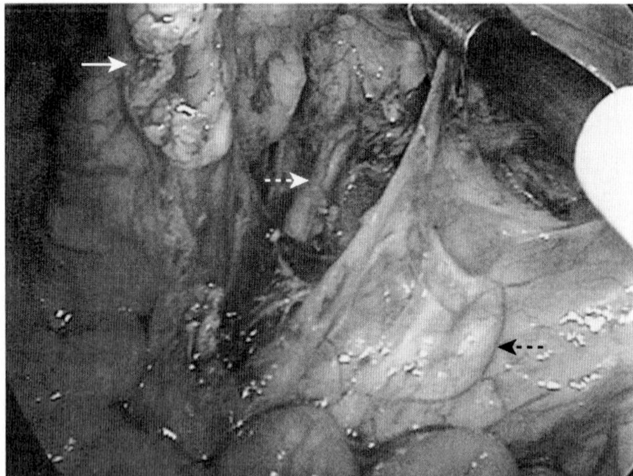

Figure 50-32. This operative photograph shows the view of the pelvis after most of the mesocolonic dissection. The sigmoid colon (*solid white arrow*) has been retracted toward the anterior abdominal wall. It is important to know the location of each ureter during this dissection. The left ureter is identified with a *white dotted arrow* and the right with a *black dotted arrow.* (From Morowitz MJ, Georgeson KE: Laparoscopic-assisted pull-through for Hirschsprung's disease. In Holcomb GW III, Georgeson KE, Rothenberg SS [eds]: Atlas of Pediatric Laparoscopy and Thoracoscopy. Philadelphia, Elsevier, 2008, pp 102-108.)

The surgeon's right hand manipulates instruments introduced through the port in the anterior axillary line in the right lower quadrant.

A hook cautery is used to devascularize the aganglionic segment of bowel. Sometimes, the ultrasonic scalpel is useful in children older than 1 year to divide the larger vessels. Care must be taken to ensure the ureters and vas deferens are not injured during this mobilization (Fig. 50-32). The legs are then elevated, and retraction sutures are placed circumferentially around the anus. A circumferential incision is made in the mucosa 5 mm above the dentate line. The endorectal dissection is done by using a cautery, scissors, and blunt dissection. As the endorectal dissection advances, the muscular cuff intussuscepts outward with traction on the mucosal sleeve. Dissection is continued to the level of the peritoneal reflection, where the muscular cuff is transected circumferentially. The colon is transected, and a watertight anastomosis is performed (Fig. 50-33).

The pneumoperitoneum is re-established, and the pull-through pedicle is inspected. A potential internal hernia space related to the vascular pedicle should be closed with interrupted sutures, preserving the vasculature to the colon. The pneumoperitoneum is evacuated, and the cannula sites are closed. The patients are usually fed on the first postoperative day and are often ready for discharge within 2 or 3 days. For further information about Hirschsprung's disease, see Chapter 35.

Pull-through Procedure for High Anorectal Malformations

Historically, high anorectal malformations have been managed with a posterior sagittal anorectoplasty.[67,68] Although the operation is elegant to perform, the incidence of postoperative fecal incontinence remains high. The laparoscopic-assisted operation for imperforate anus was developed to avoid dividing the levator

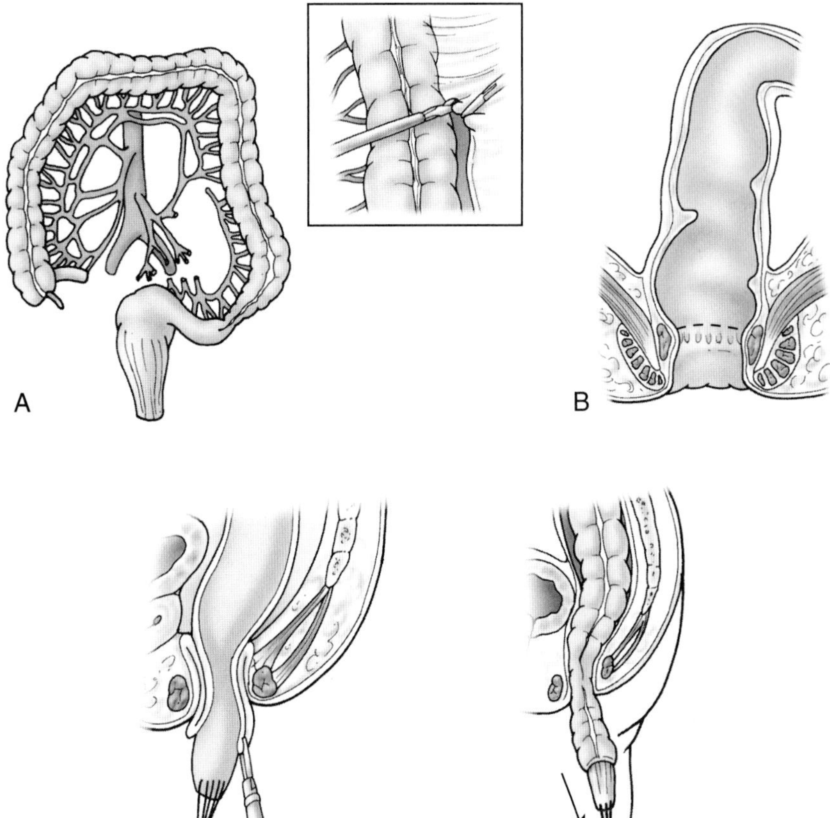

Figure 50-33. **A,** The aganglionic colon is stripped of its mesentery close to the colon wall. When needed, a pedicle is developed, and the fusion fascia is divided laterally (*inset*). **B,** The mucosectomy is performed transanally, beginning about 3 to 5 mm above the dentate line. **C,** When the muscular sleeve of the rectum prolapses, the peritoneal cavity is entered posteriorly. **D,** The aganglionic bowel is removed through the anal opening, and the neorectum is secured to the anal mucosa at the dentate line.

ani muscles and external sphincter muscles.[69,70] Conceptually, this operation approximates the operation for low anorectal malformations, in which the rectal fistula is redirected through the external sphincter complex.

A proximal sigmoid colostomy should be performed at birth. Several months later, the infant is positioned transversely across the operating table. Four cannula sites are used for the laparoscopic-assisted anorectal pull-through procedure. The position of these cannulas is identical to that used for the operation for Hirschsprung's disease. Dissection of the rectum is begun right at the level of the peritoneal reflection using the hook cautery. Injury to both ureters and to the vasculature of the rectosigmoid colon is assiduously avoided. The dissection is continued circumferentially around the rectum down to the rectourethral fistula. It is important to maintain the dissection precisely on the muscle of the rectum and fistula to avoid injury to other structures. The dissection is continued to the junction of the fistula and the urethra or bladder neck. As this point, the rectum begins to taper in size (Fig. 50-34). The fistula is divided 3 to 4 mm proximal to the urethra. A loop ligature is used to secure the urethral side of the fistula (Fig. 50-35). After division of the fistula, the pelvic floor can be clearly visualized (Fig. 50-36A).

Electrical stimulation is used to map the location of the external sphincter complex. A 1-cm incision is made vertically in the gluteal cleft over the identified

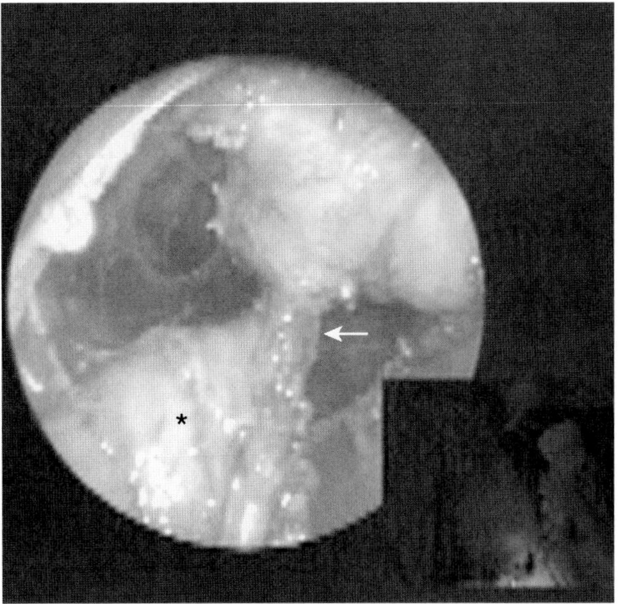

Figure 50-34. The rectum (*asterisk*) is seen tapering in size to the rectourethral fistula (*arrow*) in the pelvis. (From Morowitz MJ, Georgeson KE: Laparoscopic-assisted pull-through for Hirschsprung's disease. In Holcomb GW III, Georgeson KE, Rothenberg SS [eds]: Atlas of Pediatric Laparoscopy and Thoracoscopy. Philadelphia, Elsevier, 2008, pp 102-108.)

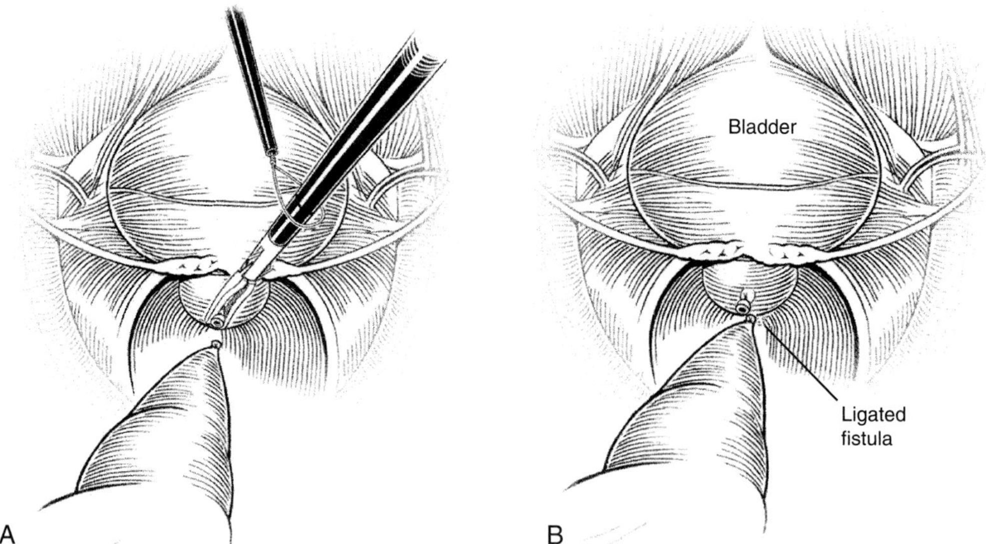

Figure 50-35. After circumferential dissection of the rectum, the fistula has been divided and the rectal end ligated with a pretied ligature. **A,** The fistula on the urethral side is grasped with a Maryland clamp preloaded with a pretied loop ligature. **B,** The ligature is tightened around the urethral side of the fistula. (From Georgeson KE: Laparoscopic-assisted anorectal pull-through. In Holcomb GW III, Georgeson KE, Rothenberg SS [eds]: Atlas of Pediatric Laparoscopy and Thoracoscopy. Philadelphia, Elsevier, 2008, pp 115-119.)

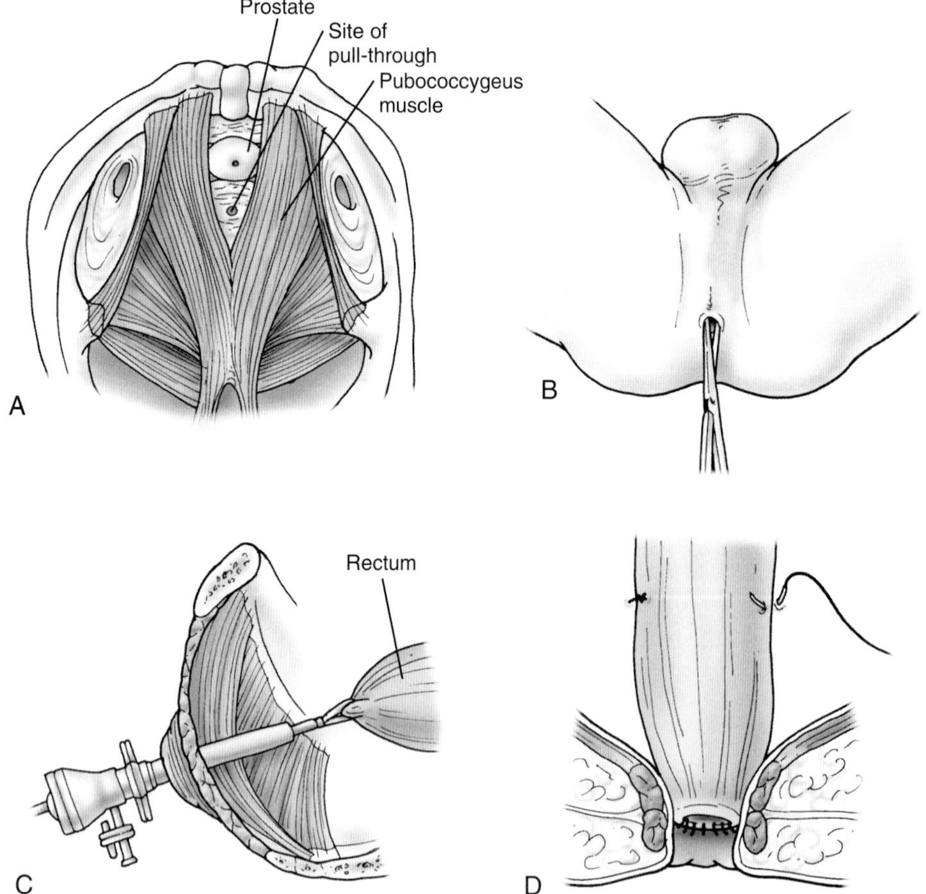

Figure 50-36. **A,** The rectourethral fistula has been divided, allowing visualization of the pelvic floor. **B,** The external sphincters are identified with electrical stimulation, and the plane inside the sphincters is developed. **C,** A Veress needle covered by an expansile sleeve is passed through the sphincter complex by using laparoscopic visualization. **D,** The tract is radially dilated with a blunt trocar, and the rectal fistula pulled down to the anal skin. The fistula is attached to the anal skin, and the rectum is hitched to the presacral fascia to deepen the anal dimple and prevent prolapse of the rectal mucosa.

external sphincter complex. Blunt dissection is used to develop the elliptical plane inside the sphincter complex. A Veress needle covered by an expandable sleeve (US Surgical, Norwalk, CT) is passed through this incision and between the two limbs of the anterior portion of the levator ani complex (puborectalis muscle). This passage is performed under laparoscopic visualization. The Veress needle and associated expanding cannula sleeve are introduced into the pelvis directly in the midline. The Veress needle is removed, and the sleeve is expanded with 5-, 10-, and sometimes 12-mm cannulas. A grasper is passed through the cannula into the pelvic cavity. The fistulous tract is grasped and exteriorized through the passage in the levator ani complex. The fistula is secured to the anal skin with a single-layer anastomosis by using absorbable suture. The rectum is retracted upward and fixed to the presacral fascia with two sutures to invaginate the anal anastomosis and lengthen the skin-lined anal canal (see Fig. 50-36D). The neoanus is dilated beginning 3 to 4 weeks after the operation. The colostomy is closed when the fistulous tract has been dilated to an adequate size.

Although the early results of this operation have been encouraging, it is obvious that many of these patients lack the basic elements of continence, such as the internal anal sphincter or innervation to the muscles of continence. In a review of nonrandomized patients in which approximately half of the patients had been operated on by the laparoscopic-assisted pull-through technique and the other half had been reconstructed using the posterior sagittal anorectoplasty operation, the laparoscopic-assisted group had a 90% incidence of a positive anorectal reflex, whereas in the posterior sagittal group, only 30% of the patients had an intact anorectal reflex.[71] Also noted in this study was that the rectum showed much better compliance in the laparoscopic group when compared with the posterior sagittal anorectoplasty group. The results of laparoscopic-assisted anorectoplasty will require years of follow-up studies to determine its role in the repair of high anorectal atresia. However, the early results are encouraging. Further information about management of anorectal anomalies is found in Chapter 36.

SINGLE-SITE UMBILICAL LAPAROSCOPY SURGERY

Although the applicability of natural orifice transluminal endoscopic surgery (NOTES) appears limited in infants and children, another approach to reduce the number of abdominal incisions is single-site umbilical laparoscopic surgery (SSULS). With this approach, the operation is performed using the umbilicus as the single site for introduction of all instruments. There are a number of approaches for single-site umbilical surgery. Two techniques are shown in Figure 50-37. In one approach, a large (15-20 mm) umbilical incision is made

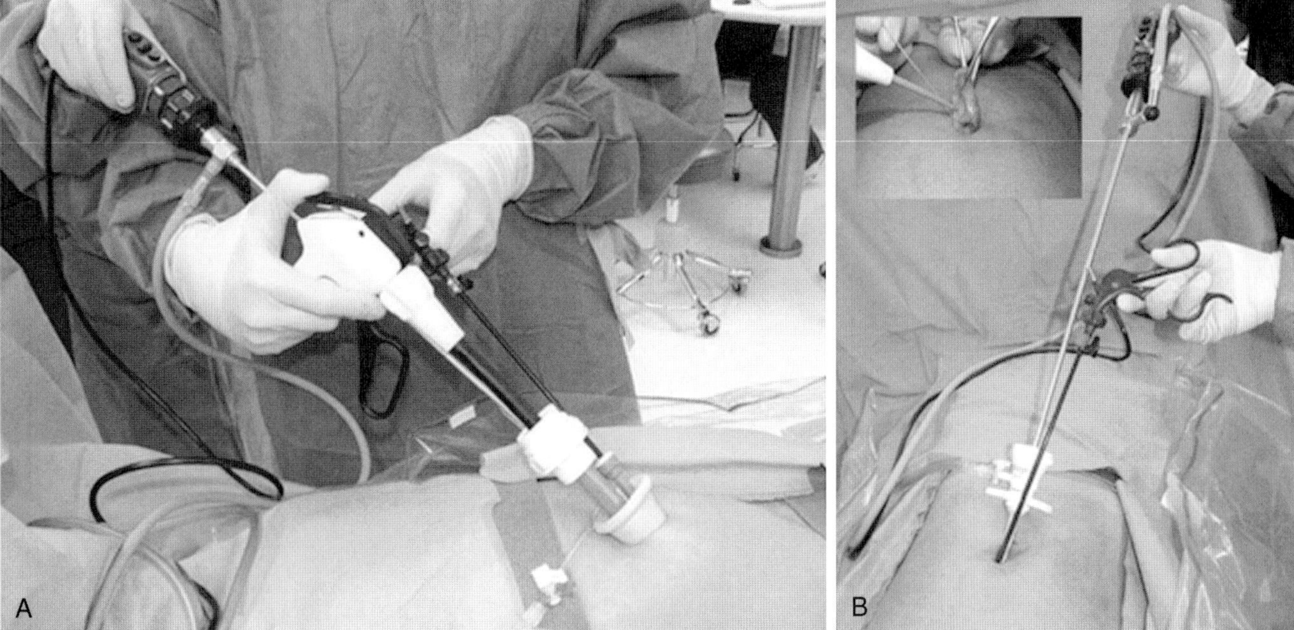

Figure 50-37. A number of techniques have been utilized for single-site laparoscopic surgery through the umbilicus. **A,** A laparoscopic appendectomy is being performed using a SILS Port placed through the umbilicus. With this technique, a 15- to 20-mm umbilical incision is necessary in order to insert the malleable port. There are three working channels in the port that can be utilized for inserting instruments. As seen, a 5-mm telescope, 5-mm grasper, and 12-mm stapler have all been introduced through this port for an intracorporeal laparoscopic appendectomy. On the right **(B),** an adolescent patient is also undergoing a laparoscopic appendectomy through a smaller umbilical incision. In this patient, a 5-mm port has been introduced in the umbilicus for the telescope and camera, and a 5-mm Maryland dissector has been inserted through a stab incision in the umbilical fascia just inferior to the cannula. The lateral peritoneal attachments to the appendix are bluntly lysed using the Maryland dissecting instrument until the appendix has been mobilized and can be brought through the umbilical incision for an extracorporeal appendectomy (see inset). In the inset, the proximal mesoappendix has been ligated with a vicryl suture and the mesoappendix distal to the ligature is being incised with the cautery. This extracorporeal technique is readily applicable for nonperforated appendicitis in which the appendix can be grasped and mobilized through the umbilicus.

through which a SILS Port (Covidien, Inc., Norwalk CT) is inserted. Instruments are then introduced down the three working channels. We have developed a technique using separate stab incisions around a single, umbilical port (see Fig. 50-37B). A 5-mm umbilical port for introduction of the telescope and camera is used. One, two, or three 3- or 5-mm instruments can be inserted through stab incisions adjacent to the 5-mm port. At the completion of the operation, the small stab incisions can be connected to the 5-mm incision, and a single fascial defect can be closed. This SSULS technique can be utilized for laparoscopic appendectomy relatively easily with a mobile appendix as the appendix can be grasped and delivered through the umbilicus, and an extracorporeal appendectomy can be performed. This technique works well for non-perforated appendicitis but is more difficult for perforated appendicitis due to increased inflammation and adhesions encountered in the peritoneal cavity. Also, laparoscopic cholecystectomy can be performed using either of these two approaches as well. The main benefit of a single umbilical site appears to be cosmesis. Currently, prospective randomized trials comparing SSULS (as seen in Fig. 50-37B) with traditional three-port laparoscopic appendectomy for nonperforated appendicitis[72] and with four- port laparoscopic cholecystectomy for gallbladder disease[73] are currently under way at our institution. In the future, the use of single-site laparoscopy will likely be more applicable to infants and children than NOTES.

section 5

INGUINAL REGION AND SCROTUM

chapter 51

INGUINAL HERNIAS AND HYDROCELES

Charles L. Snyder, MD

Inguinal hernia repairs are one of the most common operations performed by pediatric surgeons, and consultations for inguinal hernia are among the most frequent reasons for pediatric surgical referral. An inguinal hernia in a child usually refers to an indirect inguinal hernia but may include a femoral hernia and, rarely, a direct inguinal hernia. The diagnosis and management of inguinal hernias and hydroceles in infants and children and the attendant complications and controversies are discussed in this chapter.

HISTORY

Inguinal hernias were first described in the Ebers Papyrus in 1550 BC.[1] Celsus is thought to have performed hernia repairs in AD 50.[2] Galen, in AD 150, described the processus vaginalis, defined hernias as a rupture of the peritoneum, and advised surgical repair.[3] Ambrose Paré advocated repair of inguinal hernias in childhood in the 16th century.[1] There was a flurry of progress in the 1800s, with Cooper's 1807 identification of the transversalis fascia and the ligament associated with his name and Cloquet's 1817 observation that the processus vaginalis is often patent at birth as well as his description of femoral hernias.[4,5] In 1877, von Czerny first described narrowing the inguinal canal and tightening the external inguinal ring,[6,7] followed by Bassini's description of internal inguinal ring tightening and reinforcement of the posterior canal in 1887.[8,9] Bassini's interest in the subject of inguinal anatomy was personal because he had sustained a groin wound with a cecal-cutaneous fistula in 1867.[6] Gross reported a 0.45% recurrence rate in a large series of hernia repairs (3874 children) in 1953.[10]

EMBRYOLOGY AND ANATOMY

The processus vaginalis is a peritoneal diverticulum extending through the internal inguinal ring into the canal. It can be seen by 3 months of fetal life.[11] The somatic base of this diverticulum is the transversalis portion of the endoabdominal fascia. The gonads form on the anteromedial nephrogenic ridges in the retroperitoneum during the 5th week of gestation. The gonads are attached to the scrotum by the gubernaculum in the male and to the labia via the round ligament in the female. Gonadal descent begins by 3 months' gestation, and the testis reaches the internal inguinal ring by about 7 months. Descent of the testis is initiated and directed by release of calcitonin gene–related peptide (CGRP) from the genitofemoral nerve (via fetal androgen release).[12] CGRP mediates closure of the patent processus vaginalis (PPV), although this process is not completely understood.[11] The testis begins to descend down the canal by the 7th month of fetal life preceded and guided by the processus vaginalis.[11-13] The processus, which is located anterior to the cord structures, gradually obliterates, and the scrotal portion forms the tunica vaginalis. The female anlage of the PPV is the canal of Nuck, a structure that leads to the labia majora. This also closes by about 7 months of fetal life, and ovarian descent is arrested in the pelvis.[11] The precise incidence of PPV in newborns is unknown and depends on gender and gestational age. The incidence has been estimated to be 40% to 60% but may be lower.[14] However, at autopsy, only 5% of adults have a PPV.[11] PPVs at birth can still close, but this becomes less likely with increasing age. It is failure of the PPV to close that results in an indirect inguinal hernia. As mentioned, the factors driving PPV closure are incompletely understood. Intra-abdominal pressure probably plays a role because disorders with increased abdominal pressure/fluid (e.g., ventriculoperitoneal shunts) are associated with an increased incidence of indirect inguinal hernia and with increased bilaterality.[15] Indirect inguinal hernias are more common on the right. The various clinical findings related to the processus vaginalis are illustrated in Figure 51-1.

The layers of the abdominal wall contribute to the layers of the testis and spermatic cord as the gonad descends. The internal spermatic fascia is a continuation of the transversalis fascia, the cremaster muscle derives from the internal oblique, and the external spermatic fascia originates from the external oblique aponeurosis. The processus vaginalis envelops the testis as the visceral and parietal layers of the tunica vaginalis.

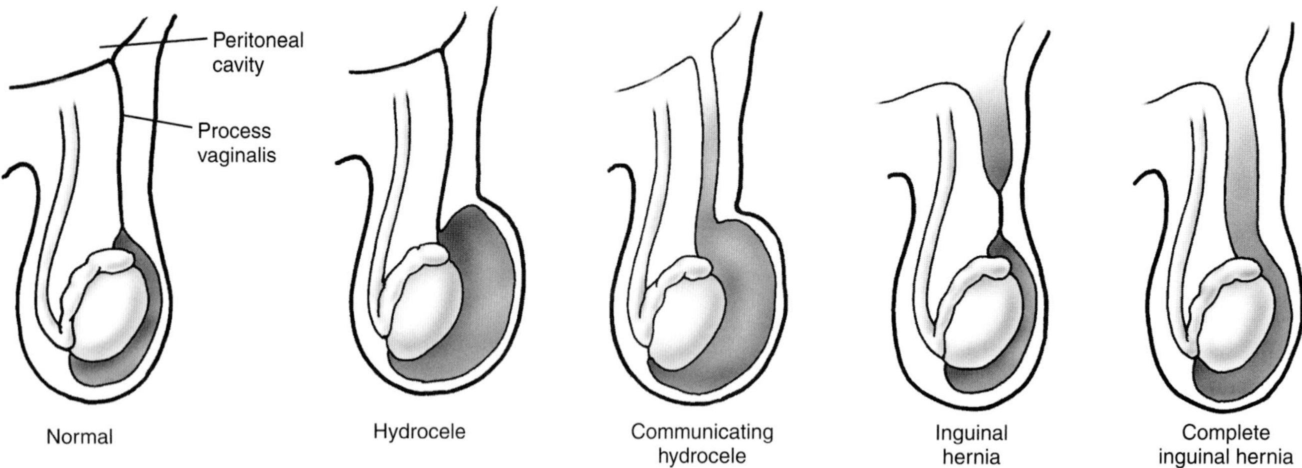

Figure 51-1. From left, configurations of hydrocele and hernia in relation to patency of the processus vaginalis.

INCIDENCE AND ASSOCIATIONS

Approximately 0.8% to 4.4% of all children will develop an inguinal hernia, with a positive family history in about 11.5%.[16] In reviewing cases at our hospital over the past 4 years, there were 15,321 general surgical operations. Within this group, there were 1991 (13%) inguinal hernia repairs. Fifteen percent were performed in infants younger than 6 months of age, 54% of patients were between 6 months and 5 years of age, and 31% were 5 years of age or older. In another series of 6361 pediatric herniorrhaphies performed by a single surgeon, the male-to-female ratio was 5:1.[17] Right-sided hernias were twice as common as those on the left. The mean age in this series was 3.3 years.

The incidence of inguinal hernia varies directly with the degree of prematurity. The overall incidence of inguinal hernia in premature infants is estimated to be 10% to 30%, whereas term newborns have a rate of 3% to 5%.[18-20] Co-morbidities such as chronic lung disease associated with prematurity may play a substantial role in the development of an inguinal hernia in this population.

Other entities associated with an increased incidence of inguinal hernia (Table 51-1) include cryptorchidism, abdominal wall defects, connective tissue disorders (Ehlers-Danlos syndrome), mucopolysaccharidoses such as Hunter's or Hurler's syndrome, cystic fibrosis, ascites, peritoneal dialysis, ventriculoperitoneal shunts, congenital hip dislocation, and meningomyelocele.

Table 51-1	Conditions Associated with an Increased Incidence of Inguinal Hernia
Prematurity	
Cryptorchidism	
Connective tissue disorders, mucopolysaccharidoses, congenital hip dislocation	
Cystic fibrosis	
Ascites, ventriculoperitoneal shunt, peritoneal dialysis	
Abdominal wall defects	
Meningomyelocele	

Patients with cystic fibrosis have an increased risk (eightfold in one report) of inguinal hernia,[21] with an incidence as high as 15%. This heightened risk may be due to elevated intra-abdominal pressure from respiratory problems, but developmental/embryologic factors may also play a role because the risk of hernia is increased in unaffected siblings and parents. Ventriculoperitoneal shunts are associated with an increased incidence of inguinal hernia as well as increased bilaterality, increased incarceration risk, and increased recurrence.[15] In a series of 430 children who underwent placement of a ventriculoperitoneal shunt, 15% developed hernias and hydroceles occurred in another 6%.[22] Injury to the shunt and shunt infection are other problems specific to these children.

CLINICAL PRESENTATION

Most hernias are asymptomatic except for inguinal bulging with straining. They are often found by the parents or by the pediatrician on routine physical examination. The diagnosis is clinical and rests squarely on the history and physical examination. Maneuvers such as having the child raise the head while supine or "blowing up a balloon" with a thumb in the mouth may be helpful in small children. Standing the child upright may also help demonstrate the hernia. The differential diagnosis includes a retractile testis, lymphadenopathy, hydrocele, and prepubertal fat. In older children, neoplasia must be considered.

A common occurrence is a normal examination in combination with a suggestive history. Some surgeons have the child return for a second examination in 2 to 3 weeks, whereas others accept a good history as an indication for operation. Although subjective and dependent on the experience of the surgeon, our preference is for the latter course. False-negative explorations should be rare. In a series of 6361 hernia repairs by a single surgeon (definitive inguinal hernia on examination was the indication for operation), there was only one false-negative exploration (0.02%).[17]

Ancillary findings such as a "silk glove sign" (feeling the thickened peritoneum of the patent processus as the cord is palpated) are of variable reliability.[23,24] Radiologic diagnostic aids are not generally necessary or helpful. Herniograms are of historic interest. Ultrasonography can be used to identify a PPV indirectly via widening of the internal inguinal ring (more than 4 to 5 mm is positive), but the technique is highly operator dependent and not in widespread use.[25,26] It is not generally necessary to restrict an asymptomatic child's activities until repair is scheduled, but prompt repair may decrease interim incarceration.

Another question that has arisen in the laparoscopic era is what to do with an incidentally discovered PPV in a child undergoing operation for an unrelated problem. A common scenario is that of unilateral or bilateral PPV discovered during the course of a laparoscopic appendectomy. A hernia repair should not be performed concomitantly in that setting. The child and the family should be informed of the findings and instructed to watch for symptoms.

OPERATIVE MANAGEMENT

Anesthesia

There are no good data comparing regional to general anesthesia for pediatric inguinal hernia repair. A 2003 Cochrane meta-analysis of available data regarding this issue in premature infants concluded: "There is no reliable evidence from the trials reviewed concerning the effect of spinal as compared to general anaesthesia on the incidence of post-operative apnoea, bradycardia, or oxygen desaturation in ex-preterm infants undergoing herniorrhaphy."[27]

Overnight stay is not necessary after inguinal hernia repair for healthy children or term infants. However, the risk of postoperative apnea and bradycardia is increased in premature infants and overnight monitoring is necessary. The postconceptual age (gestational age + chronologic age) is commonly used to decide which infants require admission. Several studies have addressed this issue.[28,29] Sixty weeks postconceptual age is used at our hospital, because a less than 1% risk of postoperative apnea was found in former premature infants of more than 56 weeks' postconceptual age in a comprehensive analysis of eight prospective studies.[30]

Timing

Because premature infants have an increased incidence of inguinal hernia, this is a common diagnosis in the neonatal intensive care unit. The incidence of bowel incarceration in premature infants is significantly increased (threefold in one large series).[17] Many institutions use 2 kg as a lower limit for repair in asymptomatic and otherwise relatively healthy newborns. We usually repair the hernia before discharge to avoid the need for readmission to repair the hernia and to decrease the risk of incarceration.[31-33] However, this decision is surgeon-dependent and often depends on other co-morbidities.

Operative Technique

Pediatric indirect inguinal hernias are usually repaired through an inguinal crease incision by splitting the external oblique aponeurosis up to the level of the internal inguinal ring. After the ilioinguinal nerve is identified, the anterior hernia sac is grasped and the vas and vessels (in the usual male hernia) are pushed away from the sac (Fig. 51-2A). The sac is clamped and divided (see Fig. 51-2B). A high ligation is performed after the sac is opened and inspected. If contralateral laparoscopic evaluation is performed, a small cannula can be gently advanced through the opened sac (see Fig. 51-2C). A 70-degree, 2.7-mm laparoscope allows examination of the contralateral side (Figs. 51-3 and 51-4).

There is an uncommon but disturbing incidence of late inguinal abscess formation related to the use of

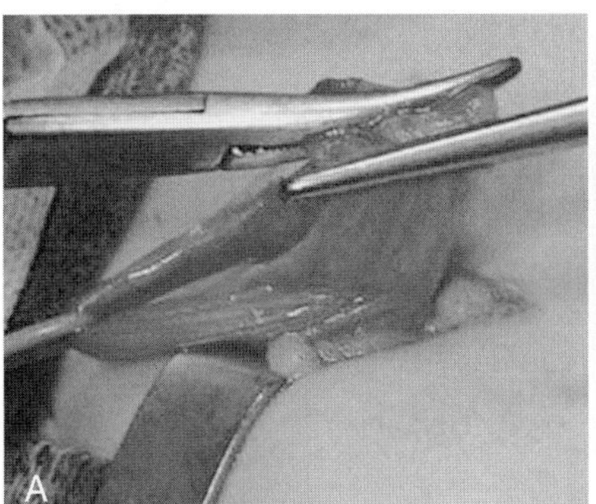

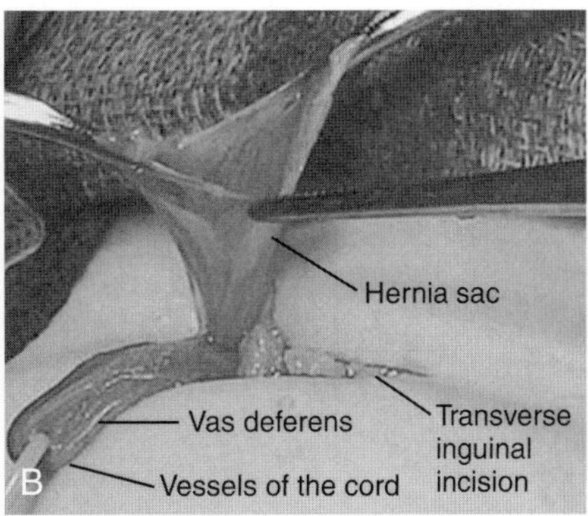

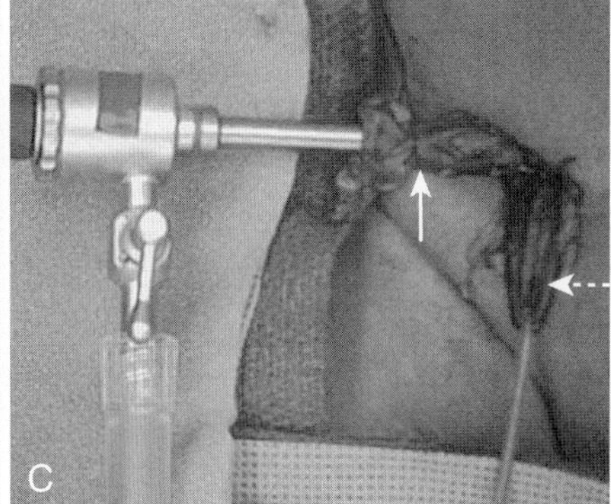

Figure 51-2. **A,** After a right inguinal incision in an infant boy, the sac has been separated from the vas and vessels by grasping the sac and "teasing" the cord structures away. The hernia sac, located anteromedial to the cord, has been carefully separated from the vas and vessels (vessel loop) and is clamped in preparation for division of the sac. **B,** In preparation for diagnostic laparoscopy to evaluate the contralateral internal ring, the sac is opened. A vessel loop is around the cord structures. **C,** A cannula has been introduced into the opened hernia sac and the sac has been tied (*solid arrow*) to keep the abdomen insufflated. The cord structures (*dotted arrow*) are retracted with the vessel loop.

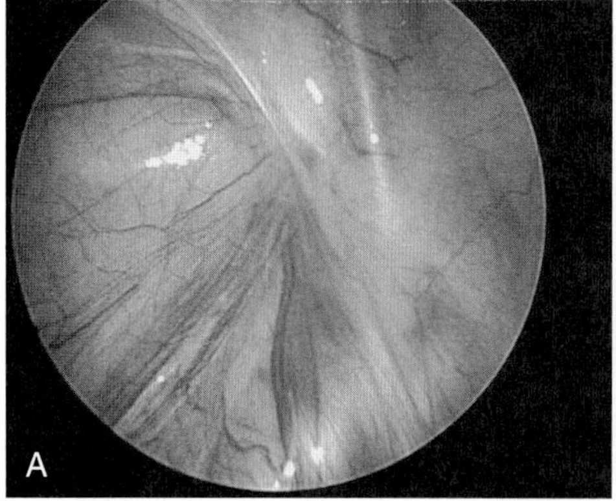

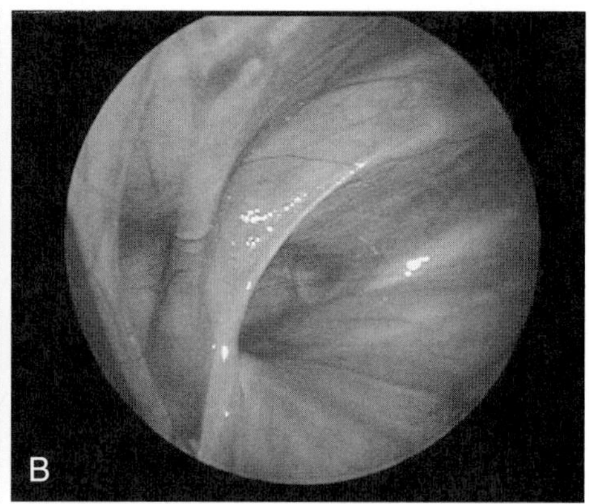

Figure 51-3. Laparoscopic evaluation of the contralateral inguinal region is used by many pediatric surgeons. **A,** A view of the left internal ring shows the inverted "V" of the laterally located gonadal vessels and the medial vas. At the apex of the "V," the left internal inguinal ring is completely closed. **B,** A right-patent process vaginalis is seen in a 7-year-old with a known left inguinal hernia.

silk suture material.[34,35] Therefore, absorbable suture material is now preferred. The sac may be twisted before ligation, but too much twisting may draw the vas and cord structures up into the base of the sac, where they risk being inadvertently ligated. It is not necessary to remove the distal sac. Removing the distal sac may increase the risk of injury to the cord structures and the testis. Distal hydroceles should be opened widely and drained. It is important to ensure that the testis is in the scrotum at the conclusion of the procedure to avoid iatrogenic cryptorchidism.

Sliding hernias are uncommon but are more frequent in females, with an incidence as high as 20% to 40%. A fallopian tube or ovary may be involved. The bladder may constitute the medial wall of the sac in infants.[36] The appendix (Amyand's hernia) may form a sliding component on the right. Distal ligation of the sac with proximal purse-string inversion is our preferred management of sliding inguinal hernias.[37]

Laparoscopic hernia repair has been used in children in both Europe and the United States.[38,39] In one recent series of 712 inguinal hernia repairs in 542 children (median age, 1.6 yr), operative times were similar to those for open procedures. A 5-mm umbilical port was inserted and two 2-mm cannulas were used for suturing. The recurrence rate was 4.1%, with a median follow-up of just over 3 years. This rate dropped to 2% in the latter part of the study. Hydroceles occurred in 0.7%.[40]

Mesh or prosthetic materials are almost never required in children. One exception may be recurrent hernias in children with connective tissue disorders or mucopolysaccharidoses.

Contralateral Hernias

Contralateral exploration for unilateral inguinal hernia in children has a long and controversial history. Meta-analyses, cost analyses, and decision-tree analyses have all been performed.[41-44] The results are discussed in more detail later, but a succinct summary of the conclusions is that routine contralateral exploration is not justified.

Surveys of pediatric surgeons have demonstrated a decrease in the practice of routine contralateral exploration over time, but laparoscopic evaluation of the contralateral side via the hernia sac has grown in popularity.[45,46] In the more recent survey, nearly half of the respondents said they would routinely explore the contralateral side in boys younger than 2 years old and

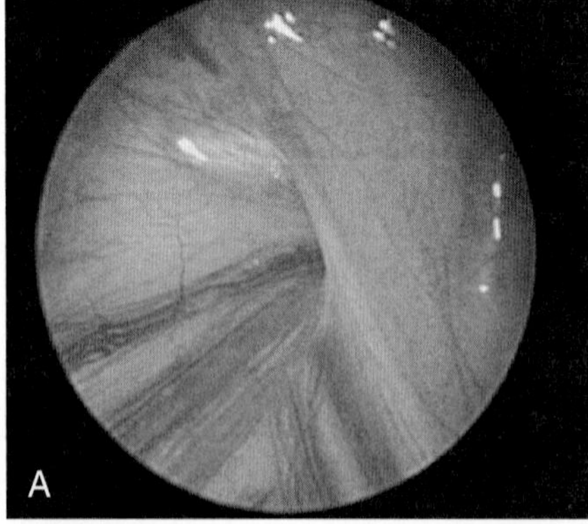

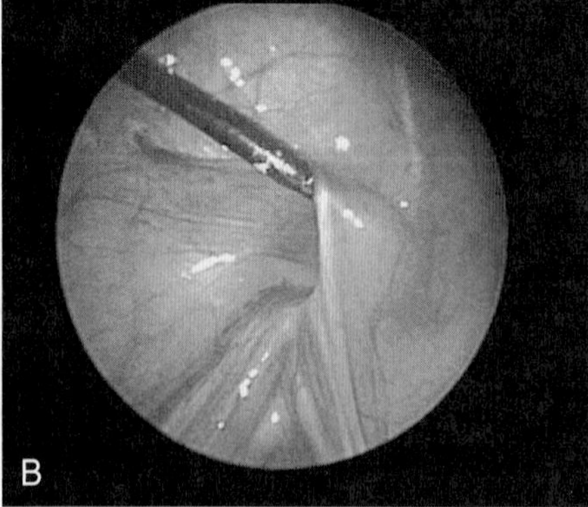

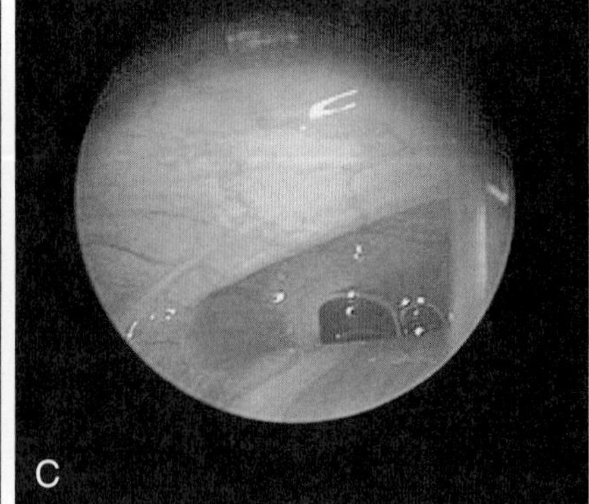

Figure 51-4. **A,** In a small percentage of cases, a veil of peritoneum will cover the contralateral internal ring and obscure the laparoscopic findings such that the surgeon is not completely certain whether a contralateral patent processus vaginalis (CPPV) is present. In this situation, a technique has been reported to retract the veil of tissue. **B,** A silver probe is introduced in the contralateral lower abdomen/flank and used to retract the veil medially so that the 70-degree telescope can then look down the possible CPPV. **C,** In this patient, a significant CPPV was visualized once the veil of peritoneum was retracted medially. (Adapted from Geiger JD: Selective laparoscopic probing for a contralateral patent processus vaginalis reduces the need for a contralateral exploration in inconclusive cases. J Pediatr Surg 35:1151-1154, 2000.)

in girls younger than 4 years old. Contralateral exploration was more likely in females. Approximately one third of surgeons performed laparoscopic evaluation of the contralateral side.

Many reports have addressed the incidence of a contralateral clinical hernia after unilateral repair.[47] A prospective study of 548 patients followed for a mean of 2 years found that 8.8% developed a contralateral hernia, with an average interval of 6 months. The incidence was higher in younger infants, premature infants, and females.[48] Another series of infants younger than 1 year of age who underwent unilateral inguinal hernia repair reported that only 7.7% developed a contralateral hernia during follow-up ranging from 5 to 10 years. Median time to occurrence was 18 months.[49] Another similar study of patients younger than 1 year of age found a 9% incidence of contralateral hernia, also after a mean of 18 months.[50] A meta-analysis of 15,310 patients in combined studies found a 7% incidence of a metachronous hernia.[43]

Although dated, a meta-analysis by Sparkman in 1962 showed 57% of children with a contralateral patent processus vaginalis at the time of unilateral hernia repair.[51] Also, perhaps the best study in terms of a controlled cohort was by MacGregor, who performed 148 unilateral inguinal hernia repairs in children younger than age 10 years over a 32-year period. Ninety-six percent of those were followed for a mean of 20 years of age. Over this length of time, he found that 28% returned with a symptomatic contralateral inguinal hernia.[52]

Left-sided initial hernia repairs may be associated with an increased risk of contralateral disease. Younger patient age and prematurity are also, albeit less frequently, identified as markers for a metachronous hernia. Although female gender carries a lower risk of contralateral exploration, and possibly a higher risk of PPV or clinical hernia, a study of 300 girls followed after unilateral herniorrhaphy found a metachronous hernia developed in only 8%.[53] Younger age, female gender, and a left-sided unilateral hernia have been used as selection criteria for diagnostic contralateral laparoscopy as well as open exploration.

The advent of laparoscopy has not clarified the situation but has added additional information. Theoretical benefits of diagnostic contralateral laparoscopy in children with unilateral hernia include identification of a contralateral PPV (and potential future hernia) without the attendant risks of contralateral open exploration. The mean additional operating time in one analysis was 6 minutes. There is some economic justification for this approach as well.[42,44]

One critical decision point is the incidence of PPV in children with a unilateral hernia. Probably the most accurate assessment is via diagnostic contralateral laparoscopy (See Figs. 51-3 and 51-4), with the caveat that (1) many of these PPVs will not develop clinically symptomatic hernias and (2) it may be difficult to distinguish a peritoneal fold from a true PPV. This technique was initially described in the early 1990s by Lobe and Holcomb.[54,55] The only significant change is that these original reports described umbilical laparoscopy rather than repair through the ipsilateral inguinal hernia sac.

Contralateral laparoscopic evaluation cannot be performed in 4% to 5% of children because of a small or thin sac or poor visualization.[23] Large combined laparoscopic series document a 30% to 40% overall incidence of contralateral PPV.[23,42] However, it remains unclear how many will develop a symptomatic contralateral hernia throughout their lifetime.

Pain Management

A randomized prospective trial of local instillation of long-acting analgesics (e.g., bupivacaine) versus caudal block for postoperative pain control after pediatric inguinal hernia repair demonstrated no significant difference in pain control.[56] Instillation of local anesthetics into the wound ("splash technique") is effective as well.

COMPLICATIONS

Incarceration

The incidence of incarceration is variable and ranges from 12% to 17%.[17,57,58] Younger age and prematurity are risk factors for incarceration.[59] The mean age of patients with incarceration is significantly lower than that of those who have elective repair.[17,60]

Symptoms of incarceration are manifested as a fussy or inconsolable infant with intermittent abdominal pain and vomiting. A tender and sometimes erythematous irreducible mass is noted in the groin. Abdominal distention is a late sign, as are bloody stools. Peritoneal signs indicate strangulation. Incarceration may be the presenting sign of the hernia. It can be difficult to distinguish a hydrocele of the cord from an incarcerated hernia. A happy infant with no tenderness suggests the former diagnosis, but if several examiners have vigorously attempted to "reduce" the hydrocele, the distinction can be difficult and ultrasonography may be helpful.

It is sometimes stated that gangrenous bowel cannot be reduced, but exceptions make this a dangerous "rule" to rely on. The presence of peritonitis or septic shock is an absolute contraindication to attempted reduction. Symptoms of bowel obstruction are a relative contraindication. Monitored conscious sedation is used after intravenous access and rehydration. Firm and continuous pressure is applied around the incarceration. Successful reduction is usually confirmed by a sudden "pop" of the contents back into the peritoneal cavity. Questionable or incomplete reductions should be explored. Once an incarcerated hernia is reduced, a delay of 24 to 48 hours to allow resolution of edema is recommended. Reliability of the family as well as clinical (very difficult reduction) and geographic considerations dictate the need for admission and observation before definitive repair. Overall, 90% to 95% of incarcerated hernias can be successfully reduced.[61] Only 8% required emergency operation in one report of 743 incarcerated hernias, and two children required bowel resection.[17]

Urgent operation is necessary if nonoperative management fails. The hernia may reduce with induction of general anesthesia. If so, the hernia sac must be opened and inspected. The presence of enteric contents or bloody fluid mandates either open exploration (separate incision or La Roque maneuver) or laparoscopic evaluation. It may be necessary to open the internal inguinal ring laterally to reduce the bowel. Some surgeons approach an incarcerated hernia via a transumbilical laparoscopy to both reduce the hernia and evaluate the bowel.[40,62,63] Intestinal injury requiring treatment is rare (1% to 2%), even with incarceration.[57] The hernia sac is often quite edematous and friable, and repair of the hernia can be quite difficult. The risk of recurrence is increased. We do not routinely perform laparoscopy on the contralateral side in patients with incarceration because of these concerns.

Within a true incarcerated hernia, the testis on the affected side is often edematous and somewhat cyanotic. Unless the gonad is frankly necrotic, it should be preserved. The parents of any boy with an incarcerated hernia should be counseled about the possibility of testicular loss or atrophy, but in most cases this will not occur. The incidence of testicular atrophy is 2% to 3%.[33,61] Incarceration of an ovary may not always impair its blood supply, but most pediatric surgeons would promptly (but not emergently) repair the hernia in a girl with an asymptomatic nontender ovarian incarceration.[62]

Recurrence

The risk of recurrence in an elective inguinal hernia repair is less than 1% in several large series.[17,63] It is higher in premature infants, in children with incarcerated hernias, and in children with associated diseases (e.g., connective tissue disorder, ventriculoperitoneal shunt).[15,64] Recurrence rates are as high as 50% in children with connective tissues disorders and mucopolysaccharidoses. A recurrent hernia even can be the presenting symptom in these diseases.[65] Recurrence rates may also be increased in teenagers.[17]

Injury to Cord/Testis

Injury to the cord/testis is a rare occurrence in elective hernia repairs, with an incidence of approximately 1 in 1000 in large surgical series.[17] The true incidence may be underestimated because, in animal models, instrument manipulation or simply touching/pinching the cord can cause microscopic injury and scarring. A recognized injury to the vas should be managed by immediate repair with fine (8-0) suture, and the family should be informed of the event. In institutions in which hernia sacs are routinely examined by a pathologist, mesonephric rests or adrenal rests are occasionally seen but do not indicate injury to the vas. However, a review of 7314 male pediatric hernia specimens over a 14-year period at a major children's hospital found either vas deferens or epididymis in 0.53% of specimens.[66]

Other Complications

Infection occurs in 1% to 3% of cases, and postoperative hematoma has a similarly low incidence. Persistent hydrocele can occur, particularly if a very large hydrocele was present preoperatively. It is important to instruct the family about this possibility before repair. Most postoperative hydroceles are simply observed for 6 to 12 months. If they do not resolve, aspiration may be tried once or twice. In our experience, aspiration is not usually permanently successful. Persistent nonresolving hydroceles usually require transumbilical diagnostic laparoscopy to exclude a recurrent hernia. In the absence of recurrence, a transscrotal exploration and obliteration of the hydrocele sac is performed.

Loss of domain due to a huge hernia in a tiny infant can occur and may even require staged repair. Death directly related to inguinal hernia or its repair is exceedingly rare.

SPECIAL ISSUES

Hydroceles

A frequent issue is whether the presence of a hydrocele in an asymptomatic infant indicates an inguinal hernia. If the hydrocele was not present at birth, or dramatically changes in size (communicating hydrocele), a PPV is present. Massive hydroceles and those extending along the length of the inguinal canal may also require operation. Static hydroceles that fail to reabsorb also indicate a PPV. Our practice is to observe these hydroceles until the child is 1 year of age.

Excision of the hydrocele sac is not necessary. The fluid is evacuated, and the distal sac is opened widely. Large or thick sacs may be everted behind the cord (Bottle procedure) if necessary.[67]

Direct Inguinal Hernias

Direct inguinal hernias are rare in children, even older teenagers. Some recurrences after indirect inguinal hernia repair (or negative contralateral exploration) are direct inguinal hernias. Pediatric direct inguinal hernias are managed with standard "adult" inguinal hernia repairs. Our preference is for a McVay repair (approximation of the transversalis aponeurotic arch and internal oblique aponeurosis to the anterior ileopubic tract and shelving edge of the inguinal ligament).

Femoral Hernias

Femoral hernias are relatively equally distributed by gender[68,69] but much less common than indirect inguinal hernias. In two combined series of over 10,000 patients, 0.2% of hernias were femoral.[70,71] Most (two thirds) are not suspected before operation (Fig. 51-5).[69,71] A mass below the inguinal ligament should alert the clinician to this possibility. Ten to 20 percent of femoral hernias are bilateral. Recurrence

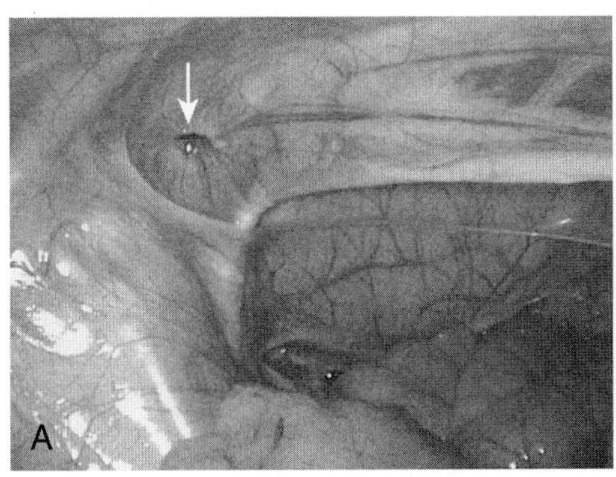
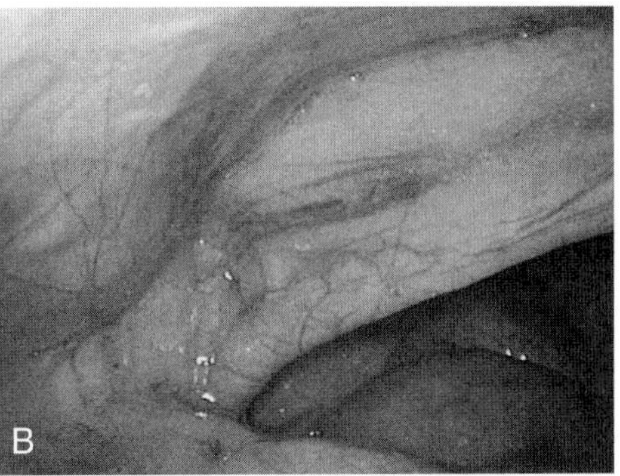

Figure 51-5. This young girl presented with symptoms suggestive, but not conclusive, of a left femoral hernia. Therefore, diagnostic laparoscopy was performed through the umbilicus to confirm the diagnosis prior to an inguinal approach and a McVay repair. **A,** The internal opening to the femoral hernia is seen. **B,** After the McVay repair, the femoral defect is closed.

is increased after femoral hernia repair compared with indirect inguinal herniorrhaphy.[68]

Absent or Atrophic Vas

Occasionally, a small or absent vas is found during inguinal hernia repair. This should prompt a workup for cystic fibrosis. Renal ultrasonography is also necessary because ipsilateral renal agenesis is associated.[72,73] Congenital absence (bilateral or unilateral) of the vas is a heterogeneous disorder, largely due to mutations in the cystic fibrosis gene. Differing genotypes are noted with congenital absence of the vas as an isolated entity versus congenital absence of the vas in association with renal anomalies.[74]

Intersex

The finding of a testis during repair of a female hernia should raise the question of congenital androgen insensitivity syndrome (CAIS) or true hermaphroditism. Some authors have reported that as many as 1.6% of female infants with inguinal hernias will have CAIS.[31] Bilateral hernias in girls are not associated with a higher risk of CAIS than is a unilateral hernia. Conversely, as many as 75% of CAIS patients present with a hernia.[75]

Laparoscopy may allow evaluation of the fallopian tube, ovary, and uterus. The gonad should be sampled. Some advocate rectal examination to attempt to palpate the uterus. Vaginoscopy is an option. In the presence of CAIS, an absent cervix will be found. Karyotyping and pelvic ultrasonography should be performed. Eventual gonadectomy will be necessary, although the timing is controversial. Further discussion is found in Chapter 63.

Other Disorders

Incidentally discovered yellow nodules along the spermatic cord or testis are due to adrenal rests and may be safely removed. Splenogonadal fusion is a very rare entity that may masquerade as a testicular neoplasm. Frozen section confirmation allows gonadal preservation.

chapter 52

UNDESCENDED TESTES AND TESTICULAR TUMORS

Hillary L. Copp, MD • Linda D. Shortliffe, MD

Numerous factors interact to affect normal testicular descent (Fig. 52-1). Any abnormality in this process can result in an undescended testis (UDT). Also known as cryptorchidism, a UDT carries fertility and malignancy implications.

EMBRYOLOGY

Testicular development and descent depend on a complex interaction among endocrine, paracrine, growth, and mechanical factors. Bipotential gonadal tissue located on the embryo's genital ridge begins differentiation into a testis during weeks 6 and 7 under the effects of the testis-determining *SRY* gene. Sertoli cells begin to produce müllerian inhibitory factor (MIF) soon thereafter, causing regression of müllerian duct structures. By week 9, Leydig cells produce testosterone and stimulate development of wolffian structures, including the epididymis and vas deferens. The testis resides in the abdomen near the internal ring until descent through the inguinal canal occurs at the beginning of the third trimester.

An important player in testicular descent is the gubernaculum testis. The gubernaculum is a mucofibrous structure with its apex at the testis and epididymis and its base in the scrotum. It undergoes two developmental phases: outgrowth and regression.[1-3] A crucial mediator of gubernacular development is the testis-secreted hormone insulin-like factor 3. Outgrowth refers to a rapid swelling of the gubernaculum. This process dilates the inguinal canal and creates a pathway for testicular descent. Mice with homozygous mutant insulin-like factor 3 have been found to have poorly developed gubernacula and intra-abdominal testes.[4] Furthermore, if a competitive inhibitor of insulin-like factor 3 is given to rats during pregnancy, cryptorchidism is induced in the offspring.[5]

During the second phase (regression), the gubernaculum undergoes cellular remodeling and becomes a fibrous structure rich in collagen and elastic fibers. Moreover, it is depleted in both smooth and striated muscle cells.[6] Mechanical and anatomic factors, including intra-abdominal pressure and a patent processus vaginalis, are required for normal testicular descent. According to this hypothesis, intra-abdominal pressure causes protrusion of the processus vaginalis through the internal inguinal ring, transmitting abdominal pressure to the gubernaculum and initiating descent. It should be noted that the gubernaculum does not provide traction on the testis to cause descent. It is not

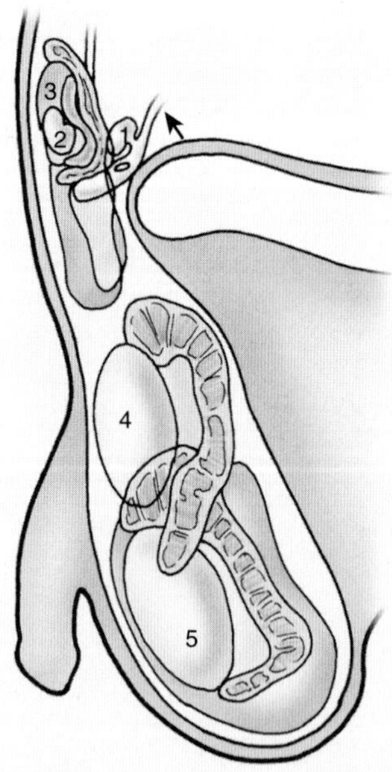

Figure 52-1. Testicular descent in males: (1) 90-mm crown-rump length (CRL) (12-24 weeks of gestational age); (2) 125-mm CRL (15-17 weeks); (3) 230-mm CRL (24-26 weeks); (4) 280-mm CRL (28-30 weeks); (5) at term. The convoluted structure is the epididymis. (Adapted from Hadziselimovic F: Embryology of testicular descent and maldescent. In Hadziselimovic F [ed]: Cryptorchidism: Management and Implications. New York, Springer-Verlag, 1983, p 23.)

anchored to the scrotum, and it does not insert onto the testis.

Androgens have also been shown to contribute to testicular descent. In humans, the frequency of UDT is increased in boys with diseases that affect androgen secretion or function.[7,8] When anti-androgens are given to pregnant rats, the rate of UDT in male offspring is 50%.[9-12] Experimentally, estradiol plays an inhibitory role in testicular descent through downregulation of insulin-like factor 3. Furthermore, maternal exposure to estrogen, such as diethylstilbestrol (DES), is associated with cryptorchidism.[13,14] In addition, growth factors such as epidermal growth factor play an active role at the level of the placenta to enhance gonadotropin release, which stimulates the fetal testis to secrete factors involved in descent such as descendin, an androgen-independent growth factor involved in gubernacular development.[1]

Other mediators of descent include MIF and calcitonin gene-related peptide (CGRP). The role of MIF is probably limited to causing resorption of müllerian structures, which may produce an anatomic obstruction to descent.[2,3] Research in animal models has shown that CGRP is excreted by the genitofemoral nerve under androgen stimulation. It causes contraction of cremasteric muscle fibers and subsequent descent of the gubernaculum, followed by the testis.[15-18] The cremaster muscle is the chief component of the gubernaculum of rats, but it is entirely distinct from the gubernaculum in humans. Therefore, the role of CGRP in human testicular descent remains controversial.[19-21]

The role of the epididymis in testicular descent also has been considered. The gubernaculum inserts into the epididymis, which precedes the testis into the scrotum. Some investigators postulate that under androgen stimulation the gubernaculum facilitates epididymal descent, indirectly guiding the testis into the scrotum.[22] Others believe that an abnormality of the paracrine function of testosterone is responsible for epididymal anomalies and UDT but that epididymal abnormalities do not cause UDT.[20] Epididymal anomalies are found in up to 50% of men with UDT.[23,24]

CLASSIFICATION

Variability in nomenclature relating to UDT has led to ambiguity in the literature and difficulty in comparing treatment results. The clearest classification divides UDT into palpable and nonpalpable.[25] A true UDT has had its descent halted somewhere along the path of normal descent. The ectopic UDT has deviated from the path of normal descent and can be found in the inguinal region, perineum, femoral canal, penopubic area, or even the contralateral hemiscrotum. A retractile testis is a normally descended testis that retracts into the inguinal canal as a result of cremaster muscle contraction. It can be manipulated down into the scrotum on examination without tension and will remain in place. Acquired UDT refers to a testis that was previously descended on examination and can no longer be brought down into the scrotum. An association between retractile testis and secondary testicular ascent has been identified.[26,27] Acquired UDT may also be due to iatrogenic causes. A previously descended testis may become trapped in scar tissue cephalic to the scrotum after inguinal surgery.

Testes may be nonpalpable secondary to an intra-abdominal location. Nonpalpable intra-abdominal testes are further classified as closed-ring and open-ring variants, depending on the status of the internal ring. The distinction between palpable and nonpalpable can be blurred by the fact that the palpable testis associated with an open ring may become nonpalpable when it falls into the abdomen through the open internal ring.

A nonpalpable testis may also be absent or vanishing due to intrauterine or perinatal torsion. This condition is known as monorchia, or anorchia if both testes are absent. Biopsy of tissue at the blind-ending gonadal vessels may reveal hemosiderin and calcification as a remnant of the previously torsed testis.

INCIDENCE

UDT occurs in 3% of term male infants and in up to 33% of premature male infants. The majority of testes descend within the first 9 to 12 months. At age 1 year, the incidence of UDT is 1%, and testicular descent after 1 year is unlikely.[28] However, 2% to 3% of boys undergo orchiopexy for UDT. An explanation for this discrepancy between higher orchiopexy rates compared with the actual incidence of the disease is the acquired undescended testis rate. In a recent retrospective review of 172 patients with 274 retractile testes, the incidence of secondary ascent was 6.9%.[27] The overall rate of secondary testicular ascent has been reported between 2% to 45%.[29]

Series documenting the location of a UDT find that two thirds to three fourths of cases are palpable, with most being palpable within the inguinal canal or distal to the external ring.[30,31] Anomalies associated with UDT include a patent processus vaginalis, epididymal abnormalities, and, uncommonly, hypospadias, posterior urethral valves, prune belly syndrome, and anomalies of the upper urinary tract.

Controversy exists as to whether the incidence of cryptorchidism may be increasing. One study found the incidence of UDT higher in Denmark versus its neighboring country of Finland.[32] Moreover, the incidence in Denmark had increased over time. The authors postulated that environmental and lifestyle exposures may predispose to cryptorchidism and contribute to this increase in incidence. However, these claims were contested by another study that showed the incidence of UDT was stable in Denmark and similar to previous reports from the 1950s.[33] It suggested that differences in the incidence between these studies were most likely due to varying definitions of what constitutes a UDT.

DIAGNOSIS

A careful history and physical examination should enable one to make a distinction between a retractile testis and a low UDT. Because the cremasteric reflex is weak or absent for the first 2 years of life, the diagnosis of a retractile testis is suggested in a boy with documentation of a scrotal testes at birth who is seen later with a suspected UDT.

The diagnosis and location of a UDT are determined by thorough physical examination performed in a warm room. The patient should be examined in both a supine and a frog-legged sitting position. In the sitting position, the boy can lean back on his hands with his knees bent outward and the soles of the feet touching or the lower legs gently crossed. The scrotum is observed for hypoplasia and examined for the presence of either testis. In cases of monorchia, the solitary testis may be hypertrophied. The first maneuver to locate the testis is to walk the fingers gently down the inguinal canal from the internal ring toward the scrotum, trying to push subcutaneous structures toward the scrotum. Lubricating gel may aid in reducing friction. Examining the patient in a squatting position may help identify the testis. Gentle pressure on the mid abdomen may help push the testis into the inguinal canal.

On physical examination, both the retractile testis and the low UDT may be manipulated into the scrotum. The retractile testis should remain in the dependent portion of the scrotum temporarily without traction, whereas the low UDT does not remain in the scrotum. With a retractile testis the ipsilateral hemiscrotum is fully developed, whereas in the other forms of UDT the hemiscrotum may be underdeveloped. Although the long-term implications of human chorionic gonadotropin (hCG) stimulation are not entirely known, hCG injections may be helpful in distinguishing the low UDT from the retractile testis.[34] In response to a total of 10,000 international units (IU) of hCG administered intramuscularly over a 1- to 3-week period, a retractile testis should descend but a low UDT will not.

If neither testis is palpable, anorchia must be differentiated from bilateral UDT. This can be determined by the hCG stimulation test. Baseline testosterone, follicle-stimulating hormone (FSH), and luteinizing hormone (LH) levels are measured before administration of 2000 IU of hCG daily for 3 days, with a testosterone level determined on day 6.[35] If the baseline FSH level is elevated (3 SD above the mean) in a boy younger than 9 years, anorchia is likely and no further evaluation is recommended. If baseline LH and FSH levels are normal and hCG stimulation results in an appropriate elevation of testosterone, testicular tissue is likely present and the patient should undergo exploration. If the testosterone level does not increase in response to hCG stimulation, testicular tissue may still be present and exploration should be performed. The hCG stimulation test does not indicate whether testes or functioning testicular remnants are present.[35]

Radiographic imaging is rarely helpful in locating a UDT. Multiple studies have shown that the experienced surgeon examiner has a higher sensitivity in locating the UDT than does ultrasonography, computed tomography (CT), or magnetic resonance imaging (MRI).[36,37] Of the options, MRI is favored, and it may be useful in obese children.[37-39] The addition of gadolinium in magnetic resonance angiography (MRA) can further improve sensitivity and specificity, because testicular tissue is particularly bright on MRA.[40] For the clinically impalpable testis, laparoscopy has a 95% or higher sensitivity for locating a testis or proving it absent.[37,41,42]

FERTILITY

A UDT and, to a lesser degree, its contralateral mate have been demonstrated to be histologically abnormal by investigators who perform bilateral testis biopsies at the time of orchiopexy. Others have found that the epididymis is often malformed.[43-45] A blunted normal testosterone surge at 60 to 90 days may result in a lack of Leydig cell proliferation and delay in transformation of gonocytes to adult dark spermatogonia. Histopathologic changes include a decrease in the ratio of spermatogonia per tubule and Leydig cell atrophy. An experimental rat model has demonstrated preservation of germ cell number and spermatogenesis in rats undergoing early orchiopexy versus hypospermatogenesis with germ cell apoptosis in rats not undergoing operation for undescended testes.[46] Furthermore, delayed orchiopexy at 3 years versus 9 months of age resulted in impaired testicular catch-up growth.[47] Clinically, patients with a history of UDT exhibit subnormal semen analyses. Despite these findings, the paternity rate of men with a history of unilateral UDT is equivalent to that of the normal population. However, bilateral UDT results in impaired fertility, with paternity rates of 50% to 65%, even if corrected early.[48-51]

RISK OF MALIGNANCY

The risk of developing testicular cancer is 5 to 60 times greater for men with cryptorchidism.[28,52] The risk of malignancy arising from a UDT varies with location and is 1% with inguinal and 5% with abdominal testes.[53-55] There are two competing theories for why this increased risk exists. The first theory rests on the carcinogenic potential of the altered environment of the undescended testis. If this theory is correct, the timing of correction could potentially influence the development of malignancy. In other words, the longer the exposure to the altered surroundings, the greater the cancer risk. This theory has been supported by a recent epidemiologic study examining 16,983 men who underwent surgical correction for UDT.[56] The relative risk of testicular cancer in patients who had orchiopexy before age 13 years was 2.23 versus 5.40 for those having surgery at 13 years or older. An additional meta-analysis showed that orchiopexy after

10 years compared with the operation before 10 years of age was associated with six times the risk of malignancy.[57] The association of orchiopexy with a decrease in cancer risk has not, however, been demonstrated prospectively. Nevertheless, orchiopexy facilitates testicular examination and cancer detection. In addition, indirect evidence supports a decreased cancer risk with early surgical intervention.

The alternate theory is that the malignancy risk may be due to an underlying genetic or hormonal etiology that causes both cryptorchidism and testicular cancer. Support for this theory is demonstrated by the fact that in those patients with a UDT, 15% to 20% of testicular tumors arise in the normally descended contralateral testis.[58] In addition, the incidence of carcinoma in situ (CIS), a premalignant lesion, is 2% to 4% in men with cryptorchidism compared with less than 1% in normal men. In the postpubertal male, CIS progresses to invasive germ cell tumors in 50% of cases within 5 years.[59] The natural history of CIS diagnosed in a young child at the time of orchiopexy, however, is less clear. It has been recommended that these patients undergo repeated testis biopsy after puberty.[60]

The risk of malignancy is highest in testes originally located abdominally. Cancers arising in uncorrected abdominal testes are most frequently seminomas. In contrast, malignancies arising after successful orchiopexy, regardless of original location, are most frequently nonseminomatous germ cell tumors.[61-63]

TREATMENT

Indications and Timing

In addition to the evidence that early scrotal placement may affect the risk of malignancy and infertility, treatment of a UDT also reduces the risk of torsion, facilitates examination of the testis, improves the endocrine function of the testis, and creates a normal-appearing scrotum (see Fig. 52-1).

The UDT is unlikely to descend after age 9 to 12 months. The recommended age for a child to undergo orchiopexy is at or near age 1 year.[64] Repair may be undertaken earlier if a symptomatic hernia is present. The risk associated with undergoing general anesthesia after 6 months is low in hospitals with dedicated pediatric anesthesiologists.

For the unilateral UDT that presents after the onset of puberty, orchiopexy or orchiectomy is recommended. The unilateral, palpable UDT in postpubertal males should be brought down surgically if the testis appears normal and orchiopexy can be easily achieved. If orchiopexy is difficult and a normal contralateral testis is present, or if the UDT is abnormally soft and small, then the UDT should be removed. Orchiectomy is the treatment of choice for management of the postpubertal, unilateral intra-abdominal UDT because of increased cancer risk. In addition, the cord length is often too short for orchiopexy. Laparoscopic orchiectomy is ideal in this setting.[65]

Hormonal Treatment

The value of hormonal therapy in the treatment of UDT is controversial. Buserelin, an LH-releasing hormone agonist or GnRH agonist, is frequently used to treat UDT in Europe. The highest success rates have been observed in cases in which the testis is at or distal to the external ring.[66-69] Trials combining buserelin and hCG have yielded success rates in the range of 60%, but the testis may not remain in the scrotum after therapy and surgical repair is required in 40% of patients.[22,69-71]

Some authors recommend low-dose hCG therapy, regardless of surgical plans, to restore a normal endocrine milieu and to enhance germ cell maturation.[72] hCG may cause virilization, although lower doses do not produce this side effect. Combined hormonal therapy is demanding and requires daily nasal administration of the LH-releasing hormone agonist for 4 weeks and several intramuscular injections. Buserelin, the LH-releasing hormone agonist, has never been approved by the U.S. Food and Drug Administration for this use.

Surgical Intervention

The surgical approach for UDT depends on whether the testis is palpable (Fig. 52-2). Unilateral and bilateral palpable UDT are treated the same way. It is important to re-examine the patient after induction of anesthesia because up to 18% of nonpalpable testes may become palpable on examination under anesthesia.[73] For unilateral and bilateral nonpalpable UDT, definitive management may be determined through a combination of inguinal exploration and diagnostic laparoscopy. We prefer to approach the nonpalpable testis first through diagnostic laparoscopy and then proceed to inguinal exploration as needed. In one retrospective review of 215 nonpalpable testes, only 34% were located distal to the internal ring. Therefore, an initial standard inguinal incision for the remaining 66% of the nonpalpable testes would have been unnecessary or would have provided suboptimal exposure. The initial implementation of diagnostic laparoscopy eliminates extensive exploration for the 10% of the cases that are intra-abdominal, vanishing testes.[73] However, some surgeons still prefer to first explore the groin and then perform laparoscopy. They argue that the only time laparoscopy is definitive is when an intra-abdominal testis is encountered. Because this occurs only 30% of the time, they believe that laparoscopy is usually an additional, unnecessary step.[74]

Palpable Undescended Testes

The mainstay of therapy for the palpable UDT is surgical orchiopexy with creation of a subdartos pouch. This may be performed through a standard, two-incision, inguinal approach or a single-incision, high scrotal approach.[75-79] With the standard inguinal approach the success rate, defined as a testis that remains in the scrotum and does not atrophy, is 95%.[80] Similar

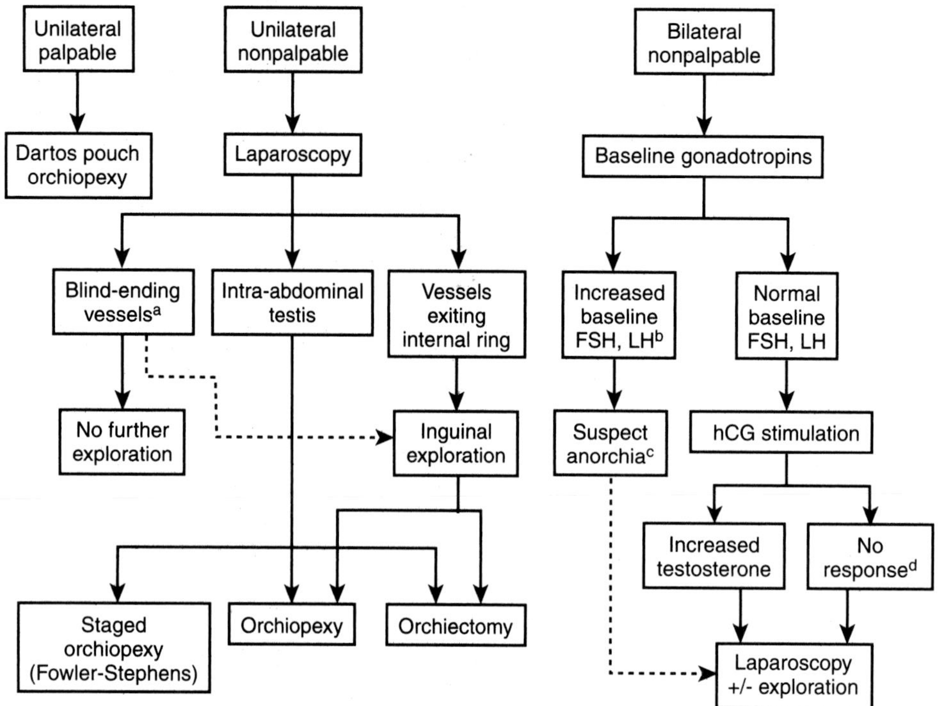

Figure 52-2. Management algorithm for undescended testis. FSH, follicle-stimulating hormone; LH, luteinizing hormone; hCG, human chorionic gonadotropin.
[a]If blind-ending vessels are unequivocally identified, then there is no need for further exploration.
[b]Baseline FSH and LH levels are elevated if values are 3 SD above the mean.
[c]Increased suspicion of anorchia with elevated baseline FSH and LH levels; however, exploration is still warranted.
[d]Testicular remnant tissue may be present despite a negative hCG stimulation test; therefore, exploration for testicular remnant tissue should still be performed.

success rates have been reported for the high scrotal approach.[78,79] With both techniques, scrotal fixation is achieved by scarring of the everted tunica vaginalis to the surrounding tissues.[81] Eversion of the tunica vaginalis also decreases the risk of torsion.[82] The placement of sutures in the tunica albuginea for scrotal fixation is generally discouraged because it causes significant testicular inflammation, increases infertility risk, and may damage intratesticular vessels, especially those in the lower pole of the testis.[83,84] Routine biopsy of the testis at the time of surgery is controversial but may provide prognostic information regarding fertility.[85,86]

A standard inguinal approach to orchiopexy with a subdartos pouch is depicted in Figure 52-3.[75-77] The operation is usually performed as an outpatient procedure under general anesthesia. The patient is supine. Intraoperative administration of an ilioinguinal nerve block with bupivacaine provides excellent postoperative analgesia. The incision should be made along one of Langer's lines, over the internal ring. The external oblique aponeurosis is incised laterally from the external ring in the direction of its fibers, avoiding injury to the ilioinguinal nerve. Once located, the testis and spermatic cord are freed. The testis and hernia sac are dissected from the canal. The tunica vaginalis is then dissected away from the vas deferens and the vessels before its division. The proximal sac is twisted, doubly suture ligated, and amputated. Retroperitoneal dissection through the internal ring may provide additional cord length for the testis to reach the scrotum.

A tunnel is created from the inguinal canal into the scrotum by using a finger or a large surgical clamp. The scrotum is bluntly enlarged. A subdartos pouch is created by placing the finger through the tunnel and stretching the skin in a dependent portion of the scrotum. A 1- to 2-cm incision is made in the skin over the finger, and a hemostat is inserted just under the skin and spread both superiorly and inferiorly to create the pouch. A clamp is then placed on the surgeon's finger in this scrotal incision, and its tip is guided into the inguinal canal by withdrawing the finger. The clamp is then used to grasp the adventitial tissue around the testis. The clamp is then pulled back to guide the testis into the pouch. One should avoid grasping the testis or vas deferens directly, because this may cause scarring. Alternatively, a testicular transfixation suture may be used to deliver the testis to the dartos pouch.

Once the testis is in the dartos pouch, a suture is used to narrow the neck of the pouch to prevent testicular retraction. This suture also may be attached to the cut edge of the tunica. Testis measurements and biopsy may be performed at this time. The scrotal skin incision is closed. The external oblique aponeurosis is

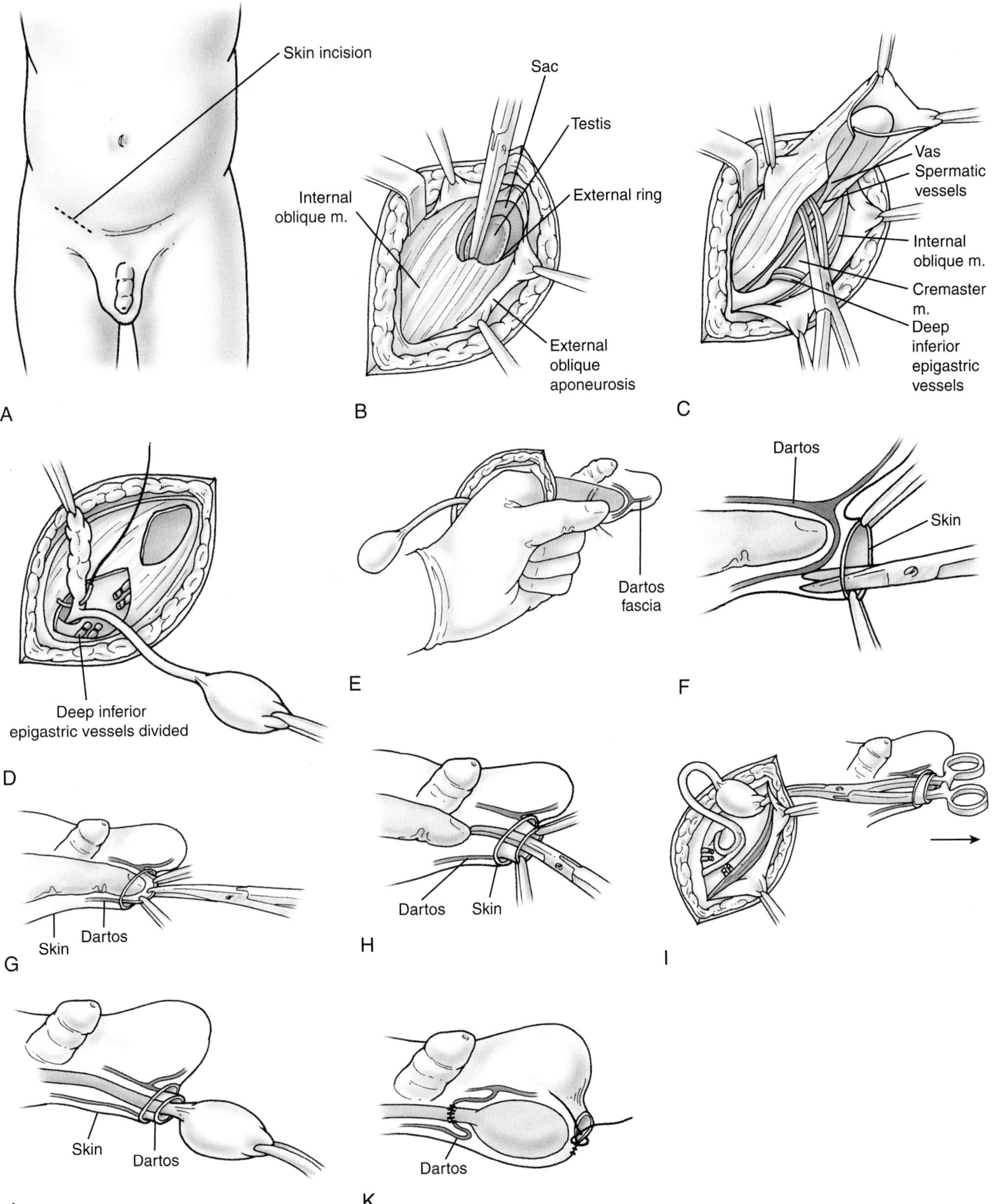

Figure 52-3. Standard inguinal orchiopexy approach. **A,** Transverse skin incision. **B,** External oblique aponeurosis is opened in the directions of its fibers, with care taken to avoid the ilioinguinal nerve. **C,** The testis is delivered, and the patent processus vaginalis is opened distally near the testis. **D,** The processus vaginalis (or indirect hernia sac) is separated from the cord structures and ligated at the internal ring. Adequate cord length is usually obtained by retroperitoneal dissection of the cord contents. If additional length is required, the inferior epigastric vessels may be ligated (Prentiss maneuver), permitting medialization of the cord. **E,** A finger is passed inferiorly into the scrotum to aid in creation of the dartos pouch. **F** to **H,** Dartos pouch creation and passage of a clamp through the scrotum into the inguinal canal. **I,** Adventitial tissue of the testis is grasped with the clamp. **J,** The testis is brought into the dartos pouch. **K,** Dartos fascia and skin are closed. (From Ellis DG: Undescended testes. In Ashcraft KW [ed]: Pediatric Urology. Philadelphia, WB Saunders, 1990, p 423.)

reapproximated with absorbable suture. The skin and subcuticular tissue are closed with interrupted subcuticular stitches. A flexible collodion or topical tissue adhesive dressing is useful in diapered boys.

The patient is seen in the outpatient clinic after a few weeks for a wound check and again several months later for testicular examination. Final position and condition of the testis should be noted. Although rare, complications include atrophy and retraction.

A single scrotal incision technique has also been applied to orchiopexy. While some authors using the scrotal incision orchiopexy technique have shown shorter operative times with similar success and complication rates to the standard inguinal approach, one group demonstrated a 3% risk of postoperative hernia when the scrotal incision method was applied.[78,87]

Unilateral Nonpalpable Undescended Testis

Depending on surgeon preference, the nonpalpable UDT may be approached through inguinal exploration or diagnostic laparoscopy. If the surgeon decides to first approach it through inguinal exploration and no testis or remnant is identified, then diagnostic laparoscopy or laparotomy may be needed to ensure the testis is not in an intra-abdominal location. If the vessels appear atretic or "blind ending" as they exit the abdomen, some surgeons have recommended no further exploration, but this is controversial.

The surgeon may also begin with diagnostic laparoscopy through an umbilical port (Fig. 52-4).[31,41] If the testicular vessels are seen exiting the internal ring, an inguinal incision is used to locate the testis or testicular remnant (Fig. 52-5). Orchiopexy is performed if a viable testis is found. If the vessels end blindly in the inguinal canal (vanishing testis), the tip of the vessels may be sent for pathologic examination. Remnants of testicular tissue or hemosiderin and calcifications are indicative of probable perinatal torsion and testicular resorption.

If diagnostic laparoscopy reveals an intra-abdominal testis, several options are available. The Fowler-Stephens orchiopexy involves ligation of the spermatic vessels, which makes the testis dependent on the vasal and cremasteric arteries for viability.[88,89] For this reason, the Fowler-Stephens approach is not a good option after prior inguinal exploration because the vascular supply to the testis may have been compromised. After ligation of the testicular vessels, which can be done laparoscopically or by laparotomy, a delay of about 6 months is recommended before orchiopexy to allow development of collateral circulation (Fig. 52-6). The success rate of this procedure in modern single-center

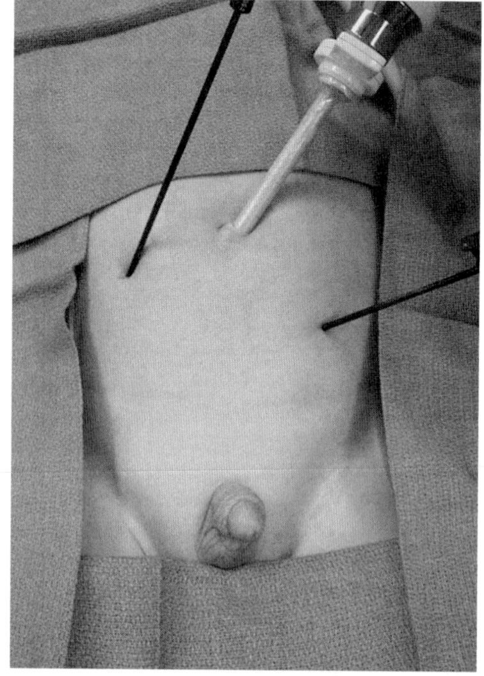

Figure 52-4. After diagnostic laparoscopy through a 5-mm umbilical cannula, if ligation and division of the testicular vessels are required, two accessory 3-mm instruments are introduced into the abdominal cavity using the stab incision technique. The surgeon should stand on the side opposite the nonpalpable testis. (From Holcomb GW III: Laparoscopic orchiopexy. In Holcomb GW III, Georgeson KE, Rothenberg SS [eds]: Atlas of Pediatric Laparoscopy and Thoracoscopy. Philadelphia, Elsevier, 2008, pp 144-148.)

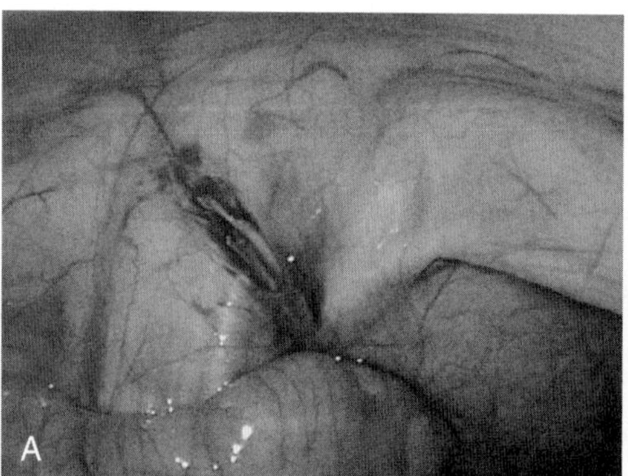

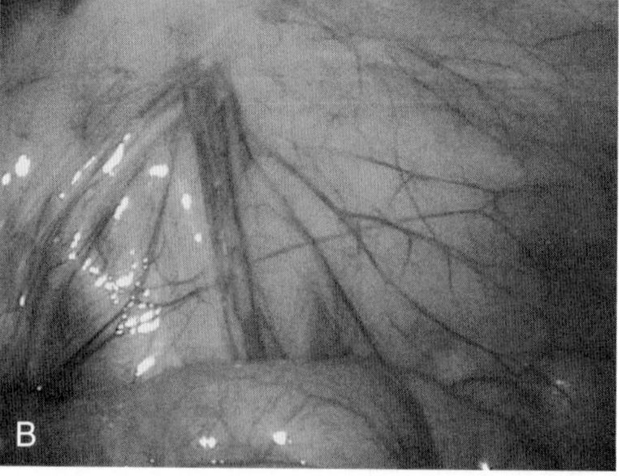

Figure 52-5. **A,** The vas deferens and testicular vessels in this patient end blindly in the retroperitoneum. The internal ring is closed. In this very unusual situation, inguinal exploration is not necessary. **B,** In the more common scenario, the testicular vessels and vas deferens are seen to enter the inguinal canal. There is no evidence for a patent processus vaginalis. The vessels and vas deferens appear to be of relatively normal caliber. In this situation, inguinal exploration is necessary. (From Holcomb GW III: Laparoscopic orchiopexy. In Holcomb GW III, Georgeson KE, Rothenberg SS [eds]: Atlas of Pediatric Laparoscopy and Thoracoscopy. Philadelphia, Elsevier, 2008, pp 144-148.)

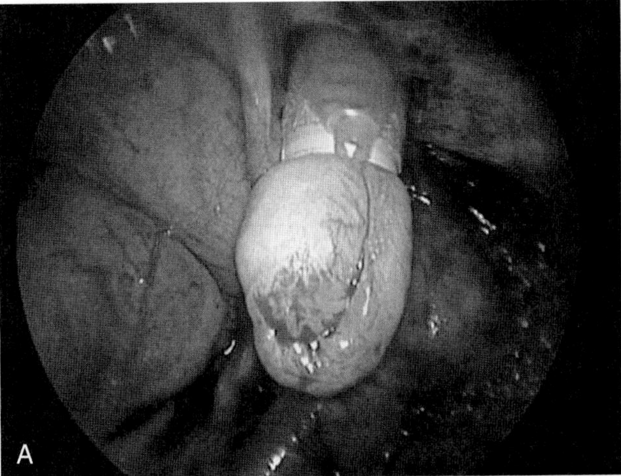

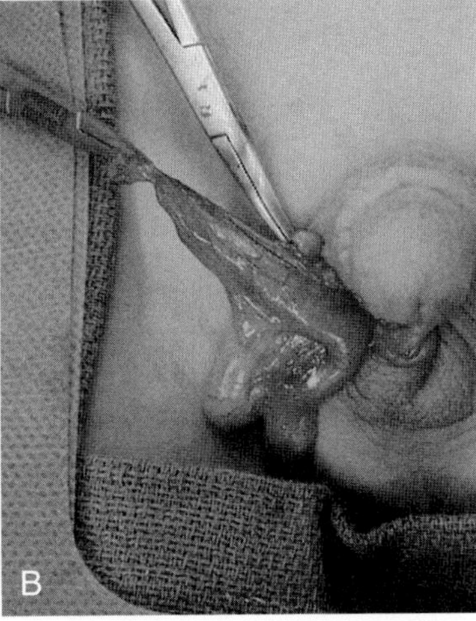

Figure 52-6. **A,** After intra-abdominal mobilization of the testis, the gubernaculum has been grasped with forceps inserted through a 10-mm cannula that has been introduced through the scrotal incision, over the pubic tubercle and into the abdomen. The testis is then withdrawn into the cannula. Often, it is not possible to place the testis entirely into the 10-mm port. **B,** The testis is delivered over the pubic tubercle and into the right hemiscrotum. (From Holcomb GW III: Laparoscopic orchiopexy. In Holcomb GW III, Georgeson KE, Rothenberg SS [eds]: Atlas of Pediatric Laparoscopy and Thoracoscopy. Philadelphia, Elsevier, 2008, pp 144-148.)

case series when defined as lack of atrophy and normal scrotal position is greater than 90%.[90-93] These success rates were maintained in studies that had a long-term mean follow-up of more than 3 years. Furthermore, a multi-institutional analysis revealed a similar 90% success rate for the two-stage laparoscopic Fowler-Stephens orchiopexy.[94] However, a higher failure rate was observed when the single-stage Fowler-Stephens orchiopexy was performed, and therefore caution is advised with this approach.

Other options for surgical management of intra-abdominal testes include microvascular orchiopexy (autotransplantation) and orchiectomy. In the hands of skilled laparoscopists, results from the two-stage laparoscopic orchiopexy compare favorably with those of open surgery.[95] Others have found that a one-stage laparoscopic orchiopexy without ligation is often possible, especially when the testis lies below the iliac vessels. Magnification and wide mobilization with laparoscopy can afford greater cord length and perhaps better preservation of collateral vascular supply.[96,97]

Bilateral Nonpalpable Undescended Testes

Diagnostic laparoscopy or laparotomy may be performed to determine surgical therapy in the same manner as for unilateral, nonpalpable UDT.

Secondary Undescended Testis

Secondary UDT is an uncommon complication of inguinal hernia repair, orchiopexy, or hydrocelectomy. When it is found, surgical dissection is different from that of primary repair because scarring from the previous procedure makes dissection difficult. The surgical technique that we have found successful for reoperative orchiopexy minimizes the risk to the spermatic cord contents (especially the vas deferens) by mobilizing the entire cord and scar en bloc along with a strip of external oblique aponeurosis.[98] The incision is made through the previous scar, and the testis, which is usually palpable near the pubic tubercle, is exposed. A traction suture is placed through the tunica albuginea in the mid-testis. Parallel incisions in the external oblique aponeurosis allow the testis/cord/aponeurosis complex to be lifted from the canal so that a plane is developed between the spermatic cord and the inguinal floor. This dissection is carried superiorly to the internal ring, where the external oblique aponeurosis is cut to allow full mobilization of the cord and testis. Dissection continues above the scar, into the retroperitoneum, to produce sufficient length to permit placement of the testis into a dartos pouch. If more length is necessary, division of the inferior epigastric vessels allows the cord to be displaced medially.

TESTICULAR CANCER

The peak incidence of pediatric testicular tumors occurs between ages 12 to 18 months, followed by a small peak during puberty. Testicular cancer is uncommon in children, accounting for 1% to 2% of all pediatric solid tumors. In contrast to the rising incidence of testicular cancer observed in adult men, the incidence of pediatric testicular germ cell tumors in U.S. children was stable from 1973 to 2000.[99] However, comparable to adults, race influenced the incidence of testicular germ cell tumors with an increased risk seen in Asian/Pacific Islanders versus whites.[100]

Germ cell tumors comprise 65% to 85% of pediatric testicular tumors. Children have a much larger percentage of benign testicular lesions than adults. Recently, the prevalence of the various histologic subtypes of testicular tumors was reviewed and found that an even higher percentage of pediatric testicular tumors may be benign. Tumor registries have reported that greater than 60% of tumors were yolk sac and approximately 20% were teratoma.[54,99] In contrast, pooled data on 98 patients from four academic medical centers found that teratomas accounted for 48% of testicular tumors, whereas yolk sac tumors (YSTs) were responsible for only 15% of testicular tumors.[101] The other main tumor types included epidermoid cysts and gonadal stromal tumors. The authors proposed that tumor registries are more prone to reporting bias because benign lesions are likely underreported compared with malignant lesions.

Presentation and Diagnosis

A testicular tumor typically presents as a painless scrotal mass. A history of trauma is often given and may be the inciting event that brings attention to the scrotal mass. Differential diagnoses include hydrocele, hernia, and tumor. Malignancy typically is nontender, does not transilluminate, and is not accompanied by an abnormal urinalysis. A hydrocele may impede adequate testicular examination. Also, a tumor arising in a UDT may undergo torsion and be seen as acute abdominal pain. Hormonally active tumors may occur with precocious puberty with or without a palpable lesion.

As part of the initial evaluation for a testicular mass, testicular ultrasonography and serum levels of tumor markers should be obtained. Ultrasonography is highly sensitive and can detect even small tumors masked by a hydrocele. Ultrasound findings of internal calcifications and a heterogeneous mass suggest teratoma. These findings may be useful in preoperative planning for testis-sparing surgery.

Serum tumor marker levels are valuable not only in the diagnosis but also in the follow-up of testicular malignancy. α-Fetoprotein (AFP) is a glycoprotein produced by the fetal yolk sac, liver, and gastrointestinal tract. It is elevated in a variety of benign and malignant diseases, including YSTs of the testis. The normal AFP value declines significantly in the months after birth.[102] The half-life of AFP is approximately 5.5 days, and the normal adult level of less than 10 ng/mL is not achieved until around 10 months of age (Fig. 52-7).[103,104] The β subunit of hCG (β-hCG) is a glycoprotein produced by embryonal carcinomas and mixed teratomas. Its half-life is 24 hours, and it is normally not detected in significant amount in boys (<5 IU/L).

Once the diagnosis of high-risk testicular cancer is made histologically, CT can be used to evaluate metastatic disease. CT has largely supplanted retroperitoneal lymph node dissection (RPLND) for the purpose of staging; however, it carries a 15% to 20% false-negative rate.[105] MRI also has been used to detect Leydig cell tumors, testicular epidermoid cysts, and Sertoli

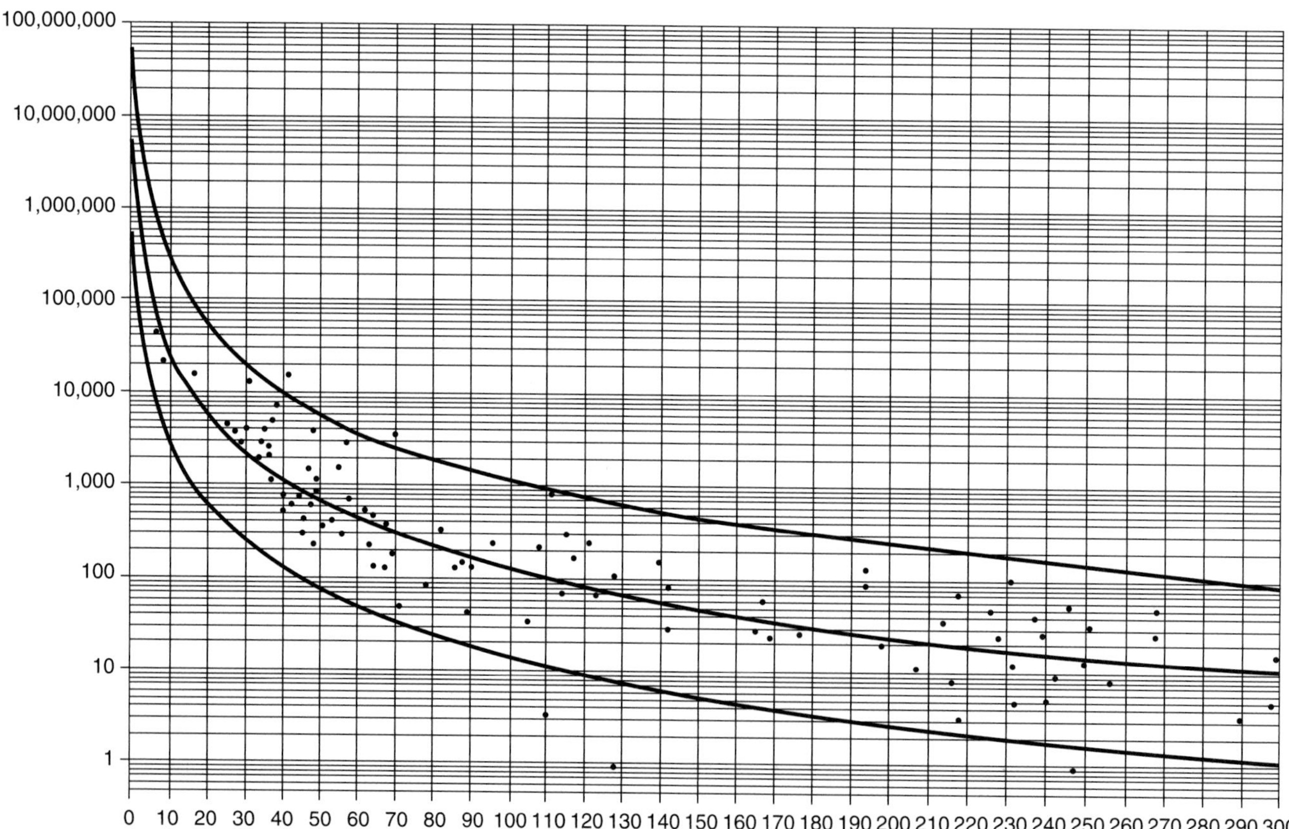

Figure 52-7. This graph displays the normal ranges of serum α-fetoprotein (AFP) in early infancy. The AFP levels in nanograms per milliliter are on the *y*-axis and age in days is on the *x*-axis. The normal range for AFP may be estimated by the middle regression line. The two flanking lines represent the 95% confidence interval. (From Ohama K, Nagase H, Ogino K, et al: Alpha-fetoprotein (AFP) levels in normal children. Eur J Pediatr Surg 7:267-269, 1997.)

cell tumors.[106-108] Information obtained can similarly guide the surgical approach, but the cost-effectiveness of MRI is unclear.

Carcinoma in Situ

CIS of the testis is a premalignant lesion. Testicular cancer is reported to develop in at least 50% of testes known to harbor CIS.[59] CIS is seen in patients with UDT and intersex disorders, conditions that are known to carry a higher risk of testicular cancer than that in the general population.[109] In addition, CIS often co-exists in the testis that harbors a known cancer.

CIS growth is stimulated by endocrinologic changes during puberty. However, the natural history of CIS in prepubertal testes is less clear.[110,111] Testicular biopsy at the time of orchiopexy is not performed routinely. However, when it is done, CIS is seen in 0.36% to 0.45%.[85,86] If biopsy of a cryptorchid testis reveals CIS, it has been recommended that the patient undergo repeated postpubertal biopsy. The prevalence of CIS in adult men with a history of UDT is 2% to 4%.[59,112,113] If CIS is identified in the prepubertal testis, it is typically managed with annual testicular examinations and testicular ultrasonography despite the reputed 50% incidence of conversion to carcinoma in adult men. In postpubertal patients, some clinicians recommend that these patients undergo biopsy of the contralateral testis and unilateral orchiectomy. If biopsy of the remaining testis also reveals CIS, they recommend 18 to 20 Gy of radiation treatment. The same investigators advocate routine postpubertal testicular biopsy in all cases of UDT. This practice has not been routine in the United States, however, and remains controversial.[114]

Germ Cell Tumors

YSTs are also known as endodermal sinus tumors, embryonal adenocarcinomas, orchidoblastomas, or Teilum's tumors.[115] Most occur within the first 2 years of life. Grossly, YSTs are firm and yellow/white. Microscopically, they are characterized by Schiller-Duval bodies and stain for AFP.[54,55,116]

Metastasis of YSTs to the retroperitoneum is uncommon in children (4% to 6%).[55] Approximately 95% of YSTs are confined to the testis. The lungs are the most common site of distant metastasis, which occurs in 20% of patients. The 5-year survival rate for YST approaches 99%.

The standard diagnostic and therapeutic procedure for all testicular tumors is radical inguinal orchiectomy. To minimize the risk of metastases during manipulation, the spermatic cord is clamped or ligated immediately on entry into the inguinal canal. The role of RPLND in children with YST is controversial. Currently, most YSTs are treated with radical orchiectomy and patients are observed for recurrence by measuring AFP levels. If the AFP level was elevated at the time of orchiectomy and subsequently returns to normal, RPLND is not performed.

Staging of YSTs requires abdominal and pelvic CT and chest radiography, pathologic examination of the radical orchiectomy specimen, and determination of serum levels of tumor markers (Table 52-1).[117] Stage I tumors are limited to the testis. They are completely resected by radical inguinal orchiectomy, after which tumor marker levels normalize. Patients with unknown or normal markers at diagnosis must have a negative ipsilateral RPLND for the disease to be stage I. Tumor marker levels are measured monthly and chest radiographs obtained every 2 months for the first 2 years. Chest and abdominal CT scans are obtained every 3 months for the first year and every 6 months for the second year. After 2 years without recurrence, follow-up may be extended to every 6 months or yearly.[55]

Stage II disease includes those tumors with microscopic node involvement discovered by RPLND. Tumors diagnosed and treated with transscrotal orchiectomy or sampled also should be considered stage II, because resection via a transscrotal incision alters the normal lymphatic drainage of the tumor. Lymphatic drainage of the testis is to the retroperitoneal nodes, whereas the scrotum drains to the inguinal nodes. If a testicular tumor is diagnosed through a scrotal incision, ipsilateral hemiscrotectomy should be considered.[110] All patients with stage II disease should receive combination chemotherapy with cisplatin, etoposide, and bleomycin (PEB). Five-year survival rates with the PEB regimen approach 100% in this patient population.[55,118] Patients with a persistent mass or elevated AFP after chemotherapy should undergo RPLND.

Stage III disease includes retroperitoneal spread seen on imaging studies and occult metastases manifest by persistent elevation of tumor markers after orchiectomy. Metastasis beyond the retroperitoneum or to any viscera defines stage IV disease. For both stage III and stage IV disease, chemotherapy follows the same protocols as described for stage II disease. RPLND is performed after chemotherapy. The overall survival approaches 100%.

Histologically, teratomas are composed of all three layers of embryonic tissue: ectoderm, endoderm, and mesoderm. Grossly, they may contain differentiated tissue such as cartilage, muscle, bone, and fat; a cystic component also may be present. Before puberty, they follow a benign course and can be managed with testis-sparing surgery.[54,55,119] Long-term follow-up at a mean of 7 years has demonstrated no tumor recurrence in the ipsilateral or contralateral gonad with a testis-sparing approach.[120] However, when a child is initially seen at or after puberty, radical inguinal orchiectomy with high ligation of the spermatic cord is indicated, because teratoma can follow a malignant postpubertal course. When immature elements are seen on frozen sections, radical orchiectomy should be performed. Overall disease-free survival after orchiectomy is excellent.[121]

Teratocarcinoma, or mixed germ cell tumor, accounts for 20% of pediatric germ cell tumors. Teratocarcinoma is more commonly seen in a previously undescended

Table 52-1 TNM Classification of Pediatric Testis Tumors

Primary Tumor (T)	
TX	Primary tumor cannot be assessed (in the absence of radical orchiectomy)
T0	Histologic scar, no evidence of primary tumor
Tis	Intratubular tumor (in situ tumor), preinvasive cancer
T1	Tumor limited to testis, including rete testis
T2	Tumor invades beyond tunica albuginea or into epididymis
T3	Tumor invades spermatic cord
T4	Tumor invades scrotum
Regional Lymph Nodes (N)	
NX	Regional nodes not assessed
N0	No regional lymph node metastasis
N1	Metastasis in a single lymph node, ≤ 2 cm in greatest dimension
N2	Metastasis in a single lymph node, > 2 cm but ≤ 5 cm in greatest dimension, or multiple lymph nodes none > 5 cm in greatest dimension
N3	Metastasis in a lymph node > 5 cm in greatest dimension
Distant Metastasis (M)	
MX	Presence of metastasis cannot be assessed
M0	No distant metastasis
M1	Distant metastasis
Serum Tumor Markers (S)	
SX	Marker studies not available or not performed
S0	Marker levels within normal limits
S1	LDH < 1.5 × normal *and* hCG < 5000 (mIu/mL) *and* AFP < 1000 (ng/mL)
S2	LDH 1.5-10 × normal *or* hCG 5,000-50,000 (mIu/mL) *or* AFP 1,000-10,000 (ng/mL)
S3	LDH > 10 × normal *or* hCG > 50,000 (mIu/mL) *or* AFP > 10,000 (ng/mL)

Normal is the upper limit of normal for the LDH assay.
LDH, lactate dehydrogenase; hCG, human chorionic gonadotropin; AFP, alpha-fetoprotein.
From AJCC Manual for Staging of Cancer, 5th ed. Philadelphia, Lippincott-Raven, 1997.

testis that has been brought down into the scrotum and may contain any mixture of YST, embryonal carcinoma, choriocarcinoma, and seminoma.[117,122] Eighty percent of teratocarcinomas are confined to the testis at presentation. Foci of choriocarcinoma confer a poorer prognosis. RPLND is usually performed even for stage I disease, and higher-stage disease is treated with chemotherapeutic protocols similar to those used for adults.

Seminoma is rare in children. This tumor is treated with radical orchiectomy and retroperitoneal radiation.[123] It is the most common tumor found in an uncorrected abdominal UDT.

Non–Germ Cell Tumors (Gonadal Stromal Tumors)

Leydig cell tumor is one of the most common non–germ cell tumors (NGCTs). The peak incidence in boys occurs from ages 5 to 9 years.[54,124] The clinical triad includes a unilateral testicular mass (90% to 93%), precocious puberty, and elevated 17-ketosteroid levels.[125] Because these tumors produce testosterone and occasionally other androgens, roughly 20% of patients may have endocrinologic signs of precocious puberty and gynecomastia.[117] Alternative explanations for precocious puberty include pituitary lesions and congenital adrenal hyperplasia. To eliminate these diagnoses, the pituitary/adrenal axis must be evaluated by assaying 17-ketosteroids and performing a dexamethasone suppression test. Reinke's crystals identified on histologic sections or on fine-needle aspirates are pathognomonic for this tumor and can be found in 35% to 40% of all patients.[126,127] However, they are rarely seen in children.[55] When the diagnosis is made preoperatively, testis-sparing enucleation through a transscrotal approach may be considered because these tumors tend to follow a benign course in boys.[128]

The granulosa cell tumor also has a benign course and may be approached with testis-sparing surgery. This tumor should be suspected in neonates with normal age-adjusted AFP levels with a complex, multiseptated, hypoechoic mass on testicular ultrasonography.[129]

The Sertoli cell tumor is a very rare form of NGCT and also is seen as a painless testicular mass. A small percentage of patients have gynecomastia. Although nonspecific, ultrasonography can show testicular microlithiasis.[130] The clinical course is usually benign, and tumors can be managed with testis-sparing surgery.

Gonadoblastoma is a form of NGCT usually seen in association with intersex disorders. The patients are typically 46XY phenotypic females with intra-abdominal testes who are seen with virilization after puberty. Up to one third of patients have bilateral gonadal lesions. Whereas the clinical course is usually benign, the germ cell component of these tumors carries a 10% risk of malignant degeneration. Early gonadectomy is recommended, especially if the patient is raised as a female.[131,132]

chapter 53

THE ACUTE SCROTUM

Charles M. Leys, MD, MSCI • John M. Gatti, MD

The term *acute scrotum* refers to acute scrotal pain with or without swelling and erythema. This presentation should always be treated as an emergency because of the possibility of testicular torsion and permanent ischemic damage to the testis. Table 53-1 lists the differential diagnoses for the acute scrotum. The etiology is generally age dependent. Most conditions are nonemergent, but prompt differentiation between testicular torsion and other causes is critical. Torsion of the appendix testis/epididymis is most common in prepubertal boys, whereas testicular torsion most commonly presents in neonates and adolescents.[1,2]

TESTICULAR TORSION

Torsion of the testis results from twisting of the spermatic cord, which leads to a compromised testicular blood supply and subsequent testicular infarction. The consequent ischemic damage affects long-term testicular morphology and sperm formation. However, there is generally a 4- to 8-hour window before significant damage occurs.[3] Table 53-2 shows that the probability of testicular salvage declines significantly beyond 6 hours. Emergent surgical treatment is indicated even beyond that window, however, because testicular viability is difficult to predict and spontaneous detorsion can occur first.[4]

Torsion may be classified as intravaginal or extravaginal. Intravaginal torsion is more common and occurs when the spermatic cord twists within the tunica vaginalis. This is predisposed by abnormal fixation of the testis and epididymis within the tunica vaginalis. Normally, the tunica will invest the epididymis and posterior surface of the testis, fixing it to the scrotum with a vertical lie. Abnormal fixation occurs when the tunica vaginalis attaches more proximally on the spermatic cord, creating a long mesorchium on which the testis can twist. The testis will then lie horizontally. In this situation, the pendulous testis is predisposed to twisting with leg movement or cremasteric contraction (Fig. 53-1). This anatomic variant is classically described as the "bell-clapper" deformity and has an incidence as high as 12% in cadaveric studies. Often, it is found in the contralateral scrotum as well.[5]

Extravaginal torsion is a perinatal event that occurs when the spermatic cord twists proximal to the tunica vaginalis. During testicular descent into the scrotum the tunica vaginalis is not firmly fixed to the scrotum, allowing the tunic and testis to spin on the vascular pedicle.

Testicular torsion typically occurs before age 3 years and after puberty. It is rare in prepubertal boys and after age 25 years. The clinical presentation of torsion classically involves the sudden onset of severe, unilateral pain in the testis, lower thigh, or lower abdomen. It is often associated with nausea and vomiting. Episodes of intermittent testicular pain may precede the acute presentation, suggesting prior incomplete torsion and spontaneous detorsion. Physical examination may reveal the involved testis retracted up toward the inguinal region with a transverse orientation and an anteriorly located epididymis. The torsed testis is usually enlarged and tender throughout. In contrast, focal tenderness at the superior pole or caput epididymis may occur with a torsed appendix testis or epididymitis. Depending on the duration of torsion, the involved hemiscrotum will show varying degrees of swelling and erythema, which may obliterate landmarks and make the examination more difficult. The cremasteric reflex is often absent with testicular torsion. However, the presence of this reflex does not reliably exclude torsion.[6-8]

Often the diagnosis of torsion is clinically apparent and is managed by immediate scrotal exploration. If

Table 53-1 Differential Diagnoses of the Acute Scrotum
Torsion of the testis
Torsion of the appendix testis/epididymis
Epididymitis/orchitis
Hernia/hydrocele
Trauma/sexual abuse
Tumor
Idiopathic scrotal edema (dermatitis, insect bite)
Cellulitis
Vasculitis (Henoch-Schönlein purpura)

Table 53-2 Duration of Torsion and Testicular Salvage Rates

Duration of Torsion (hr)	Testicular Salvage (%)
<6	85-97
6-12	55-85
12-24	20-80
>24	<10

Data from Smith-Harrison L, Koontz WW Jr: Torsion of the testis: Changing concepts. In Ball TP Jr, Novicki DE, Barrett DM, et al (eds): AUA Update Series. Vol. 9 (lesson 32). Houston, American Urological Association Office of Education, 1990.

the diagnosis is uncertain, adjunctive diagnostic studies may aid in determining the etiology of the acute scrotum. A urinalysis revealing pyuria and bacteriuria is more indicative of infectious epididymitis/orchitis but can be found with torsion. Testicular blood flow can be examined using either high-resolution ultrasonography with color flow Doppler or radionuclide imaging. These imaging studies are most useful to help confirm the presence of testicular blood flow when a diagnosis other than torsion is suspected. Ultrasonography has become the more popular study at most institutions because it allows determination of blood flow, is less time consuming, is more readily available, and does not expose the patient to ionizing radiation.[9,10] In experienced hands, color flow Doppler ultrasound imaging has a sensitivity of 89.9%, a specificity of 98.8%, and a false-positive rate of 1%.[11] Doppler ultrasonography may detect coiling of the spermatic cord, indicating torsion, even with normal blood flow within the testis.[12] It is important that ultrasonography is used only when the diagnosis is equivocal. If torsion is strongly suspected clinically, further studies will only delay emergent surgical exploration.

If testicular torsion is suspected but a delay to the operating room is unavoidable, manual detorsion can be attempted. Detorsion should be performed in a medial to lateral, "open book" rotation, because this will be the correct direction in two thirds of patients.[13] If successful, the testis will typically drop lower in the scrotum and the patient will report sudden relief of pain. If the initial attempt is not successful, an attempt in the reverse direction may be performed.[14] Although these maneuvers may decrease the degree of ischemia, prompt surgical exploration and fixation remains mandatory because the detorsion may not be complete and recurrent torsion can occur.

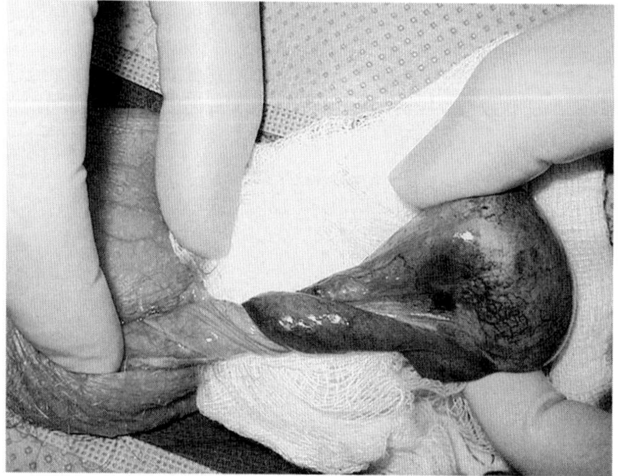

Figure 53-1. Bell-clapper deformity. The tunica vaginalis inserts very high on the spermatic cord, which predisposes to testicular torsion.

Exploration is typically performed using a median raphe incision in the scrotum. The symptomatic hemiscrotum is entered first and the testis delivered, detorsed, and placed in warm, moist sponges while the contralateral hemiscrotum is explored. The unaffected testis must be fixed to the scrotal wall with nonabsorbable suture in at least three points, excluding the tunica vaginalis by excising a portion or tucking it back in the scrotum. Excluding the tunica vaginalis allows better fixation of the testis to the scrotum, as with dartos pouch fixation used in newborn scrotal fixation.[15,16] Attention is then turned back to the affected testis. If the testis appears clearly nonviable, it should be removed to avoid potential damage to the contralateral testis. Animal studies have demonstrated contralateral testicular damage mediated by antisperm antibodies formed in response to testicular damage in the torsed gonad.[17,18] As a result, some surgeons suggest removal of all testes that have experienced significant ischemic injury. However, it is questionable whether such antibody formation is physiologically significant in humans. Therefore, our practice is to remove the testis only if it appears nonviable. If the torsed testis becomes reperfused or bleeding is noted from a cut surface, it should be fixed in the same fashion as the contralateral testis. Although bilateral fixation reduces the probability of torsion in the future, this procedure does not absolutely guarantee against this possibility, because cases of torsion after fixation have been reported.[19] Therefore, any patient with a presentation suggestive of testicular torsion should be evaluated and treated with the same diligence, regardless of whether previous fixation has been performed.

Intermittent Testicular Pain

A number of boys who present with testicular torsion will describe prior episodes of acute testicular pain that spontaneously resolved. Although intermittent testicular pain is not an unusual complaint in adolescent males, these episodes may represent intermittent torsion with spontaneous resolution.[20] This diagnosis should be strongly considered in adolescent males who report significant testicular pain that has resolved, especially with multiple episodes. This suspicion is reinforced if the testis has a transverse orientation or excess mobility. Ideally, the diagnosis could be proved with Doppler ultrasound imaging while symptomatic, although this may be difficult to obtain in a timely fashion. If clinical concern remains, even with a normal physical examination, elective scrotal exploration looking for a "bell-clapper" deformity may be warranted. Scrotal ultrasonography before elective exploration is useful to evaluate for an occult testicular lesion.

Perinatal Testicular Torsion

The term *perinatal torsion* is applied to both prenatal and postnatal events, with most (75%) occurring prenatally.[21] It may be difficult to distinguish between the two types of perinatal torsions, but the difference is important because it may affect the timing of operative management. Prenatal torsion classically presents as a hard, nontender scrotal mass noted at birth, usually with underlying dark discoloration of the skin and fixation of the skin to the mass. These findings suggest infarction of the testis secondary to a prior torsion. Postnatal torsion presents as a more classic, acutely inflamed scrotum with erythema and tenderness. The scrotum may be reported as normal at delivery, suggesting an acute postnatal event. This diagnosis requires emergent exploration with detorsion and bilateral fixation. If the timing of the torsion is in question, prompt exploration is the best course unless other medical conditions make general anesthesia exceptionally risky. Doppler ultrasonography may be helpful in uncertain cases.

The timing of exploration for prenatal torsion has been controversial. The classic teaching has been that surgical exploration is not indicated because of negligible salvage rates and increased neonatal anesthetic risks.[22] However, this has been challenged by reports of asynchronous torsion with devastating loss of the remaining contralateral testis.[23-25] Furthermore, if the torsion were to happen at or just prior to delivery, salvage may be possible. One series of 30 neonatal torsions explored within 6 hours of birth found two testes that could be salvaged and demonstrated normal growth 1 year later.[26] Therefore, many surgeons have become more aggressive with earlier exploration of these infarcted testes to fix the contralateral side and prevent potential bilateral torsion.

Unless other medical conditions preclude general anesthesia, our practice has been early exploration. This has the added benefit of ensuring the correct diagnosis because a testicular teratoma or a hernia sac filled with meconium or blood can mimic prenatal torsion. Postnatal torsion clearly mandates emergent exploration because salvage rates have been reported as high as 40% to 50%, which is similar to torsion later in life.[27] Surgical exploration is performed through an inguinal incision because a testicular tumor may be encountered in rare instances. In such a situation, a scrotal incision could lead to inguinal nodal spread.[28,29] Contralateral exploration is accomplished through a transverse scrotal incision, with placement of the testis in a dartos pouch between the external spermatic fascia of the scrotum and the dartos fascia. This technique is less traumatic to the small, delicate neonatal gonad and probably provides better fixation than sutures.[15,16]

CONDITIONS MIMICKING TESTICULAR TORSION

Torsion of Testicular Appendages

Torsion of the appendix testis or appendix epididymis is the most common cause of an acute scrotum and is frequently misdiagnosed as acute epididymitis or epididymo-orchitis. Morgagni is credited with the first description of an appendix testis in Padua, Italy, in 1761.[30] Torsion of the appendage was first reported by Colt in 1922 in Scotland.[31] The testicular appendage represents a vestigial remnant of the müllerian duct, and the epididymal appendage is of wolffian duct origin. Torsion of these appendages occurs most commonly between ages 7 and 10 years. It is thought that a prepubertal hormonal boost stimulates these structures, producing an increase in size and making them susceptible to twisting.[32]

Torsion of testicular appendages can mimic testicular torsion, with sudden onset of pain, and can be associated with nausea and vomiting. Results of urinalysis are normal. Early in the course, the appendage can be palpated and is exquisitely and focally tender. The examiner may be able to elicit differential tenderness between the upper and lower poles of the affected testis. Classically called the "blue dot" sign, the inflamed and ischemic appendage may be seen through the scrotal skin as a subtle blue-colored mass (Fig. 53-2).[33] As inflammation increases, however, the epididymis, testis, and scrotal tissues become edematous and erythematous and the diagnosis becomes more difficult. Ultrasonography can be diagnostic early in the presentation and demonstrates a discrete appendage. However, later, it may only show increased blood flow to the adjacent epididymis and testis or, possibly, a reactive hydrocele, resulting in the misdiagnosis of acute epididymitis or epididymo-orchitis.[34]

Torsion of these appendages is self-limited and is best treated with nonsteroidal anti-inflammatory medications and comfort measures such as restricted activity and warm compresses. The pain resolves as the appendage infarcts and necroses. It may then become a calcified free body within the tunica vaginalis. The syndrome can recur because there are

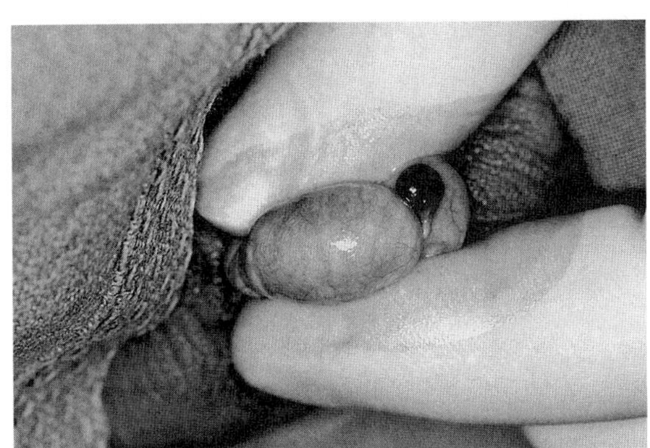

Figure 53-2. A torsed and gangrenous appendix testis is shown. This is the cause of the "blue dot" sign.

potentially five anatomic sites of appendages that can undergo torsion (appendix testis, appendix epididymis, paradidymis/organ of Giraldes, and superior and inferior vas aberrans of Haller) (Fig. 53-3).[35-37] Surgical exploration is indicated when the diagnosis of testicular torsion cannot be reliably excluded or when the symptoms are prolonged and fail to resolve spontaneously. The torsed appendage can be easily excised through a small scrotal incision with immediate symptom relief.

Epididymitis

True bacterial epididymitis is quite rare in children, accounting for 10% to 15% of patients with an acute scrotum. It is commonly employed as an inaccurate, generalized diagnosis in a patient with scrotal pain without evidence of testicular torsion. Bacterial infection extends from the bladder and urethra to the epididymis in a retrograde direction via the ejaculatory ducts and may be associated with a clinical urinary tract infection or urethritis. The scrotal pain and swelling typically have a slow onset, worsening over days rather than hours. Examination reveals induration, swelling, and tenderness of the hemiscrotum. The edema will make palpation of the testis itself very difficult. A positive urinalysis and culture, or urethral swab in sexually active adolescents, suggests the diagnosis. *Neisseria gonorrhoeae* and *Chlamydia* are classically found in sexually active boys, but common urinary pathogens, including coliforms and *Mycoplasma* species, are more likely in younger children. When studies suggest a bacterial infection, appropriate antibiotic therapy is initiated and adjusted according to culture results. If acute epididymitis is found on scrotal exploration, cultures should be obtained, but the contralateral side should not be opened to avoid spreading the infection. As with any urinary tract infection in a boy, a renal bladder sonogram and voiding cystourethrogram should be obtained after the infection has resolved. Vesicoureteric reflux is the most common finding, but other abnormalities such as an ectopic ureter (to the vas, ejaculatory duct, or seminal vesicle), ejaculatory duct obstruction, or urethral valves can also be found.

Viral infections are believed to be a common cause for acute epididymitis but are usually diagnosed presumptively. Mumps orchitis occurs in approximately one third of postpubertal boys affected by the virus and fortunately is rare in the modern era of immunization.[38] Adenovirus, enterovirus, influenza, and parainfluenza virus infections have also been found. Management is supportive, antibiotics are not indicated, and the pain is generally self-limited. Aggressive testing is usually not warranted, but viral cultures and serologic studies may be useful in clustered familial or community cases.[39]

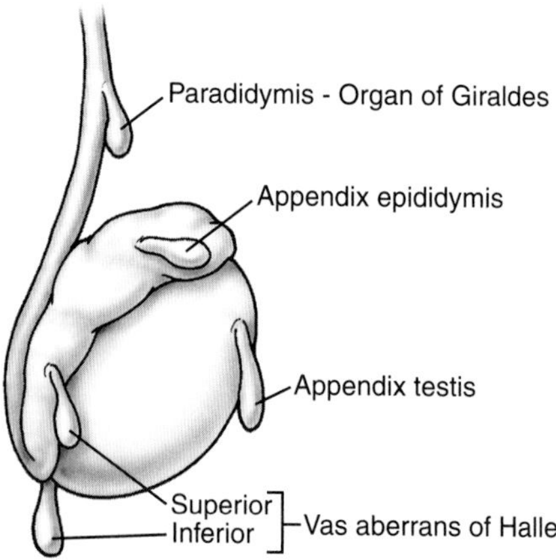

Figure 53-3. Testicular appendages. (From Rolnick D, Kawanoue S, Szanto P, et al: Anatomic incidence of testicular appendages. J Urol 100:755-756, 1968.)

Idiopathic Scrotal Edema

Scrotal swelling of unknown etiology is termed *idiopathic scrotal edema* and usually affects boys between the ages of 5 to 9 years. The syndrome is characterized by the insidious onset of swelling and erythema that typically begins in the perineum or inguinal region and spreads to the hemiscrotum. The condition may be associated with pruritus but is usually not painful. The testis is not tender on examination. Ultrasonography will show normal testicular blood flow and is not usually helpful. Many cases due to contact dermatitis, insect bites, and minor trauma are undoubtedly given this diagnosis. Evaluation should seek to exclude cellulitis from an adjacent infection (inguinal, perirectal, or urethral). The patient is managed with comfort measures, with antihistamines or topical corticosteroids possibly providing relief. If cellulitis is a concern, oral antibiotics can be administered.[40]

Voiding Dysfunction

Voiding dysfunction is a common cause of scrotal pain, especially when it is bilateral, and is not commonly recognized unless the diagnosis is sought. The pain is the result of bladder instability causing high pressure voiding against a voluntarily closed external sphincter. Dilation of the posterior urethra ("spinning-top urethra") is commonly seen on a voiding cystourethrogram in patients with voiding dysfunction. Urine may be forced up the ejaculatory duct, resulting in local inflammation and a "chemical" epididymitis or epididymo-orchitis.[41] A renal bladder sonogram may show a thickened bladder wall and is also useful to evaluate for ureteral ectopia to the ejaculatory duct or vas deferens as a potential cause in recurrent cases. There is no pathognomonic test for voiding dysfunction. However, a thorough history will often reveal urinary urgency, incontinence, a staccato urinary stream indicative of inappropriate sphincter activity, and occult constipation. Effective treatment strategies include timed voiding regimens, dietary modification, an aggressive bowel regimen to control constipation, and anticholinergic or α-antagonist medication when appropriate.

Henoch-Schönlein Purpura

Henoch-Schönlein purpura is a vasculitic syndrome that can involve the skin, joints, and gastrointestinal and genitourinary systems. Up to one third of patients may develop pain, erythema, and swelling of the scrotum and spermatic cord, most commonly in boys younger than 7 years of age. Although this condition may mimic testicular torsion, a Doppler ultrasound study will reveal normal blood flow to the testis. A thorough history and physical examination may reveal other systemic symptoms, such as skin purpura, joint pain, and hematuria. Supportive measures are typically adequate, although systemic corticosteroids may be helpful.[42,43] Despite the rarity of coincident diagnoses, cases of concurrent Henoch-Schönlein purpura and testicular torsion have been reported.[44]

TESTICULAR TRAUMA

Testicular trauma in children is rare. The diagnosis can be made by taking a complete history, with careful attention to factors that may indicate sexual abuse. Examination of an injured testis will reveal swelling and marked tenderness, associated with swelling and bruising of the scrotum. The most common injury is a hematoma of the testis. Ultrasonography should be obtained to evaluate for rupture of the tunica albuginea, which is an indication for operative repair. Repair is particularly important in postpubertal boys because of the potential for autoimmune injury to the opposing testis. A large hematoma in the space between the tunica vaginalis and the tunica albuginea should be evacuated to avoid pressure necrosis of the testis. Epididymal injuries can occur, including disruption of the epididymis from the testis, with a poor outcome likely after repair.

OTHER CONDITIONS

Other causes of the acute scrotum include an incarcerated inguinal hernia, hydrocele, and neoplasia. Testicular tumors may occur in the neonatal period and early childhood, although they are usually not associated with pain or scrotal wall changes. They are usually firm on examination and should be further evaluated with ultrasonography. Management is tailored to the diagnosis. See Chapter 52 for more information about testicular tumors.

section 6

UROLOGY

chapter 54

DEVELOPMENTAL AND POSITIONAL ANOMALIES OF THE KIDNEYS

Hsi-Yang Wu, MD • Howard M. Snyder III, MD

Anomalies of renal formation and position result in interesting radiographs, but their clinical importance lies in their associated conditions. For example, the multicystic dysplastic kidney often involutes, yet the initial evaluation aims to determine that the contralateral kidney is not at risk from vesicoureteral reflux (VUR) or ureteropelvic junction (UPJ) obstruction. Whereas no therapy is needed for unilateral renal agenesis, the link between a solitary kidney and the VACTERL (vertebral, anal, cardiac, tracheoesophageal fistula, renal, limb) and Mayer-Rokitansky (vaginal agenesis) syndromes is the main reason for further evaluation. Hydronephrosis is often seen in abnormalities of position and rotation but does not necessarily mean that obstruction is present. Therefore, anomalies of renal formation and position often pose more of a diagnostic problem than a surgical one.

RENAL EMBRYOLOGY

The pronephros, which has no adult function, induces the mesonephros to differentiate into the mesonephric duct during the 4th to 8th weeks of fetal life. The mesonephric duct is the basis of the wolffian system, which develops into the seminal vesicles, vas deferens, epididymis, and efferent ductules of the testis in boys and into the epoöphoron and paroöphoron (vestigial remnants between the fallopian tube and ovary) in girls. The ureteral bud branches off the mesonephric duct, contacts the metanephric blastema bud between weeks 9 and 12 of fetal life, and induces the entire collecting system of ureter, renal pelvis, calyx, and collecting tubules. The kidney develops via induction of the metanephric blastema by the ureteral bud into Bowman's capsule, the convoluted tubules, and the loop of Henle.[1] Figure 54-1 illustrates the progression of development from pronephros, mesonephros, to metanephros.

The kidneys begin at the upper sacral level with the renal pelvis facing anteriorly. The kidneys ascend either because the lumbar and sacral regions grow faster than the cervical and thoracic regions between 4 to 8 weeks or because there is active migration. As the kidneys ascend, the renal pelvis rotates medially by 90 degrees, leading to the normal configuration of the renal pelvis lying medial to the parenchyma. During this time, the blood supply shifts from the inferior branches of the aorta to more cephalad branches, with the final renal artery being located at about L2. Failure of normal ascent leads to the persistence of a low-lying blood supply.[1]

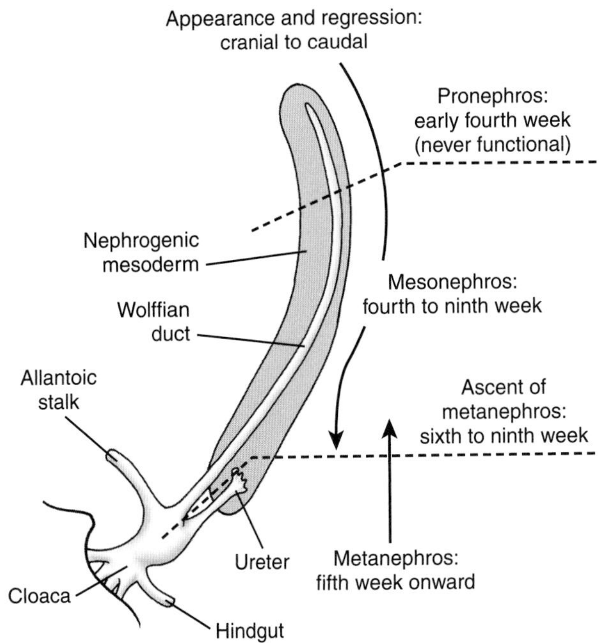

Figure 54-1. Development of the kidney. (Redrawn from Gray SW, Skandalakis JE: Embryology for Surgeons. Philadelphia, WB Saunders, 1972, p 444.)

RENAL DYSPLASIA AND HYPOPLASIA

Because the development of the kidney depends on proper interaction between the ureteral bud and the metanephric blastema, it should not be surprising that an abnormality in the location of the ureteral orifice is associated with abnormally induced renal tissue.[2] Examination of the thickness of the renal parenchyma and number of glomeruli associated with normal and ectopic ureters in fetal specimens suggests that it is the initial interaction between bud and blastema that determines whether normal renal tissue will develop, rather than subsequent obstruction or VUR.[2] Figure 54-2 shows how a ureter that arises in the proper trigonal location (see Fig. 54-2A, E, F) is associated with normal renal parenchyma, whereas a ureter arising from a more cranial location (see Fig. 54-2B-D) or caudal location (see Fig. 54-2G, H) is associated with progressively less normal renal parenchyma.

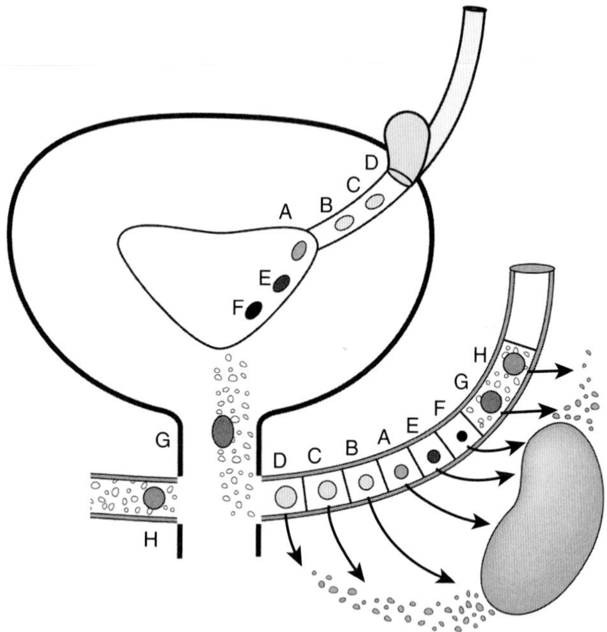

Figure 54-2. **Relation of ureteral orifice location and associated metanephric tissue.** (Redrawn from Mackie GG, Stephens FD: Duplex kidneys: A correlation of renal dysplasia with position of the ureteral orifice. J Urol 114:274-280, 1975.)

Renal dysplasia and hypoplasia can be considered errors in renal induction. Figure 54-3 shows varying changes, progressing from agenesis, dysplasia, and perhaps hypoplasia of the kidney. Although *dysplasia* is technically a histologic term, it refers to kidneys that contain primitive tubules either focally or diffusely. These ducts are lined by epithelium and surrounded by sworls of primitive collagen. No treatment is necessary for the dysplastic kidney, but there is a 14% risk of reflux in the contralateral kidney.[3] Hypoplastic kidneys are small, normal kidneys with a decreased number of nephrons. Dysplasia can also occur in hypoplastic kidneys. Whereas secondary hypoplasia can occur due to infection or obstruction, two types of hypoplastic kidneys are clinically important: the oligomeganephronic type and the Ask-Upmark kidney. In oligomeganephronia, there is a decrease in the number of nephrons with an associated hypertrophy of the ones that are present. Patients present with polyuria and failure to concentrate their urine but no hypertension. Imaging with ultrasound reveals small kidneys. Medical management with protein restriction and high fluid and salt intake is undertaken. Once the glomerular filtration rate drops significantly, dialysis is required.[4] The Ask-Upmark kidney was initially believed to be a developmental problem but is now believed to represent reflux nephropathy. The key finding is a small kidney with segmental hypoplasia, probably secondary to ascending pyelonephritis. VUR and hypertension are usually present. Most patients are older than 10 years of age with a 2:1 female-to-male ratio. If the disease is unilateral, nephrectomy may cure the hypertension. Bilateral disease is managed medically.[5]

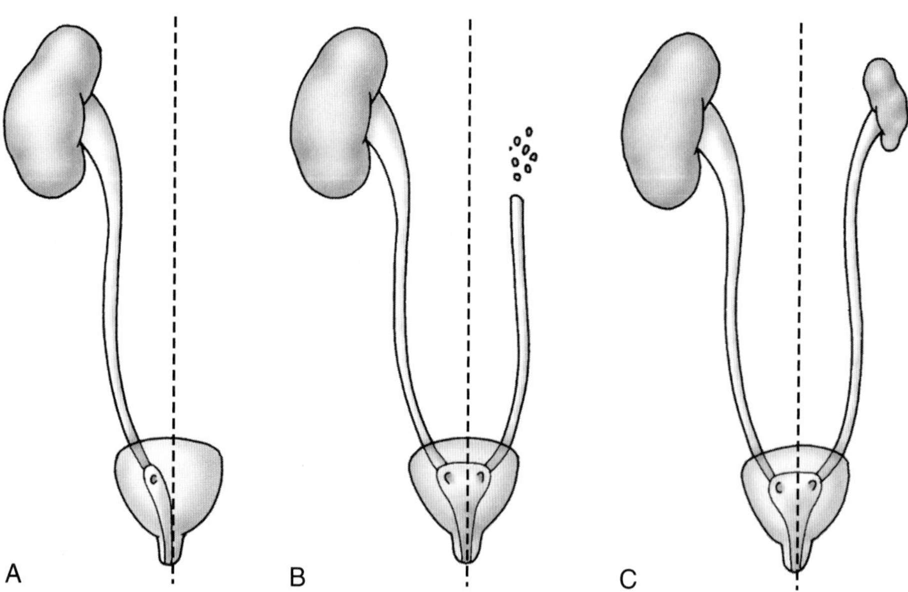

Figure 54-3. Renal agenesis **(A)**, dysplasia **(B)**, and hypoplasia **(C)**. (Redrawn from Gray SW, Skandalakis JE: Embryology for Surgeons. Philadelphia, WB Saunders, 1972, p 455.)

RENAL AGENESIS

Absence of a kidney may be due to abnormal induction of the metanephric blastema or involution of a multicystic dysplastic kidney. The presence or absence of the ureter is helpful in suggesting the cause of renal agenesis. Absence of a hemitrigone implies that the ureteral bud failed to form properly. A normal trigone with some evidence of a ureter leading to a nubbin suggests involution of a multicystic dysplastic kidney.

Unilateral renal agenesis occurs in 1:1000 live births with a 2:1 male predominance.[6,7] Unilateral renal agenesis can result in compensatory hypertrophy of the contralateral kidney. The left kidney is more likely to be affected in unilateral renal agenesis.[8] Because unilateral renal agenesis is asymptomatic and eventual renal function is normal, the diagnosis is usually made on prenatal ultrasonography or it is incidentally found during imaging for other abdominal symptoms. Sometimes it can be suspected on plain abdominal films if the colon is medially deviated at the splenic or hepatic flexure.[9] These patients should consider obtaining a medical alert bracelet so that in case of traumatic injury, the solitary kidney is not inadvertently removed.

In a neonate with the prenatal diagnosis of unilateral renal agenesis, physical examination at the time of birth should be focused on detecting the anomalies present in the VACTERL association.[10] A voiding cystourethrogram (VCUG) should also be obtained because approximately 30% of patients with unilateral renal agenesis will have VUR in the contralateral kidney.[10]

Males with unilateral renal agenesis are at risk for abnormal wolffian structures. The vas and seminal vesicle may be absent, or the seminal vesicle may be present as a cyst while the ipsilateral testis will be normal. Because the seminal vesicle develops as a separate bud from the wolffian duct at 12 weeks, it can be present in cases of unilateral renal agenesis due to regression of a multicystic dysplastic kidney. Seminal vesicle cysts that are causing symptomatic obstruction are usually removed via a transvesical approach. Conversely, if a vas is found to be abnormal or absent during a hernia repair or orchiopexy, the kidneys should be evaluated postoperatively with ultrasonography.

Females with unilateral renal agenesis should have their genital anatomy evaluated because up to 30% will have an abnormality of the müllerian duct due to the Mayer-Rokitansky syndrome (müllerian, uterine, upper vaginal duplications with or without obstruction, or vaginal agenesis).[11,12] The abnormal induction of the mesonephric duct is believed to cause partial or complete nonunion of the paired müllerian ducts.[13] Conversely, 40% of patients with abnormalities of the müllerian organs will have unilateral renal agenesis or ectopia.[14] In patients with duplicated vaginas and unilateral vaginal agenesis, the side without a vagina is also the side without a kidney.[13]

If the diagnosis of Mayer-Rokitansky syndrome is not made prenatally, the patients can present either as infants with hydrocolpos or as adolescents with lower abdominal pain after the onset of menses due to an obstructed vagina or uterus (with or without duplication). Magnetic resonance imaging (MRI) is useful in delineating the pelvic anatomy in these cases. In vaginal agenesis, the vagina is only present as a shallow pouch. There is a wide variety of abnormalities of the vagina, uterus, and fallopian tubes (Fig. 54-4), but the ovaries are embryologically normal.

Bilateral renal agenesis occurs in 1:4800 live births and has a 3:1 male predominance.[15] Infants affected with bilateral renal agenesis present with oligohydramnios, pulmonary hypoplasia, Potter's facies (low-set ears, broad flat nose, a prominent skin fold beginning over the eye and running to the cheek), and the great majority die soon after birth of their pulmonary hypoplasia. The renal arteries and ureters are usually absent and the bladder is underdeveloped. The vas is usually present, but female genital structures are usually abnormal.[16,17] The adrenals are usually present but appear round, instead of flattened, owing to the lack of compression by the kidneys.[15] Prenatal diagnosis is useful in determining that heroic efforts at extracorporeal membrane oxygenation or hemodialysis are not indicated after delivery.

SUPERNUMERARY KIDNEY

This is a rare condition in which a completely separate kidney is found in addition to two normally positioned kidneys. The additional kidney has its own blood supply and parenchyma and usually is found caudad to the normal kidney. It is usually smaller than the normally positioned kidney. This additional kidney represents abnormal induction of metanephric blastema by an abnormally directed ureteral bud, either as a separate ureteral bud from the mesonephric duct or as part of a "Y" duplication. If the supernumerary kidney is located craniad to the normal kidney, the ureter is usually completely separate and may enter the bladder ectopically. Presumably this is a result of a completely separate ureteral bud inducing the metanephric blastema and migrating very low on the mesonephric duct, separate from the normally positioned kidney.[18,19] If the ureter ends ectopically, it may present as incontinence in a girl or as infection in a poorly functioning renal unit. The diagnosis can be difficult to make.[20] Stone disease and hydronephrosis can be found in up to 50% of patients. Treatment should be reserved for these problems, because the presence of a supernumerary kidney itself is not worrisome.[19] Like other ectopic kidneys, these kidneys may be more subject to trauma, so a medical alert bracelet may be important.

RENAL ECTOPIA

Failure of rotation, while not strictly ectopia, usually results in a kidney in which the renal pelvis is anteriorly directed. In the unusual situation in which hyper-rotation occurs, the renal pelvis can actually point posteriorly. The renal vessels are normally positioned. The renal pelvis and calyces will often appear abnormal due to their unusual orientation, which

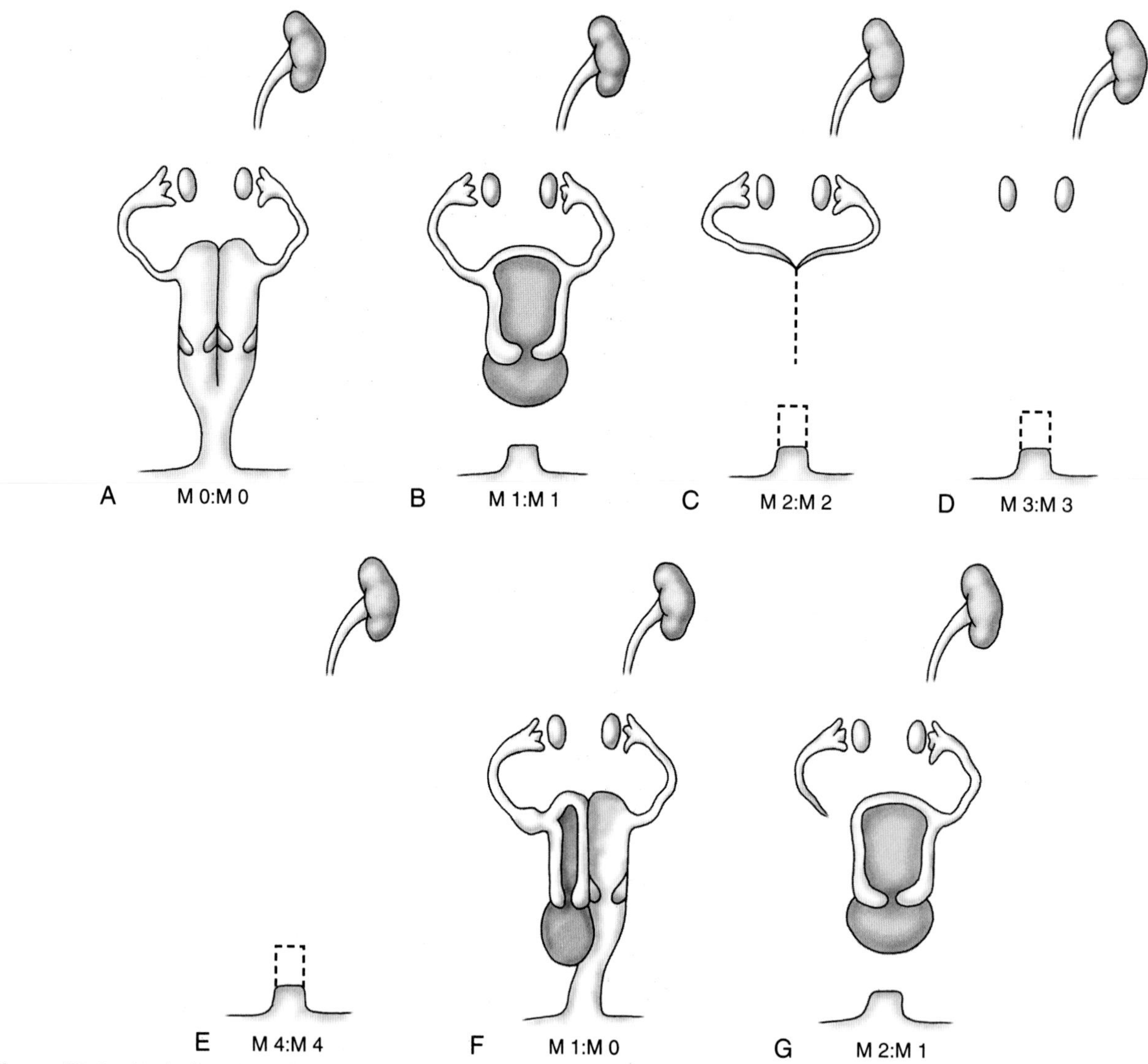

Figure 54-4. Variations in müllerian anatomy in Mayer-Rokitansky syndrome. M0, Right or left vagina and uterus, or duplex vagina and uterus with partial or complex septum. M1, Partial or complete absence of vagina. M2, Absence of vagina and uterus. M3, Absence of vagina, uterus, and fallopian tube. M4, Absence of vagina, uterus, fallopian tube, and ovary. (Redrawn from Tarry WR, Duckett JW, Stephens FD: The Mayer-Rokitansky syndrome: Pathogenesis, classification and management. J Urol 136:648-652, 1986.)

results in an interesting intravenous urogram. With oblique views the anatomy can be established and does not usually require repair, even in poorly functioning units. The best method to localize even poorly functioning ectopic renal tissue is with a nuclear medicine study. There are two technical factors to be considered in interpreting renal scans in ectopic kidneys. First, the radionuclide in the bladder can overlap a pelvic kidney so a catheter may need to be inserted for the study. Second, the pelvic kidney is located farther anterior than orthotopic kidneys and the function may be artificially lowered by the distance of the kidney from the camera. Placing the patient prone may result in a more accurate assessment.

Simple ectopia results in a kidney that is located anywhere from the pelvis to the diaphragm. The incidence is 1:1000 live births with a 3:2 male predominance.[21] The contralateral kidney often also has an abnormality of rotation or ectopia. The development of the ipsilateral adrenal is unaffected. A "thoracic kidney" is actually subdiaphragmatic, although it may lie in the chest through a focal eventration of the diaphragm. It is not associated with a true congenital diaphragmatic hernia.[22] An ectopic "abdominal kidney" is above the iliac crest, the "lumbar kidney" is anterior to the iliac vessels at the sacral promontory, and the "pelvic kidney" is below the aortic bifurcation and opposite the sacrum. All of these ectopic kidneys are more susceptible to trauma because they are not as well protected by the lower rib cage and are anterior in position. It may be advisable for these patients to avoid contact sports in which there is a risk of abdominal trauma.

Most ectopic kidneys are asymptomatic and are detected either on prenatal ultrasonography or incidentally on other imaging studies. Ectopic kidneys are at higher risk for UPJ obstruction, VUR, and stone formation. The anatomy can include an extrarenal pelvis and infundibulum and a high insertion of the ureter into the pelvis. This anatomic arrangement can mimic a UPJ obstruction, so careful evaluation is necessary to avoid unnecessary surgery.[23] More than half will have a dilated renal pelvis. Of these, 50% are due to obstruction, 25% are due to reflux, and 25% are merely dilated without UPJ obstruction.[24] For repair of UPJ obstruction with a high insertion of the ureter, a side-to-side ureteropyelostomy or ureterocalycostomy to a dilated lower pole calyx is sometimes required to obtain dependent drainage.

Although endoscopic techniques for treatment of UPJ obstruction have been used in children,[25] the presence of anomalous vessels suggests that either an open or laparoscopic approach would be safer than endoscopic incision of a UPJ obstruction in an ectopic kidney. The advent of computed tomography (CT) angiography and magnetic resonance urography (MRU) has made the assessment of anomalous vessels in ectopic or horseshoe kidneys easier and more noninvasive.

FUSION DEFECTS

Horseshoe Kidney

A horseshoe kidney is found in 1:400 live births and has a 2:1 male predominance.[26] The kidney is usually lower than normal, since the lower poles fuse in the midline and drape anteriorly over the spine. The isthmus can be fibrotic or contain parenchyma. This anomaly is believed to occur at between 4 to 6 weeks of life, because the orientation of the renal pelvis is anterior. It is proposed that as the kidneys "hurdle" the iliac vessels during ascent they come into contact at the lower pole and fuse (Fig. 54-5). Other variations of upper pole and mid-pole contact are possible but much less common than the usual lower pole fusion. The kidney is usually low owing to its inability to ascend past the inferior mesenteric artery. Each renal moiety retains its ureter, which is draped over the isthmus. The renal pelvis is usually anterior. The arterial supply varies from the normal single vessel to each moiety to vessels arising from any conceivable nearby blood supply. Horseshoe kidneys are more commonly found in patients with sacral agenesis, high cloacae, and Turner's syndrome (45,XO gonadal dysgenesis).[27] They are associated with a higher risk of renal cell carcinoma and Wilms' tumor.[28-30] In one study the presence of a horseshoe kidney in the setting of a Wilms' tumor was not suspected preoperatively in 13 of 41 patients despite imaging studies.[30]

One third of patients with a horseshoe kidney have no symptoms. The patients with symptoms often complain of vague abdominal or back pain. Ten percent have ureteral duplication, 50% have VUR, and 33% have UPJ obstruction.[27,31,32] Repair of UPJ obstruction in a horseshoe kidney requires placement of the anastomosis to avoid a secondary kinking at the UPJ. Division of the isthmus is not required. Treatment of kidney stones in horseshoe kidneys can be accomplished by extracorporeal shock wave lithotripsy, ureteroscopy, or percutaneous nephrolithotomy. Percutaneous approaches are sometimes difficult because the kidneys do not reside next to the body wall, making access to the collecting system difficult. However, percutaneous approaches result in a higher stone-free rate than ureteroscopy or shock wave lithotripsy.[33,34] Although there is no increase

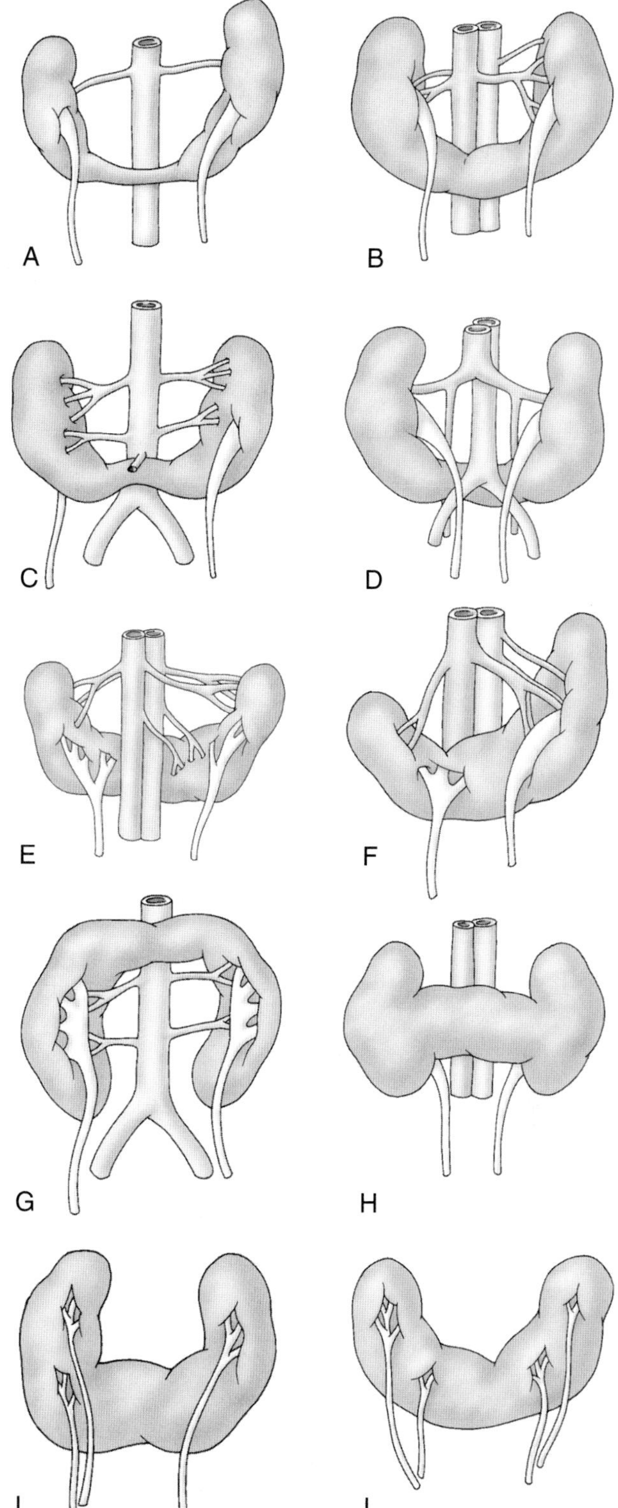

Figure 54-5. Variations of horseshoe kidney. (Redrawn from Banjamin JA, Schullian DM: Observations of kidneys with horseshoe configuration: The contribution of Leonardo Botallo. J Hist Med Allied Sci 5:315, 1950, after Gutierrez, 1931.)

in the rate of metabolic abnormalities in patients with horseshoe kidneys and kidney stones, suggesting that stasis in an extrarenal pelvis contributes to the formation of kidney stones,[35] patients with a horseshoe kidney and kidney stones are more likely to have hypocitraturia than other patients with kidney stones.[36]

Cross-Fused Renal Ectopia

This anomaly is more common than crossed, nonfused renal ectopia and is more common in boys. The lower pole of one kidney crosses the midline to fuse with an orthotopically placed contralateral kidney. Usually the left kidney crosses the midline. Presumably during ascent, the left kidney encounters a roadblock, rotates, and fuses with the lower pole of the right kidney. The ureters insert in the normal position in the bladder. This has been described as an "S" or "L" shaped kidney. Diagnosis can be made using intravenous pyelography (IVP), CT, or MRU. Solitary crossed ectopia (unilateral renal agenesis, contralateral kidney crossed to opposite side) is a rare finding. Multicystic dysplasia, obstruction, and VUR can be found in the ectopic kidney.

CYSTIC RENAL DISEASE AND CYSTIC TUMORS

Autosomal Recessive Polycystic Kidney Disease

Autosomal recessive polycystic kidney disease (ARPKD) was formerly called infantile polycystic kidney disease, which is inaccurate because it can present in older patients. Although it occurs in 1:40,000 live births, many patients die soon afterward. The kidneys are bilaterally enlarged, with very small cysts radially oriented throughout the parenchyma (Fig. 54-6). The cysts represent dilated collecting tubules. Periportal hepatic fibrosis also occurs in varying degrees and can lead to portal hypertension. The hepatic involvement appears to be inversely proportional to the renal involvement. The disease has been classified into four forms.[37] The severe perinatal form (>90% renal involvement) leads to death by 6 weeks from pulmonary hypoplasia. The neonatal form (60% renal involvement) is usually lethal by 1 year. The infantile form (25% renal involvement) results in hepatosplenomegaly, with survival up to 10 years. The juvenile form (<10% renal involvement) has severe periportal fibrosis. Some patients survive up to 15 years, but the development of portal hypertension is usually lethal. Because this is an autosomal recessive disease, screening of the family should be undertaken to determine which siblings are carriers.

A prenatal ultrasound evaluation showing bilaterally enlarged, echogenic kidneys suggests ARPKD. The IVP or CT shows a classic striated "sunburst" pattern. Unfortunately, the prognosis is poor for the perinatal or neonatal forms of ARPKD. The patients who survive the neonatal period seem to do well with some degree of renal insufficiency. Eventually, dialysis is usually required. In older patients, the kidneys become smaller as renal failure develops. The overall treatment for ARPKD is supportive, with renal transplantation being the ultimate therapy.

Autosomal Dominant Polycystic Kidney Disease

Although autosomal dominant polycystic kidney disease (ADPKD) tends to clinically present in the third to fifth decades, it has been diagnosed in the ultrasound

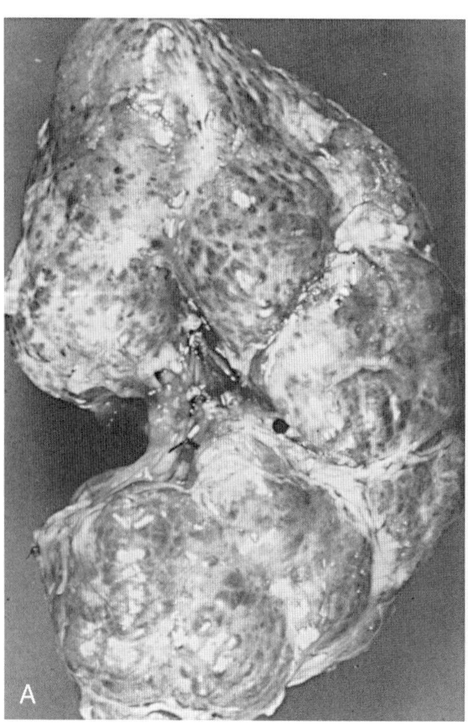

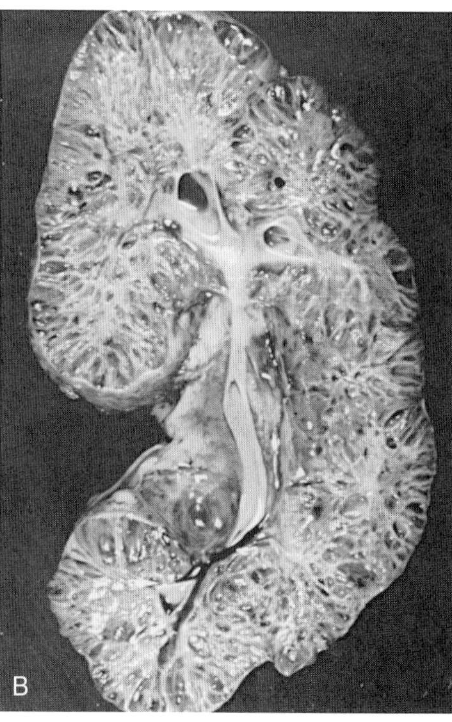

Figure 54-6. Gross pathology of autosomal recessive polycystic kidney disease.

era in asymptomatic children as well. The cysts in ADPKD are different in configuration, being few and scattered in distinction to those seen in ARPKD. This condition occurs in 1:500 patients.[38] Patients usually present with flank pain, hematuria, hypertension, and possibly renal failure, if there are extensive bilateral cysts. Neonates can present with renal enlargement, although children from affected families who are screened usually only have a few cysts. Failure to see cysts on screening ultrasonography in a child at risk for ARPKD does not exclude the disease because the cysts can develop later in life. Linkage analysis of the loci on chromosome 4 and 16 is more sensitive.[39] The cysts are located throughout the cortex and medulla, although the fetal form seems to affect the glomeruli predominantly. Hepatic involvement is limited to biliary cysts. Associated findings include cysts in the spleen, pancreas, and lungs; mitral valve prolapse; colon diverticula; and berry aneurysms of the circle of Willis.

Hypertension is commonly found in these children and may be part of the presentation. Renal failure in childhood is very rare. Periodic evaluation of blood pressure and proteinuria during childhood is recommended.[40,41] Unlike ARPKD, there is no increased risk of renal cell carcinoma. Renal transplant candidates can obtain organs from family members who have been screened for the disease.

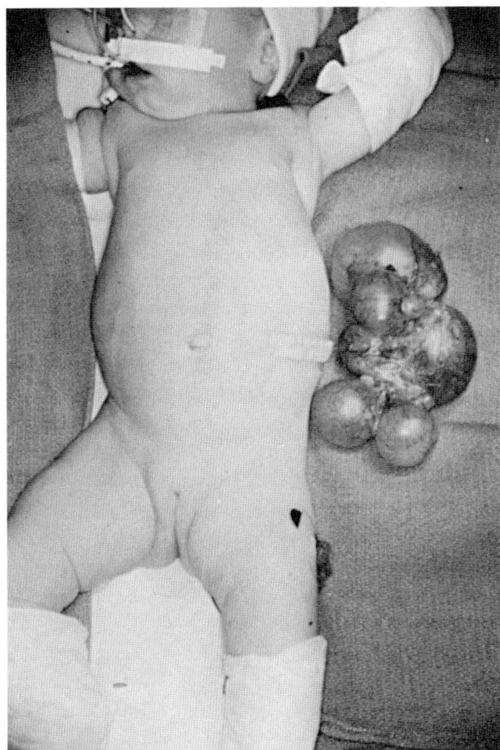

Figure 54-7. Resected multicystic dysplastic kidney.

Multicystic Dysplastic Kidney

The multicystic dysplastic kidney (MCDK) is believed to be caused by severe early ureteral obstruction or a failure in ureteral bud/metanephric blastema induction.[42,43] The main differential diagnosis is severe hydronephrosis due to UPJ obstruction. Radiographically, this occurs when the peripheral cysts surround a dominant central cyst mimicking the renal pelvis ("hydronephrotic" form of MCDK). The classic ultrasound appearance shows cysts randomly distributed throughout the kidney without a dominant medial cyst or evidence of communication between cysts. The parenchyma, if present, has abnormal echogenicity and is seen between the cysts, instead of being arranged on their periphery. A renal scan will show no function in an MCDK. The affected area may be the upper pole of a duplicated collecting system or one half of a horseshoe kidney.

The MCDK is the most common renal cystic mass in the newborn. Currently, most are detected on prenatal ultrasonography. Bilateral forms are not compatible with life. Postnatal evaluation consists of a VCUG to look for VUR in the contralateral kidney, which occurs 30% of the time.[44] If there is significant hydronephrosis (caliectasis) in the contralateral kidney (this occurs 12% of the time), then a diuretic renal scan may be necessary. Contralateral UPJ obstruction or VUR is more likely with a smaller MCDK or a lower ureteral atresia ipsilateral to the MCDK.[45,46] There are reports of malignancy arising from an MCDK, although it is unclear whether the affected kidneys were truly MCDK.[47] Hypertension has also been reported in association with MCDK, although resection is not always curative and the rate does not appear to be any higher than in the general population.[48] An MCDK usually involutes, but it can occasionally grow.[48] The follow-up is repeat imaging with ultrasonography every 6 months for the first 2 years of life. It is not usually feasible to monitor a patient indefinitely for an MCDK. We have taken an operative approach at 18 to 24 months of life if the MCDK is not involuting or if parenchyma remains visible on the sonogram. Although the indications are controversial, the kidney can be removed at that age via a small incision as an outpatient procedure (Fig. 54-7). Occasionally, the MCDK can involute prenatally, leaving a ureter with a small nubbin of tissue in the renal fossa. These were previously called "aplastic" kidneys but are now believed to represent the remnants of an MCDK.

Cystic Nephroma

Formerly called a "multilocular cyst," this is a well-demarcated tumor of cysts with an overall round configuration, lined with epithelium and septa that contain tubules.[49] It is considered to be the benign end of a spectrum progressing from cystic Wilms' tumor, cystic partially differentiated nephroblastoma, to cystic nephroma. It usually is found in boys younger than age 4 (male-to-female ratio 2:1) or women older than 30 (female-to-male ratio 8:1). It is rarely bilateral and is cured by partial nephrectomy, shelling out the tumor by following the plane of the pseudocapsule. There is a risk of sarcomatous degeneration in adults if it is not removed.[50]

Cystic Partially Differentiated Nephroblastoma

This lesion was formerly called a multilocular cystic nephroma. It is radiologically identical to the cystic nephroma and can only be diagnosed pathologically. The majority of patients are boys younger than 2 years old or women in their third to fourth decades. A classic (but not diagnostic) radiologic finding is herniation of a parenchymal mass into the renal pelvis.[22] The tumor is usually well circumscribed. Hemorrhage and calcification are usually absent. Pathologically, it differs from the cystic nephroma in that there is blastema found in the septations.

Patients usually present with an asymptomatic flank mass and, occasionally, hematuria. Surgical treatment consists of partial nephrectomy as for cystic nephroma, since the tumors rarely recur and are not multifocal. No chemotherapy is required for stage I (limited to capsule, fully resected) tumors. Although experience is limited, stage II (outside renal capsule but fully resected) tumors are usually treated with vincristine, dactinomycin, and doxorubicin. Four-year survival for both stages is 100%.[51,52]

Simple Cysts and Calyceal Diverticula

The simple renal cyst on ultrasonography has the following characteristics: distinct wall, no internal echoes, and posterior enhancement. If these criteria are not met, a CT scan is obtained to confirm that the fluid does not enhance. The differential diagnosis is a calyceal diverticulum or hydrocalyx, both of which communicate with the collecting system and in which the fluid should enhance on either IVP or CT. Ultrasonography is able to detect milk of calcium layering within a diverticulum. Calyceal diverticula require treatment when they harbor stones or infection. In the IVP era, 40% of calyceal diverticula were believed to be symptomatic.[53] In the ultrasound era, with its greater number of incidental findings, it is not clear how often calyceal diverticula require treatment. Minimally invasive approaches such as percutaneous, laparoscopic, and ureteroscopic ablation appear to be equally successful.[54]

Simple cysts reside in the cortex and are lined by simple columnar epithelium. They can grow, resorb, or remain the same size. They are usually asymptomatic and are found incidentally. Once they are found, we usually follow the patient with ultrasonography at 3- to 6-month intervals to determine if the cyst is growing. The underlying concern is whether this cyst is the first sign of ADPKD. A family history of renal cystic disease, renal failure, or death in the neonatal period from unknown causes should be sought. Biopsy to rule out tumor, followed by drainage, or unroofing should be undertaken only if the cyst characteristics are other than those listed for a simple cyst or if the cyst becomes symptomatic due to obstruction of an infundibulum or the UPJ. Minimally invasive approaches such as percutaneous puncture with instillation of sclerosing agents (absolute alcohol, bismuth, povidone-iodine[55]) or laparoscopic decortication[56] may shift the threshold for treatment of large asymptomatic simple cysts.

chapter 55

URETERAL OBSTRUCTION AND MALFORMATIONS

Tyler Christensen, MD • Douglas E. Coplen, MD

Hydronephrosis and ureteral malformations are among the most common abnormalities of the urinary tract in children. Historically, these anomalies were first identified during evaluation of urinary tract infections, abdominal pain, or incontinence. However, with the increasing use of fetal and neonatal ultrasonography, they are now often detected before symptoms develop. Urinary tract dilation is present in 1 in 100 fetuses, but significant uropathy is found in only 1 in 500.[1] Thus, the surgeon must critically evaluate these findings to determine their clinical significance and whether intervention is required.

URETEROPELVIC JUNCTION OBSTRUCTION IN CHILDREN

With ureteropelvic junction (UPJ) obstruction, there is inadequate drainage of urine from the renal pelvis into the ureter, resulting in hydrostatic distention of the renal pelvis and intrarenal calyces. The combination of increased intrapelvic pressure and stasis of urine in the collecting ducts results in progressive damage to the kidney.

Historically, the incidence of UPJ obstruction has been estimated at 1 in 5000 live births. However, with the advent of antenatal ultrasonography, the prevalence of dilation has been found to be much higher. Recent retrospective reviews have shown that although the incidence of detected dilation has increased, the actual number of operations for UPJ obstruction has been relatively constant at 1:1250 births.[2,3] UPJ obstruction is more common in boys (2:1), and two thirds occur on the left side. Bilateral UPJ obstruction occurs in 5% to 10% of patients and is much more frequently seen in younger children.[4,5]

Etiology

During development of the upper ureter, the lumen of the ureteral bud solidifies with ureteral lengthening and later recanalization.[6] Failure to recanalize adequately is thought to be the cause of most intrinsic UPJ obstructions. Other causes of intrinsic UPJ obstruction include ureteral valves, polyps, and leiomyomas.[7]

At operation, the most common observation is ureteral narrowing of a variable length that joins the renal pelvis above the expected dependent position.[8] This "high insertion" of the ureter causes an angulation with respect to the renal pelvis. At low-volume states, peristaltic waves of urine cross the UPJ. However, as the flow increases beyond a threshold, the renal pelvis dilates.[9] The dilated pelvis may functionally kink the ureter further, increasing the pelvic pressure.[10] In 20% to 30% of patients, the ureter is draped over a lower-pole vessel, producing an extrinsic UPJ obstruction. This aberrancy may be secondary to incomplete renal rotation that is associated with a normal segmental vessel.[11,12]

Histologic evaluation reveals a decrease or complete absence of smooth muscle fibers at the UPJ.[8,13] Electron microscopy may show an increase in collagen deposition between the muscle fibers that is, most likely, a response to the obstruction as opposed to the cause.[14] Fibrosis and interruption of the smooth muscle continuity block transmission of the peristaltic wave while defective innervation also may play a role.[15,16] UPJ obstruction can be acquired. It has been observed in late follow-up of high-grade vesicoureteral reflux (VUR), after cutaneous ureterostomy, and after decompression of the dilated urinary tract. In these cases, the obstruction is caused by extrinsic scarring and adhesions that cause fixed deformation and distortion of the UPJ. VUR is present in 14% of patients with UPJ obstruction.[17,18]

Clinical Presentation

Most renal dilation and obstruction is now detected prenatally (Fig. 55-1). Less frequently, it is detected because of an abdominal mass, urinary tract infection, association with other anomalies (i.e., VACTERL syndrome), or abnormalities seen during contrast or

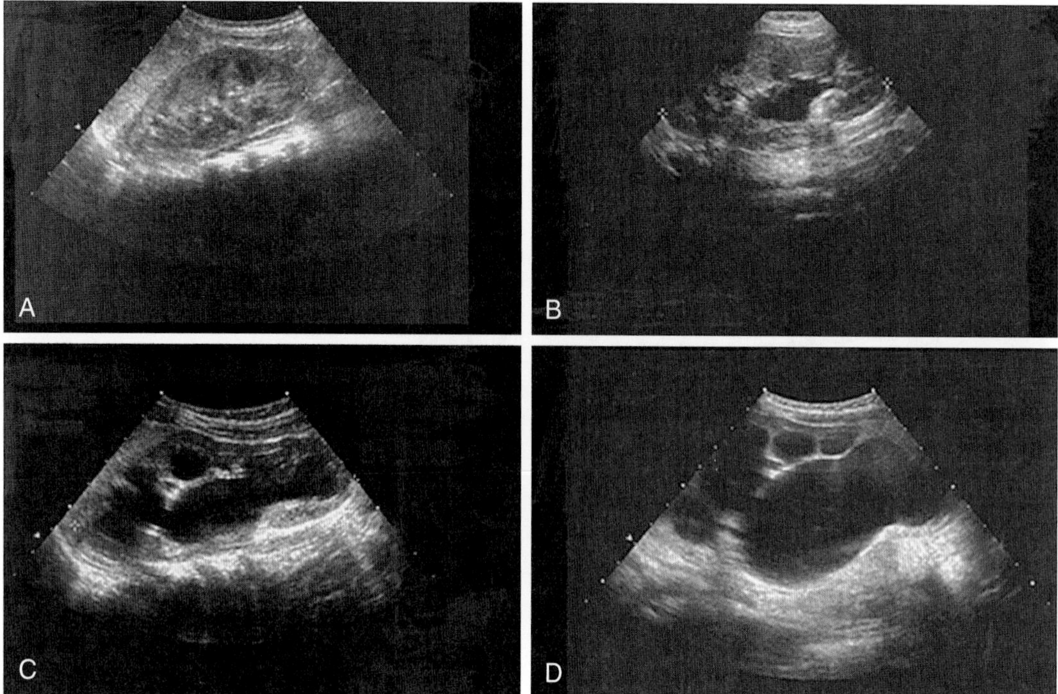

Figure 55-1. These neonatal ultrasound images were performed in infants noted to have renal pelvic dilation found on prenatal ultrasonography. **A,** The findings here are essentially normal. There is a dark renal pyramid and no renal pelvic dilation. **B,** This image shows renal pelvic dilation with minimal caliectasis. **C,** Note diffuse caliectasis and mild cortical thinning. **D,** Severe hydronephrosis with cortical thinning is evident.

radionuclide radiography. In older children, vague, poorly localized, cyclic, or acute abdominal pain associated with nausea is common. Some of these children are initially seen by gastroenterologists. The cause for the intermittent obstruction is unclear, but renal function is almost always preserved. Hematuria after minor trauma or vigorous exercise may be a presenting feature, most likely secondary to rupture of mucosal vessels in the dilated collecting system.[4] Episodic flank pain associated with diuresis is a common presenting feature in young adults but is uncommon in children.

Diagnosis

When the antenatal diagnosis of UPJ obstruction is made, the initial postpartum evaluation should be performed at 10 to 14 days of life to avoid false-negative studies resulting from neonatal dehydration. Bilateral UPJ obstruction is rarely associated with significant enough obstruction to cause oligohydramnios and warrant antenatal intervention. The neonate is placed on preventive amoxicillin (10 mg/kg once a day), pending the results of the studies. Ultrasonography confirms the presence of pelvic and calyceal dilation, with variable thinning of the renal parenchyma (see Fig. 55-1). The presence of corticomedullary junctions is indicative of preserved function.[19] Ultrasound is used to evaluate the contralateral kidney, the bladder, and the distal ipsilateral ureter to avoid confusion with a ureterovesical junction (UVJ) obstruction, but it will not provide functional information.

A voiding cystourethrogram (VCUG) was previously indicated in all patients being evaluated for UPJ obstruction. VUR increases the chance that infection will occur, even in a partially obstructed system. However, with a larger percentage of dilation now being seen with prenatal ultrasonography, it is clear that a VCUG is not required in all children with dilation because only 5% to 30% will have reflux and the majority will spontaneously resolve without infectious complications.[20] Children with isolated pyelectasis and no ureteral dilation have a very low incidence of reflux and may not require a screening VCUG. VUR that leads to kinking of the UPJ may be the primary disease process in some cases (Fig. 55-2).

The diuretic isotopic renogram is the most useful technique in the evaluation of hydronephrosis, differential renal function, and drainage of the kidneys. In this study, the transit of an injected radioisotope through the urinary tract is monitored by a gamma camera. The early uptake of the tracer indicates the split renal function, while the washout, augmented by the administration of a diuretic, is evaluated and plotted by a computer to demonstrate drainage.[21,22] The study is obtained with either technetium-99m–labeled diethylenetriamine pentaacetic acid (^{99m}Tc-DTPA), whose renal clearance is by glomerular filtration, or with ^{99m}Tc-mercaptoacetyltriglycine (^{99m}Tc-MAG3), whose clearance is predominantly via proximal tubular secretion. ^{99m}Tc-MAG3 is more efficiently excreted than ^{99m}Tc-DTPA and gives better images, particularly in patients with impaired renal function.[21,22]

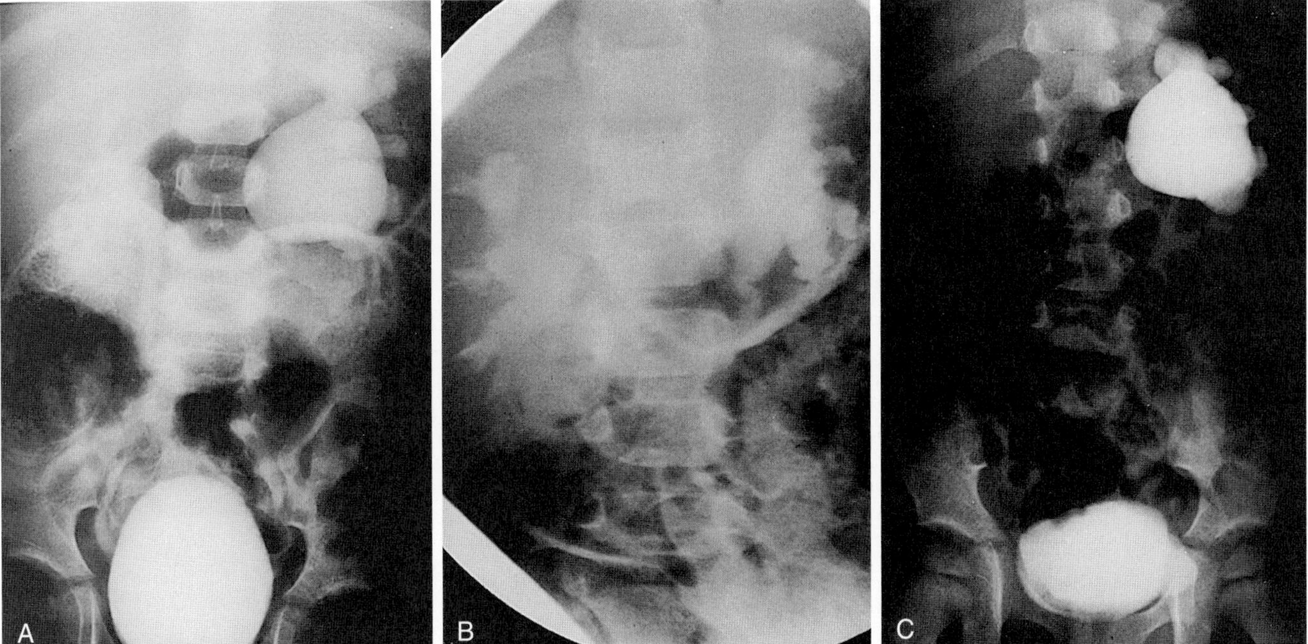

Figure 55-2. Vesicoureteral reflux and secondary ureteropelvic junction (UPJ) obstruction in a 4-year-old boy first seen with urosepsis. **A,** Intravenous pyelogram (IVP) with a full bladder shows typical findings of calyceal blunting and renal pelvic dilation. Visualization of the distal ureter suggests reflux. **B,** Cystogram shows bilateral reflux. Note the marked discrepancy in left-sided anatomy between the IVP and cystogram and the kink just distal to the UPJ on the left side. **C,** Delayed film after a cystogram shows stasis and apparent obstruction on the left side. Subsequent furosemide wash-out renal scan with a bladder catheter showed no evidence of obstruction, and the child has done well after bilateral ureteral reimplantation.

The technique for diuretic renography is standardized.[23] Patients should be hydrated intravenously (15 mL/kg) 15 minutes before injection of the radionuclide. An indwelling catheter maintains an empty bladder and monitors urine output. The diuretic (1 mg/kg furosemide, up to 40 mg) is not administered until the activity in the hydronephrotic kidney and renal pelvis peaks. The tracer activity is then monitored for an additional 30 minutes, and a quantitative analysis is performed. Historically, persistence of more than 50% of the tracer in the renal pelvis 20 minutes after diuretic administration ($t\frac{1}{2} > 20$) is diagnostic of obstruction, although the applicability of this cutoff in pediatric patients is widely debated. False-positive results may occur when the immature neonatal kidney fails to respond to diuretic, when the patient is dehydrated, when the bladder is distended, or when the pelvis is significantly dilated.

Magnetic resonance (MR) urography can be used at any age. T2-weighted images are independent of renal function, and hydronephrosis is readily detected. The anatomic images are excellent, but a good ultrasound image often gives the same information. Enhanced MR images with gadolinium can give information regarding differential function if one kidney is anatomically and functionally normal.[24]

Intravenous pyelography (IVP) has limited use in the neonate because the neonatal kidney does not concentrate contrast medium well enough to provide adequate visualization of obstructed kidneys. It also is subjective with respect to the differential renal function and degree of obstruction. This test may be indicated when more information is required regarding preoperative pelvic anatomy or to define better the level of obstruction when it is not clear from other studies.[5] In the child with intermittent flank pain, IVP may be diagnostic when performed during an episode of pain (Fig. 55-3).

Rarely, when imaging is equivocal, invasive pressure flow studies may be indicated.[25] These tests assume that obstruction produces a constant restriction to outflow that necessitates elevated pressure to transport urine at high flow rates. However, not all obstructions are constant. If the obstruction is intrinsic, a linear relation exists between pressure and flow. However, in some cases, the test results reflect only the response of the renal pelvis to distention and may be positive in the absence of obstruction.[10] These methods require general anesthesia in children and have limited applicability.

Retrograde urography at the time of surgical correction is helpful if uncertainty exists regarding the site of obstruction. This is rarely required because a well-performed ultrasound evaluation and radionuclide study will exclude distal obstruction.[26] Because risks exist when using instruments in the infant male urethra and the ureteral orifice, the routine use of retrograde studies is not recommended.

Management

Indications for Surgical Intervention

Intermittent obstruction and pain are probably the most reliable indication for surgery. However, there is no absolute or perfect definition of obstruction.

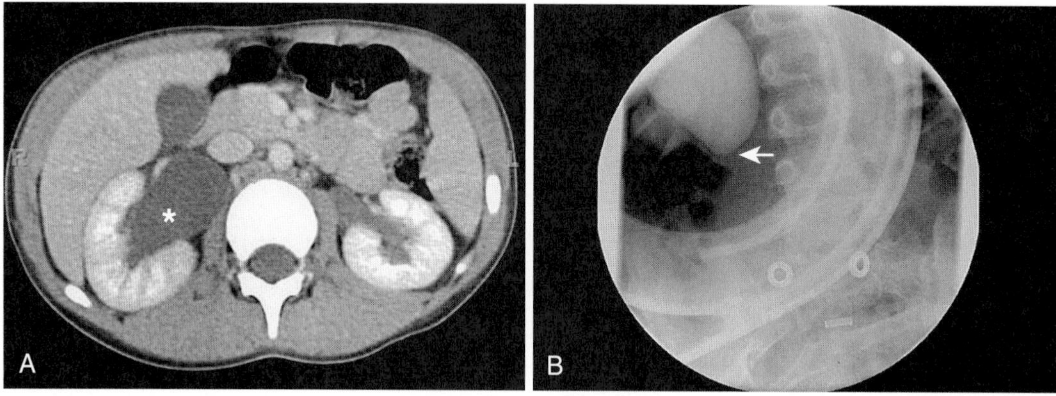

Figure 55-3. A prenatal ultrasound image of a male fetus showed left renal dilation. The left dilation resolved by age 3. On prior ultrasound images, the right kidney was always normal in appearance. **A,** A noncontrast CT scan was obtained in this patient at 5 years of age because of severe right-sided abdominal pain. A dilated renal pelvis (*asterisk*) is identified without urolithiasis. **B,** Intravenous pyelogram confirms a dilated renal pelvis and a kink (*arrow*) at the junction of the ureter and the renal pelvis.

Diminished function, delayed drainage, progression of dilation on ultrasound imaging, and loss of renal function are all potential indicators of obstruction. Randomization to surgical and observational arms is complicated by a difficult decision that a parent has to make for the asymptomatic child.[27-30] Relying on the morphologic appearance of a dilated renal pelvis by using excretory urography or ultrasonography is an insufficient basis on which to proceed with operation because many of these apparent abnormalities will completely resolve without surgical intervention (Fig. 55-4).[31] Neonatal hydronephrosis can be explained by physiologic polyuria and natural kinks and folds in the ureter.[32,33]

The ongoing debate in the management of neonatal UPJ obstruction centers on the definition of significant obstruction.[28-30] Diuretic renography has limitations in the neonate, although using the "well-tempered" approach increases its value.[24] The accumulation of the isotope in the dilated collecting system is quite variable so that the timing of the diuretic can be premature or delayed. The standard half-time of 20 minutes for obstruction in the neonate is misleading in many cases.

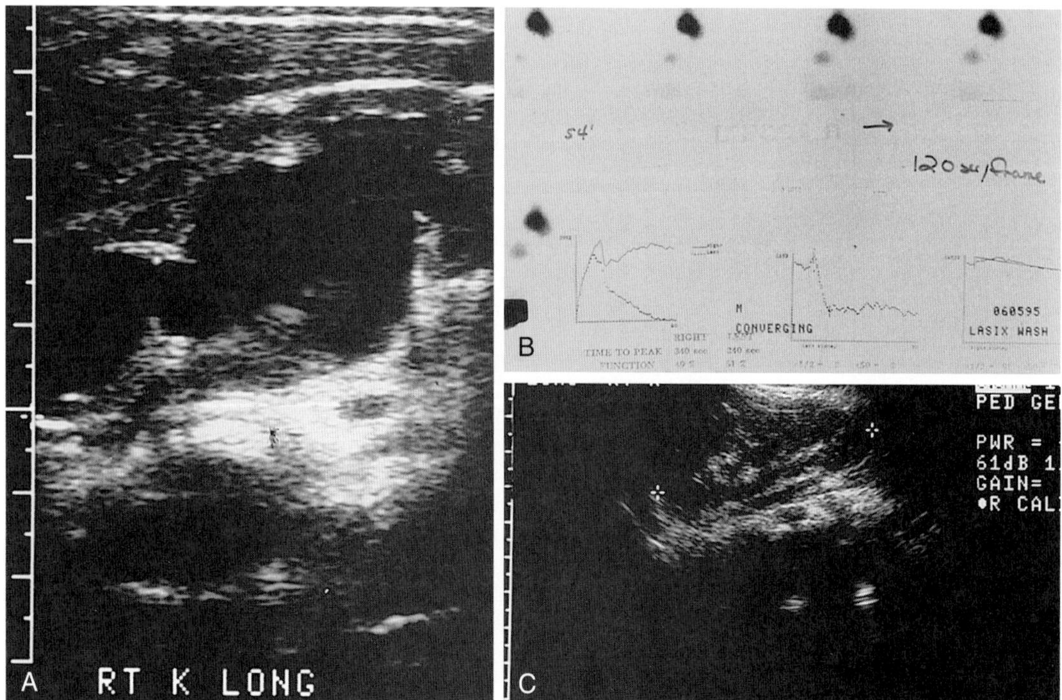

Figure 55-4. Neonatal ureteropelvic junction (UPJ). **A,** Ultrasonography shows cortical thinning, caliectasis, and renal pelvic dilation consistent with UPJ obstruction. **B,** Furosemide washout renal scan. Computer analysis is on the bottom: Time to peak function shows symmetric uptake in the first 2 minutes. Radionuclide drains out of the left kidney before the administration of diuretic. The drainage half-time from the right kidney is prolonged and was calculated to be 81 minutes. On the basis of good renal function, observation was elected. **C,** Follow-up sonogram 1 year later is normal. Renal scan at that time showed symmetric function with normal washout (5 minutes).

Differential renal function or individual kidney uptake is the most useful information obtained during renography.[22-24] An indication for operative treatment is diminished renal function in the presence of an obstructive pattern on renography. The cutoff point is arbitrary, but most centers believe that less than 35% to 40% function in the hydronephrotic kidney warrants surgical correction. However, one series of patients with dilated kidneys and no more than 25% total renal function were found to improve to more than 40% of total function in all cases without surgical treatment.[31] Long-term studies of kidneys with greater than 40% function have shown that fewer than 15% to 20% will require surgical treatment for diminishing function, urinary tract infections, or unexplained abdominal pain.[34,35] Some of these kidneys will regain some of the lost function.

The ultimate concern with an observational approach is that delaying surgical intervention until measurable deterioration of renal function occurs is suboptimal. In the past, urinary stasis (infection, calculi, hypertension, pain) was the indication for correction. Whether more emphasis should be placed on stasis and less emphasis on differential renal function is an unanswered question.[36] Pyeloplasty can be safely performed in the infant.[37,38] Early intervention eliminates the indefinite period of surveillance. The decision to follow neonates nonoperatively requires vigilance and parental cooperation to avoid unnecessary complications.

If the child is first seen with acute pain or infection, it is advisable to wait 1 to 2 weeks to allow the inflammation to resolve. Percutaneous drainage for sepsis is rarely required preoperatively. It should be strictly avoided in the absence of infection because of the inflammation that a tube in the renal pelvis induces. Exploration of a poorly functioning kidney requires assessment of the renal parenchyma. If the parenchyma is grossly dysplastic or frozen-section analysis shows only dysplasia, then nephrectomy should be performed. No test accurately predicts recovery of function. Thus, nephrectomy is rarely performed in the infant with UPJ obstruction.

Operative Techniques

Because the flank approach is the most difficult, and it is easy to commit errors of position and rotation, the anterior extraperitoneal approach or posterior lumbotomy approach is preferred. The anterior approach involves a transverse incision from the edge of the rectus to the tip of the 12th rib.[39] The retroperitoneum is entered and the UPJ is exposed, with the kidney left in situ. In infants, this is a muscle-splitting incision with low morbidity. The posterior lumbotomy also can be easily performed in infancy and provides direct access to the UPJ.[40] The kidney does not require mobilization, and the ureter and renal pelvis can usually be brought up into the incision. In bilateral cases, the child does not need to be repositioned. The lumbotomy approach should not be used with a malrotated kidney or a kidney that has an intrarenal pelvis. Also, it is more difficult in a very muscular patient. An anterior or flank approach is always preferred for reoperation.

The result of any pyeloplasty is a funnel-shaped, dependent UPJ complex. Older techniques, including the Foley YV-plasty and the Culp spiral flap, were designed to maintain the continuity of the ureter and the pelvis.[41,42] These techniques are used in unusual cases of malrotation, fusion anomalies, or long, stenotic segments. The dismembered technique consistently provides the best results (Fig. 55-5). With this approach, the renal pelvis and upper ureter are mobilized and the ureter is divided just below the obstructing segment. It is spatulated on its lateral border through the aperistaltic segment. If the segment is particularly long, this is identified before the renal pelvis is reduced, and a flap of renal pelvis can be created. Usually, it is necessary to resect some of the renal pelvis to avoid postoperative obstruction.

Gentle handling of the pelvic and ureteral tissue is important. Excessive manipulation of these tissues increases edema. Pyeloplasties are frequently performed without diversion, so it is important to be as gentle as possible. Fine chromic stay sutures allow atraumatic manipulation of the ureter and renal pelvis. A retractor is placed only after dissection is completed so that the pyeloplasty can be more appropriately designed. The anastomosis is performed with 6-0 polydioxanone or 6-0 polyglycolic acid. The anastomosis begins at the most dependent portion of the pyeloplasty with placement of interrupted everting sutures that do not bunch the tissues and cause obstruction. After the anastomosis to the dependent portion of the pyeloplasty is completed, the remainder of the ureter and pelvis can be approximated with continuous suture, taking care to irrigate any clots from the pelvis before the closure is completed. It is not necessary to pass a catheter distally into the bladder because preoperative studies should have excluded a distal obstruction.

Pyeloplasty can be safely performed without nephrostomy tubes or stents.[43] Even if leakage from the anastomosis occurs, a satisfactory outcome can usually be expected. A Penrose drain is left near the anastomosis and can usually be removed within 48 hours.

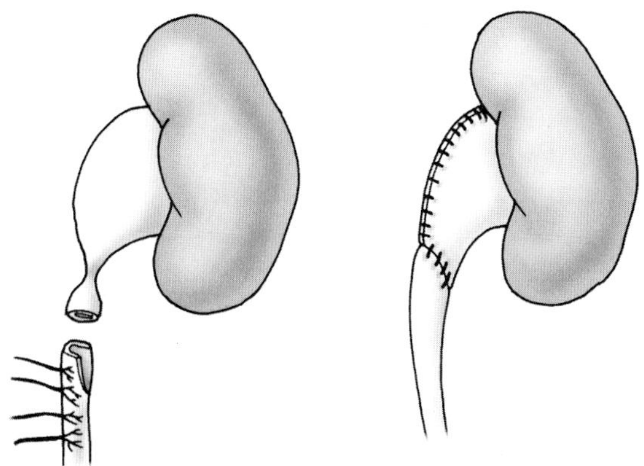

Figure 55-5. Dismembered pyeloplasty showing reduction of the renal pelvis and spatulation of the ureter (see text).

If drainage is prolonged, the child can be discharged with the drain in place.

Nephrostomy tube drainage is indicated when simultaneous bilateral pyeloplasties are performed. In small children, the ureter may be a thin diaphanous structure, in which case nephrostomy decompression will reduce the chance of postoperative obstruction. A stent (theoretically holding the ureter open and preventing synechiae formation) is usually not required. When the patient has poor preoperative renal function, a nephrostomy provides postoperative decompression and will allow a low-pressure study of the anastomosis before its removal. Once free flow across the anastomosis is demonstrated, it is unlikely that future obstruction will occur. This is reassuring when postoperative pyelography or diuretic renography is difficult to interpret because of reduced function. In reoperation, a nephrostomy is always placed because it is technically more difficult to achieve a watertight anastomosis.

Extrinsic UPJ obstruction associated with an aberrant lower-pole vessel requires division of the ureter at the UPJ and performance of a standard dismembered pyeloplasty after transposing the ureter to a nonobstructed position. In the case of an intrarenal pelvis or when significant scarring exists at reoperation, a ureterocalicostomy is a useful adjunctive technique.[44] Amputation of the lower pole is required to prevent a postoperative stricture. The ureter is spatulated and anastomosed to a calyx in the lower pole.

Endoscopic approaches to UPJ obstruction have been routinely used in adults for the last 10 to 15 years but have now been largely replaced by laparoscopic approaches.[45,46] Endoscopic relief of UPJ obstruction in children can be performed either percutaneously or retrograde by using a cutting current across the aperistaltic segment.[47] An indwelling ureteral stent is left for 4 to 6 weeks. The best results in children do not approach the near 100% success of open pyeloplasty. Endopyelotomy clearly has a role in recurrent UPJ obstruction, in which the success approaches 100%.[47]

The first laparoscopic pyeloplasty in a child was reported in 1995 by Peters.[48] The first series was published by Tan in 1999.[49] Laparoscopic pyeloplasty has been reported in children as young as 2 months.[50] Some pediatric urologists have been hesitant to adopt this technique owing to the difficulty of intracorporeal suturing and the increased operative time. The introduction of robotic surgery with articulating instruments and three-dimensional visualization has made intracorporeal suturing easier and more precise. The success rate with minimally invasive techniques are similar to open procedures and vary from 87% to 100%.[51] The benefits of laparoscopic and robotic surgery over an open approach include a decreased length of hospitalization, decreased analgesic requirements, improved cosmesis, and quicker return to normal activity.[52]

Laparoscopic pyeloplasties are mostly performed using the Anderson-Hynes dismembered technique. They can be performed through either a transperitoneal or retroperitoneal approach with a similar technique once access and exposure is obtained. With both transabdominal and retroperitoneal approaches, the child is placed in a flank or modified flank position.

UPJ Obstruction in a Duplex Kidney

The lower pole of a duplex kidney is most commonly affected because the segment in the upper pole lacks a true pelvis.[53] Ultrasonography may not be reliable for diagnosis because the duplex nature of the kidney may not be identified. A pyelogram or renogram will show a small nonobstructed upper segment.

The anatomy of the duplication influences the operation. If the ureter is incompletely duplicated and a long lower-pole ureteral segment is found, a standard dismembered pyeloplasty can be performed. If a high bifurcation with a short distal segment is found, then the end of the renal pelvis can be anastomosed to the side of the upper-pole ureter. These options can be assessed after the kidney and pelvis are exposed.

Surgical Results and Complications

The results of surgical correction have been uniformly successful[26,34,43] when performed at children's hospitals. The rate of recurrent UPJ obstruction is less than 1%, and the nephrectomy rate is less than 2%. The most common early complications are prolonged urinary extravasation and delayed drainage through the anastomosis. When an anastomotic leak persists beyond 14 days, continuity of the renal pelvis and ureter must be assessed with an antegrade or retrograde pyelogram. If a significant leak is present, either a stent or a percutaneous nephrostomy tube should be inserted. Once diversion is instituted, the leak will usually cease within 48 hours. Late scarring at the anastomotic site is common in these situations.

Delayed opening of the anastomosis is seen most commonly when a nephrostomy tube is used. When this occurs, patience is important because 80% of these will open in 3 months. Secondary obstruction or failure of the primary procedure occurs due to scarring or fibrosis, a nondependent anastomosis, ureteral angulation secondary to renal malrotation, or ureteral narrowing distal to the anastomosis. Revision can be performed via an open incision with the same principles outlined for the initial procedure[54] or by using endoscopic approaches.[47]

A postoperative functional assessment of the anastomosis should be obtained in 2 to 3 months. Further evaluation is recommended 12 to 24 months after surgery. Problems are uncommon after this time in the absence of symptoms.

URETERAL ABNORMALITIES

Embryology

Ureteral development begins during the fourth week of gestation when the ureteral bud arises from the mesonephric duct.[55] The bud elongates, grows cephalad, and forms the ureter, renal pelvis, calyces, and collecting tubules. The distal end of the mesonephric duct from the ureteral bud to the vesicourethral tract is called the common excretory duct and expands in trumpet fashion into the bladder and urethra to form half of the trigone. The attachment of the ureter to the mesonephric duct switches from a posterior to an anterolateral location. With expansion and absorption of the common excretory duct into the urinary tract, the orifices of the ureteral bud and mesonephric duct become independent and move away and settle in the bladder and urethra, respectively.

Alterations in bud number, position, and time of development result in anomalies. VUR results from caudal displacement of the ureteral bud, whereas ureteral ectopia and obstruction result from cranial displacement. Renal development and dysplasia are related to the ureteral orifice location.[55,56]

Ureteral Duplication

Duplication is the most common ureteral anomaly. Both sides are equally affected, and girls are affected twice as often as boys. The autopsy incidence is approximately 1%, but the incidence is 2% to 4% in clinical series in which pyelograms were obtained for urinary symptoms.[55,56] Infection was historically the most common reason for presentation, but the majority are now detected prenatally. Many of the duplicated units show congenital dysplasia (scarring) and hydronephrosis.[57] Histologic evaluation of the kidneys shows an increased incidence of pyelonephritis and dysplasia. There is an increased incidence of infection because both VUR and obstruction are much more common in duplicated systems.[56]

A partial or complete duplication of the ureter occurs when a single bud branches prematurely or when two ureteral buds arise from the mesonephric duct. A bifid renal pelvis is the highest level of bifurcation and occurs in 10% of the population. Other incomplete duplications occur throughout the ureter (Fig. 55-6). When the bifurcation is near the bladder, urine can pass down one limb of the duplication and then back up the other side of the Y.[58] This may lead to stasis with ureteral dilation or infection. Treatment involves either ureteral reimplantation or ureteropyelostomy at the renal level.[59] An inverted-Y ureter is the rarest of all branching anomalies.[60] This is presumably the result of separate ureteral buds that fuse before entering the metanephros. Treatment is directed at problems caused by the ectopic limb.

In complete duplications, reflux in the lower renal moiety is the most common cause of renal disease. The more caudal ureteral bud ends up laterally and cranially deviated in the bladder and has a shorter intramural tunnel. The upper-pole ureter enters the bladder adjacent or distal to the lower ureter, as defined by the Weigert-Meyer law.[61] These children are initially seen either prenatally or with urinary tract infections, and reflux is identified in up to two thirds of children with duplicated systems that appear with infection.[62] Reflux may occur into the upper-pole ureter if the ureteral orifices are immediately adjacent or if the upper ureter is distally located at the level of the bladder neck without any submucosal support (Fig. 55-7).

The treatment of VUR in duplicated ureters follows the same principles as that in the single system. Initial treatment includes preventive antibiotics and radiographic monitoring. Low grades of VUR are associated with the same rate of spontaneous resolution as the single system. The distal ureters share a common blood supply, so reimplantation involves mobilization and reimplantation of the common sheath.[63] If an associated lower-pole UPJ obstruction is noted, ipsilateral end-to-side pyeloureterostomy is an effective simultaneous management for both obstruction and reflux.[64] Even if significant scarring is present in the lower pole, reimplantation usually suffices, unless major ureteral dilation is present. In the latter case, lower-pole nephroureterectomy may be indicated.

Ureteral Triplication

This is one of the rarest anomalies of the upper urinary tract and results from either several ureteral buds or early branching. In most cases all three ureters drain

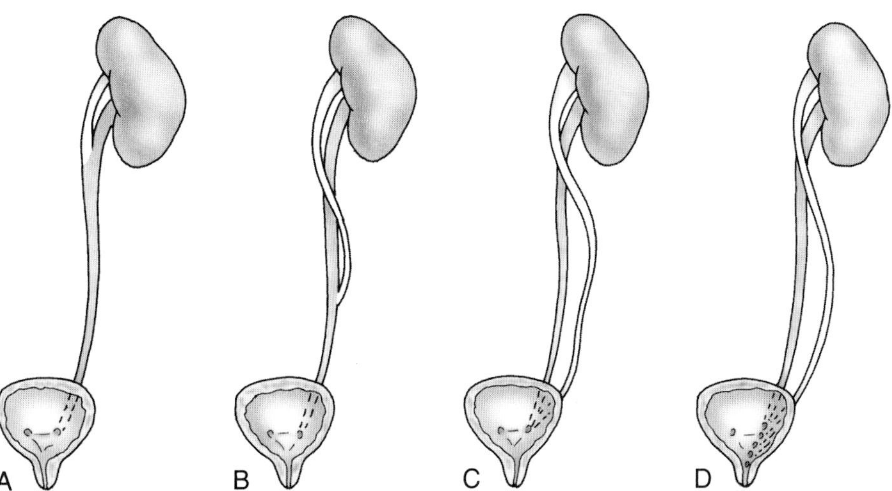

Figure 55-6. Types of duplication. **A,** Bifid pelvis. **B,** "Y" ureter. **C,** "V" ureter. **D,** Complete duplication with various ectopic orifices.

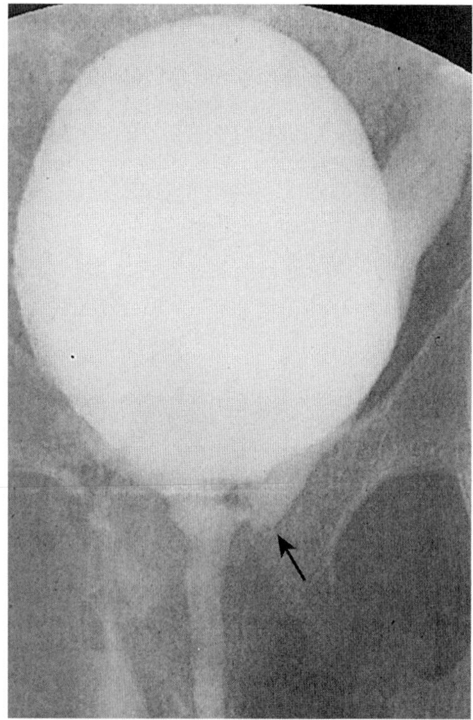

Figure 55-7. Reflux is seen into an ectopic upper pole ureter (*arrow*) that inserts into the proximal urethra in a girl first seen at age 2 months with urosepsis.

into a single orifice.[65] Triplication occurs with incontinence, infection, and symptoms of obstruction and is associated with both ectopia and ureteroceles.[66,67] Surgical treatment is individualized. Ureteral quadruplication has also been described.[68]

Retrocaval Ureter

The retrocaval or circumcaval ureter is a right ureter that passes behind the vena cava.[69] This is a result of a developmental error in the formation of the vena cava. The supracardinal vein (vena cava) lies dorsal to the developing ureter, whereas subcardinal veins lie ventral to the ureter. If the subcardinal vein persists as the vena cava, the ureter passes behind the vena cava and anterior to the iliac vein. If both veins persist, the ureter passes between the duplicated vena cava.[70]

Even though this is a congenital abnormality, symptoms are related to chronic ureteral obstruction and infection, and rarely occur in children.[71] The radiographic appearance depends on the level of obstruction. The more common distal obstruction appears as a "reversed J" on IVP.[72] Less commonly, the ureter crosses at the level of the UPJ. Both of these can be confused with UPJ obstruction and should be suspected when pyelectasis and dilation of the upper third of the ureter are seen.

Treatment is required only when significant obstruction or symptoms are present. Reconstruction is essentially a dismembered ureteroplasty with division of the ureter and anastomosis anterior to the vena cava. The other option is division and reconstruction of the vena cava, which is more problematic.

Megaureter

Megaureter is not a diagnosis but a descriptive term for a dilated ureter. Normal ureteral diameter in children is rarely greater than 5 mm. Ureters greater than 7 mm can be considered megaureters.[73] The ultrasonographic appearance of the dilated and tortuous ureter is usually striking (Fig. 55-8). Pelvicalyceal dilation and parenchymal scarring or thinning depend on the primary disease process.

These ureters can be classified as refluxing, obstructed, and nonrefluxing, nonobstructed.[74] Some ureters also have reflux and simultaneous obstruction.[75] Table 55-1 gives clinical examples of each classification. Any normal ureter will dilate if the volume of urine exceeds emptying capacity. Moreover, bacterial endotoxins and infection alone can cause dilation that will resolve after treatment of the infection.[76,77]

Primary obstructive megaureter is most commonly caused by a distal adynamic ureteral segment, but ureteral valves[33] and ectopic ureteral insertion also cause obstruction. Proximal smooth muscle hypertrophy and hyperplasia are seen. A normal-caliber catheter will

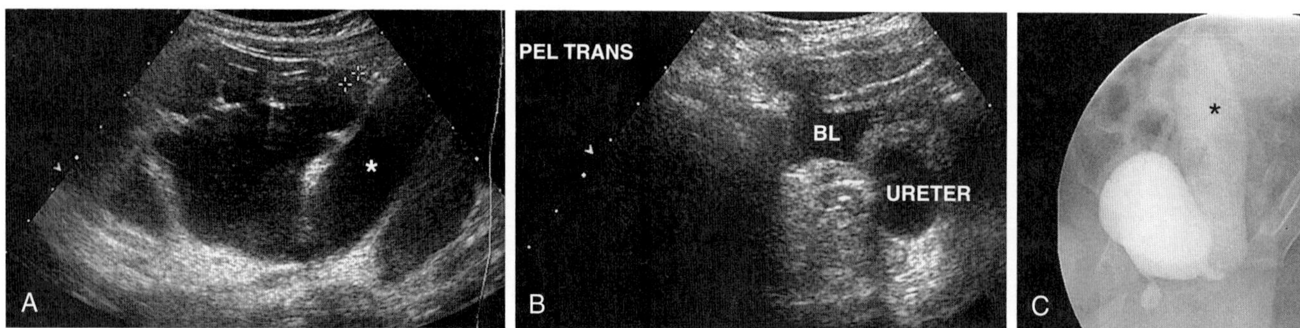

Figure 55-8. This patient has congenital megaureter. **A,** Renal ultrasound image shows diffuse caliectasis and cortical thinning with a markedly dilated left ureter (*asterisk*). **B,** Ultrasound image of the bladder confirms the markedly dilated ureter adjacent to the bladder (BL). A MAG-3 scan was performed and showed preserved renal function on the left side. **C,** The voiding cystourethrogram shows reflux into the markedly dilated left ureter (*asterisk*). Note that the contrast agent in the ureter is diluted (compared with the bladder), which is indicative of partial obstruction on that side.

Table 55-1 Classification of Megaureter
Refluxing Megaureter
Primary (congenital reflux)
Secondary (urethral valves, neurogenic bladder)
Obstructed Megaureter
Primary (adynamic segment)
Secondary (urethral obstruction, extrinsic mass, or tumor)
Nonrefluxing, Nonobstructed Megaureter
Primary (idiopathic, physiologically insignificant adynamic segment)
Secondary (polyuria, infection, postoperative residual dilation)

Modified from Khoury A, Bagli DJ: Reflux and megaureter. In Wein AJ, Kavoussi LR, Novick AC, et al (eds): Campbell-Walsh Urology, 9th ed. Philadelphia, WB Saunders, 2007, p 3468.)

usually pass through the distal 3- to 4-mm segment, but the peristaltic wave does not propel urine across this area. This absent peristalsis is not a result of a ganglionic abnormality as seen in megacolon.[78] The distal ureter has a variety of histologic appearances, but the common finding is a disruption of muscular continuity that prevents muscular propulsion of urine.[14,79-81]

As with UPJ obstruction, the majority of megaureters are now detected prenatally, although infection may also be a presentation for refluxing and obstructed megauters.[82-84] Megaureter is now the second most common urinary tract abnormality detected prenatally.[2] These children are typically asymptomatic without any physical findings or laboratory abnormalities.

Despite the variety of possibilities, standard imaging allows classification and appropriate management. The diagnosis of a nonobstructed, nonrefluxing megaureter is the hardest to make and is established only when the secondary causes of megaureter have been excluded and diagnostic tests do not show obstruction. For years it was assumed that a dilated ureter that did not reflux was obstructed,[85] but developmental ureteral dilation can occur in ureters that are not obstructed.[86]

Diagnostic imaging begins with an ultrasound study, which almost always distinguishes megaureters from UPJ obstruction. The degree of distal ureteral dilation is often much more pronounced than the degree of renal pelvic dilation or caliectasis. A VCUG should be obtained in all patients. If significant reflux is found, delayed drainage films must be obtained to exclude simultaneous obstruction with a normal-caliber distal ureteral segment. In a partially obstructed system, the contrast density in the ureter is decreased because of dilution related to stasis in the ureter (see Fig. 55-8).

Diuretic renography is used to assess function and drainage. The markedly dilated ureters can be a significant source of stasis, and determination of drainage half-time can be difficult. Diuretic administration must be delayed because the system is so capacious and may take 60 to 90 minutes to fill. A washout time of longer than 20 minutes is historically indicative of obstruction.

Treatment

Nonoperative management is based on clearance half-time and relative renal function of the hydronephrotic and contralateral kidneys. If observation is chosen, the children are given preventive antibiotics and followed with serial ultrasound and renal scans. Neonatal megaureter with obstruction suggested by renography but with preserved function can be safely observed. Most ureters will become radiographically normal over time.[82,83,87,88] Surgical correction for decreasing function or recurrent infections will be needed in only 10% to 25% of patients at age 7 years. Evidence of delayed obstruction after normalization of radiographs has not been seen in these children.

The initial attempts at surgical repair resulted in significant reflux and recurrent infections. Now, it can be performed with a high expectation of success and low morbidity.[89] Ureteral excisional tapering with preservation of the ureteral blood supply was popularized in the early 1970s.[85,90] A longitudinal segment of ureter is excised and then closed over a 10- to 12-Fr catheter. When the ureter is tunneled submucosally, the suture line is positioned against the detrusor to decrease the chance of fistula formation. Initial repairs involved tailoring the entire ureter, but this was found to be unnecessary because the upper ureteral tortuosity and dilatation often disappears after tapering the distal ureter alone.[91] Ureteral folding techniques have been popularized because they theoretically decrease the risk of ischemic injury while achieving the decreased intraluminal diameter necessary for a successful reimplant.[92,93] The increased bulk is usually not a technical problem. Although dissection is usually both intravesical and extravesical, solely extravesical reimplants have been described and may be associated with lower morbidity.[94] A vesicopsoas hitch is a useful adjunct that helps achieve a longer submucosal tunnel length without risking ureteral kinking, although excisional tailoring usually eliminates the need for this adjunctive procedure. A nonrefluxing, nonobstructed reimplantation can be achieved in 85% to 95% of patients with megaureters.[84,93] Recognized complications include persistent obstruction, reflux, and urinary extravasation. Most of these can be managed nonoperatively with drainage tubes. Lower grades of postoperative VUR will often resolve.

Primary reconstruction is preferred when indicated, but temporary cutaneous diversion may be beneficial in a neonate or infant in whom the chance of successful reimplantation of a bulky ureter into a small bladder is diminished. Diversion may decrease the ureteral diameter and decrease the need for tailoring at the time of reimplantation. An end-cutaneous ureterostomy is preferred because a high diversion may require two or more procedures for correction.

Ectopic Ureter

An ectopic ureter is defined as one that opens at the bladder neck or more caudad rather than on the trigone. Embryologically, this results from a cranial

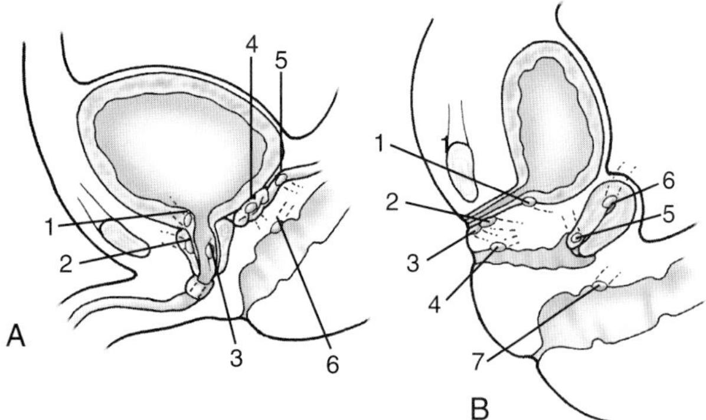

Figure 55-9. **A,** Ureteral ectopia in a boy. Possible sites are above the external sphineter (1-3), or into the seminal vesicle (4-5), or anorectal (6). **B,** Ureteral ectopia in a girl may be located at the blader neck (1), or beyond the continence mechanism in the urethra (2), or on the perineum (3). Uterine or vaginal insertion (4-6) may also cause incontinence. Anorectal insertion (7) can also occur.

insertion of the ureteral bud on the mesonephric duct that allows distal migration with the mesonephric duct as it is absorbed into the urogenital sinus.[95]

The incidence of ureteral ectopia is approximately 1 in 2000.[96] Eighty percent of ectopic ureters are reported in association with a duplicated renal system. Because clinical problems are more common in girls with ectopia, only 15% of ectopic ureters have been reported in boys.[95] Ectopia is bilateral 20% of the time.[96] Single ectopic ureters are rare but are more common in boys.[97]

Ectopic Ureter in Girls

The fundamental difference between ureteral ectopia in boys and girls arises from ureteral insertion distal to the continence mechanism in girls (Fig. 55-9). Approximately one third of ureters open at the level of the bladder neck, one third are in the vestibule around the urethral opening, and the remainder empty into the vagina, uterus, or cervix. All of these insertions are along the course of the mesonephric duct remnant (Gartner's duct).

One half of girls initially have continuous urinary incontinence in spite of what appears to be a normal voiding pattern.[95,96] If the system is markedly hydronephrotic and functions poorly, leakage may occur only in the upright position and may be confused with stress incontinence. Persistent foul-smelling vaginal discharge can suggest an ectopic ureter. When the ectopic ureter is present in the urethra or the bladder neck, both obstruction and reflux are frequently present. Although prenatal diagnosis is the most common presentation, a urinary tract infection and/or sepsis may be the presenting symptom.

The diagnosis of an ectopic ureter may be obvious or can be difficult. When genital ectopy is present, the kidney may not visualize on ultrasonography if the moiety is small and atrophic and is not associated with hydronephrosis. Often significant hydronephrosis is present in the upper pole of a duplicated kidney and the ultrasound image may show a dilated ectopic ureter behind the bladder. However, the upper pole may be simply an echogenic focus (Fig. 55-10). A scan with dimercaptosuccinic acid (DMSA) is a good test for localizing a small ectopic kidney when an orthotopic kidney is not identified on standard imaging and there is a high suspicion of genital ectopy. MR urography may be the most precise method for making this diagnosis.[98] A VCUG should be obtained in all patients to exclude occult reflux.[99]

The diagnosis is confirmed with physical examination, panendoscopy, and retrograde pyelography. Dyes used to stain urine may have a role. Urine in the bladder changes color, whereas the poorly concentrated urine is evident as persistent clear leakage. Meticulous examination of the area around the urethral meatus and vagina will often reveal an asymmetry or bead of fluid coming from an opening that can be probed and injected in retrograde fashion (see Fig. 55-10). Vaginoscopy with attention to the superior lateral aspect of the vagina may reveal a large ectopic orifice.

Ectopic Ureter in Boys

The most common sites of ectopic ureteral insertion in boys are the posterior urethra (40% to 50%) and the seminal vesicle (20% to 60%), depending on the age

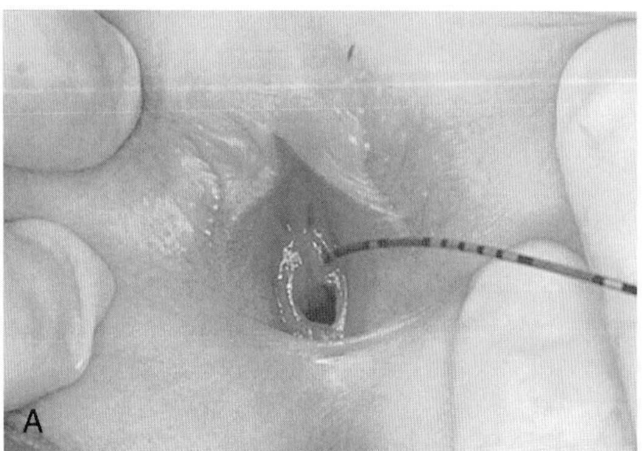

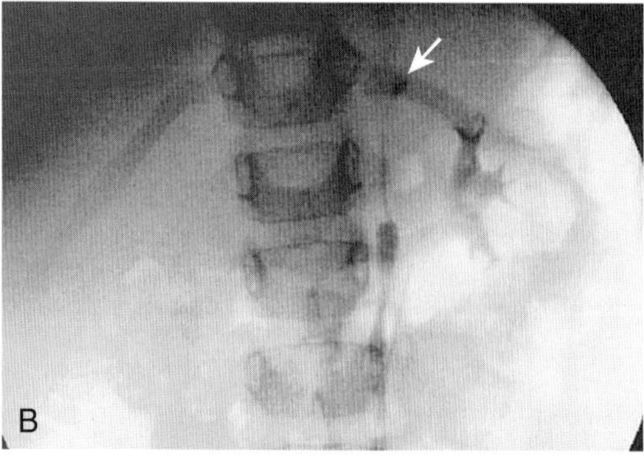

Figure 55-10. This 3-year-old girl had continuous urinary incontinence despite a normal voiding pattern. The renal ultrasound image was essentially normal on both sides with no evidence of hydronephrosis or an echogenic upper pole. **A,** A ureteral catheter has been inserted into an ectopic left ureter. **B,** The retrograde ureterogram shows a very small upper left ureter and a small cystic calyx (*arrow*) in the left upper pole medial to the lower pole collecting system that was opacified through an orifice on the trigone. The patient was continent after a laparoscopic left upper pole partial nephroureterectomy.

at presentation.[100] Symptoms in boys may not occur until after the onset of sexual activity and include prostatitis, seminal vesiculitis, or an infected seminal vesical cyst causing painful bowel movements. The genital insertion accounts for the common presentation with epididymitis. The boy may initially have post-void dribbling secondary to pooling of urine in the prostatic urethra, but incontinence is never as pronounced as in the girl.

Diagnostic testing is similar to that used in girls. Ectopic ureters in the boy are more commonly obstructed and hydronephrotic so ultrasound examination is often more useful. If the ectopic site of insertion is outside the urethra, it is rarely identified on endoscopic examination.

Surgical Management of Ectopic Ureters

Surgical treatment is dependent on the associated parenchyma.[101,102] Single-system ectopia to the genital system usually has poor function, and nephroureterectomy is appropriate. When the ectopic ureter is associated with a duplication, the function in the upper pole is usually poor, and an open or laparoscopic partial nephroureterectomy has historically been the most common surgical approach. The distal stump is left open. A ureteroureterostomy can then be performed to drain the ectopic system in the true pelvis. There are potential concerns regarding the size discrepancy of the ureters and injury to the recipient ureter, but large series show excellent success with a very low complication rate. This approach avoids potential injury to the lower pole of the kidney and can be performed through a small inguinal incision. The obstruction, dilation, and incontinence usually resolve with this approach. Even if the upper pole is poorly functioning, it should not cause any long-term problems. A common sheath ureteral reimplantation can be performed with tailoring of the ureter in the upper pole, but the increased morbidity and complication rate associated with ureteral tapering limit the utility of this approach.

The distal stump rarely causes a problem in genital ectopia. However, if urethral or bladder neck insertion of the ectopic ureter and reflux into the ureter is identified preoperatively, excision is indicated,[102] but can be tedious. If the dissection plane is kept immediately adjacent to the ureter behind the bladder, the bladder neck and sphincter should not be damaged. The stump is ligated at this point. In a postpubertal girl, this dissection can be performed transvaginally. Small stumps can be obliterated by using a Bugbee electrode.

Bilateral Single Ectopic Ureters

This is a rare abnormality in which the altered ureteral embryologic development is associated with failure of normal bladder neck development.[103] Genital and anal anomalies are commonly present. Girls have ureteral insertion in the distal urethra and are first seen with infection or are noted to have continuous urinary leakage. The bladder is usually poorly developed because it has never stored urine. Boys have somewhat larger bladders because some urine will have entered the bladder. However, because the bladder neck is not formed normally, they also have some degree of urinary incontinence.

The child who is incontinent with bilateral single ectopic ureters presents a major reconstructive challenge that may include ureteral reimplantation, bladder neck reconstruction, and bladder augmentation if the bladder capacity is insufficient.

URETEROCELES

Ureteroceles are cystic dilatations of the terminal, intravesical ureter that usually have a stenotic orifice.[104-106] In children, ureteroceles are most commonly associated with the upper pole of a duplex system (80%) and an ectopic orifice (60%) in the urethra. In adults, they are usually part of a completely intravesical single system. Ureteroceles occur four to seven times more frequently in girls and are more common in whites. Bilateral ureteroceles are found 10% of the time.

A single embryologic theory does not explain all ureteroceles. The most popular theory involves persistence of Chwalla's membrane at the junction of the wolffian duct and urogenital sinus.[107] Incomplete breakdown of the ureteral membrane causes an obstruction resulting in dilation. This theory explains the majority of ureteroceles but does not account for the development of ureteroceles with patulous ureteral orifices in the urethra or of ureteroceles associated with multicystic dysplasia and atretic ureteral segments or for the presence of ectopic ureters without ureterocele formation.[108] This clinical finding supports a more general developmental abnormality of the ureter.

It is likely that a ureterocele is the result of an abnormal induction of the trigone and distal ureter by many of the genes and growth factors that are important in renal and ureteral growth and development. Histologic studies support this concept.[108] Histologic analysis of the intravesical portion of ureteroceles shows deficiencies in the trigonal musculature of patients with ureteroceles that were not present in ectopic ureters without ureterocele formation. This field defect results in pseudodiverticulum (ureterocele eversion) and reflux into laterally displaced, poorly supported ureters. This is supported by the clinical observation of multicystic dysplasia and the absence of hydronephrosis in association with a ureterocele.

The classification of ureteroceles can be confusing. Pathologic classification describes four types: stenotic, sphincteric, sphincterostenotic, and cecoureterocele.[108] The current recommended nomenclature classifies ureteroceles as either intravesical (entirely within the bladder) or ectopic (some portion is situated permanently at the bladder neck or in the urethra).[109]

Presentation and Diagnosis

Although presentation with an infection in a system with high-grade obstruction is common, antenatal imaging is now the most common method of diagnosis

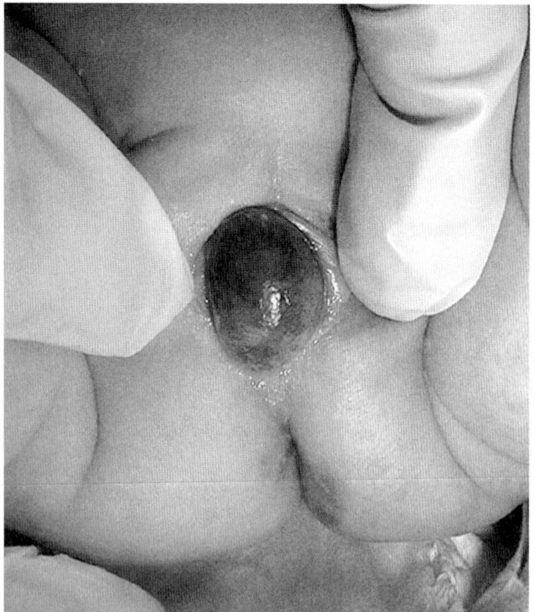

Figure 55-11. This 2-week-old presented with sepsis and was found to have this prolapsing ectopic ureterocele. The ureterocele was aspirated with return of purulent debris and underwent prompt decompression. Recovery was uneventful.

(60%).[110-113] The obstructed renal unit may be palpable in these asymptomatic infants, but most have no clinically apparent abnormality. Bladder outlet obstruction is rare because most ureteroceles decompress during micturition, but the most common cause of urethral obstruction in girls is urethral prolapse of a ureterocele (Fig. 55-11).

Abdominal ultrasonography reveals a well-defined cystic intravesical mass that is associated within the posterior bladder wall (Fig. 55-12). This can be followed to a dilated ureter in the bony pelvis and to upper-pole hydroureteronephrosis in a duplication. The thickness and echogenicity of the renal parenchyma are often consistent with dysplasia and poor function.

During cystoscopy, the bladder should be examined when both full and completely empty because compressible ureteroceles may not be evident in a full bladder or may appear as a bladder diverticulum. The dilated lower end of an ectopic ureter or megaureter may elevate the trigone, creating the cystoscopic, radiographic, and ultrasound appearance of a ureterocele, a so-called pseudoureterocele.[114]

Treatment Options

The goals of ureterocele management include control of infection, preservation of renal function, protection of normal ipsilateral and contralateral units, and continence. The natural history of an asymptomatic ureterocele is unknown. There is a subset of ureteroceles associated with multicystic dysplasia, no hydroureter, and no reflux. The multicystic moiety usually involutes and the ureterocele rarely causes symptoms and can be observed.[108] Up to 10% to 15% of prenatally identified ureteroceles have these clinical findings. Neonates given preventive antibiotics rarely develop a febrile urinary tract infection.[111,112] If significant hydroureteronephrosis is found, it should be assumed that there is significant urinary tract obstruction and preventive antibiotics should be started.

Traditional treatment of duplex ectopic ureteroceles includes upper-pole heminephrectomy through a separate flank incision, ureterocele excision, and ipsilateral lower-pole ureteral reimplant via a lower incision. The bladder-level operation may require repair of a sizable defect in the bladder base and tapering or plication of the lower ureter. The distal extent of the ureterocele and its mucosa can often be dissected through the bladder neck. Incomplete excision may result in an obstructing urethral flap. Resection of the entire ureterocele risks damaging the continence mechanisms of the bladder neck. Experienced surgeons report excellent results with low rates of reoperation (<10%) and low complication rates (<10%).[115-117] These approaches assume that ureterocele excision is an essential component of management. However, because the distal ureter and bladder defect may resolve without being removed or repaired, an absolute indication to proceed with a simultaneous bladder operation is rarely present. In older children, when absence of function is noted on the affected side (upper and lower pole), nephroureterectomy and reconstruction of the bladder is the initial treatment of choice.

Primary upper-pole partial nephroureterectomy may avoid bladder-level reconstruction and its potential risks.[110,118,119] Nearly all of the ureter can be removed through the flank incision, and the distal

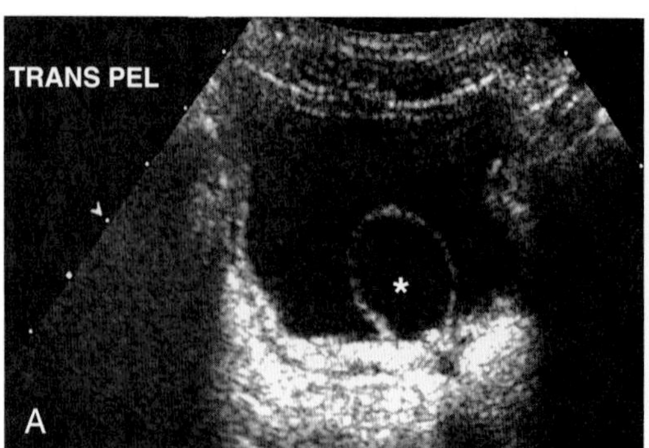

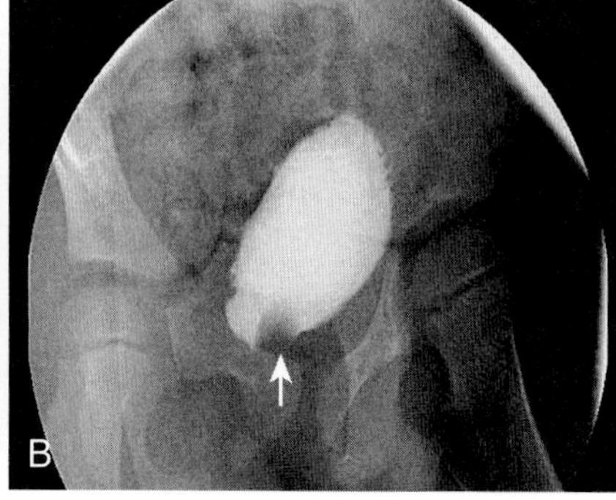

Figure 55-12. **A,** Ultrasound image of the bladder demonstrates a ureterocele (*asterisk*). **B,** The ureterocele appears as a nonopacified filling defect (*arrow*) at the base of the bladder on the cystogram.

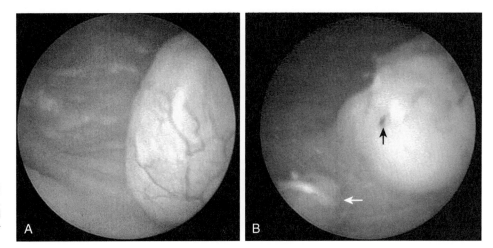

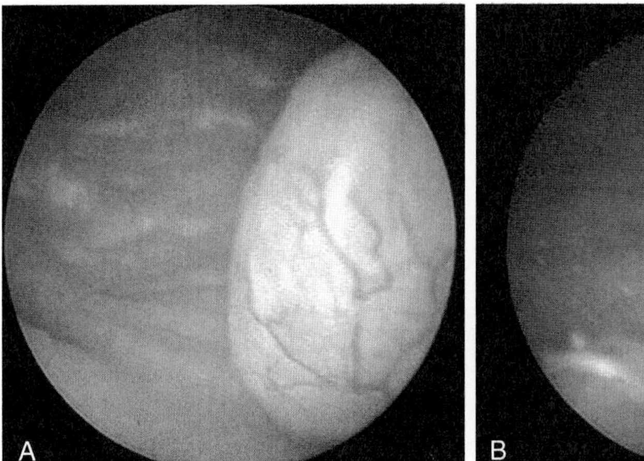

Figure 55-13. **A,** This intravesical ureterocele was found at cystoscopy. **B,** The ureterocele was punctured (*black arrow*) and decompressed using a 3-Fr electrode (*white arrow*).

ureter is left open to facilitate decompression. The need for subsequent bladder-level excision and reconstruction varies between 10% and 62%.[110,112,119] Although up to 45% of ipsilateral and contralateral VUR will resolve after ureterocele decompression, persistent VUR is the most common indication for bladder-level reconstruction.[110] Other indications for bladder-level reconstruction include ureterocele eversion acting like a diverticulum or externally compressing the bladder neck, reflux into the ureterocele, or intraluminal obstruction of the bladder neck by a cecoureterocele. The need for bladder-level intervention is directly related to the number of renal moieties that have either a ureterocele or VUR.[112]

Most partial nephrectomy specimens show dysplasia, but some may show only inflammatory and obstructive changes.[119,120] In cases with preserved function, a pyeloureterostomy or ureteroureterostomy (high or low) may be performed, along with distal ureterectomy and ureterocele decompression.[101] These procedures potentially place the lower-pole system at risk to salvage what may be a small percentage of total renal function.

Ureterocele incision is the least invasive technique for upper-pole preservation. "Unroofing" of the ureterocele is advocated only as a drainage procedure for an infected system before a definitive procedure because it invariably results in reflux.[121,122] Using a 3-Fr Bugbee electrode to drain the ureterocele just above the bladder neck is the recommended technique because reflux is not inevitable (Fig. 55-13).[111] Although the ureterocele opening is in the bladder, to be successful the surgeon must also drain the ectopic urethral portion to prevent an obstructing lip at the level of the bladder neck.

Endoscopic incision successfully decompresses the ureterocele 85% of the time.[111,120,123,124] It is the definitive procedure in more than 90% of infants with intravesical ureteroceles. However, subsequent reconstructive surgery is required in 50% to 90% of patients with ectopic ureteroceles. Reflux into the ureterocele moiety is the most common indication for reconstruction in these infants. Previous decompression of the system makes this reconstruction easier.[111]

Ureterocele incision should probably be the initial procedure in most neonates because reflux into other moieties is usually present (>50%). Even when ultrasonography shows little renal parenchyma, incision can be performed. The decompressed system may require no further treatment if iatrogenic upper pole reflux does not develop. In older children, incision is best selected when associated functioning renal parenchyma is found, the ureterocele is intravesical, or the kidney is drained by a single system.

Single-system ureteroceles are more commonly seen in older children and adults and are associated with better function and less hydronephrosis than is found in duplex kidneys. Most often, they are incidental findings that require no treatment. Antenatally detected single-system ureteroceles may not show significant obstruction on a furosemide washout renal scan. Clinically, these behave like nonobstructed megaureters and can be safely followed with preventive antibiotics. If treatment is required, endoscopic incision can be the definitive procedure nearly 100% of the time.

chapter 56

URINARY TRACT INFECTION AND VESICOURETERAL REFLUX

Eugene Minevich, MD • Curtis A. Sheldon, MD

URINARY TRACT INFECTION

Urinary tract infections (UTIs) are common and a major source of morbidity in children. They constitute a significant health burden, although the actual costs are not known.[1]

Diagnosis

Although clinical signs and symptoms are important indicators for childhood UTI, confirmation of the diagnosis by microscopic examination and quantitative culture of a properly collected specimen is imperative. Signs and symptoms of UTI are age dependent, and combinations of findings are more useful than individual signs and symptoms in identifying children with a UTI.[2] Neonates rarely present with findings specific to the urinary tract. Nonspecific symptoms such as lethargy, irritability, temperature instability, anorexia, emesis, or jaundice predominate. Bacteremia is common with neonatal UTI, and urine culture is an important part of the evaluation of neonatal sepsis.[3] Older infants often present with nonspecific abdominal discomfort, emesis, diarrhea, poor weight gain, or fever. Malodorous or cloudy urine may be reported. Older children frequently present with dysuria along with urinary frequency, urgency, and enuresis. Table 56-1 outlines the incidence of UTI symptoms as a function of age.[4,5] Because the symptoms can be quite obscure, it is important that care providers have a high index of suspicion for UTIs in children.

Analysis of a properly collected urine sample is the cornerstone of the diagnosis of UTI.[6] Errors in diagnosis most commonly result from failure to confirm a clinically suspected UTI by culture or by reliance on a specimen that has been inadequately collected or mishandled. Specimens may be obtained by bag collection, clean-catch, urethral catheterization, or suprapubic aspiration. Although invasive, urethral catheterization (or suprapubic aspiration) clearly offers the lowest risk of contamination (false-positive culture results).[7] The results of a bag specimen or clean-catch specimen are helpful only if negative.[8] Positive findings should be confirmed using a catheter or aspiration specimen unless the clinical presentation is unequivocal. The accuracy of positive findings from a bag specimen in infancy has been estimated at 7.5%.[9] The accuracy of midstream collected specimens varies with age: 42% when younger than 18 months of age and 71% from 3 to 12 years of age.[10] Specimens should be either analyzed and plated immediately or placed on ice to minimize bacterial multiplication before testing.

The standard for diagnosis of a UTI remains the quantitative urine culture. The accepted criterion for diagnosis is greater than 10^5 colony-forming units per milliliter of a single bacterial species.[11] The accuracy of such a positive finding on culture is estimated at 80% (single specimen) and 96% (confirmed by second culture). Table 56-2 outlines the probability of infection as a function of colony count and method of collection that we use in children.[12] However, one must avoid applying these criteria too strictly because the colony count varies as a function of hydration (dilution) and urinary frequency (bacterial multiplication time). One study of six untreated children with proven bacteriuria found colony counts to vary from 10^3 to 10^8 over a 24-hour period.[13]

Although clearly most accurate, urine culture results cannot provide an immediate diagnosis, and, as a result, initial treatment is generally guided by the urinalysis. Microscopic evaluation of a urine specimen should be done immediately on collection. This practice minimizes misleading ex-vivo bacterial multiplication and deterioration of cellular elements. The identification of bacteria in an unspun urine specimen is very suggestive of significant bacteriuria.[13] Pyuria (more than 10 leukocytes/mm^3) is suggestive[14] but may also be seen in such instances as vaginitis, dehydration, calculi, trauma, chemical irritation, gastroenteritis, and viral immunization. Urine Gram stain was found to be reliable in detecting UTI in young infants.[15]

A popular and indirect measurement of bacteriuria employs nitrite and leukocyte esterase analysis.

Table 56-1 Presenting Symptoms in 200 Children with Urinary Tract Infection as a Function of Age

	Age			
Symptom	*0-1 mo*	*1-24 mo*	*2-5 yr*	*5-12 yr*
Failure to thrive, poor feeding	53%	36%	7%	0
Jaundice	44%	0	0	0
Screaming, irritability	0	13%	7%	0
Foul-smelling, cloudy urine	0	9%	13%	0
Diarrhea	18%	16%	0	0
Vomiting	24%	29%	16%	3%
Fever	11%	38%	57%	50%
Convulsions	2%	7%	9%	5%
Hematuria	0	7%	16%	6%
Frequency, dysuria	0	4%	34%	41%
Enuresis	0	0	27%	29%
Abdominal pain	0	0	23%	44%
Loin pain	0	0	0	12%
Male-to-female ratio	1:2	1:13	1:10	1:10

From Smellie JM, Hodson CJ, Edwards D, et al: Clinical and radiological features of urinary tract infection in childhood. BMJ 2:1222, 1964; Bickerton MW, Duckett JW: Urinary tract infections in pediatric patients. AUA Update Service, Lesson 26. Vol 4:4, 1985.

Nitrate, normally present in urine, is converted to nitrite in the presence of bacteria. A positive colorimetric reaction between nitrite, sulfanilic acid, and α-naphthylamine is thus indicative of bacteria with specificity and a positive predictive value approaching 100%.[16] The nitrate-to-nitrite reaction requires a relatively long incubation period. Thus, urinary frequency and hydration may produce a false-negative result. Inadequate dietary nitrate and infection caused by nitrite-negative organisms may also cause false-negative reactions.[17] The combination of nitrite and leukocyte esterase is more sensitive and specific than either by itself.[18] Overall the combination of dipstick analysis and microscopic examination for bacteria have a sensitivity of and a negative predictive value approaching 100%.[16]

Classification

Classification of UTIs helps to determine the need for hospital admission and parenteral antibiotic therapy as opposed to outpatient oral antibiotic therapy. An attempt is made to distinguish between upper tract (pyelonephritis) and lower tract infections. Fever, flank pain or tenderness, and leukocytosis suggest pyelonephritis and require parenteral antibiotics to minimize the risk of renal injury. Additional findings supporting parenteral antibiotic therapy include age (< 3 months), unusual pathogens, or significant urinary anomalies. After the initial stabilization, we often complete the course of parenteral antibiotics on an outpatient basis, employing our home-based nursing service.

Laboratory studies designed to distinguish lower tract from upper tract UTI include antibody-coated bacteria assay, β_2-microglobulin excretion, antibodies to Tamm-Horsfall protein, and urinary lactic dehydrogenase assay and procalcitonin.[19,20] These tests are not sufficiently reliable for routine clinical use. Although cumbersome, direct culture by ureteral catheterization or percutaneous puncture is reliable and represents excellent options in complicated clinical problems. We have found the most usable study for localizing infection to the kidney to be an isotope image during presentation of the patient with infection (Fig. 56-1).

Another important consideration regarding classification is the distinction between reinfection and relapse. Reinfection with a new organism is very common. Relapse with the same organism, although less common, is very important because it usually implies either an ineffective therapy or a structural abnormality, such as a stone or other obstruction.

Epidemiology

Figure 56-2 outlines the age- and gender-related incidence of UTIs. At all ages, with the exception of the neonatal period, the incidence of UTI is greater in the female than in the male. In both males and females, the incidence increases with advanced age. Although the male has one early peak in the newborn period, the female has two peaks: one is at 3 to 6 years, and the other is at the onset of sexual activity. The actual incidence of infection as a function of age and gender is difficult to determine from the literature. Table 56-3 summarizes the available data.[12]

Pathophysiology

Host Factors

The establishment of clinical infection and its consequent injury to the urinary tract results from a complex interplay between host resistance and bacterial

Table 56-2 Criteria for Diagnosis of Urinary Tract Infections

Method of Collection	Colony Count (Pure Culture)	Probability of Infection
Suprapubic aspiration	Gram-negative bacilli: any number	>99%
	Gram-positive cocci: a few thousand	>99%
Catheterization	$>10^5$	95%
	10^4-10^5	Likely
	10^3-10^4	Suggestive
	$<10^3$	Unlikely
Clean voided (male)	$>10^5$	Likely
Clean voided (female)	3 specimens > 10^5	95%
	2 specimens > 10^5	90%
	1 specimen > 10^5	80%

Modified from Hellerstein S: Recurrent urinary tract infection in children. Pediatr Infect Dis 1:275, 1982.

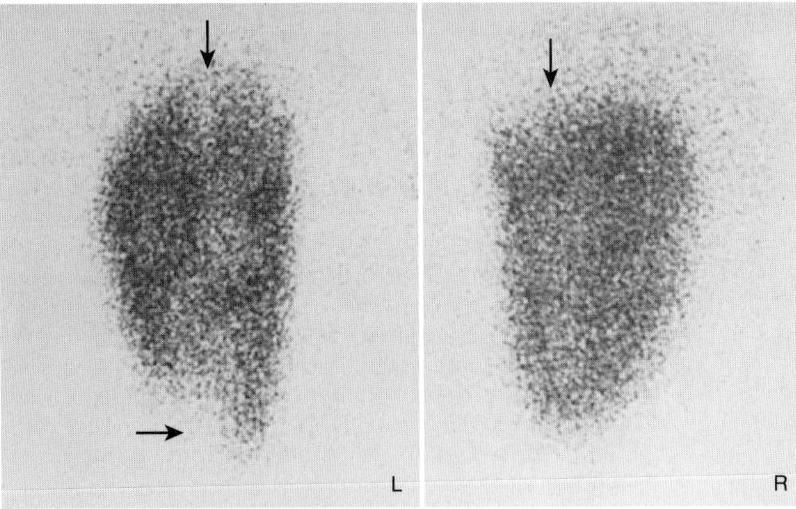

Figure 56-1. Technetium-99m dimercaptosuccinic acid (DMSA) scan. The magnified view of the left kidney (L), seen by using a pinhole collimator, demonstrates defects in both poles that extend deep into the renal parenchyma (*arrows*), suggestive of acute pyelonephritis. The right kidney (R) has an upper pole defect (*arrow*) that may represent either acute or chronic pyelonephritis. (Courtesy of Michael J. Gelfand, MD.)

virulence. As a general rule, UTI-causing organisms originate from the feces of their host. Conceptually, four levels of defense are identifiable: periurethral, bladder, ureterovesical junction, and renal papillae.[5] These concepts are illustrated in Figure 56-3.

Bacteria generally possess an ability to adhere to vaginal mucosal cells in order to readily establish infection.[21] The resultant periurethral colonization then allows replication and migration, which ultimately lead to transurethral invasion to the bladder. Healthy girls have low bacterial colonizations of the periurethral region. UTI-prone girls experience more heavy colonization, especially prior to a new episode of UTI. Furthermore, the cultivated organism from the introital region belongs to the same strain as that from the urine during the UTI that ensues. Periurethral bacterial colonization is correspondingly low in UTI patients after cessation of recurrent UTIs.[22] A similar mechanism may apply to bacterial adherence in the prepuce of males.[23] This may explain why 92% of male infants younger than 6 months old with a UTI are uncircumcised.[24]

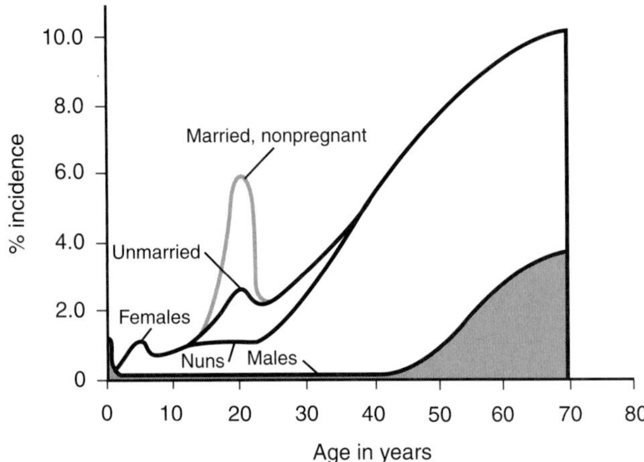

Figure 56-2. The age and gender distribution of urinary tract infection incidence. (From Devine CJ, Stecker JF: Urology in Practice. Boston, Little, Brown, 1978, p 444.)

Table 56-3 Incidence of Urinary Tract Infection as a Function of Age, Gender and Presence of Symptoms

	Symptomatic		Asymptomatic	
Age	*Male*	*Female*	*Male*	*Female*
Newborn	0.15%		1.0-1.4%*	
Preschool	0.7%	2.8%	0.2%	0.8%
School age			0.03%	1.0-2.0%

*2.4% to 3.4% in premature infants.

Data compiled from multiple sources by Hellerstein S: Recurrent urinary tract infections in children. Pediatr Infect Dis 1:271, 1982.

A number of bladder defense mechanisms help maintain sterile urine. The most critical is the act of regular and complete voiding. The healthy bladder is capable of eliminating 99% of instilled bacteria and leaves a small residual urine that minimizes the inoculum at the onset of the following cycle.[25] High intravesical pressure dynamics may also potentiate infection in children. In the absence of an elevated residual urine, uninhibited bladder contractions are associated with a high risk of recurrence of UTI, which is lessened by anticholinergic therapy.[26] Dysfunctional elimination syndrome with abnormal voiding habits and constipation can affect the development of UTI as well.[27] The acid pH of urine, as well as its osmolality, further discourages bacterial growth.[28] The uroepithelial cells of healthy individuals suppress bacterial growth and are capable of killing bacteria. The uroepithelial cells secrete a mucopolysaccharide substance that, upon coating the surface of the uroepithelium, provides an additional barrier to uroepithelial adherence.[25] Glycosaminoglycans are continuously shed and thus function to entrap and eliminate bacteria.

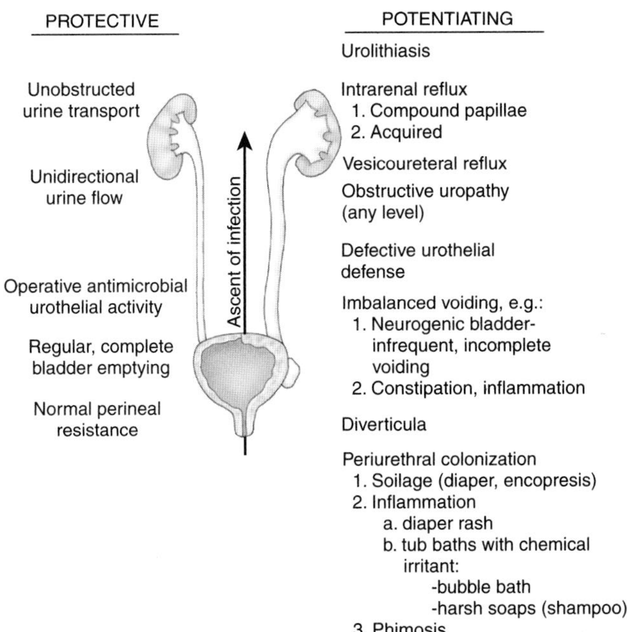

Figure 56-3. Host factors that protect the urinary tract from infection and abnormalities that potentiate the establishment of invasive bacterial infection.

Abnormalities of the ureterovesical junction and altered ureteral peristalsis may allow vesicoureteral reflux (VUR), which potentiates but is not always necessary for upper tract invasion. Distortion of the renal pyramids permits renal parenchymal invasion, which results in irreversible renal injury. The anatomy of the renal papillae usually prevents intrarenal reflux (Fig. 56-4). The papillary ducts commonly open onto the papillae with slit-like orifices that occlude with elevated intracalyceal pressure, preventing intrarenal reflux. The more circular duct orifices of compound papillae fail to accomplish this goal, allowing intrarenal reflux. The fact that compound papillae tend to occur in the upper and lower calyces and that intrarenal reflux in very young children may occur at a relatively low pressure may explain the observed polar distribution of scarring and predilection to scarring noted in these children.[5] Structural abnormalities that potentiate infection include phimosis, obstructive uropathy at any level, VUR, diverticula, urinary calculi or foreign bodies, and an abnormal renal papillary structure.

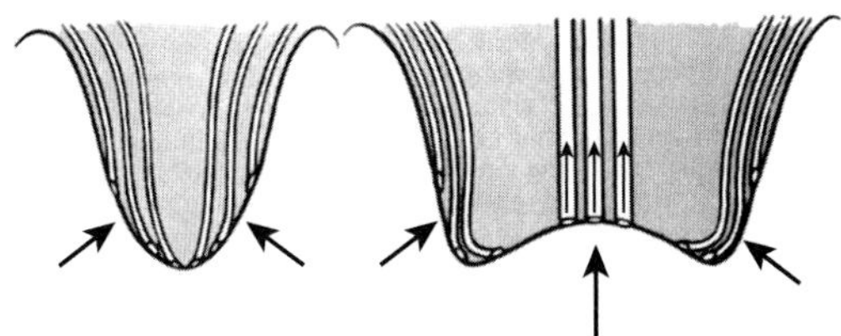

Figure 56-4. The normal oblique insertion of the collecting ducts onto the surface of simple papillae prevent intrarenal reflux (*left*). Collecting duct insertion onto the surface of compound papillae may allow intrarenal reflux (*right*). (From Ransley PG: Intrarenal reflux: Anatomic, dynamic and radiological studies. Urol Res 5:61, 1977.)

Table 56-4 Bacterial Factors Potentiating Infection

O antigens (lipopolysaccharides)
Primarily O_1, O_2, O_4, O_6, O_7, O_{11}, O_{18}, O_{35}, O_{75}
Responsible for systemic reactions (e.g., fever, shock)
K antigens
Primarily K_1, K_5
Adhesive properties
Low immunogenicity
H antigens (flagella)
Bacterial locomotion
Chemotaxis
Hemolysins (bacterial enzymes)
Tissue damage
Facilitates bacterial growth
Urease
Alkalinizes urine
Facilitates stone formation
P fimbriae—adherence
Mannose sensitive (MS)
Mannose resistant (MR)

Bacterial Factors

Several bacterial factors may potentiate urinary tract infection and are outlined in Table 56-4.[5,29] O antigens are lipopolysaccharides that are part of the cell wall. They are thought to be responsible for many of the systemic symptoms associated with infection. Of the more than 150 strains of *Escherichia coli* identified by O antigens, 9 are responsible for the majority of UTIs.

K antigens are also polysaccharides, and their presence on gram-negative bacterial capsules is considered to be an important virulence factor. They are thought to protect against phagocytosis, to inhibit the induction of a specific immune response, and to facilitate bacterial adhesion. Bacterial strains causing UTI exhibit considerably more K antigen than those isolated from the feces. Urease, a virulence factor especially prominent with *Proteus* species, allows the breakdown of urea to ammonium. This process alkalinizes the urine and facilitates stone formation. Such bacteria are generally incorporated into the stone structure, making eradication extremely difficult. Mannose-resistant pili are important adherence factors. They promote adherence to uroepithelial cells as well as renal epithelial cells. This factor appears to counter the normal cleansing action of urine flow and allows tissue invasion and bacterial proliferation. That these factors truly are associated with virulence is shown in Figure 56-5.[29]

Increasingly invasive urinary infections are associated with bacteria with a high incidence of virulence factors. Figure 56-6 demonstrates the pathophysiologic changes of renal injury that may occur in the absence of significant host factors. Colonization of the feces with a virulent organism allows periurethral colonization and, ultimately, bladder entry. Uroepithelial adherence promotes bacterial proliferation and tissue invasion. This series of events is facilitated by the presence of one or more host factors (see Fig. 56-3).

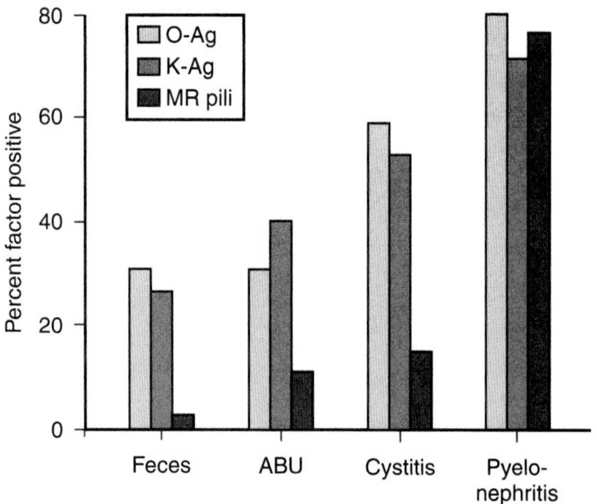

Figure 56-5. Presence of bacterial virulence factors as a function of the clinical setting. More-invasive infections are associated with a high incidence of virulence factors, implicating these factors in pathogenesis. MR, mannose resistant; Ag, antigen; ABU, asymptomatic bacteriuria. (From Mannhardt W, Schofer O, Schulte-Wisserman H: Pathogenic factors in recurrent urinary tract infection and renal scar formation in children. Eur J Pediatr 145:330, 1986.)

Investigation

Although many patients with UTI are not severely affected, the pediatric surgeon and urologist must be cognizant of several important facts. Urinary abnormalities can be found in approximately 50% of children up to the age of 12 years who present with UTI. VUR is found in up to 35% and obstructive lesions in 8%. Nonobstructive, nonrefluxing lesions are found in 7%.[30]

Also, although renal scars develop in about 13% of girls and 5% of boys with unspecified infection,[31] they develop in up to 43% of kidneys involved in acute pyelonephritis.[32] Pyelonephritic scarring is responsible for 11% of cases of childhood hypertension.[33,34] Although hypertension is most common with bilateral scarring, it is also seen with unilateral scarring.[35] Pyelonephritic scarring is also an important cause of end-stage renal failure in childhood and may require specific pretransplantation treatment, especially if associated with reflux.[36] Additionally, approximately 50% of patients will suffer from recurrent UTIs.[29]

Consequently, not only infants[37] but older children as well of either gender should be studied at the time of their initial infection.[38] Although controversial, we investigate children with UTI with initial screening ultrasonography and cyclic voiding cystography.[39] Males require contrast voiding cystourethrography (VCUG), and females are adequately evaluated by isotope VCUG that allows a lower radiation exposure to the ovaries.[40] The exception is the infant girl or the girl with suspected neurogenic bladder, ectopic ureter, or ureterocele by ultrasonography. In this case, a contrast VCUG is obtained. Radionuclide scanning using technetium-99m–labeled dimercaptosuccinic acid (^{99m}Tc-DMSA) is readily available and is used to diagnose acute pyelonephritis[41] and to detect renal scarring.[42]

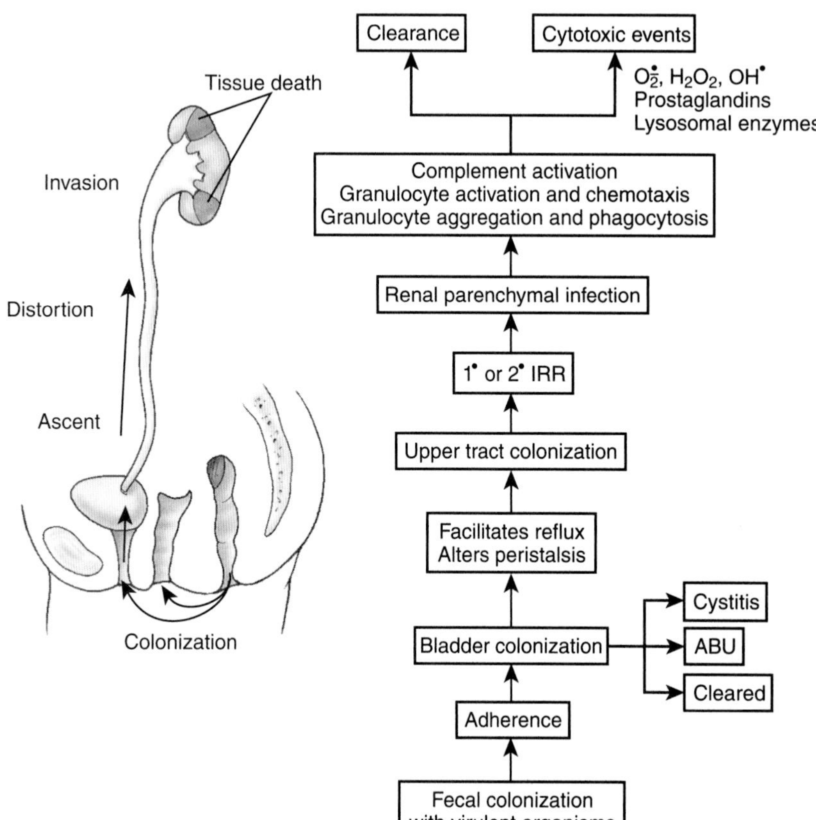

Figure 56-6. The pathogenesis of destructive infection is shown. The process is facilitated by, but does not require, defects in the host protective factors outlined in Figure 56-3. IRR, intrarenal reflux; ABU, asymptomatic bacteriuria.

Treatment

The treatment of an acute UTI is dependent on the clinical presentation. Patients with pyelonephritis should be treated immediately and aggressively. Prompt, effective treatment is the most important factor in preventing permanent renal injury.[43] We prefer to initiate therapy with intravenous ampicillin and an aminoglycoside after obtaining a reliable urine culture. Further therapy is dictated by the culture and sensitivity findings. Patients may require admission to the hospital initially. Once afebrile for 24 to 48 hours, patients with otherwise uncomplicated infections with sensitive organisms may complete a 7- to 14-day course with oral antibiotics.[44] Patients with resistant organisms or those with obstructions may finish the course with nursing-supervised home administration of intravenous antibiotics. Patients with obstruction or abscess who do not become afebrile undergo drainage percutaneously or, rarely, operatively.

Short treatment courses appear to be insufficient for treatment of childhood UTI.[45] Therefore, we prefer a 7- to 10-day course dictated by culture and sensitivity results.[46] Urinary retention due to a fear of voiding or dysuria is managed with phenazopyridine and hydration and allowing the child to void while sitting in a tub of warm water.

Patients who have recurrent UTIs or those who are managed nonoperatively for VUR require long-term suppressive antibiotics. The urothelial injury from recurrent UTIs takes several months to fully recover. As a result, irritative voiding symptoms, such as dysuria, incontinence, and frequency, may persist despite the finding of sterile urine. A propensity for recurrent UTI may also be present. Such patients generally require a minimum of 4 to 6 months of antibiotic suppressive therapy to break the cycle. Table 56-5 outlines the characteristics of the drugs we most commonly employ for suppression.

VESICOURETERAL REFLUX

VUR refers to the retrograde passage of urine from the bladder into the ureter. Although VUR was first observed in the late 1800s, its clinical importance has only been recognized in the past 5 decades. Hutch's studies, reported in 1952, demonstrated the pathophysiologic changes of VUR in the paraplegic patient. This report and the observations of Hodson in 1959, regarding the association between VUR, UTI, and pyelonephritic scarring, set the stage for the modern era of reflux management.

Although most commonly diagnosed during the evaluation of the pediatric patient with UTI, VUR may also be diagnosed during evaluation of the patient with hypertension, proteinuria, voiding dysfunction, or chronic renal insufficiency or during the evaluation of a sibling with VUR.

Pathophysiology

Figure 56-7 depicts the various anatomic components of the competent ureterovesical junction (UVJ) as well as the abnormalities most often implicated in the genesis of VUR. The normal UVJ is characterized by an oblique entry of the ureter into the bladder and a length of submucosal ureter providing a high ratio of tunnel length to ureteral diameter. This anatomic configuration provides a predominantly passive valve mechanism.[47,48]

As the bladder fills and the intravesical pressure rises, the resultant bladder wall tension is applied to the

Table 56-5 Characteristics of Commonly Used Urosuppressive Antibiotics

Drug	Therapeutic Dose	Suppressive Dose	How Supplied	Comments
Nitrofurantoin	2 mg/kg PO qid	1 mg/kg PO qd	Suspension (5 mg/mL) Capsule (25, 50 mg)	Avoid in patients < 1 mo of age Not effective if CrCl < 40 mL/min Nausea common with suspension; sprinkling macrocrystals may avoid this
Trimethoprim-sulfamethoxazole	4 mg/kg trimethoprim + 20 mg/kg sulfamethoxazole PO bid	2 mg/kg trimethoprim + 10 mg/kg sulfamethoxazole PO qd	Suspension (8 mg trimethoprim + 40 mg sulfamethoxazole per mL Tablet (80 mg trimethoprim, 400 mg sulfamethoxazole)	Avoid in patients <1 mo of age Contraindicated with hyperbilirubinemia May cause blood dyscrasias and Stevens-Johnson syndrome
Trimethoprim (Primsol)	5 mg/kg PO bid	2 mg PO qd	Oral solution 50 mg/5 mL	Avoid in patients < 2 mo of age
Amoxicillin	10 mg/kg PO tid	10 mg/kg PO qd	Suspension (25, 50 mg/mL) Drops (50 mg/mL)	Good alternative for neonates
Cephalexin	25 mg/kg PO bid	25 mg/kg qd	Suspension 125 mg/5 mL or 250 mg/5 mL	Alternative for neonates

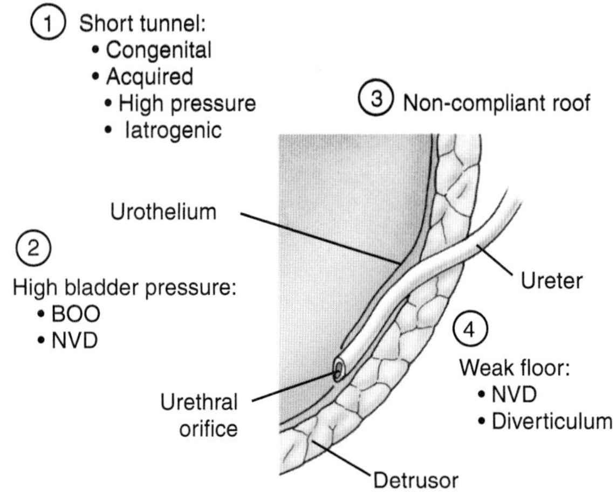

Figure 56-7. Components of the competent ureterovesical junction. Those abnormalities most often implicated in the etiology of vesicoureteral reflux are outlined. BOO, bladder outlet obstruction; NVD, neurovesical dysfunction.

roof of the ureteral tunnel. The result is a compression of the ureter, which closes this structure to the retrograde passage of urine. Intermittent increases in bladder pressure, such as the act of voiding, upright posture, activity, and coughing, are met with an equal and immediate increase in resistance to retrograde urine flow. This effect is supplemented by the active effects of ureterotrigonal muscle contraction and ureteral peristalsis.[48,49]

Marginal tunnels can be made to reflux during infection owing to UVJ distortion, loss of compliance of the valve roof, and intravesical hypertension. Excessively high intravesical pressure as with neurovesical dysfunction (NVD) or bladder outlet obstruction (BOO) may also potentiate reflux, as may a neurogenically or structurally (e.g., diverticulum or ureterocele) weak detrusor floor. Because the submucosal ureter tends to lengthen with age, the ratio of tunnel length to ureteral diameter increases and the propensity for reflux may disappear.[47,48]

Of critical importance is the concept of intrarenal reflux (IRR), which has been demonstrated clinically[50] and experimentally.[51] The usually oblique entry of the papillary ducts onto the surface of simple papillae inhibits IRR. In contrast, the papillary duct entrance onto compound papillae facilitates IRR (see Fig. 56-4). The critical pressure for IRR is considered to be about 35 mm Hg in compound papillae.[51,52]

Experimentally, this same pressure may cause scar formation in the absence of infection.[51,53,54] When occurring intravesically, this pressure has been associated with an increased risk of renal deterioration. Higher pressure is thought to be necessary to induce IRR in simple papillae.

The combination of infection and IRR is particularly devastating. Focal scarring appears to be explained by the different susceptibility of renal papillae to IRR. The polar distribution of compound papillae corresponds closely to the predominant occurrence of renal scarring in the upper and lower poles of the kidney.

Classification

Many attempts at classification have been advanced. Reflux has been described as low pressure (occurring during the filling phase of the VCUG) or high pressure (occurring only during voiding). Reflux due to a congenitally deficient UVJ is referred to as *primary* reflux, whereas reflux due to a BOO and neurogenic bladder is referred to as *secondary* reflux. Further classification includes simple reflux and complex reflux. Complex reflux would include the refluxing megaureter, the refluxing duplicated ureter, the refluxing ureter associated with a diverticulum or ureterocele, and the occasional refluxing ureter associated with ipsilateral ureteropelvic or ureterovesical obstruction. The most clinically pertinent classification systems, however, have attempted to quantitate the degree of reflux. At the present time, VUR is graded according to the international classification system depicted in Figure 56-8.[55] This classification system is based not only on the proximal extent of retrograde urine flow and ureteral and pelvic dilatation but also on the resultant anatomy of the calyceal fornices.

Grade I VUR refers to the visualization of a nondilated ureter only, whereas grade II VUR refers to visualization of a nondilated renal pelvis and calyceal system in addition to the ureter. Grade III reflux involves mild to moderate dilatation or ureteral tortuosity with mild to moderate dilatation of the renal pelvis and calyces. The fornices, however, remain sharp or only minimally blunted. Once the forniceal angle is completely blunted, grade IV reflux has developed. Papillary impressions in the majority of calyces can still be appreciated. Loss of the papillary impressions along with increased dilatation and tortuosity is referred to as grade V reflux.

Epidemiology

The incidence of VUR in otherwise normal children has been estimated to be approximately 1%.[56] Also apparent from these data is the fact that the incidence of VUR is also small in neonates and infants.

A much higher incidence of VUR (between 30% to 40%) is reported in patients undergoing evaluation for UTI.[57-59] This incidence rises with decreasing age.[60]

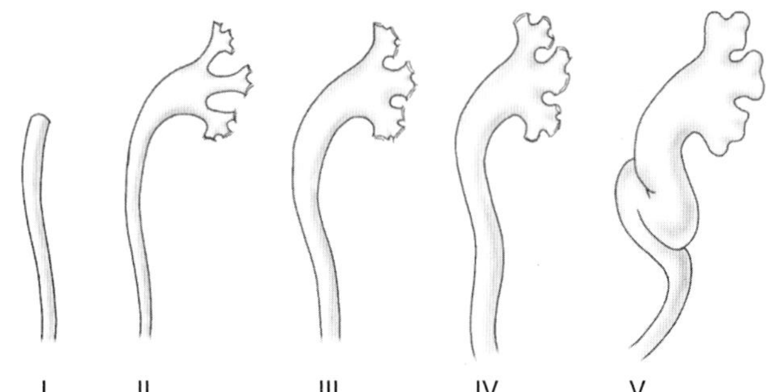

Figure 56-8. The international grading system for vesicoureteral reflux. See text for description. (From The International Reflux Committee: Medical versus surgical treatment of primary vesicoureteral reflux. Pediatrics 67:396, 1987.)

Thus, the infant who is most vulnerable to the combination of UTI and VUR is precisely the pediatric patient in whom this combination is most likely to occur.

Although the majority of reflux patients are female, a few important characteristics of males with VUR require consideration. Although males account for approximately 14% of patients with VUR,[61] an increased incidence of VUR (30%) is found in those males presenting with UTI.[58] Boys with VUR tend to present at a relatively young age (25% if younger than 3 months), and younger children tend to have the most severe degrees of reflux.[61]

Multiple studies have documented a significant risk of VUR in family members of children with reflux. The reported risk of sibling reflux ranges from 27% to 34%,[62-64] whereas as many as 66% of offspring of women with reflux also have VUR.[65] As a result of these studies, it has been suggested that siblings, especially those younger than 2 years of age, undergo screening investigation.

A particularly important subset of patients with reflux includes those who have secondary reflux. Most have NVD or BOO as their primary disease. Many patients, however, have reflux not because of increased bladder pressure alone but rather because UVJ problems appear to be part of the spectrum of their congenital deformity. Examples include imperforate anus,[66] ureterocele,[67] and bladder exstrophy. Although a significant incidence of NVD exists in patients with imperforate anus, this is not a prerequisite for VUR.[68] The diagnosis of VUR in imperforate anus thus assumes a critical importance to the pediatric surgeon. Not only may the association of NVD potentiate an increased severity of reflux and the development of infection, the presence of a rectourethral or rectovesical fistula provides the opportunity for severe urinary contamination. Consequently, we believe that the patient with a rectovesical or rectourethral fistula should be managed with a completely diverting colostomy. Although many infants with posterior urethral valves have reflux due to or exacerbated by high intravesical pressure, the incidence of VUR in these patients is only approximately 50%. Many have congenitally abnormal ureteral insertions into the bladder.[69]

In addition to these structural associations, important functional problems exist as well, including florid NVD, as seen in myelodysplasia,[70] and a variety of more subtle voiding disturbances.[71-73] A particularly important subset of VUR patients are those who have uninhibited detrusor contractions (UDCs). There are three important components needed for successful toilet training. Growth in bladder volume, development of volitional control over the striated muscle sphincter, and control over the smooth muscle in the bladder are required for the infantile bladder, which empties as a simple spinal reflex, to mature. Many children with reflux and recurrent UTI have UDCs. Such involuntary or uninhibited bladder contractions are not caused by neurologic disease. Intense voluntary constriction of the striated sphincter occurs in an attempt to ensure continence and results in excessively high intravesical pressures. Pressures exceeding 150 cm H_2O have been seen with resultant intravesical distortions, such as diverticula, saccules, trabeculations, and abnormal ureteral orifices.[74] Reflux occurred in almost half of the children studied with UDC and UTI. Abnormal ureteral orifices were seen in 30% of children without reflux.

All patients with VUR must be screened for frequency, urgency, and incontinence, all of which suggest UDCs. Vincent's curtsy, a squatting maneuver spontaneously employed to prevent incontinence, is particularly suggestive.[73] That these UDCs may cause reflux is suggested by an enhanced resolution of reflux with anticholinergic drug therapy. Equally important is the potential for UDCs to cause a false-negative cystogram. During the performance of a VCUG, the child is generally encouraged to void when the urgency to do so occurs. In the presence of UDCs, voiding may occur prematurely, and VUR, which might otherwise occur under conditions of volitional detrusor-sphincter dyssynergia, may be masked.

Diagnostic Evaluation

The diagnosis of VUR is made by a cyclic VCUG, with either contrast medium or isotope.[75,76] Great care is taken to avoid technical factors that may themselves produce or enhance reflux. Body temperature contrast material, which is not excessively concentrated, is instilled into the bladder through a small catheter by gravity flow of modest pressure in a nonanesthetized child.

Imaging of the upper tracts is extremely important and may be accomplished by ultrasonography and/or isotope renography. All may detect scarring, but isotope renography is particularly sensitive in our experience. Ultrasonography is helpful in quantitating renal growth or atrophy.

Patients with frequency, urgency, incontinence, and Vincent's curtsy should be considered strongly for urodynamic studies. The presence of UDCs or detrusor-sphincter dyssynergia should be resolved before consideration is given to antireflux surgery.

Natural History

The natural history of VUR is extremely variable, from spontaneous resolution to clinically silent scar formation to hypertension and end-stage renal failure. Numerous factors may contribute to the potential for resolution, including the patient's age, the grade of reflux, the appearance of the ureteral orifice, the length of the ureteral submucosal tunnel, and the intravesical dynamics. The American Urological Association (AUA) Pediatric Vesicoureteral Reflux Guidelines Panel analyzed 26 reports, comprising 1987 patients with conservative follow-up, to estimate the probability of reflux resolution (Fig. 56-9).[77] In general, a lower reflux grade correlated with a better chance of spontaneous resolution.

Younger children are thought to have better prognoses for resolution of reflux. This tendency for resolution may be due to the trigonal growth, but the

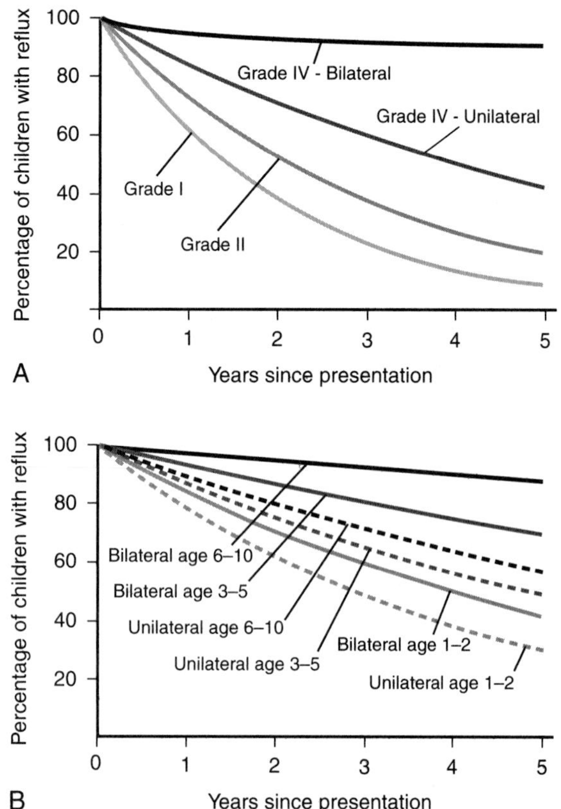

Figure 56-9. A, Percentage chance of reflux persistence, grades I, II, and IV, for 1 to 5 years after presentation. B, Percentage chance of reflux persistence by age at presentation, grade III, for 1 to 5 years after presentation. (From Elder JS, Peters CA, Arant BS, et al: Report on the Management of Primary Vesicoureteral Reflux in Children. Baltimore, American Urological Association, 1997.)

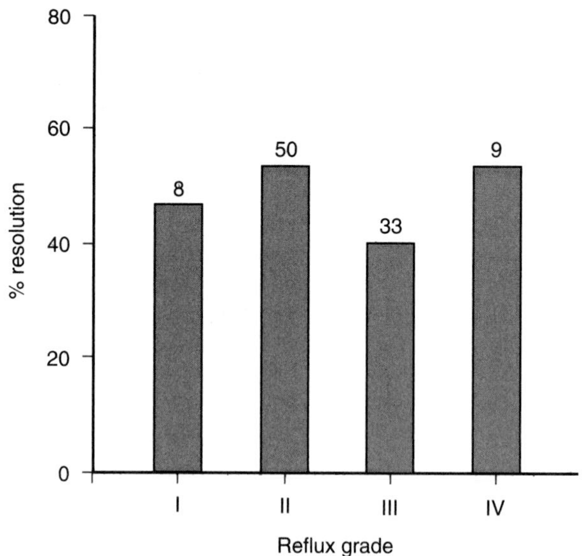

Figure 56-10. The rate of spontaneous resolution of secondary vesicoureteral reflux as a function of reflux grade. (From Cohen RA, Roston MG, Belman AB, et al: Renal scarring and vesicoureteral reflux in children with myelodysplasia. J Urol 144:541, 1990.)

diminishing prominence of UDCs with age is also important. Spontaneous resolution is relatively independent of grade in secondary reflux, implicating management of the primary bladder dysfunction as the primary prognostic variable (Fig. 56-10).[78]

Renal injury due to VUR may take the form of focal scarring, generalized scarring with atrophy, and failure of renal growth.[79] As a result, kidneys drained by refluxing ureters should be observed not only for scarring but also for renal growth.[80] Reflux-induced renal injury is usually a result of the association of VUR with UTI.[81] It is generally considered that such injury is most likely in children younger than the age of 2 years.[60] It is now clear, however, that the risk of renal injury from VUR extends well beyond this age.[59,81-83] Reflux appears capable of causing renal injury in the absence of UTI, because of the pressure effects from NVD and BOO. The ability of high intravesical pressure, when associated with VUR, to cause renal injury has been confirmed experimentally.[84]

Infants have been seen, however, with significant renal injury in the absence of BOO, NVD, and UTI.[85] The ureteral bud theory states that VUR associated with displacement of the ureteral orifice is associated with anomalies of renal differentiation.[86] Such ureters probably do not arise from the appropriate segment of wolffian duct and consequently make ectopic contact with the nephrogenic cord, resulting in abnormal renal development. Although such a mechanism may be present in some patients, it is now clear that congenital VUR-associated renal injury in the absence of BOO, NVD, and UTI may occur in the presence of a normally positioned ureteral orifice.[87] This finding implies that in-utero VUR may injure the developing kidney.

In a longitudinal study of 923 children, high-pressure bladder dynamics, severity of reflux, and frequency of UTIs were the chief contributing factors in the development of new scars or the worsening of old scars.[83]

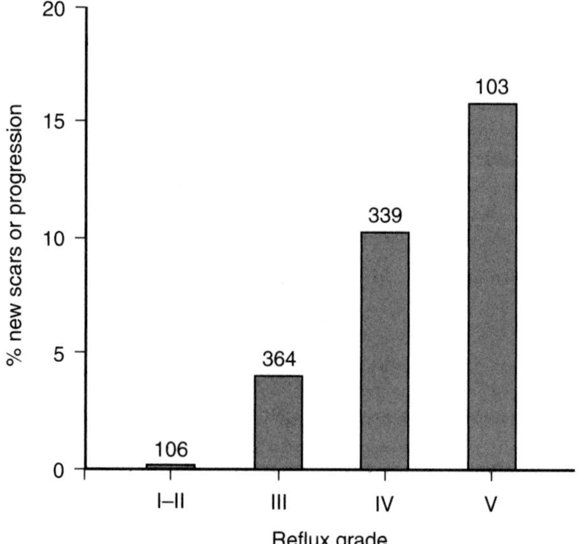

Figure 56-11. The risk of development of new scars or progression of old scars increases with increasing grades of vesicoureteral reflux. The number of ureters in each grade is indicated numerically.[83]

Children with low-grade VUR were relatively unlikely to develop progressive renal injury as compared with those children with grades IV and V reflux (Fig. 56-11). A similar relationship is seen in pediatric patients with secondary reflux (Fig. 56-12). When monitoring such children for progression of renal injury as an indicator of success of a therapeutic regimen, one must be aware that radiographic evidence of new renal injury may take up to 8 months to manifest.

Beyond the silent progression of renal scarring lies a spectrum of symptomatic nephropathy, most notably renal parenchymal hypertension and end-stage renal disease. The significance and predominance of reflux nephropathy as a cause of renal parenchymal hypertension has been reviewed.[88] Thirty to 65 percent of childhood hypertension is associated with reflux nephropathy. Reflux nephropathy is an important cause of end-stage renal failure in children and adults.[89-91] Many patients so affected will not have had recognized prior infection or will have the first recognized infection at or near the time of diagnosis of end-stage renal disease.[89] Because histologic evidence of chronic pyelonephritis is found, preceding infection is likely, underscoring the silent progressive nature of reflux nephropathy and the need for meticulous long-term follow-up of children with VUR. Much data exist to suggest that glomerular lesions play an important role in the progression of reflux nephropathy. There is a clear association between reflux nephropathy, "heavy" proteinuria, and glomerular lesions that resemble focal segmental glomerulosclerosis.[92] Although the mechanisms of this disease remain uncertain, immunologic injury, macromolecular trapping with mesangial injury, vascular alterations with hypertension, and glomerular hyperfiltration have been implicated. The latter theory of glomerular hyperfiltration is presently favored.

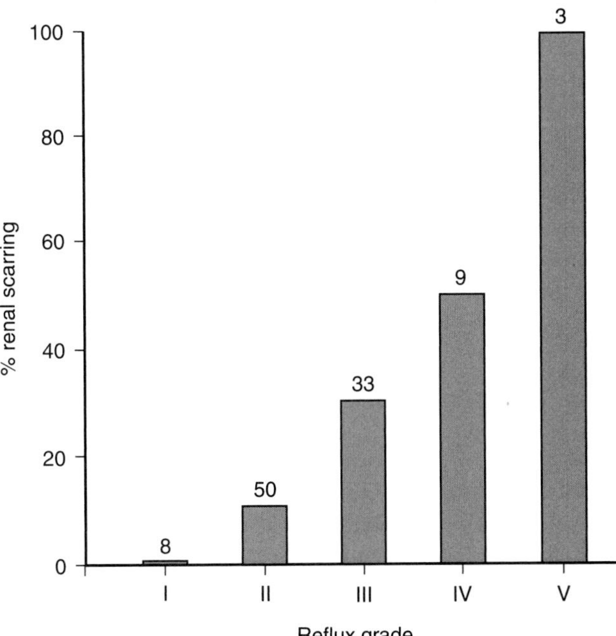

Figure 56-12. The prevalence of renal scarring as a function of reflux grade in patients with secondary reflux. Risk of renal scarring increases with increasing grades of reflux. The number of ureters in each grade is indicated numerically.[83]

Treatment

Nonoperative management of VUR (Table 56-6) is successful in the majority of patients. Such management may be considered in four stages: (1) diagnostic evaluation, (2) avoidance of infection, (3) voiding dysfunction treatment, and (4) surveillance. Diagnostic evaluation has been previously reviewed. However, it

Table 56-6 General Guidelines for the Nonoperative Management of Vesicoureteral Reflux

Treatment
Hydration
Hygiene
Perineal hygiene
Avoid:
Harsh soaps during tub baths
Bubble baths
Shampoos
Bowel management
Avoid constipation
Treat encopresis
Suppressive antibiotics
Observation without antibiotics
Anticholinergics, spasmolytics
Surveillance
Urine culture
Monthly for 3 mo after last UTI
Thereafter, every 2 to 3 mo
Renal imaging every 6 to 12 mo
Renal size (ultrasound, IVU)
Focal scarring (renal scan, IVU)
Voiding cystourethrography (yearly)
Radiographic VCUG
Initial (male, female suspected NVD)
Follow-up (NVD)
Isotope VCUG
Routine surveillance
Record growth yearly (height, weight)
Blood pressure
Routine (yearly)
Renal scarring (quarterly)
Renal function tests
BUN, creatinine (yearly if bilateral RN)
GFR estimated (yearly if azotemic)
$\frac{\text{height (cm)} \times 0.55}{\text{serum creatinine}} = \text{GFR (mL/min/1.73 m}^2\text{)}$
Maximum urine osmolality (yearly if bilateral RN)
Cystoscopy
Done at time of antireflux surgery; otherwise rarely necessary
Urodynamic evaluation
History of voiding dysfunction

BUN, blood urea nitrogen: GFR, glomerular filtration rate: IVU, intravenous urogram; NVD, neurovesical dysfunction; RN, reflux nephropathy; UTI, urinary tract infection; VCUG, voiding cystourethrogram.

is important to stress that evaluation and treatment of voiding dysfunction and BOO are imperative. Patients with problematic uninhibited detrusor contraction should undergo suppression therapy. We employ oxybutynin in the majority of these pediatric patients. NVD with retentive characteristics may require intermittent catheterization. Good hydration, perineal hygiene, and bowel management are crucial and apply to all patients. With the exception of the older boy with low-grade reflux, most children require suppression antibiotics (see Table 56-5). Although antibiotics are generally well tolerated, the long-term implications of chronic suppression remain incompletely investigated.

Once a nonoperative regimen is selected, the patient is committed to long-term, strict surveillance. Renal imaging is performed every 6 to 12 months, depending on the age at diagnosis and the stability of the disease. Attention is directed at both renal growth and focal scarring. Voiding cystourethrography is generally performed yearly. The child's growth, renal function, and blood pressure are monitored. The role of urodynamics has been previously outlined. Cystoscopy is rarely necessary except at the time of antireflux surgery when it is done to exclude urothelial inflammation and to confirm the position and number of ureteral orifices.

Although the actual decision to perform antireflux surgery must be carefully individualized, we feel the absolute indications for surgical correction of VUR are (1) progressive renal injury, (2) documented failure of renal growth, (3) breakthrough pyelonephritis, and (4) intolerance or noncompliance with antibiotic suppression. Other relative indications for surgical correction of VUR are grade IV-V reflux, pubertal age, and failure to respond to 4 to 5 years of suppression therapy.

The AUA Pediatric Vesicoureteral Reflux Guidelines Panel published their recommendations for management of VUR in children (Table 56-7).[77] There is still no consensus on the management of VUR in patients aged 10 or older or on the length of time that the clinician should wait before recommending surgery. The actual decision must be carefully individualized.

The established surgical principles of successful ureteral reimplantation include (1) adequate ureteral exposure and mobilization, (2) meticulous preservation of the blood supply, and (3) creation of a valvular mechanism whose submucosal tunnel length to ureteral diameter ratio exceeds 4:1. These goals can be attained by a variety of procedures, as shown in Figure 56-13.

Important differences exist between these operative procedures. Variables include (1) presence or absence

Table 56-7 AUA Recommendations for Treatment of Vesicoureteral Reflux[77]

Clinical Presentation (Age at Presentation)		Treatment Recommendations for Children without Scarring at Diagnosis					
		Initial (Antibiotic Prophylaxis or Open Surgical Repair)			Follow-up[*] (Continued Antibiotic Prophylaxis, Cystography, or Open Surgical Repair)		
VUR Grade Laterality	*Age (Yr)*	*Guideline*	*Preferred Option*	*Reasonable Alternative*	*Guideline*	*Preferred Option*	*No Consensus*[†]
I-II Unilateral or bilateral	<1	Antibiotic prophylaxis					Boys and girls
	1-5	Antibiotic prophylaxis					Boys and girls
	6-10	Antibiotic prophylaxis					Boys and girls
III-IV Unilateral or bilateral	<1	Antibiotic prophylaxis			Bilateral: Surgery if persistent	Unilateral: Surgery if persistent	
	1-5	Unilateral: Antibiotic prophylaxis	Bilateral: Antibiotic prophylaxis			Surgery if persistent	
	6-10		Unilateral: Antibiotic prophylaxis	Bilateral: Antibiotic prophylaxis			
			Bilateral: Surgery			Surgery if persistent	
V Unilateral or bilateral	<1		Antibiotic prophylaxis		Surgery if persistent		
	1-5		Bilateral: Surgery	Bilateral: Antibiotic prophylaxis	Surgery if persistent		
			Unilateral: Antibiotic prophylaxis	Unilateral: Surgery			
	6-10	Surgery					

(Continued)

Table 56-7 AUA Recommendations for Treatment of Vesicoureteral Reflux[77]—*Cont'd)*

Treatment Recommendations for Children with Scarring at Diagnosis							
Clinical Presentation (Age at Presentation)		Initial (Antibiotic Prophylaxis or Open Surgical Repair)			Follow-up* (Continued Antibiotic Prophylaxis, Cystography, or Open Surgical Repair)		
VUR Grade Laterality	*Age (Yr)*	*Guideline*	*Preferred Option*	*Reasonable Alternative*	*Guideline*	*Preferred Option*	*No Consensus*†
I-II Unilateral or bilateral	<1	Antibiotic prophylaxis					Boys and girls
	1-5	Antibiotic prophylaxis					Boys and girls
	6-10	Antibiotic prophylaxis					Boys and girls
III-IV Unilateral	<1	Antibiotic prophylaxis			Girls: Surgery if persistent	Boys: Surgery if persistent	
	1-5	Antibiotic prophylaxis			Girls: Surgery if persistent	Boys: Surgery if persistent	
	6-10		Antibiotic prophylaxis		Surgery if persistent		
III-IV Bilateral	<1	Antibiotic prophylaxis			Surgery if persistent		
	1-5		Antibiotic prophylaxis	Surgery	Surgery if persistent		
	6-10	Surgery					
V Unilateral or bilateral	<1		Antibiotic prophylaxis	Surgery	Surgery if persistent		
	1-5	Bilateral: Surgery	Unilateral: Surgery			Surgery if persistent	
	6-10	Surgery					

Recommendations were derived from a survey of preferred treatment options for 36 clinical categories of children with vesicoureteral reflux (VUR). The recommendations are classified as follows:

Guidelines, Treatments selected by eight or nine panel members, given the strongest recommendation language.

Preferred options, Treatments selected by five to seven of nine panel members.

Reasonable alternative, Treatments selected by three to four of nine panel members.

No consensus, Treatments selected by no more than two of nine panel members.

*For patients with persistent uncomplicated reflux after extended treatment with continuous antibiotic therapy.

†No consensus was reached regarding the role of continued antibiotic prophylaxis, cystography, or surgical treatment.

From American Urological Association: Report on the Management of Primary Vesicoureteral Reflux in Children. Baltimore, American Urological Association Pediatric Vesicoureteral Reflux Clinical Guidelines Panel, 1997.

of ureteral anastomosis, (2) need for detrusor closure, (3) transgression of urothelium, and (4) whether the neohiatus is fashioned by an appropriately sized detrusor incision or by closing the detrusor muscle around the ureter.

Performance of a ureteral anastomosis increases the risk of postoperative obstruction, whereas the need for detrusor closure increases the risk of diverticular development. Table 56-8 outlines the specific advantages and disadvantages of some of the procedures. Three of the most commonly employed operations for primary VUR are diagrammed in Figures 56-14 through 56-16.

In general, excellent results are attained with the majority of open procedures. A review of 86 reports, including 6472 patients (8563 ureters), found overall operative success to be 96%.[77] Resolution of the reflux was achieved in 99% with grade I, 99.1% with grade II, 98.3% with grade III, 98.5% with grade IV, and 80.7% with grade V.

We prefer the extravesical detrusorrhaphy approach.[93-95] Because the lumen of the bladder is not entered, there is minimal postoperative hematuria, few bladder spasms, and a short postoperative hospitalization. The absence of a ureteral anastomosis decreases the risk of postoperative obstruction. No ureteral stents, suprapubic tubes, or drains are utilized. The bladder catheter is removed on the first day after unilateral correction and the second day after a bilateral procedure. The extravesical approach for bilateral ureteral reimplantation has been questioned because of a reportedly high incidence of postoperative urinary retention.[96] In our experience with a large group of patients, we found acceptable rates of postoperative urinary retention (4%), which is transient and has minimal morbidity.[97] The use of extravesical detrusorrhaphy has been successfully expanded to include megaureter repair,[94] reimplantation of the ureters associated with paraureteral Hutch diverticula,[98] as well as

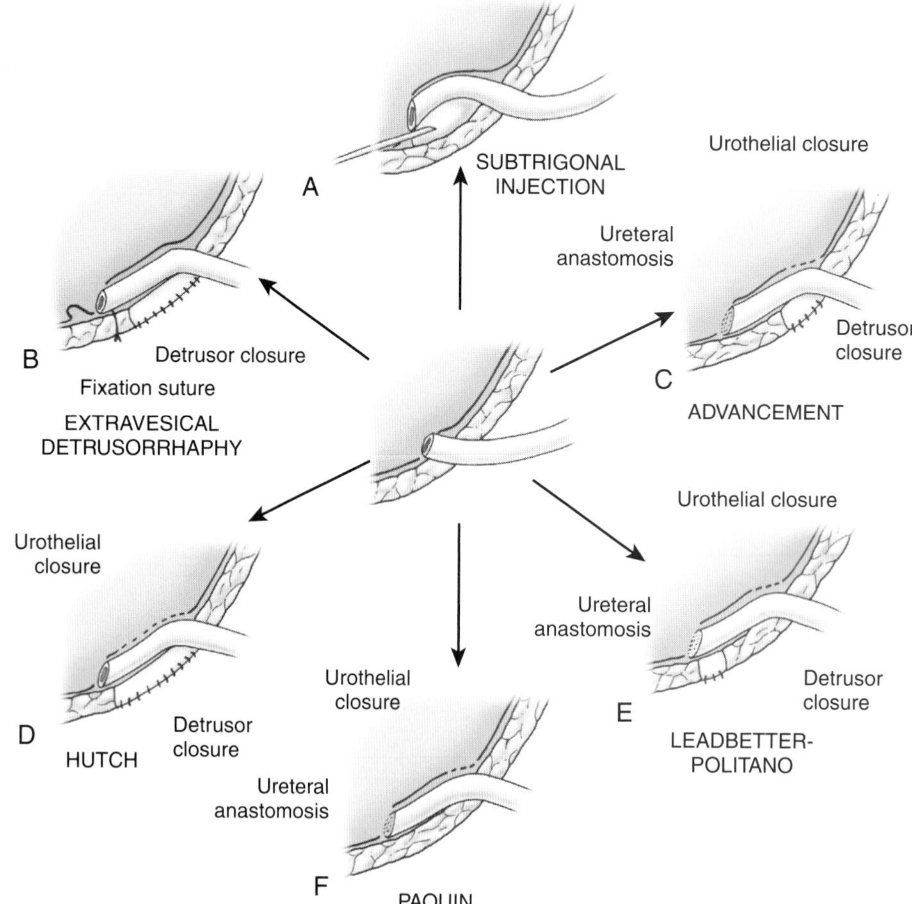

Figure 56-13. Conceptual comparison of techniques to correct reflux. A common theme is the achievement of a long length of intravesical ureter based on a strong detrusor floor and covered with compressible urothelium.

Table 56-8 Specific Advantages and Disadvantages of Commonly Performed Antireflux Procedures

Procedure	Advantages	Disadvantages
Subtrigonal injection	Endoscopic procedure	Material injected: Teflon: migration, granuloma formation Collagen: uncertain durability
Extravesical detrusorrhaphy	Bladder never opened No hematuria No ureteral anastomosis Minimal bladder spasms Endoscopically accessible ureteral orifices	
Advancement Cohen (transtrigonal) Glenn-Anderson	Avoids complications of neohiatus formation in Leadbetter-Politano reimplantation	Transtrigonal: difficult to access ureter endoscopically Glenn-Anderson: limited length of tunnel achievable
Hutch	No ureteral anastomosis Good alternative with large associated congenital diverticulum	
Leadbetter-Politano	Excellent ureteral tunnel dimensions with endoscopically accessible ureteral orifices	Risk of ureteral obstruction Risk of sigmoid colon injury with left reimplantation
Paquin	Versatility, extremely useful during complex reconstructive procedures	

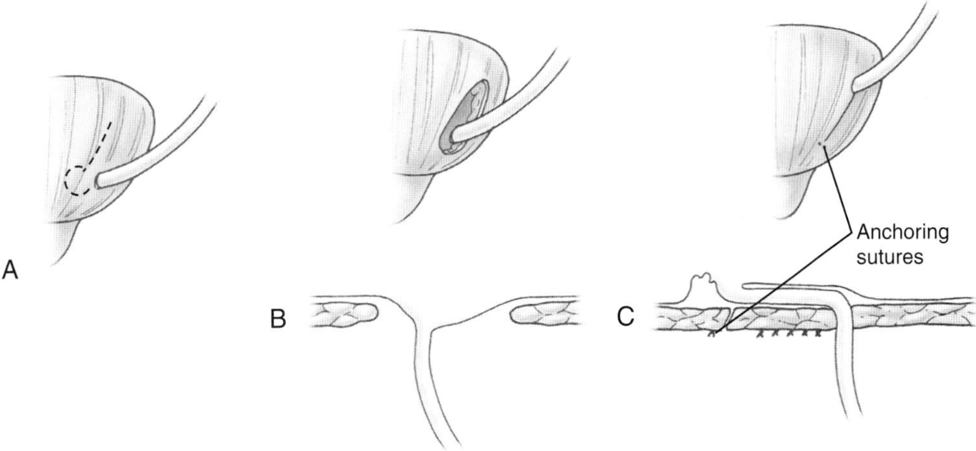

Figure 56-14. The extravesical detrusorrhaphy antireflux technique conceptually viewed from behind the bladder. **A,** The detrusor is incised. **B,** The dissection is continued until the plane between urothelium and muscle has been developed. **C,** The ureter is advanced and fixed into position with anchoring sutures. The detrusor is closed.

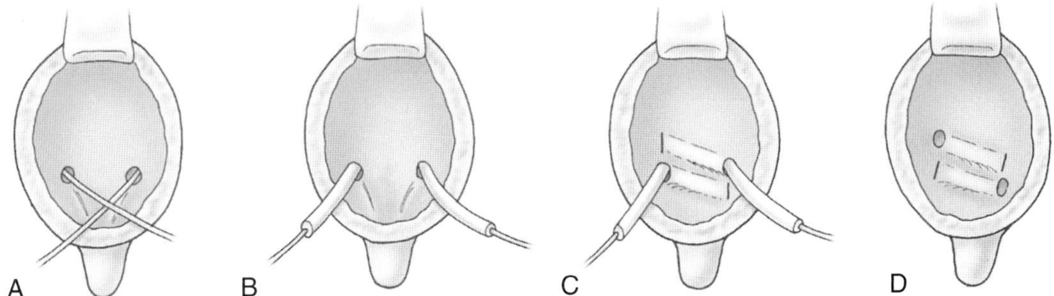

Figure 56-15. The Cohen cross-trigonal ureteral reimplantation. **A,** The ureter is intubated and the mucosa is incised circumferentially around the ureteral orifice. **B,** The ureters are dissected from the muscular attachments and mobilized until free within the retroperitoneum. **C,** Cross-trigonal tunnels are created by scissor dissection. **D,** The ureteral anastomoses are completed.

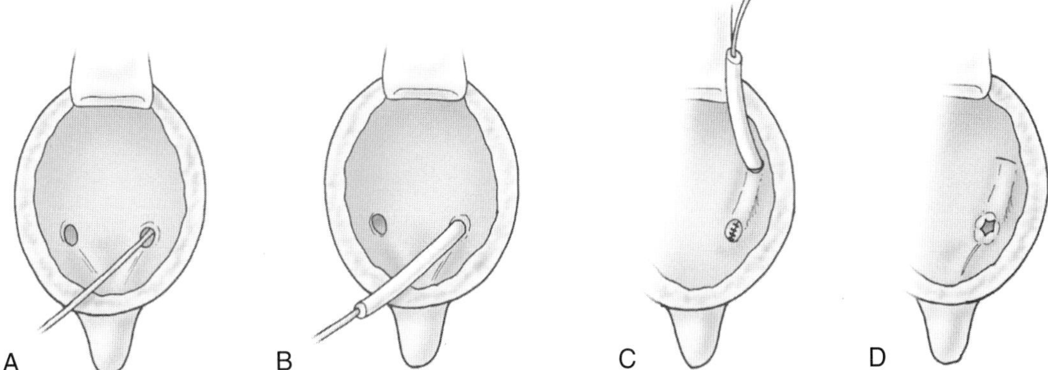

Figure 56-16. The Leadbetter-Politano ureteral reimplantation. **A,** The ureter is intubated. **B,** The ureter is mobilized. The hiatus is dilated, and the retroperitoneal ureter is mobilized. Under direct vision the peritoneum is reflected from the outer surface of the bladder. **C,** The neohiatus is created, and the ureter is internalized into the bladder. The tunnel is created by scissor dissection, and the original hiatus is closed. **D,** The ureteral anastomosis is completed.

correction of VUR associated with duplicated collecting systems.[99] The four major principles of a successful extravesical detrusorrhaphy are (1) complete encirclement and mobilization of the ureter, (2) distal fixation of the ureter with long acting absorbable sutures, (3) wide mobilization of the muscular flaps to enable firm approximation of the detrusor over the ureter, and (4) development of sufficient tunnel length.

Complications of ureteral reimplantation are not common.[77,100] The most common complication is de novo contralateral reflux,[101] whereas the most common technical complications are ureteral obstruction, persistent reflux, and diverticula formation. Persistent reflux may be caused by an insufficient tunnel length/ureteral diameter ratio. However, the greatest risk of postoperative reflux is related to the high-pressure voiding dynamics due to uninhibited bladder contraction, detrusor sphincter dyssynergia, and urinary retention. Ureteral obstruction may be due to ureteral kinking (at the neohiatus or obliterated umbilical artery), an excessively high placed neohiatus, construction of a tight neohiatus, twisting, anastomotic stricture, devascularization, and a tight tunnel. With attention directed toward the avoidance of technical complications and the selection of a procedure associated with the lowest complication rate, ureteral reimplantation remains a safe and highly successful operation.

Since the initial report in 1984 of successful endoscopic subureteral injection of polytetrafluoroethylene for correction of VUR,[102] this endoscopic technique has been widely used worldwide with different injectable materials.[103-105] This ambulatory procedure performed under a brief general anesthetic has the lowest morbidity and children return to full activity the next day. The only injectable substance with U.S. Food and Drug Administration approval is dextranomer/hyaluronic acid copolymer (Deflux, Q-Med Scandinavia, Princeton, NJ).[106] This substance is biodegradable, has no immunogenic properties, and seems to have no potential to cause malignant transformation. Results vary, but most studies indicate a success rate of around 80% for curing VUR.[106-109] Long-term reflux resolution rates are not known because it is difficult to re-study patients who are doing well, but there appears to be a low recurrence rate after 1 year.[110] However, recent studies suggest long-term recurrence of VUR may be more common than originally thought.[111]

chapter 57

BLADDER AND URETHRA

Patrick C. Cartwright, MD • Brent W. Snow, MD • M. Chad Wallis, MD

ANATOMY AND PHYSIOLOGIC FUNCTION

The lower urinary tract consists of the bladder and urethra, which normally function as a coordinated unit to store and discharge urine from the body. Both structural and functional disorders of the bladder or urethra may be responsible for bleeding, incontinence, infection, discomfort, pain, and obstruction that can cause upper tract deterioration to the point of compromising renal function. In this chapter we focus on the major diseases and dysfunctional states of the bladder and urethra as a unit and on the management of such problems.

The bladder and upper urethra are composed of bundles of smooth muscle fibers arranged in a reticular lattice, the outermost bundles being more circular and the inner bundles more longitudinal in orientation at the bladder neck.[1] The smooth muscle bundles blend into the striated muscle of the external urethral sphincter, which is derived from the pelvic diaphragm. The bladder is lined by transitional epithelium, which is sensitive to irritants such as bacterial toxins and various urinary crystals. The urethra and trigone are especially sensitive, and the presence of any irritant in these areas can create significant discomfort.

Normal innervation and bladder function are intimately related. Proper function of the lower urinary tract depends on intact autonomic and somatic nervous innervation. The detrusor muscle of the bladder proper is innervated by both sympathetic and parasympathetic fibers. Storage functions are mediated by the sympathetic component, which arises from spinal levels T10-L1 and descends through the sympathetic chain to reach the bladder. The chemical mediator of this storage process is norepinephrine, which acts on α-adrenergic receptors in the fundus of the bladder and causes muscle relaxation to aid in low-pressure storage of urine. The same sympathetic stimulus acts on predominantly α-adrenergic receptors of the trigone, bladder neck, and proximal urethra to provide an increase in internal sphincter activity and further promote continence during the storage process by maintaining outlet resistance.[2,3] The external urinary sphincter, innervated by the pudendal nerve, maintains progressively increasing tone as the bladder fills. This "guarding" provides an additional continence mechanism during the storage of urine.[4] As the child develops, the external sphincter may be consciously contracted at times of urgency or stress to prevent the unwanted passage of small amounts of urine. Properly coordinated function of the external urinary sphincter relies on an intact sacral reflex arc (afferents, sacral micturition center, pudendal efferents). This should be intact and well developed in normal infants, but is variably functional in infants with spinal cord or pelvic lesions.

The sensation of bladder fullness initiates a response in mature humans that causes them to seek an appropriate location for the discharge of urine. When ready, the parasympathetic nervous system, with acetylcholine as the mediator, causes cholinergic fibers of the detrusor to contract, resulting in a widened and shortened proximal urethra, eliminating its resistance to outflow. When coupled with relaxation of the volitional external sphincter, the bladder empties by sustained and complete contraction of the detrusor, leaving a residual urine volume in the bladder of less than 5 mL.

Spinal pathways connect the sacral micturition center with three centers in the brain stem, collectively called the *pontine micturition center.*[5] This center functions to inhibit urination during the storage phase and to produce external sphincter relaxation when sustained detrusor contraction occurs during the voiding phase. Above this level are areas of cerebral cortex, which oversee and modulate the autonomic process. It is the mature, integrated function of all these components that produces urinary continence.

Conscious control of the bladder (toilet training) is, in large part, a learned phenomenon. It requires adequate recognition by the brain that micturition would be inconvenient or socially unacceptable in a given situation. As the child grows older, the bladder gains capacity, allowing for longer intervals between voiding. The approximate bladder volume in ounces may be estimated in a child as age in years plus 2. It may also be calculated by a more precise formula if needed.[6] It has been observed that the young infant voids 20 times per day, which decreases to about 10 times per day by age 3 years.[7] Along with this change, the child also learns to resist the urge to void by voluntary contraction of the external sphincter until the detrusor contraction passes and the bladder once again relaxes. Thus, toilet training depends on the development of voluntary detrusor sphincter dyssynergia, which at times can persist as a pathologic process.[8] Finally, full bladder control relies on the child developing volitional control over the spinal micturition reflex so that he or she can initiate or inhibit detrusor contractions. The majority of children have attained day and night continence by 4 years of age.

The inappropriate discharge of urine (enuresis) may be in part due to immaturity of the bladder and its nervous system connections. The usual sequence of bladder development is linked to that of the bowel development and is as follows:

1. Control of bowel at night
2. Control of bowel during the day
3. Control of bladder during the day
4. Control of bladder at night

Many lesions interfere with the ideal storage and emptying functions of the bladder. The application of appropriate diagnostic measures can lead to appropriate management decisions, which ultimately lead to continence and to preservation and protection of the upper urinary tract.

CHILDHOOD INCONTINENCE

Incontinence is the term used for the unintentional loss of urine beyond toilet training. The following definitions are clinically useful[9]:

Enuresis or *nocturnal enuresis:* intermittent incontinence while sleeping

Primary nocturnal enuresis: never been continent at night

Secondary nocturnal enuresis: night-time incontinence after a dry period of at least 6 months

Daytime incontinence: daytime wetting after toilet training

Stress incontinence: urine leakage due to physically stressful activities such as coughing

Urge incontinence: unintentional loss of urine when bladder urgency occurs

The discussion of incontinence is divided into sections on nocturnal enuresis and daytime incontinence, realizing that some children have both. The current recommendation for children with nocturnal enuresis and daytime incontinence is to focus on daytime treatments first followed by nocturnal enuresis treatments.

NOCTURNAL ENURESIS

Fifteen to 20 percent of children at 5 years of age continue to have bed wetting.[10-12] Because so many children still wet the bed at night before this age, it is considered within the range of normal and not termed nocturnal enuresis. Night wetting, thereafter, resolves at the rate of about 15% each year, and by age 15 years, 99% of children remain dry.[13]

Etiology

Children with monosymptomatic nocturnal enuresis are, in general, physically and emotionally similar to their peers. The difference lies in their inability to awaken during sleep when their bladder is full or contracts. The etiology of this disorder is likely complex, and several factors should be considered.

Genetic

Family history is often strong, with multiple members having had childhood nocturnal enuresis. If both the parents have a history of bed wetting, 77% of their offspring will also. If only one parent had the problem, then 44% of the offspring exhibit the behavior. When neither parent has a history of nocturnal enuresis, then only 15% of their children have this problem.[14]

Psychological

Psychological stress is observed to induce nocturnal enuresis in certain children. Secondary nocturnal enuresis often raises this concern. Common factors are divorce, changing of homes, birth of a new sibling, trouble at school, or just starting school.

Developmental

As children grow, bladder capacity increases significantly each year at a proportion greater than urine volume produced.[15,16] Volitional control over the bladder and sphincter also may mature at variable rates and may be related to subtle delays in perceptual abilities or fine motor skills.[17]

Urodynamic

Studies show that enuretic episodes simulate normal awake voiding when the bladder is full.[16] Although patients with nocturnal enuresis have more night-time unstable bladder contractions than do non-enuretic patients, the contractions are at low pressure and do not cause leakage.

When observed scientifically, night-time wetting appears to occur in three scenarios: wetting associated with significant restlessness with visceral and somatic activity (deep respirations); wetting with a quick contraction and minimal movement; and wetting with no central nervous system response (parasomnia).

Sleep Disorders

Parents of children with nocturnal enuresis are generally convinced that these children sleep deeply and are difficult to arouse. However, controlled studies consistently find this not to be true. Enuretic patients sleep no more deeply than age-matched controls, wet in all stages of sleep, and show no difference in awakening patterns. Wetting episodes occur as the bladder fills throughout the night.[18]

Antidiuretic Hormone

Antidiuretic hormone (ADH) is released from the pituitary in a circadian rhythm so that levels are higher at night, and thus urine output is deminished. Some children appear to undersecrete ADH at night. Therefore, by not concentrating their urine at night, urine volume may overwhelm the bladder capacity and bed wetting results.[19-22] Although some patients follow this pattern, others do not. The altered circadian patterns appear to normalize with maturation.[23]

Evaluation

Children usually are seen by their pediatrician when either the child becomes socially embarrassed or the parents are either "fed up" or worried that a pathologic process is present. The screening evaluation should include a history, physical examination, and, always, urinalysis. If these results are normal, then no other evaluation is needed because organic disease rarely causes monosymptomatic nocturnal enuresis. Routine radiographic evaluation or cystoscopy is not necessary. Children with an associated anomaly or problem such as urinary tract infection (UTI), evidence of sacral anomalies, or complex enuresis patterns often warrant medical imaging.

Treatment

The treating physician should recognize enuresis as a symptom and not a disease. Realizing that there may be more than one cause permits the physician to consider more than one treatment option. Specific treatment is generally discouraged before the age of 7 years. Certain measures are sensible in all patients with nocturnal enuresis: void just before getting into bed, avoid huge fluid loads during the evening hours, and avoid caffeine after 3:00 PM.

Enuretic Alarms

Wetting alarms are devices that fit in the underwear of the patients. When the device is moistened, an electrical contact is made and the alarm is sounded. This is conditioning therapy requiring a motivated patient and parents. A variety of products are available with an audio alarm, a vibrating alarm, or both. In our experience, the best alarm is simply one that is easy to set up and is able to awaken the child when it goes off. The parent may need to help arouse the child, take him or her to the bathroom, and reset the alarm. This may occur multiple times each night.

A compilation of 16 published series showed an initial cure rate of 82%.[24] The average length of treatment to achieve dryness varied between 18 nights and 2.5 months. Relapse does occur in 20% to 30% of children, but re-treatment can be successful.[25] In a 1995 study, 1 year after instituting nocturnal enuresis treatments, wetting alarms were shown to give the best long-term results as compared with other treatments.[26] A more recent review confirms these findings.[27]

Imipramine

Tricyclic antidepressants such as imipramine have been used for many years to treat bed wetting. The exact mechanism of action is unknown. Initial success has been reported in the 50% range. However, a 2003 Cochrane review found that only one fifth of children became dry during treatment and the relapse rate was 96% after cessation of treatment.[28] Clinical practice reveals that the longer the initial treatment, the more benefit before the effect wanes. It is suggested that the medication be weaned slowly rather than stopped abruptly.

Side effects include anxiety, insomnia, dry mouth, nausea, and personality changes. An imipramine overdose can cause fatal cardiac arrhythmias and conduction blocks that are untreatable. Therefore, medication safety in the home becomes a significant issue.[29] Some suggest that imipramine may improve response rates with the enuretic alarm.

Desmopressin

Desmopressin is an analog of ADH that mimics its urine-concentrating activity without the vasopressor effect.[19] It is currently given orally. The effect of desmopressin is dose dependent, usually requiring 20 to 40 g/day for success.

Complete dryness rates vary with desmopressin therapy and may be highest in patients with a strong family history of bed wetting. In three multicenter trials in the United States, response rates were reported in 24% to 35% of children who had failures associated with other forms of treatment.[30] In a study in which dose titration was watched closely, 70% dryness was reported.[31] Desmopressin may occasionally have side effects, including electrolyte changes, nasal irritation, and headaches. It remains available as a nasal spray, but this formulation of the medication lost its indication for treating nocturnal enuresis owing to a higher incidence of severe hyponatremia. Parents should be warned to limit the amount of fluids a child drinks during the evening of treatment to avoid this side effect.

Anticholinergics

Oxybutynin is the most common drug used in this category for enuresis. It is effective when daytime and night-time wetting occur in the same patient but has no benefit over placebo when night-time wetting is the only symptom.[32]

General Approach

Although many parents consider bed wetting a problem, they often do not consider it significant enough to treat, especially when medications are being considered. If therapy is desired, it is often most reasonable to begin with an enuretic alarm. This has the highest response rate, no side effects, and the lowest relapse rate. Combination therapy with imipramine may be considered when use of the alarm is unsuccessful. If desmopressin has proved successful in a specific patient, the patient and family may choose to keep it available and use it only on specific nights when dryness is especially desired (e.g., sleepovers, campouts). Some patients do not respond to therapy, and time, reassurance, and a caring approach are all that can be offered.

DAYTIME INCONTINENCE

Daytime incontinence is the undesired loss of urinary control while awake. The patient history is of paramount importance in sorting out the various categories of daytime incontinence.[33,34] The physical examination and evaluation should always assess for an abdominal mass or tenderness, distended bladder, normal genitalia, signs of spina bifida occulta, perineal sensation, sacral reflexes, gait, lower extremity reflexes, and urinalysis. Radiographic evaluation, usually voiding cystourethrogram (VCUG) and renal ultrasonography, are necessary in patients with UTI or complex incontinence patterns.

Bladder Instability

Bladder instability is by far the most common diagnosis in children with persistent daytime wetting.[35] These children are usually toilet trained but later develop increasing "accidents" associated with urgency. They describe not knowing that the bladder contraction was coming. They dash to the bathroom or try to "hold it in." Boys grab and compress the penis, and girls often cross their legs and dance around or squat with the heel compressed over the perineum (Vincent's curtsy). In our experience, children with hyperactivity disorders or a willful disposition appear prone to this dysfunctional voiding pattern.

By urodynamic studies, these children demonstrate significant unstable contractions during bladder filling that cause leakage before sphincter contraction (or posturing) can control it. Because these unstable contractions or spasms occur frequently during the day, a retentive pattern develops by using the external sphincter to "hold on." When these children do get to the bathroom and try to void, the sphincter relaxes poorly or only intermittently, with resultant stop-and-go voiding, difficulty initiating a urinary stream, straining, and poor emptying, which is described by the term *voiding dysfunction.* The elevated pressure during voiding and the poor emptying may result in secondary vesicoureteral reflux (VUR) and UTI. Finally, the overactivity of the urinary sphincter may carry over to the function of the anal sphincter, making stool retention and encopresis commonly associated findings.

Treatment

Treatment rests on managing all aspects of this condition simultaneously. Mild encopresis is treated with dietary changes, fiber, laxatives, or mineral oil after initial bowel clean out. Recurring UTIs are managed with prophylactic antibiotics. Bladder instability is treated with timed voiding at frequent intervals (an alarm watch for the child is helpful) and with anticholinergics such as oxybutynin or tolterodine.[36-38]

Biofeedback has gained in popularity for the treatment of the voiding dysfunction that often accompanies bladder instability. Electrodes placed on the perineum near the genitourinary diaphragm can be attached to monitors, an audio signal, or a computer display so the child can learn to relax the external sphincter voluntarily, resulting in better voiding coordination.[39,40] The process typically requires 4 to 8 visits on a weekly basis with follow-up sessions as needed. As acceptance of this treatment modality has grown, it is becoming more available.

Unfortunately, initial success with any treatment program is often followed by later relapse. If initial treatment is unsuccessful, it may be successful if tried again later. Patients older than age 8 years who fail treatment should be considered for urodynamic testing. Secondary VUR may be present due to elevated bladder pressures and is managed in the usual manner with a high probability for resolution (80%) as bladder function improves.[41] The unstable bladder of childhood is almost always outgrown, and adults generally do not demonstrate this type of wetting problem.

ISOLATED FREQUENCY SYNDROME

A separate, and much less common, group of children present with fairly acute onset of urinary frequency. They appear healthy, are normal on examination, and have normal urinalysis and culture. They do not have true urgency or any wetting but feel that they must urinate frequently, sometimes every 5 to 10 minutes. They void a very small amount each time. Most sleep through the night and void a large amount on awakening. The pattern may come and go over weeks or months.

The cause is unclear but may relate to emotional stress in many cases. Careful assessment is crucial, and reassurance to the parent and child is paramount. Sometimes, setting an alarm to progressively lengthen voiding intervals with a reward for success is helpful. This condition is benign and self-limited, although it may persist intermittently for months. Anticholinergics have no benefit, and further evaluation is not required.

INFREQUENT VOIDER/UNDERACTIVE BLADDER

On the other end of the voiding spectrum are those children who void only once or twice daily and may not urinate until the afternoon.[42] These children have developed urinary retentive behavior without any bladder instability and have dilated, high-capacity, low-pressure bladders.[43] Some show an aversion to bathrooms or exhibit excessive neatness, whereas many others appear reasonably adjusted. They may be somewhat prone to UTIs and stress incontinence.

Evaluation must demonstrate no neurologic cause and no structural obstruction to emptying. Ultrasonography may show good emptying if performed before and after voiding. A timed voiding regimen is usually required to get these children to void regularly if problems are occurring. This pattern tends to improve with maturation.

CONTINUOUS INCONTINENCE

Patients who present with total incontinence and constant dribbling of urine have a higher probability of urinary tract anomaly pathology, and require radiographic and possibly urodynamic evaluation.

HINMAN'S SYNDROME

A small number of children demonstrate persistent incontinence, repeated febrile UTIs, reflux, high bladder storage pressures, and very poor emptying.[44] This appears to be a deeply ingrained "learned" disorder of severe voluntary detrusor-sphincter dyssynergia. In these patients, the urinary tract has the appearance of that in a patient with neurogenic bladder. There is hydronephrosis, a trabeculated bladder, reflux, and sometimes progressive loss of renal function (Fig. 57-1).

Aggressive therapy with prophylactic antibiotics, anticholinergics, urodynamic biofeedback training, timed voiding, or intermittent catheterization may be needed.[45] Some recalcitrant cases may require bladder diversion or augmentation to avoid renal failure. As with many "functional" disorders, the severity of Hinman's syndrome tends to wane with maturation, but progressive deterioration may not allow the surgeon to wait.

NEUROGENIC BLADDER

True neurogenic dysfunction of the bladder in childhood results from acquired or congenital lesions that affect bladder innervation. Acquired lesions may occur from trauma to the brain, spinal cord, or pelvic nerves, or as a result of tumor, infection, or vascular lesions affecting these same structures. Congenital lesions include spina bifida and other neural tube defects (most common), degenerative neuromuscular disorders, cerebral palsy, tethered cord, sacral agenesis, imperforate anus, VACTERL (*v*ertebral, *a*nal, *c*ardiac, *t*racheal, *e*sophageal, *r*enal, and *l*imb) syndrome, and other causes.[46]

The most practical way to classify neurogenic bladder abnormalities is by a simple functional system: failure to store, failure to empty, or a combination of both.[47] Failure to store urine may be caused by the detrusor muscle itself or by the bladder outlet. Detrusor hyperactivity or poor compliance during bladder filling causes elevated bladder pressures and incontinence on this basis. Inadequate outlet resistance secondary to an incompetent bladder neck or urethral sphincter mechanism can cause failure to store urine even if storage pressures are reasonable. Failure to empty can suggest either a bladder muscle or bladder outlet etiology as well. The hypotonic, neurogenic bladder may not generate enough pressure with detrusor contraction to empty. Alternatively, the outlet may exhibit increased resistance secondary to striated or smooth muscle sphincter dyssynergia. The advantage of this classification is that treatment can be based on urodynamic data.

Myelomeningocele

The most common cause of a neurogenic bladder in childhood is the group of neural tube defects, which ranges from occult spinal dysraphism to myelomeningocele.[48,49] Myelomeningocele is the most severe and the most common, reported in about 1 in 1000 live births with notable geographic variations and a

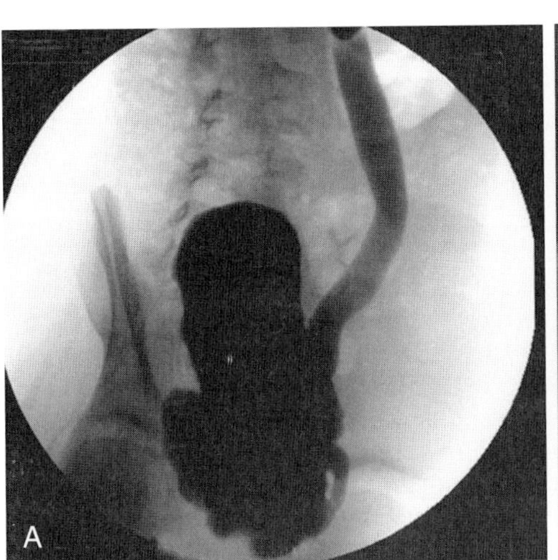

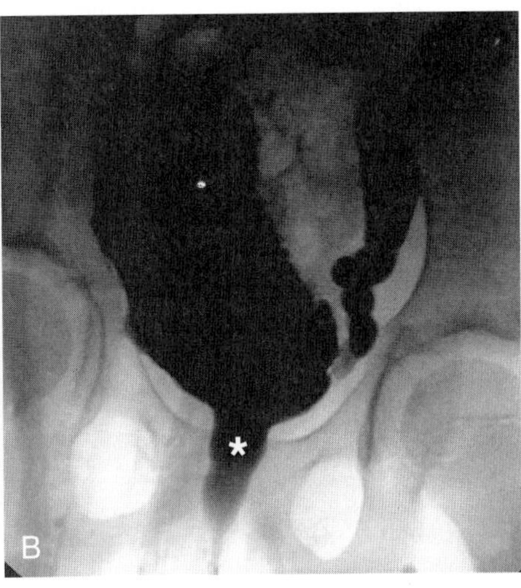

Figure 57-1. A, This cystogram shows the typical findings in a patient with Hinman's syndrome: trabeculated bladder and severe reflux. **B,** This voiding study in the same patient demonstrates dilation of the posterior urethra *(asterisk)* as a result of chronic contraction of the external sphincter during voiding.

declining occurrence over the past decade.[50,51] The etiology is multifactorial, with a clear familial association (2% to 5% sibling risk) and evidence that periconceptual folic acid supplementation (0.4 mg/day) reduces the risk by 60% to 80%.[52] Improved care of the neurosurgical aspects of this lesion since the late 1970s has increased the survival rate of children with this condition. Thus, continued urologic care is very important. Ninety percent of neonates with myelomeningocele have normal upper tracts. However, if no care is administered to the bladder, at least half of these patients show signs of upper tract deterioration or reflux within 5 years.[53] It is therefore critical that early urologic evaluation of children with myelomeningocele is undertaken.[54,55]

Evaluation of the Neonate with Myelomeningocele

There have been reports over the past decade from centers performing fetal closure of myelomeningocele recognized by prenatal ultrasonography[56-58]. Unfortunately, there has been little to suggest that this has improved lower extremity, bowel, or bladder function for these patients, but the need for ventriculoperitoneal shunting may be reduced by 50%. A multi-institutional randomized controlled trial is under way in the United States, and further outcomes will be watched with interest.

Generally, the neonate with myelomeningocele has had a thorough neurologic assessment, closure of the back defect, and possibly even ventriculoperitoneal shunting before any evaluation of the urinary tract. The level of the bony defect does not predict the functional cord level because lesions may be partial and patchy. Before discharge, a renal and bladder ultrasound evaluation should be performed to evaluate parenchymal quality, the presence of hydronephrosis, and the size and emptying ability of the bladder. About 5% of patients have an abnormality on ultrasonography, in which case a VCUG and an evaluation of upper tract function and drainage by renal scan should be performed. If the ultrasonogram is normal, other studies can probably be delayed a few months, although we prefer to proceed with VCUG before hospital discharge mainly for logistical reasons. About 10% of these patients have reflux. Children are placed on amoxicillin prophylaxis (10 mg/kg once daily), and the serum creatinine concentration is followed during the initial hospitalization period. Many children experience poor emptying for a few days or weeks after the initial back closure, and postvoid residuals should be measured before discharge from the hospital. Intermittent catheterization is begun if the residual urine is consistently greater than 15 mL. Credé's maneuver should be avoided because it is ineffective in emptying the bladder and magnifies the detrimental effects of high intravesical pressure if reflux is present.

Neonatal urodynamic evaluation has since been shown to have prognostic value in determining which children are likely to develop upper tract dilation and VUR. Children with bladder pressures higher than 40 cm H_2O at the point of urinary leakage and those with detrusor-sphincter dyssynergia are much more likely to show upper tract deterioration or VUR.[2,54] Other factors shown to indicate bladder "hostility" include the presence of reflux, hyperreflexic contractions, and poor detrusor compliance.[55] Therefore, early urodynamic evaluation (typically by 12 weeks of age) is useful for determining the frequency of follow-up studies and the timing of initiation of bladder therapy programs.

If the radiographic evaluation is normal and no infection is present, the patient can be managed by spontaneous voiding into the diaper, especially if leak-point pressures are low. Follow-up studies are planned with a urine culture and renal ultrasound evaluation at 6 months. If leak-point pressures are high or sphincter dyssynergia is present, a VCUG again at 6 months is reasonable. Ultrasonography and urine cultures should be repeated yearly if the urinary tract is stable, with or without VCUG, depending on the relative risk of the upper tract as determined by urodynamics. If reflux or upper tract deterioration occurs at any time, intervention with clean intermittent catheterization (CIC), anticholinergic therapy, or temporary cutaneous vesicostomy may be warranted.

Childhood Management

Periodic reassessment of the anatomy and function of the urinary tract is important because the clinical and urodynamic picture may change with growth and spinal cord re-tethering.[59] Initiation of a bladder management program is generally undertaken when there is worsening reflux, upper tract dilation, deterioration of urodynamics, or infection. If the urinary tract is stable, such management may be delayed until social continence is desired.

The cornerstone of treatment programs for neurogenic bladder in most children is CIC. Popularized in the early 1970s, CIC has revolutionized the treatment program for these children.[60] The purpose of CIC is to provide periodic low-pressure emptying of the bladder, which can prevent or improve existing deterioration of the upper tracts, including that secondary to reflux.[61,62] In younger children, this task is performed by the caretaker. As children become older and more responsible, they can assume the task themselves. Motivation is important in adhering to a good bladder program. Therefore, it is sometimes better to wait until social pressures influence the child's desire for continence before initiating a bladder program, unless it is required for the treatment of bladder deterioration.

CIC is associated with a high incidence of bacteriuria (when followed with serial culturing), varying greatly in different series.[63,64] Bacteriuria is eventually found in about 60% of cases, with most patients becoming culture positive within 1 year, often with one or two symptomatic episodes per year.[61] In patients with no reflux and with normal intravesical pressure, asymptomatic bacteriuria appears to have little clinical significance. However, in patients with high storage pressures, reflux, or a combination of the two, the potential for upper tract deterioration increases significantly with bacteriuria.[65] Infection with urea-splitting organisms (usually *Proteus* species) is of concern, owing to the potential for struvite stone formation.

Pharmacologic therapy for neurogenic bladder is usually coupled with CIC and is aimed at decreasing the pressures in the hypertonic, noncompliant bladder or increasing bladder outlet resistance to improve continence. Anticholinergic drugs, such as oxybutynin, propantheline, or tolterodine,[66] are used to lower bladder storage pressures by blocking hypertonic detrusor activity. Imipramine may also be useful alone or in combination with the anticholinergic agents because it can both relax detrusor and tighten the outlet. Inadequate vesical outlet resistance may also respond to α-adrenergic medications such as pseudoephedrine. Often, the combination of anticholinergics, α agonists, and CIC is required to gain adequate continence. Side effects of the anticholinergics may sometimes limit their use. Tolterodine and extended-release oxybutynin are purported to cause fewer side effects than other anticholinergics. Instillation of oxybutynin dissolved in water directly in the bladder can lessen the side effects and still maintain a therapeutic response. The recently developed oxybutynin cutaneous patch may offer an improved therapeutic index to these patients as well.[67] Finally, cystoscopic injection of botulinum toxin type A has recently been applied to children with neurogenic bladder in an effort to decrease bladder pressures and increase compliance. The effects of the injection are short-term, and repeated injections are required.[68,69]

Urodynamic assessment helps the clinician select medications and other modalities for the neurogenic bladder and to monitor their effects.[3] This study may be elaborate in certain situations, but is more often a simple measurement of the pressure-volume relationship of the bladder during filling. It is performed using a double-lumen catheter in the bladder and usually involves simultaneous assessment of external sphincter function with a perineal electrode patch. Urodynamic assessment can be performed with contrast material and monitored fluoroscopically to add information. Noting parameters such as bladder compliance, hyperreflexic contractions, leak-point pressure, stress leak-point pressure, and sphincter dyssynergia can be extremely valuable in helping to choose among treatment options. Figure 57-2 demonstrates the effect of anticholinergics in shifting the pressure-volume curve to the right and thus permitting the bladder to store more urine at any given pressure. Figure 57-3 shows the effect of α-adrenergic receptors on raising the leak-point pressure and thus permitting storage to a higher pressure.

It is crucial to understand that when bladder pressures remain greater than 35 to 40 cm H_2O, ureteral peristalsis does not effectively empty the upper tracts. Hydronephrosis and eventual renal insufficiency result. Thus, coupling cystometric data with a particular patient's estimated (or measured) hourly output permits the clinician to decide what CIC interval would keep bladder pressures in a safe range. Medications

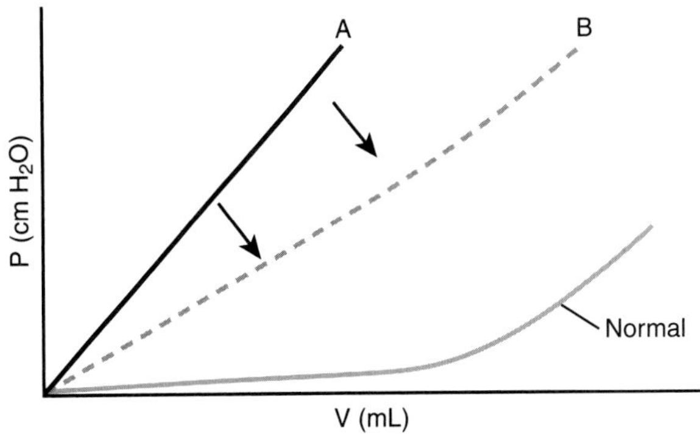

Figure 57-2. Bladder filling pressure-volume curve in a patient with a neurogenic bladder. Note the shift of the curve to the right (A to B) when anticholinergics relax the detrusor, allowing lower pressure at any given volume.

can then be sensibly adjusted to extend CIC intervals, achieve dryness, and avoid development or progression of hydronephrosis.

Transurethral electrical stimulation of the bladder has been used in several treatment centers in an effort to produce conscious urinary control in the patient with neurogenic bladder.[70] It is a time-consuming treatment program with sometimes hundreds of sessions required before a response. Although some series have shown variably encouraging results, especially concerning the improvement in bladder compliance,[70-71] others have found the results disappointing.[72,73] More experience is necessary, but this technique may be applicable in selected children. Selective sacral nerve root rhizotomy and electrical stimulation of the sacral nerve roots may also have some limited potential for treatment in certain children.[74-76]

In children with high bladder storage pressures and deterioration of the upper tracts that cannot be managed by CIC or pharmacologic therapy, temporary diversion with cutaneous vesicostomy may be necessary.[77,78] Protection of the upper urinary tracts from high bladder pressures is thus accomplished until such time that other treatments can be initiated. We reserve this treatment for infants who have serious deterioration of the upper tract and those who, for social, medical, or anatomic reasons, cannot be

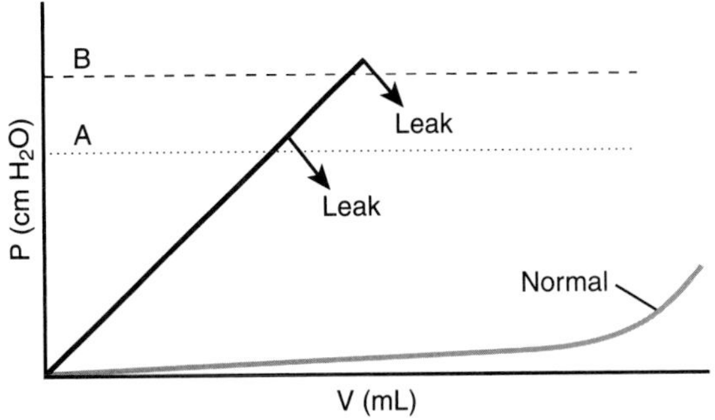

Figure 57-3. Bladder filling pressure-volume curve demonstrating a higher leak point pressure (from A to B), sometimes achieved with α-adrenergic agents such as pseudoephedrine and imipramine. The effect is to decrease incontinence at lower pressures.

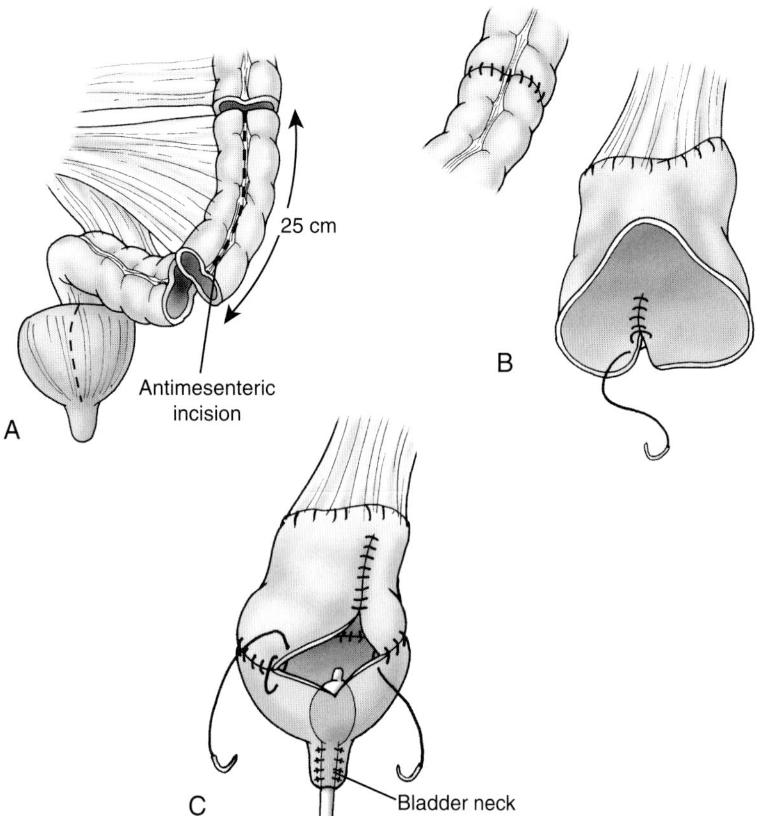

Figure 57-4. Bladder enlargement by enterocystoplasty (sigmoid) and bladder neck reconstruction. Enterocystoplasty enlarges the bladder nicely but has significant potential complications, including occasional perforation, first seen as acute abdominal pain.

managed with the other aforementioned forms of medical treatment. As an alternative, some advocate urethral dilation in girls to diminish the leak-point pressure. A surprising persistence of benefit has been noted in some series.[79]

Surgical Treatment

Although most patients with neurogenic bladder can be managed adequately without surgical intervention, those with reflux, a poorly compliant bladder, or refractory incontinence may benefit from operative intervention.

Treatment of reflux in the neurogenic bladder is much the same as that for the normal bladder.[80] It is imperative, however, that the bladder be adequately treated for poor compliance and hyperreflexia (CIC and anticholinergics) before and after surgical intervention to diminish the high recurrence risk.[81]

In other clinical circumstances, bladder augmentation or enlargement may be required. Bladder augmentation is designed to create a reservoir with good compliance and adequate capacity to store urine until it can be emptied by CIC at socially appropriate intervals. Detubularized segments of large or small bowel employed as a patch and detubularized cup on the widely opened bladder (enterocystoplasty) are the current standards for augmentation (Fig. 57-4). Other techniques for bladder augmentation include gastrocystoplasty, which has been repopularized since 1988.[82,83] It is a technically acceptable procedure and shows advantages over enterocystoplasty with respect to a decrease in mucus formation, a possible decrease in infection rate, and maintenance of electrolyte balance in patients with renal insufficiency. Unfortunately, the hematuria-dysuria syndrome may affect up to one third of patients, and limits its applicability.[84] This and other complications of enterocystoplasty such as metabolic derangements secondary to the absorption of urine by the gastrointestinal tract, excessive mucus production, stone formation, and even an increased risk of bladder cancer have led to a search for different approaches.

Bladder autoaugmentation or detrusorectomy is an alternative augmenting technique that may prove useful in selected patients (Figs. 57-5 and 57-6).[85] The procedure involves removal of the detrusor muscle over the superior portion of the bladder, leaving the underlying bladder mucosa intact. This creates a large compliant surface, essentially a large diverticulum, which decreases bladder pressures and increases bladder capacity on filling. The advantage of this technique is that the bladder epithelium is preserved and not replaced with gastrointestinal epithelium as in bowel augmentation. This change eliminates the problems associated with the secretory and absorptive functions of bowel mucosa. Long-term follow-up data on large numbers of children are lacking, but this technique appears to be a viable alternative for use in bladders with a reasonable capacity and mainly poor

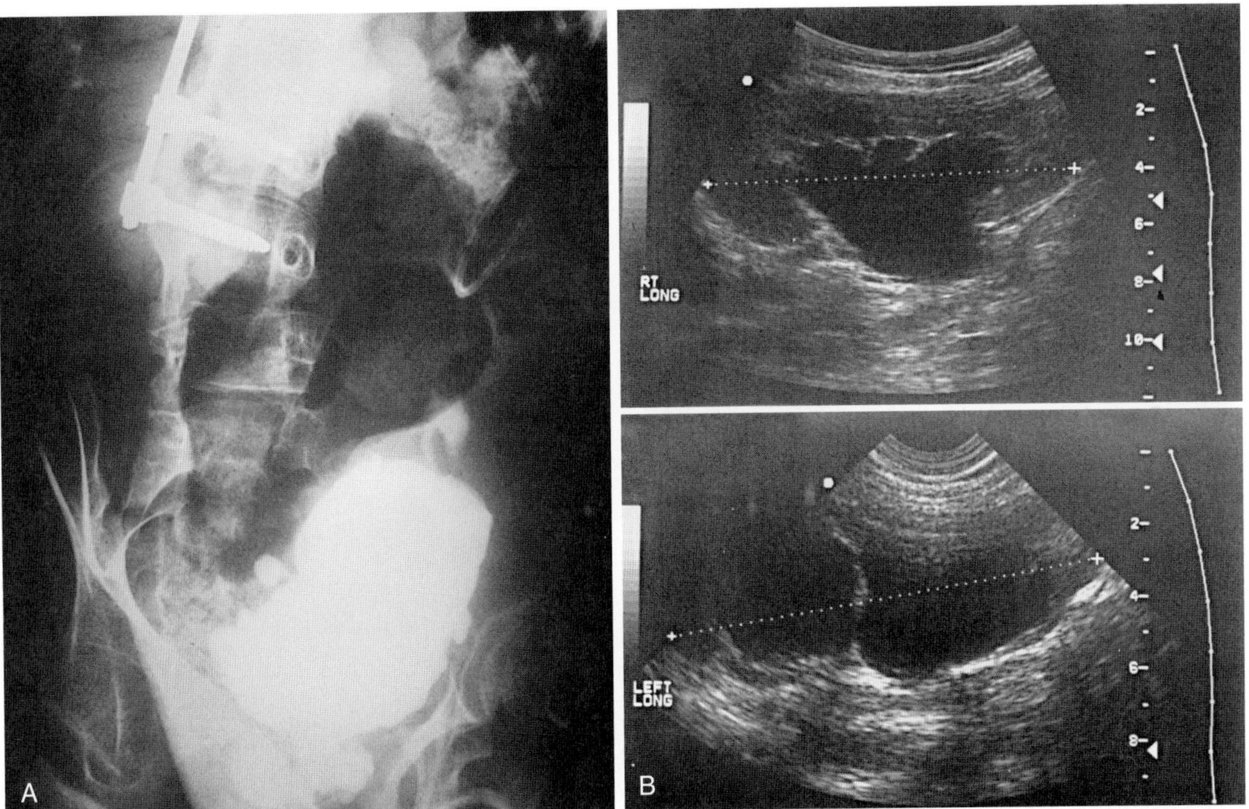

Figure 57-5. Radiographic (**A**) and ultrasonographic (**B**) images of a patient with spina bifida showing a small, poorly compliant bladder and worsening hydronephrosis (**B**).

compliance.[86] The concept has been extended to create "composite" bladders by placing demucosalized bowel or stomach patches over the urothelial bulge created in autoaugmentation.[87,88] This concept of urothelial preservation during augmentation is carried forward by current innovative approaches to replace the bladder wall with biodegradable scaffolds, typically seeded with urothelial and detrusor smooth muscle cells.[89] The future of bladder reconstruction may be greatly enhanced by these efforts.

Persistent incontinence, despite adequate treatment of the bladder to lower pressures and increase compliance and capacity, may require surgery on the bladder outlet to increase resistance. Bladder neck reconstructions of the Young-Dees type, which lengthens the urethra by infolding and tubularizing the trigone of the bladder, have generally lost favor but still have some advocates.[90] Kropp's procedure uses a tubularized anterior bladder strip reimplanted in the submucosa of the trigone to gain continence by a flap valve mechanism.[91] Continence is commonly achieved, but catheterization is sometimes difficult.[92] The Pippi-Salle procedure creates a similar (but easier to catheterize) flap valve by onlaying an anterior bladder wall flap onto a posterior incised strip up the middle of the trigone.[93] Owing to the lack of the popoff mechanism in both these procedures, if the bladder becomes overfilled, the potential for bladder rupture of an augmented bladder or for upper tract deterioration due to high pressures is increased.

One of the more popular forms of increasing urethral resistance in the neurogenic bladder is by the pubovaginal or puboprostatic fascial sling.[94-98] This procedure has many advocates and involves securing a rectus fascial strip (or other material) around the urethra and suspending it from the anterior rectus fascia or pubis. This elevates and compresses the urethra to increase outlet resistance. Suprapubic bladder neck suspension with periurethral sutures is also advocated but has a lower success rate than the fascial sling technique, especially in the urethra that is widely open with little resistance.

The artificial urinary sphincter works by way of a fluid-filled pressurized cuff around the urethra, which can be deflated by a pump-reservoir device that permits the urethra to open and the bladder to drain (Fig. 57-7). This artificial sphincter can also be used in higher-pressure bladders in conjunction with bladder augmentation.[99] The main disadvantage is that it is a mechanical device that can erode into the urethra and malfunction over time. If the devices are left in place long enough, virtually all eventually need revision. Thus, we prefer to use autologous tissue techniques in children, when possible.

The periurethral injection of dextranomer/hyaluronic acid copolymer (Deflux), Teflon, or polydimethylsiloxane represents a simple, safe technique for enhancing urethral resistance in selected patients with poor intrinsic sphincter tone. It appears to be most applicable in patients requiring only a minimal increase in stress leak-point pressure. Long-term

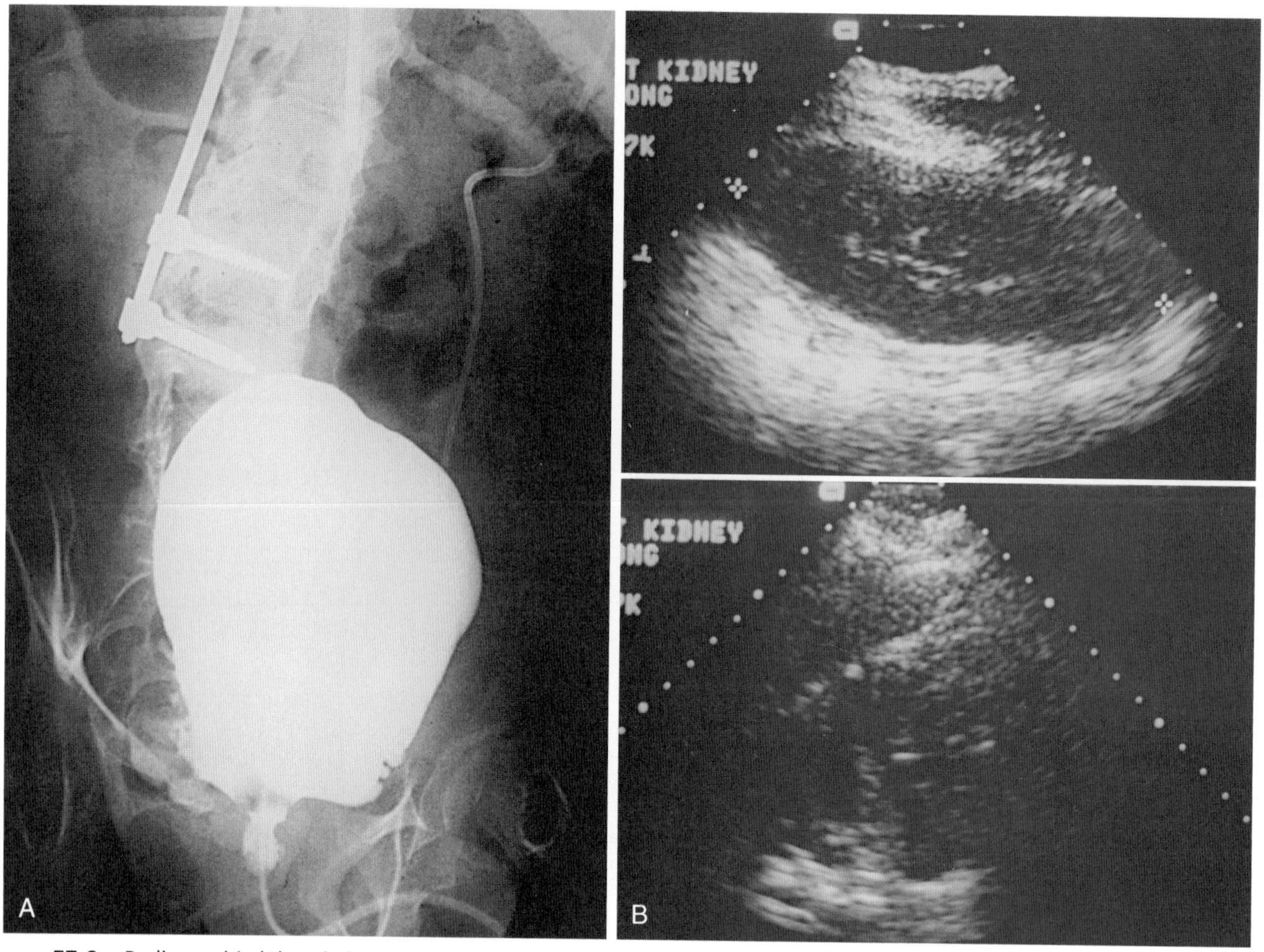

Figure 57-6. Radiographic (**A**) and ultrasonographic (**B**) images in the patient shown in Figure 57-5 after bladder autoaugmentation, demonstrating improved bladder capacity and better compliance, which resulted in continence and diminished hydronephrosis (**B**).

improvement rates are disappointing, and the usefulness of this approach in children is questionable.[100,101] With all procedures to enhance resistance at the bladder outlet, it is crucial that the storage pressures of the bladder be considered as well. When the bladder outlet is tightened but the bladder is unable to store increasing volumes at low pressure, hydronephrosis or reflux results. When the surgeon is considering bladder outlet surgery, it may be necessary to occlude the bladder neck with a urinary balloon catheter during preoperative urodynamic assessment to determine how much the bladder can hold and what the storage pressures are. This maneuver helps judge whether augmentation is needed simultaneously.

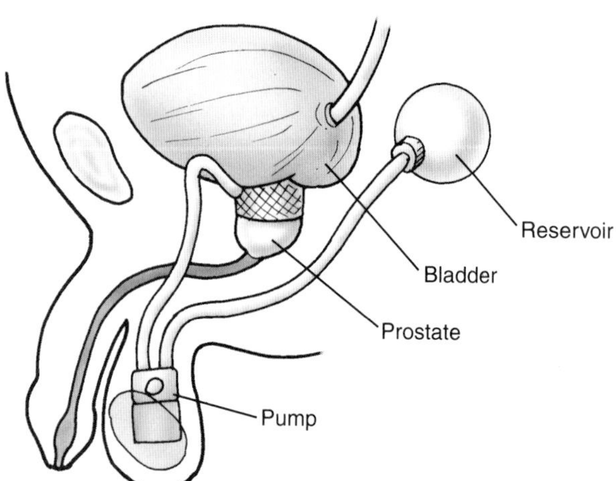

Figure 57-7. Typical artificial urinary sphincter. The scrotal pump moves fluid from the cuff to the reservoir to permit bladder emptying.

One surgical adjunct of great benefit in patients unable to self-catheterize the urethra (e.g., owing to spinal deformity, discomfort, or false passage) is the creation of a continent catheterizable stoma. This may be performed using the appendix or another small tubularized structure implanted into the bladder and anastomosed to the skin (Mitrofanoff principle).[102,103] The implanted conduit can be hidden at the base of the umbilicus (Fig. 57-8), and CIC may then be carried out through this segment.[104] The appendix may alternatively be left in continuity with the cecum and brought to the skin as a catheterizable channel for irrigation/enemas of the neurogenic colon. In this circumstance, a small segment of ileum may be refashioned as a catheterizable Monti-Yang stoma.[105] This has been a great adjunct to simplify catheterization for wheelchair-bound patients.

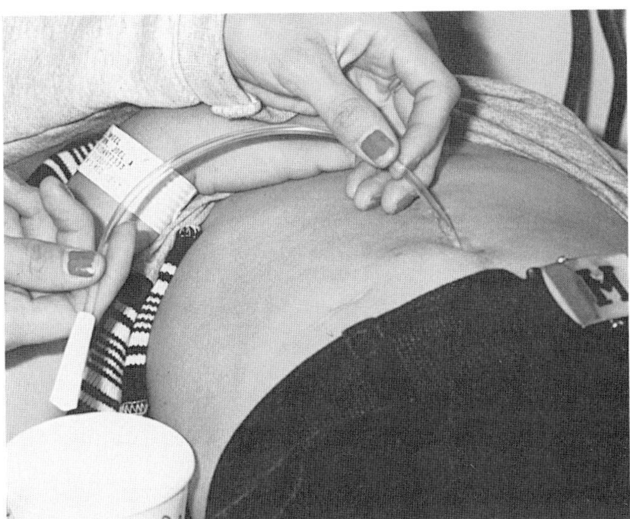

Figure 57-8. Umbilical positioning of an appendicovesicostomy permits easy access for clean intermittent catheterization. Some patients can remain in their wheelchairs and drain the bladder into the toilet through a catheter extender.

Cutaneous urinary diversion by ileal or colon conduit or by cutaneous ureterostomy is considered a last resort option in these children. Long-term deterioration of the upper tracts is well documented in refluxing ileal conduits.[106] Some protection of the upper tracts is afforded by a nonrefluxing colon conduit, but the prognosis beyond 2 decades is uncertain.[107] Therefore, avoidance of diversion, if possible, is the best course in children with neurogenic bladders. All reasonable efforts should be made to maintain ureteral drainage into the bladder, if possible.

Continent urinary diversion has evolved over the past several years as a popular alternative in treating incontinence. The intestinal segments for urinary reconstruction in children with neurogenic bladders generally are of neurogenic bowel as well. These children may not tolerate a loss of large segments (especially ileocecal segments) without developing loose stools. In children who are dependent on constipated stools for fecal continence, loose stools may be more devastating than the original urinary incontinence.

URETHRAL DISORDERS

Urethral Prolapse

Urethral prolapse occurs in girls at a mean age of 5 years, with those of African descent being particularly prone to this disorder.[108] Urethral prolapse presents as dysuria, blood spotting of the underwear, and a bulging concentric purplish ring of prolapsed urethra seen at the urethral meatus (Fig. 57-9). Mild prolapse can be treated with an antibiotic ointment or estrogen cream applied to the area several times a day along with sitz baths. There are times when a urinary catheter is needed temporarily. In unusual persistent cases, excision of the prolapsing tissue with reanastomosis of the skin edges is needed. Also, simple ligation of the prolapsing urethral epithelium over a urinary catheter, permitting necrosis, is another option.

Meatal Stenosis

Meatal stenosis is the narrowing of the male urinary meatus after circumcision. It is thought to be due to exposure and irritation of the meatus in the diaper.[108,109] For reasons that are uncertain, the stenosis is always on the ventral aspect of the meatus, causing dorsal deflection of the urinary stream that is fine and forceful. It is important for the physician to not only examine the meatus but also watch the child void. If the stream is not narrow in caliber or is not dorsally deflected, then the meatal stenosis is not physiologically significant enough to require treatment. Occasionally, voiding causes the web to tear, resulting in dysuria or a drop of blood after urination. Some patients will have ongoing inflammation around the meatus that will respond to topical corticosteroid application (betamethasone 0.05%).

Meatotomy may be necessary and can be performed under general anesthesia or as an office procedure. In the office, topical lidocaine/prilocaine cream can be applied topically, covered with a bio-occlusive dressing, and left in place for 1 hour before meatotomy with oral midazolam for sedation in selected patients. This has resulted in a painless office procedure.[109] Following tropical, local, or general anesthesia, the ventral web is clamped with a hemostat for 1 minute, which results in adequate hemostasis. The ventral web is

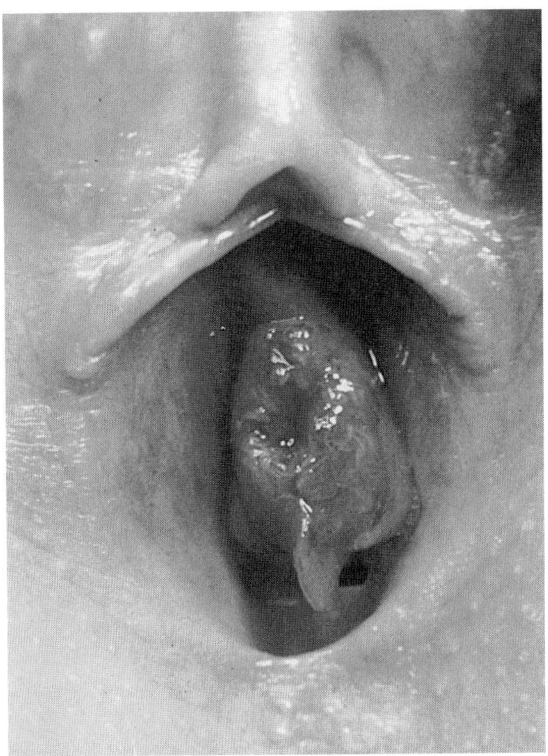

Figure 57-9. Urethral prolapse is usually seen as a circumferential, purplish bulge at the meatus.

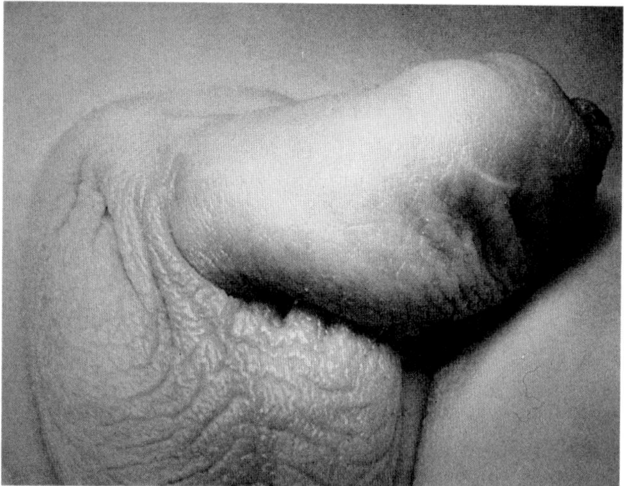

Figure 57-10. A scaphoid megalourethra is seen in a boy with prune-belly syndrome.

then incised one half the distance to the coronal margin. Parents are asked to spread the meatus and apply ointment several times daily for 2 to 3 weeks. Meatal stenosis rarely recurs. Imaging studies and cystoscopy are not needed in these boys.

Megalourethra

Megalourethra is a rare genital anomaly causing a deformed and elongated penis occurring in two forms: fusiform and scaphoid (Fig. 57-10). These differ in embryology and appearance. Megalourethra is seen more commonly in patients with prune-belly syndrome and has been reported in association with the VACTERL complex.[110]

The less severe and most common form of this anomaly is the scaphoid variety, in which spongiosal tissue fails to invest the urethra.[111] The more severe fusiform variety is caused by failure in the development of the penile mesoderm, so that there is neither spongiosal tissue nor properly formed corpora cavernosa within the penis.[112] The fusiform type of megalourethra has been reported in patients with severe forms of prune-belly syndrome, stillborn fetuses, and patients with cloacal anomalies.[113,114] Associated urologic anomalies have been described, including megaureter, megacystis, reflux, bladder diverticula, and renal dysplasia.[114] Upper tract assessment is indicated in all cases. Repair of the megalourethra relies on hypospadias techniques that tailor the urethra to a more normal size.

Urethral Duplication

Urethral duplications occur in a wide variety of forms and can be broadly classified as dorsal or ventral to the normal meatus.[115-117] Duplication may be complete, but incomplete forms predominate. Occasionally, side-by-side duplications occur, usually associated with a duplicated phallus and bladder. Most commonly, the two channels form in the sagittal plane. The urethral channel closest to the rectum is generally the more functional channel, having more normal spongiosal tissue and sphincter mechanism.[118] The more dorsal urethra is often small and poorly developed and will commonly be in an epispadiac position and associated with a dorsal chordee. Partial duplications that course along the penile urethra have been called *Y-type duplications*.[119] When the duplicated opening is in the perineum, it has been termed an *H-type duplication*.[120]

The treatment of a urethral duplication must be individualized. When only a minor septum is present, cystoscopic division of the septum has been successful. Traditionally, with more significant duplications, efforts have been made to lengthen the ventrally placed urethra to the tip of the penis using various hypospadias reconstruction techniques. Progressive dilation of the dorsal urethral channel to make it functional has also been advocated.[121]

Congenital Urethral Fistula

A congenital urethral fistula may occur in the anterior urethra where incomplete development of the spongiosum has occurred, permitting a small diverticulum to form that can rupture antenatally.[122] These are uncommon and difficult to repair due to the lack of spongiosal tissue surrounding the fistula.

Urethral Strictures and Stenosis

Most urethral strictures are acquired. Instrumentation and catheter passage by medical personnel, trauma, and inflammatory diseases are common causes. Congenital urethral stenosis is rare and generally focal. These stenoses are usually in the bulbar urethra, within the area of embryologic joining of the bulbous urethra arising from genital folds and the posterior membranous urethra arising from the urogenital sinus. If this junction is misaligned or incompletely canalized, a discrete stricture may develop.[122]

Both of these conditions can be treated with an internal urethrotomy, resection and end-to-end anastomosis, or a pedicle flap/free graft urethroplasty. Recent data would suggest a single internal urethrotomy for short strictures followed by an open repair for failures as best therapy.[123]

Urethral Atresia

When urethral atresia occurs, in order to be compatible with life, a patent urachus must be present. Reconstruction can be difficult. A vesicostomy with a subsequent catheterizable stoma may be the best alternative.[102]

Urethral Diverticulum or Anterior Urethral Valve

A urethral diverticulum occurs ventrally if the spongiosum is absent or has been thinned. The distal lip of the diverticulum functionally serves as an anterior urethral valve, blocking the urinary stream as it flows antegrade (Fig. 57-11). The diverticulum progressively fills and further compresses the urethra during

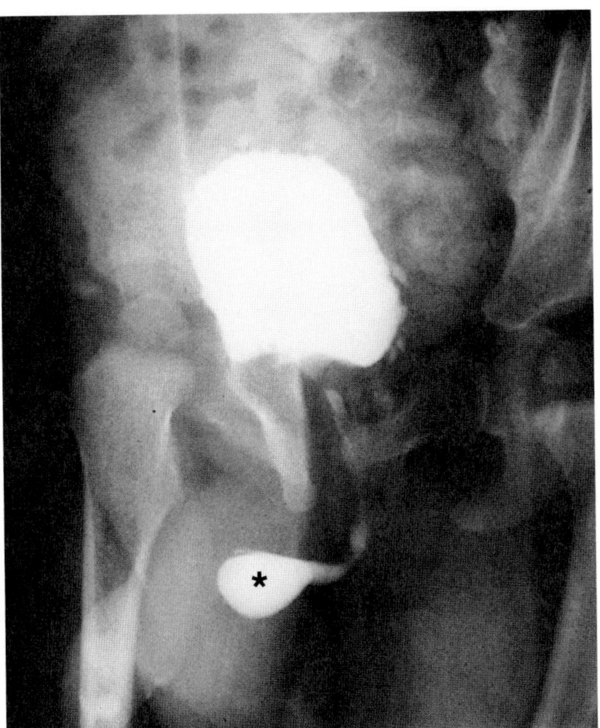

Figure 57-11. This voiding cystogram shows an anterior urethral diverticulum *(asterisk)* that functions as a valve, causing outflow obstruction. Note the bladder trabeculation.

urination. This valvular effect can cause marked proximal dilation.[124-126] In some cases, there is a diverticulum with a narrow neck that does not function as a valve. Such a diverticulum may allow stasis of urine and may be a site of urethral infection.

The diagnosis is made either by urethrogram or cystoscopy. Treatment can be accomplished by endoscopic incision of the distal lip of the neck of the diverticulum or, if more pronounced, by open excision and closure of the urethral defect.[127]

Cowper's Duct Cyst

Cowper's glands are a pair of 5-mm glands located within the urogenital membrane. The ducts from these glands course distally and enter the ventral wall of the proximal bulbar urethra. These are the homologs of the female Bartholin gland. Occasionally, these ducts can become occluded, producing bulbar urethral filling defects and, rarely, modest obstruction.[128] Cystoscopically, this appears to be a thin membrane over a fluid-filled cyst, sometimes called a *syringocele*.[129] If contrast medium enters a Cowper duct, tubular characteristic channels can be seen coursing parallel to the bulbar urethra. Treatment of Cowper's duct cysts is endoscopic unroofing and is unnecessary unless the radiographic finding is associated with clinical symptoms.

chapter 58

POSTERIOR URETHRAL VALVES

Jack S. Elder, MD • Ellen Shapiro, MD

Posterior urethral valves (PUV) comprise the most common congenital anomaly causing bladder outlet obstruction in boys, with an incidence of 1 in 5000 to 1 in 8000 male births. Although the majority of boys with PUV are diagnosed before birth, in 24% to 45% renal insufficiency will develop during childhood or adolescence. PUV are the most common obstructive cause of end-stage renal disease in children.

EMBRYOLOGY AND ANATOMY

At 5 to 6 weeks' gestation, the orifice of the mesonephric duct normally migrates from an anterolateral position in the cloaca to Müller's tubercle on the posterior wall of the urogenital sinus. This event occurs simultaneously with the division of the cloaca. Remnants of the mesonephric duct normally remain as small distinct, paired lateral folds termed the *inferior urethral crest* and *plicae colliculi.* When the insertion of the mesonephric ducts into the cloaca is anomalous or too anterior, normal migration of the ducts is impeded and the ducts fuse anteriorly. This results in the formation of abnormal ridges, which are the PUV. Valves with a smaller aperture between the leaflets cause more obstruction and upper tract damage than do those with a larger aperture and a less prominent anterior component.[1]

Three distinct types of PUV have been described. The type I valve is an obstructing membrane that radiates distally and anteriorly from the verumontanum toward the membranous urethra (the segment of urethra that traverses the urogenital diaphragm or striated sphincter), fusing in the midline. Approximately 95% of PUV are type I, in which the valves are thought to be a single membranous structure with the opening positioned posteriorly near the verumontanum. The type III valve appears as a membranous diaphragm with a central aperture at the verumontanum. The obstructing tissue also has been termed a *congenital obstructing posterior urethral membrane.*[2] It is thought that instrumentation with a urethral catheter might disrupt the posterior aspect of the membrane, resulting in the appearance of a type I valve. Type II valves are prominent longitudinal folds of hypertrophied smooth muscle that radiate cranially from the verumontanum to the posterolateral bladder neck, but these are nonobstructive and clinically insignificant.

PRENATAL DIAGNOSIS, MANAGEMENT, AND OUTCOMES

About 10% of prenatally diagnosed obstructive uropathy is due to PUV, and approximately two thirds of PUV are diagnosed prenatally. Typical findings include bilateral hydroureteronephrosis, a distended bladder, and a dilated prostatic urethra, called a "keyhole" sign.[3] Discrete focal cysts in the renal parenchyma are diagnostic of renal dysplasia. Amniotic fluid volume is variable. Those with normal or slightly reduced amniotic fluid have a better prognosis. In contrast, oligohydramnios suggests significant obstructive uropathy or renal dysplasia (or both) and pulmonary hypoplasia is common. The gestational age at which hydronephrosis is recognized also influences prognosis. In one study, fetuses with PUV and normal-appearing renal anatomy after 24 weeks were much more likely to have normal renal function than were those with hydronephrosis recognized before 24 weeks.[4] Prenatally, PUV, prune-belly syndrome, urethral atresia, and bilateral high-grade vesicoureteral reflux (megacystis-megaureter syndrome) may have a similar appearance. The presumptive diagnosis of PUV cannot be confirmed until postpartum radiologic studies are performed.

In the fetus with suspected PUV and normal amniotic fluid volume, serial fetal sonograms are necessary to monitor the status of the hydronephrosis and amniotic fluid volume. If oligohydramnios develops, prenatal drainage of the bladder may be beneficial. It is thought that oligohydramnios prevents normal fetal movement, chest mobility, and lung development in utero. Pathologically, this process results in reduced branching of the bronchial tree and reduced numbers and size of alveoli.[5]

In the fetus with suspected PUV, a karyotype should be obtained because chromosome abnormalities occur in about 12% of fetuses with bilateral hydroureteronephrosis and bladder distention.[6] Moreover, it is important to verify that the fetus is a male. Fetal renal function also must be assessed. Discrete renal cysts are diagnostic of renal dysplasia. Assuming renal cysts are absent, fetal urinary electrolytes and β_2-microglobulin provide the most accurate means of evaluating fetal renal function. Normally, fetal urine is hypotonic, with sodium less than 100 mEq/L, chloride less than 90 mEq/L, and osmolality less than 210 mEq/L.[3] Elevated fetal urine electrolytes and β_2-microglobulin levels are an indication of irreversible renal dysfunction. Sequential bladder aspiration every 48 to 72 hours should be performed, because the initial sample may be stale and new urine that forms more accurately reflects the function of the fetal kidneys.[7,8]

If fetal urine is hypotonic, and oligohydramnios is present, then fetal intervention should be considered, with a goal of preventing life-threatening pulmonary hypoplasia. This procedure has been performed in the first trimester,[9] although the majority of fetuses are in the second trimester. No evidence exists that drainage of the fetal bladder obstructed by PUV will improve renal or bladder function. Therefore, the family should understand that even if the drainage procedure is successful the infant may have limited renal function or end-stage renal disease. If the gestational age of the fetus is 32 weeks or more, early delivery is advisable. If the fetus is less than 32 weeks' gestation, however, the urine may be diverted into the amniotic fluid with a percutaneously placed vesicoamniotic shunt, which has a pigtail on each end. In a few centers, in-utero cutaneous vesicostomy or ureterostomy has been performed.[10] Percutaneous in-utero endoscopic ablation of PUV also has been reported,[11-13] but few centers have the instrumentation or technical expertise to perform this procedure.

Vesicoamniotic shunts have limitations.[5,6] They become obstructed or displaced in 25% of cases, necessitating additional procedures that increase morbidity to the mother and fetus and a 5% procedure-related rate of fetal loss. In addition, omental or bowel herniation through the fetal abdominal wall may occur. Despite adequate bladder drainage, renal function may be so limited that the amniotic fluid volume remains low. In one study of high-risk fetuses identified in the first trimester with severe bilateral hydroureteronephrosis, bladder distention, and oligohydramnios managed with a vesicoamniotic shunt, a 60% overall survival rate and a 33% incidence of renal failure were found.[14] In a review of 14 fetuses with proven PUV and favorable fetal urinary electrolytes undergoing fetal intervention at a mean gestational age of 22.5 weeks, six deaths occurred before term delivery and 8 survived, with a mean follow-up of 11.6 years.[10] Of these 8 neonates, 3 had end-stage renal disease, and the other 5 had an elevated serum creatinine value. In a more optimistic study of 20 boys with "lower urinary tract obstruction" managed by in-utero vesicoamniotic shunt, the overall 1-year survival was 91%. In this study, the mean birth weight was 2574 g, 40% had acceptable renal function, 20% had mild renal insufficiency, and 30% required dialysis.[15] Of this group, 7 had PUV and 7 had prune-belly syndrome, a nonobstructive condition. Clearly, patient selection is highly important. Consequently, when counseling families, one must emphasize that intervention may assist in keeping the fetus viable to term but will most likely not prevent the long-term sequelae of severe renal dysplasia associated with PUV.

CLINICAL PRESENTATION

Neonates with PUV who are not diagnosed before birth may appear in the nursery with delayed voiding or a poor urinary stream.[5] Respiratory distress secondary to pulmonary hypoplasia may be the only manifestation of severe urethral obstruction. Other common signs and symptoms include a palpable abdominal mass, failure to thrive, lethargy, poor feeding, urosepsis, and urinary ascites. A urinary tract infection (UTI) often develops in infants. Older boys may have persistent diurnal incontinence or abdominal distention as their only manifestations. Physical examination in the newborn typically discloses a palpable walnut-sized bladder, which corresponds to the hypertrophic detrusor muscle. If urinary ascites is present, significant abdominal distention is typical.

RADIOGRAPHIC EVALUATION

Postnatal ultrasonography usually shows significant bilateral hydronephroureteronephrosis. Demonstration of the corticomedullary junction is a favorable prognostic sign regarding renal functional potential (Fig. 58-1). Conversely, finding echogenic kidneys or subcortical cysts and the inability to see the corticomedullary junction on the initial and follow-up ultrasound studies are unfavorable signs. Suprapubic or perineal ultrasonography may demonstrate a dilated prostatic urethra, which is pathognomonic for PUV.

The voiding cystourethrogram (VCUG) remains the only radiographic study that definitively establishes the diagnosis of PUV (Fig. 58-2). The valve appears as a sharply defined perpendicular or oblique lucency in the distal prostatic urethra. The posterior urethra is dilated and elongated and has the appearance of a shield. The bladder is trabeculated with clear delineation of the bladder neck, which appears as a thick muscular collar because of hypertrophy. Vesicoureteral reflux (VUR) is present in 50%.

Renal nuclear scintigraphy with a technetium-99m–labeled dimercaptosuccinic acid (^{99m}Tc-DMSA) or mercaptoacetyltriglycine (^{99m}Tc-MAG3) scan should be performed if either kidney shows thin or abnormal parenchyma. These functional studies are useful in demonstrating baseline differential renal function. However, if renal function is poor, visualization of the kidneys is poor and the study should not be obtained. An alternative to renal scintigraphy is dynamic

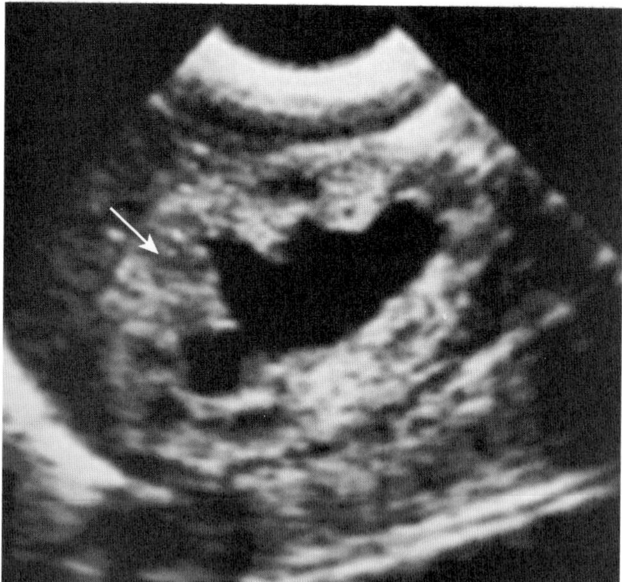

Figure 58-1. This renal sonogram demonstrates a hydronephrotic kidney with intact corticomedullary junction (*arrow*) in an infant with posterior urethral valves.

contrast-enhanced magnetic resonance urography. This study is being performed at a few pediatric urology centers and provides high-resolution renal images and assessment of differential renal function.[16]

INITIAL MANAGEMENT

The initial treatment of neonates suspected of having PUV is to decompress the urinary tract with a 5- or 8-Fr feeding tube passed transurethrally during the first ultrasound study immediately after birth. The catheter can be difficult to pass because of significant dilation of the prostatic urethra and hypertrophy of the bladder neck. A catheter coiled in the prostatic urethra will result in the majority of urine draining around the catheter. Ultrasonography confirms the placement of the catheter within the bladder. Insertion of a Foley catheter is discouraged because the inflated balloon can obstruct the ureteral orifices when the thick-walled bladder is decompressed, and it can cause severe bladder spasm that can obstruct the intramural ureters. Ampicillin or cephalexin prophylaxis should be initiated. Renal function, electrolytes, and fluid status should be monitored carefully. The serum creatinine concentration at birth reflects maternal renal function. With satisfactory newborn renal function, the creatinine value should gradually decrease to 0.3% to 0.4 mg/dL. However, with limited renal function, the creatinine value may increase, even with bladder drainage. Metabolic acidosis and hyperkalemia are common complications if renal function is impaired. Co-management of the patient with the pediatric nephrology service is often beneficial.

Neonates with respiratory distress may require immediate pulmonary resuscitation with endotracheal intubation and positive-pressure ventilation, which may cause a pneumothorax or pneumomediastinum. In rare cases, extracorporeal membrane oxygenation (ECMO) may be needed to support life until the diagnosis and prognosis are clearly defined.[17] If urinary ascites is seen, paracentesis may be necessary to correct fluid and electrolyte imbalance.

Renal ultrasonography and a VCUG should be performed expeditiously to determine whether the patient has PUV. Circumcision should be performed to reduce the risk of a UTI.

Primary Valve Ablation

Endoscopic valve ablation is performed after the neonate is stabilized medically. Well-lubricated infant urethral sounds should be passed gently to calibrate and stretch the urethra slightly. The neonatal male urethra usually accepts an 8-Fr endoscope. Overly aggressive dilation of the urethra to pass a larger instrument may lead to urethral trauma with subsequent stricture formation and should be avoided. Vigorous dilation may result in iatrogenic hypospadias due to splitting of the glans to the subcoronal level.[18]

An 8- or 9-Fr cystoscope typically is used with a Bugbee electrode on low cutting current inserted through the operating channel. The valve leaflets should be incised by using a low cutting current at the 5- and

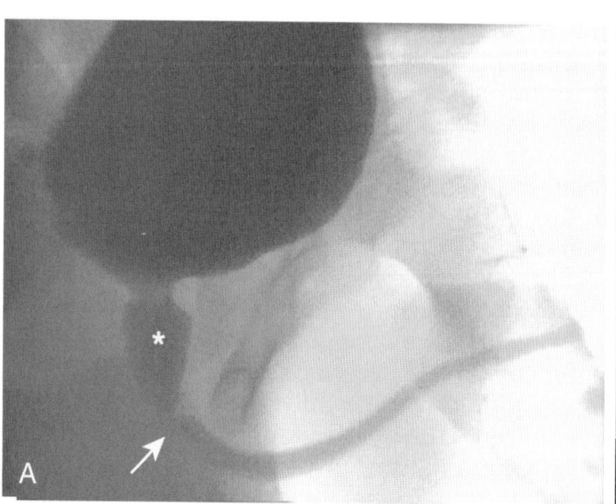

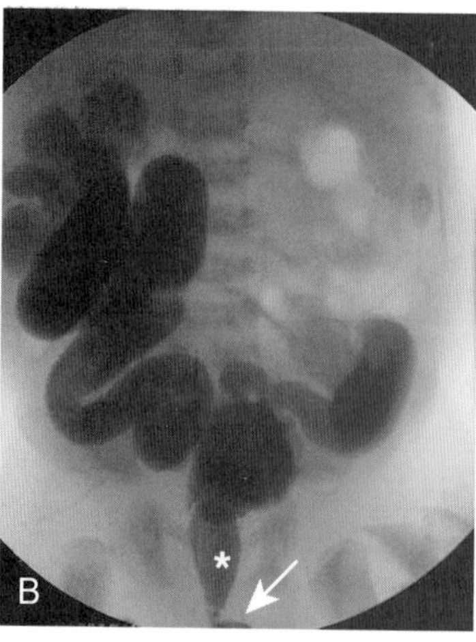

Figure 58-2. These two voiding cystourethrograms show varying degrees of obstruction from posterior urethral valves. In both studies the location of the valves is marked with an *arrow* and the posterior urethra is identified with an *asterisk*. **A,** There is no evidence of vesicoureteral reflux. **B,** There is massive, bilateral grade V reflux.

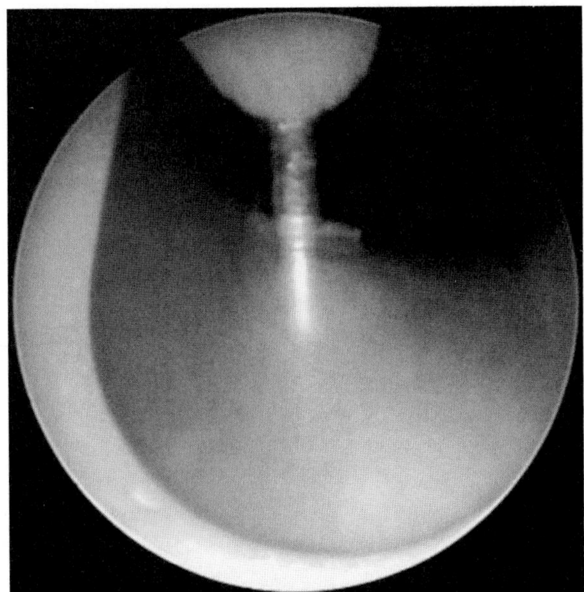

Figure 58-3. This cystoscopic view shows valve ablation with an electrode placed through the operating channel of the cystoscope.

7-o'clock positions (Fig. 58-3). Incision at the 12-o'clock position where the valve leaflets fuse also may be helpful. An alternative method of PUV ablation is to use the neodymium:yttrium-aluminum-garnet (YAG) laser.[19] In a premature or small neonate, a cystoscope as small as 6.9 Fr may be used, although the visualization of the PUV may be suboptimal. In a large infant, a pediatric resectoscope may be used. If urethral bleeding occurs, coagulation should be performed carefully, because urethral injury may occur with overzealous cautery. After valve ablation, a pediatric feeding tube is left indwelling for 1 to 2 days. In premature or small neonates, a temporary perineal urethrostomy for passage of the cystoscope or resectoscope may be helpful. Valve ablation also may be performed antegrade through a percutaneous cystostomy.[20]

A VCUG and renal sonogram should be obtained 2 to 4 weeks after ablation to confirm satisfactory valve disruption. In addition, renal function should be monitored carefully. PUV ablation is successful in more than 90% of patients. The most common complication is incomplete valve ablation, in which case repeat cystoscopy and valve incision is necessary. Urethral stricture is uncommon with the use of smaller endoscopic instrumentation and better optics.

One recent prospective study suggested that incision of the bladder neck at the time of valve ablation may be beneficial.[21] Boys who underwent bladder neck incision had a significantly lower rate of detrusor overactivity and a lower maximum voiding detrusor pressure when compared with age-matched boys who underwent valve ablation alone. Whether long-term differences will remain and whether these boys will experience retrograde ejaculation in adulthood is uncertain. Furthermore, these results need to be confirmed with other reports.

Temporary Urinary Diversion

An alternative to primary valve ablation is cutaneous vesicostomy (Fig. 58-4). This approach is appropriate in a small or premature neonate when the pediatric cystoscope is too large for valve ablation or if severe

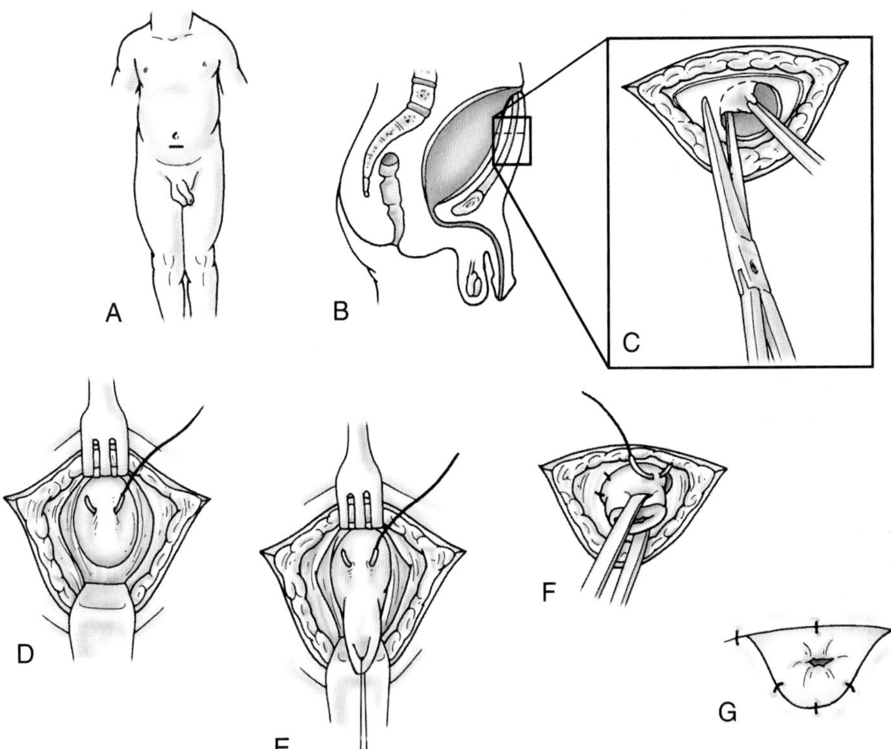

Figure 58-4. Technique of cutaneous vesicostomy. **A** to **C,** Transverse incision is made midway between the umbilicus and pubic symphysis. **D** and **E,** Traction sutures are placed through the bladder, and it is mobilized superiorly to the dome of the bladder. **F,** The detrusor should be fixed to the rectus fascia. The bladder is opened, and the mucosa is sutured to the skin. **G,** Completed vesicostomy should be calibrated to 24 Fr.

hydroureteronephrosis, urinary ascites, or high-grade reflux with poor renal function is present. In these cases, optimal drainage is necessary to maintain existing renal function. The most popular technique was described by Blocksom and popularized by Duckett.[22] A small transverse incision is performed midway between the umbilicus and pubic symphysis, and the dome of the bladder is brought to the skin. The vesicostomy should calibrate to 24 to 26 Fr to avoid stenosis. Daily dilation of the stoma with a plastic medicine dropper helps prevent contraction of the stoma. The vesicostomy drains into the diaper, and no urinary collection device is necessary. Complications include stomal stenosis, if the stomal size is less than 24 to 26 Fr, and prolapse, if the anterior wall of the bladder is exteriorized rather than the bladder dome.

When a cutaneous vesicostomy is performed, valve ablation should not be performed simultaneously because the urethra may remain dry and urethral stricture is likely. A vesicostomy allows the bladder to cycle and grow with voiding at low pressure through the stoma and does not reduce bladder capacity. These neonates should be maintained on antibiotic prophylaxis.

In the past, proximal high diversion with cutaneous pyelostomy or cutaneous ureterostomy was advocated for neonates and infants with severe hydronephrosis and a persistent elevated creatinine after catheter drainage.[22a] Theoretically, proximal diversion provides better renal drainage than does a vesicostomy, particularly with ureterovesical obstruction, and optimizes the potential for ultimate renal function and somatic growth. However, this form of therapy has not been shown to prevent end-stage renal disease, because at least 85% of these patients have renal dysplasia.[23] In addition, by diverting the urine away from the bladder, regular cyclic vesical filling and contraction does not occur and results in a smaller, less compliant bladder.[24] Consequently, proximal diversion is reserved for the rare case in which valve ablation or vesicostomy fails to improve upper tract drainage or if urosepsis occurs secondary to pyelonephritis.

The preferred method of proximal diversion is the Sober-en-T ureterostomy, in which the proximal ureter is divided and brought out to the abdominal wall (Fig. 58-5). The proximal end of the distal ureteral segment is then anastomosed to the renal pelvis. The advantage of this form of diversion is that it allows some urine to drain into the bladder and thus allows bladder cycling, while providing excellent upper tract drainage.[25] In one retrospective study of 36 boys who underwent bilateral Sober ureterostomies, the mean duration of diversion was 55 months. Bladder compliance was normal in 69%, and bladder capacity was normal in 80%.[26]

Total urinary reconstruction with valve ablation, ureteroneocystostomy, and excision of large bladder diverticula is another option in the initial management of the PUV patient. However, this approach is rarely indicated because significant improvement often occurs in VUR and bladder diverticula after ablation of the obstructing valve leaflets.

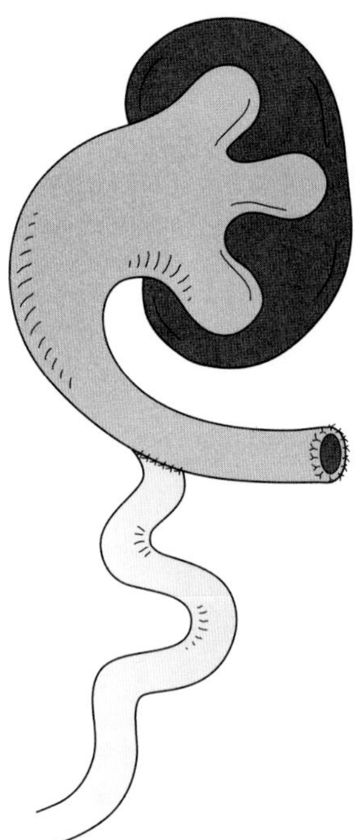

Figure 58-5. This diagram describes the Sober-en-T cutaneous ureterostomy, which is the authors' preferred method for proximal diversion in patients with posterior urethral valves. The proximal ureter is divided and exteriorized on the abdominal wall. The proximal end of the distal ureteral segment is then anastomosed to the renal pelvis.

Urinary Extravasation

A special management issue is urinary extravasation, which occurs in 5% to 15% of neonates with PUV.[27,28] Forniceal rupture or renal parenchymal blowout with transperitoneal transudation or intraperitoneal leakage after bladder rupture may occur. Some infants develop a perirenal urinoma, whereas others have urinary ascites (Fig. 58-6). In one recent retrospective series of urinomas in boys with PUV, there was no increased risk of end-stage renal disease or VUR compared with unaffected boys.[28] Moreover, the differential renal function of involved and uninvolved kidneys was similar. However, with urinary ascites, significant electrolyte abnormalities may result from urinary reabsorption and respiratory compromise may occur. The goals of initial management are to determine the site of extravasation and the level of function of the kidneys.

Evaluation for extravasation begins with ultrasonography, VCUG, and renal scintigraphy. The early uptake phase of a ^{99m}Tc-MAG3 renal scan often demonstrates which kidney is extravasating. Inserting a 5- or 8-Fr feeding tube into the bladder may decompress the bladder and upper urinary tract sufficiently that the forniceal extravasation stops. If the VCUG shows a bladder rupture, a cutaneous vesicostomy may be necessary. If the urinoma or ascites increases in volume, if the serum creatinine concentration continues to increase, or if respiratory compromise, infection, hypertension, or significant parenchymal compression is seen, percutaneous aspiration is needed. If extravasation continues,

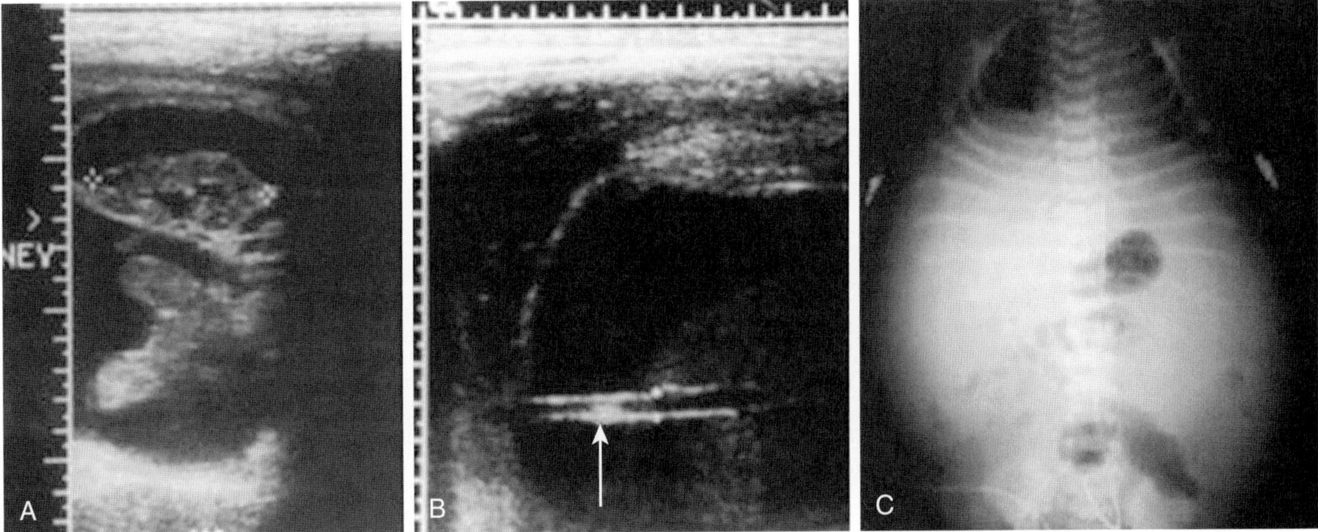

Figure 58-6. Posterior urethral valves and ascites. **A,** Prenatal ultrasound image demonstrating a perirenal urinoma around the right kidney, which is not hydronephrotic. **B,** Prenatal ultrasound image showing ascites and stretched umbilical vessels *(arrow)*. **C,** Plain radiograph of the abdomen in a neonate with a distended abdomen from ascites.

an upper tract procedure is usually required. If extravasation from a hydronephrotic kidney occurs, insertion of a percutaneous nephrostomy often solves the problem. Unfortunately, with forniceal extravasation, typically the kidney is decompressed. In these cases, the involved kidney should be explored through a small flank incision. The renal parenchyma should be inspected for evidence of rupture, and the parenchymal disruption should be repaired. In most cases, the kidney will be intact, indicating that the extravasation is from one of the calyceal fornices. A temporary cutaneous pyelostomy or ureterostomy may be performed to decompress the kidney. However, in most cases, mobilizing the kidney, separating it from the adjacent peritoneum, and leaving a Penrose drain in the retroperitoneum will allow the leak to resolve, provided PUV ablation or a cutaneous vesicostomy has been performed to decompress the lower urinary tract.

Follow-up after Initial Therapy

Antibiotic prophylaxis should be continued until the upper tract dilation improves, which may take several years. In addition, if the child has reflux, antibiotic prophylaxis should be continued until the VUR resolves spontaneously or is corrected surgically. Most patients benefit from long-term urologic management and nephrologic care initiated at birth. Common clinical problems include significant polyuria secondary to an inability of the kidneys to concentrate urine, metabolic acidosis (which may complicate somatic growth), renal insufficiency with hypocalcemia and hyperphosphatemia, and hypertension. If the patient remains clinically well with good somatic growth, periodic follow-up with ultrasonography, measurement of electrolytes, blood urea nitrogen, and creatinine, urinalysis, and blood pressure evaluations will ensure satisfactory growth and development.

PROGNOSIS AFTER INITIAL THERAPY

The prognosis for satisfactory renal function may be predicted from several factors. A serum creatinine concentration less than 0.8 mg/dL 1 month after initial treatment or at age 1 year is associated with favorable ultimate renal function.[29] Others have shown that the serum creatinine level after 4 to 5 days of catheter drainage is also predictive of long-term renal function.[30] Visualization of the corticomedullary junction on renal ultrasonography has been associated with a favorable outcome (see Fig. 58-1).[31] This radiologic finding may not be present on the initial ultrasound study but may become apparent during the first few months of life. Achieving diurnal continence by the age of 5 years indicates that minimal or no bladder dysfunction is present and is a favorable parameter.[32] Another favorable prognostic feature is the presence of a pressure pop-off mechanism such as massive reflux into a nonfunctioning kidney (termed *the VURD syndrome:* valves, unilateral reflux, dysplasia), urinary ascites, or a large bladder diverticulum (Fig. 58-7).[33] The concept is that the high intravesical pressure is dissipated, allowing more normal renal development. Although short-term studies have suggested that these mechanisms may allow more normal renal development, at age 8 to 10 years only 30% of boys with the VURD syndrome had a normal serum creatinine value.[34] One important favorable prognostic sign is a normal appearance of the contralateral kidney at diagnosis. These boys had no UTIs or incontinence with long-term follow-up.[35] Finally, absence of reflux on the initial VCUG is a favorable sign.

Adverse prognostic factors include bilateral VUR, persistence of the serum creatinine higher than 1.0 mg/dL after initial therapy,[36] identification of small subcapsular renal cysts (indicative of renal dysplasia), renal echogenicity,[37] and failure to visualize the corticomedullary junction.[31] In addition, failure to

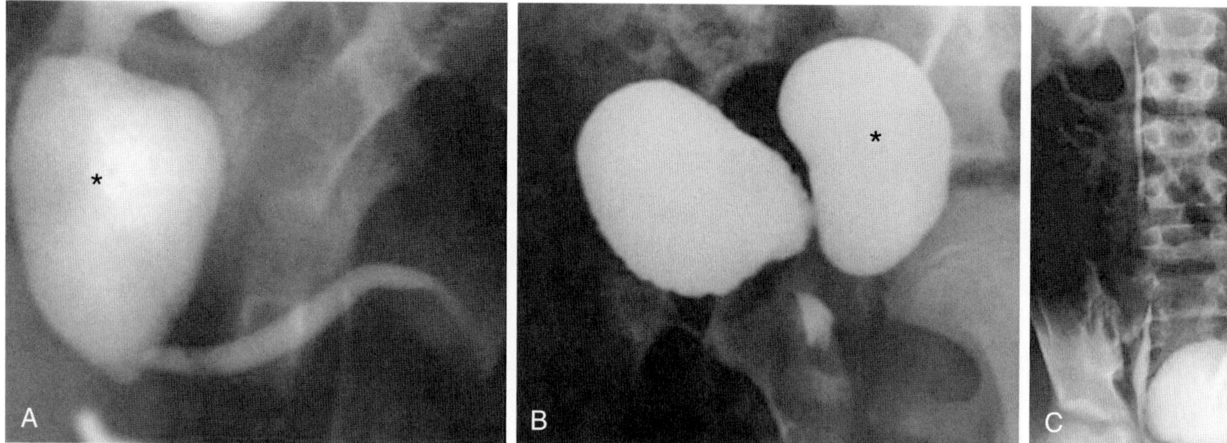

Figure 58-7. The VURD syndrome. A 7-year-old boy was found to have posterior urethral valves and a bladder diverticulum. **A,** The voiding cystourethrogram demonstrates a large, dilated posterior urethra (*asterisk*) secondary to the valves. **B,** The lateral view of this study shows a trabeculated bladder with a large bladder diverticulum (*asterisk*). **C,** The excretory urogram shows normal upper urinary tracts and deviation (*arrow*) of the distal left ureter due to the large bladder diverticulum. This boy underwent endoscopic valve ablation, excision of the bladder diverticulum, and left ureteroneocystostomy.

achieve diurnal continence is an indication of instability and detrusor sphincter dyssynergia, which can result in elevated upper urinary tract pressures and gradual deterioration in renal function and is associated with poor renal function.[2,26] Another adverse prognostic factor is the presence of the D allele in the angiotensin-converting enzyme genotype. These patients had a higher risk of renal scarring and breakthrough UTI.[38]

Review of studies of long-term renal functional outcome is difficult because of variable follow-up among study patients. In one report of 27 boys diagnosed between 1956 and 1970 with 31- to 44-year follow-up, 18% died at an early age and 11% were lost to follow-up.[39] Of the remaining surviving men, 32% were uremic, 21% had moderate renal insufficiency, and 40% had signs of bladder dysfunction. This study does not reflect the impact of early diagnosis with prenatal ultrasonography. For example, in a study of 79 cases of PUV prenatally diagnosed between 1987 and 2004, 65 had live births and all were managed with primary valve ablation. In follow-up, only 17% had renal failure and 76% of toilet-trained children were completely continent.[40] Early gestational age at diagnosis and presence of oligohydramnios were negative prognostic factors. In a prospective study of 46 cases of PUV, half were diagnosed prenatally and renal outcome was similar among those with prenatal versus postnatal diagnosis.[41]

The impact of late diagnosis also has been studied. In two large retrospective reports of late diagnosis of PUV (after age 5 years in one study and after age 2 years in the other), those with late diagnosis had a significantly higher creatinine concentration but bladder function was similar among the two groups.[42,43]

VESICOSTOMY CLOSURE

The decision to close the cutaneous vesicostomy should be made carefully. If breakthrough febrile UTIs have been noted, vesicostomy closure is important because it will reduce the risk of bacterial contamination of the urinary tract. In other patients, it may be necessary as a prerequisite to renal transplantation. In most cases, vesicostomy closure is performed after the upper urinary tracts have stabilized and the child is large enough to undergo simultaneous valve ablation, generally between ages 6 months and 3 years. Preoperatively, a VCUG should be obtained through the vesicostomy to assess whether significant vesicoureteral reflux is present and to evaluate the bladder appearance. In selected cases, urodynamics are helpful to assess bladder compliance.[44] If significant reflux is seen and the child is quite young, it is usually safe to simply close the vesicostomy and delay reflux correction until the child is older and the bladder is larger. After closure of the vesicostomy, the upper tracts should be monitored carefully to ascertain whether hydronephrosis is worsening and to be certain that the child is emptying the bladder satisfactorily.

VESICOURETERAL REFLUX

VUR is present in approximately 50% of boys with PUV at presentation, with half being bilateral and half unilateral. After valve ablation, nearly all patients will show improvement in reflux grade 1 year later.[24,45] Approximately 25% develop spontaneous resolution of the reflux. However, the reflux may not resolve for as long as 3 years after initial treatment, and resolution of high-grade reflux is unlikely.[46] Antibiotic prophylaxis is continued, and periodic upper tract imaging and cystography should be performed. Renal deterioration without infection may be a sign of bladder dysfunction. Lower tract evaluation with videourodynamics is important.

Reflux should be repaired surgically if breakthrough infections occur or if it remains high grade. The efficacy of endoscopic injection therapy has not been proved, but its use remains an option. Most pediatric

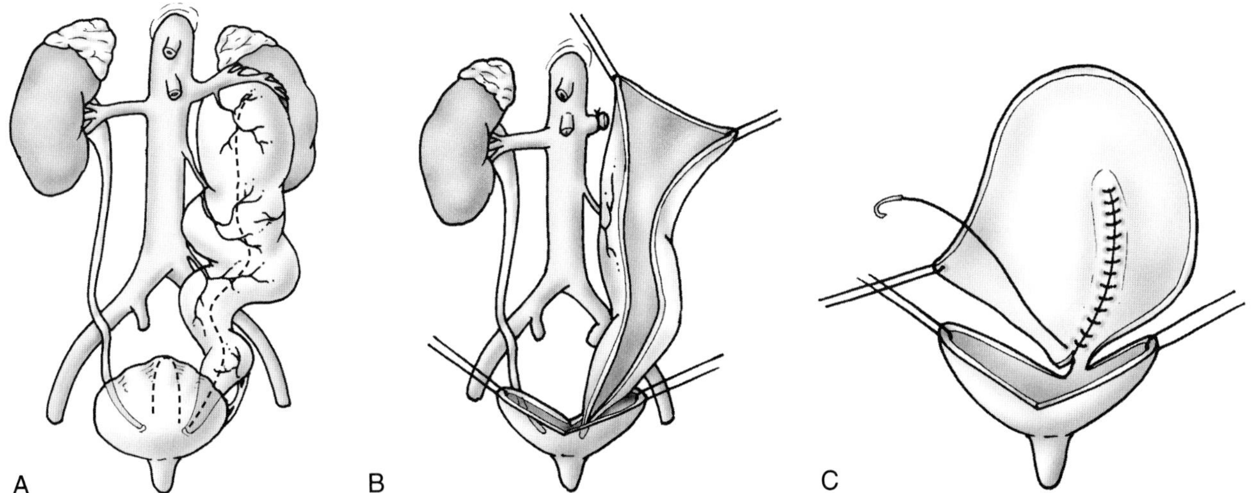

Figure 58-8. Technique of ureterocystoplasty. **A,** Left nonfunctional kidney and ureter is exposed. **B,** After the left kidney is removed, the ureter is spatulated medially. **C,** Left ureter is folded into a "U" and sutured to opened bladder.

urologists are adept at performing ureteral reimplantation surgery, but reimplanting thick, dilated ureters into the abnormal valve bladder can be most challenging. A 15% to 30% complication rate has been reported, most often persistent reflux or ureteral obstruction.[47,48] If bilateral high-grade VUR is found, a transureteroureterostomy may be performed in conjunction with a single, long, tapered reimplant and a psoas hitch. However, if the single reimplanted ureter becomes obstructed, the upper tracts may deteriorate rapidly. If unilateral high-grade reflux into a kidney with reasonable function occurs, transureteroureterostomy into the nonrefluxing ureter is an option.

In boys with the VURD syndrome, a nephrectomy should be performed at some point. The ureter should be removed, unless the bladder is small and/or poorly compliant. In this case, a ureterocystoplasty can be considered (Fig. 58-8). After this procedure, the remaining kidney should be monitored carefully for the development of hydronephrosis because the pressure "pop-off" mechanism has been removed.

BLADDER DYSFUNCTION AFTER INITIAL THERAPY

The prognosis for boys with PUV depends on the status of the kidneys and the bladder at the time of diagnosis and the method of bladder management as the child grows. In as many as 40% with PUV, end-stage renal disease or chronic renal insufficiency develops, and the vast majority of these boys have voiding dysfunction.[32] Many boys with PUV have a spectrum of urodynamic abnormalities that change. For example, in a study of 16 prepubertal boys seen before age 1 year and observed from ages 4 to 14 years, initial bladder instability was observed.[49] Over time, however, the instability improved and the bladder capacity increased. In this study, postpubertal boys had high-capacity bladders with low contractility, causing difficulties in detrusor emptying. Other groups have reported similar findings.[50,51]

The cause of the bladder dysfunction is incompletely understood, but experimental evidence suggests that fetal urethral obstruction causes irreversible changes in the smooth muscle cells of the bladder[52,53] and results in deposition of type III collagen in the bladder wall. The bladder abnormalities are manifested as incontinence or persistent hydronephrosis (or both). Boys with significant urodynamic abnormalities are most likely to experience severe renal functional impairment.[54]

As many as half of boys with PUV have ongoing daytime incontinence into late childhood.[32,55] In the past, it was thought that incontinence resulted from sphincteric incompetence from urethral maldevelopment or injury to the sphincter during valve ablation. However, it has become apparent that significant urodynamic abnormalities may persist after very satisfactory relief of bladder outlet obstruction.

Several potential causes for urinary incontinence are known in boys with PUV,[18,56] including the following:

1. Detrusor abnormalities such as (a) an overactive bladder secondary to uninhibited detrusor contractions, (b) overflow incontinence, (c) poor compliance, and (d) myogenic failure
2. High-pressure voiding secondary to incomplete valve ablation
3. Detrusor-sphincter dyssynergia in which the sphincter muscle fails to relax during bladder contraction
4. Polyuria secondary to a concentrating defect as a result of long-standing obstructive uropathy that causes renal tubular damage
5. Valve bladder, which is a bladder with poor compliance resulting from fibrosis secondary to long-standing obstruction. This clinical situation may cause secondary ureteral obstruction with worsening hydronephrosis if the bladder pressure is greater than 35 cm H_2O pressure.

Consequently, long-term therapy for the boy with PUV includes management of the bladder as well as attention to renal function.

Table 58-1 Pathophysiologic Changes in the Valve Bladder Syndrome

Organ	Pathologic Process	Clinical Effect
Kidney	Dysplasia, renal tubular dysfunction	Poor renal function; polyuria
	Urine concentrating defect (polyuria)	Rapid filling of bladder, causing persistent hydroureteronephrosis and incontinence
	Renal tubular acidosis	Impaired somatic growth, bone demineralization
Ureters	Dilated with poor peristalsis	Large dead space Increased risk of urinary tract infection
	Fibrosis secondary to previous surgical procedures or infection	Poor drainage of upper tract Possible obstruction after ureteral reimplantation
Bladder	Poor compliance; small volume	High bladder pressure most of the time
	Reduced sensation to high pressure	Progressive renal functional damage Incontinence
	Myogenic failure	Progressive renal and bladder damage
Bladder neck	Hypertrophy	Poor bladder emptying Voiding dysfunction Incontinence

From Close CE: The valve bladder. In Gillenwater JY, Grayhack JT, Howards SS, et al (eds): Adult and Pediatric Urology, 4th ed. Philadelphia, Lippincott Williams & Wilkins, 2002, pp 2311-2318.

The Valve Bladder

An understanding of the pathophysiology of the obstructed bladder allows one to develop an effective therapeutic approach to treatment. Several factors are present in patients with persistent hydroureteronephrosis after valve ablation: (1) the hydroureteronephrosis is associated with a noncompliant thick bladder wall; (2) most have diurnal incontinence; (3) incontinence is secondary to increased urine output and decreased bladder compliance; (4) acquired diabetes insipidus is the cause of the high urine output; and (5) the high urine output contributes to the hydroureteronephrosis.[57]

In 1982, the valve bladder syndrome was described.[58,59] In one series of 70 boys with PUV, 16 had polydipsia, polyuria, incontinence, hydroureteronephrosis without VUR, poorly sensate bladders, and poorly compliant bladders with high pressure at low urine volumes.[58] Normally the bladder stores urine at low pressure, allowing unimpeded drainage from the kidneys. With a poorly compliant bladder, however, as the bladder fills, the intravesical pressure increases quickly, causing a functional barrier to upper tract drainage, resulting in progressive hydroureteronephrosis. This high intravesical pressure contributes to the gradual deterioration in renal function.

The spectrum of physiologic abnormalities in boys with the valve bladder syndrome is shown in Table 58-1. The obstructed kidney often develops an irreversible urinary concentrating defect secondary to tubular injury. Despite fluid restriction, an enormous obligate urine output can be seen and may be as high as 3 L/day. This polyuria causes decompensation of the bladder, incontinence, and persistent backpressure on the upper urinary tracts, with persistent hydroureteronephrosis.

Persistent ureteral dilation causes inefficient ureteral wall coaptation and poor peristalsis, which predisposes to UTI. Fibrosis from previous infection or previous ureteral surgery may result in inefficient ureteral peristalsis and increases the risk of obstruction after ureteral reimplantation. In the past, persistent hydroureteronephrosis was thought to result from ureterovesical junction obstruction. Upper tract pressure/volume (Whitaker test) studies with the bladder empty and full have demonstrated that in the vast majority of cases unimpeded drainage into the bladder occurred with the bladder empty. As the bladder filled, with increasing intravesical pressure, increasing hydroureteronephrosis and increasing renal pelvic pressure were found.[58] Consequently, ureteral reimplantation in these patients with the goal of relieving ureterovesical junction obstruction has a high risk of failure and worsening hydronephrosis. In a recent series of 71 boys with PUV, persistent hydroureteronephrosis was noted in 20 patients (28%).[60] All of the patients with persistent hydroureteronephrosis had abnormal urodynamic findings, primarily poor compliance and instability. Aggressive treatment showed dramatic improvement or complete resolution of upper tract changes and urodynamic parameters.

Boys with a poorly compliant or unstable bladder often tolerate high intravesical pressures without discomfort. As a result, they delay voiding and experience overflow incontinence. Because of the high intravesical pressure, ongoing renal functional damage occurs. In addition, polyuria causes volume stress and contributes to chronic overdistention of the bladder. Effective bladder emptying is difficult to accomplish because of poor detrusor function and rapid refilling of the bladder. Double or triple voiding often is necessary to empty the bladder and the upper tracts, but compliance with this regimen often is not very good.

Bladder neck hypertrophy is a component of the overall detrusor hypertrophy that results from bladder outlet obstruction. After valve ablation, significant residual muscular hypertrophy may persist, resulting in functional bladder outlet obstruction with poor emptying. In the past, YV-plasty of the bladder neck was performed, but incontinence and upper tract changes persisted because of the aforementioned factors. In addition, a late complication of this procedure is retrograde ejaculation. Consequently, bladder neck surgery should be avoided unless urodynamic and radiographic documentation of intractable bladder neck obstruction is found.

Can the Valve Bladder Be Prevented?

Several clinical observations allow one to formulate a treatment plan to try to minimize the risk of developing a valve bladder. One factor relates to the primary form of therapy. In many boys with PUV, severe hydroureteronephrosis and an elevated serum creatinine concentration are present. In the past it was thought that performing cutaneous pyelostomies in the most severe cases would result in optimal upper tract decompression and give the kidneys the best chance of having unimpeded drainage. Indeed, evidence was found that these boys had better somatic growth compared with boys who underwent valve ablation alone.[22] However, it is difficult to document any case in which cutaneous pyelostomies have prevented end-stage renal disease. In addition, it became apparent that boys with proximal diversion ultimately had a small bladder that required augmentation cystoplasty. On the other hand, after valve ablation or cutaneous vesicostomy, the bladder typically grows satisfactorily, presumably because of urinary growth factors and ongoing cycling of the bladder.[61-63]

Management of Bladder Dysfunction

Close follow-up is important after valve ablation. A VCUG should be performed to document that bladder outlet obstruction has been relieved. Serial renal sonograms and serum creatinine and electrolytes are necessary. Renal scintigraphy is necessary if evidence of renal dysfunction on either side is found. If VUR is present, serial VCUGs are necessary until the reflux is minimal or absent. Urodynamic evaluation is important with persistent hydroureteronephrosis to confirm that resting and filling bladder pressures are in a safe range, less than 30 cm H_2O. Furthermore, detrusor instability or hypocontractility can be documented. In addition, uroflowmetry and sonographic assessment of postvoid residual urine volume are helpful. Having these patients followed by a pediatric nephrologist is invaluable because renal tubular acidosis, renal insufficiency, end-stage renal disease, and somatic growth abnormalities are common.

If significant polyuria and incontinence are found, timed voiding every 1 to 2 hours is beneficial. In addition, double or triple voiding provides more efficient emptying of the bladder and upper urinary tracts.

If a poorly functioning or nonfunctioning hydronephrotic kidney is noted, nephrectomy or nephroureterectomy should be performed. Usually this procedure can be performed laparoscopically. Before proceeding, however, the potential need for lower urinary tract reconstruction should be assessed because the dilated ureter can be used to augment the bladder. This augmentation procedure can be incorporated into the overall reconstruction.

If urodynamic studies demonstrate detrusor instability, anticholinergic therapy is necessary. Several medications may be used. Oxybutynin chloride suspension or tablets are effective but may cause side effects such as dry mouth, facial flushing, constipation, and blurring. The medication lasts 4 to 6 hours and generally is administered three times daily. The maximum dosage is 1 mg per year of age, three times daily, with a maximum of 5 mg, three times daily. Sublingual hyoscyamine also may be effective, has fewer side effects than oxybutynin, but is given four times daily. In recent years, tolterodine has been useful in children older than age 6 years, given in doses of 1 to 2 mg twice daily. Tolterodine has fewer side effects than oxybutynin chloride. There are also long-acting forms of oxybutynin and tolterodine with fewer side effects.

If bladder hypocontractility is present, clean intermittent catheterization usually is necessary. Learning this technique initially may be difficult for boys and their families. With persistence and support from the medical team, however, most adapt to intermittent catheterization, particularly if it improves or cures their incontinence. Intermittent catheterization tends to reduce bladder instability and improves bladder compliance.[51] In some cases, a continent appendicovesicostomy (Mitrofanoff procedure) can be performed to allow intermittent catheterization with less patient discomfort.

If detrusor-sphincter dyssynergia with inadequate bladder neck relaxation is found, treatment with an α-adrenergic blocker may be beneficial. In a study of 55 children with a variety of causes of non-neuropathic voiding dysfunction, administration of doxazosin, 0.5 to 2.0 mg daily, resulted in a significant improvement in urine flow rate, reduction in postvoid residual urine volume, and improvement in incontinence.[64] Few had significant side effects.

An important recent concept is that some of the changes that result in the valve bladder syndrome result from bladder overdistention at night, secondary to polyuria and failure to empty the bladder regularly during sleep. To address this issue, overnight catheter drainage has been used with moderate success, resulting in significant improvement in hydroureteronephrosis and improved voiding dynamics during the day.[65,66] This therapy should be strongly considered in boys with valve bladder syndrome.

If urodynamic studies demonstrate a poorly compliant or small-capacity bladder (or both), then augmentation cystoplasty is indicated. This procedure may alter voiding dynamics. Moreover, the addition of a noncontractile patch to the bladder in a boy who is emptying satisfactorily may result in a situation in which clean intermittent catheterization is necessary. In boys with PUV who undergo ureterocystoplasty, most need to perform intermittent catheterization after the operation.

Consequently, creation of a "back-up" continent stoma (appendicovesicostomy) in conjunction with an augmentation cystoplasty should be considered.

Several options exist for augmentation cystoplasty. Ureterocystoplasty results in the fewest long-term complications, but a dilated ureter is a prerequisite for this procedure (see Fig. 58-8). Ureterocystoplasty generally is performed in conjunction with removal of a nonfunctioning kidney. In these cases, the entire ureter can be used to augment the bladder. If both kidneys have satisfactory function, another option is to use the lower half of the dilated ureter for bladder augmentation and to perform a proximal transureteroureterostomy. The ureter is opened on its medial border through the ureterovesical junction. If the dilated ureter is long, then it may be folded onto itself in the shape of a "U" and sutured to the opened bladder. Although long-term results with this procedure are favorable, in one recent series 23% subsequently needed an ileocystoplasty.[67] If a dilated ureter is unavailable or the bladder needs more significant augmentation, then ileocystoplasty is the best option, assuming renal function is relatively normal.[68] Electrolyte abnormalities from absorption through the small bowel patch are uncommon. However, a generous amount of mucus is produced and regular bladder irrigation is necessary to prevent bladder calculi. Other potential long-term complications include chronic or recurrent bacteriuria and spontaneous bladder perforation from chronic overdistention. If renal function is limited, gastrocystoplasty should be considered. The advantage of this procedure is that the gastric patch secretes the hydrogen ion, and metabolic acidosis can be reversed or improved with the operation. In addition, unlike with small bowel, the patch is not absorptive. Furthermore, because the pH of the urine is low, the risk of UTI is reduced. The disadvantages of gastrocystoplasty include the need to extend the incision superiorly to the xiphoid process and the risks of severe metabolic alkalosis. In addition, some patients develop the hematuria/dysuria syndrome, characterized by intermittent severe dysuria and hematuria.[69] Furthermore, if the child has incontinence, a significant chance exists that he will experience a burning sensation where the urine leaks. Despite these potential problems, however, the long-term results with gastrocystoplasty are favorable.[70] Another option in patients with limited renal function is bladder augmentation with a patch of both ileum and stomach (gastroileocystoplasty), which avoids most of the problems associated with gastrocystoplasty.[71]

RENAL TRANSPLANTATION

Despite optimal management of boys with PUV, end-stage renal disease develops in 30% to 40%.[32] In many cases, impaired renal function can be stabilized during childhood. However, during adolescence, there is insufficient renal reserve and dialysis or renal transplantation becomes necessary. Retrospective studies of boys with PUV undergoing renal transplantation have suggested that the valve bladder may have a detrimental effect on graft survival. For example, in one study, a significantly worse 5-year graft survival was noted for patients undergoing transplantation for valve-related renal failure than was found in patients with nonobstructive abnormalities.[72] Other recent studies, however, demonstrated no difference in graft survival or serum creatinine levels between boys with PUV and children with nonobstructive causes of renal failure.[73,74] These data suggest that with intensive management of bladder function, a favorable long-term outcome can be expected.

FERTILITY

Few long-term studies have evaluated the reproductive status of men who were born with PUV. Theoretically, prostate function might be affected because of elevated urethral pressure during embryonic development and ongoing voiding dysfunction. In addition, some boys with PUV also undergo orchiopexy for cryptorchidism, which is associated with reduced fertility. Finally, in the past, some men have undergone YV-plasty of the bladder neck, which results in retrograde ejaculation. In one study of eight adolescents, sperm count was satisfactory in five, but most had abnormal sperm agglutination and a higher percentage of immotile sperm.[75] Three of the eight failed to ejaculate. In a long-term study, the ability to father children was dependent on whether the man was uremic.[39] In another study of 10 men, sperm counts were within the fertile range in all, but only 3 had initiated pregnancies.[76]

chapter 59

BLADDER AND CLOACAL EXSTROPHY

Michael Mitchell, MD • Richard Grady, MD

The exstrophic anomalies, often referred to as the exstrophy-epispadias complex,[1] are considered a spectrum of embryologic abnormalities related by certain anatomic features, including:

- *Epispadias*—considered the least severe anomaly in this spectrum; the urethra is a partial or complete open plate on the dorsal surface of the phallus.
- *Classic bladder exstrophy*—the most common of these unusual anomalies; the bladder is an open plate on the low abdominal wall and the urethra is epispadial.
- *Cloacal exstrophy*—the bladder and the ileocecal junction of the bowel are an open plate on the lower abdomen. This condition, commonly associated with other malformations, is also known as the omphalocele/exstrophy/imperforate anus/spinal defect (OEIS) complex.
- *Exstrophy variants*—partial manifestations are seen of the above anomalies.

Bladder exstrophy occurs at a rate of 1 per 10,000 to 1 per 50,000 live births.[2,3] This anomaly has long been recognized to occur more commonly in males than females, with a ratio of 3 to 6:1 reported in the literature.[4,5] Cloacal exstrophy occurs even more rarely, with an incidence of 1 in 200,000 to 1 in 400,000 live births[6] but is higher in stillborns at 1 in 10,000 to 1 in 50,000.[7]

BLADDER EXSTROPHY

Definite historical descriptions of bladder exstrophy date back to at least 1597 with von Grafenberg's description of this congenital defect. Possible depictions of exstrophy also exist on Assyrian tablets from 2000 BC. Chaussier first coined the term *exstrophie* to describe this defect in 1780 after detailed descriptions of it by Mowat in 1748. The natural history of bladder exstrophy is well known. The anomaly is not lethal, although it is associated with significant morbidity. Since the 19th century, various efforts to manage this condition have been described. Because exstrophic conditions are rare, these approaches were empirical and often unsuccessful. Until the 20th century, no effective surgical remedy was available to consistently ameliorate the morbidity associated with bladder exstrophy.

Bladder exstrophy occurs because the anterior portion of the bladder and/or urethra and the abdominal wall structures are deficient. Also, the pubic symphysis is widely separated from the midline in the majority of exstrophy anomalies. Initially, the bladder and urethra are herniated ventrally. The deformity has been described as "if one blade of a pair of scissors were passed through the urethra of a normal person. The other blade was used to cut through the skin, abdominal wall, anterior wall of the bladder and urethra, and the symphysis pubis; and the cut edges were then folded laterally as if the pages of a book were being opened" (Fig. 59-1).[8] Most of the exstrophic defects are typically found in isolation. Other organ systems are infrequently affected. However, children with bladder exstrophy typically have an anteriorly located anus. Female genital anatomy is altered with a more vertically oriented vaginal opening after closure and a wider and shorter vagina than normal. The anterior component of the penis is also foreshortened in males compared with the general population.

Currently, this spectrum of birth anomalies represent some of the most complex that pediatric urologists and surgeons manage. Although great strides in management have been made, many challenges still exist.

Diagnosis

The diagnosis of bladder exstrophy can be made antenatally, although many affected fetuses are not suspected to have exstrophy before birth.[9] Ultrasonography can reliably detect exstrophy before the 20th week of gestation.[10,11] Absence of the bladder is the hallmark of exstrophy. Other ultrasound findings include:

- A semisolid mass protruding from the abdominal wall[12]
- An absent bladder

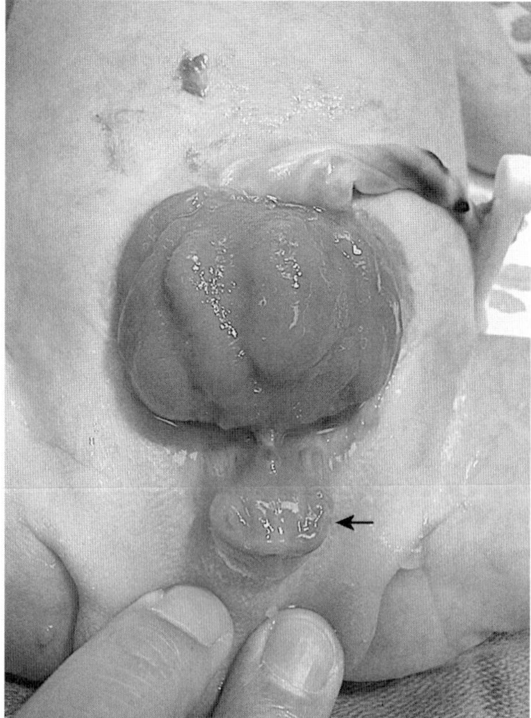

Figure 59-1. Bladder exstrophy in a male. The urethral mucosa is marked with the *arrow.* The corporeal bodies lie posterior to the urethral mucosa.

- A lower abdominal protrusion
- An anteriorly displaced scrotum with a small phallus in male fetuses
- Normal kidneys in association with a low-set umbilical cord[13]
- An abnormal iliac crest widening[10]

Subtle findings such as low umbilical cord insertion and the location of the genitalia will be seen only if the fetus is examined in a sagittal alignment with the spine.[14] Because exstrophy affects the external genitalia, the diagnosis is easier to make in males than females. Iliac crest widening can also be seen during the routine prenatal evaluation of the lumbosacral spine performed to evaluate for myelomeningocele. The iliac angle will be about 110 degrees rather than the 90 degrees that is normally seen.[14] Because urine production is normal for these fetuses, amniotic fluid levels should be normal.

Prenatal diagnosis allows optimal perinatal management of these infants. The infant can be delivered near a pediatric center equipped to treat neonates with this unusual anomaly. As importantly, prenatal diagnosis also allows the parents the opportunity to discuss early management of the patient. Prenatal counseling should include the expertise of a pediatric urologist or surgeon experienced in the treatment of bladder exstrophy. The overall prognosis for these children can be quite good if they are treated at medical centers with experience with this condition.[15]

In many areas of the developing world, early treatment remains problematic due to lack of health care infrastructure and resources to care for these patients. As a result, early diagnosis may not result in early treatment in these regions of the world. Management of these patients often includes delayed closure and adds another level of challenge to achieve optimum outcomes in this patient group. A recent overview from the KwaZulu-Natal region of South Africa highlights this problem.[16] Fifty-eight percent of the patients presented in a delayed fashion, and mortality rates approached 42% owing to concomitant medical conditions and poor primary health care.

Pathogenesis

In the scientific era, the cause of exstrophy was attributed to trauma to the unborn child causing ulceration of the abdominal wall down to the bladder. Today, we know that the developing human embryo does not normally pass through a stage that corresponds to exstrophy. This knowledge excludes arrested development as the cause and implicates an error in embryogenesis involving the cloacal membrane.[17] This membrane serves to separate the coelomic cavity from the amniotic space in early development and can be identified during development at 2 to 3 weeks of gestation. By the fourth week, it forms the ventral wall of the urogenital sinus with the unfused primordia of the genital tubercles sitting cephalad and lateral to it. With further development, the primordia grow and fuse in the midline and the mesoderm grows toward the midline, creating an infraumbilical abdominal wall. Simultaneous to this process, the urorectal septum develops medially and caudally to separate the cloaca into the urogenital sinus and rectum.[18]

One theory suggests exstrophy occurs because of a persistent cloacal membrane during fetal development.[19] Persistence of the membrane would create a wedge effect that keeps the medially encroaching mesoderm from fusing in the midline.[17] To further study this hypothesis, an animal model of cloacal exstrophy using the developing chick embryo was created. By placing a plastic graft in the region of the tail bud, cloacal exstrophy develops, perhaps due to persistence of the cloacal membrane.[17]

Other experimental models implicate the cloacal membrane in the pathophysiology of exstrophy as well but postulate that early disruption rather than persistence causes exstrophy. A model of cloacal exstrophy in the developing chick embryo created by using a CO_2 laser to create an early dehiscence in the tail bud caudal to the omphalomesenteric vessels suggests that exstrophy may be caused by failure of the mesodermal ingrowth between the ectoderm and endoderm of the cloacal membrane, which later ruptures to produce exstrophy. They hypothesize that such an event could be caused by early hypoxemic infarction in the region of the tail bud with subsequent cellular loss of the mesoderm and herniation of the developing bladder or cloaca.[20] This type of ischemic injury has been implicated as the cause of gastroschisis and could explain the spectrum of the exstrophy/epispadias complex.

Other proposed theories for exstrophy include caudal displacement of the paired primordia of the genital tubercles. According to one theory, exstrophy occurs when the primordia of the genital tubercles fuse caudal to their usual location relative to where the urorectal fold divides the cloaca into the urogenital sinus and rectum.[21] This theory readily explains the spectrum of variation seen in the exstrophy/epispadias complex. However, it fails to explain the higher incidence of bladder exstrophy compared with epispadias. One would anticipate a higher incidence of epispadias if caudal displacement were the underlying cause of exstrophy/epispadias because it would represent the least severe form of this phenomenon.[8]

A new maldevelopment theory was put forth recently for cloacal exstrophy based on a suramin-exposed chick model.[22] When these chick embryos were examined at 1 or 2 days after pericardial injection of suramin, approximately 8% were noted to have a midline infraumbilical opening into the cloaca and allantois, abnormal leg bud abduction, hypoplastic tail and allantois, broad infraumbilical pelvic region, and large aneurysmal dilation of the paired dorsal aortae at the level of the leg buds. The aortic dilation is transient, resolving 2 to 3 days after drug exposure but leaving maldevelopment. These authors implicate the aneurysmal paired dorsal aortae as the primary defects leading to cloacal exstrophy in this animal model. Pelvic maldevelopment has also been implicated in the pathogenesis of bladder exstrophy and explains both the bony abnormalities as well as soft tissue anomalies involved in this defect.[23]

The chick model to study bladder exstrophy has inherent limitations. Chicks normally possess a cloaca. Therefore, this precludes the creation of a bladder exstrophy versus a cloacal exstrophy. Other animal models to study bladder exstrophy have been difficult to create. In an exstrophy sheep model, a significant increase in the ratio of collagen to smooth muscle was noted in exstrophic versus normal control bladders ($P < .05$). There was no significant difference in the ratios of types I and III collagen in the two groups of sheep bladders. These histologic changes are similar in part to changes seen in human bladder exstrophy tissue.[24,25]

To date, the underlying cause of human exstrophy remains in question regarding whether the inciting event is related to an environmental exposure, an infectious pathogen, or another cause in genetically susceptible individuals. Epidemiologic studies, in fact, implicate a role for inherited susceptibility. Because of the associated physical anomalies with this condition, patients with bladder exstrophy often have to overcome significant obstacles to reproduce. Men may need to resort to assisted reproductive techniques (e.g., intracytoplasmic sperm injection[26]) because their seminal emissions drain from their ejaculatory ducts located at the base of their bladder plate, if at all. Furthermore, sexual intercourse due to the accompanying deformity of the phallus can be difficult for some of these patients, although the majority have the capacity for satisfactory sexual relations.

In the 1800s, males with bladder exstrophy were considered incapable of sexual activity because of the associated deformities of the penis.[27] Women with exstrophy are prone to uterine prolapse and miscarriage. Difficulty with conception and pregnancy are still a problem today despite in-vitro fertilization and careful obstetric care.[28,29] When combined, these issues may explain, in part, why familial patterns of inheritance of exstrophy-epispadias complex are noted infrequently. To date, 37 familial cases of bladder exstrophy have been reported, the most recent of which describes a mother and son with bladder exstrophy.[30] Five cases of an affected parent-child pair have been reported.[30-32] Another 18 cases with bladder exstrophy have been reported in twin pairs.[30] In 1984, a survey of pediatric urologists and surgeons reported 9 cases related to 2500 index cases of bladder exstrophy. This same series also reported on cases of twins and noted discordance in both fraternal as well as identical twinships.[32] Furthermore, in a study population of greater than 6 million births with 208 reported cases of exstrophy, no case had a family history for this anomaly.[33]

Current recommendations on counseling about the risk of recurrence in a sibling of a patient with exstrophy cite an estimate of about 1% and a 1:70 chance of transmission to the progeny of an affected parent.[31] A Florida population-based study found multiple births had a 46% increased risk of birth defects, with bladder exstrophy being the fifth highest adjusted relative risk.[34] These findings support a multifactorial etiology with evidence for genetic predisposition. More recently, an epidemiologic survey of families with bladder exstrophy found no link between exstrophy and parental age, maternal reproductive history, or periconceptional maternal exposure to alcohol, drugs, chemical noxae, radiation, or infections. Periconceptional maternal exposure to smoking was noted to be significantly more common in patients with cloacal exstrophy.[35]

Principles of Reconstruction

Current objectives for reconstruction in the treatment of exstrophy may be placed broadly in the categories seen in Table 59-1. Although these goals are straightforward and often interconnected, their successful achievement can be elusive. Many of the secondary goals address complications that can arise as a result or complication of surgical procedures used to treat exstrophy. Numerous operations have been devised for the treatment of bladder exstrophy in an effort

Table 59-1 Goals of Reconstruction

Primary Goals	Secondary Goals
Preservation of kidney function	Minimization of urinary tract infections
Urinary continence	Adequate pelvic floor support
Low pressure urine storage reservoir	Minimization of the risk for malignancy associated with the urinary tract
Volitional voiding	Minimization of the risk for urinary calculi
Functionally and cosmetically acceptable external genitalia	Adequate abdominal wall fascia

Table 59-2 Primary Pathophysiology of Bladder Exstrophy and Complications that Occur in Relation to its Management

Primary Pathophysiology (If Untreated)	Complications (Associated with Management of Exstrophy)
Malignancy (related to chronic exposure of the bladder plate)	Malignancy (related to the use of intestine in bladder reconstruction)
Pyelonephritis	Pyelonephritis
Kidney stones	Kidney and bladder stones
Total urinary incontinence	Stress or urge urinary incontinence
Chronic bladder irritation	Hydronephrosis
Pelvic floor insufficiency	Cystocele, uterine prolapse
Abnormal hip dynamics, back pain	Abnormal hip dynamics, back pain
Symphyseal diastasis, pelvic flattening	Urinary outlet obstruction
Abdominal wall defect	Absent umbilicus
Ventral and inguinal hernias	Incisional hernias
Severe penile shortening with dorsal chordee	Inadequate phallus in males with subsequent social and psychological sequelae

to achieve the goals above. The goals of surgery have expanded since the first operations were proposed and attempted in the 19th century. These objectives address the primary pathophysiology of exstrophy and the problems associated with this anomaly and its management (Table 59-2).

Natural History and Early Attempts at Treatment

Exstrophy anomalies are not fatal. Some untreated patients with classic bladder exstrophy have lived into their eighth decade.[36] However, significant morbidity exists with these conditions if they are left untreated, including total urinary incontinence, bladder and kidney infections, skin breakdown, and tumor formation in the bladder plate. The surrounding skin around the exposed exstrophic bladder is often inflamed secondary to urine contact dermatitis, loss of skin integrity from constant wetness, and secondary infection. Untreated inguinal hernias can be life threatening, and organ prolapse is especially challenging to manage later in this patient group. These patients are often social pariahs as well because of odor and hygiene problems. In contrast, when these patients receive effective surgical and medical treatment, they can lead productive, healthy lives with minimal morbidity from their underlying urologic abnormality.

Early forms of treatment were largely directed at protecting the bladder plate and controlling urinary leakage.[27] The morbidity associated with untreated exstrophy led physicians to develop empirical operative approaches for this anomaly, such as urinary reconstructive or diversion procedures. Initial efforts were directed at partial reconstruction of the abdominal wall to allow the application of a urinary receptacle to collect urine. Others performed urinary diversion through the creation of a ureterosigmoid fistula. These early results were poor. One patient died of peritonitis in the immediate postoperative period, and the other died of renal failure secondary to chronic pyelonephritis.[27] These early efforts were undertaken without an understanding of urinary tract and bladder physiology or how these operations would affect urine storage and emptying, kidney function, electrolyte homeostasis, the propensity for urinary tract infection, or urinary calculus formation.

Current Operative Approaches

A wide range of operations has been devised and performed to repair bladder exstrophy. These procedures lump themselves into two groups: (1) urinary diversion and (2) anatomic reconstruction. Surgeon preference and experience, patient anatomy, previous surgical procedures, timing of reconstruction, availability of tertiary care facilities, and access to medical care and resources all play a role in which operative procedures are chosen for a particular patient. Even in the 21st century, no standard of care exists for this patient population. However, with the complexity of care and the rarity of this congenital defect, specialists with an interest in the exstrophy-epispadias complex usually manage these patients most effectively.

Early surgical treatment remains particularly problematic in many areas of the developing world owing to lack of a uniform health care infrastructure and resources. As a result, early diagnosis may not result in early operative correction in these regions. Management in this setting often includes delayed closure, which adds another level of challenge to achieve optimum outcomes.

Urinary Diversion

Urinary diversion is not commonly used in the United States or most parts of Europe. This approach has generally been abandoned for an anatomically based approach. However, continent urinary diversion techniques can provide a more consistent degree of urinary continence with less surgical intervention than that achieved with functional reconstruction.[37] Reported rates of continence after primary reconstruction vary widely. Some urodynamic studies demonstrate low urine flow rates and poor contractility in patients after primary bladder reconstruction.[38,39]

Internal or incontinent urinary diversion avoids the complications associated with functional reconstruction, including urinary retention and subsequent kidney damage, and potential later dependence on clean intermittent catheterization (CIC) to empty the bladder. Advocates of early urinary diversion also cite a decreased risk of epididymitis and obstruction of the vas deferens by the creation of a receptacle with a suprapubic window at the level of the prostatic urethra. Diversion can also be combined with cosmetic and functional reconstructive operative procedures for the external genitalia.

Urinary diversion is also useful to achieve urinary continence in patients who have failed multiple attempts at functional reconstruction. Some also advocate primary urinary diversion for patients with bladder plates deemed too small to close. However, because we cannot accurately predict which bladder plates will increase significantly in size after primary closure, we do not use this as a criterion for primary diversion and do not divert the urine primarily in exstrophy patients.

Because of the difficulties encountered with functional bladder reconstruction in exstrophy, advocates of early urinary diversion argue that their approach achieves the primary goals of surgical intervention for bladder exstrophy with fewer operations and higher success rates than are achieved with bladder closure and urethral reconstruction. In fact, because of the dismal results associated with primary bladder reconstruction well into the 1970s, urinary diversion remained the treatment of choice for exstrophy in most of the world and still remains the treatment of choice in some regions today.

Given the successes with this approach, why abandon it? Long-term complications associated with ureterosigmoidostomy are significant and include hyperchloremic metabolic acidosis, chronic pyelonephritis, and a 250- to 300-fold increased risk of adenocarcinoma at the site of anastomosis.[40] Because of these complications, ureterosigmoidostomy was subsequently replaced by incontinent urinary diversions such as colonic and ileal conduits. A significant disadvantage to these forms of urinary diversion is the incontinent abdominal stoma associated with them. The popularization of CIC allowed the development of continent urinary diversions, which are now the preferred methods of nonorthotopic urinary diversion in areas of the world with access to medical supplies. Modifications to the ureterosigmoidostomy (described later) are currently used as well. Ultimately, any intestinal segment used for urinary storage confers a risk of bladder calculi, metabolic abnormalities, and malignancy that may be avoided with successful anatomic reconstruction.[41,42] As a consequence, although anatomic reconstruction may produce less consistent results, it has become the standard approach when possible.

Rectal Reservoirs

The Mainz II pouch and the Sigma pouch represent significant improvements to the ureterosigmoidostomy.[43,44] A rectal reservoir permits urinary continence without reliance on CIC. Renal preservation rates in children treated primarily with a urinary rectal reservoir (Mainz II pouch since 1991) approach 92%. Continence rates in school-age children approach 97% using this technique.[37] The Heitz-Boyer-Hovelaque procedure involves isolation of a rectal segment for ureteral implantation followed by posterior sagittal pull-through of the sigmoid colon to achieve both urinary and fecal continence. A small series using this procedure reported continence rates of 95% with acceptable complication rates.[45] Complications of this form of diversion continue to include fecal-urinary incontinence in patients with impaired anorectal sphincter control. Metabolic electrolyte imbalances can be treated with complete and frequent emptying of the rectal reservoir, which reduces the contact time between urine and the absorptive rectal mucosa. Oral bicarbonate replacement is also important. However, a significant risk of malignancy remains with using a rectal urinary reservoir. Various modifications of the rectal reservoir to prevent admixture of feces and urine may decrease the incidence of adenocarcinoma if the risk is due to conversion of urinary nitrates into carcinogenic nitrites by fecal bacteria.[46] Long-term results are not yet available. Methods to construct urinary diversions can be seen in Table 59-3.

Table 59-3 Surgical Options for Urinary Diversion

External Diversion (Continent Urinary Reservoir)	Internal Diversion (Rectal Sphincter–Based Continence)	Incontinent Diversions
Indiana pouch (cecal reservoir with ileal catheterizable channel)	Sigma pouch	Ileal conduit
Mainz pouch	Ghoneim reservoir	Colon conduit
Penn pouch (ileocecal reservoir with appendiceal catheterizable channel)	Gersuny	Ileocecal conduit
Kock pouch	Heitz-Boyer-Hovelacque	
	Rectal bladder with proximal colostomy	
	Ureterosigmoidostomy	
	Ileocecal ureterosigmoidostomy	

Anatomic Reconstruction

The first efforts at anatomic reconstruction of the exstrophic bladder were unsuccessful but did set the stage for an anatomic approach. In 1881, Trendelenburg described an exstrophy closure emphasizing the importance of pubic reapproximation in front of the reconstructed bladder to achieve continence and prevent dehiscence.[47] However, because of discouraging results, anatomic reconstruction was largely replaced by urinary diversion in the early part of the 20th century, although functional reconstruction was not entirely abandoned. Successful attempts at reconstruction did occur during this time.[48,49] Other primary reconstructive efforts also showed promise.[50,51] However, several large series of patients who underwent single-stage reconstruction in the 1960s and 1970s reported continence rates of only 10% to 30%.[52-57] Renal damage was as high as 90% in these series, generally because of bladder outlet obstruction.[52]

Because of these complications and the low rate of urinary continence with single-stage approaches, reconstructive surgical efforts were subsequently directed toward planned staged bladder reconstruction, an approach pioneered and advocated in the 1970s and further refined to what is now known as the modern staged repair of exstrophy (MSRE).[48,58-60] Recent advances in single-stage reconstruction for neonatal and older exstrophy patients have been advocated, and the complete primary repair for exstrophy (CPRE) has gained favor.[61]

All approaches aim to reconstruct and achieve anatomic and functional normalcy with minimal surgical morbidity. In the subsequent section, two currently popular surgical techniques, the CPRE and the MSRE, are detailed. Closure of the female with bladder exstrophy is somewhat similar in the CPRE and MSRE methods, with the end result being closure of the bladder, urethra, and abdominal wall. The difference is a more aggressive mobilization of the vagina and urethral plate into the pelvic diaphragm in the CPRE technique. In contrast, closure of the male with bladder exstrophy is quite different in the CPRE and MSRE. The CPRE closes and repositions the bladder and entire urethra at one stage. In contrast, the MSRE closes and repositions the bladder and posterior urethra at the first stage with the remainder of the urethra closed at a later date.

Preoperative Care

After delivery, to reduce trauma to the bladder plate, the umbilical cord should be ligated with silk suture rather than a plastic or metal clamp. A hydrated gel dressing may be used to protect the exposed bladder from superficial trauma. This type of dressing is easy to use, keeps the bladder plate from becoming desiccated, and stays in place to allow handling of the infant with minimal risk of trauma to the bladder. A plastic wrap is an acceptable alternative. Dressings should be replaced daily and the bladder should be irrigated with normal saline with each diaper change. A humidified air incubator may also minimize bladder injury.[62]

We routinely use intravenous antibiotics in the preoperative and postoperative period to decrease the risk for infection after reconstruction. We also perform preoperative ultrasonography to assess the kidneys and establish a baseline examination for later ultrasound studies. Preoperative spinal ultrasound examination should be considered if sacral dimpling or other signs of spina bifida occulta are noted on physical examination.

Operative Considerations

Ideally, the primary exstrophy closure is performed in the neonatal period. If the bladder template is amenable, early exstrophy closure has several advantages. A prompt closure begins the road toward anatomic normalcy. Early closure also decreases bladder exposure, which can lead to such histologic changes as acute and chronic inflammation, squamous metaplasia, cystitis glandularis and cystitis cystica, and muscular fibrosis, which may adversely impact ultimate capacity and compliance.[63] Electron microscopy has shown that the neonatal exstrophy bladder is "immature" when compared with that of control neonates,[64] having fewer small nerve fibers,[65] less smooth muscle, and a threefold increase in type III collagen content.[66] Although it is unclear whether these changes are a part of the primary pathologic process or secondary to the lack of bladder cycling in utero, it is conceivable that prompt closure could also "mature" the bladder by restoring bladder cycling. Similarly, clinical data have verified the importance of immediate postnatal bladder exstrophy closure. Infants undergoing closure before 7 days of age required fewer bladder augmentations to achieve eventual continence.[67]

Bladder template assessment is subjective. Even a small bladder template, if distensible and contractile, can enlarge to a useful size once closed. However, some choose to defer immediate surgery and reevaluate the bladder at 4 to 6 months of age with the neonate under anesthesia if the bladder template appears too small and stiff on initial assessment.[68] If at this date, the bladder continues to appear inadequate for primary closure, a nonrefluxing colon conduit may be used in combination with abdominal wall closure and epispadias repair. This can be converted later to a continent diversion or anastomosed to the rectosigmoid colon.

We routinely use general anesthesia. However, nitrous oxide should be avoided during primary closure because it may cause bowel distention, which decreases operative exposure during the operation and increases the risk of wound dehiscence. Some advocate the use of nasogastric tube drainage to decrease abdominal distention in the postoperative period, although we do not routinely use it postoperatively.[69] We also routinely place an epidural catheter to reduce the inhaled anesthetic requirement during the operation. Tunneling the catheter may reduce the risk for infection if it is left for prolonged periods after surgery.[70]

For patients older than 3 days, or neonates with a wide pubic diastasis, we perform anterior iliac osteotomies. In fact, we perform osteotomies in most patients unless the pelvis is very pliable. Robust neonates will often require osteotomy to optimize as low tension a closure as possible. Osteotomies assist closure and enhance anterior pelvic floor support, which may improve later urinary continence.[58,71]

Factors that appear to be important in the operative period include[72,73]:

- Use of osteotomies in selected cases and for neonatal closures more than 72 hours after birth to decrease the tension on the repair
- Ureteral stenting and bladder drainage catheters placed intraoperatively for use in the postoperative period to divert urine
- Avoidance of abdominal distention
- Use of intraoperative antibiotics

Complete Primary Repair for Exstrophy

Complete primary reconstruction of the exstrophied bladder is best done in the neonatal period. Primary reconstruction in the neonatal period is technically easier than in an older child. If one considers that the stimulus for bladder development is dependent on bladder cycling, then early complete closure offers the advantage of "normal" bladder development and the potential for urinary continence. The bony pelvis remains pliable in the neonatal period so that osteotomies may occasionally be avoided in some cases—usually if closure can be performed within the first 72 hours of life.

Clinical experience with patients with posterior urethral valves suggests that early restoration of nonobstructive emptying and filling of the bladder allows the bladder to regain some or all of its normal physiologic and developmental potential.[74] This implies that the bladder progresses through developmental milestones that occur in the first few months of life and that may be irreversibly lost if missed. Precedence for this form of organ development is found in the brain with the acquisition of language and visual perception. This is also true for skeletal and neuromuscular development. Finally, early primary bladder reconstruction creates a more normal appearance, which may foster improved bonding between the parents and their infant.

With the CPRE (or Mitchell operation),[61] the bladder, bladder neck, and urethra are moved posteriorly within the pelvis. This movement positions the proximal urethra within the pelvic diaphragm in an anatomically more normal position to maximize the effect of the pelvic muscles and support structures in the achievement of urinary continence. Posterior movement of the bladder neck and urethra also facilitates reapproximation of the pubic symphysis, which, in turn, helps prevent anterior migration of the urethra and bladder neck and provides a more anatomically normal muscular pelvic diaphragm.

Total penile disassembly reduces anterior tension on the urethra because it is separated from its attachments to the underlying corporeal bodies. These attachments otherwise pull the urethral plate anteriorly, preventing posterior placement of the proximal urethra and bladder neck in the pelvis. Tension reduction theoretically decreases the risk of bladder dehiscence and also temporarily reduces the dorsal tension on the corporeal bodies that may contribute to dorsal chordee in males. Combining the epispadias repair with primary closure allows for the most important aspect of primary closure—division of the intersymphyseal ligament or band located posterior to the urethra in these patients. Neonatal closure employing this technique optimizes the chance for early bladder cycling and consequent normal bladder development. It may also obviate the need for a multiple-staged repair of the exstrophied bladder, including further bladder neck reconstruction (BNR), bladder augmentation, and penile reconstructive surgery. This operation or its principles are also useful in some reoperative repairs or delayed repairs for exstrophy.

CPRE Surgical Technique: Boys

After standard preparation of the surgical field, transversely oriented traction sutures are placed into each of the hemiglans of the penis. The lines of dissection are marked (Fig. 59-2). Care is taken in marking these lines to exclude dysplastic tissue at the edges of the exstrophic bladder and bladder neck. This is particularly important at the bladder neck, where dysplastic tissue left in continuity may impair later bladder neck function. Following this, 3.5-Fr umbilical artery catheters are placed into both ureters and sutured in place with 5-0 chromic sutures. Bladder polyps are removed before beginning the dissection because these will act as space-occupying lesions after the bladder is reconstructed. Initial dissection begins superiorly and proceeds inferiorly to separate the bladder from the adjacent skin and fascia because it is usually easiest to identify tissue planes in this location. We use the tungsten fine-tip electrocautery during this dissection to reduce blood loss. The umbilical vessels may be ligated if necessary. We also incise the periumbilical skin circumferentially at this time. The umbilicus will be moved superiorly to a more anatomically normal location and will be used later as the location to exteriorize the suprapubic catheter.

Penile/Urethral Dissection. Traction sutures placed into each hemiglans of the penis aid in dissection at this point in the operation. The sutures will rotate to a parallel vertical orientation because the corporeal bodies will naturally rotate medially after they are separated from the urethral wedge (urethral plate plus underlying corpora spongiosa). We begin the penile dissection along the ventral aspect of the penis as a circumcising incision (Fig. 59-3A). This step precedes

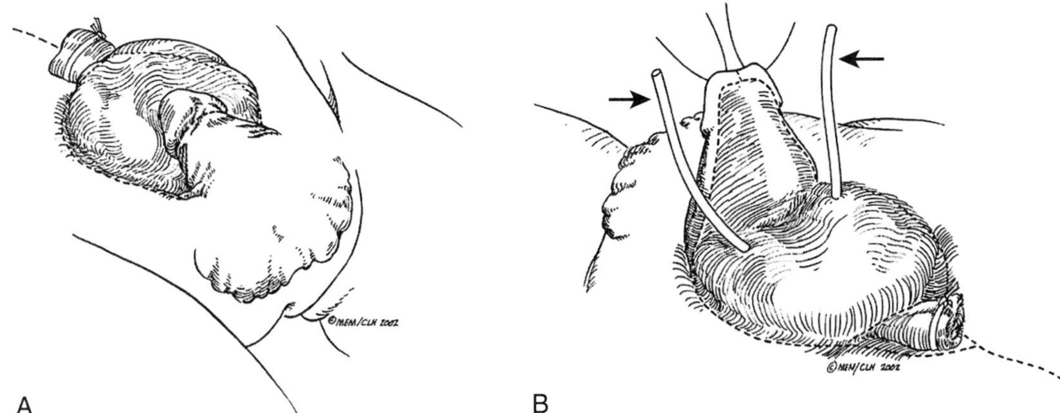

Figure 59-2. In a male undergoing complete primary repair for bladder exstrophy, the outlines of the planes of dissection are seen in these drawings. **A,** Ventral view. **B,** Dorsal view. The ureteral stents are marked with *arrows.*

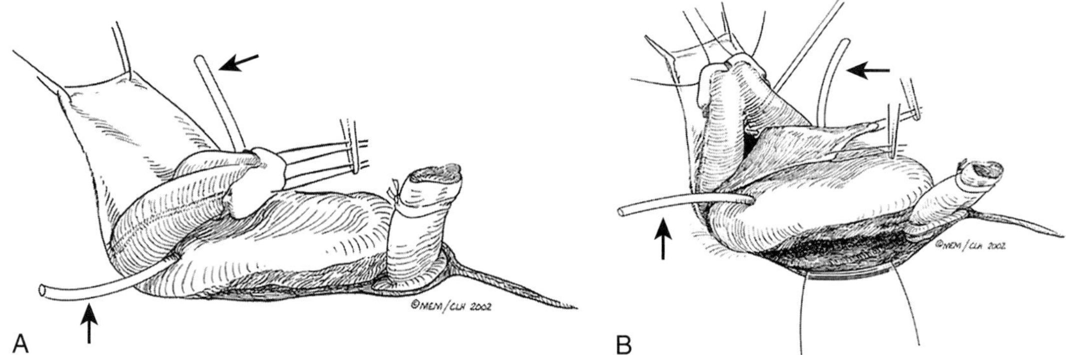

Figure 59-3. These two diagrams show early portions of the ventral subcoronal and corporeal dissection. **A,** Initiation of the subcoronal dissection is seen. This is typically the easiest plane to initiate dissection. **B,** Corporeal dissection proximally and dorsally is shown. Initiation of corporeal separation is easiest to establish proximally. Note the ureteral catheters (*arrows*), which have been introduced into the ureteral orifices.

dissection of the urethral wedge from the corporeal bodies because it is easier to identify the plane of dissection ventrally above Buck's fascia. Buck's fascia is deficient or absent around the corpora spongiosa. As the dissection progresses medially to separate the urethra from the corpora cavernosa, the plane shifts subtly from above Buck's fascia to just above the tunica albuginea. It is important to recognize this shift. Failure to adjust the plane of dissection will carry the dissection into the corpora spongiosa, which will result in excessive, difficult-to-control bleeding during the deep ventral dissection of the urethral wedge from the corporeal bodies.

Applying methylene blue or brilliant green to the urethra can help identify the plane between urothelium and squamous epithelium. We routinely inject surrounding tissues with 0.25% lidocaine and 1:200,000 U/mL epinephrine to improve hemostasis. Shallow incisions are made laterally along the dorsal aspect of the urethra to begin the dissection. Sharp dissection is required to develop the plane between the urethral wedge and the corporeal bodies. Careful dissection will preserve urethral width and length. This is particularly important because the urethra is often too short to reach the glans penis once the bladder has been located into the pelvis.

Careful lateral dissection of the penile shaft skin and dartos fascia from the corporeal bodies will avoid damaging the laterally located neurovascular bundles on the corpora of the epispadial penis. The lateral dissection on the penis should be superficial to Buck's fascia because of this lateral position of the neurovascular bundles.

Complete Penile Disassembly and Deep Dissection. Once a plane is established between the penis and the urethral wedge, the penis may be disassembled into three components: (1) the right and (2) left corporeal bodies with their respective hemiglans and (3) the urethral wedge (urothelium with underlying corpora spongiosa).[75] This is done primarily to provide exposure to the intersymphyseal band and to allow adequate proximal dissection. We have found the easiest plane of dissection to completely isolate the corporeal bodies to be proximal and ventral. The plane of dissection should be carried out at the level of the tunica albuginea on the corpora (see Fig. 59-3B). After a plane is established between the urethral wedge and the corporeal bodies, this dissection is carried distally to separate the three components from each other (Fig. 59-4A). Complete separation of the corporeal bodies increases exposure to the pelvic diaphragm for deep dissection. The corporeal bodies may be completely separated from each other because they exist on a separate blood supply. It is important to keep the underlying corpora spongiosa with the urethra. The blood supply to the urethra is based on this corporeal tissue, which should appear wedge-shaped after its dissection from the adjacent corpora cavernosa. The urethral/corpora spongiosa component will later be tubularized and placed ventral to the corporeal bodies. Paraexstrophy skin flaps should not be used with this technique because this maneuver will place the blood supply to the distal urethra at risk. Because the bladder and urethra are moved posteriorly in the pelvis as a unit (with a common proximal blood supply), division of the urethral wedge is counterintuitive to the intent of the repair. In some cases, a male patient will be left with a hypospadias that will require later surgical reconstruction. The urethra and corporeal bodies do not always have to be separated. Occasionally the urethra is long enough and the bladder mobile enough to preserve the connection between them while still effectively carrying out the deep pelvic dissection that is integral to this repair.

After separating the components distally, the urethral dissection is carried proximally to the bladder neck. Exposure to the pelvic diaphragm is optimized by complete separation of the urethra and corporeal bodies (see Fig. 59-4B). This creates the surgical exposure to perform the deep incision of the intersymphyseal band required to move the bladder and urethra posteriorly (Fig. 59-5). When dissecting the urethral wedge from the corporeal bodies medially, the dissection plane is on the tunica albuginea of the corpora cavernosa. This medial dissection should be carried down through the intersymphyseal band (the condensation of anterior pelvic fascia and ligaments).

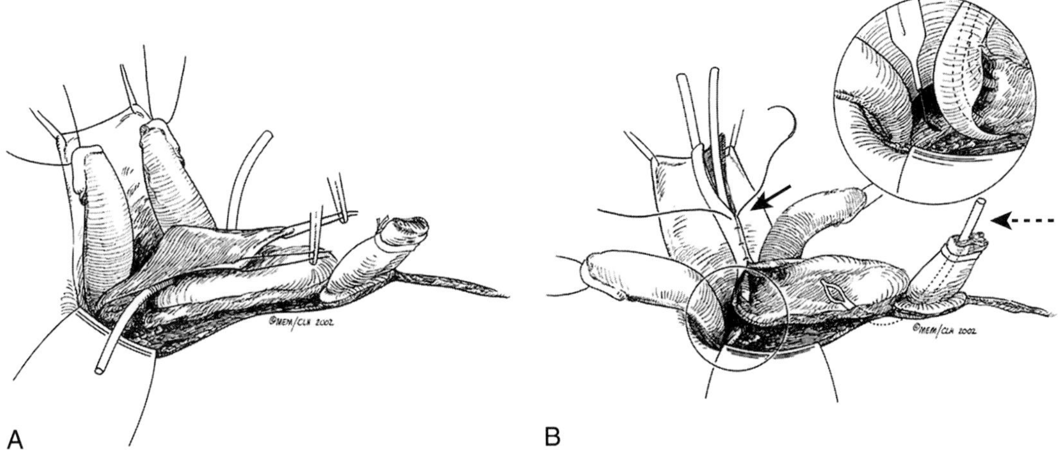

Figure 59-4. **A,** Separation of corporeal bodies and urethra. **B,** Deep pelvic dissection. Note the division of the intersymphyseal band (*inset*) is critical to allowing placement of the bladder in the pelvis. Also note the tubularization of the neourethra over the urethral catheter (*solid arrow*) and the suprapubic tube in the still-open bladder (*dotted arrow*).

Deep incision of the intersymphyseal band posterior and lateral to each side of the urethral wedge is absolutely necessary to allow the bladder and bladder neck to achieve a posterior position in the pelvis. This dissection should be carried until the pelvic floor musculature becomes visible. Failure to adequately dissect the bladder and urethral wedge from these surrounding structures will prevent posterior movement of the bladder in the pelvis and create anterior tension along the urethral plate (see Fig. 59-5).

Primary Closure. Once the intersymphyseal band is adequately incised and the bladder and urethral wedge are adequately dissected from the surrounding tissues, bladder closure and urethral tubularization can be initiated. This portion of the repair is straightforward and anatomic (Fig. 59-6A). To provide urinary drainage, a suprapubic tube is used. The bladder may be closed using a three-layer closure with monofilament absorbable suture. The urethra is tubularized using a two-layer running closure with monofilament and braided absorbable suture. Because of the previous deep dissection, we can position the tubularized urethra ventral to the corpora in a tension-free fashion. If the urethra cannot be positioned ventrally without creating tension, it is likely that a deeper incision is required into the intersymphyseal band and pelvic fascia.

The pubic symphysis is reapproximated using two No. 1 polydioxanone-interrupted sutures placed in a figure-of-eight fashion (see Fig. 59-6B). Knots are left anteriorly to prevent suture erosion into the bladder neck. Rectus fascia is reapproximated using an interrupted or running 2-0 polydioxanone suture. We also place interrupted 6-0 polydioxanone sutures along

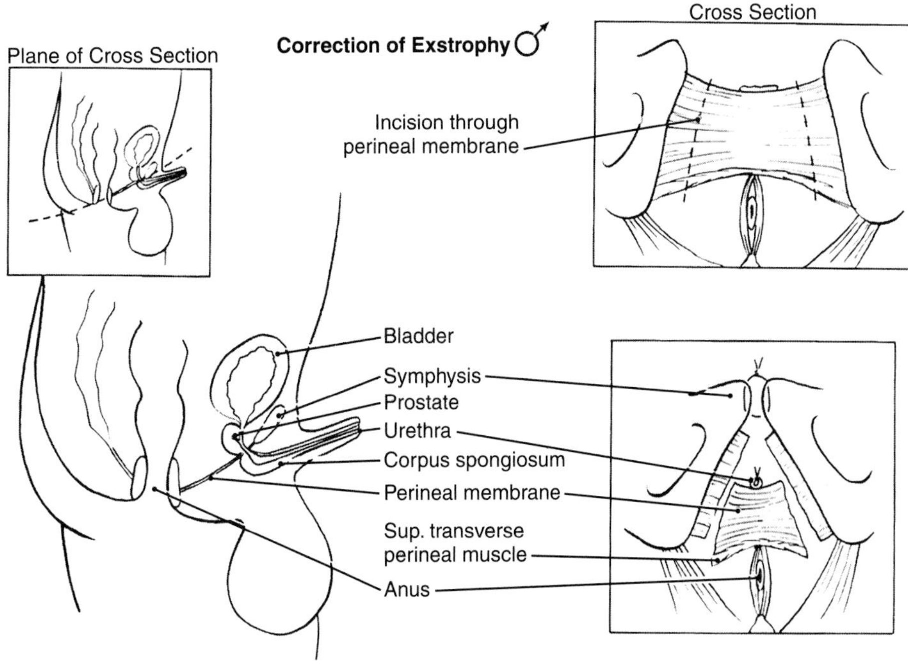

Figure 59-5. Cross-sectional view of repair of bladder exstrophy in a male.

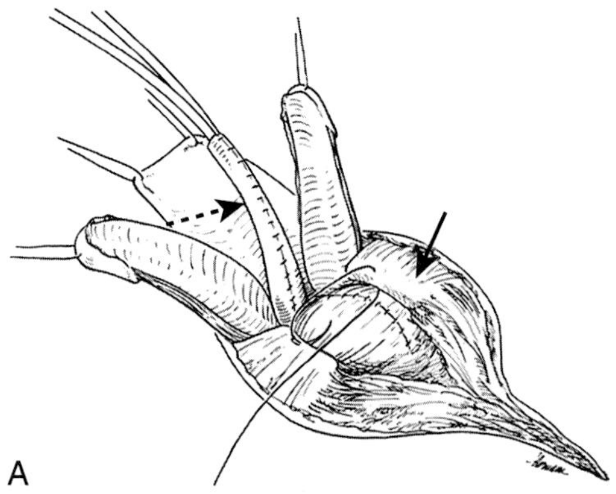

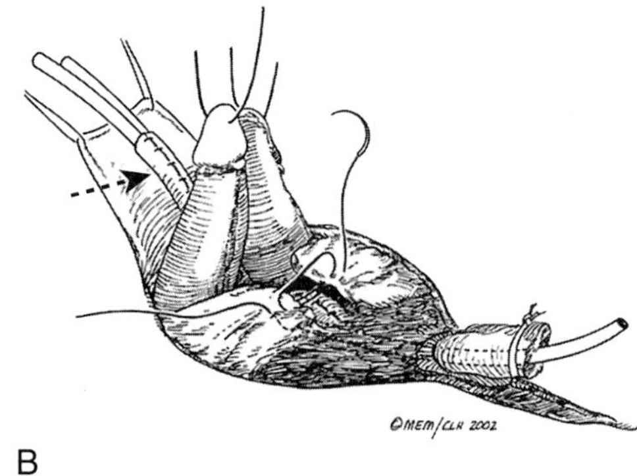

Figure 59-6. Once the intersymphyseal band is adequately incised and the bladder and urethral wedge are dissected from the surrounding tissues, bladder repair and urethral tubularization can be performed. **A,** The bladder is being closed in three layers using monofilament absorbable suture (*solid arrow*). The urethra has been tubularized using a two-layer running closure with monofilament and braided absorbable suture (*dotted arrow*). **B,** This schematic depicts closure of the pubic symphysis with two No. 1 polydioxanone interrupted sutures placed in a figure-of-eight fashion. The knots are placed anteriorly to prevent suture erosion into the neck of the bladder. The urethra (*dotted arrow*) has been placed ventral to the corpora.

the dorsal aspect of the corporeal bodies to reapproximate them. Penile skin coverage is provided using either a primary dorsal closure or reversed Byars flaps if needed. Skin covering the abdominal wall is reapproximated using a two-layer closure of absorbable monofilament suture.

The corporeal bodies will rotate medially with closure. This rotation will assist in correcting the dorsal deflection and can be readily appreciated by observing the new vertical lie of the previously horizontally placed glans traction sutures. Occasionally, significant discrepancies in the dorsal and ventral lengths of the corpora will require dermal graft insertion to correct chordee.

If there is adequate urethral length, the urethra may be brought up to each hemiglans ventrally to create an orthotopic meatus. The glans is reconfigured using interrupted mattress sutures of polydioxanone suture followed by horizontal mattress sutures of 7-0 monofilament suture to reapproximate the glans epithelium. The neourethra is matured with 7-0 braided polyglactin suture similar to our standard hypospadias repair. When needed, glans tissue reduction may also be performed to create a conical-appearing glans and to eliminate the furrow between the glans halves. Tacking sutures are placed ventrally and dorsally to prevent penile shaft skin from riding over the corporeal bodies and "burying" the penis.

The urethra may lack enough length to reach the glans in about half the cases. In this situation, it is matured along the ventral aspect of the penis to create a hypospadias (Fig. 59-7). This can be corrected at a later date as a second-stage procedure. Redundant shaft skin may be left ventrally in these patients to assist in later penile reconstructive procedures.

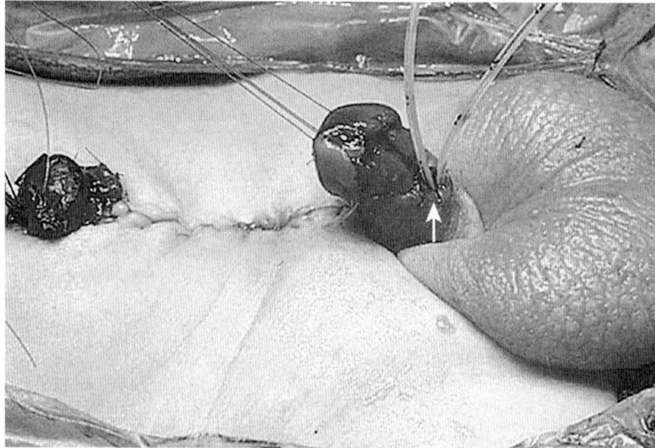

Figure 59-7. If the urethra does not have adequate length to reach the glans (which occurs in about half of the cases), it is matured along the ventral aspect of the penis to create a hypospadias (*arrow*), as seen in this operative photograph. The hypospadias will be corrected at a later date.

The Primary Repair Technique: Girls

The principles of this single-stage technique are similar in boys and girls (Fig. 59-8). After preoperative antibiotics are given, the patient is prepared and draped in a sterile field. We mark the planned lines of incision with the bladder neck, urethra, and vagina

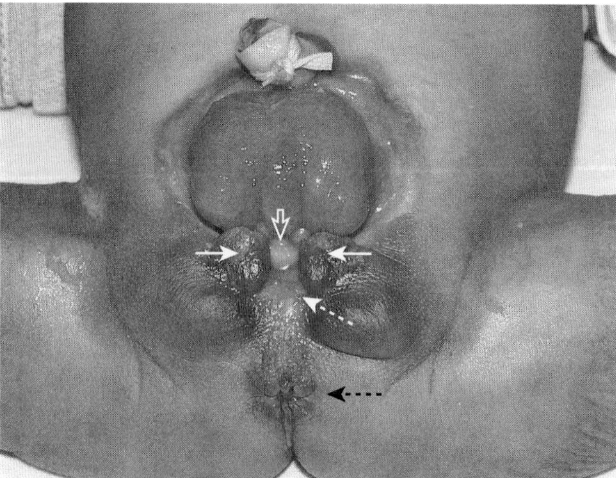

Figure 59-8. Bladder exstrophy in a female infant. The epispadial urethra is marked with an *open white arrow.* The bifid clitoris is marked with *solid white arrows,* and the vagina is marked with a *dotted white arrow.* The anus is noted with a *dotted black arrow.*

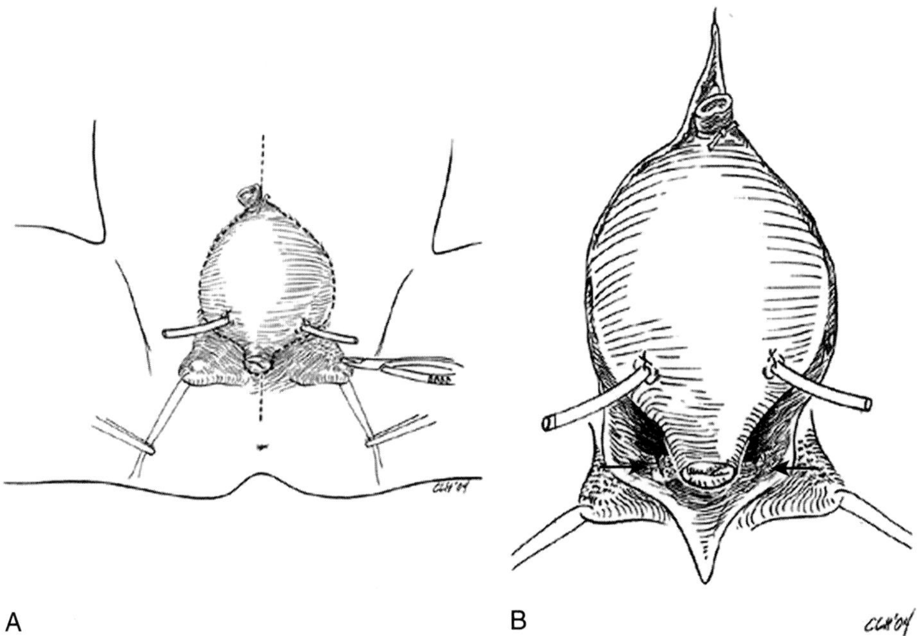

Figure 59-9. In a female infant, the bladder neck, urethra, and vagina are mobilized as a unit. **A,** The lines of incision are seen. **B,** The dissection is carried down dividing the intersymphyseal band (*arrows*). Note the ureteral catheters in both drawings.

mobilized as a unit (Fig. 59-9). Again, we perform this dissection with the tungsten-tip electrocautery to minimize tissue damage while achieving hemostasis. The appropriate plane of dissection is found anteriorly along the medial aspect of the glans clitoris and proceeds posteriorly along the lateral aspect of the vaginal vault (Fig. 59-10A). The vagina is mobilized with the urethra and bladder neck. Dissection along the vaginal wall extends quite laterally. Placement of a hemostat in the vaginal vault will help with retraction to identify the plane of dissection. The urethra and bladder neck should not be dissected from the anterior vaginal wall because this will compromise the blood supply to the urethra. During the posterior and lateral dissection, the intersymphyseal band will be encountered and should be deeply incised to allow the urethra and bladder neck to move posteriorly. The posterior limit of the dissection is reached when the pelvic floor musculature is exposed and the bladder, bladder neck, and urethra can move into the pelvis without tension.

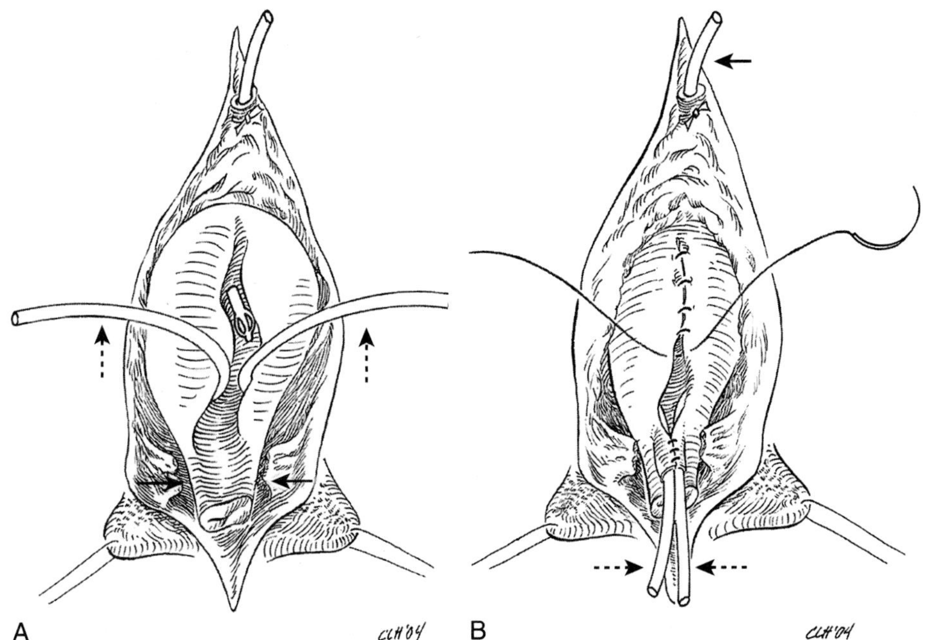

Figure 59-10. **A,** The appropriate plane of dissection is found anteriorly along the medial aspect of the glans clitoris and proceeds posteriorly along the lateral aspect of the vaginal vault. The vagina is mobilized with the urethra and bladder neck (*solid arrows*). **B,** The bladder and urethra are closed in multiple layers, and the suprapubic tube (*arrow*) is brought out superiorly. Note the ureteral catheters (*dotted arrows*) in both drawings.

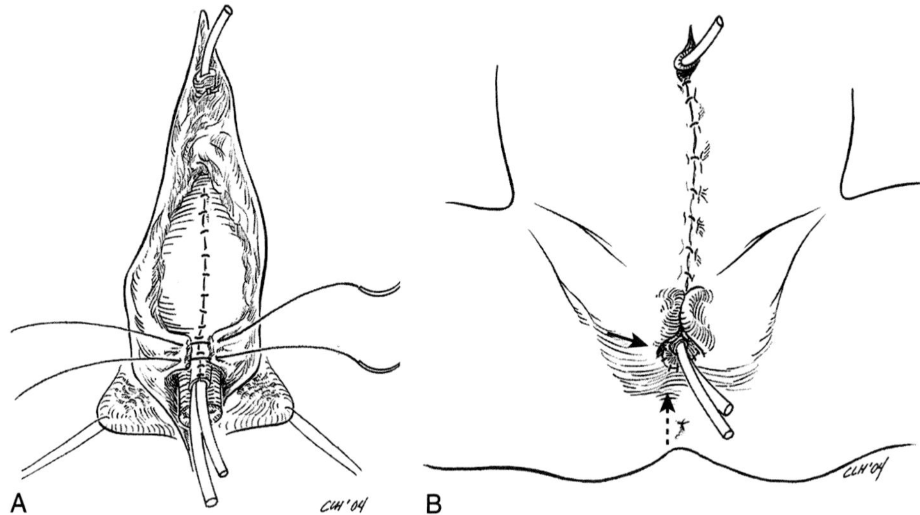

Figure 59-11. **A,** Pelvic positioning of the bladder and vagina and closure of the pubic symphysis with figure-of-eight No. 1 polydioxanone sutures. **B,** Repair of the vaginal introitus (*solid arrow*) is depicted. The labia majora are advanced posteriorly to the perineum at this time (*dotted arrow*).

After adequate dissection, the vagina, urethra, and bladder neck are moved posteriorly using a YV-plasty if the vagina is anteriorly located. The urethra is then tubularized using a two-layer closure of absorbable suture (see Fig. 59-10B). Before the urethral closure, we routinely place a suprapubic tube to provide postoperative urine drainage. The pubis symphysis is reapproximated using two figure-of-eight No. 1 polydioxanone sutures (Fig. 59-11A). Osteotomies may be necessary when a wide pubic diastasis prevents a low-tension reapproximation of the pubic symphysis or if the patient is older than 48 to 72 hours old. We use anterior iliac osteotomies in these situations. The rectus fascia can then be closed in the midline. We mature the neourethra with 5-0 polydioxanone sutures and reapproximate the bifid clitoris by denuding them medially so that they fuse together after suturing with 7-0 polydioxanone suture. The labia majora should be advanced posteriorly to the perineum at this time as well (see Fig. 59-11B). A Z-plasty aids in skin closure. A simplified mons plasty technique provides a satisfactory aesthetic result to the introital area and can be applied at the time of the primary repair.[76]

Modern Staged Repair of Exstrophy

A staged approach for bladder exstrophy repair was developed in response to high reported rates of renal damage seen in single-stage approaches in the 1970s. The sequence for staged reconstruction initially consisted of bladder and posterior urethral closure at birth, BNR at 2 to 3 years of life, and epispadias repair later.[77] However, this order shifted when bladder capacity was noted to increase with the added resistance from early epispadias repair.[78] Currently, MSRE, as described by the Johns Hopkins group, consists of bladder and posterior urethral closure at birth or soon thereafter (stage 1), epispadias repair at 6 to 12 months of life (stage 2), and BNR when the bladder capacity is adequate and the child is showing interest in toilet training (usually at 4 to 5 years of life) (stage 3).[79] Occasionally, epispadias repair and BNR ± ureteral reimplantation are combined.[80,81]

MSRE Stage 1: Initial Early Bladder Exstrophy Closure

In this first stage, the surgical objectives include (1) closure and repositioning of the bladder and urethra (posterior urethra in males and entire urethra in females) inside the pelvic ring and (2) approximation of the pelvic ring with closure of the abdominal wall. In male patients, at the end of stage 1, this closure technique ideally produces a result that mimics complete epispadias with incontinence and balanced posterior outlet resistance, which stimulates bladder growth while preserving renal function.

Male MSRE Bladder and Posterior Urethral Closure Technique. In stage 1 of the MSRE in the male child, ureteral catheters are inserted and secured. A traction suture is placed in the glans penis. The posterior urethra is developed by incising a 2-cm wide strip of mucosa from the distal trigone to below the distal verumontanum. Initial dissection begins at the umbilicus and is continued circumferentially, incising around the bladder plate. The two umbilical arteries are ligated and divided. The underlying detrusor muscle is mobilized from the rectus sheath to expose the peritoneum. The peritoneum is dissected from the dome of the bladder to allow bladder mobilization. Extraperitoneal dissection lateral to the bladder exposes the retroperitoneal space and caudally leads the dissection in the correct plane at the level of the bladder neck. At this level, the rectus fascia meets the pubis and the urogenital diaphragm fibers meet the posterior urethra/bladder neck. The urogenital diaphragm fibers and the intersymphyseal band must be completely taken down from the pubic subperiosteum bilaterally to the pelvic floor. Otherwise, the posterior urethra and bladder will not be recessed within the deep pelvis.

At this point, the posterior urethra is assessed. If the child has severe chordee and a short urethra that inhibits attempts at penile lengthening, an incision in the urethral plate may be necessary but only after extensive mobilization of the bladder and prostatic plate from the rectus fascia, the pubic bones, and the inferior ramus of the pubis. After aggressive division of the urogenital diaphragm fibers from the posterior urethra/bladder neck area, the prostatic urethra can be displaced posteriorly into the pelvis. Lack of urethral plate length can be managed by dividing the prostatic plate distal to the verumontanum in a "V"-shaped fashion. After corporeal mobilization and midline reapproximation, the penile urethral plate is fashioned from a lateral rotational flap generated after a single lateral incision in the paraexstrophy skin. Paraexstrophy skin flaps should be used with great caution because of the high complication rate associated with their use.[53,82,83]

The corporeal bodies are not sewn together at this time because this will be performed after the urethra has been transposed beneath the corpora at the time of epispadias closure. Adequacy of dissection can be assessed by compressing a urethral sound on the posterior urethra while manually approximating the pelvis.

After a silicone Malecot suprapubic tube has been placed, the umbilicus is excised and the bladder is closed in the midline in multiple layers with a running 3-0 polydioxanone suture. The posterior urethra is also closed onto the base of the penis, sizing it to accept a 12- to 14-Fr sound. It is important to perform a horizontal mattress closure of the pubic bones with long-lasting suture, planning for the knot to be placed on the anterior surface of the pubis. This technique prevents the suture or knot from eroding into the urethra or bladder neck. Once the suture is placed but not tied, three surgical personnel are used to reapproximate the pubis symphysis. One individual applies pressure over each greater trochanter to push the pubic rami to the midline. A second individual depresses the posterior urethra and bladder neck. The third individual ties the suture. If the rectus fascia is strong, a second suture is placed just above the symphysis. The abdominal wall, subcutaneous tissues, and skin are then closed in multiple layers with neoumbilical construction at or above the level of the iliac crests.

Female MSRE Bladder and Posterior Urethral Closure Technique. In stage 1 of the MSRE of the female child, the surgical technique of bladder, pelvic ring and abdominal wall closure are identical to that described for the male. However, the closure in the female differs from the male closure in that the female urethra is completely reconstructed at stage 1.[1,84] The urethral plate mucosal incision is 2 cm wide, traversing from the distal trigone to the vaginal orifice in the female. Paraexstrophy skin flaps are unnecessary in female exstrophy closure.[85] The medial aspect of each hemiclitoris is de-epithelialized to permit approximation of the two glans clitori and reconstruction of the mons. The bladder and female urethra are closed in a two-layer polyglactin closure, and the pubic bones, abdominal wall, subcutaneous tissue, and skin are closed as outlined in the male. The mons plasty and genitoplasty are then performed.

Postoperative Care of Stage 1 MSRE. Adequate urethral caliber and minimal postvoid residuals are assessed before suprapubic tube removal at 4 weeks. The status of the upper urinary tracts is assessed before discharge and is followed by ultrasonography at 3 months and every 6 months to 1 year. Antibiotic prophylaxis for vesicoureteral reflux (VUR) is also used. Increasing hydronephrosis, worsening VUR, retained urine in the bladder, and recurrent urinary infections should prompt further evaluation for suture erosion or outlet obstruction. Between the ages of 1 to 3 years, yearly cystograms under anesthesia are performed to assess the degree of reflux and, more importantly, to assess the growth of the bladder (ideally, 60 to 85 mL by this age).

MSRE Stage 2: Epispadias Repair

Epispadias repair is now typically performed at 6 to 12 months of age via the modified Cantwell-Ransley technique. The goals of epispadias repair include a straight penis and urethra, easy urethral catheterization, normal erectile function, and a cosmetically satisfactory phallus. These goals allow the patient to stand while voiding and to have intromission during intercourse.

Preoperative Considerations. Before performing the epispadias repair, some surgeons use topical or intramuscular testosterone to increase the size of the phallus and the phallic skin. Intramuscular testosterone enanthate in oil (2 mg/kg) can be administered at 5 and 2 weeks before epispadias closure. Penile lengthening can usually be achieved at this time by division of all remnants of the suspensory ligament and scar tissue as well as further release of the crura from the inferior pubic rami. In some situations, further urethral lengthening may require free skin grafts, buccal mucosal grafts, ureteral grafts, or pedicle skin flaps. These same maneuvers can be used to repair the scarred or stenosed posterior urethra.

The Modified Cantwell-Ransley Technique

Cantwell first described mobilization of the urethra and moving it ventrally for epispadias repair. The technique has subsequently been modified.[83,86] A stay suture is first placed into the glans penis. A reverse meatal advancement and glanduloplasty (MAGPI), or IPGAM, procedure at the distal urethral plate allows advancement of the urethral meatus onto the glans. Incisions are then made on the lateral edges of the urethral plate and around the epispadial meatus. This plate is dissected from the corporeal bodies up to the level of the glans distally and to the prostatic urethra proximally. Glans wings should be developed distally as well. The corporeal bodies are then separated from each other to allow medial rotation. The urethra is then tubularized over a 6- or 8-Fr urethral catheter, using running 6-0 absorbable suture. The corporeal bodies are rotated over the urethra and reapproximated using 5-0 absorbable suture in an interrupted fashion. Cavernosotomies may be performed before reapproximating the corporeal bodies to help correct persistent chordee. These are performed at the point of maximal angulation. The neurovascular bundles may require mobilization to avoid injuring them if cavernosotomies are performed. The glans wings are then closed over the urethra using interrupted 5-0 absorbable suture. Penile shaft skin can be trimmed and tailored to cover the penis using interrupted 5-0 or 6-0 absorbable sutures. Z-plasties at the level of the pubis may decrease the chance of a dorsal retractile scar at the base of the penis. Postoperative care includes bladder antispasmodics, broad-spectrum antibiotics, and removal of the urethral catheter at 2 weeks.

In the event of a significantly delayed primary closure or an initial bladder closure failure, a simultaneous closure of the exstrophy bladder and the epispadias can be performed.

Bladder Neck Reconstruction

Preoperative Assessment

In incontinent children after CPRE or MSRE, a continence procedure is indicated when (1) the urethra is stricture free and capable of catheterization, if necessary; (2) under anesthesia, the bladder capacity has achieved a minimum volume of 60 to 85 mL; and (3) the child is mature enough to participate in the postoperative voiding program.[87] This is typically around age 4 to 5 years. Cystoscopy and gravity cystography provide information regarding bladder capacity and the status of any previous repairs. Advocates of staged reconstruction emphasize the importance of achieving adequate bladder capacity before performing BNR. A bladder capacity less than 60 mL under anesthesia or during urodynamic evaluation decreases the success of BNR. BNR requires adequate bladder capacity because some volume is lost during the procedure. Factors that increase the potential for the bladder to achieve adequate capacity before BNR include:

- Avoidance of urinary tract infections
- Complete bladder emptying with institution of CIC if bladder emptying is incomplete
- Epispadias repair
- Avoidance of bladder prolapse

Preoperative urodynamic evaluation should be considered because it allows detection of detrusor hyperactivity or atony as well as assessment of functional bladder capacity and leak-point pressures. However, the urethra of these patients may be difficult to catheterize. In these situations, a urodynamic catheter can be placed suprapubically at the time of the cystourethroscopic examination to be used later that day for the urodynamic evaluation.

Ureteroneocystostomy may be required at the time of BNR to correct VUR and to move the ureters from the lower bladder where BNR will occur. The Cohen technique is often employed. However, others have described a cephalotrigonal technique that is particularly applicable to exstrophy patients because of the angle of ureteral entry into the bladder.[88] The Marshall-Marchetti-Krantz (MMK) bladder neck suspension or a bladder neck wrap using rectus muscle or fascia or gracilis may be combined with BNR as well. Osteotomies may also be necessary to stabilize the intersymphyseal bar and improve continence at the time of BNR.

The following section describes the most commonly employed BNR techniques, including the modified Young-Dees-Leadbetter and the Mitchell repairs.

MSRE Stage 3: Modified Young-Dees-Leadbetter BNR

The modified Young-Dees-Leadbetter (YDL) BNR technique[89] and the transtrigonal/cephalotrigonal bilateral ureteral reimplantation[88] are the surgical techniques employed in MSRE stage 3. The combined thoughts of several surgeons spanning an 82-year period have led to the modern YDL BNR.[87] To perform a modified YDL procedure,[89] the bladder neck is extensively dissected and a vertical cystotomy is made. Occasionally, a portion of the intersymphyseal band must be divided completely for good visualization. After transtrigonal/cephalotrigonal bilateral ureteral reimplantation, a strip of bladder mucosa 1.5 to 1.8 cm wide and 3.0 to 4.0 cm long is generated and the lateral bladder triangles are demucosalized. Use of an epinephrine-soaked sponge during this dissection aids in hemostasis and visualization. The bladder neck may be funneled further with small vertical incisions along the cut edge of the lateral bladder walls. The neourethra is tubularized over an 8-Fr stent using interrupted or running polyglycolic acid sutures (4-0 or 5-0). The two triangular regions of demucosalized detrusor muscle are then closed over the mucosal tube in a two-layer "vest over pants" double-breasted technique using 3-0 polyglycolic acid sutures. This reinforces the neobladder neck, decreases the risk of fistula, and augments the outlet resistance.[90] The sutures in the third layer are not cut because they are used in the MMK bladder neck suspension.[87]

Some surgeons recommend avoidance of a urethral catheter in the postoperative period because of concerns that it may adversely affect later urinary continence. Urinary drainage is achieved by the use of bilateral ureteral catheters and suprapubic tube drainage. Ureteral stents are removed at 2 to 3 weeks, and voiding trials are begun in the third week. The urethra is calibrated with a soft 8-Fr catheter, and voiding trials are begun with the suprapubic tube in place after the urine has been sterilized. If no urine is passed, cystoscopy and urethral stenting may be required for a short period of time. A bladder readjustment period may span several months before day and, subsequently night, continence is achieved.

BNR: The Mitchell Repair

This repair employs a modification of the Leadbetter procedure technique described previously.[89] In this modification, a full-thickness transverse incision is made in the anterior urethra and is extended cephalad. After cross-trigonal ureteral reimplantation, the urethral strip is tubularized in two layers using polyglycolate or monocryl suture (4-0 or 5-0) over an 8- or 10-Fr urethral catheter depending on the size of the patient. The bladder may be closed in continuity with the urethral closure. This procedure effectively narrows and lengthens the urethra. It also moves fibrotic tissue at the level of the original bladder neck away from the new bladder neck. After the closure, dissection around the new bladder neck may be performed if a combined bladder neck wrap or sling will also be created.

Postoperatively, urine is drained through a combination of ureteral stents, a suprapubic tube, and a 6-Fr urethral catheter. The urethral catheter is removed 7 to 10 days after the operation. Ureteral stents are removed at 10 to 14 days after surgery. The suprapubic tube remains for 3 weeks. Voiding trials are performed with measurement of postvoid residual urine volumes to assess for urinary retention before removing the suprapubic tube. As with any BNR procedure (without augmentation), several months of adjustment will be required before the patient develops adequate bladder awareness, capacity, and control to achieve prolonged intervals of urinary continence.

Occasionally, trigonal tubularization must be combined with bladder augmentation because of small bladder capacity as most BNRs decrease bladder capacity because a portion of the bladder is used to create the continence mechanism.[91] Stomach offers the best potential to preserve spontaneous volitional voiding in this group but places these children at risk of hematuria-dysuria syndrome, which can be especially troubling in the presence of persistent urinary incontinence and normal sensory innervation.[92] Other intestinal segments may also be used depending on surgeon preference. If augmentation is required, appendicovesicostomy or another form of the Mitrofanoff operation can be simultaneously performed if the urethra is difficult to negotiate because of the likelihood that the patient will require intermittent catheterization to empty the bladder after BNR.

Results

Exstrophy Results

Complications can occur with any form of exstrophy closure. The most commonly reported complication is urethrocutaneous fistula formation (at the penopubic angle dorsally) in males. These fistulas will often close spontaneously. They may initially be managed conservatively by providing urinary diversion via catheter drainage. If the fistula does not close after conservative management, the bladder and urethra should be examined cystoscopically for the possibility of obstruction at the bladder neck or urethra.

If a child develops chronic bladder and kidney infections after exstrophy closure, he or she should be evaluated for possible outlet obstruction. We routinely maintain our patients on suppressive antibiotic therapy because of the high incidence of VUR in this population.

In the long term, patients are also concerned with fertility. For men, the vas deferens and ejaculatory ducts are normal at birth. However, fertility may be compromised as a consequence of surgery they may have had in the region of the bladder neck and posterior urethra. Most men can experience orgasm but some cannot effectively ejaculate. Intracytoplasmic sperm injection can be useful in this setting. Women with bladder exstrophy can become pregnant but are prone to develop uterine prolapse, especially after pregnancy. This is thought to be due to further stress and damage to the already abnormal pelvic musculature.

Epispadias Results

Outcomes reveal urethrocutaneous fistula rates ranging from 5.5% to 42%. Complications seem more common in those patients who undergo correction as part of an exstrophy closure versus isolated epispadias.[93] Other complications include atrophy of the corpora cavernosa and urethra. These complications can occur if the blood supply to the corporeal bodies or urethral wedge is damaged during dissection or closure.[94] Similar complications have been described after the initial stage of a staged reconstruction as well as after the use of the complete penile disassembly technique.[95] In experienced hands, such complications are unusual and underscore the importance of involving surgeons experienced in the surgical management of these patients.

BNR Results

After BNR, surgical success is defined as a dry interval of more than 2 to 3 hours and spontaneous voiding without catheterization. YDL BNR and its variants have yielded surgical success with urinary continence rates of 30% to 80% or more for patients with bladder exstrophy.[89,96-98] Many factors influence the outcome of surgery. For instance, an initial failed bladder closure or prior failed BNR reduces the chance to achieve subsequent urinary continence.[99] A preoperative bladder capacity of more than 85 mL portends a greater continence rate after YDL BNR.[100] Use of osteotomies to provide a tension-free anastomosis and patient immobilization through the use of spica casting or Bryant's traction in the postoperative period increases the success of bladder closure and subsequent continence. Delayed bladder closure increases the likelihood for the eventual need for bladder augmentation due to inadequate bladder capacity that, in turn, reduces the chance for volitional voiding.

Long-term studies have reported that 8 of 13 patients with initially successful bladder closures and BNR required further surgery in their second decade of life because of poorly compliant, low-capacity bladders that caused urinary incontinence.[101] Surgeons who care for these patients must be committed to the long-term follow-up of this complex group of patients because late complications may develop.

Adjunctive Aspects of the Repair

Inguinal hernias are commonly associated with exstrophy in both male and female patients.[102,103] The majority of these are indirect hernias. They arise as a consequence of enlarged internal and external inguinal rings combined with compromised fascial support and lack of obliquity of the inguinal canal.[104] In a review of patients from the Hospital for Sick Children in Toronto, 56% of classic male exstrophy patients and 15% of classic female exstrophy patients developed inguinal hernias over a 10-year period.[62] The authors recommended that these hernias should be repaired at the time of primary bladder closure to prevent incarceration that could affect up to 50% of these patients in the first 2 years of life. Reinforcement of the transversalis and internal oblique fascia during hernia repair decreases the later development of direct inguinal hernias. Umbilical hernias, as a contiguous defect with the bladder plate, also uniformly occur with exstrophy and are corrected at the time of the primary repair.

Because of the high incidence of VUR, we use low-dose suppressive antibiotic therapy for all neonates after bladder closure. This is continued until either the VUR is corrected or resolves spontaneously. Some surgeons perform neoureterocystotomies at the time of initial closure. The results of this approach have not been reported.

Osteotomies

Approximation of the open pelvic ring eases abdominal wall closure and diminishes the rate of bladder and abdominal wall dehiscence.[72,105] This allows the construction of an intrapelvic urethra and reapproximates the pelvic floor musculature, likely contributing to long-term continence.[58,105] Therefore, pelvic ring reapproximation is useful at initial bladder closure and at later stages of reconstruction if satisfactory reapproximation was not achieved initially. However, beyond this age or at this time, if the pelvis is not sufficiently malleable, osteotomies are performed at the time of closure.

Osteotomies offer several advantages to the anatomic approach to exstrophy closure, including (1) optimizing pubic symphysis apposition; (2) diminishing tension on the fascial closure; (3) optimizing anatomic placement of the bladder, bladder neck, and urethra in the pelvis; (4) improving the reapproximation of the corporeal and clitoral bodies; and (5) possibly decreasing the chance for later uterine prolapse because the anterior closure brings the pelvic diaphragm into a more normal anatomic position that offers better support.

The need for osteotomy is typically assessed under general anesthesia. Indications for osteotomy include patients more than 72 hours old, neonates with a wide pubic diastasis, neonates with cloacal exstrophy, and patients who have had a previously failed closure. Osteotomies are usually performed at the same setting as bladder closure to help secure the closure.

Several operative approaches can be used for osteotomies. Posterior iliac osteotomies are performed with the patient in the prone position, after which the patient is then repositioned for the bladder closure. However, complications involving increased blood loss and occasional malunion of the ilium have led to using other approaches. Anterior iliac osteotomies offer the advantage of a single position (supine) and sterile field preparation. Compared with posterior iliac osteotomies, an anterior approach also has been shown to result in less blood loss and better apposition and mobility of the pubic rami. Anterior approaches include an anterior diagonal approach or a combination of bilateral combined anterior innominate and vertical iliac osteotomies, which have had excellent initial and long-term results compared with anterior iliac osteotomies alone in some series.[71,106] Both osteotomies can be performed through the same anterior skin incision on each side with minimal blood loss and 4% complication rate.[107,108] The use of a diagonal mid-iliac osteotomy performed through the same incision as the exstrophy closure has also been described.[109] Division of the superior pubic ramus has also been performed. However, it is not as effective as the other methods described but can be used in the neonatal period.[110,111]

To avoid osteotomies, a technique has been developed that secures the pubic symphyseal closure with deeply placed polyglactin sutures through the bone followed by placement of a miniature metal plate that may be removed later. Initial results are promising.[112] Use of radical soft tissue mobilization for exstrophy (the Kelly technique) also may allow the surgeon to avoid the more routine use of osteotomies seen with the CPRE and MSRE techniques for exstrophy closure.

The patient must be immobilized to decrease lateral stresses on the closure after the primary reconstructive procedure. Choice of immobilization techniques remains controversial with a variety of options. Current approaches include (1) Bryant's traction, (2) use of an external fixator, (3) spica casting, and (4) mummy or mermaid wrapping. Likely, the most important variable with these techniques is familiarity of the user because they all have learning curves associated with them that increase the complication rates of those not familiar with their use. We prefer to use a spica cast for 3 weeks to prevent external hip rotation and optimize pubic apposition (Fig. 59-12). Modified Buck's traction has been used by many groups with success. A posterior lightweight splint can be used in neonates when the child is out of traction to maintain hip adduction. We have stopped using Buck's traction because spica casts are easier for the families to manage at home. External fixation devices have also been used successfully.[106] Fixator pins for these devices should be cleaned several times a day to reduce the chance for infection. Internal fixation may be necessary in older patients. Femoral nerve palsy is a possible complication with fixation that must be monitored and can be reduced with gradual tightening of the fixator. The osteotomies are secured by intrafragmentary pins, external fixation (4 weeks for neonates; 6 to 8 weeks for older patients), and light Buck's traction for 2 to 4 weeks.

CLOACAL EXSTROPHY

Although cloacal exstrophy has been recognized for several hundred years, in 1965 Spencer reported the first successful repair and survival of an infant with this anomaly.[113] Mortality rates for infants with cloacal exstrophy remained high for years after this initial

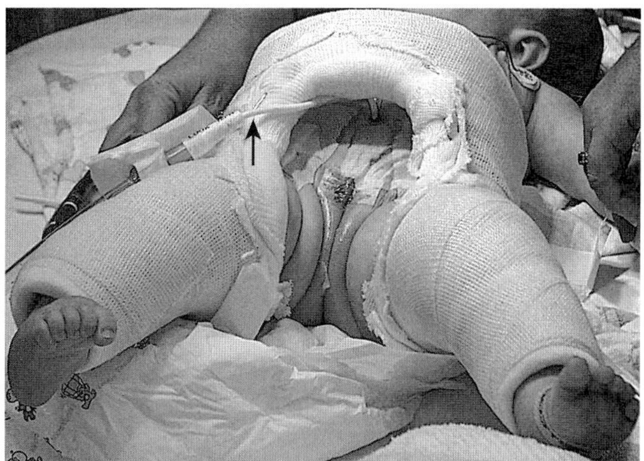

Figure 59-12. In order to immobilize the patient to decrease lateral stresses on the closure after the primary reconstructive procedure, a number of immobilization techniques are possible. This photograph shows a spica cast that was applied to prevent external hip rotation and optimize pubic apposition in the early postoperative period. Note the suprapubic bladder catheter (*arrow*).

success because affected infants routinely died of malnutrition and sepsis. With continuing improvement in total parenteral nutrition and neonatal management, mortality rates currently are less than 10%.[114] Issues of quality of life are now paramount in this patient group.

The bladder plate associated with cloacal exstrophy is divided in half by the hindgut plate, which represents the deformation in the development of the colon that occurs with cloacal exstrophy. Ileum enters and intussuscepts into the middle of the hindgut, creating the "trunk of an elephant's face" appearance with appendiceal appendages located laterally to give the impression of "tusks on the face of the elephant" (Fig. 59-13).[115]

With cloacal exstrophy, the bladder neck (internal urethral sphincter) and external urethral sphincter are not fully developed owing to the failed development of the bladder and urethral remnant located on the anterior and dorsal surfaces of the body wall and penis, respectively. However, because the innervation to these structures may be intact, anatomic closure theoretically offers the possibility of achieving urinary continence. The urethral plate is characteristically short as well.

Associated Anomalies

Kidneys and Upper Urinary Tract

Renal anomalies are much more common with cloacal exstrophy than with bladder exstrophy. They include anomalies of location such as pelvic kidneys or crossed fused ectopia. Horseshoe kidneys, renal agenesis, and ureteropelvic junction obstruction may occur as well.

Genitalia

In cloacal exstrophy, the penis is often separated into two hemiphalluses due to the wide pubic diastasis. This can make subsequent reconstructive efforts technically more challenging if a male phenotype is preserved. Cryptorchidism is the rule with cloacal exstrophy.

For girls, in addition to the genital pathology described previously with bladder exstrophy, uterus didelphys and other fusion anomalies of the müllerian duct structures are seen in up to two thirds of cloacal exstrophy patients. Vaginal agenesis occurs in a third of these girls as well.

Anorectal and Intestinal Abnormalities

Associated intestinal abnormalities specific to cloacal exstrophy include imperforate anus, foreshortening of the midgut, bowel duplication, malrotation, intestinal atresia, and Meckel's diverticulum. These are in addition to the exstrophy of the hindgut, ileal intussusception, and exposed appendices that are considered part of the primary pathology of cloacal exstrophy.

Skeletal Abnormalities

In addition to the features seen with bladder exstrophy, patients with cloacal exstrophy can have other skeletal abnormalities. Skeletal anomalies are seen in as many as half of patients with cloacal exstrophy.

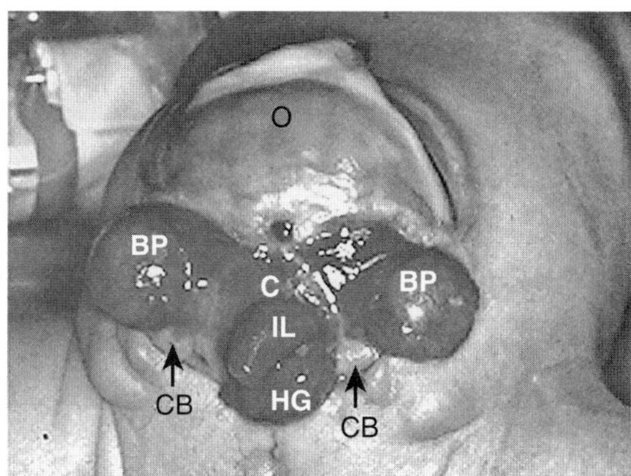

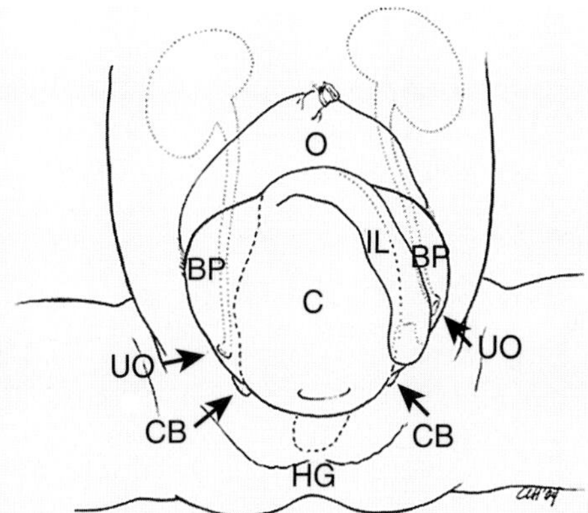

Figure 59-13. Photograph and schematic drawing of a neonate with cloacal exstrophy. O, omphalocele; IL, ileum; BP, bladder plate; C, colon plate; HG, hindgut; CB, corporeal body; UO, ureteral orifice.

Anomalies include congenital hip dislocation, talipes equinovarus, and a variety of limb deficiencies.[116]

Fascial Abnormalities

The fascial anomalies associated with cloacal exstrophy include those described previously for bladder exstrophy. In addition, an omphalocele is often associated.[117,118] This omphalocele can be closed during the initial bladder closure if it is small. If the omphalocele is large, it may require closure as a primary procedure with the reapproximated bladder halves acting as a silo to decompress the increased intra-abdominal pressure. Alternatively, the omphalocele can be treated with antiseptic paint to promote skin overgrowth. Our preference is to proceed with staged surgical correction of the omphalocele and primary reconstruction of the bladder at a later date. In our opinion, the degree of increased intra-abdominal pressure after omphalocele closure determines whether we can proceed with primary bladder closure at the same time as the omphalocele repair or whether these operations should be staged. Aggressive one-stage closure of a cloacal exstrophy can lead to organ ischemia from the increased intra-abdominal pressure. Rupture of an omphalocele clearly requires immediate attention and would take precedence over other considerations. Fortunately, this occurs rarely.

Neurologic Abnormalities

Neurologic involvement of the lower spinal cord in the cloacal exstrophy population is reported to occur in 50% to 100% of patients.[117,119,120] Most patients have lumbar or sacral cord involvement, but thoracic level myelodysplasia has been reported as well.[117] Management of cloacal exstrophy in these situations must be coordinated with the closure of the neural tube defect.

Operative Correction

Perioperative Management

Cloacal exstrophy patients are best cared for by a team of experienced physicians, including a pediatric urologist, surgeon, orthopedist, gastroenterologist, endocrinologist, and neurosurgeon. Given that many infants are diagnosed prenatally by ultrasonography, this multisystem care can often be coordinated before the infant's birth. Advances in neonatal care, intravenous nutrition, and the surgical management of these children have markedly reduced the mortality and morbidity of this disease. Nonetheless, the management of these children remains challenging.

In the neonatal period, the bladder and hindgut plate should be covered (with Saran Wrap or Vigilon [Bard Medical Division, Covington, GA]) to protect these structures. The umbilical cord should be ligated with a silk suture to prevent an umbilical clamp from abrading the bladder or hindgut plate. Antibiotic prophylaxis should be given because of the high incidence of renal abnormalities.

Preoperative studies include ultrasonography, abdominal radiographs, and karyotyping. Ultrasound examination allows the evaluation of the upper urinary tracts, internal genital structures, and spinal cord. Because the genital anomalies associated with cloacal exstrophy may make it difficult to accurately identify the gender of the neonate, karyotyping is indicated to define the chromosomal gender in situations in which the gender is unclear.

Considerations for Closure

Each cloacal exstrophy patient is unique and requires an individualized surgical plan. Because of the broad spectrum of this problem, a flexible treatment strategy is important. In general this would incorporate the following components: (1) closure of the omphalocele with reapproximation of the posterior bladder halves, tubularization of the cecum, and incorporation of the hindgut into the gastrointestinal tract (functionally this creates the anatomy of classic bladder exstrophy) and (2) repair of the exstrophic bladder and genitalia. If the neonate's condition is stable, the initial reconstructive procedures should be performed within the first 48 hours of life, thus taking advantage of the pliable bony pelvis for possible closure of the entire defect. However, spina bifida is present in many children and may need attention, delaying the ventral abdominal wall closure. In addition, the omphalocele, seen in most (88%) infants,[121] may require immediate care to prevent rupture. The size of the omphalocele, the size of the hindgut plate and bladder plates, the extent of the pubic diastasis, and the extent of co-morbidities largely dictate the timing and staging of closure. A large omphalocele containing liver may preclude any attempt at complete closure. If the large omphalocele cannot be closed because of increased abdominal pressure or tension, a Silastic silo or biosynthetic materials can be used to cover the abdominal contents.

In the past an ileostomy was routinely performed, but the metabolic consequences can be significant. Currently, management decisions focus around the use of the exstrophic cecal plate and the terminal blind-ending hindgut. Options for the cecal plate include retaining it in the bladder closure as a bladder augmentation versus separating it and reconstructing it for the fecal stream (Fig. 59-14A). To improve bowel length and water resorption, current recommendations are to tubularize the cecal plate, making the terminal ileum, cecum, and the blind-ending hindgut segment all in continuity for the fecal stream. The hindgut segment can be anastomosed either in an isoperistaltic or antiperistaltic fashion and exteriorized as a colostomy. In some cases, there are hindgut duplications. No segment of bowel should be discarded unless absolutely unusable, because it might be usable in the future for reconstruction of the bowel, bladder, or vagina. Similarly, appendiceal segments should be preserved for possible use in later reconstruction of the urinary tract. Because of altered innervation to the pelvis, only a few patients with cloacal exstrophy are candidates

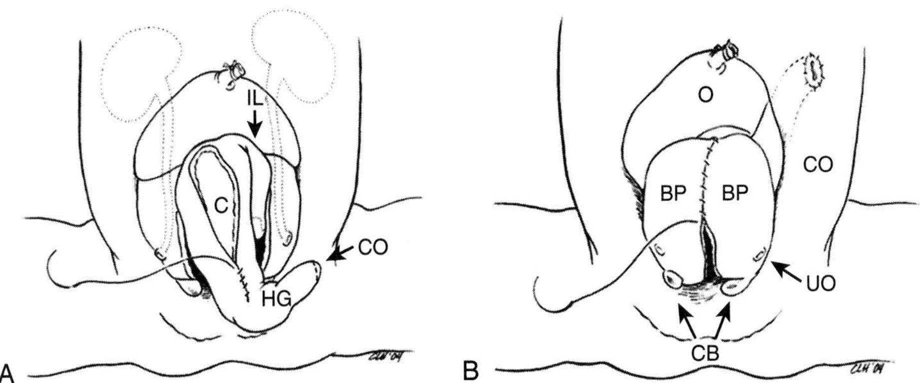

Figure 59-14. **A,** Depiction of removal and tubularization of the cecal plate. **B,** Reapproximation of the bladder plates. IL, ileum; HG, hindgut; CO, colostomy site; C, colon; BP, bladder plate; UO, ureteral orifice; CB, corporeal body; O, omphalocele.

for an anal pull-through procedure. These are infants with an anal fistula and preserved innervation.

Operative Repair

Ureteral catheters are inserted in the ureteral orifices and secured with 5-0 chromic suture. The omphalocele repair is begun with the initial dissection beginning superiorly. The umbilical vessels are ligated and the bladder plates separated from the adjacent skin as described in the CPRE and MSRE techniques. The medial cecal hindgut plate is separated from the paired bladder plates and is tubularized. After the hindgut has been reconstructed, the bladder halves are reapproximated in the midline (see Fig. 59-14B). If found, inguinal hernias should be repaired. Primary bladder closure may be performed at this time if the intra-abdominal pressure remains low after omphalocele closure. This can be determined clinically by assessing ventilatory effort. A one-stage closure of cloacal exstrophy (closure of the omphalocele, cecal plate tubularization, creation of a colostomy, bladder and urethral closure, reconstruction of the external genitalia, and osteotomies) should be performed *only* under optimal anatomic conditions.

The decision to proceed with one-stage closure versus staged reconstruction spanning a period of months must be weighed carefully. After forced closure, increased abdominal pressure may result in organ ischemia, excessive tension to the midline closure, or compromised lower extremity blood flow. The importance of including surgeons experienced in the care of these patients cannot be overemphasized. Thus, the reconstruction can be staged by converting the cloacal exstrophy into a classic bladder exstrophy. A colostomy is then created with the previously described caveats in mind.

If staging is required, once the infant has recovered sufficiently to tolerate another surgical procedure, the remaining steps of reconstruction of the bladder, bladder neck, and genitalia using the CPRE technique[122] (Fig. 59-15) or MSRE technique are performed as previously described. Deep pelvic diaphragm dissection with division of the intersymphyseal band is crucial for appropriate posterior positioning of the bladder and urethra. After the bladder and urethra are positioned within the pelvis, reconstruction of the bladder, genitalia, abdomen, and pelvis is anatomic.

Osteotomies are almost always necessary to assist in closure and posterior positioning of the urinary tract, given that the pubic diastasis is usually more severe than in classic bladder exstrophy. Before incision, the need for osteotomies is assessed under anesthesia by watching for ischemia of the lower extremities and external genitalia during pubic reapproximation. The Hopkins group recommends bilateral combined anterior innominate and vertical iliac osteotomies with gradual approximation of the bones over 1 to 2 weeks via the external fixator and interfragmentary pins.[123,124] The Seattle group prefers iliac osteotomies. Other authors prefer to avoid the use of osteotomies because they believe that osteotomies make the abdominal closure more difficult.[125] This has not been our experience. Fewer wound dehiscences and ventral abdominal wall hernias have been noted with the use of osteotomies.[124]

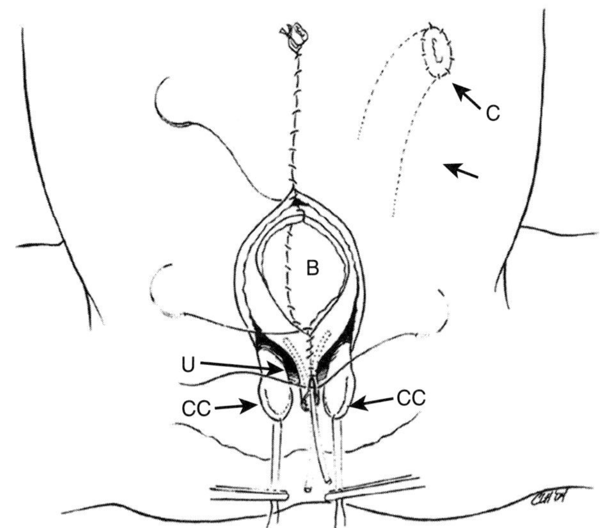

Figure 59-15. Diagram showing use of the complete primary repair of exstrophy technique for bladder reconstruction. B, bladder; CC, corpora cavernosa; U, urethra; C, colostomy.

Late procedures may be required on the urinary tract to achieve continence, including BNR, bladder neck closure, bladder augmentation with stomach, ileum, or hindgut, and creation of a continent catheterizable stoma.[117,126-129] Given nearly all of these children will be dependent on CIC to achieve dryness, surgical reconstruction must be individualized to meet the needs of their limitations.

Genital Reconstruction and Gender of Rearing

Gender assignment for patients with cloacal exstrophy is currently under scrutiny both by the medical profession and lay public. Traditionally, male patients underwent gender conversion in infancy because of concerns that the small, paired male hemiphalluses in these patients were inadequate for reconstruction. This approach was supported by anecdotal data of unsatisfied patients after reconstruction of the male phallus.[117] These observations, in conjunction with the prevailing notion that humans were gender neutral at birth and could undergo sex conversion safely in infancy, have recently come into question.[130] Gender identity now appears to be a much more complex issue than previously thought.

Currently, we reconstruct males with cloacal exstrophy as males whenever technically possible. Many gender-reassigned individuals will later identify themselves in a male gender role in adolescence and adulthood.[130] Technically, however, reconstruction of external male genitalia in the cloacal exstrophy population can be quite difficult. The wide pubic diastasis and small phallic size add to the technical complexity because these findings make it more difficult to bring the two phallic halves together. In some cases, if one phallic half is diminutive, the small one can be removed and the reconstruction performed using only the larger phallic half.

Female genital reconstruction is complex as well. In genetic females, complete müllerian and vaginal duplication often leads to attempted midline reapproximation. However, if one system appears more substantial, excision of the lesser unit may be prudent. In genetic males raised female, neovaginal reconstruction is typically delayed and may require use of hindgut segment or perineal skin.

Gastrointestinal Reconstruction

Short gut syndrome is usually present in patients with cloacal exstrophy at birth, even in those with a normal bowel length. The effects of malabsorption and fluid loss from the short bowel length appear to be clinically most significant early in life.[131] Many such children require parenteral nutritional support in early infancy.[132,133] Because of this, we share the belief that the hindgut should be constructed and placed in continuity with the intestine during initial reconstruction. This may improve nutrition and also preserves intestinal tissue that can be used in later reconstruction of the urinary tract or the vagina, if needed.

chapter 60

HYPOSPADIAS

J. Patrick Murphy, MD

Hypospadias is a developmental anomaly characterized by a urethral meatus that opens onto the ventral surface of the penis, proximal to the end of the glans. The meatus may be located anywhere along the shaft of the penis, from the glans to the perineum.

Chordee, which is ventral curvature of the penis, has an inconsistent association with hypospadias. The degree of chordee is ultimately more significant in the surgical treatment of hypospadias than is the initial location of the meatus. A subcoronal hypospadias with little or no chordee is much less complicated to repair than is one with significant chordee and insufficient ventral skin. For this reason, when discussing the degrees of hypospadias, it is more appropriate to use the clinically relevant and common classification system that refers to the meatal location after the chordee has been released (Table 60-1).[1]

Normal phallic development occurs in weeks 7 to 14 of gestation. By 6 weeks of gestation, the genital tubercle is formed anterior to the urogenital sinus. In the next week, two genital folds form caudad to the tubercle and a urethral plate forms between them. Under the influence of testosterone from the fetal testes, which begins to be produced at about 8 weeks of gestation, the inner genital folds fuse medially to form a tube that communicates with the urogenital sinus and runs distally to end at the base of the glans. The formation of the penile urethra is thus generally completed by the end of the first trimester.[2]

Table 60-1	Hypospadias Classification According to Meatal Location after Release of Chordee
Anterior (65%-70% of cases)	
Glanular Coronal Distal penile shaft	
Middle (10%-15% of cases)	
Middle penile shaft	
Posterior (20% of cases)	
Proximal penile shaft Penoscrotal Scrotal Perineal	

Classically, the glanular urethra is thought to form as an ectodermal ingrowth on the glans. This ingrowth deepens to meet the distal urethra that has formed from the closure of the endodermal genital folds. The capacious junction of these two structures is the fossa navicularis.[3] Recently, this theory has been challenged by the endodermal ingrowth theory. It suggests that the entire urethra forms from the urogenital sinus, which is endoderm. This endoderm differentiates into stratified squamous epithelium.[4] The formation of the glanular urethra is the last step in the formation of the completed urethra. This sequence probably accounts for the predominance of glanular and coronal hypospadias.

Dorsal to the developing urethra, mesenchymal tissue forms the paired corporeal bodies. These are the major erectile tissue components and are invested by the tunica albuginea. Mesenchyme also forms Buck's fascia, the dartos fascia, and corpus spongiosum.

The corpus spongiosum is the supportive erectile tissue that normally surrounds the urethra and communicates with the erectile tissue of the glans. Buck's fascia is the deep layer of fascia that surrounds the corporeal bodies and invests the spongiosum. The dorsal neurovascular bundles are deep to this layer. Superficial to this layer is the dartos fascia, which is the loose subcutaneous layer that contains the superficial veins and lymphatics. These structures form subsequent to completion of the urethra by medial fusion of the outer genital folds, proceeding from the proximal to the distal aspect of the penis. This development accounts for how a fully formed urethra can have a poorly formed spongiosum with thin overlying skin and ventral tethering, despite the meatus being located at the tip of the glans. Finally, the prepuce is formed, originating at the coronal sulcus. It gradually encloses the glans circumferentially.

Arrested development of the urethra may leave the meatus located anywhere along the ventral surface of the penis. Typically, this would lead to foreshortening of the ventral aspect of the penis distal to the meatus and to failure of the prepuce to form circumferentially.

However, in the megameatus form of hypospadias, the prepuce may form normally.

HISTORICAL PERSPECTIVES

The first description of hypospadias and its surgical correction was reported in the 1st and 2nd centuries by the Alexandrian surgeons Heliodorus and Antyllus. They described the defect of hypospadias and its relation to problems with urination and ineffective coitus. They further described a surgical treatment consisting of amputation of the glans distal to the hypospadiac meatus.[5,6]

Little progress was made in the surgical treatment of hypospadias until the 19th century, when two Americans, Mettauer and Bush, described techniques using a trocar to establish a channel from the meatus to the glans. Dieffenbach also described a similar technique in the 1830s. None of these methods was very successful.[5]

In 1874, Theophile Anger reported the successful repair of a penoscrotal hypospadias using the technique described in 1869 by Thiersch for the repair of epispadias in which lateral skin flaps were tubularized to form the neourethra. Anger's report initiated the modern era of hypospadias surgery characterized by the use of local skin flaps.[7,8] Duplay soon described his two-stage technique.[6] In the first stage, the chordee was released; in the second stage, a ventral midline strip of skin was covered by closure of the lateral penile skin flaps in the midline. Duplay did not believe that it was necessary to form the urethral tube completely because he thought that epithelialization would occur even if an incomplete tube were buried under the lateral skin flaps. Browne used this concept in his well-known "buried strip" technique, which was widely used in the early 1950s.[9] In the late 1800s, various other surgeons reported on penile, scrotal, and preputial flap techniques for multistage procedures. Several of them used the technique of burying the penis in the scrotum to obtain skin coverage, similar to the technique described by Cecil and Cuip in the late 1950s.[10] In 1913, Edmonds was the first to describe the transfer of preputial skin to the ventrum of the penis at the time of release of chordee. At a second stage, the Duplay tube was created to complete the urethral closure. Byars popularized this two-stage technique in the early 1950s.[11] Smith further improved on the procedure by denuding the epithelium of one of the lateral skin flaps to give a "pants-over-vest" closure and thus reduce the risk of fistula formation.[12] Belt devised another preputial transfer, two-stage procedure that was popularized by Fuqua in the 1960s.[13]

Nove-Josserand, in 1897, was the first to report the use of a free, split-thickness skin graft in an attempt to repair hypospadias.[14] Over the next 20 years, various other tissues were used as free grafts, including saphenous vein, ureter, and appendix. With none of these procedures was consistent success attained. McCormack used a free, full-thickness skin graft in a two-stage repair.[15] In 1941, Humby described a one-stage technique using the full thickness of the foreskin.[16] Devine and Horton later popularized this free preputial graft technique with very good results.[17]

In 1947, Memmelaar reported the use of bladder mucosa as a free graft technique in a one-stage repair.[18] Marshall and Spellman, in 1955, used bladder mucosa in a two-stage technique.[19] Urologists in China also experienced success with a primary repair using bladder mucosa. This technique was developed independently during the period of scientific and cultural isolation in China.[20] Buccal mucosa from the lip was used for urethral reconstruction in 1941 by Humby[16] and has recently gained renewed attention as a free graft technique.[21]

Improved techniques in preputial and meatal-based vascularized flaps since the 1970s to 1980s have greatly advanced hypospadias repair. Through the contributions of surgeons such as Mathieu, Barcat,[1] Mustarde,[22] Broadbent,[23] Hodgson,[24] Horton and Devine,[17] Standoli,[25] and Duckett,[26] the single-stage repair of even the most severe forms of hypospadias has become commonplace.

CLINICAL ASPECTS

Incidence

The incidence of hypospadias has been estimated to be between 0.8 and 8.2 per 1000 live male births.[27] The wide variation probably represents some geographic and racial differences, but of more significance is the exclusion of the more minor degrees of hypospadias in some reports. If all degrees of hypospadias, even the most minor, are included, then the incidence is probably 1 in 125 live male births.[28] With the most quoted figure of 1 per 250 live male births, it can be assumed that more than 6000 boys are born with hypospadias each year in the United States.[29]

Etiology

A defect in the androgen stimulation of the developing penis, which precludes complete formation of the urethra and its surrounding structures, is the ultimate cause of hypospadias. This defect can occur from deficient androgen production by the testes and placenta, from failure of testosterone to convert to dihydrotestosterone by the 5α-reductase enzyme, or from deficient androgen receptors in the penis. Various disorders of sexual differentiation can cause deficiencies at any point along the androgen-stimulation axis. These are discussed in Chapter 63.

The origin of hypospadias not associated with disorders of sexual differentiation is unclear. An endocrine cause has been implicated by some reports that show a diminished response to human chorionic gonadotropin in some patients with hypospadias, suggesting delayed maturation of the hypothalamic/pituitary axis.[30,31] Other reports have shown an increased incidence of hypospadias in monozygotic twins, suggesting an insufficient amount of human chorionic gonadotropin production by the single placenta to accommodate the two male fetuses.[32]

Environmental causes also have been implicated. A higher incidence of hypospadias has been noted in winter conceptions.[32] A weak association between hypospadias and the maternal ingestion of progestin-like agents has been noted.[33,34] No association has been found between hypospadias and oral contraceptive use before or during early pregnancy.[35]

Genetic factors in the etiology of hypospadias are indicated by the higher incidence of the anomaly in first-degree relatives of hypospadiac patients.[27,34,36] In one study that evaluated 307 families, the risk of occurrence of hypospadias in a second male sibling was 12%. If the index child and his father were affected, the risk for a second sibling increased to 26%. If the index child and a second-degree relative were affected, rather than the father, the risk of the sibling being affected was only 19%.[36] This pattern suggests a multifactorial mode of inheritance, with these families having a higher than average number of influential genes for creation of the anomaly.[36] A combination of the endocrine, environmental, and genetic factors ultimately determines the potential for developing the hypospadias complex in any one individual.[31]

Anatomy of the Defect

The clinical significance of the hypospadias anomaly is related to several factors. The abnormal location of the meatus and the tendency toward meatal stenosis result in a ventrally deflected and splayed stream. This fact makes the stream difficult to control and often makes it difficult for the patient to void while standing. The ventral curvature associated with chordee can lead to painful erections, especially with severe chordee. Impaired copulation and thus inadequate insemination is a further consequence of significant chordee. In addition, the unusual cosmetic appearance associated with the hooded foreskin, flattened glans, and ventral skin deficiency frequently has an adverse effect on the psychosexual development of the adolescent with hypospadias.[37-41] All of these factors are evidence that early surgical correction should be offered to all boys with hypospadias, regardless of the severity of the defect.

The distal form of hypospadias is the most common (see Table 60-1). Frequently, little or no associated chordee is present (Fig. 60-1). The size of the meatus and the quality of the surrounding supportive tissue as well as the configuration of the glans are variable and ultimately determine the surgical procedure. Well-formed, mobile perimeatal skin and a deep ventral glans groove may allow local perimeatal flaps to create the urethra (Fig. 60-2). In contrast, atrophic and immobile skin around the meatus may require tissue transfer from the preputium to form the neourethra.

An unusual variant of the distal hypospadias is the large wide-mouthed meatus with a circumferential foreskin (the megameatus/intact prepuce variant) (Fig. 60-3).[42] Owing to the intact prepuce, this variant is often not identified until a circumcision has been done. If clinicians discover hypospadias during circumcision, they should stop and preserve the foreskin, even if the dorsal slit has been created.

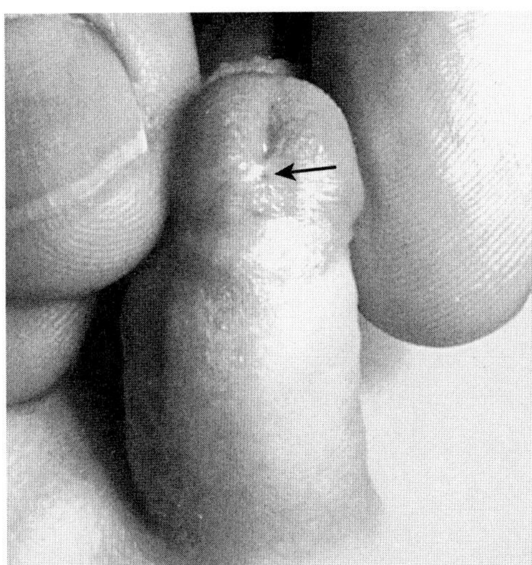

Figure 60-1. Distal hypospadias with a stenotic meatus (*arrow*) located on the glans with no chordee. This patient is a good candidate for a meatal advancement and glanuloplasty (MAGPI) procedure or a tubularized incised urethral plate (TIP) operation.

At times, the distally located meatus may be associated with significant chordee, sometimes of a severe degree (Fig. 60-4). The release of the chordee places the meatus in a much more proximal location, requiring more complicated transfers of tissue to bridge the gap between the proximal meatus and the tip of the glans.

When the meatus is located on the penile shaft, the character of the urethral plate (midline ventral shaft skin distal to the meatus) is important in determining what type of repair is possible. A well-developed and elastic urethral plate suggests minimal, if any, distal ventral curvature (Fig. 60-5). However, a thin atrophic urethral plate heralds a significant chordee. The proximal

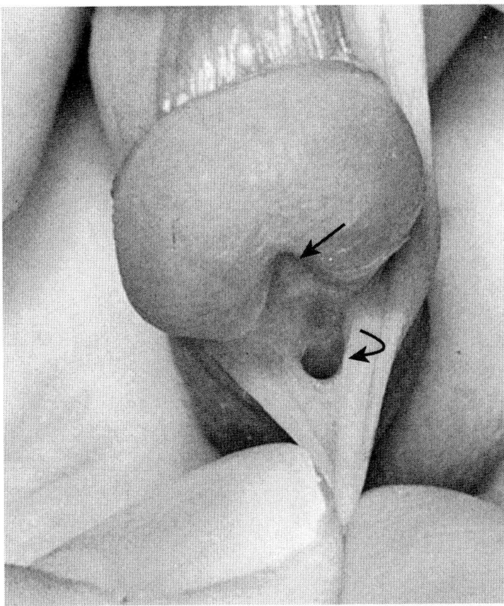

Figure 60-2. Patulous, subcoronal meatus (*curved arrow*) with mobile perimeatal skin and deep ventral glans groove (*straight arrow*). This is a good variant for a meatal-based flap procedure, glans approximation (GAP), or tubularized incised urethral plate (TIP) repair.

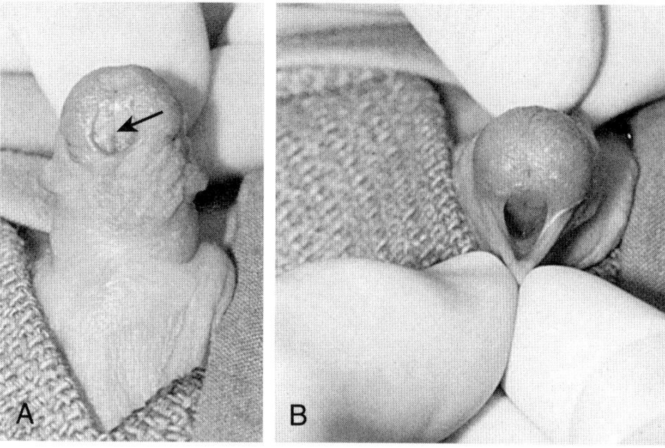

Figure 60-3. **A,** Previously circumcised penis with megameatus (*arrow*) and intact circumferential prepuce. **B,** Large wide-mouthed meatus in the same penis as shown in **A.**

supportive tissue of the urethra also is important. If there is a lack of spongiosum proximal to the hypospadiac meatus, this portion of the native urethra is not substantial enough to use in the repair (Fig. 60-6). Therefore, the neourethra must be constructed from the point of adequate spongiosum.

The position of the meatus at the penoscrotal, scrotal, or perineal location is usually associated with severe chordee, which requires chordee release with an extensive urethroplasty (Fig. 60-7). This type is usually more predictable in the preoperative period as to the choice of repair than are some of the more distal types previously discussed.

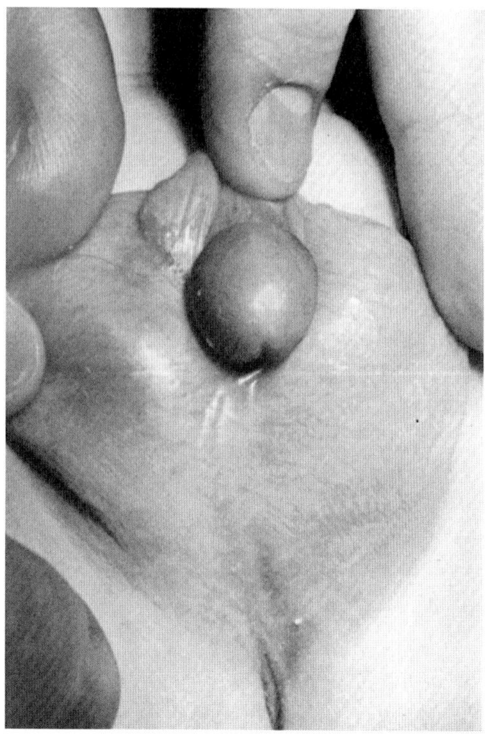

Figure 60-4. Scrotal hypospadias with severe chordee and marked penoscrotal transposition is seen in this infant.

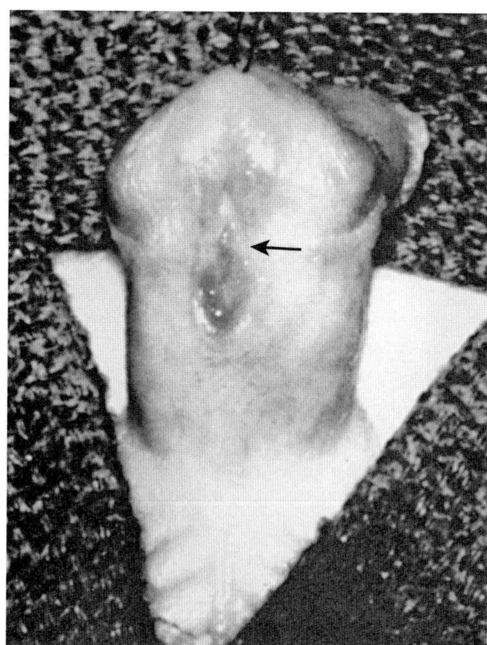

Figure 60-5. Midshaft hypospadias with elastic, well-developed urethral plate distal to the meatus (*arrow*). No significant chordee is present. This is a good variant for an onlay island flap procedure or possibly a tubularized incised urethral plate operation.

Other anatomic elements of the anomaly that are important to consider include penile torsion, glans tilt, penoscrotal transposition, and chordee without hypospadias. These are discussed more completely later.

Associated Anomalies

Inguinal hernia and undescended testes are the most common anomalies associated with hypospadias. They occur from 7% to 13% of the time, with a greater incidence when the meatus is more proximal.[43-45] An enlarged prostatic utricle also is more common in posterior hypospadias, with an incidence of about 11%.[44] Infection is the most common complication of a utricle, but surgical excision is rarely necessary.[46] Several reports have emphasized significantly high numbers of upper urinary tract anomalies associated with hypospadias,[47-50] suggesting that routine upper tract screening is necessary. However, when the association is studied selectively, it can be shown that the types of hypospadias that are at risk for surgically significant upper tract anomalies are the penoscrotal and perineal forms and those associated with other organ system abnormalities.[43,45] When one, two, or three other organ system anomalies occur, the incidence of significant upper tract anomalies is 7%, 13%, and 37%, respectively. Associated myelomeningocele and imperforate anus carry a 33% and 46% incidence, respectively, of upper urinary tract malformations. In isolated posterior hypospadias, the incidence of associated upper tract anomalies is 5%.[45]

In middle and distal hypospadias, when not associated with other organ system anomalies, the incidence is similar to that in the general population.[43,45,51] Therefore, it is recommended that screening for upper

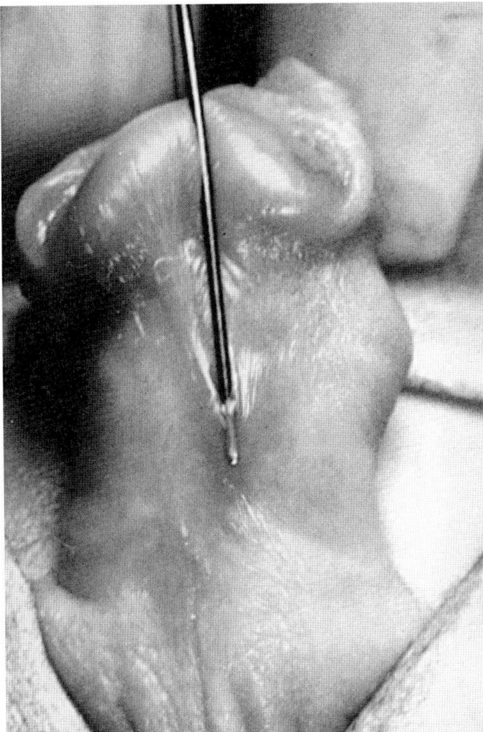

Figure 60-6. Midshaft hypospadias with a lack of spongiosum support proximal to the meatus. The urethra should be opened back to an area of good spongiosum support at the penoscrotal position.

urinary tract anomalies by voiding cystourethrogram and renal ultrasonography be done in patients with penoscrotal and perineal forms of hypospadias and in those with anomalies associated with at least one additional organ system. Screening should be done in patients with other known indications, such as a history of urinary tract infection, upper or lower tract obstructive symptoms, and hematuria, and in those boys having a strong family history of urinary tract abnormalities.[52]

Disorders of sexual differentiation are also potentially associated with hypospadias. This association is rare in the routine forms of hypospadias. Failure of testicular descent, micropenis, penoscrotal transposition (see Fig. 60-4), or bifid scrotum (see Fig. 60-7) when associated with hypospadias are all signs of potential disorders of sexual differentiation and warrant evaluation with karyotype screening.[27,53,54]

TREATMENT

The advent of safe anesthesia, fine suture material, delicate instruments, and good optical magnification has allowed virtually all types of hypospadias to be repaired in infancy. Generally, the repair is done on an outpatient basis. To deny a child the benefit of repair because the defect is "too mild" or the risk of complication is "too high" is inappropriate. The chance to make the phallus as normal as possible should be offered to all children, regardless of the severity of the defects.

Age at Repair

The technical advances over the past few decades have made it possible to repair hypospadias in the first 6 months of life in most patients.[55-57] Some surgeons have suggested delaying repair until after the child is age 2 years.[52,58-60] However, most surgeons who deal routinely with hypospadias prefer to perform the repair when the patient is 6 to 12 months old.[53,54,56,57,61,62] One study compared the emotional, psychosexual, cognitive, and surgical risks for hypospadias. The "optimal window" recommended for repair was age 6 to 15 months (Fig. 60-8).[63] Unless other health or social problems require delay, we believe the ideal time to complete penile reconstruction in the pediatric patient is about age 6 months.[64] The anesthetic risk is low and, at this age, postoperative care is much easier for the parents than it is when the child is a toddler.

Objectives of Repair

The objectives of hypospadias correction are divided into the following categories:

1. Complete straightening of the penis
2. Locating the meatus at the tip of the glans
3. Forming a symmetric, conically shaped glans
4. Constructing a neourethra uniform in caliber
5. Completing a satisfactory cosmetic skin coverage

If these objectives can all be attained, the ultimate goal of forming a "normal" penis for the child with hypospadias can be accomplished.

Straightening

Curvature of the penis is difficult to judge, at times, in the preoperative period. Artificial erection, by injecting physiologic saline in the corpora at the time of

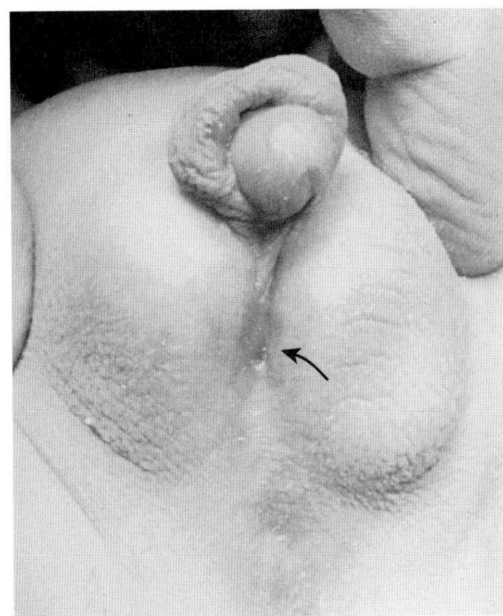

Figure 60-7. Perineal/scrotal hypospadias (*arrow*) with severe chordee and a bifid scrotum.

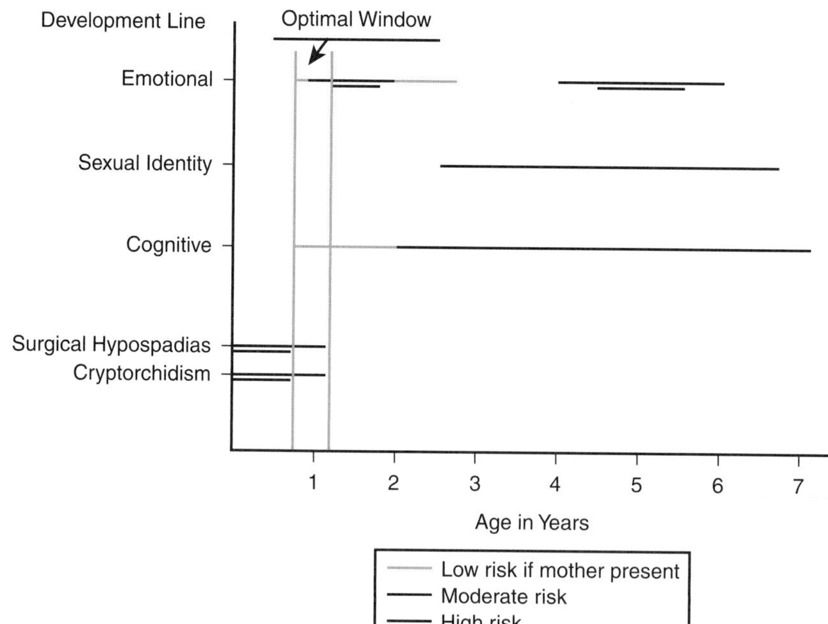

Figure 60-8. Evaluation of the risk for hypospadias repair from birth to age 7 years. Optimal window is 6 to 15 months of age. (From Schultz JR, Klykylo WM, Wacksman J: Timing of elective hypospadias repair in children. Pediatrics 71:342-351, 1983.)

operation, allows determination of the exact degree of curvature.[65] This curvature may be caused only by ventral skin or subcutaneous tissue tethering, which is corrected with the release of the skin and dartos layer.[66,67] Infrequently, the curvature may be secondary to true fibrous chordee, which requires division of the urethral plate and excision of the fibrous tissue down to the tunica albuginea.

Sometimes, even after extensive ventral dissection of chordee tissue, a repeated artificial erection still reveals the presence of significant ventral curvature. This finding is usually secondary to the uncommon problem of corporal body disproportion, which is caused by a true deficiency of ventral corporal development. This problem can be treated by making a releasing incision in the ventral tunica albuginea and inserting either a dermal or a tunica vaginalis patch to expand the deficient ventral surface.[68,69] Others have suggested the use of small intestinal submucosa as an off-the-shelf substitute for the autologous grafts.[70] Another technique is to excise wedges of tunica albuginea dorsally with transverse closure to shorten this dorsal surface and straighten the penis.[71,72] Other surgeons have had success with dorsal plication without excision of tunica albuginea.[73,74] Anatomic studies suggest that this plication should be done in the midline dorsally.[75] Still others advocate corporal rotation dorsally with or without penile disassembly to correct severe chordee.[76,77]

Axial rotation of the penis, or penile torsion, is another aspect of penis straightening that must be managed. This problem can generally be corrected by releasing the dartos layer as far proximal as possible on the penile shaft. This allows the ventral shaft to rotate back to the midline and corrects the torsion. Chordee or torsion can also occur without hypospadias. The management of these boys encompasses the entire spectrum of techniques as when hypospadias is involved (Fig. 60-9).[78,79]

Locating the Meatus

Locating the meatus at the tip of the glans has not always been standard in hypospadias repair. Historically, the risk of complications was thought to be too great to recommend procedures that would locate the meatus beyond the subcoronal area. Multistage repairs popular in the 1950s and 1960s were designed to attain only a subcoronal location of the meatus. Surgical techniques since then have improved sufficiently so that glans-channeling and glans-splitting techniques are used with minimal complications, making the distal tip meatus possible.

In glanular and subcoronal variants, the configuration of the meatus is the factor for determining what technique is used to move the meatus distally on the glans. Meatoplasty with or without dorsal advancement, distal urethral mobilization and tubularization, or meatal-based flaps are the methods selected in most cases of distal hypospadias.[80,81] In the more proximal forms, creating the neourethra with local vascularized skin flaps or free grafts allows placement of the urethra at the end of the penis. Alternatively, glans channeling or glans splitting allows placement of the meatus at the tip of the glans.[1,17,22,26,82,83]

Glans Shape

Creation of a symmetric, conically shaped glans is the objective of the glansplasty component of the repair. Approximating the lateral glanular tissue in the midline ventrally over a meatoplasty or meatal advancement corrects the flattened glans appearance to the more anatomically normal, conically shaped glans. Similarly, approximation of well-developed glans wings to the midline over a neourethra in a split glans restores the glans to its normal conical shape.

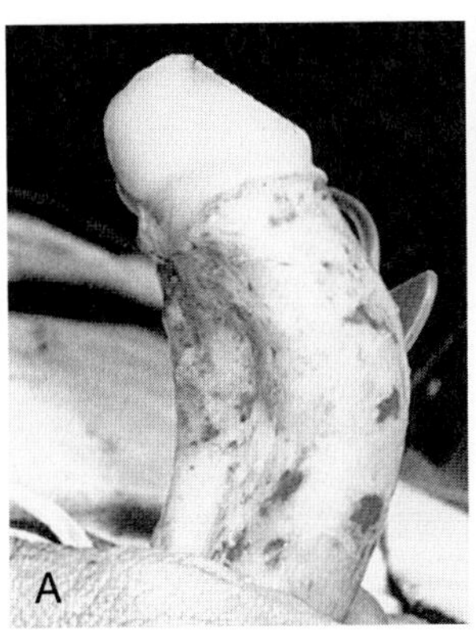

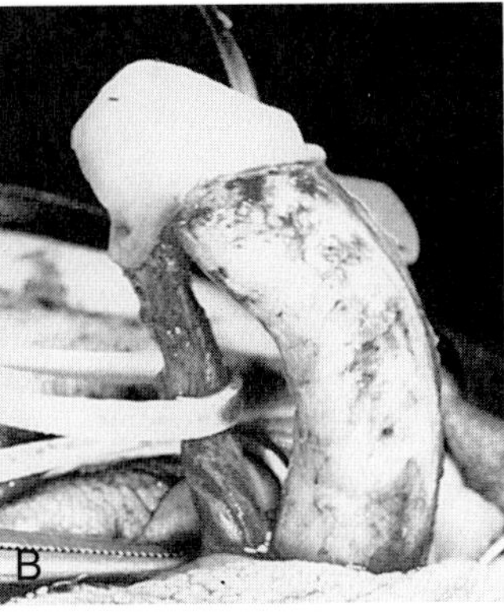

Figure 60-9. **A,** Chordee without hypospadias. The meatus is located at the tip of the glans with marked ventral curvature. **B,** Fibrous ventral tissue is all released. The urethra is mobilized, but curvature persists, indicating corporeal body disproportion. This requires a ventral patch or dorsal plication (see text).

Urethral Construction

Formation of the neourethra can be accomplished with local skin flaps, various types of free grafts, or vascularized pedicle flaps. Local skin flaps may be formed from in situ skin or dorsal skin transferred to the ventrum in a previous stage. In either case, it is important to avoid making these flaps too narrow or thin because their vascular supply may be compromised. The hypospadiac urethral plate has been shown on histologic studies to consist of epithelium covering well-vascularized connective tissue without fibrosis.[84] This finding supports the clinical findings that urethral plate preservation is helpful for successful urethroplasty. Free grafts depend on an adequately vascularized bed for survival. Therefore, they should not be placed in a scarred channel. Well-vascularized subcutaneous tissue and skin must cover them to allow adequate neovascularization and survival of the graft.[17]

Mobilized vascularized flaps of preputium have a more reliable blood supply than do free grafts. Therefore, if they are available, these flaps are the choice of most surgeons.[24,26,83,85] They may be used as patches onto a strip of native urethral plate to complete the urethra, or they may be tubularized and used as bridges over the gap between a proximal native urethra and the end of the glans.[26,86] A watertight closure of the well-vascularized neourethra is formed, with care being taken to make it uniform in caliber and of appropriate size for the age of the child. This closure helps avoid stricture and the formation of saccules, diverticula, and fistulas.

Cosmesis

Creating cosmetically appealing, well-vascularized skin coverage of the penile shaft after urethroplasty can sometimes be challenging. Transfer of vascularized dorsal preputial skin to the ventrum can be accomplished in several ways.

Buttonholes of the dorsal skin allow the penis to come through this defect, draping the distal preputium over the ventral surface of the penis.[19] This maneuver has the advantage of transferring well-vascularized skin over the repair, but it is not as appealing cosmetically.

A more satisfactory method of transferring skin to the ventrum is by splitting the dorsal skin in the midline longitudinally and advancing the flaps around on either side to meet in the ventral midline. This technique allows a midline ventral closure, which simulates the median raphe. Moreover, it allows a subcoronal closure to the preputial skin circumferentially, which simulates the suture lines of a standard circumcision.[87,88] Another adjunct is to advance lateral flaps of inner preputial skin from each side to the ventral midline of the penis at the time of glansplasty or closure of glans wings.[89] Approximating these flaps in the midline gives the appearance of an intact circumferential preputial collar, further enhancing the potential for an anatomically normal skin closure (see Fig. 60-14).

Some patients, particularly those in European countries, prefer the appearance of a noncircumcised penis. In distal repairs, reconstruction of the preputium for a noncircumcised appearance can be accomplished in certain cases.[90] Correction of the more significant degrees of penoscrotal transposition is often necessary to avoid the feminizing appearance. In select cases, this step can be done at the time of the original repair. However, when using vascularized pedicle flaps for the repair, it is usually safer to correct significant penoscrotal transposition with rotational flaps at a later time.[91-94]

Surgical Procedures

Because of the wide variation in the anatomic presentation of hypospadias, no single urethroplasty is applicable for every patient. At times, a final decision regarding the degree of curvature and the ultimate location of the meatus cannot be made until the operation has started and an artificial erection is performed. The surgeon who repairs hypospadias must be adaptable and experienced to deal with all variants of the defect. Versatility and experience with all options of surgical treatment are the keys to successful management. By recognizing the sometimes subtle nuances of meatal variation, glans configuration, and curvature character, the experienced surgeon can make the best choice as to the type of repair to use (Fig. 60-10).

Anterior Variants

Some glanular variants are amenable to the meatal advancement and glansplasty (MAGPI) type of repair (Fig. 60-11).[95] A stenotic meatus with good mobility of the urethra and a fairly shallow ventral glanular groove are the anatomic characteristics best suited for the MAGPI. A wide-mouthed meatus is not amenable to the MAGPI repair. The meatal-based flap repair may be used effectively in this situation, assuming no chordee is present and mobile, well-vascularized skin exists proximal to the meatus (Fig. 60-12).[96,97] This repair works well when there is a moderately deep ventral groove, allowing the urethra to be placed deep in the glans and a conically shaped glans to be created after

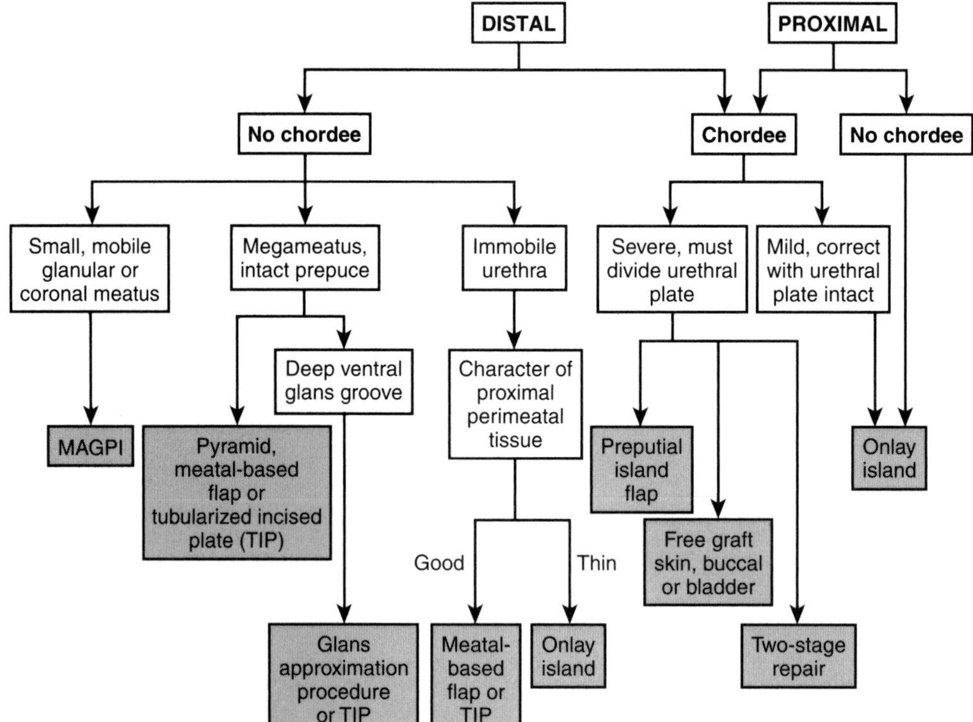

Figure 60-10. Flow diagram for types of repair in variants of hypospadias. MAGPI, meatal advancement and glansplasty. TIP, tubularized incised plate urethroplasty.

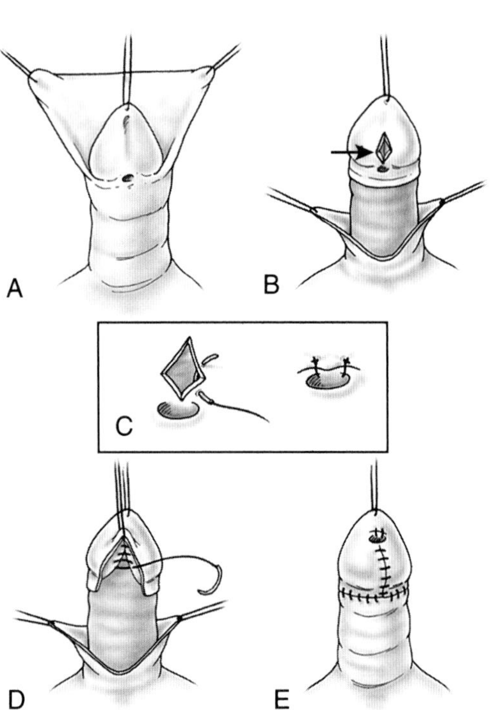

Figure 60-11. Meatal advancement and glansplasty. **A,** Circumferential subcoronal incision to deglove the penile shaft skin. **B,** Longitudinal incision through the ventral groove of glans (*arrow*). **C,** Transverse closure of glans groove incision to advance dorsal urethral plate and to open stenotic meatus. **D,** Glans tissue approximated ventrally in the midline to restore conical configuration to glans. **E,** Completion of the skin closure.

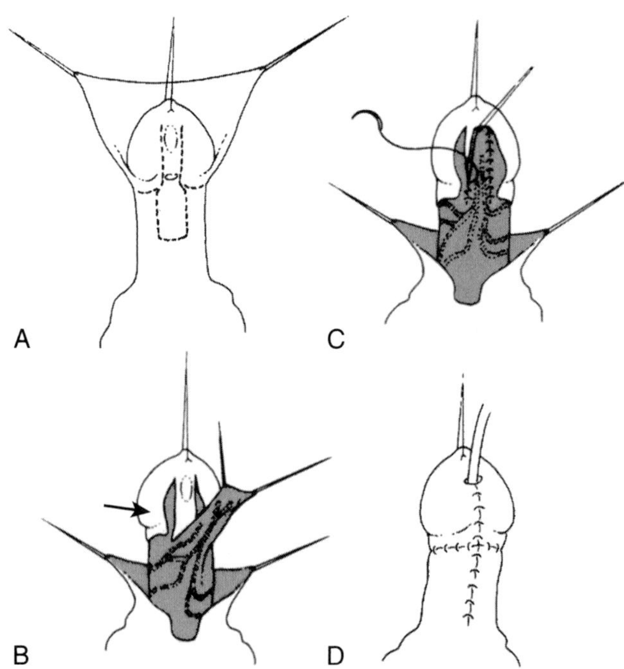

Figure 60-12. Meatal-based flap repair. **A,** Parallel incisions along ventral groove distal to the meatus and formation of meatal-based flap proximal to meatus. **B,** Glans wings developed on either side of the urethral plate (*arrow*) to close over the neourethra later. Meatal-based flap is mobilized distally maintaining good vascular and tissue support. **C,** Flap is anastomosed to bilateral edges of the urethral plate to form neourethra. **D,** Glans wings are closed over the neourethra in the midline, giving conical glans configuration. Penile shaft is covered with dorsal foreskin advanced ventrally.

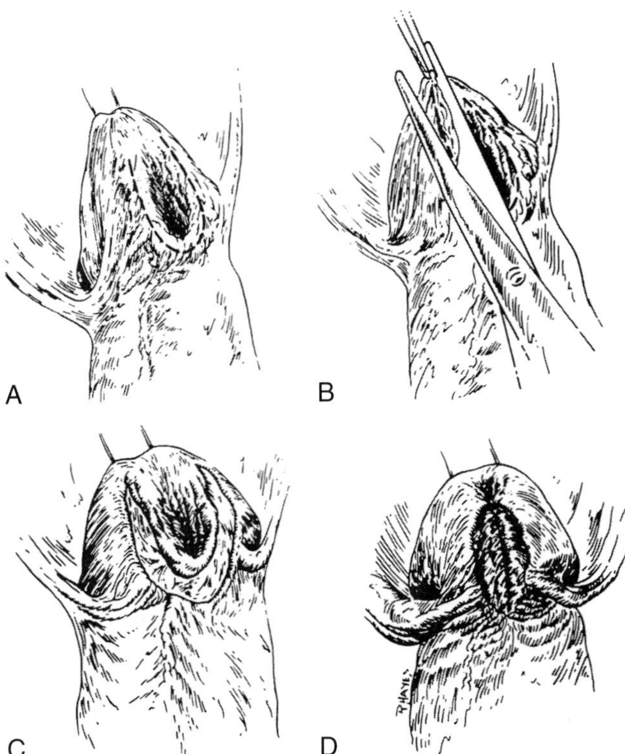

Figure 60-13. Glans approximation procedure. **A,** Deep ventral groove and patulous, coronal meatus with outline of proposed incision. **B,** Skin is excised along previously marked "U"-shaped line. **C,** De-epithelialized glans with the urethral plate intact. **D,** Two-layer closure of the glanular urethra with glans skin still open. (From Zaontz MR: The GAP [glans approximation procedure] for glandular/coronal hypospadias. J Urol 141:359-361, 1989.)

closure of the glans wings. The glans approximation procedure is sometimes useful when a wide-mouthed proximal glanular meatus exists with a very deep groove (Figs. 60-13 and 60-14).[98] The pyramid procedure is well suited for the fish-mouth type of meatus seen in the megameatus/intact prepuce variant.[42] These repairs give a very good cosmetic result when done in the proper situation.

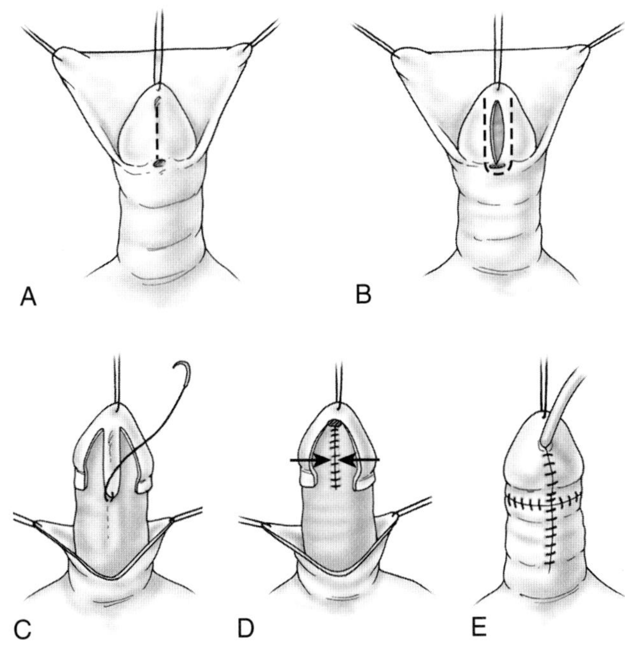

Figure 60-15. Tubularized incised urethral plate (TIP) technique. **A,** Urethral plate is incised longitudinally. **B,** Glans incisions are made longitudinally, wide enough to leave two strips of epithelium for 10-Fr size neourethra. **C,** Neourethra is tubularized in the midline with multiple layers and dartos flap to reinforce. **D,** Glans wings are closed in the midline. **E,** Skin closure is completed and the urethral stent is in place (optional).

The tubularized incised plate urethroplasty (TIP) is a modification of the Thiersch-Duplay tubularization, which involves a deep longitudinal incision of the urethral plate in the midline (Fig. 60-15). This allows the lateral skin flaps to be mobilized and closed in the midline without tension. This procedure also allows the wide-mouthed meatus variant with a flat, shallow ventral groove to be repaired without the need for additional flaps.[99] The TIP urethroplasty has gained wide acceptance in recent years. Its durability and long-term success have been demonstrated even in some of the more proximal variants.[100-102]

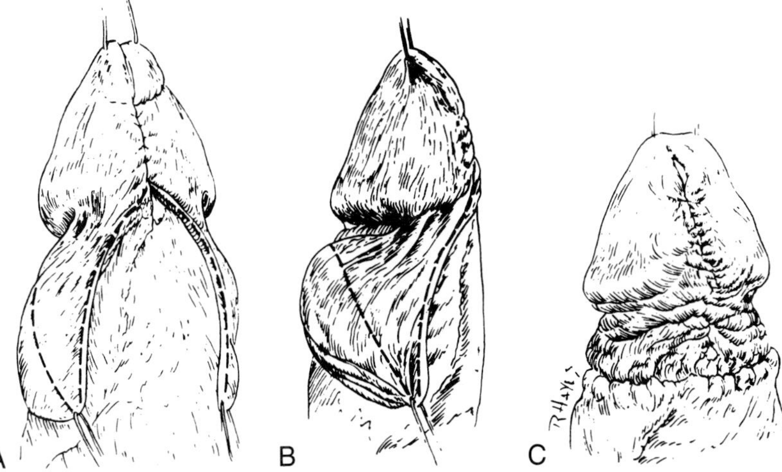

Figure 60-14. **A,** Glanular skin approximated and lateral wings of inner preputial skin outlined. **B,** Lateral view of outline for preputial collar. **C,** Lateral preputial wings closed in midline to give circumferential preputial collar. (From Zaontz MR: The GAP [glans approximation procedure] for glanular/coronal hypospadias. J Urol 141:359-361, 1989.)

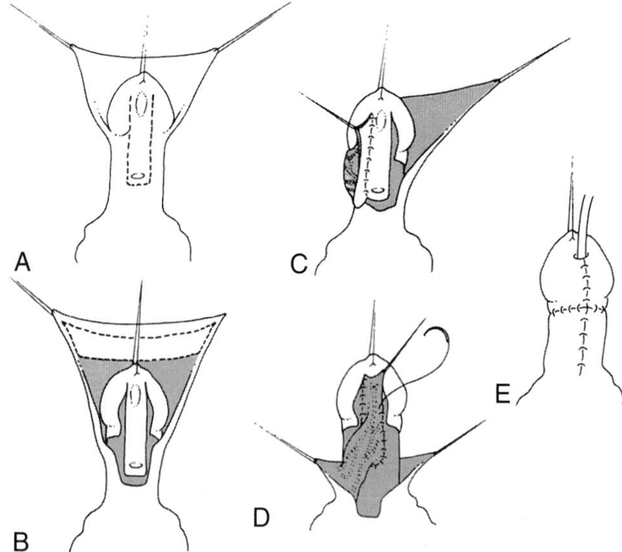

Figure 60-16. Onlay island flap repair. **A,** Outline of incisions along the well-developed urethral plate with no chordee. **B,** Mobilization of glans wings and shaft skin with urethral plate intact distal to meatus. Outline of inner preputial island flap that will be transposed ventrally for onlay completion of neourethra. **C,** Island flap transposed ventrally on pedicle. The first part of the anastomosis is completed. **D,** Remainder of anastomosis to complete neourethra to tip of glans. **E,** Glans wings are approximated over the neourethra in the ventral midline. The penile shaft is covered with the ventral advancement of dorsal foreskin.

Middle Variants

The amount of ventral curvature generally dictates the type of repair in middle- and distal-shaft hypospadias. When no significant chordee is present, the TIP repair or the meatal-based flap can sometimes be performed. Another technique is the onlay island flap repair (Fig. 60-16).[86] This procedure involves mobilizing an inner preputial flap on its pedicle and rotating it ventrally to lay on the well-developed ventral urethral plate to complete the tubularization of the neourethra. This technique is applicable to many forms of penile shaft hypospadias.

In milder degrees of chordee, the curvature can be corrected without dividing the urethral plate by taking down tethering bands lateral to the urethral plate or by dorsal plication techniques.[74,75] This allows the onlay island flap technique to be used instead of the tubularized pedicle flap or free graft, which have a higher incidence of complications.[54] If significant chordee is present, division of the urethral plate may be necessary. This moves the meatus more proximal and requires treatment as described for proximal variants.

Proximal Variants

Many of the scrotal and perineal forms of hypospadias are associated with significant chordee, which requires division of the urethral plate and results in a gap to be

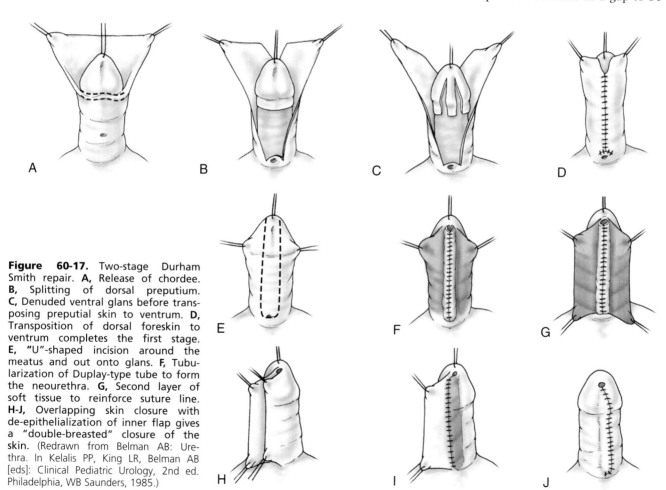

Figure 60-17. Two-stage Durham Smith repair. **A,** Release of chordee. **B,** Splitting of dorsal preputium. **C,** Denuded ventral glans before transposing preputial skin to ventrum. **D,** Transposition of dorsal foreskin to ventrum completes the first stage. **E,** "U"-shaped incision around the meatus and out onto glans. **F,** Tubularization of Duplay-type tube to form the neourethra. **G,** Second layer of soft tissue to reinforce suture line. **H-J,** Overlapping skin closure with de-epithelialization of inner flap gives a "double-breasted" closure of the skin. (Redrawn from Belman AB: Urethra. In Kelalis PP, King LR, Belman AB [eds]: Clinical Pediatric Urology, 2nd ed. Philadelphia, WB Saunders, 1985.)

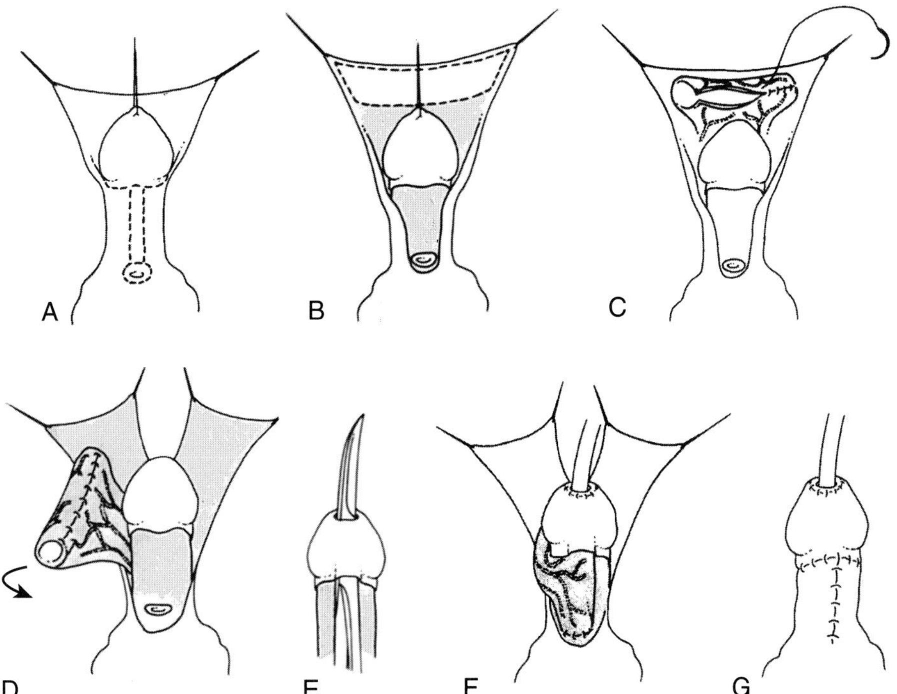

Figure 60-18. Transverse preputial island flap tube repair. **A** and **B**, Release of chordee and degloving of penile shaft skin. **B**, Outline of inner preputial island flap. **C**, Tubularization of inner preputial island flap. **D**, Transposition of the tubularized island flap to the ventrum, maintaining pedicle blood supply. **E**, Creation of a channel through glans tissue with sharp incisional and excisional technique. **F**, Island tube anastomosed to proximal native urethra, brought through glans channel and anastomosed to epithelium at tip of glans. **G**, Penile shaft covered with dorsal foreskin advanced ventrally. Skin closure is completed.

bridged between the proximal native urethra and the tip of the glans. This can be done with staged procedures in which coverage of the ventral penile shaft is attained by rotation of dorsal flaps to the ventrum, with later tubularization to form the neourethra (Fig. 60-17).

Another method is the tubularized free graft anastomosed to the native urethra proximally and extended to the end of the glans by a tunneling or splitting technique. The most commonly used free grafts are full-thickness skin, bladder mucosa, or buccal mucosa. Preputial skin is much preferred to extragenital skin.[17,103] If genital skin is not available, buccal mucosa may be the next best tissue.[21,104,105] Vascularized flaps are a more physiologically sound alternative to free grafts. The transverse inner preputial island flap that is tubularized and transposed ventrally to form the neourethra is the preferred type of vascularized flap[106] (Fig. 60-18). In contrast to free grafts, it provides good preputial skin with a reliable blood supply that does not rely on neovascularization for healing of the neourethra. Occasionally, the length of the prepuce alone may not be adequate to bridge the defect to a very proximal meatus. In this case, the shiny non–hair-bearing skin around the meatus can be tubularized (Fig. 60-19), moving the proximal urethra to the penoscrotal junction. The preputial vascularized tube graft can then be used to bridge the remaining distance to the end of the penis.[53]

In some cases, the penile shaft may be deficient enough to cause concern about ventral coverage after formation of the neourethra. The double-face island flap can solve this problem.[24] This technique leaves some of the outer preputial skin attached to the pedicle after tubularizing the inner preputial layer. This outer preputium is transferred to the ventrum with the pedicle and supplies the skin coverage of the ventral shaft. However, the complications associated with the double-face island flap are numerous, and it has few advocates.[55]

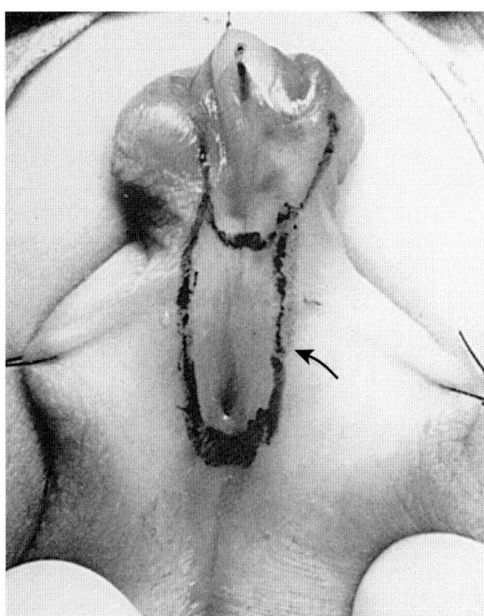

Figure 60-19. Outline of non–hair-bearing skin distal to scrotal meatus (*arrow*) that will be tubularized to move the meatus to the penoscrotal junction. Island flap tube will complete the repair to the end of the glans.

I prefer the transverse island flap in a one-stage procedure in most cases of proximal hypospadias with chordee.[106] In the rare case in which the skin deficiency is so severe that a vascularized pedicle cannot be used or in which the chordee is so severe that a dermal or tunica vaginalis graft is required to correct disproportion, a two-stage repair may be better.[107-109]

Technical Perspectives

Optical Magnification

Most surgeons agree that optical magnification is indispensable in hypospadias surgery. Standard operating loupes, ranging from 2.5× power to 4.5×, are generally thought to be ideal for the magnification needed for this type of surgery. Some workers advocate the use of the operating microscope and suggest an improved result with this technique.[110] Most surgeons have not believed that this degree of magnification is necessary for obtaining excellent results. The microscope may be overly cumbersome for the small improvement in visualization it may provide.[111]

Sutures and Instruments

Fine absorbable suture is chosen by most surgeons to close the neourethra. Polyglycolic or polyglactin material is probably the most common suture choice. However, some surgeons prefer the longer-lasting polydioxanone suture.[110] Permanent sutures of nylon or polypropylene, in a continuous stitch that is pulled out 10 to 14 days after surgery, are recommended by some.[12,56]

The type of optical magnification also determines the size of the suture. Generally, 6-0 or 7-0 suture is preferred. With the microscope, 8-0 or 9-0 may be used. Skin closure is usually accomplished with either fine chromic (6-0 or 7-0) or plain catgut suture. Small suture-sinus tracts may occur along these suture lines as they dissolve. I have used a subcuticular closure with either 6-0 chromic or polydioxanone for the past 10 years and have mostly eliminated the problem of these suture-sinus tracts.

The delicate instruments of ophthalmologic surgery are well designed for the precise tissue handling required in hypospadias repair. Small, single-toothed forceps or fine skin hooks allow tissue handling with minimal trauma. Standard microscopic tools are necessary for those who prefer the microscope over loupe magnification.

Urinary Diversion

The goal of the surgeon in any urinary diversion procedure in hypospadias repair is to protect the neourethra from the urinary stream for the initial healing phase. In theory, this diversion should decrease the complication rate, particularly fistula formation. The more traditional perineal urethrostomy and suprapubic cystostomy are uncomfortable and cumbersome to manage in the postoperative period. Small indwelling 6- or 8-Fr polymeric silicone (Silastic) tubes left through the repair and just into the bladder allow drainage of the urine into the diaper in infants (Fig. 60-20).[111] This technique greatly facilitates the outpatient care of these patients. These stents are well tolerated by the babies. Problems with the stents becoming plugged or dislodged are uncommon.

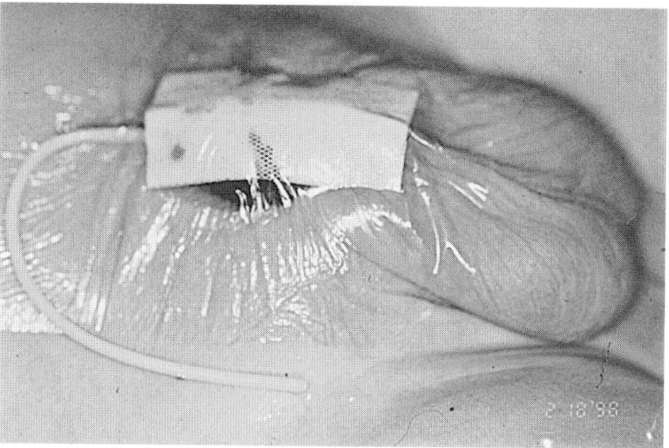

Figure 60-20. Occlusive dressing of transparent adhesive material in sandwich fashion on the abdominal wall, with a 6-Fr soft polymeric silicone (Silastic) indwelling tube inserted for urinary diversion.

Some surgeons favor a stent that traverses the repair but is not indwelling in the bladder.[110] The patient is allowed to void, but the stent protects the repair. I prefer the indwelling stent, used for 5 to 14 days, depending on the complexity of the repair. In older children who would not tolerate wearing a diaper, a 6- or 8-Fr Foley catheter may be used in the simpler distal repairs and a suprapubic cystostomy is used in the more complex repairs. Suprapubic drainage should be used in complex reoperations or in any repairs requiring a free graft. Studies have suggested that no diversion is required for simpler distal procedures, such as MAGPI, meatal-based flap, or distal Duplay tubes. Simple small fistula repairs can be accomplished without diversion.[112,113]

Dressings

Hypospadias dressings should apply enough gentle pressure on the penis to help with hemostasis and to decrease edema formation, without compromising the vascularity of the repair. Various dressings accomplish this purpose. A silicon-foam dressing, which can be placed around the penis in a liquid state that transforms to solid later, leaves a soft, mildly compressive dressing that is waterproof.[114] This dressing can be removed without difficulty several days after operation. Other dressings include transparent adhesive dressings wrapped around the penis or fixed to the abdominal wall in a sandwich-like fashion (see Fig. 60-20).[68] A DuoDerm (ConvaTec, Skillman, NJ) dressing can be applied around the penis as an alternative, before using a transparent adhesive dressing.[110] Two prospective studies have shown that the type of dressing does not influence healing or complication rates.[115,116] I have continued to use a transparent dressing against the abdominal wall for the hemostatic effect in the first 12 postoperative hours.

Analgesia

Postoperative pain is generally controlled with oral analgesics. Bladder spasms caused by indwelling catheters can be managed with propantheline bromide and opium suppositories or by oral oxybutynin. A dorsal penile nerve block performed intraoperatively with bupivacaine can help control postoperative pain.[117]

A caudal block is my preferred method for postoperative pain control. In most cases, the patients are comfortable for the entire day and evening of surgery and are easily cared for at home with only oral analgesia.[118]

Complications

The type and incidence of complications vary with the particular form of repair. Attention to detail and meticulous technique are imperative to keep the incidence of all complications to a minimum. The following is a discussion of some of the general complications that can occur with all repairs.

Bleeding

Intraoperative bleeding can, at times, be troublesome. However, with the judicious use of the point tip cautery, it can be generally be kept to a minimum. Tourniquets or cutaneous infiltrations with dilute concentrations of epinephrine can be helpful, but they should not replace careful technique. Postoperative bleeding is generally prevented by mildly compressive dressings. Subcutaneous hematomas may occur but generally do not need to be drained.

Infection

Wound infection is a rare problem in hypospadias repair, especially in the prepubertal patient. As long as good viability of tissue is maintained, infection should be a minor problem. Perioperative antibiotic prophylaxis is favored by some surgeons.[119] This is probably a reasonable precaution in an extensive repair, especially in the postpubertal patient. Urinary suppression with oral antibiotics is recommended with indwelling catheters that are open to drainage in the diaper.[68,120,121]

Devitalized Skin Flaps

If sloughing of the skin coverage occurs, it is usually on the ventral surface of the penis where dorsal skin has been transposed. When the devascularized skin is over a well-vascularized bed of tissue, such as with a pedicle flap, primary healing generally occurs without sequelae. If the slough is over poorly vascularized tissue, such as a free graft, the result can be the breakdown of the repair. Careful attention to transposing well-vascularized tissue for coverage of the neourethra in all repairs is critical to avoid this problem.

Fistulas

A urethrocutaneous fistula is the most commonly reported complication of hypospadias surgery. It results from failure of healing at some point along the neourethral suture line and can range in size from pinpoint to large enough for all voided urine to exit at this site. Fistulas also may be associated with stenosis or distal stricture. Occasionally, small fistulas seen in the early postoperative period may close spontaneously. Surgical closure should be postponed until complete tissue healing has occurred, which requires at least 6 months.[122,123] A small fistula may be closed by local excision of the fistula tract followed by closure of the urethral epithelium with fine absorbable suture. Approximating several layers of well-vascularized subcutaneous tissue over this closure is important to prevent recurrence. Urinary diversion is usually not necessary in small fistula repairs. Larger fistulas may require more complicated closures, with mobilization of tissue flaps or advancement of skin flaps to ensure an adequate amount of well-vascularized tissue for a multilayered closure.[122-124] Urinary diversion is often necessary with more complicated closures.

Strictures

Narrowing of the neourethra may occur anywhere along its course. However, the most common sites of stricture formation are at the meatus and at the proximal anastomosis. Most cases of meatal narrowing can be managed as an office procedure by gentle dilation in the first few postoperative weeks. Occasionally, meatotomy or meatoplasty is needed, especially when associated with a proximal fistula or neourethral diverticulum. More proximal strictures can generally be treated with dilation or a visual internal urethrotomy.[125] However, open urethroplasty may sometimes be required, with excision of the stricture and primary urethral anastomosis or patch graft urethroplasty.[122,123,126]

Diverticulum

Saccular dilation of the neourethra may result from distal stenosis causing progressive dilation, contained urinary extravasation from the breakdown of the repair, or initial creation of an oversized segment of the neourethra. Classic bulging of the urethra ventrally with voiding is evident with significant diverticulum formation (Fig. 60-21). Urinary stasis with chronic inflammation is common. Obstruction can result from kinking of the urethra when the diverticulum distends with voiding. Repair requires excision of the redundant neourethra with primary closure to restore a uniform caliber to the urethra.[127] Special attention should be paid to any narrowing of the neourethra distally, just as in fistula repair.

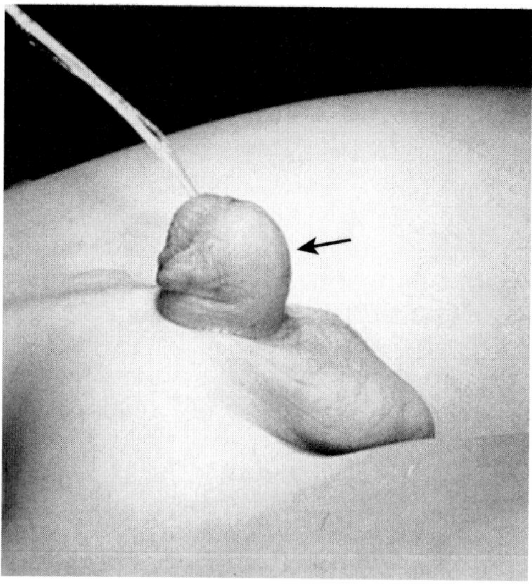

Figure 60-21. A neourethral diverticulum is seen to be bulging ventrally with voiding (*arrow*).

Retrusive Meatus

Retraction of the meatus from its original position at the tip of the glans to a proximal glanular or subcoronal position can occur with any repair. A retrusive meatus is caused by the failure of the glansplasty closure or the breakdown of devascularized distal neourethra. Retraction is a common problem when the MAGPI procedure is used in patients whose meatus is too proximal or when too much tension is placed on the glansplasty closure.[128] Correction can usually be accomplished by a repeat glansplasty or a meatal-based flap procedure.[122,128]

Persistent Chordee

Residual ventral curvature after hypospadias repair can be a troublesome problem. It is usually related to inadequate release of chordee at the original procedure. Increased ventral curvature occurring as the penis grows is at least a theoretical possibility. The artificial erection has made this complication much less common. Treatment of the problem is similar to the treatment of chordee without hypospadias. Degloving of the penis and takedown of any ventral tethering tissue is accomplished by using the artificial erection technique to guide dissection. Dorsal plication, ventral excision with patching, and division of the urethra may all be necessary.[123,129]

Recurrent Multiple Complications

Patients with recurrent multiple complications generally have experienced multiple failed repairs that have resulted in a combination of severe complications. Extensive fibrosis of the urethra with fistulas, strictures, diverticula, and residual chordee may be present. The successful outcome of further repair depends on thorough evaluation of each complication and the use of all the techniques available to the surgeon experienced in hypospadias repair. If tissue is available, vascularized flaps or staging procedures are preferable to free grafts in a scarred phallus.[130] If a free graft must be used, it is important to obtain the most vascularized bed possible in which to place the graft. Buccal mucosa is probably the best tissue for a free graft in this type of situation.[21,54,123] In patients with severe scarring and ventral skin loss, a split-thickness skin graft may be used for ventral coverage. This tissue may then be tubularized at a second stage.[131]

Sexual Function

Long-term results of hypospadias repair with regard to erectile function, ejaculation, and fertility are not available for the children who have undergone repairs at a younger age over the past decade. Historically, sexual difficulties after hypospadias repair have been reported. These were thought to be secondary to psychosexual factors related to surgery in childhood rather than to anatomic problems.[36,41] Fertility has been assessed by semen analysis in patients after hypospadias repair.[38] Higher rates of oligospermia are reported. These lower sperm counts generally occur in patients with associated anomalies such as cryptorchidism, chromosome abnormalities, varicoceles, or torsion. In a patient with an anatomically successful hypospadias repair and no associated anomalies that might affect fertility, a high potential for fertility and an adequate sexual function are expected.[132] Only close observation of pediatric patients into their adulthood after hypospadias repair early in life will reveal the true incidence of sexual dysfunction and fertility problems.

Results

A summary of the incidence of certain complications for commonly used procedures is seen in Table 60-2. Also, a personal series of mine is included that represents those patients who underwent operation over a 20-year period (1987 to 2007) with a minimum follow-up of 6 postoperative months.

Table 60-2 Complications of Various Types of Repairs

Study	No. of Cases	Meatal Stenosis (%)	Retrusive Meatus (%)	Stricture (%)	Fistula (%)	Diverticulum (%)	Total (%)
MAGPI							
Issa & Gearhart[128]	142	—	5 (3.5)	—	—	—	5 (3.5)
Keating & Duckett[54]	225	—	—	—	—	—	(<1)
Duckett & Snyder[133]	1100	—	7 (0.6)	—	5 (0.4)	—	12 (1.1)
Murphy	370	—	4 (1.2)	—	—	—	4 (1.1)
Meatal-Based Flap							
Retik et al[134]	294	1 (0.5)	—	—	1 (0.5)	—	2 (1.0)
Wacksman[97]	125	—	—	—	1 (0.8)	—	1 (0.8)
Hakim et al[112]	336	—	—	—	9 (2.7)	—	9 (2.7)
Murphy	285	4 (1.4)	—	—	3 (1.1)	—	7 (2.5)
Thiersch-Duplay (w/o Incised Plate)							
Kass & Chung[135]	308	—	—	—	28 (9.1)	2 (0.6)	30 (9.7)
Zaontz[98]	24	—	—	—	1 (4.1)	—	1 (4.1)
Murphy	214	—	—	—	3 (1.4)	—	3 (1.4)
TIP (distal)							
Snodgrass et al[100]	148	3 (2.0)	—	—	5 (3.4)	—	8 (5.4)
Cheng et al[102]	514	2 (0.3)	—	—	3 (0.6)	—	5 (1.0)
Jayanthi[138]	110	—	—	—	1 (0.9)	—	1 (0.9)
Baccala et al[150]	101	3 (3.0)	—	—	2 (2.0)	—	5 (5.0)
Murphy	328	1 (0.3)	—	—	2 (0.6)	—	3 (0.9)
TIP (proximal)							
Braga et al[151]	35	—	—	—	—	—	18 (51.4)
Snodgrass & Yucei[152]	65	—	—	—	14 (21.5)	—	14 (21.5)
Onlay Island Flap							
Elder et al[86]	50	—	—	—	1 (2.0)	—	1 (2.0)
Hollowell et al[73]	66	—	—	—	—	—	(8.0)
Keating & Duckett[54]	43	—	—	—	—	—	(9.0)
Weiner et al[136]	58	2 (3.4)	—	1 (1.7)	10 (17.0)	—	13 (22.4)
Braga et al[151]	40	—	—	—	10 (25.0)	—	10 (25.0)
Gearhart & Borland[137]	61	—	1 (1.6)	—	3 (5.0)	—	4 (6.6)
Murphy	273	3 (1.1)	—	1 (0.4)	7 (2.6)	4 (1.5)	15 (5.5)
Tube Island Flap							
Duckett[26]	100	—	—	—	—	—	(10.0)
Wacksman[97]	94	—	—	—	—	—	7 (7.4)
Keating & Duckett[54]	34	—	—	—	—	—	(18.0)
Hollowell et al[73]	85	—	—	—	—	—	(15.0)
Perovic & Djordjevic[77]	75	4 (5.3)	—		2 (2.7)	3 (4.0)	9 (12.0)
Weiner et al[136]	74	3 (4.0)	—	7 (9.4)	10 (13.5)	9 (12.2)	29 (39.1)
Murphy	57	5 (8.8)*	—	—	2 (4.0)	6 (10.5)*	8 (14.0)

MAGPI, meatal advancement and glansplasty; TIP, tubularized incised urethral plate.
*Same patients with meatal stenosis and diverticulum.

Table 60-2 Complications of Various Types of Repairs—cont'd

Study	No. of Cases	Meatal Stenosis (%)	Retrusive Meatus (%)	Stricture (%)	Fistula (%)	Diverticulum (%)	Total (%)
Free Graft (Preputium)							
Devine & Horton[17]	20	—	—	—	6 (30.0)	—	6 (30.0)
Hanna[139]	27	—	—	1 (3.7)	4 (14.8)	1 (3.7)	6 (22.2)
Hendren & Horton[140]	103	3 (2.9)	—		6 (5.8)	—	9 (8.7)
Robert et al[141]	81	—	—	7(8.6)	28 (34.6)	—	35 (43.2)
Stock et al[142]	77	2 (2.5)	—	3 (3.8)	10 (12.9)	—	15 (19.5)
Bladder Mucosa							
Koyle & Ehrlich[104]	16	1 (6.2)	—	—	1 (6.2)	—	2 (12.5)
Ransley et al[143]	47	9 (19.1)	—	1 (2.1)	10 (21.3)	—	20 (42.5)
Ehrlich et al[144]	79	—	—	8 (10.1)	2 (2.5)	4 (5.0)	14 (17.7)
Mollard et al[145]	76	14 (17.4)	—	15 (19.7) †	—	—	29 (38.1)
Li et al[146]	113	6 (5.3)	—	8 (7.0)	—	—	14 (12.4)
Buccal Mucosa							
Fichtner et al[147]	62	1 (1.6)	—	—	7 (11.3) ‡	—	8 (12.9)
Carr[148]	30	—	—	—	—	—	10 (33.3)
Hensle et al[149]	47	—	—	—	—	—	13 (27.7)

†Three of these 15 were failed grafts.
‡Three of these were failed grafts.

chapter 61

CIRCUMCISION

Stephen C. Raynor, MD

Circumcision is the removal of the prepuce or foreskin and is one of the most frequently performed surgical procedures in the world. Indications for circumcision include the treatment of disease, perceived benefits of prophylactic circumcision, and social or religious concerns. There is a wide variability in the rate of circumcision among different populations. A lack of consensus regarding the function of the foreskin as well as often strident debate concerning the benefits of circumcision have led to much controversy as to the appropriateness of the procedure.

EMBRYOLOGY

The development of the prepuce begins during the third month of gestation as a fold of skin at the base of the glans. With growth, this skin extends distally, with the dorsal portion growing at a more rapid rate than the ventral component. The proper development of the prepuce is dependent on the presence of androgen and androgen receptors. The closure of the ventral portion of the prepuce is completed by the fifth month of gestation after closure of the glanular urethra. Keratinization of the glans and inner epithelial surface of the prepuce then follows. Initially, the inner surface of the prepuce and the epithelium of the glans are fused. Lacunae then begin to form between the two surfaces, resulting in an eventual complete separation. This process of separation is a gradual one and typically remains incomplete at birth.[1]

As a result of this incomplete keratinization, the foreskin can be completely retracted in less than 5% of neonates. The adherence between the glans and prepuce may not allow visualization of the meatus in about half of neonates. The natural separation of the two surfaces continues with growth of the child. Separation of the prepuce from the glans progresses with growth. A completely retractable foreskin is present in 60% of boys aged 11 to 15 years.[2] All foreskins should be retractable by age 17.[3] Until this natural process of separation is complete, there is usually no need for forceful retraction of the foreskin and cleaning of the glans.

HISTORY AND INCIDENCE

Circumcision has been practiced since ancient times. Evidence of circumcision has been found in the study of ancient Egypt, with the identification of circumcised mummies as well as the depiction of circumcision in bas relief on an ancient tomb.[1,4] Columbus found the New World natives to be circumcised.[1] Circumcision may also have developed as a mark of defilement or slavery.[4]

A common rationale given for the decision to proceed with circumcision is religious beliefs. The Bible declares circumcision to be the sign of the covenant between God and the people of Israel.[5] In the Muslim faith, circumcision is recommended but not obligatory.[6] There is a high rate of circumcision in Jewish and Muslim populations, and circumcision is quite common in the United States. Areas of Africa, Australian aborigines, and people of the Near East also practice ritual circumcision.[7,8] In contrast, routine circumcision is rarely performed in Europe, China, the Far East, and Central and South America.[7] This wide variation in incidence is probably reflective of religious and cultural differences, as well as strong disagreement regarding the value of routine neonatal circumcision.

THE PREPUCE

The prepuce is the anatomic covering of the glans. Contributing to the debate concerning the appropriateness of routine circumcision is a lack of clear understanding of the function of the prepuce. The prepuce is a specialized junctional mucocutaneous tissue that provides adequate skin and mucosa to cover the entire penis during erection. The somatosensory innervation is by the dorsal nerve of the penis and branches of the perineal nerve. Autonomic innervation is from the pelvic plexus. There are encapsulated somatosensory receptors, both mechanoreceptors and nociceptors in the prepuce. This innervation of the prepuce differs from the glans, which is primarily innervated by free nerve endings and has primarily protopathic sensitivity. As a result of these differences, the inner mucosa of the prepuce is believed to be a part of the normal complement of the penile erogenous tissue.[9]

MEDICAL INDICATIONS

The inability to retract the foreskin of a neonate is a result of the incomplete keratinization of the glans and is not pathologic. Phimosis is the inability to retract the foreskin due to narrowing of its opening. True phimosis is associated with a white, scarred preputial orifice, which is uncommon before 5 years of age. It is most common just before puberty and is an indication for circumcision.[10] Balanitis xerotica obliterans is a ring-like distal sclerosis of the prepuce with whitish discoloration or plaque formation that may involve the prepuce, glans, or urethral meatus and is an indication for circumcision.[11] Paraphimosis occurs when the foreskin has been retracted behind the corona but is able to be brought back over the glans with great difficulty or not at all. This is also an indication for circumcision, although ardent opponents of circumcision would offer preputial stretching, preputial plasty, or topical corticosteroid creams as alternative therapy.[12-15] Balanitis is an infection of the glans, and posthitis is an infection of the prepuce. Recurrent infection with scarring of the prepuce is an accepted indication for circumcision.[8,16]

ROUTINE NEONATAL CIRCUMCISION

The appropriateness of routine circumcision of healthy male neonates is an emotional and contentious issue. Confounding the argument is the lack of a clear understanding as to the precise function of the prepuce.[17] Opponents of circumcision have represented the procedure as a symbol of the "therapeutic state"[18] and as a mutilating procedure[19] and have questioned the legality of routine neonatal circumcision.[20] Circumcision is done on the eighth day in the Jewish faith, traditionally performed by a mohel, a member of the Jewish faith trained in ritual circumcision. In Islamic countries, circumcision is considered traditional but not obligatory, with a wide variability in age at time of circumcision.[6,21] Proponents for routine neonatal circumcision generally cite three advantages: the prevention of urinary tract infections (UTIs) in infants, the prevention of sexually transmitted disease, and the prevention of penile cancer.

As rates of circumcision diminished in the United States, reports appeared demonstrating an increased rate of UTIs in uncircumcised male infants. An initial report of infant UTIs showed a male predominance in infants younger than 3 months of age, with a disproportionate number of these being uncircumcised.[22] A subsequent large retrospective analysis of infants of families in the armed services suggested that uncircumcised infants have a 12-fold increased risk for UTI as compared with circumcised infants.[23-25] A 10-fold increase in the cost of managing UTIs in uncircumcised infants as compared with circumcised infants was also shown.[26]

The increased incidence of infection is believed to be secondary to adherence of pathogenic bacteria to the prepuce.[27] It has also been suggested that there is an increased risk of UTIs in uncircumcised young adults.[28] Proponents of circumcision point out that the 10% incidence of concurrent bacteremias and the long-term sequelae of renal scarring are factors to be considered in the circumcision debate.[29] Critics have been quick to note that these studies have been retrospective analyses and therefore are subject to significant bias.[30,31] Others have suggested that colonization of the prepuce by nonmaternal uropathic bacteria could be prevented by strict rooming-in with the mother.[32]

There have been many studies examining the relationship between circumcision status and sexually transmitted diseases (STDs). Studies have shown that patients who are not circumcised have an increased risk of chancroid, syphilis, gonorrhea, candidiasis, genital warts, and genital herpes.[33-36] However, other studies have found little support for or have refuted these findings altogether.[37,38] There is also evidence that circumcision is associated with a decreased risk of cervical cancer in women with high-risk sexual partners as a result of the reduced risk of human papillomavirus infection in the male partner.[35] It is possible that the protective effect of circumcision against STDs may differ between developed and developing nations with poor hygiene.[38] Possible mechanisms for differing rates of STDs in relation to circumcision status include a more easily traumatized mucosa and epithelium of the uncircumcised phallus, the environment of the foreskin being more conducive to certain infectious agents, or nonspecific balanitis in uncircumcised men predisposing to certain STDs. Behavior and sexual practice still represent the greatest risk factors in the transmission of STDs.[35]

Epidemiologic studies of human immunodeficiency virus (HIV) infection and acquired immunodeficiency syndrome (AIDS) have raised another argument for prophylactic circumcision. There has been a substantial amount of evidence linking uncircumcised men with an increased risk of HIV infection. This increased risk of HIV infection is independent of the increased risk of genital ulcers in uncircumcised men.[39] In Africa, there are regional differences in the rate of circumcision. As the HIV/AIDS epidemic has emerged on the continent, an increased rate of HIV/AIDS has been observed in areas with low circumcision rates.[40] An analysis of 30 epidemiologic studies from Africa concluded that there was enough evidence that circumcision was associated with reduced HIV infection rates to consider male circumcision as a viable strategy to reduce HIV transmission.[32] Three randomized trials in Africa showed an estimated 50% to 60% reduction in the relative risk of HIV infection with circumcision.[41,42] A similar association between circumcision status and HIV has been noted in the United States, with uncircumcised homosexual men having a twofold increase in the risk of HIV infection.[43] If a male partner is uncircumcised, there appears be an increased risk of transmission of HIV to heterosexual contacts.[44]

Another reason espoused for routine circumcision is as a protective measure against invasive penile cancer. The lack of circumcision has been strongly associated with invasive penile cancer in multiple case series.[39] The etiology of penile cancer is unknown, but there appears to be an association with human papillomavirus (HPV).[45] The incidence of penile cancer in the United States is approximately one case per 100,000, with nearly all cases occurring in uncircumcised men.[31,46] This protective effect against penile cancer is diminished or lost when circumcision is done after the neonatal period.[8,46,47] Other factors associated with invasive penile cancer include smoking, a history of genital warts, penile rash or tears, multiple sexual partners, and poor penile hygiene.[39,47] Critics of circumcision cite equally low rates of penile cancer in developed countries with low circumcision rates. These epidemiologic data, combined with the extremely low incidence of penile cancer and the probable viral etiology, have led some authors to conclude that the impact of routine neonatal circumcision against penile cancer does not justify its widespread practice.[30,45]

There are many strong feelings but no definitive answer to the question of the appropriateness of routine neonatal circumcision. Taken together, studies do not provide conclusive evidence for or against it. Males not circumcised at birth have between a 2% and 10% likelihood of needing circumcision in the future.[15,19] A longitudinal study comparing circumcised with uncircumcised males showed a higher risk of penile problems in infancy in the circumcised group.[48] However, there was a higher rate of problems in the uncircumcised group after infancy. By 8 years of age, the uncircumcised group had experienced 1.5 times the rate of penile problems.

The most recent circumcision policy statement from the American Academy of Pediatrics in 1999 acknowledges the potential medical benefits of neonatal male circumcision, but does not recommend it as a routine procedure.[39] Its interpretation of the data, as well as this recommendation, has been questioned.[49] On their review of the data, the Canadian Pediatric Society stated that the risks and benefits of routine neonatal circumcision were evenly balanced and concluded that routine neonatal circumcision was not recommended.[45] In the United States, the decision regarding neonatal circumcision seems to be based more on social as opposed to medical reasons.[50]

SURGICAL TECHNIQUE

Circumcision has been practiced for centuries and there have been numerous techniques developed. Common to all methods, the goal is removal of an adequate amount of the prepuce to uncover the glans, treat or prevent phimosis, and eliminate the possibility of paraphimosis. Whichever method is chosen, the surgeon must be familiar with and adept at the procedure with a resultant low complication rate. Informed consent should always be obtained before any circumcision.[51]

Neonatal Circumcision

Circumcision represents the most frequently performed male operation in the United States, with close to 64% of male neonates circumcised in 1995.[39] Neonatal circumcision is most frequently performed with a circumcision device. These various devices may be a shield, which is used in the traditional Jewish circumcision, a Mogen clamp, a Gomco clamp, or a Plastibell.[7] Before the procedure, the penis should be inspected for any contraindication to circumcision. Contraindications to circumcision in the neonate include a short or small phallus, hypospadias, chordee with no hypospadias, hooded prepuce, dorsal penile cutaneous hump, penile curvature or torsion, penoscrotal fusion, or large hernias or hydroceles that engulf the penis.[52]

There is general agreement as to the need for adequate analgesia when performing neonatal circumcision. Studies have shown that infants circumcised without analgesia have a stronger pain response to vaccination at 4 and 6 months of age as compared with those who received analgesics.[53] Effective relief of circumcision pain has been found with acetaminophen, topical lidocaine-procaine cream, and local nerve blocks.[54-57] One study showed a subcutaneous ring block with 1% lidocaine without epinephrine to be the most effective pain relief.[39] Sucrose on a pacifier can also provide added pain control.[58]

Even though many circumcisions are performed outside the operating room, antisepsis is critical because infection is a serious potential complication. In performing a Gomco circumcision, the field is sterilely prepped and then the adhesions between the glans and inner surface of the prepuce are bluntly separated. The extent of foreskin to be excised is then marked, either with a marking pen or with a crush of the dorsal prepuce done with a straight mosquito clamp. A dorsal slit allows the appropriate-sized bell to be placed over the glans, inside the prepuce (Fig. 61-1). The bell and foreskin are then brought through the opening in the base of the clamp, placed in the yoke, which is tightened, followed by excision of the foreskin distal to the base of the clamp. Electrocautery must never be used to excise the foreskin because transmission of the electrical current to the shaft of the penis will occur. The bell is then released and removed, taking care not to disrupt the weld between the shaft skin and the remnant of the inner surface of the prepuce.

A Plastibell differs from the Gomco clamp in that the distal foreskin is strangulated, with a resulting slough of that tissue. After sterile prep and dorsal slit, the appropriate-sized Plastibell is placed over the glans inside the prepuce (Fig. 61-2). A string is then tied around the prepuce and positioned in a groove in the bell. The excess foreskin is trimmed and the handle is broken off the bell. The foreskin remnant and bell are expected to slough off in 7 to 12 days.

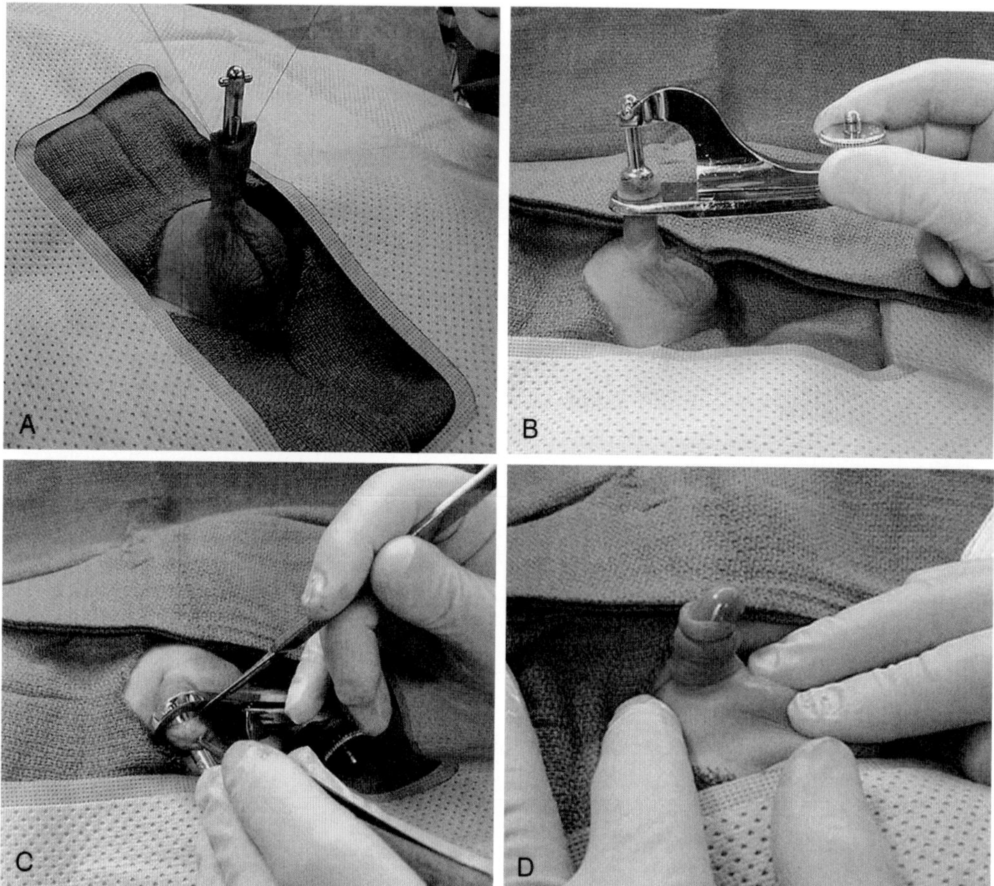

Figure 61-1. The Gomco technique. **A,** A short dorsal slit has been performed to allow an appropriate sized bell to be placed over the glans and inside the prepuce. **B,** Next, the prepuce to be excised along with the bell have been brought through the opening in the base of the clamp and placed in the yoke. **C,** The yoke has then been tightened to coapt the skin edges. After waiting for 5 to 7 minutes, the excess prepuce is excised. Electrocautery must never be used to excise the foreskin because transmission of electrical current to the shaft of the penis will occur. **D,** The bell has been released, and the circumcision is completed.

Freehand Circumcision

In older patients, circumcision is usually performed in the operating room. Circumcision devices seem to be less adequate for the older patient, and sleeve resection of the foreskin is preferable. As shown in Figure 61-3, after prepping the operative field, any remaining adhesions between the glans and foreskin are bluntly lysed.

After marking the subcoronal sulcus, the foreskin is incised along the base of the glans with the foreskin in its normal position. Less skin is excised from the ventral surface. Dissection is carried down to Buck's fascia. The prepuce is then retracted and an incision made in the subcoronal sulcus, leaving a generous cuff of subcoronal skin. Injury to the urethra must be avoided. The collar of foreskin that has been isolated is then

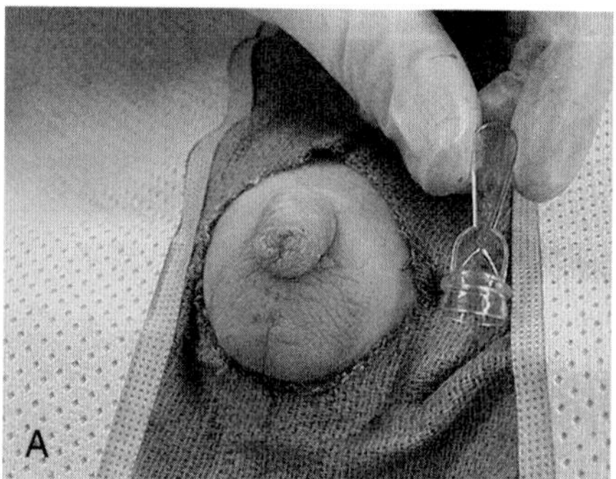

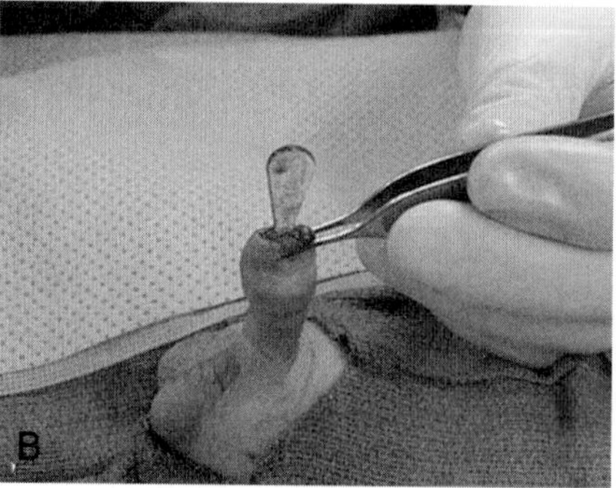

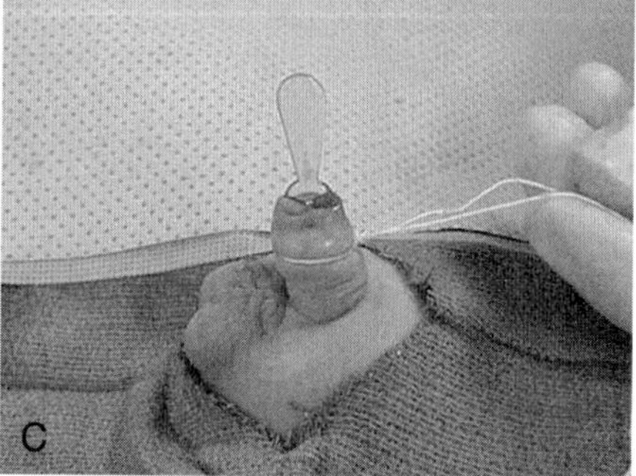

Figure 61-2. Similar to the Gomco technique, in the Plastibell technique, adhesions between the glans and inner surface of the prepuce are bluntly separated. **A,** An appropriate-size Plastibell has been selected. **B,** The Plastibell is placed over the glans inside the prepuce. **C,** A string is then tied around the prepuce and positioned in the groove of the bell. The excess foreskin is trimmed and the handle is broken off the bell. The foreskin remnant and bell are expected to slough in 1 to 2 weeks.

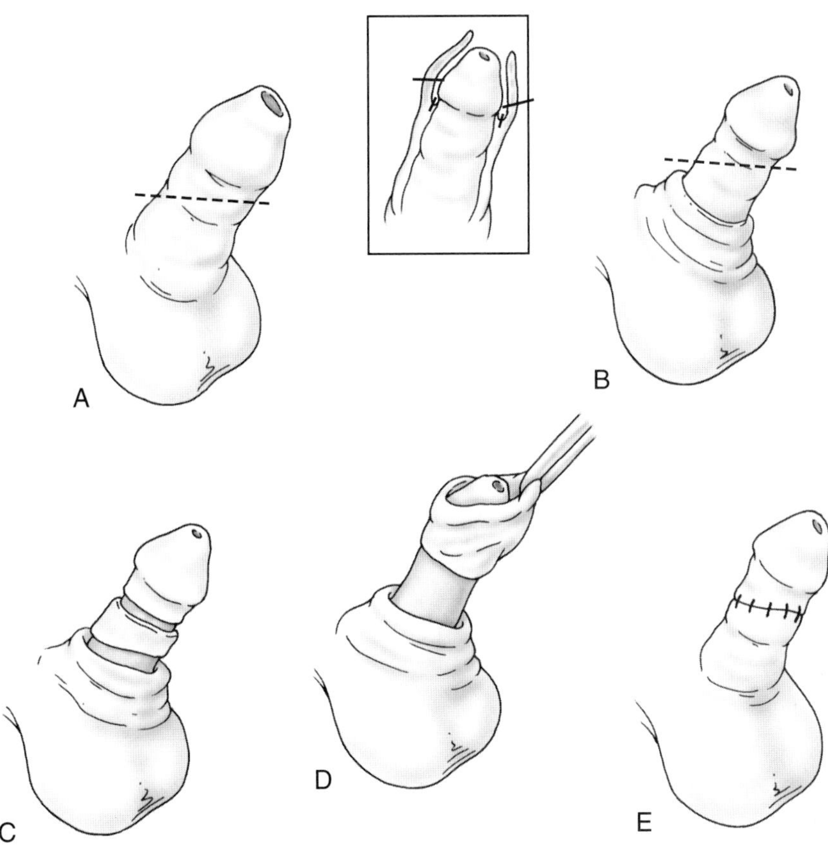

Figure 61-3. **A,** For a freehand circumcision, the initial incision is made in the shaft skin, leaving more skin ventrally. **B,** A second incision is then made in the subcoronal sulcus, leaving a generous cuff. The *inset* shows the amount of foreskin to be excised. The isolated foreskin (**C**) is then excised (**D**), and the shaft skin is sutured to the subcoronal skin (**E**).

excised, and electrocautery is used to obtain meticulous hemostasis. The shaft skin is then approximated to the subcoronal skin using absorbable sutures.

COMPLICATIONS

When performed by experienced surgeons under sterile conditions, circumcision has a low complication rate of between 2% and 10%.[45] Bleeding is the most frequent complication and is generally minor. Infection is the second most common complication and is generally minor. Although adhesions between the foreskin remnant and the glans are common, many of these will resolve with time.[59] However, serious problems can result, including necrotizing fasciitis, sepsis, Fournier's gangrene, and meningitis.[8] There can be excision of too much or too little of the foreskin, with resultant postoperative phimosis or concealed penis. Revision of the circumcision may sometimes be necessary later in childhood.[60] Other complications include skin bridges, inclusion cysts, iatrogenic hypospadias or epispadias, partial amputation of the glans, and the catastrophic loss of the penis when electrocautery is used with a metal circumcision device.

chapter 62

PRUNE-BELLY SYNDROME

Romano T. DeMarco, MD

In 1839, Frohlich first reported a neonate born with congenital absence of his abdominal musculature.[1] Years later, Parker described the accompanying genitourinary tract abnormalities of hydroureteronephrosis, megacystis, and undescended testes associated with deficiency of the abdominal wall musculature.[2] In 1901, Osler described a child with this condition, likening the abdomen to that of a prune, and coined the term prune-belly syndrome (PBS) (Fig. 62-1).[3] Subsequently in 1950, Eagle and Barrett published an exhaustive review of the syndrome and detailed the characteristic features and constellation of anomalies found in affected children.[4] These features include congenital absence or deficiency of the abdominal wall musculature and urinary tract abnormalities including a large hypotonic bladder (megacystis), dilated ureters, dilated prostatic urethra, and bilateral undescended testes. Also associated with this syndrome are renal, cardiac, pulmonary, gastrointestinal, and orthopedic anomalies (Table 62-1).[5]

Other names that have been used to describe this syndrome include Eagle-Barrett, triad, and abdominal musculature deficiency syndromes.[5,6] The use of these monikers has been encouraged by some to lessen the potential psychological impact to the affected child and family.[7] However, the designation prune-belly syndrome is still the most widely accepted term to describe the child with classic findings.

INCIDENCE

The incidence of prune-belly syndrome is estimated to be 1 in 30,000 to 1 in 50,000 live births.[8,9] The current incidence may be less, as the Malformations Surveillance Program at Brigham and Women's Hospital led to elective termination of 31% of children diagnosed prenatally with prune-belly syndrome from 1974 to 1994.[10] Children with incomplete forms of the condition may present with typical abdominal wall changes but no urologic or testicular manifestations. Also, children may present with classic bladder and ureteral features with little to no involvement of the abdominal musculature.[11,12] The female patient with characteristic abdominal wall and urologic findings is also considered to have an incomplete form of the condition and appears to make up less than 5% of reported cases.[11,13,14]

GENETICS

Although population-based studies provide a hint that gene factors may play a role in the etiology of prune-belly syndrome, no specific gene defect for the disorder has been identified. Recent work studying a consanguineous union of parents with two male offspring found to have prune-belly syndrome and three with posterior urethral valves point to two loci, 1q and 11p, as the likely causative gene(s).[15] Whereas previous studies suggested that the genetic mechanism involved in the phenotypic presentation of prune-belly syndrome was potentially an X-linked recessive mutation,[16,17] an X-linked inheritance is not supported by this recent report.[15] Sporadic cases have also been associated with other chromosomal abnormalities, including Turner's syndrome and trisomies 13 and 18.[18-20] Multiple familial cases have also been published, including twins found to have deficiency of the abdominal wall musculature.[21,22] However, no specific genetic abnormalities have been noted in these reports. In one study, maternal cocaine use was found to be associated.[23] Therefore, spontaneous genetic mutations or a combination of genetics and environment likely play a significant role in the phenotypic expression of prune-belly syndrome.

EMBRYOLOGY

A variety of hypotheses have been proposed to explain the common constellation of findings seen in prune-belly syndrome.[24] Although there is no consensus of opinion about the etiology of prune-belly syndrome, the most widely accepted specific mechanism for development of this condition is bladder obstruction.[25] According to this theory, urethral obstruction occurring early in development leads to

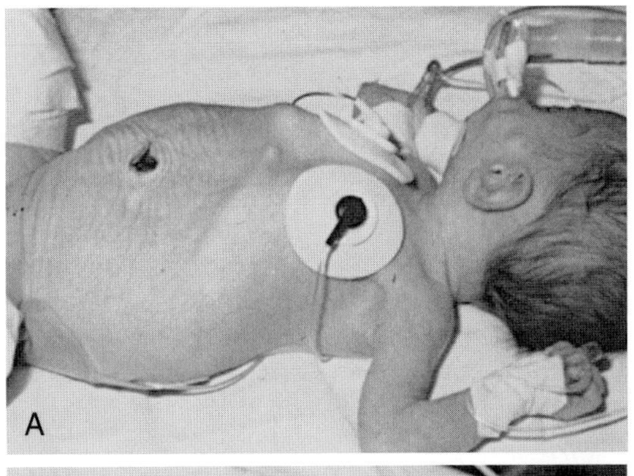

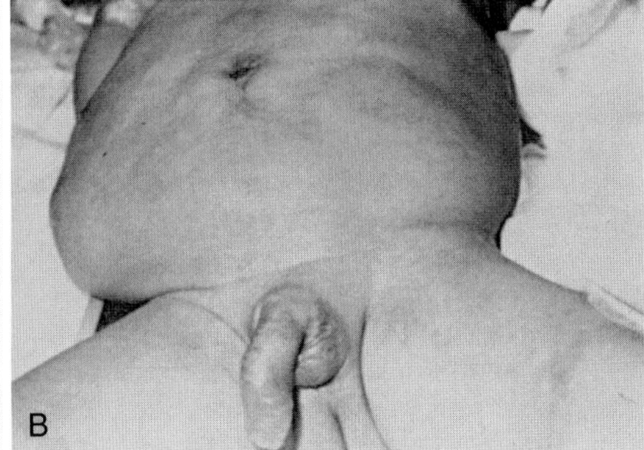

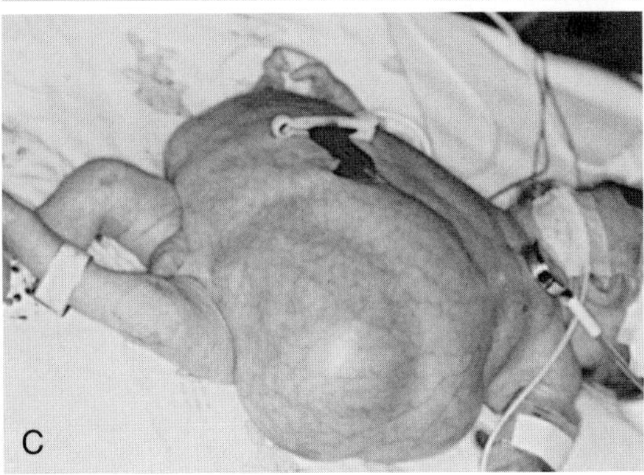

Figure 62-1. Variable degrees of abdominal wall laxity can be seen in patients with prune-belly syndrome. **A,** Subtle wrinkling in a less severely affected infant. **B,** Typical appearance. **C,** Severely affected neonate. (**C** courtesy of D. M. Joseph, MD.)

massive distention of the bladder and ureters. This obstruction may be anatomic,[26] but others have proposed a functional etiology, potentially related to hypoplasia of the prostate.[27] Whatever the source of the urethral obstruction, subsequent bladder distention leads to the abdominal wall muscle and skin changes. The high-grade urethral obstruction and secondary bladder changes can then lead to renal dysplasia and potentially oligohydramnios and bronchopulmonary dysplasia seen in many children with prune-belly syndrome. To tie in all the characteristic findings of prune-belly syndrome with this theory, the massively distended bladder prevents the normal descent of the testes, which leads to their intra-abdominal position.

The other most commonly accepted hypothesis involves a primary mesenchymal defect occurring early in embryogenesis. This defect leads to incomplete differentiation or failure of migration of the lateral mesoderm. This failure of migration is thought to lead to the characteristic myopathology and abdominal wall appearance.[28] Although this mesenchymal defect can account for the abdominal wall findings, the weakness in this theory is that it cannot explain the urinary tract and testicular abnormalities. To account for the classic triad of anomalies, researchers proposed that a primary defect of the intermediate and lateral plate mesoderm in prune-belly syndrome would also affect embryogenesis of the mesonephric and paramesonephric ducts.[29] This mesodermal error may also explain the posterior urethral abnormalities occasionally seen in this condition.

Table 62-1	Commonly Associated Anomalies in Prune-Belly Syndrome
Cardiac	
Patent ductus arteriosus	
Ventricular septal defect	
Atrial septal defect	
Tetralogy of Fallot	
Gastrointestinal	
Intestinal malrotation	
Intestinal atresia	
Omphalocele	
Imperforate anus	
Hepatobiliary anomalies	
Hirschsprung's disease	
Orthopedic	
Congenital hip dislocation	
Scoliosis	
Pectus excavatum and carinatum	
Varus deformities of feet	
Severe leg maldevelopment	
Pulmonary	
Hypoplasia	
Pneumothorax	
Pneumomediastinum	
Lobar atelectasis	
Miscellaneous	
Splenic torsion	
Adrenal cystic dysplasia	

CLINICAL FEATURES

Genitourinary Anomalies

Bladder

The bladder is usually very large and irregular with a patent urachus found in approximately 25% of patients.[4,30] The bladder wall is typically smooth, with an increased ratio of collagen to muscle fibers.[31] In some patients with severe muscle loss, the bladder will bulge and give the impression of a pseudodiverticulum most commonly seen at the dome of the bladder (Fig. 62-2).[7] The trigone is typically enlarged with displaced ureteral orifices laterally and superiorly, which likely contributes to the high incidence of vesicoureteral reflux.[5,7] The bladder neck is usually poorly defined and opens widely into a dilated prostatic urethra. Patients with prune-belly syndrome typically have a very large capacity, compliant bladder, with delay in first sensation to void.[32] The ability to empty the bladder is variable and thought to be due to relative outlet resistance. Many patients will void efficiently, but these patients must be followed closely because their ability to empty the bladder well can deteriorate.[33]

Ureters

The ureters are typically dilated and tortuous. The degree of ureteral pathology is variable and can be segmental. However, the proximal ureter is usually less dilated and appears to have more normal smooth muscle than the distal ureter.[34,35] Collagen fibers and connective tissue have been found to be abundant between muscle bundles containing few muscle cells,[36] particularly refluxing ureters.[37] Vesicoureteral reflux is found in 75% of patients with prune-belly syndrome (Fig. 62-3).[38] Obstruction, either at the ureteropelvic or ureterovesical junction, is rare.[11,39]

These large and dilated ureters have ineffective peristalsis. The propulsion of urine is hindered owing to poor contractile properties of the ureter. The decreased ureteral myofibrils, separated by patches of collagen, ineffectively transmit urine, leading to upper tract stasis.[40]

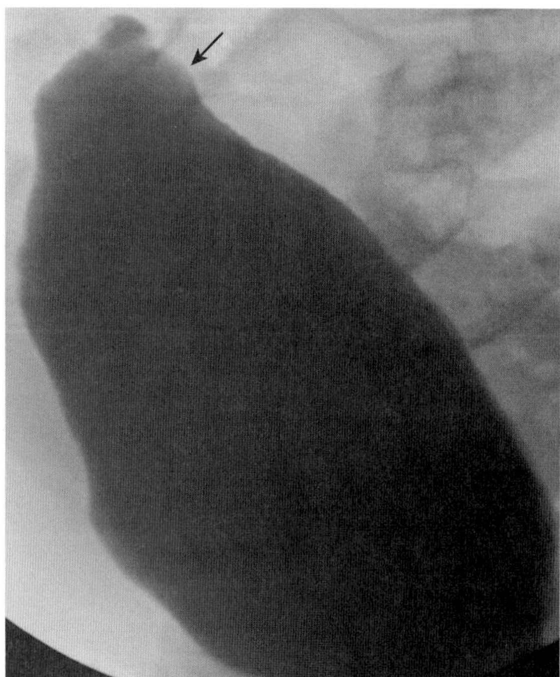

Figure 62-2. A large bladder and pseudodiverticulum (*arrow*) at the dome of the bladder is often seen in children with prune-belly syndrome.

Kidneys

Renal abnormalities span a large spectrum in children with prune-belly syndrome. Children can present with severe dysplasia or have completely normal kidneys. Patients can have significant laterality of the dysplasia, with one kidney severely affected and the other kidney normal.[39] Whereas both antenatal bladder outlet obstruction and abnormal ureteral bud-metanephric blastema interaction have been implicated in the genesis of the dysplasia,[41] the exact mechanism is uncertain.

Hydronephrosis is typically seen. The degree of hydronephrosis can be quite variable with preservation of the calyceal morphology in the presence of severe ureteral and renal pelvic distention.[38] Although primary or secondary ureteropelvic junction obstruction can occur in children with prune-belly syndrome, nonobstructive hydronephrosis is usually seen[42] without significant correlation between the degree of hydroureteronephrosis and parenchymal injury.

Posterior Urethra, Prostate, and Accessory Sex Organs

The posterior urethra is extremely dilated in children with prune-belly syndrome (Fig. 62-4). This dilation is thought to be due to generalized hypoplasia of the prostate epithelium with replacement of the normal smooth muscle anteriorly with connective tissue. While obstructive lesions are rare findings in the distal posterior urethra,[40,43] several investigators have described valve-like obstructive tissue in the posterior urethra.[44]

The loss of smooth muscle support alters the configuration of the prostate gland, leading to its widened appearance.[25] An abnormal epithelial-mesenchymal interaction has been proposed as the cause of this anomaly.[45] This lack of normal prostatic parenchyma is thought to play a role in ejaculatory failure.[44]

Retrograde ejaculation is also commonly seen in patients with prune-belly syndrome and is thought to be related to bladder neck incompetency. The vas and seminal vesicles are typically affected. Atresia of these structures is common. Conversely, some patients present with dilation of both of these structures.[29]

Anterior Urethra

Typically, the anterior urethra is normal. However, atresia of the bulbar or membranous urethra has been reported, occurring in 18% of patients in one review.[46]

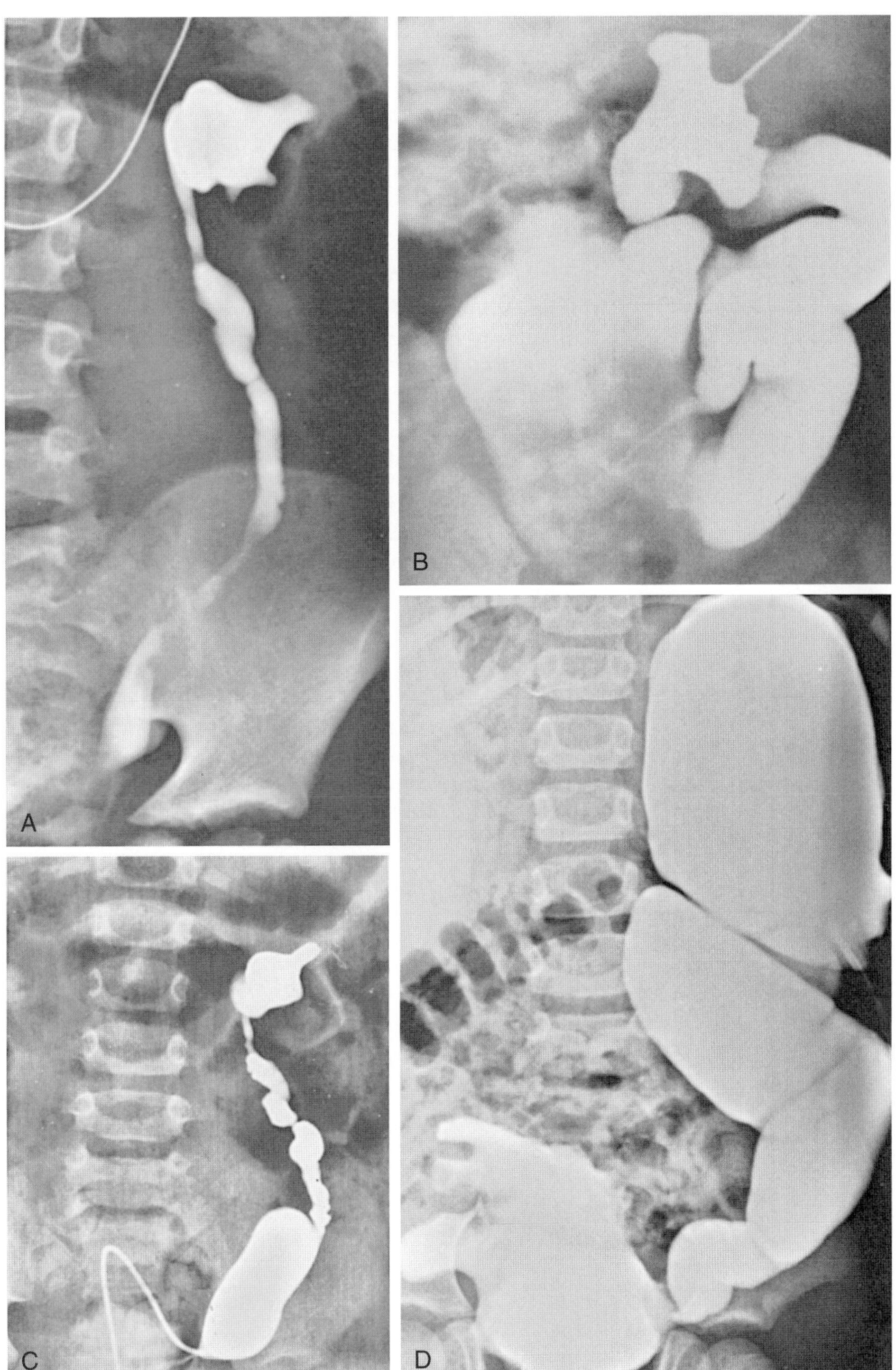

Figure 62-3. Variable degrees of dilation and dysmorphism of the upper urinary tract are seen in prune-belly syndrome. **A,** Dysmorphic renal pelvis with mild ureteral dilation. **B,** Calyceal clubbing and a tortuous "wandering" ureter. **C,** Dysmorphic pelvis with exaggerated dilation of the distal ureteral spindle. **D,** Bizarre appearance of the collecting system as well as the bladder.

In babies with urethral atresia, urachal patency, spontaneous bladder rupture with either cutaneous, vaginal, or rectal fistula formation, or in utero vesicoamniotic shunt placement are necessary for survival.

PBS is also associated with two variations of megalourethra.[47] The scaphoid megalourethra is the most common and less severe form. The scaphoid variety is associated with a deficiency of the spongiosum with preservation of the normal glans and corporeal bodies (Fig. 62-5). The fusiform type has a deficiency of not only the spongiosum but also of the corpus cavernosum.[48] With voiding, the entire phallus dilates in patients with the fusiform variety, whereas those children with the scaphoid form have dilation of only the anterior urethra.

Testes

Bilateral intra-abdominal testes are the most typical findings in children with prune-belly syndrome. The testes are commonly found near the ureterovesical

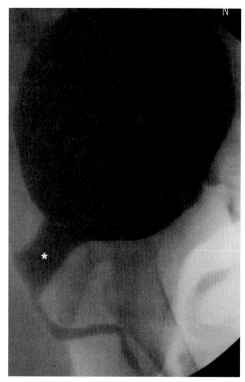

Figure 62-4. Posterior urethral dilation (*asterisk*) is often found in children with prune-belly syndrome. This dilation is similar to that seen in boys with posterior urethral valves.

junction but can be located in more proximal locations as well.[5,7] Infants with prune-belly syndrome have been reported to have essentially normal testicular histology as compared with age-matched controls.[7] Other series have documented present but diminished spermatogonia with Leydig cell hyperplasia in comparison with normal controls.[49] This suggests that the histologic findings are caused by more than the cryptorchid state. Azoospermia is the rule in adult patients with prune-belly syndrome, with no reported cases of a natural paternity.[50]

Extragenitourinary Anomalies

Abdominal Wall

The most characteristic clinical finding in neonates with prune-belly syndrome is the wrinkled and floppy appearance to the abdominal wall and bulging flanks associated with crisscrossed and creased skin. Older patients have a more potbelly appearance once the amount of cutaneous abdominal adipose tissue increases. The degree of the "pruned" appearance can vary significantly from patient to patient as can the degree of the deficiency of the abdominal wall musculature. While rarely completely absent,[39] the medial and inferior aspect of the abdominal wall is most severely involved, with normal or near-normal musculature in the periphery of the abdominal wall.[51,52] The most affected individual muscle is the transversus abdominis, followed in decreasing frequency by the rectus abdominis inferior to the umbilicus, internal oblique, external oblique, and superior aspect of the rectus.[11,39] While the innervation of the abdominal muscle appears unaffected, light and electron microscopy have demonstrated multiple abnormalities of the abdominal wall muscle. These abnormalities include variations in or decreased muscle fiber size, excessive collagen accumulation, and myofilamentous disarray and loss.[53]

Cardiac Anomalies

Cardiac anomalies occur in approximately 10% of patients with prune-belly syndrome. The most common cardiac findings include patent ductus arteriosus, atrial and ventricular septal defects, and tetralogy of Fallot.[54]

Pulmonary Anomalies

Pulmonary abnormalities are common and typically related to the degree of renal dysplasia and associated oligohydramnios. Because of the high likelihood of having pulmonary hypoplasia, neonates exhibiting pulmonary distress should be presumed to have hypoplasia and hyaline membrane disease.[11] Additionally, these children are at increased risk for both pneumonia and spontaneous pneumothorax not necessarily related to the degree of hypoplasia.[55] Older patients may be found to have significant restrictive lung disease thought to be related to musculoskeletal abnormalities rather than parenchymal lung disease.[56]

Gastrointestinal Anomalies

The most common gastrointestinal anomaly is intestinal malrotation.[39,52] The risk for malrotation is thought to be due to an incomplete rotation of the

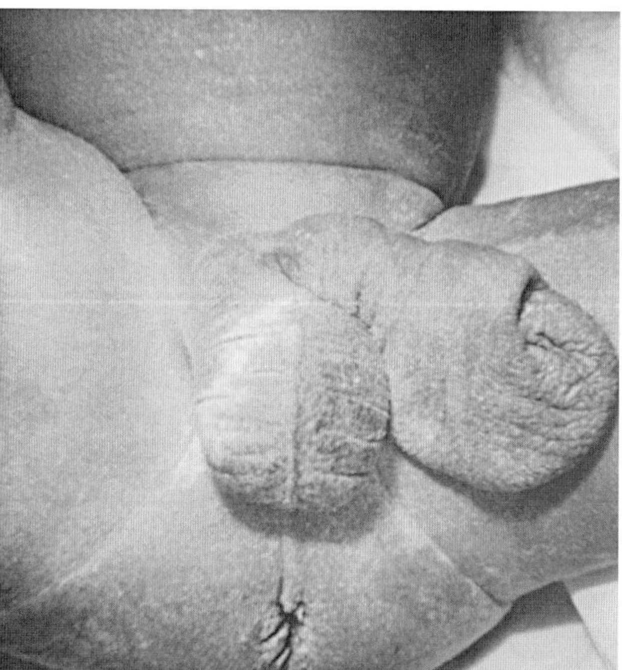

Figure 62-5. Gross appearance of scaphoid megalourethra in a child with prune-belly syndrome.

midgut leading to a wide mesentery, allowing for increased bowel mobility.[13] Other intestinal abnormalities associated with prune-belly syndrome include persistent cloaca,[13] gastroschisis,[21] imperforate anus,[57] colonic atresia,[52] and volvulus.[52] Additionally, reports of splenic torsion and biliary tract abnormalities occurring in children with prune-belly syndrome have been published.[58,59] Chronic constipation can be a lifelong issue and is secondary to the inability to generate significant intra-abdominal pressure owing to the lax abdominal wall. An acquired megacolon is sometimes encountered.[60]

Orthopedic Anomalies

Musculoskeletal abnormalities are common, occurring in approximately 50% of children with prune-belly syndrome.[61,62] Abnormalities of the hip joint, most commonly subluxation or dislocation, are frequently reported.[61] The most common orthopedic deformity is clubfoot, with an incidence of at least 25%. About 50% of patients have bilateral disease.[62] Other findings include congenital scoliosis, talipes equinovarus, and pectus excavatum.[60,62] The specific mechanisms leading to the orthopedic issues are unknown. Green and colleagues proposed that because of the unilaterality of most of the orthopedic deformities, oligohydramnios is the likely cause.[63] Others have attributed a distended bladder or a common mesenchymal error as the cause of these anomalies.

CLINICAL PRESENTATION

Antenatal Diagnosis and Management

Antenatally, a fetus with prune-belly syndrome behaves similarly to a fetus with posterior urethral valves or other causes of bladder outlet obstruction. The typical antenatal ultrasound findings include bilateral hydroureteronephrosis, a distended bladder, and an irregular abdominal wall circumference.[64] These findings are not specific for this condition, and other diagnostic possibilities should also be considered. Reports of antenatal diagnosis as early as 11 to 14 weeks have been described.[65,66] However, the more classic findings are seen early in the third trimester.

In-utero intervention has been proposed by several authors in patients with prune-belly syndrome who have met certain criteria with no appreciable benefit.[67,68] At this time it would be the rare patient who is considered a candidate for antenatal therapy. Most pregnancies are carried to term, with rare instances of dystocia or worsening oligohydramnios leading to early delivery.[69] Pregnancy termination is typically considered only in those fetuses with early and severe oligohydramnios and evidence of significant renal dysplasia.

Table 62-2 Classification System for Prune-Belly Syndrome

Category 1
Pulmonary hypoplasia and/or pneumothorax
Oligohydramnios
Renal dysplasia
Urethral atresia
Clubfeet
Category 2
Typical physical features
Renal dysplasia common but less severe than category 1
No pulmonary hypoplasia
Can progress to renal failure
Category 3
Incomplete or mild physical features
No renal dysplasia
No pulmonary dysplasia
Stable renal function

Postnatal Diagnosis

Neonatal Presentation

The appearance of a neonate with a wrinkled abdominal wall usually suggests the diagnosis of prune-belly syndrome. Another easily appreciated finding includes bilateral nonpalpable testes. Children with more significant oligohydramnios may present with some element of Potter's features, limb abnormalities, and pulmonary/chest anomalies.

Neonatal Evaluation

The initial management entails a rapid and complete evaluation of all organ systems. To help guide clinicians regarding the prognosis of children with prune-belly syndrome, a classification system has been described (Table 62-2) with three categories.[70] Category 1 patients have the worst prognosis. Although this classification system can be a helpful prognostic aid, prune-belly syndrome is a condition with a wide spectrum of severity.

The initial concern in a child born with prune-belly syndrome is that of the pulmonary and cardiac systems. Thorough initial assessment of these systems is essential and includes the physical examination, a chest radiograph, and an appropriate laboratory evaluation. Directed and further care for the cardiac and respiratory systems is determined by the neonatology, cardiology, and pulmonary consultants.

On physical examination, particular attention should be paid to whether the kidneys and bladder are palpable. Initial assessment of renal function should be used as a baseline, but initial postnatal creatinine levels are most reflective of the mother. The electrolyte and creatinine trend over the early postnatal period is more predictive of long-term renal function. A nadir creatinine concentration of greater than 0.7 mg/dL in a term infant is a poor prognostic sign that has been noted by several groups.[55,71,72]

Once the neonate is stable, renal and bladder ultrasonography is recommended to assess the renal parenchyma and degree of upper and lower tract dilation. Voiding cystourethrography is performed to assess bladder emptying and the bladder outlet in addition to evaluating for vesicoureteral reflux. Any instrumentation of the urinary tract should be undertaken with strict attention to sterile technique. Prophylactic or periprocedural antibiotics are recommended to decrease the possibility of bacterial inoculation and urinary tract infection. Nuclear renography is typically performed at 4 to 6 weeks of age to assess renal function and drainage. Earlier examinations would not account for neonatal physiologic transitioning and have less sensitivity for assessing obstruction.

MANAGEMENT

Controversy exists regarding which treatment approach is best for the child with prune-belly syndrome. Aggressive surgical management of the urinary tract has been advocated by some and historically was performed in the neonatal period.[40] This approach usually entails ureteral reimplantation with ureteral tailoring and reduction cystoplasty with the hope of eliminating obstruction and eliminating reflux to help prevent pyelonephritis and further renal loss. Now, even those surgeons who strongly agree with early reconstruction recommend waiting until the child is at least several months old to allow for improved pulmonary function.[40]

An alternative approach centers on limited surgical intervention. This treatment plan involves close surveillance with aggressive medical management. Surgical intervention is reserved for those young children with recurrent or persistent infection or proven obstruction. Advocates of this approach cite previous experience demonstrating that some patients can be maintained infection free and without worsening of their bladder dynamics and renal function using this approach.[73,74] Additionally, those advocating for a more minimalistic approach point to the fact that surgery has not been proved to slow progression of renal dysfunction. In many children with severe renal dysplasia, no approach will alter the ultimate renal outcome. Most pediatric urologists currently seem to favor the limited surgical approach, particularly within the first year of life, with intervention reserved for infection or obstruction. Elective lower urinary tract reconstruction is more controversial for the older stable child.

The goal of either management approach is to keep the child infection free. Acquired renal scarring secondary to pyelonephritis can occur often in children with PBS.[39] Antibiotic prophylaxis is recommended in all neonates, even those without reflux. Particular attention to urinary stasis, either at the bladder level or more proximally, is required. The combination of infection and stasis/obstruction can lead to worsening renal function and both factors need to be addressed aggressively.

Surgical Management

The surgical management of the patient with prune-belly syndrome focuses on addressing three main systems: the urinary tract, the undescended testes, and the abdominal wall.

Cutaneous Vesicostomy

Urinary diversion may be a necessary temporary procedure in the setting of a neonate with bladder outlet obstruction. The Blocksom technique, as modified by Duckett, is the recommended method with attention paid to creating a capacious stoma.[75] If a large diverticulum is encountered during creation of the vesicostomy, it can be excised.

Supravesical Diversion

In rare situations of either upper or lower ureteral obstruction or stasis, a proximal diversion is required. A cutaneous pyelostomy is the recommended form of diversion because it provides the best form of upper tract drainage. Percutaneous nephrostomy tubes may be placed as a temporary form of drainage and then used as a gauge to determine if a pyelostomy would be beneficial.

Internal Urethrotomy

Internal urethrotomy should be considered in the older child with increased bladder outlet resistance that is clinically manifesting as poor bladder emptying and a large postvoid residual. The procedure involves an incision through the distal prostatic urethra with careful avoidance of the urinary sphincter. Reports have demonstrated an improvement in urinary flow rates, overall radiographic appearance, and lower post-void residual urine.[32,73]

Anterior Urethral Reconstruction

Megalourethra is best treated with penile degloving, excision of the redundant urethra, and urethral tailoring and reconstruction. Urethral atresia is commonly treated in the neonatal period with a temporary cutaneous vesicostomy. Achieving a functional urethra usually requires a formal urethroplasty involving complex skin flaps and/or grafts. Progressive dilation of the hypoplastic urethra has been reported as an alternative in select patients.[76]

Reduction Cystoplasty

Poor bladder contractibility and incomplete emptying is common in the child with prune-belly syndrome. Several authors reported methods to reduce the bladder size and create a more normal, spherical bladder in hopes of improving bladder emptying. These approaches range from excision of the urachal diverticulum to more complex reconstructive surgeries involving detrusor plication or the creation of overlapping bladder flaps. Although early postoperative results seemed to be encouraging, long-term results have noted recurrence of the large bladder capacity and poor bladder emptying.[77] Currently, reduction cystoplasty is performed at the time of ureteral reconstruction to aid with the lower urinary tract reconstruction and is rarely performed as a primary procedure or to facilitate bladder emptying. Better options to improve bladder emptying include clean intermittent catheterization through the urethra or via a continent catheterizable channel.[78]

Ureteral Surgery

Ureteral tailoring and reimplantation is usually undertaken in those children with recurrent UTIs. As previously noted, routine and early postnatal ureteral reconstruction has generally been abandoned. The severity of the reflux and ureteral distention are not the sole indications for ureteral reconstruction. When performed, meticulous ureteral dissection is required. In most cases, the distal, redundant, and ectatic ureter is discarded and common ureteral tailoring techniques are used to decrease the size of the ureter. Reimplantation into a prune-belly syndrome bladder can be very difficult. Fixation of the large, floppy bladder with a psoas hitch may be required to prevent "J"-hooking and possible postoperative ureterovesical obstruction.

Orchiopexy

The timing of orchiopexy is dependent on the child's overall health and clinical status and the need for scrotal positioning of the undescended testes at a young age. In the healthy child, bilateral orchiopexy is typically performed via a transabdominal approach at about 6 months of age. Those infants requiring temporary or reconstructive surgery earlier usually have the orchiopexies performed as a conjunctive procedure. The flaccid abdomen allows for excellent exposure, and ligation of the internal spermatic vessels is usually not required for children younger than 2 years of age.[79] In older children or those with high intra-abdominal testes, a primary or staged Fowler-Stephens approach is best. With the recent advancements in laparoscopy, a minimally invasive procedure shows promise, particularly in older children and those who do not need other operations.[80,81]

Abdominoplasty

The management of the abdominal wall in children with prune-belly syndrome is determined by the severity of the condition. In children with very mild degrees of deformity, observation is usually the rule, with some having spontaneous improvement in their appearance. In those with more significant degrees of abdominal wall laxity, abdominoplasty is usually recommended, because the cosmetic and psychological benefits are believed to outweigh the risks of the surgery. Improvement in pulmonary, bladder, and bowel function after abdominoplasty may be improved but is not well substantiated.[60,82] The timing of abdominoplasty is dictated by the child's general health and need for future reconstructive surgery. Children as young as 6 months have undergone abdominal wall reconstruction at the same setting as orchiopexy or bladder reconstruction.

Several methods with modifications have been described for abdominal wall reconstruction. Popular techniques today include those described by Monfort[83] and Ehrlich.[84] The Ehrlich technique utilizes a transabdominal approach through a vertical midline incision with preservation of the umbilicus on a vascular pedicle via the inferior epigastric artery.[84] The skin and subcutaneous tissues are then elevated off the underlying fascia and muscle followed by a pants-over-vest buttressing of the more normal lateral fascia and abdominal muscle. The excess abdominal skin is then removed, and the skin is reapproximated longitudinally in the midline (Fig. 62-6).

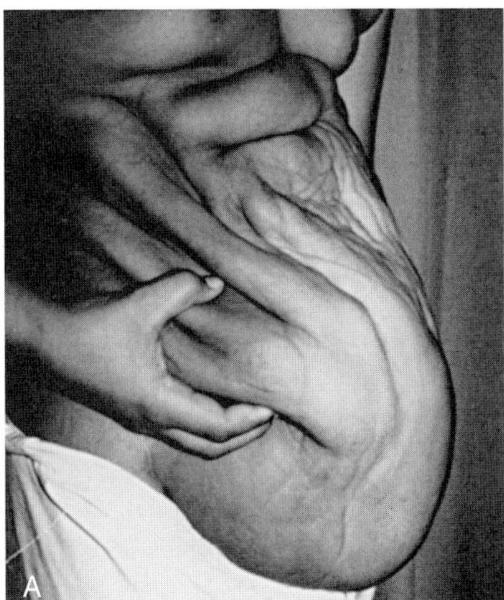

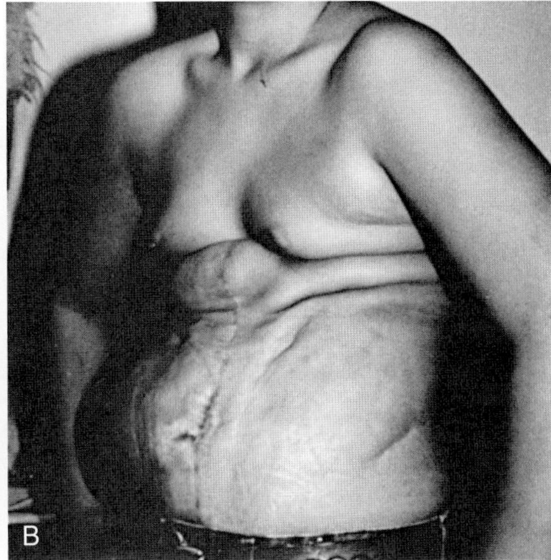

Figure 62-6. The Ehrlich technique was used in this patient. The preoperative appearance of the abdominal wall is seen on the left (**A**) and the postoperative view is on the right (**B**).

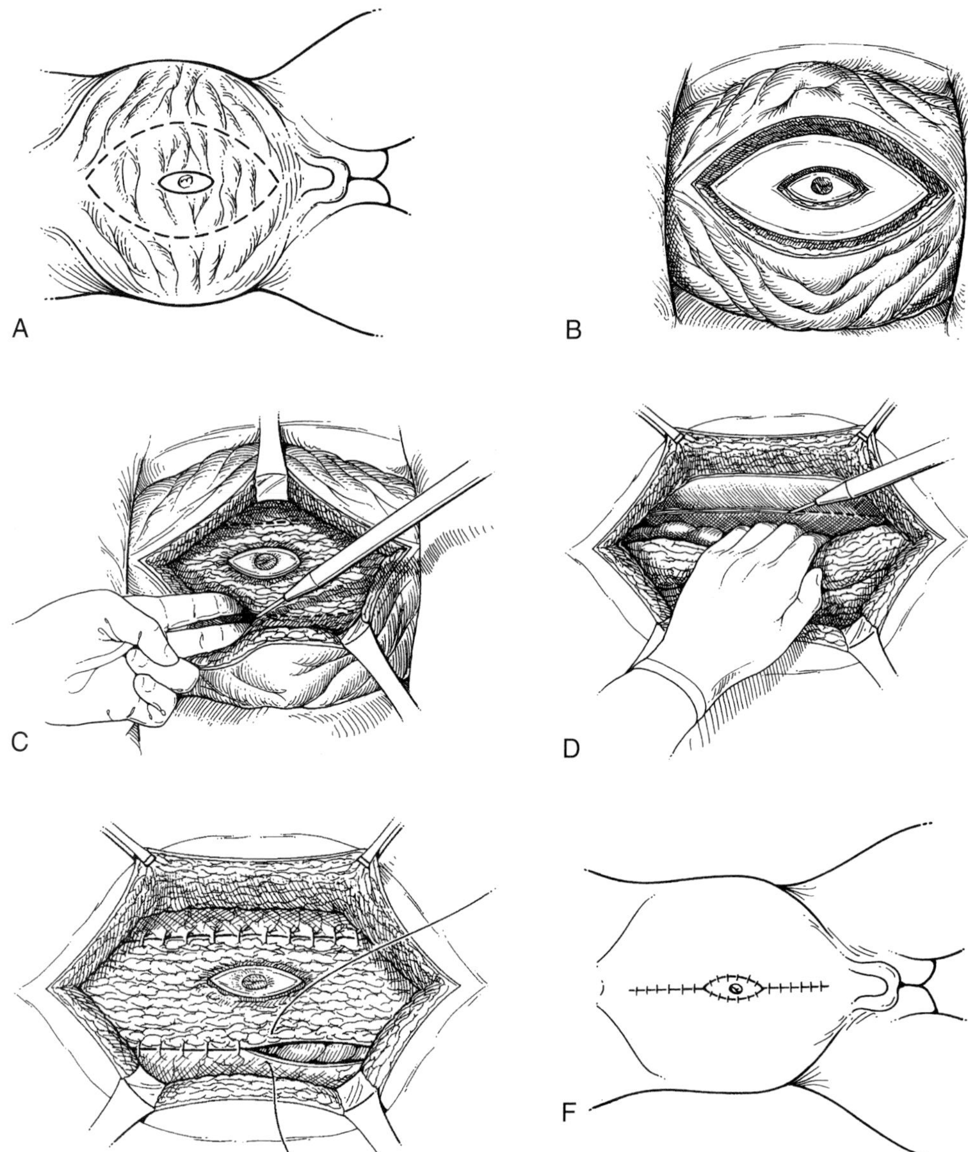

Figure 62-7. The Monfort abdominoplasty is depicted. **A,** Skin incisions circumscribe the umbilicus and define areas of adjacent abdominal wall redundancy to be removed. **B,** Excision of skin (epidermis and dermis alone) by using electrocautery. **C,** Abdominal wall central plate is incised at the lateral borders of the rectus muscle on either side, creating a central musculofascial plate. **D,** The parietal peritoneum overlying the lateral abdominal wall musculature is scored with electrocautery. **E,** Edges of the central plate are sutured along the scored line. **F,** Excess skin is removed, and the midline approximation envelops the previously isolated umbilicus.

Monfort's technique also employs a vertical incision. However, his modification uses an elliptically oriented incision as a means of excising the redundant skin (Fig. 62-7). The incision usually extends from the tip of the xiphoid down to the pubis. A second elliptical incision is then made around the umbilicus for its preservation. Similar to the Ehrlich technique, the skin is dissected off the fascia and muscle laterally to at least the anterior axillary line. However, the Monfort procedure includes making vertical relaxing fascial incisions lateral to the superior epigastric arteries, allowing mobilization of the lateral fascial flaps over a central fascial bridge. Durable functional results have been reported with this technique.[85,86] Recently, other authors have described alternative techniques for abdominal wall reconstruction, which include extraperitoneal dissection, fascial folding, or laparoscopic-assisted approaches.[87,88]

RENAL TRANSPLANT

Close follow-up and monitoring of renal function is essential in patients with prune-belly syndrome. Approximately 30% of patients presenting with renal insufficiency will develop chronic renal failure during childhood or in their adolescent years. In those requiring renal transplantation, both cadaver and living-related donor kidneys transplanted in the patient with prune-belly syndrome have equal long-term function as compared with well-matched controls.[89,90] In young children, peritoneal dialysis can be used temporarily until the child is of adequate size to accept a transplant.

chapter 63

DISORDERS OF SEXUAL DIFFERENTIATION

John M. Gatti, MD

Disorders of sexual differentiation (DSD) resulting in what have previously been referred to as intersex disorders are among the most fascinating conditions confronting the pediatric urologist and surgeon. Our understanding of these conditions and their causes continues to evolve, but many questions remain. Even with a better understanding of the underlying etiology of these different conditions, optimal gender assignment and the timing of surgical reconstruction continue to be controversial.

NORMAL GENDER AND SEXUAL DIFFERENTIATION

An understanding of these conditions builds on a working knowledge of normal sexual differentiation. The most commonly accepted paradigm, described by Jost,[1] involves a stepwise process to gender and sexual development. The primary determinant is the chromosomal gender, which is established at fertilization when the sperm provides an X or Y chromosome to the ovum's X chromosome. Chromosomal gender determines gonadal gender, with XX resulting in ovarian development and XY resulting in testicular formation. Finally, the gonadal function determines the phenotypic gender, including internal and external physical and psychological features. Although this paradigm is a helpful cascade to explain gender development, as the actual genes and locations have been elucidated, the simple Y = male, No Y = female equations are not always valid.

Chromosomal Determination

The chromosomal gender determination is based on the Y chromosome. In the 1950s, research characterizing the male phenotype of Klinefelter's syndrome with a 47,XXY karyotype, and a female phenotype of Turner's syndrome with a 45,XO karyotype, discovered that the presence of the Y chromosome causes male gonadal development and the lack of a Y chromosome results in ovarian formation.[2,3] This was irrespective of a complete X chromosomal content. The theorized gene that was responsible for male gonadal development was termed the *testis-determining factor* (*TDF*).

Gonadal Development

The location of *TDF* was further elucidated with molecular techniques by studying individuals with chromosomes discordant with their phenotype: 46,XY females with a deletion of the *TDF* region and 46,XX males with Y chromosomal and *TDF* genetic material, presumably through gene translocation or other means. *TDF* was cloned and, based on genome mapping, its location was isolated to the short arm of the Y chromosome near the centromere at the distal aspect of the Y-unique region.[4] *TDF* was found to be a 35-kilobase pair sequence on the 11.3 subband of the gender-determining region of the Y chromosome (*SRY*). Interestingly, *SRY* appears to be expressed by the somatic cells from the urogenital ridge and not from germ cells.

The *SOX9* gene, located on the long arm of chromosome 17, has been identified as an additional gender-determining gene. It has been noted that a translocation involving the *SOX9* gene results in campomelic dysplasia, characterized by skeletal abnormalities and associated with 46,XY gender reversal. The *SRY* gene is thought to regulate the *SOX9* gene. Despite the presence of a functional *SRY* gene in this syndrome, a female phenotype develops in the majority of chromosomal males.[5,6]

In addition to the *TDF* and *SOX9* genes, other genes are also involved in gonadal development. The Wilms' tumor gene (*WT1*) appears to play a key role not only in renal development but also in testicular development. It is theorized that *WT1* regulates the interaction between the mesonephric ducts and germ cells, with early alteration of gene function resulting in testicular agenesis and later dysfunction resulting in aberrant testicular development (streak gonad or dysgerminomas). This tumor suppressor gene has been implicated in Denys-Drash syndrome involving testicular (mixed gonadal dysgenesis) and renal (Wilms' tumor) abnormalities.[7,8]

Fushi-Tarzu factor-1 (FTZ-F1) exerts its effect on gonadal development through its regulation of steroidogenic factor-1 (SF-1). The *SF1* gene is involved with steroid hormone production and the production of müllerian-inhibiting substance (MIS) by the Sertoli cells of the testis that causes regression of the müllerian ductal system. Although FTZ-1 and SF-1 are also expressed in ovarian tissues, the timing and intensity of their effect are critical for normal gonadal development.[7,9]

Finally, the lack of an *SRY* gene alone does not impart normal female phenotypic and gonadal development, based on studies of 46,XY females with intact *SRY* regions. The *DAX1* gene, located on the short arm of the X chromosome, appears to be essential for the development of the ovary. The *DAX1* gene product appears to compete with the *SRY* gene product for a steroidogenic regulatory protein (StAR). Also, a dosage-sensitive element is important. Normally, the single *SRY* gene has a greater impact than a single *DAX1* gene and causes upregulation of StAR. In those chromosomal abnormalities in which more than one *DAX1* gene is present, however, downregulation of StAR occurs, testicular development is inhibited, and ovarian formation is promoted. As in the case of Turner's syndrome, however, these primordial ovaries develop into streak gonads. Likely, other genes are also important for normal ovarian development.[10-12]

Phenotype Development

Development of the internal ductal structures is dependent on hormone secretion by the developing gonads (Table 63-1). In the absence of functioning testicular tissue, the female internal müllerian duct structures develop. The presence of a functioning testis results in male internal wolffian duct development. This differentiation is mediated by the production of testosterone from the testis. Testosterone promotes wolffian duct development along with MIS, which results in regression of the müllerian duct structures. This is a paracrine effect and therefore results in gonad specific ipsilateral ductal differentiation. This effect is likely dependent on high concentrations of androgen produced by the physically proximate gonad. Decreased levels of MIS by an abnormal testis or streak gonad result in ipsilateral müllerian development. This occurs despite regression of the müllerian ducts on the contralateral side with normal testicular MIS production. Conversely, systemic administration of androgen does not result in male ductal development in a female fetus.

Table 63-1 Derivation of the Urogenital System

Wolffian Duct (Mesonephric Duct)	Urogenital Sinus	Müllerian Duct (Paramesonephric Duct)
Male:	*Male:*	*Male:*
Epididymis	Bladder	Appendix testis
Vas deferens	Prostate	Prostatic utricle
Seminal vesicles	*Female:*	*Female:*
Female:	Bladder	Vagina (upper third)
Epoöphoron	Distal vagina	Uterus
Gartner's ducts		Fallopian tubes

MIS functions as a suppressor of müllerian duct development. It is thought that MIS acts by inhibiting the effect of growth factors on the müllerian ducts. MIS is produced by the Sertoli cells in the testis and is a specific marker for functioning testicular tissue in infancy. At puberty, MIS production in the male declines, but it increases in the female. In its absence, the müllerian structures develop by default. The concentration and timing of MIS secretion appear to be critical. Secretion occurs during week 7 of gestation. By week 9, the müllerian ducts become insensitive to MIS.[11]

External genital development follows a similar path (Fig. 63-1). In the absence of testosterone and, more important, its metabolite dihydrotestosterone (DHT), the external genitalia develop into the female phenotype. The male and female phenotypes are identical until week 7. In the male, testosterone production by the testicular Leydig cells surges at 7 weeks and remains elevated until week 14 of gestation. Testosterone is converted to DHT by 5α-reductase in the tissues of the genital skin and urogenital sinus. The testosterone-binding receptor has a four to five times higher affinity for DHT than testosterone and serves to amplify the effect of testosterone on the developing external genitalia. In the absence of 5α-reductase, the internal wolffian ducts are preserved but the external structures are feminized.

After birth, neonatal testosterone levels in a male surge in response to the loss of feedback inhibition by maternal estrogens and the subsequent rise in neonatal luteinizing hormone (LH) production. This testosterone production peaks around the second to third month of life. By 6 months, the levels remain identical in males and females until puberty. Through these surges, it appears that androgen imprinting may occur on susceptible tissues, including those of the genital organs, but also on sensitive tissues in the brain related to male-type behaviors and gender orientation. This early exposure may determine how these tissues respond to subsequent androgen exposure during puberty and adulthood.

ABERRANT GENDER DEVELOPMENT

Incidence

In North and South America and Western Europe, congenital adrenal hyperplasia (CAH) is the most common cause of neonatal ambiguous genitalia, accounting for approximately 70% of cases.[13,14] The overall incidence is approximately 1 in 15,000 live births. The rate is much higher in stillborns and in certain regional populations (Yupic Eskimos and the people of La Réunion, France).[15] In the United States, mixed gonadal dysgenesis is the next most common intersex disorder, with ovotesticular DSD (true hermaphroditism) the third most common. In other areas of the world, different disorders predominate. Ovotesticular DSD is the most common intersex disorder in South Africa.[16]

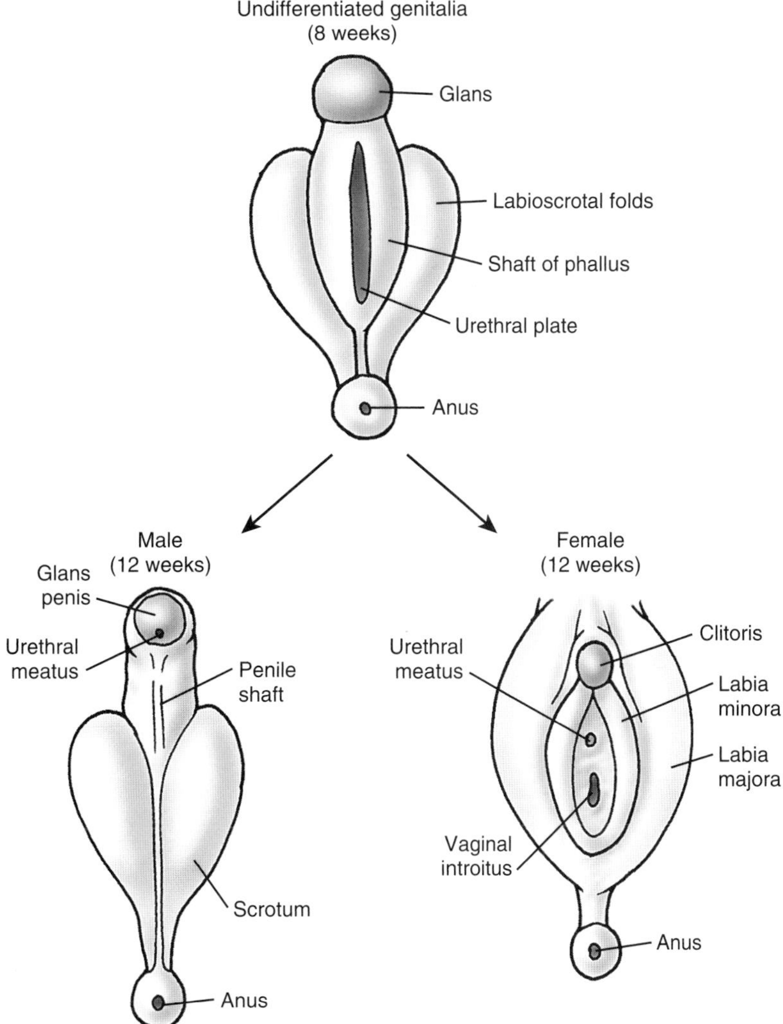

Figure 63-1. Differentiation of the external genitalia.

Classification

The most commonly used classification system was proposed by Allen in 1976.[17] This system categorizes the most common DSD well. However, as our understanding of the less common syndromes evolves, they do not fit as neatly into this paradigm. The five categories are based primarily on gonadal histology:

1. Female pseudohermaphrodite (ovarian tissue only)
2. Male pseudohermaphrodite (testicular tissue only)
3. True hermaphrodite (both ovarian and testicular tissue)
4. Mixed gonadal dysgenesis (testicular tissue and a streak gonad)
5. Pure gonadal dysgenesis (two streak gonads)

More recently, in 2006, a consensus statement was released from the International Consensus Conference on Intersex proposing new nomenclature for these disorders. This new classification system incorporates an evolving understanding of the molecular basis of these disorders and replaces more offensive gender-based labels. For instance, intersex disorders are now called disorders of sexual differentiation. The new terminology for the more familiar previous categories is summarized in Table 63-2. To facilitate this transition, both terms will be used where applicable in this chapter.[18]

Table 63-2 Nomenclature for Disorders of Sexual Differentiation (DSD)

Current	Classic
46,XX DSD	Female pseudohermaphrodite
46,XY DSD	Male pseudohermaphrodite
Ovotesticular DSD	True hermaphrodite
45,XX/46,XY Ovotesticular DSD	Mixed gonadal dysgenesis
46,XX Complete gonadal dysgenesis	Pure gonadal dysgenesis (common form)

46,XX DSD (Female Pseudohermaphrodite)

The majority of neonates with external genital ambiguity fall into this category. All patients have a 46,XX genotype and exclusively ovarian tissue in nonpalpable gonads. Simplistically, the cause of the gender ambiguity is an excess of androgen. More than 95% are due to CAH, with the remainder due to maternal androgen exposure. These patients have a normal female müllerian ductal system with an upper vagina, uterus, and fallopian tubes (see Table 63-1). They also have normal regression of the wolffian ducts. The level of virilization is largely dependent on the timing and magnitude of androgen exposure to the external genitalia. The phenotype can range from mild clitoromegaly to full masculinization.

Virilization in CAH is due to the inability of the adrenal gland to form cortisol. The precursors above the enzymatic defect are shunted into mineralocorticoid or sex-steroid pathways. Also, the end products generally have some, albeit weak, glucocorticoid function. The lack of cortisol for negative feedback inhibition of adrenocorticotropic hormone (ACTH) production by the pituitary leaves this pathway unchecked. Excess androgen is produced and is responsible for the virilization. The corticosteroid synthetic and alternative pathways are diagrammed in Figure 63-2. The most common form of CAH is 21-hydroxylase deficiency (21-OHD), which accounts for more than 90% of CAH.[19] 21-OHD has been mapped to the short arm of chromosome 6. The variable location of the adrenal defect and relative function of the gene results in salt-wasting and non–salt-wasting forms.[20-22] Type 1 (21-OHD) results in virilization but no salt wasting. The gene defect affects only the fasciculata zone of the adrenal, resulting in blocking cortisol production. However, the gene is normally expressed in the glomerulosa zone with preservation of mineralocorticoid production. In type 2 (21-OHD), also called the classic type, the gene abnormality affects both zones of the adrenal. Salt wasting results in dehydration or vascular collapse, and hyperkalemia develops because of the block in mineralocorticoid production.

11β-Hydroxylase deficiency (type 3) is a less common cause of CAH. This gene has been mapped to the long arm of chromosome 8. This abnormality results in virilization associated with hypertension. This effect is related to the level of the synthetic block below deoxycorticosterone (DOC). DOC has potent mineralocorticoid function. Its excess results in sodium resorption, fluid overload, hypertension, and hypokalemic acidosis.

Finally, 3β-hydroxylase deficiency (type 4) is a rare form of CAH. It results in severe salt wasting, and survival is rare. It is the only type of CAH to occur in both genders.

Rarely, virilization of the female fetus can be caused by exogenous androgen exposure from the mother. This occurs primarily with the use of progesterone, commonly used as an adjunct to assist with fertility and with in-vitro fertilization. Previously, androgenic compounds also were administered to expectant mothers with a history of repeated spontaneous abortion as a preventive measure.

Endogenous androgen exposure due to virilizing maternal ovarian tumors also has been reported as a cause of 46,XX DSD.[23] Fortunately, these tumors are usually virilizing to the mother and the fetus is unaffected. Virilizing tumors include arrhenoblastoma, hilar cell tumor, lipoid cell tumor, ovarian stromal cell tumor, luteoma of pregnancy, and Krukenberg's tumor.[24]

Diagnosis

The diagnosis of CAH is based on the previously described clinical and electrolyte abnormalities in addition to elevated 17-hydroxyprogesterone levels. DOC and deoxycortisol levels also aid in determining which enzymatic defect is present. The physical examination is notable for the absence of palpable gonads

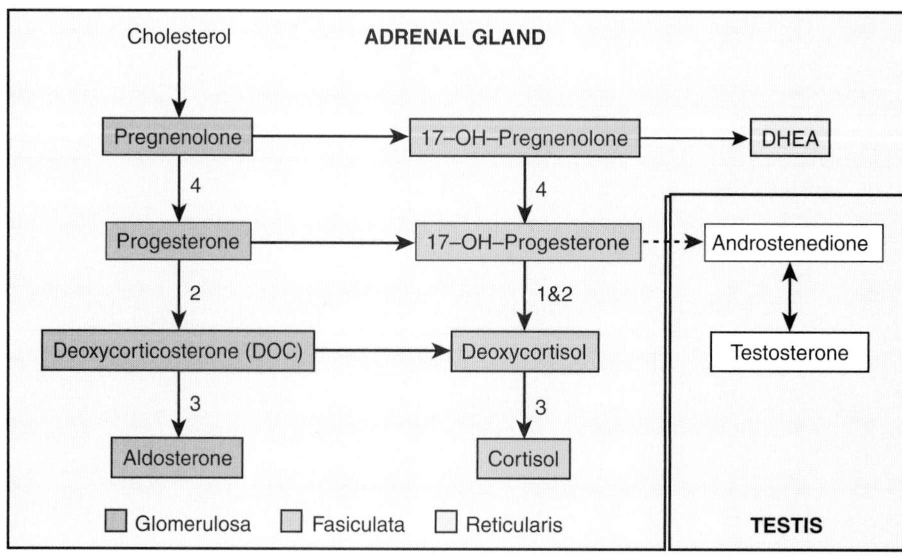

Figure 63-2. Pathways of steroid biosynthesis. The numbers correspond to CAH type and the location of the enzyme defect (see text).

and the presence of a cervix on rectal examination. Also, bronzing of the skin may be noted from excess ACTH cross-reactivity with melanocyte-stimulating hormone receptors. Palpation of a gonad virtually excludes the diagnosis of 46,XX DSD. The genitogram and an ultrasound study mirror these findings, revealing müllerian structures with a variable-length urogenital sinus.

Treatment

Because all forms of CAH are inherited in an autosomal recessive manner, genetic counseling is recommended. Although it is controversial, in families with a history of CAH, maternal treatment with dexamethasone before week 10 of gestation can eliminate or improve the level of fetal virilization and is generally well tolerated.[25] Postnatally, cortisol replacement with hydrocortisone is the mainstay of therapy, with the addition of fluorohydrocortisone if salt wasting is present. Supportive management of fluid and electrolyte abnormalities may be best provided in a neonatal intensive care unit.

With regard to gender identity, the vast majority of patients with CAH identify as female.[26] In this subgroup, gender assignment is uniformly female and is congruous, given a 46,XX karyotype and normal ovaries imparting the potential for fertility. Surgical reconstruction, a feminizing genitoplasty, generally involves three elements: clitoroplasty, monsplasty, and vaginoplasty.

46,XY DSD (Male Pseudohermaphrodite)

This group is the most heterogeneous in the classification system. All patients have a 46,XY genotype and testicular gonadal tissue only. The gonads are sometimes palpable. The condition can be simplistically thought of as a deficit of either production or reception of androgen.

The androgen deficit may result from a defect in synthesis. Several rare enzyme deficiencies have been implicated, including those of 3β-hydroxylase, 17α-hydroxylase, and 20,22-desmolase (cholesterol side-chain cleavage deficiency). All three adrenal enzymes are involved in the steps from cholesterol to androstenedione and testosterone and are associated with severe CAH and often death. 3β-Hydroxylase and 20,22-desmolase deficiencies are associated with cortisol and aldosterone deficits with hyponatremia, hyperkalemia, and metabolic acidosis. In 17α-hydroxylase deficiency, mineralocorticoid production is preserved, resulting in excess salt and water retention, hypertension, and hypokalemia. In the male, the phenotype is variable, ranging from the appearance of a proximal hypospadias with cryptorchidism to that of a phenotypic female with a blind-ending vagina.

Defects in 17,20-desmolase and 17β-hydroxysteroid oxidoreductase act at the testicular level to convert androstenedione to testosterone. Because the adrenal is unaffected, CAH does not occur. The phenotype can be quite variable, but those with complete feminization may escape detection at birth and be reared as female. In the latter disorder, however, progressive virilization is related to excess gonadotropin production at puberty, which may partially compensate for the lack of testosterone synthesis. Phallic growth and the development of male secondary sex characteristics create a conundrum with regard to gender reassignment when the diagnosis is made later in life.[27]

Despite adequate production of androgen, receptor defects can render cells blind to the virilizing effects of the hormone. The phenotype is variable and depends on the degree of insensitivity of the receptor for androgen.

The extreme is normal female external genitalia resulting from complete androgen insensitivity syndrome (CAIS). The incidence of this syndrome is approximately 1 in 40,000. It usually results from a point mutation in the androgen receptor gene, located on the X chromosome.[28,29]

Receptor defects seen in CAIS (also termed *testicular feminization*) result in normal female external genitalia and a blind-ending vagina. Testes are present but may be nonpalpable. MIS production is intact, so no müllerian ductal structures are present. These patients usually are initially seen at puberty with amenorrhea, but may be encountered earlier with the finding of a testis at the time of inguinal hernia repair.

Partial androgen insensitivity is associated with a large spectrum of phenotypic variation (e.g., Gilbert-Dreyfus, Lub's, and Reifenstein's syndromes). It can be a sporadic or inherited condition, and gender assignment and treatment are individualized.[30]

Testosterone is converted to DHT by 5α-reductase, type 2. DHT is a much more potent androgen with regard to virilization of the external genitalia and prostate. The phenotype is ambiguous, but virilization occurs at puberty related to the increased testosterone production and peripheral conversion by nongenital 5α-reductase, type 1. Unfortunately, the virilization is incomplete, and a small phallus and infertility are likely.

Diagnosis

Metabolically, the diagnosis is made similar to that of CAH in the 46,XX DSD patient, noting excess steroid levels above the enzymatic block and elevated levels of ACTH. The physical examination confirms absence of a cervix on rectal examination. Bronzing of the skin may be noted from excess ACTH as well. Palpation of a cryptorchid or descended testis is possible. The genitogram and ultrasound study mirror these findings, revealing no vagina or uterus, but a prominent utricle may be present that lacks a cervical impression at its apex. In CAIS, testosterone levels are elevated post-pubertally but the diagnosis in the prepubertal child may require human chorionic gonadotropin (hCG) stimulation and genital skin fibroblast androgen receptor studies. Receptor assays can delineate a quantitative versus qualitative receptor defect. LH levels are elevated, related to the loss of testosterone feedback

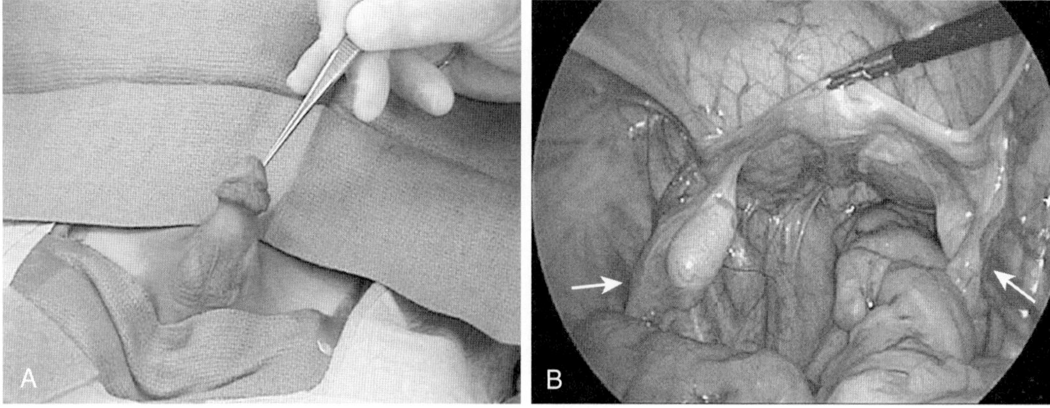

Figure 63-3. A 2-year-old boy presented with nonpalpable testes. A karyotype showed XY. **A,** External genitalia were male. **B,** Laparoscopy revealed bilateral gonads that were testes on longitudinal biopsy. Müllerian structures (*arrows*) were also seen. Note the rudimentary uterus (being held by the grasping forceps). This patient had abnormal MIS-receptor function.

inhibition, which requires normal receptor hormone interaction. 5α-Reductase deficiency is confirmed by an elevated testosterone-to-DHT ratio and an abnormal 5α-reductase type 2 gene.[31]

Treatment

In CAIS, the gender assignment is always female. CAIS patients who are assigned as female in infancy later identify themselves as female.[32] Because the androgen receptor defect is ubiquitous, virilization of the brain does not occur. Orchiectomy is required, given the low but present risk of malignant degeneration, but this is often deferred until after puberty.[33] The testis synthesizes estradiol, facilitating feminine development at puberty. Orchiectomy before puberty necessitates hormone replacement for normal pubertal development.

Gender assignment in partial androgen insensitivity syndrome (PAIS) is largely based on the response of the external genitalia to exogenous testosterone. A significant virilization response argues for the male gender. If there is no response, the female gender is favored. This subgroup is the most variable and has the least consensus with regard to gender assignment. There are reports of gender reassignment at puberty.[34,35] Dissatisfaction with the gender of rearing occurs in approximately 25% of PAIS patients, whether raised male or female.[36] In 5α-reductase deficiency syndrome, the brain is normally virilized and these individuals identify with the male gender. Thus, male gender assignment is recommended.[37]

Müllerian Inhibitory Substance Deficiency

MIS is produced by the Sertoli cells in the testis and causes regression of the müllerian ductal structures. In this rare syndrome of abnormal MIS production or MIS-receptor abnormality, wolffian ductal development is unimpaired but the müllerian ducts also persist. Because the infant has a normal male phenotype, this syndrome is rarely encountered in the neonatal period. The most common presentation to the pediatric surgeon is that of finding a fallopian tube adjacent to an undescended testis in the hernia sac at the time of orchiopexy (hernia uterine inguinale).[38]

If this scenario is encountered, a biopsy of the gonad should be performed, the hernia repaired, and all structures left intact until completion of a full evaluation with karyotype and MIS levels. Apparent males can also present with bilateral nonpalpable testes, and müllerian structures are found at laparoscopy (Fig. 63-3). Abnormal MIS-receptor gene assays also can be helpful for verifying the diagnosis in those with a normal MIS level. Subsequent management is primarily orchiopexy. This, however, may be extremely difficult because the vas deferens can be closely adherent to the fallopian tube or uterus. Excision of discordant ductal structures may be attempted, but, given the relatively low risk associated with leaving these structures, the risk of damage to the vas during this dissection likely outweighs the benefit of removal. Despite normal testosterone levels, impaired spermatogenesis is often the case.[39-41]

Leydig Cell Abnormalities

Because the Leydig cell is responsible for testosterone production in the testes, impaired testosterone production can also manifest from Leydig cell hypoplasia, agenesis, or abnormal Leydig cell gonadotropin receptors. These disorders are rare. Although the karyotype is 46,XY, the phenotype tends to be female, with a blind-ending vaginal pouch and absence of internal müllerian structures. These patients usually are seen initially in the pubertal period with amenorrhea and, therefore, are reared as female. Management is similar to that for CAIS, with orchiectomy and estrogen replacement.[42,43]

Ovotesticular DSD (True Hermaphrodite)

Ovotesticular DSD exists when both ovarian and testicular tissue are present. The gonadal configuration also can be quite variable, with the ovary/ovotestis combination being most common in the United States. Ovary and testis, bilateral ovotestes, and testis/ovotestis combinations also occur. Ovotestes are usually polar with an ovary at one end and a testis at the other, but the distribution can be longitudinal, requiring deep longitudinal biopsy to sample the gonad adequately. Because of the paracrine effect of the gonad, the ipsilateral internal duct structures correlate with the type of gonad present. Ovotestes are associated with a variable duct structure, but usually fallopian tubes prevail. A decisively müllerian or wolffian duct structure is usually present rather than an ipsilateral combination.[44]

Ovotesticular DSD can be associated with a variety of karyotypes, with 46,XX being the most common. In the United States, the majority with this karyotype are African American, but different chromosomal content has been correlated with different races. It is thought that a translocation of the *SRY* gene or associated genes to an X chromosome or autosome explains the development of testicular tissue in the 46,XX karyotype. It is more difficult to explain ovarian tissue in a patient with a 46,XY karyotype. Likely, key genes to the ovarian development are present, but undetected to complement the normal X chromosomal content. An unappreciated mosaicism could also have occurred.

The phenotype covers the entire spectrum, with ambiguity and asymmetry the rule, but with a tendency toward masculinization. Although it is unusual for ovaries to be found in the labioscrotum, testes and ovotestes are often found descended. Fertility has been described in those raised as female, but testicular fibrosis makes this unlikely in those raised as male.[29,45]

Diagnosis

The diagnosis of ovotesticular DSD is suggested by a mosaic karyotype or ductal structures, but is confirmed by the presence of ovarian and testicular tissue by biopsy.

Treatment

Gender assignment in ovotesticular DSD is quite variable and should be based on the functional potential of the phenotype. In either case, the discordant gonads should be removed early. Retained testicular tissue will cause virilization in the female. In males, the testicular tissue is preserved and orchiopexy is performed. A 1% to 10% incidence of testicular tumor development is found in males, predominantly gonadoblastomas and dysgerminomas, so long-term surveillance is needed.[46] Hypospadias repair also is required in the male, and feminizing genitoplasty is performed in the female. Males tend to require hormonal replacement because of the progressive testicular fibrosis, but females usually do not. Fertility is possible in those raised as female. Females should, however, be screened for testosterone levels, which can signal inadequate resection of testicular tissue.[47]

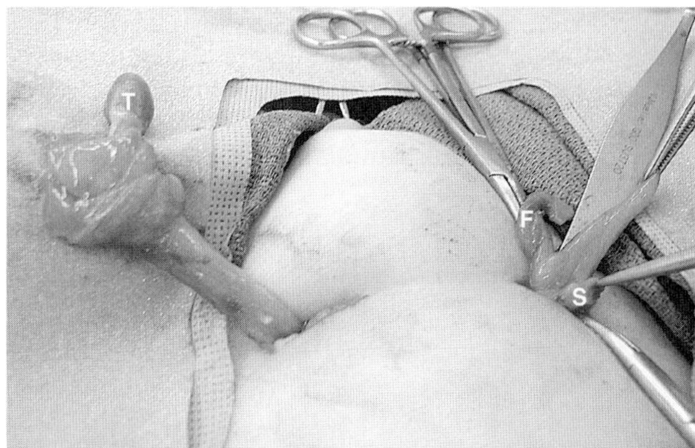

Figure 63-4. Mixed gonadal dysgenesis. The left testis was descended, and the right streak gonad was intra-abdominal. T, testis; F, fallopian tube; S, streak gonad. (Photo taken from head of table.)

Mixed Gonadal Dysgenesis

Mixed gonadal dysgenesis (MGD) is the second most common form of neonatal ambiguous genitalia. The patient will have a testis on one side and a streak gonad on the other, characterized by microscopically normal ovarian stroma without oocytes (Fig. 63-4). The internal duct structure mirrors the ipsilateral gonad, with the streak associated with a fallopian tube and uterus resulting from the lack of MIS. The karyotype is generally a mosaic of 45,XO/46,XY, and the stigmata of Turner's syndrome are variably present. The phenotype is ambiguous, but masculinized, and the testis may be descended but more commonly is not.[48]

The risk of gonadal tumor development, usually gonadoblastoma, is as high as 20%, and tumors can develop in either the testis or streak gonad.[49] An increased risk of Wilms' tumor also is present in MGD. The Denys-Drash syndrome occurs in approximately 5% of patients with MGD and is classically described as ambiguous genitalia, Wilms' tumor, and glomerulopathy, which is often seen with hypertension.[50]

Diagnosis

The diagnosis is suggested by the physical stigmata of Turner's syndrome on examination (webbed neck, shield chest) and 45,XO/46,XY karyotype. The finding of a testis and streak gonad, however, confirms the diagnosis.

Treatment

The majority of patients with MGD have been raised as female because of the short stature conferred by Turner's syndrome and the malignant risk of the retained testis. Females undergo early gonadectomy and feminizing genitoplasty. Males require early excision of the streak gonad, orchiopexy or orchiectomy, and hypospadias repair. Infertility is the rule despite adequate testicular endocrine function. Because of the increasing concern regarding testosterone imprinting on the brain, more masculinized patients are being raised as male. If individuals are raised as male, close surveillance of the testis is necessary, unless elective orchiectomy and hormone replacement are chosen. Testicular biopsy at the time of puberty to exclude dysgenetic elements is generally recommended.[46] If carcinoma in situ is identified, low-dose radiation therapy is curative.

Pure Gonadal Dysgenesis

Pure gonadal dysgenesis (PGD) is characterized by streak gonads bilaterally. The external phenotype and internal duct structures are female. These patients generally are seen at puberty with primary amenorrhea. The chromosomal makeup is classically 46,XX. PGD is an autosomally recessive trait, so genetic counseling is warranted. This implies that the condition can be caused by abnormalities in the X chromosome or supporting autosomal genes involved in gender differentiation. The gonads do not carry risk of malignant degeneration.

Other conditions are also closely related to bilateral streak gonads. The chromosomal makeup is quite variable and can be 46,XY (XY sex reversal, Swyer's syndrome, or male Turner's syndrome), 45,XO, or a mosaic. Variants with a Y chromosome differ in that they carry a high rate of malignancy in the retained streak gonads. The phenotype is as described earlier, but these patients may be first seen in infancy with gonadoblastomas or dysgerminomas, or with germ cell tumors that become more common in adolescence. The stigmata of Turner's syndrome are often present. Multiple chromosomal deletions and mutations have been described causing this syndrome.

Diagnosis

The finding of a female external phenotype and an internal duct structure with bilateral streak gonads confirms the diagnosis. Follicle-stimulating hormone and LH levels are generally elevated, and estrogen and testosterone levels are decreased. The diagnosis may be suggested by the physical stigmata of Turner's syndrome on examination (e.g., webbed neck, shield chest).

Treatment

With the presence of a Y chromosome, gonadectomy should be performed, given the high incidence of malignancy. In classic 46,XX PGD, the gonads can be left in situ because there is no malignant potential. In either case, hormonal replacement at puberty is required because the streak gonads provide no endocrine function.

Other Syndromes of Aberrant Sexual Differentiation

Several syndromes worth mentioning do not neatly fit into the described classification systems.

Vanishing testis syndrome is characterized by a 46,XY karyotype but absent testes bilaterally. This generally results in virilization to the point of normal external genitalia and internal duct structure but absent testes. The testes were thought to have produced androgen at some point, resulting in this masculinization, but subsequently vanished related to torsion or regression. Patients are generally raised as boys, and hormonal supplementation at puberty is required.[51]

Klinefelter's syndrome is characterized by a male karyotype containing two or more X chromosomes (47,XXY; 48,XXXY; etc.). Although phenotypically male prepubertally, these patients acquire abnormal male secondary sexual characteristics (tall stature with disproportionately long legs, sparse facial hair, decreased muscle mass, and a feminine fat distribution) and infertility. The testes are small and hard, with decreased androgen production and elevated estradiol levels related to primary hypergonadotropic hypogonadism. Gynecomastia often occurs with an increased risk of breast cancer.[52] Fertility has been reported but requires assisted means, such as intracytoplasmic sperm injection.[53]

46,XX Testicular DSD (XX sex reversal) is characterized by a male phenotype with a 46,XX karyotype. Most commonly this occurs from translocation of Y chromosomal material to the X chromosome, but it also can occur from mutation of the X chromosome or from mosaicism. The phenotype and management are similar to those of Klinefelter's syndrome, with the exception of shorter stature.[54]

Mayer-Rokitansky-Küster-Hauser syndrome is characterized by a 46,XX karyotype with normal female external genitalia but a short, blind-ending vagina. Normal ovaries and fallopian tubes are present, but the uterus is generally rudimentary. Patients are seen initially with primary amenorrhea but may have cyclical pain related to functioning endometrium. Treatment is geared toward vaginal reconstruction to allow menses or intercourse, or both.[55]

EVALUATION OF THE NEWBORN WITH AMBIGUOUS GENITALIA

The diagnosis of ambiguous genitalia is extremely disconcerting to the family and should be addressed as a medical emergency. Usually, genital ambiguity is obvious, but the finding of any degree of hypospadias in association with any undescended testis or of a normal penis with bilateral nonpalpable testes merits an intersex evaluation. In this population, a high rate of intersex conditions is found despite the absence of classic ambiguity.[56] Table 63-3 indicates other abnormal

Table 63-3 Abnormal Physical Examination Findings for Disorders of Sexual Differentiation

Apparent Female	Unsure	Apparent Male
Clitoral hypertrophy	Ambiguous	Impalpable testes
Fused labia		Severe hypospadias
Palpable gonad		Hypospadias and cryptorchidism

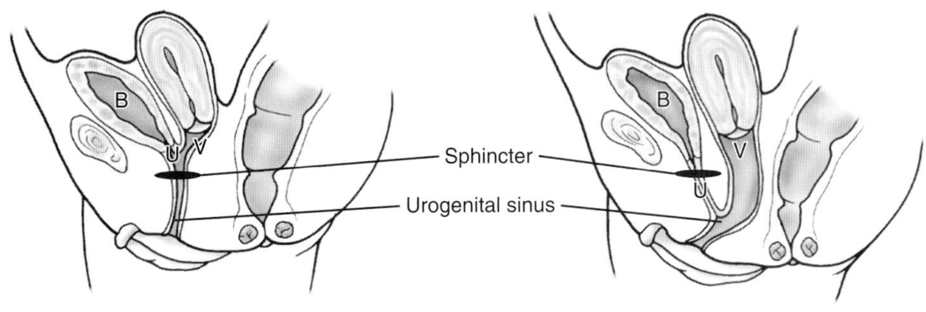

Figure 63-5. High versus low urogenital confluence. B, Bladder; U, urethra; V, vagina.

physical examination findings that warrant consideration for DSD.

The family history may reveal maternal hormone exposure, previous fetal death, or a history of genital ambiguity.

The physical examination should focus on the genitalia. Assessment for palpable gonads is important, because a palpable gonad represents a testis or ovotestis and rules out 46,XX DSD, in which only ovaries are present, or PGD, in which only streak gonads are present. If both gonads are palpable, this generally indicates 46,XY DSD. One palpable gonad is generally associated with MGD or ovotesticular DSD. Phallic stretched length, clitoral size, and the position of the urogenital sinus should be noted. A rectal examination may reveal a palpable uterus. The physical examination should include assessment for the stigmata of Turner's syndrome associated with MGD and PGD. Bronzing of the areola or scrotum can suggest elevated ACTH production in CAH.

The initial metabolic evaluation should include a karyotype or fluorescent in-situ hybridization to identify X and Y chromosomes. 17-OH progesterone levels should be obtained after 3 or 4 days of life, by the time spurious elevations resulting from the stress related to birth have subsided. Electrolyte levels should be monitored closely in the interim to identify salt wasting with CAH. Testosterone and DHT levels are important for evaluating 5α-reductase deficiency. An elevated LH level and a low MIS level suggest testis dysgenesis or absence. ACTH or hCG stimulation tests can be performed but are more controversial.[38]

Early imaging studies include pelvic ultrasonography, which should identify a uterus if one is present. Although a gonad may be seen, ultrasonography is not useful in differentiating a testis, ovotestis, or ovary. A genitogram performed by retrograde contrast injection into the urogenital sinus is helpful in identifying the level of confluence of a vagina and urethra and its relation to the urethral sphincter (Figs. 63-5 and 63-6).

Gonadal biopsy is often required for diagnostic purposes, but the diagnosis of CAH can be made by metabolic evaluation alone. Endoscopy is not usually required for diagnosis, but is essential in characterizing the internal duct structure, level of confluence of the urogenital sinus, and planning for and performing the reconstructive surgical procedures.[29]

At my institution, a gender-assignment team including a pediatric urologist/surgeon, endocrinologist, geneticist, neonatologist, psychologist, and social worker together evaluate any newborn with ambiguous genitalia. This information is synthesized by the team and presented to the parents in a combined care conference. The goals of gender assignment and management should include preservation of sexual function and any reproductive potential with the least number of operations, appropriate gender appearance with a stable gender identity, and psychosocial well-being.[57]

RECONSTRUCTIVE GENITAL SURGICAL PROCEDURES

Controversies and Considerations

For more than 20 years, largely based on the work of John Money and the "John/Joan Case," the overwhelming bias was that gender identity was largely inducible and loosely dependent on chromosomal constitution. The focus was on one of two twin boys who was reassigned to the female gender early in life after a demasculinizing circumcision injury. The child reportedly developed normally from a psychosocial

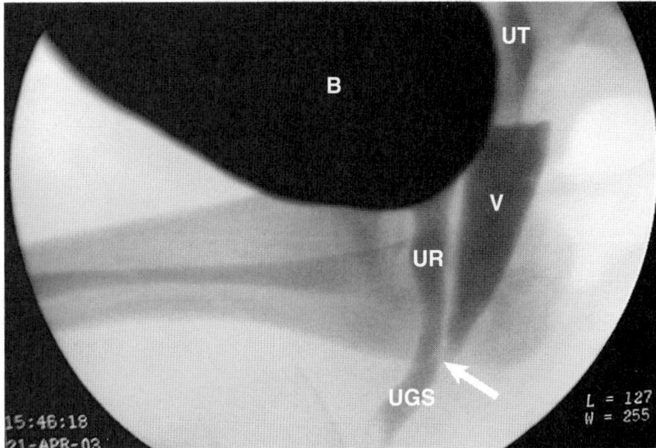

Figure 63-6. Genitogram, lower confluence. *White arrow,* level of the confluence of urethra and vagina to become the urogenital sinus. B, Bladder; UT, uterus; V, vagina; UR, urethra; UGS, urogenital sinus.

standpoint, well adapted to life as a girl.[58] Only with extended follow-up into adulthood was it discovered that the individual converted back to male gender after severe dissatisfaction with a female identity (including attempted suicide).[59] This rattled the fundamental concepts on which gender assignment had been based for decades and brought to the forefront a tremendous controversy regarding the appropriate management of children with ambiguous genitalia and possible gender reassignment.

Because reconstruction is rarely done in response to any life-threatening issues, support groups for individuals with intersex conditions have advocated delaying any reconstruction until the child can express his or her wishes regarding gender assignment.[60] Although this would decrease the likelihood of a mismatch between physical and psychological gender, the period of genital ambiguity could be quite challenging for a child in our society. Despite the controversy, the International Consensus Panel on Intersex stated that, currently, the evidence is insufficient to abandon the practice of early genital reconstruction.[18] However, all these options must be discussed thoroughly with the family before embarking on any reconstructive efforts.

In general, if surgical reconstruction is thought to be appropriate, it is planned in the first 3 to 6 months of life. For feminizing reconstruction, the vaginal tissue is thicker as a result of maternal hormonal influence and the distance from the vagina to perineum is shorter at this age. Because parents have a great degree of anxiety surrounding the gender of their child, earlier repair may help reduce this anxiety and encourage parent/child bonding.[61]

Male Gender Assignment

Reconstructive efforts for the male gender of rearing include orchiopexy or orchiectomy, when appropriate, and hypospadias repair. These techniques are described elsewhere in this text. It bears mentioning, however, that orchiopexy may be extremely difficult because the vas deferens can be closely adherent to müllerian duct remnants, such as a fallopian tube or uterus. A portion of these structures may be left in situ if the risk of damage to the vas deferens or testicular vasculature is significant, but this adherence may severely limit mobility of the testis and preclude orchiopexy.

Methods of total penile reconstruction in cases of aphallia, demasculinizing penile trauma, or female-to-male gender reassignment by using a radial forearm or osteocutaneous fibula flap have been described with some reasonable success.[62,63] These corrective efforts are usually undertaken in adulthood, and their description is beyond the scope of this discussion.

Female Gender Assignment

Feminizing genitoplasty includes three major components: monsplasty, clitoroplasty, and vaginoplasty (Figs. 63-7 and 63-8). The timing of the vaginoplasty depends on the level of confluence of the urogenital sinus. For a low confluence, it is performed in the neonatal period with monsplasty and clitoroplasty. If the confluence is high, this may be approached simultaneously. However, because vaginal dilation is often necessary after repair, this may better be deferred until the patient is peripubertal and more capable and interested in this requirement. Cystoscopy is invaluable for this assessment. We generally introduce a Fogarty balloon catheter in the vagina and a catheter in the urethra and bladder to define the confluence during dissection.

The procedure is initiated by placing a traction suture in the glans, and a dorsolateral circumcising incision is made, leaving a 4- to 5-mm distal preputial cuff, much like is done in a hypospadias repair. The lateral borders of the mucosalized plate are incised, taking this back adjacent to the urogenital sinus. The shaft of the phallus is then degloved of skin superficial to Buck's fascia. Fascial incisions are then made lateral to the neurovascular bundles. A plane is created just beneath Buck's fascia from the level just proximal to the glans back to the pubic symphysis. The mucosalized plate is elevated on the ventrum and preserved

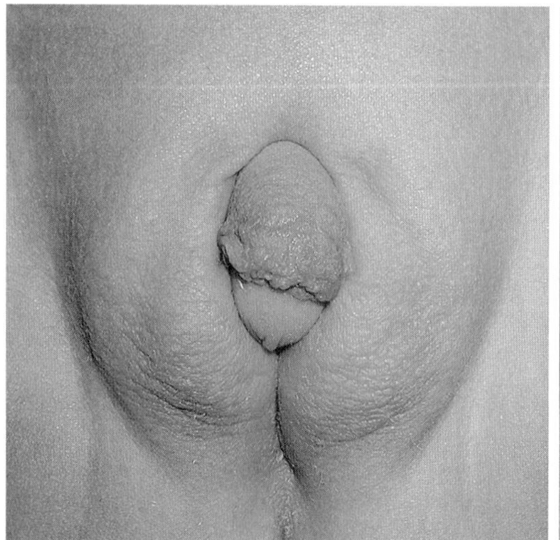
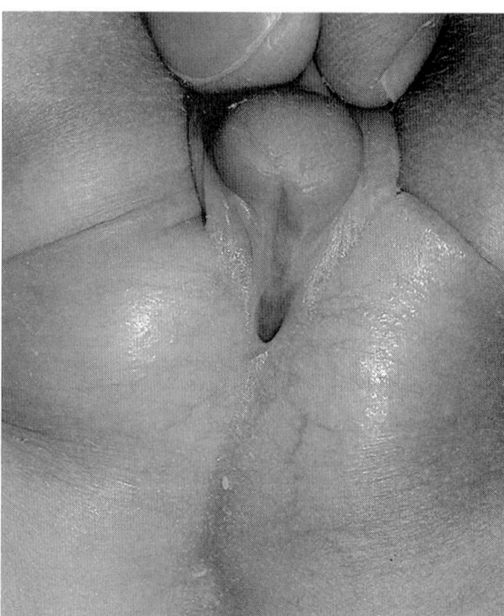

Figure 63-7. Ambiguous genitalia. The patient has congenital adrenal hyperplasia, 21-hydroxylase deficiency.

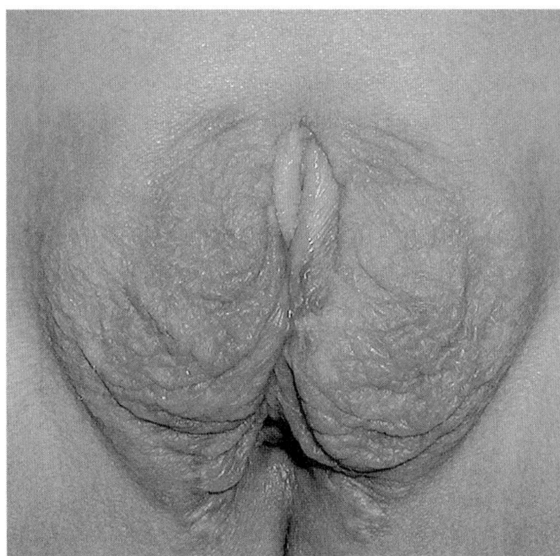
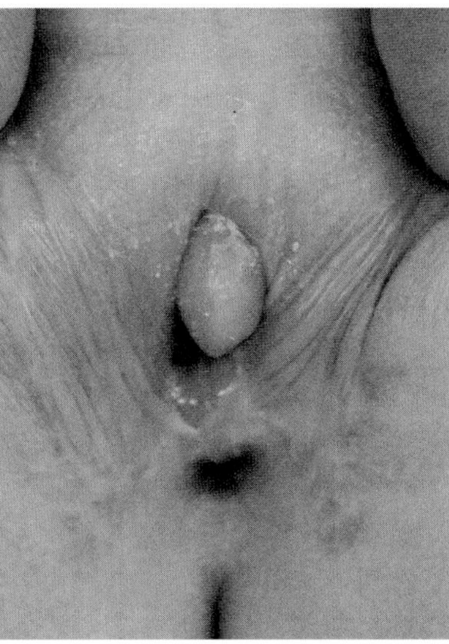

Figure 63-8. Same patient as in Figure 63-7. Appearance of genitalia 6 months after undergoing a feminizing genitoplasty.

to fill naturally the void between the urethral meatus and clitoris. The dorsal pedicles, including the neurovascular bundles, are preserved. The corporeal bodies are suture ligated at their base at the level of the pubic symphysis, and the distal corporeal tissue is excised. An alternative technique preserving the corporeal bodies has been described to maintain the potential for reversibility, but long-term functional outcome is pending.[64]

I do little to reduce the size of the glans clitoris because I believe that even when it is markedly enlarged, it can be recessed and has a quite normal appearance in adulthood. By not trying to reduce the size of the clitoris, nerve injury is limited. However, alteration in sensation is more commonly associated with clitorectomy rather than clitoral reduction.[65] The clitoris is anchored to the corporal stumps to secure its position, being sure not to compromise the dorsal neurovascular pedicle.

A posterior inverted "U"-shaped flap is then made from the level of the ischial tuberosities to just posterior to the urogenital meatus. For a very low confluence, dissection is carried along the posterior aspect of the urogenital sinus to the level of the confluence, the posterior wall is incised until the vaginal introitus is normal in caliber, and the "U"-flap is advanced to complete the posterior vaginal wall (Fig. 63-9). With higher confluences, my colleagues and I have favored total urogenital mobilization.[66-68]

For total urogenital mobilization, the urogenital sinus is incised circumferentially and mobilized as one unit to the level of the confluence (Fig. 63-10). At this point, the vagina can be carefully separated from the urethra under direct vision and the defect in the urethra is closed. The urogenital sinus can then be incised at the dorsal midline and folded back onto itself to make up the anterior vaginal wall. By using local skin flaps for the dorsolateral defects, a lengthy distance can be bridged.

Total urogenital mobilization is attractive in that one can approach even the high urogenital confluence in the neonatal period without vaginal substitution or grafting, but the family must be appropriately cautioned. Although early results are favorable, descent of the bladder neck is counterintuitive when considering our knowledge of adult female stress incontinence and long-term continence may be an issue. To complete the monsplasty, the dorsal phallic shaft skin is incised vertically, a preputial hood is formed for the clitoris, and the majority of this tissue is used to construct the labia minor with "V"-shaped advancement flaps (Fig. 63-11).

Other techniques for the high urogenital sinus include a posterior approach dividing the rectum and

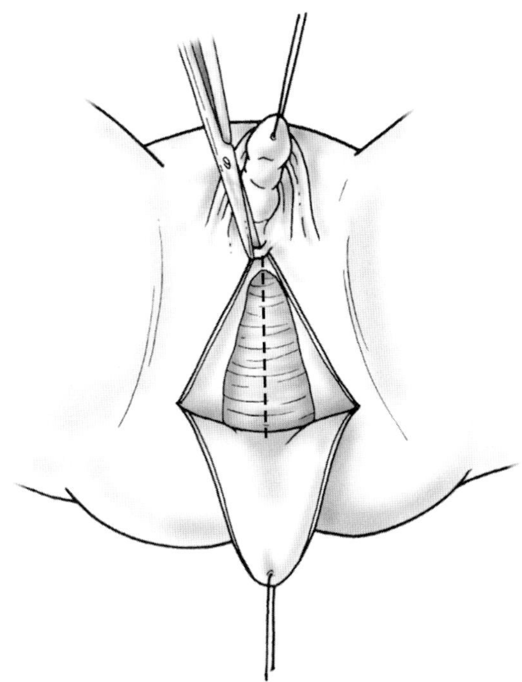

Figure 63-9. Vaginal cutback procedure for the low urogenital confluence.

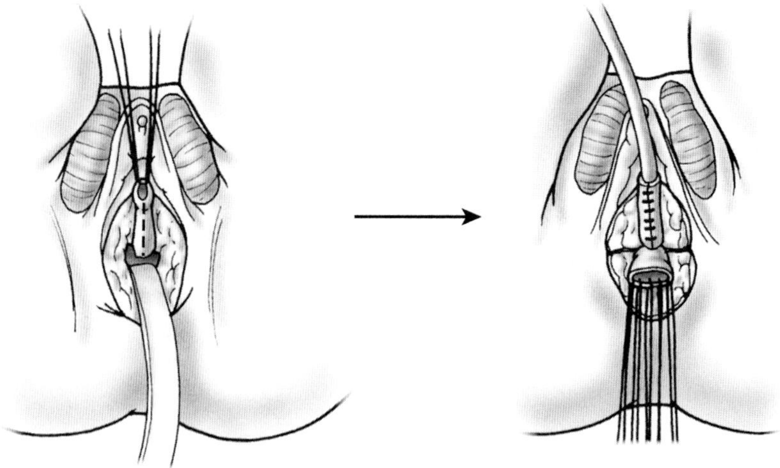

Figure 63-10. Total urogenital mobilization. The urogenital sinus is mobilized as a unit, bringing the confluence toward the perineum. Once visualized, the vagina is then detached and the urethral defect is closed.

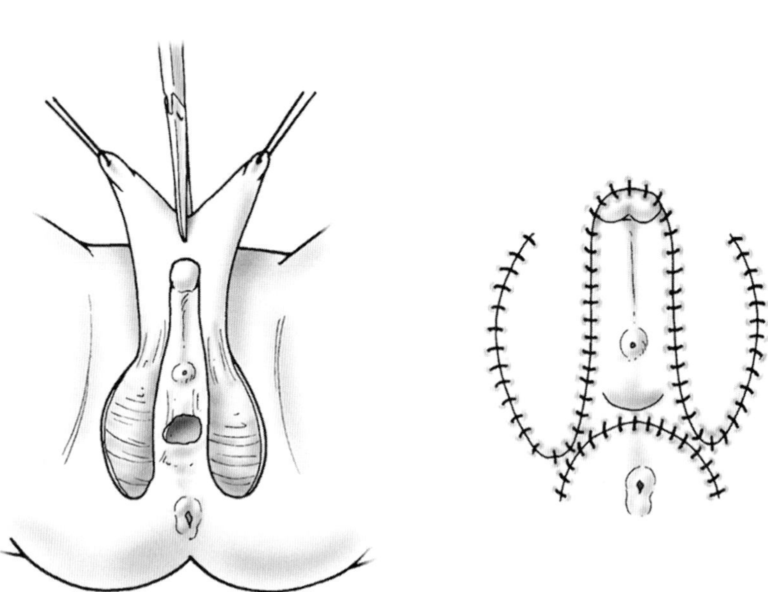

Figure 63-11. Mons plasty. Dorsal shaft skin is degloved from the phallus and incised. These flaps are then advanced to become the labia minora. (Shown before and after excision of the corporeal tissues and clitoropexy.)

an anterior transvesical approach.[69,70] These methods have not been used extensively at my institution.

In some patients with a high urogenital confluence, I have delayed vaginal reconstruction until the peripubertal period, just before menarche. The techniques described are still used, but in some patients, especially those who are obese, these methods are insufficient. I have favored vaginal substitution with a colonic segment, but ileal substitutions and split-thickness skin grafts also have been advocated. The benefit of vascularized bowel substitution is less vaginal stenosis and the natural formation of lubricating mucus, but this may require wearing a pad if there is excessive mucus production. Colonic segments appear to have a lower rate of stenosis than do ileal segments.[71] Conversely, skin grafts have a tendency toward long-term stenosis and may require frequent dilation and revision, but long-term satisfaction also has been described.[72] The barrier function to sexually transmitted diseases is likely superior with skin grafts when compared with intestine.[73]

In cases of vaginal agenesis (e.g., Mayer-Rokitansky-Küster-Hauser syndrome), the substitution techniques described are often used. However, if a rudimentary vagina or depression exists, sequential dilation with the technique described by Frank and modified to a dilating seat by Ingram may be successful.[74,75]

chapter 64

UROLOGIC LAPAROSCOPY

Craig A. Peters, MD

Laparoscopy is an adjunct to the surgical armamentarium of the pediatric urologist. As new technologies such as robotically assisted approaches emerge to augment the potential for minimally invasive procedures, they should be seen as additional tools to assist in the care of children. Uncontrolled enthusiasm may lead to inappropriate use, and unbridled skepticism about their value may lead to unrealized promise.[1,2] The focus of this discussion is to review the current applications and future horizons of laparoscopy and robotics as they apply to pediatric urology.

Diagnostic laparoscopy is the most common current application in pediatric urology and has become well integrated with operative laparoscopic orchiopexy. Renal, ureteral, and bladder surgical procedures have become common in many practices but have not fully supplanted conventional surgery and continue to evolve dynamically. Robotically assisted procedures are rapidly emerging as a viable means to achieve equivalent results in reconstructive procedures, particularly pyeloplasty. These are discussed in terms of the appropriate application, approaches, and results.

DIAGNOSTIC LAPAROSCOPY

Nonpalpable Testis

Laparoscopy in pediatric urology began with the diagnosis of undescended testes (UDTs). Over time, the interpretation of the findings and the integration with therapeutic laparoscopy have been well developed.

Because imaging studies used to locate a nonpalpable testis have repeatedly failed to demonstrate an intra-abdominal or inguinal testis in all cases, reliance on these studies might result in leaving an intra-abdominal testis in the abdomen. Given the increased risk of malignancy in these testes if undetected, the need for 100% accuracy is the foundation for using diagnostic laparoscopy. Diagnostic laparoscopy has become the most widely used method to provide information as to the presence and location of the nonpalpable testis. Although numerous studies have shown this approach to be safe and probably more accurate than open exploration,[3-5] some controversy still persists.[6-8] The predominant argument for initial inguinal incision is that it can be diagnostic and therapeutic for an inguinal testis. However, the same applies to laparoscopy for the testis located in the abdomen.

Indications and Preparation

Diagnostic laparoscopy for UDT is reserved for the boy with a nonpalpable testis and is usually performed between ages 6 and 12 months. Those with bilateral nonpalpable testes should have gonadotropin and müllerian-inhibiting substance (MIS) levels determined preoperatively. The role of the human chorionic gonadotropin (hCG) stimulation test is unclear because it is not definitive in proving testicular absence due to false-negative results, but it does provide some data as to the functional potential of the testis before any manipulation. Even if no laboratory evidence of testicular tissue is found, it has been my practice to perform laparoscopy, recognizing the existence of false-negative findings with the hCG stimulation test and lack of substantial experience with MIS. Patients are placed on a clear liquid diet for 24 hours before the procedure and given a rectal suppository that night to evacuate the rectum. A rectal tube is introduced before preparing the patient, and a bladder catheter is inserted in the sterile field. The abdomen is entirely prepped to allow placement of working ports for laparoscopic orchiopexy or for open exploration in the rare occurrence of a major injury.

Technique

Access

A 3-mm incision is made in the inferior aspect of the umbilicus, and the subcutaneous tissues are spread to reveal the fascia. The Veress needle is aimed inferiorly about 15 degrees off vertical, while the abdominal wall is "tented" by the surgeon and assistant. Elevating the abdominal wall can aid in preventing the preperitoneal placement of the needle. Excessive lifting, however, may allow preperitoneal placement as the needle skims along the peritoneum rather than puncturing it. Usually two distinct "pops" (the fascia and the peritoneum) are felt as the needle is passed. Without moving the needle, a syringe half full of saline is attached to the needle and aspirated. If no return occurs, the saline is instilled and re-aspirated to confirm the position of the needle in the peritoneal space and not in a viscus. With the syringe off, the abdomen is lifted and the water level should drop into the peritoneum. With insufflation to pressures between 8 and 12 mm Hg, flow should be free with low pressure initially. If not, the needle may be preperitoneal.

If fluid returns on the first aspiration, especially if dark, it is presumed that the intestine has been entered. In this case, the needle is withdrawn slightly until no fluid is aspirated. The peritoneum is then insufflated, and the telescope is inserted to look for the site of puncture. It should be just below the umbilicus. The umbilical fascia is enlarged and a laparoscopic grasper can be passed along the laparoscope. The intestine that has been punctured is grasped and brought out to be inspected, cleaned, and oversewn. Alternatively, the puncture can be identified and repaired laparoscopically by using two additional ports. Although a simple Veress needle puncture of the small bowel can be usually safely ignored, I prefer to repair it.

Diagnosis

Once flow has been established through the Veress needle and a pneumoperitoneum established, the needle is withdrawn and a Step cannula (Covidien, Phillipsburg, NJ) with a blunt trocar is introduced through the sleeve. The telescope is passed through the umbilical cannula. In the case of a unilateral UDT, the normal side is inspected first to provide a comparative image for reference to the opposite side (Fig. 64-1). The affected side is then inspected, with attention first placed on establishing landmarks: the iliac vessels, the

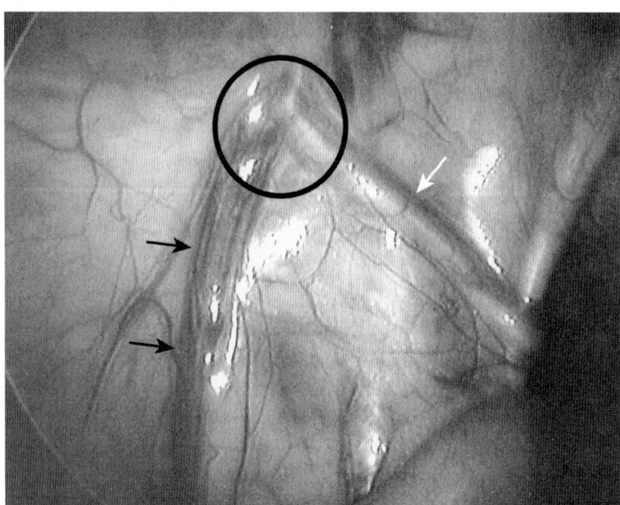

Figure 64-1. Laparoscopic view of the internal inguinal ring on the left, showing the vas deferens (*white arrow*) and spermatic vessels (*black arrows*) converging at the ring (*circle*), just lateral to the inferior epigastric vessels.

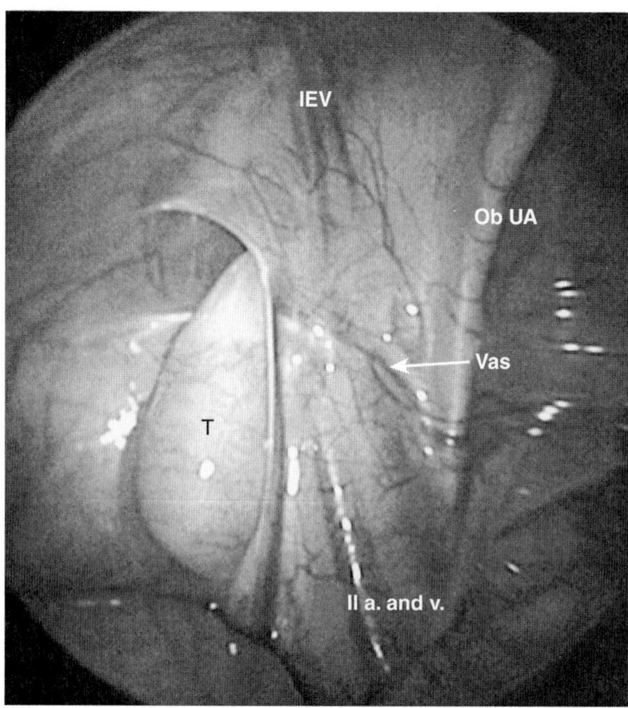

Figure 64-2. Intra-abdominal left testis (T) adjacent to the internal inguinal ring. The vas deferens is indicated by the *arrow*. Il a. and v., Iliac artery and vein; Ob UA, obliterated umbilical artery; IEV, inferior epigastric vessels.

inferior epigastric vessels, and the obliterated umbilical artery (Fig. 64-2). The vas is often first seen, but the vessels must be visualized for an accurate diagnosis. Smaller than normal vessels in the usual position are often observed with an atrophic testis in the inguinal canal. It may be necessary to retract the colon to confirm the location of the vessels. In some cases, especially on the left side, when the testis is intra-abdominal, the vessels are more medial and hidden by the colon. Usually the vessels can be seen by using the Trendelenburg position or rotation of the table. Rarely, I have placed a second port to permit mobilization of the colon. The vas deferens can be helpful in locating an intra-abdominal testis, but it must be remembered that the vas and testis can be separate. The testis, if present, will be located by following the vessels. In some cases, gubernacular structures may resemble spermatic vessels disappearing into the inguinal ring from a testis located higher in the abdomen.

If the appearance of the vessels on the affected side differs from the normal side, further exploration is necessary. A vanishing testis is readily recognized by the blind-ending vas deferens and spermatic vessels (Fig. 64-3). Under these circumstances, no testicular tissue is present and further exploration is unnecessary. Although true testicular agenesis occurs, its frequency is small because I have not seen a patient in whom the vessels and vas were completely absent in more than 300 diagnostic laparoscopic procedures.[3,9] The diagnosis of testicular agenesis requires visualization of the retroperitoneum to the level of the lower pole of the kidney because I have seen testes located well above the level of the aortic bifurcation. In most

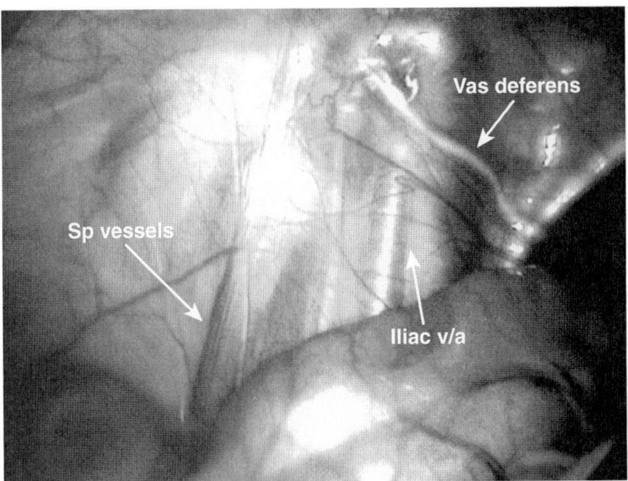

Figure 64-3. Laparoscopic view of vanishing testis with both vas deferens and spermatic vessels (Sp vessels) visible but dwindling away before the inguinal ring. Iliac v/a, iliac vein and artery.

cases, the very high testes are suggested by abnormal vessels or gubernacular structures between the testis and the internal ring.

Laparoscopic demonstration of vas and vessels exiting the abdomen into the internal inguinal ring ("canalicular" vas and vessels) suggests the testis has descended into the inguinal canal or scrotum. If the testis is not palpable, it is likely atrophic. These boys need inguinal exploration to confirm that no testis is present, especially if the child is obese. The appearance of normal canalicular spermatic vessels may suggest the presence of an ectopic testis. Canalicular vessels associated with an atrophic testis are usually, but not reliably, smaller.[9] I have occasionally seen nonpalpable perineal ectopic testes detected in this way. Five percent of atrophic testes in the scrotum or canal contain viable germ cells and should be removed. Whether these atrophic testes pose a real malignancy risk is unclear. Inguinal exploration may obviate laparoscopy, but approximately 50% of UDT patients will not need inguinal exploration for either diagnosis or treatment.

An intra-abdominal testis may require some effort to find but is easily recognizable when seen. Those located medial to the iliac vessels may be the most elusive. Some are on a long spermatic cord and drop deep into the pelvis, even along or behind the bladder.

The final component of the diagnostic laparoscopy is to determine the location of the UDT relative to the internal inguinal ring to determine the most appropriate surgical intervention: vessels-intact laparoscopic orchiopexy (VILO) or two-stage Fowler-Stephens orchiopexy (FSO). After placing the working ports, a small ruler is inserted and the distance is measured.

DISORDERS OF SEXUAL DEVELOPMENT (INTERSEX)

Diagnostic and therapeutic laparoscopy has a significant role in the child with a disorder of sexual development.[10-12] The appearance of streak gonads, uterine tissue, and inappropriate müllerian structures is readily recognized laparoscopically. The appearance of a streak gonad, as distinct from an ovotestis, is usually clear, but biopsy is needed to confirm the presence of an ovotestis (Fig. 64-4). Definition of the müllerian structures may be more precise with laparoscopy than with many imaging modalities, including ultrasonography. Removal of dysgenetic gonadal or müllerian tissue is readily accomplished.

THERAPEUTIC LAPAROSCOPY

Orchiopexy

Laparoscopic orchiopexy is one of the most developed applications of laparoscopy in children. Several reports have demonstrated its efficacy, and perhaps even its superiority to open orchiopexy.[13] However, this conclusion is limited by the fact that the true outcome of any orchiopexy, adult fertility, has never been assessed.[14]

Indications

Laparoscopic orchiopexy is used for the intra-abdominal testis. This is almost always performed under the same anesthesia as the diagnostic laparoscopy that identifies the testis and determines its location. Testes high in the inguinal canal have been subjected to laparoscopic orchiopexy,[15,16] but it is unclear whether this represents an advantage, and I have not used laparoscopy for testes located in the canal. However, intra-abdominal dissection and mobilization of the spermatic vessels might be a useful adjunct to subsequent open orchiopexy for such cases.

Laparoscopic orchiopexy can be a single-stage VILO or a two-stage FSO. The latter should be reserved for testes that cannot be brought into the scrotum with the spermatic vessels intact. In those boys, the spermatic vessels are initially occluded with a clip, suture, or fulguration and the testis is left in situ. At a second procedure 4 or more months later, the spermatic vessels are

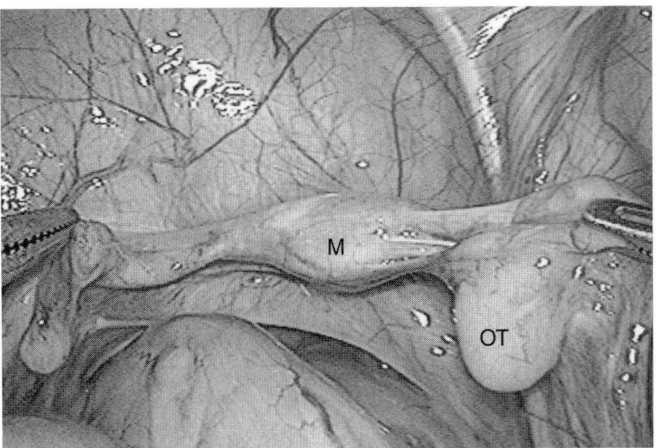

Figure 64-4. Laparoscopic view of the right ovotestis (OT) and müllerian structures (M) in a 7-year-old with ovotesticular disorder of sexual development (formerly true hermaphroditism). Removal of the ovarian tissue and orchiopexy was performed.

divided and the testis is brought into the scrotum on a pedicle of the vas deferens and peritoneum. The vasal artery provides the blood supply to the testis. Discerning which testis is best treated with which procedure is the major challenge of laparoscopic management of the intra-abdominal testis.

Some have recommended FSO for all boys with an intra-abdominal testis.[17] However, because many testes can be brought into the scrotum from the abdomen with the vessels intact, this does not seem uniformly appropriate. Preserving the major blood supply to the testis is intuitively more appealing. Placing the UDT into the scrotum based on the spermatic vessels also avoids a second anesthetic and surgical procedure. A single-stage FSO procedure has been advocated by some as well, but a high incidence of testicular atrophy without the interval period of collateral vascular development makes this approach unacceptable and cannot be recommended.[18]

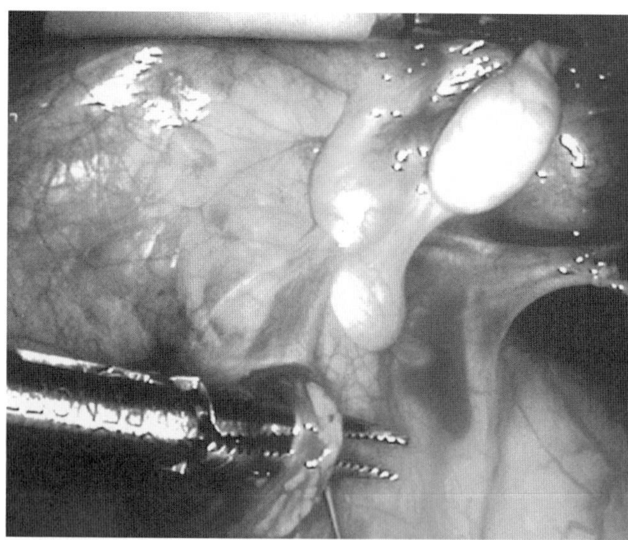

Figure 64-6. First stage of a Fowler-Stephens orchiopexy with dissection of the spermatic vessels before ligation. The testis is not manipulated.

Technique

Position

The patient's position is adjusted to a moderate Trendelenburg position with the ipsilateral side rotated upward about 30 to 45 degrees. Insufflation pressures are maintained at 12 mm Hg in most patients.

Ports

The initial umbilical port for the diagnostic portion of the laparoscopy is maintained for the laparoscopic orchiopexy. Although using 2-mm instruments is feasible, I have found these instruments too flexible. Thus, I prefer larger, more rigid instruments, either 3.5 or 5 mm (for a clip applier, if needed). Working ports are placed in the ipsilateral upper quadrant and the contralateral lower quadrant. The ipsilateral port should not be placed too low, because it will be ineffective in mobilizing the proximal testicular vessels (Fig. 64-5). The cannulas are inserted under direct vision. A fascial closure stitch is placed before cannula placement to facilitate fascial closure at the end of the procedure.

If a two-stage FSO is indicated based on testicular location or age of the patient (>2 years), the vessels are occluded with a surgical clip after creating a window in the peritoneum 1 to 2 cm proximal to the testis (Fig. 64-6). This can be performed with only one working port in the contralateral lower quadrant.

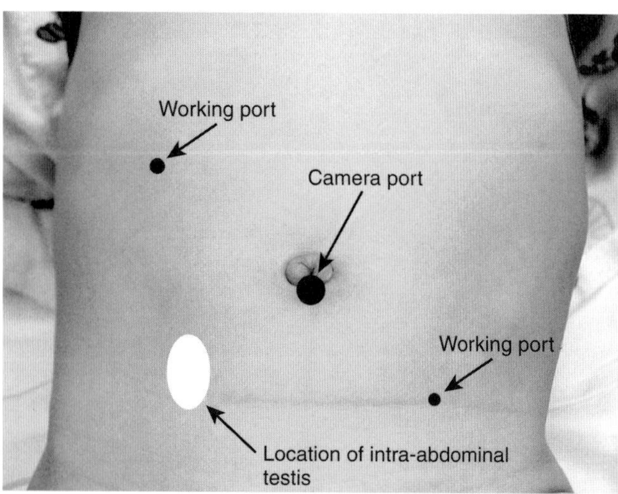

Figure 64-5. Port location for laparoscopic orchiopexy is seen on the right. Approximate position of the intra-abdominal testis is also depicted.

Instruments

For the first stage of the FSO, I use a 5-mm clip applier. For the laparoscopic orchiopexy, I use a 3.5-mm cauterizing scissors and a curved dissector. The curved dissecting instrument is used to create the passage from the pelvis into the scrotum, and a long, curved vascular clamp is then passed retrograde by locking onto the tip of the curved dissecting instrument.

Procedure

For orchiopexy, dissection begins by incising the peritoneum lateral to the spermatic vessels and testis and dissecting it to the level of the inguinal ring. The gubernacular attachments are identified at the level of the ring and carefully transected, leaving enough gubernacular tissue attached to the testis to grasp for retraction and for delivery into the scrotum. Care must be taken to avoid injury to a looping vas deferens. Cephalad retraction of the testis will expose the vas so that it can be protected throughout the procedure. Lateral dissection continues cephalad along the spermatic vessels toward their origin from the iliac vessels. The testis and the spermatic vessels are bluntly freed from the pelvic sidewall medially. The peritoneum on the lateral and inferior side of the vas deferens is incised over the obliterated umbilical artery and into the pelvis, approaching the bladder. This leaves a triangular web of peritoneum between the vas and the vessels with the testis at the apex. Some surgeons recommend leaving this peritoneum intact to preserve the blood supply of the vas, but it definitely hinders mobilization of the testis. I therefore incise it and mobilize the spermatic vessels proximally.

At this point, the testis is grasped and moved to the opposite side of the pelvis. When it can reach the opposite inguinal ring, it has adequate mobility to be brought over the pubic tubercle. The pathway from the abdomen to the scrotum is then developed. A dartos pouch is first created in the usual manner. A curved dissecting instrument is passed from the abdomen over the pubic tubercle, medial to the obliterated umbilical artery and lateral to the bladder, by using direct vision and finger palpation. The tip of the dissector is guided into the scrotal sac and pushed through an incision in the dartos fascia. A long, curved vascular clamp is then passed retrograde by grasping the tip of the dissecting instrument or a heavy silk suture. The clamp can be spread to open the tract for passage of the testis.

The gubernacular stump is then grasped, and the testis is brought into the scrotum. The testis can be fixed in place by using the dartos-pouch technique or with a button with a pull-out suture, or both. Excessive tension on the spermatic vessels may result in avulsion of the vessels or spasm. Further proximal dissection of the vessels may be necessary to prevent vascular insufficiency.

The determination of whether to perform a VILO or FSO remains incompletely defined. Initially I performed VILO if the testis "appeared" mobile enough before any dissection, but I found that those higher in the abdomen did not always move into the scrotum easily and some showed postoperative atrophy. Correlating the initial UDT position with the postoperative result, it became evident that when the testis was more than 2.5 cm from the internal inguinal ring, postoperative testicular atrophy occurred at an unacceptable rate. I also found that testes medial to the iliac vessels were more difficult to mobilize into the scrotum, even if located at the level of the internal inguinal ring. Therefore, testes more than 2.5 cm proximal to the internal inguinal ring or medial to the iliac vessels are managed with the FSO technique.

We have also observed that children older than age 2 years nearly always require a FSO. The second-stage FSO is performed by using identical port positions and ligating and then dividing the spermatic vessels just distal to the original clip. The stumps of vessels are used for retraction, and the testis is mobilized on the triangular web of peritoneum surrounding the vas deferens. The testis is moved into the scrotum and fixed in a dartos pouch. Indeed, the ease of the second stage has encouraged some surgeons to use the FSO technique in all patients with an intra-abdominal testis, but this seems inappropriate, considering the higher success rate of a VILO.

Robotic technology has been used for an abdominal testis but does not appear to offer any advantages except as a learning tool for the device. I have not used this approach.[19]

Postoperative Care

Patients may be discharged the same day if they are able to retain oral intake. The child is examined in 6 weeks and undergoes a scrotal Doppler ultrasound evaluation in 9 months to assess blood flow and testicular size.

Results

There are several reports of outcomes after laparoscopic orchiopexy, all with good results.[13,20-25] It is important to recognize that outcome parameters are based on perceived testicular viability and not on sperm production. These assessments are not really different from those used to assess open orchiopexy. No truly long-term functional assessment has ever been performed after any of the techniques for orchiopexy. The length of follow-up is important, because some testes in my patients appeared healthy at 6 months but showed a reduction in size at 12 months. Doppler ultrasound imaging has been used to assess testicular size and blood flow and seems to correlate well with physical examination.

Without any real standards of assessment of initial location or of postoperative outcome, it is difficult to stratify patients and correlate to outcome. However, it is probably reasonable to consider a success rate of about 95% for intra-abdominal testes undergoing VILO and about 90% for those undergoing FSO. Although this may be better than for open orchiopexy, correlation with the initial testicular position is undefined.

RENAL SURGERY

Nephrectomy

Simple nephrectomy for benign conditions was the first major laparoscopic procedure performed in children and is now well established and routine.[26-35] The indications are similar to those for open nephrectomy. The initial approach to nephrectomy was transperitoneal, with very good outcomes. These initial cases were performed in infants by using three 10-mm cannulas (some surgeons used four ports), and no major complications were reported.[36,37] In most cases, patients were discharged the next morning.

An interesting response emerged with publication of a series in which open nephrectomy for multicystic dysplastic kidney (MCDK) through a dorsal lumbar incision was performed on an outpatient basis.[38] Although one can remove a dysplastic kidney through a small lumbar incision, exposure is limited and compromised to the extent that, in one case, an inadvertent appendectomy was performed.

Retroperitoneal endoscopic access was developed for children with similarly good results and with smaller instruments as they became available.[39-41] Two basic access approaches were used: lateral and prone.[42] Both work well, and each has advantages in selected situations.

Indications

The indications for a laparoscopic nephrectomy include benign disease that has resulted in a nonfunctioning renal unit with the potential for infection, hypertension, or pain. I remove MCDKs only when parents insist. The contraindications to a laparoscopic nephrectomy include severe acute coagulopathy, uncontrolled sepsis, or very severe adhesions from prior laparotomy. These are uncommon in children. Laparoscopic nephrectomy has also been shown to be feasible in higher risk patients, such as those with renal failure before transplant.[43,44]

Laparoscopic nephrectomy for large malignancies has not been performed in children because of the large size of the tumors. In time this may change, particularly if preoperative chemotherapy is used to shrink a tumor or if partial nephrectomy is elected for small tumors, and anecdotal reports have appeared.[45] These principles for laparoscopic nephrectomy are well established in adults with renal tumors and will likely be appropriate for children as well.

The choice of transperitoneal or retroperitoneal nephrectomy largely depends on the experience of the operator and the associated procedures needed. If the entire ureter must be removed, or if an intra-abdominal testis is present, transperitoneal nephrectomy may be preferred. Subtotal resection of the ureter is readily done via the retroperitoneal access. The prone approach is less suited to ureteral resection but may be more efficient for access to the hilum.

Robotic technology has been used for nephrectomy, although the advantages are limited. As with cryptorchidism, it is best used as a learning approach for nephrectomy.[46]

Technique

Transperitoneal

Patients are prepared with a liquid diet for 24 hours preoperatively and a rectal suppository is given the night before. A bladder catheter and rectal tube are placed after the induction of anesthesia and before the skin is prepped. The ipsilateral side is elevated on a soft roll, and the patient is secured to the table (Fig. 64-7). The table is rotated so that the abdomen is flat for peritoneal access and port placement and then rolled back with the ipsilateral side up for the procedure. Positioning the patient with the flank up helps the surgeon reflect the colon away from the kidney. This position permits rapid return to the supine position if emergency open access is needed.

The initial port is in the umbilicus with working ports in the ipsilateral lower quadrant in the midclavicular line and just to the ipsilateral side of the midline between the xiphoid and umbilicus. For right nephrectomy, a liver retractor placed laterally on the right or contralaterally on the left may be useful. I have used 3.5-mm or 5-mm instruments and endoscopes. A 5-mm port is needed for the clip applier.

The kidney is exposed by incising the lateral peritoneal reflection of the colon and mobilizing the colon medially. The ureter is identified near the lower pole of the kidney (or occasionally at the level of the iliac vessels), transected, and used for traction to lift the kidney for identification of the renal hilum. If vesicoureteric reflux is present, the ureter should be dissected at least to the level of the bladder and ligated, because clips are unreliable for closure of a thick ureter. Blunt or cautery dissection are used to expose the lower pole and hilum. The artery is divided first if possible, preferably away from the hilum to limit the number of branches that must be controlled. It is divided between clips, usually leaving two on the proximal side. The vein is similarly controlled, avoiding any lumbar veins. The gonadal vessels should be preserved. Superiorly, the adrenal vessels should be avoided. The upper pole is mobilized with cautery because small vessels are frequently adjacent to the capsule. Lateral and posterior mobilization is usually rapid with blunt or cautery dissection. The kidney is removed through the umbilical port, which can be easily enlarged without increasing the size of the scar. The operative field is inspected, and the ports closed with preplaced fascial sutures.

Patients usually stay overnight but may occasionally be ready for discharge on the day of the procedure. Transperitoneal nephrectomy seems to induce more ileus than retroperitoneal nephrectomy, but the difference is minor.

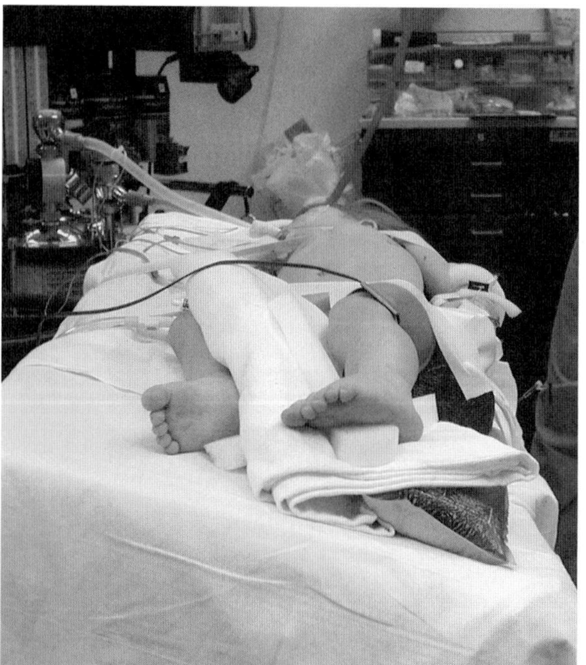

Figure 64-7. Patient and table positioning for transperitoneal laparoscopic renal surgery. The patient is placed on a 30-degree ipsilateral wedge and secured to the table at the chest and hips. The table can then be rotated so that the abdomen is flat for port placement (shown) and rotated in either direction depending on the operative exposure that is desired.

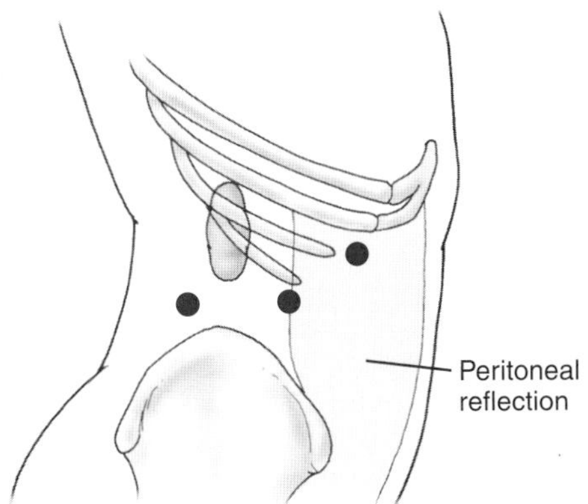

Figure 64-8. Lateral retroperitoneal port placement for right renal surgery. Approximate location of the posterior peritoneal reflection (*shaded*).

Lateral Retroperitoneal

Patients are prepared similar to a transperitoneal nephrectomy but are positioned in a nearly full flank-up position. Initial access is gained just below the tip of the 12th rib with a 1- to 1.5-cm incision and blunt dissection through the muscle layers (Fig. 64-8). The perinephric fascia of Gerota is identified and entered. At this point, a dissecting balloon can be placed or the cannula can be positioned so that the endoscope is used bluntly to develop the working space. In both approaches, the port is secured with a purse-string fascial suture, which also provides a gas seal for insufflation. Pressures are maintained between 12 and 15 mm Hg. Once the position of the kidney is defined, the posterior port is placed. This may not be possible under direct vision, although a 30-degree telescope can facilitate insertion. The anticipated trajectory of the cannula is observed to avoid injury. The peritoneal reflection is identified and bluntly pushed medially. This can be accomplished with an instrument or the endoscope, but care must be taken to avoid disrupting the peritoneum. The medial port is then introduced, either in-line with the other two or inferiorly in a triangular fashion. Fascial sutures in a box-stitch pattern are placed before the cannulas are inserted to act as retention sutures for the cannula during the procedure and to close the fascia at the completion of the operation.

If a small tear is made in the peritoneum, the operative field will be compromised by intraperitoneal insufflation. The peritoneum can be decompressed by placing a small angiocatheter through the abdominal wall to let the peritoneal gas escape. Alternatively, the peritoneal tear can be enlarged so that the peritoneum does not separately trap carbon dioxide. It is rarely necessary to abandon the procedure and convert to an open operation because of entry into the peritoneum.

Exposure of the renal hilum is the key step for retroperitoneal nephrectomy, and it is important to prevent the kidney from falling onto the hilum. This can be facilitated by maintaining the anterior attachments of the kidney so that it falls forward with the peritoneum, exposing the posterior aspect of the hilum. Even so, it may be necessary to use one instrument to retract the kidney as the hilum is exposed, limiting the surgeon's dissecting ability, which becomes one handed. If the pelvis is large, it will need to be retracted to adequately expose the vessels. This may be accomplished by transecting the ureter near the lower pole. The artery is encountered posteriorly and divided between clips. The vein also is divided between clips, and the rest of the mobilization is accomplished as with a transperitoneal approach. Near the upper pole, the peritoneum can be torn so care must be taken to stay close to the kidney.

If the ureter is to be removed, the lateral approach permits efficient access to the distal ureter, usually below the iliac vessels. If no reflux is present, the distal ureteric stump can be left open, whereas the stump of a refluxing ureter must be ligated as close to its junction with the bladder as possible.

The kidney is removed through the larger of the ports, usually the one at the tip of the 12th rib. If it needs to be morcellated with scissors, a laparoscopic specimen-retrieval bag is helpful. Most kidneys are small enough to be removed intact. Occasionally, removal of the specimen can be facilitated by placing it into the finger of a surgical glove as a miniature retrieval bag and then exteriorizing through the port site. All port sites are closed with the preplaced fascial sutures.

Prone Retroperitoneal

The prone approach has evolved from the dorsal lumbotomy technique and offers direct access to the kidney and hilum. The patient is in the full prone position with an indwelling bladder catheter. In small children, it is helpful to have the lower end of the table turned down, with the surgeon standing at the patient's feet. This allows the surgeon to be in-line with the working instruments. The initial port is placed at the costovertebral angle by using a 1-cm incision (Fig. 64-9). Blunt dissection through the posterior muscle layers

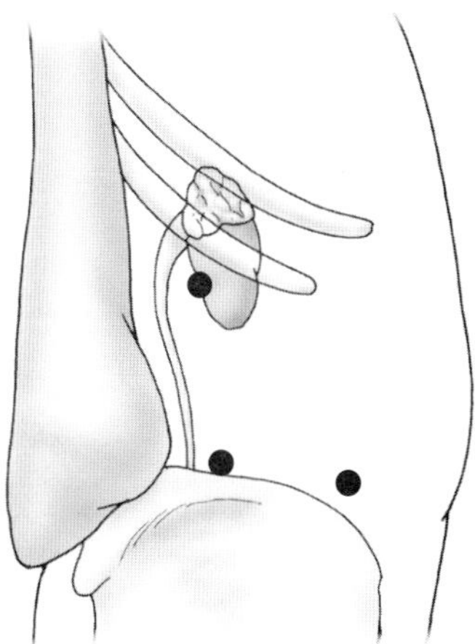

Figure 64-9. Port positions for the prone retroperitoneal approach to the right kidney.

reveals the posterior aspect of the perinephric fascia, which is entered. A lumbar fascial suture is placed for later closure. A dissecting balloon is used to develop the working space. A 5-mm cannula is inserted followed by a 3.5-mm telescope. The telescope can be moved to other ports during the dissection and at the time of placing vascular clips as needed. The endoscope is inserted as the retroperitoneum is insufflated. This should reveal the posterior aspect of the kidney, and further blunt dissection can be performed with the scope. Occasionally, the developed space is anterior to the kidney, making it difficult to immediately locate the kidney. This possibility must be considered, and the upper (posterior) abdominal wall inspected. The secondary (3.5-mm) ports are then placed, followed by insertion of 3.5-mm instruments.[39]

In the prone position, the kidney falls forward, revealing the hilum (Fig. 64-10). The vessels are controlled first, unless the ureter is needed for aid in mobilization of the kidney. Again, the vessels should be exposed somewhat away from the kidney to avoid the need to control multiple branches. It is important to maintain a consistent camera orientation to permit accurate identification of the vascular structures. The exposure can be so wide that the vena cava is readily seen, and this structure may seem smaller than expected because of the pneumoperitoneum. It has occasionally appeared to look like the renal vein, based on size and direction, when the telescope was not oriented correctly.

Once the vessels are secured and divided, the ureter is ligated and divided. The kidney is then mobilized to control the small upper pole vessels, with care being taken to avoid entering the peritoneum and to avoid the adrenal vessels. The kidney can be removed through the initial port, with the camera being moved to the inferior working ports.

If the ureter needs to be excised with the kidney, the instruments are reversed in direction and the ureter traced inferiorly as far as possible. This is usually to the level of the iliac vessels. Postoperative care is similar to that with the other techniques of laparoscopic nephrectomy.

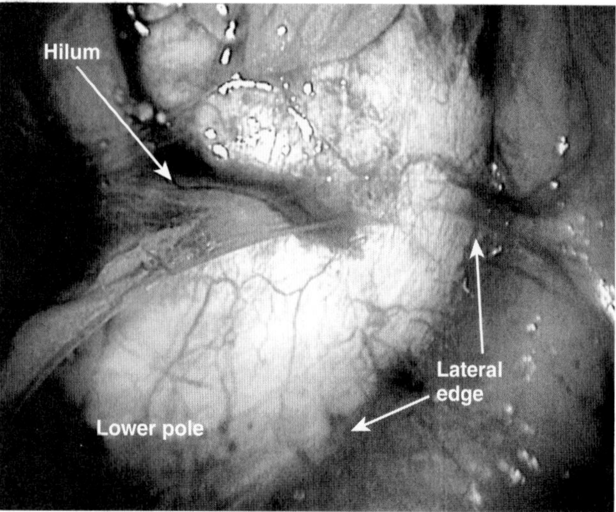

Figure 64-10. Posterior laparoscopic view of the right kidney after initial exposure. The hilum is on the left of the field. The entire kidney is exposed with its lateral edge to the right.

Results

Complications have been reported in several series but are usually limited to minor occurrences, such as entry into the peritoneum or subcutaneous emphysema.[26,47] Conversion to an open procedure is reported in fewer than 2% of the pediatric series and is usually the result of bleeding that cannot be effectively controlled laparoscopically. Conversion rates are very much operator dependent and are not likely an inherent feature of the technique.[48] Injury to other organs is the major concern and has been reported (as it has for open nephrectomy in children). These are fortunately uncommon and usually involve liver, bowel, or occasionally great vessel injuries.

Partial Nephrectomy

It has become clear that laparoscopic partial nephrectomy may be one of the most beneficial procedures to emerge from the early experience with laparoscopic nephrectomy.[49-52] Open partial nephrectomy is best performed through a flank incision, which has an appreciable morbidity, even in infants. Precise vascular control is essential, along with accurate visualization of the normal and abnormal renal moieties. Injury to the remnant pole is a significant complication and may be more likely to occur in an infant due to the mobilization required to expose the hilum. With the laparoscopic approach, the hilum can be exposed without significant mobilization of the remnant pole, theoretically reducing the risk of vascular spasm and injury, although a recent report contradicts this proposed advantage.[53] Robotic technology has been applied to partial nephrectomy as well. The robotic advantages of precise manipulation as applied to identifying, separating, and controlling what may be delicate vessels without injury to the remnant pole vessels may be advantageous. If the remnant collecting system is entered, it can be more readily controlled. Closure of the polar defect with mattress sutures can also be accomplished efficiently. I have begun using robotic technology for all partial nephrectomies in children.[54]

For conventional laparoscopy, my preferred access to the kidney is retroperitoneal and usually prone.[39] However, this limits the ability to remove the ureter, which is required in those unusual cases of obstruction combined with reflux. In such cases, the lateral approach is used or a small inguinal counterincision is made to remove the ureter to the level of the bladder neck. With simple reflux and no obstruction, total removal of the distal ureteral stump is not considered essential. The prone position allows excellent exposure of the posterior aspect of the kidney, and the delineation between the poles is usually readily evident. The ureter to be removed is identified at the level of the lower pole and separated from the remaining ureter. The ureter draining the nonfunctioning pole is transected and used for traction to mobilize the hilum. The hilar vessels are identified, and the vessels of the affected pole are isolated and divided. If the vessels are not clearly defined, dissection of the nonfunctioning pole is started, whereupon the vessels will usually become evident. Division of the renal parenchyma can be performed by using either cautery or the ultrasonic scalpel. It is not a problem if the affected collecting system is entered as long as the entire collecting system is removed. However, if the remnant pole collecting system is entered, it should be repaired and drained. Placement of a ureteral catheter in the remnant pole and injection of indigo carmine dye to confirm closure have been advocated by some. This is useful in adult partial nephrectomy without duplication but is probably not necessary with duplication anomalies because the separation is usually quite clear.

No attempt is usually made to suture the edge of the remnant pole, but this can be accomplished robotically if desired. This maneuver should ensure hemostasis and limit the risk of leakage. I have not typically drained the operative area in small children but would recommend drainage in older children or in complex cases. A bladder catheter can be left overnight, although some of these children can be discharged on the same day.

Robotic partial nephrectomy is performed transperitoneally using an umbilical camera port, a midline port between the xiphoid and umbilicus, and an ipsilateral lower quadrant port. For right-sided upper pole nephrectomies, a fourth retraction port to lift the liver is placed in the contralateral upper quadrant in the midclavicular line. The affected ureter is mobilized and used as a traction handle to dissect the renal hilum and control the vessels. These can be ligated with clips or suture. The kidney is divided by defining the plane between the collecting systems. Using cautery or the ultrasonic scalpel, the parenchyma is transected. The cut surface is closed with two or three mattress sutures with a fat pad placed in the defect for compression. Any leak or injury to the remnant pole collecting system is repaired.[54,55]

The limited number of reports of laparoscopic partial nephrectomy does not allow definite conclusions regarding its ultimate potential, but the efficiency and the reduction in morbidity seem to argue strongly in favor of its further development.[49-53,56-59] Several reports of polar urinomas have appeared, suggesting that closure of the polar defect may be important in limiting this occurrence.[52,56,57]

URACHAL CYSTS

Several reports of urachal cyst resections have been published, although it is unclear if the laparoscopic approach is advantageous.[60-63] It transforms a preperitoneal procedure into an intraperitoneal one. The conventional incision through the umbilicus is a very small incision with minimal scar. Laparoscopically, two other small incisions are needed.

Currently, I do not recommend using this approach, although I performed several initially. The situation in which this might be advantageous would be in the child with umbilical drainage of uncertain etiology. If the drainage is due to an omphalomesenteric duct or omental hernia, then laparoscopic diagnosis and subsequent therapy are efficient, including if the diagnosis is a urachal anomaly. A large inflamed mass due to an infected urachal cyst might be removed laparoscopically with some benefit, although the risk of peritoneal contamination should be considered.

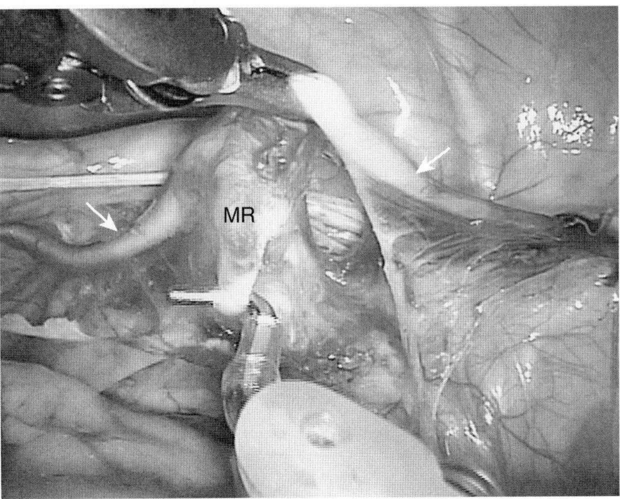

Figure 64-11. Laparoscopic robotic exposure, dissection, and resection of a müllerian remnant (MR) in a boy with right gonadal dysgenesis and the ring-Y chromosomal defect with recurrent epididymitis in the left epididymis. The *arrows* point to the vas deferens on each side.

GONADECTOMY AND MÜLLERIAN REMNANTS

In various disorders of sexual development and genital maldevelopment syndromes, laparoscopic biopsy or resection, or both, of inappropriate gonadal or müllerian structures is possible.[64,65] This is particularly advantageous when the remnant is located in the deep retrovesical pelvis, a difficult area to access with an open procedure. Although they are not strictly intersex conditions, abnormal müllerian structures such as seminal vesicle cysts also are well managed with the laparoscopic or robotic approach (Fig. 64-11).[66,67]

RECONSTRUCTIVE SURGERY

Pyeloplasty

Laparoscopic pyeloplasty in children is emerging as a common procedure using conventional laparoscopic and, increasingly, robotic techniques.[68-71] Their use in infants has also increased, although less rapidly due to the efficacy of conventional techniques.

The widespread use of laparoscopy or robotics for pyeloplasty in children is still in the future.

Both transperitoneal and retroperitoneal access have been described. Most surgeons prefer the retroperitoneal approach for conventional laparoscopy, whereas robotic approaches are largely transperitoneal. Current methods as well as robotic options are discussed.

Conventional Laparoscopic Pyeloplasty

Port placement for transperitoneal pyeloplasty is similar to that for nephrectomy, with an umbilical port, an ipsilateral upper quadrant port just lateral to the midline, and an ipsilateral lower quadrant port. A fourth port for retraction can be placed laterally if needed. Retroperitoneal access is with three ports in a line along the lower edge of the 12th rib. Prone access is possible with a similar in-line port layout.

The operation is similar to the open procedure with exposure of the renal pelvis but is facilitated by the placement of a traction suture (hitch stitch) to stabilize the pelvis. The pelvis is transected above the ureteropelvic junction and used for traction to permit spatulation of the lateral upper ureter without grasping the tissue to be included in the anastomosis. Alternatives include placing a small traction stitch on the ureter distal to the ureteropelvic junction after it is transected or leaving a bridge of pelvic tissue on the medial aspect to stabilize the ureter. The amount of pelvis removed should be limited, even in severe hydronephrosis, because the pelvis may retract and make the repair more difficult. It is not usually necessary to perform a significant pelvic resection, because this will usually shrink on its own after relief of the obstruction. For the anastomosis, most surgeons use a continuous suture anteriorly and posteriorly and use a 5-0 or 6-0 absorbable suture. A stent can be left in place if desired. I prefer using a double-J stent, which eliminates the need for a drain.

Reported outcomes are no better (or worse) than those with the open approach. Postoperative hospitalization and morbidity seems reduced, particularly for older children. Failures, primarily persistent ureteropelvic junction obstruction, have been limited to very small children (younger than 6 months) or those with massive hydronephrosis. This observation may account for the lack of enthusiasm for laparoscopic pyeloplasty in infants, who seem to recover rapidly after open surgical procedures.

Robotic Pyeloplasty

The ability to perform delicate and precise fine suturing using the DaVinci (Intuitive Surgical Corp., Sunnyvale, CA) Surgical System has allowed the advantages of laparoscopy with smaller incisional morbidity and tissue trauma but without the challenges of suturing. The ability of the robotic system to facilitate precise use of 7-0 and 6-0 suture, particularly with pyeloplasty, has moved robotic pyeloplasty in children to an equally effective method with open surgery. Age has not been a limiting factor except in the rare neonate needing an urgent pyeloplasty. I have used the robotic system in children as young as 3 months.[72,73]

Method

A double-J stent can be placed cystoscopically before the procedure. However, this can decompress the pelvis and make operative identification of the pelvis more difficult. The curl of the stent should be positioned just below the ureteropelvic junction, but this is not always easily accomplished. The advantage of preplacement is having an extraction string on the double-J stent to permit withdrawal without a general anesthesia. Alternatively, a stent can be inserted antegrade during the procedure (see later).

Access is through similar port sites as with laparoscopic pyeloplasty, but the size and position of the renal pelvis should guide the position of the lower port. If the lower port is too close to the ureteropelvic junction, movement of the lower instrument may be limited. Therefore, in smaller children, the inferior port is moved medially and more caudad. Most children with a left-sided ureteropelvic junction obstruction are approached transmesenterically to limit the need for dissection of the perinephric space when the colon is mobilized. On the right, the kidney is exposed by reflecting the colon. Once the pelvis is exposed, a hitch stitch is placed through the abdominal wall using a 3-0 monofilament suture that is passed through the anteromedial aspect of the pelvis and then back out the abdominal wall where it is secured with a small clamp. Tension on the suture is adjusted to provide optimal exposure. The hitch stitch allows exposure, stability, and lifting of the pelvis from the inevitable pool of urine and blood. In obese patients this stitch can be tied intracorporeally. As with conventional laparoscopic pyeloplasty, the pelvis is dismembered, the ureter spatulated, and the anastomosis performed (Fig. 64-12). Before completing the anastomosis, the extra pelvis is removed and extracted from the abdomen.

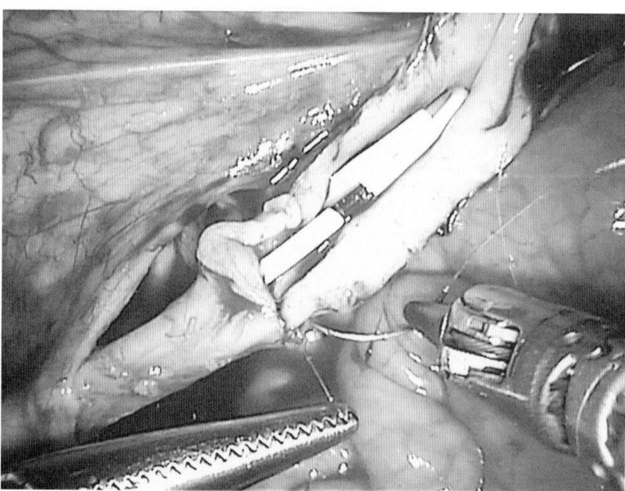

Figure 64-12. Robotically assisted laparoscopic dismembered pyeloplasty showing renal pelvic closure using 5-mm instruments and 6-0 monocryl suture. The internal double-J stent is visible inside the renal pelvis.

Antegrade stent placement is performed after the back wall of the anastomosis is completed. An angiocatheter is passed through the abdominal wall and a 0.035-inch guide wire is introduced through the angiocatheter and guided into the ureter. While this is being done, the angiocatheter is removed and the appropriate-sized stent is passed over the wire, through the abdominal wall, and into the ureter. If there is uncertainty about positioning, blue dye may be instilled into the bladder to indicate when the stent is in place. However, I have not found this step necessary. After stent placement, the anterior wall of the pyeloplasty is performed.

A nearly identical strategy may be used to perform a ureteroureterostomy or ureteropyelostomy for duplication anomalies in which the upper pole is to be preserved. Whether this is preferable to partial nephrectomy when there is limited function is debatable, but both techniques are able to be performed readily with robotic assistance.[46,74]

Several reports of robotically assisted laparoscopic pyeloplasty in children have been published.[73,75-78] Ages have ranged from 3 months to teenage years, and both transperitoneal and retroperitoneal approaches have been described. Results have been excellent to date, but caution should be observed before completely accepting these initial observations. The advantages when compared with open surgery are less obvious in infants than in older children. The clear advantage in terms of morbidity and recovery in older children argues that there is likely some benefit even in younger children. Reoperative pyeloplasty has been reported in children using the robotic system as well.[79]

Antireflux Procedures

Initial attempts at laparoscopic antireflux urologic procedures were frustrating. Using the extravesical Lich-Gregoir technique,[80] these were successful but far too time-consuming to be advantageous. After initial interest, few other attempts were made.[81,82] Interest returned with a reasonably successful series,[83] but the advantages were not clearly evident because catheterization time and hospitalization were no better than with the open approach. Robotic technology has further raised interest, and several reports of robotic extravesical procedures have been published.[46,84] Intravesical procedures, both conventional and robotic, have also been reported.[85-88] It remains uncertain if these procedures are sufficiently advantageous over open surgery to justify the investment in learning and technology. However, it is likely that efficiencies will improve with further refinement.

Method

The reimplant is similar for both the laparoscopic or robotic approach and is performed transperitoneally, exposing the distal ureter. The antireflux tunnel is created by incising the detrusor muscle from the ureterovesical junction along the axis of the ureter down to the submucosa of the bladder. Care is taken not to injure the mucosa or enter the bladder lumen. The muscularis is dissected in an inverted-"Y" manner around the ureteral hiatus. The detrusor muscle is closed over the ureter to create the antireflux tunnel. No attempt at ureteral advancement is made. Suturing the detrusor over the ureter has been the most challenging aspect of the procedure, mainly because of the angle of approach. Robotic assistance greatly facilitates this part of the operation (Fig. 64-13).

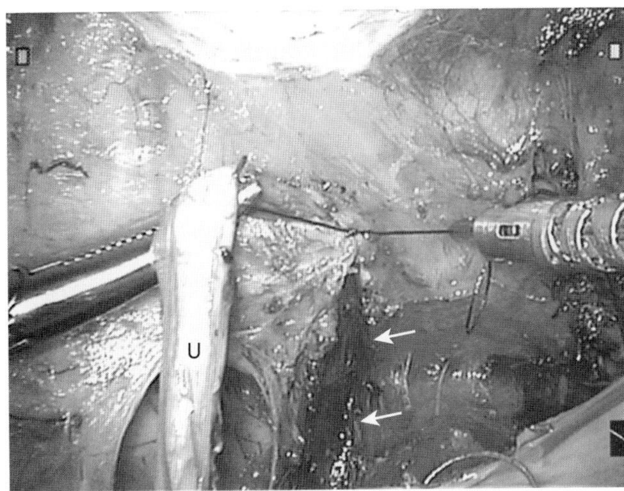

Figure 64-13. Closure of the detrusor tunnel (*arrows*) over the mobilized ureter (U) during a robotically assisted extravesical ureteral reimplant for vesicoureteral reflux. The ureter is being lifted by the left instrument while the first suture of the tunnel is being tied. This keeps the ureter in the tunnel as the subsequent sutures are placed.

In performing bilateral procedures, it is important to limit the amount of damage to adjacent nerves that presumably affect bladder function. Although it has been reported that these nerves can be identified and spared, this can be difficult. In my experience, the best approach is to stay as close to the ureter as possible during dissection. A risk of transient retention is possible, but this appears to be very low.[84]

Results

Success seems to be close to that seen with open surgical procedures. With robotic assistance, larger series have been reported with good results. Hospital stays are slightly shorter than with open methods, but outpatient open extravesical and transvesical reimplantations have been reported with good outcomes as well.[89] Demonstrating an objective clinical advantage over an open approach is challenging. The value of developing techniques for bladder reconstructive procedures using minimally invasive technologies justifies continued attention.

Intravesical Antireflux Procedures

Intravesical antireflux repair has recently emerged as an alternative to the extravesical approach. Advantages include the avoidance of urinary retention with bilateral extravesical procedures and avoiding peritoneal entry.[87,90] Several earlier attempts with the Gil-Vernet approach of bringing the ureters together in the midline, without mobilization, did not prove to be effective.[91] Recent reports of a transvesical approach to the Gil-Vernet procedure have been successful.[92] The most widely used approach to date has been that of an intravesical, transtrigonal reimplantation with insufflation of the bladder (pneumovesicum).[85,87,93] The major technical challenges include obtaining and maintaining access to the bladder without dislodging the cannulas, leaking carbon dioxide into the paravesical space, mobilizing the ureter, creating the submucosal tunnel, and the suturing to implant the ureter. Performing this procedure efficiently may be feasible in only a few highly skilled hands. Robotic assistance has been reported as well but remains challenging, primarily because of the large ports required.[86] Demonstrating a clinical advantage will be difficult.

Continent Diversion and Augmentation

Major reconstructive operations such as bladder augmentation, continent diversion, and vaginal reconstruction carry substantial morbidity with an open approach. It may be that laparoscopic procedures for reconstruction and diversion will prove most beneficial for all age groups. The creation of an appendiceal continent catheterizable stoma (Mitrofanoff) has been reported, including the use of robotic assistance.[94,95] Laparoscopically assisted mobilization with a limited open incision to complete the procedure has been advocated in several reports, with excellent results.[96,97] Laparoscopically assisted reconstruction may be the most practical approach for the present as robotic methods begin to be developed.[98]

The ability to perform an entire reconstruction, including augmentation and continent stoma formation, is technically possible today[99-101] but is not going to be of practical value until more efficient means of suturing are developed. Tissue glues or the use of robotically assisted suturing may permit more widespread use of total laparoscopic methods in complex reconstruction. It also will require novel algorithms for harvesting bowel segments to use in the reconstruction.[98]

chapter 65

RENOVASCULAR HYPERTENSION

James A. O'Neill, Jr., MD

The incidence of hypertension in children is 2% to 10% in all age groups, with the higher figure representative of adolescence. However, because blood pressure is not routinely measured in children, particularly infants, the diagnosis of hypertension is often delayed. Table 65-1 lists the common causes of hypertension in children according to the organ system involved. In this chapter, the focus will be on renovascular causes of hypertension, most of which are correctable.

In 1934, Goldblatt and coworkers described the relationship between coarctation of the aorta and renal artery stenosis with hypertension.[1] However, it was not until the 1960s that a relationship was established between renal ischemia and hypertension resulting from activation of the renin-angiotensin system, which leads to the release of renin and the production of angiotensin II (Fig. 65-1). Subsequently it has been shown that diminished renal perfusion pressure has direct effects on sodium excretion, sympathetic nerve activity, nitric oxide production, and intrarenal prostaglandin concentrations, which result in renovascular hypertension.[2] Recent studies have demonstrated different fractional angiotensin elevation patterns in children with renovascular hypertension as compared with essential hypertension.[3]

With regard to the natural history of renovascular hypertension, once it is established that the disease is progressive, there is often late recurrence of renovascular lesions in sites other than those originally identified. The progressive nature of this disorder is the best justification for an aggressive approach to correction. Second, sustained hypertension may result in left-sided heart failure and chronic renal failure based on chronic ischemic nephropathy. Also, patients with malignant forms of renovascular hypertension have a high incidence of heart failure and renal failure.

The most common cause of hypertension between birth and 20 years of age is essential hypertension in approximately 60% of patients. However, the incidence of correctable hypertension is much higher in patients younger than 15 years. In previous studies by our group, the incidence of correctable hypertension in the birth to 5-year age group was around 80%; in the 6- to 10-year age group, 45%; and in the 11- to 15-year and 16- to 20-year age groups, 20%.[4] Although a variety of causes were identified, the vast majority were renovascular. Renovascular disease comprises 8% to 10% of all forms of hypertension in children while it is 1% of all forms in adults. Additionally, long-term follow-up of patients with renovascular hypertension clearly indicates that patients who have had successful repair of their lesions have much longer survival than those who do not. Moreover, the younger the patient, the better the result.[5] Such studies support an aggressive approach to correction of identified renovascular lesions in young patients.

ETIOLOGY

Renovascular hypertension may be congenital or acquired. Congenital causes include arterial hypoplasia or aplasia; neurofibromatosis involving the renal artery; and Williams syndrome, which includes manifestations of supravalvular aortic stenosis, peripheral vascular stenosis (particularly in the subclavian and renal arteries), hypercalcemia, and elfin facies.[6] Renal involvement by tuberous sclerosis tumors has been reported as well. The most common acquired form of renovascular hypertension is fibromuscular dysplasia (FMD), which may be either localized to one or both renal arteries or appear as a more generalized type of disease, such as Takayasu's arteritis and subisthmic abdominal coarctation, now more commonly referred to as the mid-aortic syndrome.[7-9] In the mid-aortic syndrome, stenoses of visceral arteries such as the superior mesenteric and celiac arteries are common.[8] Other less common forms of acquired renovascular hypertension are renal artery trauma or thrombosis, thrombosis secondary to antithrombin deficiency, Kawasaki disease, and an anastomotic stenosis, as is seen occasionally in renal transplants.[10]

Overall, the vast majority of children with renovascular hypertension have what has been referred to as FMD or hyperplasia. Previous studies have suggested that this lesion has a congenital origin, but there is evidence to the contrary as well, because the

Table 65-1 Causes of Hypertension in Children

Essential hypertension	
Renal	Glomerulonephritis, pyelonephritis, renal hypoplasia, polycystic kidney, Wilms' tumor, neuroblastoma, arteritis, aneurysms, trauma
Cardiovascular	Aortic coarctation, Takayasu's arteritis, neurofibromatosis, tuberous sclerosis, renovascular stenosis, collagen vascular disease
Central nervous system	Encephalitis, intracranial mass with increased pressure, dysautonomia
Endocrine	Pheochromocytoma, aldosteronoma, adrenogenital syndrome, Cushing's syndrome
Secondary hypertension	Lead and mercury poisoning, glucocorticoid drugs, oral contraceptives

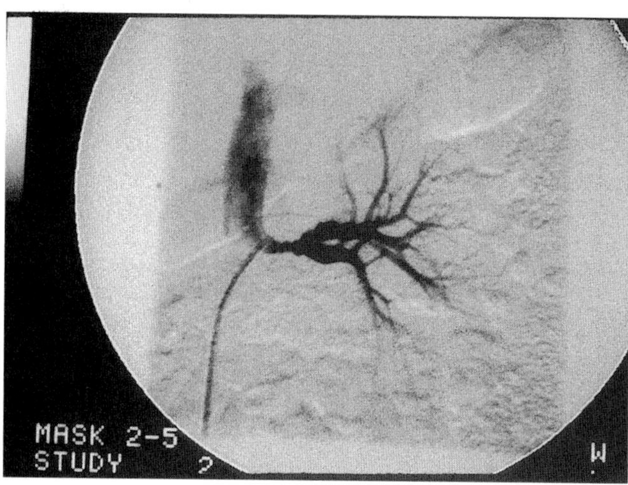

Figure 65-2. This selective renal arteriogram performed in a neonate with congestive heart failure caused by severe hypertension demonstrates significant narrowing of the left renal artery. The cause is probably congenital.

disease appears to have an acquired pattern in young adults.[6] FMD appears to coexist with neurofibromatosis, Williams syndrome, and pheochromocytoma. Because arterial and aortic hypoplasia and aplasia are seen in neonates, it is assumed that some of these lesions are congenital (Fig. 65-2).[11] Conversely, the majority of patients are initially seen at several years of age, usually with an inflammatory phase followed by a quiescent phase of arteritis.[4,7] Although it was initially thought that FMD might be an autoimmune disease, recent evidence suggests that T-cell–based immune mechanisms, macrophages, and antigen-presenting cells are mainly responsible for renovascular arteritis and a variety of other arteritides as well.[12] The pathology of the vascular lesion seen in the renal artery and aorta reveals medial and perimedial fibroplasia, which has inherent implications about approaches to treatment, particularly angioplasty. Although FMD is a systemic, occlusive arteriopathy potentially involving the entire abdominal aorta and its branches, the renal arteries are the predominant vessels involved.[13]

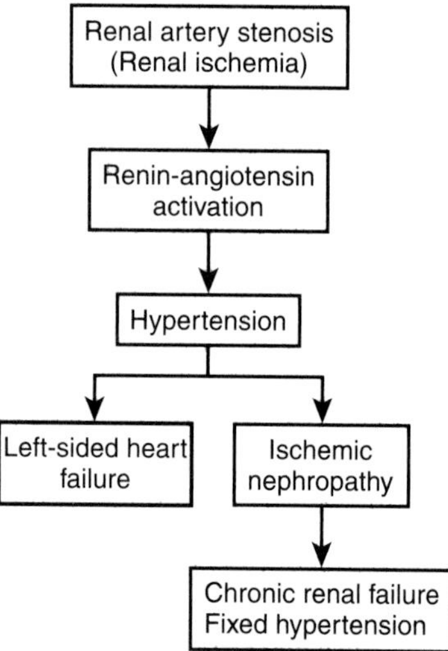

Figure 65-1. The consequences of renal ischemia from renal artery disease are depicted.

CLINICAL PRESENTATION

Children with renovascular hypertension come to attention in one of two ways in most instances. Approximately 70% of patients are asymptomatic. Commonly, an asymptomatic young child undergoing an elective surgical procedure, such as a hernia repair, is found to be hypertensive on anesthetic evaluation. Repeated measurements verify the chronic nature of this problem, which leads to diagnostic evaluation. Approximately one half of these asymptomatic patients will be found to have correctable hypertension. The remaining 30% of patients are symptomatic with headaches, vision problems, encephalopathy, congestive heart failure, oliguric renal failure, and, occasionally, leg claudication. Physical findings may indicate the presence of heart failure with enlargement of the liver and heart as well as retinopathy and retinal hemorrhage. In cases of mid-aortic syndrome, blood pressure and peripheral pulses may be diminished in the lower extremities. Although an abdominal bruit could probably be heard in the majority of instances of renal artery stenosis, it is not commonly found until a diagnosis is suspected. It is usually not known how long the hypertension has been present.

In contrast to adults with FMD, in whom women predominate, gender incidence is equal in children. Both renal arteries are simultaneously involved in approximately 70% of patients. Also, in occasional patients with unilateral lesions, FMD may develop in the opposite renal artery a number of years later. Renovascular causes of hypertension are more common in children younger than 10 years, as evidenced by an average age of 7 years in one of our studies.[5] In infants and toddlers, malignant forms of hypertension with encephalopathy and retinopathy are more likely to develop than in older children.

DIAGNOSIS

Before any invasive diagnostic studies are undertaken, clinical manifestations of severe hypertension such as headache, irritability, abdominal pain, heart failure, and seizures should be controlled with medications.

Laboratory Studies

Renovascular hypertension cannot be diagnosed by any specific laboratory study. Most laboratory studies are performed to document the patient's overall clinical status and particularly the status of the renal function. Erythrocyte sedimentation rate (ESR) is important to assess whether the patient is in the inflammatory or the quiescent phase of the arteritis. Urinary catecholamines are studied to exclude the common endocrine causes, particularly in patients with manifestations of neurofibromatosis, such as café-au-lait spots. I have not found plasma renin or captopril-stimulated renin studies to be helpful in young children. Technetium-labeled pentetic acid (DTPA) radionuclide fractional-flow studies may indicate unilateral renovascular disease, but they are not useful when bilateral disease is present. Captopril renography has the same limitation.

Imaging

Although a number of imaging studies exist, currently it is my policy to perform aortography and selective arteriography in all children with significant hypertension. Minimal complications have been encountered with these studies, even in very small patients. With appropriate hydration, even patients with some degree of oliguric renal failure can undergo aortography and selective arteriography by using low-osmolar or nonionated contrast agents in limited amounts. For patients with a distal or intrarenal vascular stenosis, nitroglycerin-enhanced selective studies promote the identification of segmental areas of ischemia in the involved kidney.

Duplex color-coded Doppler ultrasonography is capable of demonstrating the renal arteries, as well as measuring flow velocity as an index of the degree of stenosis.[14] However, Doppler ultrasound studies, whether performed preoperatively or postoperatively for follow-up, have limitations in terms of demonstrating precise anatomic detail, particularly in small vessels. The same is true of captopril scintigraphy. Magnetic resonance angiography (MRA) and computed tomographic angiography (CTA) are capable of demonstrating the renal arteries and the aorta and its branches better than Doppler ultrasonography, but there are resolution issues in small subjects.[14,15] MRA is less accurate than CTA, and the volume of contrast material for CTA is often as much as with aortography with selective angiography, so no advantage accrues from the standpoint of nephrotoxicity. If one takes the point of view that the prime purpose of an imaging study is to select the most suitable therapeutic method, aortography with selective arteriography is the most definitive study and the one most capable of demonstrating precise anatomic detail (Fig. 65-3). Doppler ultrasonography, MRA, and CTA are now considered best as screening or follow-up studies in children.

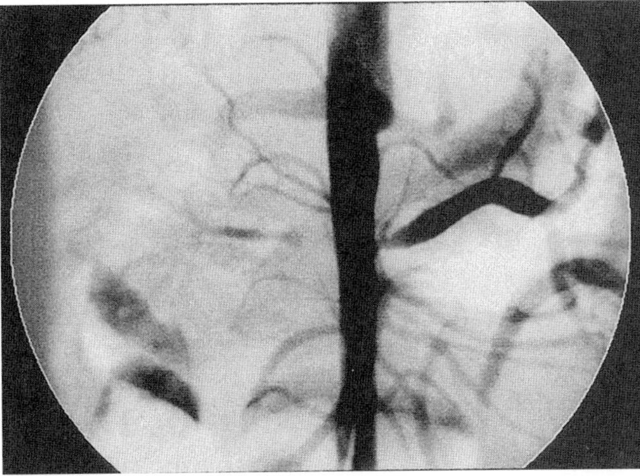

Figure 65-3. This 6-year-old boy was found to have severe hypertension when screened for an elective hernia repair. Aortography revealed marked narrowing of the left renal artery, some narrowing of the mid-aorta, and virtually complete occlusion of the right renal artery which fills late from collateral vessels. This is the typical appearance of fibromuscular dysplasia or hyperplasia.

The diagnostic approach to children, who usually have bilateral renal artery stenosis associated with FMD, is simpler than the workup in adults, who primarily have atherosclerotic lesions. Consequently, many of the noninvasive tests designed for adults with renovascular hypertension are not useful in children. For example, it was recently reported that the preoperative calculation of a high renal resistance-index value derived by Doppler ultrasonography is a predictor of the lack of success of operative correction of renal artery stenosis.[16] However, because successful revascularization in children routinely results in alleviation of hypertension, such studies are superfluous. The same is true for renal vein renin studies because renal artery stenosis in children with hypertension is always significant. On the other hand, renal vein renin studies may be useful in determining the significance of distal stenoses or aneurysms of renal artery branches or postoperative anastomotic stenoses.

Because FMD is a systemic, occlusive arteriopathy, it is necessary to survey the entire lower thoracic and abdominal aorta to delineate those patients who have not only renal artery stenosis but also the mid-aortic syndrome, visceral artery stenosis, or other forms of renovascular hypertension.[8,13,17] Thus, full angiography is needed so that an appropriate single-stage operation can be performed. It is interesting to note that hypertensive children without co-morbid conditions, who have renal artery stenosis, usually have a single, focal branch artery stenosis.[15]

TREATMENT

Medical Treatment

Antihypertensive medications are needed to control blood pressure before undertaking any invasive procedure, including arteriography. Drug therapy is not an alternative to surgical care but an integral part of patient management, not only preoperatively but also intraoperatively and postoperatively. Most patients referred for surgical or interventional treatment have severe hypertension with symptoms that are most effectively managed with intravenous drugs, gradually phasing to oral medications. In severe cases, I prefer to use nitroprusside initially. Either concurrently or sequentially, intravenous labetalol or nifedipine or both are useful drugs. The same three medications are extremely useful in the postoperative management as well, because hypertension is often exacerbated after the temporary ischemia associated with the revascularization procedures. For long-term and outpatient treatment, propranolol, atenolol, minoxidil, and oral diuretics in various combinations are useful. I prefer to use long-acting drugs whenever possible, because patient and parent compliance are better when once-daily medications are utilized. Angiotensin-converting enzyme (ACE) inhibitors such as captopril are very effective antihypertensive drugs, but they must be used with great caution in patients with renovascular hypertension because of the potential for drug-induced renal ischemia and possible oliguric renal failure.[5,18] Thus, if a decision is made to use ACE inhibitor medication, renal function must be monitored closely.

Another consideration related to the use of medical therapy is in the management of infants with severe hypertension related to renal artery stenosis. In these instances, because of the great risk for thrombosis with repair of the tiny vessels, it may be best to administer antihypertensive drugs until the renal arteries are close to adult size, if possible (ages 5 to 8 years). After revascularization, it may take up to 6 to 12 months for the hypertension to resolve or improve, so the antihypertensive drugs must be weaned gradually.

Interventional Procedures

Balloon angioplasty with and without stenting has been the subject of many reports with atherosclerotic disease as well as with FMD.[14,19] The results in patients with FMD have been more favorable in instances in which the orifice of the renal artery is not involved by the process. Balloon dilatation for orifice lesions has generally been unsuccessful, except for short periods. Experience reported in children with balloon angioplasty, which parallels my experience, indicates that balloon dilatation of orifice lesions is as ineffective as it is in adults, but it is very successful in providing long-term relief from stenosis of the main renal artery or its branches.[20,21] Nonetheless, there are a number of reports in the interventional radiology literature that promote percutaneous transluminal angioplasty (PTA) for children with all forms of renal artery stenosis, and even describe the placement of stents in very small children. Unfortunately, very few of these reports describe long-term outcomes. Tobin and colleagues have recently proposed cutting balloon angioplasty in children with resistant renal artery stenosis, although that technique may be even more risky than surgical repair.[22] In one long-term follow-up report by Shroff and coworkers, PTA and stenting in a series of 33 children with a mean age of 10 years was associated with a high rate of restenosis, one procedure-related death, and a number of complications.[19] These results are not as good as with surgical repair. McTaggart and colleagues reported that PTA was ineffective for patients with neurofibromatosis lesions of the renal artery because of the fibrotic nature of the disease.[21] Lacombe and Ricco pointed out that when patients sustain complications of PTA such as dissection, rupture, or thrombosis, surgical repair may then be difficult.[23] Because of the relatively greater degree of fibroplasia seen in children with FMD, it is not surprising that a much greater incidence of intimal dissection and thrombosis occurs in children, who most often have lesions at the ostia. Because children are growing, and because so many of these children are young, averaging 6 years of age, there is a reluctance to insert stents into these lesions after balloon dilatation for fear of inducing intimal hyperplasia or of creating obstruction as the child grows. However, dissolvable stents may possibly prove useful in the future in some pediatric patients.

In the rare instances of distal segmental renal artery lesions resulting in segmental renal infarction, interventional infusion of ethanol for ablation may be curative as an alternative to segmental resection.

Surgical Treatment

Effective surgical treatment for renovascular hypertension in children is preferable. The method selected must be based on the etiology and distribution of the lesions causing stenosis.[14,24]

Nephrectomy and partial nephrectomy should be avoided unless no other choice is available. For example, it may be necessary to perform nephrectomy in infants with uncontrollable hypertension who have unilateral renal involvement, particularly when severe hypoplasia is found. Partial nephrectomy has been used primarily in those instances of renal atrophy, with diffuse vascular involvement, or when the vessels are too small for successful reconstruction. It is my preference to attempt revascularization because partial or total nephrectomy is available as a last resort if the vascular repair fails. Additionally, because FMD may involve the opposite kidney many years later, nephrectomy is undesirable if revascularization is possible.

Although children with FMD have a predominance of ostial lesions, sufficient involvement of the renal artery and wall of the artery exists that the extent of the lesion is greater than what might be apparent on the arteriogram. Thus, patch angioplasty is only rarely effective. Reimplantation of the renal artery into another site on the aorta is the most effective approach, but its success depends on the aortic wall being normal where the new orifice is to be created and on sufficient renal artery length to reach without tension. Although autotransplantation is an alternative under these circumstances, it is more complicated because both arterial and venous anastomoses are needed. Reimplantation is contraindicated in patients with mid-aortic syndrome in which the aortic wall is involved with FMD. Also, direct anastomosis to the aorta is not an option for patients with branch vessel lesions, which must be treated with balloon dilatation, bypass, or partial nephrectomy for distally placed lesions. It is unfortunate that reimplantation is so rarely possible in this group of patients because it provides the best and most durable results.[5]

Because of the complicating factors mentioned previously, aortorenal bypass is usually the best option for revascularization. Bypass from the aorta to the side of the renal artery distal to the stenosis was often used in the past. For the past several years, it has been my preference to divide the diseased artery from the aorta and perform an end-to-end anastomosis between the bypass graft and the distal renal artery, spatulating the end of the distal renal artery and fashioning the distal end of the bypass graft obliquely, so that a so-called cobra hood anastomosis is performed. Depending on the size of the anastomosis, either a continuous suture technique, interrupted several times, or an interrupted suture technique for the anastomosis is appropriate. The anastomosis of the bypass graft to the aorta can usually be performed with continuous suture that is interrupted at least three times. The opening in the aortic wall is made with an appropriate-sized punch instrument rather than a simple incision. I prefer 6-0 polypropylene sutures for the aorta-to-graft anastomosis, whereas 7-0 polypropylene is used for the distal graft-to-renal artery anastomosis. In instances of mid-aortic syndrome in which such severe coarctation exists that an aorto-aortic bypass is needed, the renal bypass grafts may be taken off the aortic bypass graft. Depending on the size of the patient, it is my preference to use 10- to 14-mm woven Dacron grafts with enough length to permit growth and yet not so much length as to result in kinking of the graft. A full intravenous heparinizing dose is administered before aortic clamping, and a half dose is given each hour during the procedure. The heparin effect is allowed to dissipate once all the anastomoses are completed. It has rarely been necessary to reverse the heparinization.

Some debate exists regarding what is the best choice of aortorenal bypass grafts. In adults, Gore-Tex (W.L. Gore & Associates, Elkton, MD) grafts are frequently used. Paty and associates described their experience with prosthetic renal artery reconstruction in adults with a high degree of success.[25] However, thrombosis occurs more commonly in prosthetic grafts than with autogenous material. Gore-Tex grafts are rarely needed in children except when autogenous grafts have failed. There is little debate that the best choice for bypass in children is autogenous hypogastric artery, provided that it is not involved with FMD and that a sufficient length of artery can be harvested for the bypass. These two factors limit the use of the hypogastric artery, even though it clearly holds up best through the years. Additionally, because 70% of patients have simultaneous bilateral renal artery stenosis, this would require both hypogastric arteries to be harvested. Certainly some concern exists about taking both hypogastric arteries in children, although the exact risks of impotence and incontinence are not known. Because of these potential complications, the hypogastric artery is not an option for many patients. Therefore, the next best option, and the one most frequently used today for arteriorenal bypass in small patients, is the saphenous vein. Because of the risk of aneurysmal dilatation in as many as 40% of patients who have such grafts placed in the visceral location, my colleagues and I developed a procedure to cover the saphenous vein bypass grafts with a loose mandrill of Dacron mesh, which has been effective over the long term.[20,26] These techniques have been in use for more than 20 years.

Another debated issue relates to a subset of patients with mid-aortic syndrome who have varying degrees of narrowing of the superior mesenteric and celiac arteries.[8,9,27] A few scattered reports of patients with visceral artery stenosis who were initially seen with severe intermittent abdominal pain or intestinal infarction are available. However, in contrast to adults with lesions of this nature, most children are rarely symptomatic. In those rare instances in which I have encountered children with signs or symptoms related to superior mesenteric or celiac narrowing, I have performed revascularization by either direct reimplantation or bypass grafting. Currently, no consensus exists about whether asymptomatic children with marked visceral artery stenosis should have preemptive repair. Certainly, concomitant visceral artery bypass carries a high risk in a patient who is already having a bilateral renal artery bypass procedure and frequently also an aorto-aortic bypass. My group and others favor selective treatment of symptomatic patients with splanchnic artery occlusive disease.[17] Because the overwhelming majority of patients with lesions of this nature are asymptomatic, and because almost all of them have a remarkable amount of collateral circulation demonstrable on aortography, I have not undertaken visceral artery revascularization in asymptomatic patients (Fig. 65-4). Observation for as long as 30 years has indicated that these patients have remained well, supporting a conservative approach.[5]

COMPLICATIONS AND OUTCOMES

A number of long-term follow-up studies of children who have had surgical repair for renovascular hypertension and its variants report a high degree of success and durable results, with cure rates ranging from 66% to 80%, improvement rates of 18% to 22%, and only occasional failures.[5,28,29] No mortality was found in our series of over 50 renal revascularization procedures.[5] No patients developed renal failure, and those who had preoperative oliguric renal failure invariably returned to normal afterward.

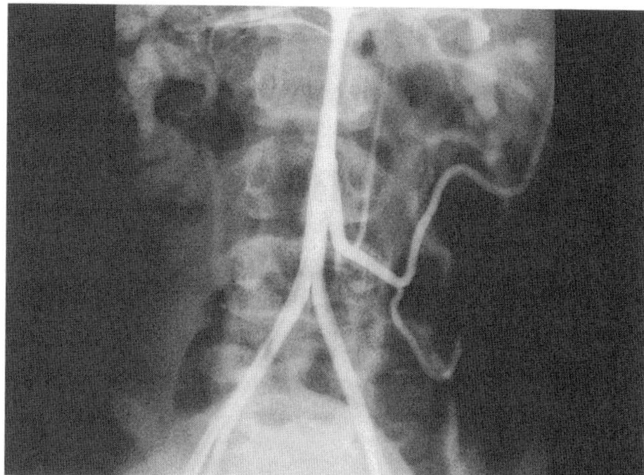

Figure 65-4. This aortogram performed on an 8-year-old boy with malignant hypertension shows the typical findings of mid-aortic syndrome or subisthmic coarctation associated with bilateral renal artery and visceral artery narrowing with collateral circulation from the inferior mesenteric artery. Aorto-aortic bypass and bilateral renal artery bypass from the aortic bypass graft were performed.

Intraoperative renal thrombosis, embolization during the procedure, and intraoperative and postoperative hemorrhage have not occurred. Postoperative graft thrombosis, because of kinking and flaws in technique, occur in fewer than 5% of renal repairs, even in small patients. However, it has always been my approach to manage patients medically, if possible, until their renal arteries are close to adult size. In those few instances in which graft thrombosis was encountered, because of the likelihood of an anastomotic problem, I have preferred immediate reoperation to the use of thrombolytic agents. Late thrombosis can occur, but the incidence is less in children than in adults because of the absence of atherosclerosis. In patients who have late thrombosis, repeat bypass grafting is preferable, but often partial or total nephrectomy is required. It is important to monitor the patient's blood pressure indefinitely in follow-up because recurrence of hypertension usually indicates a problem with the vascular reconstruction or recurrent disease. Iliorenal bypass has been used in selected high-risk patients as a remedial operation with good results.[30]

Postoperative Imaging

Recurrent hypertension after revascularization procedures is due to either recurrent FMD or an anastomotic stenosis. I have encountered two instances of late narrowing of the distal renal graft anastomosis. As with renal transplant arterial stenosis, balloon dilatation has been curative for 20 and 23 years, respectively. For follow-up of patients, it is best to have the family monitor the child's blood pressure frequently at home with at least 6-month follow-up visits initially. The patient's blood pressure should remain normal, even with exercise, although some patients may require medication to keep their blood pressure within the normal range. In the asymptomatic patient, noninvasive imaging such as CTA or MRA is suggested every 5 years, with definitive selective angiography performed if any question exists.

Even when complicated, complete revascularization can be performed at a single operation and results are excellent. Whether patients have aortorenal bypass to either one or both kidneys, or whether they also have aorto-aortic bypass procedures, 80% of children in our series have been cured of their hypertension without the need for medications and 18% are markedly improved, needing minimal antihypertensive medications.[5,8] Only about 2% of our patients are unchanged after operation. In the absence of a demonstrated vascular lesion, these patients probably have sustained hypertension because of ischemic nephrosclerosis.

section 7

NEOPLASMS

chapter 66

PRINCIPLES OF ADJUVANT THERAPY IN CHILDHOOD CANCER

Daniel von Allmen, MD • Stephan Shochat, MD

The significant improvement in cure rates for pediatric malignancies over the past 30 years could not have occurred without the development of multimodality therapy and the cooperative efforts of surgeons, pediatric oncologists, and radiation therapists across the country. In the 1940s, with the use of wide surgical excision, about 20% of children with localized solid tumors were cured of their malignancies. However, with the discovery of effective chemotherapeutic agents, pediatric oncologists joined with surgeons and radiation therapists in cooperative groups and developed a scientific approach to the study of these agents, rapidly improving on these statistics. Even in the earliest days of cancer therapy, it was the rare child who was not treated with the optimal standardized therapy, from which information was obtained and applied to the next generation of protocols. This carefully developed multimodality approach to the total care of the child with cancer led to the implementation of similar systems in the treatment of adult malignancies and has led to the fact that almost 85% of children with cancer will outlive their malignancy.[1]

HISTORY OF PEDIATRIC ONCOLOGY

The first demonstration that chemotherapy could be effective therapy for childhood malignancies occurred in 1948 when Sidney Farber[2] reported temporary remissions in children with acute lymphoblastic leukemia (ALL) when the folic acid antagonist aminopterin was given. Several years later, another folic acid antagonist, methotrexate, produced cures in choriocarcinoma.[3] As additional chemotherapeutic agents were developed, these were combined in multidrug regimens that demonstrated significantly improved response rates and response duration compared with single agents. This was first demonstrated in children with ALL and confirmed in those with Wilms' tumor.[4,5]

The treatment of Wilms' tumor also served as a model for the successful use of multimodality therapy.[6] The adjuvant use of vincristine, dactinomycin, and regional radiation therapy after surgical resection produced substantial improvements in cure rates. Similar approaches were adopted for the treatment of rhabdomyosarcoma, Ewing's sarcoma, lymphoma, and other solid tumors. The efficacy of chemotherapy in improving survival in patients with nonmetastatic osteosarcoma after surgical therapy was demonstrated in a randomized cooperative group trial. Patients who received adjuvant chemotherapy had a 66% disease-free survival, as compared with a 17% disease-free survival in the patients who received surgical intervention alone.[7] This use of "adjuvant" chemotherapy to control micrometastases has now become standard practice for most solid tumors in children.

Many advances in pediatric oncology have occurred since these early discoveries. Most of them are attributable to the continued collaboration of pediatric oncologists, surgeons, and radiation therapists within cooperative groups. With the development of improved supportive care measures, dose-intensive chemotherapy programs have been successful in improving outcome for patients with Burkitt's lymphoma, neuroblastoma, and other advanced-stage solid tumors.[8-10] Further improvements in outcome have been made by altering the schedule of chemotherapy administration, either by alternating effective groups of chemotherapeutic agents to overcome or prevent resistance,[11] or by administering agents by continuous infusion rather than bolus.[12] Most recently, noncytotoxic biologic therapies have been developed specifically to target biologic pathways. These agents include signal transduction inhibitors, various tissue growth factor receptor inhibitors, anti-angiogenesis agents, tumor-targeted antibody therapies, and adoptive immunotherapy techniques.[13] Also, improvements in radiation therapy have led to the development of intraoperative radiation therapy and radiosurgery techniques. All these advances in treatment have led to profound improvements in the quality of life and survival of children with solid tumors.

EPIDEMIOLOGY AND SURVIVAL STATISTICS FOR CHILDHOOD CANCER

When compared with the adult incidence rates of cancer, the incidence of cancer in children is very small. However, whereas childhood cancer accounts for only 2% of all reported cancer cases, it accounts for 10% of all deaths among children and is the leading cause of death from disease among children.[14]

The distribution of the types of cancer in childhood is very different from that in adults. Whereas the majority of all cancers in adults are of epithelial cell origin, fewer than 10% of childhood cancers fall into this category. Table 66-1 displays the distribution of cancer in children younger than age 15 years.[15]

The incidence rates for specific cancers vary by age, gender, and race. Overall, the annual incidence rate for all types of childhood cancer is 133.3 per million children younger than age 15 years. The peak incidence for childhood cancer is before the age of 2 years, with an incidence rate of more than 200 cases per million. The incidence then decreases to a low of 82.5 cases per million at age 9 years, at which point it begins to climb again through the adolescent years. Before age 2 years, central nervous system (CNS) malignancies, neuroblastoma, acute myeloid leukemia (AML), Wilms' tumor, and retinoblastoma account for the majority of diagnoses. Between ages 2 and 4 years, ALL is the most common childhood cancer. After age 9 years, the incidence of Hodgkin's disease, osteosarcoma, and Ewing's sarcoma begins to increase sharply.[14]

According to the Surveillance, Epidemiology, and End Results (SEER) program, the average annual incidence of childhood cancer increased 10.8% between reporting year 1973-74 and 1989-90[16] but has been fairly stable for the last decade. The change in reported incidence may be accounted for by improved reporting of cancer cases, improved identification and diagnosis of

Table 66-1 Distribution of Cancer in Children Younger than Age 15 Years

Type of Cancer	Distribution (%)
Acute lymphoblastic leukemia	23.2
Central nervous system tumors	20.7
Neuroblastoma	7.3
Non-Hodgkin's lymphoma	6.3
Wilms' tumor	6.1
Hodgkin's disease	5.0
Acute myeloid leukemia	4.2
Rhabdomyosarcoma	3.4
Retinoblastoma	2.9
Osteosarcoma	2.6
Ewing's sarcoma	2.1
All other cancers	16.4

(Data from Gurney J G. Severson R K, Davis S, et al: Incidence of cancer in children in the United States. Cancer 75:2186-2195, 1995.)

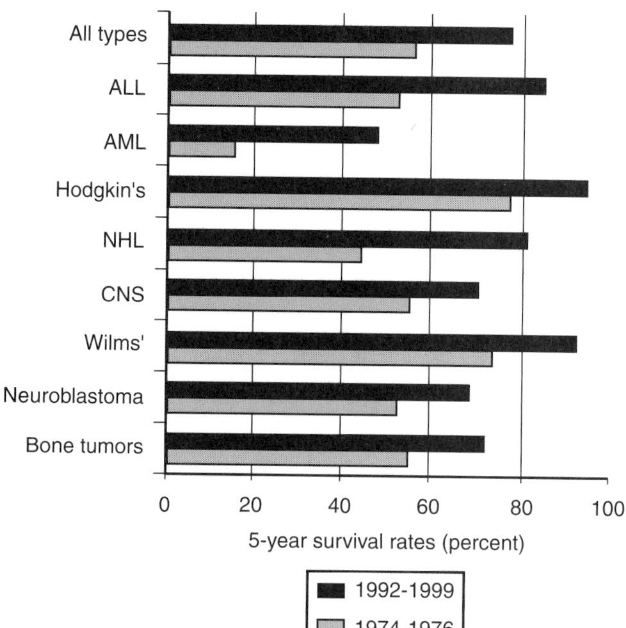

Figure 66-1. Comparison of patient survival during the period 1974 to 1976 versus 1992 to 1999 for the common childhood malignancies. (Data from SEER Cancer Statistics Review 1975-2000. Bethesda, MD, NCI, 2003. Available at http://seer.cancer.gov/csr/1975_2000.)

cancer, or a random fluctuation in the number of cases for the years studied.[17] Concern has been raised regarding the impact of environmental exposures resulting in increased cancer cases, but studies to date have not provided conclusive evidence for this assumption.

Survival from childhood cancer has improved so much over the past 30 years that the overall cure rate for childhood cancer is approaching 85%.[18] One in every 900 people between the ages of 16 and 44 years is a survivor of childhood cancer.[1] There has been a near 40% decline in mortality from childhood cancer between 1975 and 1995.[19] Figure 66-1 compares the survival statistics for specific cancers from 1974 through 1999.[20]

IMPORTANCE OF PATHOLOGY OF CHILDHOOD TUMORS IN SELECTING CHEMOTHERAPY

Unlike adult malignancies, which are primarily carcinomas, fewer than 10% of solid tumors of childhood are epithelial malignancies.[16] Although the spectrum of malignancies in childhood is more limited than in adults, the exact diagnosis is often more difficult because of the prevalence of "small round blue cell" tumors in childhood. These very primitive or embryonal malignancies often lack morphologically distinguishing characteristics. As a result, Ewing's sarcoma, neuroblastoma, lymphoma, small cell osteosarcoma, and primitive neuroectodermal tumors may appear quite similar by light microscopy. An error in diagnosis of Ewing's sarcoma in a patient who actually has a lymphoma of bone would lead to vastly different therapy and a poor outcome.

The exact diagnosis in pediatric cancer patients is crucial because chemotherapy for childhood malignancies is carefully tailored to each specific tumor type. This has become even more important over the past 2 decades as pediatric oncologists have continued to define better the prognostic subgroups for many tumors that help dictate the best therapy and the dose intensity of the therapy required for cure. Whereas the survival rate for patients with stages 1 to 3 Wilms' tumor with favorable histology is more than 90%[21] with standard therapy consisting of vincristine and actinomycin, with or without doxorubicin, a diagnosis of a Wilms' tumor with diffuse anaplasia carries a far worse prognosis and requires more intensive therapy for cure.

The initial step in the accurate diagnosis of a tumor is the availability of adequate material with which to make the diagnosis. Therefore, it is crucial that during the initial surgical procedure, whether it is a biopsy or resection, an adequate quantity and quality of tissue is obtained. The amount of tissue required for diagnostic purposes should be discussed with the surgeon, the pathologist, and pediatric oncologist before the procedure to ensure the proper handling of the specimen (e.g., the need for fresh tissue, frozen samples, and fixed specimens for histologic and biologic diagnostic use). Whereas light microscopy remains the primary tool of pathologists, they can now rely also on immunohistology, electron microscopy, DNA content of tumor, cytogenetic abnormalities, and specific tumor gene expression to establish a diagnosis.

TUMOR BIOLOGY: UNDERSTANDING CHILDHOOD CANCER AND TREATMENT PRINCIPLES

Cancer is a genetic event. Genetic alterations within a single cell, those that can be identified as a cytogenetic abnormality, the activation of an oncogene, or the loss of a tumor-suppressor gene can all lead to the accumulation of cells lacking the ability to respond to growth-regulating signals and the subsequent development of cancer.

Understanding normal cell growth and regulation is a prerequisite to understanding both the genetic basis for the development of childhood cancer and the mechanisms of action of chemotherapeutic agents designed to kill rapidly proliferating cancer cells. Normal cell growth occurs by the regulated progression of the cell through the cell cycle of DNA replication and mitosis, separated by two intervening growth phases called G_1 and G_2. Cells can temporarily leave the cell cycle and enter a resting state called G_0 (Fig. 66-2). Cells are instructed to proceed through the cell cycle by a series of external and internal stimuli. Binding of proteins (growth factors) to cell-surface receptors stimulates a cascade of cytoplasmic signaling proteins (membrane kinases and signal transducers) that carries the stimuli to the nucleus. Other proteins (transcription factors) then bind to the DNA, resulting in the expression of growth-regulating genes. When functioning normally, these genes promote or prevent cell division, direct the

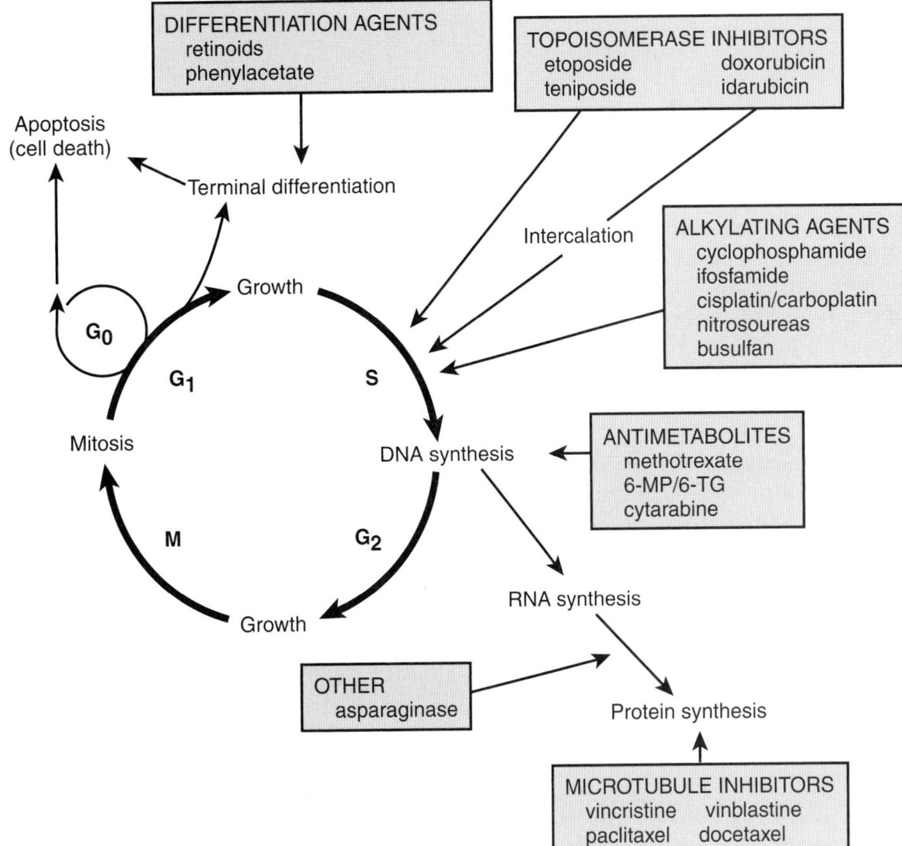

Figure 66-2. The cell cycle. Normal cell growth proceeds through DNA replication (S) and mitosis (M), separated by two growth phases (G_1 and G_2). Cells leave the cell cycle to enter a resting phase (G_0) to differentiate or to die. Chemotherapy agents act at specific sites along the cell cycle, as indicated. (Adapted from Balis FRM, Holcenberg JS, Poplack DG: General principles of chemotherapy. In Pizzo P, Poplack D [eds]: Principles and Practice of Pediatric Oncology, 3rd ed. Philadelphia, Lippincott-Raven, 1997, p 219.)

cell to differentiate, or initiate apoptosis, the process of programmed cell death.

Alterations in one or several of these signaling proteins can lead to the unregulated cell growth characteristics of cancer cells. Oncogenes result from mutation or overexpression of the normal growth-promoting proto-oncogenes. Tumor suppressor genes are normally present in cells and function as negative regulators to slow the process of proliferation and allow time for cellular repair. When oncogenes become activated or tumor suppressor gene function is lost, cells lose their ability to respond to the usual regulatory protein stimuli and proliferate rapidly. Rapid cell proliferation leads to accumulation of more genetic defects, activation of additional oncogenes, and loss of more negative regulators as the cells become increasingly more malignant. Through the study of chromosomal aberrations, more than 100 oncogenes and 25 tumor suppressor genes have now been identified.

CANCER CYTOGENETICS: A DIAGNOSTIC TOOL

The association of a consistent chromosomal aberration with a specific cancer was first made in 1960 with the discovery of the minute "Philadelphia chromosome" (9;22)(q34;q11) in chronic myeloid leukemia (CML).[22] With the discovery of chromosomal banding techniques in the 1970s, cancer cytogeneticists were first able to identify subchromosomal deletions, inversions, and translocations occurring in cancer cells. Study of these aberrant regions led to the identification of oncogenes and tumor suppressor genes, a process that is continuing today.

The presence of consistent cytogenetic abnormalities associated with a specific childhood leukemia or solid tumor helps in both cancer diagnosis and assignment of prognosis. Specific cytogenetic aberrations have been identified in rhabdomyosarcoma, Ewing's sarcoma, synovial sarcoma, germ cell tumors, medulloblastomas, neuroblastomas, retinoblastomas, and Wilms' tumors.[23] Chromosomal aberrations also can help predict prognosis. The finding of a chromosome 1q deletion, the presence of double minute chromatin bodies, or the presence of homogeneous staining regions in neuroblastoma confers a poor prognosis.[24]

The treatment of Wilms' tumor based on risk stratification determined by multiple tumor characteristics that impact prognosis, including loss of heterozygosity at 1p and 16q, is now being studied in the cooperative group setting. The process of using specific translocations for diagnostic purposes is enhanced by the use of the techniques of fluorescent in situ hybridization, which allows the localization and visualization of a single gene on a chromosome by using fluorescent DNA probes. Unlike standard cytogenetic analysis, which requires 5 to 14 days for the cancer cells to proliferate in culture before a karyotype can be obtained, this technique can be performed directly on tumor cells.[25] In the future, specific tumors may be identified by a specific "fingerprint" determined by microarray analysis that can simultaneously analyze expression of thousands of genes on a single "chip."[26] The ability to tailor therapy to individual patients based on the genetic characteristics of their particular tumor is quickly becoming a reality.

CHEMOTHERAPY PRINCIPLES IN PEDIATRIC ONCOLOGY

The goal of cytotoxic chemotherapy treatment for childhood malignancy is to maximize tumor kill while maintaining acceptable side effects. Clinical trials have led to the development of standard combination chemotherapy regimens for most childhood cancers. Adjuvant therapy (after local control measures) has remained the mainstay of cancer therapy, but neoadjuvant chemotherapy (before definitive local control measures) has proved to be effective in patients with metastatic disease and, in localized tumors, to begin to control microscopic metastatic disease immediately.

In the clinical development of promising anticancer agents, the first step is to define a tolerable dose. Phase I clinical trials are designed as dose-escalation studies to determine the maximally tolerated dose of a new drug given as a single agent. The dose of the agent is slowly increased in successive cohorts of patients until dose-limiting toxicity is consistently observed. The dose level immediately lower than the dose resulting in consistent toxicity is then selected to begin phase II trials. In a phase II trial, a consistent dose of the agent is tested for efficacy in a variety of tumor types to establish the spectrum of activity of the agent. Once an agent has demonstrated activity in a specific cancer, this agent is tested for efficacy when combined with other known active agents in that tumor system.

"Standard" therapy for a specific tumor type is established through phase III clinical trials. Classically, phase III trials use a prospective randomized design to compare two previously established effective chemotherapy combinations. At the conclusion of the trial, the chemotherapy regimen with the greatest efficacy and the least toxicity is selected as the standard regimen for that tumor system. Subsequent phase III trials then compare new regimens with this established standard therapy. It is through the development of phase I through III clinical trials within national cooperative groups that advances in cancer treatment are made.

Combination chemotherapy remains the mainstay of treatment of childhood cancer. In the 1960s, the benefit of combining several drugs together was demonstrated first for ALL. Complete remission by using single agents could be expected in only about half of the patients, whereas the combination of four or five drugs produced remission rates of more than 95%.[27]

Several biologic models have been devised to attempt to explain this observation. The most well known is the Goldie-Coldman hypothesis, which proposes that the response of any individual tumor to a chemotherapeutic agent is dependent on both the sensitivity of that tumor to the agent and the inherent tendency of that tumor to accumulate mutations that will make it chemotherapy resistant. This hypothesis predicts that once a single tumor cell develops resistance to a chemotherapeutic agent, the tumor cannot be cured using that agent alone. Therefore, the best chance to cure a tumor is to give all available active agents simultaneously, after local control measures, when the tumor burden is as low as possible and the chance of any tumor cells having acquired resistance is minimal.[28]

This principle of designing combination chemotherapy regimens by using non–cross-resistant agents with nonoverlapping toxicities has been successfully used for childhood solid tumor treatment for the past 25 years. The improvement in survival rates over this period for neuroblastoma, Ewing's sarcoma, anaplastic Wilms' tumor, and osteosarcoma can be directly linked to effective combination chemotherapy treatment.

ADJUVANT AND NEOADJUVANT CHEMOTHERAPY

The use of adjuvant chemotherapy is supported by the finding that fewer than 20% of sarcoma and lymphoma patients with initially nonmetastatic solid tumors can be cured by surgical therapy or radiation therapy alone (or even combined).[29] In the majority of these patients, recurrence is at a distant site, lending strong support to the hypothesis that micrometastatic disease exists at the time of presentation for the majority of patients with clinical nonmetastatic disease. In Wilms' tumor, as many as 40% of patients can be cured with surgical therapy or radiation therapy alone. However, survival can be increased to 90% with the addition of adjuvant combination chemotherapy.[30]

Because the goal of adjuvant chemotherapy is to prevent the appearance of metastatic disease, it is vital that chemotherapy begin as soon as possible after local control measures are completed. For this reason, most current chemotherapy regimens for childhood solid tumors recommend that chemotherapy is given within 2 weeks of initial surgical treatment.[31] In Wilms' tumor, assessment of tumor biology and risk stratification must be made by postoperative day 14 for inclusion in ongoing Children's Oncology Group studies. One approach to prevent delays in instituting chemotherapy in patients with nonmetastatic disease is to delay surgical resection until after several courses of chemotherapy can be administered. This is referred to as neoadjuvant chemotherapy, in which only a biopsy of the tumor is performed for diagnosis. Therefore, chemotherapy can begin as soon as the diagnosis is established at a time when the distant tumor burden is at its lowest. This approach has become standard in the treatment of Ewing's sarcoma and osteosarcoma and has the theoretical advantage of minimizing the appearance of chemotherapy resistance.[11,32,33] Furthermore, delayed surgical intervention may allow a more complete or less morbid resection and pathologic assessment of tumor responsiveness to the chemotherapy agents on an individual patient basis. For example, diagnostic biopsy followed by neoadjuvant chemotherapy and delayed resection of the primary tumor for complex neuroblastoma reduces the operative complication rate without compromising survival.[34] Treating the tumors on the front end with chemotherapy reduced intraoperative blood loss and the need for nephrectomy. However, neoadjuvant chemotherapy is beneficial only for tumors for which a known highly effective combination chemotherapy program limits the risk of tumor progression at the primary site.

SCHEDULE OF ADMINISTRATION

Children often tolerate chemotherapy better than adults because they have a superior and more rapid recovery from the toxic effects of treatment. Standard pediatric solid tumor chemotherapy protocols call for the administration of chemotherapy courses every 21 days to allow time for hematologic and organ recovery. Most combination chemotherapy programs are given over the first 1 to 5 days of the 21-day cycle. Historically, the next course of chemotherapy was withheld until the absolute neutrophil count was greater than $1000/mm^3$ and the platelet count was greater than $100,000/mm^3$. The recent trend has been to maximize dose intensity and begin the next course when the absolute neutrophil count is greater than $750/mm^3$ and the platelet count greater than $75,000/mm^3$, as long as mucositis or diarrhea (or both) induced by the chemotherapy has resolved. When these criteria are adhered to, the toxic death rate for standard combination chemotherapy programs is less than 5%.

Recently, changes in schedule of chemotherapy administration have led to improved efficacy of some agents. Etoposide is an epipodophyllotoxin that has been extremely effective in most pediatric solid tumors and in some epithelial cancers in adults.[35,36] The mechanism of action is inhibition of topoisomerase II. Classically, etoposide has been given with an alkylator and infused over a 1-hour period. However, it has been demonstrated that continuous intravenous exposure to etoposide for 3 to 21 days is superior to a 1- to 24-hour infusion.[37,39] In pediatric brain tumor patients, daily oral etoposide for 21 days was well tolerated and produced significant responses in patients with recurrent tumors.[37] Continuous exposure to etoposide has the theoretical advantage of maintaining a continuous blockage of topoisomerase II and thus preventing tumor cell repair, ultimately leading to more effective tumor kill. Similarly, prolonged exposure to combination chemotherapy agents in neuroblastoma and AML has led to improved responses.[38,39]

The duration of chemotherapy programs for most pediatric solid tumors has classically been 1 year. As the dose intensity of chemotherapy programs has increased, the duration of therapy has decreased. The National Wilms' Tumor Study IV demonstrated that 6 months of therapy was as effective as and could be administered at a lower total treatment cost compared with 15 months for patients with high-stage disease.[21] In neuroblastoma, when intensive induction therapy is followed by consolidation with autologous stem cell transplant, the total duration of treatment is now 6 months.[40] As dose intensity of therapy increases, duration of chemotherapy may continue to decrease.

CHEMOTHERAPY DOSE INTENSITY

To develop an effective combination chemotherapy program, it is important to select not only the correct combination of agents but also the correct dose of each agent. The trend for the past 10 years in pediatric oncology has been to increase chemotherapy dose intensity, with the goal of maximizing efficacy. In designing dose-intensive programs, the individual toxicities of the agents to be intensified must be considered. The best agents to use in high doses are those with limited organ toxicity and whose toxicity profile is mainly hematologic.

Most chemotherapeutic agents have a sigmoidal dose-response curve with a steep linear phase followed by a plateau phase. The principle of chemotherapy dose intensity is to administer the maximal tolerated dose of the agent that falls within the linear phase of the dose-response curve in the shortest possible interval while maintaining tolerable toxicity.[41,42] Dose intensity is defined as the amount of drug delivered per unit time, expressed as milligrams per square meter per week.[43] Therefore, dose intensity can be increased by giving higher doses of a chemotherapeutic agent, giving the agent more frequently, or both.

It has been demonstrated in animal systems that a 2-fold increase in administered cyclophosphamide dose can lead to a 10-fold increase in tumor cell kill,[44] whereas a decrease in dose intensity of as little as 20% in an osteosarcoma animal model can decrease the cure rate by 50%.[45] Similar clinical observations have been made in childhood leukemia and osteosarcoma. A prospective clinical trial of high-risk ALL patients revealed that patients receiving less than 94% of the planned dose of chemotherapy during the intensive portion of therapy had a 5.5-fold increased risk of relapse.[44] In osteosarcoma, patients receiving less than 80% of the proposed chemotherapy doses had a 3-fold increased risk of relapse.[45]

The positive impact of increasing the dose intensity on improving the response rate and survival duration has been demonstrated for Burkitt's lymphoma, osteosarcoma, Ewing's sarcoma, testicular cancer, breast cancer, and advanced ovarian cancer.[8-10,41,46-48] This finding has had a significant impact on the design of clinical trials for childhood solid tumors. Efforts have focused on identifying the most effective agents to intensify and then maximizing the supportive care to allow dose escalation.

Increasing the dose intensity of active chemotherapy agents in pediatric clinical trials has been possible because of recent advances in supportive care to decrease or minimize the toxic effects on normal tissues that occur from higher-dose chemotherapy. The use of cytokines to speed recovery of white blood cells and platelets (granulocyte colony-stimulating factor [G-CSF] and interleukin-11 [IL-11])[49,50] and the use of cardioprotectant agents to allow a higher cumulative dose of doxorubicin to be used have helped in the development of new dose-intensive therapy for solid tumors.[51]

Many pediatric studies have demonstrated that collection of peripheral blood progenitor cells (PBPCs) from children as small as 10 kg is feasible.[52] The infusion of PBPCs has been effective in engrafting pediatric patients after myeloablative chemoradiotherapy.[53,54] In myeloablative therapy, "supralethal" doses of chemotherapy are given and hematopoietic recovery will occur only if a stem cell source (either PBPCs or bone marrow) is infused into the patient after completion of the myeloablative regimen. PBPCs also are effective in enhancing recovery after sub-myeloablative chemotherapy.[55,56] In sub-myeloablative regimens, hematopoietic recovery usually occurs in 3 to 4 weeks when combined with growth factor or PBPC support but would ultimately occur without this support in 6 to 10 weeks. The feasibility of repetitive collection, storage, and infusion of PBPCs for use with multiple-cycle dose-intensive chemotherapy in newly diagnosed neuroblastoma patients has been demonstrated in a Children's Cancer Group study.[57]

Myeloablative chemotherapy with total body irradiation as preparation for autologous stem cell transplant has been demonstrated to be an effective method of dose-intensive consolidation treatment after induction therapy in high-risk neuroblastoma. In a randomized Children's Oncology Group trial, high-risk neuroblastoma patients who received an autologous bone marrow transplant had an improved 3-year event-free survival compared with patients who proceeded to consolidation chemotherapy alone.[58] Given the success of increasing chemotherapy dose intensity by using a single myeloablative transplant in high-risk neuroblastoma, several investigators have performed pilot studies looking at the feasibility of performing two or even three consolidative stem cell transplants.[59,60]

CHEMOTHERAPEUTIC AGENTS

The rational design of combination chemotherapy programs requires an understanding of the mechanism of action, the site of metabolism, the rate of drug clearance, and the toxicity profile for each drug. Most chemotherapy agents work by interfering with DNA or RNA synthesis, transcription, or repair. Unfortunately, these agents are not selective for cancer cells. The same metabolic pathways are disrupted in normal cells, leading to the toxic effects observed with chemotherapy treatment.

It is important to understand the normal cell cycle to understand how each chemotherapy agent interferes with the normal cell growth and repair processes. A normal cell proceeds through the four phases of the cell cycle in an orderly fashion. Checkpoints are in place to slow growth and allow needed repairs to prevent the accumulation of DNA or RNA errors. Malignant cells are usually lacking in some or most of these checkpoints. As a result, these cells may be more susceptible to the toxic effects of chemotherapeutic agents. Figure 66-2 illustrates the normal cell cycle and indicates the site of action of the major chemotherapeutic agents.

Chemotherapy agents can be divided into classes by their mechanism of action. The classes of agents include alkylating agents (cisplatin and its analogs) antimetabolites, topoisomerase inhibitors, antimicrotubule agents, differentiation agents, miscellaneous nonclassified agents, and biologic agents. Understanding the individual mechanisms of action helps in the design of drug combinations with additive or synergistic antitumor effects. The most common agents from each class, their mechanism of action, common side effects, and tumors in which they are active are listed in Table 66-2.

Acute Chemotherapy Toxicity and Supportive Care

Most acute toxicities in childhood solid tumor therapy are reversible. Toxicity is greatest in the normal cells with the highest rate of turnover. Therefore, normal bone marrow cells, mucosal lining cells, liver cells, and hair cells are frequently affected. The most common side effects from combination chemotherapy include nausea and vomiting, myelosuppression, hair loss, mucositis, diarrhea, liver function test abnormalities, and allergic reactions.

Myelosuppression is an expected side effect of almost every treatment program for childhood solid tumors. Transfusions of packed cells and platelets are frequent. Of greatest concern is the risk of severe life-threatening bacterial or fungal infections that occur during episodes of neutropenia. In dose-intensive regimens, more than 75% of chemotherapy courses result in hospitalization for fever, with the incidence of bacteremia ranging from 10% to 20% per course.[61]

Several chemotherapeutic agents have very specific toxicities. For example, vincristine and doxorubicin are vesicants and can cause severe skin and tissue necrosis if the drug extravasates into the subcutaneous tissue. Doxorubicin and related anthracyclines have cumulative cardiotoxic effects. The total lifetime anthracycline dose must be limited for each patient to minimize the risk of developing congestive heart failure. Cisplatin has toxic renal effects and is often combined with another nephrotoxic agent, ifosfamide, in treatment of osteosarcoma and neuroblastoma. Cisplatin also can cause hearing loss, especially in high doses. Vincristine and vinblastine can cause cumulative peripheral neuropathies, and drug doses frequently must be altered to prevent significant morbidity. These toxicities must be considered when designing therapeutic programs.

Some of the success in improving outcome for children with cancer is attributable to advances made in supportive care. Routine use of hematopoietic growth factors, specifically G-CSF, results in more rapid granulocyte recovery and shorter hospitalizations for fever and neutropenia.[49] IL-11 enhances platelet recovery, decreases the depth of the platelet nadir, and decreases platelet transfusions requirements.[50,62,63] It has been well tolerated in children and is very beneficial in combination regimens that induce severe thrombocytopenia.[64,65]

The gastrointestinal tract is injured by certain chemotherapy agents, specifically cytarabine, anthracyclines, and high-dose methotrexate. Leukovorin, a folate derivative, can be given to "rescue" normal mucosal and bone marrow cells from the effects of high-dose methotrexate. No rescue is known for the mucositis and diarrhea that occur with other agents. Use of IL-11, in addition to enhancing platelet production, may help speed recovery from gastrointestinal injury after chemotherapy.[66]

Renal toxicity can occur from the use of cisplatin, ifosfamide, and high-dose methotrexate. Cisplatin causes renal tubular damage, leading to elevation of levels of blood urea nitrogen and creatinine. Often this is reversible. Both ifosfamide and cisplatin cause renal electrolyte wasting, called Fanconi's syndrome, in which hypokalemia, hypocalcemia, hypophosphatemia, and hypomagnesemia can occur. Renal injury from these agents can be improved by hyperhydration and forced diuresis. Ongoing studies with the organic thiophosphate compound amifostine show promise in preventing cisplatin-induced renal injury. Amifostine also may have protective effects against neurologic and cumulative bone marrow toxicities.[67] Mesna can prevent hemorrhagic cystitis resulting from cyclophosphamide and ifosfamide by binding to the bladder-toxic acrolein metabolites.[64]

It is anticipated that supportive care measures will continue to improve. In the future, some of the toxic effects of chemotherapy on bone marrow may be ameliorated by the use of gene therapy to transfer chemotherapy resistance genes into normal hematopoietic progenitor cells. This would allow higher doses of chemotherapy to be given without myelosuppression. Preliminary in vitro and animal studies have shown that hematopoietic progenitor cells can be made more resistant to nitrosoureas.[65]

LONG-TERM SIDE EFFECTS OF CANCER THERAPY IN CHILDREN

In light of the fact that 1 of every 900 adults will soon be a survivor of childhood cancer,[1] emphasis on diagnosis, treatment, and prevention of late effects of childhood cancer therapy has become essential.

In general, tissues with the highest cell-turnover rate are the most susceptible to acute toxicities of chemotherapy. Tissues that replicate slowly or that can no longer regenerate may be susceptible to long-term or late effects of therapy. Children are more susceptible to certain late effects of therapy than are adults because their tissues are still growing. Damage to these tissues may affect growth, fertility, and neuropsychological development.

All aspects of combined-modality treatment can contribute to the late effects of childhood cancer therapy. Chemotherapy agents have been associated with specific late toxicities (see Table 66-2). Radiation

Table 66-2 Chemotherapeutic Agents

Class of Agent	Mechanism of Action	Antitumor Activity	Acute Toxicities
Alkylating Agents			
MUSTARDS			
Nitrogen mustard	Alkylation, DNA crosslinking	Hodgkin's disease	Myelo, N/V, A, mucositis, phlebitis, vesicant
Melphalan	Alkylation, DNA crosslinking	Rhabdo; for BMT: Ewing's, NB	Myelo, mucositis, N/V, A, VOD (HD)
Cyclophosphamide	(Prodrug) alkylation, DNA crosslinking	Rhabdo; Wilms'; NB; Ewing's	Myelo, immuno, N/V, A, cystitis, SIADH, cardiac (HD), lung (HD), VOD (HD)
Ifosfamide	Alkylation, DNA crosslinking	Ewing's; rhabdo; osteosarcoma; NB	Myelo, N/V, A, hepatic, renal, cystitis, neuro
Busulfan	Alkylation, DNA crosslinking	Leukemia	Myelo, skin, lung, A
NITROSOUREAS			
BCNU	DNA crosslinking	CNS tumors; lymphoma	Myelo, N/V, A, lung, renal
CCNU	DNA crosslinking	CNS tumors; lymphoma	Myelo, N/V, A, lung, renal
TETRAZINES			
Dacarbazine (DTIC)	DNA methylation	Hodgkin's; sarcomas; NB	Myelo, hepatic, flulike illness, N/V, A
Temozolomide	DNA crosslinking	Brain tumors	Myelo, N/V, diarrhea, constipation, rash, lethargy, hepatic
OTHER ALKYLATORS			
Thiotepa	Alkylation, DNA crosslinking	CNS tumors; for BMT: sarcomas, NB	Myelo, N/V, A, diarrhea, mucositis, skin, VOD (HD)
Procarbazine	(Prodrug) methylation; free radical formation	Hodgkin's; CNS tumors	Myelo, N/V, rash, allergy, mucositis
PLATINUM AGENTS			
Cisplatin	DNA/platinum adduct formation; DNA crosslinking	Osteosarcoma; NB; hepatoblastoma; germ cell tumors; CNS tumors	N/V (severe), A, myelo, renal, neuro, mucositis, ototoxicity
Carboplatin	DNA/platinum adduct formation; DNA crosslinking	NB; CNS tumors; retinoblastoma; sarcomas in HD	Myelo, N/V (mild), renal and ototoxicity rare
Antimetabolites			
Methotrexate	Inhibitor of dihydrofolate reductase; interferes with folate metabolism	Leukemia; lymphoma; osteosarcoma in HD	Myelo, rash, mucositis, hepatic, renal (HD)
5-Fluorouracil	(Prodrug) inhibits thymidine synthesis	Hepatoblastoma; carcinomas	Myelo, N/V, mucositis, diarrhea, hyperpigmentation, neuro
Cytarabine	(Prodrug) incorporated into DNA; inhibits DNA replication	Leukemia; lymphoma	Myelo, malaise, N/V, mucositis, diarrhea, neuro (HD), eye (HD), skin (HD)
6-Mercaptopurine, 6-Thioguanine	(Prodrugs) inhibit purine synthesis	Leukemia	Myelo, N/V, hepatic, mucositis
Gemcitabine	Inhibitor of DNA synthesis	Hodgkin's disease, in phase II testing in leukemia	Myelo, rash, fluid retention, hepatic, N/V
Topoisomerase Inhibitors			
EPIPODOPHYLLOTOXINS			
Etoposide	Non–DNA-binding topoisomerase II inhibitor; stabilizes DNA double-strand breaks	NB; Ewing's; rhabdo; germ cell; leukemia; CNS tumors; lymphoma	Myelo, N/V, rash, allergy, low BP, A, mucositis, hepatic (HD)
Tenoposide	Same as etoposide	NB; leukemia	Myelo, N/V, rash, allergy, low BP, A, mucositis, hepatic (HD)

Table 66-2 Chemotherapeutic Agents—cont'd

Class of Agent	Mechanism of Action	Antitumor Activity	Acute Toxicities
ANTHRACYCLINES			
Doxorubicin	DNA intercalation; free radical formation; topoisomerase II inhibitor	Wilms'; Ewing's; NB; lymphoma; leukemia	Myelo, N/V, A, mucositis, diarrhea, phlebitis, vesicant, hepatic, cardiac
Daunorubicin	Same as doxorubicin	Leukemia; lymphoma	Myelo, N/V, A, mucositis, diarrhea, phlebitis, vesicant, hepatic, cardiac
Dactinomycin	Same as doxorubicin	Wilms'; rhabdo; Ewing's	Myelo, N/V, A, mucositis, hepatic, vesicant
Bleomycin	DNA intercalation; free radical formation	Germ cell; Hodgkin's; lymphoma	Myelo, skin, allergy, mucositis, lung
CAMPTOTHECIN ANALOGS			
Topotecan	Topoisomerase I inhibitor	Rhabdo, neuroblastoma	Myelo, N/V, A, mucositis, diarrhea, hepatic
Irinotecan	Topoisomerase I inhibitor	In phase II testing in rhabdo	Diarrhea, myelo, N/V, hepatic
Antimicrotubule Agents			
VINCA ALKALOIDS			
Vincristine	Binds tubulin; prevents microtubule formation; blocks mitosis	Sarcomas; leukemia; Hodgkin's; constipation, neuro, vesicant, Wilms'; lymphoma;	SIADH
Vinblastine	Same as vincristine	Hodgkin's; germ cell	Myelo, mucositis, vesicant
TAXANES			
Paclitaxel (Taxol)	Binds microtubules; blocks microtubule depolymerization; blocks mitosis	Ovarian carcinoma	Myelo, A, mucositis, paresthesias, hypersensitivity
Docetaxel (Taxotere)	Same as paclitaxel	In phase II testing in sarcomas and other solid tumors	Myelo, A, skin, hypersensitivity, fluid retention, paresthesias, mucositis
Differentiation Agents			
RETINOIDS			
Cis-retinoic acid	Binds to retinoic acid receptor; induces differentiation	NB	Skin, mucositis, eye, pseudotumor, hepatic, electrolyte
All-*trans*-retinoic acid	Same as *cis*-retinoic acid	APML; in phase II testing in Wilms'; NB	Skin, mucositis, eye, pseudotumor, hepatic, electrolyte
Fenretinide	Still being investigated; induces cell death, not differentiation	Phase II testing in NB	Dry skin/lips, loss of night vision, increased triglycerides, hepatic, N/V
Miscellaneous Nonclassified			
Corticosteroids	Lympholysis; multiple other effects not well classified	Leukemia (ALL); lymphoma	Weight gain, high BP, high glucose, mood change, many others
L-Asparaginase, PEG-asparaginase	Asparagine depletion; inhibition of protein synthesis	Leukemia (ALL); lymphoma	Anorexia, hepatic, pancreatitis, coagulopathy, neuro

ALL, acute lymphoblastic leukemia; PEG, polyethylene glycol; rhabdo, rhabdomyosarcoma; BMT, bone marrow transplant; NB, neuroblastoma; CNS tumors, central nervous system tumors; HD, high dose; A, alopecia; myelo, myelosuppression; N/V, nausea and vomiting; VOD, veno-occlusive disease; neuro, neurologic toxicity; SIADH, syndrome of inappropriate antidiuretic hormone; BP, blood pressure; IT, intrathecal; APML, acute promyelocytic leukemia.

Data from Balis FM, Holcenberg JS, Poplack DG: General principles of chemotherapy. In Pizzo P, Poplack D (eds): Principles and Practice of Pediatric Oncology, 3rd ed. Philadelphia, Lippincott-Raven, 1997, pp 215-272; Ratain M, Teicher B, O'Dwyer P, et al: Pharmacology of cancer chemotherapy. In DeVita V, Hellman S, Rosenberg S (eds): Cancer: Principles and Practice of Oncology. Philadelphia, Lippincott-Raven, 1997, pp 375-385; Dorr R, Von Hoff D: Drug monographs. In Dorr R, Von Hoff D (eds): Cancer Chemotherapy Handbook. Norwalk, CT, Appleton & Lange, 1994, p 129.

therapy can significantly inhibit further growth of bone, muscle, heart, and kidney within the radiation field and also affect fertility.

Growth retardation is the late effect unique to children. The degree of impairment depends on the dose of chemotherapy or radiation and the age of the child at the time of therapy. The younger the child at the time of the insult, the more severe the sequelae. More than 50% of childhood brain tumor patients treated with 3000 cGy or more to the whole brain will have severe growth retardation, with adult height being less than the fifth percentile.[68] Cranial irradiation can lead to growth hormone deficiency, which will result in poor linear growth unless growth hormone replacement is given. Patients who have received total-body radiation or spinal radiation may not be able to achieve their full height potential because the irradiated bones have limited growth potential, even with growth hormone stimulation.[69]

In addition to poor overall growth, adjuvant therapy can cause other musculoskeletal problems, including scoliosis, avascular necrosis, osteoporosis, and atrophy or hypoplasia of tissues. Radiation therapy to the head and neck results in hypoplasia of the jaw, orbit, or neck, with associated atrophy of the soft tissues. Associated endocrine, dental, and psychological consequences also may occur.[70] Aseptic necrosis of bone may affect as many as 10% of high-risk patients with ALL as a result of prolonged use of corticosteroids. Osteoporosis occurs as a result of corticosteroid treatment and from high-dose irradiation, as used for sarcoma therapy.

Most children who receive chemotherapy for solid tumors do not experience neuropsychological dysfunction. However, patients treated for brain tumors and those receiving cranial radiation for ALL are the exception and can experience a severe decline in IQ.[71,72]

Specific organs are often affected by chemotherapy. Heart, liver, lung, thyroid, and gonadal function can be impaired. Gonadal dysfunction (azoospermia, amenorrhea) frequently results from alkylator treatment. Therapy with mechlorethamine, vincristine, prednisone, and procarbazine has resulted in azoospermia in 80% to 100% of all male patients.[73] Combination chemotherapy programs for childhood Hodgkin's disease have been adjusted to replace mechlorethamine with cyclophosphamide and eliminate dacarbazine from standard treatments to attempt to decrease the infertility risk. It should be noted that the children of childhood cancer survivors are not at an increased risk for congenital anomalies.[74]

Cardiotoxicity from anthracycline antibiotics has been a problem in the treatment of Ewing's sarcoma, osteosarcoma, and lymphomas. Use of continuous-infusion anthracycline can decrease the risk of cardiac muscle damage and subsequent congestive heart failure.[75] Another new strategy has been the use of the cardioprotectant dexrazoxane to prevent anthracycline-induced cardiotoxicity.[51] Until a safe dose of anthracycline given with dexrazoxane can be defined, the cumulative lifetime dose of anthracycline continues to be limited to 450 mg/m^2, a level at which fewer than 5% of patients experience clinical congestive heart failure.[76] Other cardiovascular late effects have been reported in childhood cancer survivors. Survivors of childhood brain tumor therapy treated with a combination of chemotherapy, irradiation, and surgery had a significantly increased risk of stroke, blood clots, and angina-like symptoms compared with their siblings.[77]

Pulmonary toxicity is a source of significant late toxicity of cancer therapy. Many alkylating agents and radiation therapy contribute to pulmonary fibrosis, resulting in decreased lung volume, lung compliance, and diffusing capacity. The nitrosoureas and bleomycin are the most common agents to cause pulmonary fibrosis.

Other significant organ-related late effects include hypothyroidism after radiation in Hodgkin's disease, chronic renal insufficiency from cisplatin therapy, chronic cystitis from cyclophosphamide or ifosfamide treatment, and prolonged hypogammaglobulinemia and T-lymphocyte dysfunction after multiple high-dose alkylators for bone marrow transplant.[78]

One of the more significant late effects of cancer therapy is the risk of secondary malignancy. As the number of childhood cancer survivors increases, this has become a major concern. In a retrospective review of 1406 childhood cancer patients, the actuarial risk of a second malignant neoplasm was 5.6% at 25 years after diagnosis.[79] The risk of second malignancy is highest in the patients who received both chemotherapy and radiation therapy. Hodgkin's disease survivors have the highest secondary malignancy rates. The estimated actuarial incidence of any second cancer was 7% at 15 years after diagnosis. Breast cancer was the most common solid tumor, with an estimated actuarial incidence in women of 35% by age 40 years. These patients are also at risk to develop leukemia, non-Hodgkin's lymphoma, and thyroid carcinoma.[80] In some series of survivors of childhood Hodgkin's disease, the cumulative estimated incidence of second malignancies at 30 years has ranged from 18% to 31%.[81,82] Patients who have received additional multimodality therapy for recurrent Hodgkin's disease have the highest risk of second tumors. Patients with soft tissue sarcomas, retinoblastoma, and Ewing's sarcoma who receive high-dose radiation to the primary lesion are at increased risk for secondary osteosarcoma within the radiation field.[83] Etoposide has been recognized as causing secondary acute myeloid leukemia, usually of the M4 or M5 subtype, with a short latency period (1 to 3 years from exposure) and a characteristic chromosomal translocation involving chromosome 11q23.[84]

BIOLOGIC TARGETED THERAPY

Over the past 20 years, many of the key genetic events that control carcinogenesis have been identified. In the past several years, rapid progress has been made in the development of rationally designed new agents to target biologic pathways specifically. These agents include signal transduction inhibitors (tissue growth factor receptor inhibitors, antiangiogenesis agents, and biologic response modifiers) individual cytokines, tumor-targeted antibody therapies, and adoptive immunotherapy techniques. Many of these agents are still in preclinical and early phase I testing, especially in pediatric oncology, although efficacy of agents from each class has been demonstrated. The development of these agents differs from those used in standard cytotoxic therapy. Whereas standard phase I studies for cytotoxic agents are designed to define the maximal tolerated dose, in biologic targeted therapy the optimal therapeutic dose is well below the maximal tolerated dose. The challenge in evaluating these agents is how to select the optimal dose and schedule, combine tumor-targeted agents with classic cytotoxic therapy, and validate the intended effect on the selected target for these biologic compounds designed to treat minimal residual disease.

Signal Transduction Inhibitors

Cellular signaling is a basic biologic function of all cells, controlling cellular proliferation and differentiation. Signaling can be extracellular (e.g., growth factor receptor tyrosine kinase) or through multiple intracellular effector and survival pathways (e.g., RAS, RAF, TP53, BCL-2). The malignant cell phenotype develops when apoptosis is inhibited or cells lose their ability to undergo normal differentiation. Specific agents have been synthesized to restore the usual cell functions by blocking aberrant signal transduction pathways.

Extracellular signaling can be accomplished via growth factor receptor proteins. Inhibition of the signaling pathways may result in decreased cell proliferation and increased apoptosis. A number of biologic agents have been developed to exploit this potential therapeutic option. Epidermal growth factor receptor (EGFR) is overexpressed in many solid tumors and is believed to play a role in tumor invasion and metastasis.[85] A specific inhibitor of EGFR, Gefitinib (AstraZeneca, Södertälje, Sweden), is an oral EGFR tyrosine kinase inhibitor that has demonstrated antitumor activity in adult phase I trials.[86] Potential use of this biologic agent in refractory neuroblastoma is currently in phase I testing in pediatric patients with solid tumors.[87] Inhibitors of the vascular endothelial growth factor (VEGF) receptor, vatalanib (PTK787/ZK22254), have been very effective inhibitors of angiogenesis, resulting in reduction in tumor size and number of blood vessels in treated patients.[88]

Multiple intracellular signaling pathways have recently been elucidated, and knowledge regarding the specific proteins involved in these pathways is now being exploited to develop specific targeted therapy. Production of farnesyl-protein transferase (FPTase) and BCL-2 inhibitors are examples of molecularly targeted drug development. The *ras* gene product plays a critical role in cell proliferation. Mutant forms of *ras* are associated with malignant transformation, and 30% of all human cancers express mutant *ras* genes.[89] Addition of a farnesyl isoprene group to the protein (farnesylation) is required for both mutant and wild-type ras function. However, other cellular polypeptides require farnesylation and also may be involved in the antiproliferative effects of FPTase inhibitors.[90]

Another class of new targeted agents includes small peptides that are designed to bind to messenger RNA (mRNA) of signal transduction proteins and inhibit their expression. One example of such an antisense oligonucleotide inhibitor is G3139(Genasense (oblimersen sodum) Injection, Genta Incorported, Berkeley Heights, New Jersey). This agent binds to the first six codons of the human BCL-2 mRNA, resulting in downregulation of expression of BCL-2. Because apoptosis is regulated by BCL-2 expression, and neuroblastomas overexpressing BCL-2 have a poorer outcome,[91] it is hypothesized that inhibiting BCL-2 expression may improve tumor response in these patients. G3139 has completed phase I and II testing in adults, both alone and in combination with cytotoxic agents. Responses have been observed, and inhibition of BCL-2 expression has been measured in peripheral blood and tumor tissue. This agent has now undergone phase I testing by the Children's Oncology Group for relapsed and refractory pediatric solid tumor patients and shows acceptable toxicities.[92] Additional studies will be needed to document efficacy.

Biologic Response Modifiers

The goal of biologic response modifiers is to stimulate the immune system to help eradicate tumors. The human immune system is designed to identify and destroy foreign cells. One of the great mysteries of oncology is why a patient's immune system is often unable to eliminate malignant cells. Studies in the mid 1990s indicated that some tumor cells may express a protein, Fas ligand, that conveys a "death signal" to T lymphocytes, causing them to undergo apoptosis.[93] The development of biologic response modifiers is a new branch of cancer therapy being developed to enhance or stimulate the natural products of the immune system (lymphocytes, antibodies, and cytokines) to better recognize and destroy cancer cells.

The immune system is composed of many cell types, but the lymphocyte has the primary role in controlling immune function. B lymphocytes function by secreting antibodies that mediate cell destruction by binding complement or causing opsonization, resulting in phagocytosis by macrophages. T lymphocytes can directly interact with specific cell-surface antigens on a target cell and cause cell lysis through cytotoxic granule release or programmed cell death. These cytotoxic T lymphocytes are involved with tumor cell killing. To initiate this response, antigens must be presented to the T cell by antigen-presenting cells (APCs) that express the antigens bound to major histocompatibility complex (MHC) proteins in the presence of stimulatory cytokines. Cytokines or interleukins (e.g., IL-2, interferon-α, tumor necrosis factor) are proteins produced by helper T lymphocytes and monocytes that help recruit other effector cells, including APCs, as well as regulate antibody production. The effector cells of the immune system (e.g., granulocytes, monocytes, macrophages, eosinophils, dendritic cells) can become tumor selective when activated by a specific antibody, a process called antibody-dependent cell-mediated cytotoxicity (ADCC).

Immunotherapy with biologic response modifiers takes advantage of all these immune functions. The goal of this therapy is to improve the immunogenicity of a tumor and allow it to be recognized and targeted for destruction by the immune system. Immunotherapy can be divided into two major categories: adoptive immunotherapy and tumor-targeted antibody therapy.

Adoptive Immunotherapy

Adoptive immunotherapy involves the use of tumor vaccines made from autologous or allogeneic tumor-associated antigens. Specific purified tumor antigens can be made more immunogenic by attachment to carrier proteins (adjuvants). The majority of all clinical trials using this type of tumor vaccine have been performed in melanoma patients.[94]

Another type of tumor vaccine in development is one designed to stimulate tumor-specific T-cell immunity to tumor peptides, resulting in the generation of cytotoxic T lymphocytes. For this type of vaccine to be successful, it is necessary to modify the tumor peptide to stimulate antigen presentation to the T cell. The presentation of the antigen is often restricted to specific MHC alleles. Neuroblastoma murine tumor cells have been modified to express exogenous MHC class II genes. In a murine model, this resulted in enhanced presentation of tumor antigens directly to T cells, producing a potent in-vivo tumor response.[95] Tumor cells also can be genetically engineered to overexpress cytokines (IL-2, granulocyte-macrophage colony-stimulating factor [GM-CSF]) that activate APCs and other immune cells.[96,97] Cytokines (GM-CSF, IL-2, IL-12, IL-1α) and other effector molecules (muramyl tripeptide phosphatidylethanolamine, disaccharide tripeptide) also are being used to stimulate an immune response in pediatric cancer patients.[13] Other forms of immunotherapy involve the use of cytokine infusions such as interferon-α, IL-2, and tumor necrosis factor to stimulate immune reaction against tumor cells.[98]

Tumor-Targeted Antibody Therapy

Passive immunity involves the use of monoclonal antibodies (mAbs) or cytotoxic effector cells produced in vitro and infused into the patient. mAbs have been tested in patients with neuroblastoma. One drawback of murine mAb therapy is that when these antibodies are repeatedly infused into humans, most patients will ultimately produce a human/anti-mouse antibody, which renders further antibody treatment useless.

Recently, chimeric human/mouse antibodies have been produced that may decrease the risk of human/anti-mouse antibody generation.[99] Recombinant chimeric antibodies are produced by linking the constant region of human antibodies to the variable combining region of a mouse mAb. These chimeric antibodies have been produced for the treatment of neuroblastoma[100] and more recently in leukemia and lymphoma with the development of anti-CD20, anti-CD52, and anti-CD33 mAbs. Rituximab (Genentech, Inc., San Francisco, CA) (anti-CD20) has been demonstrated to produce tumor responses in adult low-grade and follicular lymphomas.[13] The field of targeted biologic therapy is still in its infancy, but the future looks bright for the continued development of new targeted therapies, fueled by rapid advances in our understanding of cellular signaling pathways and immune mechanisms.

LOCAL TUMOR CONTROL

Control of local disease is critical to favorable outcomes in pediatric oncology. Metastatic disease is more readily eradicated in young patients than in adults when the primary lesion has been adequately treated. Advancements in techniques utilized to obtain local control (other than complete surgical excision) are constantly changing as advances in technology offer more and more opportunity to effectively treat the disease locally while minimizing morbidity.

Radiation Oncology

Radiation therapy implies the use of ionizing radiation to control malignant cells. An understanding of the biologic principles of radiation therapy in childhood cancer is important because radiation therapy plays an important role in the treatment of numerous pediatric tumors. There are several mechanisms of action through which radiation impacts tumor growth. Radiation may have a direct impact on the cellular DNA, resulting in impaired cell division. Alternatively, the radiation may result in the production of reactive free radicals that indirectly damage genetic material and interfere with the reproductive capacity of normal or malignant tissues. In most cases, the majority of the radiation effect is through production of these free radicals.

The sensitivity of normal cells and malignant cells to radiation varies widely between cell populations. Ionizing radiation initially results in sublethal damage to cells. The therapeutic effect of radiation therapy exploits the differences between a normal cell's ability to repair this sublethal damage and the slower response of radiosensitive tumor cells. Fractionated dosing allows normal cells to recover while having a cumulative effect on tumor cells. The effect of ionizing radiation on tumors depends on the number of actively reproducing cells at the time of exposure and on the length of the cellular regeneration cycle. Because most of the damage is indirect and focused on reproduction, malignant lesions usually show a delayed effect to radiation therapy. The tumor may begin to shrink or eventually disappear weeks to months after treatment. At some dose of therapy, the response of the malignant tissues becomes exponential, but further damage to normal adjacent cells also may occur.

Acute reactions to ionizing radiation depend on this balance between replication and cell death. They seem to be affected by increased intervals between dose fractions that allow enhanced cellular re-population. The radiation fraction size has a small impact on what volume of cells are immediately destroyed. Conversely, the long-term effects of therapy depend primarily on the total exposure dose and the size of each treatment fraction. The therapeutic ratio may be enhanced by exploiting the difference between the early and late radiation effects. Techniques may be used that reduce the late effects by lowering the dose per fraction and increasing the number of fractions delivered over the conventional treatment time.

Radiation therapy may be combined with surgery in a strategic manner to deliver the highest effective dose to a well-defined site, yet minimizes the dose to surrounding normal structures.[101] Preoperative radiation therapy may permit a smaller treatment area because the operative bed has not been manipulated. In larger tumors, its use may reduce the lesion volume sufficiently to allow a subsequent resection. In addition, potential tumor seeding during operative removal may be reduced because the cells that may be surgically disseminated have been rendered incapable of reproducing. On the other hand, preoperative radiation may delay the surgical procedure and alter the staging information obtained at operation.

For these reasons, many combined strategies use postoperative radiation such that the treatment fields and doses are determined after surgical resection and histologic assessment.[102] Higher doses can be delivered postoperatively when the target volumes have been more accurately defined. Doses to the periphery of the tumor can be fine-tuned, depending on the presence of gross, microscopic, or no residual disease. However, postoperative delivery may require a wider treatment area after extensive surgical manipulation.

Soft tissue sarcoma provides a model for the adjunctive role of radiation therapy. Surgery is the primary method of obtaining local control, but radiation therapy is effective when clear surgical margins are not possible.[103] Combined therapy has resulted in dramatically improved survival over the past 20 years.[104] In extremity lesions, radiation also allows more conservative resection with limb sparing. Although local tumor control rates of 75% to 98% have been achieved, with limb salvage rates greater than 80%, wound complications occur in as many as 40% of patients. Neoadjuvant radiation at more modest doses (30 Gy total) has decreased the complication rate while maintaining excellent (>95%) 5-year local control and ultimate limb salvage.[103] Postoperative radiation therapy also may be advantageous.[105] In that study, the wound complication rate was less than 10%. The use of brachytherapy offers potential advantages in obtaining local control while minimizing short and potentially long-term side effects.[106]

Several aspects of radiation treatment in pediatric patients deserve special consideration. Attention must be paid to the issues of immobilizing or sedating children so ionizing doses can be targeted to the desired area without inappropriate exposure of surrounding tissues. Pediatric radiation oncologists may use lower treatment doses and accept a higher recurrence rate to ensure lower toxicity, especially in critical developing organs such as the brain. The normal "tolerance" of organs or tissues may be adversely affected when chemotherapeutic agents are also used. The long-term effects of combined-modality therapy must be considered in regard to musculoskeletal and dental tissues, CNS and neuropsychological sequelae, and endocrine and gonadal dysfunction, as well as direct effects on the heart, lungs, or kidneys.[107] The following sections describe techniques that allow safe, efficacious doses of radiation to be delivered, often in combination with surgical excision, to produce the maximal therapeutic benefit.

BRACHYTHERAPY

Brachytherapy is radiation treatment in which the ionizing source is in contact with the lesion, usually within the initial tumor volume. Catheters are placed in the tumor during surgery and may be loaded with temporary or permanent implant sources. Remote afterloading may decrease radiation exposure to personnel and family members and can be performed in the patient's room or on an outpatient basis. Low-dose-rate sources, such as cesium, provide about 1 cGy/min, whereas high-dose-rate sources, such as iridium, provide about 100 cGy/min.

Because interstitial implants allow continuous-dose delivery over a much shorter time, they offer a radiobiologic advantage in high-grade tumors with rapid cell growth kinetics. Close cooperation between surgeon and radiation oncologist during the procedure is critical to ensure the most effective mapping of the tumor bed target.

Pediatric patients with soft tissue sarcomas can benefit from specialized radiation treatment strategies. If children have microscopic residual disease after surgery, radiation produces excellent local tumor control.[108] High-dose-rate brachytherapy has been successfully used in pediatric patients (Fig. 66-3). Low-dose-rate techniques require sedation, immobilization, long exposure times, and hospitalization, even with low-energy sources. High-dose-rate therapy is delivered in a few minutes, which is particularly helpful in young children. The short therapy duration also allows rapid reinstitution of systemic chemotherapy. The morbidity is usually related to skin or mucosal reactions, which may progress as a "recall" phenomenon in patients treated with radiosensitizing agents such as anthracyclines.[109] It has been shown that brachytherapy alone or in combination with external-beam irradiation provides a high rate of local tumor control in pediatric soft tissue sarcomas.[110-112]

Unfortunately, radiation therapy carries a significant morbidity risk. Radiation to the CNS may cause necrosis, arteritis, leukoencephalopathy, or radiation-induced tumors. Benign meningiomas have developed in children who received initial high-dose cranial radiation for malignant brain tumors.[113] The carcinogenic

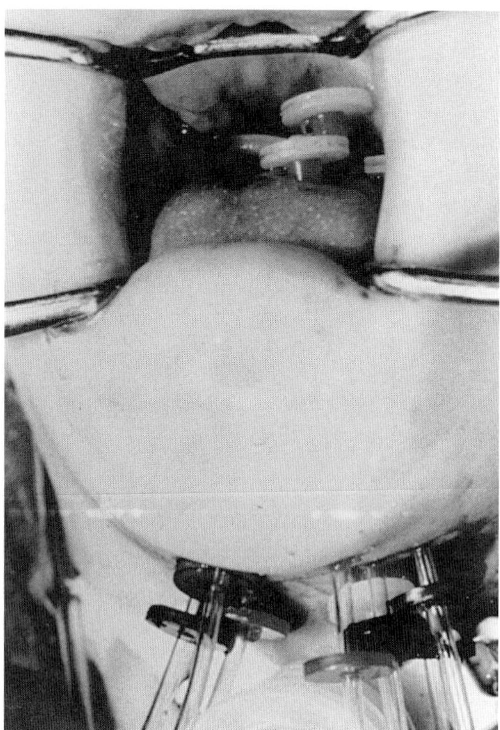

Figure 66-3. A 3-month-old infant with rhabdomyosarcoma in the base of the tongue. Eight high-dose-rate brachytherapy catheters were placed, delivering 36 Gy in 12 fractions over an 8-day period. The child is alive and disease free and has a good cosmetic result 7 years after treatment. (Courtesy of Subir Nag, MD, Chief of Brachytherapy, Ohio State University, Columbus, OH.)

effect of radiation therapy on brain tumors also has been theorized in more than 100 cases of malignant intracranial tumors.[114,115]

Intraoperative Radiation

Intraoperative radiation therapy (IORT) can be an important adjunctive measure to external-beam irradiation for local tumor control of advanced adult cancer.[116] IORT allows the radiation dose to be directly applied to the target area while shielding adjacent structures. Whenever disease remains in surgically inaccessible areas, IORT may be an effective adjunct. Most applications of IORT in children have been in patients with unresectable disease at diagnosis, delayed primary or second-look procedures, residual lesions, or local tumor recurrence. Phase I/II studies have demonstrated that IORT can be done safely in the pediatric population,[117] and preliminary outcomes suggest that this modality may be beneficial.[118,119]

IORT for retroperitoneal tumors can lead to urologic complications. In six patients treated with IORT and external-beam therapy, three patients required surgical intervention for fibrotic ureteral strictures or renal artery stenosis. In two cases, the injured structures were within a supplemental external-beam treatment field. In two children, neuropathies developed, one transiently after IORT alone and one permanently after combined therapy with external-beam irradiation. Nevertheless, all patients were survivors for up to 42 months' follow-up.[120] Other studies suggest that with more extensive dissection of normal structures and avoidance of overlapping radiation fields, the complication rate can be minimized.[118]

Intensity-Modulated Radiation Therapy

Techniques continue to evolve to improve the impact of radiation therapy on tumor response while minimizing the dose of radiation imparted to surrounding normal tissues. Stereotactic radiation therapy is sometimes used for CNS tumors.[121-129] Imaging systems, treatment-planning software, and delivery systems have undergone dramatic advancements that allow sophisticated delivery of more precise courses of radiation treatments. Intensity-modulated radiation therapy (IMRT) is an advanced form of three-dimensional conformal therapy that uses non-uniform radiation beam intensities that have been determined by using various computer-based optimization techniques. Experience with IMRT in the pediatric population is growing. Initial reports of mixed tumor cases, including pediatric patients, suggest that the technique will be effective in reducing treatment-related morbidity and allow dose escalation to the target volume.[130,131] Significant reductions in radiation exposure to critical structures has been shown for intracranial, cervical, and abdominopelvic lesions.[132]

INNOVATIVE ADJUNCTIVE TECHNIQUES

Cryosurgery

The basic principle involved in cryosurgery is the in-situ destruction of tissue by the freeze/thaw process. As the frozen tissue thaws, the circulation returns and, for a brief period, the tissue may appear almost normal. However, as endothelial cell damage, thrombosis, edema, and vascular stasis develop, the microcirculation progressively fails and cell death ensues.[133] The mechanism of tissue response is multifactorial and highly dependent on the rate of cooling. When this technique is applied to cancer, the goal is to devitalize the same volume of neoplastic tissue by freezing as would have been excised with a local resection. The most important tumoricidal mechanism appears to be the rapid freezing, slow thawing, and immediate repetition of this cycle.[134]

Intraoperative ultrasonography now allows precise placement of vacuum-insulated cryoprobes into the center of tumors. These probes can monitor the progression of the freeze margin in real time.[135] Liquid nitrogen is circulated through the tip of the probe, achieving temperatures in the range of −160°C to −180°C. When used for liver tumors (both primary and metastatic), survival has ranged from 12% to 38% at 18 months to 5 years of follow-up.[136-139] The incidence of major complications in most series is less than 5%. Hepatic enzyme elevation to about twice normal usually occurs and spontaneously resolves within the first postoperative week. Pleural effusion, myoglobinuria, hemorrhage, biliary leak, or abscess formation are rare.

Cryosurgery has been successfully used for aneurysmal bone cysts,[140] aggressive benign bone tumors, or low-grade malignancies.[141] Although cryosurgery offers the advantage of preserving supportive function of bone in these skeletal tumors, complications do occur. Most important, intraoperative venous gas embolism may rarely produce hemodynamically significant events.[142]

Radiofrequency Ablation

Radiofrequency ablation (RFA) is a technique that applies thermal energy via a probe that results in coagulation necrosis of the target tissue. The technique involves image-guided application of the probe primarily using ultrasound guidance. The probe can be introduced percutaneously, laparoscopically, or using an open exposure. The most common applications for the technique in adults have been for primary or metastatic hepatic lesions, renal lesions, and pulmonary lesions.[143-149]

Treatment of pediatric tumors with RFA is largely anecdotal. A small series reporting the use of percutaneous RFA on fetuses with sacrococcygeal teratoma reported a 50% fetal mortality rate.[150] In one child treated prenatally with RFA, a severe soft tissue defect and sciatic nerve destruction were noted at birth.[151]

Chemoembolization

The regional delivery of chemotherapy for hepatic tumors is possible because the liver has a dual blood supply, with the hepatic artery contributing approximately 25% of the parenchymal flow to normal cells, whereas malignant hepatic lesions derive nearly all of their blood supply from this source. This allows a selective delivery of cytotoxic agents to tumor. In addition, the liver can withstand regional dose escalation because of its ability to detoxify through "first-pass" kinetics. Whereas foreign body embolization produced temporary arterial occlusion and transient palliative effects, the most durable responses were achieved when chemotherapeutic agents were infused distal to the ligated hepatic artery.[152] This therapeutic strategy involves infusing high concentrations of chemotherapy and prolonging the dwell time with a variety of embolic materials (Fig. 66-4). Multiple adult series have shown tumor reduction using chemotherapy delivery via embolic materials.[153-157] A prospective randomized trial for unresectable hepatocellular carcinoma compared chemoembolization against conservative therapy.[157] Although a trend favored survival with chemoembolization, the difference was not statistically significant. Of note, in 60% of the patients in the treatment arm, liver failure developed, which parallels previous experience.

The pediatric experience with chemoembolization is quite small, although isolated cases with limited success have been described.[158,159] This technique also has been extended to hepatic malignancies in infancy.[160] Two reports of chemoembolization experience in childhood liver tumors have been reported.[161,162] In one series,[161] a suspension of cisplatin, doxorubicin, and mitomycin-C mixed with bovine collagen and radiopaque contrast material was used in 11 children with unresectable or recurrent lesions. Six hepatoblastoma patients had initial partial response, as measured by imaging and α-fetoprotein levels. Three patients underwent subsequent surgical resection, but 1 progressed and died, whereas 2 survived more than 15 months. The other 3 also eventually died of known progressive disease. Of the 3 children with hepatocellular carcinoma, 1 underwent surgical resection and was a long-term survivor for more than 65 months, 1 was alive with disease for more than 36 months, and 1 (with cirrhosis) died of progressive liver failure with no evidence of malignancy. In the other series,[162] 14 children received 50 courses of intra-arterial chemotherapy with cisplatin or doxorubicin (Adriamycin) or both, followed by Gelfoam embolization for hepatoblastoma (7 patients) or hepatocellular carcinoma (7 patients). Six of the 14 subsequently underwent orthotopic liver transplant, and 3 of the 6 died of metastatic disease. In 7 of the remaining patients, progressive disease

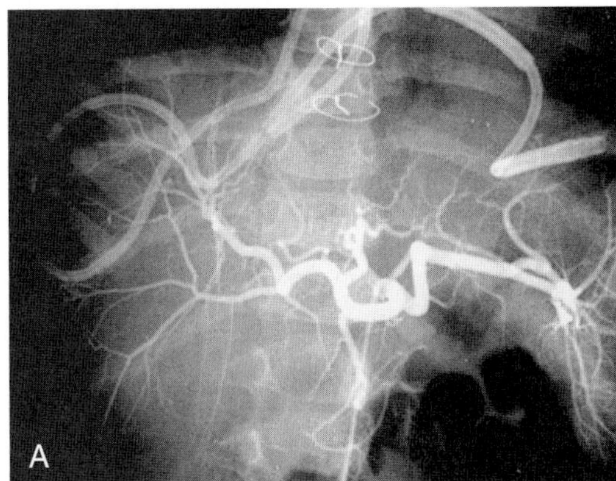

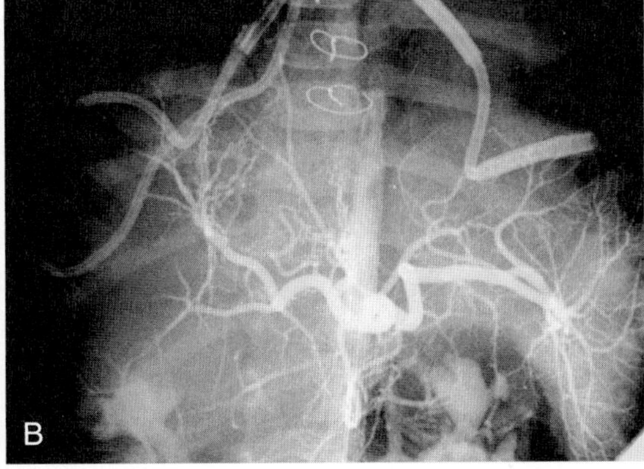

Figure 66-4. **A,** Celiac axis injection before embolization showing slight tortuosity of distal branches of the anterior superior segment of the right lobe, the middle hepatic artery, and the medial segment of the left lobe. **B,** Postembolization injection of celiac axis showing marked peripheral attenuation of the branches of the right and left lobes secondary to deposition of collagen laden with chemotherapy agent. (A and B, courtesy of Philip Stanley, MD, Pediatric Hematology-Oncology, UCLA School of Medicine, Los Angeles, California.)

developed, and 1 patient was awaiting transplant at the time of the report.

Overall, hepatic chemoembolization is feasible in young patients, with tolerable toxicity. This option represents a reasonable therapeutic alternative in persistent, unresectable, or recurrent hepatoblastoma, or in nonmetastatic hepatocellular carcinoma.

Lymphatic Mapping

Accurate staging of regional disease continues to be important in pediatric and adult tumors. The initial draining lymph node, the so-called sentinel node, is reportedly predictive of regional nodal metastases in a variety of tumors.[163] Although lymph node mapping has been applied to a number of tumors, it is most commonly used to predict nodal status of patients with melanoma or breast cancer. The technique has been refined and validated as it has evolved. In most cases, a combination of technetium-labeled sulfur colloid and lymphazurin blue dye is used to localize the sentinel node. Preoperative lymphoscintigraphy provides information regarding draining nodal basins in truncal and head and neck cases. Intraoperative lymphatic mapping is accomplished by injecting the technetium-labeled sulfur colloid at the primary tumor site 1 hour before surgery. Just before incision, the blue dye is injected at the primary tumor site and a gamma probe is used to identify areas of high counts. The underlying tissue is then examined for lymph nodes containing the blue dye. If the sentinel node has no histologic evidence of metastases, the related regional lymphatic bed is highly likely to be tumor free, and the morbidity of lymphadenectomy can be avoided.

Lymphoscintigraphy is a reliable indicator of lymphatic drainage from cutaneous melanoma of the head, neck, and trunk. In one study, a radiolabeled tracer of ^{99}Tc sulfur colloid or human serum albumin was injected before wide local excision of the primary lesion.[164] Of 297 patients reviewed, 181 underwent elective dissection of the lymph node basins identified by the lymphoscintigraphy and 27% had melanoma detected within the dissected basin. The other 116 patients were observed. In 14%, lymph node metastases developed as their first sign of recurrence. Only 1 of these patients, in whom rapidly progressive disease developed, had lymph node metastases in an area not predicted by the scan. Overall, 70 of 71 patients had documented lymphatic metastases occur in a predicted lymph node bed, confirming that cutaneous lymphoscintigraphy can be reliably used to guide therapy in high-risk melanoma. Lymph node localization by gamma probe scanning also has been extended to breast cancer management.[165]

The implications of sentinel lymph node mapping are important in pediatric tumors such as rhabdomyosarcoma. In the Intergroup Rhabdomyosarcoma Studies I and II, the incidence of positive regional lymph nodes was 12% to 17%. However, most of these patients did not undergo lymph node sampling. More recently, when the majority of patients actually did have a lymph node biopsy, the incidence of detecting disease increased to 40%.[166] These findings also were confirmed subsequently in the Intergroup Rhabdomyosarcoma Study III, which demonstrated that when regional lymph nodes were sampled, 39% contained metastatic disease.[167] Patients with positive nodes underwent radiation therapy to the involved lymph node bed, resulting in improved survival, documenting the need for accurate lymph node staging.

The technique of lymph node mapping has been successfully applied to a small series of pediatric patients.[168] On the day before operation, the patient is injected around the palpable lesion or the previous incision site with 0.2 to 0.5 mL of ^{99}Tc sulfur colloid. Immediately before surgery, the same area is injected with 0.5 to 1.0 mL of vital blue dye. When a handheld gamma probe is used, signal localization parallels the presence of the blue dye in the lymphatic channels leading to the sentinel lymph node, which is stained blue and scans positive. An excisional biopsy is performed for histologic assessment, which should predict involvement of the remaining lymphatic bed. No therapy is necessary for negative biopsies. Histologically positive tissue leads to lymph node dissection and regional lymphatic radiation.

chapter 67

RENAL TUMORS

Robert C. Shamberger, MD

Renal tumors are the second most common abdominal tumor seen in infants and children after neuroblastoma. They represent a wide spectrum of tumors from benign to extremely malignant. Advances in the management of these tumors have been significant over the past 4 decades since Sidney Farber first administered dactinomycin (Actinomycin D) for advanced-stage Wilms' tumors.[1] Much of what we know about renal tumors today has resulted from two cooperative group organizations, the National Wilms' Tumor Study Group (NWTSG) and the Société Internationale d'Oncologie Pédiatrique (SIOP). Together they have performed multiple randomized therapeutic trials, which have established the basis for how these tumors are treated. Central pathologic review of the specimens of patients enrolled in these studies has provided the current pathologic classification and staging, which could never have been established without multi-institutional participation because of the relative rarity of pediatric renal tumors. In this chapter, the early history of this tumor is described, followed by a discussion of the etiologic factors in tumor formation, pathologic subtypes and premalignant syndromes, and treatment algorithms for Wilms' tumors and other tumors of the kidney.

WILMS' TUMOR

History

The first descriptions of Wilms' tumor have been variably attributed to either Rance in 1814 or Wilms' in 1899.[2] Ironically, however, the first known specimen of this tumor was preserved by the British surgeon John Hunter between 1763 and 1793, when he was collecting specimens for his museum.[3] To this day, this specimen of a bilateral tumor in a young infant remains in the Hunterian Museum of the Royal College of Surgeons in London. Wilms' name became indelibly fixed to the mixed embryonal tumor of the kidney occurring in children after publication of his comprehensive monograph on mixed tissue tumors of the kidney in 1899.[4]

William E. Ladd and Robert E. Gross[5,6] described the principles of surgical therapy for Wilms' tumor, including transperitoneal exposure and early ligation of the renal pedicle. They stressed the need to remove the perirenal fat to include lymphatic extensions and to avoid rupture of the renal capsule, principles we continue to follow today. Adoption of their techniques significantly reduced the operative mortality of nephrectomy in children. Gross and Neuhauser[3] later proposed the routine addition of abdominal radiation to the therapy of Wilms' tumors and reported an estimated 47% frequency of cure. Under Gross's tutelage, pediatric surgeons in North America generally performed primary resection of Wilms' tumors, while in Europe the Paris school led by Schweisguth and Bamberger reported early success with preoperative irradiation, establishing a precedent for preoperative therapy.[7]

From 1931 to 1939, survival from surgical resection alone, involving ligation of the renal pedicle before removal, was 32% at The Children's Hospital in Boston.[1] Beginning in 1940, most of the patients received postoperative irradiation to the renal fossa, which decreased the local recurrence rate but did not significantly affect the frequency of pulmonary metastases or improve the long-term survival. Dactinomycin was the first active agent identified for the treatment of Wilms' tumor. Of the 53 patients who had no demonstrable metastases on admission treated with combined therapy of operation, local radiation, and dactinomycin from 1957 to 1964, an 89% 2-year disease-free survival was reported, a very reasonable survival even today.[1] In patients with metastases identified at presentation, 18 (58%) of 31 were alive and free of disease more than 2 years later. Subsequently, vincristine sulfate was identified as an active agent against Wilms' tumor and was added to the standard therapy.[8]

Wilms' tumor was the first malignancy in which the importance of adjuvant treatment was recognized. This principle was espoused by Sidney Farber decades before it would be applied to other pediatric and adult solid tumors. The concept of adjuvant therapy "was based upon the supposition that in the children with Wilms' tumor who died, the tumor must have metastasized already at the time of discovery of the primary tumor" although no evidence of spread was available.[1]

Incidence and Etiology

Wilms' tumor is the most frequent tumor of the kidney in infants and children. Its incidence is 7.6 cases for every million children younger than 15 years, or one case per 10,000 infants.[9] Its frequency varies by race. It is less common in East Asian populations than in whites but more frequent in black children.[10] In just under 10% of cases, it is associated with several congenital syndromes, including sporadic aniridia, isolated hemihypertrophy, the Denys-Drash syndrome (nephropathy, renal failure, male pseudohermaphroditism, and Wilms' tumor), genital anomalies, Beckwith-Wiedemann syndrome (visceromegaly, macroglossia, omphalocele, and hyperinsulinemic hypoglycemia in infancy), and the WAGR complex (Wilms' tumor with aniridia, genitourinary malformations, and mental retardation). All these associations suggested a genetic predisposition to this tumor.[11,12] Wilms' tumor also is reported in individuals with Simpson-Golabi-Behmel syndrome, another overgrowth syndrome similar to Beckwith-Wiedemann syndrome in many respects.[13] These congenital disorders have now been linked to abnormalities at specific genetic loci implicated in Wilms' tumorigenesis.

Genetic Origins

The identification of a large chromosomal deletion of band p13 of chromosome 11 in children with the WAGR syndrome led to a search at this site for a gene producing the Wilms' tumor. Subsequent molecular studies of children with Wilms' tumor demonstrated a deletion at this site in some cases.[14] This deletion includes the aniridia gene (*PAX 6*) and a putative Wilms' tumor suppressor gene (*WT1*). It should be recognized that children can lack the *PAX6* gene but not the *WT1* gene and not be at increased risk for the development of Wilms' tumors. In fact, from the Danish aniridia registry, 44 of 144 cases of aniridia were sporadic. Of these sporadic cases, 5 patients had a deletion of the *WT1* gene but only 2 developed a Wilms' tumor.[15] None of the patients with the familial cases lacked the *WT1* site. Therefore, for patients with aniridia, the risk appears low, but in the children with sporadic aniridia, it is estimated that the risk of developing a Wilms' tumor is 67 times higher than in a normal population. This risk is entirely attributable to the small proportion who lack the *WT1* gene. Finally, it is estimated that between 45% and 57% of children with the WAGR syndrome will develop a Wilms' tumor.[16,17]

The protein product of the *WT1* gene is a developmentally regulated transcriptional factor of the zinc-finger family, which regulates the expression of other genes, including growth-inducing genes such as those encoding early growth response, insulin-like growth factor-2 (IGF-2), and the platelet-derived growth factor A chain.[18,19] Suppression of these growth-associated genes may explain the tumor suppressor role of *WT1*. Recently, the *WT1* gene product has been found to bind physically to the TP53 protein.[20] Children with the WAGR syndrome have constitutional deletions of band 11p13, and virtually all patients with Denys-Drash syndrome carry point mutations in *WT1* in their germline.[14] These result in a dominant negative oncogene and more severe somatic abnormalities than those seen in the WAGR syndrome, attributed to the inhibition by the mutated protein on the action of the normal "wild-type" protein produced by the normal chromosome.[21] The second *WT1* allele is lost in the Wilms' tumor cells in patients with WAGR. Similarly, the tumors in children with Denys-Drash syndrome have loss of the remaining "wild-type" allele.[22] Excluding aniridia, the most common phenotypic abnormality in the WAGR syndrome is cryptorchidism, which is found in 60% of male patients, whereas abnormalities of the internal reproductive organs including streak ovaries and bicornuate uterus are seen in 17% of females. Mental retardation was found in 70% of children and renal failure in 29%, which occurred due to both nephrectomy and glomerulonephritis, predominantly focal segmental glomerulosclerosis. Studies have demonstrated that children with WAGR syndrome more frequently have bilateral tumors (17% vs. 6%) and are younger at diagnosis (22 vs. 39 months) than children without WAGR.[23]

Dysregulation of imprinted genes at chromosome 11p15 that control prenatal and childhood growth are believed to be the cause of the Beckwith-Wiedemann syndrome.[24] These include isolated hypomethylation of a differentially methylated region known as KvDMRI in approximately 50% of cases.[25,26] At the *WT2* site, there are several imprinted genes that are expressed preferentially from one of the parental alleles.[27] Some children with Beckwith-Wiedemann syndrome have overexpression of a gene normally expressed by only one of the parental alleles, paternal uniparental disomy in 20% of the cases. In some cases, a constitutional duplication of the paternal 11p15 chromosomal fragment has been identified (trisomy at 11p15).[28] These findings led to speculation that the Beckwith-Wiedemann gene is expressed only by the paternal allele and that these genetic abnormalities that lead to the presence of two paternal alleles would double the expression of this gene and may result in the overgrowth.

Loss of expression of *H19*, a tumor suppressor gene, also has been reported in Wilms' tumors.[29] The *H19* gene is expressed from the maternal allele. With loss of heterozygosity (LOH), the cell may lose the maternal (active) copy and hence its tumor suppressor function.[30]

Children whose manifestations of the Beckwith-Wiedemann syndrome include hemihypertrophy appear to have a greater risk for the occurrence of malignancy than do those who do not. In a series reported by Wiedemann, cancer was reported in 7.5% of all children with the syndrome but was found in more than 40% of children with both the syndrome and hemihypertrophy.[31]

The Simpson-Golabi-Behmel syndrome is a sex-linked syndrome linked to Xq25-27. It is an overgrowth syndrome phenotypically similar to the Beckwith-Wiedemann syndrome comprising macroglossia, coarse facial features, and visceromegaly. The less frequent manifestations of diaphragmatic and heart defects and polydactyly are unique to Simpson-Golabi-Behmel syndrome. The protein product glypican-3 may interact with the IGF-2 receptor.[32,33]

Familial cases of Wilms' tumor account for only 1% to 2% of cases and have not been associated with these syndromes. Analysis of two kindreds revealed a link with chromosome band 17q12-21, and the putative tumor gene at this locus has been named *FWT1*.[34] Recent studies in five kindreds have demonstrated an inherited Wilms' tumor predisposition gene at 19q13.3-q13.4, called *FWT2*.[35,36] In addition, LOH was seen at 19q in tumors from individuals from two families whose predisposition is not due to the previously defined 19q locus, suggesting that alterations at two distinct loci are critical rate-limiting steps in the etiology of these familial Wilms' tumors involving both germline-predisposing mutations and somatic alteration at a second focus.

In marked contrast to the *MYCN* gene in neuroblastoma, *WT1* and *WT2* do not appear to have any prognostic significance for children with Wilms' tumor. They also appear in a small percentage of children with Wilms' tumor who have the associated syndromes. Recent studies have suggested that LOH on chromosome 16q in Wilms' tumors (observed in 15% to 20% of cases) was associated with a 3.3 times greater incidence of relapse and a 12 times greater incidence of mortality as compared with those in children without these chromosomal changes.[37] This region of loss has now been localized to an area of 6.7 megabases that contain three recognized tumor suppressor genes. One of them, *E-cadherin*, has been shown to have reduced expression in Wilms' tumors with LOH at 16q.[38] A similar trend was seen for children with LOH for 1p, which occurs in approximately 10% of Wilms' tumors, but these trends were not statistically significant. One of the primary goals of the fifth NWTS study is to assess whether identified chromosomal abnormalities are of prognostic significance in Wilms' tumor (see later).

Identification of increased expression of the TP53 protein has also been associated with advanced stage at presentation and increased disease relapse.[39]

Routine radiographic screening of children with syndromes associated with Wilms' tumor has been recommended. Ultrasonograms are generally obtained every 3 months until the children are 5 years old. No prospective studies, however, have been performed to evaluate the cost-effectiveness or efficacy of this recommendation.[40,41] Retrospective reviews of routine ultrasound screening report conflicting results on the purported benefits of prospective screening, as assessed by the stage distribution at presentation or the outcome of the children.[42,43]

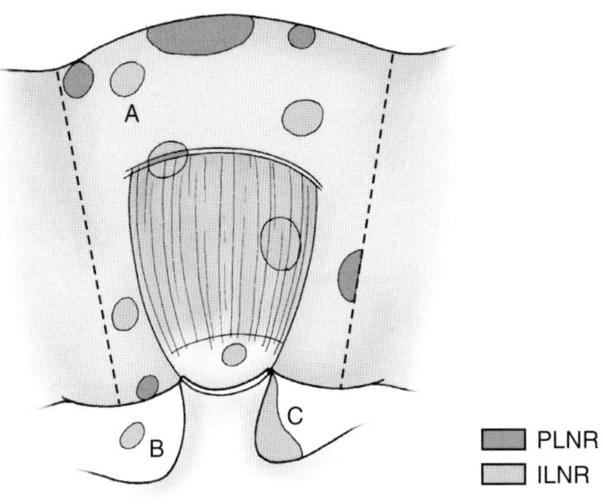

Figure 67-1. Diagram of a renal lobe and adjacent calyx and intervening sinus with potential sites of distribution of perilobar (PLNR) and intralobar (ILNR) nephrogenic rests. (From Beckwith JB, Kiviat NB, Bonadio JF: Nephrogenic rests, nephroblastomatosis, and the pathogenesis of Wilms' tumor. Pediatr Pathol 10:1-36, 1990.)

Pathologic Precursors: Nephrogenic Rests, Nephroblastomatosis, and Multicystic Dysplastic Kidneys

The presence of nephrogenic rests (NRs; persistent metanephric tissue in the kidney after the 36th week of gestation) has been associated with the occurrence of Wilms' tumor. These rests may occur in a perilobular (PLNRs) or intralobular (ILNRs) location and may be single or multiple (Fig. 67-1). In children with aniridia or the Denys-Drash syndrome, the lesions are primarily ILNRs, whereas children with hemihypertrophy or the Beckwith-Wiedemann syndrome have predominantly PLNRs.[44] The presence of multiple or diffuse nephrogenic rests is termed *nephroblastomatosis*.

The frequency of NRs was established in an autopsy series of infants younger than 3 months. Nine (0.87%) of 1035 infants had PLNRs, and ILNRs occurred in only 2 (0.1%) of 2000 cases.[45] When identified, most NRs are sclerosing, an apparently indolent or involutional phase. The vast majority will spontaneously resolve without the appearance of a tumor, because the incidence of NRs is about 100 times greater than that of Wilms' tumor (1/10,000 infants).

NRs are classified histologically as incipient or dormant NRs, regressing or sclerosing NRs, and hyperplastic NRs (Fig. 67-2).[46] Incipient or dormant rests are composed predominantly of blastemal or primitive epithelial cells, resembling those in the embryonic kidney and Wilms' tumor, but are microscopic with sharp margins from adjacent renal parenchyma. In infants and young children, the term *incipient* is used, whereas *dormant* is used in older children. Regressing or sclerosing rests demonstrate maturation of the cellular elements and progress to obsolescent rests, which are composed primarily of hyaline stromal elements. Hyperplastic NRs are problematic, in that they are often difficult to distinguish from small Wilms' tumors. They contain diffuse or synchronous proliferation of components throughout the rest. This uniform growth leads to preservation

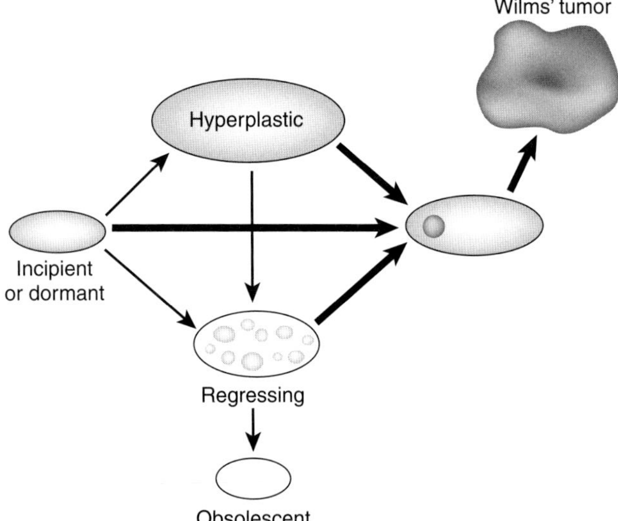

Figure 67-2. Diagrammatic depiction of nephrogenic rests and their classification. *Thick arrows* indicate tumor induction. (From Beckwith JB: Precursor lesions of Wilms' tumor: Clinical and biological implications. Med Pediatr Oncol 21:158-168, 1993.)

of the original shape of the rest, in contrast to neoplastic proliferation of a single cell, which produces a more spherical expanding nodule within the rest. It is almost impossible for even the most sophisticated pediatric pathologist to distinguish a hyperplastic NR from a Wilms' tumor based on an incisional or needle biopsy specimen that does not include the margin between the rest and the remaining kidney. Preservation of the shape of the original rest is the most obvious clue that one is dealing with a hyperplastic, rather than a neoplastic, change.[46] Most hyperplastic nodules lack a pseudocapsule at their periphery, whereas most Wilms' tumors will have one. Often this is the most helpful histologic finding in distinguishing these two lesions. Thus, biopsy specimens that do not contain the lesion and its margin will rarely adequately differentiate between these two lesions.

NRs are frequently found in association with Wilms' tumors despite their relatively rare occurrence. In a review of cases of Wilms' tumors reported in the NWTS-4, 41% of the unilateral Wilms' tumors were associated with NRs,[44] whereas in children with synchronous bilateral Wilms' tumor, the incidence of NRs was 99%. These were primarily PLNRs, possibly because these lesions are much more prevalent than the ILNRs. Similarly, an increased incidence of NRs is seen in children with the syndromes associated with Wilms' tumor (Table 67-1).[46]

It has been demonstrated that magnetic resonance imaging (MRI) can be particularly helpful in monitoring children with nephroblastomatosis. Rohrschneider and co-workers later confirmed that MRI or contrast-enhanced computed tomography (CT) was preferable to ultrasonography in this setting.[47,48] Alterations in imaging characteristics of the lesions may suggest a transition from NRs to Wilms' tumor, as does growth of isolated lesions.

Diffuse hyperplastic perilobar nephroblastomatosis (DHPLN) is a distinct entity that must be distinguished clinically from Wilms' tumor. Infants with DHPLN may initially have large unilateral or bilateral flank masses (Fig. 67-3). A characteristic radiographic finding is massively enlarged kidneys that maintain their normal configuration and lack evidence of necrosis. As with the isolated NRs, proliferation of the thin rind of NRs on the periphery of the kidney will preserve the normal configuration of the kidney, but with marked enlargement of its size. This is in contrast to Wilms' tumor, in which the normal renal configuration and collecting system is generally distorted. Nephrectomy is not required in cases of DHPLN. Chemotherapy, however, has been used to control the proliferative element of the NRs. Its use may accelerate resolution of the size of the masses and decrease the respiratory compromise they may produce. However, it has not been established that treatment with chemotherapy will decrease the risk of malignancy arising in these lesions. A recent review of 52 cases of DHPLN revealed a mean age of 16 months at diagnosis. Involvement was bilateral in 49 children. Thirty-three patients had biopsy and adjuvant therapy. Eighteen (55%) developed Wilms' tumors at a mean of 35 months. Sixteen patients had initial nephrectomy and adjuvant therapy, and 3 (19%) developed a Wilms' tumor at a mean of 36 months from diagnosis. All 3 patients who did not receive adjuvant therapy developed Wilms' tumors by 10 months after diagnosis. In total, 24 of 52 children developed Wilms' tumors that were single in 13 and multiple in 11 children. Eight of the 24 children had anaplastic tumors, an extremely high proportion.[49]

An increased risk of Wilms' tumors arising in multicystic dysplastic kidneys has been suggested. In the past, many of these lesions were resected to prevent the occurrence of Wilms' tumor. Narchi summarized 1041 infants and children with multicystic dysplastic kidneys reported in the world's literature from 26 series and found no case associated with a Wilms' tumor.[50] He concluded that nephrectomy was not required for

Table 67-1 Association of Nephrogenic Rests with Wilms' Tumor and Associated Syndromes

Population	PLNR (%)	ILNR (%)
Unilateral Wilms' tumor	25	15
Bilateral Wilms' tumor (synchronous)	74-79	34-41
Bilateral Wilms' tumor (metachronous)	42	63-75
Beckwith-Wiedemann/ hemihypertrophy & Wilms' tumor	70-77	47-57
Aniridia and Wilms' tumor	12-20	84-100
Denys-Drash and Wilms' tumor	11	78

Adapted from Beckwith JB: Precursor lesions of Wilms' tumor: Clinical and biological implications. Med Pediatr Oncol 21:158-168, 1993.)
PLNR, perilobar nephrogenic rests; ILNR, intralobar nephrogenic rests.

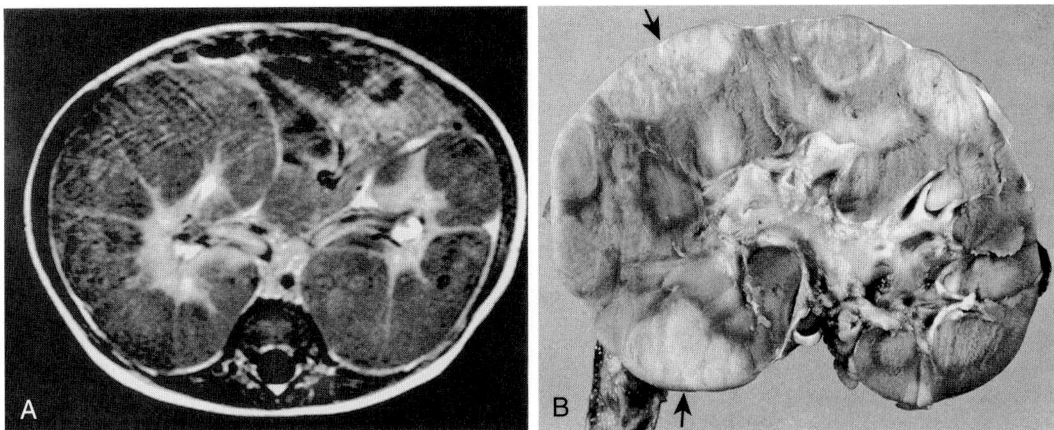

Figure 67-3. **A,** MR image of a 10-month-old infant who presented with large bilateral flank masses demonstrates a picture characteristic of diffuse hyperplastic perilobar nephroblastomatosis (DHPLN) with extensive involvement of the entire cortex of the kidney with no evidence of necrosis and general preservation of the shape of the kidney. **B,** Photograph of a kidney resected with a similar pattern of DHPLN reveals extensive involvement of the periphery of the cortex by severely hypertrophied nephrogenic rests (*arrows*). Resection of such kidneys should be avoided because, in most cases, the hypertrophy will resolve and the kidney will have excellent preservation of its function. (**B** courtesy of J. B. Beckwith by permission.)

this condition. The frequency of NRs in multicystic dysplastic kidneys has been estimated to be 4%, approximately five times the prevalence in a random autopsy population of infants younger than age 3 months.[51] If one were to estimate the frequency of Wilms' tumor in these kidneys, the standard risk of 1 in 10,000 infants might be increased to 1 in 2,000. Review of the NWTS pathology files, however, identified only three cases of dysplastic kidneys in more than 7000 children with Wilms' tumor over a 26-year interval and only 1 case in more than 1500 referral cases sent to Dr. Beckwith from around the world. Although it is impossible to estimate the number of children at risk from Wilms' tumors in remaining dysplastic kidneys, it must be concluded that this risk of developing a Wilms' tumor or congenital obstruction must be extremely low and does not justify nephrectomy to avoid the development of tumors. It has been suggested that because all of the reported Wilms' tumor cases in multicystic dysplastic kidney occurred before 4 years of age, then ultrasound surveillance up to that age should be recommended.[52]

Pathology

The collection of large numbers of renal tumor specimens by the cooperative group trials has facilitated the development of accurate pathologic classifications in a much shorter period than would ever have been feasible without these trials. Early reports of Wilms' tumors and the initial cooperative group trials included essentially all renal sarcomas under this rubric. With time and experience, however, several subgroups of tumors have now been identified as having a particularly high risk of recurrence and adverse outcome.[3,53] In NWTS-1, anaplastic and sarcomatous variants comprised only 11.5% of the tumors, yet they accounted for 51.9% of the deaths due to tumor. Unfavorable histology proved to be the most important factor in patient outcome in NWTS-1, and this finding continues through the current trials. Wilms' tumors are currently divided into those with "favorable" histology and those with "unfavorable" histology (Table 67-2). The latter group includes tumors with focal or diffuse anaplasia.[54,55] Clear cell sarcoma of the kidney and malignant rhabdoid tumors of the kidney were initially grouped with the unfavorable-histology Wilms' tumors. They are now considered distinct entities from Wilms' tumor, based on their pathologic appearance and response to quite different therapies.[56,57]

The staging system used by the NWTSG is a pretreatment surgical staging system (Table 67-3). It must be carefully distinguished when comparing treatment results with children treated on the SIOP protocols in which the staging information is obtained after preliminary treatment of the tumors (Table 67-4). The intensity of adjuvant treatment in the NWTSG protocols is determined by such factors as regional lymph node involvement and penetration of the renal capsule by tumor. These prognostic variables cannot be accurately determined by radiographic studies. The staging criteria are continually adjusted during the course of the NWTSG studies as the prognostic significance of criteria are established.[58]

Table 67-2	Pathologic Classification of Renal Tumors
Wilms' tumor	
Favorable histology	
Unfavorable histology	
Diffuse anaplasia	
Focal anaplasia	
Clear cell sarcoma	
Malignant rhabdoid tumor of the kidney	
Renal cell sarcoma	
Renal adenocarcinoma	
Renal neurogenic tumors	
Renal teratoma	

Table 67-3 Staging System Utilized by the National Wilms' Tumor Study Group

Stage	Description
Stage I	Tumor limited to the kidney and completely excised without rupture or biopsy. Surface of the renal capsule is intact.
Stage II	Tumor extends through the renal capsule but is completely removed with no microscopic involvement of the margins. Vessels outside the kidney contain tumor. Also placed in stage II are cases in which the kidney has been sampled before resection or where there is "local" spillage of tumor (during resection) limited to the tumor bed.
Stage III	Residual tumor is confined to the abdomen and not from hematogenous spread. Also included in stage III are cases with tumor involvement of the abdominal lymph nodes, rupture of the tumor with "diffuse" peritoneal contamination extending beyond the tumor bed, peritoneal implants, and microscopic or grossly positive resection margins.
Stage IV	Hematogenous metastases at any site
Stage V	Bilateral renal involvement

The SIOP classification was recently revised based on a review of the outcomes of children relative to the histologic appearance of the tumors at resection and after initial chemotherapy.[59] Tumors are now classified as completely necrotic (low-risk tumor), blastemal (high-risk tumor), and others (intermediate-risk tumors). The prognostic implications of this classification will be assessed in the current study, as will the potential for decreasing extent of therapy of the more favorable groups. Wilms' tumor is characterized as a triphasic embryonal neoplasm with blastemal, stromal, and epithelial components (Fig. 67-4).[3] Each of these components can express several patterns of differentiation, which define the histologic subgroups of Wilms' tumors. One particular subtype, the fetal rhabdomyomatous nephroblastoma, has been associated with a poor response to chemotherapy but a generally favorable prognosis.[60] In contrast, the diffuse blastemal subtype is associated with presentation at an advanced stage but also with a rapid response to chemotherapy. The anaplastic tumors are characterized by large, pleomorphic, and hyperchromatic nuclei with abnormal multipolar mitotic figures. Anaplasia can occur in the epithelial, stromal, or blastemal populations or any combination of these three. Anaplasia occurs primarily in children older than 2 years. In NWTS-1, 66.7% of the patients with anaplasia experienced relapse and 58.3% died of their tumor.[53] Even in this early report, the distinct implications of the "diffuse" versus the "focal" pattern were appreciated, with a higher frequency of relapse and death in the "diffuse" subgroup. This was confirmed in review of the NWTS-2 and NWTS-3 data. Whereas children with stage I anaplastic tumors generally did well, children with stage II to IV tumors did poorly. The severity of dysplasia was not a predictive factor. However, anaplasia in extrarenal tumor sites and a predominantly blastemal tumor pattern were both adverse prognostic factors.[61]

Approximately 1% of children initially seen with a unilateral tumor will develop contralateral disease. In 58 of 4669 (1%) children registered in the first four NWTSG studies, metachronous disease developed.[62] Analysis of this cohort by a matched case-control study demonstrated that the children with NRs had a significantly increased risk of metachronous disease, particularly those with PLNRs. This finding was especially true for young children, in whom a Wilms' tumor occurred in 20 of 206 children younger than 12 months, in comparison with none of 304 children older than 12 months. These infants younger than 12 months with Wilms' tumor and NRs, as well as the syndromic patients, require regular surveillance for several years for the development of contralateral disease. This increased risk for metachronous tumors in children with Wilms' tumor and nephrogenic rests has been confirmed by others.[63]

Clear cell sarcoma of the kidney (CCSK) is a highly malignant tumor with an unusual proclivity for bony metastasis. It generally appears as a large unifocal and unilateral tumor with homogeneous mucoid, tan, or gray/tan cut surface, often with foci of necrosis or prominent cyst formation.[3,64] This tumor invades surrounding renal parenchyma rather than compressing the margin into a pseudocapsule, as seen in Wilms' tumor. Its classic appearance is that of a deceptively bland tumor with uniform oval nuclei with a delicate chromatin pattern, a prominent nuclear membrane,

Table 67-4 Staging System Utilized by the Société Internationale d'Oncologie Pédiatrique (Based on Findings after Preoperative Therapy)

Stage	Description
Stage I	Tumor limited to the kidney, complete excision
Stage II	Tumor extending outside the kidney, complete excision
	Invasion beyond the capsule, perirenal/ perihilar
	Invasion of the regional lymph nodes* (stage II N1)
	Invasion of extrarenal vessels
	Invasion of ureter
Stage III	Invasion beyond the capsule with incomplete excision
	Preoperative or perioperative biopsy
	Preoperative/perioperative rupture
	Peritoneal metastases
	Invasion of para-aortic lymph nodes†
	Incomplete excision
Stage IV	Distant metastases
Stage V	Bilateral renal tumors

*Hilar nodes and/or periaortic nodes at the origin of the renal artery.
†Para-aortic nodes below the renal artery.

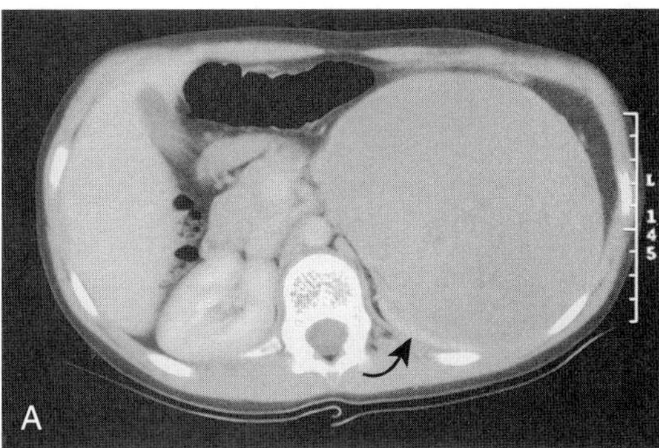

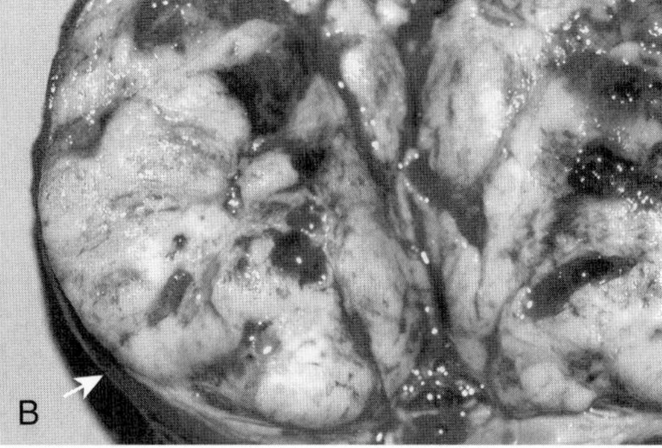

Figure 67-4. **A,** CT scan of a 10-year-old boy who presented with a large left upper quadrant abdominal mass identified on a routine "well child examination" demonstrates the characteristic findings of Wilms' tumor. The tumor mass is well circumscribed and can be seen with a margin of renal parenchyma along the periphery (*arrow*). **B,** The gross pathologic specimen shows the lobular nature of this standard histology Wilms' tumor. Again, the tumor can be seen extending from the normal renal parenchyma (*arrow*).

and sparse, poorly stained vacuolated "water-clear" cytoplasm with indistinct cell membranes. Although the cells often appear in cords or nests divided by an arborizing network of vessels and supporting spindle cell septa, nine major histologic patterns have been identified.[64] The cell of origin of this tumor is not known. In addition to osseous metastases, clear cell sarcomas also have a significant incidence of metastases to the brain. Late recurrences also are seen with this tumor, with 30% of the relapses occurring more than 2 years after diagnosis.[65] For this reason, clinical trials must consider results after an extended interval of follow-up.

Malignant rhabdoid tumors of the kidney occur in young infants with a median age of 11 months, and 85% of the cases occur within the first 2 years of life.[57] A characteristic involvement of the perihilar renal parenchyma is seen. Histologically, rhabdoid tumors are characterized by monomorphous, discohesive, rounded to polygonal cells with acidophilic cytoplasm and eccentric nuclei containing prominent large "owl eye" nucleoli reminiscent of skeletal muscle, but lacking its cytoplasmic striations, ultrastructural features, and immunochemical markers.[3] A large periodic acid–Schiff (PAS)-positive hyaline cytoplasmic inclusion occurs in a variable population of tumor cells and is a hallmark of this tumor.[66] Ultrastructural examination reveals parallel cytoplasmic filamentous inclusions packed in concentric whorled arrays, a distinctive feature of this tumor, which suggests a neuroectodermal origin. The tumor tends to infiltrate surrounding renal parenchyma rather than to compress it. These tumors are notable for the occurrence of second primary neuroglial tumors in the midline of the brain, resembling medulloblastoma.[67] A consistent deletion of 22q11-12 has been described in both renal and extrarenal rhabdoid tumors.[68,69] These deletions delineate an area of overlap at the site of the *hSNF5/INI1* gene and tumors have biallelic alternations or deletions of this gene.[70,71]

The occurrence of primitive neuroectodermal tumors (PNET) of the kidney is well documented.[72] It is clearly distinct from Wilms' tumor and the other variants previously discussed and demonstrates spread to lymph nodes, lung, bone, liver, and bone marrow, as occurs from PNET at other anatomic locations.[73] Treatment including resection, chemotherapy, and irradiation must follow that of PNETs and not that of other renal tumors.

Clinical Presentation

The classic presentation of a Wilms' tumor is the identification of an asymptomatic flank mass in an otherwise healthy toddler. It is often noted during a bath or by the pediatrician at a routine visit, and the mass may be of considerable size. This is in marked contrast to neuroblastoma, which is seen in the same age group but frequently presents as pain, often from osseous metastasis. Wilms' tumor also may be associated with hematuria, but with a much lower frequency than is seen with renal cell carcinoma. Uncommon presentations include hypertension or fever. Occasionally a child may have abdominal trauma and demonstrate pain and an abdominal mass out of proportion to what is expected. Radiographic examination will reveal a mass that cannot be attributed to the trauma alone.

Treatment

As a result of the work that demonstrated the role of adjuvant therapy in this tumor, all children treated on the early protocols of the NWTSG and SIOP received chemotherapy. Only in the past decade has adjuvant therapy been avoided in a small proportion of children with an extremely low risk of local recurrence and metastasis. Optimal chemotherapy regimens have been established by a series of well-designed randomized studies performed primarily by the NWTSG in the United States and Canada and SIOP in Europe. Despite advances in chemotherapy, surgery continues to play a critical role in the treatment of Wilms' tumor. Accurate staging and safe and complete resection of the tumor are key elements in achieving cure. Local control is rarely achieved with chemotherapy and radiation therapy alone.

Table 67-5 Randomization for Favorable Histology Wilms' Tumors on NWTS-3

Stage	Treatment	Results	
		4-Year DFS	*4-Year OS*
Stage II	Vcr, Dac	87.4%	91.1%
	Vcr, Dac + XRT (20 Gy abd)	NS	NS
	Vcr, Dac, Dox	NS	NS
	Vcr, Dac, Dox + XRT (20 Gy abd)	NS	NS
Stage III	Vcr, Dac + XRT (10 Gy abd)	Improved survival with addition of doxorubicin	
	Vcr, Dac + XRT (20 Gy abd)		
	Vcr, Dac, Dox + XRT (10 Gy abd)	82.0%	90.9%
	Vcr, Dac, Dox + XRT (20 Gy abd)	No difference in local recurrence between 10 and 20 Gy	
Stage IV	Vcr, Dac, Dox	79.0%	80.9%
	Vcr, Dac, Dox, Cyclo	NS improvement from the addition of cyclophosphamide	
	All abd XRT 20 Gy & pulmonary XRT 12 Gy		

Data from D'Angio GJ, Breslow N, Beckwith JB, et al: Treatment of Wilms' tumor: Results of the Third National Wilms' Tumor Study. Cancer 64: 349-360, 1989.)

Vcr, vincristine; Dac, dactinomycin; XRT, radiation therapy; abd, abdomen; Dox, doxorubicin; Cyclo, cyclophosphamide; DFS, disease-free survival; OS, overall survival; NS, not statistically significant.

Chemotherapy

Wilms' tumor was the first malignant pediatric solid tumor with a demonstrated response to dactinomycin.[1] Many additional effective agents have been subsequently identified: vincristine, doxorubicin, cyclophosphamide, ifosfamide, and etoposide. Children with stage I tumors were treated on the third NWTSG protocol (NWTS-3) with an 11-week regimen composed of vincristine and dactinomycin, without abdominal irradiation, based on the results of the initial two studies. The 4-year relapse-free survival (RFS) and overall survival (OS) were 89.0% and 95.6%, respectively.[74] The other three stages were treated on a regimen that involved randomization of two or four arms (Table 67-5). This study supported the addition of doxorubicin to the treatment of children with stage III tumors but did not demonstrate any benefit from the addition of doxorubicin or radiation therapy for children with stage II tumors or benefit from the addition of cyclophosphamide to the treatment of children with stage IV tumors.

NWTS-4 built on the lessons learned from the prior studies and addressed the issue of whether dose intensification could be safely used to decrease the number of visits for chemotherapy and yet maintain the favorable results previously achieved. Dactinomycin and doxorubicin were administered in single moderately high doses, compared with the traditional divided dose regimens for each drug. This study also evaluated the use of two time intervals for the administration of chemotherapy: a short course (18 to 26 weeks, depending on the regimen and stage) versus a long course (54 to 66 weeks). The findings in this study were that the pulse-intensive regimens actually produced less hematologic toxicity than the standard regimens, allowing greater dose intensity with comparable outcomes.[75,76] The second randomization demonstrated no benefit in any of the stages to the long interval of therapy over the short interval.[60]

A recent analysis of patients with stage II and III Wilms' tumors with favorable histology treated on NWTS-3 and NWTS-4 assessed the efficacy of the addition of doxorubicin.[77] Whereas no benefit was seen in the stage II patients, a decrease in the 8-year event-free survival (EFS) and OS of randomized patients was seen for those with stage III disease who received doxorubicin, dactinomycin, and vincristine (84% and 89%) compared with those who received dactinomycin and vincristine alone (74% and 83%). When a large group of nonrandomized patients were added to the analysis, the beneficial effect on OS was not seen. Unfortunately, this addition of nonrandomized patients added some question of bias.

The goal of NWTS-5 was to evaluate preliminary findings from pilot studies that LOH for chromosomes 1p and 16q were associated with an adverse prognosis. To most efficiently address this question, this was the first study from NWTSG that did not involve randomization of treatment. This study demonstrated that LOH at either site in children with favorable-histology stage I and II disease was predictive of decreased EFS. Also, in children with stage III and IV disease, the presence of LOH at both sites was predictive (Fig. 67-5).[78] A subsequent analysis has suggested that expression of telomerase RNA may also be an adverse prognostic factor for favorable-histology Wilms' tumor, but confirmatory studies will be required.[79]

Two additional components of the NWTS-5 study have been reported for favorable-histology patients. Fifty-eight children with initial stage I and II disease experienced relapse after treatment with vincristine and dactinomycin.[80] Their relapse therapy included alternating courses of vincristine/doxorubicin/cyclophosphamide and etoposide/cyclophosphamide along with surgery, if feasible, and radiation therapy. The lung was the only site of relapse in 31 children. These patients did fairly well with an EFS at 4 years of 71.1% and OS of 81.8%. Those with only pulmonary relapse

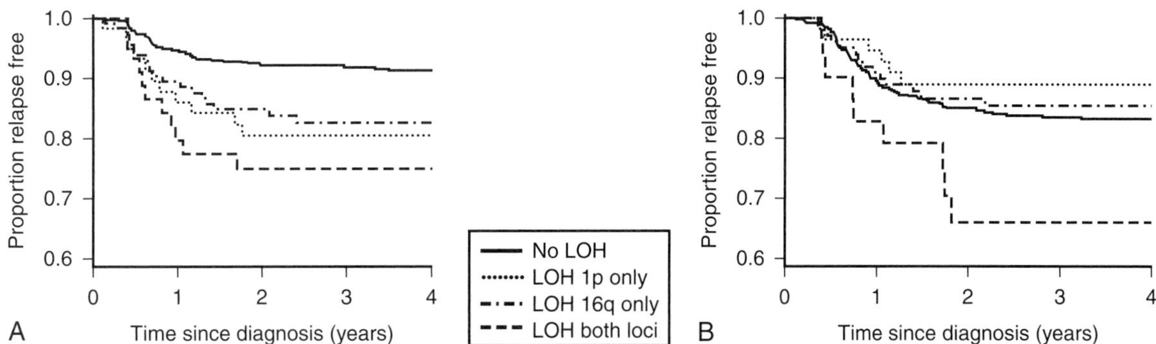

Figure 67-5. A, Relapse-free survival with loss of heterozygosity (LOH) at chromosomes 1p and 16q for patients with stage I/II Wilms' tumor of favorable histology. **B,** Relapse-free survival for patients with stage III/IV Wilms' tumor with favorable histology and LOH at chromosome 1p and 16q. (From Grundy PE, Breslow N, Li S, Loss of heterozygosity for chromosomes 1p and 16q is an adverse prognostic factor in favorable-histology Wilms' tumor: A report from the National Wilms' Tumor Study Group. J Clin Oncol 23:7312 -7321, 2005, with permission from the American Society of Clinical Oncology.)

were similar with an EFS of 67.8% and an OS of 81.0%. Sixty patients on NWTS-5 relapsed after initial therapy with vincristine, dactinomycin, and doxorubicin along with radiation therapy for stage III and IV disease.[81] Their relapse therapy included alternating cycles of cyclophosphamide/etoposide and carboplatin/etoposide along with surgery and radiation therapy. The lung was the sole site of relapse in 33 patients. EFS in these patients at 4 years was 42.3% and OS was 48.0%, whereas it was 48.9% and 52.8%, respectively, for those with only pulmonary relapse. The lower survival in this cohort could be due either to intrinsically more aggressive disease or to the significant prior treatment of the tumors.

Treatment of children with anaplastic tumors with standard therapy has resulted in a high rate of failure. Thus, in sequential studies, therapy has been intensified. Review of the NWTS-3 and NWTS-4 studies demonstrated that children with focal anaplasia had an excellent outcome when treated with vincristine, doxorubicin, and dactinomycin.[55] The addition of cyclophosphamide to this regimen improved the 4-year EFS in children with diffuse anaplasia with stages II to IV disease from 27.2% to 54.8%. Subsequent studies in NWTS-5 have further intensified therapy with the use of doxorubicin, cyclophosphamide, vincristine, and etoposide for 24 weeks plus flank/abdominal irradiation in children with stages II to IV disease. Patients with stage I disease were treated with vincristine and dactinomycin for 18 weeks. The 4-year EFS and OS of stage I patients were 69.5% and 82.6%, respectively, compared with the same survivals for stage I favorable histology of 92.4% and 98.3%.[82] The EFS progressively declined for increasing stage from 82.6% for stage II, 64.7% for stage III, and only 33.3% for stage IV disease. Clearly, even with this intensification of therapy, patients with anaplasia do not fare well.

Doxorubicin was found to be particularly effective in the treatment of clear cell sarcoma of the kidney.[83,84] However, the results have remained below those of standard-histology Wilms' tumors. No benefit was seen to pulse-intensive administration of the agents, and no difference in survival was noted at 5 and 8 years between patients treated for 6 or 15 months.[85] Treatment consisted of vincristine/doxorubicin/cyclophosphamide alternating with cyclophosphamide/etoposide for 24 weeks on NWTS-5 with local radiation therapy. Five-year EFS and OS of 79% and 89% respectively were achieved, but results remained very stage dependent with survival by stage I of 100%; II, 87%; III, 74%; and IV, 36%.[86] The most frequent site of relapse was the brain in 11 of 21 cases.

The rhabdoid tumors have remained the most resistant of all pediatric renal tumors. Current studies have used an intensive therapy with carboplatin, etoposide, and cyclophosphamide. Analysis of 142 children treated on NWTS-1 to NWTS-5 showed an overall survival of 23.2% at 4 years.[87] Survival was stage dependent and children with stage I/II disease had a 41.8% 4-year survival, while children with stage III, IV, or V tumors had a 15.9% 4-year survival. Survival was also clearly related to the age at presentation, with the 4-year survival worst for those birth to 5 months of age at diagnosis (8.8%) and best for those older than 2 years of age (41.1%). NWTS-5 used an intensive therapy with carboplatin, etoposide, and cyclophosphamide. Unfortunately, no improvement in survival occurred with the series of treatments from NWTS-1 to NWTS-5 and no survival benefit was demonstrated with the use of doxorubicin.

SIOP has promoted the use of preoperative treatment of children with Wilms' tumor with radiation therapy or chemotherapy since the early 1970s. Histologic confirmation of the diagnosis before therapy is not routinely performed in SIOP protocols. This approach has several risks. One is the potential for administration of chemotherapy for benign disease. Second, modification of tumor histology by the chemotherapy may occur. Third, staging information may be lost. Fourth, a malignant rhabdoid tumor of the kidney or clear cell sarcoma, if present, will not respond to standard therapies. Treatment without an initial diagnosis is difficult to sustain when NWTSG and SIOP studies have demonstrated a 7.6% to 9.9% rate of benign or altered malignant diagnosis in children with a prenephrectomy diagnosis of Wilms' tumor.[88,89] The histologic diagnosis after preoperative treatment in a group of children followed by NWTSG did not appear impacted by treatment, but it is less certain if staging is altered.[90]

The major driving force for the use of preoperative therapy by SIOP was the high rate of operative tumor rupture that occurred in their early series, in which patients did not receive preliminary treatment. The rupture rate decreased from 33% (20 of 60) to 4% (3 of 72) with preoperative abdominal irradiation (20 Gy) in the first randomized SIOP study of renal tumors (SIOP-1), begun in 1971.[91] It must be noted, however, that 33% is an extremely high frequency of rupture. Survival was not improved by the decrease in operative rupture, and the incidence of local recurrence was not reported. In NWTS-1 and NWTS-2, operative rupture occurred in 22% and 12% of children, respectively.[88,92] In a subsequent SIOP randomized study of Wilms' tumors begun in 1977 (SIOP-5), the rate of rupture was essentially the same for children receiving abdominal irradiation (20 Gy) and dactinomycin (9%, 7 of 76) or a combination of vincristine and dactinomycin (6%, 5 of 88).[93,94] Radiation therapy after resection was based on the stage of the tumors, with stage I patients receiving no postoperative irradiation and stage II and III patients receiving 15 Gy in the group treated initially with radiation therapy and 30 Gy in those treated initially with chemotherapy. In SIOP-6, begun in 1980, all patients received initial preoperative chemotherapy (vincristine and dactinomycin). Radiation therapy was performed after resection to those children with stage II N1 (stage III disease). Children with stage II N0 (lymph node negative) were randomized to receive either 20 Gy of radiation therapy or no radiation to the tumor bed. All children received vincristine and dactinomycin for 38 weeks. After pretreatment, 52% of cases were stage I, and a low frequency of rupture was noted (7%). The radiation therapy randomization was halted after 108 children were randomized, 58 to radiation therapy and chemotherapy and 50 to chemotherapy alone. Six local recurrences occurred in the 50 children who did not receive radiation therapy versus no recurrences in the group that did. This suggested that prenephrectomy treatment altered the pathologic findings that would have led to a diagnosis of stage II N1 (stage III disease: lymph node involvement or capsular penetration) and to the standard administration of local irradiation. Extended follow-up studies of these children showed ultimately no statistical difference in survival, because those who experienced relapse had more treatment alternatives.[95,96] The SIOP-6 protocol also extended chemotherapy to infants older than 6 months.[97] The overall favorable outcome was not improved, and an unacceptable toxicity occurred in the young infants. For the SIOP-9 study, a reduced dose in infants was recommended.

In the SIOP-9 study initiated in 1987, a randomization was performed between 4 and 8 weeks of preoperative therapy with dactinomycin and vincristine to determine whether the additional 4 weeks of therapy produced a larger proportion of stage I tumors.[98] This study also replaced postoperative radiation therapy in stage II N0 children with administration of an anthracycline (epirubicin or doxorubicin). Preoperative treatment consisted of four weekly courses of vincristine and two 3-day courses of dactinomycin every 2 weeks versus 8 weeks of the identical therapy for patients without distant metastasis. No advantage was seen from the extended therapy in terms of staging at resection between the 4-week and 8-week courses: stage I, 64% versus 62%, or of intraoperative tumor rupture, 1% versus 3%. Therapy after resection was based on the pathologic findings. Children with stage I disease and favorable or anaplastic histology received vincristine and dactinomycin for 17 weeks. Those with stage II and III tumors with favorable histology received vincristine, dactinomycin, and epirubicin (an anthracycline) for 27 weeks, with no abdominal irradiation for stage II N0 disease or with 15 Gy of abdominal irradiation in cases of stages II N1 and III disease. This therapy resulted in a 2-year EFS of 84% versus 83% for the 4- and 8-week therapies and OS of 92% and 87%, respectively. For cases with metastatic disease, children received 6 weeks of therapy including weekly vincristine, three courses of dactinomycin, and two courses of epirubicin on weeks 1 and 5. The tumor size decreased by more than 50% in 52% of the cases. During the second 4 weeks of therapy, there was another 50% reduction in 33% of the cases (Fig. 67-6). Inappropriate preoperative therapy was given to 5.5% of the cases, including 1.6% who proved to have benign lesions or malignant lesions not expected to respond to the therapy, including neuroblastoma, lymphoma, malignant rhabdoid tumors of the kidney, and renal cell carcinomas. In a recent report, the United Kingdom Children's Cancer Study Group (UKCCSG) identified 12% of cases that were clinically and radiographically consistent with Wilms' tumor but had other diagnoses established by biopsy.[99]

In SIOP-9, the surgical procedure–related complications were reported to be 8%.[100] In this treatment regimen, patients with post-therapy stage II disease received an anthracycline, whereas in the NWTS studies, patients with stage II disease received vincristine and dactinomycin alone. In SIOP-9, an evaluation of children with completely necrotic tumors at the time of resection demonstrated that they had an extremely favorable prognosis.[101] Complete necrosis was seen in 10% of 599 children enrolled into the study. In total, 37 children in this cohort had stages I to III disease and 22 had stage IV disease. Disease-free survival was 98% at 5 years versus 90% for the other patients on SIOP-9. The only death in the stage I to III group was related to chemotherapy, and survival was 100% in the stage IV group.

The goal of both NWTSG and SIOP has been to decrease the intensity of therapy and yet achieve the maximal long-term survival. Both groups have decreased the amount of radiation therapy used during the course of their studies. Among the children with unilateral nonmetastatic Wilms' tumors of favorable histology, 24% of those enrolled in NWTS (275 of 1160) were given radiation therapy and 18% of those in SIOP (81 of 447) have received irradiation in the most recent studies.[102] SIOP has elected, however, to

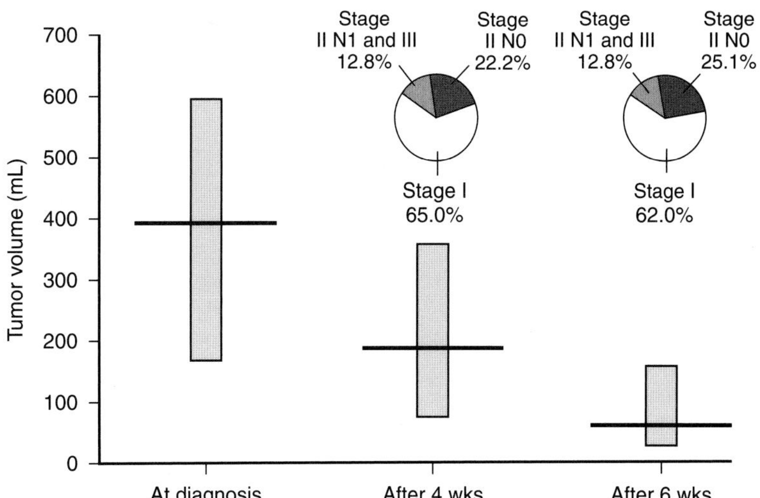

Figure 67-6. Diagram of the results from the GPOH subgroup of SIOP-9 demonstrates the progressive decrease in the volume of the renal tumors after 4 and 6 weeks of preoperative chemotherapy. The pie charts demonstrate the distribution of tumor stages that reveal an increase in low stage I tumors compared with historical controls (not shown). (From Graff N, et al: The role of preoperative chemotherapy in the management of Wilms' tumor: The SIOP studies. Urol Clin North Am 27:443-454, 2000.)

use an anthracycline rather than irradiation for their postchemotherapy stage II N0 patients in whom excessive local relapse occurred without additional therapy. This results in about 48% of patients in SIOP studies with unilateral nonmetastatic tumors of favorable histology receiving an anthracycline, which is significantly greater than the 24% of comparable patients on NWTSG regimens.

Significant complications have occurred in some children treated with doxorubicin, particularly that of cardiomyopathy.[103,104] In children treated on NWTS-1 to NWTS-4, the cumulative frequency of congestive heart failure was 4.4% at 20 years after diagnosis for those treated initially with doxorubicin, although recent estimates of the 20-year risk of congestive heart failure for children treated on NWTS-3 and NWTS-4 is now reported as 1.2%.[77] The relative risk was increased in female subjects, by cumulative dose, lung irradiation, and left-sided abdominal irradiation. Subclinical echocardiographic abnormalities have been demonstrated in children who received as little as 45 mg/m^2 of doxorubicin.[105] Only long-term follow-up of children who have received doxorubicin will document what dose, if any, is free of long-term implications.

Second malignant neoplasms also are a concern. NWTSG reported a 1.6% incidence of second malignant neoplasms at 15 years after treatment.[106] Second malignancies correlated with prior treatment of relapsed tumor, the amount of abdominal radiation, and the use of doxorubicin. Acute myelogenous leukemia was seen in patients whose treatment included either doxorubicin or etoposide.[107]

Whereas renal failure can be produced by bilateral nephrectomy, it also results from the nephropathy associated with several of the genetic syndromes. A significant incidence of renal failure most frequently developed from focal segmental glomerulosclerosis in children with WAGR syndrome and from diffuse mesangial sclerosis in children with Denys-Drash syndrome. The cumulative incidence of end-stage renal failure at 20 years after diagnosis of unilateral Wilms' tumor was 74% for 17 patients with the Denys-Drash syndrome, 36% for 37 patients with WAGR, 7% for 125 males with hypospadias or cryptorchidism, and 0.6% for 5347 patients without any of the other conditions (Fig. 67-7).[108] In children with bilateral tumors, all of these incidences are increased: 50% for the Denys-Drash syndrome, 90% for WAGR, 25% for associated genitourinary abnormalities, and 12% for those without associated conditions.

Other complications identified in patients after treatment for Wilms' tumor include diffuse interstitial pneumonitis, loss of stature, and difficulties with pregnancy primarily related to abdominal and pelvic irradiation.[109-112]

Current guidelines for radiation therapy in the North American protocols are determined by the histology and stage of the tumor. All patients receive a relatively low dose of radiation (1200 cGy) to the lung if pulmonary metastases are present, although the SIOP studies have recently excluded pulmonary irradiation in many of these children. The current protocol of the Children's Oncology Group has made two significant changes with regard to patients with pulmonary disease. First, lesions seen by CT scan only will be considered to have pulmonary metastasis unless biopsy proven not to have metastatic disease. In past protocols this has been based on standard radiographs of the chest. Second, in an attempt to spare pulmonary radiation in those children who appear to have responsive disease, children will not receive radiation therapy if the pulmonary lesions radiographically resolve by CT scan after 6 weeks of chemotherapy.

Abdominal irradiation (1080 cGy) is employed for all patients with Wilms' tumor of favorable histology who have stage III disease in the abdomen. Recent long-term results from NWTS-3 and NWTS-4 have shown that increasing the dose of radiation therapy to the flank from 10 to 20 Gy will decrease the frequency of flank relapse. Overall survival of the patients is not improved because of the lower postrecurrence mortality among nonirradiated patients.[113] Current doses employed are 1080 cGy for stage I to III focal anaplasia, stage I and II diffuse anaplasia, and stage II and III clear cell sarcoma of the kidney. Higher doses of 1980 cGy

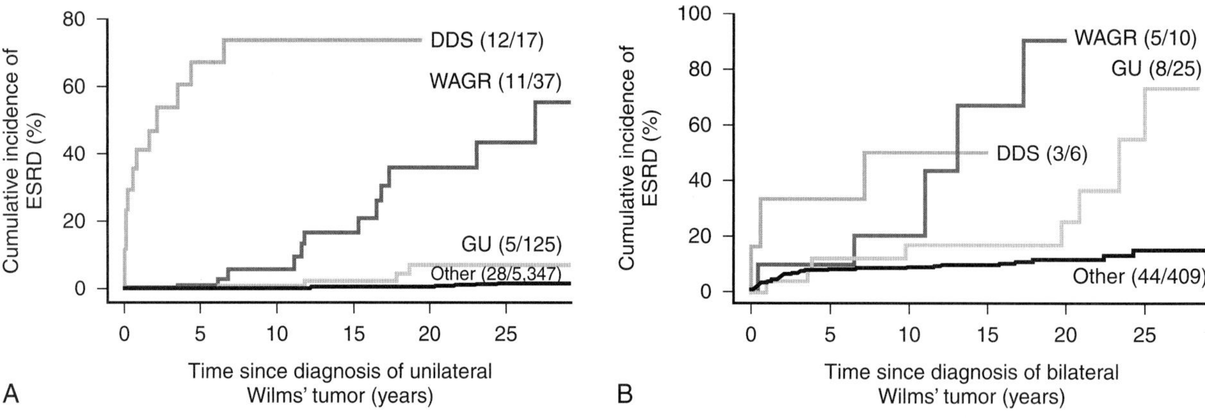

Figure 67-7. **A,** Cumulative incidence of end-stage renal disease (ESRD) in children with unilateral Wilms' tumor with Denys-Drash syndrome (DDS), WAGR syndrome, associated genitourinary anomalies (GU), and other anomalies (Other) over time. **B,** Similar plot of children with bilateral Wilms' tumors. In both groups of children, a very significant incidence of ESRD is documented. (From Breslow NE, et al: End stage renal disease in patients with Wilms' tumor: Results from the National Wilms' Tumor Study Group and The United States Renal Data System. J Urol 174:1972-1975, 2005, with permission from the American Urological Association.)

are utilized for stage III diffuse anaplasia, and for rhabdoid tumor of the kidney in infants 12 months and older. Younger infants still receive 1080 cGy.

Surgical Procedures

The NWTSG has advocated initial resection of the tumor in all of its protocols. Although most Wilms' tumors are first seen as a large mass, resection is generally feasible (Fig. 67-8). Wilms' tumor, in contrast to neuroblastoma, is much less likely to invade surrounding organs and lymph nodes. Children undergoing initial nephrectomy in the NWTS-3 study had a complication rate of 19.8% in a group that was very closely monitored.[106] The most frequent complication was intestinal obstruction, occurring in 6.9% of the

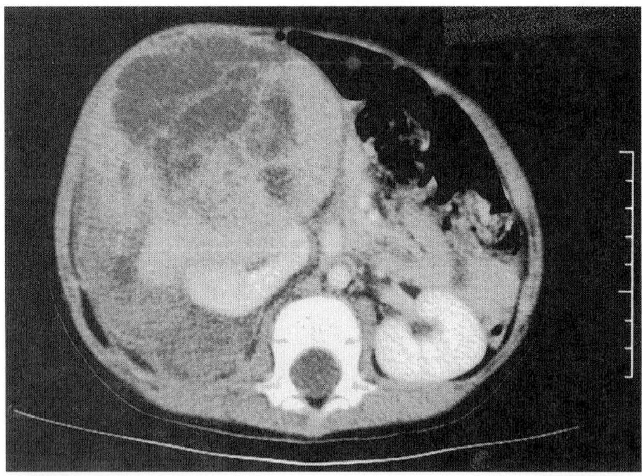

Figure 67-8. CT scan of a 3-year-old boy who presented with a history of abdominal pain, fever, and a right flank mass. The tumor is very large with extension outside the renal capsule into the retroperitoneal tissues posterior to the kidney. Despite its size, this lesion was able to be completely resected. Lymph nodes and specimen margins were negative for tumor. This tumor was therefore stage 2, and the infant was able to avoid both anthracycline therapy and abdominal irradiation because of the complete resection.

children, followed by extensive intraoperative hemorrhage (>50 mL/kg) occurring in 5.8%.[114] Injuries to other visceral organs (1%) and extensive vascular injuries (1.4%) were much less frequent. Nine deaths in the series were attributed to surgical complications (0.5%), only one of which was intraoperative. The factors associated with an increased risk of surgical complications were advanced-stage local disease, intravascular extension of the tumor, and resection of other organs. The latter were often found not to be invaded by the tumor but rather compressed, distorted, or adherent, without actual tumor infiltration. Extensive resection involving removal of other organs or operations that are of a magnitude to be life threatening should be aborted. In some cases, tumor biopsy and biopsy of the regional lymph nodes should be performed, followed by administration of chemotherapy before a second attempt at resection (Fig. 67-9). With the use of this algorithm, 93% of 131 children enrolled in NWTS-3 who were initially judged to have unresectable disease at operation or by imaging studies successfully underwent resection after initial chemotherapy or irradiation or both.[115] Only 8 children with tumors that grew or failed to respond did not undergo subsequent nephrectomy.

Complications in the NWTS-4 study have also been assessed.[116] In this study, surgeons were discouraged from performing extensive operations involving resection of adjacent organs or massive tumors. Complications occurred in 12.7% of a random sample of 534 of the 3335 patients treated in this study. Again, intestinal obstruction was the most frequent complication (5.1%), followed by extensive hemorrhage (1.9%), wound infection (1.9%), and vascular injury (1.5%). The factors associated with an increased risk of complications were again assessed. Intravascular tumor extension into the inferior vena cava or atrium and nephrectomy performed through a flank or paramedian incision were both significant factors. Tumor diameter of 10 cm or larger also was associated with increased complications. Finally, the risk of complications was

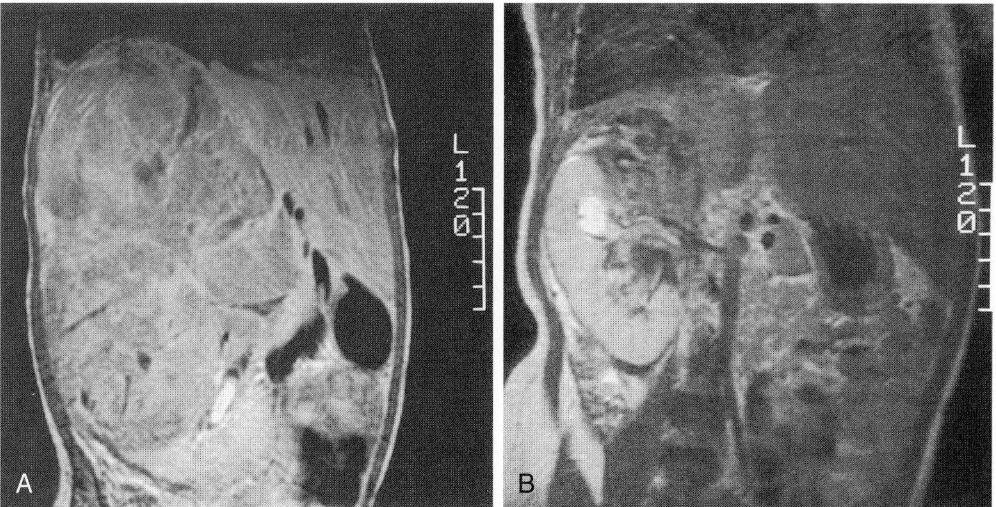

Figure 67-9. **A,** MR image of a 2 1/2-year-old girl who presented with a massive right-sided abdominal mass. Chest radiograph revealed pulmonary nodules. Because of the massive size of the primary and metastatic disease, she received initial chemotherapy after a needle biopsy demonstrated a standard risk tumor (diffuse blastemal subtype). She received three courses of dactinomycin, vincristine, and cyclophosphamide, which achieved some shrinkage of the tumor. At surgery, there was a very extensive tumor that was densely adherent to the posterior aspect of the liver and the vena cava. It was clear that resection of a portion of the liver would be required with the nephrectomy. Efforts at resection were terminated. Repeat biopsies again demonstrated a standard histology Wilms' tumor with tumor invasion into the liver. She was treated on a new protocol involving cisplatin and etoposide as well as abdominal and thoracic radiation. **B,** MR image, after additional therapy, showed remarkable shrinkage of the tumor, allowing a much easier and safer resection.

increased if the resection was performed by a general surgeon rather than a pediatric surgeon or pediatric urologist. In a recent study involving 598 patients registered on SIOP-9, a complication rate of 8% was reported. These patients were pretreated with vincristine, dactinomycin, and epirubicin or doxorubicin before nephrectomy.[75] The most frequent events were small bowel obstruction (3.7%) and tumor rupture (2.8%). The latter is not reported as a complication in the NWTS reviews. Other complications occurred in 2.0% of patients.

Surgical Details

Radiographic imaging is critical before surgical resection of a renal tumor (Fig. 67-10). The most important factors to assess in these imaging studies are the presence of two functioning kidneys, presence of contralateral tumor, and evidence of intravascular extension of the tumor. Intraoperative identification of intravascular extension has been associated with an increased incidence of surgical complications.[117] The organ of origin of the tumor can be determined in most cases, with the differential diagnosis generally between neuroblastoma and Wilms' tumor. This can generally be determined by the configuration of the kidney and the mass. In neuroblastoma, the mass will generally indent the kidney, whereas in Wilms' tumor the mass will arise from within the kidney and distort its internal configuration. Often a thin lip of renal parenchyma can be seen extending over the neoplasm in Wilms' tumor (see Fig. 67-4A). Intra-abdominal staging has been difficult to assess radiographically unless extensive lymph node involvement

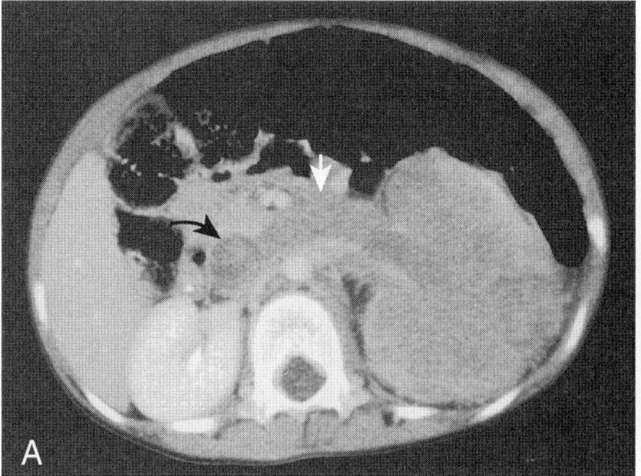

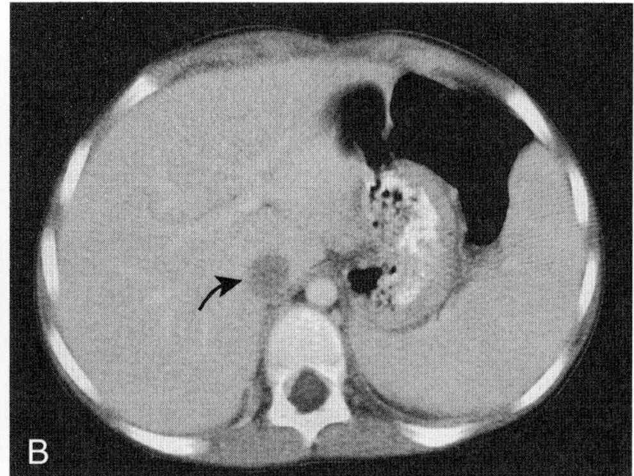

Figure 67-10. **A,** CT scan of a 7-year-old boy who presented with a left-sided abdominal mass demonstrates tumor extending through the left renal vein (*white arrow*) into the inferior vena cava (*black arrow*). **B,** Higher levels on the CT scan demonstrated tumor completely occluding the intrahepatic inferior vena cava (*black arrow*).

or intrahepatic metastases are present. A radiograph of the chest and CT scan will help determine the presence of pulmonary metastases. If the lesions are seen on the radiograph, their malignant nature must generally be assumed. Smaller lesions seen only on the CT scan should generally be sampled to confirm their malignant nature because recent studies demonstrated that these lesions were malignant in 82% of cases if the lesion was isolated and 69% if there were multiple lesions present.[118] Bone scans and brain scans are routinely performed only if the renal tumor proves to be a clear cell sarcoma or rhabdoid tumor.

Renal tumors must be resected through an adequate subcostal or thoracoabdominal incision. Struggling through an inadequate incision will often result in rupture of the tumor, increasing both the stage of the tumor and the risk for intra-abdominal recurrence.[119] A flank incision should not be used for resection in pediatric renal tumors because of the limited exposure it allows.

Initial exploration of the abdomen should be performed, including inspection for hepatic metastases or intraperitoneal spread. The vena cava, if it is accessible, also should be palpated to assess for intravascular extension of tumor. Exploration of the contralateral kidney with opening of Gerota's fascia was recommended by the NWTSG based on the 5% occurrence of synchronous lesions. In NWTS-2 and NWTS-3, contralateral involvement was not detected by intravenous pyelography (IVP) or CT in approximately one third of the children with bilateral tumors.[36] Review of children with bilateral tumors treated on NWTS-4 identified 9 of 122 children in whom the diagnosis of bilateral disease was missed by the preoperative imaging studies (CT, ultrasonography, or MRI).[120] All but one of these lesions were small: five were smaller than 1 cm, and three were 1 to 3 cm in diameter. Recent review of this material, however, has suggested that some of the small lesions on the contralateral kidney that were initially thought to be small Wilms' tumors would now be more correctly defined as hyperplastic NRs.[121] The overall outcome of children with these small lesions was also extremely favorable with no recurrences. Current studies by the Children's Oncology Group do not require examination of the contralateral side if there is no suggestion of involvement on the preoperative radiographic studies.

After initial evaluation, the colon is then mobilized off the anterior aspect of the kidney and the renal mass. Although early descriptions of the operative technique recommended initial control of the renal hilum, this is often not feasible with extremely large tumors and must await mobilization of the mass to allow safe exposure of the hilum. Premature attempts at vascular control, particularly of left-sided tumors, may result in ligation of the superior mesenteric artery.[122] Biopsy of the renal mass should not be performed unless the decision is to not proceed with a complete resection. Biopsy will produce contamination of the peritoneum and increase the stage of the tumor to stage III.

Biopsy of lymph nodes in the renal hilum and along the vena cava or aorta is critical for adequate staging. Even in children with stage IV disease, local staging is critical because it will determine whether abdominal radiation therapy is used in children treated on Children's Oncology Group protocols. Studies have demonstrated that the surgeon's gross evaluation and assessment of lymph nodes does not reliably correspond with the pathologic involvement of tumor with false-negative and false-positive rates of 31.3% and 18.1%, respectively.[123] An increased incidence of local recurrence was seen in children enrolled in NWTS-4, in whom biopsy of lymph nodes was not performed, particularly stage I cases.[119] This suggested that undertreatment of local disease in these children due to inadequate staging resulted in an increased frequency of local recurrence. Although grossly involved lymph nodes are generally resected, an extensive retroperitoneal lymph node resection has not been demonstrated to improve local control.[92]

As the tumor is being mobilized, the ureter is resected close to the bladder to avoid a "diverticulum" on the bladder, which might produce recurrent urinary tract infection, but primarily to make certain that any extension of tumor into the ureter is entirely resected. Gross hematuria in children with Wilms' tumor is infrequent, but its occurrence suggests extensive involvement of the renal pelvis with possible extension down into the ureter. Cystoscopy should be considered in these children to identify extension of the tumor into the bladder and to avoid transection of the tumor thrombus during division of the ureter. Ureteral extension that is entirely resected does not increase the local stage of the tumor. If the tumor involves the upper pole, the adrenal gland is generally resected to provide adequate margins around the tumor and also to obtain periaortic or pericaval lymph nodes. With lower-pole lesions, the adrenal gland may be preserved.

The factors associated with an increased risk of local recurrence are stage III disease, unfavorable histology (especially diffuse anaplasia), and tumor rupture during operation.[119] Tumor rupture is the only factor that the surgeon can impact. Multiple regression analysis adjusting for the combined effects of histology, lymph node involvement, and age reveal that tumor spillage remained significant and was greatest in children with stage II disease who received less intensive therapy. Most tumor ruptures occur during mobilization of the posterior aspects of the tumor where it is adherent to the diaphragm. This can be best prevented by the use of an adequate incision for exposure and resection of a segment of the adherent diaphragm, if necessary.

Resection of adjacent organs (liver, spleen, or pancreas) or resection of massive Wilms' tumors are discouraged in the recent NWTSG and Children's Oncology Group studies based on reviews of complications. Such extensive resections are associated with a significant increase in surgical complications.[116] Only in this situation should the surgeon sample the primary tumor along with perihilar and periaortic/caval lymph nodes.

Preoperative evaluation of children with renal tumors should also include studies of coagulation. An "acquired" von Willebrand's disease has been seen in children with Wilms' tumor. This coagulopathy can produce problems with hemostasis if it is not identified and corrected before operation.[124]

Preoperative Therapy

Preoperative adjuvant treatment of Wilms' tumor is generally accepted in certain circumstances: the finding of Wilms' tumor in a solitary kidney, bilateral renal tumors, tumor in a horseshoe kidney, intravascular extension of the tumor above the intrahepatic vena cava, and respiratory distress from extensive metastatic tumor. In such cases, pretreatment biopsy should be obtained. Percutaneous biopsy is often used, although needle-tract seeding has been reported.[125] The aim of treatment (before surgical resection in the bilateral tumors and tumor in a horseshoe or solitary kidney) is to preserve maximal renal parenchyma and function. The anatomy of the kidney has not been recognized before surgical exploration in many of the cases of Wilms' tumor arising within a horseshoe kidney.[126] This is often due to the large size of the tumor distorting the anatomy. An increased incidence of urine leak and ureteral injury occurs in this situation because of the aberrant anatomy of the collecting systems.

Although growth of the remaining kidney has been documented (achieving 180% volume augmentation), the occurrence of focal segmental glomerulosclerosis has been reported in children with a unilateral kidney.[127,128] In the NWTS-1 to NWTS-4 population, the incidence of renal failure after unilateral nephrectomy was only 0.25%.[98] Studies from Europe on pretreatment of unilateral Wilms' tumor have demonstrated that, in most instances, a nephrectomy is still required, rather than a partial nephrectomy, because of the extent of tumor involvement in the kidney at presentation.[129]

The efficacy of preoperative chemotherapy in allowing the safe performance of partial nephrectomy for Wilms' tumor has been evaluated by several centers. In Toronto, percutaneous biopsy in 37 children with Wilms' tumor was followed by multiple-agent chemotherapy for 4 to 6 weeks. A partial nephrectomy was then performed in 9 children (4 with unilateral and 5 with bilateral tumors).[130] Two children had intra-abdominal relapse. Only 4 (13.3%) of the 30 unilateral tumors were amenable to a partial nephrectomy. Another analysis of the feasibility of partial nephrectomies was performed at St. Jude Children's Research Hospital.[131] Preoperative CT scans of 43 children with nonmetastatic unilateral Wilms' tumor were reviewed retrospectively. Criteria used to determine whether a partial nephrectomy would have been feasible were involvement by the tumor of one pole and less than one third of the kidney, a functioning kidney, no involvement of the collecting system or renal vein, and clear margins between the tumor and surrounding structures. With these criteria, only two (4.7%) of 43 scans suggested that partial nephrectomy was feasible. The primary concerns regarding the use of preoperative chemotherapy to create "resectable" small tumors is that these children with small tumors at presentation may be curable with surgical resection alone without subjecting them to the toxicity of additional treatments.[102,103] Whereas the role of partial nephrectomy has been suggested in children with Beckwith-Wiedemann syndrome or hemihypertrophy in whom smaller tumors may be identified by prospective screening, the efficacy of this approach has not been established.[132]

One additional indication for the use of preoperative chemotherapy has been suggested in those patients with contained retroperitoneal rupture.[133] The concern expressed is that primary resection will result in rupture of the hematoma and require total abdominal radiation therapy. In two reported cases, preoperative chemotherapy allowed resorption of the rupture and resection without positive margins or contamination of the peritoneal cavity. This indication for preoperative chemotherapy will have to be confirmed in a larger number of patients.

Bilateral Wilms' Tumor

Children with bilateral tumors are generally younger than those with unilateral lesions, with a mean age of 25 versus 44 months.[134] Preservation of renal parenchyma is a critical issue for these children. In the NWTSG review of renal failure in 55 children from NWTS-1 to NWTS-4, 39 children had bilateral tumor involvement. Increasing efforts to preserve renal parenchyma in bilateral cases in the sequence of the NWTSG studies resulted in a decline in the incidence of renal failure from 16.4% in NWTS-1 and NWTS-2 to 9.9% in NWTS-3 and 3.8% in NWTS-4.[135] Although the incidence may increase in the more recent studies as children age, this declining frequency also is due in part to increased attempts to save part of the kidney by initial treatment of the tumor with chemotherapy. Preliminary treatment in most cases after biopsy and staging will produce shrinkage of the tumor and facilitate its resection with preservation of a portion of the kidney. It is important to perform biopsies of all tumors because "discordant" pathology does occur, with a favorable lesion on one side and unfavorable lesion (generally anaplastic) on the other. Bilateral lesions are rarely seen in association with clear cell sarcoma or rhabdoid tumors of the kidney. Ninety-eight children with bilateral Wilms' tumors underwent a partial nephrectomy of 134 kidneys during NWTS-4.[136] Complete resection of gross disease was accomplished in 118 (88%) of the 134 kidneys. A higher incidence of positive surgical margins (16%, 19 of 134) and local tumor recurrence (8.2%, 11 of 134) was seen in this group of children. These were justified by the attempt to preserve renal tissue and avoid renal failure. Overall, portions of 72% of the kidneys were preserved, and the 4-year survival rate was 81.7%. The UKCCSG also reported attempts at maximal preservation of renal parenchyma with preoperative chemotherapy.[137] Survival was equivalent for those with initial resection versus preoperative chemotherapy, but greater preservation of renal parenchyma was seen in those treated with initial chemotherapy. The presence of rhabdomyomatous histology has been associated with a poor response to preoperative chemotherapy, as defined by a decrease in size on radiographic evaluation, but it has been found to be associated with favorable survival.[138] Irradiation has been advocated to prevent relapse in children with partial nephrectomy for bilateral disease, but it may impair the ability of the kidney to grow.[139,140]

Intravascular Extension

Intravascular extension of a tumor thrombus occurs in 4% of children with Wilms' tumor. Identification of vascular extension by preoperative radiographic studies or early in the surgical exploration is critical to avoid a tumor embolus during mobilization of the kidney. Ultrasonography is probably more sensitive for detecting vascular extension than CT. The presence of intravascular extension does not affect the prognosis of the tumor as long as it is successfully resected.[141] Traditionally, intravascular extension has been managed by nephrectomy with resection of the tumor thrombus into the renal vein or vena cava. Cardiopulmonary bypass has been required for children with atrial extension of the tumor thrombus but is associated with a significant incidence of complications (70%).[117,142]

In an NWTSG report of intravascular extension of Wilms' tumor, 30 children (15 with caval and 15 with atrial extension) were treated initially with chemotherapy after biopsy of the renal mass. After treatment, a decrease in the size of the intravascular extension was noted in 23 children and complete resolution of the tumor thrombus was seen in 7 children.[143] Of the 15 children with tumor initially extending into the atrium, a complete or marked response occurred, and the tumor was removed transabdominally without bypass. Tumor embolism did not occur during chemotherapy. Fibrosis of tumor to the caval wall developed in some cases, and in two cases occlusion of the inferior vena cava occurred postoperatively. A similar review of children treated in the United Kingdom with extensive intravascular involvement also demonstrated a decrease in the extent of vascular involvement in 16 of 21 children and showed that children receiving preoperative chemotherapy had a better outcome.[144]

More recently, a review of all of the children treated on the NWTS-4 protocol described 165 of 2731 patients with intravascular extension into the inferior vena cava (134 patients) or atrium (31 patients).[145] Sixty-nine of these patients received preoperative chemotherapy (55 with inferior vena cava extension and 14 with atrial extension). Five complications were encountered during preoperative chemotherapy, including tumor embolism and tumor progression in 1 patient each, and 3 patients with adult respiratory distress syndrome, one of whom died. Intravascular extension of the tumor regressed in 39 of 49 children with comparable pre- and post-therapy radiographic studies, including regression in 7 of 12 in whom the tumor regressed from an atrial location, avoiding the need for cardiopulmonary bypass. A high frequency of surgical complications occurred in these patients: 36.7% in the children with atrial extension and 17.2% in those with extension to the inferior vena cava. The frequency of surgical complications was 26% in the primary resection group versus 13.2% in children with preoperative therapy. When all the complications were considered, including those that occurred during preoperative chemotherapy (1 of these 5 patients also had a surgical complication), the incidence of complications among those receiving preoperative therapy was not statistically different from the incidence among those who underwent primary resection. However, most of the severe complications occurred in the primary resection group. Also, preoperative therapy clearly facilitated surgical resection by decreasing the extent of the tumor thrombus.

Resection Alone for Select Favorable Wilms' Tumors

A small group of children with Wilms' tumor may require only resection of the primary tumor and kidney without adjuvant treatment. The outcomes of children younger than 2 years with stage I tumors weighing less than 550 g who have been registered in the NWTSG studies were reviewed.[146] The 4-year RFS for children meeting these criteria exceeded 90%, suggesting that they could be selected for treatment with resection alone. A similar review by the UKCCSG, in which children with stage I tumors received only vincristine "monotherapy," also demonstrated that infants younger than 2 years of age had particularly favorable 4-year EFS and OS of 93.2% and 98.1%, respectively.[147]

A pathologic review of children treated on NWTS-4 also demonstrated that age younger than 2 years and specimen weight of less than 550 g was highly associated with the absence of adverse microsubstaging variables.[148] A prospective pilot study looking at this question was performed at Children's Hospital in Boston. Eight children with stage I disease who were younger than 2 years of age with unilateral, favorable-histology tumors with a combined tumor and kidney weight under 550 g underwent tumor resection and were followed without adjuvant therapy.[149] In one child, a metachronous tumor was cured by resection and chemotherapy. Continued follow-up of patients in this series has not shown any episodes of local recurrence.[150]

One component of NWTS-5 was a trial of operation only for children younger than 2 years with small (<550-g tumor and kidney) stage I tumors of favorable histology. Seventy-five infants were enrolled in this study.[151] In 3 infants, metachronous, contralateral Wilms' tumors developed, and 8 patients experienced relapse 0.3 to 1.05 years after diagnosis. The sites of relapse were pulmonary (five cases) and operative bed (three cases). The 2-year disease-free (relapse and metachronous) survival including both relapse and metachronous tumors was 86.5%. The 2-year survival rate was 100%, with a median follow-up of 2.84 years.

The 2-year disease-free survival, excluding metachronous contralateral Wilms' tumor, was 89.2%, and the 2-year cumulative risk of metachronous contralateral Wilms' tumor was 3.1%. The stopping rule for the study required closure after these 75 infants were enrolled, but continuing evaluation of this cohort has demonstrated that they have done very well with a high rate of salvage for recurrence, perhaps because they had not been treated with chemotherapy. Further studies of these infants will be required to establish their optimal therapy. Treatment by surgery alone should be utilized only in patients enrolled in prospective studies.

Neonatal Wilms' Tumor

Wilms' tumor occurs rarely in the neonate. A review of the 3340 children entered into the NWTS studies from 1969 to 1984 revealed only 27 (0.8%) neonates (30 days old or younger) with renal tumors.[152] More than half of the neonates (18) had mesoblastic nephroma, and 4 others had non-neoplastic lesions. One infant had a malignant rhabdoid tumor, and 4 had Wilms' tumors. All of the Wilms' tumors had favorable histology and had not metastasized. The neonates did well, receiving a variety of treatments ranging from resection alone to 15 months of three-drug therapy. A subsequent report of 15 cases of Wilms' tumor occurring in neonates in the first 30 days of life again demonstrated tumors of favorable histology and the absence of metastatic disease.[153] Ten of these infants received postoperative chemotherapy, and 5 were observed without additional treatment. Only one of these 5 children had recurrence in the renal fossa and lungs and ultimately died of her disease at age 16 months. The other children are all disease free at a median follow-up of 31 months.

Extrarenal Wilms' Tumor

An extrarenal site of primary Wilms' tumor is uncommon. These extrarenal tumors behave identically to tumors arising within the kidney and should be treated both locally and systemically based on the same criteria.[154,155] Common sites of occurrence of extrarenal Wilms' tumors include the retroperitoneum, inguinal canal, scrotum, and vagina. Less common sites are the uterus, cervix, ovary, and presacral space.

RENAL CELL CARCINOMA

Children with renal cell carcinoma are generally older than those with Wilms' tumor and frequently initially have symptoms of flank pain and gross hematuria.[156] Renal cell carcinoma in children displays gross and microscopic pathologic features similar to those seen in adults. Clinical stage at the time of diagnosis is the most important prognostic factor, and the identification of renal vascular invasion did not appear to be an adverse predictor. Radical nephrectomy and regional lymphadenectomy have been the primary modality for cure, and children with distant spread have a grave prognosis. In a study of 22 children, the mean age at presentation with renal cell carcinoma was 14 years.[157] Overall survival is much worse than for Wilms' tumor, with a 5-year survival in a recent series of only 30%. Analysis of multiple factors including age, tumor size, location, and histology failed to demonstrate that they were predictors of survival. Only stage and successful complete tumor resection were meaningful prognostic factors. Survival was 60% in children with complete resection of the primary tumor and zero in those with only partial resection. Survival was stage dependent: 92.5% for stage I, 84.5% for stage II, 72.7% for stage III, and 12.7% for stage IV. It should be noted, however, that those with positive nodes but no distant metastasis had survival rates three times that of adult historical controls.[158]

Renal cell carcinoma is remarkably resistant to chemotherapy, preventing cure in most children with metastatic disease.[159] Ten to 20 percent of patients have nodal involvement identified at operation but lack evidence of distant metastatic disease. No benefit has been found for adjuvant therapy in children.[158]

Nephron-sparing resection has been used in adult patients with small polar lesions in whom no evidence of a multicentric tumor is found. In these selected cases with tumors smaller than 4 cm and a normal contralateral kidney, the risk of local recurrence is reported to be 2% or less, which is comparable to the frequency of metachronous recurrence in the contralateral kidney after unilateral radical nephrectomy.

The occurrence of late relapses long after nephrectomy, prolonged stability of disease in the absence of systemic therapy, and rare cases of spontaneous regression of tumors have led to an interest in immunotherapy comparable to that used for melanoma. Trials of immunomodulating therapy with interferon-alfa and interleukin-2 (IL-2) have demonstrated some efficacy, but maintenance of a durable cure has been elusive.[160] A trial with 294 patients with advanced-stage renal cell carcinoma randomized to receive placebo or 9 months of subcutaneous lymphoblastoid interferon demonstrated similar recurrence rates of the two groups and worse survival than those randomized to placebo alone.[161] With the significant toxicity involved with immunotherapy, demonstration of improved survival in randomized trials will be required before this can be adopted as standard therapy.

MESOBLASTIC NEPHROMA

Congenital mesoblastic nephroma, also referred to as fetal renal hamartoma or leiomyomatous hamartoma, is the most common renal tumor identified in the neonatal period. Although it was initially diagnosed and treated as a congenital Wilms' tumor, mesoblastic nephroma was defined as a distinct entity in 1967.[162] Mesoblastic nephromas appear most frequently in the neonatal period as a palpable flank mass, which can be massive. Additional symptoms seen at presentation include hematuria, hypertension, vomiting, and jaundice.[163]

Mesoblastic nephroma accounted for 2.8% of 1905 renal tumors submitted to the early NWTSG studies. Grossly, these tumors have a homogeneous rubbery appearance resembling a uterine fibroid in color and consistency (Fig. 67-11). Microscopically they are composed of sheets of fibrous or mesenchymal stroma, within which bizarre and dysplastic tubules and glomeruli are irregularly scattered.[164] The tumor can invade intact renal parenchyma, and extrarenal infiltration into the perihilar connective tissues is common. The histologic subtypes of this tumor include the classic type (24% of cases), the cellular type (66%), and the mixed type (10%). The pluripotency of these tumors is revealed by their differentiation into angiomatoid patterns, cartilaginous nests, and their elicitation of intratumoral hematopoiesis in addition to the tiny nephroblastic epithelial foci.

Recently, a characteristic chromosomal translocation, (t12;15)(p13;q25), was described. It results in fusion of the *ETV6* (also known as *TEL*) gene from 12p13 with the *NRTK3* neurotrophin-3 receptor gene (also known as *TRKC*) from 15q25.[27,29] This results in a chimeric RNA, which is characteristic of both infantile fibrosarcoma and the cellular variant of congenital mesoblastic nephroma. This may be helpful in differentiating the cellular variant from other lesions that must be considered in the differential diagnosis, including clear cell sarcoma and rhabdoid tumors. It also suggests a close relation between infantile fibrosarcoma and the cellular variant of mesoblastic nephroma.[64]

This generally benign tumor usually can be cured with nephrectomy alone. This should include generous margins around all gross tumors to avoid local recurrence. Particular attention should be paid to the medial aspect of the kidney, including the hilum and great vessels, because of the tumor's proclivity to have extensions into these perirenal soft tissues. Several children have been reported with local recurrence[165] or metastases to the brain, bones, lungs, and heart.[166-169] In some of these cases, the histology has revealed an unusual degree of mesenchymal cell immaturity and hypercellularity, suggesting a more aggressive tumor.[164] These rare occurrences, however, support the concept that mesoblastic nephroma cannot be considered a simple hamartoma and that complete nephrectomy with negative pathologic margins for tumor is critical in all cases.

In a series of 51 children with mesoblastic nephroma identified in the NWTSG series, adequate operative excision was achieved in 43 of 51 children, whereas 8 had local extension and 10 had tumor spillage during resection.[163] The use of adjuvant therapy in these cases depended on the era in which the children were treated. Twenty-three infants treated principally since 1978 had surgical resection alone. Prior to 1978, 24 had operation plus chemotherapy, and before 1976, 4 children also received irradiation. Survival was excellent in this entire group, and only 1 child died of sepsis during chemotherapy. One child's tumor recurred at 6 months despite receiving dactinomycin and vincristine. The tumor was surgically re-excised, and the child was treated with cyclophosphamide and doxorubicin and remained without disease 18 months later.

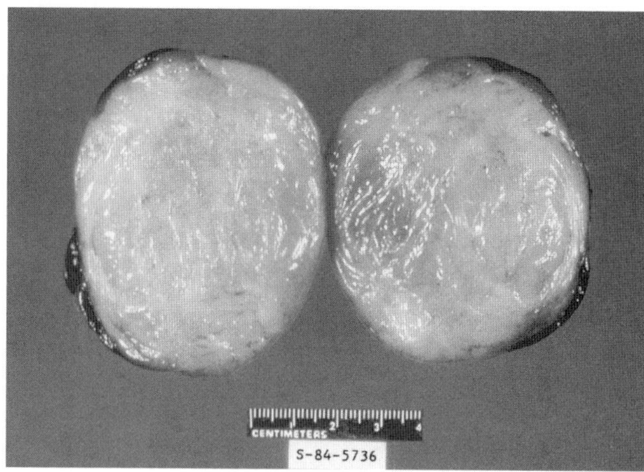

Figure 67-11. Cross section of a mesoblastic nephroma identified in an infant on a neonatal examination. Note the rubbery appearance of this tumor, which resembles a fibroid tumor of the uterus with a very thin margin of normal renal parenchyma around the periphery.

A SIOP report of 29 children with mesoblastic nephroma confirmed the early age at which this tumor is seen. Only 5 infants were older than 4 months at presentation in the series.[170] Five children with the cellular type of tumor received some chemotherapy. Two infants in this series died of sepsis after surgical treatment, but the remainder are alive and free of disease 4 years later. A proclivity for this tumor to infiltrate the renal hilum or perirenal tissue was seen again. Treatment of a neonate with an extensively infiltrating tumor with eight weekly courses of vincristine before resection is reported.[171] Shrinkage of the tumor occurred with treatment, facilitating its eventual resection and cure.

Beckwith reported the largest cohort of children with recurrent or metastatic lesions from his large collected series.[166] Twenty-four cases of aggressive tumor were seen in a series of 330 mesoblastic nephromas. Of these cases, 8 had metastatic disease, 17 had relapse in the peritoneum or retroperitoneum, and 6 of the infants have died of persistent disease. Recurrences occurred in children after initial chemotherapy or irradiation, which suggests that conventional adjuvant therapy may not decrease the incidence of recurrence. Histologic criteria were not helpful in predicting outcome. Beckwith supports aggressive surgical attempts to remove all gross tumor. He also stresses the need for close monitoring for 1 year after resection because relapse in 23 of the 24 cases was apparent within 11 months of resection. Ultrasonography of the local site is adequate, and scans for metastatic disease are unrewarding.

CYSTIC NEPHROMA

Cystic nephroma is indistinguishable grossly and radiographically from its malignant neoplastic "cousins," cystic partially differentiated nephroblastoma (CPDN) and cystic nephroblastoma. All lesions are composed of purely cystic masses characterized by multiple

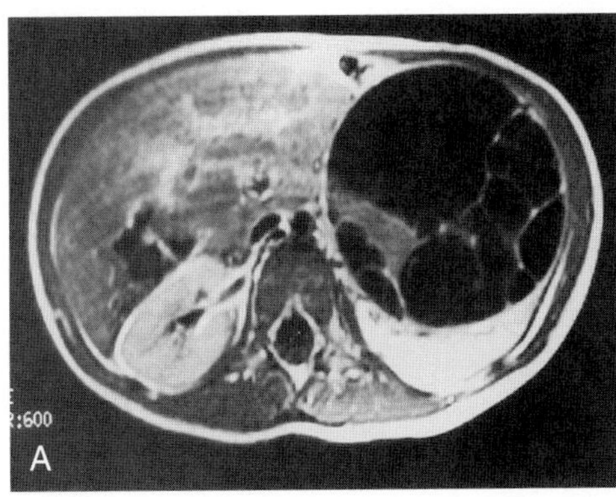

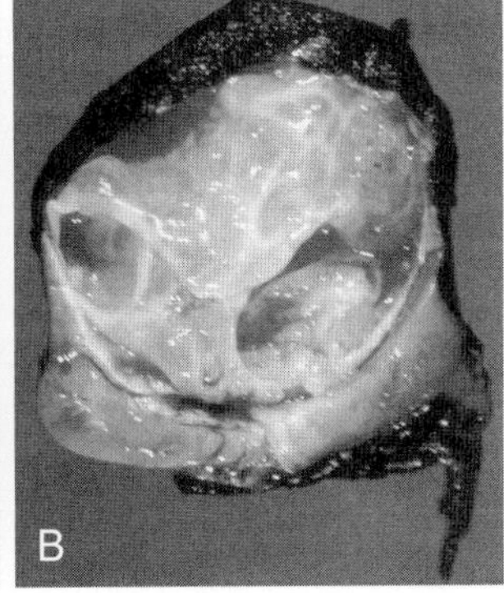

Figure 67-12. **A,** MR image obtained in a 2-year-old infant with an asymptomatic left flank mass. Note the multilocular cystic mass extending out from the normal renal tissue posteriorly. **B,** Cross section of the tumor and kidney reveals thin-walled septa within the mass. Histologic examination of this tumor revealed a cystic partially differentiated nephroblastoma.

thin-walled septations (Fig. 67-12). In cystic nephroma, the septations are lined by flattened, cuboidal or hobnail epithelium and are composed entirely of differentiated tissues without blastemal or other embryonal elements that are the distinguishing characteristics of CPDN.[172] Although the term *multilocular cyst of the kidney* has been used, *cystic nephroma* is preferred because the lesion appears to be neoplastic and not congenital. In the cystic nephroblastoma or cystic Wilms' tumor, solid nodules on the septa of blastemal or embryonal elements are characteristic of Wilms' tumor. An unexplained synchronous occurrence has been reported between cystic nephroma and pleuropulmonary blastoma.[173,174]

These lesions should not be confused with cystic clear cell sarcoma, cystic mesoblastic nephroma, or multicystic dysplastic kidney.[172] Cystic nephroma, CPDN, and cystic nephroblastoma can be distinguished from multicystic dysplastic kidney because they are confined to only a portion of the kidney with normal renal parenchyma being identified, whereas the cystic changes of multicystic dysplastic kidney almost always involve the entire kidney (its cause is early in utero urinary tract obstruction). Contralateral renal anomalies are frequent in dysplastic kidneys, including ureteropelvic junction obstruction and reflux. A multicystic dysplastic kidney is often identified antenatally or in the neonatal period, whereas the other lesions occur later.

Generally, nephrectomy will be curative in both cystic nephroma and CPDN.[175] Twenty-three children with these cystic lesions were identified in the NWTSG series: 5 with cystic nephroma and 18 with CPDN. Only one patient with CPDN had local recurrence, and no distant metastases were found. A more recent review of the NWTSG and SIOP files of the CPDN cases has again confirmed that primary resection appears to be adequate for all lesions removed intact.[176,177] In cases in which the lesion is isolated to one pole of the kidney, a partial nephrectomy may be considered. However, it must be remembered that these tumors can resemble cystic variants of clear cell sarcoma of the kidney, which carry an entirely different prognosis.[178,179] This is the major concern regarding the use of nephron-sparing surgery, as suggested by some authors for these cystic lesions.[180]

OSSIFYING RENAL TUMOR OF INFANCY

Ossifying renal tumor of infancy is a relatively rare tumor occurring entirely in infancy. In many cases, children with this lesion initially have gross hematuria, although a palpable mass may be present.[144] These lesions are attached to a renal papilla but are seen primarily within the lumen of the calyx and may extend into the renal pelvis. They have been confused occasionally with staghorn calculi. Histologically, they contain osteoid, osteoblastic cells, and spindle cells. Their true histogenesis has not been proved, although it has been suggested that they represent hyperplastic ILNRs. Metastasis or local spread of these tumors has not been reported. Renal-sparing procedures may be reasonable, although this may not result in significant ipsilateral renal function.[181,182]

chapter 68

NEUROBLASTOMA

Andrew M. Davidoff, MD

Neuroblastoma (NB) is the most common solid extracranial malignancy of childhood and the most common malignant tumor in patients younger than 1 year of age.[1] Its incidence is 1 per 100,000 children in the United States. In addition, NB represents 7% to 10% of all malignancies diagnosed in pediatric patients younger than 15 years of age and is responsible for approximately 15% of all pediatric cancer deaths.[2] However, NB is a heterogeneous disease.[3] Tumors can spontaneously regress or mature, or can display a very aggressive, malignant phenotype. Because of these unique characteristics, NB has been of great interest to both clinicians and basic scientists. Progress in molecular and cellular biology in the past 20 years has contributed greatly to a better understanding of this disease. However, this progress has not significantly altered the clinical outcome for patients with advanced-stage NB. Although the prognosis for these patients has improved somewhat in the past 2 decades, the long-term outcome still remains very poor.

The etiology of NB is currently unknown, and no environmental factors have been convincingly linked to its development. The disease generally occurs sporadically, but familial NB does occur in about 2% of cases. Interestingly, however, substantial biologic and clinical heterogeneity is often observed in familial cases.[4] Recently, the germline mutation associated with hereditary NB has been identified: activating mutations in the tyrosine kinase domain of the anaplastic lymphoma kinase (ALK) oncogene on the short arm of chromosome 2 (2p23).[5] These mutations can also be somatically acquired, although the prevalence of ALK activation in sporadic NB remains to be determined. NB has also been reported in infants with Beckwith-Wiedemann syndrome, Hirschsprung's disease, fetal alcohol syndrome, and in the offspring of mothers taking phenytoin for seizure disorders.[6-9]

The treatment of NB requires a multidisciplinary approach. Although surgical resection may be the only therapy required for patients at "low risk" of disease recurrence, the surgeon provides but one element of the modern multimodal treatment of children with "high-risk" disease. Pediatric oncologists, radiation therapists, and bone marrow transplantation (BMT) specialists are among the other important members of the pediatric oncology team. The therapy for patients with NB, as for children with other malignancies, is generally driven by clinical research protocols. Many of these protocols are sponsored by the Children's Oncology Group (COG) or by the larger children's hospitals, working individually or in small groups.

PATHOLOGY

NB is an embryonal tumor of the sympathetic nervous system. These tumors arise during fetal or early postnatal life from sympathetic cells (sympathogonia) derived from the neural crest. Therefore, tumors can originate anywhere along the path that neural crest cells migrate, including the adrenal medulla, paraspinal sympathetic ganglia, and sympathetic paraganglia such as the organ of Zuckerkandl. The German pathologist Rudolph Virchow is generally credited with being the first to describe the histologic appearance of what is now known as NB in his 1864 article entitled, "Hyperplasia of the Pineal and Suprarenal Glands."[10] The first to use the term *neuroblastoma* was James Homer Wright, who, in 1910, described the classic appearance of rosettes of tumor cells around central neural fibrils. He also noted the association between the common sites of tumor development and the pattern of migration of primitive neural cells.[11]

As one of the "small, round blue cell" tumors of infancy and childhood, NB, particularly when undifferentiated, must be distinguished from other neoplasms of this group (e.g., Ewing sarcoma family of tumors, non-Hodgkin lymphoma, and rhabdomyosarcoma). NB can be distinguished histologically by the presence of neuritic processes (neuropil) and Homer-Wright rosettes (neuroblasts surrounding eosinophilic neuropil). Scattered ganglion cells or immature chromaffin cells may also be seen. The appearance of the tumor cells may vary from undifferentiated cells to fully mature ganglion cells. In addition, NBs have variable degrees of schwannian cell stroma, which is reactive non-neoplastic tissue recruited by the tumor cells. This stroma is intermixed, to a greater or lesser degree, as

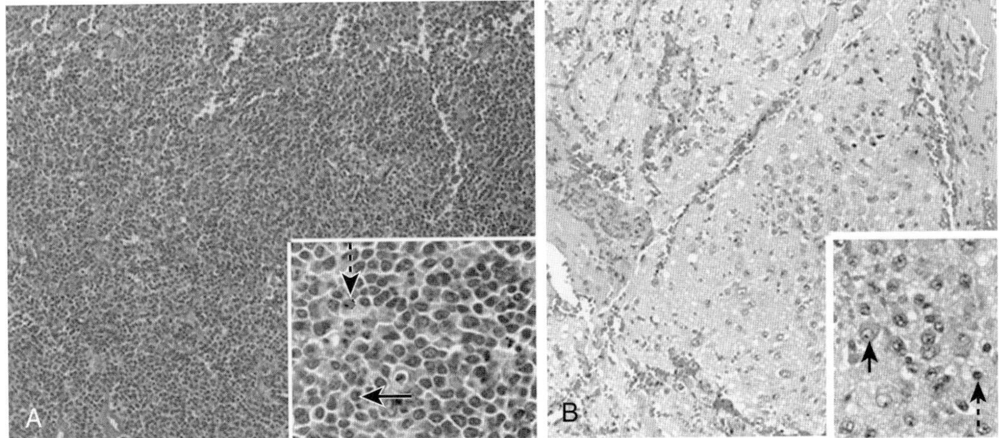

Figure 68-1. Characteristic histologic appearance of neuroblastoma. **A,** Histologic appearance of an NB with a high MKI (×10). A clump of karyorrhectic tumor cells (*dotted arrow*) and a tumor cell undergoing mitosis (*solid arrow*) are shown in the *inset* (×60). **B,** A differentiating NB with a low MKI (×10). A primitive neuroblast (*dotted arrow*) and a differentiating tumor cell (*solid arrow*), with features of differentiation in both the nucleus and cytoplasm, are shown in the *inset* (×60). Abundant neuropil is also seen. (Courtesy of Jesse Jenkins, MD, and Christine Fuller, MD, St. Jude Children's Research Hospital, Memphis, TN; reprinted from Davidoff AM: Neuroblastoma. In Oldham KT, Colombani PM, Foglia RP, Skinner MA [eds]: Principles and Practice of Pediatric Surgery. Philadelphia, Lippincott Williams & Wilkins, 2005.)

wavy bundles and sheets of spindle cells throughout the tumor and produces antiproliferative and differentiation-inducing factors that are crucial to neuronal differentiation.[12,13] In addition, the schwannian stroma appears to produce a variety of anti-angiogenic factors, including pigment epithelium–derived factor (PEDF)[14] and secreted protein acidic and rich in cysteine (SPARC).[15] Histopathologic variables among neuroblastic tumors include the degree of differentiation, maturation, lymphoid infiltration, calcification, anaplasia, necrosis, mitotic activity, neurofibrillary material (neuropil), and the presence of multinucleated cells. Finally, immunohistochemical analysis usually generates positive staining when antibodies to NB-specific antigens such as synaptophysin, neuron-specific enolase, and chromogranin are used and is negative when antibodies to actin, desmin, cytokeratin, leukocyte common antigen, vimentin, and CD99 are used.

NB is characterized by several unique clinical behaviors, including the secretion of catecholamine products and the potential to regress or mature, either spontaneously or in response to treatment. Small nodules of primitive neuroblasts are routinely found in the developing adrenal gland, even during the early postnatal period. Beckwith and Perrin described microscopic nodules that they referred to as "neuroblastoma in situ" in the adrenals of infants undergoing autopsy after death from non–malignancy-related causes.[16] The incidence of this finding was more than 200-fold greater than the clinical incidence of NB, which suggests that perhaps many NBs spontaneously regress or mature into lesions that never become clinically apparent. The process of involution is well described during embryonic life, especially in the developing central and peripheral nervous systems. Although initially thought to be mediated by the immune system, the process of involution may be the result of withdrawal of neurotrophic maintenance factors such as nerve growth factor (NGF). Clinically apparent NB can also regress or spontaneously mature, but the mechanism(s) of NB maturation and regression remain unknown.

CLASSIFICATION

In 1984, Shimada and colleagues first developed an age-linked classification system of neuroblastic tumors based on tumor morphology in which NBs were divided into two prognostic subgroups: favorable histology and unfavorable histology.[17] In 1999, the International NB Pathology Classification (INPC) was devised.[18] It was then modified in 2003[19] and is an adaptation of the original Shimada system. The INPC is based mainly on morphologic changes associated with the maturational sequence of neuroblastic tumors. It remains an age-linked classification that depends on the differentiation grade of the neuroblasts, the cellular turnover index (mitosis-karyorrhexis index [MKI]), and the presence or absence of schwannian stroma. The INPC classifies neuroblastic tumors into three morphologic categories: NB, ganglioneuroblastoma, and ganglioneuroma (Fig. 68-1).

NBs are, by definition, schwannian stroma poor (<50% of the tumor tissue) and can be subtyped as undifferentiated (requires supplemental diagnostic methods such as immunohistochemistry, electron microscopy or cytogenetics; and neuropil is not present) (see Fig. 68-1A); poorly differentiated (<5% of tumor cells have features of differentiation, and neuropil is present); or differentiating (>5% of tumor cells show differentiation toward ganglion cells) (see Fig. 68-1B). To classify a cell as a differentiating neuroblast, there must be synchronous differentiation of the nucleus (an enlarged, eccentric nucleus with a vesicular chromatin pattern and a single prominent nucleolus) and eosinophilic cytoplasm.[18]

Additional factors that contribute to the prognostic NB as favorable or unfavorable subtypes include

Table 68-1 Prognostic Evaluation of Neuroblastic Tumors According to the International Neuroblastoma Pathology Classification

International Neuroblastoma Pathology Classification		Prognostic Group
Neuroblastoma	Schwannian stroma-poor	
<1.5 yr	Poorly differentiated or differentiating and low or intermediate MKI tumor	Favorable
1.5-5 yr	Differentiating and low MKI tumor	
<1.5 yr	(a) Undifferentiated tumor or (b) high MKI tumor	Unfavorable
1.5-5 yr	(a) Undifferentiated or poorly differentiated tumor or (b) intermediate or high MKI tumor	
≥5 yr	All tumors	
Ganglioneuroblastoma, intermixed	Schwannian stroma-rich	Favorable
Ganglioneuroblastoma, nodular	Composite schwannian stroma-rich/stroma-dominant and stroma poor	Unfavorable or favorable (based on nodule histology)
Ganglioneuroma	Schwannian stroma-dominant	Favorable
Maturing		
Mature		

MKI, mitosis-karyorrhexis index.

Adapted from Shimada H, Ambros IM, Dehner LP, et al: The International NB Pathology Classification (the Shimada System). Cancer 86:364-372, 1999.

the MKI, which is defined as the number of tumor cells in mitosis or karyorrhexis per 5000 neuroblastic cells (i.e., low MKI, < 100 cells; intermediate, 100-200 cells; high, > 200 cells) and the patient's age (<1.5 years, 1.5-5 years, > 5 years) (Table 68-1). The favorable-histology subgroup of NBs includes poorly differentiated and differentiating tumors with low or intermediate MKI in patients younger than 1.5 years of age and differentiating tumors with low MKI in patients ages 1.5 to 5.0 years. The unfavorable-histology subgroup includes undifferentiated tumors or those with high MKI in patients of any age, poorly differentiated tumors or those with intermediate-MKI tumors in patients ages 1.5 to 5.0 years, or any tumor in a patient older than 5 years. The age of the patient appears to be a crucial component of the prognostic assessment of the INPC. It has been hypothesized that neuroblastic cells with maturational potential require an in-vivo latent period before demonstrating histologic evidence of differentiation. Therefore, there is a certain allowance for mitotic and karyorrhectic activities of neuroblastic cells in tumors in infants and younger children.[20]

The importance of this histopathologic classification was confirmed in a large, retrospective analysis reported by Shimada and associates.[21] The INPC classification of tumor histology provided independent prognostic information that was able to distinguish patients with tumors of favorable histology (probability of 5-year event-free survival [EFS], 90.8%) from those with tumors of unfavorable histology (EFS, 31.2%). More recently, the INPC classification has been shown to add independent prognostic information beyond the prognostic contribution of age.[22] Therefore, histopathology remains in the current multifactorial risk stratification for patients with NB. This determination is particularly important in patients who are older than age 1 year and have localized disease. Because the histopathologic pattern within a tumor can be heterogeneous, Shimada has recommended analyzing representative sections from at least 1 cm^3 of viable, non-necrotic tissue to determine histopathologic classification. The prognostic value of assessing the histopathology of a NB after chemotherapy or radiation therapy has not been validated.

Stroma-rich neuroblastic tumors are classified as either ganglioneuroblastomas or ganglioneuromas (Fig. 68-2). Ganglioneuroblastomas contain cells that are transitioning toward differentiation but are not completely differentiated/mature and have residual microscopic foci of neuroblastic cells (<50% of the total volume) distributed throughout the tumor. Ganglioneuroblastomas can be further divided into "intermixed" and "nodular" subtypes, depending on the distribution of the neuroblastic cells. This distinction is important because of the significantly worse prognosis associated with the latter subtype. In this subtype, the neuroblastic clones that comprise grossly distinct nodules appear to be responsible for the aggressive phenotype for this subtype.[20] Ganglioneuromas contain either maturing cells (i.e., those that contain a minor component of scattered differentiating neuroblasts not forming distinctive nests), or mature cells, which lack any neuroblastomatous component. Most stroma-rich tumors (ganglioneuroblastoma, intermixed; ganglioneuroma, maturing subtype) are classified as "favorable" by the INPC. However, the pathologic/prognostic classification of the ganglioneuroblastoma, nodular subtype is based on the morphologic evaluation of the neuroblastomatous nodule(s), and can, therefore, be unfavorable. Tumors that fit the criteria for ganglioneuroma, mature subtype, with abundant schwannian stroma and fully mature ganglion cells, in the absence of neuroblasts, are considered benign and are generally not considered for enrollment in protocols for neuroblastic tumors.

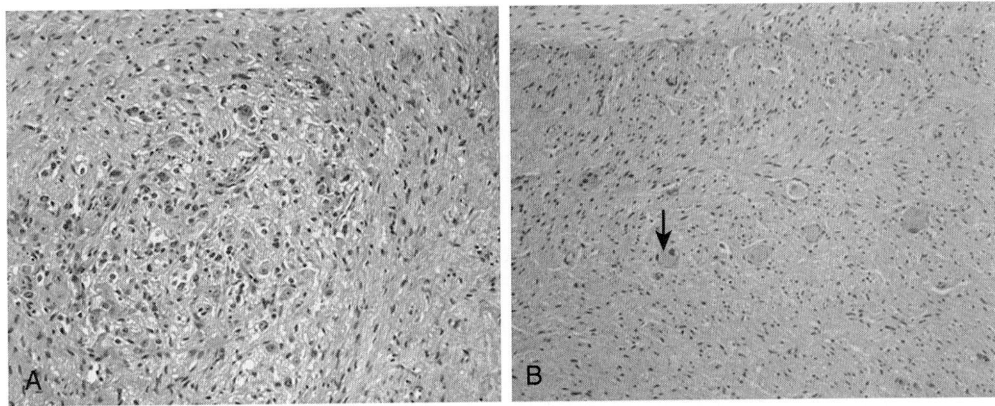

Figure 68-2. More mature neuroblastic tumors. **A,** A stroma-rich ganglioneuroblastoma with infrequent neuroblasts intermixed within abundant schwannian stroma and ganglion cells (×10). **B,** A stroma-rich ganglioneuroma with ganglion cells (*arrow*) (×10). Infiltrating lymphoid cells are also seen, but no neuroblasts are present. (Courtesy of Jesse Jenkins, MD, and Christine Fuller, MD, St. Jude Children's Research Hospital, Memphis, TN; reprinted from Davidoff AM: Neuroblastoma. In Oldham KT, Colombani PM, Foglia RP, Skinner MA [eds]: Principles and Practice of Pediatric Surgery. Philadelphia, Lippincott Williams & Wilkins, 2005.)

MOLECULAR BIOLOGY

Advances in molecular biology research in the past 2 decades have resulted in an increased understanding of the genetic events in the pathogenesis and progression of many human malignancies, including those found in children. NB, in particular, has served as a model for a molecular approach to treating patients with cancer, highlighting the utility of genetic analysis for diagnosis, risk stratification, and treatment planning. Chromosomal structural changes play a role in NB, particularly those that result in the loss of tumor suppressors or gain of oncogenes, gene amplification, and activating or inactivating mutations of relevant genes or their regulatory elements. The end result of alterations in these genetic elements, regardless of their specific mechanisms, is the disruption of the normal balance between cell proliferation and cell death. NB is characterized by marked clinical and biologic heterogeneity, which is also evident at the genetic level. Although there is no single genetic abnormality or initiating event common to all NBs, a number of different genetic alterations have been identified that provide powerful prognostic information and play crucial roles in risk assessment and treatment planning.

DNA Content

Normal human cells contain two copies of each of 23 chromosomes. Thus, a normal diploid cell has 46 chromosomes. The majority (55%) of primary NBs are triploid or "near-triploid/hyperdiploid" and contain between 58 and 80 chromosomes. The remainder (45%) are either "near-diploid" (35-57 chromosomes) or "near-tetraploid" (81-103 chromosomes).[23] The "DNA index" of a tumor is the ratio of the number of chromosomes present to a diploid number of chromosomes (i.e., 46). Therefore, diploid cells have a DNA index of 1.0, whereas near-triploid cells have a DNA index ranging from 1.26 to 1.76. NBs that are near-diploid or near-tetraploid usually have structural genetic abnormalities, most frequently chromosome 1p deletion and *MYCN* amplification. Near-triploid or hyperdiploid tumors are characterized by three almost complete haploid sets of chromosomes with few structural abnormalities. Importantly, patients with near-triploid tumors typically have favorable clinical and biologic prognostic factors and excellent survival rates when compared with those patients who have near-diploid or near-tetraploid tumors.[24] This association is most important for infants with advanced disease.[25] The prognostic significance of tumor ploidy appears to be lost in patients older than 2 years.

Amplification of MYCN

Investigation of the molecular biology of NB began with the cytogenetic characterization of tumor-derived cell lines. These studies showed the frequent presence of extrachromosomal double-minute chromatin bodies (DMs) and chromosomally integrated homogeneously staining regions (HSRs) characteristic of gene amplification (Fig. 68-3).[26] Since that time, it has been shown that the amplified region was derived from the distal short arm of chromosome 2 (2p24) and contained the *MYCN* proto-oncogene. *MYCN* encodes a 64-kD nuclear phosphoprotein MYCN that forms a transcriptional complex by associating with other nuclear proteins expressed in the developing nervous system and other tissues.[27] Enforced expression of MYCN increases the rates of DNA synthesis and cell proliferation and shortens the G_1 phase of the cell cycle.[28] *MYCN* can also function as a classic dominant oncogene that cooperates with activated *RAS* to transform normal cells.[29] Targeted expression of *MYCN* in transgenic mice results in the development of NBs.[30]

Overall, approximately 25% of primary NBs in children have *MYCN* amplification, with *MYCN* amplification being present in 40% with advanced disease but only 5% to 10% with low-stage disease.[31] The copy number, which can range from 5- to 500-fold amplification, is usually consistent among primary and metastatic sites and at different times during tumor evolution and treatment.[32] This finding suggests that

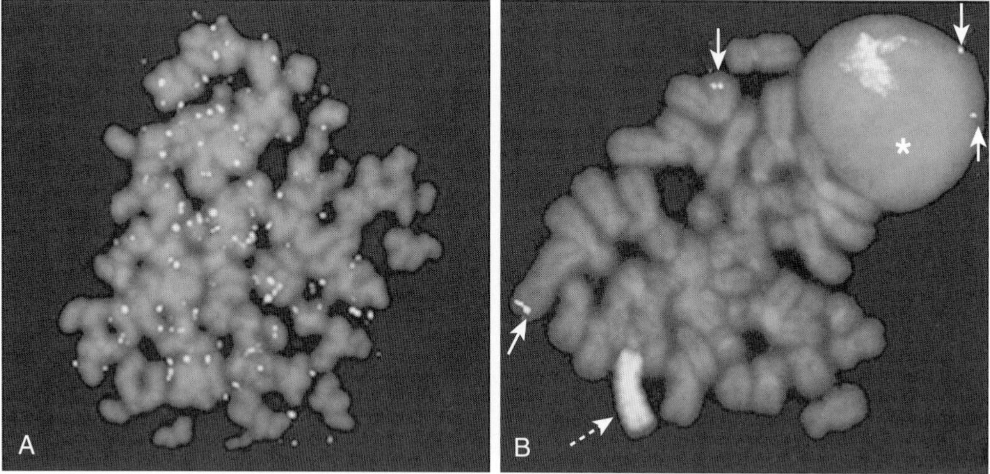

Figure 68-3. FISH analysis of a neuroblastoma. **A,** Chromosomes in metaphase. The bright spots are double-minute chromatin bodies. **B,** The metaphase chromosomes are again seen. An intact interphase nucleus is marked with an *asterisk.* The normal two copies of the *MYCN* gene are marked with *solid arrows.* Homogeneously staining regions (HSRs) are also seen. One is seen in the interphase nucleus, and the other is marked with a *dotted arrow.* (Courtesy of Marc Valentine, St. Jude Children's Research Hospital, Memphis, TN.)

MYCN amplification is an early event in the pathogenesis of NB. Amplification of *MYCN* is associated with advanced stages of disease, rapid tumor progression, and poor outcome. Therefore, it is a powerful prognostic indicator of biologically aggressive tumor behavior.[31,33] Amplification can be detected either by routine metaphase cytogenetics or fluorescent in situ hybridization (FISH). Current therapeutic NB protocols have incorporated the presence or absence of *MYCN* amplification into their risk stratification schema.

Chromosomal Changes

Also noted on early karyotype analyses of NB-derived cell lines were frequent deletions of the short arm of chromosome 1.[34] Deletions of genetic material in tumors suggest the presence (and subsequent loss) of a tumor suppressor gene. Although no individual tumor suppressor gene has been confirmed on chromosome 1p, recent data have identified CHD-5 as the strongest candidate tumor suppressor gene that is deleted from 1p36.31 in NB.[35] Functional confirmation of the presence of a 1p tumor suppressor gene came from the demonstration that transfection of chromosome 1p into a NB cell line results in morphologic changes and ultimately cell senescence.[36] Twenty to 35 percent of primary NBs exhibit 1p deletion, as determined by FISH, with the smallest common region of loss located within region 1p36.[37] About 70% of advanced-stage NBs have 1p deletions.[38] Molecular studies have shown that there is a strong correlation between 1p deletion and *MYCN* amplification and other high-risk features such as age older than 1 year and advanced-stage disease.[37] In one study it was demonstrated that 1p deletions are independently associated with a worse outcome in patients with NB.[39] Deletions of the long arm of chromosome 11 (11q) and 14 (14q) also appear to be common in NBs. Both are inversely related to *MYCN* amplification.[39,40]

Comparative genomic hybridization (CGH) studies have shown that gain of genetic material on the long arm of chromosome 17 (17q) is perhaps the most common genetic abnormality in NBs, occurring in approximately 75% of primary tumors.[41] Gain of 17q most often results from an unbalanced translocation of this region to other chromosomal sites, most frequently 1p or 11q. The term *unbalanced* implies that extra copies of 17q are present in addition to normal copies of chromosome 17. Currently, it is unclear how extra copies of 17q contribute to the malignant phenotype of NB and which genes on 17q are the critical ones. Gain of chromosome 17q is strongly associated with other known prognostic factors, but it may be a powerful independent predictor of adverse outcome.[42] Finally, more recently, a genome-wide association study has demonstrated that a common genetic variation at chromosome band 6p22 is associated with susceptibility to NB.[43]

Other Molecular Abnormalities

Neurotrophins and their tyrosine kinase receptors are important in the development of the sympathetic nervous system and have been implicated in the pathogenesis of NB. Three receptor-ligand pairs have been identified: TrkA, the primary receptor for nerve growth factor (NGF); TrkB, the primary receptor of brain-derived neurotrophic factor (BDNF); and TrkC, the receptor for neurotrophin-3 (NT-3).[44] TrkA appears to mediate differentiation of developing neurons or NB in the presence of NGF ligand, and of apoptosis in the absence of NGF.[45] High TrkA expression is associated with favorable tumor biology and a good outcome[46] and is inversely correlated with *MYCN* amplification.[47] Conversely, the TrkB/BDNF pathway appears to promote NB survival through autocrine or paracrine signaling, especially in *MYCN*-amplified tumors.[48] TrkB is expressed in about 40% of NBs, usually advanced-stage disease. TrkC is expressed in approximately 25% of NBs and is strongly associated with TrkA expression.[49] Although the exact function of the

Trk receptors in the pathogenesis of NB is unknown, they remain attractive therapeutic targets.

Other molecular abnormalities frequently detected in NB include inactivation of caspase 8, expression of CD44, and overexpression of multidrug-resistance genes. Recent studies have demonstrated inactivation of caspase 8, a component of the Fas death-signaling complex, in *MYCN*-amplified NBs.[50] It has been proposed that inactivation of caspase 8 renders tumor cells resistant to apoptotic signals. CD44 is a cell surface glycoprotein that appears to play a role in tumor cell adhesion.[51] In NBs, CD44 expression is inversely correlated with *MYCN* amplification and is undetectable in most disseminated NBs.[52] Multidrug resistance–associated protein (MRP) is an efflux pump whose expression in NB appears to be correlated with *MYCN* amplification and poor prognosis.[53,54] The presence of MRP may explain the common clinical situation in which NBs initially respond well to chemotherapy but subsequently become resistant.

CLINICAL PRESENTATION

Patients with NB usually present with signs and symptoms that reflect the primary site and extent of disease, although localized disease is often asymptomatic. Because 75% of NB occurs in the abdominal cavity (50% occur in the adrenal gland, 25% occur elsewhere in the retroperitoneum), an abdominal mass detected on physical examination is a common clinical feature, as is the complaint of abdominal pain. Other primary sites of NB include the posterior mediastinum (20%), the cervical region (1%), and the pelvis (4%) (organ of Zuckerkandl) (Fig. 68-4). Respiratory distress or dysphagia may be a reflection of a thoracic tumor. Altered defecation or urination may be caused by mechanical compression of a pelvic tumor or by spinal cord compression from a paraspinal tumor. Spinal cord compression may also present as an altered gait. A tumor in the neck or upper thorax can produce Horner syndrome (ptosis, miosis, and anhidrosis), enophthalmos, and heterochromia of the iris. Acute cerebellar ataxia has also been observed, characterized by the dancing-eye syndrome, which includes opsoclonus, myoclonus, and chaotic nystagmus. Two thirds of these cases occur in infants with mediastinal primary tumors.[55,56] Additional signs and symptoms that reflect excessive catecholamine or vasoactive intestinal polypeptide secretion include diarrhea, weight loss, and hypertension.

The distribution of NB at presentation by age and stage is shown in Table 68-2. More than 40% of patients have metastatic disease at diagnosis. These patients are often quite ill and have systemic symptoms caused by widespread disease. In older patients, NB has a pattern of metastatic disease in which metastases to the bone marrow, lymph nodes, and bone predominate. The frequency of involvement of distant sites is shown in Table 68-3. These metastases may manifest as bone pain (bone metastases) or anemia (bone marrow infiltration). The brain, spinal cord, heart, and lungs are rare sites of metastases, except with advanced, end-stage disease. Metastatic disease may be also associated with "black eyes" (also referred to as "raccoon eyes") as a result of retro-orbital venous plexus spread

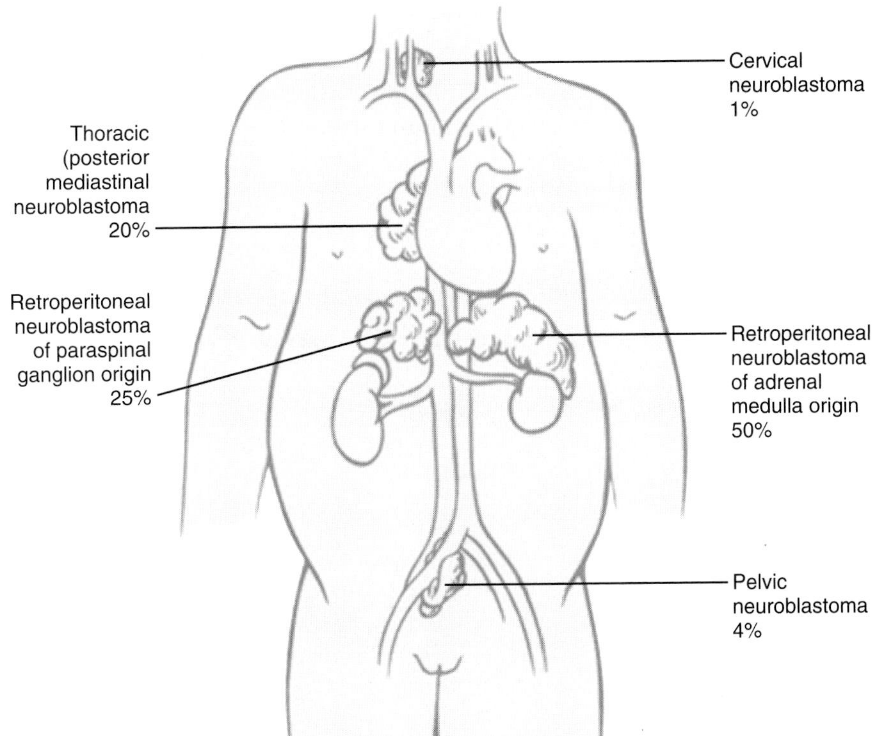

Figure 68-4. Primary sites for neuroblastoma are depicted in this anatomic drawing. (Reprinted from Davidoff AM: Neuroblastoma. In Oldham KT, Colombani PM, Foglia RP, Skinner MA [eds]: Principles and Practice of Pediatric Surgery. Philadelphia, Lippincott Williams & Wilkins, 2005.)

Table 68-2 Percentage Distribution of Neuroblastoma Cases by Age and Evans Stage

Age	Stage I	II	III	IV	IV-S	Total
<1 yr	10.5	9.5	5.1	9.5	7.5	42.2
≥1 yr	7.1	8.5	8.8	33.3	0	57.8
TOTAL	17.7	18.0	13.9	42.9	7.5	

Adapted from Bernstein ML, Leclerc JM, Bunin G, et al: A population-based study of NB incidence, survival, and mortality in North America. J Clin Oncol 10:323, 1992.

(Fig. 68-5A). This is an ominous physical sign, as is the presence of a limp in children without a history of head or extremity trauma. Infants with metastatic NB may have stage 4S disease, which, by definition, is a localized primary tumor in patients younger than 1 year, with dissemination limited to skin, liver, or bone marrow (<10% of nucleated cells). These patients may present with "blueberry muffin" cutaneous lesions (see Fig. 68-5B), respiratory distress secondary to massive hepatomegaly, and anemia secondary to bone marrow disease. The diagnosis of NB is generally made by histopathologic evaluation of primary or metastatic tumor tissue, or by the demonstration of tumor cells in the bone marrow, together with elevated levels of urinary catecholamines.

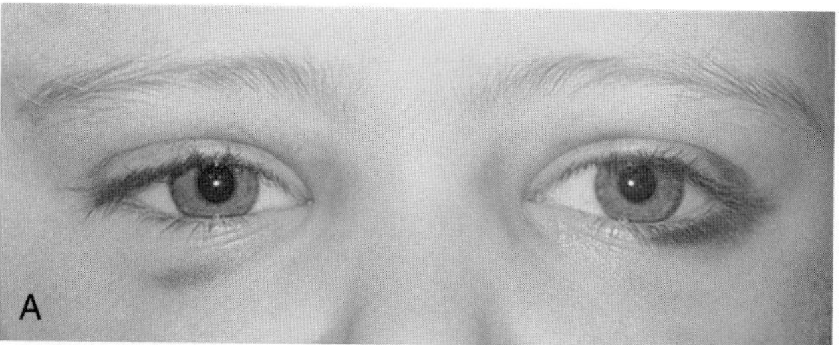

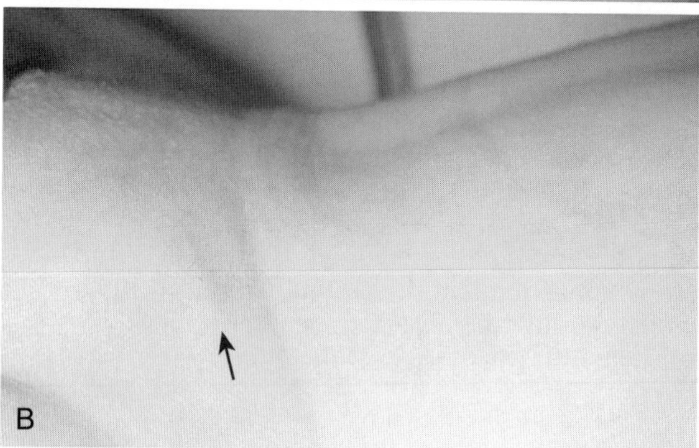

Figure 68-5. Clinical evidence of metastatic neuroblastoma. **A,** "Raccoon eyes," characteristic of metastatic neuroblastoma in the posterior orbital venous plexus, are seen in a child with stage 4 disease. **B,** "Blueberry muffin" spot (*arrow*) in the skin, characteristic of metastatic NB, is seen in the suprapubic region of an infant with a 4S NB. (Courtesy of Stephen Shochat, MD, St. Jude Children's Research Hospital, Memphis, TN).

DIAGNOSIS

Laboratory Findings

Lactate Dehydrogenase

Despite its lack of specificity, serum lactate dehydrogenase (LDH) can have great prognostic significance. High serum levels of LDH reflect high proliferative activity or large tumor burden.[57] Moreover, an LDH level higher than 1500 IU/L appears to be associated with a poor prognosis.[58] Thus, LDH can be used to monitor disease activity or the response to therapy.

Ferritin

High levels of serum ferritin (>150 ng/mL) may also reflect a large tumor burden or rapid tumor progression. Elevated serum ferritin is often seen in

Table 68-3 Sites of Metastases at Diagnosis for Patients with Evans Stage IV-S and Stage IV

	Stage IV-S (%)	Stage IV < 1 year (%)	Stage IV ≥ 1 year (%)	Total (%)
Bone marrow	34.6	57.1	81.3	70.5
Bone	0	48.9	68.2	55.7
Lymph node	8.6	28.6	35.7	30.9
Liver	80.2	53.4	12.9	29.6
Intracranial/orbit	0	25.6	19.6	18.2
Adrenal	6.2	13.5	6.0	7.6
Skin	13.6	8.3	0.9	4.0
Pleura	0	4.5	3.7	3.4
Lung	0	2.3	4.1	3.2
Peritoneum	0	3.8	2.1	2.2
Other	0	3.8	1.6	1.9
Central nervous system	0	0	0.9	0.6

Adapted from Dubois SG, Kalika Y, Lukens JN, et al: Metastatic sites in stage IV and IVS NB correlate with age, tumor biology, and survival. Pediatr Hematol Oncol 21:181-189, 1999.

advanced-stage NBs and indicates a poor prognosis.[59] Levels often return to normal during clinical remission.

Neuron-Specific Enolase

Neuron-specific enolase (NSE) is another useful prognostic marker of advanced-stage NB. The incidence of elevated NSE levels increases with stage.[60] A serum level of NSE greater than 100 ng/mL is associated with a poor outcome. NSE has been reported to correlate with tumor burden,[61] suggesting its reliability as a marker for treatment efficacy.

Catecholamine Metabolites

NB is characterized by the relatively unique capacity for secretion of catecholamine products, the metabolites of which, vanillymandelic acid and homovanillic acid can be detected in the urine of more than 90% of patients with NB. Thus, a urine specimen is of clinical value in diagnosing NB and determining the response to therapy. Documentation of elevated urinary catecholamines is required if the diagnosis of NB is being made solely by the identification of neuroblasts in the bone marrow. Urinary levels of these two catabolites can also be used as markers of tumor progression or relapse and can serve as a surrogate prognostic indicator. Random urine samples are preferable to 24-hour urine estimations for younger children.[62]

Imaging

Radiography

Chest radiography can be a useful tool for demonstrating the presence of a posterior mediastinal mass, which is usually a thoracic NB in a child. A Pediatric Oncology Group (POG) study demonstrated that a mediastinal mass was discovered on incidental chest radiographs in almost half of the patients with a thoracic NB who had symptoms seemingly unrelated to their tumors (Fig. 68-6A).[63] Abdominal radiography is less often the modality by which an NB is discovered. However, as many as half of abdominal NBs are detectable as a mass with fine calcification.

Ultrasonography

Although ultrasonography is the modality most often used during the initial assessment of a suspected abdominal mass, its sensitivity and accuracy are less than that of computed tomography (CT) or magnetic resonance imaging (MRI) for diagnosing NB.[64] These latter modalities are generally used after screening with ultrasonography to assist in generating a differential diagnosis and for further anatomic definition once the presence of a mass has been confirmed. Ultrasonography can demonstrate tumor involvement with major vessels and organs. It can provide real-time three-dimensional information regarding their relation to the tumor. Color Doppler imaging can supply further information about vascular encasement within a tumor.[65]

Computed Tomography

CT remains a useful, commonly used modality for the evaluation of NB (see Fig. 68-6B). It can demonstrate calcification in almost 85% of NBs, and intraspinal extension of the tumor can be determined on contrast-enhanced CT.[66] Overall, contrast-enhanced CT has been reported to be 82% accurate in defining NB extent, with the accuracy increasing to nearly 97% when performed with a bone scan.[67] Although some consider CT to have been supplanted by MRI, others still consider it to be the image modality of choice for patients with NB, especially when used in conjunction with bone scintigraphy.[68]

Magnetic Resonance Imaging

MRI is becoming the most useful and most sensitive imaging modality for the diagnosis and staging of NB.[69,70] MRI appears to be more accurate than CT for detection of stage 4 disease. The sensitivity of MRI is 83%, and that of CT is 43%. The specificity of MRI is 97%, and that of CT is 88%.[70] Metastases to the bone and bone marrow, in particular, are better detected by MRI, as is intraspinal tumor extension (Fig. 68-7).[70] When considering skeletal metastases alone, MRI and bone scan have been shown to be equivalent.[70] Encasement of major vessels can be better defined by MRI than CT, especially with the use of MR angiography

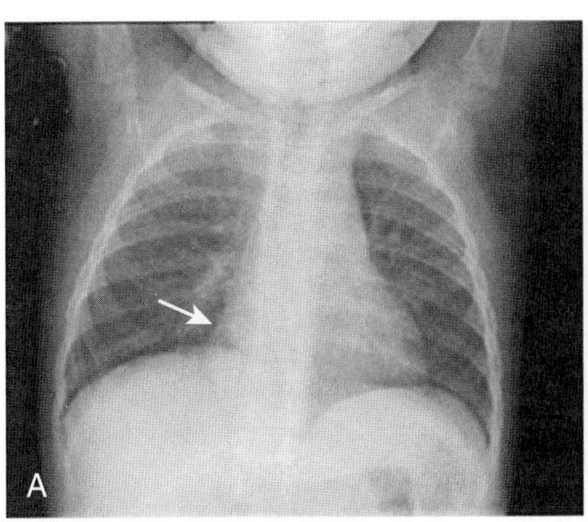

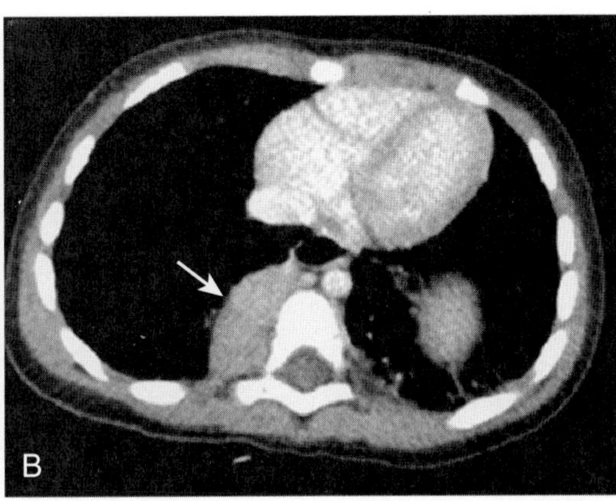

Figure 68-6. A posterior mediastinal/thoracic neuroblastoma (*arrows*) is seen on chest radiograph (**A**) and chest CT scan (**B**).

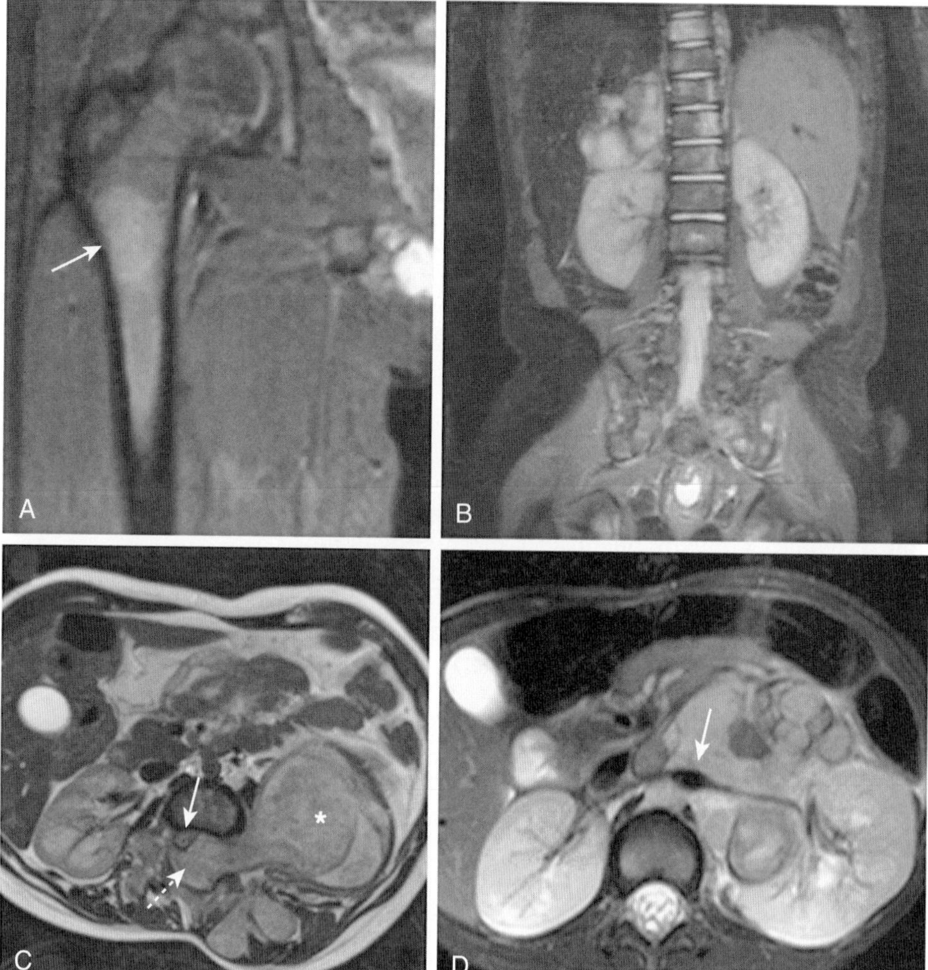

Figure 68-7. These MR images highlight several characteristics of high-risk neuroblastoma. **A,** Bone metastasis in femur (*arrow*). **B,** Bone marrow metastases in the vertebral bodies. **C,** Intraspinal tumor extension (*dotted arrow*). Note displacement of spinal cord (*solid arrow*) from a large tumor (*asterisk*). **D,** Encasement of major intra-abdominal vessels (*arrow* points to the aorta and left renal artery).

(see Fig. 68-7D). MRI in the coronal plane is suitable for routine assessment of the whole body from the neck to the pelvis. Evaluating the utility of whole-body MRI, perhaps performed in conjunction with a functional imaging study such as positron-emission tomography (PET), is being considered for future clinical staging protocols. CT and MRI are not very accurate for staging localized disease. However, the sensitivity of T1- and T2-weighted MR images is 100% for detecting NBs in infants identified by mass screening.[65]

Scintigraphy

Metaiodobenzylguanidine (MIBG) is transported to and stored in the distal storage granules of chromaffin cells in the same way as norepinephrine. MIBG has been used for scintigraphic imaging of NB. The MIBG scintiscan is the imaging study of choice in evaluating the involvement of bone and bone marrow by NB (Fig. 68-8). This imaging study has largely replaced technetium-99m methylene diphosphonate (^{99m}Tc-MDP) bone scans, which are generally inferior to MIBG in detecting NBs with skeletal or extraskeletal involvement. In addition, monitoring MDP-avid NBs by bone scintigraphy often results in false-positive imaging for months after tumor remission. Thus, ^{99m}Tc-MDP bone scanning is a second choice if MIBG imaging is not available or does not visualize known disease.[71,72] Iodine-131 (^{131}I) or iodine-123 (^{123}I) can be used to label MIBG. ^{123}I-MIBG provides a reduced absorbed radiation dosage and superior spatial resolution.[73] The reported sensitivity of MIBG in the detection of NB with metastases to the bone and bone marrow is 82%, and the specificity is 91%.[74] Primary tumors and lymph node metastases are also detectable. MIBG can demonstrate more sites of tumor involvement in the bone and bone marrow than either bone scintigraphy or standard radiography.[74] However, false-negative MIBG scans have been seen in cases in which the bone scintigraphy was positive.[72]

Bone Marrow Examination

Bone marrow biopsy has been regarded as a routine and important method for detecting bone marrow involvement with NB. Both aspiration and biopsy should be performed, although the latter has better diagnostic value. To collect more accurate information, taking specimens from multiple sites is recommended. Immunohistochemical staining with antibodies such as antiganglioside G_{D2}, S-100, NSE, and ferritin is also useful for reducing the number of false-negative

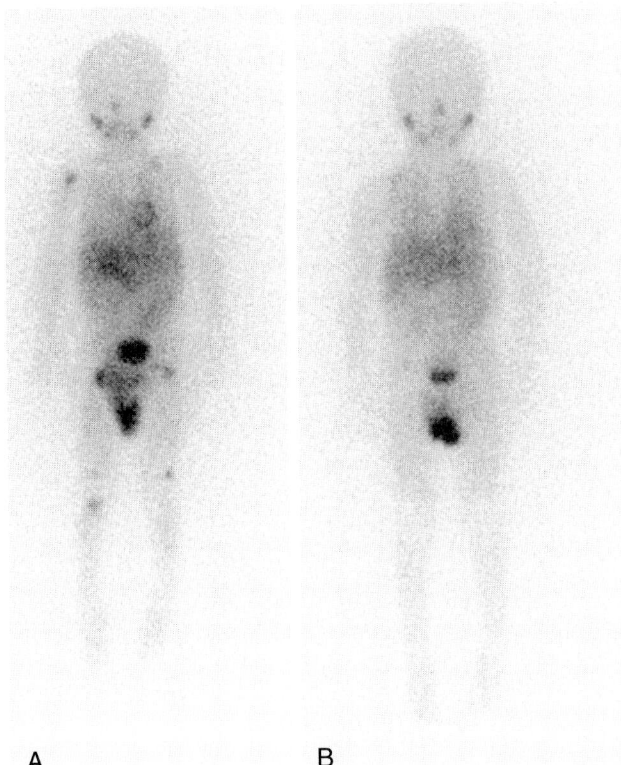

Figure 68-8. Imaging of neuroblastoma with MIBG scintigraphy. **A,** Scan obtained at presentation of a patient with metastatic NB. There is diffusely abnormal activity throughout much of the skeleton including the proximal right humerus, both proximal and distal femurs, and the proximal right tibia. There is also a focus of activity in the right upper retroperitoneum at the site of the primary tumor. **B,** Scan obtained of the same patient after completion of therapy shows no scintigraphic evidence of MIBG-avid NB.

cases.[75] Because a bone marrow biopsy is invasive and painful, noninvasive alternatives are being tested. Studies have suggested the superiority of MRI[76] and MIBG scintigraphy[77] over bone marrow biopsy in detecting bone marrow infiltration by NB. However, the specificity of these modalities requires further evaluation.

Differential Diagnosis

Making a correct clinical diagnosis of NB can be difficult because patients present with such diverse symptoms. For example, acute cerebellar ataxia with opsoclonus-myoclonus can be mistaken for a primary neurologic disease. Widespread bone involvement may resemble non-neoplastic bone disease such as osteomyelitis or rheumatoid arthritis or be associated with systemic inflammatory changes. Symptoms referable to vasoactive intestinal polypeptide secretion (i.e., diarrhea) can be misinterpreted as symptoms of an enteric infection or inflammatory bowel disease.

Histologically, undifferentiated, small blue round cell NB may be hard to distinguish from rhabdomyosarcoma, primitive neuroectodermal tumors, Ewing sarcoma family of tumors, or non-Hodgkin lymphoma. Use of a panel of specific antibodies,[76] as mentioned previously, can facilitate histologic differentiation.

Tumor Staging

In the past, two primary systems have been used to stage NB. These were the Evans classification, used by the former Children's Cancer Group (CCG) institutions,[78] and the St. Jude Children's Research Hospital classification, used by the former POG institutions.[79] The Evans classification emphasized tumor extent, as determined radiographically. In particular, it was important whether the tumor extended beyond the organ or structure of origin, and if it crossed the midline. The St. Jude classification relied on surgicopathologic staging, emphasizing lymph node involvement. Both staging systems had prognostic value, but differences and discrepancies between the two systems presented obstacles to population studies of NB. In an attempt to incorporate elements from both of these widely accepted systems and to have a single staging system, the International NB Staging System (INSS) was created (Table 68-4).[71] Evaluation of the primary tumor and involvement of metastatic sites in the INSS system depends largely on imaging studies (CT or MRI) (Table 68-5), although pathologic involvement of lymph nodes and bone marrow continue to be

Table 68-4 International Neuroblastoma Staging System Criteria

Stage	Definition
1	Localized tumor with complete gross excision, with or without microscopic residual disease; representative ipsilateral lymph nodes negative for tumor microscopically (nodes attached to and removed with the primary tumor may be positive)
2A	Localized tumor with incomplete gross excision; representative ipsilateral nonadherent lymph nodes negative for tumor microscopically
2B	Localized tumor with or without complete gross excision, with ipsilateral nonadherent lymph nodes positive for tumor. Enlarged contralateral lymph nodes must be negative microscopically.
3	Unresectable unilateral tumor infiltrating across the midline,* with or without regional lymph node involvement *or* Localized unilateral tumor with contralateral regional lymph node involvement *or* Midline tumor with bilateral extension by infiltration (unresectable) or by lymph node involvement
4	Any primary tumor with dissemination to distant lymph nodes, bone, bone marrow, liver, skin, or other organs (except as defined for stage 4S).
4S	Localized primary tumor (as defined for stage 1, 2A, or 2B), with dissemination limited to skin, liver, and bone marrow† (limited to infants younger than 1 yr)

*The midline is defined as the vertebral column. Tumors originating on one side and crossing the midline must infiltrate to or beyond the opposite side of the vertebral column.

†Marrow involvement in stage 4S should be minimal (i.e., <10% of total nucleated cells identified as malignant on bone marrow biopsy or on marrow aspirate). More extensive marrow involvement would be considered to be stage 4. The metaiodobenzylguanidine scan (if performed) should be negative in the marrow.

Table 68-5 International Neuroblastoma Staging System Staging Investigations

	Recommended Tests
Tumor Site	
Primary tumor	CT or MRI with 3D measurements; MIBG scan, if available.
Metastatic Sites	
Bone marrow	Bilateral posterior iliac crest marrow aspirates and trephine (core) bone marrow biopsies required to exclude marrow involvement. A single positive site documents marrow involvement. Core biopsies must contain ≥ 1 cm of marrow (excluding cartilage) to be considered adequate.
Bone	MIBG scan; ^{99m}Tc scan required if MIBG scan is negative or unavailable, and plain radiographs of positive lesions are recommended.
Lymph nodes	Clinical examination (palpable nodes), confirmed histologically
	CT scan for nonpalpable nodes (3D measurements)
Abdomen and liver	CT or MRI with 3D measurements
Chest	Anteroposterior and lateral chest radiographs
	CT and MRI necessary if chest radiograph is positive or if abdominal mass/nodes extend into chest

MIBG, metaiodobenzylguanidine.

important components. MIBG scanning is also recommended as part of the initial evaluation of new patients and, subsequently, for monitoring tumor response to therapy.

One drawback to the INSS is that the degree of initial surgical resection can have a significant impact on the staging of a tumor. Hence, the aggressiveness and skill of a surgeon can influence the stage and, ultimately, the therapy given to a particular patient. For example, disease in which there is a tumor that infiltrates across the midline (stage 3) but is completely resected, would be considered stage 1, and no further therapy would be given. In order to have a more uniform system for staging disease at presentation, children with localized NB who are enrolled on a COG protocol will have "image-defined risk factors" assessed by central review of diagnostic imaging studies. This will be performed to determine whether these factors are more prognostically relevant than INSS staging for patients with localized NB. These image-defined risk factors (Table 68-6) were proposed by the European International Society of Pediatric Oncology Neuroblastoma Group and generally reflect the presence of encasement of major vessels or nerves or the infiltration of adjacent organs/structures by locoregional tumor. In 2005, a report noted that the presence of one or more of these image-defined surgical risk factors was associated with a lower complete resection rate and a greater risk of surgery-related complications when attempting an initial resection of a localized NB.[80]

BIOLOGICALLY BASED RISK GROUPS AND THERAPY

As previously mentioned, one of the notable characteristics of NB is the substantial heterogeneity of the disease, which ranges from spontaneous regression or maturation, even without therapy, to a highly malignant, aggressive phenotype poorly responsive to current intensive, multimodal therapy. Increasing evidence indicates that the biologic and molecular features of NB are highly predictive of clinical behavior. Therefore, NB has served as a paradigm for phenotypic risk assessment and treatment assignment.

Current treatment of children with NB is based not only on stage but also on risk stratification that takes into account both clinical and biologic variables predictive of disease relapse. The two most important clinical variables appear to be the child's age at the time of diagnosis[81] and the stage[82] at diagnosis. The most powerful biologic factors at this time appear to be *MYCN* status,[31,33] ploidy[83] (for infants), and histopathologic classification.[21] However, additional biologic and molecular variables continue to be evaluated. Two variables, the allelic status at chromosomes 1p36 and 11q23, are currently being used to define the duration of therapy for certain patients. Taken together, these variables

Table 68-6 Image-Defined Risk Factors for Primary Resection of Localized Neuroblastoma

Neck

1. Tumor encasing major vessel(s) (e.g., carotid artery, vertebral artery, internal jugular vein)
2. Tumor extending to base of skull
3. Tumor compressing the trachea
4. Tumor encasing the brachial plexus

Thorax

1. Tumor encasing major vessel(s) (e.g., subclavian vessels, aorta, superior vena cava)
2. Tumor compressing the trachea or principal bronchi
3. Lower mediastinal tumor, infiltrating the costovertebral junction between T9 and T12 (may involve the artery of Adamkiewicz supplying the lower spinal cord)

Abdomen

1. Tumor infiltrating the porta hepatis and/or the hepatoduodenal ligament
2. Tumor encasing the origin of the celiac axis and/or the superior mesenteric artery
3. Tumor invading one or both renal pedicles
4. Tumor encasing the aorta and/or vena cava
5. Tumor encasing the iliac vessels
6. Pelvic tumor crossing the sciatic notch

Dumbbell tumors with symptoms of spinal cord compression: Any location

Infiltration of adjacent organs/structures: Diaphragm, kidney, liver, duodenopancreatic block, and mesentery

Adapted from Cecchetto G, Mosseri V, DeBernardi B, et al: Surgical risk factors in primary surgery for localized neuroblastoma: The LNESG1 study of the European International Society of Pediatric Oncology NB Group. J Clin Oncol 23:8483-8489, 2005.

Table 68-7 Children's Oncology Group Risk Stratification for Children with Neuroblastoma

Risk Stratification	INSS Stage	Age	Biology
Low			
Group 1	1	Any	Any
	2A/2B (>50% resected)	Any	*MYCN*-NA, any histology/ploidy
	4S	<365 days	*MYCN*-NA, FH, DI > 1
Intermediate			
Group 2	2A/2B (<50% resected or biopsy only)	Birth-12 years	*MYCN*-NA, any histology/ploidy*
	3	<365 days	*MYCN*-NA, FH, DI > 1*
	3	>365 days to 12 years	*MYCN*-NA, FH*
	4S (symptomatic)	<365 days	*MYCN*-NA, FH, DI > 1*
Group 3	3	<365 days	*MYCN*-NA, either UH or DI = 1*
	4	<365 days	*MYCN*-NA, FH, DI > 1*
	4S	<365 days	*MYCN*-NA, either UH or DI = 1*; or unknown biology
Group 4	4	<365 days	*MYCN*-NA, either DI = 1 or UH
	3	365 to < 547 days	*MYCN*-NA, UH, any ploidy
	4	365 to < 547 days	*MYCN*-NA, FH, DI > 1
High			
	2A/2B, 3, 4, 4S	Any	*MYCN*-amplified, any histology/ploidy
	3	≥547 days	*MYCN*-NA, UH, any ploidy
	4	365 to > 547 days	*MYCN*-NA, UH or DI = 1
	4	>547 days	Any

*If tumor contains chromosomal 1p LOH or unbalanced 11q LOH, or if data are missing, treatment assignment is upgraded to next group.
MYCN-NA, *MYCN* not amplified; FH, favorable histology; UH, unfavorable histology; DI, DNA index.

currently define the COG risk stratification (Table 68-7) for therapeutic approach. On the basis of these clinical and biologic prognostic variables, infants and children with NB are categorized into three risk groups predictive of relapse: low, intermediate, and high risk. The probability of prolonged disease-free survival for patients in each group is more than 95%, more than 90%, and less than 30%, respectively. Other factors such as chromosome 17q gain, caspase 8 inactivation, and TrkA/B expression are still being evaluated and may help further refine risk assessment in the future.

Low-Risk Disease

This classification includes all patients with stage 1 disease or patients with stage 2A/2B disease that is not *MYCN* amplified and in which the tumor has undergone a greater than 50% resection. Also included in the low-risk group are infants with stage 4S disease who have favorable histology, without *MYCN* amplification, and a DNA index greater than 1. The treatment of patients with low-risk disease is generally surgical resection alone, even in the presence of microscopic residual disease (stage 1), gross residual disease (stage 2A), or gross residual disease with ipsilateral lymph node involvement (stage 2B), if the tumor has favorable biologic characteristics (i.e., is without *MYCN* amplification). Infants with stage 4S disease who are not experiencing substantial symptoms may undergo an initial biopsy and observation only if the tumor has favorable biologic factors.

This "surgery alone" treatment plan for patients with low-risk disease was established on the basis of the prior experiences of both CCG and POG. The POG 8104 study found that 2-year survival was 89% for patients with POG stage A (INSS stage 1) disease despite microscopic residual disease, when patients were treated with surgery alone.[84,85] In a similar cohort of patients, the CCG 3881 study found 3-year EFS and overall survival to be 94% and 99%, respectively, for patients with Evans stage I disease.[86] That study also found that although patients with Evans stage II disease (similar to INSS 2A/2B) had a 3-year EFS of 81% irrespective of the extent of surgical resection and subsequent treatment, the overall survival for these patients was 99%.[86] This finding suggests that even if these patients experience disease relapse, most can be salvaged with additional therapy. Therefore, neither adjuvant chemotherapy nor radiation therapy appears to be necessary for the initial management of most patients with low-risk disease.

On the basis of these data, a group-wide COG study (P9641) was conducted from 1998 to 2006 to evaluate primary surgical therapy for biologically defined low-risk NB. The overall strategy of this study was to treat patients with low-risk NB with surgery and supportive care only. Adjuvant therapy was given only when less than 50% of the tumor was resected or when symptoms that were life- or organ-threatening developed. A probability of 3-year survival more than 95% was predicted for these patients with low-risk disease. Although the final published results from this study are still pending, the current recommendation continues to be that patients with low-risk NB are treated with surgery alone.

Intermediate-Risk Disease

This classification includes patients age birth to 12 years with stage 2A/2B disease that is not *MYCN* amplified and in whom the tumor has undergone less than 50% resection (or biopsy only), patients age birth to 1.5 years with stage 3 disease whose tumors are not *MYCN* amplified, patients age 1.5 to 12 years with stage 3 disease whose tumors are not *MYCN* amplified and are of favorable histology, infants with stage 4 disease whose tumors are not *MYCN* amplified, and patients age 1 to 1.5 years with stage 4 disease whose tumors are not *MYCN* amplified and have favorable histology and a DNA index greater than 1. Also included in this group are infants with stage 4S disease who are symptomatic from their tumor and the tumor biologic characteristics are either of unfavorable histology or the DNA index equals 1, or if no tissue was obtained at presentation for evaluation.

Intermediate-risk NB was initially defined through the analyses of CCG 3881 and POG 8742/9244 protocols. Based on these data, a group-wide COG study (A3961) was conducted from 1998 to 2006 to further refine therapy for patients with intermediate-risk disease. The overriding aim of this study was to maintain or improve survival while minimizing both acute and long-term morbidity in this group of patients. Patients received four of the most active agents for NB therapy: cyclophosphamide, doxorubicin, carboplatin, and etoposide, given for either four cycles (favorable biology) or eight cycles (unfavorable biology). Cycles were given every 3 weeks. This regimen was selected to maintain the dose intensity of CCG 3881 but to decrease therapy duration and cumulative doses, thereby reducing morbidity. Radiation therapy was not given unless there was progressive disease or an unresectable primary tumor with unfavorable prognostic features at the end of chemotherapy. Although the final published results from this study are still pending, 3-year event-free and overall survival appear excellent, at more than 85% and more than 95%, respectively.

The current COG protocol (ANBL0531), which opened in October 2007, seeks to further refine the minimal therapy needed to achieve these excellent outcomes (Fig. 68-9). As such, patients with favorable clinical and biologic factors will receive a further reduction in therapy. However, those patients in whom there is loss of heterozygosity (LOH–loss of one of the two normally paired chromosomal regions) at chromosome 1p or 11q (unbalanced) will not be eligible for this dose reduction because these events have been shown to be independently associated with decreased progression-free survival in patients with low- and intermediate-risk disease.[39] As with protocol A3961, patients will receive cycles of cyclophosphamide, doxorubicin, carboplatin, and etoposide given every 3 weeks. The duration of therapy (i.e., the number of cycles) will depend on which of three intermediate-risk groups the patient is enrolled, with group stratification again being based on clinical and biologic risk factors.[87-89] For almost all intermediate-risk patients, regardless of group (except group 4, stage 4 infants), this represents a reduction in therapy,[90,91] either shortening the duration (groups 2 and 3) or downgrading from high-risk therapy (group 4) (see Table 68-7).

The overall surgical goal in intermediate-risk patients is to perform the most complete tumor resection possible, consistent with preservation of full organ and neurologic function. This may necessitate leaving residual disease adherent to critical anatomic structures. If a primary tumor is judged by the surgeon to be unresectable, a diagnostic biopsy is generally obtained and chemotherapy initiated. Delayed surgery is performed after the prescribed number of cycles, as dictated by the group assignment. A reduction in surgical therapy is being evaluated for infants with stage 4S disease because it is no longer required that they undergo resection of their primary tumor. In addition, if they are too unstable at presentation, it is no longer required that they undergo an initial biopsy to be eligible for enrollment in the current COG study.

Radiation will be administered only to symptomatic intermediate-risk patients when there is a risk of organ impairment due to tumor bulk that does not respond to initial chemotherapy. This will most often be encountered, albeit rarely, in infants with stage 4S disease, and in patients with epidural disease and symptoms of spinal cord compression.

Patients older than 12 years of age are excluded from ANBL0531 because there is increasing evidence that adolescent patients with localized tumors have an indolent clinical course but ultimately have an unfavorable outcome.[92,93]

High-Risk Disease

This classification includes patients of any age with *MYCN*-amplified tumors unless the tumor is localized and is grossly resected with ipsilateral lymph nodes being uninvolved (stage 1), patients older than 1.5 years with stage 3 tumors who have unfavorable histology, patients 1 to 1.5 years of age with stage 4 disease who have either unfavorable histology or a DNA index equal to 1, and patients older than 1.5 years with stage 4 disease regardless of tumor biology. Although not a part of the risk classification schema, the metastatic pattern of NB correlates not only with age but also with EFS.[94]

For patients with advanced NB, chemotherapy has been the mainstay of multimodality treatment. NB is generally a chemotherapy-sensitive tumor, and multiple-agent chemotherapy is usually effective in achieving a complete, or at least partial, response in older children with disseminated disease. However, this approach rarely effects a cure. The vast majority of these patients ultimately succumb to chemotherapy-resistant disease, despite the use of increasingly intensive chemotherapy. Several general principles of chemotherapy have been applied when treating patients with high-risk NB (as well as most of the other pediatric malignancies):

1. Combination chemotherapy is used to overcome drug resistance to individual agents and to achieve antitumor synergy using agents with different mechanisms of action.

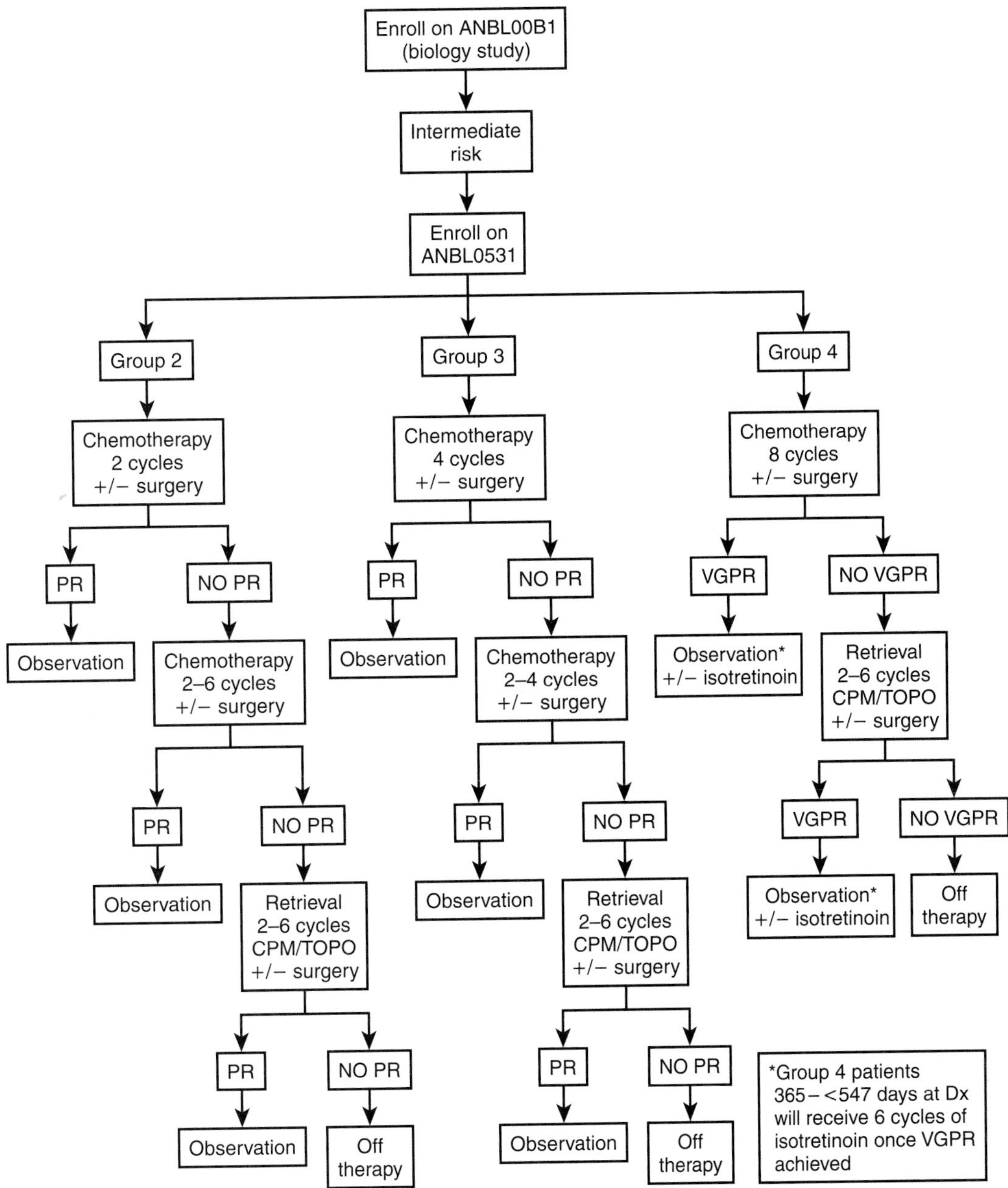

Figure 68-9. Schema for intermediate-risk neuroblastoma chemotherapy on Children's Oncology Group trial ANBL0531. PR, partial response; VGPR, very good partial response; CPM, cyclophosphamide; TOPO, topotecan.

2. Chemotherapeutic agents are administered at maximal dose intensity (the maximum tolerated dose [MTD] in the shortest time interval), because most of these drugs have a steep dose-response curve. This is why dose reduction due to organ dysfunction can have a potentially detrimental influence on disease outcome and why the risks and benefits of aggressive surgery should be carefully considered. The efficacy of MTD scheduling has been questioned recently, however, by the recognition of the importance of angiogenesis inhibition as an antitumor strategy. The recovery period that follows an MTD may permit recovery of the endothelial cells involved in the neovascularization required to support tumor growth and spread, whereas continuous, low-dose therapy more effectively inhibits angiogenesis, which in turn inhibits tumor growth, even when the tumor cells are resistant to the direct effects of a chemotherapeutic agent.[95]
3. Chemotherapy appears to be most effective when administered in the adjuvant setting to patients who have minimal residual disease. This is an extension of the Goldie-Coldman hypothesis, which predicts that the development of drug resistance is the result of a random genetic event that is less likely to occur when treating minimal residual disease with simultaneous administration of all active drugs.[96]

The general approach to treating patients with high-risk NB has included intensive induction chemotherapy,

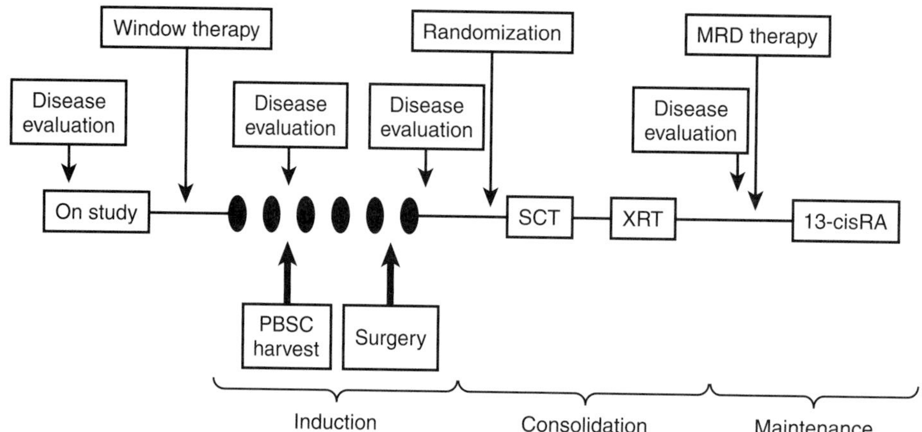

Figure 68-10. General schema of multimodal therapy for treating children with high-risk neuroblastoma. Variations include the testing of new drugs or combinations during "window therapy," the use of different "induction" regimens, randomizing patients to receive different consolidation therapy, and testing different approaches for treating minimal residual disease. Patients generally undergo PBSC harvest after two cycles of induction therapy and undergo delayed resection of the primary tumor (and locoregional disease) after five cycles of induction therapy. SCT, stem cell transplant; XRT, radiation therapy; MRD, minimal residual disease; RA, retinoic acid; PBSC, peripheral blood stem cell.

myeloablative consolidation therapy with stem cell rescue, and targeted therapy for minimal residual disease. Stem cell harvest is typically performed after the first two cycles of induction therapy, and resection of the primary tumor and bulky metastatic sites is attempted after the fifth cycle (Fig. 68-10). The CCG 3891 protocol enrolled patients with high-risk NB between 1991 and 1996. This study was designed to assess whether myeloablative therapy, in conjunction with autologous BMT, improved EFS when compared with chemotherapy alone, and whether subsequent treatment with 13-*cis*-retinoic acid, a differentiating agent, would further improve EFS.[97] The results from this double-randomization study demonstrated that the 3-year EFS was significantly better in patients who underwent BMT during the first randomization (34%) than in those who did not (22%; $P = .034$). In the second randomization, those who received 13-*cis*-retinoic acid after BMT experienced a significantly better 3-year EFS (46%) than those who did not receive the retinoid (29%, $P = .027$). Unfortunately, the long-term survival advantage for these patients is becoming less apparent. Nevertheless, autologous stem cell transplantation and 13-*cis*-retinoic acid are now part of most current high-risk NB protocols.

The first cooperative group high-risk NB protocol (COG A3973) opened in February 2001. It began with intensified induction therapy based on an analysis suggesting that increased dose intensity may improve remission rates and survival in these patients.[98] The induction therapy chosen, a dose-intensive combination of cyclophosphamide, vincristine, and doxorubicin alternating with cisplatin and etoposide, was based on the Memorial Sloan-Kettering Cancer Center (MSKCC) N7 protocol, which had a reported rate of remission of 90%.[99] Although the toxicity of the regimen was substantial, including the development of therapy-related myelodysplastic syndrome (MDS) and acute myelogenous leukemia (AML), the myelosuppression, fever, neutropenia, and mucositis were not dose limiting. After the sixth cycle of induction chemotherapy, patients were re-evaluated. Those with at least a partial response continued on the protocol and received myeloablative consolidation therapy (based on the results of CCG-3891) with stem cell support. Those patients not eligible for myeloablative therapy received maintenance therapy using topotecan and cyclophosphamide. Patients eligible to receive myeloablative therapy were then randomized to receive either unpurged or purged autologous stem cells. The rationale for this randomization and primary study question was that, although there has been some evidence that tumor cells contaminating reinfused autologous stem cells contribute to tumor relapse in patients with NB, it is uncertain whether the removal of the tumor cells by purging the stem cell product would influence relapse rates.[100,101] This protocol was closed early (March 2006), however, because an interim analysis showed no difference in outcome for children who received either the purged or the unpurged stem cell product.

The current COG high-risk NB protocol (ANB0532) opened in November 2007. Its primary goal is to test whether further intensification of myeloablative therapy will improve the cure rate. Randomization to either one myeloablative consolidation with a carboplatin/etoposide/melphalan preparative regimen or two myeloablative consolidations, in which the initial regimen includes thiotepa and cyclophosphamide, will occur at the completion of induction chemotherapy.

Another aim of this study is to determine whether additional radiation therapy delivered to gross residual disease improves local control. Four to 6 weeks after stem cell transplantation, radiation therapy is administered to the region of the primary tumor site, including involved adjacent lymph nodes. The target volume is the area of residual disease, which is determined radiographically, after induction chemotherapy but prior to delayed surgical resection, with an additional 1.5-cm margin added, even if a complete resection

Table 68-8 International Neuroblastoma Staging System Response Criteria

Response	Primary Tumor	Metastatic Sites*
CR	No tumor	No tumor; catecholamines normal
VGPR	Decreased by 90%-99%	No tumor; catecholamines normal; residual ^{99m}Tc bone changes allowed
PR	Decreased by > 50%	All measurable sites decreased by > 50% Bones and bone marrow: number of positive bone sites decreased by > 50%; no more than one positive bone marrow site allowed
MR	No new lesions	>50% reduction of any measurable lesion (primary or metastases) with < 50% reduction in any other; < 25% increase in any existing lesion
NR	No new lesions	<50% reduction but < 25% increase in any existing lesion
PD	Any new lesion	Increase of any measurable lesion by > 25%; previous negative marrow positive for tumor

*One positive marrow aspirate or biopsy allowed for PR if this represents a decrease from the number of positive sites at diagnosis.
CR, complete response; MR, minimal response; NR, no response; PD, progressive disease; PR, partial response; VGPR, very good partial response.

was ultimately achieved. Sites of persistent active metastatic disease prior to stem cell transplantation (i.e., positive sites on MIBG scan or those that do not show diminished enhancement on serial bone scans) are irradiated at the same time and with the same dose as the primary site.

Total-body irradiation is often used as part of the myeloablative therapy for bone marrow infusion.[102] In a review of CCG 3891, it was found that, in combination with external-beam radiation to the primary tumor site, the addition of 10 Gy of total-body irradiation as a component of high-dose chemotherapy with stem cell rescue improved local control compared with conventional chemotherapy without total-body irradiation.[103] Results from this study also suggested a dose-response relationship for local radiation therapy with limited short-term toxicity. Based on these results, patients treated on ANB0532 whose primary site has achieved a complete response at the end of induction therapy will receive 21.6 Gy to the site of primary locoregional disease while areas with gross residual disease will be treated with an additional boost of 14.4 Gy (36 Gy total).

A third aim of ANB0532 is to test the use of a dose-intensive topotecan-containing induction regimen, substituting two cycles of dose-intensive cyclophosphamide and topotecan for the first two cycles of induction used in COG A3973. Secondary surgical objectives embedded in this protocol include (1) a determination of whether resection completeness is predictive of local control rate or EPS, (2) a prospective tabulation of the complications related to efforts at local control, and (3) a description of the neurologic outcomes in patients with paraspinal primary tumors.

Assessment of Therapeutic Response

Precise evaluation of the therapeutic response of primary and metastatic sites to treatment is essential for confirming the efficacy of therapy, predicting disease outcome, and planning the next therapeutic modality. The International NB Response Criteria[71] was presented in 1988 and has since been revised (Table 68-8).[18] The determination of response should be based on the volume of the primary tumor and large metastases measured by three-dimensional imaging such as CT or MRI. Normalization of urinary catecholamines is included in the determination of the response of metastatic sites. Whether MIBG scans provide useful assessment of therapeutic response is currently being evaluated.

Other Treatment Approaches to High-Risk Neuroblastoma

In addition to the group-wide COG protocol, other institutional protocols for treating patients with high-risk NB are being tested. In addition, several universities and children's hospitals have formed a consortium funded by the National Cancer Institute to test promising new therapies for NB. The New Approaches to NB Therapy (NANT) consortium was formed to organize closely collaborating investigators whose laboratory programs are developing novel therapies for high-risk NB. NANT currently conducts clinical trials that test new drugs and new combinations of drugs against high-risk NB. Those with promising results will be considered for more extensive national testing.

Recurrent High-Risk Neuroblastoma

Patients with recurrent high-risk NB have a uniformly dismal outcome. Several group-wide, NANT, and institutional phase I and phase II trials are currently open and are testing new treatment strategies for these patients. However, although a few patients with relatively limited initial disease can be cured with salvage therapies at the time of relapse, disease recurrence portends a dismal outlook for most stage 4 patients (<5% survival). Radiation therapy can be used for the treatment of refractory sites of metastatic disease and for palliation of painful sites of metastatic disease, with some success in providing pain relief and disease control.[104]

Future Approaches

In an attempt to improve the poor prognosis for patients with high-risk NB, newer chemotherapeutic agents continue to be tested as single agents in patients with refractory or recurrent disease, or in phase II "upfront window" trials involving patients with previously untreated high-risk NB. This latter approach may give a more accurate assessment of a drug's efficacy because these patients are not already chronically debilitated by extended treatment. It is important to note that, at present, there is no evidence of worsening response rates to standard multidrug induction chemotherapy in children treated with an initial phase II window designed to assess the anti-NB efficacy and toxicity of a new drug.[105,106] As more information regarding diagnostically and prognostically useful genetic markers for NB become available, therapeutic strategies will change accordingly. There may ultimately be individualized treatment regimens for children with NB based on the molecular biologic profile of a patient's tumor. In addition, this profiling will not only identify patients whose tumors show a more aggressive biologic profile but also identify patients with tumors that do not have this aggressive biologic profile. Regimen toxicity, including late effects of therapy, is particularly important in the pediatric population. Therefore, treatment will be designed so that patients with biologically high-risk tumors receive intensified regimens and patients with biologically low-risk tumors benefit from the lower toxicity of less intensive therapy while maintaining cure rates.

SURGICAL TREATMENT

Complete resection of a tumor offers definitive therapy with generally excellent outcome for patients with localized NB. The value of complete tumor removal may be overestimated, however, because of the possibility that localized NB may undergo spontaneous maturation or even regression. The role of surgery is even less clear in the curative treatment of patients with high-risk NBs. Unfortunately, more than half of patients with NB present with advanced local or metastatic disease, which requires intensive multimodal therapy in addition to surgery. It is crucial that surgeons consider the heterogeneous nature of NB and the molecular and biologic characteristics associated with good or bad prognoses when determining the role of surgery for any specific case.

Localized Tumors

Most localized NBs have favorable biologic features and are successfully treated with operation alone.[84,91,107-110] In addition, studies suggest that a subset of localized tumors will spontaneously regress and that these patients can be observed without any treatment.[111-114] Local recurrences, when they rarely occur, can generally be managed surgically.[115] Thus, complete resection of a localized NB may be the only therapy required for some patients.[116] However, currently, biopsy of ipsilateral and contralateral lymph nodes is required for accurate staging, risk assessment, and therapy assignment for patients with an abdominal primary site. Lymph node evaluation is less important for patients with a thoracic primary site. Biopsy of contralateral lymph nodes is rarely feasible in patients with a thoracic primary tumor. Moreover, evaluation of ipsilateral lymph nodes, which may potentially influence staging, rarely changes the risk classification and treatment. Regardless of the presence of microscopic or even gross residual disease with positive ipsilateral lymph nodes, no further therapy is given to patients with low-risk disease. Therefore, all patients with INSS stage 1 tumors, stage 2A/2B tumors without *MYCN* amplification (and > 50% resection), or stage 3 tumors of the midline that undergo gross total resection with negative lymph nodes are treated with surgical resection alone.

Several reports have indicated that the extent of surgery for localized disease is a significant predictor of outcome. One study reported a 2-year disease-free survival of 93% in patients with nonmetastatic disease and complete tumor resection, as compared with 54% for those undergoing a subtotal resection.[117] Another study reported a 77% long-term survival for patients with Evans stage III disease who had a complete resection at some point during therapy, compared with 28% long-term survival for those unable to have a complete resection.[118] The MSKCC experience suggests that for all patients with nonmetastatic disease and a single copy of *MYCN*, surgery alone is adequate treatment, even if residual disease is present or locoregional lymph nodes are positive.[119]

In most instances, performing a biopsy before resection is unnecessary in patients with localized tumors that are likely to be NB, appear to be easily resectable (based on diagnostic imaging), and have had a negative metastatic workup. This is especially true for those patients whose primary site is thoracic because the patients with low-risk disease will not receive adjuvant therapy. Even for patients with intermediate- or high-risk disease who will receive adjuvant chemotherapy, earlier removal of bulky disease may be feasible and may potentially decrease the likelihood of developing drug-resistant tumor clones.[120] However, primary resection in these patients should be attempted only if it can clearly be accomplished safely, without injury to adjacent organs or blood vessels and without delaying the initiation of chemotherapy. In all cases, if there is any question of resectability, a pre-resection risk determination should be performed because this may influence the surgical plan. An assessment of the *MYCN* status can be performed on a minimal amount of tumor tissue, including tumor cells in the bone marrow. *MYCN*-amplified tumors, unless stage 1, are all high risk. To determine the histopathologic status, the COG protocols currently require 1 cm^3 of tissue. Therefore, an "open" tumor biopsy (or potentially a laparoscopic biopsy) is recommended, as opposed to a percutaneous core biopsy, which generally provides smaller samples. However, the only situation in which histopathology is important for accurate determination of tumor biology in a patient with localized disease is in a child between 1.5 to 12 years of age with an unresectable tumor that infiltrates across the midline (stage 3). In this circumstance, the histopathology will distinguish between intermediate- and high-risk disease (if the tumor is not *MYCN* amplified).

As mentioned previously, an alternate approach to treating patients with localized NB is taken at MSKCC. At that institution, all patients with nonmetastatic disease are treated initially with operation alone. Adjuvant therapy is reserved for patients who suffer a relapse. This approach is supported by the high success rate of salvage therapy using intensive chemotherapy and antiganglioside G_{D2} immunotherapy.[121]

Locoregional Disease in Patients with Metastatic Disease

More than 80% of patients who are older than 1 year of age and have metastatic NB will have tumor in the bone marrow.[122] The presence of disseminated NB is often suggested by a patient's ill appearance, anemia, "raccoon eyes," bone pain, or a limp and can be confirmed by demonstrating neuroblasts in the bone marrow and elevated levels of catecholamines in the urine. Therefore, most of these patients can have the diagnosis of NB confirmed by bone marrow aspirate/biopsy and the demonstration of elevated catecholamines in the urine. A surgical biopsy is required only if there is no involvement of the bone marrow, if the histopathology of the tumor is important in determining the risk classification (the patient is between 1 and 1.5 years of age with disseminated disease, and tumor cells in the bone marrow are neither *MYCN* amplified or have a DNS index = 1), or to obtain sufficient tissue to support biologic studies. Most patients with disseminated disease should receive neoadjuvant chemotherapy before attempted resection of the primary tumor and involved locoregional lymphadenopathy.

Delayed Surgical Intervention of Locoregional Disease

The role of surgery in the management of children with high-risk NB is controversial. Several reports have suggested that patients with INSS stage 3 or 4 disease who undergo gross total resection of their primary tumor and locoregional disease experience improved local tumor control and increased overall survival. However, other reports have not confirmed these observations. In one study, patients with stage 4 disease who were older than 1 year at the time of diagnosis had an improved outcome with gross total resection of the primary tumor, though the influence of resection was not independent of chemotherapy intensity.[123] A more recent paper from the same group provided further data suggesting that local control and overall survival are correlated with gross total resection of the primary tumor in high-risk NB and should be the goal in current clinical trials.[124] Similarly, another study supported the use of aggressive surgery for patients with metastatic disease in an attempt to improve outcome.[118] Also, improved survival in patients with metastatic disease who underwent complete resection of the primary tumor during delayed second-look procedures has been found.[125] Finally, a large meta-analysis of the outcomes for patients with stage 3 and 4 disease and a review of the impact of the extent of primary site resection on EFS, overall survival, and local recurrence in high-risk NB for patients treated on COG A3973 were both presented at the recent Advances in Neuroblastoma Meeting (Chiba, Japan, 2008). A 90% or greater resection was found to be associated with a significant decrease in local recurrence, with a slight but sustained improvement in both event-free and overall survival, although this was not statistically significant.

In contrast, several studies have found that the extent of surgical resection does not affect the final outcome.[126,127] Another study found that the extent of surgical resection affected only certain subgroups of patients with high-risk disease.[128] In addition, substantial complication rates have also been reported after aggressive attempts at removing all gross tumor from the retroperitoneum.[129] Another report noted that the outcome for patients with stage 4 NB depended more on the biologic characteristics of the tumor than on the extent of surgical resection.[130] This conclusion is further highlighted by the results of the CCG 3881 study, which showed that, at least in infants with stage 4 disease and single-copy *MYCN* tumors, survival was excellent, regardless of whether gross total resection (3-year EFS, 91%) or incomplete resection (3-year EFS, 94%) was performed. However, survival was poor if the tumor was *MYCN* amplified, again, regardless of the extent of surgery. Three-year EFS after total resection was 14%, and 3-year EFS after incomplete resection was 10% ($P = .18$).[131] The role of cytoreduction by surgical resection is unclear. However, resection of as much gross tumor as possible in patients who receive autologous or allogeneic BMT in combination with high-dose chemotherapy and total-body irradiation may be of some benefit.[132]

Despite the uncertainty of the role of surgery, the COG high-risk protocol currently recommends attempting gross total resection of the primary tumor and locoregional disease in patients with high-risk NB. Most children undergo delayed surgery after the completion of the fifth cycle of induction chemotherapy, even though tumor volume reduction plateaus after the second or third cycle of chemotherapy.[133] Other groups are performing surgery as soon as locoregional disease appears, radiographically, to be resectable.[134] Although initial surgical resection is often not appropriate for patients with NB, the principle of resection at the earliest feasible time should be considered. Because no prospective, randomized studies have been performed, the influence of the extent of surgical resection is unknown. However, in considering aggressive surgical resection, the risks involved, including vascular injury and significant bleeding, kidney or bowel infarction, infection, delay in chemotherapy, and long-term complications (e.g., renal atrophy and diarrhea) need to be weighed carefully against the uncertain benefits of extensive surgery. Certainly removal of kidneys or other organs is to be avoided because this may hinder or delay the ability to give potentially effective chemotherapy.

The age of the patient and the tumor biology are of critical importance when planning surgery. For example, survival of infants with stage 4, single-copy *MYCN* disease is greater than 94%, regardless of the extent of surgical resection of locoregional disease. This favorable outcome for patients with stage 4, single-copy *MYCN* disease probably includes patients up to 18 months of age if the tumor's Shimada histology is also favorable. Clearly, the excellent prognosis for these patients should not be jeopardized by overly aggressive surgery. The extent of surgery also did not appear to significantly affect the survival of infants with *MYCN*-amplified tumors in this nonrandomized trial because the outcome for those patients was very poor (<15%). Perhaps, infants with stage 4 disease and *MYCN*-amplified tumors would benefit from more aggressive surgery despite the attendant risks, given that current adjuvant therapy is unlikely to provide a cure.

Surgery for Recurrent Disease

Surgery may have a limited role in the management of patients with relapsed NB in whom the recurrence has been documented to be localized and refractory to available chemotherapeutic agents.

Operative Principles

More than half of NBs arise in the abdominal cavity. Tumor size, the extent of vascular encasement, and the exact tumor location should be considered in selecting the approach for a retroperitoneal NB. Options available for the abdominal incision include a transverse incision, bilateral subcostal (chevron) incisions, or a midline incision. A transthoracic (intercostal), transdiaphragmatic extension can be added to either incision for excision of NBs with either thoracoabdominal extension or extensive periaortic or celiac axis encasement. The tumor and adjacent lymphadenopathy should be carefully exposed to determine the relation between the tumor and normal organs and vessels. If encasement of major vessels such as the aorta, vena cava, or their branches is found, tumor dissection must be performed to free the vessels completely. Use of the ultrasonic dissector in selected patients may allow for better tumor dissection from the major vessels, with less blood loss and fewer complications.[135] Use of the argon beam coagulator and lasers[132] also helps to achieve complete or near-complete resection and reduces operative complications.[136]

For a major abdominal resection, several principles are helpful[137]:

1. Approach the operation as a vascular-type operation in which identification and skeletonization of the major intra-abdominal vessels is critical. Generally, the tumor can be separated from the vessel by dissecting in a subadventitial plane.
2. The tumor should be removed piecemeal. In particular, excessive torque on the renal artery in an effort to clear tumor from behind the renal hilum in one piece may result in injury to the intima of the artery with vessel spasm and/or thrombosis, leading to renal ischemia.
3. Dissection begins distal to the lower edge of the tumor, generally along the common or external iliac artery, and proceeds proximally to encounter the tumor along the aorta identifying the major arterial branches (and left renal vein). With deliberate dissection of the tumor from the mesenteric and renal vessels, injury to the liver, bowel, spleen, and kidneys can be avoided (Fig. 68-11), although this frequently results in piecemeal division and excision of the tumor.
4. Right-sided tumors are managed similarly and are generally less complicated unless intimately involved with the structures in the porta hepatis.

Pelvic tumors may involve the sacral plexus in addition to the iliac vessels. Thoracic tumors are usually more easily cleared of the vascular structures but often extend into the intervertebral foramina. Extraction of tumor from this location is of uncertain benefit and can be associated with significant complications. A standard posterolateral thoracotomy (with or without a muscle-sparing approach) can be used to expose tumors of the posterior mediastinum, and cervical incisions can be used to approach tumors of the neck.

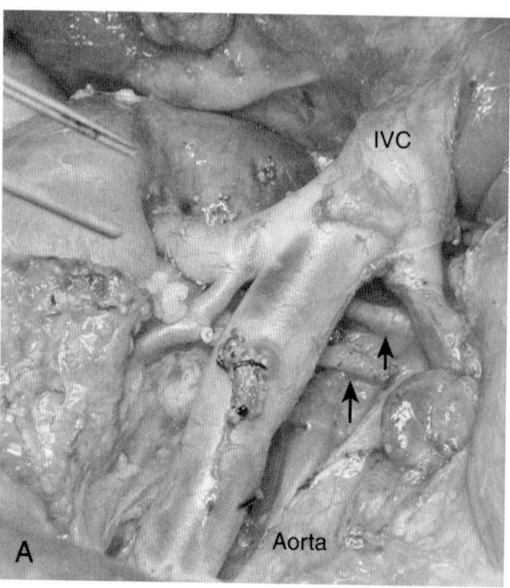

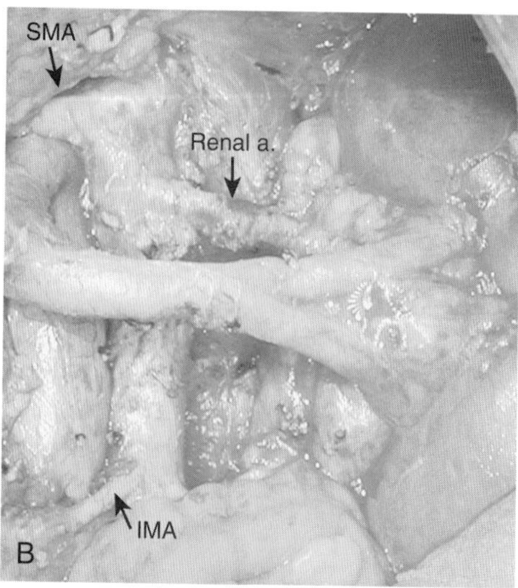

Figure 68-11. Intraoperative photographs after resection of retroperitoneal neuroblastomas. **A,** Right-sided dissection: note the presence of two right renal arteries coming from the aorta (*arrows*). **B,** Left-sided dissection: seen are the skeletonized aorta, mesenteric arteries, and left renal artery and vein. IVC, inferior vena cava; SMA, superior mesenteric artery; IMA, inferior mesenteric artery.

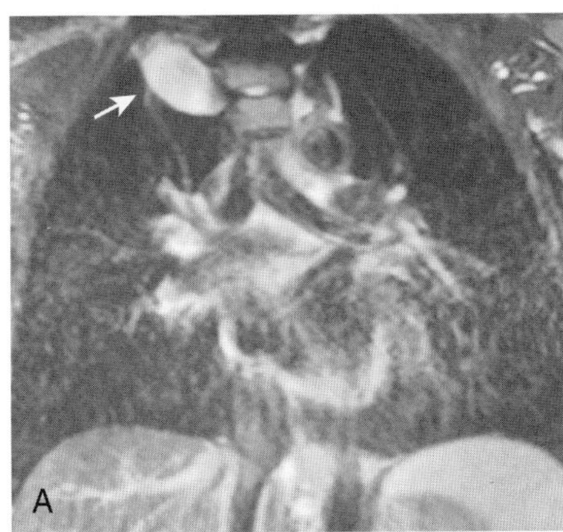

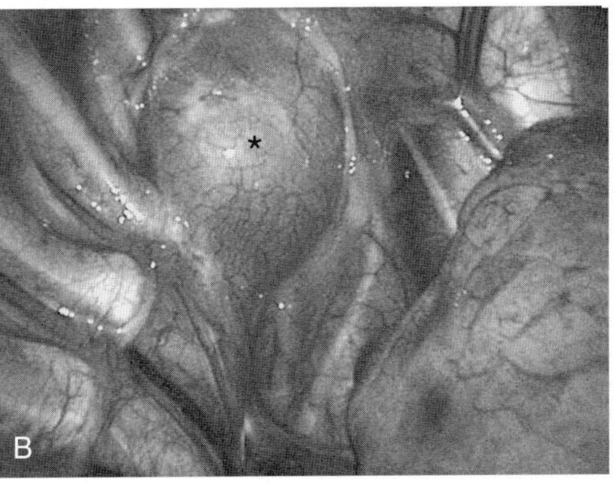

Figure 68-12. This child presented with ptosis in his right eye. **A,** MRI revealed a neurogenic tumor (*arrow*) in the superior mediastinum on the right side. **B,** At thoracoscopy, the tumor (*asterisk*) is seen. This tumor was able to be removed completely, although the ptosis persisted.

A minimally invasive laparoscopic or thoracoscopic approach may be used for resection of selected NBs in the abdomen and thorax (Fig. 68-12).[138,139]

Operative Complications

Because of the extensive surgery often required, intraoperative and postoperative complications are not uncommon.[140-143] As many as 80% of patients will experience significant blood loss during surgery that requires transfusion of blood and blood products either in the operating room or in the early postoperative period. Up to 10% will suffer an injury to a major vascular structure (aorta, vena cava, or renal vessels). Injury to other viscera (stomach, bowel, liver, spleen, or kidney) occurs in approximately 5% of cases. On occasion, this necessitates removal of injured organs, with the kidney being the most common. Postoperative complications vary widely. Wound complications and postoperative bowel obstruction occur in 1% to 5% of the patients. In addition, hypertension, chyle leak into the thorax or abdomen, pleural effusion, infection and sepsis, diarrhea, and a prolonged total parenteral nutrition requirement have been known to occur.

SPECIAL MANAGEMENT SITUATIONS

Screening for Neuroblastoma

Because the two most important clinical variables for predicting outcome in patients with NB are tumor stage and patient age at the time of diagnosis, it was hypothesized that earlier detection of NB through mass population screening might significantly impact NB-associated mortality. In Japan in the 1980s, mass screening of NB was performed in infants by quantitating urinary vanillylmandelic acid (VMA) and homovanillic acid (HVA). Initially, the mass screening showed very encouraging results.[144] However, subsequent population-based studies with concurrent control groups in Germany and North America found that although the incidence of NB increased, the additional cases were largely early-stage, favorable-biology, low-risk tumors.[145,146] Because the overall mortality of patients with NB was not affected, the implication of these studies was that mass screening most likely detected tumors that would have undergone spontaneous regression and would not have been detected clinically. Thus, there currently appears to be no role for screening infants for NB.

Small, localized NBs in young infants tend to regress spontaneously. Based on this observation, the COG protocol ANBL00P2 includes an arm of expectant observation in patients with these lesions to further define their natural history. This study is designed to prove the hypothesis that close biochemical and ultrasonographic observation can be used for safe clinical management of infants with small adrenal masses. Surgical resection is reserved for those rare cases in which there is evidence of continued growth. To be eligible, infants with an adrenal mass must be younger than 6 months of age when the mass is first identified. Also, the mass must be less than 16 mL in volume if solid or less than 65 mL if at least 25% cystic. Finally, disease must be limited to the adrenal gland.

Stage 4S Disease

In 1971, D'Angio and colleagues reported a number of patients with a "special" variant of metastatic NB termed IV-S (now referred to as 4S).[147] These patients were infants who typically had a single, small primary tumor. However, these infants often had extensive metastatic disease in the liver, resulting in significant hepatomegaly, skin nodules ("blueberry muffin" lesions), and small amounts of disease in the bone marrow (<10% of the mononuclear cells). Patients with 4S NB were quite remarkable because the large amount of disease generally underwent spontaneous regression, even without treatment, and the infants ultimately were found to have no evidence of disease.

Only supportive therapy has been recommended for this stage of NB because of the high incidence of spontaneous regression and the resultant good prognosis.[148] Most of these patients have tumor with favorable biology (single-copy *MYCN,* favorable Shimada histology, and DNA index > 1). Therefore, they are assigned to the low-risk classification and receive no therapy. However, despite the generally benign course of their malignancy, these infants can die of complications caused by the initial bulk of their disease. Limited chemotherapy, local irradiation, or minimal resection can be used to treat infants with life-threatening symptoms of hepatomegaly. Operative placement of a Silastic pouch as a temporary abdominal wall patch can be used for those with significant liver enlargement that causes either respiratory compromise secondary to diaphragmatic elevation or obstruction of the inferior vena cava. This procedure may help to avoid life-threatening events until shrinkage of the liver is achieved by either spontaneous regression or therapy. The rare infant with 4S disease and either unfavorable Shimada histology or a DNA index of 1 (or if the biology is not known) will be treated as for intermediate-risk disease (group 3). Those with 4S disease that is *MYCN* amplified will be treated as for high-risk disease.

Intraspinal Extension of Neuroblastoma

In a subset of patients with paraspinal NB, tumor growth may extend into the spinal canal ("dumbbell" tumors). If neurologic symptoms result, urgent treatment is required to prevent permanent injury caused by compression of the cord. Each of the three main therapeutic modalities (surgery, radiation therapy, and chemotherapy) has been used in the past. A POG report showed similar rates of neurologic recovery in patients treated with surgery or chemotherapy, but significant orthopedic sequelae were seen more commonly in patients treated with surgery.[149] Although chemotherapy is probably considered most appropriate for the initial management of these patients, improvements in neurosurgical techniques, including the use of laminotomy instead of laminectomy to access the intraspinal tumor, may lead to reconsideration of this approach, especially in those patients with acutely progressive symptoms.

The appropriate approach for patients with asymptomatic intraspinal tumor extension is also uncertain. For patients with low- or intermediate-risk disease, the risks of attempting to remove the intraspinal component of a paraspinal tumor probably outweigh the benefits. This situation most commonly arises in patients with thoracic primary tumors. The intrathoracic component is resected, and gross residual disease remains in the spinal canal. Care should be taken to minimize surgical complications such as leakage of cerebrospinal fluid or uncontrollable intraspinal bleeding. Because residual foraminal disease rarely grows to a symptom-developing size, the importance of conservative therapy in this circumstance should be emphasized. In the absence of metastatic disease or unfavorable tumor biology, these patients' disease will be classified as stage 2A/B, low risk, and they have a very favorable prognosis with no further therapy. For patients with high-risk disease, the importance of resecting gross intraspinal disease is uncertain.

Opsoclonus-Myoclonus Syndrome

The opsoclonus-myoclonus syndrome (OMS) consists of myoclonic jerks and random eye movements or progressive cerebellar ataxia. OMS occurs in as many as 4% of patients, usually infants with thoracic primary tumors. Although the exact etiology of this syndrome is not known, the presence of cross-reactive autoantibodies to neural antigens in some of these patients suggests that it is mediated by the immune system.[150] Although patients generally have a good prognosis with regard to their tumor, neurologic symptoms often persist after successful removal of the tumor and can be quite debilitating.[55,56] Some symptomatic relief may be attained by high doses of corticosteroids or adrenocorticotropic hormones. Some studies have suggested that chemotherapy, intravenous IgG therapy, or both may improve the long-term neurologic outcome for these patients.[151,152] COG is currently testing this approach in a prospective clinical trial.

NEW TREATMENT STRATEGIES

Differentiating Agents

Retinoids are derivatives of vitamin A. 13-*cis*-Retinoic acid (isotretinoin) is a synthetic derivative of the naturally occurring all-*trans* retinoic acid. These retinoids decrease the proliferation and expression of *MYCN* from NB cell lines in vitro and induce morphologic differentiation.[153-156] Because of these attractive characteristics and the observation that resistance to chemotherapy does not result in resistance to 13-*cis*-retinoic acid, retinoids have been tested clinically. The CCG 3891 clinical trial randomized patients with high-risk NB treated using chemotherapy or autologous BMT into two groups who received either 13-*cis*-retinoic acid for 6 months or no further therapy. The 3-year EFS of patients who received 13-*cis*-retinoic acid (46%) was significantly higher than that of patients who received no further therapy (29%; $P = .027$) and was independent of the initial randomization to either chemotherapy or autologous BMT.[97] Because of this result, all patients on the current COG high-risk protocol receive oral 13-*cis*-retinoic acid twice daily for 2 weeks followed by 2 weeks without. This treatment is continued for six cycles (6 months total). Group 4 patients, age 365 to 574 days, being treated on the current COG intermediate-risk protocol will also receive 13-*cis*-retinoic acid.

Targeted Therapy

As more information regarding diagnostically and prognostically useful genetic markers of NB become available, therapeutic strategies will change accordingly. In addition, molecular profiling will lead to new drug development designed to induce differentiation of tumor cells, block dysregulated growth pathways, or reactivate silenced apoptotic pathways. One of the most exciting prospects for improving the therapeutic index, as well as overcoming the problem of tumor resistance to therapy, involves targeted therapy. Information about the molecular profile of a given tumor type, specifically mechanisms of tumorigenesis and proliferation control, can be assembled using a variety of molecular methods. This information can then be translated into new drug development designed to induce differentiation of tumor cells, block their growth pathways, and cause tumor cell death. These new agents can be used in concert with traditional regimens, and some may be used independently. Elucidation of the complex molecular pathways involved in tumorigenesis will also encourage the production of targeted anticancer agents with high specificity, efficacy, and therapeutic index. Two examples of this are the use of agents that act on impaired apoptosis pathways and neurotrophin receptor pathways in NB.

Caspase 8 is a cysteine protease that regulates programmed cell death. The gene that encodes caspase 8 is frequently inactivated in NB. DNA methylation and gene deletion mediate the complete inactivation of caspase 8, which occurs almost exclusively in NBs with *MYCN* amplification.[50] Caspase 8–deficient NB cells are resistant to death receptor–and doxorubicin-mediated apoptosis in vitro. These deficits are corrected by enforced expression of the enzyme. This finding suggests that caspase 8 acts as a tumor suppressor in NBs with *MYCN* amplification and may be of significant clinical importance.[50] Brief exposure of caspase 8–deficient NB cells to low levels of interferon-γ results in the re-expression of caspase 8 and the resensitization of the cells to chemotherapeutic drug-induced apoptosis. This finding indicates that a targeted approach using interferon-γ, perhaps in combination with doxorubicin, may be useful in patients with *MYCN*-amplified NB.

Different neurotrophin-receptor pathways probably mediate the signal for both cellular differentiation and malignant transformation of sympathetic neuroblasts to NB cells. As previously discussed, three tyrosine kinase receptors for these neurotrophins have been identified. Studies are ongoing to test agonists of TrkA in an attempt to induce cellular differentiation. Conversely, blocking the BDNF/TrkB signaling pathway with Trk-specific tyrosine kinase inhibitors, such as CEP-751, may induce apoptosis by blocking crucial survival pathways.[48,157-159] This targeted approach has the attractive potential for increased specificity and lower toxicity than conventional cytotoxic chemotherapy.

Immunotherapy

Several characteristics of NB suggest that the immune system can be successfully recruited for the treatment of this tumor. For example, the incidence of NB in situ far exceeds that of the actual disease and the tumors in infants often spontaneously regress. Both occurrences are potentially mediated by the immune system. NB is derived from embryonic neuroectoderm and, therefore, expresses antigens not widely detected in normal tissues. In addition, a substantial amount of innate, IgM-mediated humoral anti-NB cytotoxicity has been detected in the sera of healthy adults.[160] Several studies have suggested that patients with NBs are likely to have lymphocytes with specific antitumor activity.[161,162]

Cellular-Mediated Immunotherapy

Efforts to recruit T-cell–dependent and T-cell–independent cytotoxic effector mechanisms have focused largely on recombinant cytokines (e.g., interleukin-2 [IL-2]) that stimulate the immune system,[163] or on agents such as interferon-γ, which may render NB cells more immunogenic to cytotoxic T cells by increasing their expression of class I MHC molecules.[163-166] Although these approaches increase cytotoxic effector function against NB cell lines in vitro, similar effects on tumor growth in vivo are uncertain.[167-171]

Humoral-Mediated Immunotherapy

NB cells are sensitive to antibody-dependent cell-mediated cytotoxicity and to complement-dependent cytotoxicity.[172] Although a particular NB antigen has not been defined, monoclonal murine antibodies have been raised against the ganglioside G_{D2}, the predominant antigen in NB cells. Targeted immunotherapy using antiganglioside G_{D2} antibodies may be a promising approach for the treatment of advanced NBs. Therapeutic responses were initially obtained in phase I and phase II studies of the murine IgG_3 antibody 3F8[173,174] and the murine IgG_{2a} antibody 14G2a.[175-177] In a phase II trial, the mouse monoclonal antibody 3F8 induced a tumor response in 40% of patients with NB resistant to chemotherapy.[178] Phase I studies of 14G2a have demonstrated significant responses in patients with refractory NBs.[176] To decrease the immunogenicity of murine antibodies, a chimeric antibody was constructed by combining the variable regions of murine IgG_3 antiganglioside G_{D2} antibody 14.18 and the constant regions of human IgG_1-κ. This chimera, ch14. 18, binds the ganglioside G_{D2} antigen with exquisite specificity and alters both complement and cell-mediated cytotoxicity of NB cells by effector cells, such as peripheral blood mononuclear cells or granulocytes.[179] Superiority of ch14.18 over 14G2a in antibody-dependent cell-mediated cytotoxicity to NB cells in vitro was supported by a phase I trial of the chimeric antibody in which a durable response was achieved in children with refractory NB.[180] Ch14.18 was tested alone[181] and in combination with granulocyte-macrophage colony-stimulating factor (GM-CSF) in POG 9347. Some therapeutic efficacy in patients with refractory disease was found, although toxicity, particularly neuropathic pain, was substantial.[182] Because the induction of antibody-dependent cell-mediated cytotoxicity with antiganglioside G_{D2} antibodies is enhanced by cytokines such as GM-CSF[182] and IL-2,[183] the current phase III anti-NB antibody trial, COG ANBL0032, is designed to determine whether treatment with ch14.18 and cytokines (GM-CSF and IL-2) together with 13-*cis*-retinoic acid improves EFS and overall survival after autologous BMT as compared with treatment with 13-*cis*-retinoic acid alone.

MIBG Therapy

Refractory NB has been treated with ^{131}I-MIBG because it is readily taken up by the tumor cells.[184] In an investigation of patients with advanced chemoresistant NBs, response rates approached 33%.[185] Studies further suggest that this treatment can be used as front-line therapy, followed by chemotherapy, without significant hematologic toxicity.[186] In addition, [130] I-MIBG may have a potential role in the intraoperative identification of sites of active disease and in guiding the extent of surgical resection.[124] I-MIBG may be an even better treatment option for NBs with micrometastases or bone marrow infiltration[187] and is being tested for the treatment of patients with "ultra-high-risk" NB (expected survival of < 15%).

Antiangiogenesis

Angiogenesis is the biologic process of blood vessel formation. In addition to occurring as part of several normal, physiologic processes, angiogenesis is an essential component of a number of pathologic conditions, including cancer. Compelling data suggest that inhibition of angiogenesis not only prevents tumor-associated neovascularization but also affects tumor growth and spread. NB growth appears to be angiogenesis-dependent and is, therefore, likely to be susceptible to antiangiogenic therapy. Animals studies have demonstrated that NB is susceptible to a variety of angiogenesis inhibitors, including TNP-470 (a fumagillin derivative),[188-190] VEGF-Trap,[191] a truncated soluble form of the VEGF receptor-2,[192,193] and pigment epithelium–derived factor.[194] In addition, standard chemotherapeutic agents, when given using a low continuous dosing schedule, appear capable of treating tumors that had been previously resistant to them by destroying the neovascularity required by a progressing tumor.[195] By avoiding a "maximal tolerated dose" scheduling of these drugs, the patient can forego the recovery time required between cycles, thereby preventing recovery of the chemotherapy-sensitive endothelial cells.

chapter 69

LESIONS OF THE LIVER

Walter S. Andrews, MD

Hepatic tumors in children are relatively rare. The most common malignant neoplasms in the liver are not primary hepatic tumors but rather metastatic lesions such as Wilms' tumor, lymphoma, and neuroblastoma.[1] Primary liver tumors comprise between 1% and 4% of all solid tumors in children. Malignant hepatic tumors occur at a rate of about 1 to 1.5 per million children per year.[1,2] However, 10 primary liver masses occur with some frequency in the pediatric age group. Five of these occur only in children: infantile hemangioendotheliomas, hepatoblastoma, mesenchymal hamartoma, rhabdomyosarcoma of the biliary tract, and undifferentiated embryonal sarcoma (Table 69-1). Among these five tumors, the age distribution is distinctive, with hepatoblastoma and infantile hemangioendothelioma occurring most commonly in the first 2 years of life and hepatocellular carcinoma and focal nodular hyperplasia occurring most commonly after age 5 years (Table 69-2).[1]

Couinaud's elegant description of the segmental anatomy of the liver has allowed hepatic surgical procedures to evolve to a level at which they can be performed with an acceptable morbidity and mortality (Fig. 69-1).[3,4] The cumulative experience with hepatic resection and hepatic transplantation has allowed the development of techniques for both subsegmental and multisegmental resections of the liver in children. With the continued expansion of knowledge about these tumors, reasonable surgical and medical management plans can be devised.[5]

BENIGN HEPATIC TUMORS

Infantile Hemangioendothelioma

Incidence

Infantile hemangioendothelioma is the most common benign solid hepatic tumor in children, comprising about 16% of all pediatric liver tumors.[1] It also is the most common liver tumor in the first year of life. Almost all children with hepatic hemangioendotheliomas are seen initially before age 6 months, and the majority are encountered in the first 2 months.[6,7] Historically, a slight female predominance has been found, but this finding has not been uniformly seen.[8]

Clinical Presentation

Hepatic hemangioendotheliomas can be either single lesions that can expand to a massive size or a multinodular infiltrative lesion. Occasionally these lesions are asymptomatic and present simply as an abdominal mass or abdominal distention. Hepatic vascular tumors can also be found in association with congenital syndromes such as Osler-Weber-Rendu, Klippel-Trénaunay-Weber, and Ehlers-Danlos. Infantile hemangioendotheliomas have also been reported in association with Beckwith-Wiedemann syndrome, diaphragmatic hernia, trisomy 21, transposition of the great arteries, and extranumerary digits.[9,10] They frequently occur with hepatomegaly, high-output congestive heart failure, respiratory distress, and anemia. In addition, these patients may also have acute thrombocytopenia, a microangiopathic hemolytic anemia, and

Table 69-1 Hepatic Tumors in Pediatric Patients, Birth to 2 Years (AFIP 1970-1999)

Type of Tumor	No.	%
Hepatoblastoma	124	43.5
Infantile hemangioendothelioma	103	36.1
Mesenchymal hamartoma	38	13.3
Nodular regenerative hyperplasia	6	2.1
Hepatocellular carcinoma	4	1.4
Angiosarcoma	4	1.4
Focal nodular hyperplasia	3	1.1
Undifferentiated embryonal sarcoma	3	1.1
Hepatocellular adenoma	0	0
Embryonal rhabdomyosarcoma	0	0
TOTAL	285	100.0

Reprinted from Stocker JT: Hepatic tumors in children. In Suchy FJ, Sokol RJ, Balistreri WF (eds): Liver Disease in Children, 2nd ed. Philadelphia, Lippincott Williams & Wilkins, 2001, p 915.

Table 69-2 Hepatic Tumors in Pediatric Patients, 5 to 20 Years (AFIP 1970-1999)

Type of Tumor	No.	%
Hepatocelluar carcinoma	96	36.6
Focal nodular hyperplasia	40	15.3
Undifferentiated embryonal sarcoma	39	14.9
Nodular regenerative hyperplasia	26	9.9
Hepatocellular adenoma	22	8.4
Hepatoblastoma	22	8.4
Angiosarcoma	6	2.3
Mesenchymal hamartoma	5	1.9
Infantile hemangioendothelioma	4	1.5
Embryonal rhabdomyosarcoma	2	0.8
TOTAL	262	100.0

Reprinted from Stocker JT: Hepatic tumors in children. In Suchy FJ, Sokol RJ, Balistreri WF (eds): Liver Disease in Children, 2nd ed. Philadelphia, Lippincott Williams & Wilkins, 2001.

a consumptive coagulopathy (Kasabach-Merritt syndrome).[11] The development of this syndrome is often life threatening and requires aggressive treatment, as well as treatment of the primary cause. Fortunately, the Kasabach-Merritt syndrome occurs infrequently and is usually associated with hemangioendotheliomas that have rapid growth to a diameter of 5 cm or more. No cases have been reported in association with smaller tumors.[12] Other associated symptoms can include jaundice, failure to thrive, respiratory difficulties, or poor feeding. It was recently found that some of these patients also have congenital hypothyroidism. The presence of severe hypothyroidism can significantly complicate the management of these patients if it is overlooked.[13]

As many as 50% to 60% of these patients will display symptoms of congestive heart failure.[14,15] Interestingly, neonates with a focal hemangioma tend to have high-output heart failure at birth, whereas infants with multifocal lesions tend to be initially seen between ages 1 and 16 weeks. A classic symptom-complex has been described in hepatic hemangioendotheliomas: hepatomegaly, congestive heart failure, and anemia or other cutaneous hemangiomas. This triad occurs in 80% of infants who have multiple hepatic hemangiomas.[6] Associated hemangiomas occur at multiple distant sites, including skin (45%), lung (10%), pancreas, lymph nodes, and bone.[16,17]

Hepatic transaminase levels and occasionally the α-fetoprotein (AFP) level can be elevated. The cause of this elevation in AFP is unclear. The AFP level can be elevated in normal neonates and does not decrease to adult levels until about age 6 months.[17] In the presence of a significant elevation of AFP, however, hepatoblastoma must be excluded by either imaging studies or by biopsy of the lesion.[18]

A significant incidence of placental abnormalities has recently been reported in very low birth weight infants (<1500 g) who presented with infantile hemangiomas.[19] These researchers discovered a variety of placental anomalies that could lead to the shedding of placental cells into the fetal circulation along with fetal hypoxic stress. This hypoxic stress could then lead to increased production of angiogenic factors that could cause increased endothelial cell or placental cell proliferation in the postnatal period with the subsequent development of a hemangioendothelioma.

Imaging

The ultrasonographic evaluation of hepatic hemangioendotheliomas can be highly variable. Solitary lesions can have a very heterogeneous echogenicity, and the Doppler spectral analysis can show a variety of flow patterns. Multifocal lesions, however, tend to be more uniform in their appearance and are seen as echolucent nodules associated with a high-flow vessel.[20] On computed tomography (CT) with intravenous contrast, classically the lesions either enhance diffusely or rim enhancement is followed by gradual filling of the center of the lesion (Fig. 69-2).[15]

Focal hemangiomas are most often described as showing the rim enhancement with an avascular center related to either hemorrhage or necrosis.[21,22] This enhancement pattern is not typical for a hemangioendothelioma and can lead to uncertainty in the diagnosis. Currently, magnetic resonance imaging (MRI) is thought to be the single most useful modality to show both the location of the hemangioma and its flow pattern and structure.[23,24] The addition of intravenous gadolinium and a gradient-recalled-echo sequence to the MRI enhances its utility in focal lesions. Recently, however, there has been a case report of a hypervascular hepatoblastoma that had a MRI pattern that was identical to a hemangioendothelioma.[25] Therefore, radiology alone cannot reliably distinguish between benign and malignant lesions.

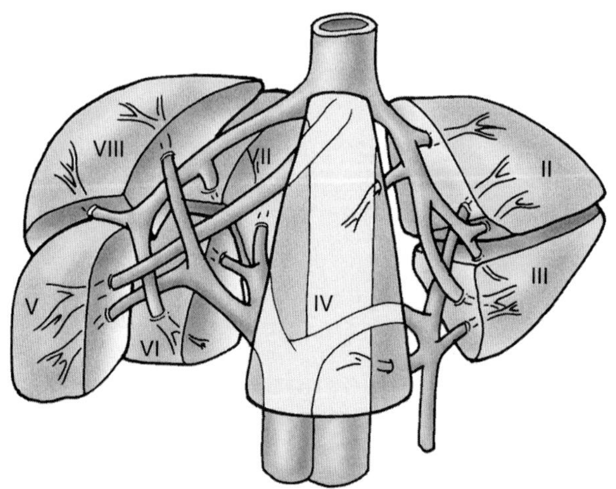

Figure 69-1. The segmental hepatic anatomy as defined by Couinaud. A comprehensive understanding of the hepatic segmental division is necessary for successful hepatic resection. (From Couinaud C: Surgical anatomy of the liver: Several new aspects. Chirurgie 112:337-342, 1986; and Couinaud C: The anatomy of the liver. Ann Ital Chir 63:693-697, 1992.)

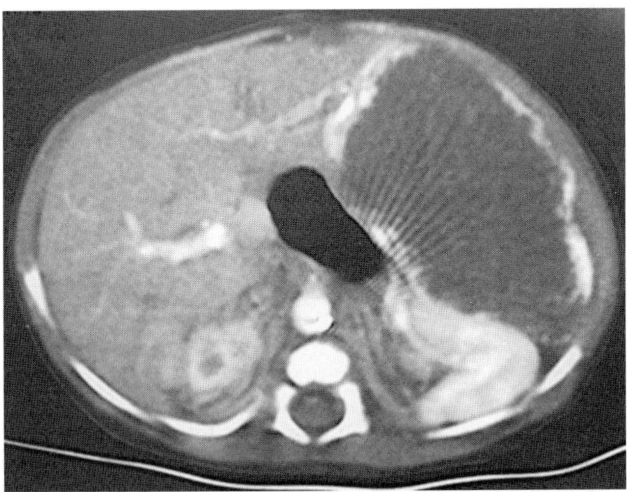

Figure 69-2. CT scan after intravenous administration of a contrast agent shows a large hemangioendothelioma with peripheral enhancement in the left lateral segment.

Another method for diagnosing hemangioendotheliomas is the use of a technetium-tagged red blood cell (RBC) blood pool scan. On delayed images (4 hours), an abnormal increase in activity is seen in the region of the hemangioendothelioma. This test is very specific and highly sensitive for hemangiomas.[26]

Hepatic hemangioendothelioma also has been seen in conjunction with focal nodular hyperplasia.[27] This association is important to remember during the radiologic evaluation of a child with multiple hepatic masses.

Pathology

Microscopically, most of these lesions consist of a single layer or, occasionally, several layers of flat endothelial cells on a supporting fibrous stroma (type 1 lesion).[28] In the type 2 lesion, seen in about 20% of the cases, the endothelial cells are pleomorphic, larger, and more hyperchromatic than those seen in type 1 tumors. Also, they are present along poorly formed vascular spaces that often show tufting or branching. It is thought that the histologic picture of the type 2 lesion is more characteristic of a rapidly proliferating process. However, the differentiation between a type 2 lesion and an angiosarcoma can sometimes be difficult.[16,29] Pathologically, infantile hemangioendotheliomas will stain positive for the marker Glut 1.[9]

Well-preserved bile ducts can often be seen near the periphery of the type 1 lesion, whereas bile ducts are absent in the type 2 lesion.

Treatment

The therapy for hemangioendotheliomas depends on the severity of the presenting symptoms and the size of the mass. In general, the natural history of these lesions is that they tend to grow over the first year of life and then begin to regress spontaneously.

Asymptomatic lesions are simply monitored, and no specific therapy is instituted until symptoms occur.[11,30] As part of the evaluation in asymptomatic patients with multifocal hemangiomas, however, imaging studies of the brain and chest should be performed to make sure no associated intracranial or pulmonary lesions are present. In addition, all patients with hemangiomas should be screened for hypothyroidism.

Patients first seen with congestive heart failure, coagulopathy, or respiratory compromise will require intervention. Mortality rates in these patients have been reported to range from 17% to 35%, with some reports of death in as many as 90% of severely symptomatic patients.[31-33] Risk factors for death include congestive heart failure, jaundice, multiple tumor nodules, and the histologic absence of cavernous differentiation.

In patients with congestive heart failure, stabilization is initiated with digoxin and diuretics. Supportive measures may be necessary in patients with respiratory compromise either from the high-output cardiac failure or from restriction of diaphragmatic movement by the abdominal mass. Coagulation factors can be administered if a coagulopathy is present.

If hemodynamic or respiratory compromise or coagulopathy becomes a problem, therapy directed toward the hemangioma is needed. The usual initial treatment for a symptomatic lesion is prednisone or prednisolone at a dose of 2 to 3 mg/kg/day. The symptomatic response rate to corticosteroids is reported to be about 45%.[34,35] If this is not effective in relieving the symptoms after 1 to 2 weeks, a trial of interferon-alfa should be instituted. Prolonged administration may be necessary for a clinical response.[36] Interferon-alfa therapy is indicated in the presence of the Kasabach-Merritt syndrome.[8] A recent report described a reduction in levels of vascular endothelial growth factor (VEGF) after administration of interferon-alfa.[37] Three cases of steroid-resistant infantile hemangioendotheliomas showed resolution by using vincristine at a weekly dose of 1 to 2 mg/m^2 for 2 weeks.[12] Surgical resection of these lesions appears to be most effective when it is confined to a single lobe. In this situation, a survival rate of 92% has been reported, even if the clinical situation is complicated by congestive heart failure.[29]

Embolization is being used more frequently, especially in patients whose condition is thought to be too unstable for surgical intervention.[38,39] With this therapy, it is important to identify and occlude as distally as possible both the arterial and portal vascular supply.[11,15] After successful embolization, a rapid improvement in the clinical course usually occurs within 5 days.[38,39]

Finally, in patients in whom other modes of treatment have failed, liver transplantation has been used as successful therapy for severe congestive heart failure or unremitting coagulopathy (or both).[40]

Regardless of the treatment modality, if the hemangioendothelioma does not completely involute, malignant transformation of an infantile hemangioendothelioma to an angiosarcoma has been reported in older children.[14,41] For this reason, patients who are asymptomatic or who become asymptomatic after therapy must be monitored for complete resolution of their hemangioendothelioma. Surgical resection of any residual lesion should be considered.

Mesenchymal Hamartoma

Incidence

Mesenchymal hamartoma is reported to be the third most common hepatic tumor and the second most common benign tumor in children.[1] Of the benign hepatic lesions that have been described, mesenchymal hamartomas account for between 18% and 29% of these tumors.[42,43] Approximately 120 cases of mesenchymal hamartomas have been described in the English literature.[44]

Epidemiology

The reason for the development of a mesenchymal hamartoma is unclear. One theory is that it results from abnormal development of the primitive mesenchyme, which appears to occur at the level of the hepatic ductal plate, causing an abnormality of the bile ducts.[45] This postulate is supported by the histologic finding of a combination of cystic, anaplastic, and proliferating bile ducts, as well as the presence of multiple portal vein branches within the tumor. It is conjectured that the tumor then develops a cystic component as a result of obstruction and dilatation of lymphatics or from occluded bile ducts (or both). The tumor enlarges during infancy as the cystic areas increase in size. Most of the proliferative growth appears to occur before or just after birth because no observable mesenchymal mitotic activity is visible on histologic sections of the tumor.[46]

A second theory is that the lesions are reactive rather than developmental.[47] It is hypothesized that an abnormal blood supply to an otherwise normal hepatic parenchyma causes ischemic necrosis, leading to reactive cystic changes within that portion of the liver. This theory is supported by the findings that hamartomas often have a necrotic center, are often attached to the liver by only a thin pedicle, and rarely are found centrally in the liver.

The third theory suggests that a mesenchymal hamartoma is a proliferative lesion. This theory is supported by several findings. Increased fibroblast growth factor-2 (FGF-2) staining has been noted in the proliferating hepatic mesenchymal cells adjacent to the mesenchymal hamartoma.[48] Both the mesenchymal cells in the liver and the mesenchymal hamartoma tissue strongly express molecules of the FGF-receptor family. It is speculated that a local increase of FGF-2 secretion could stimulate the growth of mesenchymal cells to form the mesenchymal hamartoma. FGF-2 also is a potent angiogenic factor that could contribute to the intense vascularization seen within some of these lesions. Cytogenetic studies in these tumors have documented balanced translocation of chromosomes 11 and 19 and 15 and 19 as well as the presence of aneuploidy.[49-52] This cytogenetic abnormality along with aneuploidy suggests that a mesenchymal hamartoma may be a proliferative lesion.

Clinical Presentation

The widespread use of prenatal imaging has led to the detection of hepatic masses before birth.[17] Cases of hepatic mesenchymal hamartoma that were diagnosed or detected prenatally have been reported.[53,54] One of the unique characteristics of a neonatal mesenchymal hamartoma is that it can be solid as well as cystic. Unfortunately, the prognosis for these neonates is often poor. Of the reported cases mentioned earlier, five experienced very rapid tumor growth, with fetal hydrops occurring in three. Two of these five fetuses died. It was believed that the rapid growth of the liver cyst caused the development of fetal hydrops. Thus, it may be best to deliver these fetuses before fetal hydrops develops.[54] Another series reported the use of repeated intrauterine aspiration of the cysts until the infants could be delivered and definitive treatment initiated.[55]

In the neonate, these lesions can have a varying presentation. High-output cardiac failure with associated pulmonary hypertension has been reported in neonates with highly vascular mesenchymal hamartomas.[56,57] Respiratory distress secondary to a large hepatic mass impinging on the diaphragm has also been described.[54]

The presentation of a mesenchymal hamartoma in the older child is usually that of progressive abdominal distention or an abdominal mass (or both). A significant right-sided predilection exists for these masses, and they tend to be somewhat more common in male than female patients. Occasionally there are associated symptoms such as nausea and vomiting that are secondary to the compression of the stomach and intestine by the expanding mass.[1]

On physical examination, abdominal distention or a palpable abdominal mass is most common. The mass tends to be nontender and fixed. Laboratory studies almost always are normal, including liver function studies. The AFP level can be moderately elevated and it will return to normal after resection. This is important because patients have been treated with chemotherapy for hepatoblastoma until a tumor biopsy was obtained.[58]

Imaging

CT, ultrasonography, and MRI have all been used for diagnosis. On CT and ultrasonography, usually a multiseptated, multicystic, anechoic mass is located in the periphery of the liver.[59,60] Occasionally the mass is pedunculated. Calcification is uncommon.[61] MR angiography has been proven useful both in the diagnosis and planning of the resection of these lesions.[62] The finding of a small round hyperechoic parietal nodule on ultrasonography is usually highly sensitive.[63]

Pathology

Mesenchymal hamartomas typically are large, well-circumscribed tumors that measure at least 8 to 10 cm in diameter (Fig. 69-3). Three of four of these tumors

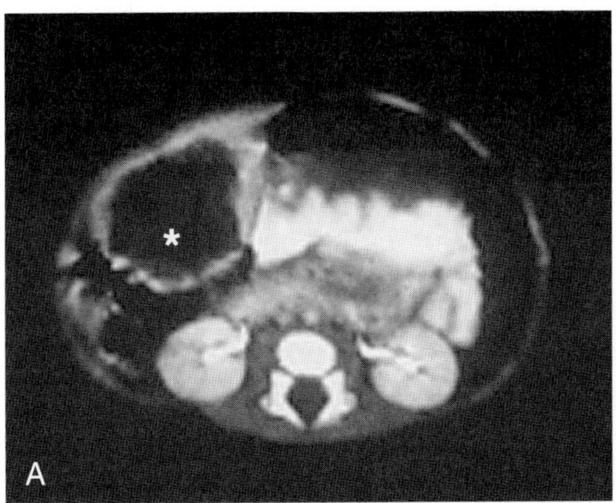

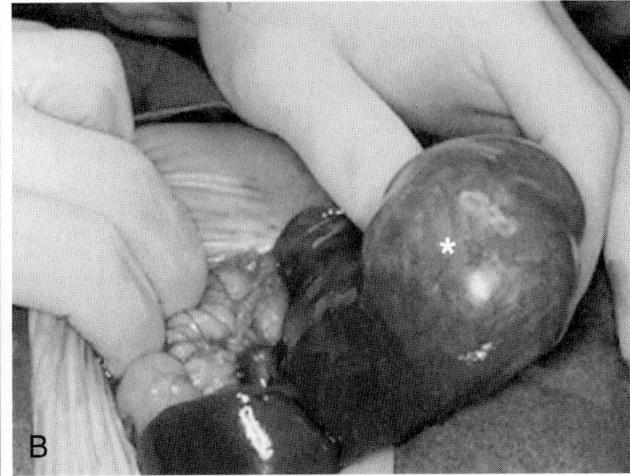

Figure 69-3. This young child presented with a palpable right upper abdominal mass. **A,** CT scan shows an anechoic mass (*asterisk*) in the periphery of the liver. **B,** At operation, the mass (*asterisk*) was found to be pedunculated and emanating from the right lobe of the liver. This hamartoma was easily removed.

occur in the right lobe of the liver, and only 3% are seen in both lobes of the liver. On cut section, multiple cysts measure from a few millimeters to 15 cm in diameter. These cysts are filled with either serous or viscous fluid separated by loose fibrous and myxoid tissue (Fig. 69-4). The surrounding tissue is yellow-tan to brown and is loose to moderately dense.

Microscopically, the tissue consists of a mixture of bile ducts, liver cell cysts, and mesenchyme. The cysts may simply be dilated bile ducts, dilated lymphatics, or amorphous fluid surrounded by mesenchyme. In older patients, the cysts may be lined with cuboidal epithelium (Fig. 69-5). Elongated or tortuous bile ducts surrounded by connective tissue are unevenly distributed throughout the mesenchyme. Typically the hepatocytes appear normal, and they are not a predominant part of the pathologic process. The bile ducts in the periphery of the lesion seem to be undergoing active proliferation.[1]

Despite the fact that the majority of these tumors are localized, there have been reports of these tumors being multifocal.[52] This may account for the occasional recurrences that are seen after resection of the primary tumor.

Treatment

Various management strategies have been used for these lesions. Because they are sometimes encapsulated, simple surgical enucleation may be possible. Very large, bilobar tumors that are not amenable to resection can be marsupialized into the peritoneal cavity, but recurrence after marsupialization has been described.[44] If a patient is to have marsupialization alone, there needs to be very careful, long-term follow-up because of the risk of recurrence or the development of undifferentiated embryonal sarcoma. Complete excision of the lesion with a margin of normal liver is usually curative (including the use of liver transplantation for large, bilobar lesions) and is the recommended therapy.[64] Spontaneous involution of these lesions has been reported, but this is unusual.[65]

There is now strong evidence that an undifferentiated embryonal sarcoma of the liver can develop within a preexisting mesenchymal hamartoma.[52,66-69] This association has occurred both synchronously and metachronously (undifferentiated embryonal sarcoma in a 6-year-old who had undergone a resection at 18 months for mesenchymal hamartoma). The evidence for a direct link between a mesenchymal hamartoma and an undifferentiated embryonal sarcoma of

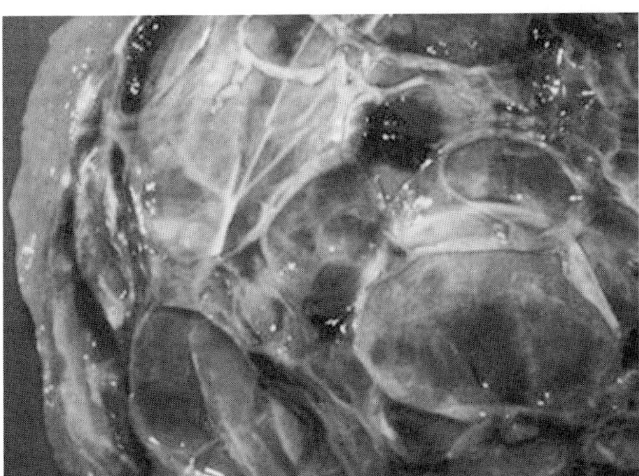

Figure 69-4. Cut surface of a mesenchymal hamartoma showing multiple cysts.

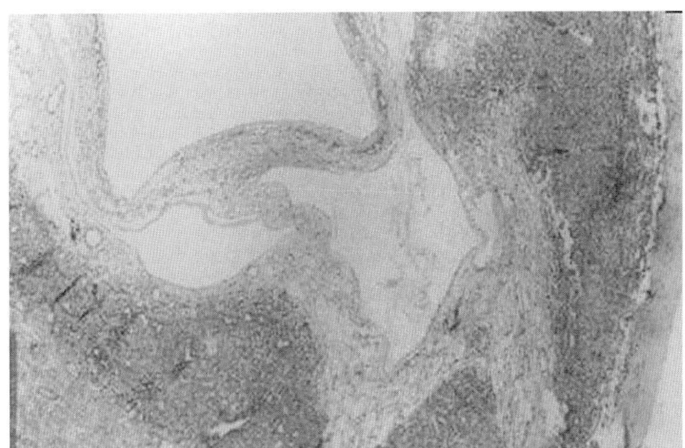

Figure 69-5. Light microscopy of mesenchymal hamartoma showing a cyst lined with cuboidal epithelium.

the liver comes from the simultaneous finding of both tumors arising within the same mass. Moreover, aneuploidy and similar chromosomal abnormalities involving chromosome 19q13 have been reported in both a mesenchymal hamartoma and an undifferentiated embryonal sarcoma of the liver.[49,50,70,71]

Focal Nodular Hyperplasia

Incidence

Focal nodular hyperplasia (FNH) accounts for about 10% of the hepatic tumors in children.[1] The reported age range is between 7 months and 16 years, with a mean of 7 years, and there is a slight female predominance.[72] The majority of these tumors are discovered incidentally.[72,73] The most common symptom is abdominal pain, but some patients describe decreased appetite, an abdominal mass, weight loss, or a combination of these. Hepatomegaly is a common finding, and liver function test abnormalities have been described.

FNH has been seen in association with a variety of different conditions and situations, including previous trauma to the liver, other liver tumors, hemochromatosis, Klinefelter's syndrome, the use of itraconazole, and cigarette smoking.[74-79]

The etiology of FNH is not certain, but the evidence suggests that it may be a congenital vascular abnormality. Pathologically, these lesions have a single feeding artery and there is an absence of bile ducts or veins in the lesion. The large artery causes a hyperperfused area of the parenchyma with subsequent growth of the liver tissue around the artery.[80] In addition, FNH has been associated with other vascular lesions such as hemangiomas, arteriovenous malformations, and hereditary hemorrhagic telangiectasia.[81,82] Further evidence that FNH is a reactive lesion secondary to vascular anomalies comes from a study in which an increase in the angiopoietin ratio (ANGPT1/ANGPT2) was seen.[83] The *ANGPT1* and *ANGPT2* genes are necessary for normal vascular development. In FNH, an overexpression of the *ANGPT1* gene and an absence of the antagonistic *ANGPT2* gene lead to uncontrolled and disorganized vascular development. Although it is not clear that this is the exact pathogenesis of FNH, it certainly suggests that this genetic imbalance may play a causative role.

Controversy exists about the relation between oral contraceptive use and the development of FNH. In a case-control study, it was noted that neither menstrual nor reproductive factors correlated with FNH risk. However, oral contraceptive use was a significant risk factor in the development of FNH.[78] Because the use of oral contraceptives also appears to be associated with hepatocellular adenomas, a history of oral contraceptive use does not help in distinguishing between these two entities.[78]

In children, an association has been noted between the congenital absence of the portal vein (Abernathy's syndrome) and FNH.[84-86] In addition, these patients have an increased incidence of other solid tumors such as hepatoblastoma, hepatocellular carcinoma, and hepatocellular adenoma. FNH also has been seen, albeit less frequently than hepatocellular adenoma, in patients with glycogen storage disease (GSD) type 1.[86] An especially interesting association was described with the development of FNH a number of years after treatment for either neuroblastoma or a variety of other small round cell tumors.[87] It was hypothesized that the chemotherapy caused microvascular alterations within the liver, resulting in the development of FNH.[88]

Therefore, it is important to remember that a liver lesion that occurs after treatment of a previous cancer does not always mean that there has been a recurrence of the primary tumor. A biopsy of the lesion should always be done before the initiation of any further therapy.[89]

Imaging

The diagnosis of FNH by radiologic means often requires the use of multiple different imaging modalities. On CT, the classic findings are early enhancement of the lesion and the presence of a central scar (Fig. 69-6).[90] Unfortunately this pathognomonic association is not often seen.[91,92] Additional imaging modalities include single-photon emission CT (SPECT) radionuclide scans with either radiolabeled sulfur colloid or hepatoiminodiacetic acid (HIDA) imaging, which demonstrates hypervascularization, increased tumor tracer uptake, and a central cold area.[93-95] Technetium-99m sulfur colloid scanning can also be useful in distinguishing between FNH and a hepatic adenoma. The colloid is taken up by the Kupffer cells in 80% of the FNH lesions but not by hepatic adenomas because they lack Kupffer cells.[96] MRI also has been useful when coupled with either gadolinium enhancement or the use of liver-specific contrast agents such as mangafodipir trisodium or iron oxide. These agents help to delineate the lesion better by specifically looking for the central scar.[97,98]

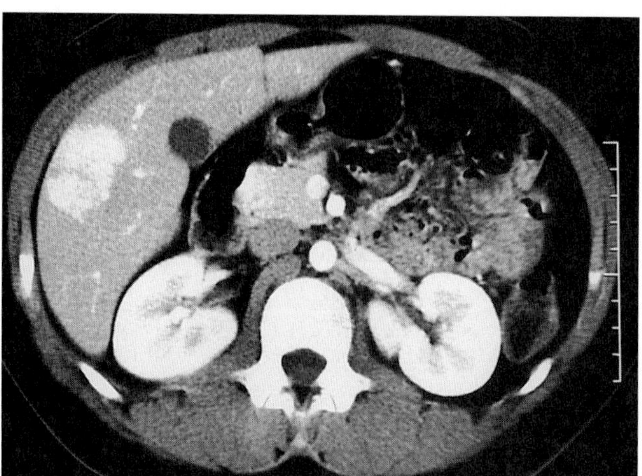

Figure 69-6. CT scan after intravenous administration of a contrast agent shows an early enhancing lesion in the right lobe with hypodense central scar consistent with focal nodular hyperplasia.

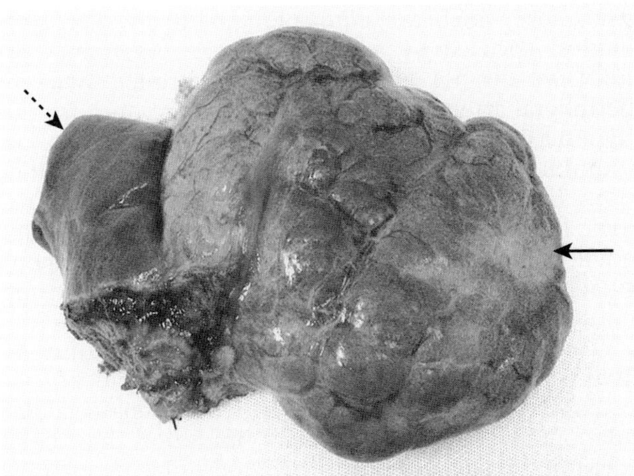

Figure 69-7. A large focal nodular hyperplasia lesion was resected. External scarring (*solid arrow*) is seen in the lesion. The *dotted arrow* points to normal liver.

Pathology

FNH classically is characterized by nodular architecture, a central or eccentric scar containing malformed vessels that resemble an arteriovenous malformation, and a variable amount of bile duct proliferation (Figs. 69-7 and 69-8).[99,100] This entity develops in the setting of a noncirrhotic liver.

Histologically, the classic form of FNH with a central scar accounts for about 80% of the lesions. Twenty percent are nonclassic where the FNH lacks either the nodular architecture or the presence of the malformed blood vessels. These lesions are subdivided into three histologic categories: the telangiectatic form, the mixed hyperplastic and adenomatous form, and the atypical form.[101] These nonclassic categories always lack a macroscopic scar. The mixed hyperplastic and adenomatous form often can be difficult to distinguish from a hepatocellular adenoma. Hepatocellular adenomas have been reported to be present in association with FNH in about 4% of the cases.[99]

Recently, there has been a case report of what appears to be malignant transformation of an FNH to a fibrolamellar hepatocellular carcinoma.[102] Also, FNH has been reported by several authors to occur in association with a well-differentiated fibrolamellar hepatocellular carcinoma.[102,103] This observation is important to remember in patients who have multiple hepatic nodules.[104,105]

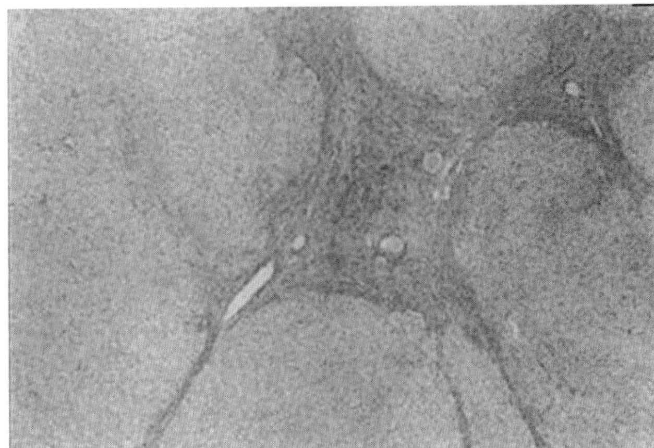

Figure 69-8. Light microscopy of a focal nodular hyperplasia showing a central scar containing abnormal blood vessels.

Treatment

The treatment of FNH depends on the clinical situation. If the diagnosis is certain, and the patient is asymptomatic, the consensus is that these patients can be followed with serial ultrasonography to make sure that no progression of the lesion occurs.[72,91] Percutaneous biopsy of these lesions has been helpful in their diagnosis.[106] However, if the patient is symptomatic, if the lesion is greater than 5 cm, if progression of the mass is seen, or if the diagnosis is unclear, then a biopsy or a resection of the lesion should be performed.[107,108] Because of the association of FNH with hepatocellular carcinoma, patients who are expectantly managed must have serial evaluations to ensure that no progression occurs. Moreover, they need to be monitored for the development of other hepatic lesions.

Several reports have noted a 40% to 50% regression rate in cases of FNH that have been monitored.[109,110] Regression of FNH is more likely if the use of oral contraceptives ceases.[111,112]

In two symptomatic patients in whom the FNH was in an area that was thought to be difficult for surgical resection, arterial embolization either with Lipiodol and absorbable gelatin foam (Gelfoam) or iodized oil and polyvinyl alcohol resulted in a significant regression in the size of the mass.[113-115]

Hepatocellular Adenoma

Incidence

Hepatocellular adenoma is a very rare hepatic tumor in children, comprising only about 4% of all solid liver tumors.[1] It is most commonly seen in women in their 20s and is associated with the use of oral contraceptives.

Clinical Presentation

In children, these lesions are often asymptomatic and are discovered during the evaluation for other problems. Occasionally, they can produce intermittent abdominal pain and rarely can spontaneously rupture, resulting in hemoperitoneum and the clinical signs of acute volume depletion.

Imaging

Hepatic adenomas are often solitary lesions in most cases, but occasionally two to three adenomas can be seen in one patient.[114,116,117] This finding carries the separate diagnosis of liver adenomatosis. On ultrasonography, these lesions can have a variable appearance, depending on the tumor composition. They can have a hyperechoic, hypoechoic, or a mixed echoic pattern depending on whether it is a simple adenoma, an adenoma with fatty metamorphosis, or an adenoma with hemorrhagic necrosis.[114]

On CT, the adenoma can either be isoattenuating relative to the normal liver or hyperattenuating (due to the presence of fat). They are usually sharply marginated and nonlobular but can be encapsulated or calcified in some patients.[118] Hyperattenuated areas often correspond to recent hemorrhage. Occasionally, on CT scan with intravenous contrast, peripheral enhancement secondary to large subcapsular feeding vessels occurs. The finding of central hemorrhage or necrosis on CT scan helps differentiate hepatocellular adenoma from FNH.

Associated Conditions

Hepatocellular adenomas were extremely rare prior to 1960, which corresponds to the year in which oral contraceptives were first introduced.[119] In women who have never used oral contraceptives, the annual incidence of hepatic adenoma is estimated to be about 1 per million. The duration of oral contraceptive use is directly related to the risk of developing a hepatic adenoma. The use of contraceptives for 5 to 7 years carries a 5-fold increased risk, and use for 9 or more years has a 25-fold increased risk.[120-122]

Hepatocellular adenomas also have been associated with galactosemia, hypothyroidism, polycythemia, diabetes, Fanconi's anemia, polycystic ovary syndrome, and the use of anabolic steroids.[123-126]

Hepatocellular adenomas can develop in patients with type 1A GSD from their teenage years into adulthood.[127,128] The estimated prevalence of adenomas in these patients is close to 50%.[129,130] These adenomas are often multiple rather than solitary lesions. Unfortunately, hepatocellular carcinoma can occur in association with hepatocellular adenomas in these patients as well. The youngest patient with GSD was 6 years old at the time of the diagnosis of hepatocellular carcinoma.[131] In several series, hepatocellular carcinoma has been found to develop in up to 18% of patients with a hepatocellular adenoma.[132-136] Direct evidence for malignant transformation of a hepatocellular adenoma into a carcinoma has been confirmed with the reporting of a hepatocellular carcinoma within a hepatic adenoma in patients with GSD.[137]

Adenomatosis (the occurrence of more than 10 simultaneous adenomas) is a rare disorder, with 38 cases reported in the literature through 2000.[138] The two forms are the massive form, characterized by multiple nodules measuring between 2 and 10 cm, and the multifocal form, in which most lesions are smaller than 1 cm, with only a few larger than 4 cm.[139] Oral contraceptive use has been seen in about half of the female patients. Interestingly, diabetes and hepatic steatosis has been noted in these patients but it is not clear whether a causative relation is present.[139,140]

Pathology

Hepatocellular adenomas histologically consist of large plates or cords of cells that resemble normal hepatocytes. These plates are separated by dilated vascular sinusoids, which are equivalent to thin-walled capillaries perfused by arterial pressure. Adenomas do not have a portal venous supply and are fed solely by peripheral arterial feeding vessels that account for the hypervascular nature of these lesions. Kupffer cells are found in reduced numbers and have little or no function. The absence of bile ducts serves as a key histologic feature that helps distinguish the hepatocellular adenoma from the FNH. Lipid accumulation is responsible for the characteristic yellow appearance on the cut surface.[1]

The exact reason for their development is unclear. Two reports have cited the mutations of the Wnt/β-catenin pathway in patients with hepatocellular adenoma.[141,142] This pathway mutation has been identified in many human hepatocellular neoplasms, although its direct contribution to carcinogenesis is not completely understood. A second mutation has been found in the *HNF1A* gene that leads to the downregulation of hepatocyte nuclear factor-1α. This downregulation has been linked to the development of hepatic steatosis and hepatic adenomas.[143] The significance of these findings in hepatocellular adenoma also is unknown.

Hepatocellular adenomas may be asymptomatic but also may be the site of hemorrhage. Larger lesions are more likely to bleed than are smaller lesions. Contained hemorrhage may result in rapid enlargement, but rupture with intraperitoneal hemorrhage may occur if the lesion is near the liver surface. Signs of blood loss or peritonitis (or both) may result.

Treatment

The treatment approach for these lesions depends on a variety of factors. In patients who are receiving oral contraceptives or androgenic steroid therapy, the first step should be withdrawal of these medications. Multiple case reports mention regression of these adenomas after withdrawal of these compounds. However, in other multiple reports, withdrawal of these agents has resulted in persistence of the adenoma.[144-146] If discontinuation is not effective, then the adenoma should be surgically resected. This removes the potential for future hemorrhage or malignant degeneration (10% of lesions).[147] If the adenoma is larger than 5 cm or if the diagnosis of the hepatic lesion is uncertain, then surgical excision is immediately recommended.[148,149]

For patients with ruptured hepatocellular adenomas, the current suggested therapy in the hemodynamically stable patient is nonoperative monitoring and hemodynamic support. Once the hemorrhage has resolved and the patient has recovered, elective resection should be performed. In patients who continue to bleed actively, hepatic arterial embolization should be performed. This not only stops the hemorrhage but also can decrease the size of the adenoma.[150] After resolution of the hemorrhage, resection is indicated. This management plan results in a decrease in size of the lesion and allows a more limited hepatic resection under controlled conditions.[151,152]

In patients with type 1 GSD in whom multiple adenomas develop, hepatic transplantation should be considered because of the significant probability of the development of a concurrent hepatocellular carcinoma. Liver transplantation not only corrects the potential hemorrhagic problem but also removes the potential for development of hepatocellular carcinoma.

MALIGNANT HEPATIC TUMORS

Hepatoblastoma

Most hepatoblastomas develop before age 3 years, with a median age of about 18 months.[153] About 4% are present at the time of birth; 69% are present by the end of 2 years, and 90% develop by the end of 5 years. Only 3% of cases are noted in children older than 15 years.[154] A definite male predominance(1.7:1) is seen.[5]

Epidemiology

Hepatoblastomas are associated with a variety of clinical conditions, syndromes, and malformations (Table 69-3). Beckwith-Wiedemann syndrome is associated most commonly with Wilms' tumor, but other tumors such as hepatoblastomas, gonadoblastomas, and adrenal carcinomas are also seen.[155,156] The association with hepatoblastoma is so strong that patients with Beckwith-Wiedemann syndrome must be monitored with serial AFP levels every 3 months until the age of 4 years and an abdominal ultrasonogram every 3 months until they reach age 8 years.[156-158] Screening studies for hepatoblastoma are also recommended in patients with familial adenomatous polyposis. These patients should be screened for the *APC* tumor/suppressor gene. If this gene is present, then these patients are at increased risk for developing hepatoblastoma.[159,160]

Another interesting association exists between hepatoblastoma and extreme prematurity (<1000 g). In the Japanese Children's Cancer Registry (JCCR), it was noted that hepatoblastomas accounted for 58% of the malignancies diagnosed in extremely low birth weight children.[161] In a recent epidemiologic study, several factors were associated with an increased risk for the development of neonatal hepatoblastoma, including birth weight less than 1000 g, maternal age younger than 20 years, use of infertility treatment, maternal smoking, and a higher prepregnancy body mass index (BMI of 25-29).[162] The time from birth to onset of hepatoblastoma in this population ranges from 6 months to 6 years.[163] Unfortunately, the tumors that occurred in this group grew rapidly and had an unfavorable biologic behavior.[164] Although the etiology for the predilection of hepatoblastomas to develop in very low birth weight infants is not known, oxygen therapy, furosemide use, and a retarded growth rate all were noted to be risk factors.[164] The highest correlation was with the duration of oxygen therapy. The risk of hepatoblastoma increased by 20% if oxygen therapy was continued for 30 days, and the risk increased by 100% in children who were treated with oxygen for 4 months.

Table 69-3 Conditions Associated with Hepatoblastoma

Conditions
Beckwith-Wiedemann syndrome
Budd-Chiari syndrome
Gardner's syndrome
Hemihypertrophy
Heterozygous α_1-antitrypsin deficiency
Isosexual precocity
Polyposis coli families
Trisomy 18
Type 1a glycogen storage disease
Very low birth weight

Cysteine has also been implicated as a contributing factor. Cysteine is an amino acid that is necessary for the production of glutathione and taurine, both of which are intracellular antioxidants. In premature infant livers, there appears to be impaired production of cysteine.[165]

Because of the complexities of treating "micropremies" through their first few months, multiple other interventions could influence the development of a hepatoblastoma.

Pathology

Hepatoblastomas tend to be unifocal lesions in most cases. Fifty percent are isolated to the right lobe, 15% are in the left lobe, and 27% are centrally located to involve both lobes (Fig. 69-9).

Histologically, the tumor can be divided into six different subtypes (Figs. 69-10 and 69-11) based on light microscopy (Table 69-4). A correlation between clinical outcome and the histologic subtypes has been suggested. The pure fetal subtype appears to be associated with the better prognosis, whereas the small cell undifferentiated subtype appears to have a very poor prognosis.[166-169] In several other studies, chemotherapy

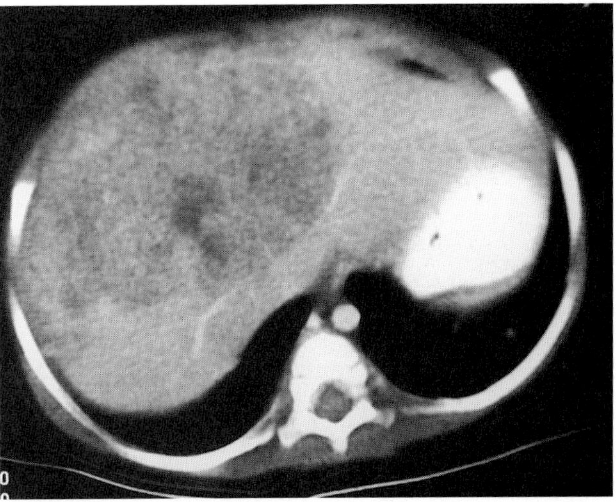

Figure 69-9. CT scan after intravenous administration of a contrast agent shows a large right lobe hepatoblastoma extending into the left lateral segment.

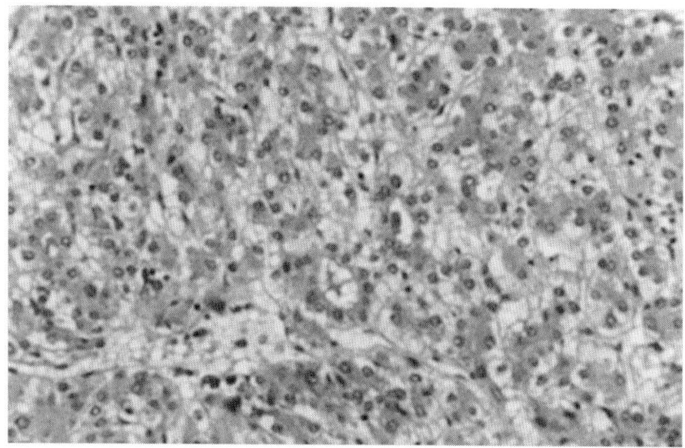

Figure 69-10. Histology of a pure fetal hepatoblastoma. Note the hepatocytes have clear glycogen-rich cytoplasm and small, regular nuclei.

was initiated before surgical intervention and likely altered the accuracy of histologic definition of the resected tumor, making it difficult to correlate histology and outcome.[170]

Biology and Cytogenetics

Thrombocytosis is common in patients with hepatoblastoma. This may be related to increased thrombopoietin levels, which have been reported in hepatoblastoma cell extracts.[170] Elevated interleukin-1b levels also have been noted in hepatoblastoma cell lines.[171] This results in an increased production of interleukin-6, which is known to stimulate thrombopoiesis and thrombocytosis.[172]

Chromosomal abnormalities have been documented in patients with hepatoblastoma.[173] The most common defects have been trisomy of chromosomes 20, 2, or 8, or a combination of these. Trisomy 18 also has been found.[174] As yet, however, no correlation has been noted between these cytogenetic abnormalities and either clinical outcome or tumor biology.

An association between hepatoblastoma and the *APC* gene was noted in patients with familial adenomatous polyposis and Gardner's syndrome.[172,175] A recent study has found an association between the activation of the Wnt/β-catenin signaling pathway and the development of carcinogenesis in hepatoblastoma and hepatocellular carcinoma.[176]

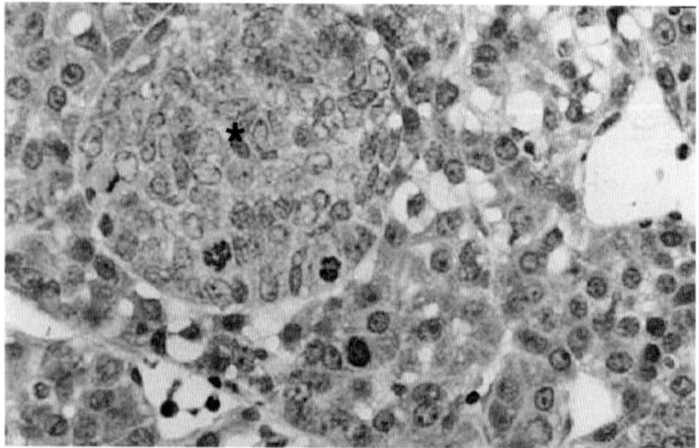

Figure 69-11. Histology of a hepatoblastoma with mixed fetal and embryonal elements. Note the large solid nest (asterisk) of poorly defferentiating cells (embryonal components). In contrast, note the surrounding trabeculae of the differentiating fetal hepatoblasts.

Table 69-4	Histologic Subtypes of Hepatoblastoma
Pure fetal	
Embryonal	
Macrotrabecular	
Small cell undifferentiated	
Mixed epithelial and mesenchymal pattern	
With teratoid features	
Without teratoid features	

Clinical Presentation

Patients with hepatoblastoma are most commonly seen with an asymptomatic right upper abdominal mass that is noted incidentally by either a parent or the pediatrician. Rarely these patients have tumor rupture, followed by significant hemorrhage and hypovolemia. Sexual precocity may be a presenting feature with hepatoblastoma, secondary to the tumor producing human chorionic gonadotropin. With large tumors, it is not unusual to see anorexia and failure to thrive. These lesions can become very large (15 cm) and can extend across the midline or down into the pelvis.

Imaging

The first diagnostic test is usually an ultrasound examination. This usually differentiates between a renal mass and a hepatic mass. An abdominal CT scan is then usually performed. In half of patients, calcification is noted within the mass.[177] Spiral CT with an intravenous bolus of a contrast agent not only is helpful in the diagnosis but also is useful in the staging of the tumor and in determining its resectability. With three-dimensional reconstruction, the location of the mass with respect to the vena cava, the hepatic veins, and the portal venous system can often be precisely delineated (Fig. 69-12). MRI is becoming an increasingly helpful modality for determining the relation of the tumor to the hepatic anatomy and in differentiating hepatoblastomas from other childhood hepatic tumors.[178] A word of caution, however, is that no current noninvasive study can always differentiate between a benign or malignant liver lesion.[25] If there is any concern about the diagnosis, a tumor biopsy should be performed.

Laboratory Studies

Anemia and thrombocytosis (platet count >500,000/mm^3) are often found in patients with hepatoblastoma.[179] However, the hallmark of hepatoblastoma is an elevated AFP level, which occurs in up to 90% of patients.[180] The serum levels of AFP can sometimes exceed 1 million ng/mL. This can lead to the

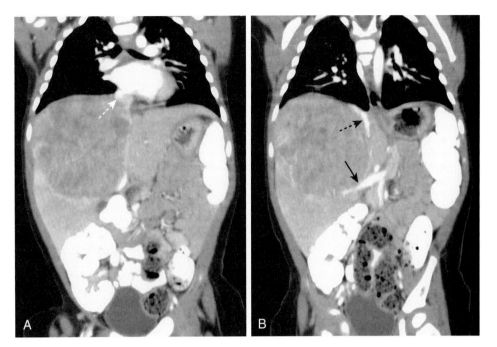

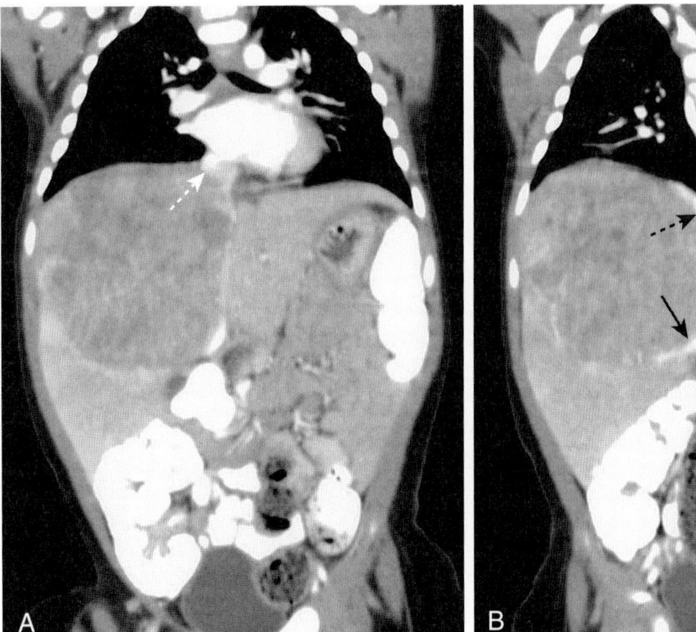

Figure 69-12. **A,** This CT scan obtained after intravenous administration of a contrast agent in a 1-year-old shows a large mass in the right hepatic lobe. On other images, the mass appears to invade or compress the medial segment of the left lobe. The middle hepatic vein (*dotted arrow*) is being compressed by the tumor. **B,** The inferior vena cava (*dotted arrow*) is being displaced medially and anteriorly by the mass, and the portal vein (*solid arrow*) is markedly displaced inferiorly.

"hook" effect in which the initially reported AFP level can be low despite the actual level being very high. If the lesion is suspicious for hepatoblastoma, a request should be made to dilute the AFP sample before retesting.[181] Serum AFP has a half-life of between 4 and 9 days, and the levels usually decrease to normal by 4 to 8 weeks after complete removal of the tumor.[182] It also is important to remember that neonates normally have an elevated AFP level (25 to 50,000 ng/mL) at birth that does not decrease to "adult" levels until age 6 months.[17] This becomes important when evaluating a neonate with a hepatic mass or when monitoring the AFP after liver resection in a neonate or infant.

AFP also has been used for monitoring purposes. In one case report, a radioimmunodetection method was used (technetium-labeled mouse antihuman monoclonal antibody to AFP).[183] After an initial decline in the AFP after liver resection, it began to increase, and an anti-AFP nuclear medicine study accurately located an active tumor in the remaining liver.

Recently, a new marker has been found for hepatoblastoma. Glypican 3 (GPC3) has been detected in hepatic stem cells and has been identified as being expressed by fetal, embryonal, and small cell undifferentiated hepatoblastomas. This marker is also shed by the tumor cells and has the potential to be used as a serum marker for hepatoblastoma.[184]

Staging

Two staging systems are currently used. In the United States, a combined histologic and surgical staging system is used by the Children's Oncology Group (COG) (Table 69-5).[185] This tumor staging system is self-explanatory and is based on information gathered before any chemotherapy is started. The second staging system, used by the International Society of Pediatric Oncology (SIOP), is based on the radiologic location of the tumor before treatment and is called the PRETEXT (Pretreatment Extent of Disease) Grouping System (Fig. 69-13).[186] Both of these staging systems are currently being used in ongoing studies so patient groups can be compared across different study groups.

In the PRETEXT system, the liver is divided into four sections: the anterior and posterior sectors on the right and the medial and lateral sectors on the left. Therefore, based on the extent of the tumor, the patient is classified as follows: PRETEXT 1, with three adjoining sectors free (tumor in only one sector); PRETEXT 2, with two adjoining sectors free (two sectors involved); PRETEXT 3, in which one sector but in two nonadjoining sectors is free (tumor involves two or three sectors); and PRETEXT 4, in which no sector is free (tumor in all four sectors). It is noted whether hepatic vein or portal vein involvement is present, if extrahepatic spread has occurred (enlargement of the hilar

Table 69-5 Children's Oncology Group Staging System and Outcomes

Stage	Description	5-Year Survival
I	Complete resection, clear margin, pure fetal histology	100%
IU	Complete resection, clear margin, unfavorable histology	98%
II	Gross total resection with microscopic residual or perioperative rupture	100%
III	Unresectable or resection with gross residual or lymph node involvement	69%
IV	Metastatic disease	37%

From Ortega J, Siegel S: Biological markers in pediatric cancer. In Pizzo P, Poplack D (eds): Principles and Practice of Pediatric Oncology. Philadelphia, Lippincott, 1989, pp 149-162, with permission.

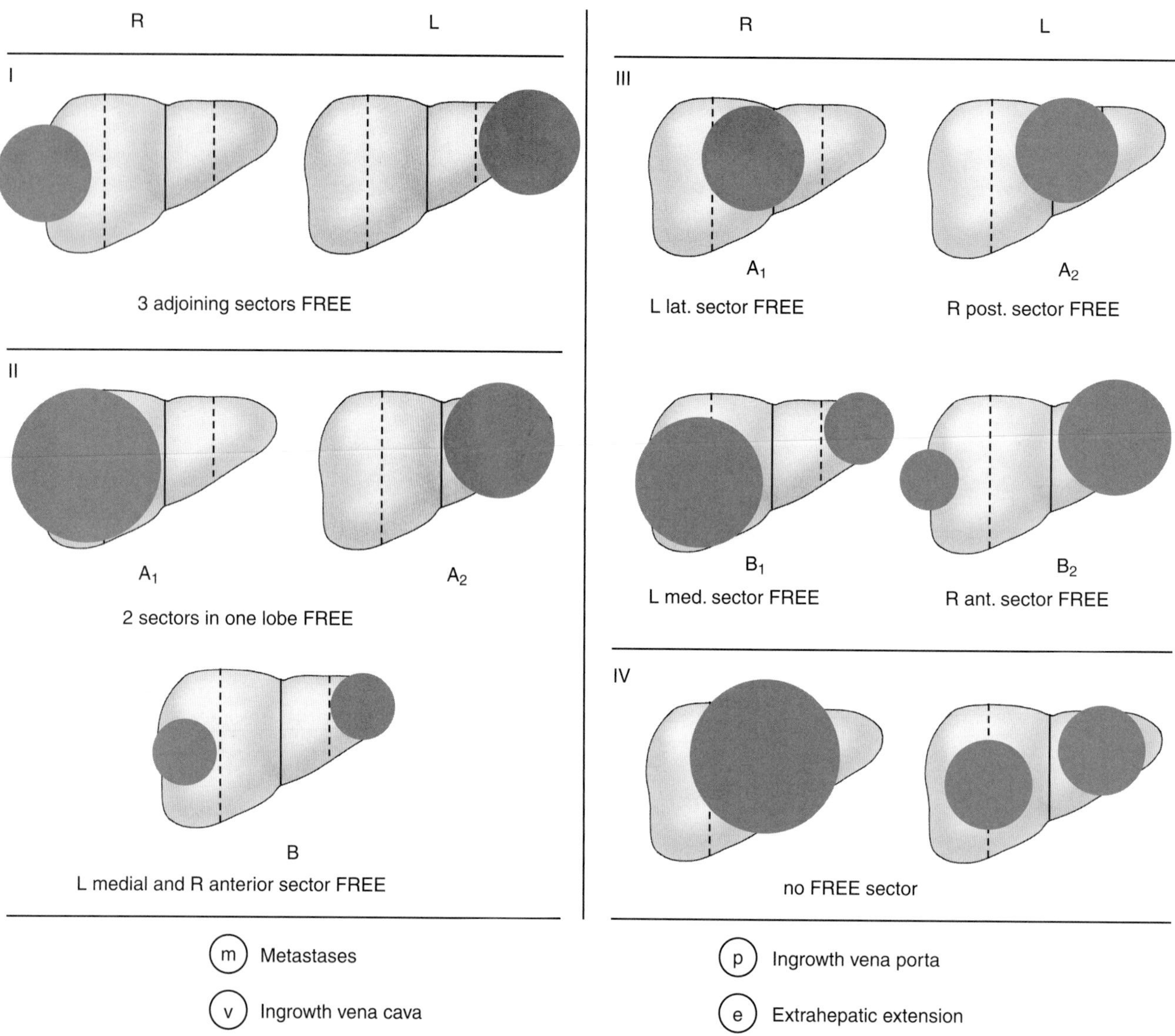

Figure 69-13. PRETEXT (Pretreatment Extent of Disease) staging system. Stage is determined by the number of liver sectors free of tumor.

lymph nodes), or if metastases are found. Both staging systems have been shown to have direct correlations with ultimate patient survival (Table 69-6).

In addition to the staging systems, in upcoming protocols the patients will also be stratified according to risk. In the COG staging system, low-risk patients will be stage I/II without unfavorable biologic features, intermediate-risk patients will be stage III or stage I/II with small cell undifferentiated histology, and high-risk patients will be stage IV or stage I, II, III with an AFP less than 100 ng/mL at diagnosis. In the SIOPEL studies, the patients are stratified into standard risk (PRETEXT I, II, III) or high risk (PRETEXT IV or any tumor with metastases, vena cava or portal vein invasion, contiguous extrahepatic disease, or tumors with an AFP < 100 ng/mL at presentation).[187]

Treatment

The treatment of hepatoblastoma requires a combined-modality approach. Except on very, very rare occasions, chemotherapy alone is unable to eradicate the tumor. The only chance for a long-term cure is complete resection of the primary tumor. This goal can be achieved by the use of either traditional hepatic resections (right lobectomy: segments 5-8; left lobectomy: segments 2-4; or left lateral segmentectomy: segments 2-3) or extended resections (right trisegmentectomy: segments 4-8; or left trisegmentectomies: segments 2-4, 5, 8). The resection can be performed

Table 69-6 SIOP PRETEXT Staging and Outcome

Stage	5-Year Survival
I	100%
II	91%
III	68%
IV	57%

SIOP, International Society of Pediatric Oncology.
From Brown J, Perilongo G, Shafford E, et al: Pretreatment prognostic factors for children with hepatoblastoma: Results from the International Society of Pediatric Oncology (SIOP) Study SIOPEL 1. Eur J Cancer 36:1418-1425, 2000.

using either open or laparoscopic techniques. There have been several case reports and two large series of laparoscopic liver resections in adults for both benign and malignant disease.[188-191] The outcomes of these laparoscopic series have been identical to the results of resections by an open approach. Obviously, a laparoscopic approach to a liver mass requires a team that has extensive expertise in both laparoscopic and hepatobiliary surgery. Unfortunately, due to the lower frequency of liver masses in children, it may be difficult to translate the excellent adult laparoscopic hepatic resection experience to the pediatric population.

The resection should be planned so that there is an anticipated margin of normal liver around the tumor. Fortunately, this margin does not need to be large (2-3 mm).[192] If it is doubtful that the tumor can be resected with a clear margin, then the patient should undergo preoperative chemotherapy to try to reduce the size of the tumor to the point where surgical resection is possible. In several studies, only between 30% and 50% of the patients were able to undergo either a complete or gross total resection of the tumor at the initial procedure.[193,194] In the COG trials, only 23% of the patients initially presented with stage I or stage II disease.[195]

If a difficult liver resection is elected, the conundrum exists as to what to do if the resection is unsuccessful and microscopic residual disease is left after a resection. The data from the COG studies, SIOPEL-1 and SIOPEL-2, indicate that microscopic residual disease after resection can be successfully treated with additional chemotherapy.[168,196,197] On the other hand, several series have reported that the most common reason for tumor recurrence is either a gross or microscopically incomplete resection.[198-201] If local recurrence of the tumor does occur, the prognosis is poor.[182,202,203] "Rescue" transplantation for local recurrence results in a survival rate of only 30%.[204] This would suggest that there must be multiple, yet to be defined, variables that determine if microscopic disease can be eradicated or if it will result in recurrent disease. In any case, there must be careful thought before undertaking a "difficult" liver resection when the possibility exists of leaving residual disease versus referring the patient directly for liver transplant evaluation.

If chemotherapy is necessary, it should be noted that there are two distinct approaches to its utilization in the treatment of hepatoblastoma. The COG approach is based on the premise that all patients who present with hepatoblastoma should be evaluated for a primary resection. If this is not possible, then the patient receives chemotherapy with the goal of shrinking the tumor to the point where it is resectable. The intent of this approach is to limit the patient's exposure to chemotherapeutic drugs that carry significant side effects (renal, cardiac, and ototoxicity). The SIOP approach is fundamentally different in that all their patients receive chemotherapy before any consideration for resection. The logic behind this approach is that chemotherapy will provide multiple benefits, such as shrinking the tumor, thereby potentially decreasing the size and risks of hepatic resection, decreasing the

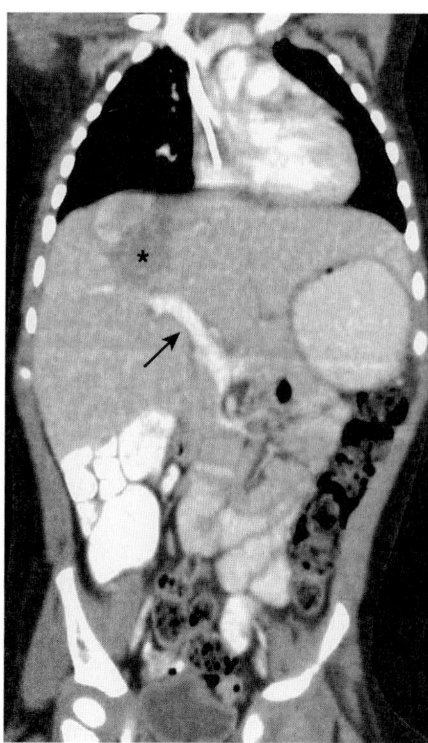

Figure 69-14. After four cycles of chemotherapy, the CT scan showed marked diminution in the size of the mass (*asterisk*). Note the portal vein (*solid arrow*) has returned to its normal anatomic position. Compare with prechemotherapy CT scan in Figure 69-12.

viability of the tumor prior to surgical manipulation, and decreasing the vascularity of the tumor. The SIOP group uses the PRETEXT staging system, but the correlation between survival and PRETEXT stage is based on the fact that all PRETEXT staged tumors (regardless of stage) have received chemotherapy. It should be noted that neither approach has been proved to be superior to the other in multiple, multicenter trials.

Multiple chemotherapy regimens have been evaluated for hepatoblastoma.[185,205] The most active chemotherapy agent for hepatoblastoma is cisplatin. This drug is then combined with either vincristine, doxorubicin, or 5-fluorouracil and used in either an adjuvant or neoadjuvant fashion. The current recommended COG chemotherapy regimen for initially unresectable hepatoblastoma is cisplatin, 5-fluorouracil, and vincristine.[206] In the patients who have had complete resection of their tumor (without preoperative chemotherapy), either four to six postoperative courses of chemotherapy are given. In those children in whom the liver tumor was deemed unresectable at the initial operation, four rounds of chemotherapy are initially given, followed by repeat imaging (Fig. 69-14). With chemotherapy and delayed or second-look surgery, the resection rate has been reported to be increased to between 69% and 98%.[5,207-209] In patients with stage 3 disease whose tumor was initially unresectable and who underwent four cycles of chemotherapy, between 51% and 60% of the patients had their tumors rendered resectable (Fig. 69-15). In patients with stage 4 disease (initially unresectable), only 40% of these

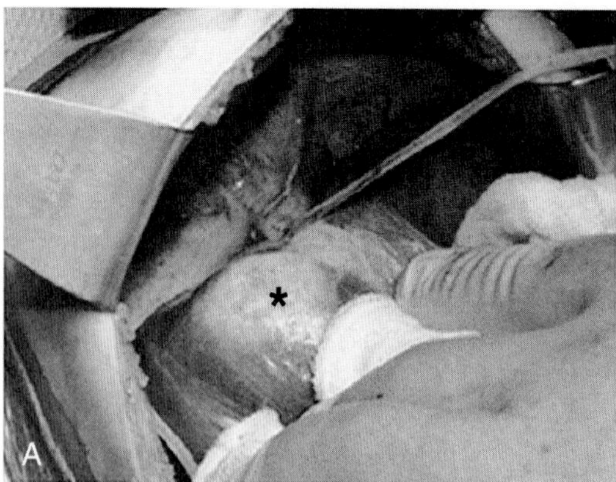

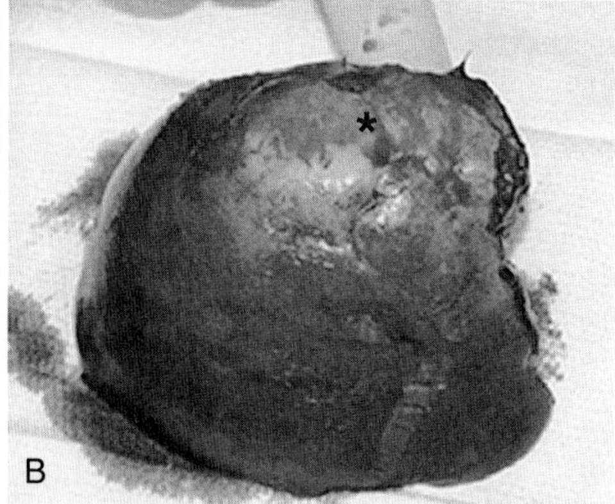

Figure 69-15. Operative findings of the patient whose CT scans are seen in Figures 69-12 and 69-14. An umbilical tape has been used to encircle the middle hepatic vein. **A,** Note the residual tumor (asterisk) in the cephalad portion of the right hepatic lobe. **B,** The right hepatic lobe containing the lesion (*asterisk*) is seen. It was possible to obtain a normal margin of liver in the left lobe, but a trisegmentectomy was needed.

tumors were rendered resectable after four rounds of chemotherapy.

Resection is then performed if it is possible. If the tumor is not resectable, then the child is referred for evaluation for liver transplant. If the child is a transplant candidate (no evidence of active extrahepatic disease), additional rounds of chemotherapy are given until a donor is found. The time to transplantation, however, needs to be as short as possible. Preferably the time between the last round of chemotherapy and transplantation should be less than 4 weeks because it is now known that up to 80% of hepatoblastomas will develop drug resistance after four to five courses of chemotherapy.[208,210]

Some newer chemotherapy agents have been investigated for hepatoblastoma. Topotecan inhibits growth and neovascularization in a mouse model.[211] In addition, the suppressive effects of the topotecan lasted several weeks after discontinuation of the agent. Irinotecan appears to have some promise in salvaging patients who have recurrent disease. This drug could potentially be added to front-line chemotherapy regimens.[212] High-dose chemotherapy with stem cell rescue has been attempted but has not been successful.

Another approach to the unresectable hepatoblastoma is the use of preoperative chemoembolization.[213] Transarterial catheterization with selective tumor chemoembolization was able to shrink the tumor by an average of 26%, which allowed subsequent complete tumor resection in every case. Interestingly, the surgical specimens showed only minimally viable or no viable tumor. It was postulated that this technique may be useful not only as a therapeutic modality for unresectable hepatoblastomas but also potentially for resectable tumors that could be made minimally viable to nonviable before surgical intervention.[214]

Another therapeutic dilemma occurs in the child first seen with a ruptured tumor. In one review, all three patients who survived the initial rupture had no evidence of recurrent disease, with a mean survival of 36 months.[215] Even though rupture of the tumor and peritoneal soiling occurred, no peritoneal growths were subsequently identified in any patient.

Outcome

Patient-outcome studies have been based on histologic type, the extent of the original tumor, or tumor response to chemotherapy.[166] Several studies have shown a good outcome with fetal histology and with complete resection of the tumor.[41,155,169,216,217] All the studies that have consistently shown a good outcome based on fetal histology have strictly limited this diagnosis to tumors with a mitotic activity less than 2 per 10 high-power fields. Conversely, several studies have consistently reported a poor outcome for those patients who have small cell undifferentiated hepatoblastoma.[167] Except for these data, no consistent correlation has been found with any of the other histologic patterns and patient outcome.

The AFP level also has been shown to have both prognostic and therapeutic implications. Patients with an AFP level less than 100 ng/mL or greater than 1 million ng/mL were found to have a worse prognosis.[218] The low-AFP group comprised patients with small cell undifferentiated tumors, suggesting that a low AFP level could be related to a very primitive and poorly differentiated tumor that was unable to make AFP.[219] Patients who had a slow decline in their AFP levels either after resection or chemotherapy had a poorer long-term prognosis than did those who had an early, very rapid decline (>99% drop in AFP levels).[220]

The best survival in patients with hepatoblastoma is in patients with stage 1 pure fetal histology who were treated with low-dose intravenous doxorubicin (100% survival). In the most recent COG study, the 3-year event = free survival (EFS) was 90% for stage I/II tumors, 50% for stage III tumors, and only 20% for stage IV tumors.[221] The European SIOPEL-2 study reported that the 3-year survival for standard risk tumors was 90% and for high-risk tumors it was 50%. These data compare favorably with those of a large German series that noted an EFS of 100% for stage 1, 80% for stage 2, and 68% for stage 3 disease.[209] None of the patients with stage 4 disease in the German trial survived. In another prospective study, the German group showed that the important prognostic factors for survival appeared to be the tumor growth pattern, vascular invasion, and serum AFP levels.[217,222]

Because the patients in the high-risk PRETEXT or COG trials have poor outcomes, despite a complete surgical resection, additional or different chemotherapy regimens are necessary to improve patient survival in these groups.[217] Currently there are ongoing studies that are evaluating the possibility of modifying different cellular or gene targets in hepatoblastoma cells that will make them more susceptible to chemotherapy.[223]

Transplantation

Once a patient has completed four rounds of chemotherapy to shrink the tumor, a decision is made to either perform a surgical resection with the goal of complete tumor excision or to refer the patient for liver transplantation. Several characteristics of hepatoblastoma have recently been reported as possible indicators of unresectability. Therefore, these patients need to be considered early for possible transplantation. Patients who were younger than 3 years of age at presentation tend to respond better to chemotherapy with greater reductions in tumor size when compared with older children.[224] Bilobar, multifocal tumors at presentation are candidates for transplantation. Despite apparent radiologic clearing of a lobe after chemotherapy, microscopic disease can persist in the liver leading to later recurrent disease.[196,225,226] Patients who present with low AFP levels (<100 ng/mL) tend not to respond to chemotherapy, so they should be considered for either upfront resection or transplantation. Patients who have tumor extension into the inferior vena cava, all three hepatic veins, or the bifurcation of the portal vein are unlikely to sufficiently shrink their tumor with chemotherapy to allow a surgical resection and therefore should be considered candidates for transplantation.[204]

Orthotopic liver transplantation is a successful treatment for unresectable hepatoblastoma.[227] A recurrence-free survival rate of between 79% and 92% has been reported.[204,228,229] In several series, an important prognostic factor that predicted good results after transplantation was a good initial response to chemotherapy. In one series, only 60% of the patients who were poor responders are currently alive, with a follow-up of less than 1 year.[228] As mentioned previously, liver transplantation for local tumor recurrence after resection is associated with a post-transplant recurrence rate of 30%. The utility of one to two post-transplant courses of chemotherapy in reducing this recurrence rate is controversial. Although post-transplant chemotherapy is frequently utilized, one multicenter review noted no significant difference in survival rates between those patients who received chemotherapy (77%) versus those who did not (70%).[201,230-232]

Patients with extrahepatic metastases found on initial evaluation can be successfully treated with liver transplantation if the metastatic disease is eradicated before the transplant. Hepatoblastoma commonly metastasizes to the lungs, and lung metastases are often present at diagnosis. Because this tumor tends to be chemoresponsive, these metastases will often disappear after the first several rounds of chemotherapy. If the pulmonary metastases do not resolve, then current data would suggest that these patients should undergo a metastasectomy for any remaining disease, either before or shortly after resection and before consideration for transplantation. This approach has been successful in increasing patient survival.[233,234] Unfortunately the data on resection of pulmonary recurrences are less optimistic. There may be a role for resection of late pulmonary metastasis in patients who presented with stage I disease. However, pulmonary relapse in stage III and IV disease portends a poor prognosis that is not changed by lung resection.

Undifferentiated Embryonal Sarcoma

Incidence

Undifferentiated embryonal sarcoma of the liver makes up about 7% of the solid liver tumors in children.[1] Unfortunately, this is a very malignant tumor with a poor outcome.

Clinical Presentation

Undifferentiated embryonal sarcoma most commonly affects children between the ages of 6 and 10 years but has been reported in a child as young as 19 months.[235] A slight male predominance has been noted. The most common clinical presentation is either right upper quadrant or epigastric pain with or without a palpable abdominal mass. Occasionally, marked hepatomegaly is seen without a definite mass. Rarely, this tumor can even masquerade as a hepatic abscess or infection.[236] Other nonspecific presenting complaints can include vomiting, anorexia, and lethargy. Laboratory studies, including AFP level, are usually normal.

Imaging

On ultrasound examination, the lesion appears predominantly solid.[237] However, on CT and MRI, the lesion appears cystic without any significant solid component (Fig. 69-16). This same type of disparity has been reported only in Wilms' tumor metastatic to the liver. Thus, it appears that such a discrepancy between the two imaging techniques would be highly suggestive of an undifferentiated embryonal sarcoma.

Pathology

Undifferentiated embryonal sarcoma is a neoplasm with a very primitive mesenchymal phenotype. These tumors tend to occur predominantly in the right lobe of the liver and to be large, with an average diameter of 14 to 21 cm.[237] In cross section, the tumors are often variegated, with white mucoid or gelatinous areas alternating with other areas of tumor necrosis and hemorrhage (Fig. 69-17). The tumor typically is well demarcated from the adjacent liver by a compressed, fibrous pseudocapsule.[235]

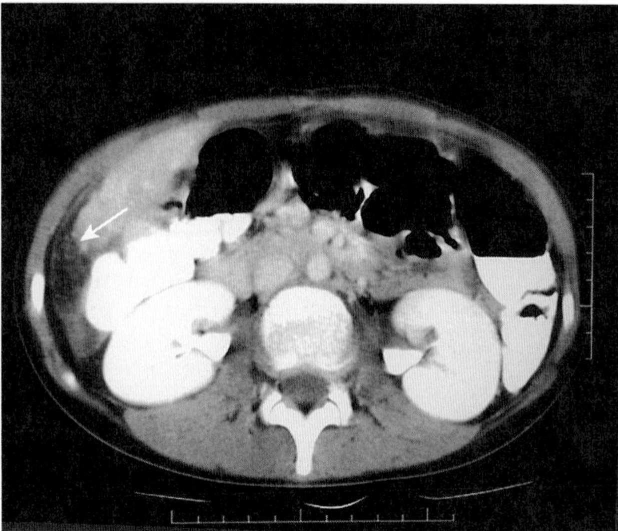

Figure 69-16. CT scan of an undifferentiated embryonal sarcoma after intravenous administration of a contrast agent shows a hypodense area (*arrow*) in the right lobe of the liver.

On microscopic section, these tumors are composed of medium to large spindle- to stellate-type cells in a variable amount of myxoid stroma (Fig. 69-18). The cells are usually densely arranged in a myxomatous background. In the periphery, entrapped bile ducts or hepatic cords have been noted.[1,235] Mitoses are frequent and usually bizarre.

No characteristic immunohistochemical stain pattern has been identified for embryonal sarcoma.[238] The only consistent cell markers have been vimentin and the "histiocytic" determinants α_1-antitrypsin and α-antichymotrypsin.[239,240]

In a cytogenetic study, extensive chromosomal rearrangements were noted to be very similar to other soft tissue sarcomas such as leiomyosarcoma, osteosarcoma, and malignant fibrous histiocytoma.[241] In only a few cytometric studies, the findings have ranged from diploidy to tetraploidy to aneuploidy.[242,243]

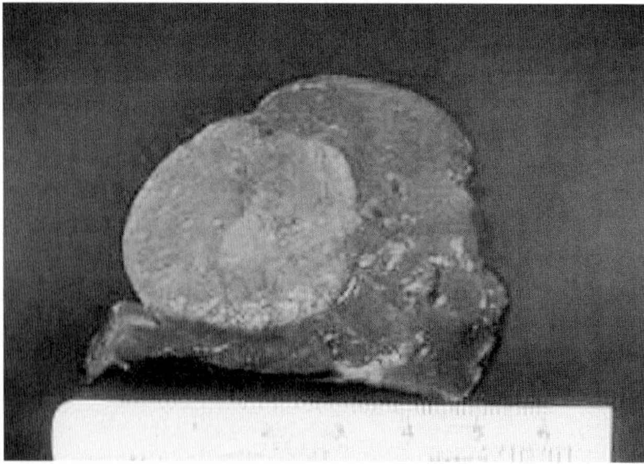

Figure 69-17. Note the variegated appearance on cut section of an undifferentiated embryonal sarcoma.

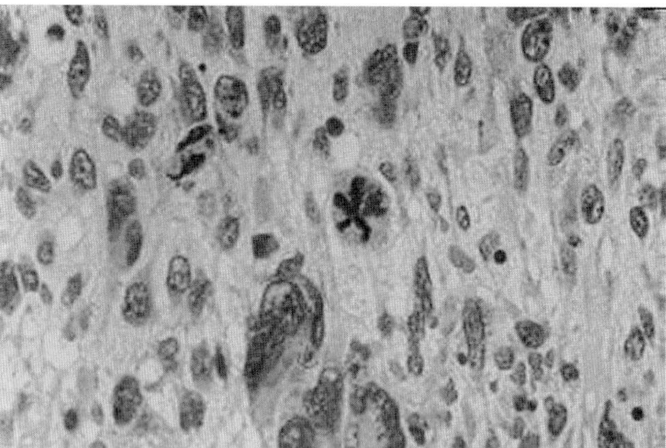

Figure 69-18. Histology of undifferentiated embryonal sarcoma shows large spindle cells with multiple mitoses.

Treatment

In addition to the highly suggestive radiologic findings, these patients can be diagnosed by fine-needle aspiration. Two separate reports have noted that the cytologic features of undifferentiated embryonal sarcoma are distinctive and different from other childhood tumors.[244,245]

The initial experience with undifferentiated embryonal sarcoma of the liver was poor. In a review of patients treated from 1950 to 1988, only 37% of the patients were noted to be alive.[243] This tumor usually proves fatal because of massive upper abdominal growth with secondary involvement of the diaphragm, stomach, abdominal wall, ribs, or pancreas rather than by metastases. Occasionally, intra-abdominal dissemination of the tumor can occur, causing diffuse matting of the small bowel. Pulmonary and pleural metastases have been noted but are much less common than the secondary involvement of the extrahepatic tissue by direct extension.[235]

The only chance for cure is radical excision.[246,247] Unfortunately, despite complete surgical resection of the tumor, many patients have recurrent disease, which suggests the need for postoperative chemotherapy.[248]

The chemotherapy regimens that have been used are based on nonrhabdomyosarcomatous soft tissue sarcoma–type protocols.[249] With these regimens, survival rates have improved to 66%, because these tumors are very chemotherapy sensitive.[250,251] This finding has led to the use of preoperative chemotherapy to shrink an unresectable tumor to a size at which a radical hepatic resection is possible.[252] This is similar to the approach used to manage an initially nonresectable hepatoblastoma.

With the ongoing improvement in chemotherapy regimens for sarcomas, the previously bleak outlook for this tumor is now much more optimistic. The use of an aggressive chemotherapy regimen, along with complete resection of the primary tumor, has resulted in a 37% survival rate in patients whose tumors initially presented as free intraperitoneal rupture.[251]

In patients in whom complete resection of the tumor is not possible despite chemotherapy, liver transplantation has been advocated as another possible means for complete excision. This aggressive approach is not completely unwarranted because these tumors are sensitive to chemotherapy. This approach is analogous to patients with hepatoblastoma who have chemotherapy-responsive tumors.

Hepatocellular Carcinoma

Hepatocellular carcinoma is a relatively rare, highly malignant tumor that is more commonly seen in adults than in children. It is the second most common pediatric liver tumor, occurring about 19% of the time, but it still comprises less than 1% of all pediatric cancers.[253] Its peak incidence seems to be between 10 and 15 years, and it is more common in boys.[254]

The predisposing factors for hepatocellular carcinoma are distinctly different between the pediatric and the adult population. In the adult population, cirrhosis seems to be the primary etiology. The cirrhosis is usually seen in patients with either hepatitis B, hepatitis C, genetic hemochromatosis, alcohol-related cirrhosis, or cirrhosis due to primary biliary cirrhosis. In a recent review, it was noted that patients in these groups were at a significantly increased risk for developing hepatocellular carcinoma.[255] Hepatic ultrasonography and serum AFP evaluations every 6 months were recommended to detect this tumor at an early stage.

In contrast, cirrhosis is often not part of the antecedent process in children. Moreover, a previous congenital or acquired disorder of the liver may be found (Table 69-7).[256] Hepatocellular carcinoma in children has been associated with a variety of metabolic, familial, and infectious disorders. Some of these metabolic disorders include tyrosinemia, α_1-antitrypsin deficiency, and hemochromatosis.[257] Patients with tyrosinemia seem to be at a particularly high risk for development of hepatocellular carcinoma. Because of this high prevalence rate, it has been suggested that liver transplantation be performed in this population before age 2 years.[258,259] Hepatocellular carcinoma also has been seen in patients with type 1 GSD. Most hepatic masses that develop in this population are hepatic adenomas, but carcinomas do present a real risk in this group.[260] A variety of other noncirrhotic liver diseases also have been associated with hepatocellular carcinoma, including familial polyposis, Gardner's syndrome, Sotos' syndrome, Blum's syndrome, neurofibromatosis, Abernathy's malformation, methotrexate therapy, and neonatal hepatitis. There is also an association with parenteral nutrition.[261-266]

Congenital and infectious disorders also are associated with this tumor, including extrahepatic biliary atresia, congenital hepatic fibrosis, Alagille syndrome, persistent familial intrahepatic cholestasis (PFIC),[267] hepatitis B, and hepatitis C. In areas where hepatitis B is endemic, it ranks fifth in the causes of childhood malignancies and outnumbers hepatoblastoma by 3:1.[268] The importance of hepatitis B and the subsequent development of hepatocellular carcinoma in children is highlighted by the aggressive hepatitis B vaccination program that began in 1984 in Taiwan.[269] When the mortality from liver carcinoma in the group from birth to age 9 years was compared between the years 1984 and 1993, a substantial and statistically significant decrease in the mortality was seen by 1993. Another study from Gambia showed similar results.[270] Hepatitis C also has been linked to the development of hepatocellular carcinoma.[271] In contrast to hepatitis B, the cirrhosis and the subsequent development of hepatocellular carcinoma in the hepatitis C population usually takes several decades to develop.[272]

Table 69-7 Conditions Associated with Hepatocellular Carcinoma in Children

α_1-Antitrypsin deficiency
Anomalies of abdominal venous drainage (Abernathy's syndrome)
Alagille syndrome
Biliary atresia
Congenital hepatic fibrosis
Familial hepatocellular carcinoma
Familial polyposis
Focal nodular hyperplasia of the liver
Gardner's syndrome
Hepatic adenoma
Hepatitis B infection
Hepatitis C infection
Hereditary tyrosinemia
Hyperalimentation
Progressive familial intrahepatic cholestasis
Methotrexate therapy
Oral contraceptives
Types I and III glycogen storage disease
Wilms' tumor
Wilson's disease

Of particular interest is the association between hepatocellular carcinoma and biliary atresia.[254,273] In a review, except for one patient first seen at age 5 months, all the other patients were older than 2 years with a mean of age 7.5 years when the hepatocellular carcinoma was discovered. These tumors were found either at autopsy or incidentally at the time of liver transplantation for biliary atresia. In those patients in whom hepatocellular carcinoma was identified at the time of transplantation, all of these patients are alive and well after transplant. This association between hepatocellular carcinoma and biliary atresia, or any other disease that would lead to hepatic cirrhosis, would suggest that a routine screening protocol every 6 months with hepatic ultrasonography and determination of AFP levels is warranted.[274]

Clinical Presentation

Most patients are initially seen with either an abdominal mass or abdominal pain. Other associated symptoms include nausea and vomiting, anorexia, malaise, and a significant weight loss.[268] As many as 10% are seen primarily with tumor rupture and hemoperitoneum.[275] More than one third of hepatocellular carcinomas appear as multiple nodules rather than a single tumor.[276]

Laboratory studies can show mild elevations in the serum glutamic oxaloacetic transaminase (SGOT) and lactic dehydrogenase (LDH) levels. The AFP is elevated in about 85% of patients but can be normal or only mildly elevated with the fibrolamellar variant.[275,277] An elevated AFP is associated with an increased risk for recurrence after resection and therefore reflects a poorer prognosis.[278,279]

Imaging

CT and MRI are both helpful for delineating the mass and for determining resectability. With the advent of spiral CT with intravenous bolus contrast administration, the hepatic veins and portal venous system can be well delineated, and any tumor involvement can be adequately assessed. The American Association for the Study of Liver Diseases has published criteria for the noninvasive diagnosis of hepatocellular carcinoma. In nodules less than 2 cm in diameter in cirrhotic livers, the diagnosis of hepatocellular carcinoma can be made without biopsy of the lesion if two coincidental dynamic imaging studies (e.g., CT/MRI) reveal arterial-phase hypervascularity followed by wash-out in the portal venous phase.[280] The fibrolamellar variant is notable as a hypodense, single or multilobed mass on CT that tends to be hypervascular as well as sometimes showing a central scar.[281] This appearance could easily be confused with FNH, and care must be taken to distinguish between these two lesions.

Pathology

Hepatocellular carcinoma can vary in size from 2 to 25 cm, and the surrounding liver can exhibit either micro- or macronodular cirrhosis in up to 60% of cases (Figs. 69-19 and 69-20).[1] Microscopically, trabeculae that are 2 to 10 cell layers in thickness are seen with the larger trabeculae sometimes displaying central necrosis. The individual cells are usually larger than normal hepatocytes, with nuclear hypochromasia and frequent and bizarre mitosis (Fig. 69-21). Vascular invasion may be prominent. Tumors less than 2 cm generally are well differentiated. Over time, as the tumor grows, the original tumor cells are replaced by poorly differentiated cell clones.[282] Moreover, as the tumor enlarges, its blood supply becomes more dependent on newly formed arterial vessels and less dependent on the portal circulation. This imbalance between the hepatic arterial and portal venous supply leads to the hypervascular pattern that is the radiologic hallmark for hepatocellular carcinoma.

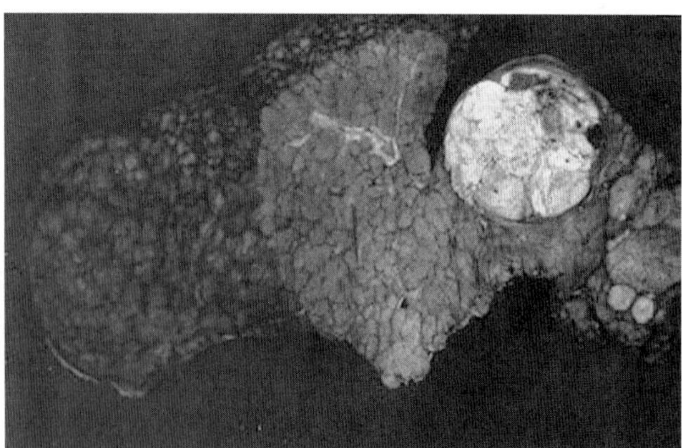

Figure 69-19. Hepatocellular carcinoma in the setting of cirrhosis.

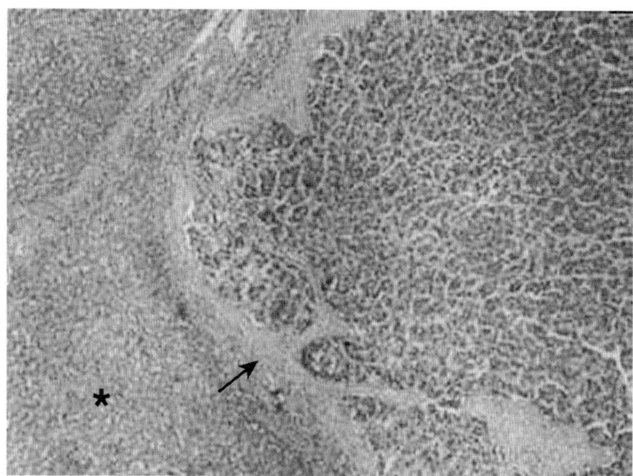

Figure 69-20. This histologic photomicrograph shows hepatocellular carcinoma with surrounding cirrhosis (*arrow*) and uninvolved liver (*asterisk*).

In the fibrolamellar variant, the hepatocytes are large, deeply eosinophilic, and embedded within a lamellar fibrosis. Clusters of cells are often separated by broad bands of laminated collagen.[1,283] The presence of large amounts of fibrosis alone is not sufficient in itself for the diagnosis of fibrolamellar carcinoma.[284]

Treatment

The treatment of hepatocellular carcinoma is surgical resection, varying from a simple anatomic resection to a liver transplant. Unfortunately, primary resection is not always possible because either the tumor is bilobar or the tumor is associated with cirrhosis. Because of the cirrhosis, concern may exist that the hepatic resection might leave the patient with insufficient functioning parenchyma.

In one pediatric report of 49 children, resection was possible in only 10%. Only 2 patients lived for more than 2 years.[268] If a complete, microscopically free, radical resection is possible, the prognosis can be good, with an 80% to 90% survival.[285] Unfortunately, the overall cure rate for this tumor in children is a dismal 15%. In the adult population, 3-year survival rates between 34% and 57% have been reported.[286,287] Multiple studies have looked at prognostic factors that influence outcome and recurrence after resection for hepatocellular carcinoma. Multiple staging systems have been proposed based on multivariant analyses of various prognostic factors. Three factors that have been repeatedly associated with improved survival and decreased recurrence rates are small tumor size (<2 cm), the number of tumor nodules, and a histologic increase in tumor microvascular density. These

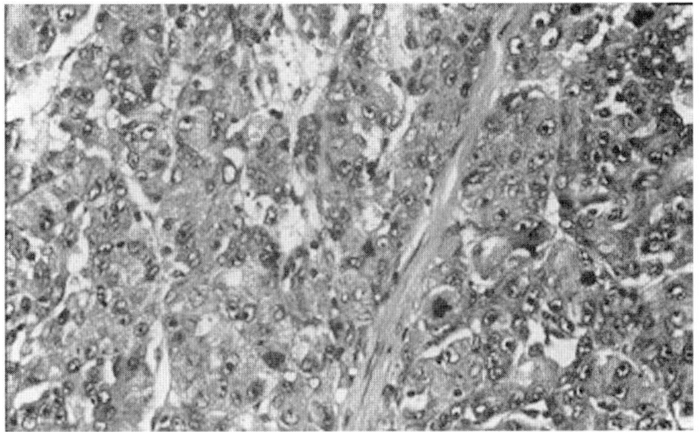

Figure 69-21. Histology of a hepatocellular carcinoma demonstrating enlarged hepatocytes and nuclear hypochromasia.

findings are highly predictive of tumor relapse after resection.[288] Unfortunately, it is rare to see patients initially with all three favorable variables. In most series, the tumors are usually larger than 5 cm in diameter at presentation.[286,289]

An important variant that should be mentioned is the fibrolamellar type. Only in the 1980s did this variant become established as a histologic and clinically distinct entity.[290] This lesion is characterized by relatively slow growth and occurs almost exclusively in a noncirrhotic liver.[283] The fibrolamellar variant usually occurs in adolescents and young adults, with a peak incidence in the second decade of life.[291,292] It accounts for between 16% and 50% of the hepatocellular carcinoma diagnosed in patients younger than 21 years of age.[293] In contrast to conventional hepatocellular carcinoma, fibrolamellar carcinoma is not associated with risk factors such as cirrhosis or chronic hepatitis B infection.[294,295] However, an association does exist between FNH and the fibrolamellar variant.

Radiologically, the fibrolamellar variant is often hypodense on noncontrast CT and can show a variable perfusion, including hypervascularity, on contrast CT. In addition, a central hypodense or hypervascular area can be seen that can mimic a central scar.[296] This can create confusion between the diagnosis of the fibrolamellar variant and FNH. MRI has been reported to be helpful in distinguishing between these two diagnoses.[297] The results after resection for fibrolamellar carcinoma in adults are very good, with 50% 5-year survivals. However, after apparent curative resections, recurrences or metastases can occur after very long disease-free intervals.[298,299] Unfortunately when the fibrolamellar variant was examined in children, there was no survival benefit to this diagnosis.[221]

Transplantation for Hepatocellular Carcinoma

Liver transplantation has been used as curative therapy for the treatment of hepatocellular carcinoma. The early experience of liver transplantation in adults for hepatocellular carcinoma was discouraging.[300] However, in a review of 344 patients who underwent liver transplantation for hepatocellular carcinoma (excluding the fibrolamellar type), three factors were associated with tumor-free survival: a unilobar tumor, a tumor smaller than 2 cm, and the absence of vascular invasion.[301] Two different pretransplant selection criteria are currently being utilized in adults (Table 69-8).

The Milan criteria are widely recognized as excellent predictors of a low recurrence rate after transplantation.[302] These criteria, however, have not been verified in the pediatric population, and their applicability in children has been questioned.[303] Because hepatocellular carcinoma can be a rapidly growing tumor, frequently by the time an organ becomes available the tumor has exceeded these criteria and the patient is no longer a candidate for transplant. The University of California at San Francisco criteria are an attempt to allow an increased pretransplant tumor burden and still have a low post-transplant recurrence rate. Several studies have supported this hypothesis.[304,305]

Currently there are two contraindications to transplantation for hepatocellular carcinoma in children: extrahepatic spread and macroscopic vascular invasion.[231] The SIOPEL-1 study reported no long-term survivors among those who failed to respond to chemotherapy.[306] Therefore, the lack of response to preoperative chemotherapy is a relative contraindication to transplantation. Despite these possible limitations, liver transplantation in children for hepatocellular carcinoma has a very good 5-year survival rate between 63% and 89%.[231,307] To transplant both adults and children quickly, patients are given additional points in the United Network for Organ Sharing (UNOS) matching system so they can be transplanted before the tumor progresses.

Interestingly, in contrast to patients with hepatoblastoma, several studies have shown that liver transplantation is an appropriate salvage procedure for patients with hepatocellular carcinoma who experience a recurrence after a resection. Their post-transplant survival is comparable to that of patients who underwent primary transplantation for hepatocellular carcinoma.[308,309]

Chemotherapy for hepatocellular carcinoma has not appeared to be beneficial in adults when given either before or after resection or transplant. Postresection chemotherapy has been uniformly ineffective in preventing or treating recurrences in the Pediatric Oncology Gray (POG), SIOPEL, and German studies.[306,310-312] New chemotherapeutic approaches are needed for this tumor, and currently studies are being planned that

Table 69-8 Milan and UCSF Transplant Criteria for Hepatocellular Carcinoma

	Milan Criteria	UCSF Criteria
Single Tumor Maximum Diameter	≤5.0 cm	≤6.5 cm
Maximum Number	3	3
Largest Tumor Size	≤3.0 cm	≤4.5 cm
Total Tumor Size	NA	≤8.0 cm

NA, not applicable; UCSF, University of California at San Francisco.

will combine chemotherapeutic agents with antiangiogenic agents. However, in two small series, chemotherapy was given to children with unresectable hepatocellular carcinomas before transplant. Eighty percent of these children had a dramatic decrease in their tumor size.[253,313] At the time of transplant, all tumors still had viable cells but only one patient after transplant had a recurrence and subsequently died.

Patients who are not surgical or transplant candidates, patients who demonstrate recurrences, or patients who are on the transplant list and their tumors have grown to the point that they exceed the Milan criteria can potentially benefit from several nonsurgical strategies, including percutaneous ethanol injection, radiofrequency ablation, or chemoembolization of the hepatic mass.[314] All of these therapies have proved efficacious in decreasing or eradicating localized tumors, treating recurrent tumors, or shrinking tumors so that the patient again falls within the transplant criteria.[315] These therapies also improved survival with this tumor, but unfortunately, none has been proved to be curative.[255]

A catastrophic presentation of hepatocellular carcinoma is spontaneous rupture. These patients present with acute right upper quadrant pain and hypovolemic shock. The diagnosis can be made with ultrasonography or abdominal CT. In the hemodynamically stable patient, the treatment is conservative with correction of volume status and correction of any coagulopathy. Then a careful assessment of the tumor needs to be made with the goal of primary resection of the tumor. If the patient is hemodynamically unstable, then transarterial embolization of the tumor should be done to control the hemorrhage. After the patient's condition has stabilized, he or she needs to be evaluated for a resection.[316]

The outcome for patients with hepatocellular carcinoma, regardless of the treatment modality, is still not as good as the outcome for hepatoblastoma. Further improvements in survival for hepatocellular carcinoma will come from advances in chemotherapy regimens that will prevent tumor recurrences.

Rhabdomyosarcoma of the Biliary Tree

Incidence and Clinical Presentation

Even though rhabdomyosarcoma is the most common sarcoma in children, it accounts for only 1% of all liver tumors and only 0.8% of all rhabdomyosarcomas in children.[1,317] Hepatobiliary rhabdomyosarcoma tends to be a disease of the young, with a median age of 3 years. It is rarely seen in children older than 15 years.[318,319] This tumor most commonly arises in the intrahepatic biliary system and then extends into the liver parenchyma itself. It also has been reported to arise from a variety of other sites, including an intrahepatic cyst, the gallbladder, the cystic duct, the ampulla of Vater, a choledochal cyst, and the hepatic parenchyma itself.[318-324]

Because it arises most commonly from the bile ducts, the most common presenting symptom is jaundice. Because the median tumor diameter at diagnosis is 8 cm, an abdominal mass is a common finding.[317]

Laboratory Findings and Differential Diagnosis

Because jaundice is a common presenting symptom, elevated direct bilirubin, alkaline phosphatase, and γ-glutamyltransferase (GGT) levels are common. The differential diagnosis for an intraductal lesion in a child would include either an inflammatory pseudotumor or a cholangiocarcinoma, but these are extraordinarily rare.[325] If the rhabdomyosarcoma is a predominantly hepatic mass with minimal bile duct involvement, then the differential diagnosis would be more dependent on the patient's age, as noted in the previous sections.

The pathology of the intraductal lesions is similar to that of rhabdomyosarcoma at extrabiliary sites. The intraductal tumor is usually either the botryoid or embryonal subtype, unless the lesion involves predominantly the hepatic parenchyma, in which the alveolar subtype predominates.[326]

Imaging

Multiple imaging modalities have been used for diagnosis. Ultrasonography typically reveals biliary dilatation and possibly a mass in the biliary system. Larger lesions may have cystic areas within them, possibly reflecting areas of partial tumor necrosis.[177] CT will often show an intraductal mass in association with areas of low attenuation within the tumor. MRI may have an advantage over CT in that it not only can show the anatomic source and location of the mass but, with the advent of MR cholangiography, also can evaluate the bile ducts by demonstrating biliary dilatation and intraductal irregularity.[327] Percutaneous transhepatic cholangiography (PTC) also can be useful in patients who have a dilated biliary system. PTC can demonstrate multiple filling defects that correspond to the intraductal tumor.[328] PTC also has the advantage of providing external drainage of the biliary system in those patients with obstructive jaundice.

Treatment and Prognosis

The best treatment for biliary rhabdomyosarcoma is a multidisciplinary approach using surgical procedures, chemotherapy, and, potentially, radiation therapy. Unfortunately, surgical resection alone is not usually possible because of spread of the tumor into the liver parenchyma or direct local extension into the duodenum, stomach, or pancreas. It is common to find lymphatic spread at the initial operation. Because of these problems, adequate resection is usually possible in only 20% to 40% of the patients.[317-319] In patients in whom primary resection is not possible, the initial approach should be biopsy and lymph node sampling, followed by standard rhabdomyosarcoma chemotherapy protocols and a second-look procedure. In a study of biliary rhabdomyosarcoma that used this multimodality approach, 4 of 10 children remained disease free after an average of 4 years.[317]

chapter 70

TERATOMAS, DERMOIDS, AND OTHER SOFT TISSUE TUMORS

Jean-Martin Laberge, MD • Pramod S. Puligandla, MD • Kenneth Shaw, MD

TERATOMAS

Teratomas are generally divided into gonadal and extragonadal types. The focus of this discussion is on those in extragonadal locations, the most common being sacrococcygeal teratomas.

Embryology and Pathology

Teratoma, from the Greek *teratos* ("of the monster") and *onkoma* ("swelling"), is a term first applied by Virchow in 1869 to "sacrococcygeal growths."[1] Teratomas are composed of multiple tissues foreign to the organ or site from which they arise.[2] Although teratomas are sometimes defined as having the three embryonic layers (endoderm, mesoderm, and ectoderm), recent classifications also include monodermal types.[2,3]

Teratomas are thought by some to arise from totipotent primordial germ cells.[3,4] These cells develop among the endodermal cells of the yolk sac near the origin of the allantois and migrate to the gonadal ridges during weeks 4 and 5 of gestation (Fig. 70-1).[5] Some cells may miss their target destination and give rise to a teratoma anywhere from the brain to the coccygeal area, usually in the midline. Another theory has teratomas arising from remnants of the primitive streak or primitive node.[5-7] During week 3 of development, midline cells at the caudal end of the embryo divide rapidly and, in a process called gastrulation, give rise to all three germ layers of the embryo (Fig. 70-2).[5] By the end of week 3, the primitive streak shortens and disappears. This theory would explain the more common occurrence of teratomas in the sacrococcygeal region. With either theory, the totipotent cells could give rise to monoclonal neoplasms. Recent evidence shows that, whereas immature teratomas may be monoclonal, mature teratomas can be polyclonal, more like a hamartoma than a neoplasm.[8] This finding is compatible with the third theory that teratomas are a form of incomplete twinning.[2,3]

The primordial germ cell is the principal but probably not the exclusive progenitor of a teratoma.[2] The recent trend is to include teratomas under the classification of germ cell tumors.[2-4] This histologic classification also includes germinomas (formerly dysgerminomas), embryonal carcinomas, yolk sac tumors, choriocarcinomas, gonadoblastomas, and mixed germ cell tumors. Gonadal and extragonadal teratomas may have a different origin, explaining the different behavior according to tumor site.

Teratomas are fascinating tumors owing to the diversity of tissues they may contain and the varying degree of organization of these tissues. Many tumors contain skin elements, neural tissue, teeth, fat, cartilage, and intestinal mucosa, often with normal ganglion cells. These tissues are usually present as disorganized islands of cells with cystic spaces. The tumor sometimes consists of more organized tissue, such as small bowel, limbs, and even a beating heart. These have been called fetiform teratomas (Fig. 70-3).[2,3,6,9,10] When the mass includes vertebrae or notochord and a high degree of structural organization, the term *fetus-in-fetu* is used. This is viewed by some as a variant of conjoined twinning but is classified as a teratoma by others, owing to the absence of a recognizable umbilical cord in its vascular pedicle.[3,11] Whether teratomas are at one end of a spectrum that includes fetus-in-fetu, parasitic twins, conjoined twins, and normal twins is the subject of controversy.[3] One certainly cannot dismiss the many reports of teratomas associated with fetus-in-fetu in the same patient and with a twin pregnancy.[2,3,12-14]

The overall tissue architecture is variable in teratomas. Moreover, a spectrum of cellular differentiation exists. Most benign teratomas are composed of mature cells, but 20% to 25% also contain immature elements, most often neuroepithelium.[2-4] The degree of histologic immaturity is of proven prognostic significance only in ovarian teratomas.[3,15] Even this concept is being questioned since one large cooperative study demonstrated that overlooked microscopic foci

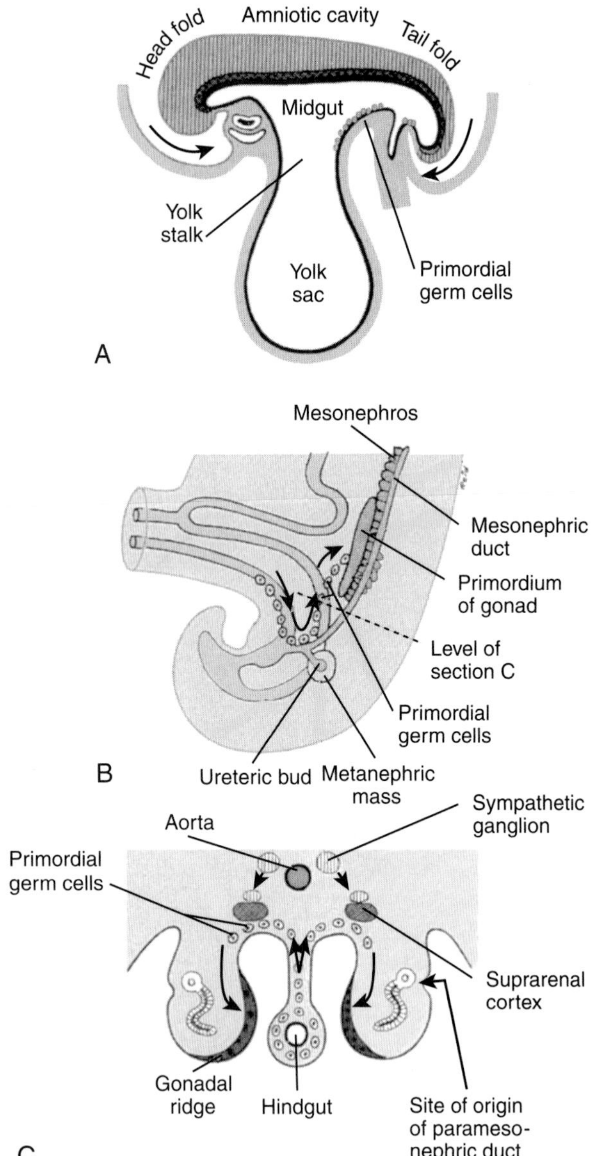

Figure 70-1. Commonly cited theory on the origin of teratomas. **A,** Drawing of embryo during week 4 (longitudinal section), showing primordial germ cells at the base of the yolk sac. **B** and **C,** During week 5, these cells migrate toward the gonadal ridges. According to this theory, some cells could miss their intended destination. (Modified from Moore KL, Persaud TVN: The Developing Human. Philadelphia, WB Saunders, 1993, pp 71, 181.)

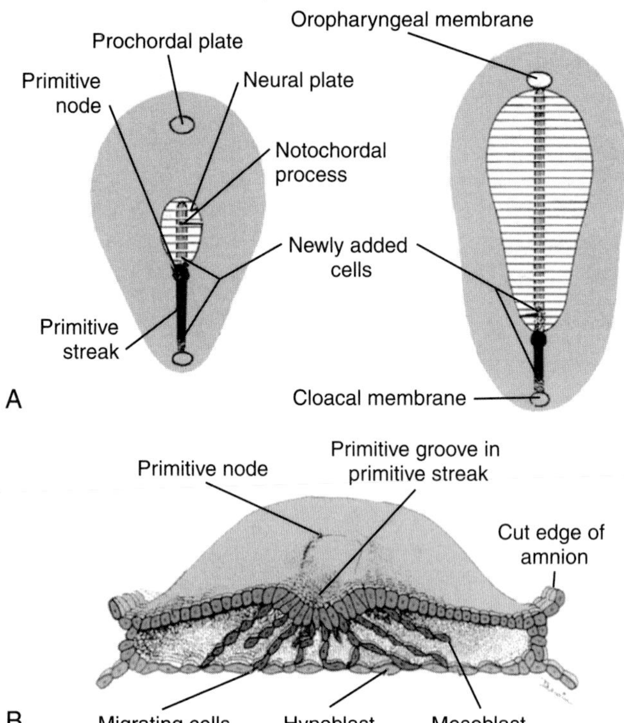

Figure 70-2. Alternate theory on embryogenesis of teratomas. **A,** Sketches of dorsal views of the embryonic disk on days 17 and 18, showing the primitive streak and primitive node. **B,** Drawing of a transverse cut of the embryonic disk during week 3. This shows that cells from the primitive streak migrate to form the mesoblast (the origin of all mesenchymal tissues) and also displace the hypoblast to form the endoderm. Hence, remnants of these pluripotent primitive streak cells could give rise to teratomas and could account for the more frequent sacrococcygeal location. (From Moore KL, Persaud TVN: The Developing Human. Philadelphia, WB Saunders, 1993, pp 55-56.)

of yolk sac tumor, rather than the grade of immaturity, was predictive of recurrence.[16] In neonatal teratoma, immature tissue is considered normal and without any influence on prognosis.[2,6] Spontaneous maturation of malignant tumors has been reported after partial excision of giant sacrococcygeal teratomas in two fetuses at 23 and 27 weeks of gestation.[17]

Teratomas may also contain or develop foci of malignancy. A malignant germ cell tumor may be found in sites typical for teratomas, such as the mediastinum or sacrococcygeal area. Whether the lesion was malignant from the onset or the malignant cells destroyed and replaced the benign teratoma component is often difficult to differentiate. The most common malignant component within a teratoma is a yolk sac tumor, also called an endodermal sinus tumor. Other malignant germ cell tumors can occur, and, rarely, malignancy of other tissues composing the teratoma, such as neuroblastoma,[18,19] squamous cell carcinoma,[20] carcinoid,[21] and others can develop. Malignancy at birth is uncommon but increases with age and with incomplete resection. An apparently mature teratoma may recur several months or years after resection as a malignant yolk sac tumor, illustrating the difficulties in histologic sampling of large tumors and the need for close follow-up.[2,3]

Most yolk sac tumors and some embryonal carcinomas secrete α-fetoprotein (AFP), which can be measured in the serum and demonstrated in the cells by immunohistochemistry.[22] This marker is particularly useful for assessing the presence of residual or recurrent disease. AFP levels are normally very high in neonates and decrease with time.[22,23] The postoperative half-life is about 6 days. Persistently high levels may be an indication for the need for further surgical procedures or chemotherapy. Other markers that may be elevated are β-human chorionic gonadotropin (β-hCG), produced by choriocarcinomas, and, rarely, carcinoembryonic antigen. Secretion of β-hCG

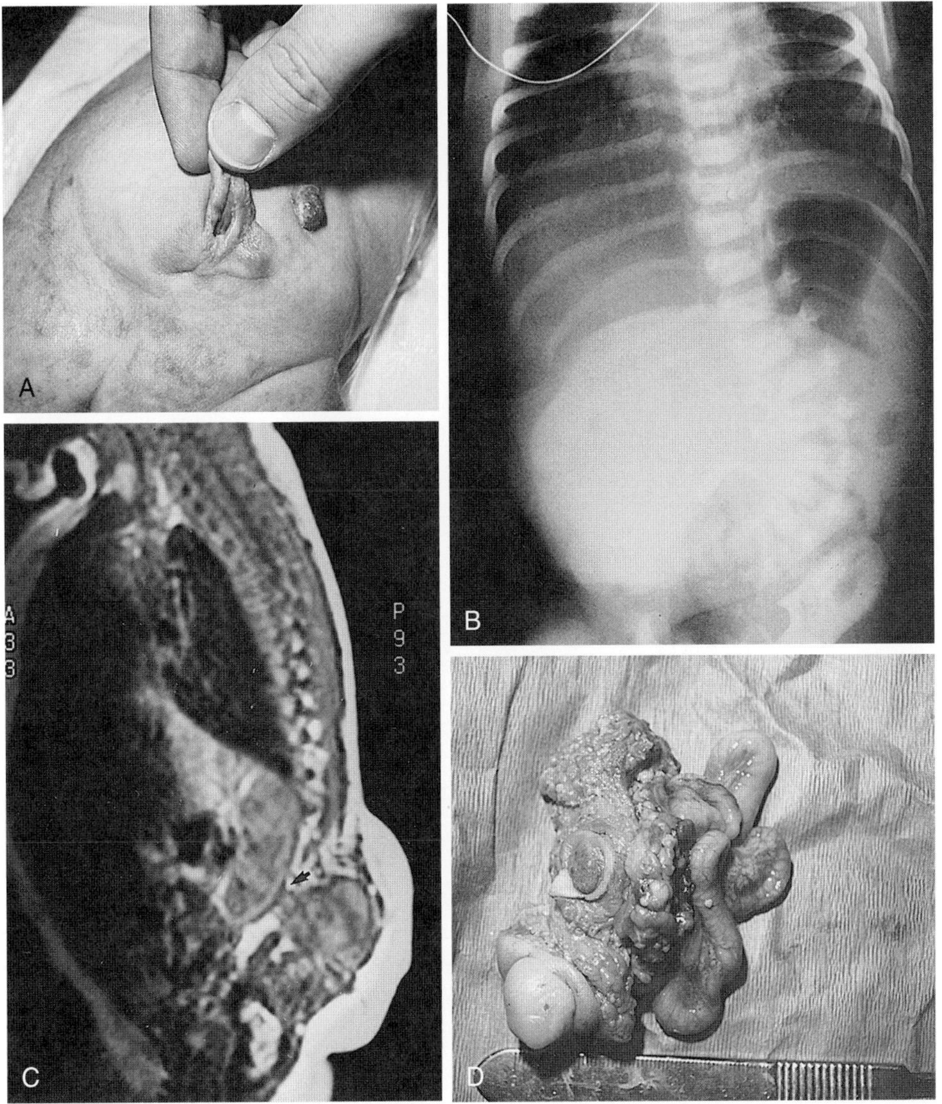

Figure 70-3. **A,** This child had a large fluctuant lumbar mass at birth. A family history of myelomeningocele existed in a great aunt. She also had an atrophic right leg with neurologic impairment below the L3 root and clubbing of the right foot. Note the ulcerated, arachnoid-looking area cranially and the pedunculated skin caudally, which had the appearance of a vulva and was oozing serous fluid. **B,** Plain radiograph shows a severe lumbosacral scoliosis with vertebral anomalies. CT confirmed the vertebral anomalies with spina bifida and demonstrated a pattern of intestine with inspissated or calcified meconium in the teratoma. **C,** MR image reveals that the mass extended into the retroperitoneum, where it was contiguous with the lower pole of the right kidney (*arrow*). **D,** At operation, normal-looking blind bowel loops were found deep to the vulva-like structure. Part of the mass extended along the spinal cord, which required dissection and untethering by a neurosurgeon. The pathologic diagnosis was a mature fetiform teratoma that contained, among many other things, two adrenals, two ovaries, renal tissue with some glomeruli and tubules, bone with bone marrow, and portions of stomach and small and large bowel. The child recovered well neurologically but required spinal instrumentation owing to progressive scoliosis at age 2 years.

by the tumor may be sufficient to cause precocious puberty.[24]

The genetic basis of teratomas is not yet understood. Most germ cell tumors appear to have an amplification, or isochromosome, in a region of the short arm of chromosome 12, designated i(12p).[3,4,25] This has been well described in adults but was not confirmed in one pediatric series in which deletions on chromosomes 1 and 6 were found instead.[26] Similarly, oncogenes and tumor suppressor genes did not appear to correlate with prognosis in one study.[27] *MYCN* gene amplification was present in immature teratomas but absent in mature teratomas in another report.[28] *BAX* mutation and overexpression correlated with survival in childhood germ cell tumors.[29] The clinical usefulness of these findings remains unclear.

Associated Anomalies

Teratomas are usually isolated lesions. A well-recognized association is the Currarino triad of anorectal malformation, sacral anomaly, and a presacral mass.[30,31] The presacral mass is usually a teratoma or an anterior meningocele. However, hamartomas, duplication cysts, and dermoid cysts have been described, as have combinations of these lesions.

An extensive review of the English and German literature published in 1989[32] found 51 cases of infants with the Currarino triad and highlighted several important facts. Twenty percent of patients were older than 12 years at the time of diagnosis, yet no reports of malignancy were found. This contrasts to a 75% malignancy rate in patients older than 1 year who had the usual sacrococcygeal teratoma.[33] Later, a case report of a child with severe anal stenosis and a presacral teratoma without a sacral bony defect described a malignant recurrence that subsequently resulted in the patient's demise at 4 years of age despite chemotherapy.[34] Subsequently, more reports of malignant transformation of a presacral teratoma in the context of the Currarino triad have appeared, and the risk of malignant transformation has been estimated at 1%.[35,36] Hence, one should not dismiss the presacral mass as always benign in these patients. The female preponderance for patients with this triad is only 1.5:1, which is less than the 3:1 ratio noted in isolated sacrococcygeal teratomas. A familial predisposition, first recognized in 1974,[37] is noted in 57% of cases and has an autosomal dominant inheritance pattern. Although all variants of anorectal malformations have been described, by far the most common is anal or anorectal stenosis. In one report, this triad was present in 38% of all patients with anorectal stenosis and in 1.6% of patients with low imperforate anus.[38]

Anal anomalies also have been reported in conjunction with a presacral mass, but in the absence of sacral defects. Hirschsprung's disease has been incorrectly diagnosed in some cases,[4,39,40] indicating the need to eliminate the presence of a presacral mass by digital rectal examination, by a metal sound when the anus is too tight, or by imaging techniques. In the screening of family members, normal plain radiographs of the sacrum are not adequate, because a presacral mass may exist in the absence of a bony defect.[41] The low incidence of malignancy has led one author to conclude that the presacral lesion in this context is a hamartoma rather than a teratoma.[42] This is supported by the demonstration of deletions or mutations of the homeobox gene *HLXB9*, located at 7q36, in several affected families.[43] In one recently reported family, no deletions of 7q could be detected, but the authors did not comment about *HLXB9* mutations.[44] However, in another family with proven *HLXB9* mutation, one affected member died at 22 years-of-age from a metastatic neuroendocrine tumor, likely originating from the presacral teratoma.[35]

Urogenital anomalies, such as hypospadias, vesicoureteral reflux, vaginal or uterine duplications, and other anomalies are associated with teratomas.[31,33,45] Congenital dislocation of the hip has been found in 7% of patients with sacrococcygeal teratomas, drawing attention to vertebral anomalies and late orthopedic sequelae (see Fig. 70-3).[46] Central nervous system lesions, such as anencephaly, trigonocephaly, Dandy-Walker malformations, spina bifida, and myelomeningocele, may occur.[2,3,47-49] Another peculiar association with sacrococcygeal teratomas is a family history of twins in as many as 10% of the patients.[37,50,51] Although not confirmed in all series, this finding, combined with reports of simultaneous twin pregnancy or sequential familial occurrences of fetus-in-fetu and teratoma, supports the theory that teratomas are just one end of the spectrum of conjoint twinning.[2,3,10,12,14]

Klinefelter's syndrome is strongly associated with mediastinal teratoma[52] and has been reported in patients with intracranial[53] or retroperitoneal tumors.[54,55] It is estimated that 8% of male patients with primary mediastinal germ cell tumors have Klinefelter's syndrome, which is 50 times the expected frequency.[52] These tumors are often malignant, are of the choriocarcinoma type, secrete β-hCG, and produce precocious puberty. Histiocytosis is also associated with mediastinal teratoma, both with[56,57] and without Klinefelter's syndrome.[58] Other hematologic malignancies, such as acute leukemias[59,60] and Hodgkin's disease,[61,62] occur rarely.

The following rare associations have been reported, most often with nonsacrococcygeal lesions: trisomy 13,[63] trisomy 21, Morgagni hernia,[64] congenital heart defects,[47,48] Beckwith-Wiedemann syndrome,[65] pterygium,[66] cleft lip and palate,[47] and rare syndromes, such as Proteus[67] and Schinzel-Giedion syndromes.[68]

Diagnosis and Management by Tumor Site

Sacrococcygeal Teratoma

Sacrococcygeal teratomas account for 35% to 60% of teratomas (gonadal included) in large series (Table 70-1).[69-71] This is the most common tumor in the newborn, even when stillbirths are considered.[47] The estimated incidence is 1 per 35,000 to 40,000 live births.[3,4]

Table 70-1 Relative Frequency of Teratomas by Site

Site	No. of Cases (%)
Sacrococcygeal	290 (45)
Gonadal	
Ovary	176 (27)
Testis	31 (5)
Mediastinal	41 (6)
Central nervous system	30 (5)
Retroperitoneal	28 (4)
Cervical	20 (3)
Head	20 (3)
Gastric	3 (<1)
Hepatic	2 (<1)
Pericardial	1 (<1)
Umbilical cord	1 (<1)
TOTAL	643 (100)

Modified from Dehner LP: Gonadal and extragonadal germ cell neoplasms: Teratomas in childhood. In Finegold M (ed): Pathology of Neoplasia in Children and Adolescents. Philadelphia, WB Saunders, 1986, pp 282-312.
Data are from five series of teratomas in children.

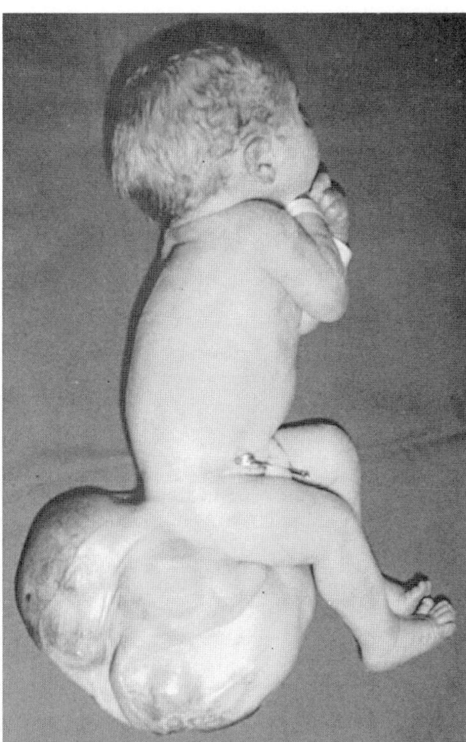

Figure 70-4. This infant has a large sacrococcygeal teratoma. The infant and attached teratoma weighed 2363 g. The teratoma weighed 675 g. After surgical excision of the tumor, the infant weighed 1688 g. The external size of such a teratoma is not a deterrent to surgical excision because the attachment in large and small teratomas is similar.

Diagnosis

In countries where prenatal ultrasonography is not readily available, most sacrococcygeal teratomas are seen as a visible mass at birth, making the diagnosis obvious (Fig. 70-4). Prenatal diagnosis has important implications and will be discussed further.

There is an unexplained female preponderance of 3:1.[33,69] The main differential diagnosis is meningocele. Typically, meningoceles occur cephalad to the sacrum and are covered by dura, but sometimes they are covered by skin. Examination of the child reveals bulging of the fontanelle with gentle pressure on a sacral meningocele, helping to establish the diagnosis before plain radiography, ultrasonography, and magnetic resonance imaging (MRI) confirm it. The co-existence of meningocele with teratoma is well recognized in the familial form, but these are usually presacral. Rarely, a typical exophytic teratoma may have an intradural extension.[72] Other lesions in the differential diagnosis of neonatal sacrococcygeal masses include lymphangiomas, lipomas, tail-like remnants (Fig. 70-5), meconium pseudocysts, and several other rare conditions.[33,73,74]

Although many neonates with sacrococcygeal teratomas do not have symptoms, some require intensive care because of prematurity, high-output cardiac failure, disseminated intravascular coagulation,[75] and tumor rupture or bleeding within the tumor.[76-78] Lethal hyperkalemia from tumor necrosis has been described.[79] Lesions with a large intrapelvic component may cause urinary obstruction. Besides looking for signs of a myelomeningocele, the physical examination should always include a rectal examination to evaluate any intrapelvic component. The most helpful imaging studies consist of plain anteroposterior and lateral radiographs of the pelvis and spine, looking for calcifications in the tumor and for spinal defects, and ultrasonography of the abdomen, pelvis, and spine. Further preoperative studies are unnecessary in most newborns.

The diagnosis of purely intrapelvic teratomas is often delayed.[33] Children develop constipation, urinary retention, an abdominal mass, or symptoms of malignancy, such as failure to thrive. Age is a predictor of malignancy in patients with testicular, mediastinal, and sacrococcygeal teratomas.[2] The risk of malignancy is less than 10% at birth but more than 75% after age 1 year for sacrococcygeal teratomas, with the exception of familial presacral teratomas. The risk of malignancy also is high for incompletely excised lesions. Complete excision of the tumor should be carried out as soon as the neonate is stable enough to undergo the operation. Serum markers should be determined before the operation for later comparison.

In recent decades, the diagnosis has often been made on prenatal ultrasonography, especially when this examination is routinely performed in the second trimester. The site of the lesion, its complex appearance, and intrapelvic extension with or without urinary tract obstruction are easily recognized. Although most small teratomas do not adversely affect the fetus in utero, the presence of a large solid vascular tumor is associated with a significant mortality rate, both in utero and perinatally.[76,77,80,81] Perinatal mortality is usually related to prematurity or tumor rupture with exsanguination (or both). Premature delivery may

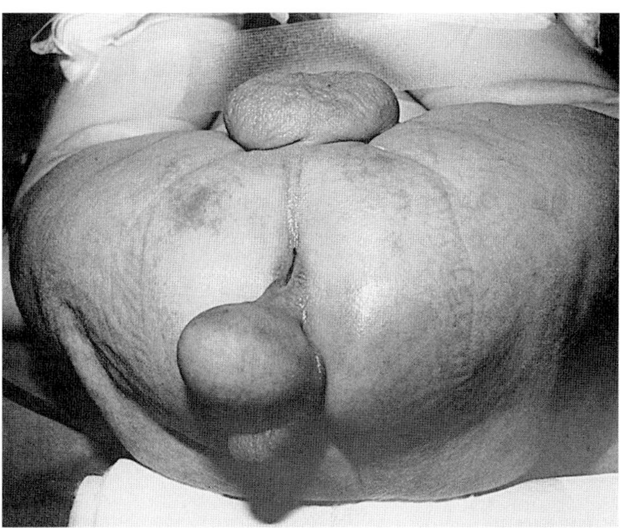

Figure 70-5. This patient had a scrotum-like perianal mass with anal stenosis at birth. An anoplasty was done with removal of the mass, which was not attached to the coccyx. Pathology showed only fibroadipose tissue with smooth muscle, vascular structures, and cartilage, consistent with a hamartomatous process or caudal vestige (also called a tail remnant).

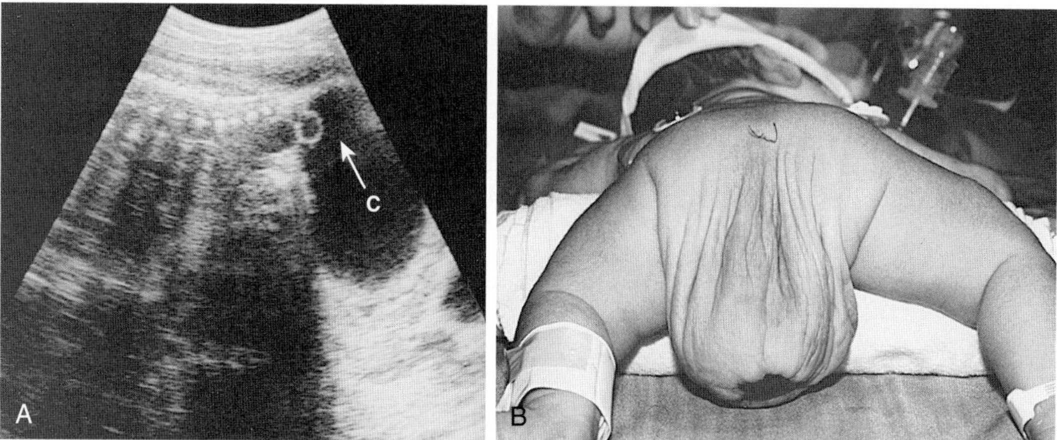

Figure 70-6. **A,** Ultrasound image of a female fetus at 38 weeks of gestation, showing a large cystic mass (C) attached to the coccyx, with tiny cysts anterior to the sacrum (*arrow*). An ultrasound evaluation at 18 weeks was normal. The cyst was gradually enlarging from an initial diameter of 9.5 cm at 31 weeks of gestation. The cyst was aspirated for 650 mL of fluid, permitting external rotation from breech to the vertex position. Two days later, when labor was induced, another 200 mL of fluid was removed to permit an uncomplicated vaginal delivery. **B,** Twenty-four hours postnatally, the lesion remained floppy with an area of skin ulceration, likely a consequence of excessive in utero distention. A mature cystic teratoma was confirmed histologically.

occur spontaneously from polyhydramnios or may be induced urgently because of fetal distress.

Repeated ultrasound assessment of tumor size is important because the fetus should be delivered by cesarean section if the tumor is larger than 5 cm or larger than the fetal biparietal diameter.[80] Dystocia during vaginal delivery is associated with tumor rupture and hemorrhage and is an avoidable obstetric nightmare. The options in managing unexpected cases with dystocia include emergency cesarean completion of the partially delivered fetus who has been intubated and ventilated after vaginal presentation of the head.[80]

Polyhydramnios with larger tumors may lead to premature labor. Tumors that are larger than the fetal biparietal diameter at diagnosis, or that grow faster than the fetus, are associated with a poor prognosis.[82] As the tumor enlarges, the fetus may develop placentomegaly or hydrops. This is a harbinger of impending fetal death and should lead to urgent cesarean delivery, especially when the maternal mirror syndrome is present.[83] Open fetal surgical excision has been performed with success in three of four cases considered too premature to deliver in one center and in two of four cases in another.[17,77] Others have reported survival after emergency delivery as early as 26 weeks of gestation.[84] Successful intrauterine endoscopic laser ablation was reported in one case.[85] Attempts at interrupting the high vascular flow have also been described by using radiofrequency ablation, with two survivors in four attempts.[86] One survivor had significant perineal damage.[87] Purely cystic teratomas occur in 10% to 15% of cases. Prenatal diagnosis allows percutaneous aspiration to facilitate delivery (Fig. 70-6),[81,88] to eradicate uterine irritability, or to prevent tumor rupture at delivery.[77] In other reports, prenatal decompression using a cyst-amniotic shunt was successfully performed to relieve the obstructive uropathy caused by the cystic teratoma.[89,90] Fetal MRI is a useful adjunct to the prenatal evaluation, providing additional information that helps in counseling and preoperative planning.[91] It also helps in the differential diagnosis when the teratoma is entirely presacral.[92]

Operative Procedure

Adequate intravenous access and the availability of blood products should be ascertained before starting the operation, especially with large tumors.

For most tumors, the major component is extrapelvic and the patient is placed in the prone position. If a significant intrapelvic or intra-abdominal component is present, it may be wise to begin with a laparotomy or laparoscopy. In our experience, most resections can be achieved completely in the prone position, especially if the internal portion is cystic. When in doubt, a safe approach is to prepare the skin from the lower chest to the toes, allowing the infant to be turned to the supine position without having to re-drape. Vaseline packing in the rectum facilitates its identification throughout the procedure (Fig. 70-7). En-bloc excision, including the coccyx, is preferable. Failure to remove the coccyx is associated with a high recurrence rate.[2-4] An acceptable gluteal crease and perineum is formed by the appropriate positioning of the perianal musculature. The use of plastic surgical principles to close the skin improves the cosmetic appearance of the scar (see Fig. 70-7, *inset*).[93]

Although the chevron incision has been used by most surgeons, a vertical incision is sometimes possible. It is preferred for smaller teratomas because it leaves a nearly normal-looking median raphe (Fig. 70-8). Resection of the excess skin at the closure gives an optimal cosmetic result.

Several techniques have been described to help in the management of giant sacrococcygeal teratomas. These include intraoperative snaring of the aorta,[78,94] laparoscopic clipping of the median sacral artery,[95] the use of extracorporeal membrane oxygenation and hypothermic perfusion,[96] devascularization and staged resection,[84] preoperative embolization, and radiofrequency ablation.[97] Autologous cord blood transfusion is a useful adjunct recently described.[98]

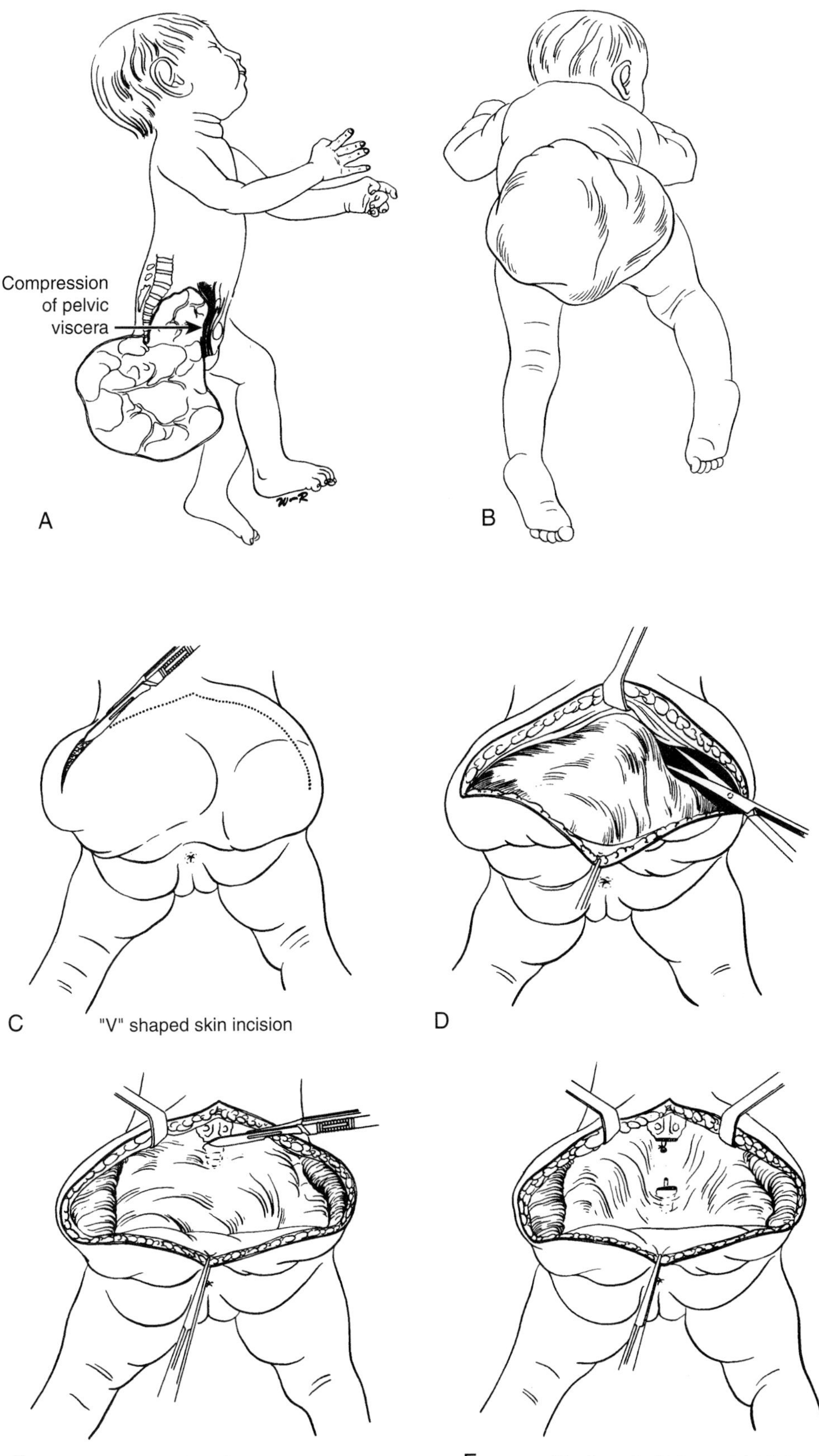

Figure 70-7. **A,** The teratomatous attachment may compress the rectum, vagina, and bladder anteriorly. **B,** The patient is placed on the operating table in a prone jackknife position, with general endotracheal anesthesia. An appropriate intravenous cannula should be placed in an arm vein. **C,** The incision is an inverted-"V" shape to allow excision of the tumor and to facilitate an eventually satisfactory cosmetic closure. The amount of skin excised is dependent on the size and shape of the tumor. **D,** The tumor is dissected from the gluteus maximus muscle. **E,** The coccyx is transected and removed in continuity with the tumor. **F,** The middle sacral artery is the major blood supply to the tumor and is ligated after transection of the coccyx.

(continued)

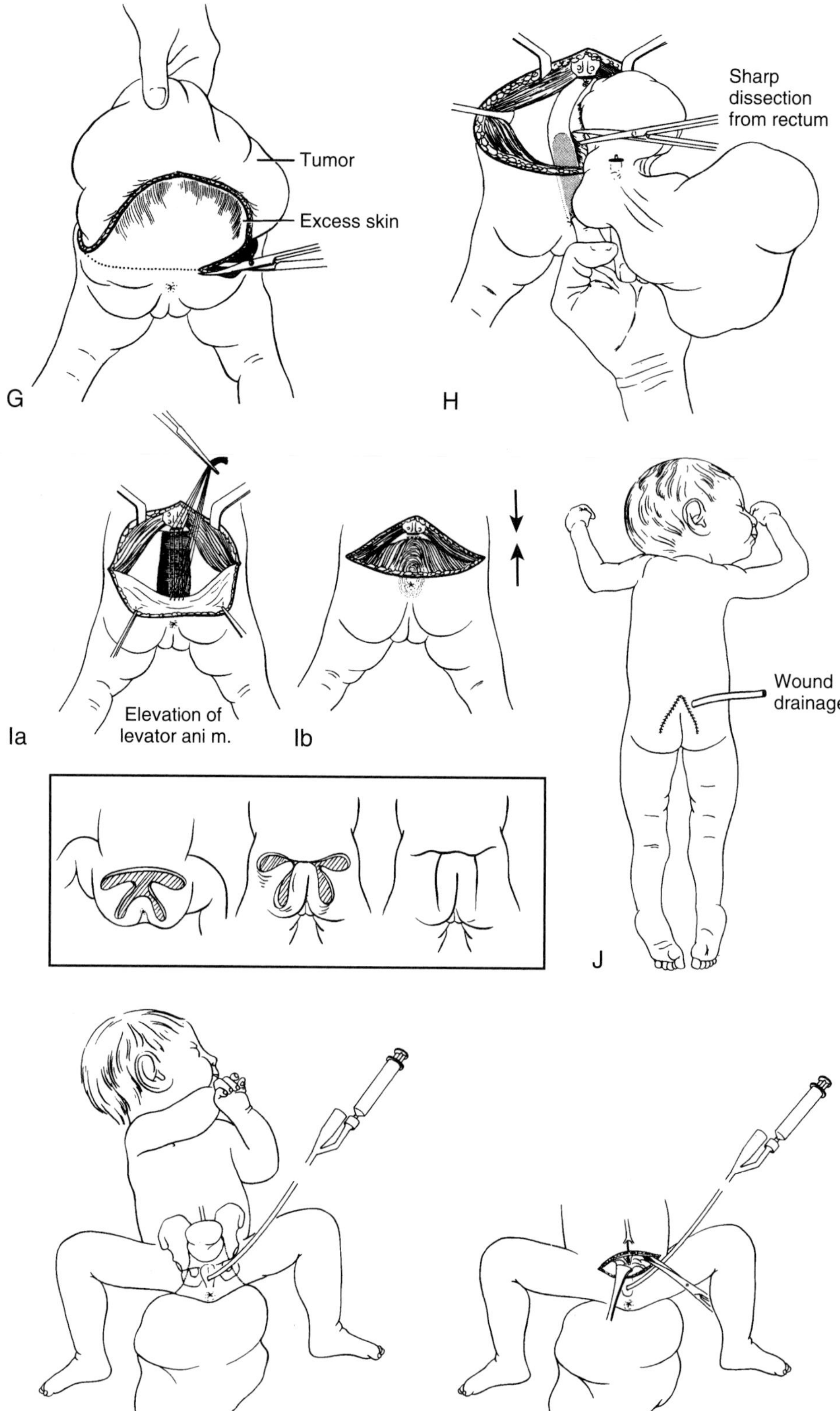

Figure 70-7, cont'd G, Excess skin is excised to facilitate closure. **H,** Because the tumor is adherent to the rectum, sharp dissection can be directed by placing a finger in the rectum. **I,** Placement of sutures between the anal sphincter and the presacral fascia (*a*). When the sutures are tied, the anal sphincter is pulled upward to the sacrum to form a gluteal crease (*b*). **J,** A drain is left in the surgical site for drainage of postoperative serosanguineous fluid. **Inset,** Recently described technique for closure after excision of large teratomas. Using plastic surgery principles, this avoids "dog ears" and places the scars along natural skin lines for a much-improved long-term cosmetic result. **K,** If the tumor extends through the bony pelvis into the retroperitoneum, a urinary bladder catheter is inserted to facilitate suprapubic dissection. **L,** Lower abdominal transverse incision allows interruption of the middle sacral artery and dissection of the tumor from the sacrum and pelvis, which is eventually removed from the perineum. (Inset redrawn from Fishman SJ, Jennings RW, Johnson SM, et al: Contouring buttock reconstruction after sacrococcygeal teratoma resection. J Pediatr Surg 39: 439-441, 2004; with permission.)

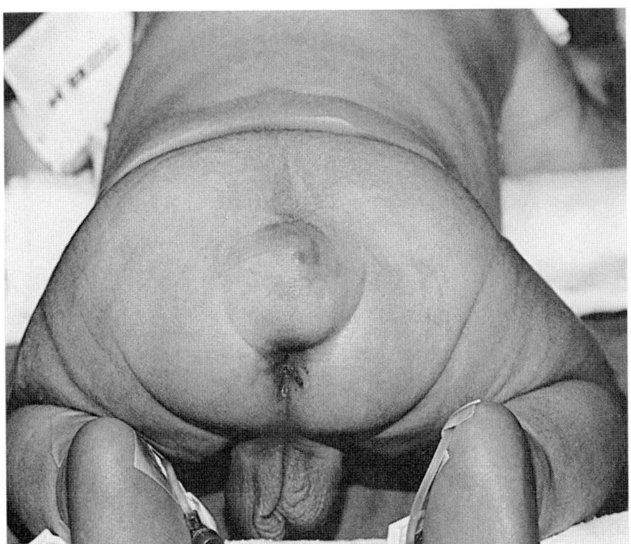

Figure 70-8. Smaller cystic teratoma at age 1 month, initially mistaken for a hemangioma owing to its soft compressible nature and bluish skin discoloration. This tumor lends itself well to a longitudinal elliptical excision with midline closure, as in a posterior sagittal anorectoplasty.

PROGNOSIS

Fetuses with tumors diagnosed in utero have a survival rate in excess of 90% if the tumors are small and discovered by routine prenatal ultrasonography. If a complicated pregnancy is the indication for ultrasound evaluation, the mortality increases to 60%. Nearly 100% of patients die when hydrops or placentomegaly occurs.[77,80,81] Dystocia or tumor rupture during delivery are likely underreported as a cause of mortality.[99] In one series, 10% of patients died during transfer, all before the widespread use of antenatal ultrasonography.[100] In a report of 24 patients with sacrococcygeal teratoma diagnosed on routine obstetric ultrasonography, 3 were aborted electively, 4 died in utero at 20 to 27 weeks of gestation, and 3 died of tumor rupture during delivery at 29 to 35 weeks of gestation (1 after vaginal and 2 after cesarean delivery).[76] The incidence of placentomegaly (none), hydrops (5%), and polyhydramnios (19%) was lower than in series in which ultrasonography was performed for an obstetric reason.[77,80,101] Tumor size, vascularity, and content were used to develop a prognostic classification from a cohort of 44 fetal sacrococcygeal teratomas. Fifty percent of infants with tumors 10 cm or greater that were highly vascular or fast growing died, whereas none died if these features were absent or if the tumor was predominantly cystic.[102]

In the absence of severe prematurity and intrapartum complications, the prognosis is dependent on the presence of malignancy and is therefore related to age at operation and completeness of resection.[103,104] When the tumor is benign and completely excised, recurrence is less common than when the tumor is large and mostly solid.[105] The recurrent tumor may be benign or malignant, and benign metastatic tissue may become evident in lymph nodes.[106] Although immature or fetal elements in gonadal teratomas are associated with a higher risk of aggressive behavior,[107] this is not considered true for sacrococcygeal teratomas.[2,6] However, a recent multicenter study identified immature histology and incomplete resection as risk factors for recurrence.[108] Although malignant recurrence of a "benign" teratoma may be as high as 10% to 15%,[7,108] the original benign diagnosis may have been due to sampling error,[16] an undetected residual microscopic focus of malignant tumor,[109] or secondary to incomplete coccygectomy at the initial operation.[34] Patients whose tumors are resected after the newborn period have a higher risk of malignant recurrence, especially when an elevated AFP level is present at diagnosis. The elevated AFP likely signifies the presence of malignancy in the original tumor.[16,110] It is important to monitor all patients with physical examination, including rectal examination and serum markers, every 2 or 3 months for at least 3 years, because most recurrences occur within 3 years of operation.[111]

Recurrent disease is usually local, but metastases to inguinal nodes, lung, liver, brain, and peritoneum can occur, including pseudomyxoma peritonei.[112] The prognosis of a malignant tumor or a malignant recurrence was dismal until the advent of platinum-based chemotherapy.[109] Survival rates higher than 80% are now achieved, but the risk of late recurrences or second malignancies persists.[110,111,113,114]

A Children's Cancer Group (CCG) review illustrates the revised prognosis.[114] The mortality was 10% in 126 patients treated in 15 institutions from 1972 to 1994. Three patients died of severe associated anomalies. Two died of hemorrhagic shock postoperatively and 6 due to combinations of severe prematurity, birth asphyxia due to failed vaginal delivery, or preoperative tumor rupture. Death from metastatic yolk sac tumor occurred in 1 patient. A second patient with metastatic disease was lost to follow-up and is presumed dead. Thus, only two deaths occurred from malignancy, despite a total of 20 yolk sac tumors (13 malignant at initial operation, 7 malignant recurrences after resection of "benign" teratomas). Owing to the effectiveness of current chemotherapy in treating recurrent disease, as well as its toxicity in young infants, it appears that a completely excised malignant yolk sac tumor does not require adjuvant therapy. These patients should be closely monitored clinically and with serial AFP measurements.[115] Similar encouraging results were seen in the German Cooperative Studies.[116]

In older patients, treatment of malignant tumors involves excision, chemotherapy, and monitoring with imaging studies and serum markers. For unresectable tumors, biopsy and chemotherapy are followed by excision of the primary tumor after adequate reduction has been obtained.[113] Radiation therapy is usually reserved for local recurrence of malignant tumors. Patients with malignant tumors should be enrolled in a pediatric cooperative study or treated according to their guidelines.

In the current era of the rather routine use of ultrasonography in pregnancy, the prognosis for patients with a sacrococcygeal teratoma is not dependent on Altman's classification[33] but rather on tumor size, physiologic consequences, histology, and associated anomalies. The prognosis of malignant tumors depends on tumor type, stage,[114] location, and patient age. Functional results in survivors have been reported as excellent in most series.[69,71,105,117] However, several reports draw attention to fecal and urinary continence problems, as well as lower limb weakness.[103,118-123] Some of these problems are clearly related to associated anomalies[100] or to the presence of large presacral or intra-abdominal tumors,[117] but they can occur after excision of purely extrapelvic benign tumors. A good outcome requires meticulous dissection along the tumor capsule, preservation and reconstruction of muscular structures, and long-term follow-up. One group advocates earlier cesarean delivery to minimize urologic sequelae in patients with large tumors causing urinary tract dilatation.[121] A poor cosmetic result was noted in more than half of the patients in another review.[124] These authors advocate early assessment of bladder, anorectal, and sexual function along with cosmetic results within a structured oncology follow-up program. The technique described by the Boston Children's group is a major step to improve cosmesis(see Fig.70-7).[93]

Thoracic Teratomas

The anterior mediastinum is the most common site of thoracic teratomas, which account for 7% to 10% of all teratomas (see Table 70-1).[2,3]

Mediastinal Teratomas

Mediastinal teratomas are diagnosed from the fetal period to adolescence and even adulthood.[2,125,126] Most are located in the anterior mediastinum, but a few have been described in the posterior mediastinum,[127] some with epidural extension.[128] In infants, respiratory distress is a common presenting manifestation,[129] but in older children the teratoma is often an incidental finding on chest radiography (Fig. 70-9).[2] Mediastinal teratomas may be first seen as a chest wall tumor and may even erode through the skin (Fig. 70-10). They also can erode into a bronchus, with hemoptysis as the initial manifestation, or rupture into the pleural cavity.[130] Secondary pericardial effusion and tamponade have also been described.[131] A strong association is found with Klinefelter's syndrome. In these cases, choriocarcinoma within the teratoma often leads to precocious puberty.[2,24,132] Histiocytosis also has been reported with mediastinal teratoma, both with and without Klinefelter's syndrome.[50,57,58,132]

Histologically, the presence of immature tissue does not affect the prognosis in children younger than 15 years.[2] After age 15 years, mediastinal teratomas have a high incidence of malignant behavior, which is usually indicated by elevated levels of AFP or β-hCG (or both).[133] The tumor should be excised through either a median sternotomy or a thoracotomy.[2,132] Smaller tumors may be approached through an anterior mediastinotomy (see Fig. 70-9) or by thoracoscopy.[134] Chemotherapy is required for malignant lesions as adjuvant therapy or preoperatively for unresectable tumors. Complete resection correlates best with event-free survival and is more often achieved with a strategy of delayed resection after preoperative chemotherapy.[133]

Intrapericardial Teratomas

Intrapericardial teratomas are most commonly seen in the newborn period or in utero, with evidence of cardiorespiratory distress or nonimmune fetal hydrops.[2,3,135] They are a leading cause of massive pericardial effusion in the neonate.[3] Delay in diagnosis can be fatal. A fetal diagnosis allows early postnatal treatment in most patients[136] or early delivery for emergency surgical excision if the infant develops signs of cardiac tamponade.[137]

On ultrasonography, a cystic or solid teratoma is located anterior to the right atrium and ventricle with attachments to the great vessels.[135] In older infants,

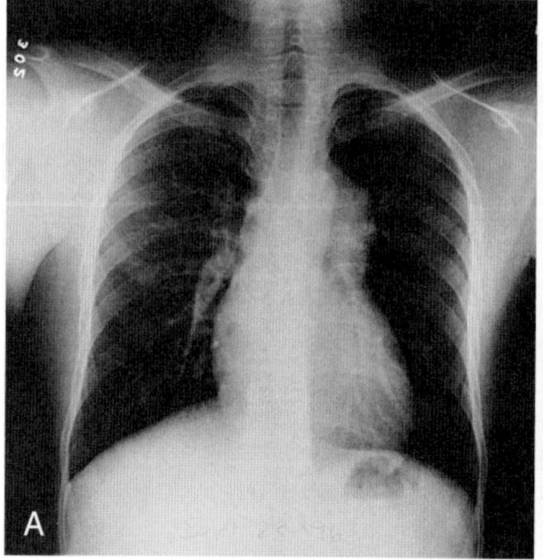

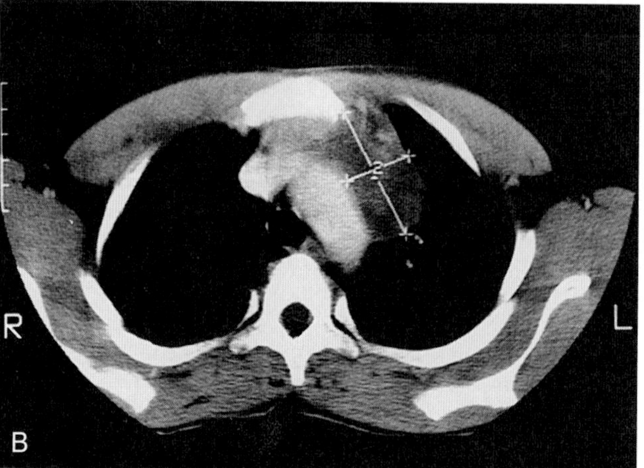

Figure 70-9. A, A 13-year-old African boy has an asymptomatic anterior mediastinal mass that was discovered on routine immigration chest radiograph. **B,** The CT scan shows a heterogeneous mass adjacent to the aorta, suggestive of a neoplasm (thymoma or lymphoma). During consideration of a fine-needle aspiration biopsy, ultrasonography was done and suggested the presence of cysts with debris (not shown). MRI (not shown) confirmed the presence of the cystic components as well as fat. A mature teratoma was excised through a small left anterior mediastinotomy, removing the left second costal cartilage.

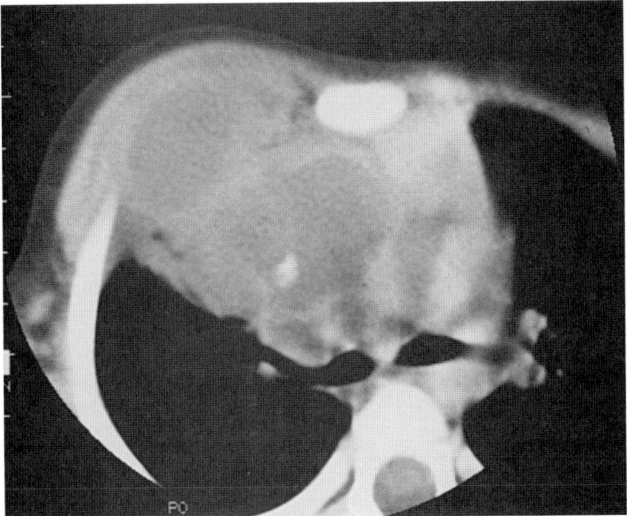

Figure 70-10. This 2-year-old was referred for a 5 × 5-cm, hard, fixed, right chest wall mass that appeared suddenly during an upper respiratory tract infection. The CT scan shows a bilobed lesion that extends through the chest wall and contains a small area of calcification. An incisional biopsy revealed pus-like material, containing ghost cells and calcified debris. Serum markers were normal. Complete excision of the mass required a right anterior thoracotomy and partial resection of an adherent right middle lobe. Pathologic examination revealed a ruptured mature teratoma with marked inflammatory reaction, containing foci of enteric, respiratory, and squamous mucosa; smooth muscle; salivary glands; pancreas; neuroglial tissue; and bone.

it may present as respiratory distress or poor feeding. Often, the tumor may be found incidentally on a chest radiograph. The only treatment is surgical excision. On histologic examination, these teratomas are usually composed of mature tissue with or without neuroglial components.[2,3]

Intracardiac Teratomas

Intracardiac teratomas are rare and arise from the atrium or ventricle. Many can be cured by surgical resection.[2]

Pulmonary Teratomas

Few cases of intrapulmonary teratoma have been described.[138,139] Symptoms included trichoptysis or hemoptysis. Lobectomy is the usual treatment.

Abdominal Teratomas

The most frequent abdominal teratomas are the gonadal teratomas, which are discussed in Chapters 52 and 76.

Retroperitoneal Teratomas

Retroperitoneal teratomas occur outside the pelvis, often in a suprarenal location. They represent about 5% of all childhood teratomas, and 75% occur in children younger than 5 years of age.[2,3] An association with Klinefelter's syndrome has been described.[55] Usually the tumor is discovered as an abdominal mass that can compress the gastrointestinal tract, causing symptoms such as vomiting and constipation.[140] Presentation with an acute abdomen from infection has also been described.[141]

Abdominal radiographs may show calcifications or bony structures within the tumor (Fig. 70-11). Ultrasonography and computed tomography (CT) are the investigations used, and assessment of serum markers is important. Surgical excision is usually straightforward, but occasionally the tumor may encase major vessels, making resection difficult.[142] Malignancy is uncommon,[2,140] but sometimes differentiation from a teratoid Wilms' tumor can be difficult.[143] The retroperitoneum is the most common location for the

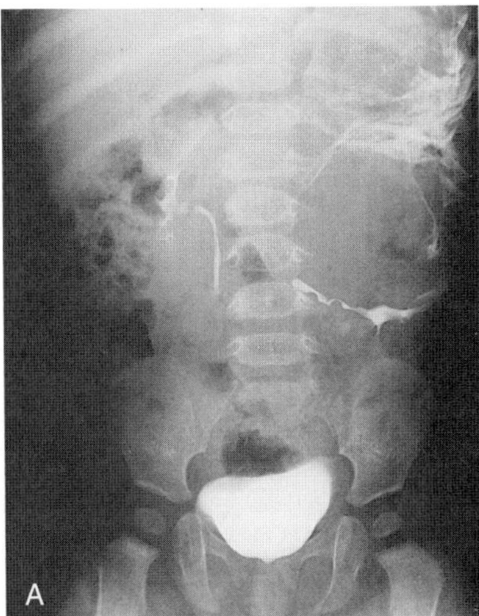

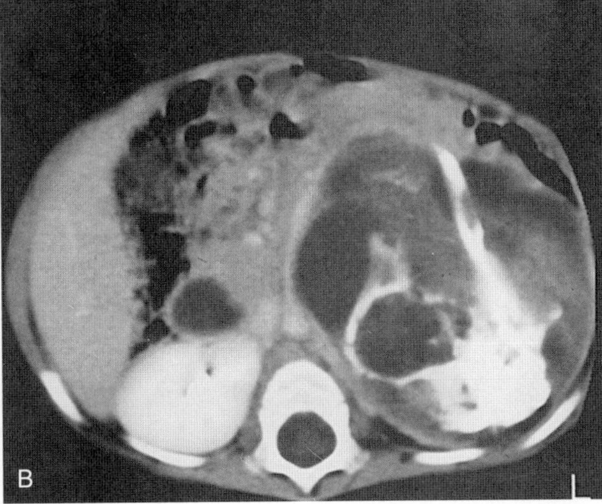

Figure 70-11. This 7-month-old girl was found to have an abdominal mass on physical examination. **A,** Plain films showed a large calcified left upper quadrant mass, which can be seen to displace the kidney inferiorly after injection of intravenous contrast. Ultrasonography (not shown) revealed multiple cystic areas. **B,** This was confirmed by CT, which also revealed areas of fat density, making teratoma much more likely than neuroblastoma. The mature teratoma contained all types of cerebral and cerebellar tissues; respiratory, transitional, and squamous epithelium; sebaceous and salivary glands; smooth muscle; cartilage; and fat. Serum markers were normal.

fetus-in-fetu malformations and intermediate fetiform teratomas.[2,3,144,145]

Gastric Teratomas

Gastric teratomas are rare lesions seen most commonly in male infants.[2,50,146,147] They account for 1% of all teratomas. Clinically, the tumors present as hematemesis or vomiting due to gastric outlet obstruction.[2,3,50,147,148] A palpable mass is common. The tumor is an exophytic mass in the lesser curvature or posterior wall of the stomach, and the whole stomach may be involved.

Most gastric teratomas are benign with primarily mature and immature neuroglial tissue. Benign peritoneal gliomatosis has been found incidentally in hernia sacs 10 months after resection of a gastric teratoma in the newborn period, illustrating the unusual behavior of some of these tumors.[149] Surgical excision is curative. Recurrence and malignancy are rare, despite local infiltration or nodal metastasis.[146,150] Regardless, periodic follow-up including AFP measurements is important.[151]

Other rare sites of abdominal teratomas include liver, gallbladder, pancreas, kidney, intestine, bladder, prostate, uterus, mesentery, omentum, abdominal wall, and diaphragm.[2,3,152-159]

Head and Neck Teratomas

More than 10% of teratomas in children originate from the neck, head, and central nervous system.[2,3,160,161] Most of these tumors are recognized at or shortly after birth and are associated with an increased incidence of stillbirth. They also can be diagnosed with prenatal ultrasonography (Fig. 70-12).[162,163]

Cervical Teratomas

Cervical teratomas represent up to 8% of all teratomas.[18,163] Large tumors can be seen in utero with ultrasonography.[162] These tumors are initially seen as a partial or completely cystic neck mass, which may compromise the airway and require immediate intubation or tracheostomy.[164,165] Large teratomas often lead to severe polyhydramnios, presumably because of esophageal compression. In turn, this may lead to premature labor. Serial amnioreduction may be required to prevent this complication. At birth, death may result from tracheal compression or deviation and the inability to intubate.[18,166-168] Prenatal diagnosis permits cesarean section and establishment of an airway by the surgical team before the cord is clamped.[167] Refinements of this technique, called the EXIT procedure (EX-utero Intrapartum Treatment), have been documented in a series of 31 patients, 7 of whom had a large cervical teratoma.[169] Extension of the tumor to the mediastinum or displacement of the trachea and carina may cause pulmonary hypoplasia, which increases respiratory morbidity and mortality.[2,3,169] The tumor is usually well defined and may contain calcifications. The differential diagnosis includes lymphangioma, congenital goiter, foregut duplication cyst, and branchial cleft cyst (see Fig. 70-12).[166,169] Investigation should include plain radiographs, ultrasonography, and measurement of AFP and β-hCG, as well as urinary catecholamine metabolites. CT and MRI may be useful to establish the diagnosis and to define the anatomic relations.

Complete excision is accomplished through a wide collar incision. The tumor is usually not difficult to separate from the strap muscles and the fascial planes, but the pretracheal fascia is sometimes very adherent. Often, the site of origin cannot be identified. In many instances, however, the tumor is firmly attached to and appears to originate from the thyroid gland. In such cases, a thyroid lobectomy should be performed. The terms *thyrocervical* and *cervicothyroidal* are often used to describe cervical teratomas.[2,3] In other instances, the tumor is adherent to the pharynx. In these cases, meticulous dissection and pharyngotomy, if necessary, are important to prevent tumor recurrence. Giant teratomas may distort the anatomy, leading to permanent sequelae (see Fig. 70-12E, F). Generally, the tumor is composed of both mature and immature neuroglial tissue, but cartilage and bronchial epithelium can also be found.[18,166,170] In 35% of cases, the tumor contains thyroid tissue.[171] Hypothyroidism can be a well-known postoperative complication.[172]

Cervical teratomas are usually benign, but malignancy has been reported, even in infants. A CCG report showed that 20% of tumors clearly contained malignant elements, most often neuroblastoma, but also teratocarcinoma, neuroblastoma-like tumor, and neuroectodermal tumor.[18] Complete excision in the neonatal period results in a survival rate of 80% to 90%. As for teratomas in other sites, one neonate was reported with a benign thyroid teratoma accompanied by neuroglial tissue deposits in cervical nodes.[173] A prognostic classification for cervical teratomas takes into account birth status, age at diagnosis, and the presence of respiratory distress.[170] In neonates without respiratory distress, the mortality rate was 2.7%, compared with 43.4% in those with respiratory compromise. Prenatal diagnosis and delivery by using the EXIT procedure can undoubtedly increase survival.[167-169]

Thyroid teratomas may be present in older children and adults and are often malignant in the latter.[174,175] Spindle epithelial tumor with thymus-like elements (SETTLE) is a malignant thyroid neoplasm that can sometimes be confused with thyroid teratomas due to their spindle cell and epithelial components.[176] These unique neoplasms have a propensity for delayed metastases, particularly to the lungs, kidney, mediastinum, lymph nodes, liver, and vertebrae.[177] Adjuvant chemotherapy and radiotherapy do not seem to have a significant impact on overall outcome for metastatic disease. In these patients, survival is poor.[176]

Craniofacial Teratomas

Craniofacial teratomas include a spectrum of lesions that may be life threatening.

Epignathus. *Epignathus* is a term used to describe teratomas protruding from the mouth (Fig. 70-13). These tumors arise from the soft or hard palate in the

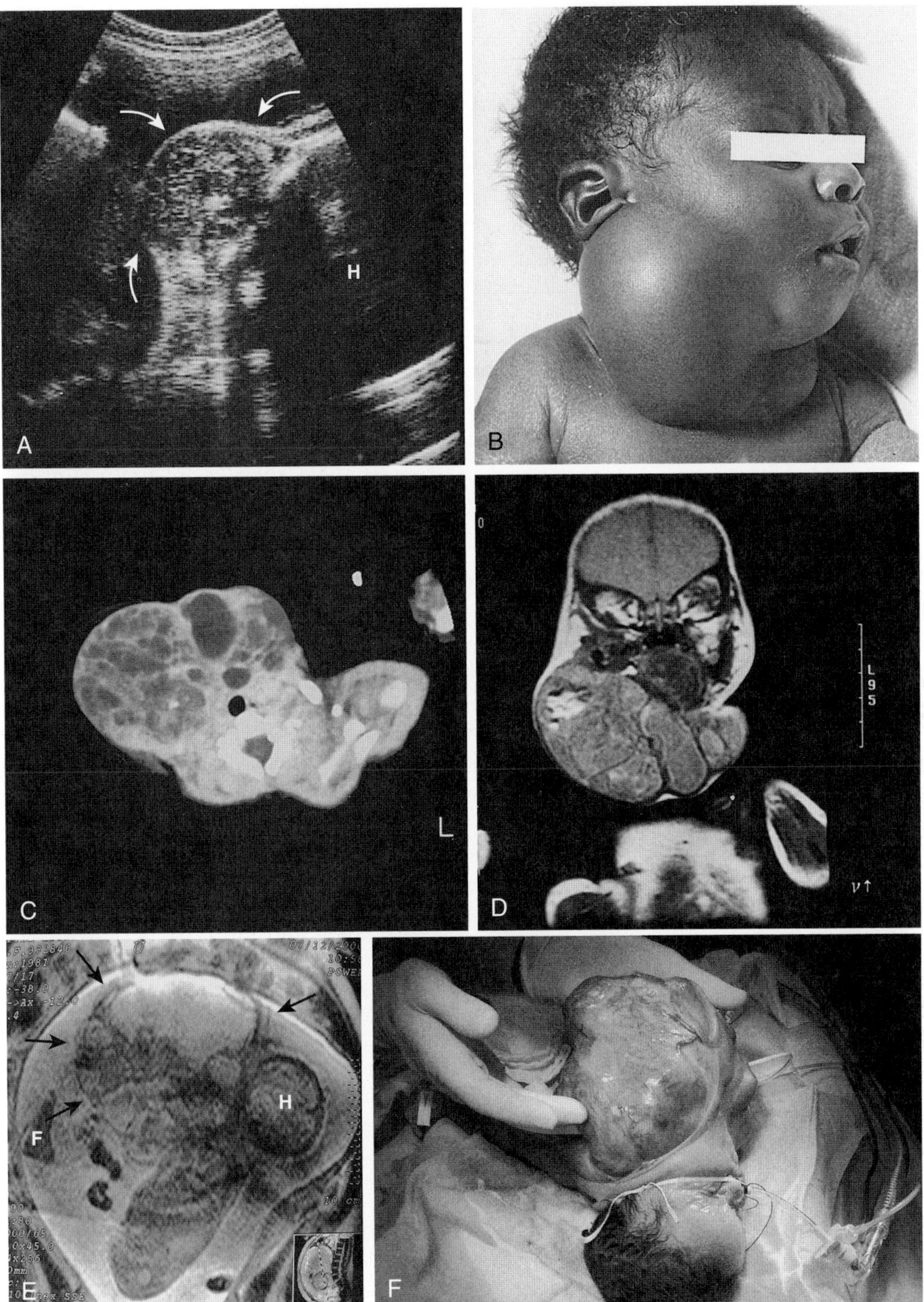

Figure 70-12. **A,** Fetal ultrasound image at 34 weeks of gestation shows a 7-cm cervical mass of mixed echogenicity, containing blood flow by Doppler (*arrows* point to the mass; H, head). **B,** After birth by cesarean section, the neonate had only mild tachypnea despite the large right cervical mass extending to the left side. Parts of the mass transilluminated, suggesting the diagnosis of a lymphangioma. **C,** CT scan of the lower cervical area shows an intact trachea and multiple cysts in the mass. **D,** MRI confirmed the presence of fat, which appears bright on T1-weighted images as well as on the proton density–weighted imaging sequence shown here. At operation, the mass appeared to originate from the right lobe of the thyroid gland. It contained epithelium-lined cysts, cartilage, bone, glandular tissue, and complex papillary structures; A predominance of neuroepithelial tissue was found with a few small areas of immature, neuroblastoma-like tissue. Preoperative vanillylmandelic acid levels were normal. The patient required postoperative thyroid hormone supplementation because of subclinical hypothyroidism (elevated thyroid-stimulating hormone with normal thyroxine and triiodothyronine levels). **E,** Another patient, with a giant cervical teratoma, seen on magnetic resonance at 30 weeks of gestation. The lesion was first diagnosed on routine ultrasonography at 18 weeks and grew much faster than the fetus. Several amnioreductions were required because of polyhydramnios, and an EXIT procedure was performed at 34 weeks of gestation (H, head; F, foot; *arrows* outline the tumor). **F,** After securing the airway during the EXIT procedure and stabilizing the neonate, resection was completed successfully. Notice the displacement of the ear. During resection, it became obvious that the left carotid artery and jugular vein entered the tumor. The left vagus nerve (hence the left recurrent nerve) was never seen, and the left glossopharyngeal nerve also was sacrificed. The tumor originated from the left pharyngeal wall. Including the fluid within the cystic parts, the teratoma weighed 1.4 kg, and the neonate weighed 1.6 kg postoperatively.

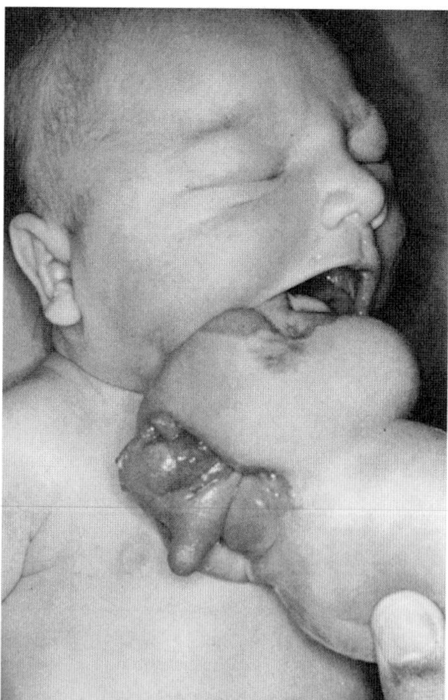

Figure 70-13. This baby was born with the epignathus protruding from his mouth.

region of Rathke's pouch.[178,179] They generally fill the oral cavity and extend out through the mouth. They can prevent fetal swallowing, which leads to polyhydramnios. Surgical excision is mandatory. They are usually benign, and recurrence is rare. A high degree of organization often gives them the appearance of a parasitic fetus.

Pharyngeal Teratomas. Pharyngeal teratomas arise from the posterior aspect of the nasopharynx. Large tumors can interfere with fetal swallowing and produce polyhydramnios, cause severe respiratory distress at birth, and lead to stillbirth.[2,180] Most pharyngeal teratomas are benign. Their treatment is surgical excision.[164]

Oropharyngeal Teratomas. Oropharyngeal teratomas represent 2% of all teratomas.[181] These tumors can originate from the tongue, sinuses, mandible, and tonsils. Airway compromise requires immediate care at the time of delivery. For oropharyngeal and nasopharyngeal teratomas, the EXIT procedure may be indicated when a large tumor detected prenatally appears to obstruct the airway. Most tumors are benign, and recurrence is uncommon after complete resection.[181] Separate tumors may occur in the same infant, and intracranial extension has been described.[182,183]

Orbital Teratomas. Orbital teratomas usually present at birth with unilateral proptosis in a normal, term neonate.[184] They grow rapidly, but the eye is intact. Occasionally, the tumor extends intracranially. The proptotic eye may rupture because of prolonged exposure. Histologically, these tumors are benign and contain mature tissue and immature neuroglial elements. Surgical resection is the treatment of choice, and the eye can usually be preserved.[2,184]

Middle Ear Teratomas. Middle ear teratomas may be difficult to differentiate from hereditary cholesteatoma. They are benign tumors, but surgical resection is difficult owing to the location of the tumor and the deformation of the middle ear. Ossiculoplasty is sometimes necessary.[185,186]

Intracranial Teratomas

Intracranial teratomas generally present with symptoms of space-occupying lesions. These lesions account for only 2% to 4% of all teratomas, but they represent nearly 50% of brain tumors in the first 2 months of life.[2,3,50,187] Most are benign in neonates, but malignancy dominates in older children and young adults.[50,187-190] These teratomas can appear in utero and cause massive hydrocephalus. A massive teratoma, causing skull rupture at delivery, has been reported.[188] The pineal gland is the most common site of origin, but intracranial teratomas may be seen in other areas, including the hypothalamus, ventricles, cavernous sinus, cerebellum, and suprasellar region.[50,189-191]

Pineal gland teratomas can secrete chorionic gonadotropin hormone, causing precocious puberty. In infants younger than 2 years, obstructive hydrocephalus is the most common clinical finding. In older children, symptoms of increased intracranial pressure are most common. The diagnosis can be made by using skull radiographs, ultrasonography, CT, or MRI.

Treatment of intracranial teratomas is difficult, and many are unresectable. The only long-term survivors are those who have the mass completely resected. Palliative shunting to reduce intracranial pressure is of little long-term benefit.[50] Perinatal mortality is high, with only a 6% survival when diagnosed in the fetus or newborn.[3,192]

Miscellaneous Sites

Teratomas have been reported in other sites, such as skin, parotid, vulva, perianal region well away from the coccyx, spinal canal, umbilical cord (possibly associated with omphalocele), and placenta.[2,3,193-197] Some of the spinal teratomas are now considered as enterogenous cysts.[198]

DERMOID, EPIDERMOID, AND RELATED CYSTS

Dermoid Cysts

Dermoid cysts are congenital cysts that are lined by skin with fully mature pilosebaceous structures.[199,200] They are the result of sequestration of skin along lines of embryonic closure. The head and neck are the sites

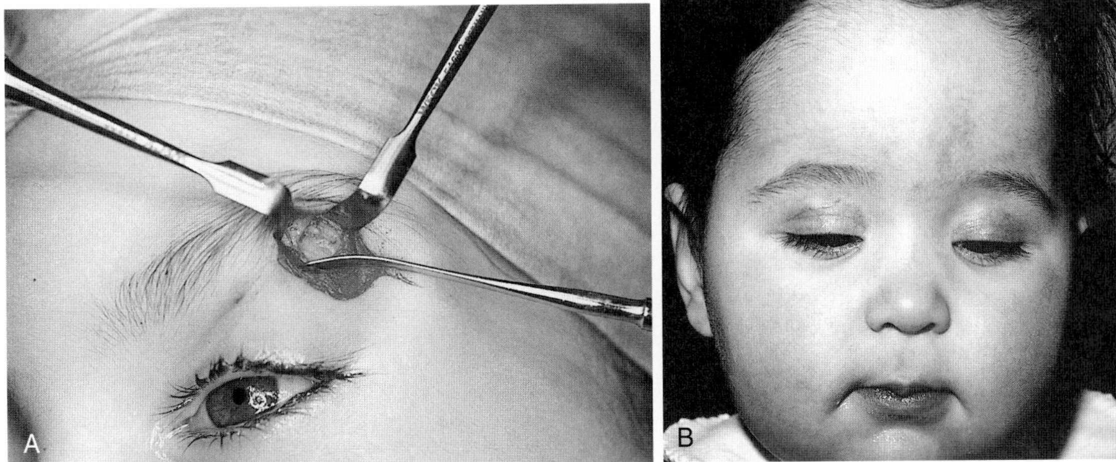

Figure 70-14. **A,** A dermoid cyst deep to the lateral part of the left eyebrow is approached through an incision made in the palpebral crease, taken through the muscle, which is then retracted upward, exposing the cyst lying on the periosteum. **B,** A different patient shown 1 month after excision of a right eyebrow dermoid through a palpebral skin incision. (A courtesy of Patricia Bortoluzzi, MD.)

of predilection, but these lesions have been described in other midline sites, including the sacral area, perineal raphe, scrotum, and presternal area.[200] The so-called dermoids of the ovary are, in fact, cystic teratomas and are discussed in Chapter 76.

Typical locations on the head are under the lateral part of the eyebrow, the scalp, the glabella, the tip of the nose, the orbit, and the palate, where they are associated with a cleft.[201] They also occur intracranially and in the spinal canal.[202]

Dermoids are usually round, soft, and often fixed to deep tissues or to bone. They usually present as a painless mass of 1 or 2 cm in diameter but can grow up to 4 cm or more if untreated. Some are associated with a sinus tract, especially those on the nose. This site is also typical for intracranial extension and a familial occurrence.[202] Dermoids in the head area are usually deep to muscles and often cause an indentation in the outer table of the skull. They can even erode through both bony tables and extend intracranially. A skull radiograph may show the defect, but it may be normal if the cyst is situated over a fontanelle or an unfused suture. CT is essential in those cases, and neurosurgical consultation is advisable.[202]

Dermoids deep to the lateral part of the eyebrow are usually approached through an incision just above the eyebrow because an incision within the eyebrow leaves a more visible scar. We have been impressed with an alternative incision through the palpebral crease(Fig. 70-14). This requires a slightly longer incision and more retraction but leaves an invisible scar (see Fig. 70-14). This approach also has the advantage of allowing access to the orbit for the rare cases in which the cyst penetrates through the orbital bone in a dumbbell fashion.

Dermoids in the cervical area are usually midline, mostly suprahyoid or submental. Because they are deep within muscles, they tend to move with swallowing, just as thyroglossal duct cysts do. On ultrasonography, they usually appear echogenic and are often misinterpreted as being solid rather than cystic. They can be differentiated intraoperatively by their yellowish appearance and their soft, buttery content with sebaceous material and hair (Fig. 70-15). This appearance alleviates the need for a hyoidectomy.

Dermoid cysts should be excised because they tend to grow and may rupture or become infected, resulting in a more difficult excision and a higher risk of recurrence.

Epidermal Cysts

Epidermal or epidermoid cysts have a wall composed of true epidermis, as seen on the skin surface and in the infundibulum of hair follicles (hence, they also are called infundibular cysts).[199] They do not contain pilosebaceous units or hair. Some have a congenital origin like dermoid cysts, whereas others are acquired, either spontaneously arising from hair

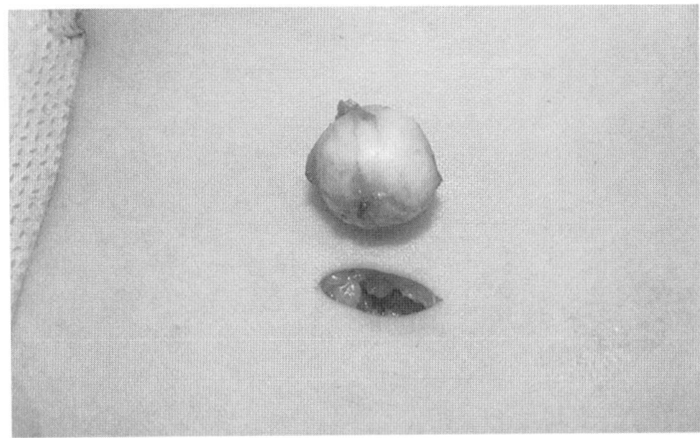

Figure 70-15. Dermoid cysts in the cervical region are found in the midline. They are usually suprahyoid or submental. This operative photograph shows a midline cervical dermoid cyst with its characteristic yellowish appearance. The cyst consists of a soft, buttery, cheesy content with sebaceous material. Preoperatively, these lesions are usually confused with a thyroglossal duct cyst. However, removal of the hyoid bone is not needed if a dermoid cyst is found.

follicles or secondary to trauma with implantation of epidermis into the dermis or subcutaneous tissue.

Epidermal cysts are slow growing and are formed by the desquamation of epithelial cells. They are round, intradermal, or subcutaneous lesions that stop growing after having reached 1 to 5 cm in diameter. They occur most commonly on the face, scalp, neck, and trunk (i.e., hair-bearing areas). They may be associated with a small sinus tract or dimpling of the skin. In the neck and infraclavicular area, they may be confused with branchial cleft remnants. Preauricular sinuses and cysts are often considered epidermal cysts. Epidermoid cysts of the spleen are discussed in Chapter 47.

Some patients may have more than one cyst, but the presence of multiple cysts, especially on the scalp and face, should raise the possibility of Gardner syndrome.[199,200] The cysts contain dry cheesy or horny material and lack skin appendages on histology. Treatment is excision, which often can be achieved under local anesthesia, even in young children.

Preauricular cysts are better excised under general anesthesia, owing to their deep attachment to the helix cartilage.[201] Spontaneous rupture of any epidermal cyst leads to an intense foreign-body reaction, and the child presents with an abscess-like mass. This may require incision and drainage but often can be treated with antibiotics and local warm compresses. This mode of presentation increases the risk of cyst recurrence after excision and often results in a wider scar than would have occurred with earlier excision. Infection of the cyst also may be caused by bacteria tracking along the small sinus tract that is sometimes present. These lesions rarely degenerate to epidermoid or basal cell carcinomas.[202] The treatment of asymptomatic preauricular sinuses is controversial, but certainly excision should be carried out in the presence of a palpable cyst or discharge of material from the sinus tract.

Epidermoid cysts of the skull and central nervous system share some similarities with dermoids, but they usually become symptomatic at an older age, between 20 and 40 years.[203] Most are thought to have a congenital origin, although iatrogenic and inflammatory mechanisms are likely for intraspinal epidermoids (caused by multiple lumbar punctures, especially when using a needle without stylet) and middle ear epidermoids (cholesteatomas), respectively.

Trichilemmal Cysts

Trichilemmal cysts, also called pilar or sebaceous cysts, are thought to arise from hair follicles.[199] Most are acquired and appear in adulthood. They often show an autosomal dominant inheritance pattern and are solitary in only 30% of the cases.[199] Some authors classify these as epidermoid or epidermal cysts.[202]

SOFT TISSUE TUMORS

Numerous soft tissue tumors have been described and are of mainly ectodermal and mesodermal origin. Some of these pediatric neoplasms are classified in Table 70-2. Only those soft tissue tumors likely to be encountered by pediatric surgeons are discussed here. More extensive discussions of soft tissue tumors are available.[204,205] Many soft tissue tumors are cutaneous or subcutaneous and are amenable to excision under local anesthesia.

Epidermal Tumors

Pyogenic Granulomas

Pyogenic granulomas are solitary polypoid capillary lesions often associated with trauma or local irritation. They are commonly found on the skin as red, raised, occasionally bleeding lesions or in the mouth in association with pregnancy.[206] They are easily treated with topical silver nitrate or liquid nitrogen or ligature of the polyp neck. Rarely, excision or electrocautery is needed.

Skin Papillomas

Skin papillomas resemble skin tags of the mucous membrane and occur at birth or in childhood.[207] Sessile variants may be called *verrucae*, whereas the

Table 70-2 Classification of Soft Tissue Tumors That Occur in Children

Tissue	Benign	Malignant
Ectoderm		
Epidermis	Dermoid cyst, calcifying epithelioma (pilomatrixoma)	Epidermoid cancer
Sweat gland	Hidradenoma	Adenocarcinoma
Sebaceous gland	Sebaceous cyst	Epidermoid cancer
Melanocytes	Nevus	Malignant melanoma
Nerve tissue	Neurofibroma	Neurofibrosarcoma
Mesoderm		
Undifferentiated	Mesenchymoma, myxoma	Malignant mesenchymoma
Fibrous tissue	Fibroma, fibromatosis, keloid	Fibrosarcoma
Vascular tissue	Hemangioma, lymphangioma, glomus	Hemangioendothelioma, Angiosarcoma
Adipose tissue	Lipoma, lipoblastoma	Liposarcoma
Muscle	Rhabdomyoma	Rhabdomyosarcoma
Synovial tissue	Giant cell synovioma, ganglion cyst, synovial cyst	Malignant synovioma

projections are termed *acrochordons*. Treatment is by simple excision.

Warts

Warts are uncommon before age 4 years but are a common pediatric complaint.[207] Various subtypes of human papillomavirus affect different body areas.[206] Verrucae spread through families, sports teams, and schoolmates and are most common on the hands and feet.[207] Topical treatment includes salicylic or trichloroacetic acid, liquid nitrogen, or fine-tip electrocautery. Excision is occasionally required.

Condylomata acuminata occur in the perineal skin and suggest, but do not prove, child sexual abuse. The virus may be transmitted by hand contact during diaper changes in infants or acquired at birth during vaginal delivery, but the lesions may take months to develop. One study suggested that sexual abuse is an unlikely source of transmission in children younger than 3 years if no other signs of abuse are present.[208] These lesions have a core of connective tissue covered in epithelium, occurring as solitary or cauliflower-like lesions. Spontaneous regression is known, but topical podophyllin may be required. Some cases may necessitate electrocautery under general anesthesia to enable a thorough rectoscopic and vaginoscopic assessment and treatment.

Aberrant Skin Glands

Aberrant skin glands appear as rough, yellow-brownish skin resembling nevi or xanthoma. Histologic examination reveals adenoid hyperplasia, but a potential for later malignant change is reported. Therefore, excision of these lesions is recommended.[207]

Calcifying Epithelioma of Malherbe

The calcifying epithelioma of Malherbe or pilomatrixoma is a solitary benign calcifying tumor of hair follicles. This is one of the most common acquired soft tissue lesions in children. Clinically, a circumscribed, firm, mobile, intracutaneous or subcutaneous nodule is palpable, with occasional yellowish or bluish coloration (Fig. 70-16). These lesions are most common before age 20 years, and 60% to 70% are found in the head and neck region.[206] Only 2% to 3% are multiple, and most are smaller than 1 cm, although lesions up to 4 cm have been reported.[206,209] They are more common than sebaceous cysts in younger patients. Local excision is indicated.[209]

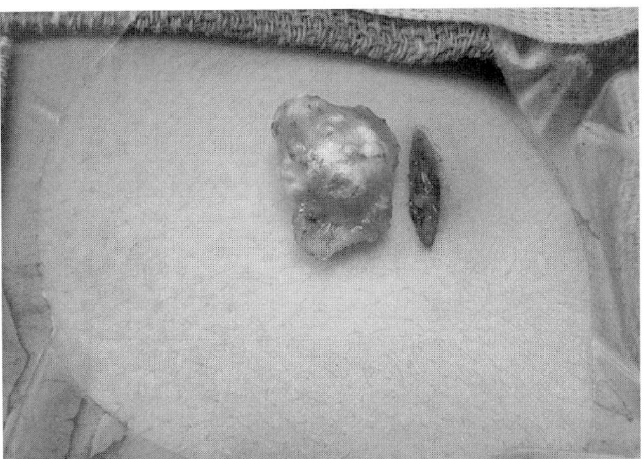

Figure 70-16. This operative photograph shows a pilomatrixoma (calcifying epithelioma of Malherbe). These lesions are circumscribed, are firm, and have a distinctive "knobby" appearance. Once removed, they are seen to have a yellowish content. Most of these lesions are found in the head and neck region.

Sweat Gland Lesions

Sweat gland pathology results from disorders of the sebaceous, apocrine, or eccrine adnexal structures of the skin. One series reported that only 1.7% of pediatric skin biopsy specimens showed these lesions.[206] Hidradenomas originate from the ductal portion of the sweat gland and are seen as multiple small flesh-colored papules on the face, neck, and upper chest during puberty and adolescence. Two subtypes are of interest: the eruptive form results in many lesions in a short period, whereas the clear cell variant causes solitary and occasionally painful lesions.[206] Sweat gland carcinomas are uncommon and are rarely differentiated enough to subtype confidently.[206] They may be locally aggressive and metastasize to the local lymph nodes. Treatment primarily involves resection with individualized adjuvant therapy.

Malignant Epithelial Tumors

Malignant epithelial tumors are rare in children.[207] General treatment principles include wide local excision and radiation therapy for prevention of recurrence.[207] Only 1% of all basal cell carcinomas occur in children. The basal cell nevus syndrome[210] is an autosomal dominant disease with basal cell lesions of the eyes, nose, and cheeks in association with anomalies of the mouth, skin, skeleton, central nervous system, eyes, and genitals. These patients may have concomitant xeroderma pigmentosum. Epidermoid or squamous cell carcinoma also is found in xeroderma pigmentosum patients.[206] Epidermoid cancers in pediatric transplant recipients also have been reported.[206]

Tumors of Nerve Tissue

Neurofibromas

A neurofibroma is a benign neoplasm of abnormal proliferation of Schwann cells, usually of peripheral nerves. When multiple fibromas are present or associated with multiple café-au-lait spots, neurofibromatosis type 1 (NF1, von Recklinghausen's disease), an autosomal dominant disorder, may be present. The *NF1* gene appears to produce a tumor suppressor product, and neurofibromatosis may be a disease to which the two-hit genetic hypothesis applies.[211] The diagnosis may be delayed, but children in affected probands are usually diagnosed earlier, even by prenatal

Table 70-3 Clinical Patterns in Neurofibromatosis

Clinical Pattern	Description
Fibroma molluscum	Hundreds or thousands of pedunculated nodules; number makes resection impractical.
Plexiform neurofibroma	Occur usually in the face and scalp, causing bony deformity by pressure erosion; resections for cosmesis may be repeated because curative resection is rare.
Elephantiasis nervorum	With neurofibromas of the extremities, these cause greatly thickened skin simulating limb hypertrophy; resection is done to manage disfigurement.
Thoracic neurofibroma	May have intraspinal extension (dumbbell tumor); has a high incidence of malignancy
Visceral neurofibroma	May affect intestine, kidney, and bladder because of the presence of associated nerves; when large, neurofibrosarcoma incidence increases.
Skeletal syndromes	Include kyphoscoliosis, pseudarthrosis of tibia and ulna
Cranial syndromes	Meningiomas, gliomas, and optic gliomas have been reported.
Endocrine syndromes	Sexual precocity, medullary thyroid carcinoma, and pheochromocytoma have been reported.
Cardiovascular syndromes	Heart is rarely involved, but coarctation of the aorta and renal artery lesions have been reported.

ultrasonography.[212,213] Neurofibromas of the mucosa are associated with multiple endocrine neoplasia type 2B and can appear in childhood before medullary thyroid carcinoma or pheochromocytoma.[214] The *NF2* gene has been associated with acoustic neuromas.

Neurofibromatosis type 1 has several clinical forms, which are summarized in Table 70-3.[215] Because operative management can not cure a genetic disorder, a multidisciplinary team supports patients and parents through decision making, treatment, rehabilitation, and developmental challenges (Fig. 70-17). Malignant degeneration to neurofibrosarcoma and associated malignancies[216] may necessitate ultrasonography, CT, or MRI studies for new symptoms. Patients with neurofibromatosis type 1 have a 7% to 12% lifetime risk of developing associated malignant peripheral nerve sheath tumors, which often arise within a plexiform neurofibroma.[217] These lesions are aggressive, metastasize widely, and portend a poor prognosis. Traditionally, clinical symptoms such as pain, rapid tumor growth, and new-onset neurologic deficit have been used to predict malignant change in previously stable neurofibroma.[217,218] Recent studies have suggested that 18-fluorodeoxyglucose positron-emission tomography (FDG-PET), in conjunction with CT or MRI, may help identify malignant lesions based on standardized uptake levels.[219]

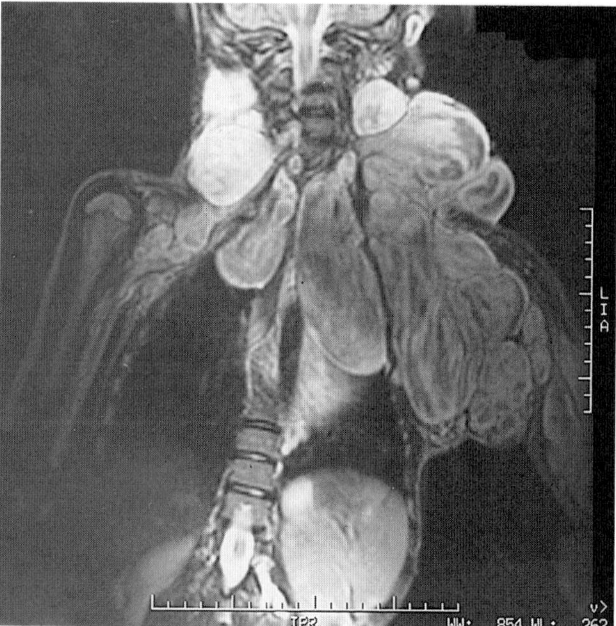

Figure 70-17. MR image of a young boy with extensive neurofibromatosis type 1 who had undergone two previous cervical laminectomies to remove plexiform neurofibromas that were causing symptomatic cord compression. The left neck mass was enlarging, causing tracheal deviation and growing along the cervical nerve roots. This boy also had increasing left arm weakness and pain. A trial of chemotherapy with vincristine and dactinomycin did not stop progression of the disease.

These imaging modalities are useful in monitoring larger or deeper neurofibromas as well. Rapid growth is an ominous sign of malignant transformation. Excision or debulking may be combined with chemotherapy and radiation therapy.[220] Radiation therapy does not appear to be useful in slowing the progression of benign disease but has been documented to cause neurofibrosarcoma.[221] Treatment with chemotherapy and interferon-alfa has been of limited value.

Xanthomas

A xanthoma is a tumor of lipid-laden histiocytes or foam cells forming yellowish skin nodules. It may be due to uncontrolled diabetes mellitus or biliary tract obstruction, which unbalances triglyceride and cholesterol metabolism, leading to accumulation in histiocytes. Xanthomas are typical features of Alagille syndrome (syndromic paucity of bile ducts) and familial hypercholesterolemia (Fig. 70-18). Correcting the underlying disorder reverses these lesions, but excisional biopsy may be indicated for bothersome lesions or for diagnostic purposes.

Tumors of Mesoderm

Undifferentiated Mesenchyme

MESENCHYMOMAS

Mesenchymoma is a mixed mesenchymal tumor of two or more cellular elements not commonly associated (not including fibrous tissue). It can occur after

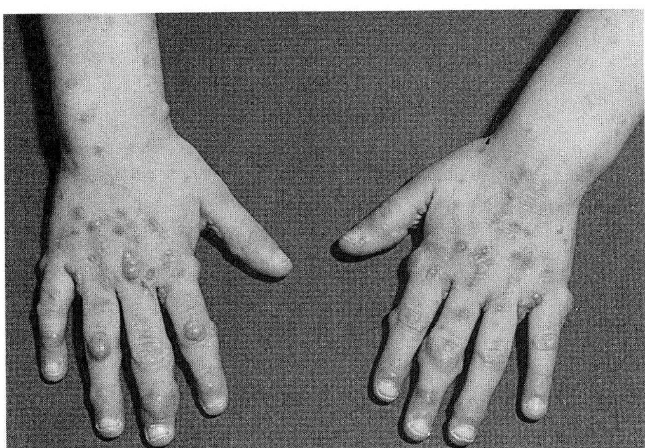

Figure 70-18. Multiple xanthomas are seen in a child with Alagille syndrome.

radiation therapy or chemotherapy.[222] These lesions are usually benign in children and occur primarily in the head, neck, and extremities. Rib lesions in neonates and liver lesions also are described.[223] Malignant mesenchymoma is the corresponding sarcoma and is rare.

Myxomas

A myxoma is a benign primitive connective tissue cell and stroma tumor resembling mesenchyme. It occurs mainly in the heart, producing symptoms by obstructing normal blood flow, and is removed by using cardiopulmonary bypass (Fig. 70-19).

Fibrous Tissue Tumors

Fibromas

A fibroma is a lesion composed of fibrous or fully developed connective tissue occurring as lytic bone lesions, breast lumps, finger swelling, and other forms.[223] Fibromatosis usually is first seen in infancy with multiple firm rubbery masses in the soft tissues, generally in the lower extremities and head and neck. When it is congenital and generalized, death may occur in the first weeks of life, due to pulmonary lesions.[223]

Nodular Fasciitis

Nodular fasciitis is the most common fibrous tissue tumor or self-limiting reactive process.[224] These tumors may be subcutaneous, intramuscular, or fascial in location and are commonly found in the head and neck of children.[224] Half of cases are associated with discomfort, and one fourth of lesions occur in patients younger than 20 years. Excisional biopsy is necessary to differentiate these rapidly growing lesions from a malignancy.

Fibrosarcomas

Fibrosarcoma is a neoplasm producing collagen that otherwise lacks cellular differentiation. Childhood fibrosarcoma has a bimodal age distribution (younger than 5 years and ages 10 to 15 years). Childhood

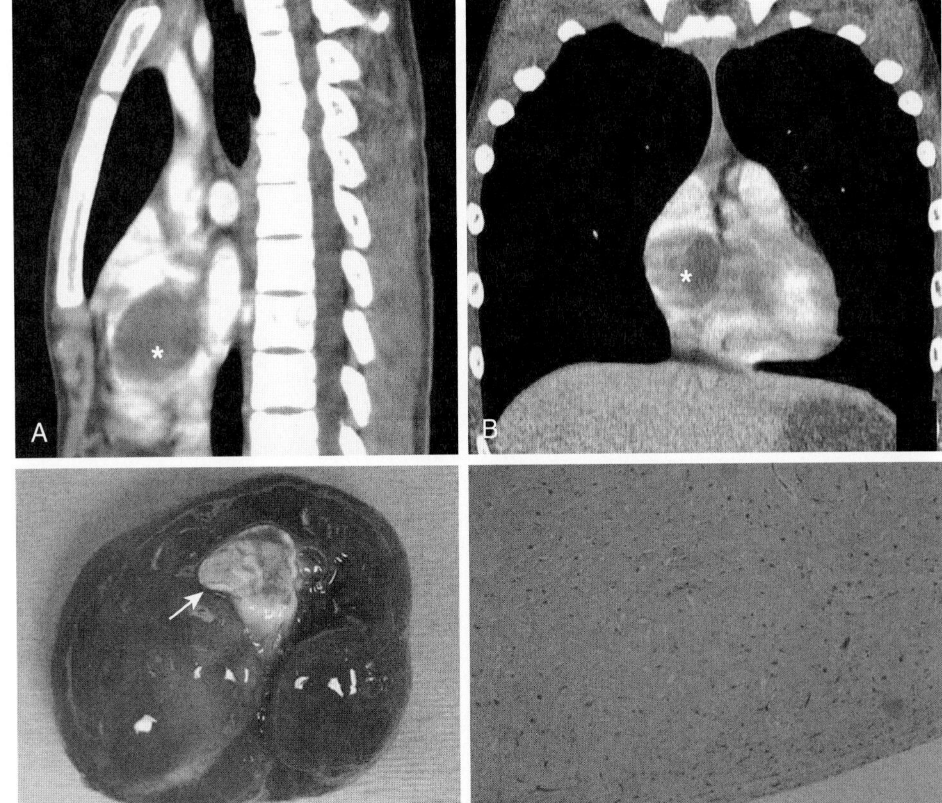

Figure 70-19. This 15-year-old presented with jugular venous distention and upper torso edema. **A** and **B,** A large (4 × 5 cm) mass (*asterisk*) was found in the right atrium on CT scan. **C,** The mass was excised in its entirety along with a full-thickness portion of the atrial septum (*arrow*). **D,** On histologic examination, the characteristics of an atrial myxoma are identified. This low-power photomicrograph shows a very hypocellular tumor with an abundant extracellular myxoid matrix.

fibrosarcoma is treated with complete excision. Adult-type fibrosarcoma is an aggressive lesion with a poor prognosis despite multimodal therapy. The two lesions may be difficult to differentiate.[225]

Congenital Epulis

Congenital epulis is a benign granular cell tumor occurring almost exclusively in girls at or immediately after birth. It originates from the maxillary dental mucosa and averages 1 to 2 cm in diameter.[226] Its exact nature is not clear. Some classify it under tumors of peripheral nerves, whereas others consider it a fibrous tumor, hence the synonym granular cell fibroblastoma. Spontaneous regression is unusual, and simple excision is curative.[226]

Keloid

A keloid is a sharply elevated, irregularly shaped, progressively enlarging scar caused by excessive collagen in the dermis during connective tissue repair. Unlike the hypertrophic scar (which does not progress), a keloid may recur after excision. Treatment with intradermal injection of corticosteroids, pressure garments (as used for burn patients), and cryosurgery may be attempted. Rarely, judicious excision with radiation therapy may be used.[227] Keloids developing after minor procedures are common. Their incidence is higher in blacks.

Desmoid Tumors

Desmoid tumors are fibrous tumors that usually arise from musculoaponeurotic tissue of the skull or abdominal cavity, hence the modern name musculoaponeurotic fibromatosis.[228] They are not encapsulated and are locally invasive, although they do not metastasize. They are associated with Gardner syndrome.

When they arise from the retroperitoneum, complete resection may be impossible without risking damage to splanchnic vessels. High-dose radiation therapy or interstitial brachytherapy may be considered for residual tumor. Chemotherapy using methotrexate and vinblastine or the tyrosine kinase inhibitor imatinib mesylate has engendered favorable reports.[229,230] Corticosteroid therapy (tamoxifen, prednisone) and nonsteroidal therapy (indomethacin and sulindac) have been used in recurrent and inoperable tumors.[231] Shrinkage of a desmoid tumor has been reported by using interferon-alfa as well.[232]

Vascular Glomus Tumors

A glomus tumor is an uncommon pediatric lesion consisting of a meshwork of fine arterioles connected to veins and intertwined with nerve tissue. Multiple tumors have a greater tendency to develop in children than in adults, possibly representing autosomal dominant inheritance.[223] The lesions on the skin are discrete blue-black spots and may be extremely painful if present under nails. Excision is the preferred treatment.

Adipose Tissue Tumors

A lipoma is a benign, soft, rubbery, encapsulated tumor of adipose tissue composed of mature fat cells occurring on the trunk, neck, and forearms. In one review of adipose tumors, lipomas represented 94%; lipoblastoma, 4.7%; and liposarcoma, 1.3%.[233] All are slow-growing tumors. Diagnosed often before age 3 years, lipoblastoma may be superficial and well encapsulated or it may be deep and infiltrative. Definitive treatment of adipose tumors is complete resection. Chemotherapy may play a role in treating residual liposarcoma. Local recurrence rates for lipoblastoma and liposarcoma are 10% to 20%.[233] Characterized by a myxoid stroma, embryonal lipoblasts, and mature fat cells, the myxoid variant of liposarcoma is similar histologically to lipoblastoma. Tumor karyotyping may be useful in differentiating these adipose tumors.[233]

Liposarcoma arises from the intramuscular fascia, where embryonal lipoblasts exhibit variable differentiation with occasional nuclear atypia. The myxoid variant is the most common and metastasizes late, if at all. The dedifferentiated subtype is highly malignant and may co-exist with spindle cell sarcoma.

Tumors of Synovial Tissue

Synovial Cysts

Synovial cysts or ganglion cysts arise from joints or tendon sheaths, resulting in firm 0.5- to 2-cm, mucin-filled lesions with a fibrous capsule. They are most common on the hand, especially on the dorsum of the wrist, but also occur on the ankle, foot, and popliteal fossa (where they are called Baker's cysts [Fig. 70-20]). One fourth of the latter occur in children younger than 6 years.[234]

Pathology texts separate synovial cysts that have a true synovial lining (e.g., Baker's cysts) from ganglia, which are thought to be degenerative and are without a synovial lining.[235,236] Clinicians, however, usually use both terms interchangeably.[237] Symptoms of pain and weakness can occur, but most children present with an asymptomatic mass. Spontaneous resolution of all types of synovial cysts is common in children. Surgical treatment is reserved for patients with persistently symptomatic lesions.[237] Classic treatment includes traumatic disruption ("strike it with the family Bible") or corticosteroid injection. Both should be discouraged because of the high recurrence risk and associated pain. The use of nonsteroidal anti-inflammatory agents, coupled with rest or wrist splinting, is usually sufficient if the cyst causes transient discomfort.

Giant Cell Synoviomas

The giant cell synovioma is a benign tumor of the tendon sheath, generally occurring before age 10 years.[223] It occurs on the volar aspect of fingers in most cases.

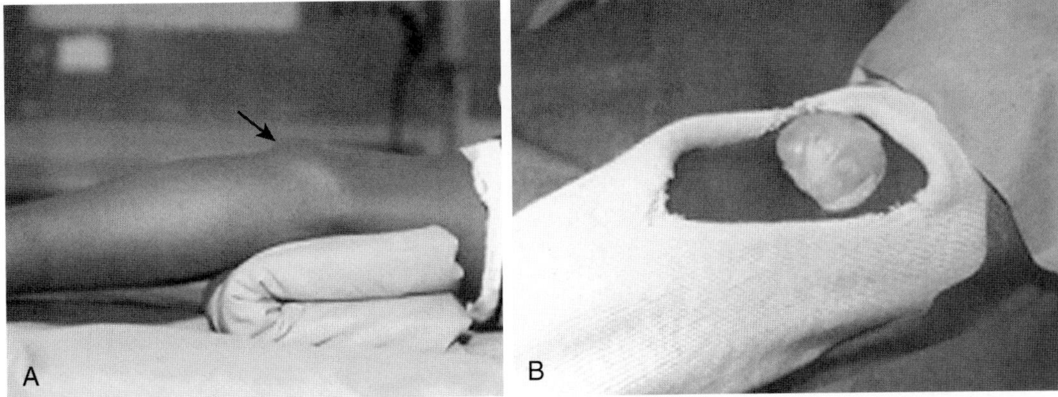

Figure 70-20. **A,** This patient has been turned in a semi-prone position and a Baker cyst (*arrow*) is readily visualized with extension of the knee. **B,** On the right, the cyst is seen bulging through the skin incision. The cyst was excised due to its large size and interference with running. The child recovered uneventfully without recurrence.

A 10% to 15% recurrence rate can be expected after treatment by resection.[223] Malignant synovioma or synoviosarcoma represents 5% to 10% of soft tissue malignancies in patients younger than 20 years.[238] Most occur near the knee, but they also are found in the head and neck, anterior abdominal wall, and inguinal area. The mass may be palpable or reveal itself as calcification on a radiograph. Cure by wide excision without chemotherapy can often be achieved, but the neurovascular anatomy related to the tumor may necessitate microsurgical reconstruction, if not amputation. The calcifying subtype has a better 5-year survival rate (83%) than the noncalcifying subtypes (25% to 50%).[239]

chapter 71

LYMPHOMAS

Karen B. Lewing, MD • Alan S. Gamis, MD, MPH

Lymphomas are a result of chromosomal alterations resulting in the uncontrolled growth of cells of lymphoid origin. Among all ages, lymphomas constitute just 4% of all cancers diagnosed annually in the United States.[1] In children, however, this percentage increases to 11%.[2] Combined, Hodgkin's and non-Hodgkin's lymphoma are the second most common childhood solid tumors (behind brain tumors and ahead of neuroblastoma). These two malignancies compose approximately 15% of all childhood solid tumors annually.

Lymphomas have classically been divided into two distinct groups: Hodgkin's disease (HD) and non-Hodgkin's lymphoma (NHL). In 2001, HD was designated Hodgkin's lymphoma (HL) by the World Health Organization (WHO) lymphoma classification system.[3] Typically, patients with both HL and NHL are initially seen with enlarged lymph nodes and may have systemic symptoms of fever and fatigue and/or extralymphatic spread. However, these two types of lymphoma also have clear differences. HL typically is seen as an indolent process, whereas NHL is most often seen in children with a rapid onset of symptoms. Because of this propensity for rapid growth, children with NHL often have associated anatomic and metabolic co-morbidities to such a degree that their recognition and need for treatment constitutes a medical emergency. With HL, treatment is based primarily on staging and less on histologic subtype. In contrast, the current treatment of NHL depends on the histologic and immunophenotypic subtypes in addition to stage.

These two lymphomas are truly a study of contrasts. This is no more evident than in the evolution of their therapy. For years, HL has been one of the most curable cancers. Now, with markedly improved treatment protocols, NHL has a nearly equivalent cure rate.[4] Owing to the historic high survival with HL, its therapy has focused on reduction in intensity. Because of its previously poor prognosis, NHL therapy has focused on intensification of therapy. The use of higher doses of chemotherapy over a short period (as compared with prior methods) has resulted in the dramatic improvement in cure and response of NHL.

Although most histologic types of HL are treated similarly, it is important to classify fully the subtype of NHL because marked differences occur in the effective therapies administered for each type. In considering the surgeon's role in the therapy for childhood lymphomas, there are no real differences between the two types of lymphomas. However, in contrast to other solid tumors of childhood, in which initial resection of the tumor is important, the primary role of the surgeon in the initial management of lymphomas is to ensure the rapid attainment of adequate and properly preserved biopsy material to allow the pathologist the opportunity to make the diagnosis of the specific type and subtype of lymphoma. Except for certain situations, attempts to resect lymphomas at the time of presentation have no role in the modern management of lymphomas.

HODGKIN'S LYMPHOMA

Thomas Hodgkin, in his classic thesis in 1832, described the gross necropsy examinations of seven patients.[5] He noted the association of generalized lymphadenopathy and splenomegaly in six patients without evidence of infection or inflammation. Histologic descriptions of the Reed-Sternberg (RS) cell, the pathognomonic multinucleated giant cell, did not occur until after the turn of the century.[6,7] Even though the etiology was unclear, therapeutic interventions began soon after the discovery of x-rays. More successful application of radiation therapy awaited the description of the disease's propensity for contiguous spread. With this knowledge, application of radiation to the involved and adjacent nodal areas (extended-field technique) resulted in improvements in survival in the late 1930s.[8] In the early 1960s, in acknowledgment of the limitations of the radiologic techniques of that era, the practice of systematic laparotomy, splenectomy, and celiac node and liver biopsy at the time of initial presentation was developed for the purpose of staging and for targeted therapy.[9] This has properly been described as the model for the careful staging of cancer as a required prerequisite to the design of therapy, which is a hallmark of oncologic practice today.[10,11] During this same time, chemotherapy combinations entered into the physician's armamentarium. With their use, remission and cure rates markedly improved. The improvement has made HL one of the most curable cancers today, with a 5-year survival of 95% for patients diagnosed between 1996 and 2002.[12] With this high expectation for cure, attention over the past decade in pediatric oncology has focused on the reduction of long-term sequelae of treatment. To this end, chemotherapy has evolved from an adjunctive role to a primary one, with the hope of eliminating the need for irradiation (and its attendant sequelae) altogether. When irradiation is needed, if used in combination with chemotherapy, the focus has been to reduce the size of the fields (from extended to involved) and the doses used. The two classic chemotherapy combinations (MOPP: nitrogen mustard, vincristine [Oncovin], procarbazine, prednisone; and ABVD: doxorubicin [Adriamycin], bleomycin, vinblastine, dacarbazine) have evolved to reduce long-term sequelae. Hybrids of these combinations are being utilized to reduce the doses delivered to the patient, with equivalent results and less toxicity.

Incidence and Epidemiology

Among all ages, 7500 individuals each year are diagnosed with HL in the United States, accounting for just 0.5% of all cancers and only 12% of all lymphomas.[1] However, in children, it is the sixth most common type of cancer, with approximately 500 children diagnosed annually.[2] This constitutes 5% of all childhood cases of cancer and 44% of all childhood cases of lymphoma. HL has an incidence of 5 cases/million children age birth to 14 years/year.[13] A bimodal distribution exists when considering all ages, but in children alone a gradual trend is seen of increasing incidence with increasing age (Fig. 71-1). HL is exceedingly rare in children younger than age 2 years and peaks in the adolescent years.[2] Beyond age 11 years, it is the most common of the two types of lymphoma and accounts for about 15% of all cancer in young adults ages 15 to 24 years.[13] A slight male predominance (1.32:1) is noted, but in the youngest children the male-to-female ratio is much larger (12 to 19:1).[2,14]

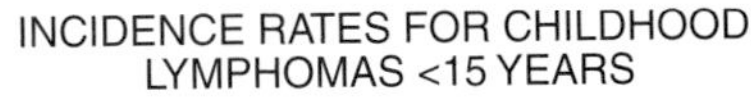

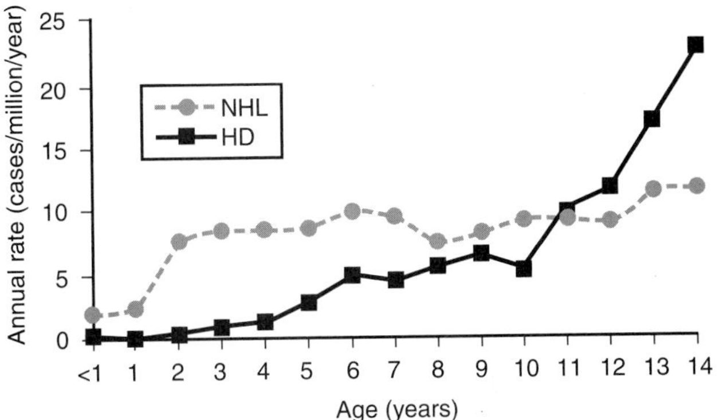

Figure 71-1. Incidence rates for lymphomas in children younger than 15 years. HD, Hodgkin's disease; NHL, non-Hodgkin's lymphoma. (From Gurney JG, Severson RK, Davis S, Robison LL: Incidence of cancer in children in the United States. Cancer 75:2186-2195, 1995.)

HL occurs more often in whites than in blacks (1.3:1).[15] Familial clusters of HL have been noted. Whether this represents risk due to environmental exposure (most often thought to be infectious) or genetics is uncertain. Monozygotic twins of HL patients have been found to be at greater risk of developing HL than are dizygotic twins,[16] strongly implicating genetics as a principal risk factor. Conversely, again in young adults, an increased risk of HL is found with higher socioeconomic status.[17] Young adults with HL come from smaller families, have fewer infectious exposures as young children, and/or have later exposure to infections than do control populations.[17,18] This correlates closely with socioeconomic status and implicates a delayed infectious exposure as a principal risk factor.

Most likely, a combination of genetic risk and infectious exposure predisposes a young adult to HL. Immunodeficiency may be the link between these two risk factors, at least in a subgroup of HL patients. HL is more prevalent in human immunodeficiency virus (HIV)-infected patients.[19-21] Also, patients with HL have a higher incidence of cellular immunodeficiency at the time of diagnosis.[22] Etiologic theories encompass these two risk factors and focus primarily on the Epstein-Barr virus (EBV). Genomic material from EBV has been found in the RS cells in up to 79% of HL cases.[23-25] This has the highest association with the mixed cellularity subtype.[26] An association with EBV is not seen in patients with the nodular lymphocyte-predominant (LP) subtype.[27] A higher risk of HL has been noted in individuals with a history of infectious mononucleosis[28-30] and with previously high titers to EBV.[31] This risk was greater when infected at an older age, and the risk lessened with time from infection.[29] In one report, epidemiologic investigations identified a median incubation time of 4.1 years between infectious mononucleosis and the development of EBV-positive HL.[30] One hypothesis that incorporates these factors suggests the following sequence: (1) a genetic, iatrogenic, or viral immunosuppression; (2) subsequently or coincidentally, an EBV infection or oncogenetic rearrangement in a lymphoid precursor cell; (3) further genetic alterations, followed by (4) clonal expansion of lymphoid cells with morphologic features of RS cells, finally resulting in (5) the clinical syndrome known as HL, diagnosed by the presence of RS cells.[32]

Classification and Histologic Subtyping

The diagnosis of classic HL requires the dual finding of the diagnostic Hodgkin's and RS cells (HRS cells) plus a reactive cellular background.[33] The RS cell is a large cell (15 to 45 mm) with an "owl's eye" appearance

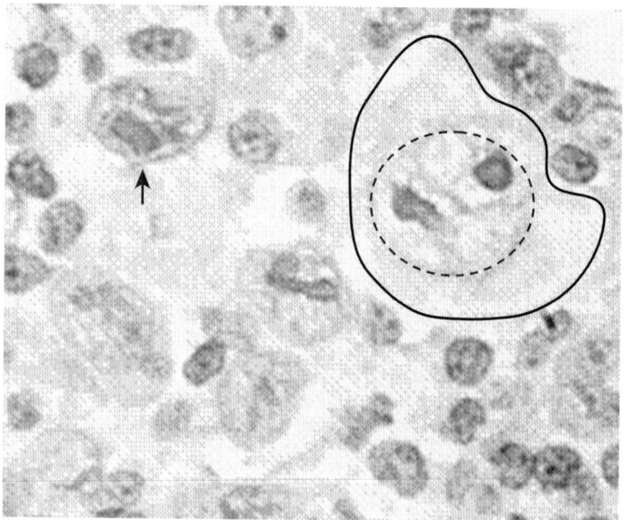

Figure 71-2. This photograph depicts a Reed-Sternberg cell, which is pathognomonic for Hodgkin's disease. On the right side of the slide, the large nucleolus is outlined by the *dotted circle* and the entire cell is outlined by the *solid line*. Note the relatively pale nuclear chromatin. The nucleolus has the appearance of an "owl's eye" from which it receives its name. The *arrow* points to a mononuclear variant of the Reed-Sternberg cell, which has reticulated nuclear chromatin surrounding an almost rectangular macronucleus.

(Fig. 71-2). It has a multilobed nucleus (or is multinucleated), each with a prominent eosinophilic nucleolus surrounded by a clear zone (halo) and an intensely stained nuclear membrane. The "owl's eye" appearance is the result of a bilobed nucleus. The RS cell often makes up no more than 2% of the involved cells. Hodgkin's cells are the mononuclear variant of RS cells. The cellular background is a reactive, pleomorphic mixture of inflammatory cells including reactive lymphocytes, histiocytes, plasma cells, eosinophils, neutrophils, and fibroblasts, with varying degrees of fibrosis and sclerosis. The HRS cell is a clonal, neoplastic cell seen in classic HL and is thought to induce the reactive background through the abundant release of various cytokines.[34] The origin of HRS cells remained elusive until recently because of its paucity in sampled tissue. However, research now indicates that they are usually derived from germinal center B lymphocytes that are clonal and have lost their immunoglobulin gene transcription ability.[35,36] Post–germinal center B-cell origin has been described, as well as a rare case of HL derived from peripheral T cells.[37-41] In classic HL, HRS cells have a unique molecular defect with clonal immunoglobulin gene rearrangement and no immunoglobulin gene transcription or expression. HRS cells typically are CD15 and CD30 positive and negative for CD45 and B-lineage antigens.[42] In contrast, the nodular LP HL cells (popcorn cells) are usually positive for B-lineage antigens, CD15 and CD30 expressions are lacking, and the immunoglobulin genes are expressed.[42]

For histologic typing, the Rye classification was commonly used for 3 decades but has been supplanted by the WHO classification. The 2001 WHO classification lists two main types of HL: classic HL and nodular LP. Classic HL is further divided into four subtypes by morphology. These subtypes include nodular sclerosis (NS, the most common), mixed cellularity (MC), lymphocyte predominant (LPHL), and lymphocyte depleted (LDHL).[3] The NS subtype is seen in 40% of younger patients and 70% of adolescents.[43] It is characterized by tumor nodules surrounded by broad sclerotic bands arising from a thickened fibrotic capsule.[33] This subtype has a strong predilection for involvement of the lower cervical, supraclavicular, and mediastinal lymph nodes. The MC subtype is found in 30% of cases and has an increased incidence in younger children.[14] HRS cells are typically increased in number. The lymph node architecture is often completely effaced by the HRS cells and their surrounding reactive cells. This subtype often is first seen with advanced, widely disseminated disease in extranodal sites. In addition to its relatively common incidence among all HL patients, it is the most common histologic type seen in HIV-infected patients.[21]

From 1978 to 1986, the National Cancer Institute (NCI)-sponsored SEER data revealed the following patient 5-year survival rates using the formerly used Rye classification histologic subtype: LP, 83.9%; NS, 82.2%; MC, 68.1%; and LD, 36.4%.[44] Reports have now shown that LPHL has a better prognosis with markedly reduced therapy needed to achieve cure.[45,46] This differentiation of therapeutic response between LPHL and the other classic HL histologic types appears to validate the distinction observed in the immunophenotyped RS cells.[47] Clinical trials are now underway to explore this difference further and to examine whether reduced therapy for nodular LPHL is possible. The worse outcome of the MC and LDHL types may reflect their typically higher stage at diagnosis.

Clinical Presentation

Children are first seen with painless enlarged lymph nodes, typically in the cervical or supraclavicular nodal groups (Table 71-1). Nodes are often described as rubbery and fixed. They may be either single or matted with other nodes. Occasionally, because of rapid growth, tenderness may be present. Tumor lysis syndrome, a result of rapid and extensive tumor growth and a common complication in children with NHL, is rarely seen in children with HL.

HL tends to spread in a contiguous manner. Therefore, at presentation, one must examine carefully the nodal groups adjacent to the initially identified nodes. More than 90% of patients have involvement of either the cervical or mediastinal nodal groups, or both.[48] Interestingly, HL tends to spread from the cervical nodes of one side of the neck to the mediastinum before it spreads to the contralateral cervical nodes. When surgical laparotomy was included in the staging process (which is no longer routinely recommended), the spleen was noted to be involved in 27% of patients.[48] When evaluating the histologic subtypes and patterns of initial involvement, it is clear from Table 71-1 that the MC and LD subtypes of HL have

Table 71-1 Hodgkin's Disease: Sites of Involvement at the Time of Initial Diagnosis

	Histologic Subtype (%)			
Nodal Sites	*NS*	*MC/LD*	*LP*	*All*
Mediastinum	73	46	8	59
Cervical	55-62	53-60	41-46	55-58
Axillary	11-15	14-16	13-14	13-14
Hilar	14-15	8-9	3-5	11-12
Upper neck	4	4	14	5
Epitrochlear	1	1	6	2
Spleen	24	35	17	27
Upper abdomen	13	18	5	14
Lower abdomen	8	17	8	11
Inguinal	1	3	10	2-3

NS, nodular sclerosis; MC/LD, mixed cellularity/lymphocyte depleted; LP, lymphocyte predominant.

Adapted from Mauch PM, Kalish LA, Kadin M, et al: Patterns of Hodgkin disease: Implications for etiology and pathogenesis. Cancer 71:2062-2071, 1993.

more widespread involvement than do the NS or LP HL subtypes.

Mediastinal disease, in addition to a predilection for certain histologic subtypes, is most common in children older than 12 years, in girls, and in those with constitutional symptoms (also known as B symptoms).[49] Mediastinal disease may appear with significant respiratory compromise due to compression of the trachea, carina, or both, including the major bronchi.[50] These patients may have dyspnea on exertion or at rest, persistent cough, or stridor. They may have recently been treated for presumed asthma or bronchiolitis, without radiographic imaging. Patients with this presentation may have a history of orthopnea and are most comfortable in an upright forward-leaning position to relieve the pressure on the airway (from the anterior mediastinal mass). The physician must be vigilant for mediastinal disease because it may be silent until a patient is sedated for a radiologic or surgical procedure. These patients may prove impossible to aerate even with intubation because of distal tracheal or bronchial obstruction. It is imperative that all patients with suspected lymphoma (HL or NHL) have a chest radiograph or chest CT scan before any sedation or procedure. These patients may also have signs of superior vena caval obstruction, including edema and cyanosis of the face and venous distention. Extralymphatic involvement can include the liver (the most common extralymphatic organ involved), lungs, bone, bone marrow, and skin, among other sites. Whereas bone marrow involvement is present in only 4% to 14% of patients overall, among those patients with stage IV disease it is present 32% of the time.[51]

Most patients have no systemic symptoms at the time of initial diagnosis. About one fourth of patients will have one or more B symptoms, defined as weight loss of more than 10% in the previous 6 months, unexplained recurrent fevers greater than 38°C, or drenching night sweats.[48] Pruritus, fatigue, and anorexia are other nonspecific symptoms seen in HL patients. Laboratory findings in patients at diagnosis are nonspecific and typically are indicative of an inflammatory process. The erythrocyte sedimentation rate (ESR), serum copper, and ferritin levels are frequently elevated and may be monitored later for evidence of relapse. A high ferritin (>142 ng/mL) level or increased ESR (>50) has been associated with a worse prognosis.[52,53] The lactate dehydrogenase (LDH) value may be elevated as well. Although not common, leukopenia may be indicative of bone marrow involvement.[51]

Diagnosis

The diagnostic evaluation should include physical examination and laboratory and radiologic studies (Table 71-2). The physical examination should be directed to the obviously involved nodal groups and also to the adjacent groups, keeping in mind the natural history of HL and its propensity for contiguous spread. The number of involved nodal groups in stage II patients (more than four) has been associated with a worse prognosis and should be carefully determined.[54] The size of the palpable nodal masses should be estimated and recorded. Bulky disease (nodes or nodal aggregates > 10 cm and/or mediastinal tumor width more than one third of intrathoracic width on a posteroanterior chest radiograph or CT) is associated with a worse outcome in low-stage patients and necessitates additional therapy to achieve equivalent outcomes.[55-57] Auscultation of the airway, palpation of the abdomen, and examination of distant nodal groups are critical as well.

Laboratory examination should include full blood cell counts and chemistries, including hepatic function tests, LDH, and ESR. Serum copper and ferritin levels also should be obtained. However, no clinical findings

Table 71-2 Hodgkin's Disease: Diagnostic and Staging Evaluation at Presentation

- Complete physical examination with documentation of involved nodal groups (including measurements of nodes), and involved extralymphatic organs
- Complete blood cell count, chemistry panel including hepatic function tests, erythrocyte sedimentation rate, copper, ferritin, lactate dehydrogenase
- Chest radiography to evaluate for possible mediastinal disease and airway compression
- CT scans of areas identified on physical examination (also include chest, neck, and abdomen)
- Positron emission tomography
- Gallium scan
- Bone scan
- Excisional biopsy of node
- Bone marrow biopsies and aspirates (bilateral)
- Lymphangiogram (optional)
- Staging laparotomy/laparoscopy (mandatory if considering radiation therapy alone) with splenectomy, nodal sampling, and wedge biopsies of hepatic lobes

are pathognomonic for HL. Ultimately, the diagnosis awaits the biopsy of involved sites, most commonly an excised lymph node. The surgeon's goal is to biopsy the most accessible nodal region to obtain adequate tissue for diagnosis. Open excision of the largest lymph node is preferred because fine-needle aspirations generally do not provide adequate tissue. Excisional biopsy is where the diagnosis is made, based on the pathognomonic finding of HRS cells within a reactive cellular background. For cytogenetic and molecular genetic evaluations, it is imperative that all tissues are placed in a sterile container for fresh samples. Formalin should never be used. For patients critically ill at diagnosis, such as those with severe airway obstruction, diagnosis by alternative methods needs to be considered. These may include nodal biopsy with local anesthesia alone, CT-guided percutaneous needle biopsy of the mass, aspiration of a pleural effusion, or a bone marrow biopsy and aspirate.

Staging

Further evaluation of a patient with HL is required to determine the extent of disease at diagnosis and thus the stage of disease (Table 71-3). The common staging system for HL was adopted in 1971.[58] This system is based on the observation of contiguous nodal spread in HL. Patients are further divided into asymptomatic (A) and symptomatic (B) subcategories. This subclassification for symptomatic patients is based on the findings of a worse prognosis for B patients and the need for a systemic therapy approach in them (i.e., chemotherapy in addition to radiation). This likely reflects the finding that patients with B symptoms are more likely to have distant, widespread disease when pathologically staged.[59]

For HL, the decision for the method and the extent or intensity of therapy rests on the staging results. Traditionally, two types of staging were used in HL patients: clinical and pathologic. Until recently, all patients underwent both methods. Clinical staging includes physical, laboratory, and radiologic evaluations. Pathologic staging requires a staging laparotomy with splenectomy, nodal sampling, and wedge biopsies of both hepatic lobes. The radiologic evaluations have been in evolution over the past decade. Lymphangiograms, once a critical component of staging in HL, have been supplanted by more modern and less invasive imaging modalities. CT examination is used most frequently.[60] For those who will be treated by irradiation alone, accurate assessment of abdominal disease is critical. Staging laparotomy with splenectomy, nodal sampling, and wedge biopsies of both hepatic lobes has been shown to increase the stage of disease in up to 35% of patients initially evaluated with CT[61,62] (i.e., the difference between clinical and pathologic staging). This would seem to indicate that abdominal exporation is important. However, again, with the use of systemic chemotherapy and the deemphasis on irradiation, this discrepancy between clinical and pathologic staging no longer appears to have a significant impact on treatment or outcome.[63,64]

For the majority of children with HL, staging is based on clinical criteria and laparotomy (or laparoscopy) is not encouraged or recommended. Abdominal staging should continue to be used in patients destined to be treated with irradiation alone (although this is now rare in children) because abdominal disease would have a significant impact on planned therapy.[65] Staging laparotomy (or laparoscopy) with splenectomy is not without its risks. These are the typical postoperative complications of abdominal surgery. Moreover, with splenectomy, there is a lifelong risk of overwhelming sepsis with encapsulated organisms and these patients require lifelong antibiotic prophylaxis.[66] An increased risk of secondary leukemia also exists in those HL patients treated with chemotherapy who have undergone splenectomy (5.9%) compared with those who have not (0.7%) as part of their staging procedure.[67-69]

Nuclear medicine scans are another modality that are increasing in HL patients. Although early studies of gallium scanning found its value suspect,[70,71] it has its greatest impact in identifying unrecognized sites of disease at presentation and in follow-up. This is especially true for patients with mediastinal disease. Patients with NS subtypes will often have persistently enlarged cervical and mediastinal nodes due to scar tissue. Although these are enlarged on CT, negative

Table 71-3 Ann Arbor Staging Classification for Hodgkin's Disease

Stage	Definition
I	Involvement of a single lymph node region (I) or of a single extralymphatic organ or site (I_E)
II	Involvement of two or more lymph node regions on the same side of the diaphragm (II) or localized involvement of an extralymphatic organ or site and its regional lymph node(s) with involvement of one or more lymph node regions on the same side of the diaphragm (II_E)
III	Involvement of lymph node regions on both sides of the diaphragm (III), which may be accompanied by involvement of the spleen (III_S) or by localized involvement of an extralymphatic organ or site (III_E) or both (III_{SE})
IV	Disseminated (multifocal) involvement of one or more extralymphatic organs or tissues with or without associated lymph node involvement or isolated extralymphatic organ involvement with distant (nonregional) nodal involvement

Adapted from Carbone PP, Kaplan HS, Husshoff K, et al. Report of the committee on Hodgkin's disease staging classification. Cancer Res 31: 1860-1861, 1971.

gallium scans (in patients in whom these sites were gallium avid at presentation) indicate a non-neoplastic cause (i.e., residual scar tissue).[72,73] It has been suggested that this is most accurately predictive in initially low-stage patients (I or II) and less so in patients with advanced disease (III or IV).[74]

In children, it is important also to recognize the phenomena of thymic rebound after therapy. This may result in both an enlarging mediastinal mass on CT and a positive gallium scan. An experienced radiologist will recognize this phenomenon by its timing (within the first 6 months after therapy has been completed) and by the normal (although enlarged) homogeneous appearance of the thymic tissue. However, false-negative interpretations can occur. Thus, close follow-up of these patients is critical. In the past, shortages of gallium have made this examination more problematic. However, fluorodeoxyglucose-labeled positron emission tomography (FDG-PET) has been found to be more sensitive and specific than either gallium or CT.[75-78] Similar to gallium scanning, it leads to a higher staging in a significant percentage of patients. FDG-PET during and after therapy has been highly predictive of patient outcome[79,80] and helps to differentiate residual scar tissue from residual lymphoma,[81] although false-positive findings with inflammatory conditions have been reported.[80] More experience with this new modality is required before it can be used alone. Finally, the bone marrow examination continues to be important, regardless of planned methods of therapy, because its involvement would upgrade the patient's disease to stage IV status and necessitate more intensive chemotherapy.

Treatment

Principles of Therapy

Several strategies have been effective in the treatment of HL. These have included radiation therapy alone, combinations of irradiation and chemotherapy, and, most recently, chemotherapy without radiation. For children in particular, four principles guide modern HL therapy. For those with early or low-stage HL (I to III), reduction of therapy duration and intensity to reduce long-term sequelae (while maintaining the current high cure rates) is a central principle in today's regimen designs. In concert with this, the reduction and eventual elimination of irradiation as a method of therapy in children with early or low-stage HL is important. The third and most recent principle is response-based therapy. This reduces therapy for those who do not require additional doses by adjusting or eliminating anticipated cycles of chemotherapy based on the tumor's response to the initial courses of therapy. Fourth, for those with advanced-stage HL (stage IV), intensification of therapy and identification of new and more effective regimens to increase relapse-free survival are needed.

Finally, advances in pediatric oncology have been substantial, primarily owing to patients being managed on protocols through the cooperative groups (COG and SIOP). Children, including adolescents, diagnosed with HL should be referred to, and their treatment coordinated through, one of the many centers associated with these groups. These children, through participation in the clinical trials, receive the most advanced and effective therapy available today (Table 71-4).

Principles of Radiation Therapy in the Treatment of Hodgkin's Lymphoma

Despite the goal of eliminating radiation from the therapeutic regimens for children with early-stage HL, it must be recognized that HL is a very radiosensitive neoplasm. A long record of efficacy exists in using radiation either alone or in combination with chemotherapy regimens for this neoplasm. Radiation therapy has traditionally been given to the sites of disease and contiguous, clinically uninvolved, areas. This is known as extended-field irradiation. Various fields of therapy have evolved and include the preauricular (Waldeyer's ring) field, the supradiaphragmatic mantle field (submandibular, submental, cervical, supraclavicular, infraclavicular, axillary, mediastinal, and pulmonary hilar nodal groups), the subdiaphragmatic field (splenic pedicle, spleen, para-aortic nodal groups), and two pelvic fields, inverted-"Y" (common iliac, external iliac, inguinal-femoral nodal groups) or spade (inverted-"Y" excluding those nodes below the common iliac group).

More recently, involved-field irradiation has become more widely used. This is a more attractive option when combined with chemotherapy. In children, involved-field irradiation has been shown to provide excellent local control (97%).[82] A study from Germany identified that not only were the remission rate and disease-free survival no different between involved-field and extended-field irradiation but the side effects (leukopenia, thrombocytopenia, nausea, gastrointestinal toxicity, and pharyngeal toxicity) were significantly reduced when using only involved-field irradiation.[83]

The use of radiation therapy alone remains an option for therapy in adults with low-stage (I to III) HL because it allows them the opportunity to avoid the toxicity associated with chemotherapy.[84-87] Even if relapse occurs in those treated with radiation only, the ability to salvage a long-term cure does not appear to be compromised by delaying the use of chemotherapy until the first relapse.

However, the severe and lifelong side effects of irradiation (cosmetic defects, growth retardation, endocrinologic sequelae, and secondary malignancy) on a growing and developing child are a compelling reason to look for alternative methods. Appreciation for these long-term effects has led to a gradual reduction in the dose and in the size of the field treated. More recently, the focus has been to eliminate irradiation completely in the treatment of children with HL. An adult study suggested that this may be possible for those individuals who achieve a complete

Table 71-4 Therapeutic Regimens for Children with Hodgkin's Disease

Chemotherapy Agents	Stage	Radiation	Radiation Dose	DFS (%)	OS (%)	Reference
None	PSI-IIB	EF	≥3500 cGy	67-82	86-96	84, 85, 86
		IF		41	95	
	CSI-IIB	IF		79-85	96-98	
MOPP	I-II	IF	<2500 cGy	96	100	76, 108
	III-IV			84	78	
	IV	EF	33-4400 cGy	69	78	
COP/ABVD	II	IF	<2000 cGy	96	96	112
	III			97	100	
	IV			85	86	
MOPP/ABVD	I-II	IF	2-4000 cGy	89		105
	III			82		
	IV			62		
MOPP/ABVD	I-III	IF	1500-2500 cGy	100	100	106
	IV			69	85	
MOPP/ABVD	IIB-IV	TNI	2100 cGy	77	91	110
MOPP/ABV	II-IV	IF	3500 cGy	93	90	111
COPP/ABV	I-IV	IF	<2500 cGy	100	100	113
OPPA	I-IIA	IF	3500 cGy	98	100	114
ABVD	III-IV	IF	21-3500 cGy	87	89	109
BEACOPP	II-IV	IF	3-4000 cGy*	87	91	100
Stanford V	I-II	IF	3600 cGy*	97		102
	III-IV			85		

*Radiation given to sites of bulky disease present at diagnosis.

MOPP, Nitrogen mustard, vincristine, prednisone, procarbazine; ABVD, doxorubicin (Adriamycin), bleomycin, vinblastine, DTIC; OPPA, vincristine, prednisone, procarbazine, doxorubicin (Adriamycin) – C, cyclophosphamide; BEACOPP, bleomycin, etoposide, doxorubicin (Adriamycin), cyclophosphamide, vincristine, procarbazine, prednisone; Stanford V, vinblastine, doxorubicin (Adriamycin)–vincristine, bleomycin, nitrogen mustard, etoposide, prednisone; EF, extended-field irradiation; IF, involved-field irradiation; TNI, total nodal irradiation; cGy, centigray (1 cGy = 1 rad); CR, complete remission; DFS, disease-free survival; OS, overall survival.

response (CR) with four cycles of chemotherapy.[88] The CCG 5942 clinical trial compared no radiation therapy to low-dose (LD) involved-field irradiation in an attempt to eliminate radiation therapy in those patients who achieved a CR after four courses of chemotherapy. Patients who received LD involved-field irradiation had an improved event-free survival (EFS), but overall survival (OS) was not different between the two groups. Currently, combined-modality therapy remains the standard of care for children and adolescents with HL.[89] Trials of patients with stage IA and IIA classic HL and nonbulky disease (low-risk HL) are underway to evaluate whether radiation can be eliminated after three cycles of a more intensively timed chemotherapy regimen.

The small subgroup of children in whom irradiation alone may still be considered for front-line therapy are the fully grown adolescent boys with localized disease (I to IIA). Circumvention of chemotherapy in this particular group avoids the impaired fertility that is a particular concern in boys and is related to the alkylating agents. Also, the adolescent's growth is complete. Therefore, irradiation will not result in permanent cosmetic deformities (i.e., arrest of bone growth). On the other hand, even for this group of boys, new regimens that no longer contain alkylating agents have shown excellent efficacy when used in combination with LD radiation therapy.[90] Because of worries about secondary breast cancer, radiation therapy alone for adolescent girls should be given only after strong consideration for the increased risk of breast cancer known to result from irradiation of the breast tissue at this critical age.[91-95]

Principles of Chemotherapy

Chemotherapy is the therapeutic backbone for children with both early and advanced-stage HL. A large number of chemotherapy combinations have been used for HL. For years, two regimens have been the most widely and effectively used combinations for patients with early-stage HL. MOPP or ABVD is administered over a 12-month period and has resulted in excellent outcomes.[96,97] However, these combinations have proven significant long-term sequelae when administered in full doses for a year. The recognition that successful treatment with chemotherapy for children with HL would have significant impact on their quality of life and ultimate survival has led to newer combinations of chemotherapy. In general, these regimens have been variations of MOPP and ABVD. These hybrids have either replaced those agents having the worst sequelae (e.g., cyclophosphamide for nitrogen mustard) or have involved the originals being given at significantly lower doses, or both.

Newer regimens in low-stage patients are now being examined with lower-dose alkylating agents, which are the causes of the majority of the long-term sequelae seen in these patients.[90] In addition, the number of cycles or overall duration has been significantly decreased as well.[57,98] Typically, a complete therapeutic protocol currently is given over 3 to 6 months. Radiation therapy sometimes remains a part of these regimens, although it is given at lower doses and encompasses smaller fields. In some studies, the chemotherapy regimens that have been given without irradiation have produced equivalent results to regimens with irradiation in patients with low-stage disease.[99-101] A trial to confirm these early results showed no difference in OS between low-risk patients who received radiation and those who did not.[89] But those patients who were given LD involved-field radiation therapy had a superior EFS. For those with high-risk HL, therapeutic regimens that are intensifying both dose and timing are showing improved outcomes over the traditional regimens, with disease-free survival (DFS) now in excess of 80%.[102-104]

Stage, Histology, and Response-Based Therapy

Until recently, therapy for HL was primarily dictated by the stage at which the child was first seen. Now histology and response to therapy are added to the equation.[45,105] Those with LPHL and low-stage disease may be considered for further reductions in chemotherapy. If the disease is completely resected via an excisional biopsy, no further treatment may be needed. A current clinical trial is attempting to confirm the results of smaller studies showing favorable outcomes with surgical resection alone in stage I patients with LPHL, a single involved lymph node, and a complete resection. Early response to therapy has been shown to identify those with superior cure rates (94% vs. 78% EFS).[105] Many regimens now incorporate this concept into their design, with fewer cycles of chemotherapy or elimination of irradiation for those with early complete responses.

Symptomatic disease at the time of diagnosis calls for therapy similar to that for higher-stage patients. Current recommendations are for patients with stage I to III disease to receive three to eight cycles of chemotherapy, with the number of cycles dependent on the presence of bulky disease (mediastinal or nodal), number of involved nodal sites (in stage II), and achievement of remission after two to four cycles. Those with adverse risk factors receive six to eight cycles of therapy. The decision to use irradiation after chemotherapy remains under study. When irradiation is used, it should be given in low doses (<2500 cGy) and to involved areas only. Male patients with bulky mediastinal disease should receive radiation in addition to systemic chemotherapy, regardless of response to therapy. Attempts are being made to eliminate irradiation in female patients with bulky disease and a rapid response to therapy. Stage IV patients should receive more intensive regimens of systemic chemotherapy and involved-field radiation.

Currently, blood or marrow stem cell transplantation is reserved for those patients whose disease is refractory to systemic chemotherapy or who have experienced relapse. Recent trials have shown that regardless of the duration of initial remission, those who are treated with high-dose chemotherapy and stem cell rescue have less treatment failure than do those treated with conventional chemotherapy.[106]

Results

Most patients treated with combinations of chemotherapy and radiation enter into CR (>90%).[107,108] Many patients, especially those with the NS subtype, may have persistent adenopathy or mediastinal enlargement for months or years after therapy. Although most prove to be cured, close monitoring of these patients is necessary. For those who do not enter remission with today's front-line chemotherapy/irradiation combinations, the prognosis is poor. Therapeutic intensification with subsequent stem cell transplant should be strongly considered.[106,109]

For stage I and II patients, combined-modality (chemotherapy and radiation) therapy typically results in greater than 90% 5-year DFS rates; for stage III patients, greater than 80% 5-year DFS rates; and for stage IV patients, the outcome was until recently greater than 60% (see Table 71-4). This last group has seen significant advances, with successful outcomes now exceeding 80% in several recent trials.[102,103]

Acute Complications

Acute complications of therapy in children with HL are due to either the tumor itself or the therapy. Because of airway compression, anterior mediastinal lymphomas can be a medical emergency. All patients suspected of having a lymphoma should have an immediate chest radiograph or CT scan to determine whether a mediastinal mass is present. Therapy with chemotherapy (preferable in children) or irradiation is effective in the immediate relief of these symptoms. The complications due to splenectomy are due to overwhelming sepsis from encapsulated organisms. This risk is increased because of the myelosuppression and immunocompromising effects of chemotherapy. Fever in the neutropenic patient necessitates hospitalization and intravenous antibiotic therapy. Bone marrow suppression may require transfusions of either red cells or platelets. Specific chemotherapy agents may have immediate complications. These include nausea and vomiting, restrictive pulmonary disease (bleomycin, irradiation), extravasation burns (nitrogen mustard, vincristine, vinblastine, doxorubicin [Adriamycin]), and chemical phlebitis (nitrogen mustard, vinblastine, DTIC). To alleviate these last risks, right atrial catheters are often placed. This also reduces the discomfort of repeated venipuncture required throughout the duration of treatment.

Long-Term Sequelae

The concern over long-term sequelae guides much of modern therapy for HL, both in adults and particularly in children. These sequelae result from both radiation therapy and chemotherapy.[110,111]

The long-term sequelae of irradiation in growing children are the overriding reason for the efforts to reduce or eliminate it from therapeutic regimens. Bone irradiation may result in shortening of the clavicles in those receiving mantle radiation or a shortened height in those receiving radiation to the spine.[112] Radiation to the neck often results in permanent hypothyroidism[113] and increases the risk of thyroid cancer.[114,115] If radiation is to be given to the pelvis of a female patient, consideration should be given to surgically moving the ovaries away from the field of irradiation.[116]

Second malignancies are a major concern after therapy for HL.[117-119] The most frequent cause of death in long-term survivors of HL is a second malignancy.[120] The relative risk of a second malignancy in HL patients has been estimated to be 5- to 11-fold that of the general population.[118,121] This represents a 15- to 25-year actuarial risk of 7% to 23%.[118,121-123] Second malignancies are more prevalent in those with HL treated before age 21 years than in the older age groups for all tumors except lung cancer.[118] These second cancers include leukemia and solid tumors. The risk of leukemia seems primarily related to the type of chemotherapy used,[121,124] with a cumulative incidence of 3.3%, with a plateau after about 10 years. However, one recent study found a decrease in secondary leukemia among those treated with the newer hybrid regimens.[123] This likely is a result of the reduction in nitrogen mustard and procarbazine (in MOPP) doses, the principal culprits in the development of secondary leukemia.[125,126] Patients treated with ABVD do not have an increased risk of leukemia. The reduction in the incidence of leukemia may be a result of the decreasing use of splenectomy in pathologic staging, because this operation has repeatedly been shown to increase the risk of leukemia in HL patients treated with chemotherapy.[125,127]

Solid tumors, including those of lung, stomach, melanoma, bone, and soft tissue, have accounted for most of the second malignancies, with a cumulative incidence of 13% to 22% at 15 to 25 years. No plateau has been appreciated.[118,121,122] This risk in HL survivors has not decreased when cohorts treated in the 1960s are compared with those in the 1980s.[118] This increased risk of solid tumors is related primarily to irradiation,[128,129] with some added risk when subsequent chemotherapy is used in relapse patients.[130] It has been recognized that radiation exposure to the breast tissue in adult women has resulted in a fourfold increase in rates of subsequent breast cancer,[91-93,131] whereas the risk of subsequent breast cancer is increased by 39-fold if the breasts are irradiated during adolescence.[94] For an adolescent, this increases the probability of developing breast cancer between the ages of 20 and 30 years from 0.04% to 1.6%[95] and may be as high as 35% by age 40 years.[118] For all types of secondary cancer, adolescents seem to be at greater risk than younger children.[115,132] Recent evidence suggests that the risk of breast cancer is slightly reduced by the premature menopause induced by the chemotherapy these patients receive.[133,134] Most patients who received chemotherapy and radiation therapy had menopause before age 41 years, whereas only 9% treated with radiation alone had premature menopause. Menopause before age 36 years had a significant impact on the reduced risk of breast cancer among those receiving radiation. Patients must be closely observed for second malignancies for decades after their therapy has been completed. No plateau in risk has yet been seen.[111,135]

Other long-term sequelae include cardiac complications secondary to mantle irradiation or the use of doxorubicin (Adriamycin in ABVD regimens), or both, that affect up to 13% of patients.[136,137] These complications are typically congestive heart failure due to myocardiopathy and secondary arrhythmias. Occasionally, restrictive pericarditis may occur as a result of radiation. Overall, the relative risk of death due to cardiovascular disease in HL survivors is elevated and especially so in those treated before age 21 years.[111] Pulmonary toxicity due to bleomycin or irradiation, (or both) affected up to 9% of children who received 12 courses of ABVD with 2100-cGy radiation.[138] This high incidence appears to be decreasing with the use of hybrid regimens and low-dose involved-field irradiation.[139]

Infertility and early menopause in women are primarily a result of ovarian dysfunction as a result of exposure of the ovaries to radiation.[140,141] When the ovaries are surgically moved out of the field of irradiation, these problems are less likely to occur.[116,142] Male patients have a 30% to 40% rate of gonadal dysfunction at the time of diagnosis before any therapy.[143] After more than three to six courses of MOPP therapy, all men are usually sterile.[144] This side effect does not follow ABVD therapy.[145] Spermatogenesis is only transiently reduced by pelvic radiation. Although spermatogenesis is significantly affected by the alkylating agents in MOPP therapy, testosterone production seems unimpaired. It is anticipated that with reduction in single and cumulative doses of chemotherapy, with older agents being replaced with less toxic ones, and with the reduction in radiation field size and dose, these long-term sequelae will be further reduced.

NON-HODGKIN'S LYMPHOMA

In contrast to the similarities between adult and pediatric HL, the types of NHL that occur in adults and children, their presentation, their treatment, and their outcome are dramatically different. Most adults with NHL have low- or intermediate-grade lymphomas. In distinct contrast, children with these types of lymphomas are exceedingly rare. Instead, virtually all children with NHL have one of four high-grade, diffuse types: Burkitt's lymphoma (formerly small, non-cleaved cell lymphoma [SNCCL]), precursor T-cell lymphoblastic lymphoma (T-LL), diffuse large B-cell lymphoma (DLBCL), or anaplastic large cell lymphoma (ALCL). Most patients will be seen initially with advanced or disseminated disease (stages III and IV).

These lymphomas typically appear as a rapidly expanding mass with a short symptomatic history. This propensity for rapid growth makes the diagnostic evaluation in a child with suspected NHL a medical urgency, if not emergency. Of all the childhood tumors, NHL has the greatest chance of acute complications at the time of presentation. Anatomic impingement of adjacent structures (mediastinal tumors on the trachea and bronchi, nasopharyngeal tumors on the orbits, bowel obstruction with or without intussusception) and metabolic derangements due to tumor lysis (before and after therapy is initiated) are not infrequent results of its very rapid growth. Better management of the initial anatomic and metabolic complications, improved methods of determining the subtypes of NHL (perhaps the most important reason for improved survival), and better chemotherapy combinations (more intensive, yet shorter) have brought the most dramatic improvements in DFS and OS for children with NHL over the past several decades.[146] Five-year relative survival was 86% for patients diagnosed with NHL from 1996 to 2002.[12] In addition to more intense therapy of shorter duration, the other major change in therapy for children with NHL is the virtual elimination of radiation from treatment regimens. This should reduce the long-term sequelae that would have otherwise resulted. For the surgeon seeing the child with suspected lymphoma, rapid evaluation and proper handling of biopsy material will have dramatic beneficial effects on the outcome for the child.

Incidence and Epidemiology

NHL accounts for 4% of all cancers in adult and pediatric patients, with nearly 53,600 new cases diagnosed annually in the United States.[1] In children, NHL patients accounted for 4.5% of childhood cancers,[12] 8.7% of all solid tumors, and 57% of all lymphomas.[2] The annual incidence is 9.9 cases/million children younger than 15 years/year.[15] Before age 11 years, it is the most common of the two types of lymphoma. A high male-to-female ratio of 3.0 is found, making it the most disproportionately occurring tumor between the two genders during childhood. This large difference is present in all ages of childhood. A 1.4 greater risk occurs in whites than in blacks.[15] This, too, is seen in all ages, with the exception of children younger than 1 year. The age distribution demonstrates two small peaks in incidence from 6 to 7 years and between 12 and 14 years (see Fig. 71-1). The 6- and 7-year olds overwhelmingly have Burkitt's lymphoma, and the teenagers typically have T-LL.

NHL of B-cell origin, either Burkitt's lymphoma or DLBCL, occurs more often in patients with prior EBV exposure, in individuals with a history of immune suppression, and in equatorial Africa.[147-149] Considerable work now convincingly reveals that, in patients with an iatrogenic (e.g., post-transplant, immunosuppressive therapy) or acquired immunodeficiency, congenital-EBV infection has an etiologic role in either the development or the predisposition to B-cell NHL.[150,151] Correlations have been made between viral load levels and the risk of post-transplant lymphoproliferative disorders (PTLDs).[152-154] Patients at greatest risk for PTLDs are those in whom their primary infection with EBV occurs within the first 3 to 4 months after transplantation. For T-LL or ALCL, no such etiologic correlations have been found.

Classification

Over the years, several classification schemes have been used.[155] Among these are the Rappaport, the Kiel, the Lukes-Collins, the WHO, the International Working Formulation, and the Revised European-American Classification of Lymphoid Neoplasms (REAL).[156] REAL was developed as an effort to eliminate the confusion surrounding the diagnosis of the lymphoma subtype caused by the prior variety of classification schemas. The REAL is a consensus classification system based on morphologic, immunologic, and cytogenetic characteristics, in addition to clinical presentation, course, and putative cell of origin.[156]

REAL is the basis for the WHO classification in current use, a comprehensive classification system published in 2001. Childhood NHL primarily consists of just four subtypes in the WHO system: (1) Burkitt's lymphoma/leukemia and Burkitt-like (mature B-cell neoplasms accounting for 39% of NHL patients[4]); (2) T-cell lymphoblastic lymphoma (28%[4]), (3) diffuse large B-cell lymphoma, and (4) mature T-cell neoplasms (ALCL). DLBCL and ALCL were previously lumped together as large cell lymphomas and comprised about one third of the NHL of childhood. With the separation of these two entities, the cases previously identified as large cell lymphoma are now divided almost equally between DLBCL and ALCL.[157] The first two classifications are part of the "small, round, blue cell tumors," which presents the pathologist with the challenge of proper identification. To differentiate these from the other three classic small round blue cell tumors (neuroblastoma, rhabdomyosarcoma, and Ewing's sarcoma) requires the presence of the immunocytochemical marker leukocyte common antigen CD45 (LCA), which is absent on the other tumor cell types.

Burkitt's lymphoma has classically been divided into Burkitt's and non-Burkitt's (Burkitt-like in the REAL classification) subtypes. These are of a mature B-cell origin, with flow cytometric immunophenotyping revealing the presence of surface immunoglobulin IgM, CD10, CD19, CD20, CD22, CD79a, and human leukocyte antigen (HLA)-DR antigens. The histologic appearance of these two types differs in the degree of pleomorphism, with Burkitt's being more uniform appearing than non-Burkitt's. Although a distinction has been made for years between Burkitt's and non-Burkitt's subtypes of diffuse SNCCL lymphomas, no clinical differences are found between these two subtypes.[158] Histologically, the cells of Burkitt's lymphoma are medium sized with round nuclei containing two to five nucleoli, abundant basophilic cytoplasm, and cytoplasmic lipid vacuoles. Owing to its extreme rates of proliferation and spontaneous cell death, a number of macrophages are seen within this monomorphic field, consuming the dying cells and giving rise to the classic "starry sky" appearance of Burkitt's lymphoma.[156]

Lymphoblastic lymphomas (LL) are distinguished by round or convoluted nuclei, finely dispersed chromatin, inconspicuous nucleoli, and scant cytoplasm. In the vast majority of these tumors, flow cytometry reveals the presence of the T-cell markers CD3 and CD7, with variable positivity for CD2 and CD5. These cells are typically Tdt positive, whereas Burkitt's lymphomas are Tdt negative. This subtype is classified as a precursor T-cell LL in the WHO classification. A small number of LL cases are B-cell precursor and express pre–B-cell antigen profiles.[157]

Large cell lymphomas are a heterogeneous group of neoplasms. Histologically, approximately half are immunoblastic, 40% are large noncleaved cell, and fewer than 5% are large cleaved cell.[159] Flow cytometry shows relatively equal frequencies of B- or T-cell origin (36% and 33%, respectively) with 30% indeterminate.[160,161] A unique subset, identified by the immunophenotype CD30$^+$ (the antigen identified by the Ki-1 monoclonal antibody),[162] is recognized morphologically by its anaplastic characteristics, including very large cells with abundant cytoplasm, atypical lobulated nuclei, and prominent nucleoli. These cells exhibit a cohesive pattern with lymph node sinusoidal invasion. In the WHO classification, this is referred to as anaplastic large cell lymphoma. In the past, this subtype has also been referred to as malignant histiocytosis. The majority (60%) of these children have a T-cell immunophenotype.[160,163] Recent studies reveal that, although it was originally thought to be uncommon in children, it accounts for 40% to 50% of the large cell lymphoma cases.[160,161,164,165]

Cell Biology

Cancer is a result of (1) the inappropriate or unregulated expression of a gene (or both) at either the wrong time in a cell's cycle or in the wrong cell; (2) abnormal combinations of genes producing proteins not normally present in cells; or (3) the loss of gene expression and their products required for cellular control. The first two categories encompass the proto-oncogenes and oncogenes, and the last comprises the tumor suppressor genes. Lymphomas arise from precursors of lymphocytes at various stages of maturation, primarily because of errors in transcriptional factor control and production as a result of proto-oncogenes and oncogenes. Early B and T cells normally splice together different segments of their immunoglobulin and T-cell–receptor (TCR) genes to generate the diverse proteins capable of binding foreign antigens.[166] In lymphoid cancers, this system goes awry because of the inadvertent splicing juxtaposition of TCR genes (proto-oncogenes) to one of these regions. This leads to the abnormal and unregulated expression of this gene (now an oncogene) and the production of its oncoprotein. This oncoprotein eventually leads to the cell's malignant transformation by a variety of mechanisms and, hence, its uncontrolled growth.[166-169] This neoplastic process typically occurs as a result of nonrandom chromosomal translocations or inversions, although deletions and insertions of DNA sequences likely also contribute to the malignant transformation.

Burkitt's lymphoma was the tumor in which this chromosomal translocation process was originally described.[170] The translocation involving chromosomes 8 and 14 was first identified in Burkitt cells in 1976.[171] As a result of this translocation, t(8;14), the *MYCC* oncogene, located on chromosome 8q24, is juxtaposed to the immunoglobulin receptor subunit gene on chromosome 14q32 (immunoglobulin heavy-chain gene). This translocation is found in both African (endemic) and American (sporadic) Burkitt's lymphoma, although the exact breakpoints on chromosome 8 differ.[172] In a smaller percentage of Burkitt's lymphoma patients, *MYCC* is juxtaposed to chromosome 2p11 (κ immunoglobulin light-chain gene), t(2;8), or 22q11 (λ light-chain gene), t(8;22).[173] It is thought that an increased pool of B cells, either through prolonged stimulation (as in the case of malaria) and/or through inhibition of cell death (as in the case of EBV) increases the chance occurrence of these translocations.[174,175] The oncoprotein MYC normally controls progression through G_1 into the S phase of the cell cycle. However, as a result of these translocations, its expression is dysregulated, leading to uncontrolled lymphoproliferation.[176]

Clinical Presentation

By Initial Site of Disease

Overall, unlike those with HL and adult NHL, children with NHL are often initially seen with extranodal disease and typically have disease that spreads by routes other than contiguous nodal pathways. In children, the abdomen is the originating site of disease in 31%; the mediastinum in 27%; and the head and neck in 29%.[4] Other sites include peripheral nodes, bone, and skin. Most abdominal disease primary lesions are due to Burkitt's lymphomas, whereas most mediastinal/intrathoracic primary lesions are due to T-LL (Table 71-5). Disease that occurs primarily in the peripheral nodes and bones is often due to large cell lymphomas, and skin involvement is primarily associated with the Ki-1$^+$ large cell lymphoma subtype (ALCL).[161,177,178] Correlating with this distribution and the known age peaks of the two types of small cell lymphomas, abdominal primary lesions occur more often in children younger than 10 years, whereas mediastinal primary lesions are more likely to occur in adolescents. Children with abdominal primary lesions may present with nausea, vomiting, abdominal pain, and changes in bowel habits. On physical examination, they may be found to have an abdominal mass in any of the quadrants. Also, they may present with an acute abdomen due to either intussusception (typically due to infiltration of Peyer's patches) (Fig. 71-3) or small bowel obstruction, perforation of an involved bowel wall, or an ileocecal mass mimicking acute appendicitis.[179]

Table 71-5 Non-Hodgkin's Lymphoma: Prevalence of Histologic Subtypes in Primary Sites						
	Abdominal	Thoracic	Head/Neck	Peripheral Nodes	Bone	Other*
SNCCL/B cell	74%	4%	48%	17%	6%	29%
LBL/T cell	3%	74%	24%	33%	31%	14%
LCL	23%	22%	28%	50%	56%	57%
Total	100%	100%	100%	100%	100%	100%

*Includes bone.

SNCCL, small noncleaved cell lymphoma; LBL, lymphoblastic lymphoma; LCL, large cell lymphoma.

Adapted from Murphy SB, Fairclough DL, Hutchison RE, Berard CW: Non-Hodgkin's lymphomas of childhood: An analysis of the histology, staging, and response to treatment of 338 cases in a single institution. J Clin Oncol 7:186-193, 1989; and Wollner N, Lane JM, Marcove RC, et al: Primary skeletal non-Hodgkin's lymphomas in the pediatric age group. Med Pediatr Oncol 20:506-513, 1992.

A child older than age 5 years with an intussusception must strongly be considered to have NHL until proven otherwise. Moreover, NHL should always be part of one's differential diagnosis when faced with a 5- to 10-year-old child with an abdominal mass. Radiographic evaluation with either CT or ultrasonography typically reveals a homogeneous mass with or without evidence of central necrosis, arising either from the retroperitoneum or from the bowel wall. Accompanying adenopathy and metastatic dissemination to the liver and spleen is often seen. The bowel loops may simply be shifted away from the mass or may show evidence of intussusception or obstruction (or both).

Children with mediastinal primary lesions may have minimal symptoms, such as a mild cough or audible wheeze, or can have impending airway obstruction. These latter patients may also have significant engorgement of the vasculature in the head, face, and upper thorax because of superior vena cava compression. Thrombosis may be present in these vessels as well. Often these patients will assume a forward-leaning position and cannot tolerate being placed in the supine position because of the anterior mediastinal mass. The patient's history may reveal orthopnea as well as shortness of breath and dyspnea on exertion. The recent onset of asthma symptoms is not uncommon. Shortness of breath also may be due to pleural effusions. A chest radiograph or chest CT scan is an essential component of the patient's initial evaluation before sedation or any procedure (Fig. 71-4). Chest radiography and chest CT will reveal the widened mediastinum

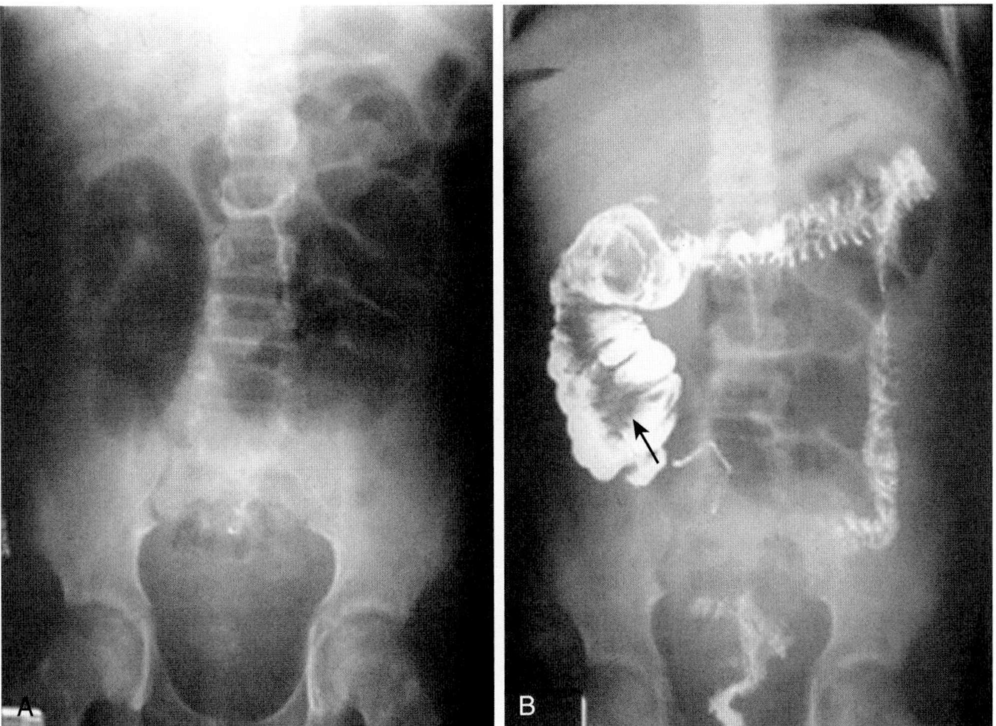

Figure 71-3. This 9-year-old presented with abdominal pain. **A,** The abdominal radiograph shows evidence of a possible small bowel obstruction. Because of the marked leukocytosis and other laboratory parameters, an intussusception due to non-Hodgkin's lymphoma was suspected. **B,** This was confirmed with a retrograde contrast study showing the intussusception (note the filling defect in the contrast medium, *arrow*) in the right colon. This was not able to be reduced radiographically and required operative reduction and intestinal resection.

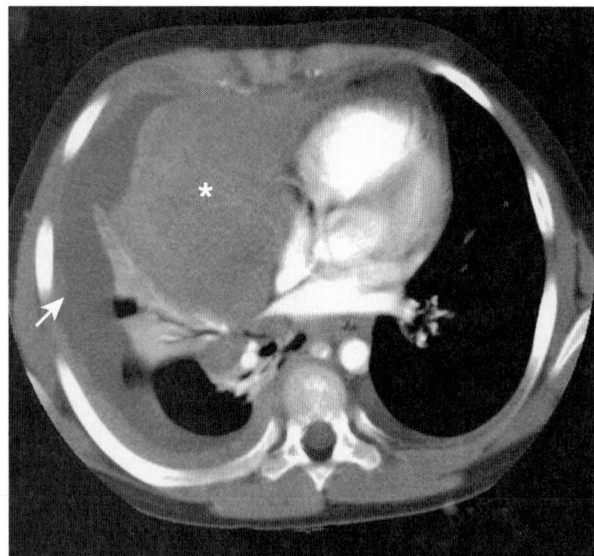

Figure 71-4. This 8-year-old presented with dyspnea. The CT scan shows a very large anterolateral mediastinal mass (*asterisk*). There is also collapse of the adjacent right lung and a rather large pleural effusion (*arrow*). The diagnosis of T cell lymphoma was made on thoracentesis.

with often dramatic narrowing of the trachea and bronchi. Pericardial effusions are often present and may be seen on CT, magnetic resonance imaging(MRI), or echocardiography.[180]

Patients with head and neck lymphomas may have a history of rapidly progressive adenopathy, recent onset of snoring at night, mouth breathing, bad breath, epistaxis, proptosis or periorbital edema, diplopia, extraocular muscle paralysis due to entrapment, cranial nerve paralysis, and sudden blindness or a combination of these symptoms. Physical examination of the nares, oral cavity, and extraocular movements is critical and may reveal signs not appreciated as abnormal by the child. The presence of asymmetric and painless tonsillar hypertrophy should also alert the clinician to the possibility of NHL.[181]

Evaluation with CT often reveals a homogeneous mass that may show destruction of the adjacent bony structures. Bone NHL primary disease is usually seen as lytic lesions found on radiographs obtained for various reasons, including localized tenderness.[182-184] Skin lesions are typically ulcerative and fail to heal but also may be completely subcutaneous.[177] Patients with central nervous system (CNS) involvement may be asymptomatic, have seizures, or have signs and symptoms related to tumor infiltration in the brain.

Laboratory findings at the time of diagnosis are dependent on the amount of tumor present (regardless of the histologic subtype). Generally, patients will have an elevated ESR or C-reactive protein (CRP) level. Those with large tumor burdens typically will have high LDH levels as an indicator of tumor lysis risk,[185,186] disease regression, and disease progression. The degree of LDH elevation has been used as an adverse prognostic factor.[4,187,188] For those with a high tumor burden at presentation, laboratory signs of tumor lysis will also include elevated uric acid, phosphorus, and potassium levels and a low calcium level. Some patients may already be in renal failure at the time of presentation and have an elevated creatinine.[185,186] Hematologic values are nonspecific, and the presence of cytopenias should raise the suspicion of marrow involvement. Cerebrospinal fluid (CSF) pleocytosis may or may not be present in those with CNS involvement.

More than 60% of patients have advanced or disseminated (stages III and IV) disease at diagnosis.[4,189] Bone marrow msetastasis is defined as greater than 5% but less than 25% involvement. Patients with more than 25% disease in the bone marrow are classified as having leukemia. Fourteen percent of patients initially have some bone marrow involvement, and 3% have CNS involvement.[4]

By Histologic Subtype

Burkitt's lymphoma was first described by the surgeon Denis Burkitt in Uganda, where he identified the common finding of enormous involvement of the nodes around the jaw.[190] Later, it was determined that, although this was a common presentation of those patients with endemic Burkitt's (African) lymphoma, those with sporadic Burkitt's (American) lymphoma more typically had presentation of disease either in the abdomen or the nasopharynx.[191] Patients with endemic Burkitt's lymphoma have accompanying abdominal disease in roughly half the cases, and patients with sporadic Burkitt's lymphoma have jaw involvement 15% to 20% of the time.[192] Patients with sporadic Burkitt's lymphoma have a higher incidence of bone marrow involvement (21% vs. 7%) but lower CNS dissemination (11% vs. 17%). Approximately two thirds of Burkitt's lymphoma patients will have disseminated or advanced disease (defined as stages III and IV) at diagnosis.[193]

T-LL patients most often are adolescents with supradiaphragmatic disease, affecting either the intrathoracic region or the head and neck. Disseminated disease is present in nearly 90% of T-LL patients at diagnosis.[193] In T-LL patients, involvement of the bone marrow has been found in approximately one fourth of children, with CNS disease at presentation in fewer than 10%.[193]

ALCL patients may present with disease in all sites but have a higher prevalence than the other two subtypes for skin, bone, and peripheral nodes.[177,184,194] ALCL may present as two distinct clinical forms: primary cutaneous ALCL and primary systemic ALCL (as fevers and weight loss and in advanced stage).[157] Disseminated disease in ALCL patients is present at diagnosis in up to 65% of patients.[193] Involvement of the bone marrow or CNS in ALCL patients is rare (Table 71-6). DLBCL may present as a mediastinal primary lesion or as nodal or extranodal disease, most commonly in the abdomen or head and neck.[157]

In Immunodeficient Patients

For patients with congenital or acquired immunodeficiency, NHL presentation will vary from polyclonal plasmacytic hyperplasia, most often localized in nasopharyngeal nodes or tonsils, to a clonal polymorphic

Table 71-6 Prevalence of Primary Sites among the Three Primary Types of Childhood Non-Hodgkin's Lymphoma

	SNCCL	LBL	LCL
Abdomen	56%	3%	25%
Intrathoracic	2%	65%	21%
Head/neck	34%	23%	29%
Peripheral nodes	2%	7%	11%
Other	5%	3%	14%
Total	100%	100%	100%

NHL, Non-Hodgkin's lymphoma; SNCCL, small noncleaved cell lymphoma; LBL, lymphoblastic lymphoma; LCL, large cell lymphoma.

Adapted from Murphy SB, Fairclough DL, Hutchison RE, Berard CW: Non-Hodgkin's lymphomas of childhood: Analysis of the histology, staging, and response to treatment of 338 cases at a single institution. J Clin Oncol 7:186-193, 1989.

lymphoma slowly arising in the lymph nodes or extranodal sites, to widely disseminated, rapidly progressive immunoblastic lymphoma.[195,196] Symptoms may be nonspecific, with fever and malaise. Hepatosplenomegaly and lymphadenopathy may be presenting signs. Gastrointestinal symptoms of longer than 14 days duration with anorexia, weight loss, and diarrhea should raise suspicion of this condition.[154] NHL has become more common with the use of very potent anti-rejection drugs after solid organ or bone marrow transplantation. Involvement of the transplanted organ is not unusual.[154,197]

Diagnosis

Children initially suspected of having NHL should be evaluated immediately because of the high risk of either metabolic or anatomic complications before therapy begins. The rapid growth of these tumors may create a life-threatening complication overnight in a child who seemed relatively healthy the previous day (Table 71-7).

No clinical findings are pathognomonic for NHL. Ultimately, the diagnosis awaits the biopsy of involved sites, most commonly an excised lymph node or percutaneous needle biopsy. Fine-needle aspirations do not provide enough tissue for the necessary subtyping, which is performed with flow cytometry, molecular genetics, and cytogenetics. It is critical for the excised tissue to be delivered quickly to the pathologist for processing. For cytogenetic and molecular genetic evaluations, it is imperative that all tissue is placed in a sterile container for fresh samples. Formalin should never be used.

For patients critically ill at diagnosis, such as those with severe airway obstruction, diagnosis by alternative methods may be required. These may include nodal biopsy with local anesthetic alone, CT- or US-guided percutaneous needle biopsy of the mass, aspiration of a pleural effusion, or bone marrow biopsy and aspirate. In the majority of cases of NHL, the role of the surgeon is to obtain adequate tissue for diagnosis. Debulking and attempts at local control are unnecessary (with one exception) because NHL is a systemic disease that requires chemotherapy. The one instance in NHL patients in which initial total resection may be considered are those patients with an abdominal mass in whom bowel resection is already required because of perforation or obstruction. In this case, total resection of the tumor should be considered. In this setting, resection reduces the stage of the patient's disease, improves survival, and reduces the amount of therapy required.[198] For all other patients, resection of the mass provides no improvement in staging or long-term cure and delays the time to initiation of chemotherapy. It should be remembered that most patients have disseminated disease at presentation. Also, it is important to note that with chemotherapy alone, more than 90% will achieve a complete remission.

Once NHL is suspected, a concerted and well-conceived plan of evaluation is important to achieve a diagnosis as quickly as possible. This should include laboratory examination to evaluate tumor burden and presence or risk of tumor lysis syndrome. The radiographic evaluation in these patients is extremely important.[60] No procedures or sedation should be attempted until a mediastinal mass has been excluded. To identify the extent of disease, CTs of the neck, chest, abdomen, and pelvis are required. An examination of the head, either CT or MRI, should be obtained in those patients with CNS symptoms, with CSF pleocytosis, or in whom the primary lesions are parameningeal based. Bone scans should typically be obtained. ^{18}FDG-PET or gallium scans are currently recommended. Gallium scans are an effective method for assessing the extent of disease at initial diagnosis, to evaluate residual disease at the end of therapy, and for ongoing monitoring for relapse after therapy.[199] A positive gallium scan at the end of therapy is a strong predictor of relapse. ^{18}FDG-PET scans are gradually replacing gallium scans in the diagnostic evaluation and monitoring of NHL

Table 71-7 Non-Hodgkin's Lymphoma: Diagnostic and Staging Evaluation at Presentation

- Complete physical examination with documentation of involved nodal groups (including measurements of nodes) and involved extralymphatic organs
- Complete blood cell count, chemistry panel (including hepatic and renal function tests), erythrocyte sedimentation rate, lactate dehydrogenase
- Chest radiography to evaluate for mediastinal disease and airway compression
- CT scans of areas identified on physical examination (also include chest, neck, and abdomen)
- Bone scan
- Gallium scan
- Excisional biopsy of node or mass with samples sent for routine pathology, molecular genetics, cytogenetics, and flow cytometry
- Bone marrow biopsies and aspirates (bilateral)
- Lumbar puncture with CSF analysis of cytocentrifuged sample

CT, computed tomography; CSF, cerebrospinal fluid.

patients. Advantages of PET over gallium include same-day imaging, improved resolution, and a higher target-to-background ratio.[200] Diagnostic PET scans are reliable (greater than 90% positive) in patients with DLBCL. Three studies of patients with HL and NHL found PET to be superior to gallium for diagnosing disease sites.[80]

Pathologic evaluation of the biopsy material should include general histochemical techniques to confirm the lymphoma and its subtype. Critical additions to the basic evaluation are flow cytometric analysis of cell-surface markers to determine the immunophenotype of the lymphoma, cytogenetic evaluation for diagnostic translocations, fluorescent in situ hybridization (FISH), and DNA analysis using either Southern blotting or the polymerase chain reaction for detection of the pathognomonic oncogenes (gene rearrangements), even in the absence of identifiable cytogenetic translocations.[201] Examination of markers in tumor cells for EBV is important in the evaluation of PTLDs. These are all essential components at the time of initial diagnosis and should be performed at an institution capable of performing all of them. Therapy differences between the subtypes of lymphoma are such that assignment to the wrong subtype due to a lack of adequate diagnostic material will adversely affect the chance of cure. These evaluations may be performed with biopsy material from any involved site, including the primary mass, enlarged lymph nodes, effusions, and bone marrow. A new technique, known as gene expression profiling, which uses DNA microarrays, has been shown to categorize patients further into specific histologic and genetic subsets of lymphoma, with much greater predictability of the clinical outcome.[202] This new technique will likely revolutionize diagnostic and prognostic characterization for NHL.

Completing the diagnostic protocol is the determination of whether or not there is CNS or bone marrow dissemination. Lumbar puncture for cytocentrifuged CSF analysis should be performed in all patients. However, in those with localized abdominal Burkitt's lymphoma, and those with large cell lymphoma, the benefit gained from this is arguable because of the low incidence of CNS disease in these subpopulations. Bone marrow evaluation should include bilateral iliac crest biopsies and aspirates.

Staging

Once the diagnosis of NHL has been made, staging permits determination of the extent of disease at presentation. This provides direction in monitoring disease response to therapy. In contrast to HL, relapse does not necessarily occur at the site of initial or previous disease in NHL. Thus, this initial staging should not limit the extent of monitoring for relapse after therapy is completed.

Staging is important in the determination of therapeutic planning. The most widely used staging schema today is the St. Jude's or Murphy system (Table 71-8).[203] This is an adaptation of the Ann Arbor scheme and is applicable to all types of childhood NHL. It divides patients into localized (stage I or II) and disseminated or advanced (stage III or IV) disease. Involvement of the CNS or bone marrow immediately places the patient in the stage IV category. Patients with more than 25% bone marrow involvement are, by definition, diagnosed with leukemia rather than with lymphoma. These would include B-cell or Burkitt's leukemia (L3 leukemia morphologic classification) and T-cell leukemia. The former patients are treated on B-cell NHL protocols with much better results than previously obtained on acute lymphoblastic leukemia (ALL) regimens. Many of the B-cell NHL protocol results reported in the literature include these patients in their stage IV populations. The T-cell leukemia patients remain on ALL protocols, but many similarities exist between these protocols and those used in T-LL therapy.

Table 71-8 St. Jude's (Murphy) Staging System for Childhood Non-Hodgkin's Lymphoma

Stage	Definition
I	Single tumor (extranodal) or single anatomic area (nodal), excluding mediastinum or abdomen
II	Single tumor (extranodal) with regional node involvement On same side of diaphragm: a) Two or more nodal areas b) Two single (extranodal) tumors with or without regional node involvement Primary gastrointestinal tract tumor (usually ileocecal) with or without associated mesenteric node involvement, grossly completely resected
III	On both sides of diaphragm: a) Two single tumors (extranodal) b) Two or more nodal areas All primary intrathoracic tumors (mediastinal, pleural, thymic) All extensive primary intra-abdominal disease; unresectable All primary paraspinal or epidural tumors regardless of other sites
IV	Any of the above with initial CNS or bone marrow involvement (<25%)

CNS, central nervous system.

Prognostic Risk Factors

When all patients are treated similarly, the stage of the lymphoma at diagnosis is a strong predictor of outcome.[4] Prediction of a patient's eventual outcome stratifies patients at high risk for relapse to more intensive or novel therapies and patients at low risk to shorter, more moderate therapies. Many prognostic factors have been evaluated over the years. All prognostic factors are dependent on the therapy subsequently given.[4] It has been definitively shown that histology-based therapy is of critical importance in the successful outcome of patients (Table 71-9).[189]

CNS involvement in both SNCCL and LBL patients has predictably worse outcomes.[189] In patients with Burkitt's lymphoma, the adverse effect of CNS disease on outcome has, in some studies, been more attributable to tumor burden at diagnosis than to the presence of CNS disease alone (i.e., those with greater tumor burden are more likely to have CNS disease).[204] Patients with Burkitt's lymphoma older than 15 years of age have a worse prognosis than patients younger than 15 years old. An LDH greater than 500 IU/L also predicts a worse outcome for patients with Burkitt's lymphoma.[205]

DLBCL and ALCL patients (historically large cell lymphoma patients) have unique prognostic characteristics that are likely to change as this entity is better described and therapy is more appropriately administered by subtype. Skin involvement at presentation in patients with large cell lymphoma has been shown to be a poor prognostic indicator.[198] In one study of patients with advanced large cell lymphoma, the presence of $CD30^+$ cells indicated a better OS.[206] However, in another study, no effect on prognosis was noted.[160] B-cell immunophenotype has been shown to improve prognosis.[160] Patients with intrathoracic primary lesions have a better prognosis than do those with primary lesions elsewhere.[206] Children with NHL arising in the bone, regardless of the histologic subtypes, have an excellent prognosis with histology-directed chemotherapy alone.[207]

Table 71-9 Selected Therapeutic Trials for Children with Non-Hodgkin's Lymphoma

Protocol/Therapy	Stage	DFS % (yr)	OS % (yr)	Reference
Small Noncleaved/B cell				
POG/ADCOMP	I-II	87 (4)	93 (5)	217
CCG 551, 501/COMP	I-II	86-98 (5)	91-98 (5)	210
CCG 551/COMP	III-IV	50 (5)	54 (5)	193
CCG 551/LSA_2L_2	III-IV	29 (5)	33 (5)	193
CCG 552/CHOP	III, LDH < 500	86 (4)	86	191
	III, LDH > 500	39	39	
	IV	38	48	
Total therapy B	III	86 (2)		226
POG/Intensified total therapy B	IV	79 (4)		212
HiC-COM	III	92 (3)		192
	IV	50		
SFOP/LMB 84	III	80 (3)	82 (3)	211
	IV	68	71	
SFOP/LMB 89	I-II	100 (1)		226
	III	89		
	IV	80		
Lymphoblastic/T cell				
POG/ADCOMP	I-II	87 (4)	93 (5)	217
CCG 551/LSA_2L_2	III-IV	64 (5)	67 (5)	193
CCG 551/COMP	III-IV	34 (5)	45 (5)	193
CCG 552/CHOP	III-IV	54 (4)	77 (4)	191
CCG 502/ADCOMP or LSA_2L_2	Localized	84 (5)		214
	Disseminated	67		
UCCSG 8503	Disseminated	65 (4)		226
St. Jude/Total therapy X-high risk	III-IV	73 (4)		226
SFOP/LMT 81	III	79		226
	IV	72		
Large Cell				
St. Jude/CHOP	I-II CD30+	75 (5)		161
	I-II CD30-	92		
St. Jude/CHOP & MACOP-B	III-IV CD30+	57	84 (5)	
	III-IV CD30-	29	27	
CCG 551/LSA_2L_2	III-IV	43 (5)	44 (5)	193
CCG 551/COMP	III-IV	52 (5)	69 (5)	193
BFM 83,86,90	I	75 (5)		165
	II	68		
	III-IV	86		
POG 87191/POG 8615	B cell/ALL	96 (3)		160
	T cell or?/ALL	67		
	B cell/III-IV	100		
	T cell or?/III-IV	69		

DFS, disease-free survival; OS, overall survival; LDH, lactate dehydrogenase.

Treatment

Therapy for childhood NHL has evolved over the past several decades, and is based on the knowledge that this tumor is extremely chemosensitive. For Burkitt's lymphoma and large cell lymphoma, the duration of therapy has become shorter, as it became apparent that most, if not all, patients were experiencing relapse within the first 6 to 8 months of therapy.[193,208] Despite reduction in therapy to 6 months or less, no increase in relapse has been seen. Relapses for the most part have occurred within the first 6 to 8 months after diagnosis and virtually all have occurred within the first 2 years.[187-189,208,209] Therapy for Burkitt's lymphoma has shown a clear improvement as methotrexate and cytarabine doses have been increased. These two agents, in addition to cyclophosphamide, vincristine, doxorubicin (Adriamycin), and prednisone (and etoposide for the stage IV patients), now play a critical role in the successful outcome of these children.[193,198,209,210] The addition of rituximab (an anti-CD20 monoclonal antibody) and rasburicase (a recombinant urate oxidase for treatment of hyperuricemia) is currently being studied.

For T-LL, the duration of therapy has been decreased to 2 years. The most effective regimens for LBL have been ones similar to the intensive T-cell ALL protocols in current use. For ALCL patients, the use of T-cell regimens without much CNS-directed therapy has been efficacious.

For Burkitt's and large cell lymphomas, it has become apparent that no benefit in DFS or OS is gained with the use of radiation for treatment, either to involved areas or to the CNS for prophylaxis.[164,177,211] Rather, prophylaxis to prevent CNS relapse is effectively accomplished with intrathecal chemotherapy.[204] Although some type of CNS prophylaxis is thought to be needed for all patients with NHL to prevent CNS relapse, in one small group of patients, it is not. Patients with localized, resected gastrointestinal primary tumors with Burkitt's or large cell lymphomas do not have CNS relapse, even in the absence of CNS prophylaxis.[208]

For patients with LBL, irradiation to areas of bulky disease has been eliminated. In the past, irradiation was used for CNS prophylaxis in patients without CNS disease at diagnosis, but recent studies substituting intrathecal chemoprophylaxis have not shown increased CNS relapses. For those patients with LBL with CNS disease at diagnosis, irradiation remains an important part of their therapy.

Several additional points deserve mention. The use of corticosteroids before a diagnostic procedure should absolutely be avoided. This can induce rapid necrosis in the lymphoma, making subtype determination difficult if not impossible, and potentially jeopardizing the patient's outcome. However, once adequate tissue has been obtained, chemotherapy including corticosteroids is an excellent method for rapid reduction of a life-threatening mass. Because of the extreme sensitivity of NHL, one can anticipate rapid reduction of tumor size once therapy is initiated. Radiation therapy is not necessary. It is not unusual to have symptoms completely resolve within 24 hours and have patients be in complete radiographic remission within 7 days. Many protocols now call for a period of reduced-dose chemotherapy for the first week to obtain a more controlled tumor reduction because of the severe tumor lysis that may accompany more rapid, therapy-induced necrosis.

NHL in immunodeficient individuals is most often a B-cell lymphoma, either small or large cell. Therapy for these patients has typically been directed toward these histologic types. For patients with ongoing iatrogenic immune suppression, a reduction of the immunosuppressive agent with or without acyclovir may be adequate to induce a remission in up to 75% of cases.[154,212] However, this may not be possible after transplant because of the risk of rejection. Interferon-alfa has been used with mixed success in these patients and may exacerbate rejection. A small proportion of patients with localized disease may be cured with operative resection of the involved nodal tissue. When the tumor is resistant to these approaches, chemotherapy regimens can be used, although mortality has been higher than that found in immunocompetent patients. In the past few years, new methods using monoclonal antibody therapy, primarily rituximab, have been used with promising results alone, but these antibodies are most efficacious when combined with chemotherapy.[213]

Results

When reviewing the outcomes of children treated for NHL, it is quickly apparent that considerable improvement in DFS and OS has occurred over the past several decades (see Table 71-9).[4] Today, typically 90% to 100% of patients will achieve complete remission.[164,208,214] Five-year relative survival rates for children ages birth to 19, diagnosed between 1996 and 2004, were 83.3%.[13] Patients with localized disease have an overall excellent prognosis, regardless of histologic subtype, with DFS typically exceeding 90% to 95%. Burkitt's lymphoma patients with advanced disease have experienced DFS exceeding 80% in the recent trials. Patients with LBL with disseminated disease are not faring as well, but DFS for these patients is exceeding 65% to 70% in most trials. Overall, when they occur, treatment failures typically happen within the first 2 years after diagnosis. Patients with Burkitt's lymphoma who experience relapse primarily do so within the first 6 to 8 months. LBL patients will have an occasional late failure after 2 years, although even in this group of patients the vast majority of failures will occur early.[214] Patients with large cell lymphoma have more late relapses. Thus, radiographic follow-up is an important modality in the ongoing post-therapeutic evaluation of NHL patients for several years. With the advent of modern radiographic techniques, second-look operations have not been beneficial to patient outcome.[198,215]

Acute Complications

Depending on the tumor burden at diagnosis, patients may initially have a constellation of significant metabolic derangements known as tumor lysis syndrome.[185,186] This includes hyperuricemia, hyperphosphatemia, hyperkalemia, and hypocalcemia. Recognition of this syndrome is critical to prevent life-threatening complications, including acute renal failure. Without treatment, the incidence of acute renal failure may be as high as 30%.[216] Tumor lysis syndrome is the result of the rapid turnover of cells within the tumor. The fraction of tumor cells in S phase at any given time can approach 27% in some patients.[217] These tumors have a high degree of spontaneous lysis at the time of diagnosis because they rapidly outgrow their blood supply. Any manipulation, including transfusion or operation, may induce a sudden worsening of this syndrome.

Therapy is primarily based on the risk of developing hyperuricemia. For those at high risk, determined by the presence of an elevated LDH, creatinine, or uric acid value, intervention is important. For most patients with little or no elevation in these values, adequate hydration (>3000 mL/m^2/day) and monitoring of blood pH (maintain between 7.0 and 7.5) is adequate, along with the initiation of allopurinol to reduce the production of uric acid through inhibition of xanthine oxidase.[218] Rasburicase, which cleaves uric acid into allantoin, a soluble by-product, has been approved for use by the U.S. Food and Drug Administration (FDA). This agent, administered daily for 1 to 5 days, dramatically reduces measurable uric acid levels to immeasurable levels, thus allowing the clinician to focus on prevention or treatment of hyperphosphatemia, which requires maintaining acidic urine.[219,220] Despite these measures, it may be necessary to place patients on dialysis either to treat oliguria/anuria or to prevent it in the presence of rapidly increasing uric acid, phosphorus (typically >10 mg/dL), or potassium (>7.5 mEq/L) levels.[193,221] In an effort to avoid this complication, some regimens have used an initial low-dose therapy (usually 1 week) to more slowly reduce the tumor burden.

Because of the much more myelosuppressive regimens required in NHL therapy, infection is a much larger risk for NHL patients as compared with HL patients.[189] In one recent study, 63% of the deaths were due to infection. Most patients require transfusion support during treatment because of the myelosuppression. The chemotherapy itself may cause acute complications, including severe chemical burns due to extravasation of certain vesicant agents (vincristine, anthracyclines). Because most children require the placement of right atrial catheters to facilitate their therapy, thrombosis of this area and the surrounding vasculature has become more frequent.[222] Mucositis is seen in a significant number of patients during therapy for Burkitt's lymphoma as well.

Long-Term Sequelae

As long-term survival has improved, the concern over lifelong sequelae has increased in these patients. With current therapy, these complications include cardiac toxicity,[137] infertility as a result of the alkylating agents used,[223] and secondary leukemias due to epipodophyllotoxins (etoposide, tenoposide) and alkylating agents used in the NHL regimens.[224] The risk for developing cardiac toxicity is related to several factors, including irradiation dose, cumulative anthracycline dose, and age at exposure. Patients are at an increased risk for anthracycline-related cardiomyopathy if they are female, have received doses greater than 200 to 300 mg/m^2, and were younger when given anthracyclines.[225]

The risk for infertility is related to the cumulative dose of the alkylating agents. Fertility is likely to be maintained in males receiving less than 4 g/m^2 of cyclophosphamide and no other alkylating chemotherapy or radiation.[225] In female survivors, the risk of infertility increases with age at the time of treatment. Prepubertal patients tolerate higher cumulative doses of alkylating agents than adult women. Survivors of childhood lymphoma must be monitored closely for early identification and proper intervention to maintain a good quality of life in these long-term survivors.

chapter 72

RHABDOMYOSARCOMA

Shinil K. Shah, DO • Peter A. Walker, MD • Richard J. Andrassy, MD

Rhabdomyosarcoma (RMS) is a soft tissue tumor originating from immature mesenchymal cells that form any tissue except bone. It is the most common type of soft tissue sarcoma in children and adolescents, accounting for approximately 50% of all soft tissue sarcomas. As a result of prospective, multicenter clinical trials conducted by the Intergroup Rhabdomyosarcoma Study Group (IRSG) (established in 1972) as well as other collaborative networks, the overall survival of patients with RMS has increased to as high as 70% with current multimodal therapies.[1]

Approximately 350 new cases of RMS are diagnosed annually in the United States, corresponding to a yearly incidence of 4.6 cases per million children aged 20 years or younger.[2] RMS is the third most common childhood extracranial solid tumor, after neuroblastoma and Wilms' tumor.[3] A bimodal age distribution is found, with approximately 65% of cases occurring in children younger than 6 years and the remaining cases occurring in children aged 10 to 18 years.[4] More than 80% of cases are diagnosed before the age of 14.[5]

Children with RMS appear to have an increased incidence of other congenital anomalies, with the central nervous and genitourinary systems being the most commonly affected.[6] In the most recent Intergroup Rhabdomyosarcoma Study (IRS-IV), 883 patients were enrolled and analyzed between 1991 and 1997.[1] The distribution of primary tumor sites was as follows: head and neck, 7%; parameningeal, 25% (nasopharynx, paranasal sinus, middle ear mastoid, pterygoid-infratemporal sites); orbit, 9%; genitourinary, 31%; extremities, 13%; retroperitoneum, 7%; trunk, 5%; and all other sites, 3%.

Histopathologically, RMS is classified with the category of small, round, blue cell tumors of childhood, a category including neuroblastoma, Ewing's sarcoma, small cell osteogenic sarcoma, non-Hodgkin's lymphoma, and leukemia. Six major pathologic subtypes of RMS are outlined by the International Classification of RMS (presented in order of decreasing 5-year survival): (1) embryonal (botryoid); (2) embryonal (spindle cell); (3) embryonal, not otherwise specified (NOS); (4) alveolar, NOS or solid variant; (5) anaplasia, diffuse; and (6) undifferentiated sarcoma. Botryoid RMS is associated with a superior 5-year survival rate of 95% and most commonly occurs in the bladder or vagina in infants and young children and in the nasopharynx in older children.[7] The most common location for spindle cell RMS is paratesticular, head and neck, extremities, or orbit.[8] Nearly 60% of all pediatric RMS, embryonal and embryonal variant RMS account for the majority of cases in younger patients.[9,10] Alveolar, anaplastic, and undifferentiated variants of RMS account for approximately 35% of all new cases and generally have the poorest prognosis. Although the embryonal subtypes are the most common type of RMS, the alveolar subtype is seen more often in patients presenting later in life, that is, during the second peak in incidence.[10] A "solid alveolar" variant lacks the characteristic alveolar septations but behaves similarly to the conventional alveolar subtype.[11]

The impact of specific histologic subtype on outcome has varied somewhat in different studies. Confounding variables in examining the importance of histologic type include different subtypes that preferentially occur in specific sites, are present as different primary tumor sizes, and have different invasiveness capabilities. For example, with extremity RMS in IRS-IV, clinical group and stage, but not histologic subtype, were important prognostic variables.[12] Other studies support that histologic subtype is an important independent prognostic factor, with embryonal RMS having a significantly favorable outcome.[11,13] In IRS-IV, 3-year failure-free survival (FFS) was 83% for embryonal, 66% for alveolar, 55% for undifferentiated, and 66% for unclassified sarcoma ($P < .001$).[1]

STAGING

Two classification schemes are currently used to categorize patients with RMS. The clinical grouping system was devised by the IRS in 1972 and is a surgicopathologic system that relies on the initial surgical assessment (Table 72-1).[10] This classification scheme demands an initial surgical approach, which may vary between institutions and surgeons. Stratification

Table 72-1 Clinical Grouping Classifications for Rhabdomyosarcoma

	Extent of Disease		
Clinical Group	*Tumor*	*Resectability/ Margins*	*Lymph Node Status*
1	Localized	Complete resection Negative margins	Negative Confined to tissue of origin
1a	Localized	Complete resection Negative margins	Negative Not confined to tissue of origin
2a	Localized	Complete gross resection Microscopically + margins	Negative
2b	Localized	Complete gross resection Microscopically + margins	Positive regional nodes
2c	Localized	Complete gross resection Positive margins	Positive regional nodes
3a	Localized/ locally extensive	Residual disease after biopsy only	
3b	Localized/ locally extensive	Residual disease after debulking of > 50% tumor	
4	Distant metastasis		

From Qualman SJ, Coffin CM, Newton WA, et al: Intergroup Rhabdomyosarcoma Study: Update for pathologists. Pediatr Dev Pathol 1:550-561, 1998.

of survival is based on the ability for complete resection. However, clinical grouping has consistently been shown to be an independent prognostic indicator predicting outcome. Overall survival curves, according to clinical group of patients enrolled in all IRS studies, are shown in Figure 72-1.[9]

More recently, the IRS, which is now part of the Sarcoma Committee of the Children's Oncology Group (COG), has implemented a pretreatment staging system based on the tumor/node/metastasis (TNM) system (Table 72-2).[14] The system is modified for RMS to incorporate known important prognostic variables, including primary tumor site, lymph node involvement, distant metastatic disease, and size. Primary tumor site is known to be an important prognostic factor with RMS. Favorable sites include the orbit, eyelid, other nonparameningeal head/neck sites, and nonbladder, nonprostate genitourinary structures (paratesticular, vaginovulvar, uterine). Unfavorable sites include extremities (including buttock), trunk, retroperitoneum, perineum, urinary bladder and prostate, and cranial parameningeal sites. IRS-IV was the first study to use this staging system to classify patients prospectively. Failure-free survival (FFS) rates for patients with local or regional tumors, according to stage, are shown in Figure 72-2. In this cohort of patients, pretreatment staging appeared to be a more accurate predictor of outcome than was the clinical grouping classification system.

MOLECULAR BIOLOGY

Further characterization of RMS tumors utilizing specific molecular fingerprints is important in establishing a definitive diagnosis in difficult cases. Additionally, specific molecular markers offer promise as prognostic indicators. One of the challenges in the treatment of RMS is to stratify patients into risk categories, ensuring that low-risk patients are not exposed to overly toxic treatment regimens and high-risk patients are not undertreated. Identification of the specific molecular pathways involved in RMS also offers potential therapeutic targets.

Globally, mutations in certain tumor suppressor genes, including *TP53*, predispose individuals to RMS. It is important to note that patients with Li-Fraumeni syndrome and neurofibromatosis type 1 are more likely to develop RMS. Also, up to 10% of patients with RMS may have one of these syndromes.[15,16]

Embryonal RMS is characterized by loss of heterozygosity (LOH) with loss of maternal genetic information and duplication of paternal genetic information at the 11p15 locus.[17] This genetic locus is the site of the insulin-like growth factor-2 (*IGF-2*) gene, which codes for a growth factor thought to play a role in the pathogenesis of RMS through one of several possible mechanisms. The LOH results in overexpression of *IGF-2*.[9,15] Another potential etiologic molecular finding is the loss of 9q22, which corresponds to a tumor suppressor gene in embryonal RMS patients.[18]

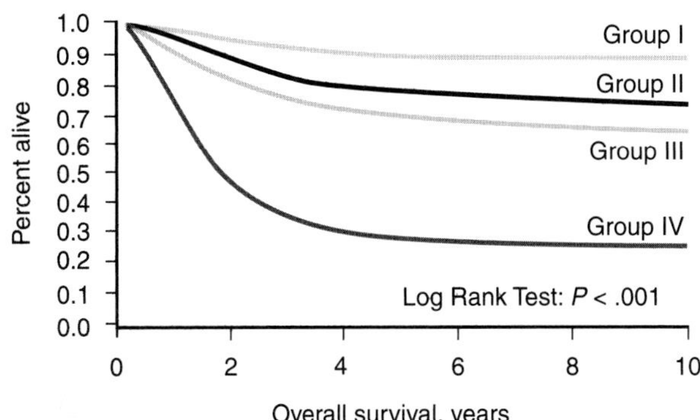

Figure 72-1. Overall survival according to clinical group assignment (Intergroup Rhabdomyosarcoma Study [IRS] I to IV). Survival of patients treated on IRS-I, IRS-II, IRS-III/IV-P (IV pilot), and IRS-IV by clinical group at diagnosis is shown. A significant difference is seen in outcome by the extent of initial surgical resection, with the best outcome among the patients with completely resected tumors (group 1), followed by those with microscopic residual (group 2) and gross residual (group 3) disease. Patients with metastatic disease (group 4) at diagnosis fare poorly. (J.R. Anderson, personal communication, 2000; from Pizzo PA, Poplack DG [eds]: Principles and Practice of Pediatric Oncology, 4th ed. Philadelphia, Lippincott Williams & Wilkins, 2002.)

Table 72-2 TNM RMS Pretreatment Staging Classification

TNM Stage	Sites	Tumor*	Size†	Node‡	Metastasis§
Stage 1	Orbit Head and neck (excluding parameningeal) Genitourinary: nonbladder/ prostate	T1 or T2	a or b	N0 or N1 or Nx	M0
Stage 2	Bladder/prostate Extremity Head and neck parameningeal Other (includes trunk, retroperitoneum, etc.)	T1 or T2	a	N0 or Nx	M0
Stage 3	Bladder/prostate Extremity Head and neck parameningeal Other (includes trunk, retroperitoneum, etc.)	T1 or T2	a b	N1 N0 or N1 or Nx	M0 M0
Stage 4	All	T1 or T2	a or b	N0 or N1	M1

*Tumor: T1, confined to anatomic site of origin. T2, extension and/or fixation to surrounding tissue.
†a, <5 cm in diameter; b, ≥ 5 cm in diameter.
‡Regional nodes: N0, regional nodes not clinically involved; N1, regional nodes clinically involved by neoplasm; Nx, clinical status of regional nodes unknown (especially sites that preclude lymph node evaluation).
§Metastasis: M0, no distant metastases present; M1, distant metastases.

In approximately 70% of alveolar RMS, a common translocation between chromosomes 2 and 13, t(2;13)(q35;q14), is present.[19] This translocation usually involves the *PAX3* gene (which regulates transcription driving neuromuscular development) and the *FOXO1* gene, which is involved in the differentiation process of myoblasts).[20] Less commonly, the translocation involves the *PAX7* gene located at 1p36 to the same location on chromosome 13.[21] The exact molecular pathway leading to the development of alveolar RMS potentially caused or exacerbated by these translocations remains to be elucidated. *PAX3/FOXO1* expression can increase *IGF-2* expression and an IGF-binding protein, providing a common pathway for both embryonal and alveolar RMS. These known molecular disturbances are just now being adopted and studied clinically. Several studies have demonstrated a worse prognosis with the presence of a *PAX3/FOXO1* fusion gene in alveolar subtypes of RMS.[15,22] Additionally, the t(2;13) translocation has been shown to characterize alveolar RMS with a poor prognosis, whereas the t(1;13) translocation is associated with improved outcome.[23] These preliminary findings and other molecular features will be examined more fully in IRS-V.

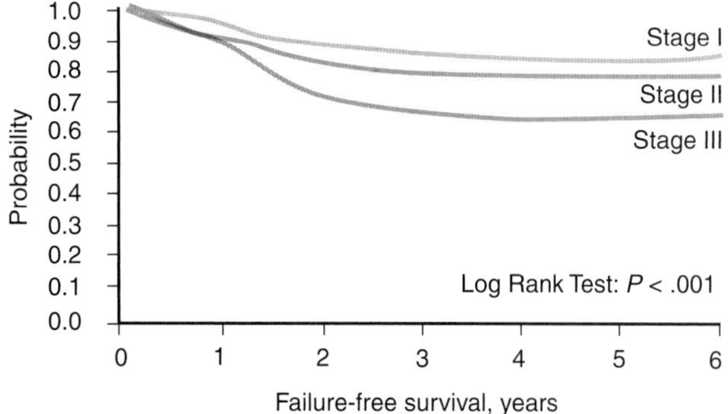

Figure 72-2. Failure-free survival for nonmetastatic disease patients according to staging classification in Intergroup Rhabdomyosarcoma Study-IV.

CLINICAL PRESENTATION

The clinical presentation of RMS is highly variable and depends largely on tumor site, patient age, and the presence and/or absence of metastatic disease. The majority of symptoms are secondary to the local mass effect. RMSs involving the head and neck region including orbits, parameningeal tissues (middle ear, nasal cavity, paranasal sinuses, nasopharynx, and infratemporal fossa), and nonparameningeal tissues (scalp, face, oral cavity, oropharynx, hypopharynx and neck) are most commonly embryonal subtype and rarely involve regional lymph nodes. Local symptoms may include proptosis, ophthalmoplegia, nasal/sinus obstruction with or without discharge, cranial nerve palsies, meningeal symptoms, or a painless, enlarging localized mass. Paratesticular RMS may mimic a hernia, hydrocele, or varicocele and present as a painless swelling in the scrotum or inguinal canal. There is a high rate of lymph node spread to the retroperitoneum. Tumors involving the bladder and/or urinary tract or prostate may cause obstruction, hematuria, constipation, and/or urinary frequency. Vaginal tumors are more common in very young patients and may present as vaginal bleeding, discharge, or a mass. Tumors involving the uterus more commonly present in older girls with extensive tumor at diagnosis.

Table 72-3	Preoperative Treatment/Evaluation of Pediatric Rhabdomyosarcoma

- History/physical examination
- Measurement of lesion (physical or imaging)
- Complete blood cell count with differential and platelets
- Urinalysis
- Electrolytes, creatinine, calcium, and phosphorus
- Liver function tests (alkaline phosphatase, lactate dehydrogenase, bilirubin, and transaminases)
- Bone marrow biopsy/aspirate
- Chest radiograph
- MRI/CT of primary lesion
- CT of chest
- MRI/CT of head (for head tumors)
- Bone scintigraphy
- Cerebrospinal fluid cytology (for parameningeal tumors)
- Electrocardiography or echocardiography (selective)

RMSs involving the extremity usually present as a mass, tend to be more aggressive with the majority being the alveolar subtype, and have a high incidence of spread to regional lymph nodes (approximately 50%). Approximately 15% of patients present with metastatic disease. Presentation in the neonate is extremely rare, with most being embryonal/botryoid/undifferentiated subtypes (0.4%).[12,24-29]

DIAGNOSIS

The diagnosis of RMS is usually made by biopsy. Depending on location, this may involve endoscopy or needle biopsy (genitourinary tumors) or excisional/incisional biopsies (trunk/extremity). Incisions made for biopsy should be placed in such a way that complete excision would be possible if subsequent wide local excision is necessary. Sentinel lymph node mapping is advised in tumors involving the trunk and/or extremities. Prior to definitive surgery, a full evaluation including imaging, laboratory work, and bone marrow evaluation should be performed (Table 72-3).[5]

SURGICAL TREATMENT

Primary Resection

It is evident from the impact of clinical grouping on eventual survival rates (see Fig. 72-1) that complete tumor resection, with no microscopic residual disease, offers the best chance for cure. However, in many sites (e.g., orbit, bladder, prostate, vagina, uterus) complete tumor resection is not feasible while still preserving function of vital organs or structures and avoiding mutilating surgical procedures. One of the major achievements in the surgical treatment of RMS over the past 30 years is the progressive increase in organ salvage rates (e.g., bladder, vagina, uterus, prostate) and a decrease in disfiguring surgery while not adversely affecting overall patient survival. The decision as to how aggressive to make the original surgical approach depends on primary tumor site, size, presence or absence of lymph node involvement, and distant metastases. These decisions must be made in the context of a multidisciplinary team, including the surgeon, oncologist, pediatric radiologist, and radiotherapist to allow optimal care for the patient. The recommended initial surgical approach is to perform a nonradical tumor resection if the primary site and tumor size is amenable and the treatment team believes that a complete resection with negative margins is feasible. Otherwise, a biopsy sufficient to provide the definitive diagnosis as well as tissue for ongoing biology studies, if applicable, is recommended.

Primary Re-excision

Primary re-excision (PRE) of a tumor is defined as a second attempt at complete resection before the initiation of any other form of therapy. PRE is recommended when an initial resection results in positive margins if this can be accomplished without sacrificing vital structures or organs, causing significant functional impairments, or resulting in a poor cosmetic outcome. A strategy of PRE has been shown to improve survival in patients with extremity tumors (who tend to have a worse prognosis secondary to histology)[30] and in perineal RMS,[14] by converting a significant proportion of patients from group IIa to group I. When the initial resection was performed for presumed benign disease, or when the margin status is not known, PRE also is recommended. The benefit of PRE was recently examined by the Italian Cooperative Study Group. They concluded that PRE was the treatment of choice for children with RMS and nonrhabdomyosarcoma soft tissue sarcoma (NRSTS) age 3 years or younger who cannot receive radiation therapy, and also for paratesticular sites.[31] PRE and postoperative irradiation showed equivalent results in achieving local control in extremity and trunk sites. PRE was not effective in tumors larger than 5 cm. As with the primary tumor resection, PRE is performed to allow a clinical group I classification (no residual), but only if this does not require a mutilating radical surgical procedure. If not feasible, reliance on adjuvant irradiation and chemotherapy is advisable.

Lymph Node Evaluation

It has become increasingly recognized that RMS frequently spreads to regional lymph nodes early, that these involved nodes can go undetected by sophisticated imaging techniques, and that lymph node involvement significantly worsens the prognosis. Because of these findings, pediatric surgeons frequently must evaluate the status of the regional lymph nodes with RMS. Any clinically or radiographically suspicious lymph node requires pathologic confirmation. It is important to note that lymph node excision serves a diagnostic purpose only. There is no therapeutic value.[5] With extremity RMS patients in IRS-IV, 37% of all patients and 50% of those in whom surgical lymph node evaluation was performed had positive regional lymph node involvement.[12] This study also found that

17% of patients with clinically negative regional nodes had positive biopsy on histologic examination. Patients with positive regional lymph nodes had a 3-year FFS of 40% versus approximately 70% in patients without nodal involvement. It is important to determine regional lymph node status accurately so that if it is positive, more aggressive treatment approaches (e.g., irradiation) can be used. Thus, these patients are recognized to be at higher risk. With perianal RMS, 46% of patients have been found to have regional lymph node involvement.[14] In this group of patients, N1 patients had a 5-year overall survival rate of 33% versus 71% in N0 patients. Regional lymph node metastases also were frequently documented with paratesticular RMS.[32] With paratesticular and perineal/perianal RMS, an increase in regional lymph node involvement is found with age older than 10 years, indicating that there should be a heightened index of suspicion in older children and adolescents with RMS.

Specific recommendations regarding regional lymph node evaluation will be reviewed according to the specific site. However, in general, a strategy of routine surgical evaluation of regional lymph node status is recommended for RMS patients with primary tumors of the extremity, perineum, and for older patients (>10 years) with paratesticular sites, even if there is no clinically apparent disease. If disease is found in the regional nodes, distal lymph nodes should be sampled to determine metastatic disease.[16] Additionally, during the course of tumor resection at other sites (e.g., genitourinary, retroperitoneum), lymph node sampling should be performed, if feasible.

Although not yet standard of care, lymphatic mapping with sentinel lymph node biopsy may allow adequate staging while limiting operative morbidity.[32,33] Most experience with this technique has been gained with extremity and truncal tumors, and with adult breast cancer and melanoma.[16] Typically, lymphoscintigraphic mapping (using technetium-labeled sulfur colloid injected at the primary tumor site with subsequent images showing the lymphatic drainage route) is performed before the planned operation (either 24 hours before or immediately before the surgical procedure). Intraoperatively, vital blue dye is injected at the primary tumor site and a radioisotope detector is used to identify the lymph node with the highest "counts." Utilizing a small incision and limited dissection, a blue sentinel lymph node(s) with evidence of radioactive tracer is excised. These techniques limit the extent of the operation and, potentially, the morbidity as compared with formal lymph node dissection as previously performed. Because the goal is to determine nodal disease for future treatment (i.e., radiation therapy), this approach may play a larger role in the future.

Second-Look Operation

The majority of patients with RMS are initially seen with tumors that do not allow complete resection to achieve either clinical group I or II status secondary to size, invasion, or location. In IRS-IV, among all patients without metastatic disease (n = 883), 62% were classified as group III (i.e., gross residual disease after biopsy only or attempted resection).[1] After intensive multiagent chemotherapy with or without irradiation, these patients usually benefit from a second-look operation. The goals of the second-look operation are to remove residual tumor and to determine pathologic response, because clinical and radiographic assessment is often inaccurate.[34] The primary benefit of a second-look operation is to resect residual tumor before additional adjuvant treatment, which has been shown to improve patient survival and/or to classify patients as complete responders.[16,35] Alternatively, a negative biopsy (i.e., no tumor) on second-look operation does not exclude or diminish the possibility of recurrence.[35,36] Moreover, there appears to be no advantage from a second-look operation in patients with a complete clinical response determined radiographically.

Surgical Treatment for Recurrent Disease

Despite the successes of primary therapy for RMS, survival after relapse remains very poor. Approximately 30% of RMS patients will experience relapse, and between 50% and 95% of these will die of progressive disease.[37] Factors associated with a better prognosis in recurrent disease include embryonal/botryoid histology and stage or group I disease.[5] In a large review of relapsed RMS patients from IRS-III, IRS-IV pilot, and IRS-IV studies (n = 605), 95% of all failures occurred within 3 years from treatment initiation.[37] Patterns of relapse were as follows: local, 35%; regional, 16%; distant, 41%; and unknown, 8%. Overall, the median survival time from first recurrence or progression was 0.8 year, and the estimated 5-year survival after recurrence was 17%. Factors in this study associated with overall higher survival after relapse included botryoid histology and initial clinical group I assignment. For embryonal RMS, local recurrence predicted improved survival compared with those with regional or distant recurrences. Unfortunately, this review did not report data regarding the effect of surgical therapy at the time of relapse on outcome. RMS patients with local relapse compose a very challenging patient population, and the results of repeated attempts at surgical resection are not fully known. Many RMS patients with locally recurrent disease are those with primary tumors of the extremities, pelvis, retroperitoneum, and other sites at which repeated surgical procedures are difficult. Such patients often require aggressive and often mutilating procedures (e.g., amputation, pelvic exenteration).

The IRSG recommends that patients with locally recurrent disease be treated according to risk stratification. For more favorably rated relapse patients, intensive multiagent chemotherapy is given, followed by radiation therapy, surgical treatment or both, when feasible.[37] For less favorably rated patients, initial dose-intensified chemotherapy and maintenance therapy with agents such as etoposide or experimental therapies may be offered. In a smaller study of RMS and NRSTS patients with first relapse (n = 44), repeated surgical resection appeared to benefit survival with embryonal RMS but not with alveolar RMS or other soft tissue sarcoma histologic subtypes.[38] A retrospective review of patients treated at MD Anderson Cancer Center for recurrent RMS over an 11-year period (n = 32) demonstrated a 37% disease-free survival (mean follow-up period of 4.9 years). Morbidity was 35%, and the percentage of operations considered aggressive was 52%. Several factors present in survivors included embryonal/botryoid histology and RMS of vaginal/paratesticular origin. Factors associated with those who died included alveolar histology and extremity and bladder/prostate disease. No carefully reviewed data are available at this time from which to make definitive surgical recommendations for patients with recurrent/relapsed RMS. Results from the Cooperative Weichteilsarkom Studiengruppe identified certain factors that may predict relapse. Three hundred thirty-seven of 1164 patients initially determined to be in remission at the end of initial therapy for RMS were analyzed to identify particular factors that predict relapse.[39] Factors identified included increased age, histology (alveolar), tumor size (>5 cm) and site, stage after surgery, and lack of radiation therapy.[40]

Surgical Treatment for Metastatic Rhabdomyosarcoma

Approximately 15% of RMS patients are first seen with metastatic disease, most commonly involving lung (39%), bone marrow (32%), lymph nodes (30%), bones (27%), or other sites. The 3-year overall survival for 129 metastatic RMS patients enrolled in IRS-IV was 39% with an FFS of 25%. In this cohort of patients, 24% had metastases isolated to the lung. The surgical management of these patients is typically restricted to biopsy to confirm the diagnosis, followed by intensive multimodality therapy in an attempt to salvage these patients. In the most recent review of metastatic RMS patients from IRS-IV, survival did not differ between patients who underwent operation and histologic confirmation of lung metastases and those diagnosed radiologically only. The value of aggressive resection of RMS pulmonary metastases has not been extensively studied, primarily because of the rarity of these patients. For other soft tissue sarcomas in children and adults, aggressive resection of isolated pulmonary metastases is thought to be beneficial for prolonged survival.[41,42]

SITE-SPECIFIC SURGICAL GUIDELINES

Head/Neck Tumors

Nonparameningeal orbital and other head and neck RMS tumors are considered favorable sites and are classified as stage 1, regardless of size or nodal status. Surgical therapy for orbital and other deep-seated head and neck RMS tumors is largely restricted to biopsy followed by adjuvant chemotherapy and radiation therapy (Fig. 72-3) (except for small lid lesions, in which

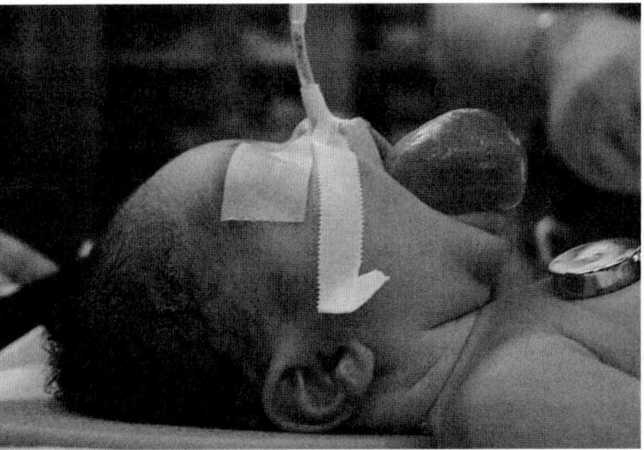

Figure 72-3. This neonate was born with this large tongue mass. Biopsy showed it to be a rhabdomyosarcoma. Tracheostomy was done to protect his airway, and gastrostomy was performed for enteral alimentation. The patient has required numerous debulking procedures in addition to chemotherapy.

wide local excision may be feasible). Parameningeal tumors have slightly poorer prognosis due to the presence of abundant lymphatics and the tendency for delayed diagnosis because these lesions tend to be somewhat hidden in presentation (as opposed to orbital RMS). Previously, extensive mutilating operations were performed. However, with more effective systemic therapy, these operations are rarely indicated and essentially never used for primary therapy. Metastatic disease to regional nodes is present in less than 3% of cases.[25] Unless there is clinical evidence of lymph node involvement, routine nodal sampling is not warranted. As discussed earlier, recurrent disease portends a much poorer prognosis. Thus, an aggressive surgical approach may be justified. Additionally, surgical intervention may be warranted when there is evidence of persistent disease after adjuvant therapy. These tumors are optimally managed by oncologic otolaryngologists and neurosurgeons, when needed. More superficial lesions, such as parotid tumors, may benefit from primary surgical resection especially when wide surgical excision is feasible (Fig. 72-4).

Tumors of the Extremities

Extremity RMS constitutes 15% to 20% of all pediatric RMS.[16,42] These tumors are considered to be in an unfavorable site and are classified as stage 2 if smaller than 5 cm and N0, or as stage 3 if greater than or equal to 5 cm or N1 status. In IRS-IV, the median age of these patients was 6 years. Most (71%) had alveolar histology, and more than 60% were classified as clinical group III or IV.[12]

Surgical evaluation of extremity RMS includes magnetic resonance imaging (MRI) and careful physical examination to determine tumor size and involvement of surrounding structures. For primary tumors smaller than 5 cm, depending on anatomic location, complete resection is the goal. The exact required surgical margin remains a matter of debate. The standard 2-cm margins are not always practical in children.

Moreover, there is no clear evidence that a larger margin decreases the chance of recurrence. After distortion of the tissues associated with resection and histopathologic processing, this actual "pathologic margin" is usually smaller. This should be taken into consideration during the operation.[44] Unfortunately, only a minority of extremity RMS patients (31 [22%] of 139 patients in IRS-IV) could be treated with complete primary surgical resection with negative margins.[12]

For patients with larger tumors, or those in unfavorable anatomic sites (e.g., popliteal or antecubital fossae or the groin), an initial incisional biopsy is recommended. The biopsy incision should be oriented longitudinally (i.e., along the long axis of the limb) so that it does not interfere with a later attempt at resection. An incisional biopsy has an increased likelihood of providing the definitive diagnosis and also provides tissue for ongoing biology studies, as compared with fine-needle or cone biopsies. After intensive multiagent chemotherapy and possibly radiation therapy, a second-look operation can be planned to resect residual disease.

A high rate of regional lymph node involvement is found with extremity RMS. Therefore, evaluation of the regional lymph drainage basin (axillary nodes in upper extremity disease, and femoral triangle nodes in lower extremity disease) is mandatory, even if there is not evidence of clinically apparent nodal disease.[16] In IRS-IV, approximately 40% of all extremity RMS patients had positive regional lymph nodes.[12] Of 139 patients overall, only 76 actually underwent surgical lymph node evaluation, and 50% of these were positive. An additional 13 patients had regional node disease diagnosed by imaging alone. Among patients with negative imaging and physical examination, but who underwent surgical evaluation of nodal status, 17% were actually positive. This implies that some patients with negative imaging who did not undergo surgical lymph node evaluation probably had undetected positive lymph nodes. Lymph node disease status is a critical component of the preoperative staging classification scheme (see Table 72-2) and has a direct impact on the treatment plan. Undetected positive nodal disease will lead to inaccurate staging and perhaps less than optimal treatment.

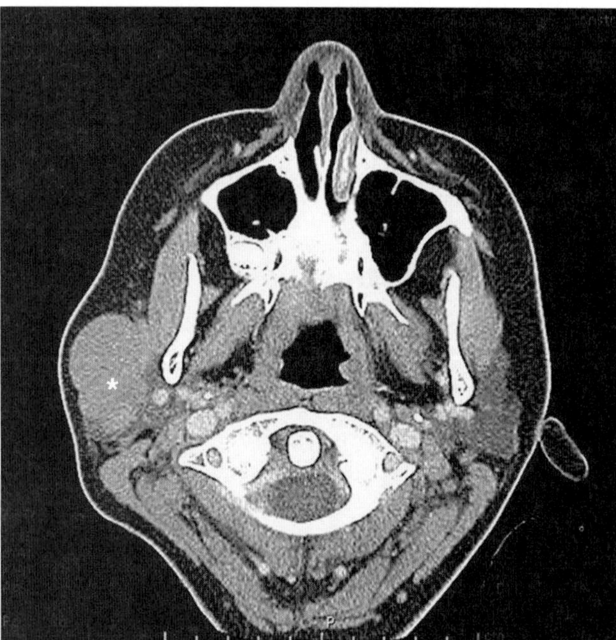

Figure 72-4. A 13-year-old presented with a large right parotid mass. CT scan shows the large mass (*asterisk*) in the right parotid gland. The patient underwent total parotidectomy and tolerated the operation well. However, metastatic disease subsequently developed.

Survival with multimodality therapy now approaches 75%, with a significantly lower rate for patients with nodal disease.[16] As reviewed previously, for extremity RMS with microscopically positive or indeterminant margins, or after an initial resection was performed for presumed benign disease, PRE is recommended and has been shown to improve survival.[30]

Genitourinary Tumors

Within the genitourinary system, RMS can arise from the vagina, vulva, uterus, paratesticular region, prostate, or bladder. Rarely, the kidney or ureter may be involved. In the IRS-IV study, genitourinary RMS accounted for 12% of all patients and more than 30% of nonmetastatic tumor patients, with bladder/prostate genitourinary primary tumors occurring most commonly.[42]

Bladder/Prostate Tumors

For these deep-seated tumors, the surgical approach is usually limited to initial biopsy. Other surgical approaches, including internal ureteral stents and/or percutaneous nephrostomy tubes, may be necessary in the presence of urinary obstruction. Suprapubic catheters are generally not advised secondary to risk of seeding the tract with tumor.[44] Historically, aggressive initial surgical resection was performed with good local control rates but with significant morbidity and low bladder salvage rates. Currently, bladder salvage is a primary goal with these patients. In selected cases in which the primary tumor involves only the dome of the bladder, complete initial resection may be feasible. However, for most bladder and prostate tumors, the primary therapy is chemotherapy and radiation therapy, followed by a more limited and conservative resection.[45] The rate of exenterative cystectomy with current approaches is approximately 30% (Figs. 72-5 and 72-6).[46-48] Even in those patients in which bladder salvage is possible, a significant percentage of patients may have bladder dysfunction.[16] It is difficult to determine the exact number of patients affected with postresection urinary dysfunction because most studies do not use urodynamics to assess this complication.[44]

For these tumors, careful consideration should be given to the type of initial biopsy. Often, laparotomy with open biopsy can be avoided, and alternative techniques such as transurethral cystoscopic needle biopsy, image-guided core needle biopsy, laparoscopic exploration with needle biopsy, or others can help to reduce morbidity.[49]

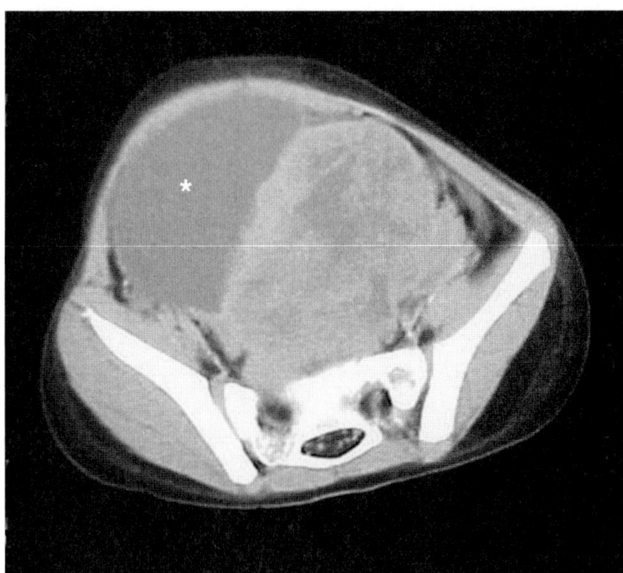

Figure 72-5. This CT scan shows a large mass emanating from the pelvis. Biopsy confirmed this mass to be a rhabdomyosarcoma. The bladder has been marked with an *asterisk.*

The estimated 5-year FFS with genitourinary nonbladder/prostate tumors is approximately 80%, indicating a favorable outcome with the conservative surgical approach.[1] If, however, these tumors fail to respond well to primary chemotherapy, as determined by surveillance imaging, a role exists for aggressive tumor resection, including anterior or total pelvic exenteration if needed to achieve local control.

Vagina, Vulva, or Uterus

These tumors are usually embryonal or botryoid histologic subtype (Fig. 72-7) and are considered to be in a favorable site (stage 1), with an overall 5-year survival rate of more than 80%.[50] Current recommendations are to perform an initial biopsy, often transvaginally, and to rely on effective primary chemotherapy. The need for complete surgical excision is rare. There is no role for initial aggressive resection such as vaginectomy or hysterectomy.[51] These patients are then best followed with routine abdominal and pelvic MRI (rather than computed tomography [CT]) to document tumor response.[52,53] A second-look operation with cystoscopy and re-biopsy is common. Lymph node involvement is uncommon. As with other pelvic RMS, relapsed or persistent disease in the vagina, vulva, and uterus is associated with a very poor outcome. In such cases, aggressive attempts at local control including radiation therapy (external-beam therapy or brachytherapy), partial or total vaginectomy, hysterectomy, or pelvic exenteration are all viable options. Unless there is direct involvement of the ovary by advanced/recurrent disease, there is no role for oophorectomy.

Paratesticular Tumors

Paratesticular RMS were found in 14% of all IRS-IV study patients.[42] Only 5% of these patients were clinical group IV after the initial surgical intervention. This is considered a favorable site, with all paratesticular patients classified preoperatively as having stage 1 disease regardless of tumor size, invasiveness, or lymph node status. The overall FFS rate for paratesticular RMS is more than 80%, with patients younger than 10 years having approximately 90% FFS.[1]

The recommended initial surgical approach for paratesticular tumors is radical orchiectomy with proximal ligation of the spermatic cord at the internal inguinal ring via an inguinal incision. A transscrotal incision for biopsy or resection is contraindicated. When done, a subsequent hemiscrotectomy may be required to resect the contaminated tumor bed. Meticulous surgical technique is extremely important. Tumor spillage upstages patients to clinical group IIa regardless of the completeness of resection.[54] When paratesticular tumors are fixed to the scrotal skin or invade the overlying scrotal skin, hemiscrotectomy is indicated. With this surgical approach, 90% to 95% of patients are able to have complete resection (groups I or II).[32]

Paratesticular RMS has a high incidence (~30%) of regional spread to the retroperitoneal lymph nodes

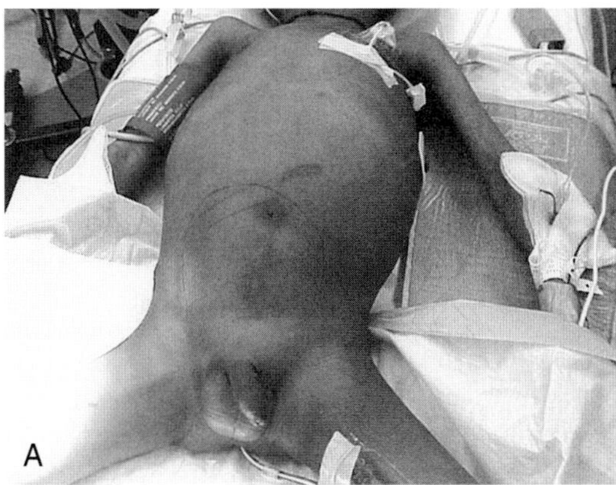

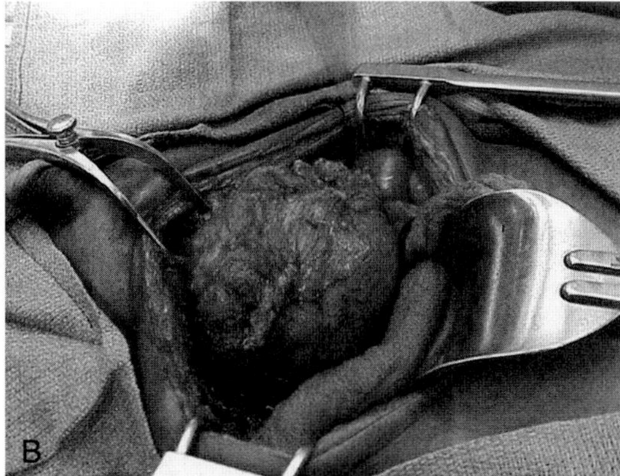

Figure 72-6. This patient's CT scan is seen in Figure 72-5. **A,** The patient presented with lower abdominal distention and a large mass that was palpable. **B,** The mass (visualized in the operative photograph) was not responsive to chemotherapy, and an attempt at complete resection was made. Most, but not all, of the mass could be excised. The patient eventually died of metastatic disease.

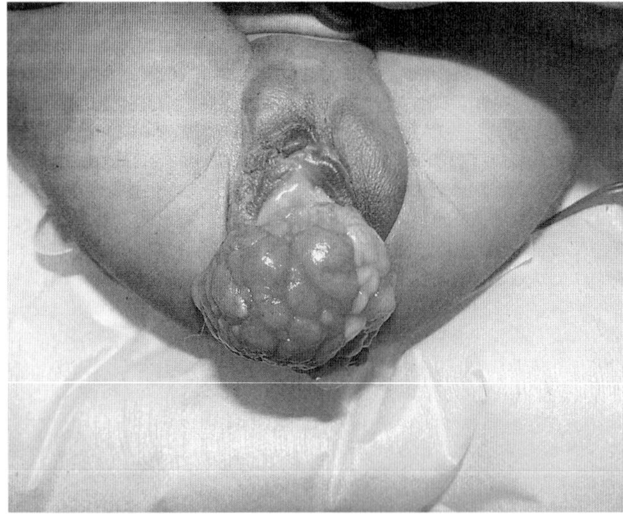

Figure 72-7. This neonate was born with this protruding mass from her vagina. Biopsy of the mass showed rhabdomyosarcoma. She underwent chemotherapy and has recovered uneventfully. Rhabdomyosarcoma of the vagina has been termed *sarcoma botryoides.*

(RPLNs). Therefore, careful evaluation of these nodes is an important part of the surgical staging workup for these patients. All patients should have thin-cut (3.8 to 5.0 mm) abdominal and pelvic CT scans to assess the retroperitoneum. Because the outcome with paratesticular RMS has been shown to be partially age dependent, as has the frequency of RPLN positivity, the treatment guidelines also vary by age.

Current recommendations for RPLN evaluation are as follows: For patients younger than 10 years, clinical group I, and with no lymph node enlargement on CT scan, no RPLN dissection or sampling is recommended. These patients are then followed with repeated CT scans every 3 months. For patients with suggestive or positive CT scans, ipsilateral retroperitoneal dissection is recommended and further therapy depends on the pathologic LN status. For all patients 10 years or older, ipsilateral RPLN dissection is recommended up to the level of the renal hilum. In this procedure, a systematic approach is used to remove lymph nodes from each station from the internal inguinal ring, along the iliac vessels and aorta, up to the renal hilum. This risk-based application of surgical RPLN evaluation is meant to ensure that underestimation of the extent of disease is minimized but also that only the higher-risk patients are exposed to these invasive surgical procedures. It is apparent in multiple studies and in multiple RMS tumor sites that CT misses 15% to 20% of patients who actually have involved lymph nodes, which are subsequently identified with surgical removal and histologic examination.[12,14,55] RPLN dissection is associated with significant morbidity, including loss of ejaculatory function and lower extremity lymphedema.[56]

RPLNs are somewhat controversial in the management of paratesticular RMS. The International Society of Pediatric Oncology (SIOP) de-emphasizes RPLN surgical evaluation, and discourages RPLN dissection, yet reports similar favorable survival rates.[57] SIOP investigators concluded that avoidance of RPLN dissection might underestimate the extent of disease in a few patients but that this does not compromise survival. Moreover, these investigators believe that avoiding this surgical intervention with known complications helps to reduce the overall morbidity burden to the patient. Additionally, SIOP investigators and others have also reported that hemiscrotectomy may not be required when a prior scrotal approach has been used, although all cooperative groups strongly recommend an initial inguinal approach.[57,58]

Other Sites

RMSs occurring in other sites are rare. However, when they do occur, they can present unique challenges to both pediatric surgeons and oncologists. Tumors arising in the trunk (paraspinal, thoracic or chest wall, including pleura, lung, or heart as a primary site), abdominal wall, intra-abdominal (including biliary), and/or pelvic/retroperitoneal areas (including perineum/perianal) were found in approximately 12% of all IRS-IV patients.[42] For truncal tumors, primary surgical resection is the preferred initial approach for tumors smaller than 5 cm in patients in whom a negative operative margin can be realistically anticipated. For larger primary tumors, initial incisional biopsy is preferred. There is a higher incidence of alveolar subtype RMS in truncal RMS, which has a worse prognosis than other sites. Additionally, especially with larger tumors, postoperative reconstructive procedures may be necessary.[16] Paraspinal masses need to be differentiated from extraosseous Ewing's sarcoma. Because of the rarity of these tumors, no data are available from which to make definitive surgical guidelines regarding regional lymph node evaluation. For many truncal lesions, the primary lymphatic drainage basin can be equivocal and preoperative lymphoscintigraphy may be helpful.

Retroperitoneal and nongenitourinary pelvic tumors are among the most difficult to manage because of the relatively "hidden" location and subsequent late presentation. More than 90% of these patients are first seen as clinical group III (gross residual disease with biopsy or attempted resection) or IV (metastatic disease) with large, invasive tumors.[43] The preferred surgical approach for these patients is generally initial biopsy, aggressive multiple-agent chemotherapy, radiation therapy, and second-look operation, if indicated. The role for debulking large retroperitoneal or nongenitourinary pelvic tumors is not entirely clear. Adding to this controversy is the finding that the subset of retroperitoneal/nongenitourinary pelvic RMS patients, with embryonal tumors who had debulking surgical procedures in IRS-IV or IV-pilot (1984 to 1991), had an improved 4-year FFS versus similar patients who underwent biopsy only (72% vs. 48%; P = .03).[59] Additionally, in IRS-IV patients (1991 to 1997) with localized retroperitoneal/pelvic RMS, debulking of 50% of the tumor prior to initiation of chemotherapy was found to reflect positively on outcome (5-year survival rate of 75% and FFS rate of 70%).[60] These findings should be viewed as preliminary data rather

Table 72-4 IRSG Study vs. Risk-Based Protocol Assignment

Risk (Protocol)	Stage	Group	Site*	Size†	Age (yr)	Histology	Metastasis	Nodes	Treatment
Low, subgroup A (D9602)	1	I	Favorable	a or b	<21	EMB	M0	N0	VA
	1	II	Favorable	a or b	<21	EMB	M0	N0	VA + XRT
	1	III	Orbit only	a or b	<21	EMB	M0	M0	VA + XRT
	2	I	Unfavorable	a	<21	EMB	M0	N0 or Nx	VA
Low, subgroup B (D9602)	1	II	Favorable	a or b	<21	EMB	M0	N1	VAC + XRT
	1	III	Orbit only	a or b	<21	EMB	M0	N1	VAC + XRT
	1	III	Favorable (excluding orbit)	a or b	<21	EMB	M0	N0 or N1 or Nx	VAC + XRT
	2	II	Unfavorable	a	<21	EMB	M0	N0 or Nx	VAC + XRT
	3	I or II	Unfavorable	a	<21	EMB	M0	N1	VAC (+XRT, Gp II)
	3	I or II	Unfavorable	b	<21	EMB	M0	N0 or N1 or Nx	VAC (+XRT, Gp II)
Intermediate (D9803)	2	III	Unfavorable	a	<21	EMB	M0	N0 or Nx	VAC ± Topo + XRT
	3	III	Unfavorable	a	<21	EMB	M0	N1	VAC ± Topo + XRT
	3	III	Unfavorable	b	<21	EMB	M0	N0 or N1 or Nx	VAC ± Topo + XRT
	1 or 2 or 3	I or II or II	Favorable or unfavorable	a or b	<21	ALV/UDS	M0	N0 or N1 or Nx	VAC ± Topo + XRT
	4	I or II or III or IV	Favorable or unfavorable	a or b	<10	EMB	M1	N0 or N1 or Nx	VAC ± Topo + XRT
High (D9802)	4	IV	Favorable or unfavorable	a or b	10	EMB	M1	N0 or N1 or Nx	CPT-11, VAC + XRT
	4	IV	Favorable or unfavorable	a or b	<21	ALV/UDS	M1	N0 or N1 or Nx	CPT-11, VAC + XRT

*Favorable, orbit/eyelid, head and neck (excluding parameningeal), genitourinary (not bladder or prostate), and biliary tract; unfavorable, bladder, prostate, extremity, parameningeal, trunk, retroperitoneal, pelvis, other.

†a, tumor size < 5 cm in diameter; b, tumor size ≥ 5 cm in diameter.

EMB, embryonal, botryoid, or spindle cell rhabdomyosarcomas or extomesenchymomas with embryonal RMS; ALV, alveolar rhabdomyosarcomas or ectomesenchymomas with alveolar RMS; UDS, undifferentiated sarcomas; N0, regional nodes clinically not involved; N1, regional nodes clinically involved; Nx, node status unknown; VAC, vincristine, dactinomycin (actinomycin D), cyclophosphamide; XRT, radiotherapy; Topo, topotecan; Gp, group; CPT-11, irinotecan.

than a recommendation for routine debulking of large retroperitoneal or pelvic tumors.

Biliary RMS generally has a good prognosis without the need for aggressive surgical resection. Most patients have the botryoid variant of embryonal RMS that responds well to chemotherapy. Biopsy followed by neoadjuvant chemotherapy frequently results in resolution of symptoms, including jaundice. Surgical intervention is fraught with complications, including the inability to resect all disease in most cases and infections associated with external biliary drains.[61]

Perineal and perianal RMSs also are rare sites that have an overall poor outcome at least in part because of late presentation.[62] From 1972 to 1997, 71 patients had perineal and perianal tumors, with a 5-year FFS rate of 45%.[14] Important surgical issues for these patients are (1) more than one third of patients are seen initially with presumed benign disease (usually infections); (2) approximately 50% have regional nodal disease, which adversely affects survival; and (3) primary re-excision frequently lowers the clinical group assignment, which improves outcome.[14]

CURRENT/FUTURE RESEARCH

The ongoing IRS-V study is divided into separate protocols for patients categorized into various risk strata or categories (Table 72-4). Low-risk patients (D9602 protocol) are estimated to have 3-year FFS rates of 88%, based on previous studies.[63] This subgroup is limited to patients with localized embryonal, botryoid, or spindle cell tumors. In general, these patients receive either VAC (vincristine, dactinomycin [actinomycin D], cyclophosphamide) or VA (vincristine, actinomycin D) chemotherapy and radiation therapy to residual tumor with resection.

Intermediate-risk patients (D9803 protocol) have a predicted FFS rate of 55% to 76% and include those with localized alveolar or undifferentiated sarcoma, stages 1 to 3; embryonal RMS stages 2 and 3 with gross residual disease; or stage 4 embryonal RMS patients younger than 10 years. In IRS-V, these patients are randomized to VAC and radiation therapy or VAC alternating with vincristine, topotecan, and cyclophosphamide and radiation therapy.

High-risk patients (D9802 protocol) have a 3-year FFS of less than 30% and include stage 4 alveolar or undifferentiated tumors and embryonal RMS patients older than 10 years. In general, these patients receive up-front chemotherapy with irinotecan followed by VAC and radiation therapy. For patients responding to irinotecan, treatment continues with four additional cycles of irinotecan and vincristine, in addition to VAC.

An important component of ongoing IRS studies is the investigation of the biology of these tumors. This aspect of the care of RMS patients must be emphasized. Its success hinges on full participation by pediatric surgeons and oncologists. All newly diagnosed or relapsed RMS patients should be considered for enrollment in ongoing biology study protocols. The surgeon should facilitate the submission of fresh tumor specimens as well as peripheral blood and bone marrow when indicated, so that continued improvements in the care of these children can be realized.

section 8

SKIN AND SOFT TISSUE DISEASES

chapter 73

NEVUS AND MELANOMA

Arlet G. Kurkchubasche, MD • Thomas F. Tracy Jr., MD

There is an increasing awareness of the importance of pigmented lesions in infants and children. Referrals for evaluation and management of pigmented skin lesions represent a significant component of the outpatient pediatric surgical experience. Also, with the increased incidence of melanoma and limited options for treatment of melanoma, early diagnosis and surgical management must adhere to the guidelines established by the American Joint Committee on Cancer (AJCC).[1]

EMBRYOLOGY AND ANATOMY OF MELANOCYTIC LESIONS

The terminology used for the description of pigmented cutaneous lesions is often confusing. Therefore, a basic understanding of the epithelial anatomy and physiology is essential to the clinical identification and correct classification of these lesions. Figures 73-1 and 73-2 depict the basic anatomy of the epidermis and dermis.

The melanocyte is a dendritic cell and neural crest derivative (Fig. 73-3). During development, the melanocyte precursors (melanoblasts) migrate to the dermis, hair follicles, leptomeninges, uveal tract, and retina. After the eighth week of development, they migrate from the dermis to the epidermis. Failure of migration results in congenital nevi and a variety of dermal melanoses, which can be considered hamartomatous lesions because they represent normal tissues in an abnormal location. Melanocytes normally reside in the basal layer of the epidermis as a single cell associated with a group of keratinocytes. Melanin is transferred in storage granules referred to as melanosomes through the dendritic arm and is internalized by the keratinocytes, which then migrate through the layers of the skin. Nevus cells are derived from melanocytes or their precursors and distinguish themselves by (1) the absence of dendrites, (2) the clustering of cells, (3) their variable location within the dermis and epidermis, and (4) their variable content of melanin. In contrast to the congenital nevi that result from failure of migration of melanocytes from the dermis to the epidermis, acquired nevi are proliferative lesions and represent benign neoplasms of the skin located within the epidermis or dermis (or both).

The term *macule* refers to a circumscribed, pigmented lesion, less than 5 mm in diameter without elevation or depression from the surrounding skin, whereas a *patch* refers to a larger area of involvement without palpable characteristics. *Papules* represent solid elevated lesions less than 5 mm in diameter, and *plaques* are raised lesions larger than 5 mm. *Nodules* arise from the dermis or subcutaneous tissues. Dermal *melanoses* are pigmented lesions resulting from the deposit of melanin in melanophages, from free melanin in the dermis, or in dermal melanocytes. *Melanocytosis* refers to an increased number of melanocytes.

The epidermis consists of multiple layers, commencing with the basal layer that is the site of mitotic activity leading to the proliferation of keratinocytes. This basal layer consists of columnar cells anchored to the basement membrane via hemidesmosomes and anchored in the dermis via penetrating fibrils (see Fig. 73-1). Interspersed between the basal cells are melanocytes, which morphologically are dendritic cells and the source of melanin (see Fig. 73-2). These cells are not secured via desmosomes or tonofilaments. There are functional units (epidermal melanin units) composed of a melanocyte and the keratinocytes that are responsible for the transfer of melanin, which ultimately results in the pigmentation of the skin. The differentiation in racial pigmentation is not based on numbers of melanocytes but instead on the variable production of melanosomes and their content and rate of degradation. Melanosomes are cytoplasmic organelles that result from the fusion of vesicles containing tyrosinase and vesicles containing structural melanosomal proteins, both of which are generated by the endoplasmic reticulum of the melanocyte. Patients with albinism lack tyrosinase, which is essential for making melanin. These melanosomes are transferred from the perinuclear area along microtubules to the dendritic tips, where these are phagocytosed by the keratinocyte. As the squamous cells differentiate, the melanosomes are degraded by lysosomal enzymes. The prickle cell layer is the next histologic layer and site of Langerhans cells, which are bone marrow–derived dendritic cells, akin to macrophages, and have antigen-presenting capacity.

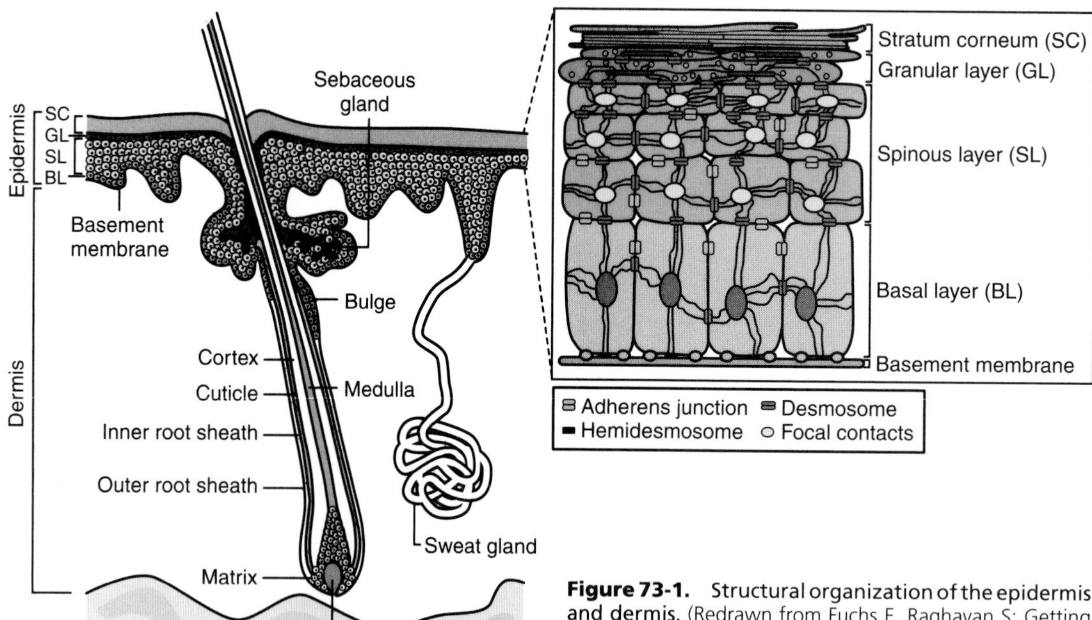

Figure 73-1. Structural organization of the epidermis and dermis. (Redrawn from Fuchs E, Raghavan S: Getting under the skin of epidermal morphogenesis. Nat Rev Genet 3:199-209, 2002.)

With further differentiation, the keratinocytes become flattened and form the granular cell layer distinguished by the presence of keratohyaline granules. These granules become the source of the fibrous protein keratin and lamellar granules (Odland bodies), which contain lipids and enzymes and are secreted into the intercellular spaces forming the cement between the epidermal cells and keratinocytes. The outermost layer is the stratum corneum or horny layer composed of devitalized keratinocytes (see Fig. 73-1).

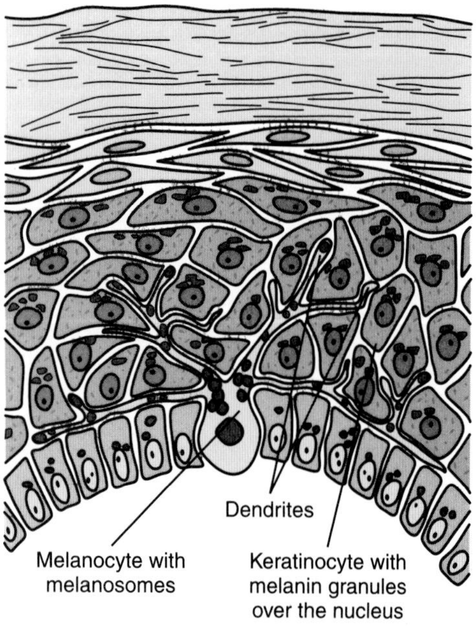

Figure 73-2. The melanocyte rests within the basal layer of the epidermis and is associated with a group of keratinocytes to which it delivers the melanosomes. (Redrawn from Gray J: The World of Skin Care. Available at http://www.pg.com/science/skincare/Skin_tws_16.htm.)

CLASSIFICATION OF NEVI

Nevi can be grossly categorized as pigmented and nonpigmented skin lesions. The basis of their designation rests on whether melanocytes are involved in the disorder, and the classification actually distinguishes between epidermal and melanocytic nevi.

Epidermal nevi refer to nonmelanocytic lesions that result from proliferation of components of the epidermis and encompass a number of variants based on the involvement of adnexal structures such as sebaceous glands, hair follicles, and apocrine glands. When large or extensive, they may be associated with important ocular, neurologic, and musculoskeletal conditions. These skin lesions must be recognized as clinically benign. However, with the hormone-induced changes during puberty, there is an association of nevus sebaceous with benign tumors as well as basal cell carcinoma.

Melanocytic nevi (also known as nonepidermal nevi or dermal nevi) can be classified according to whether they involve disorders of melanocyte migration or proliferation. These lesions are most commonly categorized based on age at presentation as either congenital or acquired (Fig. 73-4). Congenital melanocytic nevi (CMN) result from failure of embryologic migration of the melanocyte precursors and form hamartomatous lesions that are evident at birth, which may evolve over time. Acquired melanocytic nevi are the result of benign proliferative disorders of nevi (melanocytic derivatives) and, therefore, constitute neoplasms.

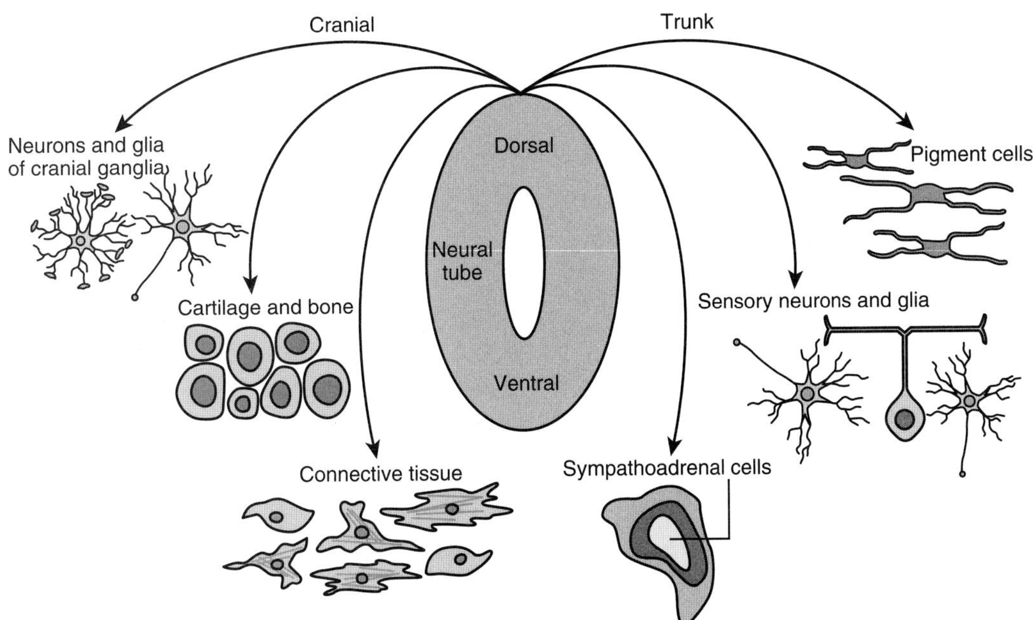

Figure 73-3. The neural crest derivation of these dendritic cells explains the association of melanocytic disorders with CNS, bony, and ophthalmic disorders. (Redrawn from www.nature.com/nrg/journal/v3/n6/images/nrg819-i1.jpg.)

They have a tendency to increase in number during childhood, adolescence, and early adulthood but then spontaneously regress with age. To identify those lesions presenting a risk for malignant degeneration, these two groups are further stratified according to the size of the lesion. The two subsets, which require greatest clinical vigilance, are (1) the giant congenital melanocytic nevi and (2) the atypical acquired nevi.

An alternate classification scheme for melanocytic nevi focuses on the relationship between the physical and histologic features of the lesion. This results in a stratification based on where the nevus resides in relation to the epidermal-dermal junction (Table 73-1). This system avoids the diagnostic reliance on an often inexact recollection of when a nevus first appeared in infancy or childhood. In this scheme, both congenital and acquired nevi can be described as being (1) junctional (situated at the junction of the epidermis/dermis), (2) compound (involving both regions), or (3) dermal (confined to the dermis). These are generic histologic terms and do not imply biologic behavior. Although this schema allows for classification of all congenital and acquired nevi, some nevi are sufficiently clinically distinct to retain specific descriptive or eponymous names. These warrant individual discussion because it is their features that may prompt referral for biopsy to exclude malignancy. Examples of these lesions include the blue nevus, Spitz nevus, and halo nevus.

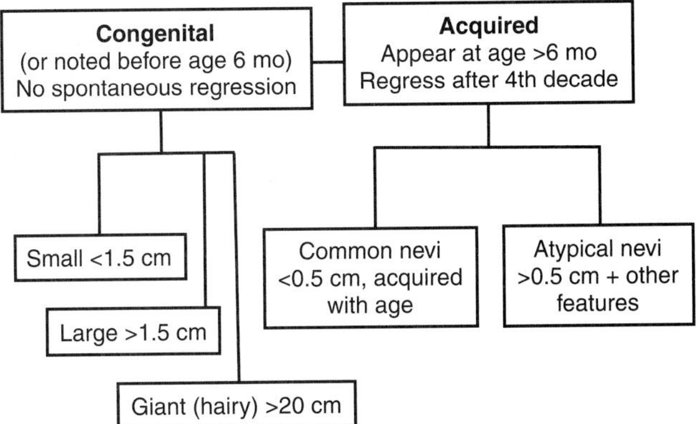

Figure 73-4. Pigmented lesions are classified based on their age at appearance and further stratified by size and other physical features to yield two subsets that require close monitoring of the patient for the development of melanoma.

NONMELANOCYTIC NEVI

Epidermal Nevi

Epidermal nevi are skin lesions not associated with the proliferation of melanocytes. Instead, these represent congenital hamartomas of ectodermal origin that are classified based on their hyperplastic element (Table 73-2). Keratinocytic lesions involve the epidermal layer only, whereas the organoid lesions involve the sebaceous, apocrine, eccrine, and follicular structures. They are clinically distinct and appear as raised, pigmented, velvety to wart-like proliferations of the dermis along dermatomal distributions. Lesions are usually apparent in infancy, but some may appear in later childhood. The incidence in newborns is estimated to be 0.3%. The most common sites involved are the scalp, face, trunk, and proximal extremities. Often a hairless patch is noted on the scalp, or a raised linear yellow-tan to orange plaque is evident on the face or trunk during infancy. With age and the hormonal changes during puberty, these lesions change in appearance and become verrucous or develop more coarse hair growth.

Table 73-1 Clinical and Histologic Features of Melanocytic Nevi

	Junctional	Compound	Dermal
Histologic Location	Junction of epidermis and dermis	Involving both dermis and junctional region	Involving dermis only
Configuration	Flat, round-oval, symmetric	Raised, become more elevated with age	Protuberant, dome shaped, pedunculated
Surface	Smooth, hairless	Smooth to verrucous, may have hair	Smooth to verrucous
Pigmentation	Uniform dark brown to black	Flesh colored or brown, may have uniform distribution of darker spots, may develop halo	Flesh colored, tan to pink, may have halo or telangiectases

AJCC, American Joint Committee on Cancer
*Only in the presence of ulceration or reticular dermal invasion.

A number of syndromes are associated with these epidermal nevi, particularly when they are large or extensive. The epidermal nevus syndromes typically involve abnormalities of the central nervous system, ocular system, and skeletal system. While the classification of these lesions and syndromes remains based on clinical findings, advances in molecular biology suggest that these disorders are based on genomic mosaicism and that future biologic classification will become possible.[2] The common variants of epidermal nevi (see Table 73-2) include:

- Nevus sebaceous (Fig. 73-5), which represent 50% of the epidermal nevi
- Keratinocytic nevi
- Nevus comedonicus (Fig. 73-6)
- Inflammatory linear verrucous nevus
- Linear Cowden nevus
- Becker's nevus (pigmented hairy epidermal nevus)

These lesions are associated with a risk for transformation. Whereas syringocystadenoma papilliferum is the most likely benign neoplasm identified, basal cell carcinoma, squamous cell carcinoma, and keratoacanthoma are known to be primarily associated with nevus sebaceous after puberty. Recommendations for excision are based on this natural history.

MELANOCYTIC NEVI

Congenital Melanocytic Nevi

CMN are variable-size pigmented lesions that present during the first few months of life. These lesions grow proportionally with the infant and are generally categorized as small (<1.5 cm), medium (1.5-20 cm), and large (>20 cm). Those especially large lesions (>40 cm

Table 73-2 Characteristics of Epidermal Nevus Variants

Primary Name	Other Names	Cutaneous Features	Histologic Features	Other Features or Associations
Linear sebaceous nevus (LSN)	Nevus sebaceous, organoid nevus, Jadassohn nevus, phakomatosis	Yellowish orange plaque, affects scalp and face, hairless, 2-3 cm diameter	Epidermal, follicular, sebaceous and apocrine abnormalities	Epidermal nevus syndrome with seizures, CNS and ocular anomalies
Linear nevus comedonicus (NC)	Comedone nevus, nevus follicularis	Firm dark papules that look like comedones in linear pattern	Keratin-plugged hair follicles	Cataracts, variable CNS and bony defects (e.g., scoliosis, fused vertebrae, spina bifida occulta, absent fifth finger)
Linear epidermal nevus (LEN)	Nonorganoid epidermal nevus	Verrucous, nonerythematous, nonpruritic hyperkeratosis	Keratinocytic changes only	Significant involvement of other organ systems, neurodevelopmental delay, seizures, movement disorders
Inflammatory linear verrucous epidermal nevus (ILVEN)	Psoriasiform hyperplasia	Linear persistent pruritic plaque, usually on limb, tends to coalesce as linear formation	Inflammatory infiltrate, hyperkeratosis	Pruritic, female predominance 4:1, uncommon musculoskeletal associations
Linear Cowden nevus	Nonorganoid epidermal nevus	Thick linear lesion	Papillomatous	Cowden disease (germline *PTEN* mutation)

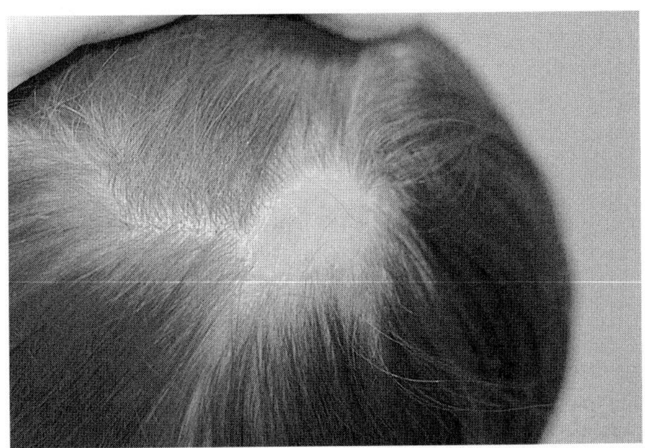

Figure 73-5. This young child has the classic appearance of a nevus sebaceous, which is a solitary yellow-orange plaque on the scalp. These lesions are well circumscribed, hairless, oval to round, and usually less than 2 to 3 cm in diameter.

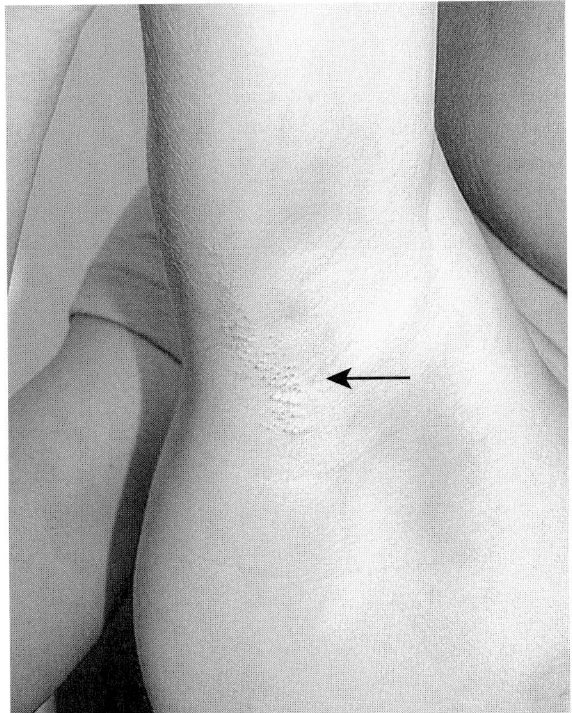

Figure 73-6. In the right axilla of this 5-year-old is a nevus comedonicus (*arrow*). This lesion is a well-circumscribed plaque that is composed of keratin-plugged hair follicles. It was present at birth and has been slowly enlarging.

in final diameter) are also referred to as garment nevus, giant hairy nevus, or bathing trunk nevus because they tend to cover large truncal areas in confluence (Fig. 73-7). Although the pigmentation and surface are initially uniform and flat, the lesions evolve into thick, dark, and often hair-covered lesions.

Histologically, the melanocytic cells in CMN are located deeper than those in acquired nevi (Fig. 73-8). The melanocytic cells can be contained (1) in the lower two thirds of the dermis, (2) between collagen bundles, or (3) in the lower two thirds of the reticular dermis or subcutis and associated with appendages, nerves, and vessels. The absence of superficial involvement may explain why transformation is often not noticed until late in its development. The incidence of transformation is greatest in the large or giant congenital nevi and low in small to medium-sized lesions.

Excision of small and medium-sized CMN can be delayed or avoided in favor of lifelong medical observation, because transformation is presumed not to occur in the prepubertal years. Biopsy may be of value in stratifying the risk of malignant degeneration. If histologic examination shows the more superficial variant, continued observation is warranted because any transformation is likely to be associated with epidermal changes that will be apparent on close follow-up or meticulous self-examination. If the histologic variant demonstrates deep melanocytes, then prophylactic excision is warranted. The estimated lifetime risk of melanoma in small to medium-sized CMN is estimated at 1% and most often occurs after puberty.

The management of large or giant CMN is more controversial. The melanoma risk for these lesions is increased and estimated to be 5% to 10% over a lifetime, with 50% of this risk during the first 5 years of life.[3,4] The highest risk lesions in this group are associated with the nevus that is situated over the posterior trunk (see Fig. 73-7), greater than 40 cm in maximal dimension, and associated with satellite nevi. Melanoma in these patients can arise from the deep dermal layer or even originate from sites distant from the skin, such as the central nervous system or retroperitoneum.[4] These patients are at risk for development of other soft tissue malignancies such as rhabdomyosarcoma or neurofibrosarcoma (peripheral nerve sheath tumor).[5] They are also at risk for neurocutaneous melanosis and central nervous system malformations such as Dandy-Walker malformation, defects of the vertebra, and skull and intraspinal lipomas. In these patients, screening magnetic resonance imaging (MRI) of the brain and spinal cord is recommended during the first 6 months of life. Two thirds of patients with neurocutaneous melanosis have giant CMN, and the others have multiple non-giant lesions. The prognosis for patients with symptomatic neurocutaneous melanosis is extremely poor even in the absence of malignancy.[6]

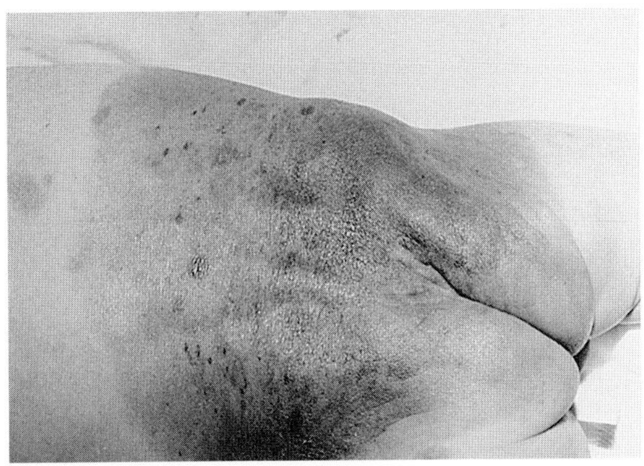

Figure 73-7. Giant congenital melanocytic nevus (garment nevus) of the back and buttock in a neonate.

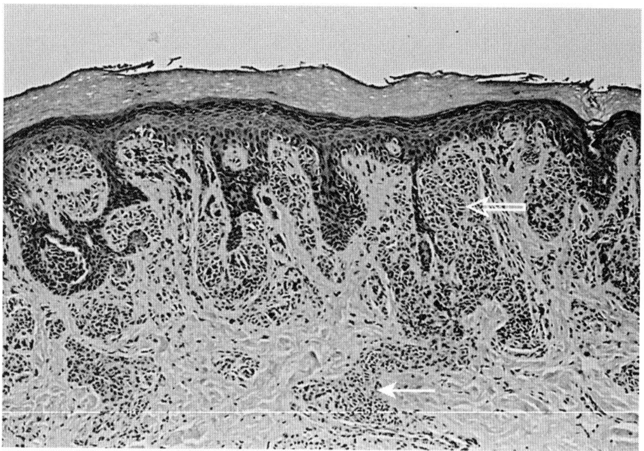

Figure 73-8. Congenital melanocytic nevus is characterized by nevus cells extending from the dermal-epidermal junction (*open arrow*) along skin appendage structures into the deep dermis (*solid arrow*).

Because operative resection of these extensive lesions is often not feasible and never completely eliminates the risk for development of melanoma, these patients must have close expert surveillance. Areas of epidermal change within the nevus should be sampled. However, caution must be exercised in interpreting the histologic results, because evidence suggests that proliferative nodules may resemble melanoma but behave in a benign manner.[7] Features useful in differentiating cellular nodules from melanoma include (1) lack of high-grade uniform cellular atypia, (2) lack of necrosis within the nodule, (3) rarity of mitoses, (4) evidence of maturation, (5) lack of pagetoid spread, and (6) no destructive expansile growth.[8]

Speckled lentiginous nevi are probably variants of CMN because they frequently present in early infancy. These nevi are evaluated and treated with the same level of concern as would be warranted for congenital nevi of similar size. A variable number of black, brown, or red-brown macules and papules are seen within a usually oval patch of tan-to-brown hyperpigmentation, which is generally 3 to 6 cm in diameter.

Common Acquired Nevi

Common acquired nevi are benign neoplasms of the skin, which appear after 6 months of age and persist through the fourth decade after which they may disappear. They are most frequently located on sun-exposed areas and are rare on the breast or buttock. Common to all these acquired nevi is that they are less than 6 to 8 mm in diameter, symmetric, with a homogeneous surface with even pigmentation and a regular outline with a sharply demarcated border. On close inspection, they may have some pigmentary stippling.

Histologically, these acquired nevi are subdivided into subtypes based on the location of the nests of nevus cells and this feature corresponds with certain clinical findings (see Table 73-1). *Junctional nevi* tend to be flat with brown to black pigmentation, and the nevus cells are located at the dermal-epidermal junction. When the nevus cells extend from the junction into the dermis, the lesion is described as a *compound nevus*. Clinically this corresponds to a lesion that is slightly raised and pigmented brown to black.

When the nevus cells migrate completely into the dermis, the lesion is an *intradermal nevus*, which is raised and typically not pigmented. In general, the deeper the nests of nevus cells, the more raised and less pigmented the lesion (i.e., dark flat lesions vs. raised tan lesions). The temporal evolutionary path of nevi was originally described by Stegmaier and explains the clinical observations of progressive change within individual nevi or their resolution.[9] New nevi tended to be small and flat (junctional) and either develop a raised profile or disappear with time as a consequence of fibrosis. In one study, when the nevi on adolescents were followed over a 4-year period, it was demonstrated that there was a net increase of 50% in total number of nevi despite complete regression of 15% of the nevi.[10] This demonstrates the degree of active turnover in individual patients. Freckling and lighter-colored skin are associated with increased numbers of nevi. In darker-skinned individuals, nevi also develop, but with a different distribution usually found on the palms and soles, unlike in individuals with a more fair complexion.

Sun exposure during childhood, especially when it is intense, intermittent, and not necessarily associated with sunburn, is a promoter for nevus development and the major environmental factor associated with the risk of melanoma. Recent evidence suggests that sunscreen use has led to a false sense of security in that it provides incomplete protection to ultraviolet (UV) rays. Sunscreen use alone does not provide sufficient protection, and expanded public health education must focus on the avoidance of midday sun and use of physical barriers such as UV protectant clothing and hats.[11-13]

The role for excision of these commonly acquired lesions is limited when they are clearly defined by their age at presentation and the features described in Table 73-1. The natural evolution and changes on these common lesions should not be mistaken for malignant progression.

Atypical Nevi

Atypical nevi, previously referred to as dysplastic nevi or Clark's nevi, are common lesions occurring in as much as 5% of the population. They may occur either in a familial pattern or sporadically. The onset of their first appearance is principally during adolescence on the sun-exposed areas of skin, and they continue to increase in number and size with age. Unlike the common acquired nevi, these lesions are usually larger than 5 mm (up to 15 mm) and have an irregular surface ranging from completely flat to flat with a raised center resembling a fried egg (Fig. 73-9). The pigmentation usually is dark and irregular, and the border of the lesion is often irregular as well. These lesions are most common in individuals with light skin and hair

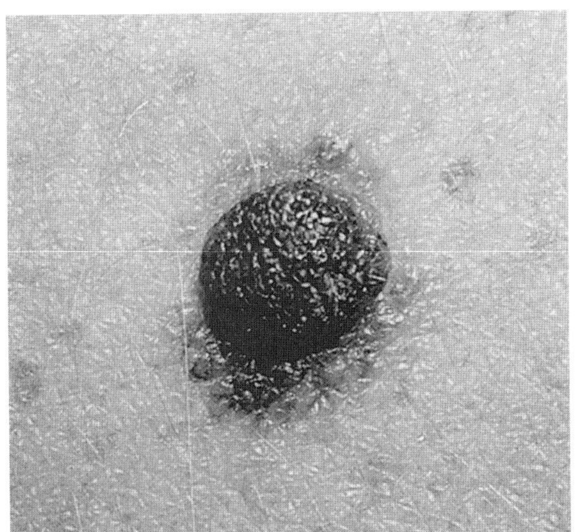

Figure 73-9. Clark's nevus (dysplastic nevus) with "fried egg" appearance.

color. UV light has been implicated in the transformation of melanocytes in these nevi.

When a patient has multiple atypical nevi or moles, they may be diagnosed with the atypical mole syndrome. While it can be normal to have up to 10 to 20 moles, people with this syndrome may have in excess of 100 moles. Individuals with 50 to 100 moles and one or more first or second-degree relatives with melanoma are considered to have the familial atypical mole and melanoma (FAMM) syndrome that identifies them at significant increased risk for the development of melanoma, which may approach 100%. The melanoma lesion may arise de novo on any part of the body and not necessarily from a preexisting atypical lesion. Simple excision of an atypical nevus therefore does not obviate the patient from close dermatologic follow-up. In families with the atypical mole syndrome, nevi arising on the scalp can be an early predictor to the atypical mole syndrome, although the scalp nevus itself may involute with time. The moles in these individuals tend to be similar in appearance, the corollary being that a new nevus that varies in appearance or location should be regarded with suspicion. The ability of nonclinicians to identify the "ugly duckling" has been found to be reliable.[14]

Atypical nevi are not necessarily removed to confirm the histologic pattern of atypia but should be sampled when the differential diagnosis includes melanoma. The biopsy specimen should encompass a 1- to 2-mm rim of normal tissue and be sufficiently deep to allow for assessment of depth of invasion in the event that melanoma is identified. The original designation of dysplastic nevus has been replaced with the term *atypical nevus,* and the pathologic description should use the term *nevus with architectural disorder* and indicate the extent of cytologic atypia. The concordance between clinically atypical nevi and the histologic findings of dysplasia is poor. Newer adjuncts to clinical examination such as dermatoscopy (epiluminescence microscopy) may assist the clinician in the future in determining which lesions require excisional biopsy. These lesions are at the heart of much of the unfortunate controversy and misinformation that surrounds patients and referring physicians with terms and descriptions of atypia and dysplasia. These descriptive features have prompted inappropriate re-excision of some lesions and sentinel lymph node biopsy for a completely benign process. Expert dermatopathologic review, as discussed in the following sections, is essential for achieving the highest standard of care.

Specific Congenital or Acquired Melanocytic Lesions Requiring Distinction from Melanoma

Several melanocytic lesions and nevi are discussed separately owing to their unique features, which frequently prompt their evaluation for malignancy. These lesions can be congenital or acquired and can be described in terms of their junctional, compound, or dermal location. A recent review by Schaffer provides some practical advice regarding these specific lesions.[11]

Halo nevi (Sutton's nevi) are unique lesions that appear between 6 and 15 years of age and are typically located on the trunk or extremities. They appear as round or oval lesions with a central area of pigmentation that may be tan to brown and is surrounded by a rim of depigmentation (Fig. 73-10). Histologically, the central nevus is usually a compound or dermal nevus surrounded by a uniform infiltrate of T lymphocytes. Pigmentation may come and go, and the role for excision is limited to those that develop atypical characteristics within the pigmented lesion itself. There is no association with malignancy, and these nevi only cause clinical suspicion because regressing melanoma may be gray or white.

A *blue nevus* is a benign proliferation of dendritic dermal melanocytes. The etiology is attributed to a dermal arrest in embryonic migration of neural crest melanocytes that fail to reach the epidermis, creating a hamartoma (normal cells in an abnormal location).

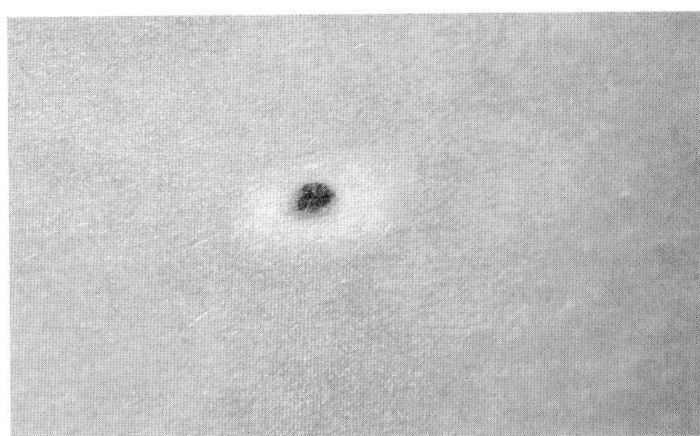

Figure 73-10. The classic appearance of a halo nevus. These small pigmented lesions are surrounded by a rim of hypopigmentation. They are typically seen in adolescents and are most commonly located over the trunk, especially on the back. Treatment is usually not needed unless the pigmented portion of the halo nevus appears atypical. In that case, excision of the entire lesion, including the halo, is recommended.

This is a lesion with large amounts of pigment within the dermis, resulting in absorption of the longer wavelengths of light and scattering of blue light known as the Tyndall effect. Two variants of blue nevi are distinguished based on size: (1) the common blue nevus, which is usually less than 5 mm, and (2) the cellular blue nevus, which measures 1 to 3 cm.

The *common blue nevus* appears in adolescence and is most often located on the head and neck, the sacrum, and the dorsal aspect of the hands and feet. These lesions are usually nodular, given their dermal location, and can be mistaken for nodular melanoma, except that there will be no history of rapid ongoing growth. Dermatoscopy shows a uniform blue-gray pigment profile that helps distinguish blue nevus from melanoma.

The *cellular blue nevus* is usually 1 to 3 cm in diameter and presents on the scalp, buttock, sacrum, and face. It may be congenital or acquired. Histologically, it is located within the deep (reticular) dermis and is a well-demarcated nodule. Cellular lesions may have occasional mitoses, but significant atypia and necrosis are absent. A potential for malignant degeneration exists only in the cellular lesions and is clinically heralded by an increase in size and ulceration.

The presence of multiple blue nevi should prompt consideration for the Carney complex of myxomas, spotty pigmentation, and endocrine neoplasia. The persistence of extensive *dermal melanoses* such as those found in mongolian spots, especially when in a ventral distribution, should prompt evaluation for lysosomal storage diseases such as Hurler's syndrome and GM_1 gangliosidosis.

Spitz nevi are raised, often light or nonpigmented lesions (light tan-red or reddish brown) that appear dome shaped with either a smooth or a verrucous surface (Fig. 73-11). Typically, these lesions are compound nevi, although pure junctional and pure dermal variants exist as well. Dermatoscopic examination shows a starburst pattern (Fig. 73-12). These lesions tend to occur on the face or lower extremities and measure 0.3 to 1.5 cm in diameter. There is a slight female predominance, with 50% of these occurring in children younger than 10 years of age and 70% in those younger than 20 years of age. The increased red coloration is in part due to increased vascularity, with telangiectasia in the superficial dermis. The vascular

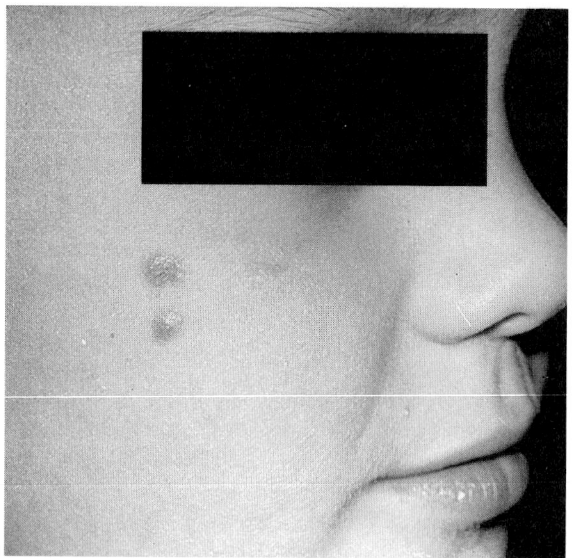

Figure 73-11. Two Spitz nevi on the face.

surface features explain why these lesions are more prone to bleeding with minimal trauma.

The pigmented variant of the Spitz nevus is known as a nevus of Reed and typically occurs on the leg of a young woman. The appearance of Spitz nevi may be quite sudden, prompting the concern for potential melanoma. Spitz nevi were previously classified as "benign juvenile melanoma," a misnomer that was responsible for the misconception that pediatric melanoma was less aggressive than the adult melanoma counterpart. Most Spitz nevi are completely benign. However, atypical clinical features such as a diameter greater than 1 cm, asymmetry, or ulceration should prompt a complete excision. Most often, a young patient who has undergone a shave biopsy is referred for complete excision of the lesion so that it may be fully evaluated by a dermatopathologist.

The histologic features of Spitz nevi can be complex, but they generally are reassuring in that the lesion is uniform and symmetric. The junctional nests of melanocytes have few or no mitoses. The nevus includes spindle cells and large epithelioid cells in variable architectural arrangements; thus, prior designations have included the "spindle and epithelioid cell nevus." Multinucleated cells may be present but should not

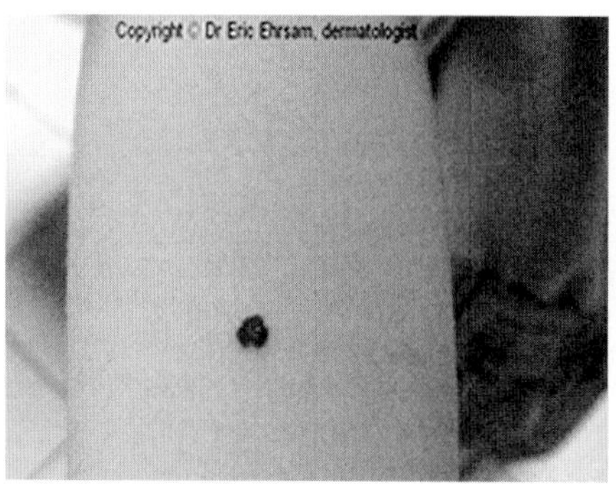

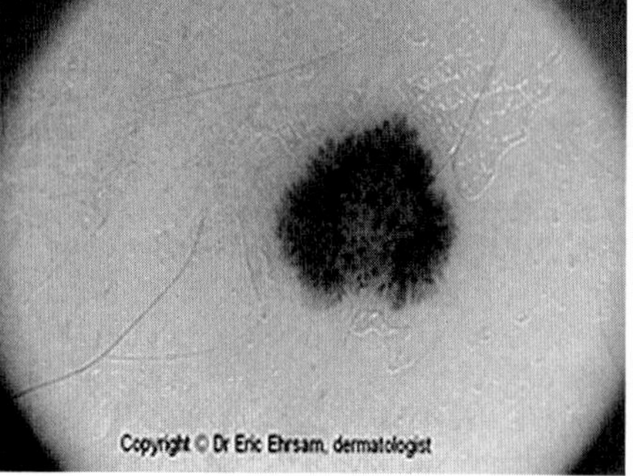

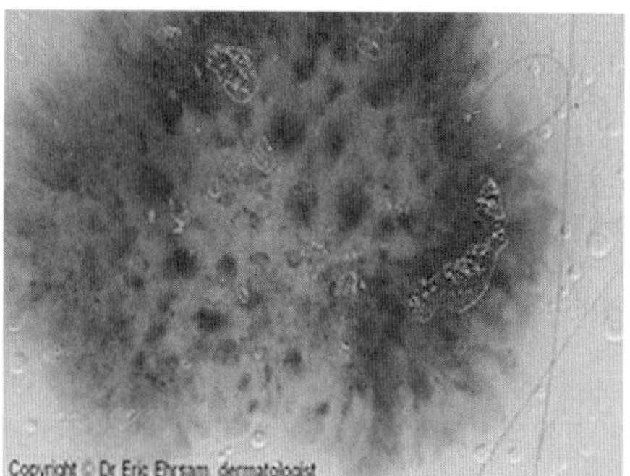

Figure 73-12. This patient has a Spitz nevus on her arm. Dermatoscopic examination shows a classic starburst pattern. (Photographs courtesy of Dr. Eric Ehrsam. Reprinted with permission.)

exhibit much pleomorphism. Nucleoli are often prominent and rounded. Some of these features in another clinical context could be reminiscent of melanoma, which requires that these lesions be evaluated by dermatopathologists with significant experience in all of the elements of this variant. Those Spitz lesions with unusual histologic features should be excised completely.

In approximately 10% of all cases, histologic features within these lesions do not permit distinction of a Spitz nevus from melanoma. These atypical Spitz nevi then become diagnostic and treatment dilemmas. In these complicated instances, one might consider the safest course of action would be to treat the lesion as equivalent to a melanoma of the same depth. Although some have advocated sentinel lymph node biopsy (SLNB) as a diagnostic tool to identify metastasizing Spitz nevi and classify them as melanoma, this approach has been strongly criticized as being unnecessarily invasive for the limited information gained. In the limited numbers of patients who have undergone SLNB and were then treated with radical lymph node dissection (RLND) and chemotherapeutic agents, there has been no recurrence of disease. This is not consistent with the normal course of "metastatic melanoma" as discussed later. The current biologic and clinical evidence demonstrates that the presence of melanocytic lymphoid infiltrate does not predict clinical behavior and may not identify metastasis or even malignancy as it does for melanoma.[15]

The *nevus of Ito* and *nevus of Ota* are congenital dermal melanocytic disorders that develop because of incomplete migration of melanocytes resulting in hamartomatous lesions. Both of these lesions are most commonly found in Asian populations. In the case of the nevus of Ota, the lesion appears along the distribution of the ophthalmic and maxillary branches of the trigeminal nerve on the face and is evident as a blue-gray patch. These nevi may also involve the ocular and mucosal surfaces. The nevus of Ito involves pigmentation over the shoulder area and is often associated with a nevus of Ota. The pigmentation becomes more prominent with age and may be amenable to laser therapy.[16] Although melanoma has been reported to arise infrequently in the nevus of Ota, the association with glaucoma must be recognized and lead to ophthalmologic referral.[17]

Nevi Occurring at Special Sites

Acral nevi are found on the palms and soles. They may have linear streaks, but if they have mottled pigmentation and are greater than 7 mm, they must be viewed with suspicion.[18] Longitudinal melanonychia are pigmented streaks emanating from the nail matrix and can be a normal variant that is most frequently seen in darker-skinned individuals. Dark bands and those lesions wider than 6 mm, associated with nail dystrophy or extending beyond the nail fold, should be sampled to exclude melanoma.[19,20] Labial melanotic macules are benign lesions on the lower lip of women that resemble freckles but do not darken with sun exposure. However, lesions in the oral cavity must be taken seriously and evaluated.[21] In young women presenting with melanotic lesions over the vulvar area, caution must be applied to not overtreat these generally benign lesions.[22]

PRACTICAL CONSIDERATIONS FOR EXCISION OR BIOPSY OF MELANOCYTIC LESIONS

The many major and minor differences in the clinical and pathologic features for the benign lesions presented thus far have led to understandable confusion about the role for excision of these lesions in infants and children. Pressure for excision from families and pediatricians is often significant and may be based on important but vague family histories of "skin cancer" despite the fact that the vast majority of those family experiences are not with melanoma. Once referred to a pediatric surgeon, many patients and families expect that a procedure will be performed rather than the start of what may be a period of observation and collaborative consultation with dermatologists and pediatricians. Before the referral, the patients are often not informed about the relative risks and benefits of excision for a young group of patients who may require anesthesia or conscious sedation. Scarring is unpredictable and should not be acceptable in the presence of a benign lesion that does not have cosmetic consequences and has no future transformation potential. The natural evolution of acquired lesions and the changes that occur with age, puberty, and exposure to UV radiation need to be taken into account. Moreover, clinical judgment and experience should guide decisions for resection. Simple considerations such as scalp pliability and the tolerance for suture or staple removal from large scalp lesions should be considered and possibly delay the resection of a large nevus sebaceous until after early puberty when this lesion first demonstrates any potential for transformation. On the other hand, one cannot overlook the dangers of transformation during the first 5 years in infants with giant congenital nevi. Staged resections and tension-relieving incisional techniques must be considered as well as the use of important techniques such as tissue expansion and rotational flaps that may be required for the best functional and cosmetic outcome. We have therefore established only general guidelines for our practice for excisional management of congenital and acquired lesions (Table 73-3).

CMN and speckled lentiginous nevi are treated by excision in a similar manner based on the size of lesion. Lesions greater than 20 cm may develop malignant transformation early and warrant consideration for excision at an early age. With a lifetime risk of melanoma at 1%, smaller and intermediate lesions must be monitored closely. Elective resection may be indicated after puberty based on a predicted later onset of potential transformation in those lesions greater than 5 cm. Complicated head

Table 73-3 General Guidelines for Excision of Congenital and Acquired Lesions

Type of Lesion	Age at Presentation, Site	Configuration, Size, Surface	Pigmentation	Biopsy Indication
Common acquired	After age 6 mo	Small (<5 mm) flat	Brown-black	None
Atypical nevus	Usually adolescence; sun-exposed areas	Irregular, 5-15 mm Uneven, maculopapular "fried egg"	Uneven, dark	Acute change*
Blue nevus	Any time; on scalp, dorsum of hands/feet	Nodular, <5 mm smooth	Dark gray to blue-black	None
Cellular blue nevus	Scalp, sacrum, buttock, face	5-15 mm	Dark gray to blue-black	Acute change*
Spitz nevus	Face, lower extremities	Dome shaped, 5-15 mm, smooth to warty	Light tan to pink, telangiectasia	Acute change*
Halo nevus	6-15 yr; back	Central nevus with halo of depigmentation, flat to slightly raised	Area of depigmentation	Acute change in center of lesion*
Becker's nevus	Adolescent male; shoulder	Variable shape, flat	Brown macule or patch of hair	Acute change*

*Based on clinical behavior.

and neck lesions present significant challenges that require a number of surgical considerations and applications.

Perhaps the greatest potential for misdirected concern remains with acquired melanocytic nevi. For the common nevi that are less than 5 mm, there are no evidence-based indications for excision. Atypical nevi defined as larger lesions (5-15 mm) with an irregular surface and a dark, irregular pigmentation warrant excision when physical changes suggest melanoma and not for prevention of transformative changes. Patients with the atypical nevus syndrome or FAMM have the highest risk for malignant melanoma. They require continuous monitoring by the team of consulting physicians and surgeons and a low threshold for biopsy for lesions that appear different from their "usual" nevi (the "ugly duckling" sign).

Blue nevus lesions are common lesions without malignant potential. The cellular blue nevus variant that is greater than 1.0 cm requires a biopsy when ulceration and physical changes become evident. Similarly, the halo nevus has no indication for excision unless suspicious changes occur in the central nevus.

Spitz nevi are often the most worrisome lesions because they can often appear rapidly with dome-shaped firm lesions, simulating a nodular melanoma. These temporal and physical characteristics, along with their variable coloration, often prompt biopsy. Demonstration of epithelioid and spindle features, with or without atypia, after shave biopsy is a common reason for referral for complete excision with a 2-mm margin. With these lesions, expert pathologic review must be available to differentiate them from melanoma and to avoid SLNB, which has no role in these lesions in young patients.

Nonmelanocytic nevi are represented by epidermal nevus variants, which have no risk for transformation other than the nevus sebaceous at adolescence. We therefore recommend excision of sebaceous nevi before the teen years and when the patient is cooperative with the removal of sutures from the often large and augmented scalp closures that result from complete excisions.

PEDIATRIC MELANOMA

Melanoma remains a rare cancer in childhood, with children representing less than 2% of all patients with melanoma.[23] There has been a worldwide increase in the incidence of melanoma in adulthood with a doubling over a period of 25 years with age-standardized incidences now at 15/100,000/year and 22/100,000/year in men and women, respectively.[24] Melanoma in children has become more prevalent, but the rates of increase are not as dramatic and primarily affect the postpubertal age group. Current estimates are an annual incidence of 0.8/million in the first decade of life. The maximal rates reported are from Australia and New Zealand where melanoma affects 30/million in the 10- to 14-age group.[25] Regardless of geographic factors, these data are indicative of an increased lifetime risk of cutaneous melanoma of children born today (1/58) when compared to children born in 1980 (1/250).[26]

Fortunately, there has also been a leveling off in the mortality associated with melanoma. This has been attributed to improved early detection, with 90% of new diagnoses involving thin, less than 1-mm melanomas. Some of this improvement in early diagnosis can be linked to the use of expert dermoscopy[27] and computer-based dermoscopy in differentiating between small melanomas and atypical moles.[28] Evidence has shown that the melanoma risk is associated with fair complexion, the presence of freckles and moles, as well as intermittent intense sun exposure, even in the absence of severe sunburns. Careful clinical surveillance of patients with risk factors for the development of melanoma is important in all age groups. Among these risk factors, the atypical mole syndrome, FAMM, and large CMN remain the most important. The most important factor for the development of melanoma is the presence of melanocytic nevi, with an eightfold increase in relative risk for those with more than 100 moles. If someone has five or more atypical nevi, they have a nearly 50-fold risk of developing melanoma.[24] If there is a family history of melanoma, the incidence approaches 100%. Recent studies based on genetic analysis of families with mutations in the melanoma predisposition gene *CDKN2A* suggest that the FAMM syndrome has a 70% lifetime penetrance of melanoma with sun exposure and mutations in the melanocortin-1 receptor further impacting its development.[29,30]

It is critical to understand that even in these patients, most (80%) lesions arise de novo and not from preexisting lesions. For example, in a series of 33 prepubertal patients with melanoma, seven cases arose from CMN (not giant nevi), two from an acquired nevus, and 24 (73%) de novo.[23] Although heritable factors and pigment traits contribute to the development of nevi, the only controllable factor for melanoma is the environmental cumulative effects of sun exposure, which is best limited with physical barriers such as clothing and hats and avoidance of midday sun. The use of sunscreen appears to be principally effective in preventing sunburn, of which blistering sunburns during childhood and adolescence have been implicated in the development of melanoma.[12]

Specific Predisposing Conditions

The diagnosis of melanoma is made in children in several discrete clinical contexts. Congenital melanoma is the least common. It can be due to transplacental transmission or may arise from a primary cutaneous lesion. The appearance of any rapidly growing, ulcerating, or bleeding lesion in the newborn must be evaluated promptly. The incidence of this clinical scenario is so low that projections about outcome are difficult to make, but the prognosis is generally considered poor. However, there are reported instances of spontaneous regression. Moreover, the presence of micrometastases do not appear to impact survival.[7,31]

Melanoma associated with CMN has been well described (Fig. 73-13) and presents a unique set of clinical issues. The lifetime risk for development of melanoma in patients with CMN lesions is variably estimated between 5% and 40%.[32] More conservative estimates indicate a 5% to 10% lifetime risk, with half of this risk distributed within the first 5 years of life.[3,33] Two recent prospective studies of patients with giant CMN showed the incidence of melanoma during the first 5 years of life was between 3.3% and 4.5%.[32, 33] Those patients with a posterior axial giant CMN and numerous satellite lesions have the greatest risk[10] when compared with those with lesions restricted to the head and extremities. These tumors may originate from deep dermal sites and are often not readily apparent based on skin changes. Despite the sometimes ominous appearance of the satellite lesions, these have not been documented as the primary site for melanoma. Proliferative nodules within giant CMN often raise the

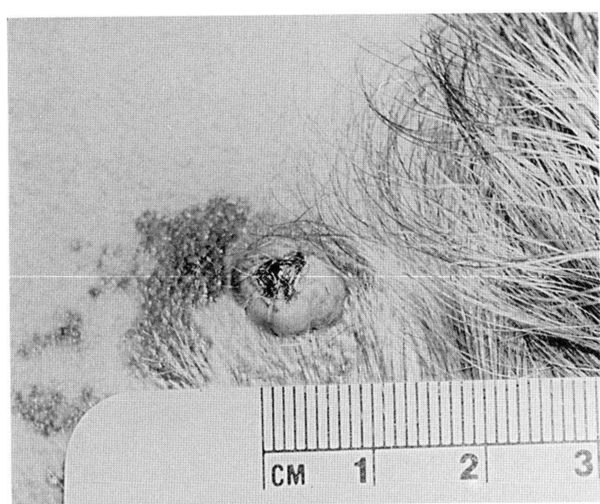

Figure 73-13. Congenital melanocytic nevus of the scalp with a melanoma arising from it (raised centrally pigmented lesion).

specter of malignancy, but numerous authors caution against hasty conclusions in this clinical scenario.[7,34] Neurocutaneous melanosis occurs in conjunction with the largest CMN and presents the opportunity for nonepithelial melanoma to occur. Although techniques for resection and reconstruction have improved such that disfiguring contour changes can be avoided with soft tissue transfers, these remain surgically challenging operations and there is no assurance of alleviation of this risk, despite full-thickness resection of the CMN. In contrast, the smallest (<1.5 cm) lesions are not clearly associated with any increased risk for melanoma. It is within the intermediate group that little data exist to help guide management. In the experience of Massachusetts General Hospital, CMN lesions up to 5 cm have not been associated with melanoma in patients younger than 20 years of age.[32] Illig and associates reported melanoma arising in CMN lesions less than 10 cm only after age 18 years.[35] Rhodes and Melski calculated a lifetime risk of 2.6% to 4.9% in persons with small CMN living to 60 years of age.[36]

While large and perhaps some intermediate CMN identify patients at risk for the development of melanoma, radical excisional therapy has been tempered by the recognition that cautious observation and selective biopsy present an alternative therapy, especially because the melanoma may arise from sites other than the CMN. When resectional therapy is considered, extensive preoperative planning allows for the optimal use of reconstructive techniques including the use of skin and tissue expanders and a variety of rotational flaps or free tissue transfers in addition to the standard use of skin grafts.

Other conditions predisposing to the development of melanoma include patients with the rare, inherited disorder xeroderma pigmentosum in whom the inability to repair UV-induced DNA damage results in a 2000-fold increased risk of skin cancer. Patients with heritable immunodeficiency syndromes are reported to have a threefold to sixfold increased risk. Pediatric patients on immunosuppression due to chemotherapy for childhood malignancies or solid organ transplantation experience an increase in total nevus counts and induction of atypical nevi. Although neonatal phototherapy for hyperbilirubinemia has been demonstrated to induce an increased number of nevi, it is uncertain whether this will escalate risk for future melanoma.[37] Despite our efforts to identify patients for screening, it is worthwhile to remember that 60% to 80% of malignant melanoma in children younger than 20 years occurs in the absence of known cutaneous risk factors for melanoma.[38]

Diagnosis

The difficulty in making the diagnosis of melanoma during childhood relates to a number of variables. The natural evolution of congenital and acquired nevi during childhood and adolescence often limits the use of criteria extrapolated from adult patients. There is limited value to the mnemonic ABCDE (Asymmetry, Border irregularity, Color variegation, lesion Diameter greater than 6 mm, and Evolution of a pigmented lesion; Fig. 73-14) because variegations and irregular shape are not infrequently associated with the atypical nevi. Specifically, the physical characteristics of giant CMN predispose to melanoma arising in the deep dermal layers and extending within the deep subcutaneous tissues, rather than becoming apparent as an epithelial change. Consequently, several authors have pointed out that childhood melanoma may present in a markedly different manner from the adult counterpart. In aggregate, these pediatric series indicate that recent growth, ulceration, or bleeding may be the most frequent presenting features. In contrast to the adult experience with diagnosis of thin (<1 mm) melanomas, pediatric melanomas are typically greater than 1.5 mm thick. This may be due to delays in diagnosis, a deeper origin within a CMN, and a higher incidence of nodular melanomas in children.[26] In a pediatric series of melanoma from St. Justine, Montreal, the most common presenting symptoms were recent growth, pain, ulceration, itching, bleeding, and change in color.[39] Three of 13 patients had lesions that resembled pyogenic granuloma. Only one patient presented with evidence of metastatic disease. Most of the melanomas were nodular (11/13), and only two were superficial spreading. The mean tumor thickness was 3.2 mm in this series.

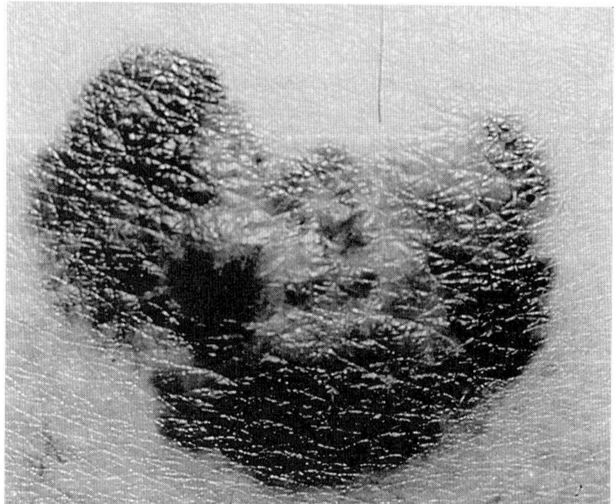

Figure 73-14. This malignant melanoma demonstrates some of the classic ABCD features for melanoma: *A*symmetry, *B*order irregularity, *C*olor variegation, and *D*iameter greater than 6 mm.

In another series, the clinical parameters that favor melanoma in children younger than age 12 years were found to be a rapid increase in size (55% of patients), bleeding (35%), or color change (23%) of a nodular lesion.[38] Less frequent signs or symptoms included a subcutaneous mass (6%), pruritus (15%), and enlargement of a regional lymph node (7%). In 7% of patients in whom a melanoma developed in association with a preexisting nevus, the patients had no clinical complaints.

A study of 33 prepubertal patients attempted to delineate the clinical features and outcomes of pediatric melanoma.[23] In this series, the sites of origin were most frequently the extremity (15 lesions), followed by trunk (10 lesions) and head or neck (8 lesions). Interestingly, about 14 of 28 patients had amelanotic lesions that were raised and resembled pyogenic granuloma. Superficial spreading (15 lesions) and the nodular subtypes (9 lesions) of melanoma were the most common lesions, and the median thickness was 2.5 mm.

The consistently thicker lesions in childhood melanoma suggest either a delay in diagnosis or reflect biologic characteristics, such as the propensity for nodular melanoma and for lesions arising from the deep dermal layers. These lesions unfortunately may be misdiagnosed initially. Only their sudden appearance and rapid growth over a few months may prompt biopsy. Therefore, despite the infrequency of this diagnosis, the pediatric clinician must consider melanoma in the differential diagnosis of cutaneous lesions.

The role of clinical dermatoscopy, computer dermatoscopy (digital epiluminescence microscopy), and even ultrasound imaging of the skin has been described for monitoring high-risk adult patients. However, there are no current reports focusing on the pediatric population.[27,40-42]

SURGICAL MANAGEMENT OF THE LESION SUSPECTED TO BE MELANOMA

Once a decision has been made to evaluate a lesion for possible malignancy, the aim is to accomplish this with the least negative impact on function and cosmesis. The clinical scenarios most often encountered are (1) a primary referral for excision of a suspicious lesion, (2) re-excision of a lesion that was previously incompletely excised and showed atypia, or (3) re-excision of a lesion with dysplastic and potentially malignant features.

In these instances, most young children benefit from excision under general anesthesia, which allows the surgeon to focus on achieving a full-thickness biopsy with an adequate margin. When the lesion is

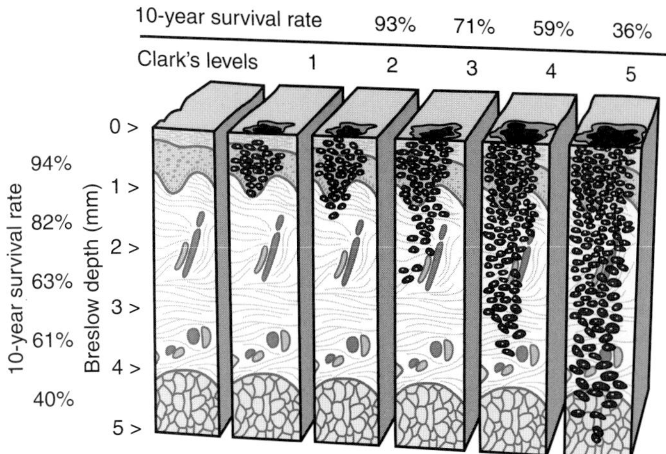

Figure 73-15. This drawing shows the 10-year survival rate for Clark and Breslow classification schemes. As is evident, excisional biopsy of lesions suspicious for melanoma must be full thickness to allow assessment of the Breslow level, which helps determine future therapy. (Redrawn from http://www.med-ars.it/various/livelli4.jpg. © 2001 Images by Med-Art.)

being excised for the first time or re-excised for atypia, it is reasonable to target a 1-to 2-mm circumferential margin. There are no prospective data to provide an evidence-based approach in this setting. In the setting of dysplastic changes or frank malignancy, the parameters set forth by the AJCC for melanoma should guide extent of margin based on the Breslow stage and Clark's level (Fig. 73-15). Sometimes a shave biopsy of such a lesion does not provide sufficient data and one should therefore plan an adequate excision that may require 1- to 2-cm margins. It is in these settings that a discussion must be held with the family regarding the consequences of resection and the option for proceeding with SLNB under the same anesthetic.

An assessment for the potential for primary closure must occur at the preoperative visit. Lesions over joints, on the distal extremities, and on the face require consideration of more advanced techniques, such as tension-relieving plastic operations, skin grafts, and rotational flaps. Despite the anxiety about a potential tumor, parents must understand that healing and scarring are unpredictable. The best results for achieving adequate margins are obtained by marking out and measuring the margins along the periphery of the lesion while it is in situ. The orientation of the incision depends on the site of the lesion and its relationship to the lines of Langer. Also, consideration should be given to the potential need for re-excision.

The deeper tissues can be excised with electrocautery to limit blood loss. Any suspicious lesion should be marked for orientation in the event that re-excision becomes necessary. Specimens should be submitted for permanent analysis. Frozen section examination has no role in this setting. Techniques for skin closure require consideration of the physical characteristics of the wound as well as the tolerance of the child for suture removal. The use of long-acting local anesthetic agents such as bupivacaine should be encouraged for postoperative analgesia in combination with appropriate oral medications. In the event of more extensive resections or resections across joints, the use of immobilizing splints should be considered.

In the presence of established malignancy, there is no doubt that a re-excision with margins is mandated. In the more common atypical nevus with dysplasia, the likelihood of malignant degeneration is low and therefore a conservative re-excision is advised. This topic is most heatedly debated in the context of a Spitz nevus with cellular atypia. Whereas most Spitz nevi can be histologically identified as benign lesions, many show atypical features that complicate their differentiation from melanoma. These histologically ambiguous melanocytic tumors have generated intense interest and controversy. A recent review provides an excellent perspective of these dermatopathologic controversies and has offered a well-designed proposal for the evaluation of pediatric patients with Spitz nevus–like melanocytic tumors when there is diagnostic controversy.[43] Expert review may lead to the recommendation for adjunct procedures, such as SLNB. The controversy regarding SNLB for all melanoma, owing to its failure to improve survival of melanoma patients across all stages, is even more dramatic in children. Whereas SLNB has been proposed as a means for differentiation between a benign and malignant lesion, it has limited effectiveness because the presence of melanocytic cells within a sentinel lymph node does not necessarily indicate the presence of metastasis. The features of the melanocytic cell and its location within the lymph node may indicate that these are benign nodal melanocytes that arrive at draining nodes by lymphatic migration or are formed in adjacent nodes during development. However, even the presence of "metastatic" cells in the sentinel lymph node does not appear to have the same biologic effect as it would in true melanoma because the frequency of recurrent disease is virtually absent in the scenario of Spitz nevi with cellular atypia.

The collective experience from organized cancer centers offering SNLB for Spitz nevi–like melanocytic tumors has shown that the rates of "positive nodes" range from 29% to 50%. With this significant number of lymph node–positive patients, one might expect the original diagnosis to have been melanoma and the clinical course to follow that of conventional melanomas. Yet, there have been no reported deaths of lymph node–positive patients with primary Spitz tumors. Although these findings underscore the irrelevance of SLNB, they do present some interesting speculations about the altered tumor biology of these melanocytic tumors in young patients. Expert dermatopathologists have developed a number of protocols to distinguish these nodal melanocytes from metastatic melanoma, but they contend that the characteristics of the original lesion are best used to arrive at an accurate diagnosis. There is no doubt that experts in defined reference laboratories must review the original tumor. As occurs in many difficult areas of experience and judgment, sporadic cases of metastases after Spitz lesions erode confidence and have had medicolegal implications.

If controversy persists, then fluorescence in situ hybridization (FISH) or comparative genomic hybridization should be performed and may lead to results that favor the diagnosis of either nevus or melanoma.[44] Again, the pediatric surgical community must be aware of the lack of correlation with survival for melanomas based on SLNB. It has been our experience that within our center and among the reference laboratories, significant controversy can still remain in a few cases. These are highly individualized cases in which the long-term follow-up will be most important, recalling that nodal melanocytes may not resolve the question for the family. The best clinical course would avoid the trap to perform SLNB or to falsely offer it as a clinical advantage in these difficult cases. SLNB is a procedure that currently adds unnecessary expense, pain, and discomfort and has no proven benefit for these fortunately rare scenarios.

When the diagnosis of melanoma is confirmed, staging and treatment protocols are derived from the adult literature. The recommendations for the extent of re-excision are based on the thickness of the tumor and generally require a 0.5-cm margin for in situ lesions, a margin of 1 cm for lesions up to 2 mm, and 2-cm margins for lesions greater than 2 mm in thickness. SLNB is advised for lesions thicker than 1 mm or for those between 0.76 mm and 1 mm with ulceration or reticular dermal invasion (Table 73-4). The new staging system of the AJCC is primarily based on (1) Breslow tumor thickness with 1, 2, and 4 mm indicating the current cutoffs for thin, intermediate, and thick lesions, respectively, and (2) histologic features such as ulceration, which is perhaps most important in the intermediate-thickness group. Clark levels are taken into account only in thin melanomas. Lymph node involvement is stratified by the number of nodes involved and whether microscopic or macroscopic metastases are present. Finally, three subgroups of distant metastases are distinguished: (1) skin and soft tissue, (2) lung, and (3) other visceral. Patients with visceral metastases have the worst prognosis. In this new classification, the serum marker lactate dehydrogenase is used to further stratify risk. If elevation of this marker is verified in the presence of either skin, soft tissue, or lung metastases, the prognosis is equivalent to that for those patients with visceral metastases.[1]

Table 73-4 AJCC Guidelines for Surgical Management of Melanoma

Lesion Depth	Margin (cm)	Sentinel Node Dissection
In situ	0.5	
<1 mm	1.0	
0.76-1.0 mm*	1.0	+
1-2 mm	1.0-2.0	+
>2 mm	2.0	+

AJCC, American Joint Committee on Cancer
*Only in the presence of ulceration or reticular dermal invasion.

The standard imaging techniques used to identify potential metastatic disease sites include computed tomography (CT), magnetic resonance imaging, and positron emission tomography (PET). Combined PET/CT has been approved for this use because it has been demonstrated to be particularly helpful in identifying developing metastases.[45] The limitations of PET continue to relate to lesion size. It cannot compete with lymph node biopsy in patients with nonpalpable lymph nodes.[46]

In adult melanoma therapy, SLNB has become a mandatory procedure in the current AJCC staging system to detect lymph node micrometastases. When the SLNB is positive, the recommendation is to proceed with an RLND. A negative SLNB, however, does not guarantee lack of distant spread. This algorithm protects against early locoregional recurrences, but it has not been shown to have an impact on overall survival. These protocols have been applied to pediatric patients with melanoma and atypical melanocytic tumors. In a review at the University of Colorado Health Sciences Center, 20 patients younger than 21 years of age underwent SLNB for melanoma or atypical nevi.[47] No complications occurred as a result of the SLNB, and results showed that positivity correlated with tumor thickness. Five of 15 patients with melanoma had a positive SLNB, as did 3 of 5 with melanocytic proliferation. Seven of 8 patients underwent completion lymph node dissection (one patient with blue cell nevus did not). Complications such as lymphedema and wound infection occurred with the completion lymphadenectomy in 4 patients.[47] When this was further explored in a subsequent study, the investigators found a higher incidence of positive SLNB in a group of patients younger than 20 years with either melanoma or melanocytic lesions (40%) as compared with a group of adults (18%).[48] None of the pediatric patients with a positive SLNB experienced a recurrence, whereas 25% of the adults did. These series and others suggest that although SLNB is feasible, it may not be of sufficient value or benefit to the patient.[49] Adjunct molecular techniques such as polymerase chain reaction assays for melanocytic enzymes such as tyrosinase or MART1 have not yet shown correlation with clinical outcomes.

Adjuvant therapies include chemotherapy, radiation therapy, and immunotherapy.[50] The use of cytotoxic agents has a limited role in current adjuvant therapy. Radiation therapy has limited applicability and is primarily reserved for palliation. Most active trials and current research focus on the use of immunomodulating agents, of which interleukin 2 (IL-2) and interferon alfa (IFN-α2b) are approved agents. In limited series, these agents have shown the ability to induce partial and even total remission. The use of high-dose IFN-α2b is limited to patients with tumors greater than 4 mm deep and/or lymph node metastases. There have been inconsistent reports as to the ability of pediatric patients to tolerate high-dose interferon regimens. While in one series no dose reduction was necessary,[51] it became necessary in 50% of patients in a second series.[52] Vaccines are also within the armamentarium for treating melanoma and consist of either polyvalent vaccines or defined melanoma antigens such as the ganglioside GM_2, which is the most immunogenic ganglioside expressed on melanoma. Furthermore, recent reports on the use of heat shock proteins as vehicles for the vaccines have been encouraging.[26,53]

OUTCOME AND PROGNOSIS

Statistics for pediatric-specific studies on melanoma are limited. The most recent report (2001) from the National Cancer Institute Surveillance, Epidemiology, and End Results database indicated that patients younger than 20 years of age had an overall 5-year survival of 93.6%. The hazard ratio of death from melanoma increased for male gender, increased age, and more advanced disease, as well as for location other than trunk or extremity.[54] This compares well with an older review that showed overall 5-year survival rates at 34% for stage 4 disease and as high as 90% for stage 1 and 2 disease.[55] The most important prognostic parameters remain the thickness of the tumor and the clinical stage of disease.

Postoperative follow-up is best performed under strict guidelines, as suggested by Garbe and Eigentler.[24] Risk-adapted, scheduled follow-up examinations in the German protocols have been validated for three monthly intervals during the first 5 years and every 6 months for the next 5 years. Most (83%) recurrences were identified on screening rather than by the patient (17%). One half were detected sufficiently early that complete surgical excision was possible. They further stratified risk by indicating that patients with thin melanoma lesions could undergo surveillance by physical examination rather than a technology-based system every 6 months. Those with lesions greater than 1 mm thick should undergo lymph node ultrasonography and determination of the S-100 tumor marker protein.[24]

Melanoma remains a challenge for diagnosis and treatment. With a concerted effort to study new modalities in the context of clinical trials, information should be derived that will allow for rational treatment of this rare and potentially lethal disorder.

chapter 74

VASCULAR ANOMALIES

C. Jason Smithers, MD • Steven J. Fishman, MD

Better understanding of vascular anomalies has come in the past several decades with improved knowledge about the growth of blood vessels (angiogenesis) and the development of a more logical classification system. Based on their biologic and clinical behavior, vascular anomalies can be broadly divided into two groups: vascular tumors and vascular malformations. Vascular tumors, of which the infantile hemangioma is the most common example, are true neoplasms that arise from endothelial hyperplasia. Conversely, vascular malformations are congenital lesions of vascular dysmorphogenesis that arise because of errors of embryonic development. These lesions exhibit normal endothelial cell turnover. Evaluation of vascular anomalies has historically been hindered by confusing and misused terminology and nomenclature. Along with the rarity and often complex nature of some of these disorders, this confusion has combined to make diagnosis and treatment of vascular anomalies inconsistent. The fact that these lesions do not fit neatly into the realm of any one medical or surgical specialty further complicates the picture. In this chapter, we outline the proper classification and nomenclature of vascular anomalies. This classification provides a basis for understanding the pathophysiology, diagnosis, and treatment of these disorders.[1-3]

CLASSIFICATION AND NOMENCLATURE

A biologic classification system of vascular anomalies has been devised based on physical characteristics, natural history, and cellular features (Table 74-1).[4,5] This system was accepted in 1996 by the International Society for the Study of Vascular Anomalies. It divides these anomalies into vascular tumors and vascular malformations. Examples of vascular tumors include infantile hemangioma, kaposiform hemangioendothelioma (KHE), and tufted angioma (TA). Vascular malformations can be divided based on vascular channel type (capillary, lymphatic, venous, arterial, or combined) or by flow (slow or fast). Examples of slow-flow lesions are capillary malformations (CMs), lymphatic malformations (LMs), and venous malformations (VMs). Fast-flow lesions include arteriovenous fistulas (AVFs) and arteriovenous malformations (AVMs).

Although now more clear, the nomenclature and classification of vascular anomalies have historically been confusing because the same or similar terms have been used to describe vastly different lesions. Unfortunately, the persistent use of the historic terms continues to confuse proper diagnosis and treatment of many patients. The various vascular anomalies often have a similar appearance whether involving the skin, mucosa, or viscera. These lesions can be flat or raised and can have pink, red, purple, or blue coloration. For centuries, these cutaneous vascular nevi were named based on their resemblance to common foods such as "cherry," "strawberry," or "port-wine stain." The term *nevus* generically refers to any circumscribed malformation of the skin, especially if colored by hyperpigmentation or increased vascularity. In the 19th century, Virchow[6] was the first to describe the histologic features of vascular nevi and initiated the term *angioma*. The term *angioma* became a base term used to describe all such nevi regardless of natural history or other clinical features. He labeled the infantile hemangioma as "angioma simplex." This same lesion has also been historically referred to as "capillary hemangioma" and "strawberry hemangioma." Virchow's "angioma cavernosum" actually was used to label two distinct lesions, infantile hemangiomas (when located deep to the skin) and VMs, because they have similar appearances on physical examination. Another example is Virchow's designation of the "angioma racemosum," which referred to what is called today an AVM and which also has been historically called an "arteriovenous hemangioma."

Wegener, a student of Virchow, described the histology of LMs, which he called "lymphangiomas."[7] The term *cystic hygroma,* referring to LMs, unfortunately also continues to have common usage. Although in the classic sense, the suffix "-oma" refers to a swelling of any cause, in contemporary usage this term connotes neoplastic tumors. Thus, both the terms *cystic hygroma* and *lymphangioma* should be abandoned in favor of LM (macrocystic and microcystic, respectively). The problems with this

Table 74-1 Classification of Vascular Anomalies

Vascular Tumors	Slow-Flow Vascular Malformations	Fast-Flow Vascular Malformations	Combined Vascular Malformations
Hemangioma	Capillary malformation (CM)	Arteriovenous fistula (AVF)	Klippel-Trénaunay syndrome, a capillary lymphaticovenous malformation (CLVM)
Kaposiform hemangioendothelioma (KHE)	Venous malformation (VM)	Arteriovenous malformation (AVM)	Parkes Weber syndrome, a capillary arteriovenous malformation (CAVM)
Tufted angioma (TA)	Lymphatic malformation (LM)		

jumble of descriptive and histologic terms are obvious. The same lesion can often have several different names, and the same name can refer to several different lesions. Use of the term *hemangioma* is the most classic case. The term *hemangioma,* combined with descriptive modifiers such as "strawberry," "cavernous," and "lympho-," is used to describe tumors, birthmarks, and vascular malformations. Thus, vascular anomalies with quite distinct features, whether congenital or acquired, whether they spontaneously regress or progress over time, become lumped under the umbrella of *hemangioma.* This faulty designation leads to improper diagnosis and treatment for patients. Moreover, it leads to misguided interdisciplinary communication and research efforts. A good example of this problem is provided by cavernous hemangiomas, which are truly VMs but which have often been treated with therapies directed at inhibition of angiogenesis, as if they were vascular tumors.

The nomenclature and the biologic classification of vascular anomalies have provided a useful clinical framework for the diagnosis and treatment of these lesions. Nevertheless, patients with vascular anomalies often provide complex exceptions to these designations. Lesions that are congenital malformations may not become apparent until adulthood, because of either anatomic location or progressive expansion over time. Likewise, neoplastic lesions, such as infantile hemangiomas, often have a premonitory cutaneous sign at birth. Additionally, hemangiomas, when they have a significant fast-flow component, can be difficult to distinguish from AVMs. Lastly, at times, vascular malformations exhibit enlargement and even endothelial hyperplasia triggered by clotting, ischemia, or partial resection. This hyperplasia leads to their propensity for recurrence after treatment. For these reasons, several regional and international centers have developed an interdisciplinary vascular anomaly team that serves as a referral center. These centers combine the medical, surgical, and radiologic expertise required to diagnose and manage effectively these often complex disorders.

VASCULAR TUMORS

Infantile Hemangiomas

Hemangiomas are the most common tumor of infancy, occurring in the skin in up to 4% to 10% of white infants, with a female-to-male ratio of 3 to 5:1.[8] The incidence may be significantly higher in premature infants.[9] They are much more common in whites than dark-skinned individuals. Infantile hemangiomas have a unique and characteristic life cycle of rapid growth in the first year of life (proliferative phase) followed by spontaneous slow regression from ages 1 to 7 years (involuting phase). Once involuted, they never recur.

Pathophysiology

The proliferating phase of hemangiomas is characterized by angiogenesis in the tumor.[10,11] The tumor is composed of plump, rapidly dividing endothelial cells, forming a mass of sinusoidal vascular channels. Enlarged feeding arteries and draining veins vascularize the tumor. Markers for mature endothelium, CD31 and von Willebrand's factor, are present on these neoplastic endothelial cells. In addition, a specific marker for endothelial cells of hemangiomas that is not found in other vascular anomalies is GLUT-1 (an erythrocyte-type glucose transporter).[12] Proangiogenic factors, such as fibroblast growth factor (FGF) and vascular endothelial growth factor (VEGF), are prominent during the proliferative phase. Increased levels of these peptides may be found in the urine of patients with hemangiomas. Additional factors that are required for angiogenesis include increased local levels of matrix metalloproteinases, which are necessary for remodeling of the extracellular matrix.

The involuting phase of hemangiomas is marked by reduced angiogenesis and endothelial cell apoptosis.[13] Levels of FGF and VEGF decrease and those of tissue inhibitors of metalloproteinases increase to suppress new blood vessel formation. The endothelial cells of the tumor flatten, the vascular channels dilate, and the tumor takes on a lobular architecture with replacement by fibrofatty stroma. In the end, with the involuted phase, all that remains is a residuum of fibrofatty tissue with tiny capillaries and mildly dilated draining vessels.

The triggers for angiogenesis and tumor formation are unknown. Viral causes have been postulated, but none have been elucidated. Human herpesvirus 8, which is associated with Kaposi's sarcoma, is not seen in hemangiomas. This polyomavirus can induce vascular tumors in mice and rats but leads to malignant growth and not to spontaneous regression. Almost certainly, some alteration occurs on a genetic level, but no specific genetic mutations have been found and no

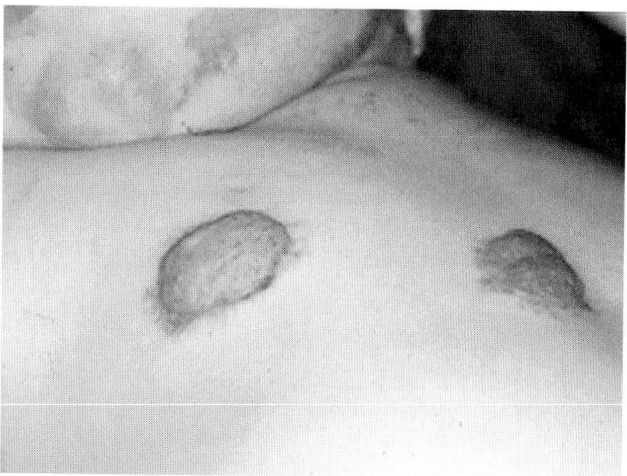

Figure 74-1. This infant has multiple cutaneous hemangiomas. Many of these patients also have internal hemangiomas in the liver, gastrointestinal tract, and brain.

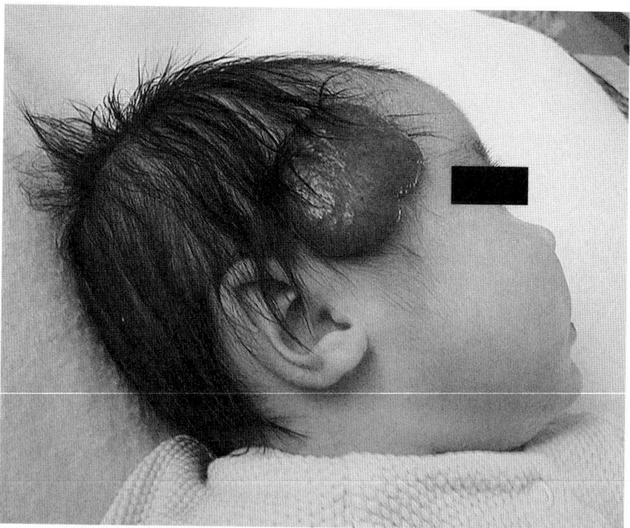

Figure 74-2. Infantile hemangioma, proliferative phase.

evidence exists for inheritance.[14,15] No animal model exists for a spontaneously regressing hemangioma, such as the common hemangioma of infancy.

Clinical Presentation

Hemangiomas first appear in the neonatal period, with a median age at onset of 2 weeks. A premonitory cutaneous sign is present at birth in 30% to 50% of cases. Hemangiomas are most often single cutaneous lesions and have an anatomic predilection for the head and neck region (60%). They occur in the trunk in 25% of cases and on the extremities in 15% of cases. Internal and visceral lesions are uncommon. Up to 20% of patients can have multiple tumors (Fig. 74-1). In these patients, internal hemangiomas can be found in the liver, gastrointestinal tract, and brain. Rare congenital hemangiomas are fully developed at birth and do not usually exhibit postnatal tumor growth. These are the rapidly involuting congenital hemangioma (RICH) and the noninvoluting congenital hemangioma (NICH).[16-19] An understanding of these recently discovered entities is still in its infancy.

The proliferative phase of hemangiomas is marked by rapid growth, for the first 6 to 8 months, which typically plateaus by age 10 to 12 months. Tumors that involve the superficial dermis are first seen as a red, raised lesion (previously named "capillary" or "strawberry" hemangiomas; Fig. 74-2). Superficial tumors that are larger or that exhibit more rapid growth can cause ulceration of the skin and bleeding in 5% of cases. Tumors in the lower dermis, subcutaneous tissue, or muscle appear bluish with slightly raised overlying skin and have frequently incorrectly been called "cavernous" hemangiomas. With experience, history and physical examination can establish an accurate diagnosis for 90% of these tumors.

The involuting phase of hemangiomas occurs from age 1 to 7 years, during which time the tumor slowly regresses, although it may grow in proportion with the child (Fig. 74-3). This phase is notable for the fading color of the tumor to a dull purple and the softening of the tumor mass. The skin usually becomes pale in the center of the tumor first, spreading outward. Both the deep color and the bulk of the tumor show continued gradual improvement until the regression is entirely complete by age 10 to 12 years. In the final involuted phase of the tumor, 50% of patients have nearly normal skin in the area of the prior lesion. Patients that had larger tumors may have lax or redundant skin and yellowish discoloration. Scars will persist if parts of the tumor were previously ulcerated.

The differential diagnosis of cutaneous hemangiomas consists primarily of other vascular anomalies. Capillary malformations that involve the skin can be mistaken for superficial hemangiomas and vice versa. Deeper hemangiomas can be confused with VMs or LMs, because they may all appear as bluish masses through the skin (Fig. 74-4). Hemangiomas with fast-flow vascularity of the tumor parenchyma could be mistaken for AVMs, but the age at onset and history generally distinguish the two. Congenital hemangiomas, such as RICH or NICH, can be confused with vascular malformations that are congenital by definition. Pyogenic granulomas are first seen in childhood, often

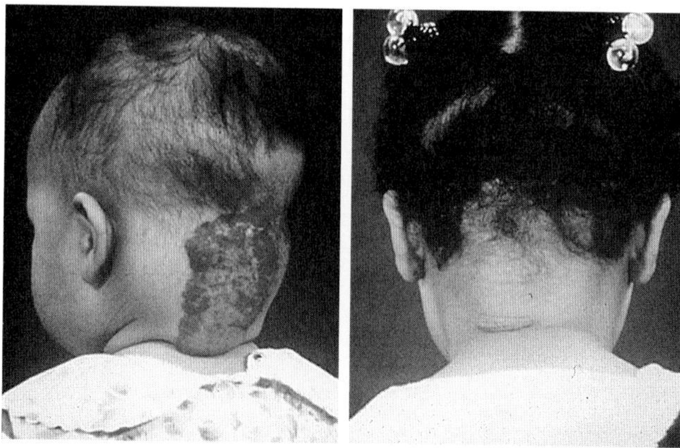

Figure 74-3. Posterior cervical hemangioma *(left)* has undergone involution *(right)*.

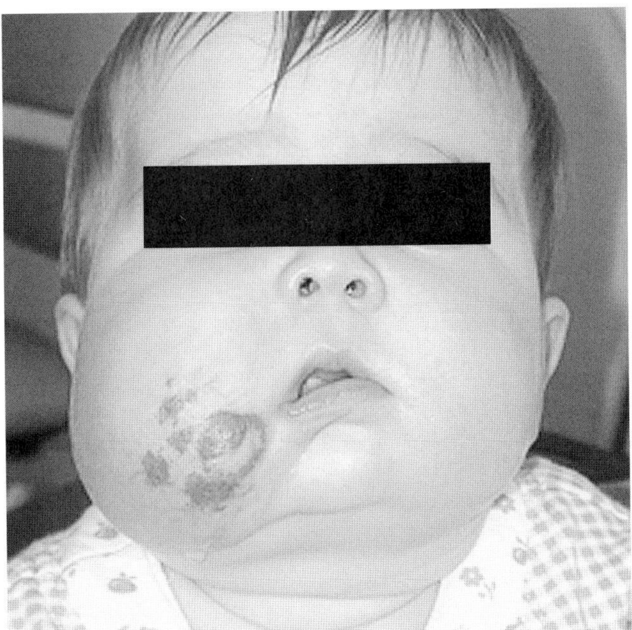

Figure 74-4. A right parotid hemangioma is seen in this infant.

associated with minor trauma, and rarely appear before age 6 months (mean age, 6 to 7 years).[20,21] Finally, other tumors such as TA, hemangiopericytoma, and fibrosarcoma should be considered.[22] If any concern exists for malignancy, further evaluation with imaging or biopsy is mandated.

The primary local complications that can occur with cutaneous hemangiomas are ulceration, bleeding, and pain. Ulceration is seen in about 5% of cases. Severe complications also are possible, depending on size and location of the tumor. Lesions of the cervicofacial region may produce airway obstruction as they grow during the proliferative phase. Very large hemangiomas, notably of the liver, can lead to high-output congestive heart failure secondary to fast flow and vascular shunting within the tumor. Facial lesions can result in tissue necrosis with cosmetic consequences when involving the eyelid, nose, lip, or ear. Periorbital and eyelid lesions also may cause visual impairment or obstruction that leads to deprivation amblyopia (Fig. 74-5). Distortion of the cornea can alternatively cause astigmatic amblyopia. Subglottic hemangiomas may occur with stridor and lead to airway obstruction with continued growth. Gastrointestinal hemangiomas are very rare but can cause gastrointestinal bleeding.

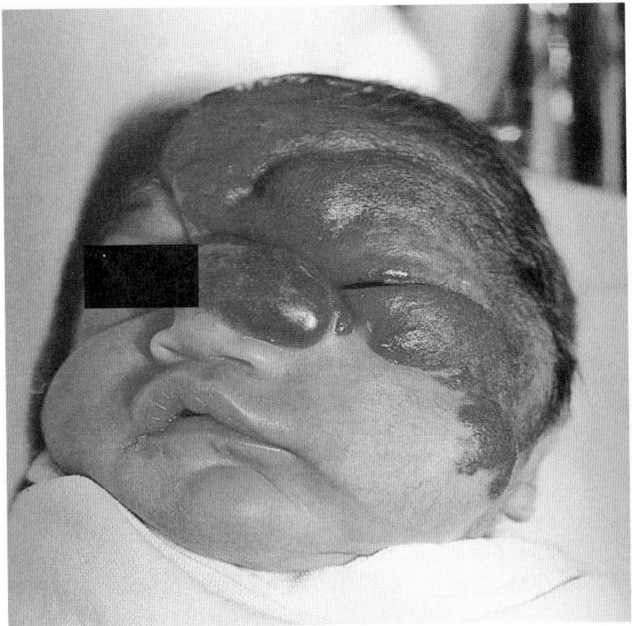

Figure 74-5. This left periorbital hemangioma was causing visual impairment.

Other Manifestations

Hemangiomatosis consists of multiple disseminated hemangiomas. The cutaneous tumors are usually tiny (<5 mm) and, when five or more are present, visceral lesions should be sought as well. Screening patients with ultrasonography or magnetic resonance imagine (MRI) or both may be indicated for these patients.

Infantile hepatic hemangiomas must be differentiated from "hepatic hemangiomas" that are first seen in adulthood.[23] Adult "hepatic hemangiomas," which are sometimes called "cavernous hemangiomas," are VMs. Conversely, hepatic hemangiomas of infancy are true tumors and have a pattern of involution similar to that of cutaneous hemangiomas. Contrary to popular belief, not all liver hemangiomas are life threatening. Indeed, the "classic triad" of heart failure, anemia, and hepatomegaly is unusual. Recently, it has been recognized that hepatic hemangiomas present in several different patterns: focal, multifocal, or diffuse.[24,25] Focal lesions are single, generally large masses on antenatal imaging studies and/or present as a mass in early infancy. They may cause moderate thrombocytopenia that generally resolves spontaneously. This is in contrast to the profound thrombocytopenia seen with Kasabach-Merritt phenomenon (KMP). These single large lesions often do not exhibit growth after birth and are thought to represent RICH lesions, which are histologically distinct from the typical hemangioma. They are fully grown at birth and regress much faster than the typical hemangioma. However, a subset of focal hepatic RICH-type hemangiomas will have macrovascular shunts from the hepatic arteries and/or portal veins to the hepatic veins. These shunts can cause a large steal, accounting for blood-flow demands above and beyond the hypervascular tumor parenchyma. This may result in high-output cardiac failure. These shunts may close as the tumor involutes. However, cardiac strain may mandate interruption of the shunts, which can be performed by embolization. A skilled pediatric interventional radiologist may be able to embolize the shunts without disrupting the major hepatic vessels.

Multifocal hepatic hemangiomas are histologically identical to the typical cutaneous hemangioma. Smaller enlarging lesions, detected by imaging stimulated by the presence of cutaneous hemangiomas, may often remain asymptomatic. However, some will also have associated macrovascular shunts that may cause cardiac failure. These shunts may close with corticosteroid therapy, but embolization may be necessary in those severe cases in which there is insufficient time to wait for involution.

The most dangerous hepatic hemangiomas are the diffuse type, presenting with innumerable compacted nodular lesions replacing normal liver parenchyma, and causing massive hepatomegaly, abdominal compartment syndrome, and respiratory compromise. Massive hemangiomas (e.g., those causing hepatomegaly) may induce profound acquired hypothyroidism.[26] Hemangiomas have been found to express type 3-iodothyronine deiodinase that inactivates circulating thyroid hormones. Lesions of sufficient size can break down active thyroid hormones more rapidly than the endocrine axis can replace them. Therefore, patients with large hemangiomas should be screened by measuring thyroid-stimulating hormone levels. When untreated, hypothyroidism in infancy will lead to severe mental retardation. For these unusual cases, aggressive exogenous thyroid replacement and close endocrinologic consultation are mandated. The condition is self-limiting after tumor involution.

The differential diagnosis of hepatic hemangiomas includes AVMs and malignant tumors such as hepatoblastoma and metastatic neuroblastoma. The diagnosis is established by imaging with ultrasonography, MRI, or computed tomography (CT). If typical imaging findings of one of the hemangioma patterns are not found, percutaneous biopsy may be indicated to ensure a malignancy is not present.

Although other congenital anomalies are rarely associated with infantile hemangiomas, a few have been reported, most commonly associated with larger or midline hemangiomas. Cervicothoracic hemangiomas can be seen in conjunction with sternal nonunion.[27] Tumors of the lumbosacral area have been noted to occur along with spinal dysraphism abnormalities such as meningocele and tethered spinal cord.[28,29] Hemangiomas of the pelvis and perineum have been reported in association with urogenital and anorectal anomalies. Craniofacial hemangiomas have been rarely associated with congenital ocular abnormalities such as micro-ophthalmia, cataracts, and optic nerve hypoplasia; posterior fossa cystic malformations; hypoplasia or absence of the carotid and vertebral vessels; and malformation of the aortic arch.[30,31]

Imaging

Proper radiologic diagnosis of vascular anomalies is dependent on specific expertise and clinical experience with the radiologic features of these lesions.[32] Ultrasonography and especially MRI are the principal useful modalities. Ultrasonography of proliferative-phase hemangiomas demonstrates a mass with dense parenchyma exhibiting fast-flow vascularity.[33,34] This distinguishes deep infantile hemangiomas from VMs that exhibit slow flow and larger blood-filled spaces. MRI of proliferating hemangiomas shows a lobulated solid mass of intermediate intensity with T1-weighted spin-echo sequences and moderate hyperintensity on T2-weighted spin-echo images. Flow voids that represent fast flow and shunting are seen in and around the tumor. For the involuting phase, MRI demonstrates decreased flow voids and vascularity with the mass, taking on a more lobular and fatty appearance.[35]

Treatment

The majority of infantile hemangiomas do not require any specific treatment other than observation and reassurance of the parents.[36] Even though the tumor may exhibit rapid growth and the skin is fiery red, these tumors will spontaneously regress with either no or minimal evidence of occurrence. Reasons for treatment or referral to a vascular anomalies center are the following: dangerous location (impinging on a vital structure such as the airway or eye), unusually large size or rapid growth, and local or endangering complications (skin ulceration or high-output heart failure). Few prognostic indicators exist for these potential complications. Regularly scheduled follow-up is essential. Serial photographs are very helpful in documenting progression and subsequent improvement.

Because hemangiomas are tumors of pure angiogenesis, pharmacologic therapy involves angiogenesis inhibition.[37] The first-line antiangiogenic therapy for hemangiomas exhibiting appropriate risk factors or complications is systemic corticosteroids.[38] Oral prednisone is used at a dose of 2 to 3 mg/kg/day. Doses up to 5 mg/kg/day have been administered for life-threatening complications with large hemangiomas causing airway obstruction or heart failure.[39] The overall response rate is 80% to 90%, with initial improvement in the color and tension of the mass usually noted within 1 week. The corticosteroids are maintained with a very gradual taper every 2 to 4 weeks, with the goal of discontinuation around age 10 to 11 months. Live vaccines such as those for polio, measles, mumps, rubella, and varicella should be withheld while children are on prednisone. Hemangiomas will demonstrate rebound growth if corticosteroids are tapered or stopped too quickly. A return to the initial dosage and a slower tapering will usually resolve this problem.

Potential complications of corticosteroid use in infants and children include impaired linear growth and weight gain in about 30% of cases. All children will have "catch-up" growth and return to pretreatment growth curves by age 14 to 24 months. Cushingoid facies occur in almost all patients and normalizes on tapering of the corticosteroids. In rare circumstances, corticosteroids may induce hypertension or hypertrophic cardiomyopathy, both of which are indications to wean or change therapy.[40]

Intralesional corticosteroids are used for hemangiomas that cause local deformity or ulceration, especially for facial lesions of the eyelid, nose, cheek, or lip.[41] A total of three to five injections (at a dose of 3 to 5 mg/kg per injection) are typically given at intervals of 6 to 8 weeks. The response rate approaches that of systemic corticosteroids. Subcutaneous atrophy is a potential complication of corticosteroid injection, but it is usually temporary. Cases have been reported of blindness after intralesional corticosteroid injection for periorbital hemangiomas. This has been presumed to be secondary to particle embolization of the retinal artery through feeding vessels.[42] Manual compression around the periphery of the tumor is recommended during injection.

Recombinant interferon, previously considered as a second-line agent, has fallen out of favor, except in very limited circumstances, because of the severe potential complication of spastic diplegia that can occur in 5% to 12% of treated infants.[43,44] Spasticity usually resolves if the drug is terminated quickly. Children receiving interferon should be monitored carefully by a neurologist. On the other hand, experience is growing with low-dose, high-frequency antiangiogenic regimens of vincristine as second-line therapy after corticosteroids. A recent report of propranolol used to treat infantile hemangioma may indeed revolutionize medical therapy.[45]

Although it has popular appeal, laser therapy is not often beneficial for infantile hemangiomas.[46] The flash-lamp pulse-dye laser penetrates the dermis to a depth of only 0.75 to 1.2 mm. Most cutaneous hemangiomas are deeper and therefore not affected by laser treatment. Additionally, laser therapy carries risks of scarring, skin hypopigmentation, and ulceration, which may lead to a poor result compared with observation alone. A few specific indications for laser treatment of hemangiomas are worth mentioning. One instance in which the laser is beneficial is the treatment of telangiectasia, which often remains during the involuted phase of hemangioma. Also, the use of an endoscopic continuous-wave CO_2 laser has been shown to be a good technique for controlling proliferative-phase hemangiomas in the unilateral subglottic location.[47] Finally, intralesional photocoagulation with bare fiber neodymium:yttrium-aluminum-garnet (Nd:YAG) laser can be useful for hemangiomas in certain locations, such as the upper eyelid, when visual obstruction is a concern.

Indications for surgical resection of infantile hemangiomas vary with patient age. During the proliferative phase in infancy, well-localized or pedunculated tumors can be expeditiously resected with linear closure, especially for tumors complicated by bleeding and ulceration. Sites that are most amenable to resection in this stage are the scalp, trunk, and extremities. Other modalities to treat ulceration in hemangiomas include wound care with dressing changes, topical antibiotics, and topical corticosteroids, which can accelerate healing.[48] Tumors of the upper eyelid that obstruct vision and that do not respond to pharmacologic therapy also may require surgical excision or debulking. Focal lesions of the gastrointestinal tract that cause bleeding and for which medical management fails also may require resection by means of enterotomy or endoscopic band ligation. Preoperative localization with capsule endoscopy or intraoperative endoscopy (or both), may be necessary to identify lesions of the small intestine.[49]

Surgical resection is considered during the involuting phase in early childhood for hemangiomas that are large and protuberant and, therefore, likely to create excess and lax overlying skin.[50] Indications are the following: (1) when it is obvious that resection would be necessary sooner or later; (2) when the surgical scar would be identical, regardless of timing of operation; and (3) when the surgical scar is easily hidden. Lesions of the nose, eyelids, lips, and ears require special expertise. It is often preferable to perform the operation for these indications in patients at preschool age before the children become aware of and focus on body differences that may lead to low self-esteem.

After complete involution of the hemangioma, cosmetic distortion is the primary indication for operative management. Fibrofatty residuum and redundant skin can be excised in staged operations, if necessary. Occasionally, extensive scarring from tissue destruction may necessitate reconstructive procedures. Finally, for the difficult-to-treat and life-threatening large hemangiomas, especially in the liver, angiographic embolization may be required to manage high-output cardiac failure.

Arterial catheterization in infants carries significant risks and generally should be limited to those situations with cardiac compromise in which the capacity and intent to perform simultaneous embolization exists. In these rare cases, antiangiogenic pharmacotherapy remains as the first line and should continue along with angiographic procedures. Repeated embolization procedures may be required. Successful embolization is dependent on occlusion of macrovascular shunts within the tumor rather than on occlusion of feeding vessels.[51,52]

Tufted Angioma and Kaposiform Hemangioendothelioma

These vascular tumors of childhood are more aggressive and invasive than are infantile hemangiomas. TA and KHE probably exist within the same spectrum, because they share many overlapping clinical and histologic features.[53,54] Both tumors typically present at birth, although they occur postnatally as well. Male and female infants are affected equally. The tumors are unifocal and are most often located on the trunk, shoulder, thigh, or retroperitoneum. TA appears as erythematous macules or plaques, and histology reveals small tufts of capillaries. KHE is a more extensive tumor with deep red-purple skin discoloration and overlying and surrounding ecchymosis. Generalized petechiae may be apparent and coincide with profound thrombocytopenia secondary to the Kasabach-Merritt Phenomenon (KMP). Imaging of KHE depicts an enhancing lesion with poorly defined margins that extend across tissue planes. This is contrasted to hemangiomas, which are well circumscribed and respective of tissue planes. Biopsy is usually not necessary, but histology reveals infiltrating sheets of slender endothelial cells.

Kasabach-Merritt Phenomenon

KMP was first reported in 1940 as a case of profound thrombocytopenia, petechiae, and bleeding in conjunction with a "giant hemangioma."[55] As with many terms in the field of vascular anomalies, the term has been often misused in connection with other varieties of coagulopathy and vascular lesions, most prominently VMs. However, the profound and persistent thrombocytopenia that occurs with KMP does not occur with either VMs or infantile hemangioma. The only known true associations are with TA and KHE.[56,57] The platelet count with this disorder is typically less than 10,000/mm^3 and may be accompanied by decreased fibrinogen levels and a mildly elevated prothrombin time (PT) and partial thromboplastin time (PTT). Bleeding can result from this platelet-trapping coagulopathy at many sites (including intracranial, gastrointestinal, peritoneal, pleural, and pulmonary). Treatment of KHE with KMP is primarily medical, because the tumor is usually too large and extensive to be resected. Corticosteroids and interferon alfa have been effective in about 50% of cases. Vincristine also is beneficial, but no single agent has been shown to be consistently successful. Platelet transfusions are ineffective and should be avoided unless active bleeding occurs. Heparin stimulates tumor growth and worsens the thrombocytopenia of KMP and should likewise be avoided. Mortality rates with KMP and KHE or TA remain high at 20% to 30%. The natural history of these tumors is one of continued proliferation into early childhood followed by subsequent but incomplete regression. These tumors usually persist, albeit in a smaller form.[58] Fortunately, they are usually asymptomatic in later stages, although they may cause musculoskeletal pain.

VASCULAR MALFORMATIONS

Pathophysiology

Vascular malformations are congenital lesions of vascular dysmorphogenesis that can be local or diffuse. They are classified, based on the appearance of the abnormal channels, as resembling capillaries, lymphatics, veins, arteries, or a combination thereof. The majority of vascular malformations are sporadic, although some rare varieties are familial.[59] They can be quite complex and associated with underlying soft tissue and skeletal abnormalities. Vasculogenesis refers to the process of blood vessel formation from mesodermally derived endothelial precursor cells. The destiny of endothelial precursors to create different types of blood vessels appears to be imprinted early in embryogenesis. Unique cell-surface markers are seen on these endothelial cells.[60] Arterial endothelial cells express ephrin-B_2, and venous endothelial cells express ephrin-B_4.[61] Although the understanding of vasculogenesis and the pathogenesis of VMs is still limited, the molecular processes are beginning to be understood. VMs probably result from genetic mutations that lead to dysfunction in the regulation of endothelial proliferation and apoptosis, cellular differentiation, maturation, and cell-to-cell adhesions.[62]

Hereditary hemorrhagic telangiectasia (HHT or Rendu-Osler-Weber disease) was the first vascular anomaly to be elucidated at the genetic level.[63] This autosomal dominant disease generally is first seen in the third and fourth decades of life with telangiectasia, AVFs, and AVMs that occur in the skin, mucous membranes, lung, liver, and brain. Two primary causative genes, both on chromosome 9, involve the binding and signaling of transforming growth factor-β. Endoglin is the affected gene for HHT type 1 and codes for an endothelial glycoprotein. HHT type 2 involves mutation of an activin receptor kinase.

Lymphatic vessels are thought to develop from preexisting veins and express a unique receptor for vascular endothelial growth factor (VEGF3 or Flt-4).[64,65] Genetic studies with mice have shown that VEGF3 knockout mice die on embryo day 9 with major venous anomalies before any lymphatic sprouting has occurred.[62] Conversely, transgenic mice that overexpress the ligand for VEGF3 (VEGF-C) develop distended lymphatic channels.[66] LMs, especially posterior cervical LMs, are one of the components of several sporadic chromosomal syndromes, including trisomies 13, 18, and 21, as well as Turner's, Roberts', and Noonan's syndromes. As with the other vascular malformations, the majority of VMs are sporadic as well. However, some families have demonstrated an autosomal dominant pattern of inheritance.[67] Studies of these families have shown a mutation in the gene for TIE-2, a receptor expressed by endothelial cells.[68] Defective smooth muscle cells in the vascular wall are thought to be responsible for some VMs. These examples support the concept of genetic mutations as being the causative mechanism for vascular malformations.

Capillary Malformations

Capillary malformations (CMs), which have been previously referred to as "port-wine stains," are present at birth as permanent, flat, pink-red cutaneous lesions (Fig. 74-6). The most common location is the

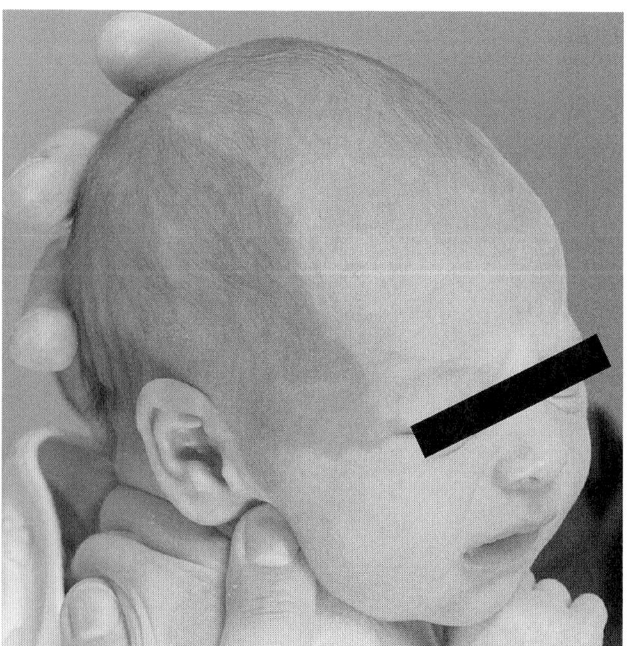

Figure 74-6. This capillary malformation is seen along this baby's right temporal lobe.

head and neck region. It is rare to have multiple CMs. These lesions can be localized or exhibit an extensive, geographic pattern. The histology of cutaneous CMs consists of dilated capillary- to venule-size vessels located in the superficial dermis. These abnormal vessels gradually dilate over time, leading to a darker color and, occasionally, nodular ectasias. In the newborn nursery, CMs can be confused with nevus flammeus neonatorum, commonly called an "angel's kiss" when located on the face or a "stork bite" when in the posterior cervical location. However, these nevi fade with time, whereas a CM does not.

CMs can be associated with underlying soft tissue and skeletal overgrowth as well as other internal abnormalities. CMs of the occiput can signal underlying encephalocele or ectopic meninges. When located over the spine, underlying spinal dysraphism is a concern. Sturge-Weber syndrome represents a classic case of underlying anomalies associated with CMs of the face. In this syndrome, facial CMs affect the trigeminal dermatomes and are associated with ipsilateral ocular and leptomeningeal vascular anomalies. Ocular lesions lead to an increased risk for retinal detachment, glaucoma, and blindness. Leptomeningeal involvement can manifest as seizures, hemiplegia, and impaired motor and cognitive function. MRI reveals the central nervous system abnormalities, showing pial vascular enhancement and gyriform calcifications.[69]

Treatment of CMs is indicated primarily for cosmetic purposes. Flash-lamp pulsed-dye laser therapy causing photothermolysis of the CM will improve the appearance by lightening the color of the lesion in 70% of patients.[70] The timing of therapy remains controversial, and repeated treatments are usually needed.[71] Ablative and orthopedic surgical procedures can be tailored to treat cosmetic and functional problems related to soft tissue and bony hypertrophy.

LYMPHATIC MALFORMATIONS

Clinical Presentation

LMs occur as a wide spectrum from localized masses to areas of diffuse infiltration to chylous fluid accumulations in various body cavities. LMs are usually noted at birth but can be seen at any age or even prenatally by fetal ultrasonography.[72,73] The skin and soft tissues are most commonly affected. LMs can involve the subcutaneous tissues, muscle, bone, and, more rarely, internal organs such as the gastrointestinal tract and lungs. Anatomic sites frequently seen are the axilla and thorax, cervicofacial region, mediastinum, retroperitoneum, buttock, and anogenital regions (Fig. 74-7). As with CMs, underlying localized soft tissue and skeletal hypertrophy can often be associated with LMs. The abnormal lymphatic spaces can be either macrocystic, microcystic, or a combination. According to previous terminology, macrocystic LMs were referred to as "cystic hygromas" and microcystic LMs

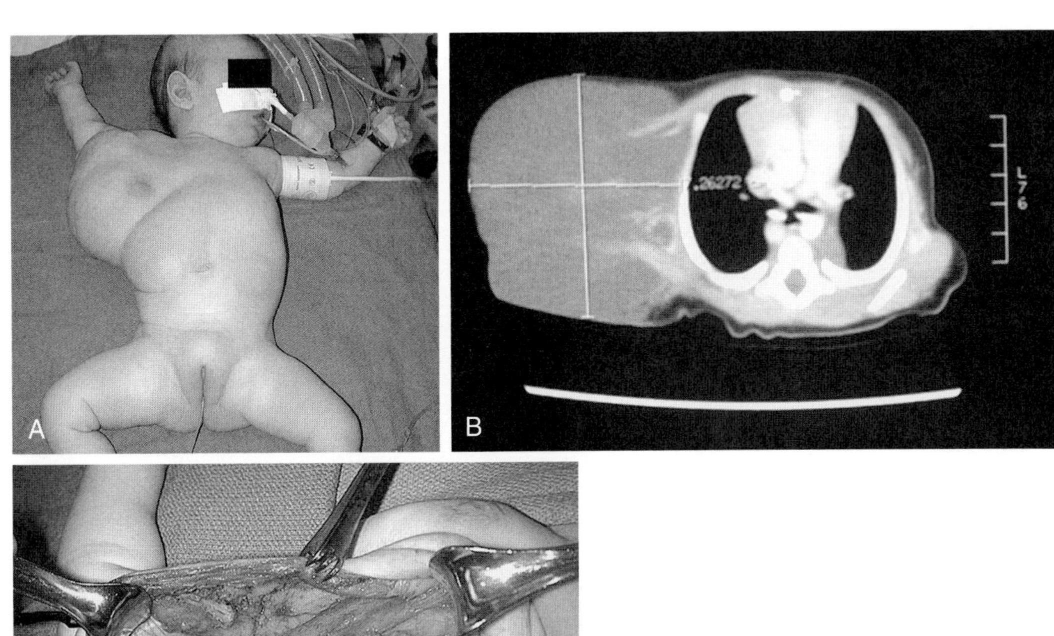

Figure 74-7. **A,** This baby has a large right axillary lymphatic malformation which is seen on the CT scan (**B**). **C,** This operative photograph shows the residual cavity after resection of the mass.

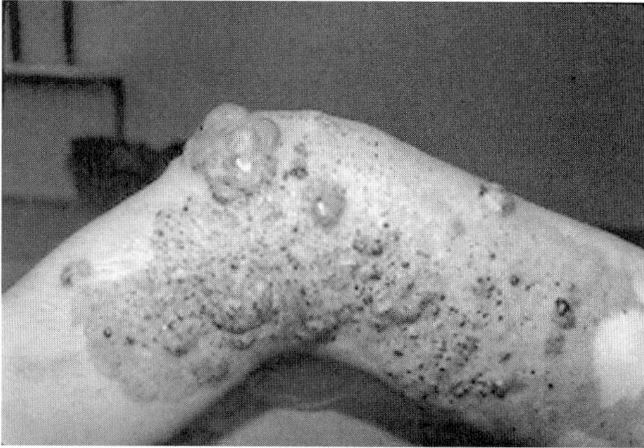

Figure 74-8. This teenager has lymphangiomatous involvement of the dermis, which produces puckering of the skin and vessels that can weep clear fluid. This is termed *lymphangioma cutis.*

as "lymphangiomas." However, these names should be abandoned.

LMs appear as soft compressible masses, similar to VMs, and may have a bluish hue, although not to the same extent as VMs. Involvement of the dermis (lymphangioma cutis) may produce puckering of the skin or vesicles that weep clear yellowish fluid (Fig. 74-8). Diffuse infiltration of the subcutaneous tissue can produce extensive lymphedema that also falls within the spectrum of LMs. One unique factor among the vascular anomalies is that LMs are at risk for infection that can lead to cellulitis or even systemic illness. Similarly, infections located elsewhere in the body or viral illnesses can cause increased size and tension of LMs. The cystic components of LMs also are subject to intralesional bleeding secondary to trauma or abnormal venous connections. The vesicles from cutaneous involvement also can leak thin sanguineous fluid or appear as red, purple, or black nodules.

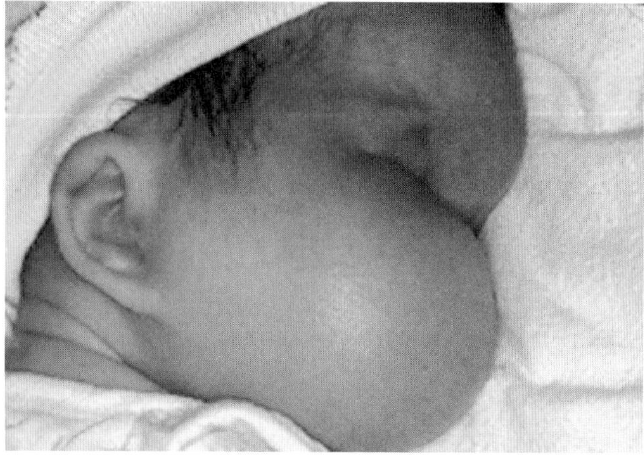

Figure 74-9. This neonate was born with a large lymphangioma of the face. This tumor is often associated with macrocheilia, macroglossia, and macromala. Staged resections are usually necessary.

LMs at various anatomic locations are prone to unique associated anomalies. Periorbital LMs can lead to proptosis. Facial LMs can cause the associated deformities of macrocheilia, macroglossia, and macromala (Fig. 74-9). Overgrowth of the mandible, sometimes massive, can be seen with cervicofacial LMs.[74] Congenital airway obstruction is rare but also possible. Lesions of the tongue and floor of the mouth, conversely, may more commonly produce obstruction of the oropharynx. LMs of the cervical and axillary regions can signal associated LMs of the mediastinum. Anomalies of the central conducting lymphatic channels, the thoracic duct and cisterna chyli, can lead to very problematic and recurrent chylous effusions that affect the pleural, pericardial, and/or peritoneal cavities. In addition, LMs of the gastrointestinal tract can lead to loss of chyle and subsequent protein-losing enteropathy. In the pelvis, associated problems include recurrent infection and bladder outlet obstruction. LMs of the extremities are seen in conjunction with overgrowth and limb-length discrepancy. A rare but very difficult problem arises with Gorham's syndrome, in which soft tissue and skeletal LMs lead to progressive osteolysis and "disappearing bone disease."[75] Pathologic fractures and vertebral instability can become manifest with this often fatal syndrome.

Imaging

Well-localized and cystic LMs are easily characterized by ultrasonography and CT (see Fig. 74-7). MRI, however, provides the most reliable diagnosis and is superior in documenting the full extent of more complex LMs as well as their macrocystic and microcystic components. LMs are hyperintense on T2-weighted sequences because of their high water content. Within the cysts, fluid-fluid levels denote layering of protein or blood, or both. Cystic rims and intralesional septa are highlighted by contrast enhancement. Adjacent enlarged or anomalous venous channels may be apparent as well. The differential diagnosis of these cystic lesions in the infant includes teratoma and infantile fibrosarcoma. For lymphatic anomalies of the thoracic duct and chylous effusions, contrast lymphangiography, although technically difficult to perform, can be helpful to locate the abnormal lymphatic channels or site of leakage.[76]

Treatment

The indications for treatment of LMs vary with the extent and location of the lesions.[77] Surgical resection provides the only method for potential "cure," but this is possible only for lesions that are well localized. Focal and macrocystic lesions are amenable to ablation by both sclerotherapy and resection. In contrast, more diffuse and predominantly microcystic LMs are difficult to eradicate by any method. For local intralesional bleeding that causes sudden enlargement of LMs and pain, conservative management with rest and pain medications is sufficient. Similarly, the enlargement of LMs that coincides with systemic viral or bacterial infections can be managed expectantly, as it usually resolves. Conversely, bacterial infections within LMs causing cellulitis require treatment with antibiotics. Infected LMs become more tense and swollen, producing erythema, pain, and toxicity. The incidence of this complication is around 17%. Treatment consists of systemic antibiotics, and hospitalization for intravenous antibiotics is often necessary. The antibiotic regimen is directed toward oral pathogens for LMs of the head and neck and toward enteric pathogens for lesions of the trunk, pelvis, and perineum.

Indications for ablative or excisional therapy include recurrent complications with infection, cosmesis, deformity, dysfunction, and leakage into body cavities or from the skin. Intralesional sclerotherapy is most beneficial for LMs with macrocystic components. The commonly used agents are ethanol, sodium tetradecyl sulfate, and doxycycline that produce scarring and collapse of the cysts. For simple, well-localized macrocystic LMs, sclerotherapy can indeed be curative. For more diffuse and complex LMs, sclerotherapy procedures are staged and can lead to significant improvement. Re-expansion of the lesions, however, is the typical course. Weeping or bleeding from cutaneous vesicles can be controlled with local injection sclerotherapy, although leakage generally resumes in 6 to 24 months. Complications of sclerotherapy to be avoided include injury to adjacent nerves, necrosis of overlying skin, and cardiotoxicity related to the overall dose.

Surgical resection for complex LMs also can be of significant benefit (see Fig. 74-7). A staged approach is often required.[78] The operations may be long and tedious and require meticulous, thorough dissection to preserve vital structures. General guidelines for surgical resection are as follows: each operation should (1) focus on a defined anatomic region, removing as much lesion as possible, including neurovascular dissection, but without injuring vital structures; (2) limit blood loss to less than the patient's blood volume; and (3) allow prolonged closed suction drainage of the resection cavity. The recurrence rate after "macroscopically complete excision" ranges from 15% to 40%. This recurrence is thought to be secondary to regrowth and re-expansion of unexcised lymphatic channels. Some have considered that sclerotherapy of the resection cavity after operation may be helpful in this regard. After resection, it is common for cutaneous vesicles to occur within the surgical scar. These can be controlled to some extent with local intravesicular sclerotherapy. Alternatively, additional staged excision, pulling uninvolved dermis over the resection bed, may prevent this annoying result.

Some other caveats of surgical treatment for LMs deserve mention. Cervicofacial LMs will often require staged orthognathic procedures to improve bite and speech impediments related to maxillary and mandibular overgrowth. Tracheostomy may be needed in cases of oropharyngeal and airway obstruction (Fig. 74-10). When considered necessary, tracheostomy should precede any attempts at sclerotherapy for cervicofacial LMs. Reactive inflammatory swelling can be dramatic in the initial period after sclerotherapy and can exacerbate partial oropharyngeal obstruction. Lesions of the cervical and axillary regions often involve the brachial plexus. Nerve stimulators can be a useful adjunct to prevent injury in these cases. Resection of thoracic and mediastinal LMs to treat recurrent pleural and pericardial effusions involves dissection and skeletonization of the great vessels and vagus and phrenic nerves. For pelvic and anorectal LMs, detailed knowledge of the anatomy of the ischiorectal fossa and sciatic nerve is paramount. Preoperative sclerotherapy to shrink lesions is often useful as well, but discernment is necessary, because scarring can impede the preservation of important nerves. Finally, for the specific type of cutaneous LM, "lymphangioma circumscriptum," wide resection and closure with split-thickness skin grafts can be curative.

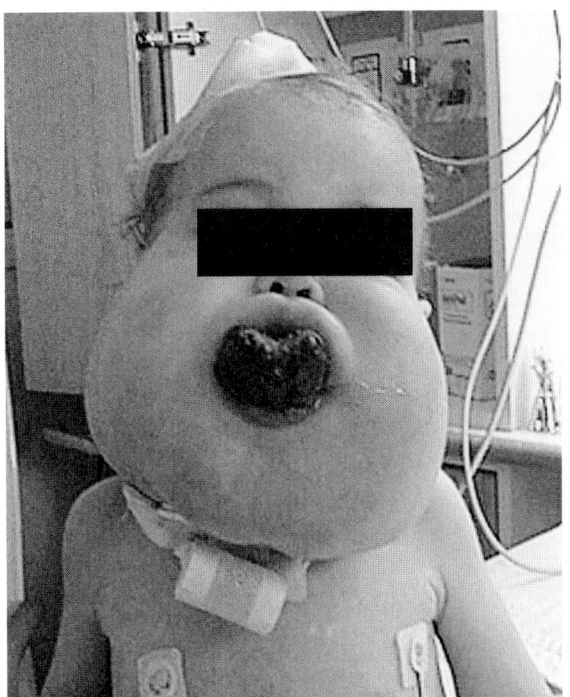

Figure 74-10. This baby has undergone a tracheostomy due to oropharyngeal obstruction from this large cervicofacial lymphatic malformation.

VENOUS MALFORMATIONS

Clinical Presentation

As one might expect from the embryonic relation of veins and lymphatics, VMs share many clinical features with LMs. VMs, often incorrectly called "cavernous hemangiomas," are slow-flow lesions consisting of venous channels that can develop anywhere in the body. They are most common in the skin and soft tissues. VMs may be seen at birth or become apparent later, depending on the anatomic location. They comprise a wide spectrum, including simple varicosities and ectasias, discrete spongy masses, and complex channels that can permeate any tissue or organ system. VMs are probably the most common of the vascular malformations, and they are more likely to be multiple

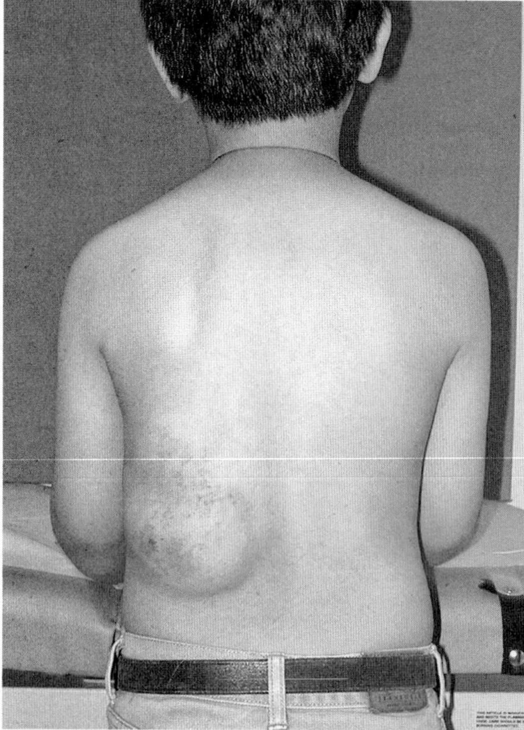

Figure 74-11. This adolescent has a venous malformation in the subcutaneous tissue of his back.

as well. They tend to enlarge slowly with normal growth of the patient but can dilate and become symptomatic at any time. As with other vascular malformations, the proportional growth that occurs may become exaggerated during puberty. On examination, these soft, bluish, compressible lesions will expand with dependent position and Valsalva maneuver (Fig. 74-11). Episodes of phlebothrombosis secondary to stasis may lead to acute pain and swelling. Associated local overgrowth and limb-length discrepancy are not uncommon. Involvement of bones and joints may lead to pathologic fractures, hemarthroses, and subsequent arthritis.

VMs of the gastrointestinal tract are often multiple and can affect every part of the tract from mouth to anus. They are more commonly found in the left colon and rectum when associated with VMs of the pelvis and perineum. Gastrointestinal bleeding, typically chronic, can result. Blue rubber bleb nevus syndrome (or Bean's syndrome) represents a specific rare disorder consisting of multifocal VMs that affect the skin and gastrointestinal tract primarily.[79] The skin lesions are unique in that they are often quite numerous and resemble tiny "blue rubber nipples." These skin lesions are classically located on the palms and soles of the feet (Fig. 74-12). As with other gastrointestinal VMs, chronic bleeding and anemia can result. Intussusception of polypoid VMs can be another presentation. Diagnosis of gastrointestinal VMs is generally based on endoscopic findings.

VMs of the liver deserve specific mention. Historically called by the misnomer "hepatic hemangiomas," these lesions typically are first seen in adulthood, most often as an incidental finding of abdominal imaging obtained for other reasons. The majority of these lesions are asymptomatic, although they can be quite large or even massive. Reported cases of spontaneous or traumatic rupture have had devastating consequences, but this is exceedingly rare. The most common indications for treatment of these VMs are persistent discomfort from very large lesions and the inability to exclude malignancy. In experienced hands, surgical resection is safe and effective. The technique of enucleation is preferred.[80]

Large VMs also can be complicated by localized intravascular coagulopathy caused by stasis and stagnation of blood within the malformation, leading to consumption of coagulation factors. The clotting profile consists of prolonged PT, decreased fibrinogen, and elevated D-dimers. The PTT is often normal. Thrombocytopenia occurs, with a typical platelet range of 100,000 to 150,000/mm^3. The distinction between this coagulopathy and KMP is important. KMP only occurs with two specific vascular tumors, TA and KHE, and has a much more profound thrombocytopenia, with a platelet range of 2,000 to 10,000/mm^3. Also, lesions causing KMP are treated with antiangiogenic agents, whereas VMs will not respond to pharmacotherapy.

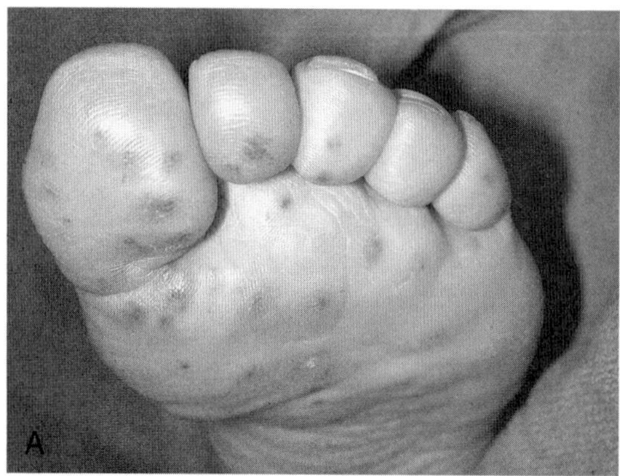

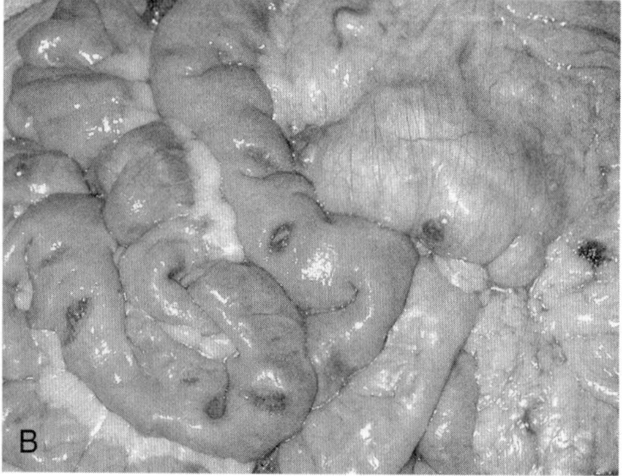

Figure 74-12. Blue rubber bleb nevus syndrome. **A,** Classic cutaneous venous malformations are seen on the sole of the foot. **B,** Venous malformations of the small intestine and colon were found at operation.

Histologically, VMs most often consist of sinusoidal vascular spaces with variable communications with adjacent veins (the dilated venous channels of VMs are thin walled when compared with normal veins). Staining with smooth muscle actin reveals abnormal smooth muscle architecture that may be responsible for the gradual expansion seen over time with these lesions. Moreover, calcified phleboliths may provide evidence of prior clot formation within the VMs. A variant of VMs, glomovenous malformation (also incorrectly called "glomangioma"), has the additional presence of ball-shaped glomus cells that line the vascular channels.

Imaging

Radiologic modalities useful for the diagnosis of VMs include ultrasonography, MRI, and venography. MRI is most informative and demonstrates hyperintense lesions with T2-weighted sequences. Contrast enhancement of the vascular spaces distinguishes VMs from LMs, as does the presence of pathognomonic phleboliths. Intralesional bleeding within LMs causing contrast enhancement can be an exception to this rule. In contrast to AVMs, VMs do not demonstrate evidence of arterial flow on MRI.

Treatment

The indications for treatment of VMs are appearance, pain, loss of function, and bleeding. Unfortunately, cure for VMs, as with LMs, is difficult to achieve for all but the most localized and therefore less problematic lesions. For extensive VMs of the extremities, conservative management with the use of graded compression stockings can achieve significant improvement in size and symptoms. Patient satisfaction with this modality depends on a proper customized fit, but can be elusive, especially for children and teenagers. To prevent phlebothrombosis of VMs with resultant pain and swelling, low-dose aspirin may be beneficial.

Intralesional sclerotherapy is the mainstay of treatment for most VMs.[81] Sclerosing agents, most commonly ethanol and sodium tetradecyl sulfate, cause direct endothelial damage, thrombosis, and scarring. For small VMs, the injection process is similar to that of simple varicosities. Larger lesions are accessed by direct puncture, and therapeutic agents are injected under fluoroscopy with the use of tourniquets and compression of venous drainage to prevent systemic administration of the sclerosants. General anesthesia is required in most instances. Staged therapy and occasional embolization of large venous channels are useful for more complex VMs. The more complex lesions are best treated by a skilled interventional radiologist who has experience with vascular anomalies. Potential local complications of sclerotherapy are blistering, skin necrosis, and damage to adjacent nerves. Systemic complications include hemolysis, sudden pulmonary hypertension, and cardiac and renal toxicity. These can usually be avoided with proper dosage and sclerosant selection. For example, ethanol is a strong sclerosant that carries a higher risk of damage to local tissues and adjacent structures.

VMs have a propensity for recanalization and, therefore, re-enlargement. Cure with sclerotherapy is rare. Results from treatment are often stated in terms of patient satisfaction from decreased pain and appearance, given that recurrence is so prevalent. Surgical resection is typically reserved for well-localized lesions but is marked by procedural morbidity and recurrence. Preoperative sclerotherapy is recommended preceding operations for extensive VMs to shrink the lesion and decrease bleeding during the resection.

Unifocal gastrointestinal lesions can be excised. Diffuse colorectal malformations causing significant bleeding may be treated with colectomy, anorectal mucosectomy, and coloanal pull-through.[82] For multifocal VMs of the blue rubber bleb nevus syndrome, complete surgical resection of the lesions, combined with endoscopy of the entire gastrointestinal tract at the time of operation, provides the only chance for possible cure. Bowel resections for these lesions are rarely indicated. Rather, wedge excision and polypectomy by intussusception of successive lengths of intestine are the preferred methods of resection.[83]

ARTERIOVENOUS MALFORMATIONS

Clinical Presentation

AVMs are fast-flow vascular malformations characterized by abnormal connections or shunts between feeding arteries and draining veins without an intervening capillary bed. These shunts define the nidus of the malformation. This lesion tends to be localized but can be extensive as well. AVMs are familiar to neurosurgeons as one of the more common vascular anomalies that occur in the central nervous system. Indeed, intracranial AVMs are more frequent than AVMs of the skin and soft tissues within the head and neck region. Other common sites of involvement are the extremities, trunk, and viscera. These congenital malformations exhibit a peculiar but characteristic natural history of progression in stages (Table 74-2). At birth, they appear as a pink cutaneous blemish that can be confused with both CMs and the premonitory sign of an infantile hemangioma. However, fast flow across arteriovenous shunts is present beneath the innocent-appearing surface. This fast flow becomes more evident in childhood, and the lesion develops into a mass. AVMs grow in proportion with the child, but puberty, pregnancy, or local trauma tends to trigger more rapid expansion. The lesion becomes more obviously warm to touch and may develop a bruit or thrill. With continued expansion, the lesion becomes more red and prominent. Because of expansion and local steal phenomenon, skin ischemia can develop, leading to pain, ulceration, and bleeding (Fig. 74-13). For large AVMs, high-output cardiac failure can result.

Table 74-2	Schobinger Clinical Staging System for Arteriovenous Malformations
Stage	**Clinical Findings**
I (Quiescent)	Pink to bluish stain, cutaneous warmth, and arteriovenous shunting by Doppler ultrasound imaging
II (Expanding)	Same as stage I, plus enlargement, pulsation, thrill, bruit, and tortuous and tense veins
III (Destructive)	Same as stage II, plus skin ulceration, bleeding, persistent pain, or tissue necrosis
IV (Decompensating)	Same as stage III, plus cardiac failure

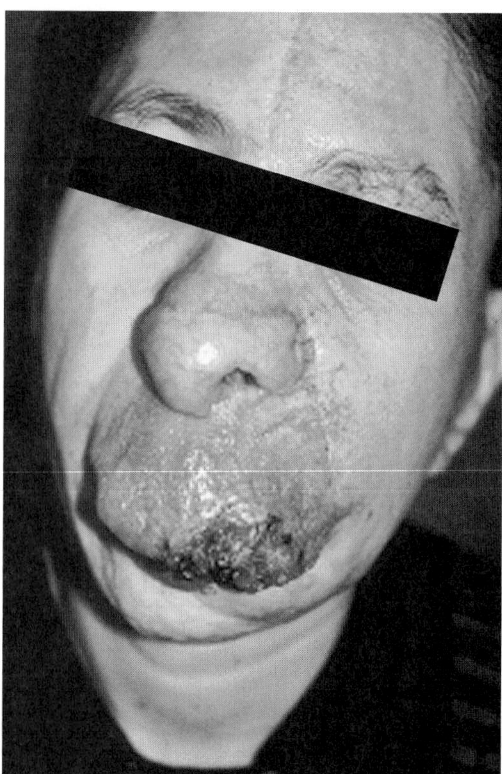

Figure 74-13. A facial arteriovenous malformation (stage III) with ulceration of the skin is seen in this patient.

Imaging

Ultrasonography and Doppler imaging are excellent tools to elucidate the fast flow of these lesions and to distinguish them from VMs. Although hemangiomas can be characterized by fast flow as well, the history and age at onset should distinguish them from AVMs. MRI and MR angiography are the most useful tools to demonstrate the full extent of these lesions. They appear as hyperintense masses with contrast enhancement and flow voids seen on flow-sensitive sequences. Superselective angiography has its role at the time when treatment is planned.

Treatment

The majority of AVMs will require treatment at some point because of the natural history of continued expansion that leads to local tissue ischemia and pain.[84,85] The mainstays of treatment for these lesions are angiographic embolization alone or in combination with surgical excision. However, in the early stages, the full extent of the AVMs may not be appreciated, such that local recurrence would complicate embolization or resection. Therefore, resection of AVMs during infancy and early childhood is rarely advocated. At the same time, the very well localized stage I AVMs may be amenable to excision. The usual recommendation is to observe AVMs in the early stages and monitor them carefully through regularly scheduled annual examinations. Intervention is delayed until symptoms develop indicative of stage III: local pain, ulceration, and bleeding. For treatment initiated at any stage, it is critical that the proximal feeding arteries *not* be embolized or ligated. Although ligation may provide temporary improvement for complications such as bleeding, these feeding arteries provide the only avenue for subsequent successful embolization. The nidus of the AVMs will recruit other nearby arteries after the primary feeding vessels are occluded, and the AVMs will recur and continue to progress.

Embolization must be directed to the nidus itself and to the AVFs at the epicenter of the lesion. Direct puncture sclerotherapy of the AVM nidus can be a useful adjunct to embolization, especially when the feeding arteries are too tortuous or have been previously ligated. Repeated and staged embolization procedures are typically necessary for these lesions but often only provide temporary improvement. The reason for this problem is the quantity and microscopic nature of the AVFs that comprise the nidus of AVMs. It is difficult to achieve complete occlusion for the entirety of these microscopic shunts. Nonetheless, patients often have significant improvement in their symptoms, and cures with embolization alone have been reported.

The preferred strategy of treatment of AVMs typically consists of surgical resection performed 2 to 3 days after preoperative embolization of the nidus. Angiographic embolization facilitates the operation by decreasing bleeding but does not reduce the extent of tissue that should be resected. Whenever possible, the goal should be complete excision to normal margins. Both the nidus of the AVMs and the involved skin are removed. The most important factor for success that should be given close attention is the decision regarding extent of resection. Review of radiologic imaging is necessary, including the earliest available MR images and angiograms before any other treatment. Intraoperatively, observation of the pattern of bleeding at the resection margins also can guide the extent of excision, as can intraoperative frozen section pathology. Primary closure is sometimes not possible without tissue transfer techniques. Vacuum-assisted closure devices also can be useful in wounds with large soft tissue loss precluding linear closure. The best results are seen with AVMs that are well localized. Yet, even for these cases it is prudent to monitor these patients for years to evaluate for signs of recurrence. Unfortunately, most AVMs are extensive and often not amenable to surgical options. For these difficult lesions, embolization is used for palliation. For difficult AVMs of the extremities, if distal in location, amputation should be considered as an option.

COMBINED VASCULAR MALFORMATIONS

As with other vascular malformations, combined malformations are classified as either slow flow or fast flow. These more complex disorders, as a rule, are associated with soft tissue and skeletal overgrowth. They tend to be named for the person or persons who first described them. However, these eponyms often create confusion because of misuse. Thus, it is preferred to use the anatomic terms that best describe the anomalous vascular channels that are present.

Klippel-Trénaunay Syndrome

Klippel-Trénaunay syndrome is a slow-flow combined vascular malformation involving abnormal capillaries, lymphatics, and veins.[86-88] This capillary lymphaticovenous malformation (CLVM) usually involves one or more extremities, most often a lower limb, and is associated with prominent soft tissue and bony hypertrophy (Fig. 74-14). This syndrome is sporadic and obvious at birth, although a wide range of severity occurs. The CM component can be multiple and typically is seen as a large geographic pattern affecting the extremity, buttock, and trunk. It is macular at birth and develops hemolymphatic vesicles over time. The lymphatic anomalies have a variable presentation, including hypoplasia, lymphedema, and macrocystic LMs. The venous component consists of anomalous lateral superficial veins in the extremity that are persistent embryonic vessels. These veins are usually dilated and have incompetent valve systems. Anomalous deep system veins may be hypoplastic or even absent. Thrombophlebitis of the anomalous veins occurs with a frequency of 20% to 45%, and pulmonary emboli are reported in 4% to 25% of cases.

Limb hypertrophy is obvious at birth and occurs in peculiar patterns. It tends to be progressive over time. The spectrum of deformities includes enlargement of hands and feet, both ipsilateral and contralateral to the limb affected by CLVMs. Although the affected extremity is generally larger, it is occasionally smaller. With CLVMs of the legs, pelvic involvement with LMs and VMs also can occur but is often asymptomatic. Alternatively, problems with recurrent infections, hematuria, hematochezia, and bladder outlet obstruction may occur. With CLVMs of the superior trunk and arms, the mediastinum or retropleural space can harbor the vascular malformations as well.

Imaging plays an important role in the evaluation of patients with Klippel-Trénaunay syndrome. Plain radiographs are used to document limb-length discrepancies serially. MRI provides the foundation for

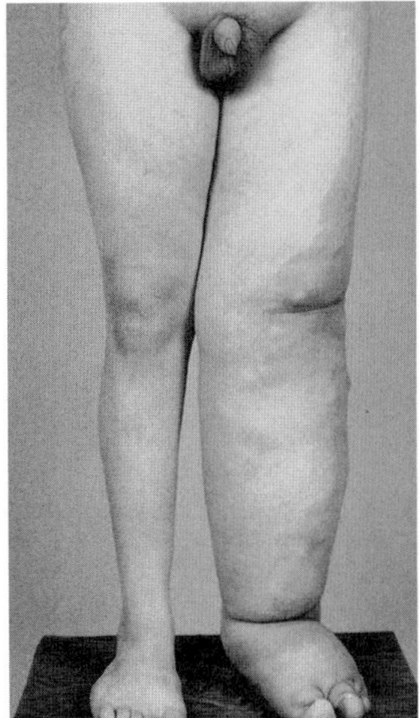
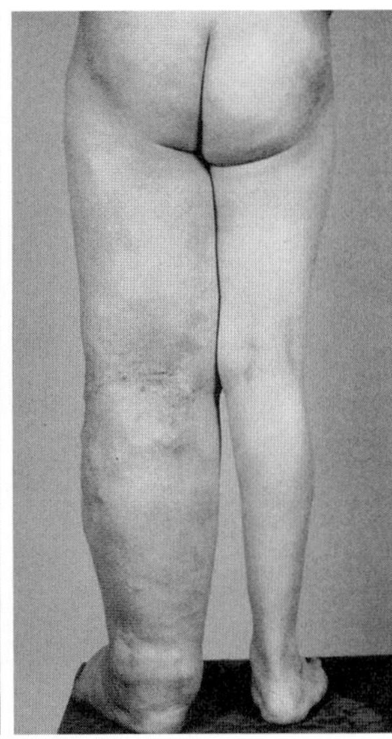

Figure 74-14. Patient with Klippel-Trénaunay syndrome or capillary lymphaticovenous malformation (CLVM) and associated soft tissue and skeletal overgrowth of the lower extremity.

describing the type and extent of each of the vascular malformation components. Hypertrophic fatty tissue is often seen on MRI in areas of overgrowth. One common pattern seen with LMs of the lower extremity is to find macrocystic lesions in the pelvis and thigh and microcystic LMs affecting the abdominal wall, buttock, and distal extremity. These LMs can be localized to the subcutaneous tissues or extend into the intramuscular compartments. MR venography can elucidate the anatomy of the deep system veins. Identification of a subcutaneous vein coursing along the lateral calf and thigh (the marginal vein of Servelle) is pathognomonic for Klippel-Trénaunay syndrome. Venography is considered for some patients to map the venous drainage of the extremity before resection of any anomalous superficial veins if concern exists regarding patency of the deep veins based on MR venography.

In general, treatment for Klippel-Trénaunay syndrome is conservative, because it is not a curable disease. However, operative therapies do have a place to manage some of the specific problems that are encountered, which are primarily overgrowth.[89] Gross foot enlargement that impairs ambulation and the ability to wear shoes requires orthopedic corrective procedures and partial amputations to permit the use of custom footwear. Leg-length discrepancy should be followed up annually by an orthopedic surgeon to document and predict severity. Shoe lifts are recommended to prevent limping and scoliosis if the discrepancy is greater than 1.5 cm at age 2 years. Sometimes, epiphysiodesis of the distal femoral growth plate is performed around age 12 years to correct overgrowth. Correction for arm-length discrepancies is unnecessary. Staged contour resection can be used to treat areas of soft tissue overgrowth and lymphedema. Symptoms of pain and deformity secondary to venous anomalies can often be improved with compression stockings. Alternatively, sclerotherapy can treat certain components of CLVMs such as focal VMs, macrocystic LMs, and bleeding capillary lymphatic vesicles. Recurrence after sclerotherapy, however, is often a problem. Surgical resection of anomalous veins producing pain or potential sources of pulmonary emboli also is an option. Perioperative management during significant resections should include consideration for anticoagulation and temporary inferior vena cava filter placement to help prevent deep venous thrombosis and pulmonary embolization.

Maffucci Syndrome

Maffucci syndrome consists of exophytic VMs of the soft tissue and bones, bony exostoses, and endochondromas. It is sporadic and not usually evident at birth. It can be unilateral or bilateral. The bony lesions and endochondromas manifest first in childhood, and the venous anomalies appear later. Spindle cell hemangioendotheliomas commonly occur and denote reactive vascular proliferation within the preexisting VMs, rather than true tumors.[90] The endochondromas can undergo malignant transformation in 20% to 30% of cases, leading to chondrosarcomas.[91] This fact suggests that a tumor suppressor gene may be involved in the pathogenesis.

Bannayan-Riley-Ruvalcaba Syndrome

Bannayan-Riley-Ruvalcaba syndrome is an autosomal dominant syndrome caused by mutations of the tumor suppressor gene *PTEN* (phosphatase tensin homolog) on chromosome 10.[92] It is primarily an overgrowth syndrome that has vascular malformations as a minor component. Typically, cutaneous CMs, VMs, or AVMs are found. The more prominent clinical features are macrocephaly, multiple lipomas, hamartomatous polyps of the ileum and colon, and Hashimoto's thyroiditis.

Proteus Syndrome

This syndrome is probably diagnosed more often than it actually occurs. It is named after a Greek god who was able to assume any shape or form.[93] This overgrowth disorder is sporadic and progressive over time. Vascular, skeletal, and soft tissue anomalies tend to be asymmetric and variably expressed. Common features include lipomas or lipomatosis, macrocephaly, and gigantism of the hands or feet or both.

Parkes Weber Syndrome

Parkes Weber syndrome is a sporadic combined fast-flow vascular malformation affecting the limb and trunk, with the lower extremity being the most common site.[94,95] Capillary arteriovenous fistulas (CAVF) and capillary arteriovenous malformations (CAVM) are combined with hypertrophy of the bone and muscle of the affected limb. CAVM is obvious at birth, appearing as overgrowth with a large geographic macular pink stain. In contrast to CLVM seen with Klippel-Trénaunay syndrome, the limb hypertrophy is symmetric along the length and substance of the extremity. The macular stain associated with CAVM has much greater cutaneous warmth than do typical CMs. The findings of bruits or thrills on examination confirm the diagnosis.

MRI demonstrates symmetric muscular and bony overgrowth, with generalized enlargement of the normal named arteries and veins within the affected limb. Angiography depicts the discrete AVFs. In rare cases, superselective embolization is used to occlude the arteriovenous shunts if symptoms of ischemia, pain, or high-output congestive heart failure occur.

chapter 75

HEAD AND NECK SINUSES AND MASSES

Stephanie Acierno, MD, MPH • John H. T. Waldhausen, MD

Lesions of the head and neck in children can be subdivided by etiology as resulting from infection, trauma, or neoplasm, or being of congenital origin. The more common benign neoplasms, including hemangiomas, lymphangiomas, and cystic hygromas, are discussed in Chapter 74. Malignant neoplasms of childhood (e.g., neuroblastoma, lymphoma, and rhabdomyosarcoma), which occur as a primary or metastatic mass in the head and neck, lesions of the thyroid and parathyroid, and traumatic injuries of the head and neck, also are discussed in other chapters. In this chapter, common congenital head and neck malformations are described and inflammatory lesions are reviewed.

LESIONS OF EMBRYONIC ORIGIN

Congenital cysts and sinuses that appear in the neck result from embryonic structures that have failed to mature or have persisted in an aberrant fashion.[1,2] Successful treatment of a child with a mass or sinus in the head or neck requires accurate identification of the lesion as well as a planned course of therapy. Both diagnosis and therapy depend on a working knowledge of the embryologic origin and differentiation of the head and neck structures.[3,4] This knowledge is particularly important because complete surgical resection of cartilaginous remnants, remnants of the branchial arch and cleft structures, and midline fusion abnormalities is imperative to avoid recurrence. Congenital lesions of the head and neck, in descending order of frequency, are thyroglossal duct cysts, preauricular pits and sinuses, branchial cleft anomalies, dermoid cysts, and median cervical clefts.

Thyroglossal Duct Cyst

One of the most common lesions in the midline of the neck is a thyroglossal duct cyst. Thyroglossal duct remnants are found in 7% of the population, although few become symptomatic.[4,5] Although they are embryonic in origin, it is rare for these lesions to be found in the newborn period.[1] More commonly, they are noted in preschool-age children.[1] Thyroglossal duct cysts also are common in young adults and, with the exception of thyroid goiter, are the most common midline neck masses in this age group.[6]

EMBRYOLOGY

The embryogenesis of the thyroglossal duct is intimately involved with that of the thyroid gland, the hyoid bone, and the tongue.[7] The foramen cecum is the site of the development of the thyroid diverticulum.[7] In the embryo, this structure develops caudal to the central tuberculum impar, which is one of the pharyngeal buds that leads to the formation of the tongue.[7] As the tongue develops, the thyroid diverticulum descends in the neck, maintaining its connection to the foramen cecum. During this time, the hyoid bone is developing from the second branchial arch. The thyroid gland develops between weeks 4 and 7 of gestation and descends into its pretracheal position in the neck.[8] As a result of these multiple events occurring simultaneously, the thyroglossal duct may pass in front of or behind the hyoid bone, but most commonly it passes through it. Usually, the duct disappears by the time the thyroid reaches its normal position by 5 to 8 weeks' gestation.[5,9] Thyroglossal duct cysts never have a primary external opening because the embryologic thyroglossal tract never reaches the surface of the neck.[8] Usually the thyroglossal tract becomes obliterated. If it persists, a cyst can be located anywhere along the migratory course of the thyroglossal tract in the neck (Fig. 75-1). Occasionally, the cysts attach to the pyramidal lobe of the thyroid or may be intrathyroidal.[10] Complete failure of migration of the thyroid results in a lingual thyroid, which develops beneath the foramen cecum at the base of the tongue.[11] In this instance, no thyroid tissue is found in the neck.[11]

CLINICAL PRESENTATION

Two thirds of thyroglossal duct anomalies are discovered within the first 3 decades of life.[5] Classically, the thyroglossal cysts are located in the midline at or just below the hyoid bone (Fig. 75-2). Suprahyoid thyroglossal cysts must be distinguished from submental dermoid cysts and from submental lymph nodes.[12]

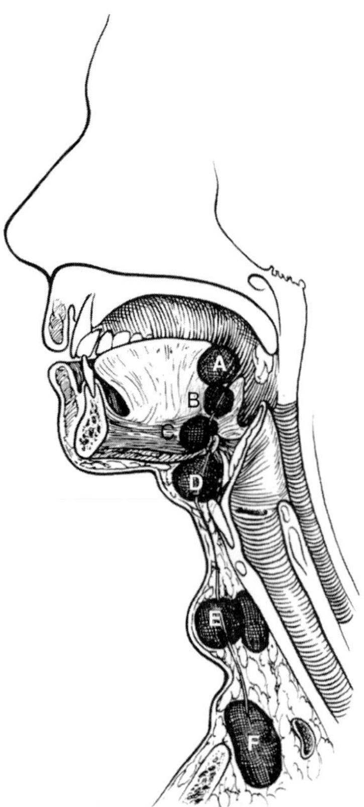

Figure 75-1. Thyroglossal duct cysts can be located anywhere from the base of the tongue to behind the sternum. A and B, Lingual (rare). C and D, Adjacent to hyoid bone (common). E and F, Suprasternal fossa (rare). (From Welch KJ, Randolph JG, Ravitch MM, et al [eds]: Pediatric Surgery, 4th ed. Chicago, Year Book Medical, 1986, p 549.)

Rarely, the cysts are suprasternal in location. The initial sign is usually a painless mass in the midline of the neck, with 66% found adjacent to the hyoid bone.[9] On physical examination, the thyroglossal duct cyst is smooth, soft, and nontender. To distinguish this lesion from the more superficial dermoid lesion, one should palpate the lesion while the child sticks out his or her tongue. Owing to its attachment to the foramen cecum, the thyroglossal duct cyst does not fully move when the tongue protrudes. This maneuver is more reliable than asking the child to swallow and determining whether the mass moves with swallowing. Owing to the communication to the mouth via the foramen cecum, thyroglossal cysts can become infected with oral flora. One third of patients will present with a concurrent or prior infection and a fourth will present with a draining sinus from spontaneous or surgical drainage of an abscess.[9] Some patients may present with a foul taste in the mouth from spontaneous drainage of the cyst via the foramen cecum.

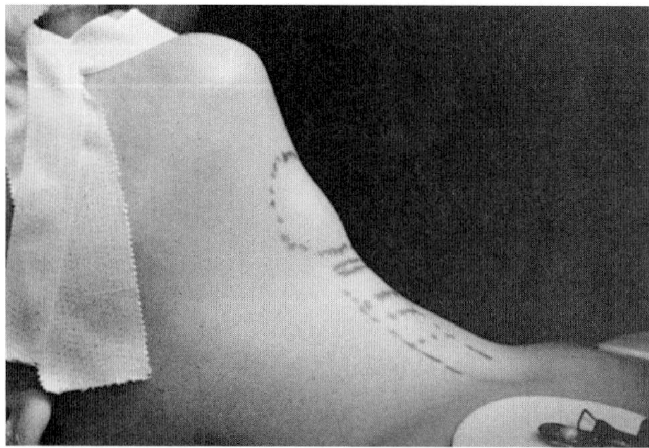

Figure 75-2. A classic thyroglossal duct cyst located in the midline just below the hyoid bone. Markings on the neck represent the thyroid, cricoid and tracheal cartilages.

The preoperative evaluation for a patient with a suspected thyroglossal duct cyst should include a complete history and physical examination. Patients with findings suggestive of hypothyroidism should undergo thyroid function testing and additional imaging to exclude a median ectopic thyroid. The incidence of ectopic thyroid tissue in or near the duct is reported to be from 10% to 45%. Some clinicians have advocated preoperative thyroid scanning or ultrasonography to eliminate the possibility of an ectopic thyroid gland masquerading as a thyroglossal duct cyst.[13-17] Ultrasonography appears to be very accurate and avoids the need for irradiation and possible sedation in younger children.[16] The anatomic location also may be useful in differentiating cysts and ectopic thyroid. Ninety percent of ectopic thyroid tissue lies at the base of the tongue, and thyroglossal duct cysts are rarely found there. Abnormal thyroid function tests, a suggestive history, or a solid mass evident on an ultrasound image should prompt a preoperative thyroid scan to ensure the lesion is not the only thyroid gland present, which occurs in less than 1% to 2% of patients with thyroglossal duct cysts.[9,15,18] If ectopic thyroid tissue is found, the management becomes controversial, but some clinicians suggest a trial of medical suppression to decrease the size of the mass.

Treatment

Elective surgical excision is advised to avoid the complications of infection and because of the small risk (<1%) of cancer developing in the cyst.[15] The cyst and its cephalad tract are completely excised to the base of the tongue (Fig. 75-3). In 1920, Sistrunk described excision of the central portion of the hyoid bone as necessary treatment to prevent cyst recurrence.[19] The operation must include resection of the central portion of the hyoid bone.[20,21] Several other studies have shown that multiple smaller tracts can connect through the hyoid bone to the floor of the mouth, requiring wide resection of tracts above the hyoid.[20-22] If these suprahyoid tracts remain, the incidence of recurrence increases.[23] The best chance for successful resection is adequate wide resection at the initial procedure.[22]

As for all neck surgery, the patient should be supine with the neck slightly hyperextended (Fig. 75-4). The thyroglossal cyst is exposed through a transverse incision. The cyst has a characteristic appearance that is distinctly different from that of thyroid tissue. The dissection should continue cephalad to the hyoid, resecting a block of tissue along the proximal tract. Transecting the hyoid is simplified by using angled scissors, similar to Potts scissors, or by using a

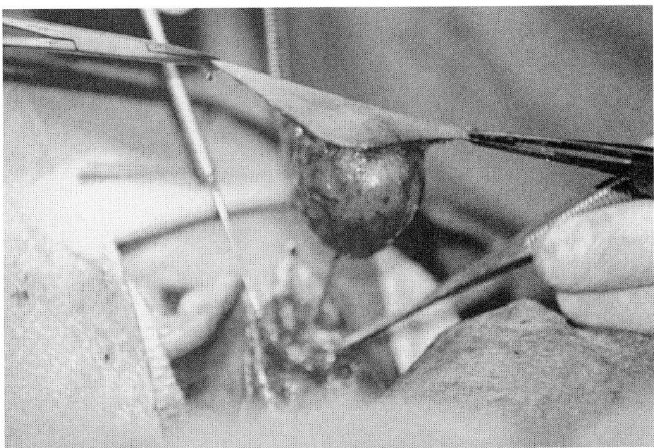

Figure 75-3. Complete excision of a previously infected thyroglossal duct cyst. Surrounding skin was removed because of changes related to a previous infection. Note the well-defined tract leading toward the hyoid bone and the floor of the mouth. The operation was completed by excising the central portion of the hyoid bone and suture ligating the tract.

side-cutting bone cutter. The base of the tract at the floor of the mouth is ligated with absorbable suture. The wings of the hyoid are not approximated. The incision is copiously irrigated, and the wound is closed in layers. If the floor of the mouth is entered inadvertently, this can be repaired with absorbable suture.

Occasionally, the dissection may be made easier by having the anesthesiologist place his or her finger at the base of the child's tongue to identify the cephalad extent of the dissection. With complete excision, including the central portion of the hyoid bone, the risk of recurrence is low, 2.6% to 5.0%.[5,9,23,24] Risk factors for recurrence include simple cyst excision alone (recurrence rates of 38% to 70%), intraoperative cyst rupture, presence of a cutaneous component, and postoperative wound infections.[5,9,25] As mentioned, the cyst is usually connected to the foramen cecum by single or multiple tracts that pass through the hyoid. On histologic examination, the duct lining is stratified squamous epithelium or ciliated pseudostratified columnar epithelium, with associated mucus-secreting glands.[9] The cyst contains a characteristic glairy mucus. Less than 1% have malignant tissue, which is most often papillary thyroid carcinoma.

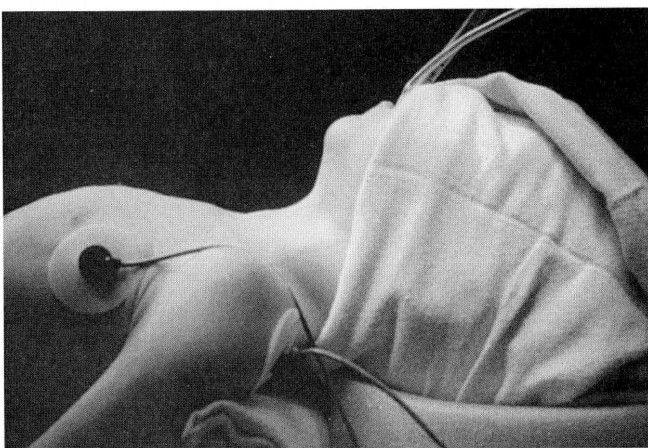

Figure 75-4. Positioning a child for a cervical operation. Hyperextension of the head with support under the shoulders and stabilization with a bean bag keeps the child in a stable position and facilitates exposure. The head of the bed should be elevated 30 degrees to decrease venous pressure in the neck.

Infected cysts or sinuses should be managed by initially treating the infection. The usual route of infection is via the mouth. Thus, the common organisms are *Haemophilus influenzae, Staphylococcus aureus,* and *Staphylococcus epidermidis.*[9] Needle aspiration may be required to decompress the cyst and allow for identification of the organism, but formal incision and drainage should be avoided. This may seed ductal cells outside of the cyst and increase recurrence rates.[9] If incision and drainage is required, the incision should be placed so that it can be completely excised during a formal Sistrunk procedure once the infection clears.

If a solid mass is found during thyroglossal duct cyst excision, it should be sent for frozen section to exclude median ectopic thyroid. If it is normal thyroid tissue and there is additional functional thyroid tissue in the normal location, a Sistrunk procedure with excision of the mass should be performed.[9] If there is no other thyroid tissue present, management is controversial. One option is to leave the tissue in situ or reposition it into the strap muscles. This is attempted to prevent the patient from becoming permanently hypothyroid. However, most patients still require thyroid hormone therapy for hypothyroidism or to control the size of the ectopic thyroid. Because of this likely need for long-term therapy and possible malignant degeneration, some surgeons advocate complete excision of the ectopic thyroid tissue regardless of the presence of additional thyroid tissue.[9]

Remnants of Embryonic Branchial Apparatus

Branchial anomalies comprise approximately 30% of congenital neck masses and can present as cysts, sinuses, or fistulas.[5,26] They are equally common in males and females and present in childhood or early adulthood.

Embryology

During weeks 4 to 8 after fertilization, four pairs of well-developed ridges (branchial arches) dominate the lateral cervicofacial area of the human embryo.[27] These four pairs are accompanied by two rudimentary pairs, which are analogous to the gill apparatus of lower forms.[2,27] No true gill mechanisms are found in any stage of the human embryo. These pharyngeal arches and clefts are formed without a true connection between the outer ectodermal clefts and the inner endodermal pharyngeal pouches (Fig. 75-5). The mature structures of the head and neck are derivatives of several branchial arches and their intervening clefts.[27,28] The branchial clefts and pouches are gradually obliterated by mesenchyme, but branchial cleft anomalies result if that process is incomplete.[26]

Each arch transforms during gestation into a defined anatomic pattern. Understanding this pattern and its relationship to normal neck structures is key in

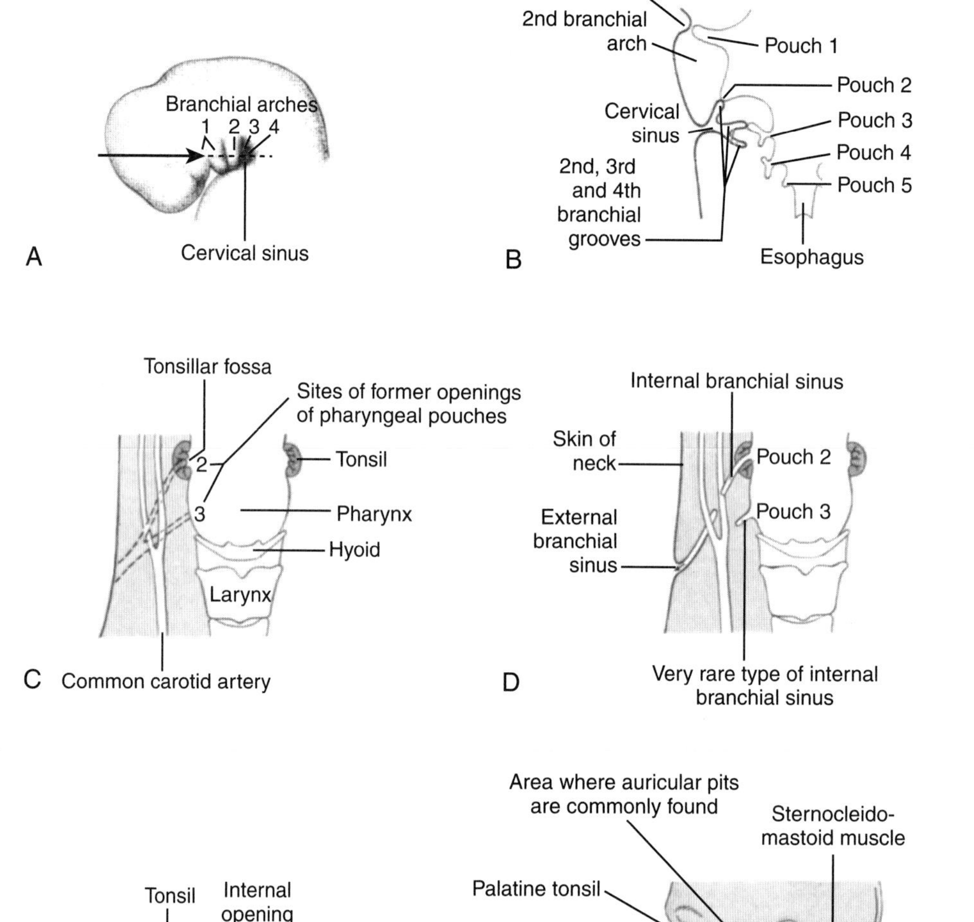

Figure 75-5. **A,** The head and neck region of a 5-week-old embryo. **B,** Horizontal section through the embryo illustrating the relationship of the cervical sinus to the branchial arches and pharyngeal pouches. **C,** The adult neck region, indicating the former sites of openings of the cervical sinus and the pharyngeal pouches. The *dotted lines* indicate possible courses of branchial fistulas. **D,** The embryologic basis of various types of branchial sinuses. **E,** A branchial fistula resulting from persistence of parts of the second branchial cleft and the second pharyngeal pouch. **F,** Possible sites of branchial cysts and openings of branchial sinuses and fistulas. A branchial vestige also is illustrated. (From Moore KL: The Developing Human: Clinically Oriented Embryology. Philadelphia, WB Saunders, 1977.)

the diagnosis and treatment of these anomalies. Each anomaly is classified by the cleft or pouch of origin, which can be determined by the internal opening of the sinus as well as its relationship to nerves, arteries, and muscles. Careful attention to these relationships is necessary to prevent injury to surrounding tissues and ensure complete resection.[26]

Pathology

Branchial anomalies are lined with either respiratory or squamous epithelium. Sinuses and fistulas usually have the former and cysts have the latter.[26] One also can see lymphoid tissue, sebaceous glands, salivary tissue, or cholesterol crystals. Squamous cell cancer has been reported in adults, but it is rare and can be difficult to distinguish a primary branchiogenic lesion from a metastatic lesion from an occult primary lesion.[5]

Clinical Presentation

Complete fistulas are more common than external sinuses. Both are more common than branchial cysts, at least during childhood.[29,30] In adults, cysts predominate.[29] By definition, all branchial remnants are truly congenital and are present at birth.[30,31] Cysts are remnants of sinuses without an external opening and usually appear later in childhood than do sinuses, fistulas, and cartilaginous remnants, which are often found at birth.[5,31] Sinuses have the persistence of the external opening only, whereas fistulas involve the persistence of the branchial groove with breakdown of the branchial membrane.[5] Commonly, the tiny external opening of the fistula and the external sinuses remain unnoticed for some time. Spontaneous mucoid drainage from the ostium along the border of the sternocleidomastoid usually heralds its presence and initiates the parent's concern and the reason for the child's referral. The first clinical presentation may be an infected mass as a result of the inability of the thick mucoid material to drain spontaneously. Infection is, however, less common in fistulas and external sinuses than in cysts.[1] The cutaneous openings are occasionally marked by skin tags or cartilage remnants. The tract itself may be palpable as a cord-like structure ascending in the neck when the child's neck is hyperextended and the skin is taut. Compression along the tract may produce mucoid material exiting from the ostium.

The evaluation of these lesions starts with a thorough history and physical examination. Palpating the tract and observing the mucoid discharge can be confirmatory. Although colored dye or radiopaque material may be injected to delineate the tract, these manipulations generally are unnecessary. Upper endoscopy can be helpful to locate the pharyngeal opening. Both the pyriform sinus and tonsillar fossas should be examined. Cysts may be more difficult to diagnose. They lie deep to the skin along the anterior border of the sternocleidomastoid muscle.[1] They can usually be distinguished from cystic hygromas, which are subcutaneous and can be transilluminated. Ultrasonography, computed tomography (CT), and magnetic resonance imaging (MRI) can help define the lesion and can be particularly helpful in narrowing the differential diagnosis, but CT is most often used and can demonstrate a fistula in 64% of cases.[32] A barium esophagogram has 50% to 80% sensitivity for third and fourth branchial fistulas.[33] Whereas fine-needle aspiration is necessary in adults to rule out metastatic carcinoma, it is not necessary in children, and incisional biopsy should be avoided.[26]

TREATMENT

The goal of treating all congenital neck sinuses, cysts, and fistulas is usually complete excision, done electively, when no inflammation is present.[34] Timing of resection is controversial, with some advocating for early resection to prevent infection while others support waiting until 2 or 3 years of age.[26,35,36] As with thyroglossal duct cysts, if the lesion is infected at clinical presentation, antibiotic therapy and warm soaks to encourage spontaneous drainage of mucoid plugs should precede definitive excision. Approximately 20% of lesions will have been infected at least once before surgery.[35] Attempts at complete excision in an inflamed, infected field increase the risk of nerve injury and incomplete resection. Aspiration or a limited incision and drainage procedure is sometimes necessary to resolve the infection. Complete surgical excision is delayed until the inflammation subsides and the surrounding skin is supple. Endoscopic cauterization of fourth branchial cleft sinuses has been described either at the time of initial abscess drainage or 4 to 6 weeks later. Recurrence with this technique seems to be uncommon.[37]

Surgical resection is performed under general anesthesia with the patient positioned as shown in Figure 75-4. A small transverse elliptical incision is made around the external opening and deepened beneath the cervical fascia. The initial dissection is along the inferior border of the incision so that the ascending tract is identified from below and is not injured. Placement of a 2-0 or 3-0 monofilament suture or probe within the tract can facilitate this dissection. Dissection proceeds cephalad, staying on the tract until visualization of the most superior portion of the tract becomes difficult. At this level, a second, more cephalad, parallel "stair step" incision or extension of the original incision may be necessary for adequate exposure. If a second, more cephalad incision is needed, the tract is pulled subcutaneously through the second incision and the dissection is continued cephalad between the bifurcation of the carotid artery to the point where the tract inserts into the pharynx. The fistula is suture ligated with absorbable suture material. The incision is closed in layers with absorbable sutures. No drains are needed if resection is complete. Recurrences are rare and imply that a portion of the epithelium-lined tract was overlooked. The incidence of recurrence is higher in cases of previously infected lesions. The specific embryology, anatomic presentation, and treatment for each type of branchial anomaly will now be discussed.

First Cleft Anomalies

The first branchial arch forms the mandible and contributes to the maxillary process of the upper jaw.[28,31,38] Abnormal development of the first branchial arch results in a host of facial deformities, including cleft lip and palate, abnormal shape or contour of the external ear, and malformed internal ossicles.[28,31] The first branchial cleft contributes to the tympanic cavity, eustachian tube, middle ear cavity, and mastoid air cells. Microtia and aural atresia occur with failure of the first branchial cleft to develop.[27,28]

First branchial anomalies are rare and account for less than 1% of branchial cleft malformations.[26] Cysts are seen as swellings posterior or anterior to the ear or inferior to the earlobe in the submandibular region. External openings, if found, are located inferior to the mandible in a suprahyoid position. One third open into the external auditory canal.[6] The tract may be intimately associated with, or course through, the parotid gland. This and the proximity of the seventh cranial nerve make resection difficult, particularly in the younger patient who is likely to have a tract deep to the facial nerve.[32] First cleft anomalies are classified as type I or type II (Figs. 75-6 and 75-7).[5,26] Type I lesions are duplications of the external auditory canal, have only ectoderm, course lateral to the facial nerve, and present as swellings near the ear. Type II consist of both mesoderm and ectoderm, can contain cartilage, pass medial to the facial nerve, and present as swellings inferior to the angle of the mandible or anterior to the sternocleidomastoid in a preauricular, infra-auricular, or postauricular position. First branchial anomalies are more common in females than males and are often misdiagnosed, leading to delay in excision.[39] Presentation can include cervical, parotid, or auricular signs.

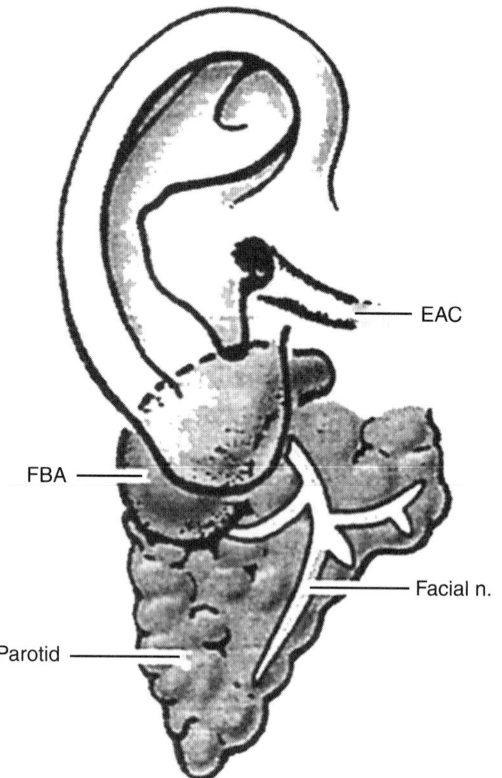

Figure 75-6. Type I first branchial cleft anomaly (FBA). Note that the anomaly, located in the parotid gland, has no connection to the external auditory canal (EAC). (From Mukherji SK, Fatterpekar G, Castillo M, et al: Imaging of congenital anomalies of the branchial apparatus. Neuroimaging Clin North Am 10:75-93, 2000.)

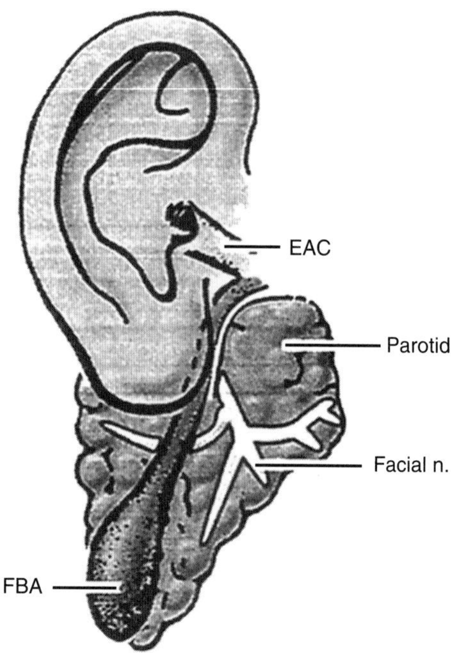

Figure 75-7. Type II first branchial cleft anomaly (FBA). The anomaly connects with the external auditory canal (EAC) and extends deep into the parotid gland. (From Mukherji SK, Fatterpekar G, Castillo M, et al: Imaging of congenital anomalies of the branchial apparatus. Neuroimaging Clin North Am 10:75-93, 2000.)

Cervical signs include drainage from a pit-like depression at the angle of the mandible. Parotid signs result from rapid enlargement due to inflammation. Auricular signs can consist of swelling or otorrhea.

Resection of first arch anomalies often requires at least partial facial nerve dissection and superficial parotidectomy. It is important to resect any involved skin or cartilage of the external auditory canal (Fig. 75-8). If it extends medial to the tympanic membrane, a second procedure may be necessary to remove the medial component. Tracts that go to the middle ear are more likely to travel deep or split around the facial nerve.[39] Recurrence is common, and more than two procedures are often required for complete resection.[40] Each repeat surgery places the facial nerve at greater risk from prior scarring, emphasizing the importance of complete resection at the first attempt.[26]

Second Cleft Anomalies

The second arch forms the hyoid bone and the cleft of the tonsillar fossa.[1,2] The second pouch gives rise to the tonsillar and supratonsillar fossa.[26] The external ostium of the second branchial cleft is along the anterior border of the sternocleidomastoid muscle, generally at the junction of the lower and middle thirds.[29] Because of its embryonic origin, the second cleft tract penetrates platysma and cervical fascia to ascend along the carotid sheath to the level of the hyoid bone. Remnants may be found anywhere along this course. The residual tract then turns medially between the branches of the carotid artery, behind the posterior belly of the digastric and stylohyoid muscles, and in front of the hypoglossal nerve to end in the tonsillar fossa (Fig. 75-9).[29] Although the internal opening can be anywhere in the nasopharynx or oropharynx, it is most commonly found in the tonsillar fossa. Figure 75-10 demonstrates the four types of second arch anomalies. Type I anomalies lie anterior to the sternocleidomastoid muscle and do not come into contact with the carotid sheath. Type II lesions are the most common, passing deep to the sternocleidomastoid and anterior or posterior to the carotid sheath. Type III anomalies pass between the internal and external carotid arteries, ending adjacent to the pharynx. Type IV lesions are medial to the carotid sheath adjacent to the tonsillar fossa.

Second branchial cleft anomalies represent 95% of all branchial cleft anomalies. About 10% of second branchial remnants are bilateral.[29] These anomalies commonly present as a fistula or cyst in the lower, anterolateral neck. Fistulas are commonly diagnosed in infancy or childhood after presenting with chronic drainage from an opening anterior to the sternocleidomastoid muscle in the lower third of the neck. Cysts usually present during the third to fifth decades of life with an acute increase in size after an upper respiratory tract infection.[5,26] The dissection of the tract follows the course as described above with care taken during the resection to protect the spinal accessory, hypoglossal, and vagus nerves. A finger or bougie in the oropharynx can help identify the opening in the

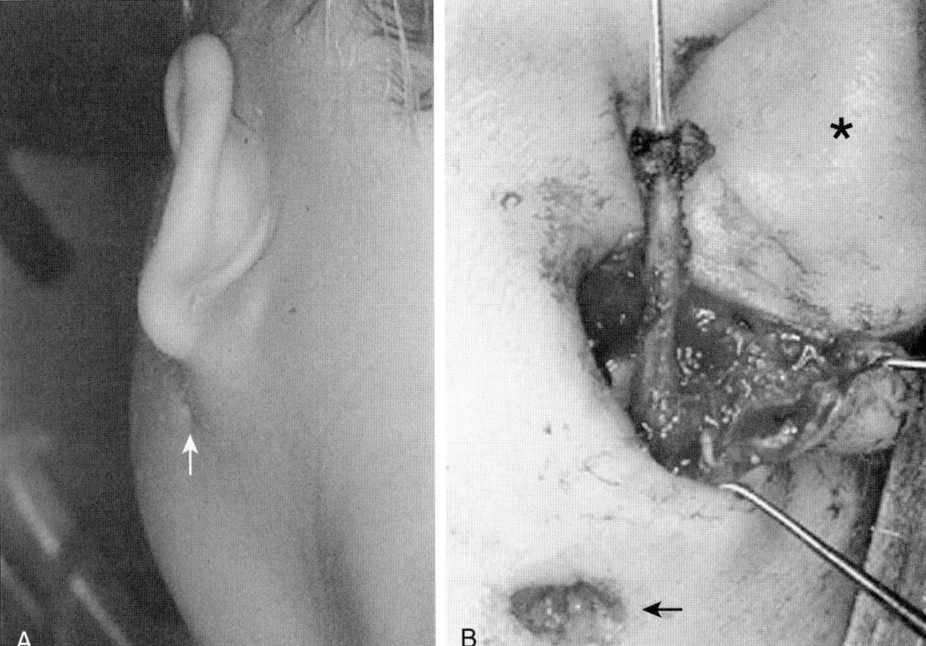

Figure 75-8. **A,** This young child presented with drainage from a first branchial cleft fistula. The ostium is marked with an *arrow*. **B,** In the operative photograph, the fistula has been dissected from its external opening (*arrow*) and is seen progressing toward the external auditory canal. The left ear (*asterisk*) has been elevated to improve visualization.

tonsillar fossa. The tract must be carefully ligated at this entry point.

Third and Fourth Cleft Anomalies

Third and fourth branchial anomalies are rare. The third and fourth pouches form the pharynx below the hyoid bone; thus, these anomalies enter into the pyriform sinus. The third cleft migrates lower in the neck to form the inferior parathyroid glands and the thymus.[7,29] The descent of the fourth cleft stops higher in the neck to form the superior parathyroid glands. The fourth pouch has added significance because its ventral portion develops into the ultimobranchial body, which contributes thyrocalcitonin-producing parafollicular cells to the thyroid gland.[7] It is unusual to find cysts and sinuses from the third branchial cleft.[2,28] When found, they are in the same area as those of the second cleft but ascend posterior to the carotid artery rather than through the bifurcation (Fig. 75-11).[28] The fistula pierces the thyrohyoid membrane and enters the pyriform sinus.

Fourth branchial fistulas are difficult to differentiate from other associated anomalies. Also, fourth pouch cysts are highly unusual and must be differentiated from laryngoceles. These tracts originate at the apex of the pyriform sinus, descend beneath the aortic arch, and then ascend anterior to the carotid artery to end in the vestigial cervical sinus of His (Fig. 75-12).[41] Other anomalies arising from the third and fourth branchial pouches may appear as cystic structures in the neck. Thymic cysts may occur as a result of incomplete degeneration of the thymal pharyngeal duct or of progressive cystic degeneration of epithelial remnants of Hassall corpuscles.[41] Most are found on the left side of the neck. Parathyroid cysts may be

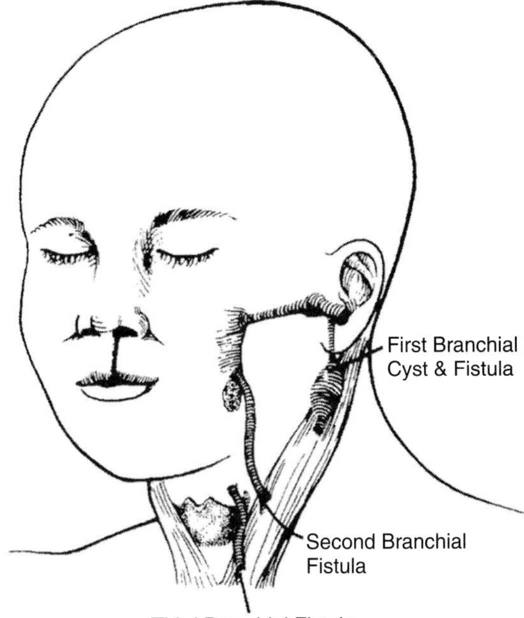

Figure 75-9. A child with a cleft lip and remnants of the first three branchial systems. Note the important relation to the sternocleidomastoid muscle and the fistula's origin. (From Welch KJ, Randolph JG, Ravitch MM, et al [eds]: Pediatric Surgery, 4th ed. Chicago, Year Book Medical, 1986, p 543.)

located anywhere around the thyroid gland or in the mediastinum. These are usually not associated with biochemical abnormalities, although reports of hyperparathyroidism secondary to functioning cysts have been seen. The etiology of these cysts is not clear, but they may be embryologic remnants of third and fourth branchial pouches or may represent cystic

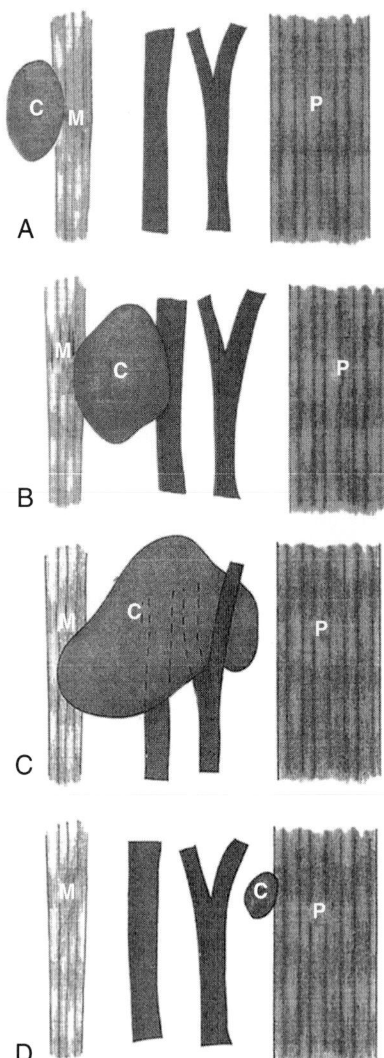

Figure 75-10. Types I to IV second branchial cleft anomalies. **A,** Type I: the cyst (C) is superficial to the sternocleidomastoid muscle (M). **B,** Type II: the cyst is adjacent to the carotid sheath. **C,** Type III: the cyst passes between the internal and external carotid arteries to the lateral wall of the pharynx (P). **D,** Type IV: the cyst is deep to the carotid sheath abutting the pharynx. (From Mukherji SK, Fatterpekar G, Castillo M, et al: Imaging of congenital anomalies of the branchial apparatus. Neuroimaging Clin North Am 10:75-93, 2000.)

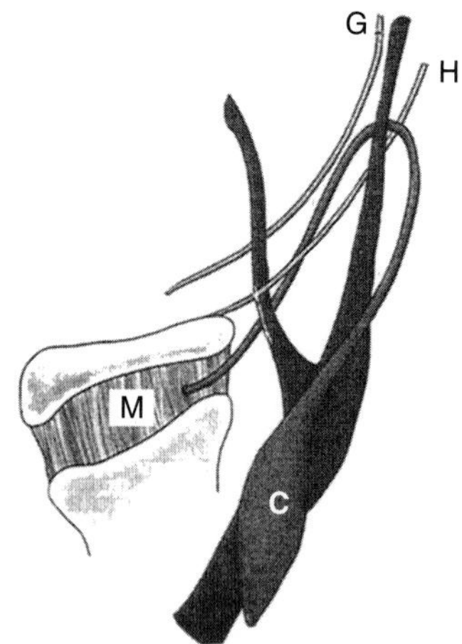

Figure 75-11. Third branchial cleft anomaly. The cyst (C) is posterior to the sternocleidomastoid muscle, and the tract ascends posterior to the internal carotid artery. It then passes medially between the hypoglossal (H) and glossopharyngeal (G) nerves. It pierces the thyroid membrane (M) to enter the pyriform sinus. (From Mukherji SK, Fatterpekar G, Castillo M, et al: Imaging of congenital anomalies of the branchial apparatus. Neuroimaging Clin North Am 10:75-93, 2000.)

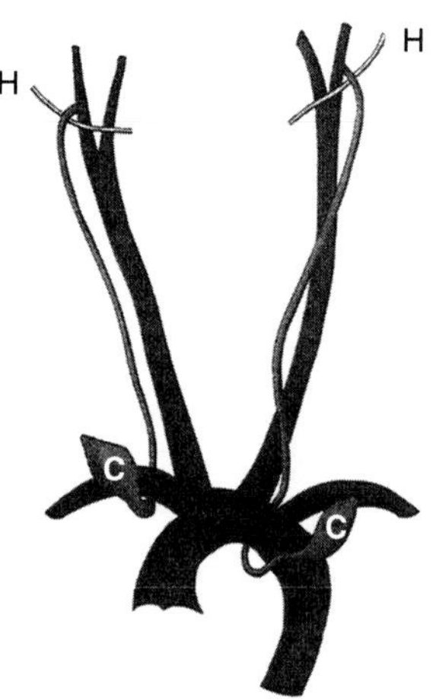

Figure 75-12. Fourth branchial cleft anomaly. The cysts (C) are located anterior to the aortic arch on either side. The tract hooks either the subclavian artery or the aortic arch, depending on the side, and ascends to loop over the hypoglossal nerve (H). (From Mukherji SK, Fatterpekar G, Castillo M, et al: Imaging of congenital anomalies of the branchial apparatus. Neuroimaging Clin North Am 10:75-93, 2000.)

degeneration of adenomas or gradual enlargement of microcysts.[41]

Both third and fourth cleft lesions can present at any age. In the neonate, both can present as tracheal compression or airway compromise owing to rapid enlargement. They can also present as cold nodules within the thyroid or as a thyroid abscess. Other initial presentations include recurrent upper respiratory tract infections or neck pain.

Surgical therapy for third and fourth arch anomalies is similar to that for anomalies of the second arch, with a few notable exceptions. Endoscopy should be used to find the pyriform sinus entry point to allow cannulation of the tract to aid with dissection. Fourth arch anomaly resections require ipsilateral hemithyroidectomy for complete excision, and partial resection of the thyroid cartilage may be necessary to expose the pyriform sinus.[42]

Preauricular Pits, Sinuses, and Cysts

Embryology

Preauricular pits, cysts, and sinuses are not of true branchial cleft origin.[43] They represent ectodermal inclusions, which are related to embryonic ectodermal mounds (auditory hillocks) that essentially form the auricles of the ear.[28,44] The sinuses are often short and end blindly. They never connect internally to the external auditory canal or eustachian tube.[43] They characteristically end in thin strands that blend with the periosteum of the external auditory canal. Some authors propose that they are a marker of teratogenic exposure.[44] Preauricular cysts are located in the subcutaneous layer superficial to the parotid fascia and may seem deeper if they become infected. These cysts and sinuses are lined with stratified squamous epithelium. They do not contain hair-bearing follicles, owing to their origin from the ectoderm associated with external ear formation.[34]

Clinical Presentation

The estimated incidence of preauricular sinuses is 0.1% to 0.9% in the United States and as high as 4% to 10% in Africa.[44] These cysts and sinuses are commonly noted at birth and are more common on the right side.[44] The parent may remark about the familial and bilateral nature of these lesions.[29] Preauricular sinuses usually do not drain. In those situations, excision is not required. However, parents may report that sebaceous-like material drains from the sinus. The presence of drainage is an indication for surgical excision. Sinuses that drain are often connected to subcutaneous cysts that have an increased likelihood of staphylococcal infection. Ideally, these lesions should be completely excised before becoming infected (Fig. 75-13). Prior infection increases the difficulty of complete surgical excision, which increases the risk of recurrence.

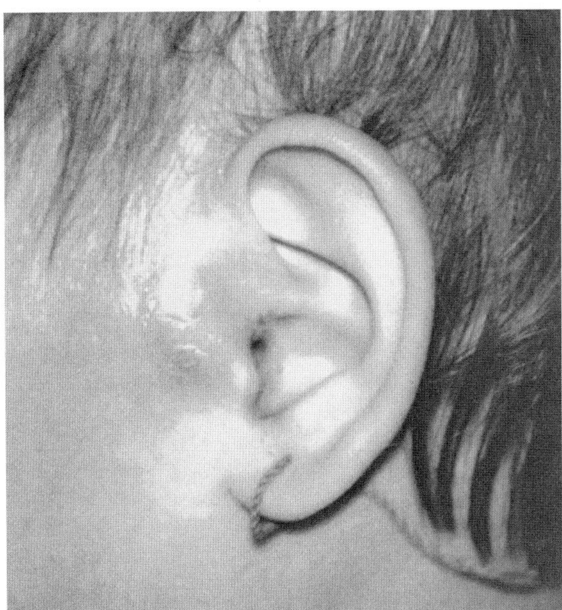

Figure 75-13. An infected preauricular cyst. The pit anterior to the helix is difficult to see. Note the swelling and skin changes anterior to the tragus. Preauricular sinuses that drain sebaceous material should be excised electively. Warm compresses and antibiotics allowed the inflammation to diminish. The cyst and sinus were then completely excised.

Treatment

Complete surgical excision of the sinus tract and subcutaneous cyst to the level of the temporalis fascia is the treatment of choice in the uninfected draining sinus. It is important to avoid rupture of the sinus and to perform a complete excision to decrease the risk of recurrence.[45] If infection supervenes, the lesion is treated with antibiotics and warm soaks to encourage drainage and control of the surrounding inflammation. Occasionally, as with infected branchial cysts, incision and drainage or needle aspiration may be required to control the infection. Surgical excision is often done through an elliptical incision with a small, chevron-shaped skin flap surrounding the sinus. The cyst is then dissected from the subcutaneous tissue and removed in its entirety.[43] The cyst or sinus may have multiple branches, making complete resection difficult. Removal of a small bit of adjacent cartilage reduces the risk of missing one of these branching tracts.[44] The incidence of recurrence is as high as 40%, owing to these multiple branches. As a result, some clinicians have advocated an extended preauricular incision to enhance exposure.[45] Postoperative wound infection also is common.

Branchio-oto-renal Syndrome

Branchio-oto-renal syndrome (Melnick-Frazier syndrome) is an autosomal dominant disorder that can occur with branchial fistulas and preauricular pits. It occurs in 2% of profoundly deaf students and has been mapped to chromosome 8q13.3, which has roles in cochlear and vestibular development and renal morphogenesis.[46] The typical phenotype includes cup-shaped pinnas; preauricular pits; branchial fistulas; conductive, sensorineural, or mixed hearing impairment; and renal anomalies ranging from mild hypoplasia to agenesis. Hearing loss and preauricular pits are the most common associations, and 50% of patients have branchial cleft fistulas.[46]

Dermoid and Epidermoid Cysts

Dermoid cysts embryologically represent ectodermal elements that either were trapped beneath the skin along median or paramedian embryonic lines of fusion or failed to separate from the neural tube.[47-50] Dermoids are differentiated from epidermoids histologically by the accessory glandular structures found in dermoids.[47] Dermoids contain sebaceous glands, hair follicles, connective tissues, and papillae.[47] Both contain sebaceous material within the cyst cavity.

Most dermoid or epidermoid cysts are diagnosed before the patient is 3 years of age.[5] The most common location for dermoids in children is along the supraorbital palpebral ridge (Fig. 75-14). This lesion commonly appears as a characteristic swelling in the corner of the eyebrow and is most commonly first noticed at birth or within the first 1 to 3 months of life. Although commonly attached to the underlying bony fascia, this lesion is movable and nontender. Occasionally, the mass may be dumbbell shaped and penetrate through the orbital bone. Dermoids may

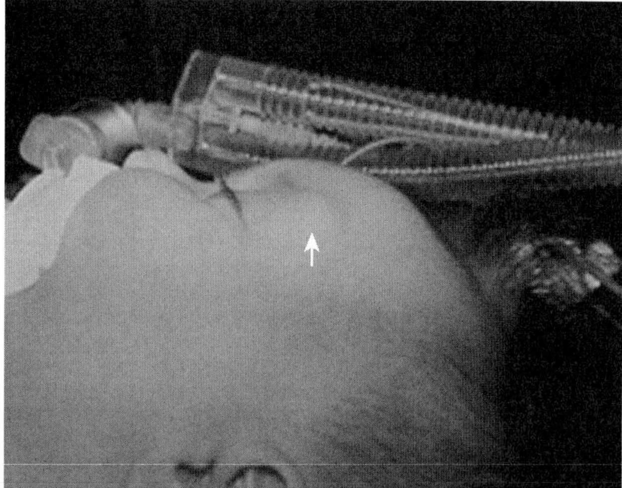

Figure 75-14. This infant presented with the classic finding of a dermoid cyst located along the supraorbital palpebral ridge (*arrow*).

occur along the midline or atypical locations such as the medial orbital wall, nose, floor of the mouth, or submental and submaxillary areas.[51] Midline cysts can be confused with midline thyroglossal duct cysts. Dermoids, however, are more superficial and remain mobile when the tongue is forcibly protruded and will lack a deep-seated tract to the hyoid bone or other neck structures. Nasal dermoids may present as a cyst or sinus anywhere from the glabella to the base of the columella.[51] Any midline scalp lesion suspected of being a dermoid should undergo preoperative radiographic evaluation to evaluate for intracranial extension. This is especially important for nasal dermoids, which have been reported to extend to the cribriform plate in 12% to 45% of cases.[51] The best way to evaluate for deep extension of a midline lesion is controversial. Both CT and MRI may be used in a complementary fashion, with CT better for evaluating bony abnormalities and MRI better for defining soft tissue structures. Some clinicians argue that CT alone is adequate; however, false-negative results have been reported.[51] Dermoids and epidermoid cysts gradually increase in size owing to the accumulation of sebum.[49] Infection is rare, but the cysts can rupture, resulting in granulomatous inflammation.[5,49] Fine-needle aspiration may also be helpful in distinguishing an infected thyroglossal duct cyst from a ruptured dermoid.[49]

Surgical excision is the treatment of choice for all dermoids and epidermoids, especially those that are symptomatic, enlarging, or have ruptured. This has been most commonly performed as an open operation, although increasing experience with removing these lesions is accruing by using endoscopic minimally invasive techniques.[52] Proponents of the open technique report good cosmetic results with minimal complications, whereas early reports with the endoscopic technique have reported a few partial facial nerve injuries especially early into the surgeon's learning curve.[53] It is important to completely remove the capsule and avoid intraoperative rupture to decrease the risk of recurrence. Infection is possible secondary to repeated local trauma. Malignant degeneration of dermoids also is possible but rare.[23] Complete surgical excision is curative.

Midline Cervical Clefts

Midline cervical clefts are rare congenital cervical anomalies that present at birth as a cutaneous ulceration with overhanging skin or cartilage tag in the anterior lower midline of the neck (Fig. 75-15). There may be a tract that extends downward into the skin connecting to the sternum or mandible, or it can end blindly. The embryologic origin is unknown but thought to be a "mesodermal fusion abnormality" involving the branchial arches.[9] Most are sporadic but can be found with cleft abnormalities of the tongue, lower lip, or mandible. Early surgical excision at the time of diagnosis is recommended to avoid neck contractures or growth deformities of the sternum or mandible. This is achieved through complete excision of the skin lesion and the subcutaneous sinus to reduce the rate of recurrence. Stair-step incisions or a series of Z-plasty incisions may be required.[9]

Torticollis

Etiology

Torticollis in childhood may be congenital or acquired. Congenital torticollis resulting from fibrosis and shortening in the sternocleidomastoid muscle is the most common type.[54-56] The shortening of the

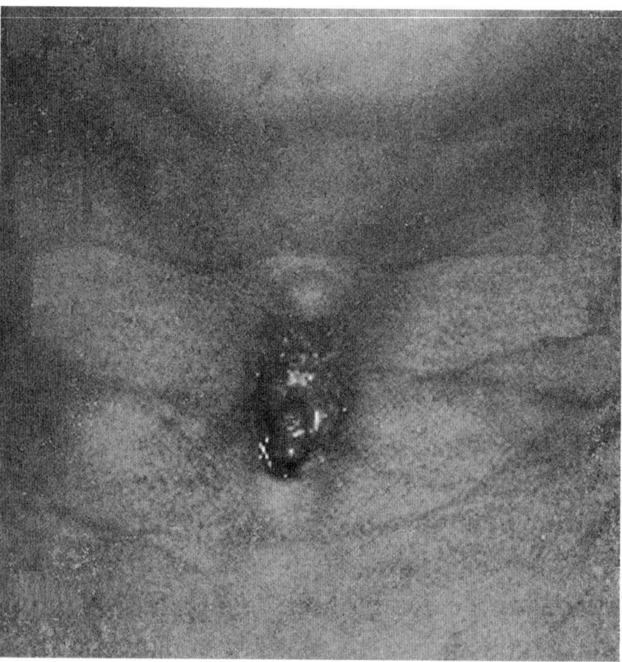

Figure 75-15. Congenital midline cervical cleft. (From Foley DS, Fallat ME: Thyroglossal duct cysts and other congenital midline cervical anomalies. Semin Pediatr Surg 15:70-75, 2006.)

sternocleidomastoid muscle characteristically pulls the head and neck to the side of the lesion. The resulting "mass" represents the fibrous tissue palpable within the muscle. The etiology of this "fibrous tumor" is debatable.[57] The significant incidence of breech presentations and other abnormal obstetric positions has been used to support both the injury and the tumor etiology. Those who favor tumor see the abnormal presentation as the result of the fixed abnormal head position, whereas those who favor trauma see the difficult extraction as the cause of injury.[55,58] No single theory completely explains this condition.

The etiology of acquired torticollis includes cervical hemivertebra and imbalance of the ocular muscles. In children in whom no identifiable muscular etiology is found, a high likelihood exists of Klippel-Feil anomalies or other neurologic disorders as the cause.[59] Acquired torticollis also should raise the suspicion of otolaryngologic infection, gastroesophageal reflux (Sandifer's syndrome), or the possibility of a neoplastic condition as the underlying cause.[60,61]

Pathologically, the basic abnormality in congenital torticollis is endomysial fibrosis—the deposition of collagen and fibroblasts around individual muscle fibers that undergo atrophy.[57] The sarcoplasmic nuclei are compacted to form "muscle giant cells," which appear to be multinucleated. The severity and distribution of fibrosis differ widely from patient to patient. Some cases of fibrosis occur bilaterally. The fact that mature fibrous tissue is present even in the neonate suggests that the disease begins well before birth and probably does not result from a difficult delivery.

Diagnosis

In a series of 100 infants with torticollis, 66% had a "tumor" in the muscle and the other 34% had fibrosis but no tumor.[24,62] A more recent series of 624 cases from China noted only 35.4% with a tumor.[63] In the typical case, the mass is not found in the neonatal period but is noted at the first "well-baby" checkup, some 6 weeks after birth. The infant has the characteristic posture, with the face and chin rotated away from the affected side and the head tilted toward the ipsilateral shoulder. Acquired torticollis may develop at any age. It is important to keep in mind the various causes of the acquired lesion. Its appearance depends on the severity of the lesion, the distribution of the fibrosis, and the child's growth pattern. With time, facial and cranial asymmetry develop and a notable flattening of the facial structures on the side of the lesion occurs. This may become irreversible by age 12 years, although there have been reports of excellent results when the surgical procedure is performed after age 10 years.[64,65]

Treatment

Experience with this condition has shown that 80% to 97% of affected infants do not require operative treatment.[63,64] The key to successful treatment is early recognition and prompt physical therapy.[56,66] The longer the shortening of the muscle persists, the more facial and cranial asymmetry develops, and the more the deeper cervical tissues become involved in the process. Ultrasonography may be used not only as a diagnostic tool but also to help determine which children may be more likely to need surgical therapy. In a study from China, the cross-sectional as well as longitudinal extent of fibrosis in the sternocleidomastoid muscle correlated well with the need for surgical intervention.[67]

In most instances, complete correction can be achieved by early range-of-motion and stretching exercises and positional changes with the infant in the crib. The parents should be taught to perform these exercises with the infant multiple times each day. One parent holds the child's shoulder down against a firm surface, and the other rotates the head toward the opposite shoulder. When the child's head is rotated toward the opposite shoulder, the muscle is gently kneaded along its entire course. Often one parent can accomplish the stretching exercises by placing the infant on his or her lap, turning the infant's head, and gently extending the head and neck over the parent's knees. An additional maneuver is rearranging the infant's room, changing objects in the crib, and encouraging the infant to look toward the side opposite the involved muscle. One study showed a mean duration of 4.7 months for successful nonoperative resolution.[68] Some clinicians have used botulinum toxin injections in select patients who have failed to improve after 6 months of aggressive physical therapy, avoiding surgery in 74% to 95% of subjects.[69,70]

Some clinicians have suggested that the criterion for operation, regardless of age, is the development of facial hemihypoplasia.[66] In children with significant torticollis, facial hemihypoplasia is invariably present, not always with a linear relation between the two conditions.[66] The muscle can be divided anywhere, but transection in the middle third, through a lateral collar incision, is the simplest and provides the most aesthetically acceptable scar.[66,71] Through this incision, one can divide the fascia colli of the neck, which is often tight and may need to be divided anteriorly as far as the midline and posteriorly to the anterior border of the trapezius. Intensive physiotherapy, including full rotation of the neck in both directions and full extension of the cervical spine, is instituted as soon as possible. Occasionally, in an older child, a splint is used to provide overcorrection and stretching of the muscle.[66,71]

INFLAMMATORY LESIONS

Cervical Adenopathy

Enlarged cervical lymph nodes are by far the most common neck masses in childhood. In most instances they are the result of nonspecific reactive hyperplasia.[1] The etiology is often viral or is related to an upper respiratory tract or skin infection. The adenitis resolves spontaneously. Many patients are initially seen with bilateral enlarged nodes. Because the anterior cervical nodes drain the mouth and pharynx, almost all

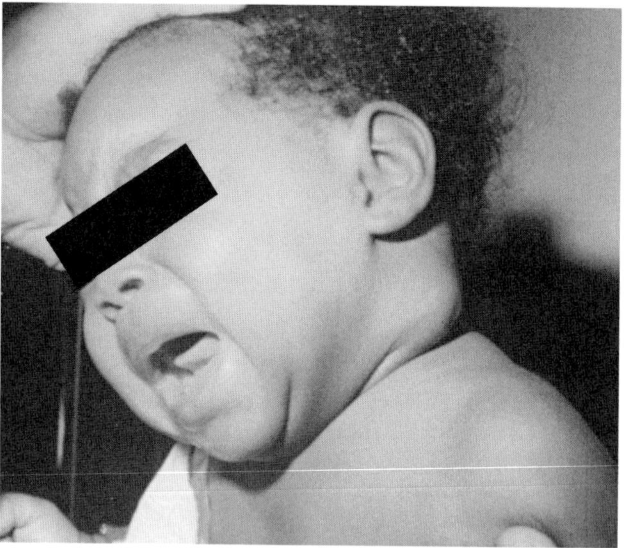

Figure 75-16. Acute suppurative cervical adenitis. Skin is shiny and taut over the centralized abscess cavity.

upper respiratory and pharyngeal infections have some effect on the anterior cervical nodes. Enlarged cervical lymph nodes are frequently palpable in children between ages 2 and 10 years. Palpable nodes are uncommon in infants. A mass in a child younger than 2 years old is more likely to be a cystic hygroma, thyroglossal duct cyst, dermoid cyst, or branchial cyst. The mass can often be diagnosed on clinical findings.[72]

Because the head contains so many structures through which bacteria or viruses may enter the body, the cervical lymph nodes frequently become involved in these cervicofacial infections and inflammatory diseases. Cervical nodes also may be the first clinical manifestations of various tumors, particularly those of the lymphoma group.[1] The most frequent inflammatory lesion of the cervical lymph nodes is suppurative lymphadenitis (Fig. 75-16). Others of importance are cat-scratch disease, atypical mycobacterial lymphadenitis, and tuberculous lymphadenitis. Less common but important considerations in the differential diagnosis of cervical adenitis include Kawasaki's disease and acquired immunodeficiency syndrome (AIDS).

Acute Suppurative Cervical Lymphadenitis

The most common cause of acute lymphadenopathy is a bacterial infection arising in the oropharynx or elsewhere in the drainage area.[73] The most common organisms are penicillin-resistant *Staphylococcus aureus* and *Streptococcus hemolyticus,* although cultures of the pus often yield a mixture of both or prove to be sterile.[73] *Staphylococcus* may be more prevalent in infants.[74] Anaerobes, although common in the oropharynx, are not common pathogens in cervical adenitis. The diagnosis is usually apparent. Fever is variable and usually mild. Initial treatment with antibiotics is often followed by resolution without suppuration. Without treatment, the node often enlarges and becomes fluctuant, eventually leading to thinning of the overlying skin and abscess formation. Needle aspiration can be both diagnostic and therapeutic. Aspiration of the purulent material confirms the diagnosis. The material obtained can be cultured (Fig. 75-17). Frequently, needle aspiration and drainage of the purulent material coupled with judicious antibiotic therapy may alleviate the necessity of formal incision and drainage. Occasionally, repeated aspirations may be necessary.

If the child appears toxic or is quite young, hospitalization and intravenous antibiotics, including a β-lactamase–resistant antibiotic, may be helpful, but formal incision and drainage is often required. The node can be incised and the cavity packed loosely with a Silastic drain. The parent can be taught to perform irrigations through the drain, which encourages drainage of the residual debris. Usually, apparent improvement is evident in 2 to 3 days, although antibiotic therapy should be continued for 10 days. Complete resolution of the adenopathy may take weeks.

Chronic Lymphadenitis

Children occasionally have impressively enlarged nodes that do not seem to be acutely infected. The nodes are not as inflamed or as tender as those in acute bacterial adenitis. Progression to fluctuation is unlikely. The child with this type of lymphadenopathy must be evaluated for tuberculosis, atypical mycobacterial infection, and cat-scratch disease. Most children should receive a full 2-week course of an oral antistaphylococcal antibiotic. The same physician should examine the child on a number of occasions to assess the results of therapy. A single dominant lymph node present for longer than 6 to 8 weeks that has not responded to appropriate antibiotic therapy, should be completely excised, fully cultured, and submitted for histologic examination to exclude the diagnosis of malignancy. Nodes present in the supraclavicular space

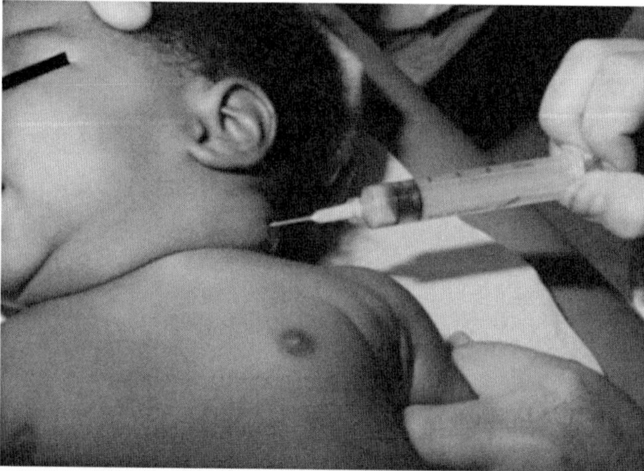

Figure 75-17. Aspiration of purulent material confirms the diagnosis of suppurative lymphadenitis. Frequently, repeated aspirations may be necessary to remove the majority of debris and can often obviate the need for formal incision and drainage.

and posterior triangle tend to be more of a concern for malignancy than those found in the submandibular or anterior triangle.

Mycobacterial Lymphadenitis

CLINICAL PRESENTATION

The prevalence and the relative incidence of infections caused by different mycobacteria vary with the success of preventive health measures in particular populations.[75] In developed countries, bovine mycobacteria have been eliminated from milk. Most mycobacterial lymphadenitis is caused by the atypical mycobacteria of the *Mycobacterium avium-intracellulare-scrofulaceum* (MAIS) complex.[75] Internationally adopted terminology defines this group of 10 to 15 mycobacteria, which produce a specific and localized form of lymphadenitis.[20,47,75] The portal of entry is primarily through the mucous membranes of the pharynx. Lymphadenitis resulting from infection with *M. tuberculosis* is thought to be an extension of a primary pulmonary infection and usually involves the supraclavicular nodes.[76] Infection with the atypical strains usually involves higher cervical nodes, most commonly the submandibular or submaxillary.[76] This finding is consistent with the etiology being a primary infection and not pulmonary disease. Infection is most commonly seen between ages 1 and 5 years; occurrence before age 1 year is rare. The disease involves unilateral nodes, and dissemination is rare. Atypical mycobacteria enter from the environment and are not contagious, although the reservoir may be the mouth and oropharynx of apparently healthy children.[74] Person-to-person spread of disease has not been documented, and isolation is not necessary.

Infection with atypical mycobacteria is generally limited to the lymph nodes. Pediatric patients with atypical mycobacterial lymphadenitis are usually asymptomatic. The nodes are usually nontender. Spontaneous regression of the atypical lymph node infection may occur but is likely to lead to breakdown of the nodes, resulting in sinus or fistula formation. Children with tuberculous scrofula usually are symptomatic. Most have pulmonary tuberculosis when the diagnosis is made.[77] It is rare for the infection to progress from cervical adenopathy to pulmonary disease if the initial chest radiographs are clear. Degeneration of nodes with abscess and fistula formation is unusual.

DIAGNOSIS

In children, tuberculous or atypical mycobacterial lymphadenitis presents as a clinical picture of chronic lymph node hypertrophy.[78] Pulmonary tuberculosis on chest radiograph helps to identify the cause of the cervical swelling. Patients with MAIS usually have a normal chest radiograph. Skin testing helps differentiate these diseases. All children with tuberculosis should show positive test results to second-strength purified protein derivative (PPD). Children with atypical mycobacterial infection have either a negative or a doubtful skin test. If the initial PPD is inconclusive, second-strength PPD may help confirm the mycobacterial etiology. A history of familial exposure to tuberculosis should suggest tuberculosis as more likely than atypical mycobacteria. Although specific skin tests for atypical mycobacteria often provide positive results, it is difficult to obtain the appropriate antigen. Final diagnosis may depend on culture results or histopathology after excision of the involved nodes.[79]

TREATMENT

It is important to distinguish tuberculous from MAIS lymphadenitis because the treatment is significantly different. In tuberculous infections, antituberculous chemotherapy is required, usually resulting in marked resolution of the lymphadenopathy within a few months. Chemotherapy is continued for 2 years.[77] Surgical intervention in a human tuberculosis infection is confined to an excisional biopsy of a node if the diagnosis cannot be made on other grounds. Most children with tuberculous lymphadenitis respond well to chemotherapy with standard drugs.

Treatment of MAIS infections is primarily surgical.[80] Careful, thorough excision of the group of affected nodes (the one or two sentinel nodes) and adjacent smaller nodes is required. This procedure should ideally be performed before extensive ulceration of the overlying skin occurs. Standard chemotherapy for tuberculosis is of no value in MAIS infections except in patients in whom a draining sinus develops after primary excision of infected nodes.[81] Children with atypical mycobacterial infection respond well to complete surgical excision without drug therapy. Some authors report successful treatment with antibiotics alone (e.g., clarithromycin, ethambutol, and rifampin) in patients whose lesions were too close to the facial nerve or other key structures.[82]

Cat-Scratch Disease

The incidence of cat-scratch disease varies greatly in different parts of the world. In developed countries, cat-scratch disease is the most common cause of nonbacterial chronic lymphadenopathy.[83] *Bartonella henselae*, a gram-negative rickettsial organism, is responsible for most cases of cat-scratch disease.[84] The disease is usually transmitted via a superficial wound caused by a cat, dog, or monkey.[85] A healthy kitten is the most frequent vector. The disease begins as a superficial infection or pustule forming in 3 to 5 days and is followed by regional adenopathy in 1 to 2 weeks. Generally, only one node is involved. Nodal involvement corresponds to the inoculation site and the nodes that drain it. The axilla is the most commonly involved area.[1] The diagnosis can be made by a commercially available indirect fluorescent antibody test for detection of antibody. Histology findings are characteristic but not pathognomonic. Polymerase chain reaction studies for *B. henselae* on a fine-needle aspirate may be useful when the diagnosis is in question, although this technique is not readily available in all hospitals.[86] Complete excision of the involved node may be needed to confirm the diagnosis. Patients usually have tender lymphadenopathy and few systemic symptoms. On rare occasions, complications include encephalitis, retinitis, and osteomyelitis. The delay between inoculation and subsequent lymphadenopathy can approach 30 days.[85] Treatment of cat-scratch disease is most often symptomatic because the disease is usually self-limited. Lymphadenopathy resolves spontaneously over a period of weeks to months with only occasional suppuration. Specific antimicrobial therapy against *B. henselae* has not proved efficacious, although it is susceptible to many common antibiotics. Azithromycin, rifampin, ciprofloxacin, and trimethoprim-sulfamethoxazole may be useful if antibiotics are needed.[87,88]

Lesions of the Salivary Glands

Surgical lesions of the salivary glands in children are unusual. In this section we address benign and inflammatory conditions in these glands.

Ranula

In children, prominent, glistening, cystic masses occasionally develop below the tongue in the floor of the mouth. These cystic lesions generally arise from the sublingual glands and are known as ranulas (Fig. 75-18).[89] Most are simple cysts that result from the partial obstruction of the sublingual salivary duct. The traditional ranula is a simple cyst lined with salivary ductal epithelium. Occasionally, the sublingual duct can become completely occluded. The duct may rupture, which leads to the formation of a pseudocyst. The pseudocyst forms because amylase-containing secretions extravasate and erode or "plunge" into the neck muscles. This leads to the condition known as "plunging ranula."[90,91] This lesion lacks a true epithelial lining.[90]

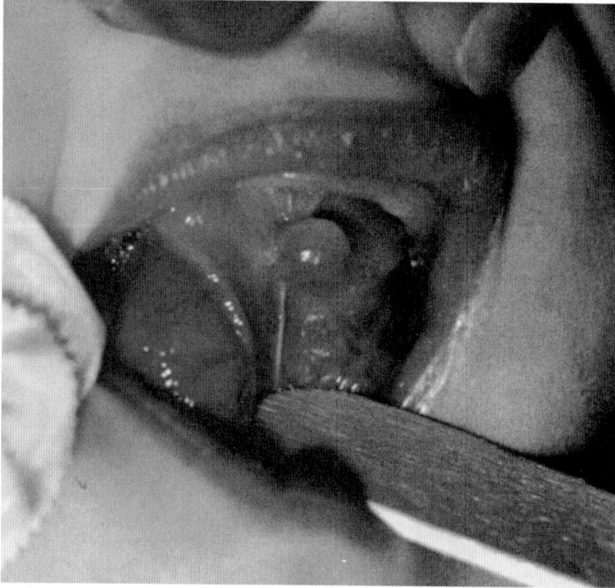

Figure 75-18. A simple cystic ranula, located below the tongue, is arising from the sublingual glands.

Many surgeons suggest marsupialization at the initial procedure for a simple ranula.[92,93] By incising the cyst and draining the contents, the mass rapidly decreases in size. Suturing the epithelium back on itself allows the partially occluded duct to drain. Marsupialization alone has a fairly high recurrence rate, and complete resection or marsupialization with packing may be preferable.[92,93] Concurrent resection of the ipsilateral sublingual gland has been shown to decrease the rate of recurrence (1.2% compared with 66%).[93,94] Recent trials with picibanil (OK-432) similar to therapy for lymphangioma have been described with some success in Japan.[95]

The complex or plunging ranula requires a more extensive dissection into the neck to totally excise the pseudocyst and the atrophied sublingual gland.[91] This may be accomplished using an intraoral approach but may require a cervical incision. Dissection may be tedious in this inflamed area because the hypoglossal and lingual nerves run beneath the sublingual gland and become entrapped in the mass.

Parotid Hemangioma

This is the most common benign neoplasm affecting the major salivary glands and is seen most often in female infants at birth or within the first few months of life.[96] It is usually confined to the intracapsular component of the gland and rarely involves the overlying subcutaneous tissues and skin. A surface sentinel lesion may be present. It appears as a spongy mass anterior to the ear. The diagnosis is usually evident on physical examination. Rarely is a cutaneous component present in the hemangioma. Growth may be rapid in the first few weeks of life. Ultrasonography is helpful, and MRI can be useful in establishing the diagnosis. Most parotid hemangiomas involute by age 4 to 6 years, and only 10% need surgical intervention. One series demonstrated that parotid hemangiomas, like other hemangiomas, respond to medical therapy with corticosteroids or interferon in 98% of cases, with surgical therapy being delayed until the involuting or involuted phase for reconstruction only.[97] Surgical resection puts the seventh nerve at risk so it must be conducted with great care.

Sialadenitis

Inflammation and swelling of the salivary glands are not common in children. Sialadenitis may appear as an acute suppurative infection, a chronic infection, or a granulomatous replacement of the gland. Acute suppurative sialadenitis is most frequently seen in infants. The organism most often involved is *S. aureus,* followed by *Streptococcus* and group D pneumococcus.[98]

The pathophysiology of chronic sialadenitis may involve duct ectasia, stricture, and sialolithiasis. Sialectasis, a saccular dilation of the small, intercalated ducts that connect acini with the striated ducts, is a common congenital abnormality of the gland. Sialolithiasis occurs much more commonly in the submandibular than in the parotid gland. Culture of material from the duct may not reveal pathogenic organisms. Recurrent bacterial infection without demonstrable obstruction is the primary problem in some cases.

Clinical Presentation

Sialadenitis is characterized by episodes of pain that may last from 1 to 7 days. Swelling and pain are isolated to the anatomic distribution of the gland and do not involve the overlying skin and subcutaneous tissue. Secretions are thick and flocculent. Bilateral involvement may occur over time, although each acute episode tends to be unilateral.

Diagnosis

Salivary gland abnormalities may follow diseases such as mumps. Tenderness may occur, with cystic or solid swelling of the gland. The pus may be seen draining from Warthin's duct. Plain radiographs are useful in detecting radiopaque stones, which are seen four times more frequently in the submandibular than in the parotid gland.[98] Sialography remains the definitive study for ductal abnormalities, although it is associated with some discomfort and may require general anesthesia in younger children. High-resolution ultrasonography may demonstrate ductal ectasia.[98] CT has been used in children to evaluate vascularity and abscess formation. MRI may be useful in imaging the course of the facial nerve through the parotid gland.[99] Incisional biopsy is rarely indicated. The utility of fine-needle aspiration is questionable.[100]

Treatment

Antibiotics may be useful in both acute and recurrent sialadenitis. Nonspecific therapy with sialagogues, with massage of the gland, may be helpful. Sialolithotomy or dilation with removal of demonstrated calculi is usually curative. Radical surgical treatment is rarely necessary in children.

section 9

SPECIAL TOPICS

chapter 76

PEDIATRIC AND ADOLESCENT GYNECOLOGY

Julie Strickland, MD

From birth through adulthood, many gynecologic conditions may come to the surgeon's attention. Acute gynecologic problems may mimic urologic or general surgical diseases. Surgeons who care for children must be equipped to diagnose and treat a variety of developmental and acquired disorders of the vulva, vagina, upper female genital tract, and ovary. It is important to begin with an understanding of the normal anatomy and developmental changes of the genital tract. Knowledge of examination techniques and modifications necessary in children to obtain diagnostic information can facilitate accurate diagnoses. Consequently, the proper use and interpretation of radiologic and endoscopic techniques is essential in the care of female children and adolescents.

NORMAL GENITAL ANATOMY

The genital tract undergoes visible morphologic changes from infancy through childhood and adolescence.[1,2] At birth, owing to the influence of maternal circulating estrogens, the labia majora are anteriorly placed and edematous. The mons pubis has a flattened triangulated look. The labia majora are thickened and cover the introital opening. The clitoral proportion is larger. The vestibule and hymen are pale and thickened and may occlude visualization of the vaginal canal without manipulation. The vagina is rugated and moist, and vaginal secretions may be present. The cervix is visible, and the uterus may contain functioning endometrial tissue, leading to the occurrence of estrogen-withdrawal bleeding in infancy.

During early childhood, the vulva remodels with thinning and attenuation of the labia majora and minora. The vestibule takes on an erythematous color with prominent vascular markings. It may now lie unopposed by the labia, allowing for easy visualization of the vaginal orifice with minimal retraction. The hymen of a prepubescent female is normally easily visualized and is thin, often translucent, and inelastic. Normal variations in the shape and amount of hymenal tissue have been described, (Fig. 76-1). Knowledge of these variations becomes important in the evaluation of penetrating injuries and anomalies[3-5] The vagina has an erythematous appearance and is inelastic and without rugations. Normally, the pH is mildly basic and a mixture of bacterial flora is present. The cervix is flush with the vaginal vault and may be difficult to identify. The uterine fundus is poorly developed, with the cervicovaginal ratio being 3:1. No endometrium is visualized on sagittal imaging.

With the onset of puberty, the mons, labia majora, and labia minora all begin to develop. The vestibule begins to lose its erythematous appearance and lies opposed by the labia majora. The hymen thickens and becomes elastic and redundant.[6] The vagina grows in length and develops rugations. The cervix develops a well-defined junction from the uterus, and the uterine fundus develops a rounded appearance. Evidence of an endometrial lining begins to be seen before menarche.

Folliculogenesis of the ovary, with small cyst formation, can be imaged as early as 16 weeks of gestation.[7] Three to 5 percent of children have small incidental ovarian cysts detected on ultrasound evaluation.[8] Follicular growth and atresia occurs throughout childhood, with increased follicular activity and size coinciding with advancing age.[9] Ovarian volume and position change with age, with the ovaries intra-abdominal in childhood and assuming a pelvic position at puberty.

GENITAL EXAMINATION

The genital examination of a child can be anxiety provoking to both the child and her parents. It is important to have a calm, professional attitude and establish rapport with the patient and her family. Examinations are not very successful if they are hurried, forced, or exceed the developmental understanding of the child. An adequate light source and proper positioning are usually all that is needed to accomplish an examination

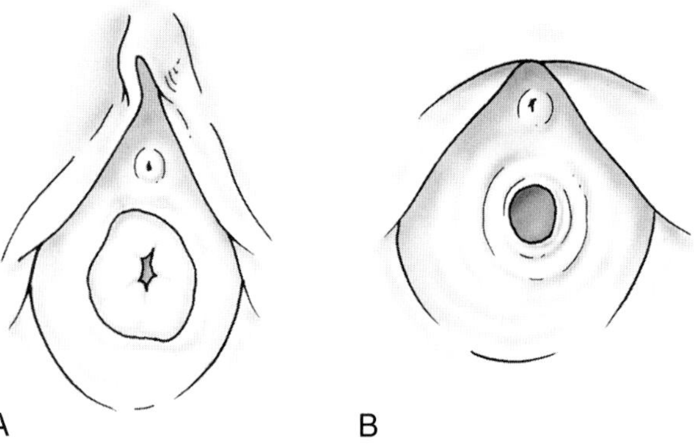

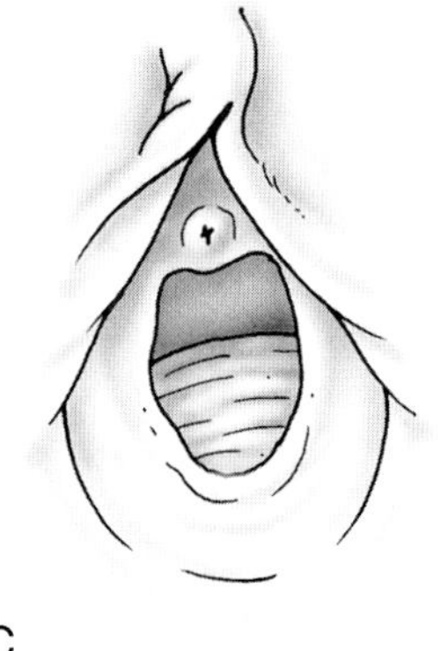

Figure 76-1. A to C, Normal anatomic variations of the hymen. (Adapted from Pokorny SF, Stormer J: Atraumatic removal of secretions from the prepubertal vagina. Am J Obstet Gynecol 156:581-583, 1987.)

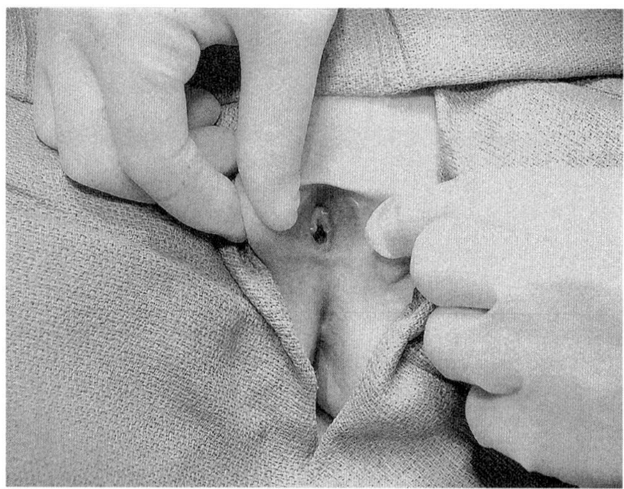

Figure 76-2. Examination of the genitalia by labial traction. Gently grasping the posterior labia majora and pulling anteriorly and superiorly allows visualization of the genital structures.

in a prepubertal child.[10] For visualization of the vulva, introital opening, and lower vagina, gentle downward traction on the labia in a lithotomy position is usually successful (Fig. 76-2). Placing the child on the mother's lap can sometimes facilitate the examination in young children. The knee-chest position may offer a clearer view of the hymen and lower vagina (Fig. 76-3).[11] A magnifying glass, colposcope, or otoscope may be helpful to see the detail of the lower vagina.[12] The office use of speculums is discouraged in prepubertal children. Comprehensive vaginal inspection, when necessary, is ideally done through endoscopic instruments under sedation.[13,14] By gently occluding the vaginal orifice, the entire vaginal canal can be visualized with hydrodistention. Speculum examinations of the vagina are usually well tolerated in postpubertal girls when a narrow-caliber straight blade speculum is gently inserted. Bimanual examinations can be accomplished through a rectal approach or, in adolescents, with a single digit inserted into the vaginal fornix. Imaging with ultrasound or, occasionally, magnetic resonance imaging (MRI) is adjuvant to examination and provides additional information on the status of the upper genital tract.[15]

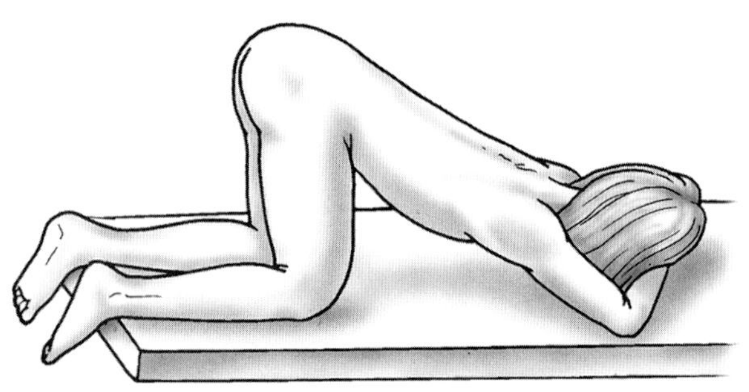

Figure 76-3. Knee-chest positioning. The lower vagina and hymen can occasionally be viewed more successfully by using the knee-chest position.

Vulvar Abnormalities

Vulvar pruritus, pain, and discharge are common complaints in children. An etiology can be obtained in most cases with careful external inspection and, if necessary, blind vaginal cultures. Biopsy is seldom indicated. Most often, symptoms involve irritation or eruption of the vulvar skin related to hygienic practices. Atopic or irritant dermatitis are the most common diagnoses.[16] Infections are more associated with acute inflammation with erythema and the presence of a vaginal discharge.[17] Common respiratory pathogens such as *Streptococcus pyogenes* and *Haemophilus influenzae* may cause acute genital symptoms.[18,19] When a bacterial infection is suspected, cultures of the vagina may be obtained by using moistened urethral swabs, feeding tubes, or catheters. A double-catheter system with a butterfly catheter within a small rubber catheter can be used to collect upper vaginal secretions.[20]

Recurrent or persistent vaginitis despite treatment should alert the clinician to the presence of a retained foreign body in the vagina. Occasionally, foreign bodies also may cause vaginal bleeding and become symptomatic as a protruding mass.[21,22] The most common foreign body is toilet paper shreds.[21] Pelvic ultrasonography may reveal the bladder-indentation sign, suggesting a foreign body.[23] When a foreign body is suspected, vaginal lavage can be attempted in the office by using warm-water saline in a venous catheter or straight urinary catheter. Vaginoscopy under sedation may be necessary to retrieve an object. Endoscopic

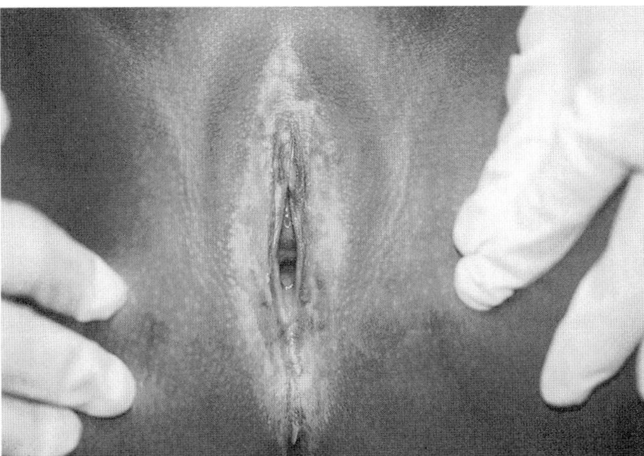

Figure 76-4. Lichen sclerosis diagnosed in a 5-year-old. A sharp demarcation of hypopigmented, thin epithelium is seen. This lesion is often associated with fissures and purpura.

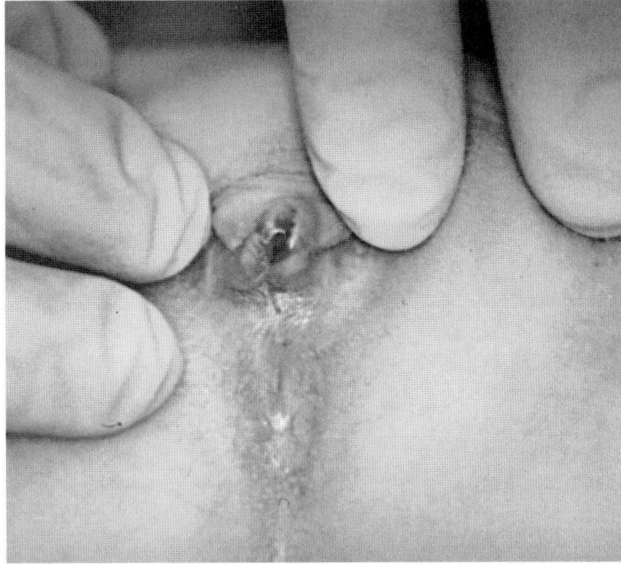

Figure 76-5. A 2-year-old child with labial (minora) adhesions is seen.

instruments such as cystoscopes or hysteroscopes allow easy location of the object with minimal trauma to the genital area.[14]

Vulvar dermatoses may lead to acute vulvovaginal symptoms. Lichen sclerosis has the hallmark characteristic of a loss of skin markings with a sharply demarcated pale epithelial ring encircling the introitus but sparing the vagina (Fig. 76-4). Signs of inflammation and trauma may be present, with purpura, fissures, and secondary infection associated with scratching. Lichen sclerosis may be confused with sexual abuse in some cases. Mainstays of treatment include avoidance of trauma with loose clothing, mild soaps, and the generous use of emollients. Early treatment with ultrapotent corticosteroids may be effective in reducing symptoms of lichen sclerosis and minimizing long-term scarring. In 20% of patients, ultrapotent corticosteroids have been shown to reverse skin changes.[24] Tacrolimus has been reported to offer similar benefit to pediatric patients.[25] Other dermatologic conditions such as psoriasis, eczema, and allergic dermatitis also may mimic vulvovaginitis.[14]

Labial agglutination or adhesions occur relatively frequently in prepubescent girls (Fig. 76-5). Adhesions are thought to occur because of irritation or trauma to the unestrogenized labia, leading to a midline fusion of the labia. Adhesions can be associated with an increase in urinary tract infections, perineal wetness, symptomatic vulvitis, and an inability to access the urethra and vaginal orifice. When symptomatic, the treatment of choice is an estrogen-based cream applied under traction to the adhesion site.[26,27] Surgical separation is seldom indicated because of the efficacy of topical hormonal therapy but may be necessary in unusually dense adhesions or those that have required previous separation.[26,27] Even with recurrent or persistent labial agglutination, estrogen therapy was effective in over one third of cases in one study.[28] Long-acting local anesthetics, such as EMLA cream, may allow office separation in some girls.[29] Manual separation of the adhesions without anesthesia should be avoided because of the discomfort and the high risk of recurrence.

Genital Bleeding

Unexplained bleeding from the genital area in a prepubescent child is always abnormal (Table 76-1). Bleeding is most commonly extragenital, resulting from hematuria, rectal fissures, and vulvar epithelial irritation. Prolapse of the urethra may occur and be associated with bleeding or even gangrenous changes. A red, granular lesion is seen protruding from the urethral meatus (Fig. 76-6). Topical treatment with estrogen-based cream usually relieves the symptoms. If symptoms persist, excision of the redundant tissue may be necessary. Vaginal bleeding may be associated with precocious puberty or autonomous production or exogenous sources of hormonal stimulation. It is important to perform a detailed physical examination searching for evidence of breast development, estrogenization of the genital tract, or the presence of an

Table 76-1	Causes of Genital Bleeding in Prepubescent Girls
Genital trauma: Accidental, sexual abuse	
Genitourinary: Urethral prolapse, urinary tract infections	
Gastrointestinal: Inflammatory bowel disease, rectal fissure, hemorrhoids	
Vulvovaginitis: Acute dermatitis, pinworms, β-hemolytic *Streptococcus, Shigella*	
Foreign body	
Vulvar dermatosis: Lichen sclerosis	
Condylomata acuminata	
Hemangiomas	
Tumors: Malignant or benign endocrine abnormalities: isosexual precocious puberty, pseudoprecocious puberty, exogenous hormonal stimulation	

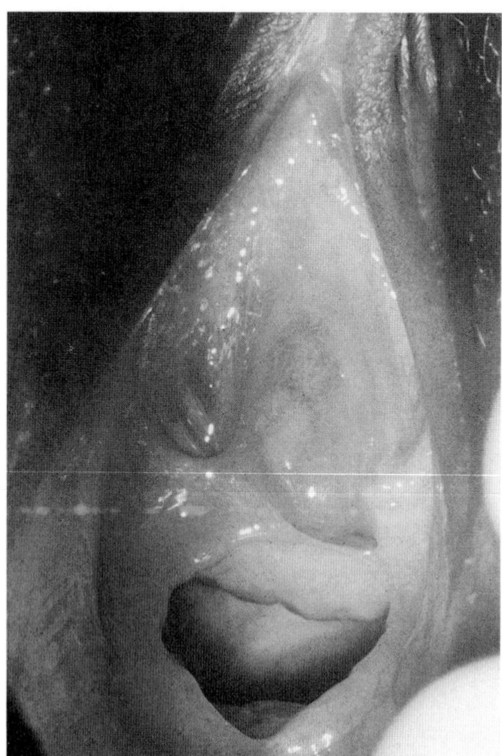

Figure 76-6. Urethral prolapse was found in this 6-year-old child with a history of recurrent painless genital bleeding.

abdominal mass. In the absence of a satisfactory explanation for the source of bleeding, vaginoscopy should be performed to evaluate the vaginal canal and cervix for the presence of a foreign body, trauma, infection or, rarely, primary and metastatic tumors of the lower genital canal.

Acute genital bleeding in children requires immediate evaluation for the presence of serious injury or sexual abuse.[30] If the source of bleeding is not readily apparent, if the entire lesion cannot be identified, or if the patient is not tolerant of the examination, vaginoscopy under sedation is indicated.[31] Straddle injuries are common during childhood from accidental falls onto blunt objects, resulting in soft tissue trauma from striking the pubic symphysis or rami. Straddle injuries are usually anterior, involving the mons, clitoris, and labia and sparing the vaginal ring or perineal body (Fig. 76-7). They may result in hematoma formation, linear lacerations, or abrasions. Vulvar hematomas can be extensive but are usually self-limited. In the absence of acute ongoing hemorrhage, small or moderate hematomas can be managed conservatively with bed rest, ice, and pain control. Evacuation of extremely large hematomas causing distortion of the pelvic midline occasionally is necessary to facilitate recovery. Evacuation with debridement should be performed with the child under anesthesia by incising the medial mucosal surface and placing absorbable sutures for hemostasis and closure of dead space.[32] Drainage of the urinary bladder may be necessary because of edema, resulting in urinary retention.

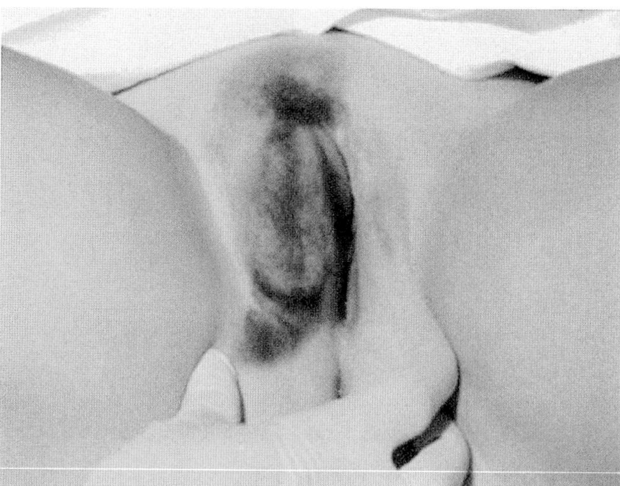

Figure 76-7. An extensive vulvar hematoma is seen after a straddle injury. (Courtesy of Diane Merritt, MD.)

Penetrating injuries can occur through accidental impalements onto irregular objects, but the possibility of sexual abuse must always be strongly considered (Figs. 76-8 and 76-9). In the prepubertal child, lacerations involving or occurring above the hymenal ring require vaginoscopy under general anesthesia. Because of the inelasticity of the vaginal epithelium, penetrating injuries can result in disruption of the vagina, with possible internal hemorrhage and hematoma formation.[33] All injuries that cannot readily be explained by the presenting history should be referred to child protection. Surgeons should familiarize themselves with the legal and social resources for sexual abuse diagnosis and care that are available within their communities.

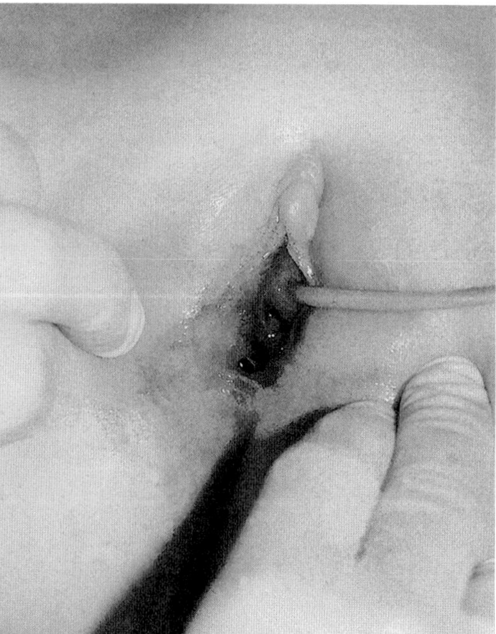

Figure 76-8. A 9-year-old girl has a penetrating posterior vaginal injury sustained after falling onto an open cabinet. A urinary catheter has been inserted in the urethra.

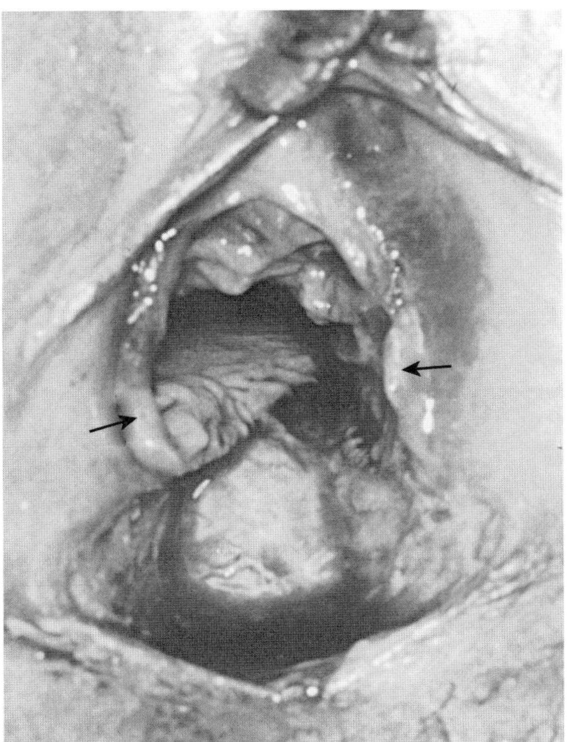

Figure 76-9. An 8-year-old victim of acute sexual assault has small bowel herniating through the apex of the avulsed vagina. Note the abundant, although transected, amount of hymenal tissue (*arrows*) present, indicating that she had not had significant stretch trauma to her hymen before this episode of rape. (From Pokorny SF, Pokorny WJ, Kramer W: Acute genital injury in the prepubertal girl. Am J Obstet Gynecol 166:1461-1466, 1992.)

Introital masses in children occasionally come to the attention of surgeons. Masses of the introitus or vagina are most commonly epithelial inclusion cysts of the hymen or lower vagina and often spontaneously resolve. In young girls, the rare possibility exists of embryonic rhabdomyosarcoma, a malignant primary tumor that appears as indolent, grape-like masses protruding from the vagina (Fig. 76-10). Other possibilities include condylomata acuminata, ectopic ureter, and an obstructive vaginal anomaly. Occasionally, the Bartholin gland or periurethral gland may occlude or form an abscess, leading to an acquired lateral mass. It is important that the origin of the mass be fully evaluated, with evaluation under anesthesia as necessary. Transperineal ultrasonography may be helpful to delineate the mass further. In cases that are unclear, biopsy or excision (or both) are essential.

UTEROVAGINAL ANOMALIES

Developmental abnormalities causing agenesis or obstruction of the genital tract can occur in children. These can often be recognized in the newborn period with routine examination, but the majority are diagnosed in the adolescent period with the lack of anticipated menses or with symptoms of obstruction.

Imperforate hymen is the most commonly diagnosed obstructive anomaly, with an incidence of less than 1%.[4,34] It arises as an isolated anomaly from failure of canalization of the urogenital sinus. Symptoms typically are first noted during late puberty with cyclic pelvic pain and introital distention, associated with the absence of menstruation. With the continued accumulation of menstrual blood, a pelvic mass and obstructive genitourinary or gastrointestinal symptoms may develop. Occasionally, presentation will be in the newborn period because of the accumulation of mucus, producing an abdominal mass (Fig. 76-11). Transabdominal ultrasonography reveals a dilated vaginal and uterine canal. If this is found during childhood and is asymptomatic, correction is usually deferred until the

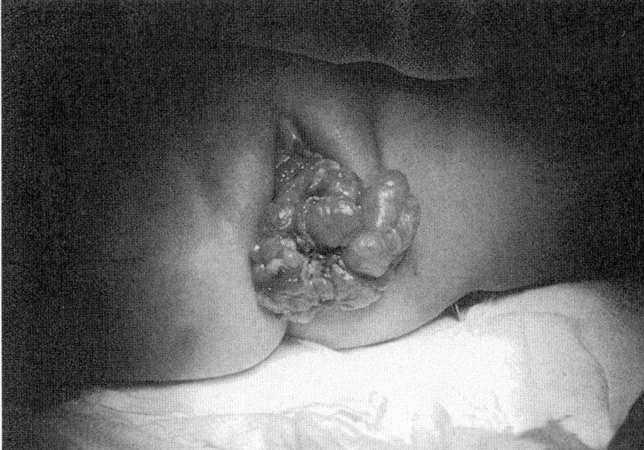

Figure 76-10. A 3-year-old with an extensive protruding vaginal mass diagnosed as embryonic rhabdomyosarcoma of the vagina. These rare tumors often begin as an indolent-appearing mass at the introitus. (Used with permission from the North American Society for Pediatric and Adolescent Gynecology, 1999.)

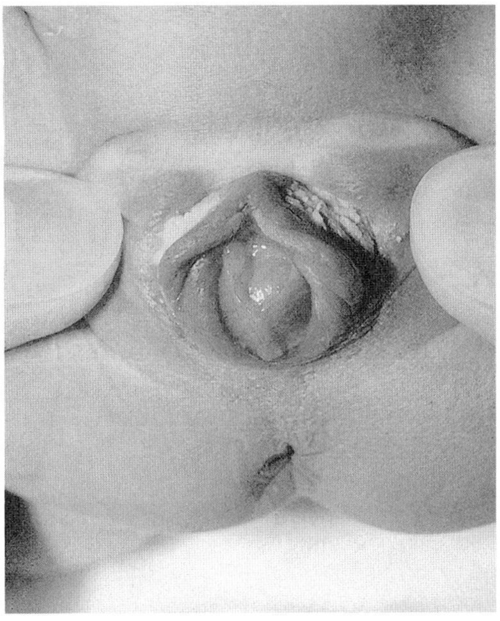

Figure 76-11. Mucocolpos, leading to urinary obstruction in a 2-day-old infant.

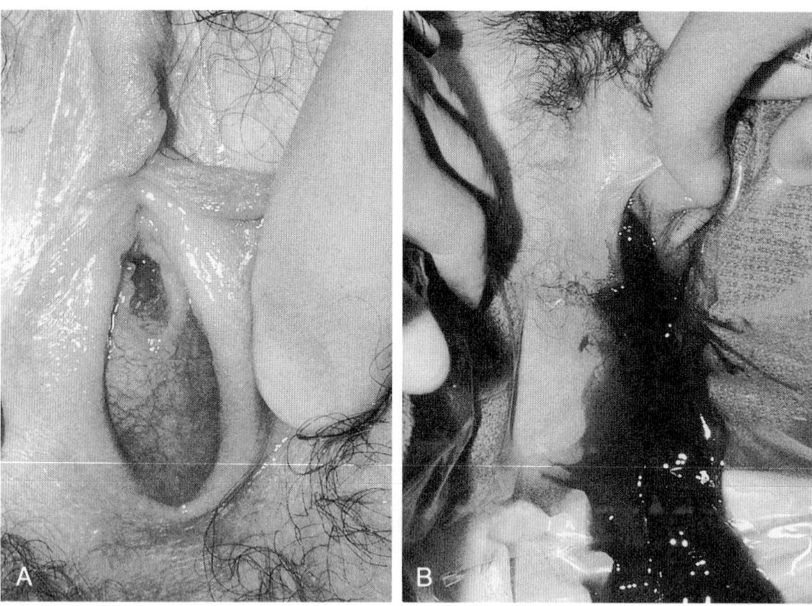

Figure 76-12. **A,** Imperforate hymen in a 12-year-old girl with a 6-month history of recurrent abdominal pain. **B,** Evacuation of the menstrual obstruction at hymenotomy.

onset of puberty. Surgical excision of the hymen with evacuation of the retained menstrual fluid provides permanent correction (Fig. 76-12). This is performed by carefully identifying the anatomic landmarks, such as the urethra and the lateral hymenal borders. It is important to recognize that significant distention of the posterior vaginal wall may cause the hymenal membrane to be located in a more superior position. A cruciate incision is made into the membrane inferior to the urethral meatus. After decompression, the individual flaps of tissue are then excised. The vaginal mucosa is sutured to the introital edge with interrupted absorbable sutures to avoid stenosis (Fig. 76-13). Needle aspiration without definitive surgical correction is contraindicated because of the possibility of bacterial seeding and abscess development.

A transverse vaginal septum also may exist at various levels of the vagina because of failure of unification

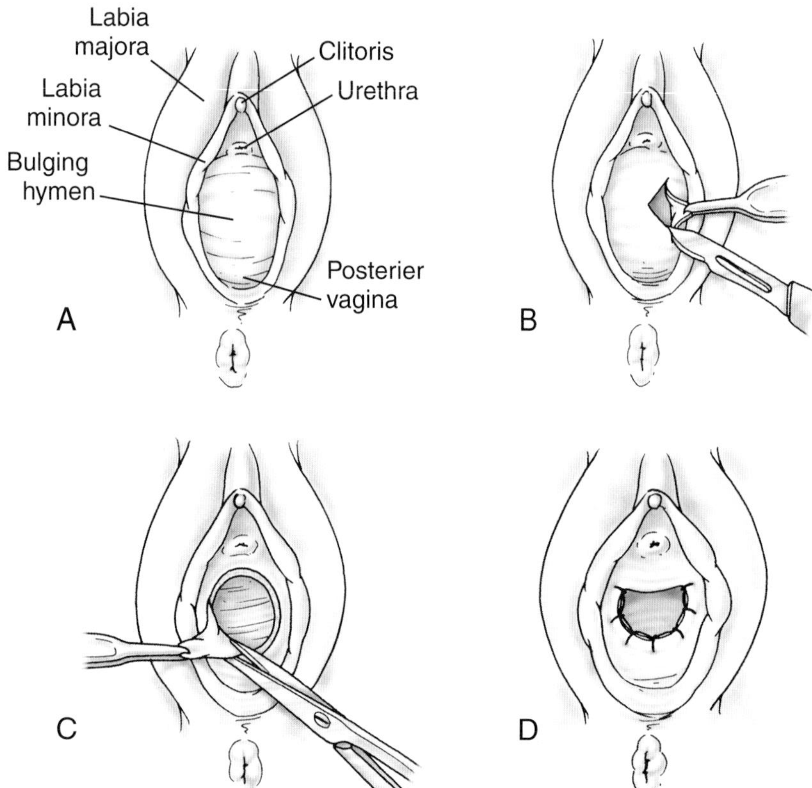

Figure 76-13. **A,** Imperforate hymen. **B,** A cruciate incision is made in the apex of the hymen after identifying the outer hymenal borders. **C,** The hymenal remnants are trimmed. **D,** Interrupted sutures are utilized for hemostasis.

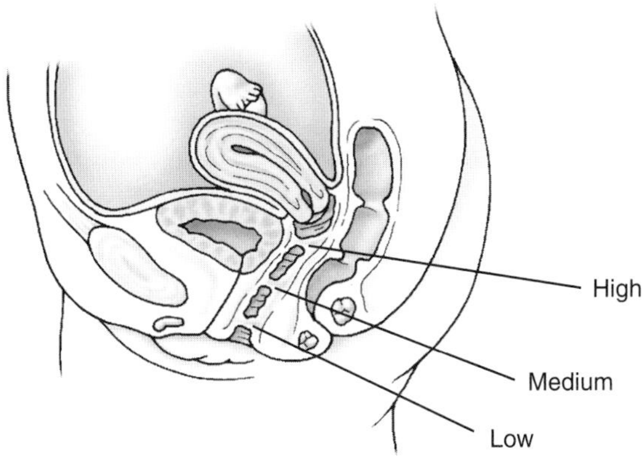

Figure 76-14. The transverse vaginal septum is the result of failed unification or canalization of the urogenital sinus and the müllerian duct. It can arise anywhere in the vagina, but is most common in the upper vagina.

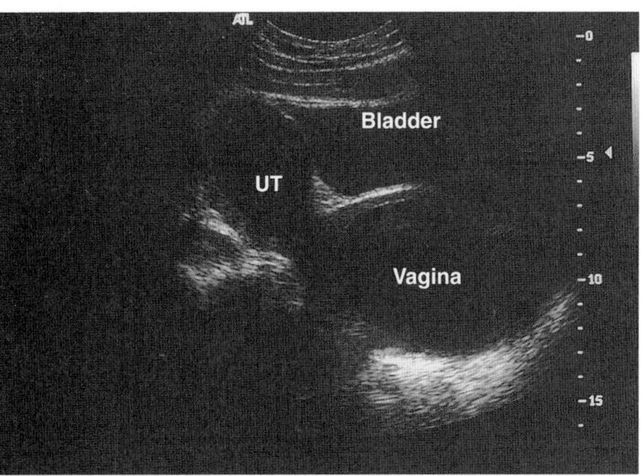

Figure 76-15. A sonographic sagittal view of the pelvis of a 16-year-old girl with cervicovaginal agenesis and a resultant hematometra. Note the dilated vagina and uterus (UT).

of the urogenital sinus and the müllerian ducts during embryogenesis. A vaginal septum may be complete or partial and may occur at any level in the vaginal canal (Fig. 76-14).[35] These lesions are most common in the upper vagina. Because the introitus may appear normal, the diagnosis may be delayed. MRI or ultrasonography is essential in defining this anomaly and indicating the thickness of the septum.[36] Before surgical exploration, it is important to ensure the presence of cervical tissue by imaging to differentiate this condition from true agenesis of the cervix. Surgical correction is dependent on the location and thickness of the septum, but most often entails excision of the septum with a vaginal-mucosal anastomosis. A thick septum may require preoperative vaginal dilation, mobilization of the upper vagina, or occasionally a skin graft to maintain vaginal patency. Circumferential stenosis is common at the anastomotic site, particularly with high or thick septa. Vaginal dilation may be required postoperatively. Occasionally, a uterine duplication is associated with hypoplasia of one cervix and obstruction. This condition is treatable with laparoscopic hemihysterectomy of the affected side.[37] True cervicovaginal agenesis is a rare disorder associated with an obstructed uterine canal, the absence of a patent cervix, and agenesis of the upper vagina (Fig. 76-15). The lower vagina may be patent. These patients are initially seen with cyclic or noncyclic abdominal or pelvic pain (or both) and a pelvic mass. This condition has a poor prognosis for reconstruction, with reports of significant morbidity from ascending infection and even death.[38] Hysterectomy is usually recommended, but the surgical creation of a vagino-uterine fistula has also been described.[39,40]

Occasionally, patients may be seen with a duplication of the uterus and cervix and a unilateral obstructing longitudinal septum of the vagina. Associated ipsilateral renal agenesis or hypoplasia is commonly found.[41] Menstruation occurs from the nonobstructed side, so the diagnosis may be made well past menarche. Pelvic ultrasonography and MRI are very reliable in distinguishing these disorders, especially when obstruction is present (Fig. 76-16).[36,42] Surgical repair through a vaginal approach is performed at diagnosis, with full excision of the vaginal septum. Care must be taken to approximate the vaginal mucosa of the two cavities.

Mayer-Rokitansky-Küster-Hauser syndrome was first described in 1961 and includes primary amenorrhea in women with normal secondary sexual characteristics, uterine hypoplasia, and congenital absence of the vagina.[43] The incidence is approximately 1 in 5000.[44] Because of failure of development of the müllerian system, the uterus, cervix, and upper two thirds of the vagina fail to form. Renal and skeletal anomalies are commonly associated with this disorder. Although patients have primary amenorrhea, pubertal development and ovarian function are normal. The diagnosis can be made clinically on the basis of a normal phenotype and the genital findings cited earlier. An absent uterus with an elevated testosterone, poor breast development, virilization, or the lack of sexual hair

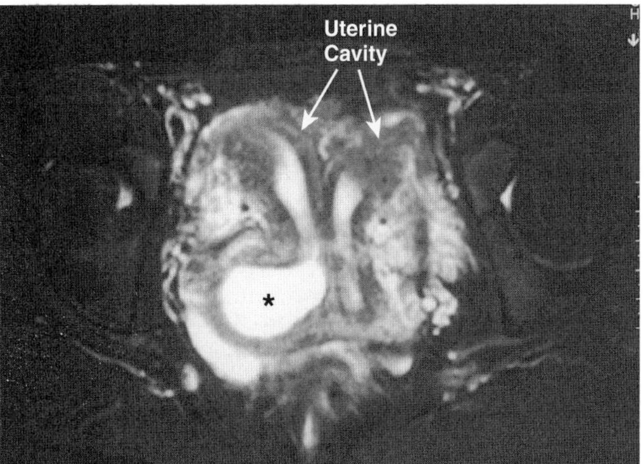

Figure 76-16. MR image of a 16-year-old girl with a complete uterine duplication and a blind right hemivagina. Note the obstructed and dilated right hemivagina *(asterisk)* and the resultant right-sided hematocolpos and hematometra.

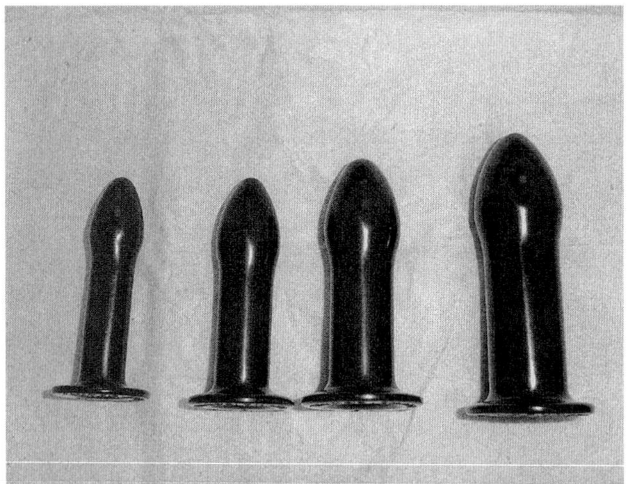

Figure 76-17. Sequential vaginal dilators are often used to create a coital pouch in individuals with vaginal agenesis.

requires a full chromosomal and hormonal evaluation for the presence a disorder of sexual development.

Therapy for this condition is centered on creation of an adequate vaginal pouch to allow normal sexual functioning. The use of Lucite dilators, first popularized in the 1930s, has provided a highly effective nonsurgical alternative for many patients with agenesis (Fig. 76-17).[45,46] Through the use of successive pressure dilators placed at the hymenal ring, the vaginal vault can be lengthened and enhanced to provide an adequate vaginal capacity. This approach has the advantage of being patient controlled and associated with extremely low morbidity. Vaginal dilation can usually be accomplished over a 2- to 3-month period or even more rapidly in highly motivated individuals. Sexual satisfaction of young women treated with dilation has been shown to be comparable with a normal population.[47] In selected patients, surgical creation of an artificial vagina may be indicated.[48] Many surgical options have been described, with the split-thickness graft vaginoplasty being advocated most often for patients with agenesis.[49] In this approach, a split thickness of skin is harvested from an aesthetic place on the buttocks and sewn, dermal side exposed, over a vaginal mold (Fig. 76-18). The potential space above the levator plate is surgically dissected, followed by placement of a skin-covered vaginal mold. The vaginal mold is sutured in place. After initial epithelialization, the mold is removed and the patient is required to dilate the vagina for several months to maintain patency. Surgical outcome and patient satisfaction remains high for this type of vaginoplasty.[50,51] Other materials such as amnion, peritoneum, and absorbable adhesion barriers (INTERCEED, Ethicon, Somerville, NJ) have been described as an alternative to skin grafting.[52,53] Novel laparoscopic techniques using these alternatives have also been described.[54] New laparoscopic methods using a transperitoneal pulley system to advance the neovagina have shown rapid correction with high success rates.[55]

The use of sigmoid bowel pedicles pulled to the introitus for vaginal creation is less commonly utilized for this problem, but also may be associated with good long-term results.[56] Although this approach has the advantage of avoiding postoperative dilation, it is occasionally associated with prolapse, chronic vaginal discharge, and vaginitis, which limit its functional result.[50,57,58] Rarely, external interposition of gracilis muscle or vulvoperineal flaps are used to create a coital pouch.

ADNEXAL DISEASE

Surgical disorders of the adnexa are common, particularly in the adolescent period. Ultrasonography has increased the level of understanding regarding the development and natural history of ovarian cysts. New less-invasive surgical techniques allow more conservative management of adnexal disease in children.

Ovarian cysts may occur at any time from fetal life to adulthood. Simple cysts in the neonate are generally follicular and originate from the influence of maternal estrogens. Complex masses in this age group may represent in-utero or neonatal torsion.[59] The risk of malignancy is extremely small, but complications requiring surgical intervention can arise from torsion, hemorrhage, or mass effect. Both simple and complex masses are likely to resolve without therapy. Percutaneous aspiration is indicated for cysts larger than 5 cm to minimize the risk of torsion.[60,61] Indications for operative intervention include the presence of a complex mass that fails to resolve in the neonatal period, the recurrence of a cyst after aspiration, the development of acute abdominal symptoms, or a combination of these complications.[61] Treatment may consist of laparoscopic fenestration of simple cysts or cystectomy, if it can be done without loss of functional tissue.[62]

In childhood, small cysts representing follicular development and atresia are common and not associated with a pathologic state.[8] Management of ovarian cysts in children is based on size, the presence of symptoms, and cyst composition. Worrisome findings include cysts of larger than 5 cm, cysts with solid or complex internal echoes on ultrasonography, and fixed masses accompanied by systemic symptoms of disease or precocious development.[63] Occasionally, cysts may be associated with breast development or vaginal bleeding (Fig. 76-19). It is important to distinguish follicular development arising from true precocious puberty from autonomously active cysts. Recurrent gonadotropin-independent cysts are most commonly associated with McCune-Albright syndrome or, more rarely, with hormonally active stromal or germ cell tumors. The diagnosis of an ovarian tumor must be considered in children, especially in those with a large, persistent complex mass that has solid components (Table 76-2). The most common ovarian tumor of childhood is the mature cystic teratoma, followed by stromal tumors [64,65] Malignant tumors are rare, comprising about 10% of all surgically treated masses.[64,66] In prepubertal girls, ovarian masses, when symptomatic or associated with worrisome radiologic signs, should undergo surgical exploration. In the absence of

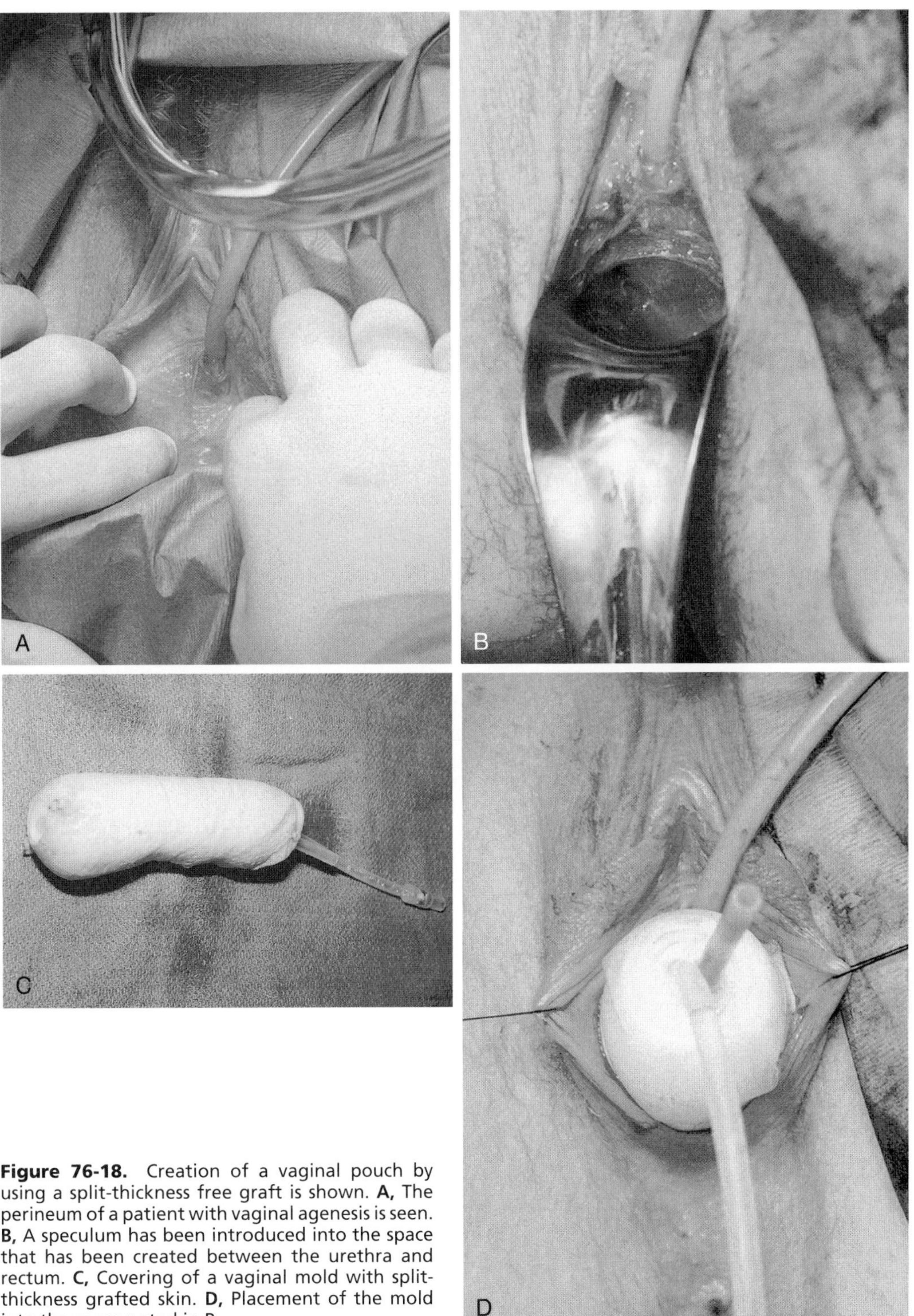

Figure 76-18. Creation of a vaginal pouch by using a split-thickness free graft is shown. **A,** The perineum of a patient with vaginal agenesis is seen. **B,** A speculum has been introduced into the space that has been created between the urethra and rectum. **C,** Covering of a vaginal mold with split-thickness grafted skin. **D,** Placement of the mold into the space noted in B.

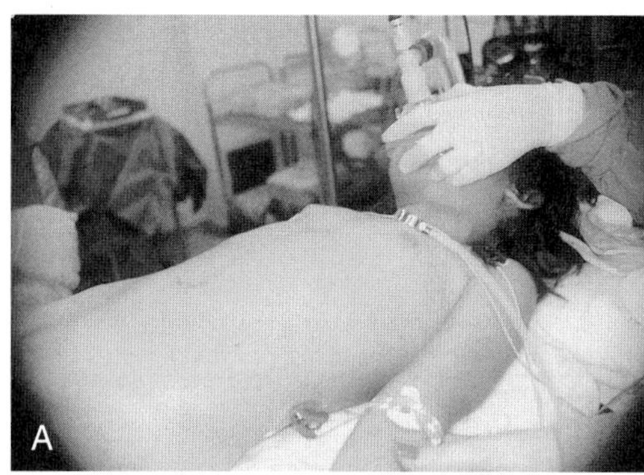

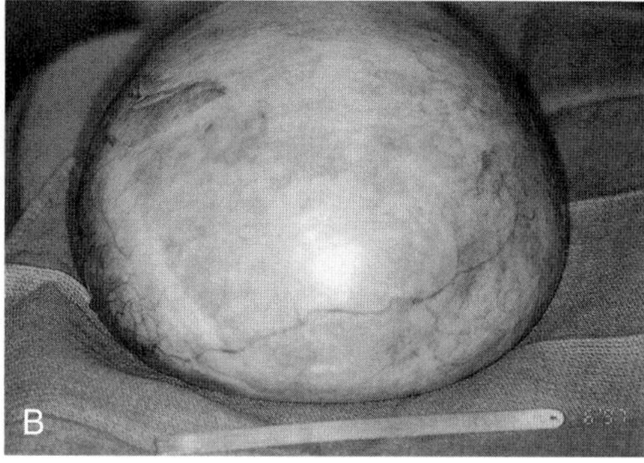

Figure 76-19. **A,** A 6-year-old girl presented with precocious puberty and a large pelvic mass. **B,** An autonomously functioning ovarian serous cystadenoma was found. All pubertal signs regressed after its removal.

Table 76-2 Neoplasms in Female Children and Adolescents

Tumor Neoplasm	Appearance	Markers	Other Information
Benign teratoma (dermoid)	Irregular, cystic and solid; or primarily cystic	None	Most common germ cell tumor 6%-8% malignant Malignant immature forms may be associated with other germ cell tumors
Dysgerminoma	Thick, white, opaque; cytologic reactivity with alkaline phosphatase	None	Inspect other ovary 15%-20% bilateral, 95% cure (stage I) Chemotherapy for advanced disease
Endodermal sinus tumor (yolk sac tumor)	Solid and cystic Schiller-Duval bodies	AFP	Primarily unilateral Surgery and chemotherapy for all stages 15% survival after stage I
Embryonal carcinoma	Smooth with areas of hemorrhage and necrosis Schiller-Duval bodies	β-hCG	Usually part of a mixed germ cell tumor 60% endocrinologically active (precocious puberty) Surgery and chemotherapy for all stages 50% survival (stage I)
Choriocarcinoma	Syncytiotrophoblasts and cytotrophoblasts	β-hCG	Rare primary tumor in pediatric age group Surgery and chemotherapy for all stages
Mixed germ cell tumor	Predominantly solid, or cystic and solid, depending on composition	AFP	Most commonly composed of dysgerminoma and endodermal sinus tumor
Sex cord stromal tumors	Granulosa-theca or Sertoli-Leydig cells	None	More common in younger patients Isosexual precocious puberty or androgenization
Juvenile granulosa-theca cell tumor	Very vascular	None	Malignancy related to percentage of granulosa cells Pure thecomas benign Surgery alone for stage I Surgery and chemotherapy for advanced disease
Sertoli-Leydig cell tumors (arrhenoblastoma)			Variable malignant potential
Epithelial tumors	Predominantly cystic		Commonly large size
Serous cystadenoma			May have borderline variants Low malignant potential
Mucinous cystadenoma	Predominantly cystic with septations		From coelomic epithelium
Serous or mucinous cystadenocarcinoma			Rare in children and adolescents
Miscellaneous Tumors			
Polyembryoma	Tissues resemble embryos with all three germ cell types (amniotic cavity, yolk sac, placental primordia)		
Gonadoblastoma			Predominantly dysgenetic gonads
Mesothelioma			
Metastatic disease			

AFP, α-fetoprotein; hCG, human chorionic gonadotropin.
From Bacon JL: Surgical treatment of adnexal pathology. In Hewitt G (ed): Operative Techniques in Gynecologic Surgery. Philadelphia, WB Saunders, 1999, vol 4, p 215.

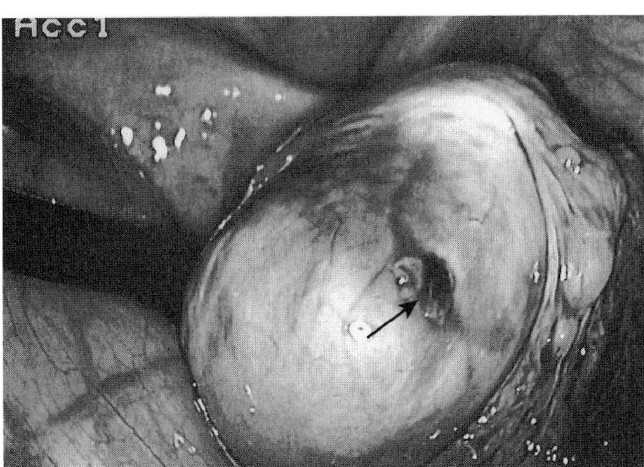

Figure 76-20. A ruptured corpus luteum cyst in a 15-year-old girl with acute pelvic pain. The site of rupture is marked by the arrow.

malignancy, conservation of ovarian tissue should be attempted, whenever possible.

Ovarian cysts are extremely common in adolescence because of persistent anovulation or ovulation dysfunction. They may be associated with rupture, pain, and hemorrhage (Fig. 76-20). A mass in the pelvis may be present, or the cyst may be found as an incidental finding at the time of radiologic studies. Mature cystic teratomas are the most common neoplasm, followed by a cystadenoma. Malignant neoplasms are seen but comprise less than 4% of all surgically excised masses.[64] In adolescents, a variety of reproductive disorders such as endometriosis, pelvic inflammatory disease, disorders of the fallopian tube, congenital uterine anomalies, or disorders of pregnancy may have the appearance of ovarian cysts (Table 76-3). It is essential to elicit a full history, including the details of menstrual function and sexual activity. Pregnancy must be excluded, and the possibility of complications of a sexually transmitted infection considered. Diagnostic imaging is very helpful in the management of ovarian cysts.[67]

The conservative approach to the management of ovarian cysts in adolescents is based on the low rate of malignancy and the high rate of functional cysts and benign germ cell tumors. Recurrent observation is recommended as an initial therapy for adolescent women. Indications for surgical intervention include cysts larger than 10 cm, persistent complex masses, acute symptoms, or a high suspicion for malignancy, based on radiologic or clinical criteria. In the absence of findings suggestive of neoplasm, minimally invasive surgical techniques such as laparoscopy should be paired with cystectomy and ovarian conservation. Cystectomy is performed by incising the ovary on the antimesenteric portion of the ovary. Blunt dissection separates the cyst from the ovarian capsule, allowing the cyst wall to be removed in toto (Fig. 76-21). Electrocautery or sutures may be needed to obtain hemostasis. Closure of the cyst wall is not necessary. Although marked distortion of the ovarian capsule may be present, rapid involution occurs. The cyst may be removed using a laparoscopic bag to prevent spillage of contents into the peritoneum. Laparoscopic management of cystic teratomas remains controversial because of concerns about the effects of rupture and spillage on long-term fertility. Recent studies, however, have found laparoscopic removal to be safe and efficient and without long-term sequelae, even in the presence of rupture and spillage (Fig. 76-22).[68,69] When malignancy is suspected, oophorectomy through a midline laparotomy incision allows proper staging with careful exploration, collection of pelvic cytology, and pelvic and periaortic lymph node sampling.

The ovaries or tubes may occasionally undergo torsion, with ischemia and ultimately necrosis of the adnexa (Fig. 76-23). Torsion of the ovary can occur at any age and is recognized by the acute onset of pain, nausea, vomiting, and a pelvic mass. Ovarian torsion is classically associated with the presence of an ovarian cyst or tumor but can be associated with normal ovaries.[70] Doppler-enhanced ultrasonography demonstrating the absence of blood flow has historically been used to predict ovarian torsion, but has been shown to be less predictive than ovarian enlargement.[71,72] Ovarian torsion is a surgical emergency. If a prompt diagnosis is made, the ovary may be salvaged with detorsion and cystectomy, even when it visually appears to have

Table 76-3 Etiology of Adnexal Masses in Adolescent Girls

Ovarian
Follicular cyst Corpus luteum Endometrioma Ovarian torsion Benign or malignant neoplasm Fallopian tube Paraovarian cyst Ectopic pregnancy
Uterus
Uterine anomaly Pregnancy Myoma
Gastrointestinal
Abscess Appendicitis Inflammatory bowel disease
Urinary
Pelvic kidney Acute urinary retention Urachal cyst
Neoplasms
Sarcoma Lymphoma Teratoma Hemangioma

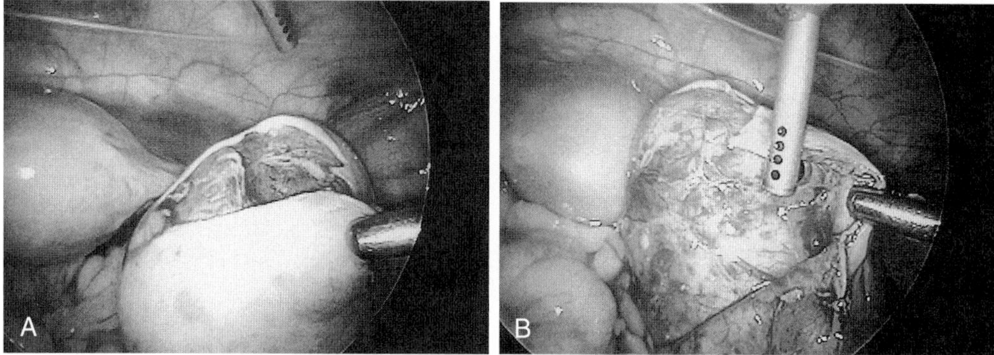

Figure 76-21. Laparoscopic ovarian cystectomy. **A,** An incision is made on the antimesenteric portion of the ovary. **B,** The capsule is separated from the ovarian cyst with blunt and sharp dissection.

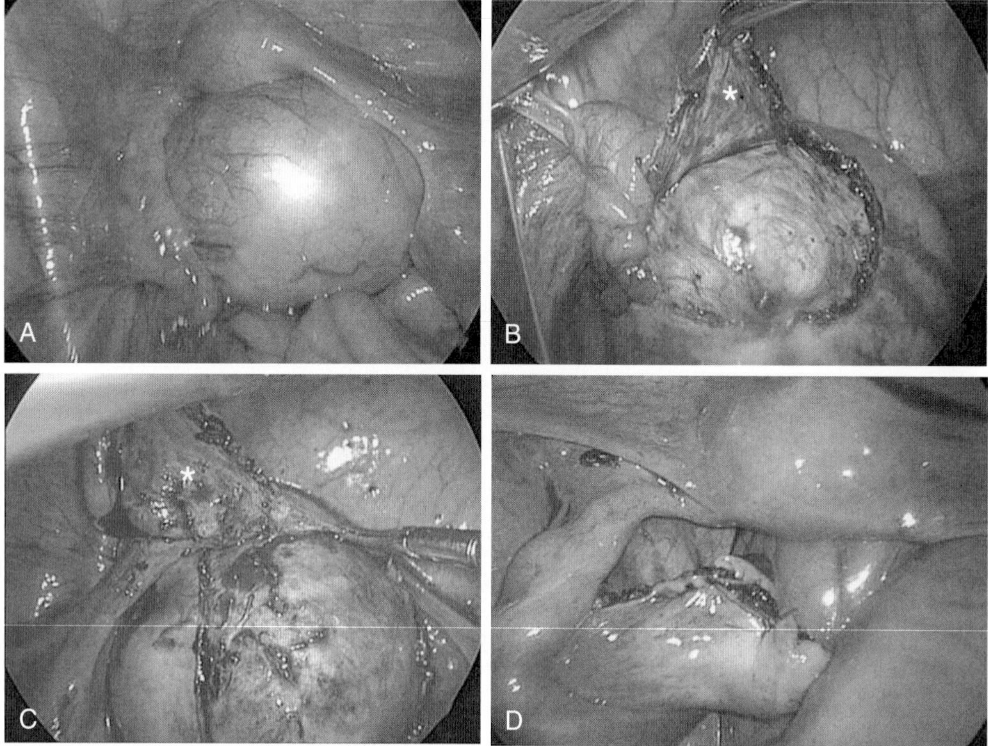

Figure 76-22. A 14-year-old presented with abdominal pain. Ultrasonography and CT showed calcifications within this left ovarian mass (**A**), indicating that it was a likely ovarian teratoma. **B,** Laparoscopic excision of the teratoma was initiated by incising the outer layer and peeling back the normal ovarian parenchyma (*asterisk*). **C,** The ovarian parenchyma (*asterisk*) has almost been completely stripped from the teratoma. **D,** The ovarian parenchyma was approximated after excision of the mass. The teratoma was placed into an endoscopic retrieval bag and exteriorized through the umbilicus after some morcellation. Histologic examination showed it to be a benign teratoma.

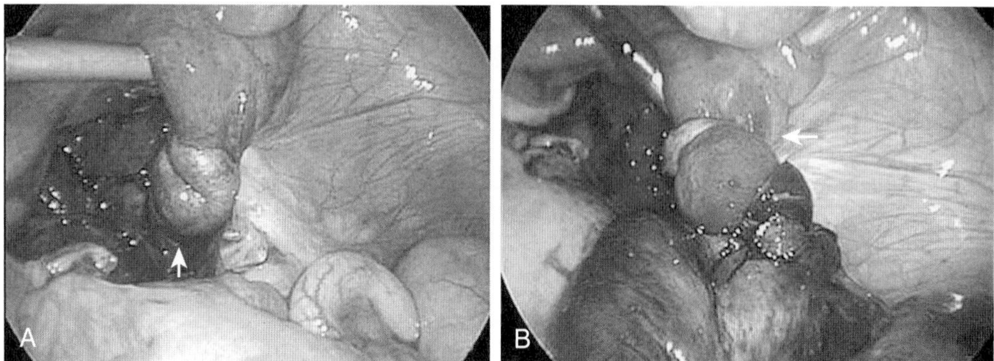

Figure 76-23. **A** and **B,** Right ovarian torsion in a 14-year-old girl with acute abdominal pain. The fallopian tube and ovarian vascular pedicle are twisted several times (*arrow*), resulting in acute venous congestion. Untwisting the pedicle allowed return of arterial flow and resolution of the venous congestion. Although the ovary appeared ischemic, it was not removed.

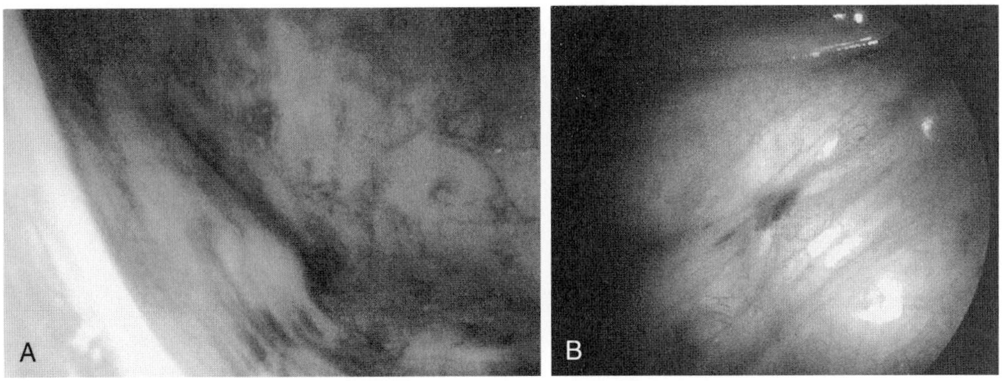

Figure 76-24. **A,** The peritoneal surface of a 14-year-old with endometriosis. Note the hypervascularity and subtle vesicular type lesions. **B,** The peritoneal surface of a 17-year-old with endometriosis. Note the classic "powder burn" appearance.

vascular compromise.[73] Oophorectomy is reserved for cases of delay associated with necrosis. Oophoropexy by side-wall fixation or shortening of the meso-ovarian ligament has been advocated by some to decrease the risk of subsequent contralateral torsion, although there is no evidence showing its efficacy.[73]

ENDOMETRIOSIS

Endometriosis refers to the presence of endometrial glands and stroma functioning outside the uterine lining. Endometriosis has been traditionally thought to be a disease of women in their 20s and 30s, but is well described in the adolescent population. Common symptoms among adolescents, such as dysmenorrhea, chronic pelvic pain, and dysfunctional uterine bleeding, have been associated with a 38% to 47% prevalence of endometriosis.[74,75] As many as 75% of symptomatic adolescents with medically refractory pelvic pain are found to have endometriosis at laparoscopy.[76] Although symptoms can suggest the diagnosis, definitive diagnosis is made by laparoscopic visualization or biopsy (or both). Because few adolescents need laparoscopy during their adolescent years, the exact prevalence of endometriosis in adolescents remains unknown. Progression of disease and the types of lesions appear to change with age. Clear, vesicular-appearing lesions and low-stage disease are more common in adolescence, with more classic hemosiderin "powder burn lesions" identified in older adults (Fig. 76-24).[77,78]

The treatment of endometriosis in adolescents is based on alleviation of symptoms and slowing the progression of disease. For patients undergoing surgical therapy, removal of all visible lesions by resection or destruction, with normalization of the pelvic anatomy, should be undertaken at the time of diagnosis. To accomplish this, CO_2 laser, cautery, coagulation, and the laparoscopic approach are all used. Menstrual suppression with oral contraceptives or progesterone-only medication (or both), along with nonsteroidal anti-inflammatory agents, are the mainstays of therapy. Gonadotropin-releasing agonists may be used on a short-term basis as an adjuvant to surgical therapy in adolescents but carries the risk of a detrimental effect on bone density. This therapy should be used cautiously in younger adolescents. Likewise, newer therapies advocated to control the symptoms of endometriosis such as the Levonorgestrel IUS (Schering Health, Berlin-Wedding, Germany) and aromatase inhibitors have not been studied in adolescents.[79,80] Noninterventional pain therapies may have a place in controlling the chronic pain associated with endometriosis. The long-term outcomes of infertility and chronic pain in those diagnosed with endometriosis as adolescents is not well described.

chapter 77

BREAST DISEASES

Don K. Nakayama, MD, MBA

The embryonic breast is formed in three steps.[1] First, the ectoderm thickens into a pair of longitudinal streaks in the ventral surface of the embryonic torso that become the primitive mammary ridges or "milk lines." Next, paired lens-shaped placodes appear as thickenings at specific locations along the milk lines, five in number in the mouse and a single pair in humans. Third, epithelial cells invaginate from the placode into the underlying mesenchyme to form the breast bud. A dense mesenchymal stroma coalesces around the bud, a situation that remains quiescent until the final stages of embryonic development. At this point epithelial cells begin to proliferate, sprouting from the mesenchyme and into a fat pad that has developed within the dermis.

Ductal branching follows entry of the bud into the fat pad forming a rudimentary ductal tree. Early lactiferous ducts are well established by 16 weeks. Ductal trees coalesce at the nipple that forms from differentiating epithelium at the skin. The nipple and areola form during late fetal development. A pigmented areola is first seen at 20 to 24 weeks, but a true nipple is not present until later in the perinatal period and is frequently inverted at birth. The buds respond to estrogenic hormonal stimulation by the maternal-placental-fetal unit during the last trimester, canalizing into ducts and enlarging en masse to form a true breast nodule during the final weeks of gestation.

Once perinatal maternal endocrine influences subside, the breast bud begins to involute in a process that resembles that seen in menopause.[2] Then it increases in size at a rate similar to somatic growth until puberty and undergoes robust branching, development of terminal duct lobular units, and stromal expansion that fills the entire mammary fat pad by adulthood.

ANATOMY AND PHYSIOLOGY

The fetus is subject to relatively high levels of placental estrogens in the perinatal period, resulting in breast enlargement in both genders at birth. A bimodal surge in hypothalamic-pituitary-gonadal axis activity, originally in the first 2 days of life with a second peak at 2 months, causes a "minipuberty of early infancy" that may explain persistence of breast enlargement well into the first few months to a year of life. At 6 months, the hormonal levels fall to prepubertal levels. A sudden fall in estrogens may allow prolactin and oxytocin secretion and the release of small amounts of milk by the infant breast ("witch's milk"). Sex hormone levels then remain low until puberty. Activation of the gonadotropin axis causes ovarian estradiol production in girls and, at a later age, testicular testosterone secretion in boys, with the resulting changes in body habitus and appearance of secondary sexual features. The testes are responsible for about 15% of estradiol production. Extragonadal aromatization then converts this compound into active estrogen.

The breast in the term neonate is a firm discrete nodule of white tissue up to 1 cm in diameter.[3] The nodule may persist well into the first year of life and may be more prominent at 6 months than earlier in infancy. The nodule begins to involute in late infancy. Throughout prepuberty, breast tissue is minimal and the nipple lies nearly flush with the skin contour in both boys and girls. The premature infant lacks this defined breast nodule and is particularly vulnerable to damage to the breast by an ill-placed surgical incision.

The onset of puberty is characterized by an increase in pulsatile secretion of gonadotropin-releasing hormone and gonadotropins, especially during sleep.[4] Thelarche is a response to the maturation of functional ovarian follicles.[5] Prolactin, glucocorticoids, and insulin have a permissive effect on breast development. With puberty, ovarian follicles initiate estrogen production. Estrogens circulate to the breast and stimulate ductal development and site-specific adipose deposition. Male adolescents fail to produce a significant breast mass, primarily because they lack significant levels of circulating estrogen. Once started, the process usually progresses smoothly to maturity in about 3 years. The breast stages; as defined by Marshall and Tanner, are as follows[6]:

Stage 1: Preadolescent; elevation of papilla only
Stage 2: Breast bud stage; elevation of breast and areola as a small mound, enlargement of areola diameter

Table 77-1 Aberrations of Normal Development and Involution of the Breast (ANDI)

Stage (Peak Ages, Adult yrs, Newborn mos)	Aberration			
	Normal Process	*Underlying Condition*	*Clinical Presentation*	*Disease State*
Early reproductive period (Adult, 15-25; Newborn, -2 to Birth)	Lobule formation	Fibroadenoma	Discrete lump	Giant fibroadenoma, multiple fibroadenomas
	Stroma formation	Juvenile hypertrophy	Excessive breast development	
Mature reproductive period (Adult, 25-40; Newborn, Birth to 2)	Cyclical hormonal effects on glandular tissue and stroma	Exaggerated cyclical effects	Cyclical mastalgia and nodularity (generalized or discrete)	
Involution (Adult, 35-55; Infant, 2-24)	Lobular involution (including microcysts, apocrine change, fibrosis, adenosis)	Macrocysts	Discrete lumps	
		Sclerosing lesions	Radiographic abnormalities (mastalgia lumps)	
	Ductal involution (including periductal round cell infiltrates)	Duct dilation	Nipple discharge	Periductal mastitis with bacterial infection and abscess formation
		Periductal fibrosis	Nipple retraction	
	Epithelial turnover	Mild epithelial hyperplasia		Epithelial hyperplasia with atypia

From Hughes LE: Aberrations of normal development and involution (ANDI): An update. In Mansell RE (ed): Recent Developments in the Study of Benign Breast Disease. London, Parthenon Publishing, 1994, pp 65-73, with permission.

Stage 3: Further enlargement of breast and areola, with no separation of their contours

Stage 4: Projection of areola and papilla to form a secondary mound above the level of the breast

Stage 5: Mature stage; projection of papilla only, resulting from recession of the areola to the general contour of the breast

The sequence of developmental changes that surround puberty is the onset of the adolescent growth spurt, breast development, appearance of pubic hair, and menarche. Thelarche has been shown to be influenced by diet (earlier among Korean girls eating a diet rich in shellfish and processed meat)[7] and environment (earlier among Mexican girls raised in valley ranches practicing modern agriculture compared with those raised in ranches using traditional methods).[8]

PATHOPHYSIOLOGY

Female breast disease in pediatric age groups can be seen as an aberration of normal development and involution (ANDI).[9] ANDI links adult breast pathology to events in early breast development. Thus, many of the same disease processes observed in adults may be present in the pediatric age group. Under the ANDI concept, a fibroadenoma is not a typical benign tumor but a disorder of normal lobular development. Excessive stroma development results in juvenile hypertrophy. Benign conditions that result from breast involution may be encountered during infancy, such as periductal mastitis, nipple discharge, and nipple retraction. The complete ANDI classification and associated pathology at each stage of breast development, modified to include events and conditions that involve the infant breast, is summarized in Table 77-1.

Breast cancer represents the extreme end of the spectrum of developmental disorders. It is a disorder of the mature breast, apparently the cumulative product of genetic and hormonal influences over time.[10] It is extremely rare in pediatric age groups, almost exclusively seen in late adolescence when encountered. Although risk factors for breast cancer certainly involve events during childhood and adolescence (e.g., early menarche) and genetic influences (e.g., familial breast cancer), breast cancer is not a childhood disease.

DISORDERS OF DEVELOPMENT AND GROWTH

Polythelia

Extra nipples and areolae may develop anywhere along the milk line from axilla to pubis. The most common location is on the chest below the actual breast.[11] In a minority, a true accessory breast develops. Unsightly structures should be removed.

Hypoplasia and Aplasia

Either breast aplasia or hypoplasia may occur in Poland's syndrome. Underlying chest wall structures, including pectoralis muscles and ribs, are absent or diminished in size. The ipsilateral upper extremity

Table 77-2	Differential Diagnosis of Breast Hypertrophy
Virginal hypertrophy	
Inflammation	
Giant fibroadenoma	
Cystosarcoma phyllodes	
Hormone-secreting tumors of the ovary, adrenal gland, or pituitary gland	
Lymphoma	
Sarcoma	
Adenocarcinoma	

From Samuelov R, Siplovich L: Juvenile gigantomastia. J Pediatr Surg 23:1014-1015, 1988, with permission.

may also be affected. Reconstruction of the chest wall and placement of a mammary prosthesis or breast reconstruction by a variety of flap techniques is usually indicated.[11,12] Adolescents with small breasts and otherwise normal pubertal development are normal, and reassurance is the most appropriate intervention. Hypoplasia with any abnormality of pubertal development requires an endocrinologic evaluation for ovarian failure, including gonadal dysgenesis and androgen excess (congenital adrenal hyperplasia or intersex-associated enzyme deficiencies).[13] Breast augmentation is a therapeutic option for these patients.

An important iatrogenic cause of breast hypoplasia is an incision at or near the infant breast, at an exit site for an indwelling central venous catheter, a thoracotomy incision, or incision and drainage of a breast abscess. Extreme care must be taken when placing these incisions, particularly in prematurely born infants in whom the breast may be barely visible.

Atrophy

Patients with atrophy of the breast who have undergone normal development should be evaluated for an underlying cause. Weight loss results in loss of fat from stroma and bilateral atrophy. Eating disorders also may be complicated by hypothalamic suppression and hypoestrogenism, further retarding breast growth.[14] In an otherwise well-nourished adolescent, endocrine disorders that result in low estrogen or increased androgens should be evaluated with appropriate hormone determinations.

Unilateral atrophy may occur in scleroderma.[14] Also, it has been reported as a complication of infectious mononucleosis.[15]

Premature Thelarche

The differential diagnosis of breast enlargement in female patients is seen in Table 77-2. Because of racial differences with thelarche, breast development is premature if it occurs before 8 years of age for white girls and 7 years for blacks and Hispanics. Premature thelarche is defined as isolated breast development without sexual hair growth, vaginal mucosal estrogenization, linear growth spurt, adult body odor, and pubertal behavioral changes. It is unilateral in 50% of cases. It has a peak incidence between 6 months to 2 years and resolves in more than half of patients.[16]

Premature thelarche is distinguished from physiologic perinatal breast development and precocious puberty. Precocious puberty has a peak incidence between 5 to 8 years, later than true premature thelarche, and is associated with other features of puberty just listed. Gentle retraction of the labia is necessary to observe the vaginal mucosa. The prepubertal vaginal mucosa is reddish and delicate, whereas an estrogenized mucosa is pink and thicker. Two or more signs of precocious puberty establish this diagnosis.

Causes of premature thelarche may involve partial activation of the hypothalamic-pituitary-gonadal axis by follicle-stimulating hormone secretion, failure of ovarian follicular involution, and gonadotropin-independent estrogen production (McCune-Albright syndrome, rarely hepatocellular carcinoma, and ovarian and adrenal tumors). Exogenous estrogens in poultry, cosmetics, and hair products have been implicated in the early sexual development as well. Xenoestrogens are compounds that bind to the estrogen receptor and include a wide variety of environmental toxins used in pesticides, cosmetics, and packaging material. Patients with precocious puberty and those in whom the diagnosis of premature thelarche is uncertain should be referred to an endocrinologist, who likely will request a bone age radiograph; ultrasound evaluation of the liver, adrenals, and ovaries; and gonadotropin stimulation tests. Those with true central precocious puberty undergo suppression of the hypothalamic-pituitary-gonadal axis with long-acting gonadotropin-releasing hormone analogs.[17]

Virginal Hypertrophy

The cause of virginal hypertrophy is probably an end-organ hypersensitivity to normal hormonal fluxes at the time of puberty.[11,18] Histologically, breasts show stromal and ductal hypertrophy with dilated ducts. Tissue necrosis and rupture of the skin may result from the sheer weight and justify reduction mammaplasty. Little experience is available with medical therapy, although some improvement has been reported with danazol therapy. Reduction mammaplasty is a safe and appropriate procedure for virginal hypertrophy. Repeated resections may be necessary as the breast may continue to grow.

Unilateral Hypertrophy

Breast asymmetry may result from unilateral hypertrophy, a condition easily distinguished from hypoplasia and aplasia. Some degree of asymmetry is normal and is detectable in many patients. Breast growth may magnify differences and may hamper the child psychologically, even though both breasts are completely clinically normal. Once Tanner stage 5 breast maturity is reached, breast reduction of the enlarged breast is reasonable.[11,19]

Gynecomastia

Excellent reviews by Braunstein[20] and Diamantopoulos and Bao[21] discuss the various causes of gynecomastia and its diagnostic workup. Gynecomastia is the benign proliferation of glandular tissue of the male breast enough to be felt or seen as an enlarged breast. Male breast enlargement occurs physiologically in the neonate, adolescent, and elder. Infant gynecomastia, discussed previously, may persist for up to 12 months in boys and 24 months in girls. Prepubertal gynecomastia (enlargement in boys) and thelarche (the equivalent condition in girls) warrants careful investigation.

Thirty to 60 percent of boys exhibit physiologic or pubertal gynecomastia. A hypothesis is that a lag in maturation in testosterone synthesis with the onset of puberty allows a relatively greater estrogen effect, but studies have failed to detect hormonal differences in boys with pubertal gynecomastia. This disorder first appears between 10 and 12 years of age. Its highest prevalence is at 13 to 14 years, corresponding to Tanner stage 3 or 4. Involution is generally complete at 16 to 17 years but may persist longer in obese boys.

Pathologic gynecomastia results from imbalances between estrogen and androgen concentrations. Testicular (germ cell, Sertoli cell, and Leydig cell tumors) and adrenal neoplasms may overproduce estrogens. Feminizing adrenal tumors are generally malignant. Increased aromatase conversion of testicular precursors into active estrogen occurs in idiopathic gynecomastia and in infants with hepatocellular carcinoma. Decreased androgen levels or androgenic effects may result from primary defects in the testis, loss of tonic stimulation by pituitary gonadotropins, or increased binding of androgens to sex-hormone–binding globulin. Displacement of androgens from their receptors by the many drugs associated with gynecomastia (Table 77-3) may result in unopposed estrogen effects in sex-hormone–sensitive tissue, including the breast.

Histologic studies in the early stages of gynecomastia show marked duct epithelial cell proliferation, inflammatory cell infiltration, increased stromal fibroblasts, and enhanced vascularity. This proliferative stage, also known as the florid stage, may explain breast pain and tenderness that are typical of the clinical presentation. Epithelial proliferation and ductal dilation then both decrease, and the stroma begins to undergo fibrosis and hyalinization. Clinical resolution of breast enlargement and pain follow in 85% of cases, a fact that must be considered when contemplating treatment.

Painful, tender gynecomastia is often seen in adolescent boys. The patient often recalls trauma to the breast; however, the injury is more likely to have brought the lump to his attention than to have caused it. On palpation, true gynecomastia is a disc of rubbery tissue arising concentrically beneath and around the nipple and areola. This distinguishes it from pseudogynecomastia, which is increased amounts of adipose tissue beneath the breast causing prominence of the area.

Table 77-3 Drugs Associated with Gynecomastia

Hormones (growth hormone, human chorionic gonadotropin, estrogens, anabolic steroids)
Androgen synthesis/androgen receptor antagonists (ketoconazole, finasteride, cimetidine, cyproterone)
Antibiotics (isoniazid, ethionamide, metronidazole, highly active antiretroviral treatment)
Anti-ulcer (cimetidine, ranitidine, omeprazole)
Abuse (alcohol, heroin, amphetamines)
Chemotherapy (methotrexate, alkylating agents, *Vinca* alkaloids, cyclophosphamide)
Cardiovascular (furosemide, spironolactone, angiotensin-converting enzyme inhibitors, nifedipine, verapamil, reserpine)
Psychiatric/neurologic (phenytoin, tricyclic antidepressants, phenothiazines, risperidone, diazepam, clonidine, selective serotonin reuptake inhibitors)
Other (theophylline D-penicillamine, cyclosporine)

From Diamantopoulos S, Bao Y: Gynecomastia and premature thelarche: A guide for practitioners. Pediatr Rev 28:e57, 2007, reprinted with permission.

Because pubertal gynecomastia is so prevalent, a thorough history and physical examination, especially of the testes, is sufficient in adolescent boys. Reassurance and follow-up examinations at 6-month intervals is suggested. Pubertal gynecomastia generally resolves within 1 year. Suggestive aspects of the personal medical history (especially drugs and medications), abnormal physical findings (particularly of the testes and genitalia), onset of gynecomastia between early infancy (not persistent from birth) and the onset of puberty, rapid increase in breast size, macrogynecomastia greater than 4 cm in diameter, and pubertal gynecomastia that persists longer than 1 year should lead to a directed endocrinologic and oncologic workup. Drugs should be discontinued, if possible, and the patient re-examined in 1 month. Imaging studies of the testes and adrenal glands are necessary if a tumor is suspected.

Indications for therapy include severe pain, tenderness, or embarrassment sufficient to interfere with the patient's normal daily activities. Subcutaneous mastectomy through a periareolar incision is definitive treatment (Fig. 77-1). Liposuction is another surgical alternative.[11,22] Pharmacologic approaches include estrogen receptor modulators or antiestrogens (tamoxifen, raloxifene, and clomiphene citrate) and aromatase inhibitors (testolactone, anastrozole, and letrozole). Tamoxifen and raloxifene improved the condition in 91% of boys in one study,[23] but anastrozole was no better than placebo.[24] It is difficult to assess the efficacy of these various medical regimens because gynecomastia undergoes spontaneous regression in a large number of cases. Side effects from these medications must be considered when employing drug therapy for pubertal gynecomastia.

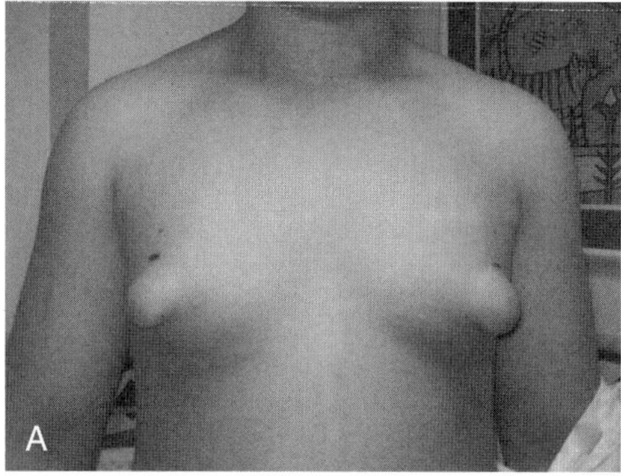

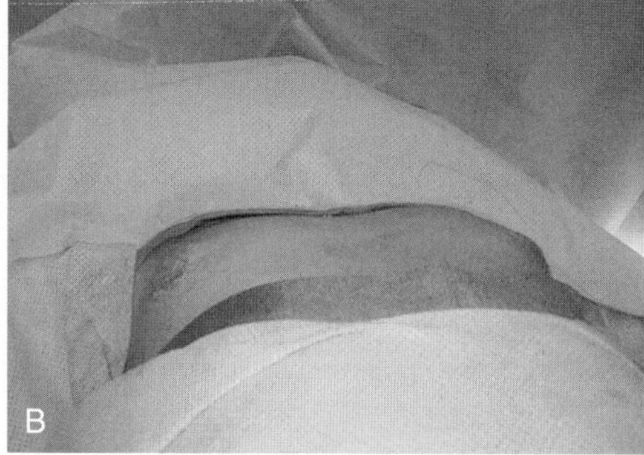

Figure 77-1. **A,** This teenager has gynecomastia, which was causing him discomfort as well as having negative psychosocial ramifications. **B,** On the operating table, the enlarged breast tissue was removed and a nice cosmetic appearance achieved.

INFLAMMATORY LESIONS

Breast Trauma and Fat Necrosis

Soft tissue injury to the breast may result from blunt and penetrating trauma. Shoulder-harness restraints have been reported to cause subcutaneous rupture of the breast. Most breast trauma is mild and self-limiting. Specific therapy is rarely required.

Fat necrosis is a benign condition that can mimic breast carcinoma. It is thought to result from breast trauma.[25] A history of antecedent trauma is present in about 40% of cases. Areas of fat necrosis are seen as single or multiple firm, round, or irregular masses, often in the center of the breast near the areola. The masses may be painless, firm, and immobile and cause skin tethering and thickening, all features that suggest carcinoma. Spiculated calcifications may be present on mammography, further suggesting the presence of a neoplasm. Patients who are seen later with painless masses require biopsy to exclude malignancy.

Mastitis and Abscess

Infections of the breast of a neonate, uncommon today, had a high mortality and caused substantial morbidity to the breast and chest wall before the antibiotic era. The disease primarily affects the neonatal breast before involution of the ductal anatomy. Eighty-four percent of these infections occur in the first 3 weeks of life. *Staphylococcus* is the causative organism in more than 90% of cases. *Streptococcus, Salmonella,* and *Escherichia coli* also may cause a breast infection.

Both genders are affected, with a female-to-male ratio of 1.8. The skin and nipple are red. Swelling and edema cause induration of the area. Fluctuance and deep discoloration to a fiery red or purple color indicate the presence of an abscess or extension of the infection beneath the fascia. Although in some infants, a small drop of pus may be expressed from the nipple, this is not sufficient drainage if an abscess is truly present. Most patients lack systemic reactions to infection, with only one fourth having a fever and fewer than 10% having other constitutional symptoms (irritability or refusal to feed). One fourth have pustular skin lesions elsewhere, usually in the inguinal region.

Mastitis and breast abscess require appropriate antibiotic therapy against *Staphylococcus, Streptococcus, Salmonella,* and *E. coli.* Areas of fluctuance or progression of inflammation while taking antibiotics suggest the presence of an abscess that requires drainage. Mastitis in neonates responds in nearly all cases to intravenous antibiotics and warm packs to the affected breast. The decision to explore the infant breast for an abscess must be made with great care to avoid unnecessary damage that may result in breast deformity later in adolescence. An initial needle aspiration of suggestive areas is a prudent first step. If no purulence is encountered, antibiotics are continued. Discovery of a true abscess requires incision and drainage. One study documented a significant decrease in breast size relative to the opposite breast in two of five patients who had undergone incision and drainage of a breast abscess as a neonate.[26]

Mastitis and abscess occur more commonly after thelarche. Causes include manipulation and breast feeding, although in many cases the cause cannot be identified. Nursing may continue in cases that develop while breast feeding. Adequate abscess drainage usually requires general anesthesia owing to loculations of pus and breast septations in the developing and mature breast.

NIPPLE DISCHARGE

Galactorrhea

Galactorrhea is inappropriate lactation that is not related to pregnancy or that continues post partum in the absence of breast feeding.[13,27] The five etiologic groups are neurogenic, hypothalamic, endocrine, drug-induced, and idiopathic. Neurogenic causes result from local breast and nipple irritation and stimulation. The most common hypothalamic cause of galactorrhea in adults is a prolactinoma, a rare tumor in childhood and adolescence. Failure of sexual maturation

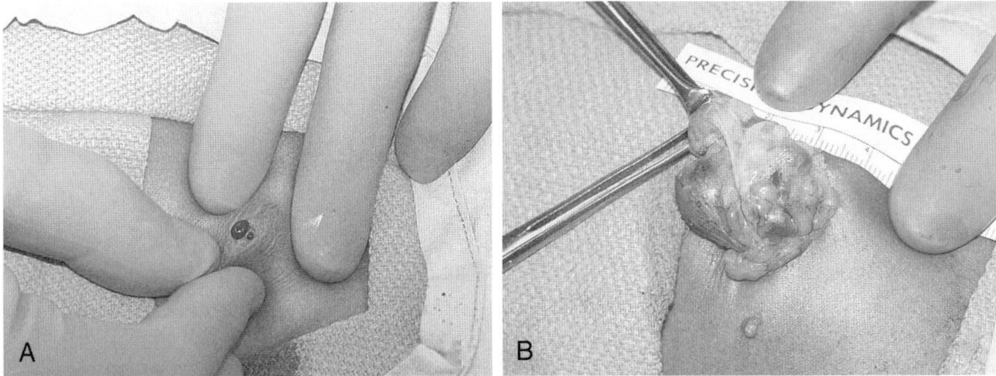

Figure 77-2. **A,** Bloody and green discharge from a 5-month-old boy is seen. **B,** Multiple subareolar epithelial cysts, which were causing the drainage, were removed.

often accompanies galactorrhea in children with these tumors.[28] Visual symptoms and headaches are rare in children as compared with adults. Cessation of oral contraceptives, polycystic ovary, adrenal tumors, and gonadal tumors are rare causes of galactorrhea in adolescents.[13] Hypothyroidism in infants and children has been reported to be associated with galactorrhea and precocious puberty. Nipple discharge ceases with correction of the underlying thyroid condition.[29,30]

Nipple discharge in boys is always abnormal, and a cause must be sought. A prolactinoma is the most common cause in young boys.[20] If prolactin levels are high and evaluation of the sella turcica is unrevealing, annual imaging of the sella is necessary until the end of puberty, even if the galactorrhea resolves.

Other Nipple Discharges

Nonmilky discharges include pus, cyst contents, and blood. Purulent discharges usually respond to antibiotics; chronic discharge may require drainage and duct excision. Serous drainage of brown to green fluid may indicate the presence of a communicating breast cyst and is usually self-limited. Bloody drainage, a sign of cancer in adults, is generally drainage from an intraductal papilloma or duct ectasia in children and adolescents.[31] Bloody nipple drainage may be culture positive for *Staphylococcus,* so drainage should be cultured and treated if positive. Excision of the abnormal duct is indicated if drainage persists or recurs (Fig. 77-2).[32]

Mastalgia

Breast pain, or mastalgia, is a poorly characterized and underreported syndrome.[33] It accounts for about one fourth of visits to adult breast clinics and is the presenting symptom of breast cancer in 15% of cases. Its prevalence in young and adolescent girls is unknown.

Initial evaluation excludes localized lesions (benign and malignant) and inflammatory conditions. Pain is then characterized as cyclic or noncyclic. The distinction is important because the likelihood of response to drug treatment differs because cyclic pain is more likely to respond. Cyclic mastalgia usually occurs in the third decade of life. It is usually characterized as bilateral, dull, burning, or aching. Pain starts 7 to 10 days before the onset of menses, building until menses, when the pain dissipates. Pain may persist throughout the menstrual cycle. Spontaneous resolution occurs in 22% of cases. Noncyclic mastalgia tends to occur a decade later and resolves in 50% of cases. Treatment includes removal of methylxanthines from the diet and reassurance. Evening primrose oil, danazol, and bromocriptine may be effective as adjunctive therapy.

BREAST MASSES

Evaluation of Breast Masses

The age of the patient affects the differential diagnosis for breast masses and hence the diagnostic approach (Tables 77-4 and 77-5). Patient age, history, and physical examination are sufficient to make the diagnosis in most cases. A retrospective review of 374 breast specimens from patients aged 20 years and younger over a 10-year period revealed only one papillary carcinoma.[31]

Table 77-4 Breast Masses in Children
Physiologic
Normal breast bud
Premature thelarche
Pathologic
Inflammatory
Mastitis
Breast abscess
Fibrosis
Fat necrosis
Benign neoplasms
Hemangioma
Cyst
Lipoma
Papilloma
Malignant neoplasms
Metastatic (e.g., rhabdomyosarcoma, lymphoma)
Secretory carcinoma

Table 77-5 Breast Masses in Adolescents
Physiologic
Thelarche
Unilateral hypertrophy
Pathologic
Inflammatory
Mastitis
Breast abscess
Fibrosis
Fat necrosis
Benign neoplasms
Fibroadenoma
Phyllodes tumor
Cyst
Fibrocystic disease
Neurofibroma
Malignant neoplasms
Primary breast cancer
Metastatic (e.g., lymphoma)

The majority were fibroadenoma (44%), gynecomastia (22%), and juvenile hypertrophy (14%). Twenty-two lesions were a variety of soft tissue tumors, including phyllodes tumor, granular cell tumor, neurofibroma, low-grade angiosarcoma, high-grade stromal sarcoma, metastatic alveolar rhabdomyosarcoma, and giant cell fibroblastoma. Because primary breast cancer is so rare in the pediatric age group, observation has little risk and often is an appropriate step in determining the clinical diagnosis.[32] It is important, however, to observe all lesions to resolution and to obtain further studies when lesions continue to grow or have features that are worrisome to the experienced clinician (e.g., hard consistency, irregular margins, fixation to chest wall or skin, regional lymphadenopathy). A directed workup in such cases may include fine-needle aspiration for cytology, mammography, ultrasound examination, and, ultimately, biopsy.

The issue of breast self-examination among adolescents is controversial.[13,34] Given the rarity of breast cancer in this age group, some clinicians recommend that time could be better used educating them about greater risks to their health, such as drugs, alcohol, and smoking. However, four in five of adolescent breast masses were detected during self-examination. A consensus statement has recommended that individuals with an inherited predisposition to breast cancer begin monthly breast self-examination between 18 and 21 years, with annual clinical breast examinations and adjunctive mammography at age 25 to 35 years.[35]

Prepubertal Breast Masses

Masses may occur in the prepubertal breast but are nearly always benign. The most important diagnosis to consider is asynchronous thelarche.[13] One breast bud may appear weeks to months ahead of the other. A breast bud is easily recognized as a disc of firm tissue beneath the areola. In such cases, biopsy is never indicated because it may lead to unilateral iatrogenic amastia.

Cysts and Fibrocystic Disease

Benign simple cysts occur throughout childhood, but they most commonly occur with the onset of breast development. They appear as soft, painless masses that are not fixed to surrounding breast tissue. Needle aspiration of the cyst results in complete disappearance. Fluid may be serous or brown. Persistence of the mass after cyst aspiration is an indication for biopsy. Fibrocystic disease is a disease of the mature breast, occurring most commonly in the fourth to fifth decades, and is generally not an issue in adolescents.[36] Masses that occur with fibrocystic disease may be asymptomatic or associated with mastalgia, often worse in the perimenstrual period.[13] Resolution of the mass may occur over the course of one or two cycles. A persisting or dominant mass should be aspirated for diagnostic and therapeutic reasons. A number of nonoperative interventions have been tried.[13] Dietary methylxanthines have been implicated as a contributing factor in fibrocystic disease, but elimination of sources of the compound (coffee, tea, cola drinks, and chocolate) may not be successful in resolving the condition. Oral contraceptives improve symptoms in 70% to 90% of individuals. Evening primrose oil has been found to be beneficial in 44%, given in a 1000-mg dose three times daily for 3 months.[13]

FIBROEPITHELIAL TUMORS

Fibroadenomas

Fibroadenomas are the most common breast mass in the pediatric age group.[31] Two variants, adult and juvenile, can affect children. Adult fibroadenomas affect older adolescents and young women (Fig. 77-3). They may be multiple in 10% to 15% of cases. The mass is usually painless and small, measuring 1 to 2 cm in diameter. It is well circumscribed, rubbery, and mobile. A true capsule is not present, but there is a well-demarcated stromal interface where the tumor comes in contact with normal tissue.[31] Areas of focal hemorrhage may be present, a feature associated with pain and rapid enlargement. Juvenile fibroadenomas affect younger adolescents around the time of puberty. In contrast to an adult fibroadenoma, the juvenile variant is much larger and may cause considerable breast asymmetry.[11,18] Fibroadenomas are considered to be benign, although adult fibroadenomas can rarely harbor a carcinoma.[37] Also, juvenile variants may be related to phyllodes tumors.[31,37] Clonal analysis shows that epithelial and stromal elements of the fibroadenoma are polyclonal, indicating a hyperplastic rather than a neoplastic process.[38] Adult fibroadenomas confer a small but definite increased risk for breast cancer development.[39] Clonal analysis in three patients in whom phyllodes tumor of the breast developed

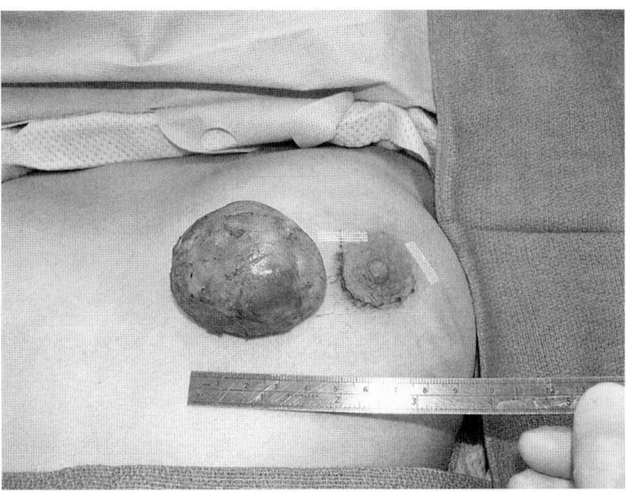

Figure 77-3. This 16-year-old developed an enlarging, painful fibroadenoma in her left breast. The lesion measured 7 × 5 × 4 cm on ultrasound examination. She underwent excision of the medially placed lesion through a circumareolar incision and tolerated the operation well. The histologic examination returned a benign fibroadenoma. Her symptoms have resolved.

after excision of a fibroadenoma suggested that the former developed from the latter.[40] A phyllodes tumor tends to be larger (>4 cm in diameter), occur in older patients (mean age, 28.5 years in fibroadenoma, 44 years in phyllodes tumor), has high density on mammography, and appears round or lobulated with posterior acoustic enhancement on breast ultrasonography compared with a fibroadenoma.[41,42] However, a considerable overlap exists between the two conditions with these criteria, and aspiration cytology or excisional biopsy is often necessary to confirm the diagnosis.[31]

Whether fibroadenomas can be safely followed without operation is debatable.[43] Some advocate nonoperative management if the lesion exhibits the expected characteristic features: 1 to 2 cm, solitary, firm, rubbery, nontender, and well circumscribed.[44] Fine-needle aspiration is useful in distinguishing fibroadenomas from carcinomas and phyllodes tumors, but differentiating fibroadenomas from other benign conditions is more difficult.[43] The probability of disappearance of the mass is 0.46 at 5 years and 0.69 at 9 years.[44] Although fibroadenoma is a long-term risk factor for breast cancer,[45] because of the rarity of breast cancer among adolescents it is reasonable to wait a period of years to see whether a small lesion will disappear. Enlarging fibroadenomas should be excised to avoid further enlargement of the mass and preserve the architecture of the remaining normal breast tissue. Rapid growth may cause impressively large lesions and require complex reconstructive surgery.[18] Excision of a fibroadenoma proceeds through an incision directly over the mass, following one of Langer's lines. The mass is held by a centrally placed suture or clamp and is removed with no more than a few millimeters of normal breast tissue. Further breast development is usually normal and symmetric because the tissue compressed by the tumor fills the defect over time.

Phyllodes Tumors

Phyllodes tumors, formerly called cystosarcoma phyllodes, are rare fibroepithelial tumors that can be benign (with significant risk for local recurrence) or malignant (with rapidly growing metastases).[46] They range in size from 1 to 40 cm. Only about 10% of phyllodes tumors occur in women younger than the age of 20 years and never in children younger than the age of 12. The clinical presentation is a rapidly growing breast mass larger than 6 cm.[34] Closely resembling a fibroadenoma, a phyllodes tumor appears well circumscribed grossly but, like a fibroadenoma, lacks a true capsule. Complete surgical excision requires a 2-cm margin of normal breast parenchyma. Fibrous areas are interspersed with soft, fleshy areas, and cysts are filled with clear or semisolid bloody fluid, all features that distinguish it from a fibroadenoma. On microscopy, both epithelial and stromal elements show hyperplasia and may have areas of atypia, metaplasia, and malignancy. Characteristics of the stroma alone, particularly mitotic activity, determine whether a phyllodes tumor is malignant (Fig. 77-4).[47] The mean age of these patients is in the fourth decade, about a decade older than that for an adult fibroadenoma.

Distinguishing a phyllodes tumor from a fibroadenoma before operation is difficult, and a definitive diagnosis may require open excisional biopsy. Fine-needle aspiration depends on the detection of a dimorphic pattern of stromal elements and benign epithelial tissue, although the technique may not yield a definitive diagnosis in all cases.[48] The mammographic appearance of phyllodes tumors resembles that of fibroadenomas, with smooth polylobulated margins.[46] Ultrasonography is useful if cysts are found within an otherwise solid mass, a characteristic of phyllodes tumor.

When the preoperative diagnosis is known, wide local excision with a 2-cm margin of normal breast tissue is recommended.[46,48] Tumors that extend to the pectoralis fascia require removal of the muscle adjacent to the tumor. Owing to the similarity in appearance between a fibroadenoma and a phyllodes tumor, the latter may be enucleated without a margin when the diagnosis is not known before operation. Because 20% of phyllodes tumors will recur when resected without an adequate margin, most authorities recommend re-excision of normal breast tissue to ensure its removal with an adequate margin. Traditionally, malignant phyllodes tumors were treated with simple mastectomy. Recently, malignant tumors have been treated by using wide local excision with 2-cm margins with acceptable results.[48,49] Lymph node metastases are not present, so lymph node dissection is not indicated. Benign tumors more than 5 cm in diameter have a higher rate of recurrence (39%) than do smaller ones (10%).[50] Both benign and malignant phyllodes tumors recur. Among recurrences in previously resected benign tumors, about 20% show malignant histologic transformation with a worse overall prognosis. Local recurrence of a benign tumor should be re-excised, whereas most authorities recommend

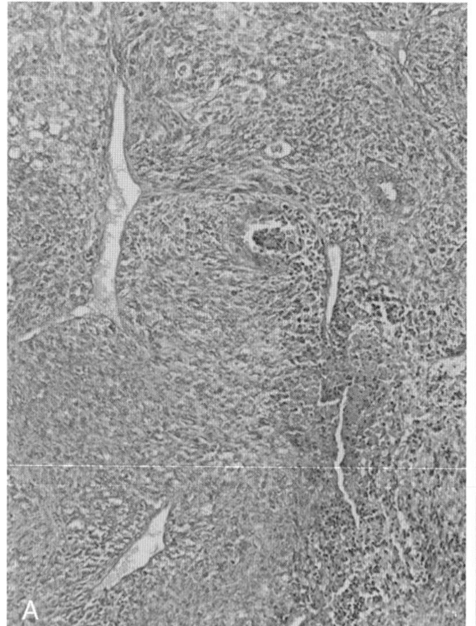

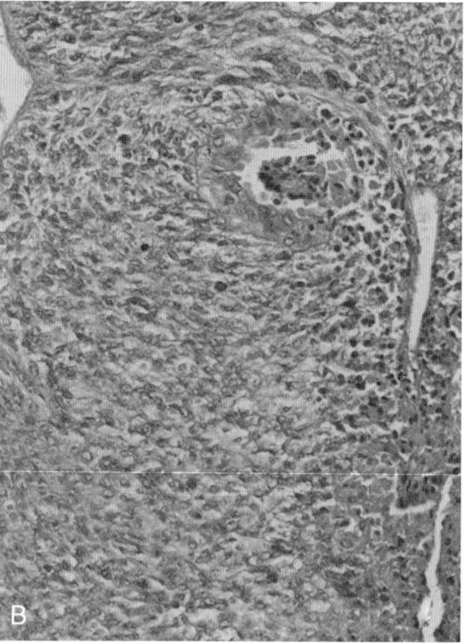

Figure 77-4. A 16-year-old girl underwent resection of a malignant phyllodes tumor. **A,** Photomicrograph shows an area of necrosis typical of rapidly growing neoplasms (×10). **B,** A higher-power view shows stromal and epithelial atypia and numerous mitotic figures (×20). (Courtesy of Edgar Pierce, MD, and Earl Mullis, MD, Medical Center of Central Georgia.)

simple mastectomy for recurrence of a malignant tumor.

Breast Cancer

Breast malignancy in children falls into three groups: primary malignancies, metastatic tumors that involve the breast, and second malignancies.[51] Primary breast cancer is extremely rare in childhood age groups. Although only 0.2% of primary breast cancers occur before age 25 years, they have been found in children younger than age 5 years and in male as well as female adolescents. More than 90% are first seen as a breast mass. On occasion, nipple discharge is a presenting sign, so a sample of fluid should be sent for cytologic examination.

Secretory carcinoma is a form that occurs relatively more frequently, but not exclusively, in children. It has a low-grade clinical behavior with a good prognosis for long-term survival after simple mastectomy.[52] Girls are affected five times greater than boys. The youngest patient reported is a 3-year-old boy.[53] Even though most tumors measure 3 cm or less, lesions of 12 cm have been described. Axillary lymph node involvement is present in about 20% of cases. Standard treatment is simple mastectomy, although some long-term survivors have been reported after excisional biopsy. Axillary node dissection is indicated if nodes are clinically involved. Recurrence after lumpectomy has been described in several reports. Long-term follow-up is imperative owing to the indolent nature of the disease and the risk for late recurrence.

Nonsecretory breast cancers are less common than secretory breast cancers in the pediatric age group. Some large children's hospitals report no primary breast cancers in their series of pediatric breast masses. A 40-year review of adolescent patients at the M. D. Anderson Cancer Center found 10 patients with primary adenocarcinoma of the breast, 4 with malignant phyllodes tumors, and 2 with metastatic tumors.[54] Ages ranged from 13 to 19 years, and 4 patients had a positive family history for breast disease. These adenocarcinomas were reported exclusively in female adolescents and young adults and probably represent the leading edge of the prevalence distribution for adult primary breast cancer. They include histologic types seen in primary breast cancers in mature women: invasive intraductal (most common), invasive lobular, and signet ring. A family history of breast cancer is a risk factor for early-onset breast cancer and was present in one fourth of these patients. The treatment regimen is the same as for adult primary breast cancer, dictated by histology, stage, presence of hormone receptors, and patient menstrual status.

The breast has been reported as the primary site for rhabdomyosarcoma, leukemia, and lymphoma, as well.[31,51] More commonly, it is the site of acute leukemic relapse. Metastatic carcinoma may involve the breast, with retinoblastoma, osteosarcoma, neuroblastoma, leukemia, lymphoma, and rhabdomyosarcoma having been reported.[31,51] Alveolar rhabdomyosarcoma appears to have a relative predilection for the breast, with 6% to 10% of cases metastasizing to the breast during its course.[55]

chapter 78

ENDOCRINE DISORDERS AND TUMORS

Jae-O Bae, MD • Michael A. Skinner, MD

THYROID GLAND

Diseases of the thyroid gland occur in 37 of 1000 school-aged children in the United States.[1] About half of these are diffuse gland hypertrophy or simple goiter. Thyroiditis is the second most common abnormality, followed by thyroid nodules and functional disorders. Malignant neoplasms are rare.

Embryology and Physiology

The thyroid gland is the first endocrine organ to mature in fetal development, arising as an outpouching of the embryonic alimentary tract at about 24 days' gestation. The developing thyroid gland descends from the base of the tongue, ventral to the hyoid bone and the larynx, to its final location by about 7 weeks' gestation. In about half of the population, a persistence of the thyroglossal diverticulum results in a pyramidal thyroid lobe. Accessory thyroid tissue may appear in the tongue or anywhere along the course of the duct. Rarely, nondescent results in a lingual thyroid.

Histologically, by week 11 of gestation, colloid begins to form and thyroxine (T_4) can be demonstrated in the embryo. Parafollicular cells, or C cells, arise from the ultimobranchial bodies and are found throughout the thyroid gland.

Thyroglobulin is recognized histologically as colloid. Thyroid hormone is synthesized at the interface between the follicular cell and the thyroglobulin. The first step in thyroid synthesis is the iodination of tyrosine molecules, which are then coupled to form the definitive thyroid hormones T_4 and triiodothyronine (T_3). When free T_4 reaches the nucleus of the target cell, the T_3 molecule interacts with the nuclear receptors. This receptor-T_3 conjugate then binds to DNA to regulate genetic transcription.[2] T_4 increases cellular oxygen consumption and the basal metabolic rate, stimulates protein synthesis, and influences carbohydrate, lipid, and vitamin metabolism.

The production and secretion of T_3 and T_4 are stimulated by thyroid-stimulating hormone (TSH) secreted by the pituitary in response to thyrotropin-releasing hormone, which is, in turn, secreted by the hypothalamus. Other peptides are present within the thyroid gland such as neuropeptide Y, substance P, cholecystokinin, and vasoactive intestinal peptide, which may assist in the production and secretion of thyroid hormones.[3]

TSH is nearly always decreased in the hyperthyroid state and elevated in hypothyroidism and is an extremely sensitive measure of this condition. The plasma free T_4 level is a measure of biologically active thyroid hormone, unaffected by protein binding. Alternatively, when total plasma T_3 and T_4 are measured, it is necessary to consider the level of thyroid-binding globulin to estimate the level of unbound biologically active hormone.

Several imaging modalities are available to assist in evaluating the thyroid gland. Radionuclide scintigraphy is probably the most commonly used test. The radiolabeled iodines ^{123}I and ^{131}I are most effective in detecting ectopic thyroid tissue or metastatic thyroid carcinoma, whereas technetium-99m pertechnetate produces superior imaging of thyroid gland nodules or tumors. Ultrasonography is useful to delineate whether a neck mass actually arises from the thyroid and whether multiple nodules are present.

Non-neoplastic Thyroid Conditions

Goiter and Thyroiditis

The causes of thyromegaly in one study are listed in Table 78-1.[4] Simple adolescent colloid goiter was the most common cause. Physiologically, diffuse thyroid enlargement may be due to a defect in hormone production, related to autoimmune diseases, or a response to an inflammatory condition. Goiters are classified as diffusely enlarged or nodular and either toxic or euthyroid. Most children with goiters are euthyroid, and surgical resection is rarely indicated.

The differential diagnosis for diffuse thyroid enlargement is seen in Table 78-2. Laboratory evaluation should begin with plasma free T_4 and TSH levels. With a simple colloid goiter, the patient is euthyroid. Ultrasonography or scintigraphy reveals uniform enlargement, and serum

Table 78-1 Etiology of Thyroid Gland Enlargement in 152 Children

Diagnosis	Frequency (%)
Simple goiter	83
Chronic lymphocytic thyroiditis	12.5
Graves' disease	2.5
Benign adenoma	1.5
Cyst	1

Adapted from Jaksic J, Dumic M, Filipovic B, et al: Thyroid disease in a school population with thyromegaly. Arch Dis Child 70:103-106, 1994.

thyroid antibody titers are normal. The etiology of this condition may be an autoimmune process.[5] The natural history of colloid goiter is not well known, but one study of adolescents found that 20 years after diagnosis nearly 60% of the glands were normal in size.[1] Exogenous thyroid hormone does not significantly enhance resolution of the goiter. In rare cases, resection may be indicated because of size or the suspicion of neoplasia.

Chronic lymphocytic (Hashimoto's) thyroiditis is another common cause of diffuse thyroid enlargement, occurring most frequently in female adolescents. This condition is part of the spectrum of autoimmune thyroid disorders. It is thought that CD4 T cells are activated against thyroid antigens and recruit cytotoxic CD8 T cells, which kill thyroid cells, leading to hypothyroidism.[6] Children are initially euthyroid and slowly progress to become hypothyroid. However, approximately 10% of children are hyperthyroid, a condition known as "hashitoxicosis." The thyroid gland is usually pebbly or granular and may be mildly tender.

Ninety-five percent of patients with Hashimoto's thyroiditis have elevated antithyroid microsomal antibodies or antithyroid peroxidase antibodies. Plasma thyroid hormone levels are normal or low, and TSH levels are elevated in 70% of patients. Thyroid imaging is usually not necessary if clinical and laboratory findings are strongly suggestive of the diagnosis. The radionuclide scan usually shows patchy uptake of the tracer and may

Table 78-2 Differential Diagnosis of Diffuse Thyroid Enlargement (Goiter) in Children

Autoimmune Mediated
Chronic lymphocytic (Hashimoto's) thyroiditis
Graves' disease
Simple colloid goiter
Compensatory
Iodine deficiency
Medications
Goitrogens
Hormone or receptor defect
Inflammatory Conditions
Acute suppurative thyroiditis
Subacute thyroiditis

mimic the findings in Graves' disease or multinodular goiter. The principal ultrasound finding is nonspecific, diffuse thyroid hypoechogenicity. Rarely, autoantibodies cannot be detected and fine-needle aspiration is needed to confirm the diagnosis. In as many as one third of adolescent patients, the thyroiditis resolves spontaneously with the gland becoming normal and the antibodies disappearing. Thus, expectant management should be considered. Exogenous thyroid hormone should be administered in the hypothyroid patient. However, in euthyroid children, it is ineffective in reducing the size of the goiter.[7]

Subacute (de Quervain's) thyroiditis, a viral inflammation of the thyroid gland, is unusual in children. The thyroid is swollen, painful, and tender. Mild thyrotoxicosis results from injury to the thyroid follicles, with release of thyroid hormone into the circulation. Serum T_3 and T_4 levels are elevated, and TSH is decreased. Because of thyroid follicular cell dysfunction, decreased radioactive iodine uptake occurs, a finding that distinguishes subacute thyroiditis from Graves' disease. Histologically, granulomas and epithelioid cells may be seen. The treatment of subacute thyroiditis is symptomatic and generally consists of nonsteroidal anti-inflammatory agents or corticosteroids. The condition typically lasts 2 to 9 months, and complete recovery can be expected.

Acute suppurative thyroiditis is a bacterial infection of the gland. The gland is acutely inflamed, and the patient is septic. Patients are usually euthyroid. Staphylococci or mixed aerobic and anaerobic flora are common causal agents. A congenital pharyngeal sinus tract may predispose the patient to infection. Management consists of intravenous antibiotics. Abscess drainage may be necessary. The thyroid gland should be expected to recover completely.

Graves' Disease

Graves' disease, or diffuse toxic goiter, is the most common cause of hyperthyroidism in childhood. The condition is an autoimmune disease caused by the presence of immunoglobulins of the IgG class directed against components of the thyroid plasma membrane, possibly including the TSH receptor. These autoantibodies have several effects. They stimulate the thyroid follicles to increase iodide uptake and cyclic adenosine monophosphate production and induce the production and secretion of increased thyroid hormone.

TSH receptor antibodies are present in more than 95% of patients with active Graves' disease. The inciting event eliciting the antibody response against the TSH receptor is unknown. Reports have demonstrated that TSH-binding sites are present in a number of gram-positive and gram-negative bacteria. It is possible that infection may elicit the production of antibodies that react with the TSH receptor.[8] An infectious etiology for Graves' disease is further supported by scattered epidemiologic reports of disease clustering.[9] Graves' disease is seen in girls about five times more often than in boys, and the incidence steadily increases throughout childhood, peaking in the adolescent years. Congenital Graves' disease, resulting from the transplacental passage of maternal antibodies, occurs in about 1% of infants born to women with active Graves' disease. The onset may be delayed until 2 to 3 weeks after birth.

In most children, the onset of Graves' disease develops over several months. Initial symptoms include nervousness, emotional lability, and declining school performance. Later, weight loss becomes evident, as does sweating, palpitations, heat intolerance, and general malaise. A smooth, firm, nontender goiter is present in more than 95% of cases. A bruit may be heard on auscultation. Exophthalmos is unusual in children, but a conspicuous stare may be evident. Laboratory evaluation generally reveals elevated free T_4 and decreased TSH levels. Ten to 20 percent of patients will have elevation of T_3 only, a condition known as T_3 toxicosis. The diagnosis of Graves' disease is definitively established by the presence of these TSH receptor antibodies.

Although the basic pathogenesis of Graves' disease is understood, no generally successful methods are available to correct the immunologic defect. The treatment of Graves' disease is palliative and is designed to decrease the production and secretion of thyroid hormone. The natural course of untreated Graves' disease is unpredictable. In some patients, the thyrotoxicosis may be persistent but variable in severity. In others, it may be cyclic, with exacerbations of varying degree and duration.

Current treatment includes antithyroid medications, ablation with radioactive ^{131}I, and surgical resection.[10] In the United States, most pediatric endocrinologists initiate therapy with methimazole or propylthiouracil, which reduces thyroid hormone production by inhibiting follicle cell organification of iodide and the coupling of iodotyrosines. Propylthiouracil also inhibits peripheral conversion of T_4 to T_3 and may be the agent of choice if rapid alleviation of thyrotoxicosis is desired. Both agents may possess some immunosuppressive activity because usually a reduction in antithyroid antibodies occurs. In most cases, methimazole is preferred because of its increased potency, longer half-life, and associated improved compliance. The initial adolescent dose is 30 mg once daily, which is reduced if the patient is younger. When the patient becomes euthyroid, as determined by normal T_3 and T_4 levels, the daily dose of methimazole should be reduced to 10 mg. T_3 and T_4 levels must be monitored. The thyroid gland decreases in size in about one half of patients. Thyroid enlargement with therapy signals either an intensification of the disease or hypothyroidism from overtreatment.

Side effects of methimazole include nausea, minor skin reactions, urticaria, arthralgias, arthritis, and fevers. The most serious reaction is an idiosyncratic agranulocytosis, occurring in less than 1% of patients. This may occur at any time during the course of treatment or even during a second course of the drug. The most common symptom of agranulocytosis is pharyngitis with fever, for which the patient should be warned to seek medical attention. In most cases, the granulocyte count increases 2 to 3 weeks after stopping the drug, but rare fatal opportunistic infections have been reported. Treatment with parenteral antibiotics during the recovery period has been recommended.

When treating Graves' disease, the goal is to allow natural resolution of the underlying autoimmune process. In general, the disease remission rate is approximately 25% after 2 years of treatment, with a further 25% remission every 2 years.[11] The resolution rate is decreased if TSH-receptor antibodies persist during and after treatment. The addition of T_4 to methimazole has had variable results in reducing disease recurrence. However, the use of T_4 cannot be recommended in pediatric patients receiving antithyroid medications.

The thyroid gland must be ablated if resistance or severe reactions to the antithyroid medications occur. Both surgical resection and ablation with radioactive ^{131}I have complications. The advantages of ^{131}I therapy include its effectiveness, safety, ease of administration, and relatively low cost.[12] Even though the disease recurrence rate is low after ^{131}I treatment, patients have a 50% to 80% incidence of long-term hypothyroidism.[13] Despite studies demonstrating no increased risk of cancer relative to the general population, concerns remain over the possibility of teratogenic or carcinogenic effects of ^{131}I in children and adolescents.[12,14]

Either a subtotal or total thyroidectomy is indicated for patients who refuse radioiodine treatment, for those children whose thyroid gland is so large that airway symptoms develop, or for those in whom medical management fails (Fig. 78-1). Antithyroid medication

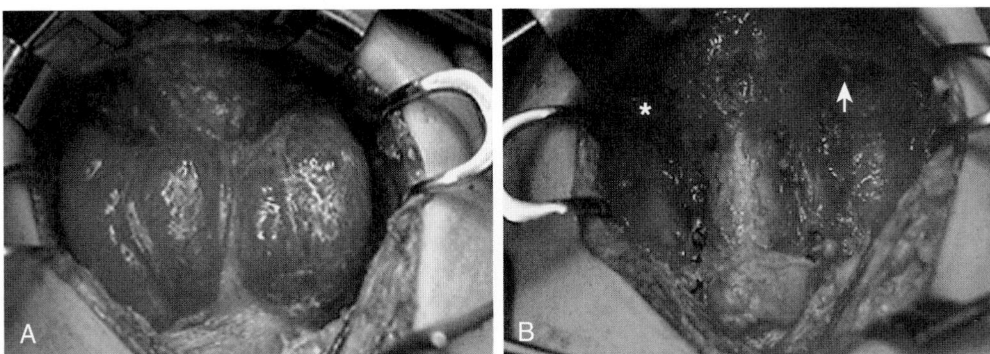

Figure 78-1. This teenage girl developed Graves' disease and her parents declined radioiodine treatment. **A,** The diffusely enlarged, hyperemic thyroid gland is visualized. **B,** The thyroid bed is seen after subtotal thyroidectomy. Each upper pole (*asterisk, arrow*) was left intact.

should be administered to decrease T_3 and T_4 levels into the normal range before operation. Alternatively, β-blocking agents, such as propranolol, may be used to ameliorate the adrenergic symptoms of hyperthyroidism. In addition, Lugol's solution, 5 to 10 drops per day, should be administered for 4 to 7 days before thyroidectomy to reduce the vascularity of the gland.

The incidence of hypothyroidism after subtotal thyroidectomy is 12% to 54%, and the hypothyroidism may be subclinical in up to 45% of children.[12] When abnormal TSH levels are considered, the incidence of hyperthyroidism or hypothyroidism is even higher. The rate of recurrent hyperthyroidism is approximately 13%. It is likely that the relapse rate increases with time after operation because approximately 30% of adult patients exhibit recurrent hyperthyroidism 25 years after their subtotal thyroidectomy.[10]

Hypothyroidism

Hypothyroidism may result from a defect anywhere in the hypothalamic-pituitary-thyroid axis and is rarely treated surgically. Approximately 90% of pediatric hypothyroidism is congenital, detected by neonatal screening programs, and results from dysgenesis of the thyroid gland. Two thirds of these infants have a rudimentary gland, and complete absence of thyroid tissue is noted in the rest of the patients. The rudimentary gland may be ectopic (e.g., the base of the tongue). Maternal thyroid hormone may prevent symptoms even in children with complete thyroid agenesis. Ectopic thyroid tissue may supply a sufficient amount of T_4 for years or may prove to be insufficient later in childhood.

Neoplastic Thyroid Conditions

Thyroid Nodules

Thyroid nodules are uncommon in children but have a relatively high likelihood of associated cancer. In children, the incidence of malignancy in thyroid nodules is about 20%.[15-17] This cancer rate is lower than has been reported in previous decades because fewer children today have been exposed to neck irradiation. Appropriate and prompt evaluation and management are important because the malignancy may be at an early curable stage. A summary of pathologic results from several large series of children who underwent operation for thyroid nodules is seen in Table 78-3. Other diagnostic possibilities for thyroid nodules include cystic hygroma, thyroglossal duct remnant, and germ cell tumor.

Girls have twice the incidence of thyroid nodules as boys.[18] Most patients are initially seen with an asymptomatic mass in the low anterior neck. It is impossible to differentiate benign from malignant lesions on clinical grounds, but a careful neck examination should be performed, especially to determine whether enlarged cervical lymph nodes are present. Thyroid imaging studies are unreliable in distinguishing benign from malignant nodules. However, if ultrasonography reveals multiple nodules, the diagnosis of thyroiditis becomes more likely. Because malignant nodules may be either solid or cystic, ultrasonography is not helpful in this regard. Similarly, thyroid scintiscan is not a reliable diagnostic modality because malignant nodules may be either functioning or nonfunctioning. A therapeutic trial of exogenous thyroid hormone to induce nodule regression is not recommended for children.

Table 78-3 Diagnosis in 251 Pediatric Patients Treated for Thyroid Nodules

No. Malignant	**42 (17%)**
Histologic subtype	
Papillary	29
Follicular	6
Mixed	2
Anaplastic	2
Medullary	2
Lymphoma	1
No. Benign	**209 (83%)**
Diagnosis	
Follicular adenoma	101
Thyroiditis	27
Thyroglossal cyst	5
Colloid nodule	59
Branchial cyst	12

Data from Desjardins JG, Khan AH, Montupet P, et al: Management of thyroid nodules in children: A 20-year experience. J Pediatr Surg 22:736-739, 1987; Hung W, Anderson KD, Chandra RS, et al: Solitary thyroid nodules in 71 children and adolescents. J Pediatr Surg 27:1407-1409, 1992; and Yip FWK, Reeve TS, Poole AG, et al: Thyroid nodules in childhood and adolescence. Aust N Z J Surg 64:676-678, 1994.

The usefulness of fine-needle aspiration cytology in children has not been well defined. Pediatric surgeons have historically recommended the removal of thyroid nodules. Few large studies have defined the natural history of cytologically benign nodules in children. In one study of 57 children with thyroid nodules evaluated with aspiration, the incidence of malignancy was 18%.[19] If these benign nodules could be accurately diagnosed without surgical removal, significant potential savings may occur in operative morbidity and cost.

Because the adolescent spectrum of thyroid disease is similar to that of adults, fine-needle aspiration may be acceptable in evaluating thyroid nodules in this population. The incidence of malignancy in thyroid nodules in patients age 13 to 18 years is approximately 11%.[18] Benign nodules in adolescent patients can be followed up with serial physical examinations and ultrasound studies. Exogenous thyroid hormone to suppress benign thyroid nodules has not been shown to alter their natural history.

Surgical resection should be performed if the nodule is malignant or has indeterminate cytology or if the size of a benign nodule increases. If a cystic thyroid lesion disappears after aspiration, surgical treatment may be deferred. If the lesion recurs, it should be removed. Even though cyst fluid can be sent for cytologic analysis, the sensitivity of this test for determining the presence of cancer in children is unknown.[20]

Thyroid nodules in prepubertal children have a higher risk of malignancy. The natural history of benign lesions in younger children is unknown, and the safety of nonoperative treatment has not been demonstrated. Based on these data, the current recommendation for management of all thyroid nodules in children younger than age 13 is surgical resection. Preoperative ultrasonography and thyroid scintigraphy aid in determining the anatomy.[16,21]

Thyroid Carcinoma

Thyroid carcinoma represents about 3% of all pediatric malignancies in the United States. The peak incidence is between ages 10 and 18 years, and it occurs more often in girls in a ratio of 2:1. Approximately 10% of all malignant thyroid tumors occur in children. In comparison to adults, pediatric patients with thyroid carcinoma present with more advanced-stage disease and with a higher incidence of lymph node and pulmonary metastases but with lower mortality.[22]

The incidence of childhood thyroid malignancy has decreased in most parts of the world since the mid 1970s owing to the reduced use of radiation to treat benign diseases. A marked increase of thyroid tumors was noted in the Republics of Belarus and Ukraine after the 1986 Chernobyl nuclear power plant catastrophe.[23] The latency period for developing thyroid cancer after radiation exposure is 4 to 6 years. In Belarus, a 62-fold increase in thyroid tumors was noted after the Chernobyl accident.

Treatment of a previous malignancy is another significant risk factor for thyroid carcinoma. Thyroid cancers constitute about 9% of second malignancies.[24] Hodgkin's lymphoma is the most common malignancy associated with a subsequent thyroid cancer. Whereas most thyroid second neoplasms follow previous radiation exposure to the neck, alkylating agents alone also predispose to thyroid cancer. The mean age at diagnosis of thyroid second neoplasms is 20 years, demonstrating the importance of careful surveillance for second tumors in children who have been successfully treated for cancer.

The diagnosis of thyroid carcinoma is impossible to determine based on clinical grounds alone. In adults, fine-needle aspiration cytology has been used as the initial evaluation of a thyroid nodule. Its use in children has not been thoroughly explored because most surgeons recommend surgical resection of all thyroid lesions because of the concern for false-negative interpretations.

Various molecular biologic events may account for the disparity in behavior of the different histologic subtypes of thyroid cancer. *RAS* proto-oncogene mutations are found in about 20% of papillary tumors and 80% of follicular tumors.[25] Other studies have reported that *RAS* is frequently activated in benign follicular adenomas, suggesting that this genetic event occurs early in the transformation process.[26] An activating mutation of the *RET* proto-oncogene is found in about 35% of papillary thyroid cancers.[27] The RET protein is a receptor tyrosine-kinase molecule, which probably functions within the cell to regulate proliferation or differentiation. This protein has been shown to be responsible for the development of medullary thyroid carcinoma (MTC). Specific point mutations are associated with the multiple endocrine neoplasia type 2 (MEN 2A, MEN 2B) syndromes and familial MTC (FMTC). In addition, as many as 40% of patients with sporadic nonfamilial MTCs possess *RET* mutations.[28]

Thyroid carcinoma usually presents clinically as a thyroid mass, sometimes with enlarged cervical lymph nodes. Regional lymph node metastases are present in three of four children when the disease is first detected (Table 78-4). The pathologic diagnosis can be established by using either fine-needle aspiration cytology or frozen section biopsy at operation. The functional status of the mass can be determined by preoperative scintiscan. Ultrasonography may be helpful in planning the operation.[21] Because pulmonary metastases are frequent, a preoperative chest radiograph should be obtained.

No clinical trial has established whether total thyroidectomy, with lymph node dissection if the regional nodes are involved, is better than subtotal thyroidectomy.[29-31] Radioiodine ablative therapy is more effective after removal of the entire gland because less functioning thyroid tissue takes up the radionuclide. Surgeons preferring a lesser resection believe that differentiated thyroid carcinoma in children is an indolent disease and that survival is not clearly related to the extent of gland removal.[32,33] Although these complications occur less commonly in recent reports, the historical incidence of recurrent laryngeal nerve injury ranges from zero to 24%, whereas permanent hypocalcemia occurs in 6% to 27% of patients undergoing total thyroidectomy.[32,34]

In one retrospective review, multivariate analysis revealed that younger age at diagnosis and the histologic type of tumor were the only factors predictive of early disease recurrence.[32] Children with follicular histology and older than 12 years at diagnosis were more likely to be cured at the initial procedure. Thus, tumor factors may be more important than treatment factors in determining the outcome.

Lobectomy with isthmus resection may be sufficient for tumors clearly isolated to one lobe. However, thyroid cancer is bilateral in up to 66% of cases. Also, about 80% of tumors exhibit multifocality. Therefore, most pediatric surgeons believe that more aggressive thyroid gland resections are indicated and recommend that either a total or near-total thyroidectomy be performed for the management of differentiated thyroid cancer.[35,36]

The recurrent laryngeal nerve should be identified and protected. When tumor invades the recurrent laryngeal nerve, the nerve can be safely preserved without compromising survival through adjuvant therapy with ^{131}I irradiation to successfully eradicate residual tumor.[37] The most reliable way to preserve parathyroid gland function is to identify and preserve the glands at the time of thyroidectomy (Fig. 78-2). If there is apparent devascularization, then one should autotransplant one or two of the glands into the sternocleidomastoid

Table 78-4 Clinical Aspects of Differentiated Thyroid Cancer in Children from Six Large Pediatric Series

	Clinical Series					
	A	*B*	*C*	*D*	*E*	*F*
Total No. of Patients	89	59	58	100	49	72
Mean Age (yr)	12.8	NA	11.9	13.3	14.0	11
Girls (%)	81	66	69	71	69	71
Histology (No.)						
Papillary	83	37	58	87	44	50
Follicular	6	19	0	7	4	21
Medullary	0	1	0	0	1	0
Other	0	2	0	6	0	0
Metastasis (%)	88	50	90	71	73	75
Median Follow-up (yr)	NA	11	28	20	7.7	13
Cancer Mortality (%)	2.2	3.4	3.4	0	2.0	17

NA, data not available.

Data from: *A,* Harness JA, Thompson NW, McLeod MK, et al: Differentiated thyroid carcinoma in children and adolescents. World J Surg 16:547-554, 1992; *B,* Samuel AM, Sharma SM: Differentiated thyroid carcinomas in children and adolescents. Cancer 67:2186-2190, 1991; *C,* Zimmerman D, Hay ID, Gough IR, et al: Papillary thyroid carcinoma in children and adults: Long-term follow-up of 1039 patients conservatively treated at one institution during three decades. Surgery 104:1157-1163, 1988; *D,* La Quaglia MP, Corbally MT, Heller G, et al: Recurrence and morbidity in differentiated thyroid carcinoma in children. Surgery 104:1149-1156, 1988; *E,* Ceccarelli C, Pacini F, Lippi F, et al: Thyroid cancer in children and adolescents. Surgery 104:1143-1148, 1988; *F,* Schlumberger M, De Vathaire F, Travagli JP, et al: Differentiated thyroid carcinoma in childhood: Long-term follow-up in 72 patients. J Clin Endocrinol Metab 65:1088-1094, 1987.

muscle or into the nondominant forearm.[38,39] If there is regional nodal metastasis, a node dissection is recommended. In patients with locally advanced disease, it is imperative to remove as much of the thyroid gland as possible to allow subsequent radioiodine scanning and treatment if the tumor recurs. Finally, after surgical resection, most investigators recommend that all patients be treated with exogenous thyroid hormone to suppress TSH-mediated stimulation of the gland.

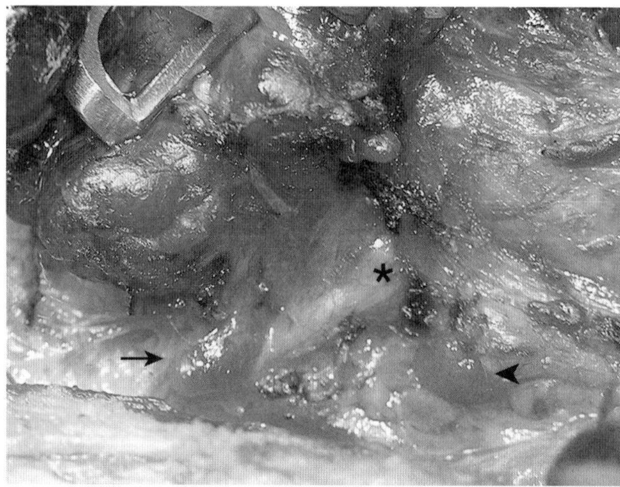

Figure 78-2. The relationship of the parathyroid glands to the recurrent laryngeal nerve during prophylactic thyroidectomy for multiple endocrine neoplasia type 2 is seen. The left recurrent laryngeal nerve is marked by an *asterisk.* The superior parathyroid gland (*arrowhead*) is typically located posterior to the nerve. The inferior parathyroid gland (*arrow*) is usually found anterior to the nerve.

The incidence of pulmonary metastases at diagnosis in childhood is about 6%, but they rarely occur in the absence of significant cervical lymph node metastases.[33,40] Pulmonary metastases require treatment with radioiodine. Plain chest films demonstrate the pulmonary disease in only 60% of cases, making scanning with radioiodine necessary. The pulmonary scintiscan may be falsely negative if significant residual thyroid gland remains in the neck.[40]

Overall survival in nonmedullary thyroid carcinoma is 98%.[22] A higher rate of recurrence has been seen in children who did not receive postoperative ^{131}I than in those who did.[22] The time to first recurrence has ranged from 8 months to 14.8 years (mean, 5.3 years), thereby emphasizing the importance of long-term follow-up for these children. Prognostic factors associated with recurrence include capsular or soft tissue invasion, positive margins, and tumor location at diagnosis (thyroid, lymph nodes, lung).[22] A whole-body ^{131}I scan should be performed approximately 6 weeks after the initial thyroid resection and followed by therapeutic doses of the radionuclide administered as necessary to ablate residual tissue and treat residual metastatic disease. Radioactive ablation has been shown to decrease the risk of local recurrence, increase the sensitivity of subsequent diagnostic whole-body scans, and improve the utility of serum thyroglobulin as a marker for recurrent or residual disease during long-term follow-up.[35]

Thyroglobulin has been shown to be a useful marker of residual or metastatic thyroid cancer. The plasma level of this protein should be measured yearly, and an elevated value should raise the suspicion of recurrent disease.[41] The diagnostic accuracy of this test is significantly decreased in children who have residual thyroid tissue or in those who are taking thyroid hormone supplementation.

MTC accounts for approximately 5% of thyroid neoplasms in children. Arising from the parafollicular C cells, MTC may occur either sporadically or in association with MEN 2A, MEN 2B, or the FMTC syndrome. MTC is usually the first tumor to develop in MEN patients and is the most common cause of death in this group. The neoplasm is particularly virulent in patients with MEN 2B and may occur in infancy.[42]

As with other pediatric thyroid neoplasms, the clinical diagnosis of MTC not associated with a known familial or MEN syndrome is usually made only after metastatic spread of the tumor has occurred to the adjacent cervical lymph nodes or to distant sites.[43] Surgical resection is the only effective treatment for MTC, underscoring the importance of early diagnosis and therapy before metastasis occurs. For this reason, current management of MTC in children from MEN 2 and FMTC kindreds relies on the presymptomatic detection of the *RET* proto-oncogene mutation responsible for the disease. Prophylactic thyroidectomy in young asymptomatic children carrying a mutated allele of the *RET* proto-oncogene in MEN 2A kindreds has been demonstrated to prevent or cure MTC. In a study of 50 children and teenagers with the *RET* proto-oncogene mutation who underwent prophylactic thyroidectomy, 66% already had foci of MTC within the thyroid gland.[44] However, no child younger than 8 years of age was found to have metastatic disease at time of surgery. Moreover, when followed for 5 to 8 years, none had evidence of persistent or recurrent disease when screened by physical examination and plasma calcitonin levels obtained after calcium and pentagastrin stimulation. Based on this information, affected children with MEN 2A should undergo total thyroidectomy at approximately age 5 years.[45-47] Because of the increased virulence of MTC in children with MEN 2B, prophylactic thyroidectomy should be performed at approximately age 1 year. Complete removal of the thyroid gland is the recommended surgical management of MTC in children because of the high incidence of bilateral disease.[48] Central lymph node dissection (i.e., removal of lymph nodes medial to the carotid sheaths and between the hyoid bone and the sternum) is likely not necessary except in older children or when gross lymphadenopathy is discovered at the time of prophylactic thyroidectomy. Early detection by DNA mutation analysis and early operative intervention result in a normal life expectancy in these children.[49]

PARATHYROID GLANDS

Embryology and Physiology

Parathyroid gland development begins about week 5 of gestation when the epithelium in the dorsal portions of the third and fourth pharyngeal pouches begins to proliferate. During week 6 of development, the inferior parathyroid glands, associated with the third pair of pharyngeal pouches, migrate caudad with the thymic primordium and come to rest on the dorsal surface of the thyroid gland low in the neck. The superior parathyroid glands arise from the fourth pharyngeal pouches and come to rest cephalad to the other glands. Mobilization of calcium from the bones is directly stimulated by parathormone (PTH), a process that also requires vitamin D.

Hyperparathyroidism

PTH is secreted as an 84–amino acid protein, which is rapidly cleaved in the liver and kidney into the carboxyl-terminal, amino-terminal, and mid-region fragments. The biologic activity of PTH resides in the amino-terminal segment, but the plasma level of this moiety is low, owing to its very short half-life in the circulation. The carboxyl-terminal fragment levels are 50- to 500-fold those of the amino-terminal fragment. Most clinical assays of PTH measure the carboxyl-terminal levels of the hormone. These assays are usually effective for the evaluation of hyperparathyroidism, but plasma levels of the carboxyl-terminal fragment may be selectively elevated if there is a component of renal failure. The laboratory hallmark of hyperparathyroidism is the finding of an inappropriately elevated plasma PTH level with hypercalcemia.

The differential diagnosis of hypercalcemia in childhood is shown in Table 78-5. Unlike hypercalcemia in adults, hypercalcemia in children is rarely related to a neoplasm. However, in rare cases, pediatric tumors may secrete a parathyroid-related polypeptide that elevates the calcium level. Reported neoplasms include malignant rhabdoid tumor, mesoblastic nephroma, rhabdomyosarcoma, neuroblastoma, and lymphoma. In these patients, the PTH level is generally normal or decreased.

Primary Hyperparathyroidism

Primary hyperparathyroidism in childhood usually results from a solitary hyperfunctioning adenoma and more rarely from diffuse hyperplasia of all four glands.[50] Hyperparathyroidism resulting from hyperplasia in all

Table 78-5 Differential Diagnosis of Hypercalcemia in Childhood

Elevated parathyroid hormone level
Primary hyperparathyroidism
Secondary hyperparathyroidism
Ectopic parathyroid hormone production
Hypervitaminosis D
Sarcoidosis
Subcutaneous fat necrosis
Familial hypocalciuric hypercalcemia
Idiopathic hypercalcemia of infancy
Thyrotoxicosis
Hypervitaminosis A
Hypophosphatasia
Prolonged immobilization
Thiazide diuretics

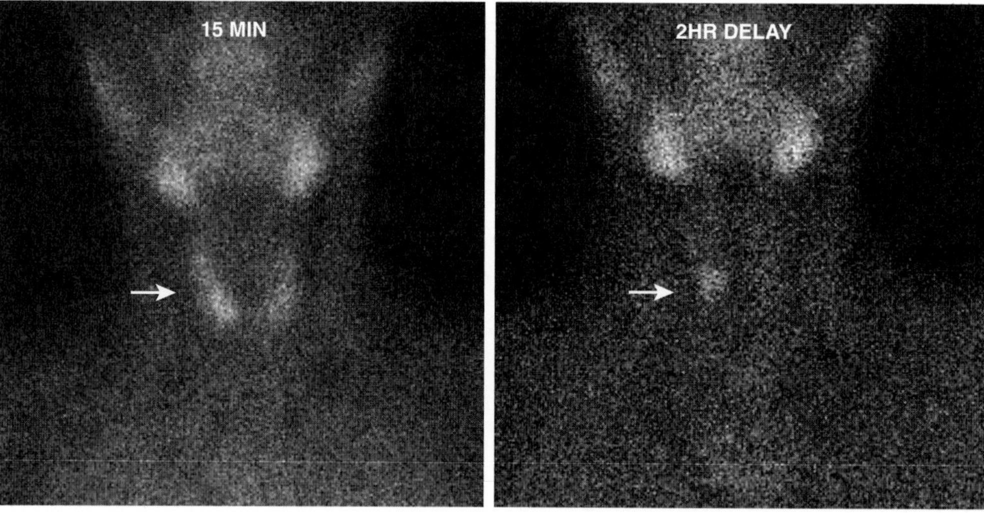

Figure 78-3. Early and delayed ^{99m}Tc-sestamibi scintigraphy in a 12-year-old boy with primary hyperparathyroidism. **A,** The image at 15 minutes demonstrates rapid uptake of the radioisotope by the thyroid gland (*arrow*). **B,** The image at 2 hours reveals that the radioisotope has been washed out of the thyroid, but a focus persists (*arrow*) that is consistent with a right parathyroid adenoma.

four glands is a feature of MEN 1. Hyperparathyroidism develops in approximately 30% of patients having MEN 2A in their second or third decade of life.[51] At the time of prophylactic thyroidectomy for MEN 2, the parathyroid glands can be identified and autotransplanted into the nondominant forearm.[38] If hyperparathyroidism develops, a portion of the heterotopic tissue may easily be removed from the forearm.

Surgical options for parathyroid gland hyperplasia involving all of the glands include either 3½ gland parathyroidectomy or total parathyroidectomy with heterotopic autotransplantation of some parathyroid tissue back into the nondominant forearm.[52] The latter approach has been shown to be safe in infants and children and has the advantage of avoiding repeated neck exploration if hyperparathyroidism should recur.[38,47] Moreover, total parathyroidectomy with heterotopic autotransplantation results in improved survival rate in infants with severe hypercalcemia.[52] Patients with total parathyroidectomy and autotransplantation require a short period of vitamin D and calcium supplementation until the heterotopic tissue begins to function.[38]

Primary hyperparathyroidism of infancy is a rare, often fatal, condition that usually develops within the first 3 months of life.[52,53] Signs include hypotonicity, respiratory distress, failure to thrive, lethargy, and polyuria. The serum PTH level always is elevated, and histologic diffuse parathyroid gland hyperplasia occurs. In about half of the cases, a familial component to the disease is found. Early recognition and treatment are essential to allow normal growth and development of the infant.

The management of primary hyperparathyroidism in children is surgical. Neck exploration with evaluation of all four parathyroid glands is the standard parathyroidectomy operation and should be employed when parathyroid gland hyperplasia or MEN is suspected. However, because a solitary hyperfunctioning adenoma accounts for the majority of primary hyperparathyroidism, less invasive parathyroidectomy procedures have gained popularity. These operations are safe and effective alternatives to traditional bilateral neck exploration when preoperative studies demonstrate a single abnormal gland.[54] Unilateral neck exploration with focused evaluation and excision relies on accurate preoperative localization studies and rapid intraoperative PTH (IO-PTH) assays to confirm that the offending gland or glands have been excised. ^{99m}Tc-sestamibi is avidly taken up by parathyroid tissue, especially adenomas (Fig. 78-3).[55] The sensitivity of detecting abnormal parathyroid glands by sestamibi scan alone is 87%; however, when in conjunction with ultrasonography sensitivity reaches 96% in detecting a parathyroid adenoma.[56,57] Unilateral neck exploration is guided by the localizing studies (Fig. 78-4). A baseline serum PTH level is obtained, followed by PTH levels drawn at 5 and 10 minutes after the presumptive abnormal parathyroid gland has been

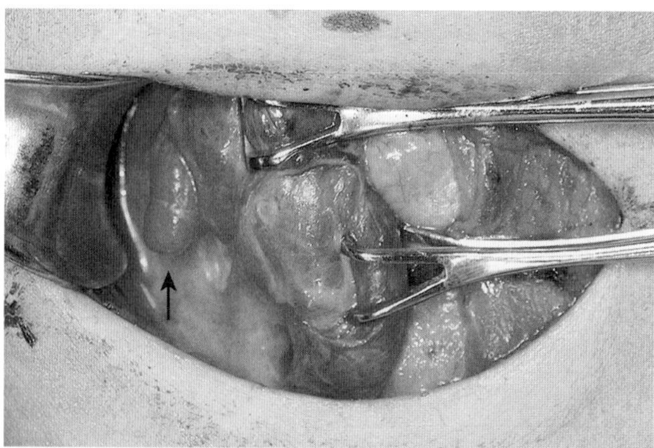

Figure 78-4. This intraoperative photograph demonstrates an enlarged right superior parathyroid adenoma (*arrow*) during unilateral neck exploration that was directed by preoperative localizing studies.

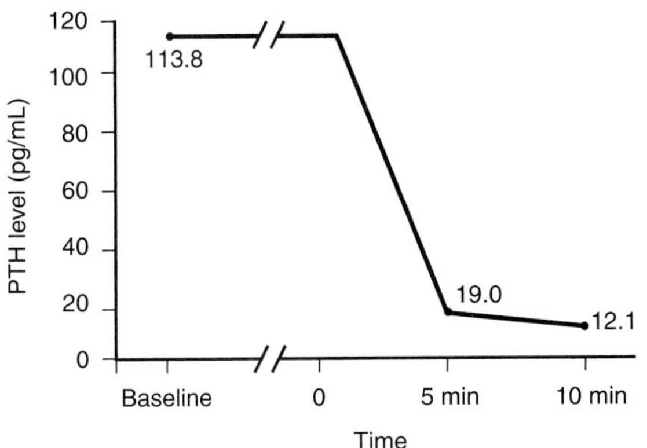

Figure 78-5. A rapid intraoperative parathyroid hormone (IO-PTH) assay during unilateral focused parathyroidectomy is depicted. Baseline plasma PTH levels have been drawn. Time 0 represents the moment of resection of the hypersecreting parathyroid gland. PTH levels are drawn at 5 and 10 minutes. A 50% decline in PTH level from baseline at 10 minutes indicates that the offending parathyroid gland or glands have been removed.

excised. Because intact PTH half-life is only a few minutes, a greater than 50% drop in IO-PTH level within 10 minutes signifies successful removal of the hyperfunctioning parathyroid tissue (Fig. 78-5).[58]

Familial Hypocalciuric Hypercalcemia

Familial hypocalciuric hypercalcemia differs from primary hypoparathyroidism in that the PTH value is normal but urinary excretion of calcium is low. Patients are usually asymptomatic with an elevated serum calcium level. The serum magnesium level also may be elevated.

The disease is inherited as an autosomal dominant disorder caused by a heterozygous mutation in the Ca^{2+}-sensing receptor gene.[59] The parathyroid glands are normal, and usually there is no benefit to parathyroidectomy. If both parents are carriers, the neonate may have severe hypercalcemia. These infants have inherited mutations in both copies of the Ca^{2+}-sensing receptor gene and often have hyperplasia of all of their parathyroid glands. These infants do benefit from parathyroidectomy with transplantation of one gland.

Secondary Hyperparathyroidism

Secondary hyperparathyroidism occurs in children with renal insufficiency or malabsorption. PTH production is increased in response to decreased calcium levels. Affected patients typically respond to medical treatment designed to decrease intestinal phosphorus absorption. In rare cases, severe renal osteodystrophy develops, manifested by skeletal fractures and metastatic calcifications. Especially severe cases of secondary hyperparathyroidism may be candidates for total parathyroidectomy with autotransplantation.[50]

Tertiary Hyperparathyroidism

Tertiary hyperparathyroidism occurs when persistent hyperfunction of the parathyroid glands occurs, even after the inciting stimulus has been removed. This is often seen in patients with chronic renal failure and secondary hyperparathyroidism who undergo renal transplantation. Tertiary hyperparathyroidism is commonly due to hyperplasia of all four glands. Children with this condition are candidates for total parathyroidectomy with autotransplantation.

ADRENAL GLANDS

Anatomy and Embryology

The primordial adrenal cortex arises from the coelomic mesoderm and becomes visible between weeks 4 and 6 of development. During development, the fetal adrenal gland contains the permanent cortex, fetal cortex, and medulla. The fetal cortex, whose function is unknown, is responsible for the large size of the fetal adrenal gland, with the fetal adrenal gland being four times the size of the fetal kidney at the fourth month of gestation. The fetal cortex begins to decrease in size within a few hours of birth and disappears by the first year of life. The cells of the permanent cortex are arranged into three separate zones: the zona glomerulosa, zona fasciculata, and zona reticularis. The zona glomerulosa gives rise to the narrowed zona fasciculata and reticularis of the adult cortex. The zona reticularis does not reach adult form until late childhood.[60]

The adrenal glands weigh 1 g at birth and grow to 4 to 5 g by late childhood. The mature adrenal gland measures 3 to 5 cm in length and 4 to 6 mm in thickness. The adrenal glands have a profuse arterial supply. One or more middle adrenal arteries arise from the aorta, six to eight superior adrenal arteries from the inferior phrenic artery, and one or more inferior adrenal arteries from the renal artery. The adrenal gland is drained by a single large adrenal vein. The right adrenal vein drains into the inferior vena cava and the left adrenal vein drains into the left renal vein.

The adrenal gland can be found in several anomalous locations. In adrenal heterotopia, the adrenal gland is situated in the normal location but lies under the capsule of the kidney (adrenal-renal heterotopia) or capsule of the liver (adrenal-hepatic heterotopia). Extra-adrenal tissue may be found anywhere in the abdominal cavity but usually is found along the anatomic derivatives of the urogenital ridge for the adrenal cortex and along the dorsal root ganglia for the medullary tissue. Accessory adrenal glands usually occur without a medullary subcomponent and have been found in 16% of 100 consecutive autopsies.[61] Another 16% had complete accessory glands.

Physiology

The adrenal cortex produces three major hormones: aldosterone, cortisol, and androgens. The zona glomerulosa is exclusively responsible for the production of aldosterone because it lacks the enzyme 17α-hydroxylase, which is necessary to produce the precursors to cortisol and androgens. The zona fasciculata and zona reticularis together produce cortisol, androgens, and small amounts of estrogens. These areas lack the enzymes necessary to produce the precursors to aldosterone.

Aldosterone

Aldosterone regulates extracellular fluid volume as well as sodium and potassium balance. Aldosterone concentrations are regulated by the renin-angiotensin system. Renin is secreted by the juxtaglomerular cells in response to decreased pressure in the renal afferent arterioles and by decreased plasma concentration that is detected by the macula densa. Renin converts angiotensinogen into angiotensin I, which is then converted to angiotensin II by the angiotensin converting enzyme in the lung. Angiotensin II is a potent vasoconstrictor and also directly stimulates the zona glomerulosa to release aldosterone. Aldosterone stimulates renal tubular reabsorption of sodium in exchange for potassium and hydrogen, thereby increasing renal fluid resorption and expanding intravascular volume.

Cortisol

The regulation of cortisol is controlled through the cortisol-releasing factor (CRF) from the hypothalamus and subsequent stimulation of pituitary adrenocorticotropic hormone (ACTH). The neuroendocrine control of cortisol results in a peak in cortisol level in the early morning and a nadir in the late evening. The metabolic effects of cortisol include stimulation of hepatic gluconeogenesis, inhibition of protein synthesis, increased protein catabolism, and lipolysis of adipose tissue. Cortisol also causes a loss of collagen, inhibition of wound healing through decreased fibroblast activity, and induction of a negative calcium balance, leading to osteoporosis.

Androgens

The adrenal androgens include dehydroepiandrosterone (DHEA) and DHEA sulfate (DHEA-S). These hormones undergo peripheral conversion to the biologically active forms testosterone and dihydrotestosterone. In the normal male, adrenal androgens account for less than 5% of the circulating testosterone. The adrenal androgens become most clinically relevant with congenital adrenal hyperplasia (CAH), a group of autosomal recessive enzyme deficiencies resulting in an accumulation of steroid precursors shuttled away from the synthesis of cortisol and/or aldosterone and into the pathway of androgens. Deficiency in the enzyme 21-hydroxylase accounts for over 90% of CAH.

Adrenal Masses

The differential diagnosis of adrenal masses is listed in Table 78-6. Neuroblastoma accounts for more than 90% of adrenal masses. Adrenal masses are being detected at a greater rate than previously described for children because of the increased use of diagnostic testing for other clinical conditions that are unrelated to adrenal disease. The significance of such adrenal masses seen by computed tomography (CT) is unknown in children. At autopsy, adrenal masses are detected in less than 1% of patients younger than age 30 years.[62] This incidence increases to 7% in patients older than 70 years. Follow-up of patients with nonfunctioning adrenal masses demonstrates that 5% to 25% increase in size by at least 1 cm, and the risk of malignancy is 1 in 1000. Patients who have an incidentally discovered adrenal mass should undergo hormone evaluation, including a 1-mg dexamethasone suppression test, aldosterone levels, and measurement of plasma free metanephrines.[62] Surgical treatment is indicated for all functional adrenal cortical tumors and pheochromocytoma. In children, most surgeons will resect these tumors regardless of size (Fig. 78-6). However, no clear evidence supports this management over conservative therapy, especially in lesions smaller than 3 cm.

Table 78-6 Differential Diagnosis of an Adrenal Mass

Functional Tumors
Adrenal adenoma
Adrenocortical carcinoma
Pheochromocytoma
Nonfunctional Tumors
Neuroblastoma
Adrenal cyst
Hemangioma
Leiomyoma
Leiomyosarcoma
Non-Hodgkin's lymphoma
Malignant melanoma
Metastatic Disease to the Adrenal Gland
Squamous cell carcinoma of the lung
Hepatocellular carcinoma
Breast cancer
Traumatic Adrenal Hemorrhage
Neonatal child abuse

Adrenal Cortex

Hypercortisolism (Cushing's Syndrome)

Hypercortisolism, or Cushing's syndrome, describes any form of glucocorticoid excess that can be caused by pituitary adenomas secreting ACTH, adrenal tumors including carcinoma and adenoma, ectopic ACTH syndrome, nodular adrenal hyperplasia, and ACTH-producing tumors (Table 78-7). Additionally, the administration of supraphysiologic quantities of ACTH or glucocorticoids can lead to iatrogenic Cushing's syndrome, the most common cause of hypercortisolism in adults and children. Cushing's disease is caused by a pituitary microadenoma or, more rarely, by a macroadenoma. It is the

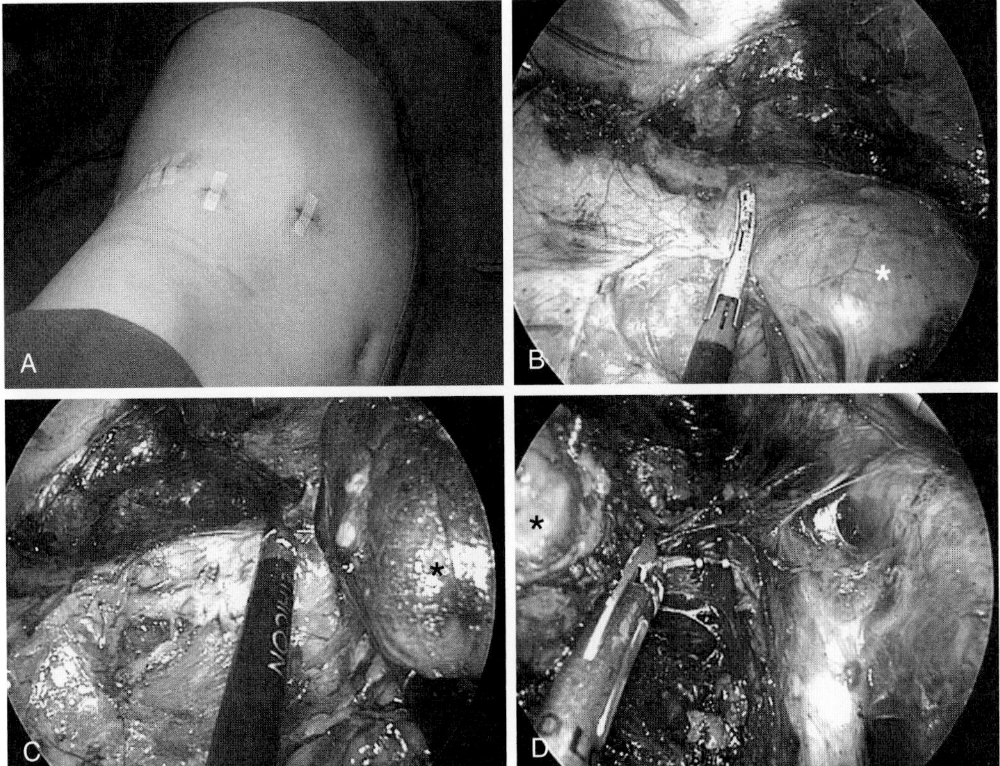

Figure 78-6. This teenager was found to have a right adrenal mass measuring 4.5 cm in greatest dimension. Preoperative evaluation did not reveal evidence of a functioning tumor. **A,** She was placed in the left lateral decubitus position for the laparoscopic right adrenalectomy. The incisions utilized for the operation are seen. **B,** The harmonic scalpel is being used to free the tumor (*asterisk*) from the lateral surrounding tissue. **C,** The tumor (*asterisk*) has been almost completely mobilized and the cephalad attachments are being lysed with the harmonic scalpel. **D,** The tumor (*asterisk*) is being retracted laterally, and the right adrenal vein is being clipped with endoscopic clips. This tumor was excised uneventfully and was found to be a nonfunctioning adrenal adenoma. The patient was discharged on her first postoperative day.

second most common cause of Cushing's syndrome in pediatric patients. Ectopic ACTH syndrome is rare in children but has been reported in infants younger than 1 year. Tumors that can produce ACTH include pulmonary neoplasms, neuroblastomas, pancreatic islet cell carcinomas, thymomas, carcinoids, MTCs, and pheochromocytomas. In children, the most frequent cause of ectopic ACTH is a bronchial carcinoid. ACTH levels are usually 10 to 100 times higher than those seen in Cushing's disease. These markedly elevated levels of ACTH lead to hypokalemic alkalosis. Additionally, ACTH-independent multinodular adrenal hyperplasia is characterized by hypersecretion of both cortisol and adrenal androgens.

Hypercortisolism is more common in children than previously recognized. In Harvey Cushing's original description,[63] the patient was a 23-year-old woman whose clinical features indicated long-standing disease. In infants and children younger than 7 years, the most common cause of Cushing's syndrome is an adrenal tumor. Among 60 infants younger than 1 year, 48 had adrenal tumors, with a 4:1 ratio between girls and boys (Fig. 78-7).[64] In adults and children older than 7 years, adrenal hyperplasia secondary to hypersecretion of pituitary ACTH predominates.

Clinical features of Cushing's syndrome can take 5 years or longer to develop. Thus, the classic cushingoid appearance may not be seen in children. The most frequent and reliable findings in children with Cushing's syndrome are weight gain and growth failure.[65] Specifically, any obese child who stops growing should be evaluated for Cushing's syndrome.

Table 78-7 Etiology of Cushing's Syndrome: Exogenous Corticosteroid Administration

ACTH-Dependent Causes
Cushing's disease (pituitary adenoma)
Ectopic ACTH production
Small cell bronchogenic carcinoma
Carcinoid tumors
Pancreatic islet cell carcinoma
Thymoma
Medullary thyroid carcinoma
Pheochromocytoma
ACTH-Independent Causes
Adrenal adenoma
Adrenocortical carcinoma
Adrenal hyperplasia

ACTH, adrenocorticotropic hormone

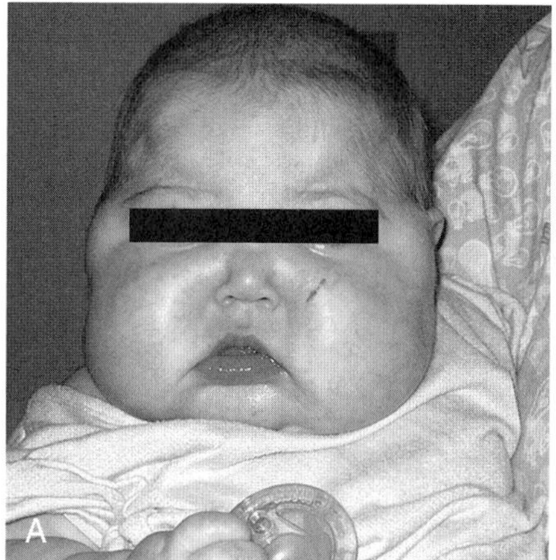

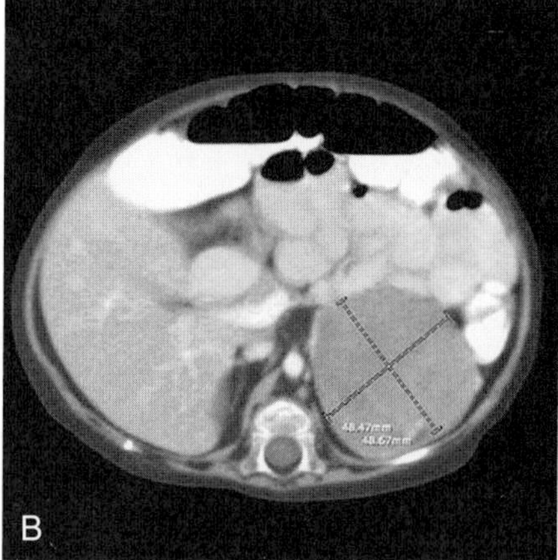

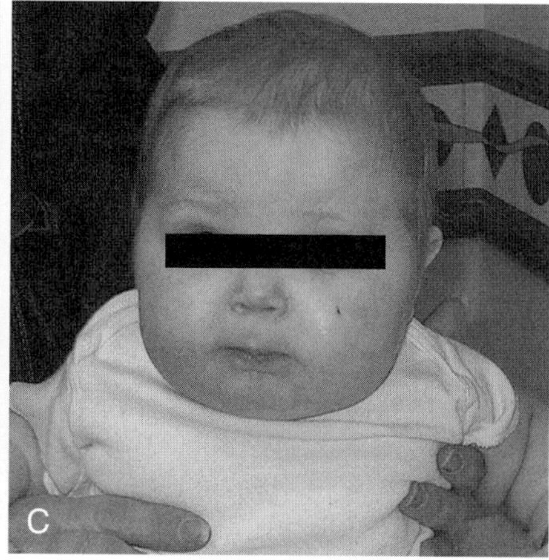

Figure 78-7. This 8-month-old was seen in the emergency department for progressive facial swelling. **A,** Examination reveals cushingoid features with moon facies. In addition, she had generalized obesity. Her plasma cortisol level was elevated and her ACTH level was suppressed. **B,** CT scan revealed a 4.3 × 4.8 × 4.8-cm left adrenal mass that was homogeneous and showed no evidence of invasion of adjacent structures. The infant subsequently underwent laparoscopic left adrenalectomy and was discharged on postoperative day 2. **C,** At 2-month follow-up, there is marked improvement in the physical manifestations of her Cushing's syndrome. (From Kim E, Aguayo P, St. Peter SD, et al: Adrenocortical adenoma expressing glucocorticoid in an 8-month-old female. Eur J Pediatr Surg 18:1-2, 2008. Reprinted with permission.)

The initial phase in the diagnosis of Cushing's syndrome is to screen for the syndrome. Next, it is necessary to determine its etiology. Screening for Cushing's syndrome can be accomplished by measuring the plasma cortisol at 8:00 AM (normal levels, <14 mg/dL) and 6:00 PM (normal levels, <8 mg/dL) to coincide with the diurnal variation in plasma cortisol. The loss of diurnal rhythm is usually the earliest reliable laboratory index of Cushing's disease. A single measurement at midnight should be less than 2 mg/dL in normal patients and more than 2 mg/dL in Cushing's disease.[66] The most sensitive screening test is the 24-hour urinary 17-hydroxycorticosteroid or free cortisol value, which is more than 150 mg/day in patients with Cushing's syndrome. The overnight dexamethasone suppression test is performed by administering 1 mg of dexamethasone at 11:00 PM and measuring the plasma cortisol level the following morning at 8:00 AM. In normal individuals, ACTH is suppressed and the cortisol level is decreased by 50% or more of baseline (<5 mg/dL). This dose of dexamethasone is insufficient to cause suppression in patients with Cushing's syndrome.

Once Cushing's syndrome is established, further tests are used to determine the specific cause. The high-dose dexamethasone suppression test is used to distinguish pituitary causes from nonpituitary causes. An oral dose of 2 mg of dexamethasone is given every 6 hours for 48 hours (or 40 mg/kg/dose for infants). Urine is then collected for 24 hours to measure free cortisol and 17-hydroxysteroids. In patients with a pituitary neoplasm, the steroid excretion levels are suppressed to 50% of baseline. In patients with an adrenal adenoma or adrenocortical carcinoma and most patients with tumors that produce ACTH, the levels are not suppressed. Plasma ACTH levels are generally low or normal with adrenal causes of hypercortisolism, modestly elevated with pituitary neoplasms, and extremely elevated with tumors producing ectopic ACTH.

Among children, 80% to 85% of those with Cushing's disease have a surgically identifiable microadenoma[67] and transsphenoidal hypophysectomy offers the best chance for cure. Twenty percent of patients experience relapse after complete resection and manifest Cushing's disease within 5 years. Alternate therapies include pituitary irradiation, adrenalectomy, and drugs that inhibit adrenal function. Of these alternate therapies, adrenalectomy is the preferred treatment when two transsphenoidal procedures fail. Mitotane, an adrenolytic agent that causes a chemical adrenalectomy, has severe side effects, including nausea, anorexia, and vomiting.

Primary Hyperaldosteronism

Primary hyperaldosteronism is defined as excess production of aldosterone from the adrenal glands with consequent suppression of renin. Most commonly, this is caused by either adrenocortical hyperplasia or an adrenal adenoma. Adrenal adenoma, or Conn's syndrome, is the most common cause of primary hyperaldosteronism in adults, whereas adrenocortical hyperplasia is the most common cause in children.[68] Rarely, adrenal carcinoma can present as primary hyperaldosteronism.

Signs and symptoms of primary hyperaldosteronism are nonspecific. Patients have hypertension, muscle weakness, polydipsia, and polyuria. Hyperaldosteronism increases the total body sodium level and consequently increases the total body fluid volume. It is characterized by hypertension and hypokalemic alkalosis. The elevated aldosterone levels suppress renin and angiotensin.

The diagnosis should be entertained in any child with hypertension and hypokalemia. Initial screening in children with hypertension involves checking a potassium level. Hypokalemia (<3.5 mEq/L) is consistent with primary hyperaldosteronism. The aldosterone level is elevated, the renin level is suppressed, and patients frequently have a metabolic alkalosis. If necessary, the diagnosis may be confirmed by performing a saline load challenge. A large volume of intravenous normal saline is infused over 4 hours. In normal subjects, the saline bolus should decrease plasma aldosterone levels below 6 to 8 ng/dL. Alternatively, an outpatient saline load test consists of administering a high-sodium diet for 3 to 5 days that fails to suppress aldosterone in patients with hyperaldosteronism. The serum aldosterone level must be determined in the morning before the patient has assumed an upright position.

After hyperaldosteronism is diagnosed, it is important to distinguish between an aldosterone-secreting adenoma and bilateral adrenal hyperplasia. A solitary adrenal mass greater than 1 cm with a normal-appearing contralateral gland on CT or magnetic resonance imaging (MRI) supports the diagnosis of an adenoma.[69] When imaging does not clearly demonstrate a solitary adrenal mass, selective adrenal vein sampling can differentiate unilateral versus bilateral aldosterone hypersecretion. Alternatively, some institutions utilize scintigraphy with ^{131}I-iodomethylnorcholesterol (NP-59), a cholesterol analog that is taken up as cholesterol in the steroidogenic pathway. Dexamethasone suppression of ACTH-dependent adrenocortical tissue is followed by NP-59 administration. An adenoma is suggested if asymmetric adrenal uptake occurs. Bilateral hyperplasia is suggested if the uptake is symmetric.

The treatment of a functional adrenal adenoma is excision. The mortality rate from operative removal is generally less than 1%, with a cure rate of 75%. Treatment of patients with bilateral adrenal hyperplasia is with spironolactone.

Adrenocortical Carcinoma

Adrenocortical carcinoma is rare. National Cancer Institute's Surveillance, Epidemiology and End Results (SEER) data report that adrenocortical carcinoma represents 1.3% of all carcinomas in children and adolescents younger than 20 years of age in the United States, accounting for only 0.1% of all childhood malignancies.[70] There is a female-to-male predominance of about 2:1. The tumors occur equally on the right and left sides and are hormonally functional in 80% to 100% of patients. In the SEER database, half of the adrenocortical carcinomas occur in children younger than 5 years of age. Around the world, there is geographic variability, with southern Brazil having a 15-fold greater incidence of adrenocortical carcinoma compared with other populations. This increased incidence has been attributed to a unique germline missense mutation.[71]

The etiology of adrenocortical carcinoma is unknown, but its association with several hereditary tumor syndromes gives insight into the molecular pathogenesis of this malignancy. Li-Fraumeni syndrome is an autosomal dominant familial disease and is characterized by the early onset of tumors, including sarcomas, osteosarcomas, breast and brain cancers, leukemia, and adrenocortical carcinoma. Germline mutations in the *TP53* tumor suppressor gene on chromosome 17p13.1 are found in 70% of affected families, and these mutations have been found in 20% to 27% of sporadic cases of adrenocortical carcinomas.[72] Beckwith-Wiedemann syndrome is a congenital overgrowth disorder in which patients are predisposed to certain embryonal tumors such as Wilms' tumor, hepatoblastoma, neuroblastoma, rhabdomyosarcoma, and adrenocortical carcinoma. Overexpression of insulin-like growth factor (IGF)-2 is believed to contribute to the tumorigenesis in Beckwith-Wiedemann syndrome.[73] Several genetic alterations such as loss of imprinting or loss of heterozygosity of the 11 p15 gene locus causing a strong IGF-2 overexpression have been demonstrated in the majority of adrenocortical carcinomas.[71,74,75] Other hereditary syndromes associated with adrenocortical tumor formation include Carney complex, MEN 1, and congenital adrenal hyperplasia. However, these adrenal tumors are mostly adenomas and rarely carcinoma.

The clinical presentation of adrenocortical carcinoma in children is usually associated with steroid overproduction. In contrast to adult tumors, most adrenocortical tumors are hormonally active. Virilization is the most frequent presenting feature (66%), whereas the remainder of children will usually first be seen with Cushing's symptoms.[76,77] Virilization is secondary to secretion of the adrenal androgens. Features include axillary and pubic hair, deepening of the voice, acne, a rapid acceleration of height, hirsutism, enlargement of the penis or clitoromegaly, and development of body odor. Feminization may occur in 2% to 25% of patients and results from an overproduction of estrogens, particularly estradiol.[78] Nonfunctional tumors in children are infrequent. Only about 5% of pediatric adrenocortical tumors produce no clinical evidence of hormone excess. Accordingly, these patients usually are first seen late in disease with abdominal pain or fullness.

Because most tumors present with virilization symptoms, evaluation should be directed toward detection of elevated androgens. Screening should include measurement of plasma testosterone, urinary and plasma DHEA, and DHEA-S. Urinary 17-ketosteroids are also important because usually two thirds of 17-ketosteroids are derived from adrenal androgens. Although the most specific assessment of adrenal androgen production is DHEA-S, 17-ketosteroids are more frequently elevated in malignant disease.[79] The clinical presentation of Cushing's syndrome is confirmed by hypercortisolism and the loss of diurnal variation. Cortisol excess is determined by elevated plasma cortisol, urinary 17-hydroxycorticosteroids, and urinary free cortisol. Adrenal malignant disease generally causes markedly greater elevations of 17-hydroxycorticosteroids and plasma cortisol than is usually seen with functioning adenomas.

Radiographic evaluation should proceed concurrently with endocrine evaluation so that surgical intervention can proceed in an expeditious manner. Plain abdominal radiographs reveal a soft tissue mass in 47% of patients, and adrenal calcification can be noted in up to 30% of patients.[80] Ultrasonography, which can detect tumors as small as 3 cm, should be used for screening the adrenal region and for postoperative assessment of recurrence. Smaller lesions are smooth and homogeneous with no pattern of hyperechogenicity or hypoechogenicity. Larger lesions usually demonstrate a "scar sign," radiating linear echoes that represent an interphase between separate areas of necrosis, hemorrhage, and neoplasm.[81] CT can detect tumors as small as 0.5 cm and also can identify malignancy in the presence of regional invasion or distant metastases in the liver, lung, or brain. MRI has an accuracy similar to that of CT with lesions larger than 1 to 2 cm.[82] MRI has the advantage of producing coronal sections that can identify 1-cm images not identified on CT scan.[83] Finally, adrenal scintigraphy using iodocholesterol-labeled analogs has shown promise in identifying and differentiating functional adrenal lesions.[84] Differentiation between hyperplasia, adenoma, and carcinoma is made possible by the inability of carcinoma to concentrate radionuclide. Bilateral symmetric images indicate hyperplasia. Unilateral uptake suggests adenoma, and nonvisualization is suggestive of carcinoma.[85]

Surgical resection offers the only chance for cure. If extensive disease is found during operation, wide en-bloc resection of the tumor, lymph nodes, and involved organs is indicated.[86] For less extensive disease, minimally invasive techniques for adrenalectomy have been advocated, although most authors cite invasive disease as a contraindication to laparoscopic resection.

Adjuvant therapy has marginal results. Survival in patients who have undergone adjuvant therapy with localized disease has been reported to be 5 years versus 2.3 years for patients who have tumor spread beyond the adrenal gland.[86] For patients who underwent further surgical procedures for recurrent disease, survival is extended 3.5 years. Pediatric series report the incidence of metastases at diagnosis as being between 5% and 64%.[72] Mitotane is an adrenolytic agent that selectively causes adrenal gland necrosis and has been the most widely used chemotherapeutic agent. It is used for metastatic disease, for incompletely excised tumors, and for the hormonal effects of the tumors. In adults, response rates of tumors to mitotane are reported to be between 10% and 60%,[72] with a mean duration of response of only 10.2 months.[87] In the pediatric literature, tumor responses have been reported between 30% and 40%.[88,89] Additional regimens that have shown some promise include the combination of cisplatin, etoposide, and taxol. The role of radiation therapy in children has not been well established. In adults, adrenocortical carcinoma is thought to be radioresistant. However, some response has been noted in small series of children with metastatic disease.[78] In one report, radiation was used to shrink an "unresectable" tumor that was subsequently completely excised.[72]

Patients who are untreated for adrenocortical carcinomas have a mean survival of 2.9 months.[90] These tumors are highly lethal, with nonfunctional tumors demonstrating a worse prognosis. A delay in diagnosis leads to a worse prognosis as well. The range of time from symptoms to diagnosis has been reported to be between 6 and 36 months.[72] The prognosis depends on the child's age and the resectability of the tumor. In one review of 55 children with adrenocortical carcinoma, the 2-year survival rates were 82% for children younger than 2 years and 29% for children older than 2 years. Survival rates were more than 67% if the tumors were completely excised, but no survivors were found after partial resection.[91]

Adrenal Medulla

Pheochromocytoma is a neuroendocrine tumor that arises from neural crest–derived chromaffin cells in the adrenal medulla. During embryologic development, chromaffin cells migrate to the adrenal medulla as well as around the paraganglia of the carotid arteries, aortic arch, abdominal aorta, and thoracic sympathetic ganglia. Any of these nests of chromaffin cells has the potential to become a tumor and they are the cause of extra-adrenal pheochromocytoma, also termed *paraganglioma*. The adrenal gland is the most common site for these tumors and accounts for 85% of adrenal and extra-adrenal pheochromocytoma in adults. Children are reported to have a higher incidence of extra-adrenal pheochromocytoma, approximately 30%,[92] and multifocal and familial disease[93] but a lower incidence of malignancy compared with adults.[94] As in adults, children with pheochromocytoma present with signs and symptoms of catecholamine excess, including hypertension, headaches, sweating, visual complaints, nausea, vomiting, weight loss, polydipsia, and polyuria. Pheochromocytoma should be considered in any child with hypertension.[95]

The evaluation of pheochromocytoma includes biochemical studies to establish the diagnosis and radiologic imaging to localize the disease. Traditionally, the biochemical diagnosis of pheochromocytoma was based on measuring urinary catecholamine levels. More recently, measurements of plasma catecholamines as well as their plasma or urinary metabolites have been widely utilized. Catecholamines are metabolized within chromaffin cells to metanephrines. This intratumoral process occurs independent of variations in catecholamine release. Therefore, measuring plasma or urinary metanephrines provides a more reliable method for diagnosing pheochromocytoma than measuring the parent amines.[96] The current guidelines, based on the First International Symposium on Pheochromocytoma, recommends that the initial testing for pheochromocytoma should include measurements of fractionated metanephrines (i.e., normetanephrine and metanephrine) in plasma, urine, or both.[97] Radiologic imaging options include MRI, CT, and ^{123}I- or ^{131}I-metaiodobenzylguanidine (MIBG) scanning. MRI has the highest sensitivity and is preferred over CT in children because of decreased radiation exposure.[93,98] Although not as sensitive, ^{131}I-MIBG scanning is the most specific imaging technique and is favored when recurrent or metastatic disease is suspected. Almost all paragangliomas are found in the abdomen and pelvis. When pheochromocytoma is suspected biochemically but not found by imaging, an intrathoracic or intracranial tumor should be suspected.

The perioperative management of patients with pheochromocytoma is critical to successful surgical outcome. These patients are in a hyperadrenergic state with vascular contraction and relatively low intravascular volume. Catecholamine blockade and intravascular volume expansion are standard preoperative strategy. An α-adrenergic antagonist (e.g., phenoxybenzamine, prazosin, doxazosin, or terazosin) is started a minimum of 2 weeks before surgery. β-adrenergic blockers may be used to treat tachycardia but must never be used until the patient has had adequate α blockade owing to the risks of unopposed α-adrenergic stimulation with β blockade alone. Alternatively, calcium channel blockers have been successfully utilized in the perioperative management of pheochromocytoma and may provide fewer fluctuations in blood pressure and may have cardioprotective effects.[94]

Pheochromocytoma resection has traditionally been performed via an open transabdominal adrenalectomy. Even with appropriate preoperative preparation, intraoperative hypertensive and hypotensive episodes are common and must be anticipated by the anesthesia and surgical team. Surgically, it is important to ligate the adrenal vein early and to minimize handling the gland itself to limit catecholamine surges during the procedure. Laparoscopic transabdominal adrenalectomy has gained significant popularity and has been validated for pheochromocytoma resections in adults.[99] Although the data in children are currently limited to small patient series, laparoscopic adrenalectomy appears equally safe and effective for select patients in experienced hands (Fig. 78-8).[100-102]

Up to 25% of pheochromocytomas are familial, and germline mutations in the following genes have been associated with pheochromocytoma: *VHL* (von Hippel-Lindau syndrome); *NF1* (von Recklinghausen's neurofibromatosis type 1); *RET* (MEN 2A or 2B); *SDHD* and *SDHB* (familial paragangliomas associated with gene mutations of the mitochondrial succinate dehydrogenase family).[93] Pheochromocytomas are more frequently associated with MEN 2 syndromes in children than those in adults. Also, pheochromocytomas associated with the MEN 2 syndrome are more likely to be bilateral and benign.

In children with familial pheochromocytoma such as in MEN 2 or von Hippel-Lindau syndrome, bilateral tumors inevitably occur. Controversy exists over management of these patients. Bilateral adrenalectomy has been suggested by some but predisposes these patients to significant morbidity secondary to corticosteroid replacement as well as complications of medication noncompliance, such as addisonian crises.[103] Cortical-sparing adrenalectomies have been proposed for patients with bilateral tumors and those that are at high risk for developing a metachronous contralateral lesion.[104]

For patients with metastatic disease, ^{131}I-MIBG scanning and chemotherapy should be considered. Current evidence supports high initial doses of ^{131}I-MIBG for all patients with metastatic lesions who have positive diagnostic ^{131}I-MIBG scans. With tumors that respond symptomatically or hormonally to treatment, survival has been reported to be 4.7 years after treatment.[105] Chemotherapy also seems to have an additive effect with ^{131}I-MIBG scanning to increase survival of these patients.[106]

PRECOCIOUS PUBERTY

In boys, precocious puberty is defined as the development of secondary sexual characteristics before age 9 years. In girls, the development of breasts (thelarche) before age 7.5 years, the development of pubic hair (pubarche) before age 8.5 years, or the onset of menses (menarche) before age 9.5 years is considered precocious. Precocious puberty can be complete or incomplete.

True, or complete, precocious puberty is due to the premature maturation of the hypothalamic-pituitary axis and results in gonadal enlargement and premature development of secondary sexual characteristics. The secondary sexual characteristics that develop in true precocious puberty are appropriate for the sex

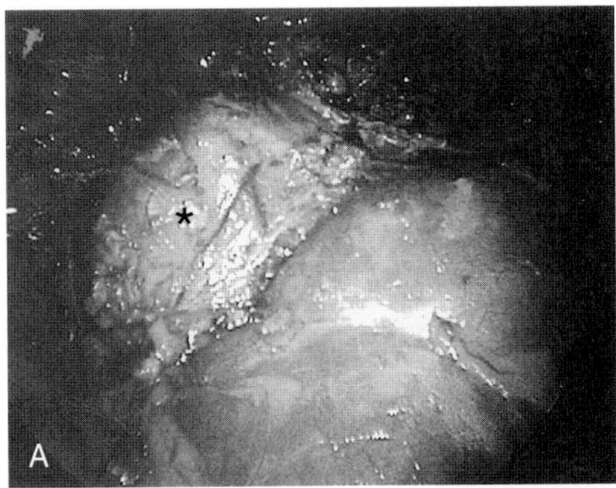

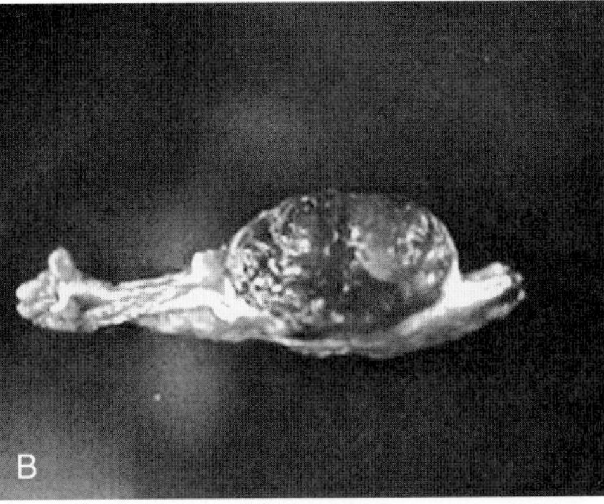

Figure 78-8. A teenage boy was found to have marked hypertension and a pheochromocytoma after a metabolic evaluation. He underwent laparoscopic left adrenalectomy and tolerated the procedure nicely. **A,** The pheochromocytoma (*asterisk*) is seen lying on the cephalad portion of the left kidney. The tumor was removed uneventfully. **B,** On the cut section of the adrenal gland, the tumor can be seen to be nicely demarcated from the normal adrenal gland.

of the child and merely occur at a younger-than-appropriate age. In incomplete or pseudoprecocious puberty, only one secondary sexual characteristic develops prematurely. Moreover, it may or may not be appropriate for the patient's gender. Pseudoprecocious puberty is not due to pituitary gonadotropin secretion. Rather, it is due to production of human chorionic gonadotropin (hCG), luteinizing hormone (LH), follicle-stimulating hormone (FSH), androgens, or estrogens, or it is due to stimulation of their receptors by the tumors.

Precocious Puberty in Girls

True precocious puberty, resulting from premature activation of the hypothalamic-pituitary axis, is idiopathic in 75% to 95% of girls. The condition may be a normal variant that is simply at the younger age of a normal distribution curve. Neurogenic disturbances can cause true precocious puberty by interfering with inhibitory signals from the central nervous system (CNS) to the hypothalamus or by producing excitatory signals. Neurogenic disorders may include hydrocephalus, cerebral palsy, trauma, irradiation, chronic inflammatory disorder, or tumors, such as hypothalamic hamartomas or pineal tumors.

McCune-Albright syndrome is an interesting disorder that can cause either true precocious puberty or pseudoprecocious puberty. Patients have a classic triad of precocious puberty, café-au-lait nevi with irregular "coast of Maine" borders, and polyostotic fibrous dysplasia. In these patients, autonomously functioning ovarian follicular cysts may develop, causing precocious puberty. Excess production of LH, FSH, or prolactin by pituitary adenomas also has been described. Other endocrine abnormalities including acromegaly, Cushing's syndrome, and hyperthyroidism have been associated with this syndrome.[107]

Generally, incomplete precocious puberty is first seen as isolated premature breast development (thelarche) or premature growth of pubic hair (pubarche). Premature pubarche is frequently caused by androgen excess. Isolated prepubertal menses is rare, and prepubertal vaginal bleeding is usually caused by a foreign body, sexual abuse, or tumors of the genital tract. Incomplete precocious puberty can be a normal variant or can be due to the production of hormones from neuroendocrine, adrenal, ovarian, or exogenous sources. In the Van Wyk-Grumbach syndrome, premature breast development is associated with hypothyroidism. Unlike most other causes of precocious puberty, growth is inhibited rather than stimulated. This syndrome may be due to the shared α-subunit of LH, FSH, and TSH. Tumors that produce excess quantities of LH or hCG can cause virilization.

Precocious Puberty in Boys

As with girls, true precocious puberty in boys may be neurogenic, constitutional, or idiopathic. However, in boys, true precocious puberty is more often neurogenic than idiopathic.

The most common CNS tumor that causes male precocious puberty is a hamartoma of the tuber cinereum. These hamartomas are ectopic hypothalamic tissue connected to the posterior hypothalamus. Because they are nonprogressive tumors and are in a surgically precarious location, they are generally treated with gonadotropin-releasing hormone (GnRH) agonists. Other disorders that can cause precocious puberty in boys are gliomas of the optic nerve or hypothalamus, astrocytomas, choriocarcinomas, meningiomas, rhabdomyosarcomas, neurofibrosarcomas, nonlymphocytic leukemia, ependymomas, neurofibromatosis type 1, and germinomas. Other space-occupying lesions or causes of increased intracranial pressure such as head trauma, suprasellar cysts, granulomas, brain irradiation, and hydrocephalus also can cause true precocious puberty. Some of these tumors or CNS conditions can cause both precocious puberty and growth hormone deficiency. In these patients, the growth rate may appear normal because the testosterone stimulates growth and compensates for the deficiency of growth hormone. However, the degree of growth is inadequate for the degree of pubertal development.

Incomplete precocious puberty can be caused by autonomous production of androgens or hCG. With many types of incomplete precocious puberty, the testes are not enlarged as they are with true precocious puberty. As with girls, the McCune-Albright syndrome can cause either true or pseudoprecocious puberty. Tumors producing hCG such as teratomas, chorioepitheliomas, hepatomas, hepatoblastomas, or germinomas of the pineal gland may lead to Leydig cell stimulation. Testotoxicosis is an autosomal recessive disorder in which premature Leydig cell maturation causes incomplete precocious puberty. The etiology in some families is due to the constitutive stimulation of the LH receptor and can cause the onset of precocious puberty at age 1 to 4 years. Ketoconazole, spironolactone, and testolactone can be used to treat testotoxicosis.

Excess androgen production causing virilization can be caused by congenital adrenal hyperplasia, specifically the 21-hydroxylase or the 11-hydroxylase enzymatic defects. During embryonic development, adrenal rests may be left in the testes. In untreated adrenal hyperplasia, ACTH stimulation may cause enlargement of these adrenal rests and the secretion of androgens. These testes have an irregular appearance. Excess testosterone production also can be caused by interstitial cell tumors of the testes. Finally, exogenous administration of androgens or hCG (for undescended testes) can cause precocious puberty.

Evaluation

For both boys and girls, evaluation of precocious puberty begins with a thorough history and physical examination. The patient's height and weight should be measured, and the growth curve should be examined. The bone age also should be determined. If the bone age and the height age correlate closely, it is likely that the presenting symptom is an extreme variant of normal. This simply requires close follow-up in 6 months to verify the diagnosis. However, if the bone age is abnormally accelerated relative to the height age, further investigation is warranted. The Tanner stage should be carefully documented. In boys, the size and shape of the testes are of utmost importance. In true precocious puberty, the testes generally enlarge symmetrically, whereas asymmetric or nodular enlargement is noted with Leydig cell tumors or adrenal rests. Feminization in boys may appear as gynecomastia.

Serum estradiol, testosterone, and DHEA levels should be obtained. In girls, a vaginal smear for estrogen effect may be more sensitive than a serum estradiol level. Significantly elevated DHEA levels are typically seen in adrenal tumors. Evidence of association with other syndromes may warrant measuring other hormone levels, including prolactin, thyroid hormone, or cortisol. A GnRH test can be useful in determining whether the patient has complete or incomplete precocious puberty. Patients with true precocious puberty respond to GnRH with a typical pubertal pattern, whereas those with pseudoprecocious puberty have a minimal response to gonadotropin. Alternatively, a sleep-related increase in plasma LH levels can be diagnostic but is more cumbersome to obtain. In patients with feminizing or masculinizing features, ultrasonography is useful to locate abdominal or pelvic masses. MRI should be used in patients with true precocious puberty to locate potential intracranial lesions.

Treatment

In general, tumors causing precocious puberty should be removed if they are surgically accessible. A number of agents have been used in the medical treatment of precocious puberty. True (gonadotropin-dependent) precocious puberty can be treated with GnRH agonists. Although initially these agents stimulate gonadotropin secretion, ultimately, GnRH receptors are downregulated, and LH and FSH secretion is subsequently decreased. Examples of GnRH agonists include deslorelin, buserelin, nafarelin, leuprolide, and triptorelin.

Other medications have been used in the medical treatment of incomplete precocious puberty. Medroxyprogesterone acetate, a progestational agent, can halt the progression of secondary sexual characteristic development and can prevent menstruation. Ketoconazole is an antifungal agent that also inhibits the synthesis of testosterone by blocking the conversion of 17-hydroxyprogesterone to androstenedione. Testolactone competitively inhibits the aromatase enzyme that converts androgens to estrogens. Androgen antagonists include cyproterone acetate and spironolactone.

CARCINOID TUMORS

Carcinoid tumors comprise less than 0.1% of tumors identified at one large pediatric cancer center.[108] These tumors arise from amine uptake and decarboxylation cells and are usually classified according to their site of origin as foregut, midgut, or hindgut carcinoids.[109] Foregut tumors account for approximately 5% of carcinoid tumors and can arise in the bronchus, stomach, or duodenum. Midgut tumors account for about 80% to 85% of carcinoid tumors. The majority of carcinoids arise from the appendix (46%), followed by the jejunum and ileum (28%), and the rectum (17%). Carcinoid tumors also have been found to arise from ovarian teratomas.

Most patients present with vague symptoms. Only 10% of patients have symptoms of carcinoid syndrome (flushing, diarrhea, abdominal pain, asthma, and right-sided cardiac valvular problems).[110] Carcinoids are detected incidentally in up to 60% of patients, usually when associated with appendiceal carcinoids.

Most pediatric patients are first seen with appendiceal carcinoids smaller than 2 cm (Fig. 78-9). These can be treated with simple appendectomy.[108] Right hemicolectomy is indicated for tumors larger than 2 cm, those close to the cecum, and those with mucin production. Metastases are extremely rare in children, but regular follow-ups with measurement of serotonin and chromogranin A should be performed.[111] Treatment of

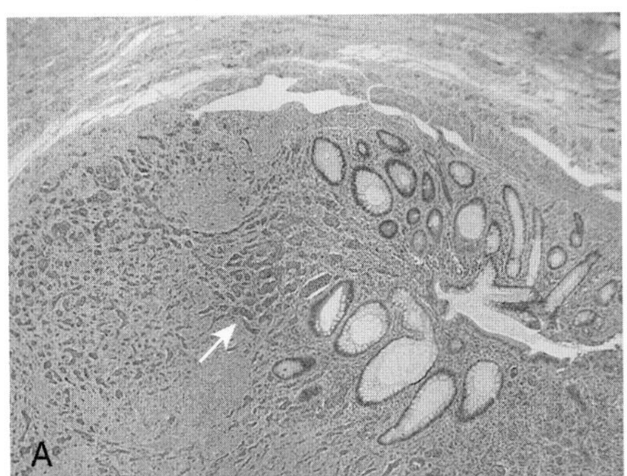

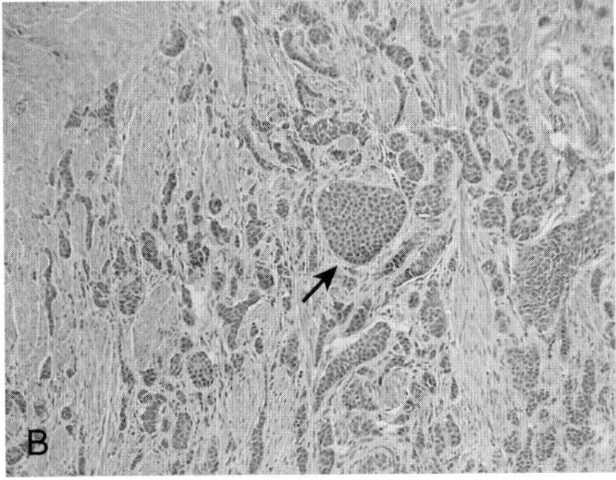

Figure 78-9. These two histologic photomicrographs depict a carcinoid tumor of the appendix. **A,** Lower-power view shows the nests of neuroendocrine cells (*arrow*) that are seen invading the muscularis mucosa. **B,** Higher-power view shows the solid islands or nests (*arrow*) of uniform oval to polygonal cells with minimal pleomorphism. There are indistinct cellular borders and round uniform nucleoli with finely granular diffuse chromatin and inconspicuous nucleoli. Mitotic figures are rare.

metastatic disease includes hepatic chemoembolization and surgical resection for isolated hepatic metastases. Long-acting octreotide or ^{131}I-MIBG is used for widely metastatic disease.[112]

Carcinoids are fairly indolent tumors. In one retrospective series of 40 children with appendiceal carcinoids, no recurrences or metastases were reported.[113] The site of origin has universally been shown to predict survival, with the appendix having the best survival and midgut or hindgut having the worst.

Of significance, the most common pulmonary tumor is the bronchial carcinoid. These most frequently appear with recurrent or persistent pneumonia secondary to obstruction of the bronchus by the tumor. Usually these tumors excrete low levels of serotonin. Children commonly present with wheezing, atelectasis, and weight loss. Also, they can have cough, pneumonitis, and hemoptysis, which are frequently seen in adults.

Bronchial carcinoids can be diagnosed by bronchoscopy. They have a characteristic pink, friable, mulberry appearance. Biopsy should not be attempted because the carcinoids have a propensity to hemorrhage and because of their classic gross appearance. If no evidence of lymph node involvement is found, segmental bronchial resection can be performed. However, lobectomy or pneumonectomy is often required for treatment. These tumors are radiosensitive and radiation therapy can be considered for unresectable disease. The prognosis after complete resection is excellent, with a 10-year survival rate of approximately 90%.[114,115]

chapter 79

BARIATRIC SURGICAL PROCEDURES IN ADOLESCENCE

Go Miyano, MD • Victor F. Garcia, MD • Thomas H. Inge, MD, PhD

Childhood obesity is an increasingly prevalent and progressive disease with few successful treatment options. Not only have increasing numbers of children and adolescents been affected over the years, but the average weight of obese individuals has soared as well. Pediatric specialists are increasingly considering alternative measures to combat the serious immediate and long-term health complications of this disease. Evidence from clinical trials show that behavioral weight management may have longer-lasting effects in younger children compared with adults, but good long-term results are rare. These conventional treatment approaches are not effective for most who suffer with severe obesity,[1-3] leading some to consider weight loss surgical options for select adolescents. A number of important factors must be considered when contemplating bariatric surgical procedures for severe obesity in adolescents. Surgical weight loss results in significant improvement, if not resolution, of most obesity-related co-morbidity in adults.[4] Preliminary results suggest that this also is true for adolescents,[5,6] but little information is available about long-term efficacy and potential adverse consequences to an adolescent with lifelong restriction of calories and certain micronutrients. The issue of recidivism and the potential multigenerational consequences of bariatric surgical treatment in children and adolescents necessitate that considerable care and deliberation be applied to decision-making concerning surgical weight management.

DEFINITIONS

Obesity specifically refers to the condition of having excess body fat. Measurement of body mass index (BMI) is a reasonably accurate method for predicting adiposity, is reproducible in the clinical setting, and can be easily used as a screening tool.[7-10] In children and adolescents, physiologic increases in adiposity, height, and weight during growth are expected. Childhood obesity is a global problem. In that context, it should be noted that there are ethnic and racial variations in onset, prevalence, and severity of the metabolic consequences of childhood obesity. Growth charts that are typically used to define obesity are age and gender specific.[11,12]

The terms *overweight* (BMI for age and gender > 85th percentile), *obese* (BMI for age and gender > 95th percentile), and *extreme obesity* (BMI for age and gender > 99th percentile) have been used to refer to the increasing weight problem in children.[13,14] The 85th and 95th percentiles of BMI for age were chosen mainly because these percentile boundaries approximate the BMI in young adults of 25 kg/m^2 (overweight) and 30 kg/m^2 (obese), respectively. Whereas more than 32% of adults in the United States are obese, about 18% of children and adolescents are obese, a prevalence that has more than tripled in the past 2 decades.[15] Regarding extreme obesity, adolescent boys and most adolescent girls younger than age 18 with a BMI of 35 kg/m^2 are above the 99th BMI percentile.[16] Increasing metabolic risks associated with higher BMI for age, especially greater than or equal to the 99th BMI percentile, have been found when compared with lower levels of obesity.[16] In addition, because all children with a BMI above the 99th percentile become obese adults (BMI $\geq$ 30 kg/m^2) and because obese adults who were obese as children have more health complications and a higher mortality,[16-18] bariatric surgical procedures in the mature adolescent may be a reasonable option for weight reduction that may well reduce the risk of obesity-related morbidity and early mortality.[19]

ANTECEDENTS AND CONSEQUENCES OF ADOLESCENT OBESITY

Adolescent obesity is a multifaceted disease with serious immediate, intermediate, and long-term consequences.[20] Critical periods exist between preconception and adolescence during which the risk of development of obesity is increased.[21] Important risk factors for childhood and adolescent obesity are (1) low birth weight,[22-25] (2) bottle feeding,[26,27] (3) early adiposity rebound,[28-32] (4) having a diabetic mother,[33,34] (5) puberty,[35-37] and (6) parental obesity.[38-40] Knowledge of these risk factors for adolescent obesity gives insight into the genetic and environmental factors that result in obesity. With few exceptions, little understanding exists of which risk factors portend the development of extreme obesity.[41-43] This lack of understanding adds to the complexity in decision-making regarding the application and timing of surgical treatment of obesity.

Associated with the remarkable increase in the prevalence of pediatric obesity is a parallel increase in the severity of obesity and in obesity-related chronic diseases. These diseases have an onset at a younger age and carry an increased risk for adult morbidity and mortality.[44,45] Childhood obesity has adverse social and economic consequences.[46-48] The most important co-morbid conditions for childhood obesity, which are used to justify the use of weight loss operations, are cited in Table 79-1.

Table 79-1	Selected Co-morbidities of Adolescent Obesity
Psychosocial	
Poor self-esteem[101-103]	
Depression[104-107]	
Eating disorders[108,109]	
Discrimination and prejudice[110,111]	
Quality of life[110-113]	
Sexual abuse[114-116]	
Neurologic	
Pseudotumor cerebri[117-121]	
Pulmonary	
Sleep apnea[122-131]	
Asthma and exercise intolerance[132]	
Cardiovascular	
Dyslipidemia[133-135]	
Hypertension[136-141]	
Coagulopathy[142]	
Chronic inflammation[143]	
Endothelial dysfunction[144,145]	
Gastrointestinal	
Gallstones[146-148]	
Nonalcoholic fatty liver disease[149-154]	
Renal	
Glomerulosclerosis[155]	
Endocrine	
Type 2 diabetes mellitus[156-161]	
Diabetic precursors/insulin resistance[158,162,163]	
Precocious puberty[48,164-166]	
Polycystic ovary syndrome[167-169]	
Hypogonadism (boys)[170]	
Musculoskeletal	
Slipped capital femoral epiphysis[171,172]	
Blount's disease[104,173]	
Forearm fractures[85,174]	
Flat feet[175,176]	
Related Issues	
Reviews of health consequences of childhood obesity[20,177-184]	
Excess health care costs[48]	

GUIDELINES FOR PERFORMING BARIATRIC SURGICAL PROCEDURES IN ADOLESCENCE

Patient Selection Criteria

National Institutes of Health (NIH) guidelines suggest that it is reasonable to consider weight loss surgery for adults with a BMI of 35 kg/m^2 or greater in the presence of severe obesity-related co-morbidities (e.g., sleep apnea, diabetes, joint disease severe enough to require joint replacement) or a BMI of 40 kg/m^2 in the presence or absence of co-morbidities.[49] Although these criteria have remained unchanged since 1991, investigators at several institutions have used lower BMI guidelines for studying the effect of weight loss surgery on adults without adverse consequences. Data would support the use of lowered BMI guidelines for patients with severe co-morbidities, such as type 2 diabetes, which are responsive to weight loss.[50]

Because less is known about the long-term risks and durability of the surgery, most pediatric specialists have supported more restrictive guidelines for operations in adolescents. Currently, we consider BMI greater than or equal to 35 kg/m^2 with significant co-morbidities or BMI of 40 kg/m^2 with other co-morbidities as factors to be used in the selection of adolescents who are most likely to benefit from bariatric surgical procedures.

Specifically, when a teenager has achieved a BMI greater than or equal to 35 kg/m^2 with serious obesity-related co-morbidity, and surgical therapy will be predictably successful in reversing the obesity and co-morbidity, it is reasonable to consider a surgical treatment before adulthood. This is the case for adolescents with type 2 diabetes mellitus, pseudotumor cerebri, sleep apnea (apnea-hypopnea index > 15), and severe steatohepatitis. For adolescents with less severe co-morbidities or risk factors for long-term diseases, for which there is no disadvantage of waiting until adulthood, we recommend a BMI of 40 kg/m^2 as a threshold for operative intervention. These co-morbidities include, among others, mild obstructive sleep apnea syndrome (OSAS), hypertension, milder forms of obstructive sleep apnea (OSA), impaired quality of life, insulin resistance, glucose intolerance, or dyslipidemia. Figure 79-1 outlines a suggested algorithm for management.

Bariatric Programs for Adolescents

For highly motivated adolescents with co-morbid conditions (Table 79-2) who have been unsuccessful with prior dedicated attempts at weight loss, bariatric surgery

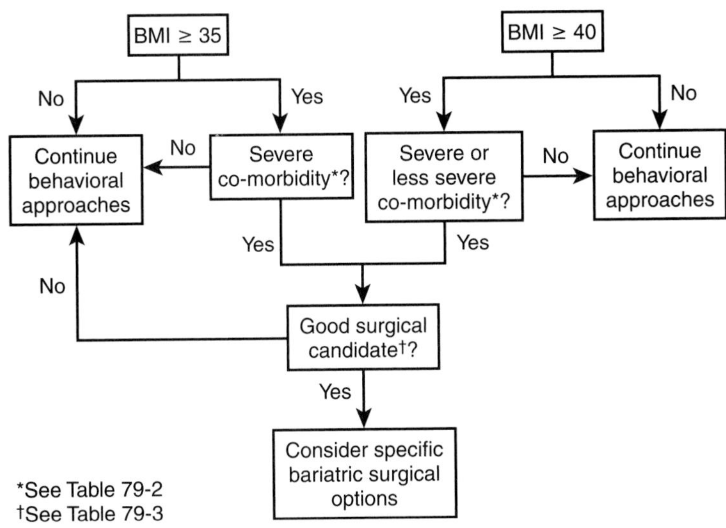

Figure 79-1. Algorithm of management strategies for the severely obese adolescent.

should be considered as a therapeutic option. Young patients being considered for bariatric surgical procedures should be referred to a specialized center with a multidisciplinary bariatric team with pediatric expertise. Such a team is equipped for the sometimes difficult patient selection decisions and can provide long-term follow-up and management of the unique challenges posed by the severely obese adolescent. Guidelines have been established by the American Society for Bariatric Surgery (ASBS) (www.asbs.org), and the American College of Surgeons (ACS) that define such multidisciplinary bariatric teams to include specialists with expertise in obesity evaluation and management, psychology, nutrition, physical activity, and bariatric surgical treatment.[51] Depending on the individual needs of the adolescent patient, additional expertise in general pediatrics, adolescent medicine, endocrinology, pulmonology, gastroenterology, cardiology, orthopedics, and ethics should be readily available. At Cincinnati Children's Hospital, the patient review process is similar to that used in our multidisciplinary oncology and transplant programs.[52] This review by a panel of experts from various disciplines results in specific treatment recommendations for individual patients, including appropriateness and timing of possible operative intervention.

Table 79-2	Obesity-Related Conditions That May Be Improved with Bariatric Surgical Procedures
Serious Conditions	
Type 2 diabetes mellitus	
Obstructive sleep apnea	
Pseudotumor cerebri	
Less Serious Conditions	
Hypertension	
Dyslipidemias	
Nonalcoholic steatohepatitis	
Venous stasis disease	
Significant impairment in activities of daily living	
Intertriginous soft tissue infections	
Stress urinary incontinence	
Gastroesophageal reflux disease	
Weight-related arthropathies that impair physical activity	
Obesity-related psychosocial distress	

Factors Influencing Timing of Surgery

Physical Maturation

The timing for surgical treatment of extremely obese adolescents remains controversial and depends, in most cases, on the compelling health needs of the patient. However, certain physiologic factors must be considered in treatment planning. There is a theoretical concern about the impact of significant caloric restriction on attainment of a genetically predetermined adult stature. Physiologic maturation is generally complete by sexual maturation (Tanner) stage 4.[53] Skeletal maturation (adult stature) is normally attained by the age of 13 to 14 years in girls and 15 to 16 years in boys.[54] Overweight children generally experience accelerated onset of puberty. As a result, they are likely to be taller and have advanced bone age compared with age-matched non-obese children.

If uncertainty exists about whether adult stature has been attained, skeletal maturation (bone age) can be objectively assessed with a radiograph of the hand and wrist.[55] If an individual has attained more than 95% of adult stature, it is unlikely that a bariatric procedure would significantly impair completion of linear growth.[56] For those who have not yet reached or nearly reached their predicted adult stature, one must balance the risks of growth delay due to caloric restriction against the potentially more significant risks of progression of obesity-related co-morbid conditions if surgery is delayed.

Psychological Maturation

Adolescent psychological development also impacts the ability to participate in surgical decision-making and postoperative dietary compliance. Cognitive development refers to the development of the ability to think and reason. At any given age, adolescents are at varying stages of cognitive, psychosocial, and biologic maturity. The more mature adolescent who can reason and think abstractly is better able to consider the consequences of taking or not taking nutritional supplements or of following and adhering to the prescribed medical and nutritional regimens that are necessary for lifelong success (e.g., maintenance of weight loss and prevention of avoidable nutritional complications) after bariatric procedures.[57]

Before any decision for surgical treatment is made, all candidates should undergo a comprehensive psychological evaluation. Goals of this evaluation include:

- To determine the level of cognitive and psychosocial development, primarily to judge the extent to which the adolescent is capable of participating in the decision to proceed with the intervention
- To identify past and present psychiatric, emotional, behavioral, or eating disorders
- To define potential support for, or barriers to, regimen compliance, the family readiness for surgical treatment, and the required lifestyle changes (particularly if one or both parents are obese)
- To assess reasoning and problem-solving ability
- To assess whether reasonable outcome expectations exist
- To assess family unit stability and identify psychological stressors or conflicts within the family
- To determine whether the adolescent is autonomously motivated to consider bariatric surgical treatment or whether any element of coercion is present
- To assess weight-related quality-of-life status.

Unfortunately, no "relative value scale" exists that would enable one to assign appropriate significance to the wealth of information (subjective and objective) obtained in the psychological evaluation. However, during a comprehensive assessment, we have found that a complete psychological assessment is very helpful for team decision-making and that generally good team agreement is reached about whether a particular patient has a majority (or conversely a minority) of the attributes of a good candidate for bariatric surgery (Table 79-3).

Table 79-3 Suggested Attributes of A "Good" Adolescent Bariatric Candidate

- Patient is motivated and has good insight.
- Patient has realistic expectations.
- Family support and commitment are present.
- Patient is compliant with health care commitments.
- Family and patient understand that long-term lifestyle changes are needed.
- Patient agrees to long-term follow-up.
- Decisional capacity is present.
- Weight loss attempts are well documented and at least temporarily successful.
- No major psychiatric disorders are evident that may complicate postoperative regimen adherence.
- No major conduct/behavioral problems are noted.
- No substance abuse has occurred in the preceding year.
- No plans for pregnancy are present in the upcoming 2 years.

SURGICAL OPTIONS

In 1991, the NIH Bariatric Consensus Development Conference established parameters that led to a more uniform application of bariatric surgical procedures for adults. After that conference, an increase in the use of these procedures was seen. This conference concluded that, at that time, insufficient data existed to make recommendations about bariatric surgical treatment for patients younger than 18 years. Fortunately, outcome data are emerging for the adolescent age group, and adolescent bariatric research is now receiving some attention at the NIH. Indeed, six studies with an adolescent bariatric focus have now been funded by the National Institute of Diabetes and Digestive and Kidney Diseases to examine various outcomes of adolescent weight loss surgery. Five of these have been based at Cincinnati Children's Hospital and one at the University of Pennsylvania. In addition, a multicenter research consortium called Teen-Longitudinal Assessment of Bariatric Surgery has also emerged that includes investigators at Cincinnati Children's Hospital, Texas Children's Hospital, Children's Hospital of Alabama, Nationwide Children's Hospital, and the University of Pittsburgh. More information about this research consortium can be obtained on the website www.cchmc.org/teen-LABS.

Of the many procedures that have been advocated for weight loss, the operations that have been used primarily can be classified as either purely restrictive or restrictive and malabsorptive (Fig. 79-2). The laparoscopic adjustable gastric band (AGB) and laparoscopic vertical sleeve gastrectomy (LSG) are purely restrictive procedures, and the degree of weight loss with these operations in adults has generally been satisfactory. The LSG is a new operation that produces significant initial weight loss with low operative risk in adult studies.[58,59] Because it likely does not affect micronutrient absorption, it may be a safe alternative with fewer nutritional risks than Roux-en-Y gastric bypass (RYGB) and also may avoid device-related long-term risks inherent in the AGB procedure.

There are good reasons to think that adolescents may be better served by purely restrictive options such as the AGB (Figs. 79-3 and 79-4) or LSG.[60] Although nutritional deficiencies are not as likely to develop from the purely restrictive operations as compared with diversionary operations (gastric bypass, duodenal switch), these operations still impair overall energy intake significantly. This may lead to impaired intake of important vitamins and minerals if not adequately

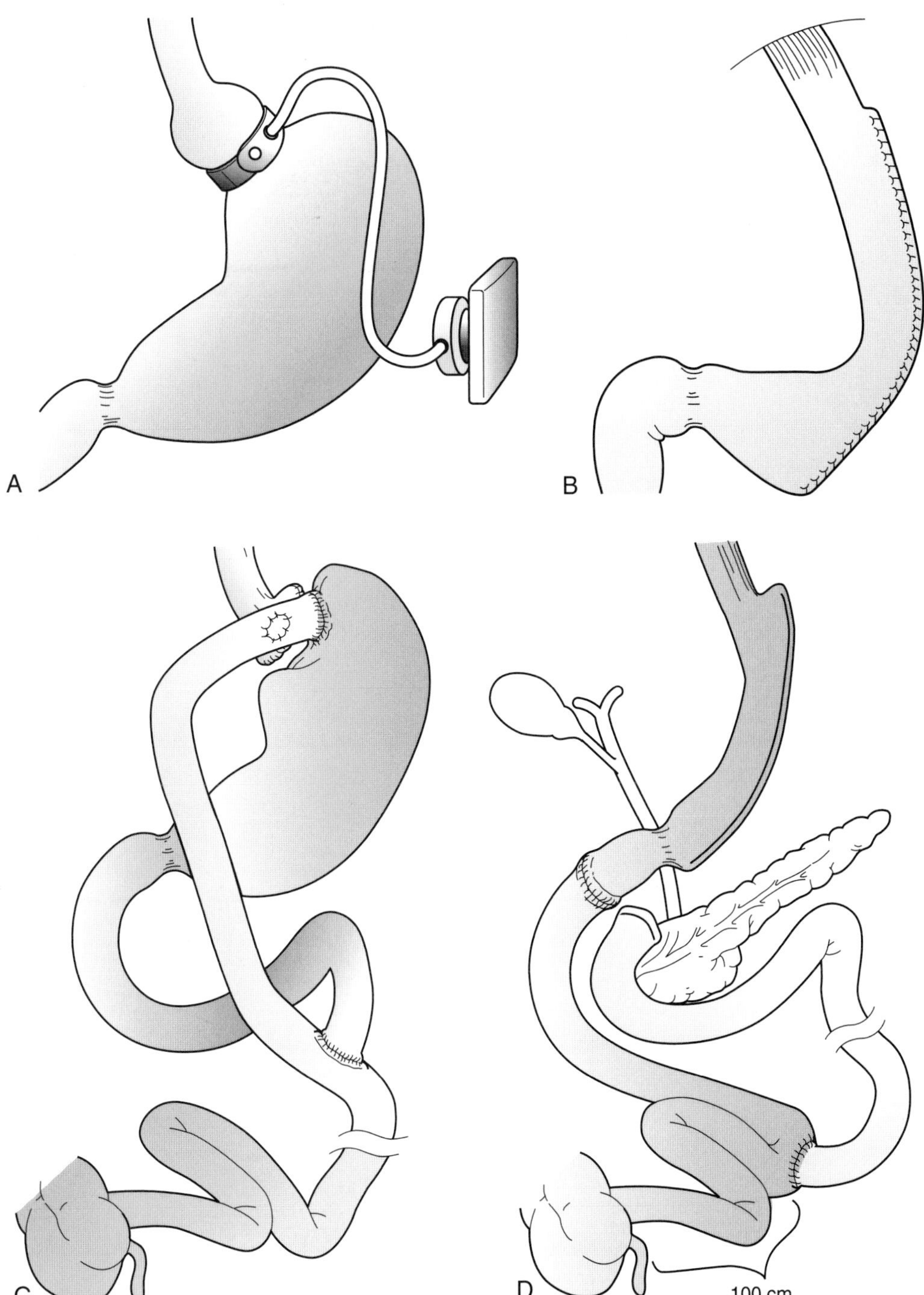

Figure 79-2. Operative procedures for weight loss that are performed laparoscopically. **A,** Adjustable gastric band (AGB). **B,** Vertical sleeve gastrectomy (VSG). **C,** Roux-en-Y gastric bypass (RYGB). **D,** Duodenal switch operation.

supplemented. With surgical procedures that do not transect the gastrointestinal tract, there is less operative risk and a reportedly lower mortality risk compared with gastric bypass.[61] A specific patient group for which one might suspect that a purely restrictive operation would be well suited is the younger adolescent, or even preadolescent, with a significant, progressive co-morbid condition (e.g., type 2 diabetes, OSAS, or pseudotumor cerebri). However, these patients have the greatest potential for noncompliance with postoperative nutritional recommendations.

The adjustable gastric band is not currently approved by the Food and Drug Administration for adolescents younger than 18 years of age. The theoretical benefits of nontransectional surgical revision are lost when considering LSG owing to the long staple line. Both the AGB and the LSG must be seen as procedures with less than adequate long-term outcome data. Any patient

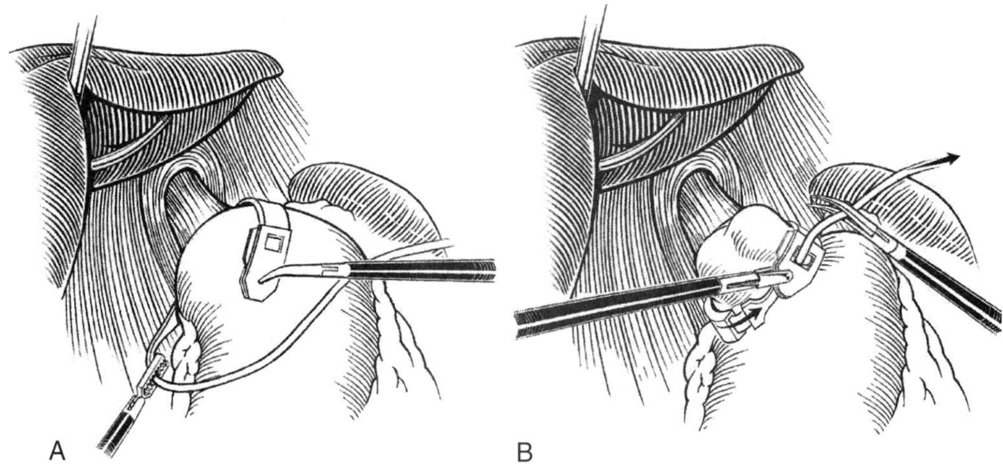

Figure 79-3. **A,** The tubing and the adjustable gastric band are being pulled behind the stomach with the grasper. The tubing is then exteriorized through one of the ports to allow manual traction on the gastric band as it dilates the narrow retrogastric tunnel. Once the thick portion of the gastric band emerges from behind the stomach, the tubing is then re-introduced into the abdomen and threaded through the hole in the buckle of the gastric band. **B,** The buckle is being locked in place.

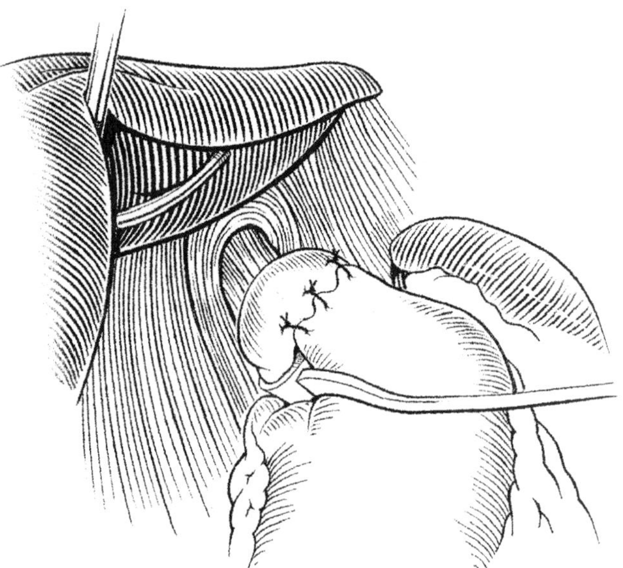

Figure 79-4. Plication of the anterior wall of the stomach over the gastric band is accomplished with three or four sutures using 2-0 permanent suture. These sutures should be deep and full thickness. It is important to remove the orogastric tube before placement of these sutures so that the tube is not incorporated in these plication sutures.

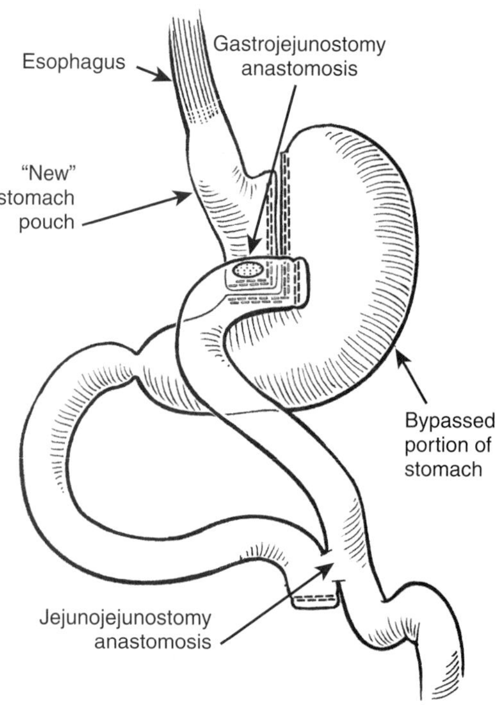

Figure 79-5. The Roux-en-Y gastric bypass consists of both a restrictive pouch size and a mildly malabsorptive component (the bypass of the stomach and duodenum). The gastric pouch is based on the lesser curve and is created using a 34-French orogastric tube as a guide. A 75- to 150-cm Roux limb is used in most patients.

undergoing these operations must be carefully counseled about the unknown long-term efficacy. Clinical outcome data should be collected prospectively to enable objective assessment of efficacy and safety.

The RYGB (Figs. 79-5 to 79-8) consists of both a restrictives pouch size and a mildly malabsorptive component (the bypass of the stomach and duodenum). Moreover, it also offers an additional negative reinforcement of "dumping syndrome" in some patients, providing excellent weight loss in adolescents and adults. The partial biliopancreatic bypass with duodenal switch is primarily a malabsorptive procedure that results in good weight loss for adults with the highest classes of obesity (generally > 60 kg/m^2 BMI), but at the expense of higher risks of operative complications and postoperative nutritional risks. Thus, the duodenal switch is not widely recommended for adolescents.

Regardless of the procedure used, surgeons and allied health personnel new to the field should, at a minimum, undergo a basic training course offered by one of the professional surgical organizations (ASBS, ACS, or the Society of American Gastrointestinal Endoscopic Surgeons). Before performing laparoscopic

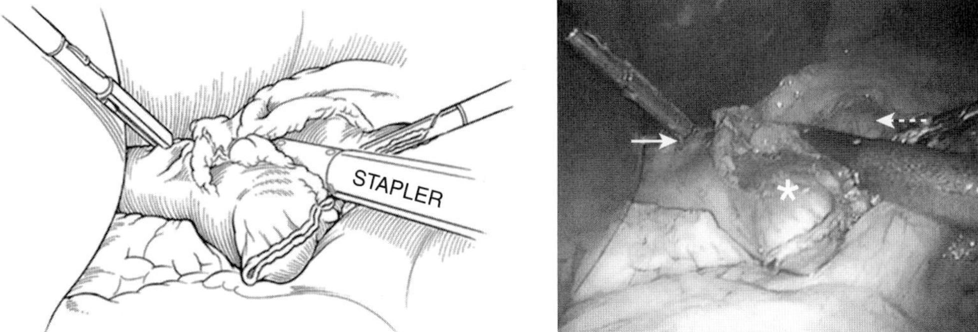

Figure 79-6. A 30-mL gastric pouch (*asterisk*) is created along the lesser curve of the stomach just beyond the gastroesophageal junction using a linear cutting stapler. The esophagogastric junction is labeled (*solid arrow*) demonstrating that the distal most portion of the pouch is typically located within several centimeters of the gastroesophageal junction. The first vertical application of the stapler that creates the distal most portion of the vertically oriented, tubular gastric pouch is being shown. Also shown is the remnant stomach (*dotted arrow*), which will be left in situ beside the gastric pouch. The Roux limb will be brought anterior to this remnant stomach.

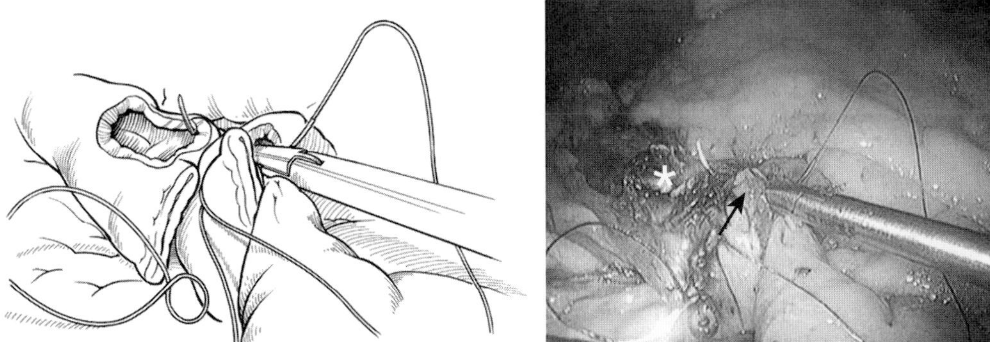

Figure 79-7. The inner posterior running layer of the gastrojejunostomy is being performed. This full-thickness suture line unites small bowel and gastric pouch tissue, resulting in a mucosa-to-mucosa approximation. The lumen of the gastric pouch is marked by an *asterisk* and the jejunal wall is indicated by the *arrow.*

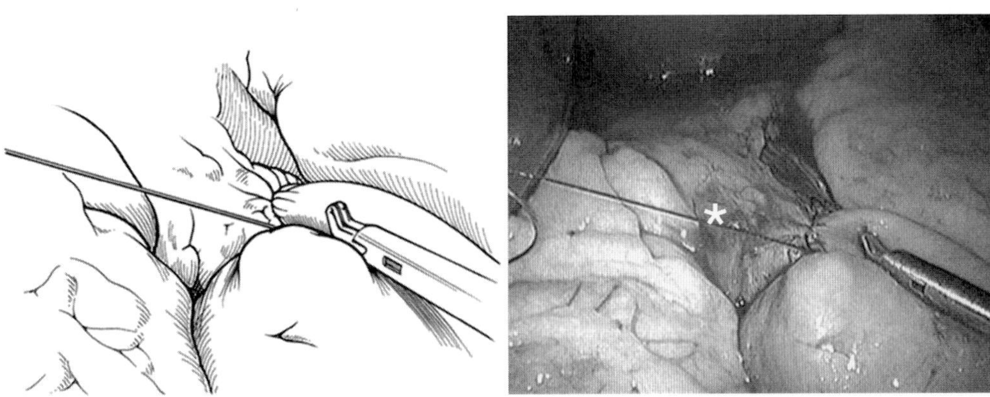

Figure 79-8. The two-layer hand-sewn gastrojejunal anastomosis has been completed. The gastric pouch is marked with an *asterisk.* An under-saline leak test is then performed using air insufflated through an orogastric tube (not shown).

bariatric operations, surgeons must meet all local credentialing requirements for the performance of bariatric procedures and advanced laparoscopic operations. Credentialing guidelines for both open and laparoscopic bariatric procedures have been outlined previously.[62-66]

PERIOPERATIVE AND SURGICAL MANAGEMENT

Preoperative Education and Management

The multidisciplinary preoperative evaluation that leads to the decision to offer surgical treatment is followed by considerable patient and family preoperative education. It is important that this process is organized and not rushed because patients must comprehend a great deal of information about the anatomic and physiologic changes that occur after surgery that impact success and the risks for the short- and long-term complications. Detailed information about the options for various surgical procedure(s), nursing care, dietary strategies, physical activity, and behavioral approaches to support adherence to the postoperative regimen is provided. Patients may also benefit from discussion with others who have undergone surgical treatment. In the weeks before the operation, a final outpatient visit for anesthesiology consultation, final informed permission (consent) discussion, and final review of the postoperative regimen is scheduled. At the conclusion of this visit, some programs require the patient to take a written test, which is scored and reviewed with the patient, as further documentation of his or her level of understanding of the procedure and known and potential adverse and beneficial consequences.

During the evaluation of a potential surgical patient, studies include serum chemistry and liver profiles, lipid profile, complete blood cell count, hemoglobin A_{1C} level, fasting blood glucose value, thyroid-stimulating hormone level, and *Helicobacter pylori* titers. If these titers are positive, a breath test is done to confirm or exclude active *H. pylori* infection. An electrocardiogram is obtained to screen for cardiac problems and dysrhythmias. For instance, prolonged QT syndrome does exist in morbidly obese adolescent patients and may be previously unrecognized. Because unrecognized sleep disorders are relatively prevalent in the severely obese, a complete sleep history is sought, including a history of snoring, irregular breathing, and increased daytime somnolence. A history suggestive of sleep apnea should prompt formal polysomnography. If the fasting glucose concentration is elevated, or if other symptoms of diabetes exist, patients should undergo a 2-hour glucose tolerance test to determine if more significant abnormalities of carbohydrate metabolism exist, including impaired glucose tolerance and type 2 diabetes.

On the day before the operation, the patients are limited to clear liquids. Preoperative medications include low-molecular-weight heparin (40 mg injected subcutaneously and continued twice daily postoperatively). A second-generation cephalosporin antibiotic is administered within 1 hour of surgery. Sequential compression boots also are used intraoperatively and postoperatively. Most patients are candidates for laparoscopic procedures, although some of the heavier and centrally obese patients may present challenges, particularly in the early portion of a surgeon's learning curve.

General Aspects of Surgical Techniques for the Morbidly Obese

In general, an open laparotomy should be avoided in morbidly obese individuals due to difficulty with adequate visualization and the higher risk of wound complications. For initial abdominal access, we have found that a laparoscopically guided technique using a transparent, bladeless, 12-mm cannula is safe and efficient. Alternatively, some surgeons prefer a blind puncture using the Veress needle in the left upper quadrant. To access the gastroesophageal junction for bariatric procedures, a wide variety of surgical instruments have been developed with the morbidly obese patient in mind. However, it should be noted that the majority of laparoscopic procedures in morbidly obese individuals can be efficiently and safely accomplished using standard adult 5-mm instrumentation. The left lobe of the liver is retracted with the Nathanson retractor (Cook Surgical, Bloomington, IN) to expose the stomach for bariatric operations. The details and nuances of the procedures used for adolescents can be obtained from a variety of excellent bariatric texts.[67]

POSTOPERATIVE MANAGEMENT

Postoperatively, the patients are placed in a monitored, non–intensive care unit setting, and maintenance fluids are administered based on lean body weight (typically 40% to 50% of actual weight). Early warning signs of complications include fever, tachycardia, tachypnea, increasing oxygen requirement, oliguria, hiccoughs, regurgitation, left shoulder pain, worsening abdominal pain, a feeling of anxiety, or acute alteration in mental status. These signs warrant aggressive attention and appropriate investigation because they may signal a gastrointestinal leak, pulmonary embolus, bowel obstruction, or acute dilation and impending rupture of the bypassed gastric remnant. Routinely, a water-soluble upper gastrointestinal contrast study is obtained on postoperative day 1 for patients who have undergone procedures that transect the gastrointestinal tract. After satisfactory passage of contrast is documented, patients are begun on clear liquids and subsequently advanced to a high protein liquid diet for the first month after operation.

Bariatric surgical treatment reduces the intake and decreases the absorption of food items rich in essential fatty acids, vitamins, and other specific nutrients, the long-term results of which are not well understood and are of legitimate concern. Poor nutrition during fetal development can result in a variety of adverse health outcomes, including future obesity, as suggested by the Dutch famine cohort.[22] Therefore, success in adolescent bariatric surgical treatment requires an expanded definition—not only sustained weight loss but also subsequent normal progression through the remainder of adolescence, adulthood, and eventually uncomplicated reproduction with normal offspring.

Nutritional and metabolic consequences of bariatric surgical procedures have been well delineated in adults.[68-79] To avoid nutritional complications, patients must adhere to procedure-specific guidelines for diet and vitamin/mineral supplementation. Restrictive operations (including gastric bypass) essentially result in a surgically enforced very low-calorie intake, thus requiring attention to an adequate (0.5 g/kg) daily protein intake to minimize lean mass loss during the rapid weight loss phase. Impaired absorption of iron, folate, calcium, and vitamin B_{12} may occur after gastric bypass.[71,80] Some obese adolescents may have vitamin deficiency even before operative intervention.[81] Even with postoperative supplementation, severe deficiencies may occur. Adolescence also may be a particular risk for thiamine deficiency.[82] In addition, poor postoperative compliance among adolescents who have undergone bariatric operations has been reported.[83] Because certain micronutrient deficiencies, such as folate and calcium, have established ramifications for the patient and potential offspring, both warrant special consideration.

Folate is a water-soluble B vitamin that is essential for growth, cell differentiation and embryonic morphogenesis, gene regulation, repair, and host defense.[84] Adequate maternal periconceptional folic acid consumption during critical periods of organ formation early in the first trimester may reduce the likelihood of fetal malformations, including neural tube defects and perinatal complications such as low birth weight, prematurity, and placental abruption and infarction. This information is particularly relevant because the majority of adolescents seeking bariatric surgical treatment are girls, many of whom will want to be mothers in the future. Thus, physicians caring for adolescents who undergo bariatric surgical procedures must stress the importance of daily folate and other B-complex vitamin intake. Moreover, patients should be monitored annually (and before planned conception) for serum vitamin levels, particularly when uncertainty about compliance exists.[84]

There are no studies examining outcomes of pregnancy after bariatric surgical procedures in the adolescent population. However, unplanned adolescent pregnancy is a legitimate concern after massive weight loss.[85] We strongly recommend that all girls and caregivers are informed about increased fertility (a physiologic change due to increased insulin sensitivity) and the likelihood for increased risk-taking after surgical weight loss. These patients should be counseled to avoid pregnancy during the 2-year period after operation and should be offered reliable contraception. The modern intrauterine devices are effective and safe and may be placed at the time of the bariatric operation.

Adolescence is a period of rapid skeletal mineral accretion and is, therefore, a window of opportunity to influence life-long bone health, both positively and negatively. While obese adolescents have higher than average bone mineral density/content, they may well have less than normal bone mineral density and content for their weight. This may translate into greater risk for fractures.[86] Furthermore, impaired accretion of bone mineral content in adolescence increases the risk for osteoporosis and results in a two-fold greater risk of fracture in later life.[87] Given the impaired absorption of both vitamin D and calcium after bariatric surgical procedures and the large individual variation in bone accretion, it is essential to monitor closely the bone mineral density of adolescents undergoing bariatric surgical treatment. Behavioral strategies can and should be used to encourage compliance with postoperative vitamin and mineral intake, which should positively influence nutritional outcomes after adolescent bariatric surgical procedures.[87]

Adolescent compliance may be enhanced by (1) visual aids, (2) focus on immediate benefit from treatment, (3) participation in self-management, (4) self-monitoring, and (5) reinforcement (Table 79-4).[88] With the alterations in eating patterns required after bariatric surgical procedures, repetitive reinforcement is needed to facilitate the formation of lifelong health-promoting habits. The adolescent bariatric surgical program should build on the best practices of other adolescent disease-management programs. Success will be based on the premise that sustained weight control for the adolescent requires ongoing behavioral intervention, structured family involvement, and continued support.[87,89,90]

Table 79-4 Strategies to Improve Postoperative Compliance

- Rehearse the dietary regimen to enable preoperative problem identification and solving before the surgical intervention.
- Use actual measuring cups, a food scale, and photographs of specific recommended food items to enhance the adolescent's ability to follow through with plans.
- Provide the adolescent with a diet diary and exercise diary with form pages to fill out, and practice this preoperatively.
- Provide a list of acceptable food items for every phase of the postoperative recovery (first week, second through fourth weeks, second through third months) including the caloric density and protein, carbohydrate, and fat content of the items to encourage label reading.
- Provide a detailed listing of micronutritional supplements needed postoperatively, including why the supplement is needed and the potential consequences of not taking it.

LONG-TERM MANAGEMENT

Postoperative follow-up visits after bariatric surgical procedures in adolescence are intensive but depend in part on the type of surgical procedure performed. For example, we see gastric bypass patients every 2 weeks for 1 month, then monthly for 3 months, and then approximately every third month for the next 18 months. Dietary advancement after the first month is a methodical process of introducing new items of gradually increasing complexity toward the goal of a well-balanced, small portion (~1 cup per meal) diet, which includes the daily intake of 0.5 to 1 g of protein per kg of ideal weight. Nonsteroidal anti-inflammatory medications should be avoided to reduce the risk of intestinal ulceration and bleeding after gastric bypass. Ursodiol and ranitidine are often prescribed for 6 months. Postoperative vitamin and mineral supplementation typically consists of two pediatric chewable multivitamins, a calcium/vitamin D supplement, and an iron supplement for menstruating females. Because of the severity of thiamine deficiency, additional B-complex vitamins beyond what is contained in multivitamin preparations should be given.[91] We routinely re-emphasize five basic "rules" with each patient encounter: (1) eat protein first, (2) drink 64 to 96 ounces of water or sugar-free liquids daily, (3) do not snack between meals, (4) exercise 30 to 60 minutes per day, and (5) always remember vitamins and minerals.

Serum chemistries, complete blood cell count, and representative B-complex vitamin levels (e.g., B_1, B_{12}, folate) are obtained at 6 months and 12 months postoperatively, and then yearly. Body composition is assessed preoperatively with either bioelectrical impedance or dual-energy x-ray absorptiometry (DEXA), and then on an annual basis after operation. DEXA not only allows for the measurement of the rate and relative amounts of fat and lean body mass loss but also provides a quantitative assessment of bone mineral density changes.

OUTCOMES IN ADOLESCENTS

Results of RYGB have been retrospectively reviewed in small series of adolescents with generally satisfactory results.[92-100] However, a 14-year follow-up of a small cohort of nine patients demonstrating considerable late weight re-gain suggests that adolescents may require different selection criteria or postoperative management than adults to achieve optimal long-term weight loss outcomes.[5] In a 2007 report, data from 17 studies that enrolled a total of 553 pediatric patients were reviewed. Eight studies reported outcomes after laparoscopic AGB, six after RYGB, two after vertical banded gastroplasty (VBG), and one after banded bypass. One study reported data separately for RYGB and VBG. A detail technology report from this review is available at http://www.hta.hca.wa.gov.

At Cincinnati Children's Hospital Medical Center, 86 adolescents have undergone laparoscopic gastric bypass between 2001 and 2007. The mean age of this group is 17 years and with a mean BMI of 59 kg/m^2. Seventy-five of these patients have been observed for more than 12 months after operation. On average, BMI in this follow-up cohort changed from 59 to 36 kg/m^2, representing a 39% (range, 16%-49%) reduction over 1 year. Despite this dramatic weight loss, precise body-composition analysis with DEXA at 1 year after surgery has suggested that lean body mass is preserved relative to fat mass loss. Satisfactory preservation of visceral protein despite extremely hypocaloric intake (typically 400 to 600 kcal per day) also is suggested by serial monitoring of serum albumin and total lymphocyte counts.

chapter 80

EVIDENCE-BASED MEDICINE

Shawn D. St. Peter, MD

"In God we trust; all others must bring data."
—W. Edwards Deming, physicist and quality improvement pioneer

Evidence-based medicine (EBM) is defined as the conscientious, explicit, and judicious use of the current best evidence in making decisions about the care of individual patients.[1] A simpler concept would be treating patients based on data rather than the surgeon's thoughts or beliefs. EBM represents the concept that medical practice can be largely dictated by *evidence* gained from the *scientific method*. Given that the practice of medicine has historically been based on knowledge handed down from mentor to apprentice, the concepts of EBM embody a new paradigm, replacing the traditional paradigm that was based on authority. In a global sense, it describes a methodology for evaluating the validity of clinical research and applying those results to the care of patients.

HISTORY

The initial groundwork forming the framework for EBM can be considered the earliest scientists who pursued explanatory truth instead of accepting beliefs. The process of discovering truth became replicable for aspiring scientists when the scientific method was outlined. No one individual can be credited for developing the scientific method because it is the result of the progressive recognition for a natural process of acquiring facts. However, the earliest publication alluding to the steps of current scientific methodology may be found in *Book of Optics* published in 1021 by Ibn al-Haytham (Alhazen).[2] His investigations were based on experimental evidence. Furthermore, his experiments were systematic and repeatable as he demonstrated that rays of light are emitted from objects rather than from the eyes. In Western literature, Roger Bacon wrote about a repeating cycle of observation, hypothesis, and experimentation in the 1200s. Influenced by the contributions of many scientists and philosophers, Francis Bacon delineated a recognizable form of the scientific method in the 1620 publication of *Novum Organum Scientificum*.[3] He suggested that mastery of the world in which man lives is dependent on careful understanding. Moreover, this understanding is based entirely on the facts of this world and not, as the ancients portrayed it, in philosophy. Nearly 400 years later, we find ourselves coming to the same conclusions in the practice of medicine and surgery. We now understand that facts and truths transcend experience and that facts about optimal care can be gained through experimentation more reliably than from beliefs generated through experience.

The establishment of the scientific method in the pursuit of proven truths was fundamental to the development of EBM as an entity. The current scientific method consists of several steps that are outlined in Table 80-1. However, the concepts of EBM are not simply encompassed by the application of these steps to attain facts but also address the ability to understand the value of the results generated from experimentation. Under the auspices of EBM, investigators are burdened with the first five steps, from inquiry to experimentation, while all caregivers must develop a deep understanding of experimental methodology, analysis of data, and how conclusions are drawn to be able to place appropriate value on published studies to influence their practice.

The movement urging physicians to utilize proven facts in the development of decision-making algorithms began in 1972 with the publication of the revolutionary book *Effectiveness and Efficiency: Random Reflections on Health Services*.[4] The author, Archie Cochrane, a Scottish epidemiologist working in the United Kingdom's National Health System, has likely had the greatest influence in the development of an organized means of guiding care through data and results. The book demonstrates disdain for the scientific establishment, devalues expert opinion, and shows that physicians should systematically question what is the best care for the patient. Most impressively, Cochrane calls for an international registry of randomized controlled trials and for explicit quality criteria for appraising published research. At the time of his passing in 1988, these aspirations had not fully materialized. However,

Table 80-1 Fundamentals of the Scientific Method

1. Establish an inquiry.
2. Develop background knowledge.
3. Develop a hypothesis.
4. Design a logical experiment to prove or disprove the hypothesis.
5. Conduct and/or repeat the experiment.
6. Analyze data.
7. Draw conclusions.
8. Communicate results.

the field of medicine is fortunate that Cochrane's prophetic ideas have precipitated the maturation of centers of evidence-based medical research that make up the global not-for-profit organization called the Cochrane Collaboration. The product of the Collaboration is *The Cochrane Library,* which is a collection of seven databases that contain high-quality, independent evidence to inform health care decision-making.[5] The most clinically utilized database is the Cochrane Database of Systematic Reviews containing reviews on the highest level of evidence on which to base clinical treatment decisions. There are now over 550,000 entries.

After Cochrane and other proponents of care guided by evidence popularized the importance of comparative data, it took over a decade for the amorphous clouds of these concepts to solidify into tangible terms and usable methods. The methodology of specifically qualifying data and judging the relative merit of available studies did not begin to appear in the literature until the early 1990s. In a paper published in 1990 by David Eddy on the role of guidelines in medical decision-making, the term *evidence-based* first appeared in the literature.[6] Much of the framework currently used to determine best available evidence was established by David Sackett and Gordon Guyatt at the McMaster University–based research group called the Evidence-Based Medicine Working Group. In 1992, *JAMA* published the group's landmark paper titled, "Evidence-Based Medicine: A New Approach to Teaching the Practice of Medicine," and the term *evidence-based medicine* was born.[7] A cementing moment in the paradigm shift occurred when the Centre for Evidence-Based Medicine was established in Oxford, England, in 1995 as the first of several centers. Over the past decade, centers or departments focusing on clinical research and EBM have been developed at universities and hospitals around the world, including our own (www.centerforprospectiveclinicaltrials.com). EBM principles are now represented in a module of the core curriculum that is integral to three of the six general competencies outlined by the Accreditation Council for Graduate Medical Education that oversees the accredited residency training programs in the United States. The concept of EBM is no longer a movement of progressive physicians but rather a basic guiding principle of medical training and practice.

LEVELS OF EVIDENCE

Utilization of evidence in guiding health care decision-making requires an understanding of the merit of the evidence and the ability to decipher whether a given course of treatment has been proven superior. The quality of evidence specifically indicates the extent to which one can be confident that an estimate of effect is correct. Systems to stratify evidence by quality have been developed by several sources. Although there are specific differences in published rankings, the generally accepted levels in a broad sense are defined as follows:

Level 1 evidence is supported by prospective, randomized trials.

Level 2 evidence is supported by cohort studies, outcomes data, or low-quality prospective trials.

Level 3 evidence comprises case-control studies.

Level 4 evidence is based on case series.

Level 5 evidence is expert opinion or beliefs based on rational principles.

The general levels are outlined in Table 80-2. However, the quality of data that is conveyed within each level and study type is clearly a wide spectrum. The complete delineation in the levels of evidence as defined by the Oxford Centre for Evidence-Based Medicine is outlined in Table 80-3.

As can be seen by the levels listed in Tables 80-2 and 80-3, the strength of evidence improves significantly by the application of prospective data collection. In clinical medicine, and particularly in the practice of surgery, there are many aspects of trial design that are not feasible such as blinding, placebo treatments, independent follow-up evaluation, and others. However, if one accepts these limitations and conducts a trial with prospective evaluation, the results remain markedly more meaningful than a retrospective case-control comparative series that compares surgeons and/or timeframes against one another.

The review of several studies can gain strength over an individual study, which is valid in many models and fields of medicine. However, one should be cautioned about the real strengths of such a meta-analysis before considering it to have a high level of evidence. The strength of these combined reviews is derived from the strength of the individual trials providing the numbers for the analysis. In the best scenario, such a combined review is composed of multiple prospective trials with similar design that each compare the effect

Table 80-2 General Levels of Evidence

Level	Type of Evidence
1	Prospective, randomized trials
2	Review of case-control or cohort studies with agreement or poor-quality randomized trials
3	Case-control studies
4	Case-series or poor-quality case-control and cohort studies
5	Expert opinion, or applied principles from physiology, basic science, or other conditions

Table 80-3 Levels of Evidence as Defined by the Oxford Centre for Evidence-Based Medicine

Level	Type of Evidence
1a	Systematic review of randomized trials displaying homogeneity
1a–	Systematic review of randomized trials displaying worrisome heterogeneity
1b	Individual randomized controlled trials (with narrow confidence interval)
1b–	Individual randomized controlled trials (with a wide confidence interval)
1c	All or none randomized controlled trials
2a	Systematic reviews (with homogeneity) of cohort studies
2a–	Systematic reviews of cohort studies displaying worrisome heterogeneity
2b	Individual cohort study or low quality randomized controlled trials (<80% follow-up)
2b–	Individual cohort study or low quality randomized controlled trials (<80% follow-up/ wide confidence interval)
2c	"Outcomes" research; ecological studies
3a	Systematic review (with homogeneity) of case-control studies
3a–	Systematic review of case-control studies with worrisome heterogeneity
3b	Individual case-control study
4	Case series (and poor quality cohort and case-control studies)
5	Expert opinion without explicit critical appraisal, or based on physiology, bench research or "first principles"

of two treatments on a specific outcome. However, in the field of pediatric surgery, multiple prospective trials with similar designs that address the same disease with the same interventions are nonexistent. Therefore, such combined reviews do not currently exist in pediatric surgery that can be considered level 1 evidence. Also, surgeons should not overvalue the influence of combined reviews derived from retrospective studies. Such reviews should be interpreted as a mosaic of the individual studies. Any attempt by authors to combine a number of retrospective studies to harness statistical power is fraught with hazard.

GRADES OF RECOMMENDATION

The quality of the evidence as defined in Tables 80-2 and 80-3 applies a score of strength for each individual contribution in the literature. However, on many topics, particularly common clinical scenarios, there is an abundance of published studies such that the appropriate care cannot be guided by a single study. The total body of available information places caregivers in the difficult position of evaluating the published principles from the multiple sources that makes up practice guidelines. The caregiver applying these clinical practice guidelines and other recommendations needs to know how much confidence can be placed in the recommendations from a conglomerate of citations. Strength of recommendation scales were born from this need.[8-12] Given that the level of evidence indicates the extent to which one can be confident that an estimate of effect is correct, the strength or grade of recommendation indicates the extent to which one can be confident that adherence to the recommendation will do more good than harm.[13] As with the levels of evidence, there are multiple published grading scales. The grading format used by the Oxford Centre for Evidence-Based Medicine is outlined in Table 80-4.

The levels of evidence are more easily assessed because each contribution falls into a given level based on study design. However, establishing the grade of recommendation can be more complex given the fact that multiple levels of evidence from different timeframes invariably exist on any given clinical topic. This is further confusing because many disease processes have multiple outcome measures. Also, each treatment option can affect different outcomes in independent ways that must be balanced against the risk or toxicity of each treatment. A working group has outlined a process for establishing grade based on the following sequential steps[14]:

1. Assess the quality of evidence across studies for each important outcome.
2. Decide which outcomes are critical to a decision.
3. Judge the overall quality of evidence across these critical outcomes.
4. Evaluate balance between benefits and harms.
5. Levy the strength of recommendation.

Currently, an accepted standard of respecting the level of evidence and assessing grades of recommendation is lacking in the pediatric surgery field.

LANDSCAPE OF PEDIATRIC SURGERY

Progress in the field of pediatric surgery regarding EBM has been hindered by its relatively young age and the size of its membership. As opposed to our adult general surgery colleagues who operate on a foundation built through centuries of work, the first American textbook in pediatric surgery, *Abdominal Surgery of Infancy and Childhood* by Robert Gross and William Ladd, was published in 1941. These men trained the initial cohort of pediatric surgeons who then developed

Table 80-4 Grades of Recommendation as Defined by the Oxford Centre for Evidence-Based Medicine

Grade	Level of Evidence
A	Consistent level 1 studies
B	Consistent level 2 or 3 studies or extrapolations from level 1 studies
C	Level 4 studies or extrapolations from level 2 or 3 studies
D	Level 5 evidence or troublingly inconsistent or inconclusive studies of any level

other training centers around the country. The total number of training sites has remained relatively small. As a result, the philosophies of only a few people have been taught to the entire practicing population of pediatric surgeons. The practice of pediatric surgery has generally progressed without extensive critical analysis. This phenomenon is pronounced in the pediatric surgery literature, which has been replete with retrospective case-control studies and case series (levels 3 and 4). There are few publications in the pediatric surgery literature that entail comparative analysis, and the majority that do are retrospective studies.

RETROSPECTIVE STUDIES

Because our field is overly represented with retrospective comparisons, it is important to recognize the natural flaws introduced by retrospective analysis. At least one of two confounding factors is present when an institution reviews and compares different therapies retrospectively. When an institution is concurrently using different treatment plans, usually the comparison between treatment plans also compares caregivers. The other possibility is that the center has changed treatment plans and then retrospectively investigates the effect of this change. Although this sounds attractive, it becomes a comparison between timeframes. Historical comparison groups are difficult to use with scientific confidence owing to the rapid ongoing changes in hospital systems. Many institutions have quality assurance programs that intend to make all patient care more consistent and efficient. Such change will impact outcomes regardless of the surgical treatment. A universal concern with retrospective studies is the assurance of reviewing the entire population and the entire dataset. It can be very difficult to accurately identify all the data desired when retrospectively collecting information. As a result, datasets are often incomplete, which decreases scientific confidence. Another issue, rarely acknowledged in retrospective studies, is the difficulty with capturing the entire population intended for study. There are many coding nuances within an institution that may exclude patients from lists when the database is searched by ICD-9 code. A specific type of patient, such as a treatment failure, can go undetected, because of being hidden under a different diagnosis code. This can create tremendous error in the published data.

CONSIDERATIONS FOR PROSPECTIVE TRIALS IN PEDIATRIC SURGERY

Although it is clear that prospective trials offer the highest scientific integrity and the best vehicle for determining superior efficacy among options, they have been underutilized in the field of pediatric surgery. Critics have postulated that consented prospective trials would have a limited role in pediatric surgery care because parents would be unwilling to enroll their children into such studies. Studies should not be conducted in any human population when there is substantial risk of harm balanced against questionable benefit. A well-designed study should offer patients the potential for a better outcome than the standard means of treatment outside the study. However, there is no example in the published literature to support the speculation that studies should not be attempted in children. Moreover, there are several prospective, randomized trials being conducted and emerging in the pediatric surgery literature now that would suggest otherwise.[15-18]

The specific details of trial development are beyond the scope of this chapter, but there are general considerations that can allow pediatric surgeons to identify situations for which a trial can be employed. Specifically, these include an understanding of equipoise or stepwise progression, the need for patient volume, an understanding of population characteristics, and the possibility of influencing practice habits.

Equipoise

There is usually a role for a trial when equipoise exists for the currently available therapeutic options. Equipoise is the assumption that two treatment plans are equal. Thus, the trial simply pits the two options head to head to identify which is superior. Each caregiver participating in a study does not need to possess true inherent equipoise without bias. Naturally, each practitioner will have biases and suppositions about which management strategy is superior, but there remains a role for a trial when each caregiver can honestly acknowledge that there is not enough evidence to prove his or her own thoughts are correct. The most obvious examples for where a role exists for a trial are circumstances in which more than one management strategy is utilized in a given institution. This usually occurs due to caregiver bias. An example would be the open operation versus the laparoscopic approach for pyloromyotomy.[15] Another would be tube thoracostomy and fibrinolysis versus thoracoscopic decortication for empyema.[17-19] If a given patient condition is treated by pathway A or B based simply on the caregivers who were on call that day when no evidence exists to support either pathway, then not only is there a role for a trial, but, in reality, there is an ethical need to conduct such a study to prevent the potential tragedy wherein half of the patients are receiving inferior care simply due to bias without evidence.

The other natural situation for prospective evaluation is when caregivers can follow the next step in the progression to simplify care but that step may be at the expense of increasing a negative outcome. As an example, if a group would like to attempt to shorten the length of any therapy, then this is clearly advantageous to the patient unless there is a greater investment that subsequently results from treatment failures. As caregivers we owe it to the patients to pursue courses of treatment that ease their investment, but we cannot compromise outcome. Parents would enjoy a shorter course of anal dilation after anoplasty for imperforate anus but not to the point that it results in a detectable increase in anal stricture. Also, caregivers contemplating fewer doses of antibiotics, shorter periods of observation for various injuries, or less invasive therapeutic options should introduce them under prospective evaluation to be sure the attenuation in care is not offset by higher negative event rates. Under this paradigm, once each study is complete, then a treatment protocol can exist that becomes simple to compare to the next advancement. Our colleagues in oncology understand this concept well. In the cooperative oncology groups, each treatment plan follows a protocol with known outcomes and is compared to a potentially better regimen. Under this plan, once survival for a given cancer becomes high enough, then stepwise progression focuses on minimizing toxicity or surgical morbidity. The surgical fields have been less effective in advancing care using this model, largely due to the individual surgeon unwilling to relinquish his or her independent plans of care.

Patient Volume

The conduction of a study requires adequate patient volume. This is easily completed for common conditions. However, acquisition of good evidence has long been difficult in pediatric surgery owing to the large number of rare conditions. When considering less common conditions, physicians often suggest to simply expand the number of institutions to overcome volume limitations. This would appear to be a reasonable suggestion, but is extremely difficult to implement because each additional institution will need to take on a tremendous workload. Moreover, not all surgeons at each institution will buy in to the study design. Also, depending on the nature of the study, not all surgeons may be able to offer treatment in both arms. For instance, one of the reasons that a prospective randomized trial failed in comparing open and minimally invasive surgical approaches for cancer in the mid 1990s was because very few of the surgeons could perform the required minimally invasive surgical procedures.[19] It remains a fact that the integrity of the study will decrease with the addition of more institutions and more caregivers because it is less likely the protocols will be followed completely.

The lack of large volumes with certain conditions can be interpreted in a different and more pragmatic way for the practicing surgeon. Instead of focusing on the attainment of a large number of patients to try to detect a difference with strong statistical power, perhaps we should investigate more reasonable sample sizes to see if a larger difference can be detected. Why would we intentionally seek a larger difference when a smaller one might be detected in a larger study? For example, if a busy group of six surgeons were to conduct a study that enrolls over 5 years, and the study fails to detect a difference in any outcome parameter, even though the calculated power may be statistically small and unconvincing by traditional trial design, the number of patients treated by the group is the equivalent volume that an individual surgeon would treat over a 30-year career. Therefore, if the difference is small enough not to be evident over an an individual surgern's career, the surgeon should not be too concerned about the relevance of the variable studied and should focus on a different treatment variable to improve patient outcome.

Population Characteristics

The most important consideration of the study population is the homogeneity of the disease. A study on two types of stomal takedown techniques would be difficult due to the large variations in reasons for stoma placement, the intestinal level of the stoma, the degree of expected adhesions, the integrity of the remaining bowel, the function of the anus, and so on. The population should provide enough patient-to-patient similarity that the outcome from one patient can be related to another.

Generalizability

A study is less useful when there are just a few surgeons who can use the results. This applies not only to technologies or techniques that very few centers can provide but also to the development of the protocol. The protocol should attempt to assimilate real-world, typical practice problems without compromising structural integrity. If the protocol is overly strict, although it provides superior ability for detection of any differences, the results may not be applicable to the typical practice. Therefore, the subsequent value of the study diminishes.

Relevance

Before developing a project that will provide an answer, the question needs to be asked as to whether a problem exists in the first place. The important parameters for relevance are event rate and burden. While a very powerful study could be done on two methods of closing the skin after an inguinal hernia, the event rate of infection or wound breakdown is so small that surgeons do not concern themselves with this aspect of their practice. The time required for skin closure is a minute or less regardless of technique. Moreover, when infection does occur, the wound is not large enough to create a clinically important problem. Therefore, the practicing surgeon is unlikely to alter his or her technical habits of hernia repair based on the results of such a study.

RESOURCES

The application of EBM practices requires a functional knowledge of how to identify, interpret, and implement the information available into care plans and practice guidelines. Although many institutions have entire departments focusing on the utilization of EBM, not all physicians have ready access to the available information. In the field of surgery, there are many examples of heterogeneous care plans within institutions and group practices despite convincing, high-level evidence. Also, there are many reasons for these often

Table 80-5 Websites that Pertain to Evidence-Based Medicine

Name of Website	Address
The Cochrane Collaboration	www.cochrane.org
The Cochrane Library	www3.interscience.wiley.com
National Guideline Clearinghouse	www.guideline.gov
Centre for Evidence-Based Medicine	www.cebm.net
Berkeley Systematic Reviews Group	www.medepi.net/meta
Clinical Evidence	www.clinicalevidence.org
Evidence-Based Medicine Resource Center	www.ebmny.org
Welch Medical Library	http://www.welch.jhu.edu/internet/ebr.html
Prime Answers	www.primeanswers.org
Evidence-Based Practice Centers	www.ahrq.gov
PubMed	www.ncbi.nlm.nih.gov/entrez/query.fcgi?db=PubMed

conflicting care plans. One is that personal bias for some providers is stronger than their ability to interpret data. Thus, they continue working in their comfort zone and are skeptical of sound data. Some of these surgeons completed training in the apprentice era, and they have continued to follow what their chief told them. Also, some physicians who understand the principles of EBM simply do not have wide access to the evolving body of EBM. To overcome some of these hurdles, several web-based support sites have been developed for both EBM tutorial and review of available studies. A few examples are listed in Table 80-5.

INDEX

Page numbers followed by f indicate figures; t, tables.

E

F

G

H

M

V